290.85

KELLEY'S
Textbook of Rheumatology

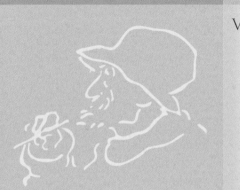

VOLUME
II

KELLEY'S
Textbook of
Rheumatology

NINTH EDITION

Gary S. Firestein, MD

Professor of Medicine
Dean and Associate Vice Chancellor of Translational
 Medicine
UC San Diego Health Sciences
La Jolla, California

Ralph C. Budd, MD

Professor of Medicine
Director, Vermont Center for Immunology and Infectious
 Diseases
The University of Vermont College of Medicine
Burlington, Vermont

Sherine E. Gabriel, MD, MSc

William J. and Charles H. Mayo Professor
Professor of Medicine and Epidemiology
Mayo Clinic College of Medicine
Rochester, Minnesota

Iain B. McInnes, PhD, FRCP, FRSE

Muirhead Professor of Medicine
Director, Institute of Infection, Immunity and
 Inflammation
College of Medical, Veterinary and Life Sciences
University of Glasgow
Glasgow, United Kingdom

James R. O'Dell, MD

Bruce Professor of Medicine
Vice Chairman, Department of Internal Medicine
University of Nebraska College of Medicine;
Chief, Division of Rheumatology and Immunology
University of Nebraska Medical Center;
Omaha VA
Omaha, Nebraska

ELSEVIER
SAUNDERS

SAUNDERS

1600 John F. Kennedy Blvd.
Ste 1800
Philadelphia, PA 19103-2899

KELLEY'S TEXTBOOK OF RHEUMATOLOGY, NINTH EDITION   ISBN: 978-1-4377-1738-9
Copyright © 2013, 2009, 2005, 2001, 1997, 1993, 1989, 1985, 1981 by Saunders, an imprint of
Elsevier Inc.

Mayo drawings © Mayo Foundation for Medical Education and Research.

**Cover image: Courtesy Thomas Deerinck and Mark Ellisman, the National Center for Microscopy and
Imaging Research, UCSD.**

Notices

Library of Congress Cataloging-in-Publication Data

Kelley's textbook of rheumatology / Gary S. Firestein ... [et al.].—9th ed.
   p. ; cm.
   Textbook of rheumatology
   Includes bibliographical references and index.
   ISBN 978-1-4377-1738-9 (hardcover : alk. paper)
   I. Firestein, Gary S.   II. Kelley, William N., 1939-   III. Title: Textbook of rheumatology.
   [DNLM: 1. Rheumatic Diseases.   2. Collagen Diseases.   3. Joint Diseases.   4. Lupus Erythematosus,
Systemic.   WE 544]
   616.7′23—dc23
                              2011036500

Executive Content Strategists: Pamela Hetherington and Michael Houston
Senior Content Development Specialist: Janice Gaillard
Publishing Services Manager: Patricia Tannian
Senior Project Manager: Kristine Feeherty
Design Direction: Ellen Zanolle

Printed in China

Last digit is the print number: 9 8 7 6 5 4 3 2 1

Sincerest thanks to my wonderful wife, Linda, and our children,
David and Cathy, for their patience and support.
Also, the editorial help of our three Cavalier King Charles puppies,
Winston, Humphrey, and Punkin, was invaluable.
Gary S. Firestein

Sincere thanks for the kind mentoring
from Edward D. Harris, Jr.,
as well as for the support of my wife, Lenore,
and my children, Graham and Laura.
Ralph C. Budd

To my three boys:
my dear husband, Frank Cockerill, and our two wonderful sons, Richard and Matthew,
for being my constant source of inspiration, love, and pride.
And to my parents, Huda and Ezzat, for their love and tireless support.
Sherine E. Gabriel

To my wife, Karin, for her patience,
understanding, and love and to our wonderful girls,
Megan and Rebecca, who continue to enlighten me.
Iain B. McInnes

Sincere thanks to my wife, Deb, for her patience and love
and to our wonderful children, Kim and Andy, Jennie and Dan, and Scott and Melissa.
I also want to thank the members of my division
who continue to support me in all my efforts.
James R. O'Dell

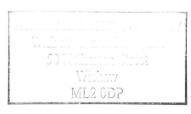

DEDICATION

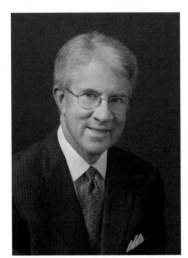

Edward D. Harris, Jr., MD
1937-2010

Edward D. "Ted" Harris, Jr., was one of the four founding editors of the *Textbook of Rheumatology*. In the late 1970s, Bill Kelley sensed the need for a text that reflected the growth of rheumatology into a mature discipline. He met with Ted, who quickly agreed, and they identified Shaun Ruddy and Clem Sledge as co-editors. A prime concern was that the new book should be grounded in the abundant information in basic science that supported our subspecialty. The standards they set were responsible for the high quality of the finished Textbook. Ted's choice of the iconic profile of Renoir, who suffered from rheumatoid arthritis, has graced the cover of nine editions of the book and served to connect us to the humanitarian aspect of our discipline.

Ted was a graduate of Dartmouth College and its medical school and of Harvard Medical School. Following his residency at Massachusetts General Hospital he moved to the National Institutes of Health (NIH), where he engaged in research on collagen. In his spare moments he also formed a jazz ensemble, with himself playing bass. Upon Ted's return to Mass General he entered a rheumatology fellowship and joined the laboratory of Dr. Stephen Krane, where Ted applied his knowledge of collagen to the inflammatory synovium of rheumatoid arthritis.

In 1970 Ted was recruited back to Dartmouth, where he built a robust connective tissue disease unit and received one of the NIH's first arthritis center awards. Along with long-time colleague Dr. Constance Brinckerhoff, Ted's group defined the role of collagenase and metalloproteinases in the rheumatoid synovium. In 1979 Ted was sole author of the seminal monograph *Rheumatoid Arthritis*, which detailed the complex interactions of the immune system with connective tissue in rheumatoid arthritis. In 1983

Rutgers Medical School recruited Ted to become Chair of Medicine, and four years later he assumed the Chair of Medicine position at Stanford, a position he held until 1995. During Ted's career he authored well over 100 peer-reviewed publications and 70 reviews, chapters, editorials, and books.

Ted served as President of the American College of Rheumatology (ACR) and, during his tenure, skillfully helped arrange an amicable separation of the ACR and the Arthritis Foundation so that each organization could better pursue its mission. He was named a fellow of the British Royal College of Physicians in 2002 and received the Presidential Gold Medal from ACR in 2007.

Ted had a remarkably perceptive intellect and a razor wit. A former English major, his writing was crisp and vigorous. His love of language elevated and animated text. Colleagues knew that an "EDH note" could be mellifluous, mirthful, and merciless all at once. As academic secretary to Stanford, Ted's amusing touches to the minutes of the Stanford Senate were legendary. He might squeeze in a quote from Dr. Seuss's *Horton Hatches the Egg*, add footnotes on faculty members' attire, or slip in sly editorial comments such as "wisely interrupted" or "introduced with appreciated brevity." As a result, Ted's words resonated and got results.

The English degree came in handy when, in 1997, Ted was named executive secretary of Alpha Omega Alpha (AOA) and editor of *The Pharos*, the society's nontechnical compendium of essays, poetry, art, and articles on medical history, ethics, and health policy. Ted breathed new life and style into the journal during his 13-year tenure as editor. Ted also created a 532-page anthology called *Creative Healers: A Collection of Essays, Reviews, and Poems from The Pharos, 1938-1998*, published by AOA in 2004. Reviewers on Amazon.com have mentioned the editor's keen eye for engaging writing, calling the volume's contents "moving" and "a tribute to the range of interests percolating around in active intellects."

Ted Harris mentored a generation of rheumatologists and taught us all by his example of dynamic creative thought and a deep humanitarian spirit. All of us involved with *Kelley's Textbook of Rheumatology* feel a profound sadness with the loss of Ted, but even here Ted would provide the appropriate perspective, with a passage he wrote in a *Pharos* editorial: "Melancholy, that gray veil that takes color out of life, can, at the same time, add to the brilliance and value of life, if we feel what it is asking of us. Melancholy and sadness, similar to love, can make those compartment walls in our minds permeable, enabling us to express empathy that is truly felt within."

Ted Harris was a consummate scholar and a great humanitarian, with a facile mind that spanned a wide array of interests from science to the arts. He was in essence a civilized man, something that has always been distinguished by its rarity.

Steven B. Abramson, MD
Professor of Medicine and Pathology
Department of Medicine, Division of Rheumatology
NYU School of Medicine
New York, New York
 Neutrophils; Eosinophils; Pathogenesis of Osteoarthritis

Kai-Nan An, PhD
Professor of Biomedical Engineering
Mayo Clinic College of Medicine;
Program Co-Director, Biomechanics and Motion Analysis Lab
Department of Orthopedic Surgery
Mayo Clinic
Rochester, Minnesota
 Biomechanics

Felipe Andrade, MD, PhD
Assistant Professor of Medicine
Department of Medicine, Division of Rheumatology
Johns Hopkins University School of Medicine;
Center for Innovative Medicine
Johns Hopkins Medicine
Baltimore, Maryland
 Autoantibodies in Rheumatoid Arthritis

John P. Atkinson, MD
Samuel B. Grant Professor of Medicine and Professor of Molecular Microbiology and Immunology
Washington University in St. Louis School of Medicine;
Physician, Barnes-Jewish Hospital
St. Louis, Missouri
 Complement System

Dominique Baeten, MD, PhD
Associate Professor of Rheumatology
Department of Clinical Immunology and Rheumatology
University of Amsterdam Faculty of Medicine
Academic Medical Center
Amsterdam, The Netherlands
 Ankylosing Spondylitis

Robert P. Baughman, MD
Profesor of Medicine
Department of Internal Medicine
University of Cincinnati College of Medicine
Cincinnati, Ohio
 Sarcoidosis

Dorcas E. Beaton, BScOT, PhD
Associate Professor
Graduate Department of Rehabilitation Science and Department of Occupational Science and Occupational Therapy
Faculty of Medicine;
Clinician-Investigator
Institute of Health Policy, Management and Evaluation;
Scientist, Health Measurement
Institute for Work and Health
University of Toronto;
Director, Mobility Program Clinical Research Unit, Li Ka Shing Knowledge Institute
St. Michael's Hospital
Toronto, Ontario, Canada
 Assessment of Health Outcomes

Robert Bennett, MD
Professor of Medicine
Oregon Health & Science University School of Medicine
Portland, Oregon
 Overlap Syndromes

Susanne M. Benseler, MD
Associate Professor of Paediatrics
Department of Paediatrics, Division of Rheumatology
Faculty of Medicine;
Clinician-Investigator
Institute of Health Policy, Evaluation and Management
University of Toronto;
Associate Scientist
Research Institute
The Hospital for Sick Children
Toronto, Ontario, Canada
 Pediatric Systemic Lupus Erythematosus, Dermatomyositis, Scleroderma, and Vasculitis

George Bertsias, MD, PhD
Fellow, Internal Medicine
Research Associate in Rheumatology, Clinical Immunology, and Allergy
University of Crete Faculty of Medicine
Heraklion, Crete, Greece
 Treatment of Systemic Lupus Erythematosus

Nina Bhardwaj, MD, PhD
Professor of Medicine, Dermatology, and Pathology
Department of Medicine
NYU School of Medicine
New York, New York
 Dendritic Cells

Johannes W.J. Bijlsma, MD, PhD
Professor and Chair, Department of Rheumatology and
    Clinical Immunology
University of Utrecht Faculty of Medicine
Utrecht, The Netherlands
    Glucocorticoid Therapy

Linda K. Bockenstedt, MD
Harold W. Jockers Professor of Medicine
Department of Internal Medicine, Section of
    Rheumatology
Yale University School of Medicine
New Haven, Connecticut
    Lyme Disease

Maarten Boers, MD, PhD, MSc
Professor of Clinical Epidemiology
Department of Clinical Epidemiology and Biostatistics
VU University Amsterdam Faculty of Medicine
Amsterdam, The Netherlands
    Assessment of Health Outcomes

Francesco Boin, MD
Assistant Professor of Medicine
Department of Medicine, Division of Rheumatology
Johns Hopkins University School of Medicine
Baltimore, Maryland
    Clinical Features and Treatment of Scleroderma

Dimitrios T. Boumpas, MD, FACP
Professor of Internal Medicine
Professor of Rheumatology, Clinical Immunology, and
    Allergy
University of Crete Faculty of Medicine
Heraklion, Crete, Greece
    Treatment of Systemic Lupus Erythematosus

†Barry Bresnihan, MD
Professor of Rheumatology
University College Dublin School of Medicine and
    Medical Science
National University of Ireland;
Consultant Rheumatologist
St. Vincent's University Hospital;
Principal Investigator
Conway Institute of of Biomolecular and Biomedical
    Research
Dublin, Ireland
    Synovium

Doreen B. Brettler, MD
Professor of Medicine
University of Massachusetts Medical School;
Director, New England Hemophilia Center
UMass Memorial Medical Center
Worcester, Massachusetts
    Hemophilic Arthopathy

Christopher D. Buckley, DPhil, FRCP
Arthritis Research UK Professor of Rheumatology
College of Medical and Dental Sciences, School of
    Immunity and Infection;
Head, Rheumatology Research Group
Institute for Biomedical Research
University of Birmingham;
Birmingham, United Kingdom
    Fibroblasts and Fibroblast-like Synoviocytes

Ralph C. Budd, MD
Professor of Medicine
Director, Vermont Center for Immunology and Infectious
    Diseases
The University of Vermont College of Medicine
Burlington, Vermont
    T Lymphocytes

Christopher M. Burns, MD
Assistant Professor of Medicine
Department of Medicine, Section of Rheumatology
Geisel School of Medicine at Dartmouth;
Staff Rheumatologist
Dartmouth-Hitchcock Medical Center
Lebanon, New Hampshire
    Clinical Features and Treatment of Gout

Amy C. Cannella, MD
Assistant Professor of Internal Medicine
Department of Internal Medicine, Division of
    Rheumatology
University of Nebraska College of Medicine
Omaha, Nebraska
    *Traditional DMARDs: Methotrexate, Leflunomide,
    Sulfasalazine, Hydroxychloroquine, and Combination
    Therapies*

Eliza F. Chakravarty, MD, MS
Associate Member
Arthritis & Clinical Immunology Program
Oklahoma Medical Research Foundation
Oklahoma City, Oklahoma
    *Pregnancy in the Rheumatic Diseases;
    Musculoskeletal Syndromes in Malignancy*

Christopher Chang, MD, PhD
Professor of Pediatrics
Chief, Division of Allergy, Asthma, and Immunology
Department of Pediatrics
Thomas Jefferson University
Philadelphia, Pennsylvania;
Associate Clinical Professor of Medicine
Department of Internal Medicine, Division of
    Rheumatology, Allergy, Clinical Immunology
UC Davis School of Medicine
Davis, California
    Osteonecrosis

Joseph S. Cheng, MD, MS
Associate Professor of Neurological Surgery, Orthopedic
 Surgery, and Rehabilitation
Vanderbilt University School of Medicine;
Director, Neurosurgery Spine Program
Vanderbilt University Medical Center
Nashville, Tennessee
 Neck Pain

Christopher P. Chiodo, MD
Chief, Foot and Ankle Service
Department of Orthopedic Surgery
Brigham and Women's Hospital;
Instructor in Orthopaedic Surgery
Harvard Medical School
Boston, Massachusetts
 Foot and Ankle Pain

Leslie G. Cleland, MBBS, MD
Clinical Professor
Department of Medicine
University of Adelaide School of Medicine, Faculty of
 Health Sciences
Head, Rheumatology Unit
Royal Adelaide Hospital
Adelaide, South Australia, Australia
 Nutrition and Rheumatic Diseases

Megan E. Clowse, MD, MPH
Assistant Professor
Department of Medicine, Division of Rheumatology and
 Immunology
Duke University School of Medicine
Durham, North Carolina
 Pregnancy in the Rheumatic Diseases

Paul P. Cook, MD
Professor of Medicine
Department of Medicine, Division of Infectious Diseases
Brody School of Medicine at East Carolina University
Greenville, North Carolina
 Bacterial Arthritis

Joseph E. Craft, MD
Paul B. Beeson Professor of Medicine and Professor of
 Immunobiology
Director, Investigative Medicine Program
Yale University School of Medicine;
Chief of Rheumatology
Yale–New Haven Hospital
New Haven, Connecticut
 Antinuclear Antibodies

Leslie J. Crofford, MD
Gloria W. Singletary Professor
Chief, Division of Rheumatology
Department of Internal Medicine
University of Kentucky School of Medicine
Director, Center for the Advancement of Women's
 Health
UK HealthCare
Lexington, Kentucky
 Prostanoid Biology and Its Therapeutic Targeting

Bruce N. Cronstein, MD
Paul R. Esserman Professor of Medicine
NYU School of Medicine
New York, New York
 *Acute Phase Reactants and the Concept of
 Inflammation*

Mary K. Crow, MD
Joseph P. Routh Professor of Rheumatic Diseases in
 Medicine
Weill Cornell Medical College;
Benjamin M. Rosen Chair in Immunology and
 Inflammation Research
Divisions of Rheumatology and Research
Hospital for Special Surgery
New York, New York
 *Etiology and Pathogenesis of Systemic Lupus
 Erythematosus*

Gaye Cunnane, MB, PhD, FRCPI
Clinical Professor
Trinity College Dublin;
Consultant Rheumatologist
St. James's Hospital
Dublin, Ireland
 Relapsing Polychondritis; Hemochromatosis

John J. Cush, MD
Professor of Medicine and Rheumatology
Baylor University Medical Center–Dallas;
Director, Clinical Rheumatology
Baylor Research Institute–Rheumatology
Dallas, Texas
 Polyarticular Arthritis

Maurizio Cutolo, MD
Professor of Rheumatology
University of Genova;
Director, Research Laboratories and Academic Unit of
 Clinical Rheumatology
Medical School University of Genova
Genova, Italy
 Endocrine Diseases and the Musculoskeletal System

Maria Dall'Era, MD
Associate Professor of Medicine
Division of Rheumatology
University of California, San Francisco
San Francisco, California
 Clinical Features of Systemic Lupus Erythematosus

Kathryn H. Dao, MD, FACP, FACR
Associate Director, Clinical Rheumatology
Department of Rheumatology
Baylor Research Institute
Dallas, Texas
 Polyarticular Arthritis

Erika Darrah, PhD
Postdoctoral Fellow
Division of Rheumatology
Department of Medicine
Johns Hopkins University
Baltimore, Maryland
Autoantibodies in Rheumatoid Arthritis

John M. Davis III, MD
Assistant Professor of Medicine
Department of Medicine, Division of Rheumatology
Mayo Clinic College of Medicine;
Consultant in Rheumatology
Mayo Clinic
Rochester, Minnesota
History and Physical Examination of the Musculoskeletal System

Jeroen DeGroot, PhD
Research Manager
Pharmacokinetics & Human Studies
TNO Quality of Life
Business Unit Biomedical Research
Zeist, The Netherlands
Biologic Markers

Clint Devin, MD
Assistant Professor of Neurological Surgery, Orthopaedic Surgery, and Rehabilitation
Vanderbilt University School of Medicine
Nashville, Tennessee
Neck Pain

Betty Diamond, MD
Investigator
Center for Autoimmune and Musculoskeletal Diseases
The Feinstein Institute for Medical Research
Manhasset, New York
B Cells

Federico Díaz-González, MD
Professor of Medicine
Department of Internal Medicine
University of La Laguna;
Staff, Rheumatology Service
University Hospital of the Canary Islands
San Cristobal de La Laguna, Tenerife, Spain
Platelets

Paul E. Di Cesare, MD, FACS
Professor and Michael W. Chapman Chair, Department of Orthopaedic Surgery
UC Davis School of Medicine
Davis, California
Pathogenesis of Osteoarthritis

Rajiv Dixit, MD
Clinical Professor of Medicine
Department of Medicine
UCSF School of Medicine
San Francisco;
Director, Northern California Arthritis Center
Walnut Creek, California
Low Back Pain

Joost P.H. Drenth, MD, PhD
Professor of Molecular Gastroenterology and Hepatology
Department of Gastroenterology and Hepatology
Radboud University Nijmegen Faculty of Medical Sciences
Nijmegen, The Netherlands
Familial Autoinflammatory Syndromes

Michael L. Dustin, PhD
Muriel G. and George W. Singer Professor of Molecular Immunology
Program in Molecular Pathogenesis
Helen L. and Martin S. Kimmel Center for Biology and Medicine, Skirball Institute of Biomolecular Medicine
NYU School of Medicine
New York, New York
Adaptive Immunity and Organization of Lymphoid Tissues

Hani S. El-Gabalawy, MD, FRCPC
Endowed Research Chair in Rheumatology
Professor of Medicine and Immunology
University of Manitoba Faculty of Medicine;
Rheumatologist, Winnipeg Health Sciences Centre
Winnipeg, Manitoba, Canada
Synovial Fluid Analyses, Synovial Biopsy, and Synovial Pathology

Keith B. Elkon, MD
Professor of Medicine and Immunology
University of Washington School of Medicine
Seattle, Washington
Cell Survival and Death in Rheumatic Diseases

Doruk Erkan, MD
Associate Professor of Medicine
Weill Cornell Medical College;
Associate Physician-Scientist and Associate Attending Physician
Barbara Volcker Center for Women and Rheumatic Diseases
Hospital for Special Surgery
New York, New York
Antiphospholipid Syndrome

Antonios Fanouriakis, MD
Professor of Rheumatology, Clinical Immunology, and Allergy
University of Crete Faculty of Medicine
Heraklion, Greece
Treatment of Systemic Lupus Erythematosus

Max Field, MD, FRCP
Associate Academic
Division of Immunology, Institute of Infection,
  Immunology and Immunity
College of Medical, Veterinary and Life Sciences
University of Glasgow
Glasgow, United Kingdom
  Acute Monoarthritis

Andrew Filer, PhD, MRCP
Senior Lecturer
College of Medical and Dental Sciences, School of
  Immunity and Infection;
Rheumatology Research Group
Institute for Biomedical Research
University of Birmingham;
Honorary Consultant Rheumatologist
University Hospitals NHS Foundation Trust Birmingham
Birmingham, United Kingdom
  Fibroblasts and Fibroblast-like Synoviocytes

Gary S. Firestein, MD
Professor of Medicine
Dean and Associate Vice Chancellor of Translational
  Medicine
UC San Diego Health Sciences
La Jolla, California
  *Synovium; Etiology and Pathogenesis of Rheumatoid
  Arthritis; Clinical Features of Rheumatoid Arthritis*

Oliver Fitzgerald, MD, FRCPI, FRCP(UK)
Newman Clinical Research Professor
University College Dublin School of Medicine and
  Medical Science
National University of Ireland;
Fellow, Conway Institute of Biomolecular and Biomedical
  Research;
Consultant Rheumatologist
St. Vincent's University Hospital
Dublin, Ireland
  Psoriatic Arthritis

John P. Flaherty, MD
Professor in Medicine–Infectious Diseases
Associate Chief and Director of Clinical Services
Division of Infectious Diseases
Department of Medicine
Northwestern University Feinberg School of Medicine;
Chicago, Illinois
  *Mycobacterial Infections of Bones and Joints; Fungal
  Infections of Bones and Joints*

Adrienne M. Flanagan, MD, PhD
Professor
Institute of Orthopaedics and Musculoskeletal Science
University College London
London;
Royal National Orthopaedic Hospital
Stanmore;
Department of Histopathology
University College Hospital
London, United Kingdom
  Synovium

Karen A. Fortner, PhD
Assistant Professor
Immunobiology Program
Department of Medicine
The University of Vermont College of Medicine
Burlington, Vermont
  T Lymphocytes

Sherine E. Gabriel, MD, MSc
William J. and Charles H. Mayo Professor
Professor of Medicine and Epidemiology
Mayo Clinic College of Medicine
Rochester, Minnesota
  Cardiovascular Risk in Rheumatic Disease

J.S. Hill Gaston, MA, BM, PhD, FRCP, FMedSci
Professor of Rheumatology
Department of Medicine
University of Cambridge;
Addenbrooke's Hospital
Cambridge, United Kingdom
  *Reactive Arthritis and Undifferentiated
  Spondyloarthritis*

Steffen Gay, MD
Center for Experimental Rheumatology
Zurich Center for Integrative Human Physiology, Life
  Science Zurich Graduate School/University Hospital
  Zurich
Zurich, Switzerland
  Epigenetics

M. Eric Gershwin, MD
Distinguished Professor of Medicine
Chief, Division of Rheumatology, Allergy and Clinical
  Immunology
Department of Medicine
UC Davis School of Medicine
Davis, California
  Osteonecrosis

Allan Gibofsky, MD, JD, FACP, FCLM
Professor of Medicine and Public Health
Weill Cornell Medical College;
Attending Rheumatologist
Hospital for Special Surgery
New York, New York
  Poststreptococcal Arthritis and Rheumatic Fever

Mark H. Ginsberg, MD
Professor of Medicine
Department of Medicine, Section of Rheumatology
UC San Diego School of Medicine
La Jolla, California
  Platelets

Mary B. Goldring, PhD
Professor of Cell and Developmental Biology
Weill Cornell Medical College;
Senior Scientist, Research Division
Hospital for Special Surgery
New York, New York
Biology of the Normal Joint; Cartilage and Chondrocytes

Steven R. Goldring, MD
Professor of Medicine
Weill Cornell Medical College;
Chief Scientific Officer
Hospital for Special Surgery
New York, New York
Biology of the Normal Joint

Yvonne M. Golightly, PT, PhD
Postdoctoral Research Associate
UNC Thurston Arthritis Research Center;
Department of Epidemiology
UNC Gillings School of Global Public Health
Chapel Hill, North Carolina
Principles of Epidemiology in Rheumatic Disease

Stuart Goodman, MD, PhD
Professor of Orthopaedics
Stanford University School of Medicine
Stanford, California
Hip and Knee Pain

Siamon Gordon, MB, ChB, PhD
Professor Emeritus
Sir William Dunn School of Pathology
University of Oxford
Oxford, United Kingdom
Mononuclear Phagocytes in Rheumatic Diseases

Walter Grassi, MD
Professor of Rheumatology
Clinica Reumatologica
Università Politecnica delle Marche
Jesi, Ancona, Italy
Imaging Modalities in Rheumatic Diseases

Adam Greenspan, MD, FACR
Professor Emeritus of Radiology
Department of Radiology, Section of Musculoskeletal Imaging
UC Davis School of Medicine
Davis, California
Osteonecrosis

Peter K. Gregersen, MD
Director, Robert S. Boas Center for Genomics and Human Genetics
The Feinstein Institute for Medical Research;
Professor of Molecular Medicine
Hofstra University School of Medicine
Manhasset, New York
Genetics of Rheumatic Diseases

Christine Grimaldi, PhD
Senior Principal Scientist
Nonclinical Drug Safety, US
Boehringer Ingelheim Pharmaceuticals, Inc.
Ridgefield, Connecticut
B Cells

Rula A. Hajj-Ali, MD
Assistant Professor of Medicine
Cleveland Clinic Lerner College of Medicine of Case Western University;
Staff Physician, Center for Vasculitis Care and Research
Cleveland Clinic
Cleveland, Ohio
Primary Angiitis of the Central Nervous System

Lorraine Harper, PhD, MRCP
Professor of Nephrology
College of Medical and Dental Sciences, School of Immunity and Infection
University of Birmingham
Birmingham, United Kingdom
Antineutrophil Cytoplasm Antibody–Associated Vasculitis

†Edward D. Harris, Jr., MD, MACR
George DeForest Barnett Professor of Medicine, Emeritus
Stanford University School of Medicine;
Academic Secretary to Stanford University, Emeritus
Stanford University
Stanford, California
Clinical Features of Rheumatoid Arthritis

Dominik R. Haudenschild, PhD
Assistant Professor in Residence
Department of Orthopaedic Surgery
UC Davis School of Medicine
Davis, California
Pathogenesis of Osteoarthritis

David B. Hellmann, MD
Aliki Perroti Professor of Medicine
Department of Medicine
Johns Hopkins University School of Medicine;
Vice Dean and Chairman, Department of Medicine
Johns Hopkins Bayview
Baltimore, Maryland
Giant Cell Arteritis, Polymyalgia Rheumatica, and Takayasu's Arteritis

Rikard Holmdahl, MD, PhD
Professor of Medical Biochemistry and Biophysics
Karolinska Institute
Stockholm, Sweden
Experimental Models for Rheumatoid Arthritis

†Deceased.

Joyce J. Hsu, MD, MS
Clinical Assistant Professor of Pediatrics
Department of Pediatrics, Division of Pediatric
  Rheumatology
Stanford University
Palo Alto, California
  Treatment of Juvenile Idiopathic Arthritis

James I. Huddleston, MD
Assistant Professor
Department of Orthopaedic Surgery
Stanford University School of Medicine
Stanford, California
  Hip and Knee Pain

Thomas W.J. Huizinga, MD, PhD
Chairman, Department of Rheumatology
Leiden University Faculty of Medicine
Leiden, The Netherlands
  Early Synovitis and Early Undifferentiated Arthritis

Gene G. Hunder, MD, MS
Professor of Medicine
Department of Medicine, Division of Rheumatology
Mayo Clinic College of Medicine;
Emeritus Consultant in Rheumatology
Mayo Clinic
Rochester, Minnesota
  *History and Physical Examination of the
  Musculoskeletal System*

Emily W. Hung, MD
Internal Medicine/Rheumatology
University of Texas Medical School at Houston
Houston, Texas
  *Rheumatic Manifestations of Human
  Immunodeficiency Virus Infection*

Robert D. Inman, MD
Professor of Medicine and Immunology
University of Toronto Faculty of Medicine;
Director, Arthritis Centre of Excellence
Toronto Western Hospital
Toronto, Ontario, Canada
  *Pathogenesis of Ankylosing Spondylitis and Reactive
  Arthritis*

Maura Daly Iversen, DPT, ScD, MPH
Professor and Chair, Department of Physical Therapy
Northeastern University Bouvé College of Health
  Sciences;
Senior Lecturer and Behavioral Scientist
Brigham and Women's Hospital/Harvard Medical School
Boston, Massachusetts
  *Introduction to Physical Medicine, Physical Therapy,
  and Rehabilitation*

Johannes W.G. Jacobs, MD, PhD
Associate Professor
Department of Rheumatology and Clinical Immunology
University of Utrecht Faculty of Medicine;
Rheumatologist and Senior Researcher
University Medical Center Utrecht
Utrecht, The Netherlands
  Glucocorticoid Therapy

Joanne M. Jordan, MD, MPH
Herman and Louise Smith Distinguished Professor of
  Medicine, Professor of Orthopaedics, and Adjunct
  Professor of Epidemiology
Chief, Division of Rheumatology, Allergy, and
  Immunology
University of North Carolina School of Medicine;
Director, UNC Thurston Arthritis Research Center
Chapel Hill, North Carolina
  *Principles of Epidemiology in Rheumatic Disease;
  Clinical Features of Osteoarthritis*

Joseph L. Jorizzo, MD
Professor and Former (Founding) Chair, Department of
  Dermatology
Wake Forest University School of Medicine
Winston-Salem, North Carolina
  Behçet's Disease

Kenton R. Kaufman, PhD, PE
Professor of Biomedical Engineering
Mayo Clinic College of Medicine;
Program Co-Director, Biomechanics and Motion Analysis
  Lab
Department of Orthopedic Surgery
Mayo Clinic
Rochester, Minnesota
  Biomechanics

William S. Kaufman, MD
Resident Physician
Department of Dermatology
Wake Forest Baptist Medical Center
Winston-Salem, North Carolina
  Behçet's Disease

Arthur Kavanaugh, MD
Professor of Medicine
Department of Medicine, Division of Rheumatology,
  Allergy, and Immunology
UC San Diego School of Medicine;
Director, UCSD Center for Innovative Therapy
La Jolla, California
  Anticytokine Therapies

Robert T. Keenan, MD, MPH
Assistant Professor of Medicine
Division of Rheumatology and Immunology
Duke University School of Medicine
Durham, North Carolina
  Etiology and Pathogenesis of Hyperuricemia and Gout

Shaukat Khan, PhD
Postdoctoral Fellow
NYU Cancer Institute
NYU Langone Medical Center
New York, New York
Dendritic Cells

Alisa E. Koch, MD
Frederick G.L. Huetwell and William D. Robinson, MD,
  Professor of Rheumatology
University of Michigan Medical School
Ann Arbor, Michigan
Cell Recruitment and Angiogenesis

Dwight H. Kono, MD
Professor of Immunology
Department of Immunology and Microbial Science
The Scripps Research Institute Kellogg School of Science
  and Technology
La Jolla, California
Autoimmunity

Deborah Krakow, MD
Professor
Department of Orthopaedic Surgery and Department of
  Human Genetics
David Geffen School of Medicine at UCLA
Los Angeles, California
Heritable Diseases of Connective Tissue

Robert G.W. Lambert, MB, FRCR, FRCPC
Professor of Radiology
Department of Radiology and Diagnostic Imaging
University of Alberta Faculty of Medicine and Dentistry
Edmonton, Alberta, Canada
Imaging Modalities in Rheumatic Diseases

Robert B.M. Landewé, MD
Professor of Rheumatology
University of Amsterdam Faculty of Medicine
Academic Medical Center
Amsterdam;
Consultant, Atrium Medical Center
Heerlen, The Netherlands
Clinical Trial Design and Analysis

Nancy E. Lane, MD
Endowed Professor of Medicine and Rheumatology
Director, Musculoskeletal and Aging Research Center
UC Davis School of Medicine
Davis, California
Metabolic Bone Disease

Carol A. Langford, MD, MHS
Director, Center for Vasculitis Care and Research
Department of Rheumatic and Immunologic Diseases
Cleveland Clinic
Cleveland, Ohio
Primary Angiitis of the Central Nervous System

Daniel M. Laskin, DDS, MS, DSc(Hon)
Professor and Chairman Emeritus, Department of Oral
  and Maxillofacial Surgery
Virginia Commonwealth University Schools of Dentistry
  and Medicine
Richmond, Virginia
Temporomandibular Joint Pain

Ronald M. Laxer, MDCM, FRCPC
Professor of Pediatrics and Medicine
University of Toronto Faculty of Medicine;
Rheumatologist
The Hospital for Sick Children
Toronto, Ontario, Canada
Pediatric Systemic Lupus Erythematosus,
  Dermatomyositis, Scleroderma, and Vasculitis

David M. Lee, MD
Head, ATI Translational Research
Autoimmunity, Transplantation and Inflammation
Novartis Institutes for BioMedical Research
Novartis Pharma, AG
Basel, Switzerland
Mast Cells

Lela A. Lee, MD
Professor of Dermatology and Medicine
University of Colorado School of Medicine;
Director of Dermatology
Denver Health Medical Center
Denver, Colorado
The Skin and Rheumatic Diseases

Tzielan Chang Lee, MD
Clinical Associate Professor of Pediatrics
Department of Pediatrics, Division of Pediatric
  Rheumatology
Stanford University
Palo Alto, California
Treatment of Juvenile Idiopathic Arthritis

Michael D. Lockshin, MD
Professor of Medicine and Obstetrics-Gynecology
Weill Cornell Medical College;
Director and Attending Physician
Barbara Volcker Center for Women and Rheumatic
  Diseases
Hospital for Special Surgery
New York, New York
Antiphospholipid Syndrome

Rik Lories, MD, PhD
Professor
Department of Musculoskeletal Sciences, Division of
  Rheumatology;
Faculty of Medicine;
Head, Homeostasis, Regeneration, and Ageing
Laboratory for Skeletal Development and Joint Disorders
Katholieke Universiteit Leuven
Leuven, Belgium
Pathogenesis of Ankylosing Spondylitis and Reactive
  Arthritis

Carlos J. Lozada, MD
Professor
Department of Medicine, Division of Rheumatology
University of Miami Miller School of Medicine
Miami, Florida
  Treatment of Osteoarthritis

Ingrid E. Lundberg, MD, PhD
Professor of Medicine
Department of Medicine;
Head, Rheumatology Unit
Karolinska Institute/Karolinska University Hospital
Stockholm, Sweden
  Inflammatory Diseases of Muscle and Other Myopathies

Raashid Luqmani, BMedSci, BM, BS, MRCP, FRCPEd, FRCP, DM
Professor of Rheumatology
Nuffield Department of Orthopaedics, Rheumatology and Musculoskeletal Science
University of Oxford
Oxford, United Kingdom
  Polyarteritis Nodosa and Related Disorders

Frank P. Luyten, MD, PhD
Chairman, Department of Musculoskeletal Sciences
Katholieke Universiteit Leuven Faculty of Medicine;
Head, Division of Rheumatology
University Hospitals
Leuven, Belgium
  Regenerative Medicine and Tissue Engineering

Reuven Mader, MD
Head, Rheumatic Diseases Unit
Department of Rheumatology
Ha'Emek Medical Center
Afula;
Associate Clinical Professor of Medicine
B. Rappaport Faculty of Medicine
Technion Institute of Technology
Haifa, Israel
  Proliferative Bone Diseases

Walter P. Maksymowych, MD, PhD, FRCPC, FACP, FRCP(UK)
Professor of Medicine
Department of Medicine, Division of Rheumatology
University of Alberta Faculty of Medicine and Dentistry
Edmonton, Alberta, Canada
  Ankylosing Spondylitis

Brian Mandell, MD, PhD
Professor and Chairman, Department of Medicine
Cleveland Clinic Lerner College of Medicine of Case Western Reserve University;
Senior Staff, Department of Rheumatic and Immunologic Diseases
Center for Vasculitis Care and Research
Cleveland Clinic
Cleveland, Ohio
  Rheumatologic Manifestations of Hemoglobinopathies

Scott David Martin, MD
Associate Professor of Orthopedics
Harvard Medical School;
Attending Staff Physician
Department of Orthopedics
Brigham and Women's Hospital
Boston, Massachusetts
  Shoulder Pain

Eric L. Matteson, MD, MPH
Professor of Medicine
Mayo Clinic College of Medicine;
Consultant in Rheumatology
Mayo Clinic
Rochester, Minnesota
  Cancer Risk in Rheumatic Diseases

Matthew J. McGirt, MD
Assistant Professor of Neurological Surgery, Orthopedic Surgery, and Rehabilitation
Vanderbilt University School of Medicine
Nashville, Tennessee
  Neck Pain

Iain B. McInnes, PhD, FRCP, FRSE
Muirhead Professor of Medicine
Director, Institute of Infection, Immunity and Inflammation
College of Medical, Veterinary and Life Sciences
University of Glasgow
Glasgow, United Kingdom
  Cytokines

Elizabeth Kaufman McNamara, MD
Dermatologist
Roanoke, Virginia
  Behçet's Disease

Ted R. Mikuls, MD, MSPH
Professor of Medicine
Department of Internal Medicine, Division of Rheumatology
University of Nebraska College of Medicine;
UNMC Physician
University of Nebraska Medical Center and Omaha VA Medical Center
Omaha, Nebraska
  Antihyperuricemic Agents

Mark S. Miller, PhD
Research Associate
Department of Molecular Physiology and Biophysics
The University of Vermont College of Medicine
Burlington, Vermont
  Muscle: Anatomy, Physiology, and Biochemistry

Kevin G. Moder, MD
Associate Professor of Medicine
Department of Medicine, Division of Rheumatology
Mayo Clinic College of Medicine;
Consultant in Rheumatology
Mayo Clinic
Rochester, Minnesota
*History and Physical Examination of the
Musculoskeletal System*

Kanneboyina Nagaraju, DVM, PhD
Professor of Integrative Systems Biology and Pediatrics
George Washington University School of Medicine and
   Health Sciences;
Director, Murine Drug Testing Facility
Center for Genetic Medicine Research
Children's Research Institute
Children's National Medical Center
Washington, DC
*Inflammatory Diseases of Muscle and Other
Myopathies*

Stanley J. Naides, MD
Medical Director, Immunology Research and
   Development
Quest Diagnostics Nichols Institute
San Juan Capistrano, California
Viral Arthritis

Amanda E. Nelson, MD, MSCR
Assistant Professor
Department of Medicine, Division of Rheumatology,
   Allergy and Immunology
University of North Carolina School of Medicine
Chapel Hill, North Carolina
Clinical Features of Osteoarthritis

Peter A. Nigrovic, MD
Assistant Professor of Medicine
Division of Rheumatology, Immunology, and Allergy
Department of Medicine at Brigham and Women's
   Hospital and Harvard Medical School;
Director, Center for Adults with Pediatric Rheumatic
   Illness (CAPRI)
Brigham and Women's Hospital;
Division of Immunology
Boston Children's Hospital
Boston, Massachusetts
Mast Cells

Kiran Nistala, MD, PhD, MRCP
Wellcome Trust Research Fellow in Paediatric
   Rheumatology
Centre for Rheumatology
University College London;
Consultant in Paediatric Rheumatology
Rheumatology Unit
Great Ormond Street Hospital
London, United Kingdom
*Etiology and Pathogenesis of Juvenile Idiopathic
Arthritis*

Johannes Nowatzky, MD
Assistant Professor of Medicine
Department of Medicine, Division of Rheumatology
NYU School of Medicine
New York, New York
Etiology and Pathogenesis of Hyperuricemia and Gout

James R. O'Dell, MD
Bruce Professor of Medicine
Vice Chairman, Department of Internal Medicine
University of Nebraska College of Medicine;
Chief, Division of Rheumatology and Immunology
University of Nebraska Medical Center;
Omaha VA
Omaha, Nebraska
*Traditional DMARDs: Methotrexate, Leflunomide,
Sulfasalazine, Hydroxychloroquine, and Combination
Therapies; Treatment of Rheumatoid Arthritis*

Yasunori Okada, MD, PhD
Professor of Pathology
Keio University School of Medicine
Tokyo, Japan
Proteinases and Matrix Degradation

Nataly Manjarrez Orduño, PhD
Center for Autoimmune and Musculoskeletal Diseases
The Feinstein Institute for Medical Research
Manhasset, New York
B Cells

Caroline Ospelt, MD
Center for Experimental Rheumatology
Zurich Center for Integrative Human Physiology, Life
   Science Zurich Graduate School/University Hospital
   Zurich
Zurich, Switzerland
Epigenetics

Mikkel Østergaard, MD, PhD, DMSc
Professor of Rheumatology
Department of Orthopaedics and Internal Medicine,
   Division of Rheumatology
Copenhagen University Faculty of Health and Medical
   Sciences/Glostrup Hospital
Copenhagen, Denmark
Imaging Modalities in Rheumatic Diseases

Bradley M. Palmer, PhD
Research Assistant Professor
Department of Molecular Physiology and Biophysics
The University of Vermont College of Medicine
Burlington, Vermont
Muscle: Anatomy, Physiology, and Biochemistry

Richard S. Panush, MD, MACP, MACR
Professor of Medicine
Department of Medicine, Division of Rheumatology
Keck School of Medicine of USC
Los Angeles, California
*Occupational and Recreational Musculoskeletal
Disorders*

Stanford L. Peng, MD, PhD
Assistant Clinical Professor
Department of Medicine, Division of Rheumatology
University of Washington School of Medicine;
Head, Rheumatology Clinical Research Unit
Benaroya Research Institute at Virginia Mason;
Physician, Section of Rheumatology
Virginia Mason Medical Center
Seattle, Washington
Antinuclear Antibodies

Michael H. Pillinger, MD
Associate Professor of Medicine and Pharmacology
Department of Medicine, Division of Rheumatology
NYU School of Medicine;
Section Chief, Rheumatology
Department of Medicine
VA New York Harbor Healthcare System, Manhattan
  Campus
New York, New York
*Neutrophils; Eosinophils; Etiology and Pathogenesis
of Hyperuricemia and Gout*

Gregory R. Polston, MD
Associate Professor of Clinical Anesthesiology
Department of Anesthesiology
UC San Diego School of Medicine;
Associate Medical Director, Center for Pain Medicine
UC San Diego Medical Center
La Jolla, California
Analgesic Agents in Rheumatic Disease

Steven A. Porcelli, MD
Murray and Evelyne Weinstock Professor of Microbiology
  and Immunology
Department of Microbiology and Immunology and
  Department of Medicine
Albert Einstein College of Medicine
Bronx, New York
Innate Immunity

Mark D. Price, MD, PhD
Assistant Professor of Orthopedics and Rehabilitation
University of Massachusetts Medical School;
Orthopedic Surgeon, Sports Medicine Center
UMass Memorial Medical Center
Worcester, Massachusetts
Foot and Ankle Pain

Johannes J. Rasker, MD, PhD
Professor Emeritus of Rheumatology
Department of Psychology and Communication of Health
  and Risk
University of Twente Faculty of Behavioural Sciences
Enschede, The Netherlands
Fibromyalgia

John D. Reveille, MD
Professor of Internal Medicine
Director, Division of Rheumatology and Clinical
  Immunogenetics
University of Texas Medical School at Houston;
Memorial Hermann-Texas Medical Center
Houston, Texas
*Rheumatic Manifestations of Human
Immunodeficiency Virus Infection*

W. Neal Roberts, Jr., MD
Charles W. Thomas Professor and Rheumatology
  Fellowship Program Director
Department of Internal Medicine, Division of
  Rheumatology, Allergy, and Immunology
Virginia Commonwealth University School of Medicine,
  Medical College of Virginia Campus
Richmond, Virginia
Psychosocial Management of Rheumatic Diseases

Monika Ronneberger, DrMed, DiplBiol
Medizinische Klinik 3 mit Poliklinik
University of Erlangen–Nuremberg
Erlangen, Germany
Enteropathic Arthritis

Antony Rosen, ChB, BSc, MB
Mary Betty Stevens Professor of Medicine and Professor of
  Pathology
Director, Division of Rheumatology
Department of Medicine
Johns Hopkins University School of Medicine
Baltimore, Maryland
Autoantibodies in Rheumatoid Arthritis

James T. Rosenbaum, MD
Professor of Ophthalmology, Medicine and Cell Biology
  and Edward E Rosenbaum Professor of Inflammation
  Research
Department of Ophthalmology
Oregon Health & Science University School of Medicine
Portland, Oregon
The Eye and Rheumatic Diseases

Andrew E. Rosenberg, MD
Professor of Pathology
Director, Anatomic Pathology
Director, Bone and Soft Tissue Pathology
University of Miami Miller School of Medicine
Miami, Florida
*Tumors and Tumor-like Lesions of Joints and Related
Structures*

Eric M. Ruderman, MD
Professor of Medicine
Department of Medicine, Division of Rheumatology
Northwestern University Feinberg School of Medicine;
Clinical Practice Director, Rheumatology Clinic
Northwestern Memorial Hospital
Chicago, Illinois
*Mycobacterial Infections of Bones and Joints; Fungal
Infections of Bones and Joints*

Merja Ruutu, MD
Postdoctoral Fellow
Diamantina Institute for Cancer, Immunology, and
    Metabolic Medicine
University of Queensland
Princess Alexandra Hospital
Queensland, Australia
    Dendritic Cells

Jane E. Salmon, MD
Professor of Medicine
Weill Cornell Medical College;
Co-Director, Mary Kirkland Center for Lupus Research;
Attending Physician, Hospital for Special Surgery
New York, New York
    Antiphospholipid Syndrome

Jonathan Samuels, MD
Instructor in Medicine–Rheumatology
NYU University School of Medicine;
Director, Clinical Immunology Laboratory
NYU Langone Medical Center
New York, New York
    Pathogenesis of Osteoarthritis

Christy I. Sandborg, MD
Professor of Pediatrics
Department of Pediatrics, Division of Pediatric
    Rheumatology
Stanford University
Palo Alto, California
    Treatment of Juvenile Idiopathic Arthritis

Caroline O.S. Savage, PhD, FRCP, FMedSci
Professor of Nephrology
College of Medical and Dental Sciences, School of
    Immunity and Infection
University of Birmingham
Birmingham, United Kingdom
    *Antineutrophil Cytoplasm Antibody–Associated
    Vasculitis*

Amit Saxena, MD
Clinical Instructor in Medicine–Rheumatology
NYU School of Medicine
New York, New York
    *Acute Phase Reactants and the Concept of
    Inflammation*

Jose U. Scher, MD
Instructor in Medicine–Rheumatology
NYU School of Medicine;
Director, Microbiome Center for Rheumatology and
    Autoimmunity;
Staff Physician
NYU Langone Medical Center Hospital for Joint Diseases
New York, New York
    Neutrophils; Eosinophils

Georg Schett, MD
Professor of Medicine
Chief of Rheumatology
Department of Internal Medicine 3
Institute for Clinical Immunology
University of Erlangen–Nuremberg;
Erlangen, Germany
    Biology, Physiology, and Morphology of Bone

David C. Seldin, MD, PhD
Professor of Medicine
Boston University School of Medicine;
Chief, Section of Hematology-Oncology
Boston Medical Center;
Director, Amyloidosis Treatment and Research Program
Boston University School of Medicine/Boston Medical
    Center
Boston, Massachusetts
    Amyloidosis

Anna Simon, MD, PhD
Clinical Investigator
Department of Medicine, Division of General Internal
    Medicine
Radboud University Nijmegen Faculty of Medical
    Sciences
Nijmegen, The Netherlands
    Familial Autoinflammatory Syndromes

Dawd S. Siraj, MD, MPH&TM
Clinical Associate Professor of Medicine
Brody School of Medicine at East Carolina University;
Director, ECU Physicians International Travel Clinic,
    Section of Infectious Diseases
Greenville, North Carolina
    Bacterial Arthritis

Martha Skinner, MD
Professor of Medicine
Director, Special Programs
Amyloidosis Treatment and Research Program
Boston University School of Medicine
Boston, Massachusetts
    Amyloidosis

E. William St. Clair, MD
Professor of Medicine and Immunology
Duke University School of Medicine;
Chief, Division of Rheumatology and Immunology
Duke University Medical Center
Durham, North Carolina
    Sjögren's Syndrome

Lisa K. Stamp, MBChB, PhD, FRACP
Associate Professor
Department of Medicine
Christchurch School of Medicine and Health Sciences
University of Otago Faculty of Medicine
Christchurch, New Zealand
    Nutrition and Rheumatic Diseases

John H. Stone, MD, MPH
Associate Professor of Medicine
Department of Medicine, Division of Rheumatology
Harvard Medical School;
Director, Clinical Rheumatology
Massachusetts General Hospital
Boston, Massachusetts
  Classification and Epidemiology of Systemic Vasculitis;
  Immune Complex–Mediated Small Vessel Vasculitis

Rainer H. Straub, MD
Professor of Experimental Medicine
Laboratory of Experimental Rheumatology and
  Neuroendocrine Immunology
University of Regensburg Faculty of Medicine;
Department of Internal Medicine I
University Hospital
Regensburg, Germany
  Neural Regulation of Pain and Inflammation

Susan E. Sweeney, MD, PhD
Associate Professor of Medicine
UC San Diego School of Medicine
La Jolla, California
  Clinical Features of Rheumatoid Arthritis

Nadera J. Sweiss, MD
Sarcoidosis and Scleroderma Clinic
University of Illinois at Chicago
Chicago, Illinois
  Sarcoidosis

Carrie R. Swigart, MD
Assistant Professor of Orthopaedics and Rehabilitation
Yale University School of Medicine
New Haven, Connecticut
  Hand and Wrist Pain

Deborah Symmons, MD, FFPH, FRCP
Professor of Rheumatology and Musculoskeletal
  Epidemiology
School of Medicine;
Director, Arthritis Research UK Epidemiology Unit
School of Translational Medicine
Musculoskeletal Research Group
University of Manchester;
Honorary Consultant Rheumatologist
Central Manchester University Hospitals NHS
  Foundation Trust
Manchester, United Kingdom
  Cardiovascular Risk in Rheumatic Disease

Zoltan Szekanecz, MD, PhD, DSc
Professor of Rheumatology, Medicine, and Immunology
Department of Rheumatology
Institute of Medicine
University of Debrecen Medical Center
Debrecen, Hungary
  Cell Recruitment and Angiogenesis

Paul-Peter Tak, MD, PhD
Professor of Medicine
Department of Clinical Immunology and Rheumatology
University of Amsterdam Faculty of Medicine
Academic Medical Center
Amsterdam, The Netherlands
  Biologic Markers

Peter C. Taylor, MA, PhD, FRCP
Norman Collisson Professor of Musculoskeletal Sciences
Kennedy Institute of Rheumatology
Botnar Research Centre
Nuffield Department of Orthopaedics, Rheumatology and
  Musculoskeletal Sciences
University of Oxford
Oxford, United Kingdom
  Cell-Targeted Biologics and Targets: Rituximab,
  Abatacept, and Other Biologics

Robert Terkeltaub, MD
Professor of Medicine
La Jolla;
Interim, Chief, Division of Rheumatology, Allergy, and
  Immunology
UC San Diego School of Medicine
San Diego, California
  Calcium Crystal Disease: Calcium Pyrophosphate
  Dihydrate and Basic Calcium Phosphate

Argyrios N. Theofilopoulos, MD
Professor and Chair, Department of Immunology and
  Microbial Science
The Scripps Research Institute Kellogg School of Science
  and Technology
La Jolla, California
  Autoimmunity

Ranjeny Thomas, MD, MBBS
Professor of Rheumatology
School of Medicine
University of Queensland Faculty of Health Sciences;
Rheumatologist, University of Queensland Diamantina
  Institute/Princess Alexandra Hospital
Queensland, Australia
  Dendritic Cells

Thomas S. Thornhill, MD
Professor of Orthopedics
Harvard Medical School;
Chief of Orthopedics
Brigham and Women's Hospital
Boston, Massachusetts
  Shoulder Pain

Karina D. Torralba, MD, MACM, FACP, FACR
Assistant Professor of Medicine
Department of Medicine, Division of Rheumatology
Keck School of Medicine of USC
Los Angeles, California
  Occupational and Recreational Musculoskeletal
  Disorders

Michael J. Toth, PhD
Associate Professor
Department of Medicine
The University of Vermont School of Medicine
Burlington, Vermont
  Muscle: Anatomy, Physiology, and Biochemistry

Peter Tugwell, MD, MSc, FRCPC
Professor of Medicine
Department of Medicine
Ottawa Health Research Institute
University of Ottawa Faculty of Medicine
Ottawa, Ontario, Canada
  Assessment of Health Outcomes

Zuhre Tutuncu, MD
Rheumatologist
Scripps Coastal Medical Center
San Diego;
Voluntary Assistant Clinical Professor of Rheumatology
UC San Diego School of Medicine
La Jolla, California
  Anticytokine Therapies

Katherine S. Upchurch, MD
Clinical Professor of Medicine
University of Massachusetts Medical School;
Clinical Chief, Division of Rheumatology
Department of Medicine
UMass Memorial Medical Center
Worcester, Massachusetts
  Hemophilic Arthropathy

Désirée M.F.M. van der Heijde, MD, PhD
Professor of Rheumatology
Department of Rheumatology
Leiden University Faculty of Medicine
Leiden, The Netherlands
  Clinical Trial Design and Analysis

Annette H.M. van der Helm-van Mil, MD, PhD
Internist/Rheumatologist
Leiden University Medical Center
Leiden, The Netherlands
  Early Synovitis and Early Undifferentiated Arthritis

Sjef M. van der Linden, MD, PhD
Professor of Rheumatology
Department of Medicine
Maastricht University Faculty of Health, Medicine and
  Life Sciences
Maastricht, The Netherlands
  Ankylosing Spondylitis

Jos W.M. van der Meer, MD, PhD, FRCP
Professor of Internal Medicine
Department of Medicine, Division of General Internal
  Medicine
Radboud University Nijmegen Faculty of Medical
  Sciences
Nijmegen, The Netherlands
  Familial Autoinflammatory Syndromes

Jacob M. van Laar, MD, PhD
Professor of Clinical Rheumatology
Musculoskeletal Research Group
Institute of Cellular Medicine
Newcastle University
Newcastle upon Tyne, United Kingdom
  Immunosuppressive Drugs

John Varga, MD
John and Nancy Hughes Professor of Medicine
Northwestern University Feinberg School of Medicine
Chicago, Illinois
  Etiology and Pathogenesis of Scleroderma

Mark S. Wallace, MD
Professor of Clinical Anesthesiology
Department of Anesthesiology
UC San Diego School of Medicine;
Program Director, Center for Pain Medicine
UC San Diego Medical Center
La Jolla, California
  Analgesic Agents in Rheumatic Disease

David M. Warshaw, PhD
Professor and Chair, Department of Molecular Physiology
  and Biophysics
The University of Vermont College of Medicine
Burlington, Vermont
  Muscle: Anatomy, Physiology, and Biochemistry

Lucy R. Wedderburn, MD, PhD, FRCP
Professor in Paediatric Rheumatology
Rheumatology Unit
UCL Institute of Child Health
University College London;
Consultant in Paediatric Rheumatology
Rheumatology Unit
Great Ormond Street Hospital
London, United Kingdom
  *Etiology and Pathogenesis of Juvenile Idiopathic
  Arthritis*

Victoria P. Werth, MD
Professor of Dermatology
University of Pennsylvania School of Medicine;
Chief of Dermatology
Philadelphia VA Medical Center
Philadelphia, Pennsylvania
  The Skin and Rheumatic Diseases

Fredrick M. Wigley, MD
Professor of Medicine
Associate Director, Division of Rheumatology
Department of Medicine
Johns Hopkins University School of Medicine
Baltimore, Maryland
  Clinical Features and Treatment of Scleroderma

Christopher M. Wise, MD
W. Robert Irby Professor of Medicine
Department of Medicine, Division of Rheumatology,
   Allergy, and Immunology
Virginia Commonwealth University School of Medicine,
   Medical College of Virginia Campus
Richmond, Virginia
   Arthrocentesis and Injection of Joints and Soft Tissue

David Wofsy, MD
Professor of Medicine and Microbiology/Immunology
Department of Medicine
UCSF School of Medicine
San Francisco, California
   Clinical Features of Systemic Lupus Erythematosus

Frederick Wolfe, MD
Director, National Data Bank for Rheumatic Diseases;
Clinical Professor of Medicine
Department of Medicine
University of Kansas School of Medicine
Wichita, Kansas
   Fibromyalgia

Frank A. Wollheim, MD, PhD, FRCP
Emeritus Professor of Rheumatology
University of Lund Faculty of Medicine
Lund, Sweden
   Enteropathic Arthritis

Robert L. Wortmann, MD
Professor of Medicine
Department of Medicine, Section of Rheumatology
Geisel School of Medicine at Dartmouth
Lebanon, New Hampshire
   Clinical Features and Treatment of Gout

Edward Yelin, PhD
Professor in Residence of Medicine and Health Policy
Department of Medicine, Division of Rheumatology, and
   Philip R. Lee Institute for Health Policy Studies
UCSF School of Medicine
San Francisco, California
   Economic Burden of Rheumatic Diseases

David Yu, MD
Emeritus Professor of Medicine
David Geffen School of Medicine at UCLA
Los Angeles, California
   *Pathogenesis of Ankylosing Spondylitis and Reactive
   Arthritis*

John B. Zabriskie, MD
Professor Emeritus
Rockefeller University
New York, New York
   Poststreptococcal Arthritis and Rheumatic Fever

Robert B. Zurier, MD
Professor of Medicine Emeritus
Department of Medicine, Division of Rheumatology
University of Massachusetts Medical School
Worcester, Massachusetts
   *Prostaglandins, Leukotrienes, and Related
   Compounds*

Anne-Marie Zuurmond, PhD
TNO Quality of Life
Business Unit Biomedical Research
Leiden, The Netherlands
   Biologic Markers

PREFACE

Rheumatology continues to evolve and inspire as a discipline that occupies the forefront of molecular medicine and novel targeted therapies. The previous edition of the Textbook built on a proud heritage of excellence but was distinguished by change: new editors, more color, new online access, and many other features. Matching the extraordinary pace of change in our field, this new edition continues a grand tradition by accelerating our commitment to excellence in the face of the changing world of publishing. The most obvious examples are the editors for this edition. Three distinguished and longtime colleagues, "The Three Amigos" who were the heart and soul of the Textbook for a generation, have stepped down: Shaun Ruddy, John Sergent, and Ted Harris. Ted passed away recently but left a legacy that will endure (see dedication to the 9th edition). Finding new editors of such high caliber was daunting, but fortunately we met the challenge when we convinced Jim O'Dell and Sherine Gabriel to join our intrepid crew. They brought incredible new strength and expertise, especially in clinical medicine, clinical trials, outcomes research, and epidemiology.

The 9th edition includes a multitude of new authors and chapters. Improved graphics and more easily accessible online content are also features of this edition. The print edition now limits the number of references because we preferred to use allotted pages for scientific content rather than long lists of articles. The complete citations are, however, still available online.

The initial preparative stages of the book occurred, like the last edition, in Costa Rica, where we slaved away for days on the Table of Contents and in selecting an outstanding group of authors. We admit that some fun and entertainment occurred as well, organized and supervised by Linda Lyons Firestein, MD. We also thank the Elsevier staff who braved the rigors of tropical paradise with us, Pam Hetherington and Janice Gaillard. But mostly we want to thank the authors who put in countless hours writing chapters and putting up with our constant haranguing out of love for our discipline, readers, and students.

We hope that you enjoy the Textbook as much as we enjoyed preparing it. The journey has been a formidable and gratifying collegial effort. Because our "Textbook of Rheumatology Costa Rica" Headquarters was sold in 2011, we are searching the globe for alternative sites when it is time to prepare the 10th edition. Although we do not yet know how the next edition will evolve, one certainty is that it will continue the tradition of excellence.

The Editors

CONTENTS

🎥 Video available on the accompanying ExpertConsult website.
📷 Supplemental images available on the accompanying ExpertConsult website.

VOLUME II

KELLEY'S
Textbook of
Rheumatology

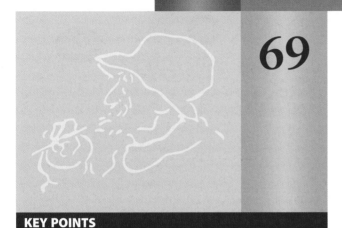

69

Etiology and Pathogenesis of Rheumatoid Arthritis ▇◂

GARY S. FIRESTEIN

KEY POINTS

Rheumatoid arthritis (RA) is a complex disease involving numerous cell types, including macrophages, T cells, B cells, fibroblasts, chondrocytes, neutrophils, mast cells, and dendritic cells.

Several genes are implicated in susceptibility to RA and severity of disease, including class II major histocompatibility complex genes, *PTPN22*, and peptidylarginine deiminases.

Evidence of autoimmunity, including high serum levels of autoantibodies such as rheumatoid factors and anticitrullinated protein antibodies, can be present for many years before the onset of clinical arthritis.

Adaptive and innate immune responses in the synovium have been implicated in the pathogenesis of RA.

Cytokine networks involving tumor necrosis factor, interleukin-6, and many other factors participate in disease perpetuation and can be targeted by therapeutic agents.

Bone and cartilage destruction are primarily mediated by osteoclasts and fibroblast-like synoviocytes, respectively.

Rheumatoid arthritis (RA) is the most common inflammatory arthritis, affecting from 0.5% to 1% of the general population worldwide. Although the prevalence is surprisingly constant across the globe, regardless of geographic location and race, there are some exceptions. For instance, in China the occurrence of RA is somewhat lower (≈0.3%), whereas it is substantially higher in other groups such as the Pima Indians in North America (≈5%). Because of its prevalence and the ready accessibility of joint samples for laboratory investigation, RA has served as a useful model for the study of all inflammatory and immune-mediated diseases. As such, the information gleaned from these studies provides new and unique insights into the mechanisms of normal immunity.

Although RA is primarily considered a disease of the joints, abnormal systemic immune responses are evident and can cause a variety of extra-articular manifestations. These manifestations clearly show that RA has features of a systemic disease that can involve many organs. In some cases, autoantibody production with the formation of immune complexes that fix complement contribute to these extra-articular findings. One of the mysteries of RA is why the synovium is the primary target, although the unique structure of its vascular bed could provide an environment that is ideal for innate and adaptive immune responses.

Although the precise causes of RA remain uncertain, environmental and genetic influences clearly participate. Clues have been provided by detailed immunogenetic studies and the observation that underlying autoimmunity antedates onset of arthritis by up to a decade. Progress in understanding the pathogenesis has been even more robust: The roles of small-molecule mediators of inflammation (e.g., arachidonic acid metabolites), autoantibodies, cytokines, growth factors, chemokines, adhesion molecules, and matrix metalloproteinases (MMPs) have been carefully defined. Synovial cells can exhibit behavior resembling a localized tumor that invades and destroys articular cartilage, subchondral bone, tendons, and ligaments. Irreversible loss of articular cartilage and bone begins soon after the onset of RA, and early interventions can probably improve long-term outcomes. Increased appreciation of how comorbidities, especially cardiovascular disease and accelerated atherosclerosis, can affect mortality has also led to attempts to suppress synovial and systemic inflammation.

ETIOLOGY AND PATHOGENESIS OF RHEUMATOID ARTHRITIS: ROLES OF INNATE AND ADAPTIVE IMMUNITY

The etiology and pathogenesis of RA are complex and multifaceted. A variety of predetermined (genes) and stochastic (random events and environment) factors contribute to susceptibility and pathogenesis. As an introduction, a summary of how these mechanisms interact to create and perpetuate RA is shown in Figure 69-1. Individual mechanisms are discussed in greater detail throughout the chapter.

The initiation of RA probably begins years before the onset of clinical symptoms. This process involves certain specific genes that can help break tolerance and lead to autoreactivity. It is likely that the earliest phases are marked by repeated activation of innate immunity (see Figure

▇◂   Video available on the Expert Consult Premium Edition website.

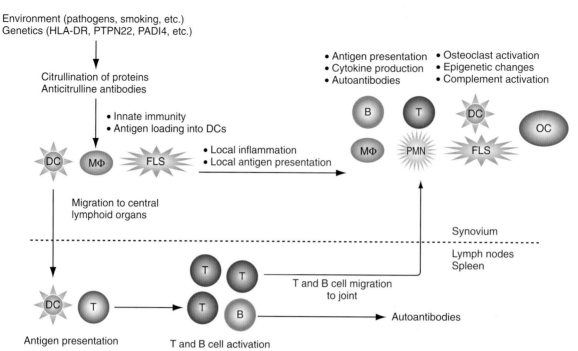

Figure 69-1   Schematic diagram of disease mechanisms that likely occur in rheumatoid arthritis. Innate immunity could activate fibroblast-like synoviocytes (FLS), dendritic cells (DC), and macrophages (MΦ) in the earliest phases in individuals with underlying immune hyper-reactivity as evidenced by the production of autoantibodies. The genetic makeup of an individual including the presence of certain gene polymorphisms in genes that regulate immune responses and environmental exposures are both required. Chronic inflammation leads to citrullination of proteins in a variety of sites including mucosal surfaces such as the lungs or the joint. In a genetically susceptible individual, a breakdown of tolerance can occur with the formation of anticitrullinated protein antibodies. DCs can migrate to the central lymphoid organs to present antigen and activate T cells, which can in turn activate B cells. These lymphocytes can migrate back to the synovium and enhance adaptive immune responses in the target organ. In addition, repeated activation of innate immunity can directly lead to chronic inflammation and possibly antigen presentation in the synovium. In the latter phases of disease, many cell types activate osteoclasts (OC) through the receptor activator of nuclear factor κB (NFκB)/receptor activator of NFκB ligand (RANK/RANKL) system, although FLS and T cells likely provide the greatest stimulus. Autonomous activation of FLS might also contribute to this process.

69-1).[1] Cigarette smoke, bacterial products, viral components, and other environmental stimuli can contribute to these responses. This process probably occurs often in normal individuals but is self-limited. In individuals, a predetermined propensity for immune hyper-reactivity or autoreactivity might lead to a different outcome. The genome of these individuals might encode for a variety of genes implicated in RA including class II major histocompatibilty complex (MHC) genes, protein tyrosine phosphatase-22 (PTPN22), cytokine promoter polymorphisms, signal transduction gene polymorphisms, population-specific genes (e.g., *PADI4* in Japanese or Koreans), and other undefined genes. Abnormal T cell selection could also contribute by allowing autoreactive T cells to escape deletion. The environmental stresses can lead to post-transcriptional modification of proteins, especially citrullination of arginine residues, in mucosal surfaces or the synovium. Although this commonly occurs without sequelae in normal individuals, people with a propensity for RA can develop antibodies against these modified proteins with production of rheumatoid factors (RFs) and anticitrullinated protein antibodies (ACPAs).

Activation of synovial innate immunity can also increase vascular leakage in the synovium, production of chemoattractants that recruit immune cells to the joint, and processing of antigens by dendritic cells. Antigen presentation can potentially occur in the synovial germinal centers or, more commonly, in central lymphoid organs after the loaded dendritic cells migrate via the lymphatics. Naïve T cells can then be activated through interactions with the T cell receptor and co-stimulatory signals. T cells can help B cells produce pathogenic antibodies and/or migrate to the joint, where they can influence other cells through the production of cytokines such as interleukin (IL)-17 or through cell contact mechanisms that do not require a specific antigen. Although it is uncertain what transforms subclinical inflammation to symptomatic arthritis, this process can take up to a decade before it reaches fruition.

Ultimately, a destructive phase proceeds, which can have antigen-dependent and -independent mechanisms and is mediated by mesenchymal elements such as fibroblasts and synoviocytes. Bone erosions are subsequently caused by osteoclasts, whereas cartilage dissolution results from proteolytic enzymes produced by synoviocytes in the pannus or synovial fluid neutrophils. Anti-inflammatory mechanisms such as soluble TNF receptors, suppressive cytokines, cytokine binding proteins, protease inhibitors, lipoxins, antioxidants, antiangiogenic factors, and natural cytokine antagonists are not present in sufficient concentrations to truncate the inflammatory and destructive process. The only way to suppress this response is through therapeutic interventions that either modulate pathogenic cells or neutralize the effector molecules produced by the rheumatoid process, or restore tolerance.

The heterogeneity of mechanisms provides an explanation for the unpredictable response to therapeutic agents and also allows clinicians to consider new therapeutic targets to either prevent RA or interfere with the immunologic, inflammatory, or destructive components as separate but interrelated entities. Each of these mechanisms is discussed in detail later. Brief summaries are also provided intermittently to help guide the reader through this complex maze.

ETIOLOGY OF RHEUMATOID ARTHRITIS

KEY POINTS

Genes play a key role in susceptibility to RA, as well as disease severity.

Class II major histocompatability genes, especially those containing a specific 5 amino acid sequence in the hypervariable region of HLA-DR4, are the most prominent genetic association.

Newly defined genetic associations including polymorphisms in *PTPN22* and *PADI4* suggest that the associations in RA are complex and involve many genes.

Although the etiology of RA remains unknown, a variety of studies suggest that the interaction of environmental and genetic factors is responsible; either one is necessary but not sufficient for full expression of the disease. The most compelling example for a genetic component is in monozygotic twins, in whom the concordance rate is perhaps 12% to 15% when one twin is affected, compared with 1% for the general population. The fact that concordance is not higher provides key evidence that other influences such as the environment, epigenetics, or even microchimerism from maternal-fetal transfer might be as important as or even more important than the genetic component. The risk for a fraternal twin of a patient with RA is also high ($\approx$2% to 5%) but similar to the rate for other first-degree relatives.

Although the immunogenetics is, at best, incompletely understood, one of the best-studied and perhaps most influential genetic risk factor is the class II MHC haplotype of an individual. *PTPN22* and *PADI4* increase risk in some racial and ethnic groups, but not all. Genome-wide screens have implicated at least 35 genes, many of which are involved with immune function. However, most have a relatively modest contribution and the susceptibility polymorphism confers only a 1.1- or 1.2-fold increase. Combinations of genes can clearly interact with one another, and a 45-fold increase in risk is conferred by a combination of *HLA-DR*, *PTPN22*, and the *TRAF1-C5*.[1] This combination, however, is found in less than 1% of individuals with RA. The RA-associated alleles identified to date contribute approximately 40% of total genetic susceptibility. Additional progress in understanding the role of genes in RA including rare variants that might be more important than some common polymorphisms will require sophisticated bioinformatics to clarify how individual alleles contribute to susceptibility, severity, and response to targeted therapies.

Role of HLA-DR in the Susceptibility to and Severity of Rheumatoid Arthritis

The structure of class II MHC molecules on antigen-presenting cells is associated with increased susceptibility and severity of RA and accounts for about 40% of the genetic influence. A genetic link between HLA-DR and RA was initially described in the 1970s with the observation that HLA-DR4 occurred in 70% of RA patients, compared with about 30% of controls, giving a relative risk of having RA to those with HLA-DR4 of approximately 4 to 5.

The susceptibility to RA is associated with the third hypervariable region of DRβ-chains, from amino acids 70 through 74. The epitope is glutamine-leucine-arginine-alanine-alanine (QKRAA), a sequence found in DR4 and DR14, in addition to some DR1β-chains. The "susceptibility epitope" (SE) on DR4β-chains with the greatest association with RA are DRB*0401, DRB*0404, DRB*0101, and DRB*1402 (Table 69-1). Up to 96% of patients with RA exhibit the appropriate HLA-DR locus in some populations.[2] In certain ethnic and racial groups, however, the association with QKRAA is not as prominent or is not associated. The QKRAA epitope might also predict the severity of established RA, with a greater prevalence of extra-articular disease and erosions in patients with two copies. Other HLA genes such as DRB*1301 contain the DERAA sequence and are associated with decreased susceptibility to RA.[3]

One intriguing possibility that could account for some patients who do not fit within this paradigm is microchimerism.[4] Maternal cells expressing the SE can survive and persist in the circulation throughout adulthood. These non-inherited maternal antigens (NIMAs) could then confer increased risk of disease in the children of SE-expressing women.

The region associated with RA (QKRAA) primarily faces away from the antigen-binding cleft of the DR molecule that determines the specificity of peptides presented to

Table 69-1 Nomenclature for HLA-DR Alleles and Associations with Rheumatoid Arthritis

Old Nomenclature (HLA-DRB1 Alleles)	Current Nomenclature	Association with Rheumatoid Arthritis
HLA-DR1	0101	+
HLA-DR4 Dw4	0401	+
HLA-DR4 Dw14	0404/0408	+
HLA-DRw14 Dw16	1402	+
HLA-DR4 Dw10	0402	−
HLA-DR2	1501, 1502, 1601, 1602	−
HLA-DR3	0301, 0302	−
HLA-DR5	1101-1104, 1201, 1202	−
HLA-DR7	0701, 0702	−
HLA-DRw8	0801, 0803	−
HLA-DR9	0901	−
HLA-DRw10	1001	−
HLA-DRw13	1301-1304	1301 associated with protection
HLA-DRw14 Dw9	1401	−

Modified from Weyand CM, Hicok KC, Conn DL, Goronzy JJ: The influence of HLA-DRB1 genes on disease severity in rheumatoid arthritis, *Ann Intern Med* 117:801, 1992.

CD4+ helper T cells. Attempts to elute peptides from the binding pocket of RA-associated alleles have not revealed a specific antigen that is either unique to or associated with RA. The precise function of the SE is uncertain, but it could also play a role in shaping the T cell repertoire in the thymus or altering intracellular HLA-DR trafficking and antigen loading. QKRAA could serve as an autoantigen due to molecular mimicry in some situations because some xenoproteins such as gp110 from the Epstein-Barr virus also include this sequence.

The shared epitope might not be an independent risk factor for RA but instead a marker for immunoreactivity and anticitrullinated protein antibodies (ACPAs).[5] In a large series of patients with early undifferentiated inflammatory arthritis, one-third of patients met criteria for RA within 1 year. Progress to RA occurred regardless of HLA-DR genotype if patients were anticitrullinated protein (anti-CP) positive. When patients were stratified according to ACPA, the shared epitope did not make an additional contribution to progression from undifferentiated arthritis to RA. The shared epitope probably contributes to immune hyperreactivity, but ACPAs are more closely associated with RA. In other studies, however, the presence of the shared epitope and ACPAs together is associated with even greater disease severity.

Additional Polymorphisms: Cytokines, Citrullinating Enzymes, *PTPN22*, and Others

The genetic influence on RA has also led to studies evaluating non-MHC genes. Single nucleotide polymorphisms (SNPs) in promoter regions, coding regions, or areas with no known function have been extensively investigated in RA with a variety of methods including genome-wide association studies. Table 69-2 shows some of the SNPs and microsatellites that have been associated with RA. The relative contribution for most is modest, and variations in technique, stage of disease, and patient populations result in some disagreement among various reports.

Given the importance of cytokines in RA (see following), it is not surprising that many studies have focused on these genes. The most intriguing evidence relates to tumor necrosis factor (TNF). This proinflammatory factor is a major cytokine in the pathogenesis of RA, and the TNF genes are located in the MHC locus on chromosome 6 in humans. Several polymorphisms of the TNF promoter including two at positions −238 and −308 can alter gene

Table 69-2 Key Genetic Associations in Rheumatoid Arthritis

Gene	Odds Ratio for Risk Alleles	Comment
HLA-DR	4-5 fold	
PTPN22	≈2 fold	Not in Asian populations
PADI4	≈2 fold	Primarily in Asian populations
TRAF1-C5	>1.2 fold; <2 fold	
STAT4	>1.2 fold; <2 fold	
TNFAIP3	>1.2 fold; <2 fold	
IL2/21	>1.2 fold; <2 fold	

Other genes with odds ratio >1.0 and <1.2: *CTLA4, CD40, CCL21, CD244, IL2Rb, TNFRSF14, PRKCQ, PIP4K2C, IL2RA, AFF3, REL, BLK, TAGAP, CD28, TRAF6, PTPRC, FCGR2A, PRDM1, CD2-CD58, IRF5, CCR6, CCL21, IL6ST, RBPJ.*

transcription. Associations among the TNF polymorphisms and RA susceptibility and radiographic progression have been reported, although there is not uniform agreement. In addition, certain polymorphisms in cytokines, especially TNF or Fc receptors, have been associated with differential response to therapy. For instance, substitution of a T for a C at position −857 in the TNF promoter might confer greater responsiveness to TNF inhibitors.[6]

Among the many noncytokine and non-MHC genetic linkages described for RA, the ones associated with peptidyl arginase deiminase (*PADI*) and *PTPN22* have the strongest effect on susceptibility. The *PADI* genes are responsible for the post-translational modification of arginine to citrulline. Four isoforms have been identified, known as *PADI1* through *PADI4*. In light of the striking associations of RA with ACPAs, several groups have investigated potential associations with these genes. The most promising is an extended haplotype in the *PADI4* gene that can lead to increased levels of PADI4 protein due to enhanced messenger RNA (mRNA) stability.[7] In a Japanese cohort, a twofold increase in risk of RA was observed with *PADI4* SNPs. Confirmatory reports have been mixed because the association has been confirmed in other Asian populations but not in Western Europe. These studies suggest that the contribution of *PADI4* to RA might be restricted, depending on the overall genetic background of the patient population.

Protein tyrosine phosphatase-22 (PTPN22) associations have been discovered in large-scale screening efforts to identify SNP associations in RA.[8] Using 12,000 SNPs in the initial screens, a novel association was discovered at position 1858 in the *PTPN22* gene that, like *PADI4*, conferred a twofold increase in risk. The allele containing thymidine leading to an amino acid substitution (R620W) was present in 8.5% of controls but was found in nearly 15% in patients with seropositive RA. Subsequent studies have demonstrated a similar association with systemic lupus erythematosus (SLE), type 1 diabetes, and several other autoimmune diseases. *PTPN22* is a phosphatase that regulates the phosphorylation status of several kinases important to T cell activation including Lck and ZAP70. The R620W allele surprisingly results in a gain of function that alters the threshold for T cell receptor (TCR) signaling. Because the *PTPN22* allele is rare in Japan, it is another gene (e.g., *PADI4*) where susceptibility is specific for particular ethnic or racial populations.

The list of genes associated with RA consistently involves immune regulation.[9] Cytokine polymorphisms such as for TNF and the IL-1 inhibitor, IL-1Ra are not surprising. Genes that regulate adaptive immune responses in T cells such as *PTPN22* and the co-stimulation receptor CTLA have also been associated with RA. Other genes associated with B cell function and/or antigen presentation such as *BTLA* (B- and T-lymphocyte attenuator), Fc receptors, and *CD40* are also implicated. Polymorphisms have also been identified in signal transduction pathways that regulate immune function such as TRAF1-C5 and STAT4. The consistent thread in this analysis is that most gene associations for RA cluster to innate immunity, adaptive immunity, and inflammation. Aside from providing insight into the mechanisms of disease, they could also potentially contribute to responses to targeted therapies.

Interactions between Genes and Environment

A number of environmental factors clearly contribute to RA susceptibility, although no specific exposure has been identified as the pivotal agent. Smoking is the best defined environmental risk factor for seropositive RA. The reason for its influence on the development of synovitis is not fully defined but could involve the activation of innate immunity and *PADI* in the airway. Citrullinated proteins have been detected in bronchoalveolar lavage samples of smokers, and this could provide a stimulus for generation of ACPAs in susceptible individuals.[10] Repeated activation of innate immunity, especially in an individual with underlying genetically determined autoreactivity, could potentially contribute to autoreactivity and the initiation of synovitis. Other environmental factors such as oral contraceptives appear to modestly protect from RA, perhaps due to changes in the hormone milieu.[11]

The interaction between HLA-DR and tobacco exposure is perhaps the best example of how genes and the environment conspire to enhance risk. Although smoking and the SE alone modestly increase the likelihood of developing RA, the combination is synergistic.[12] An individual with a history of cigarette smoking and two copies of the SE increases the odds of developing RA by up to 40-fold. The mechanism of the interaction is not known, but it could potentially relate to the increase in protein citrullination in smokers and increased ability of SE-containing HLA-DR molecules to bind some citrullinated proteins. The extent of smoking is also predictive, with the greatest risk seen with at least 20 pack-years. The risk declines slowly with cessation of smoking, taking more than a decade to begin approaching nonsmokers.[13] Alcohol consumption can decrease this risk, and exposure to other inhaled irritants like silica dust increases risk, demonstrating the complexity of environment and human behavior on understanding disease susceptibility.

Gender

RA is one of many chronic autoimmune diseases that predominates in women. The ratio of female-to-male patients is 2:1 to 3:1, which in not as high as Hashimoto's thyroiditis (25:1 to 50:1) or SLE (9:1). The gender effect is often observed in some animal models of autoimmunity such as the NZB/NZW model of SLE, in which female mice have more severe disease. Estrogens are one obvious explanation, and some data support the concept that these hormones modulate immune function.[14] For example, autoantibody-producing B cells exposed to estradiol are more resistant to apoptosis, suggesting that autoreactive B cell clones might escape tolerance. The effect on T lymphocytes is harder to reconcile with the female preponderance in RA because estrogens tend to bias T cell differentiation toward the Th2 phenotype. The cytokines produced by this subset such as IL-4 and IL-13 are usually considered anti-inflammatory in animal models of arthritis and are present in only limited amounts in the RA synovium. Estrogen receptors are expressed on fibroblast-like synoviocytes (FLS) and increase production of metalloproteinases. In macrophage cell lines, estrogen can enhance production of TNF. Nulliparity has also been suggested as a risk factor in early studies, but more recent reports do not support this notion. Thus the effects of estrogens are complex, and the specific mechanisms responsible for the female preponderance of RA are not fully understood.

Pregnancy is often associated with remission of the disease in the last trimester. More than three quarters of pregnant patients with RA improve in the first or second trimester, but 90% of these experience a flare of disease associated with a rise in RF titers in the weeks or months after delivery. The mechanism of protection is not defined but might be due to the expression of suppressive cytokines such as IL-10 during pregnancy, production of α-fetoprotein, or alterations in cell-mediated immunity. One intriguing finding is that fetal DNA levels in the maternal peripheral blood correlate with the propensity for improved symptoms in pregnant RA patients. It is not certain whether the DNA itself contributes or whether it is a marker for increased leakage of fetal cells into the maternal circulation.[15] Immune responses directed against paternal HLA antigens can occur and lead to the production of alloantibodies in the maternal circulation. Maternal-fetal disparity in human leukocyte antigen (HLA) class II phenotypes can correlate with pregnancy-induced remission. More than three-fourths of pregnant women with maternal-fetal disparity of HLA-DRB1, DQA, and DQB haplotypes have significant improvement, whereas disparity is only observed in one-fourth of women whose pregnancy is characterized by continuous active arthritis.[16] Therefore suppression of maternal immune responses to paternal HLA haplotypes might be protective. This question remains unsettled because another study failed to find a correlation between the HLA disparity and clinical improvement during pregnancy.[17]

Epigenetics

Epigenetics describes phenotypic or gene expression properties caused by mechanisms other than changes in the underlying DNA sequence. Modification of CpG DNA sequences by methylation, for example, can suppress gene expression, and it plays a role in cell differentiation. Histone acetylation also alters accessibility of DNA for transcription factors and RNA polymerases. microRNAs can bind to DNA and suppress expression of key genes involved with the inflammatory process. Some epigenetic information such as DNA methylation can be transferred from one generation to the next, thereby providing an alternative mechanism for rapidly altering disease susceptibility in a population due to the environment.

Most information on epigenetics in RA comes from studies of RA synovium or cultured synoviocytes. Some evidence of imprinting is available in the latter, with evidence of global DNA hypomethylation.[18] Only low levels of a key DNA methylase, Dnmt1 are expressed in RA synovium, suggesting a molecular basis for this observation. Because this enzyme is carried by gametes, the methylation pattern can be transgenerationally maintained. One particular CpG site in the IL-6 promoter of peripheral blood mononuclear cells has decreased methylation, and this is associated with higher levels of IL-6 production.[19] Dietary influences such as ingestion of methyl donors such as folate, or even exposure to methyl donors in utero, can profoundly alter DNA methylation and adaptive immune functions and affect susceptibility to autoimmune disease.

The histone deacetylase HDAC1 is overexpressed in RA FLS. When this gene is suppressed, synoviocyte proliferation decreases and expression of tumor suppressor proteins such as p53 increases. HDAC inhibitors are also effective in collagen-induced arthritis, markedly delaying the onset of disease and decreasing bone erosions. Finally, analysis of synovioyctes shows that some individual microRNAs such as microRNA-124a are decreased in RA compared with osteoarthritis (OA) cells. This particular microRNA can suppress cell cycling and chemokine genes. Increasing microRNA-124a levels in RA synoviocytes decreased the production of the chemokine MCP-1.[20] Forced expression of microRNA-203 increases metalloproteinase and IL-6 expression by synoviocytes as well.[21]

The role of epigenetics in RA is not understood. It is not clear whether these observations occur before the onset of disease, are involved with the transition from asymptomatic autoimmunity to clinical disease, or participate in the destructive phase in established RA. Environmental stress plays a major role in disease susceptibility, perhaps greater than DNA polymorphisms. The mechanisms probably involve epigenetic deregulation of gene expression leading to decreased thresholds for autoreactivity in the adaptive immune system.

Changing Epidemiology of Rheumatoid Arthritis

The history of RA reveals the surprising observation that it is a relatively new disease in Europe and Northern Africa. Examination of ancient skeletal remains in Europe and Northern Africa fails to reveal convincing evidence of RA, even though other rheumatic diseases such as OA, ankylosing spondylitis, and gout are readily discernable. In contrast, typical marginal erosions and rheumatoid lesions are present in the skeletons of Native Americans found in Tennessee, Alabama, and Central America from thousands of years ago. The first clear descriptions of RA in Europe appeared in the seventeenth century, and the disease was distinguished from gout and rheumatic fever by Garrod in the mid-nineteenth century. Although still controversial, the disease might have migrated from the New World to the Old World coincident with opening the trade and exploration routes. Because genetic admixture was relatively limited, an undefined environmental exposure potentially caused RA in susceptible Europeans. The most obvious explanation would, of course, be that an infectious agent is responsible. However, other environmental influences like tobacco smoking were also introduced to the Old World at the same time and could play a role.

Equally intriguing, the severity and incidence of RA appeared to decrease in the late twentieth century (Figure 69-2).[22] In certain well-defined populations including Native Americans, the incidence of RA has gradually declined by as much as 50% over the past half of the twentieth century. Changes in hygiene and other lifestyle modifications related to industrialization might contribute, and an infectious agent might be less prevalent secondary to these societal changes, as with many other infectious diseases. Recent data from 1995 to 2007 suggest that the incidence might be rising again in women, but not in men.

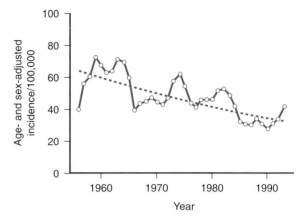

Figure 69-2   Population studies in Minnesota demonstrated a gradually decreasing incidence of rheumatoid arthritis from 1960 to 1990. Similar results have been observed in Native American populations. *(From Doran MF, Pond GR, Crowson CS, et al: Trends in incidence and mortality in rheumatoid arthritis in Rochester, Minnesota over a forty-year period, Arthritis Rheum 46:625–631, 2002.)*

Dissecting the environmental exposures will be key to understanding how the susceptibility to disease varies over time.[23]

PATHOGENIC MECHANISMS IN RHEUMATOID ARTHRITIS

> **KEY POINTS**
>
> Although an etiologic link has not been established, pathogens such as viruses, retroviruses, bacteria, and mycoplasma have been associated with RA.
>
> A single specific "RA pathogen" is unlikely.
>
> Repeated inflammatory stress, especially through specialized receptors that recognize common molecules produced by pathogens, in a genetically susceptible individual might contribute to breakdown of tolerance and subsequent autoimmunity.

Considerable effort has been expended to assess the role of infectious agents in RA (Table 69-3). A potential pathogen could initiate disease through a variety of mechanisms including direct infection of the synovium, activation of innate immunity by pattern-recognition receptors that bind to components of the agent, or through molecular mimicry that induces an autoreactive adaptive immune response.

Infectious Agents: Direct Infection and Innate Immune Responses

Toll-like Receptors and the Inflammasome in the Joint

Infectious agents could contribute to the initiation or perpetuation of RA through a variety of mechanisms. Some arthrotropic microorganisms could potentially infect the synovium and cause a local inflammatory response. There is increasing awareness that the innate immune system could also directly affect the onset and course of synovitis.

Table 69-3 Etiology of Rheumatoid Arthritis: Possible Infectious Causes

Infectious Agent	Potential Pathogenic Mechanisms
Mycoplasma	Direct synovial infection; superantigens
Parvovirus B19	Direct synovial infection
Retroviruses	Direct synovial infection
Enteric bacteria	Molecular mimicry (QKRAA, e.g., in bacterial heat shock proteins)
Mycobacterium	Molecular mimicry (proteoglycans, QKRAA), immunostimulatory DNA (Toll-like receptor 9 activation)
Epstein-Barr virus	Molecular mimicry (QKRAA in gp110)
Bacterial cell walls	Toll-like receptor 2 activation

Pathogen-associated molecular pattern receptors, especially the Toll-like receptors (TLRs), are expressed by sentinel cells in the host that provide a first line of defense. These receptors recognize preserved structures in bacteria and other infectious agents and permit rapid release of inflammatory mediators, activation of antigen-presenting cells, and enhancement of adaptive immune responses.

At least 11 TLRs exist in humans such as TLR2 (binds peptidoglycans), TLR3 (binds double-stranded RNA [dsRNA]), TLR4 (binds lipopolysaccharide), and TLR9 (binds bacterial DNA containing CpG motifs). Many of these pattern recognition receptors are expressed by rheumatoid synovial tissue and cultured FLS including TLR2, TLR3, TLR4, and TLR9. Exogenous TLR ligands such as bacterial peptidoglycan and DNA, as well as endogenous ligands (e.g., heat shock proteins, fibrinogen, and hyaluronan), are present in arthritic joints (see later). Engagement of these receptors participates in certain animal models of arthritis and can exacerbate synovial inflammation. TLR3, which recognizes viral dsRNA and activates the antiviral response, is also expressed by synovial cells in the intimal lining. Necrotic debris containing mRNA from RA synovial fluid cells activates TLR3 signaling and proinflammatory gene expression in synovitis.

The role of innate immunity in RA led to the notion that repeated engagement of TLRs in the synovium could help initiate disease. This hypothesis could explain why specific pathogens have been difficult to identify in the joint. In contrast, a genetically susceptible individual could potentially break tolerance if the TLRs are repeatedly engaged and permit autoimmune responses against articular antigens. Several animal models of disease require TLR ligands for initiations such as TLR9 in adjuvant arthritis. TLR2 is required for streptococcal cell wall arthritis, and the chronic T cell–dependent phase of that model requires TLR4. Mice lacking TLR4$^{-/-}$ have significantly less joint damage induced by IL-1 overexpression, even though synovial inflammation is still robust.[24] These data suggest that endogenous TLR ligands play a key role in matrix regulation independent of inflammatory responses.

A second mechanism that regulates innate immunity involves a novel structure called the inflammasome. This complex includes several proteins involved in recognition of "danger signals" and pathogens such as muramyl dipeptides and uric acid. One central component is cryopyrin, also called NALP3, which is linked to caspase 1 (IL-1 convertase) by adapter proteins. When the inflammasome is engaged, caspase 1 is activated and IL-1 is produced.

Mutations in this pathway, especially in cryopyrin, have been associated with autoinflammatory disorders such as Muckle-Wells syndrome and familial cold autoinflammatory disease. Inflammation induced by uric acid crystals or ATP uses this pathway and can be abrogated by IL-1 inhibitors. Cryopyrin is abundant in RA synovium and is constitutively expressed by FLS and macrophages. Expression in cultured FLS is markedly increased by TNF. Although the role of the inflammasome in RA has not been fully defined, its ability to induce cytokine production by exposure to bacterial products and other danger signals suggests that it participates in IL-1 and IL-18 regulation.

Bacteria, Mycobacteria, Mycoplasma, and Their Components

Active infection of synovial tissue by pyogenic bacteria is an unlikely cause of RA, and extensive searches for a unique or specific organism in synovial tissue or joint effusions have been negative. Antibodies to certain organisms such as *Proteus* are reportedly elevated in the blood of patients with RA, but this could represent an epiphenomenon or a nonspecific B cell activation. Most RA and reactive arthritis patients contain bacterial DNA sequences in their synovium. The bacteria identified are not unique and generally represent a cross-section of skin and mucosal bacteria including *Acinetobacter* and *Bacillus* spp. It is possible that the synovium functions as an adjunct to the reticuloendothelial system in arthritis, allowing local macrophages to accumulate circulating bacterial products.

In addition to prokaryotic DNA, bacterial peptidoglycans have been detected in RA synovial tissue (Figure 69-3). Antigen-presenting cells containing these products express TLRs and produce proinflammatory cytokines such as TNF. It is not known whether the peptidoglycans activate cells in situ or whether phagocytic cells from other sites or the blood engage the molecules and then migrate to the joint. In either case, it is not difficult to imagine how they can contribute to synovial inflammation.

Several animal models of arthritis are dependent on TLR2, TLR3, TLR4, or TLR9. For instance, rodents injected with streptococcal cell walls (TLR2 ligand) develop severe polyarticular arthritis. The initial phase of disease resolves and is then followed by a chronic T cell–dependent phase that resembles RA. The arthritogenicity of complete Freund's adjuvant in the rat adjuvant arthritis model is dependent on mycobacterial DNA that binds to TLR9 and activates an adaptive immunity. Endogenous TLR4 ligands such as heat shock proteins and fibrinogen also play a role in immune complex models such as passive K/BxN arthritis.[25]

Mycoplasma-derived superantigens such as from *Mycoplasma arthritidis* can directly induce T cell–independent cytokine production by macrophages and can exacerbate or trigger arthritis in mice immunized with type II collagen. There is also a higher prevalence of antimycoplasma pneumoniae IgG antibodies in RA patients than matched controls. Despite this and other circumstantial evidence, most efforts to identify *Mycoplasma* and *Chlamydia* organisms or DNA in joint samples have been negative, and there is no direct evidence to support these organisms as etiologic agents.

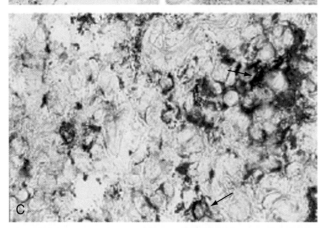

Figure 69-3 Accumulation of bacterial peptidoglycan in rheumatoid synovium. **A** and **B,** Immunohistochemistry shows synovial cells containing peptidoglycan *(red).* **C,** Double staining studies show that bacterial peptidoglycan accumulates in synovial macrophages *(arrow).* These bacterial products can activate Toll-like receptors and stimulate cytokine production. *(From Schrijver IA, Melief MJ, Tak PP, et al: Antigen-presenting cells containing bacterial peptidoglycan in synovial tissues of rheumatoid arthritis patients coexpress costimulatory molecules and cytokines,* Arthritis Rheum *43:2160, 2000.)*

Epstein-Barr Virus, dnaJ Proteins, and Molecular Mimicry

Epstein-Barr virus (EBV) is a polyclonal B lymphocyte activator that increases the production of RF, and rheumatoid macrophages and T cells have defective suppression of EBV-induced proliferation of human B cells. Rheumatoid patients have higher levels of EBV shedding in throat washings, an increased number of virus-infected B cells in the circulating blood, higher levels of antibodies to normal and citrullinated EBV antigens, and abnormal EBV-specific cytotoxic T cell responsiveness compared with controls. Defective elimination of EBV-transformed lymphocytes in RA has fueled speculation that a specific immune defect contributes to initiation of disease.

Additional intriguing data implicating EBV in RA are derived from sequence homology between the susceptibility cassette in HLA-DR proteins and the EBV glycoprotein gp110. Like DRB*0401, gp110 contains the QKRAA motif and patients with serologic evidence of a previous EBV infection have antibodies against this epitope. Hence T cell recognition of EBV epitopes in some patients with the SE might cause an immune response directed at innocent bystander cells through "molecular mimicry." This hypothesis could potentially account for disease perpetuation in the absence of active infection in patients with a specific MHC genotype. However, the data are circumstantial and gp110 is only one of many xenoproteins such as the *Escherichia coli* heat shock protein dnaJ that contain QKRAA. RA T cells, especially synovial fluid T cells, have increased proliferative responses to gp110, perhaps supporting the molecular-mimicry link between a variety of QKRAA-containing proteins and arthritis.

Parvovirus

Antecedent infection with parvovirus B19 has been implicated in some patients with RA based on serologic evidence including the nonstructural protein NS1. However, only about 5% of patients have evidence of recently acquired parvovirus B19 infection at the time of disease onset. Of interest, 75% of RA synovium samples contain B19 DNA compared with about 20% of non-RA controls. Immunohistochemical evidence of the B19 protein VP-1 was detected in patients with RA but not other forms of arthritis. However, evidence of the B19 genome in RA joint samples was not found in other studies.

The mechanisms of B19-induced synovitis, when it does occur, could be related to alterations in the function of FLS.[26] In a cell-culture model of synoviocyte invasion into cartilage, infection with the parvovirus significantly increased the migration of cells into the matrix. Mice that are transgenic for the B19 protein NS1 were more susceptible to collagen-induced arthritis and developed high titers of anti–type II collagen antibodies. These data suggest that the B19 genome might not cause arthritis but can enhance an arthritogenic response to other environmental stimuli.

Other Viruses

Because rubella virus and the rubella vaccine can cause arthritis in humans, the virus has attracted some attention as a possible triggering agent. Live rubella virus can be isolated from synovial fluid of some patients with chronic inflammatory oligoarthritis or polyarthritis without clinical evidence of rubella. However, most rubella patients do not have the classic polyarticular involvement and display an oligoarthritis involving large joints. As with B19 infection, it is possible that a small subset of patients with chronic polyarthritis that are called RA actually have direct infection with wild-type or attenuated rubella virus.

Studies of synovial tissue in a variety of inflammatory and noninflammatory arthropathies have also demonstrated DNA of other viruses such as cytomegalovirus and herpes simplex, but not adenovirus or varicella-zoster. As with bacterial DNA, parvovirus, and EBV, the localization of viral DNA to the inflamed joint might be related to the migration of inflammatory cells containing the viral genome or other nonspecific mechanisms rather than an active infection. Although the hypothesis that one or more of these viral infections might serve as a triggering agent in the genetically susceptible host is both appealing and intellectually satisfying, the pathogenic role of these agents is unlikely.

Retroviral infections have been suggested as a cause of RA. Extensive searches for potential agents have not been fruitful. Endogenous retroviruses are abundant in inflamed and normal synovium, and certain transcripts are expressed in RA cells. In one study, higher levels of HERV-K10 gag protein from a common endogenous retrovirus were detected more often in RA compared with OA and normal peripheral blood mononuclear cells. Some indirect studies are suggestive of retroviral infection such as the demonstration of zinc-finger transcription factors in cultured synoviocytes that can increase signaling through enzymes like p38 mitogen-activated protein (MAP) kinase. In addition, the pX domain of one human retrovirus, human T lymphotropic virus-1 (HTLV-1), causes synovitis in transgenic mice, and synoviocytes from patients infected with HTLV-1 have increased cytokine production. Other studies failed to demonstrate increased expression of human retrovirus-5 proviral DNA in rheumatoid synovium. There is still no direct evidence that retroviruses cause RA, but some viral products could activate TLR3 or TLR7 to enhance cytokine and chemokine production.

Autoimmunity

> **KEY POINTS**
>
> Evidence of autoimmunity can be present in RA many years before the onset of clinical arthritis.
>
> Autoantibodies such as RFs and anticitrullinated protein antibodies are commonly associated with RA.
>
> Autoantibodies in RA can either recognize joint antigens such as type II collagen, or systemic antigens such as glucose phosphate isomerase.
>
> These autoantibodies can potentially contribute to synovial inflammation through several mechanisms including local activation of complement.

The idea that aberrant immune responses are directed toward self-antigens in RA was recognized with the discovery of RF in the blood of patients with the disease. Initially described by Waaler and later by Rose, it was not until the mid-1950s that Kunkel and colleagues firmly established that RF is an autoantibody. Although our understanding of autoantigens has changed over the years and the relative contributions of cellular and humoral immunity have been debated, emphasis on the role of autoantibodies in RA has enjoyed a resurgence over the past few years. Clinical improvement can be associated with decreases in levels of RFs or ACPAs, although the changes tend to be modest and are inconsistent.

Rheumatoid Factor

The identification and characterization of RF as an autoantibody that binds to the Fc portion of IgG was the first direct evidence that autoimmunity might play a role in RA. For many years, immune complexes comprising RF and other immunoglobulins were thought to play a primary role in the pathogenesis of synovitis (see Chapter 56). Even today, the

presence of RF and its resultant pathogenic consequences are still considered cardinal features of RA. Longitudinal studies show that production of RF and other autoantibodies can precede the onset of RA by many years (Figure 69-4).[27] Although some patients are initially "seronegative" for RA and subsequently convert to "seropositive," this is rather unusual and seroconversion typically occurs during the first year of disease activity.

The role of RF and other autoantibodies in the pathogenesis of RA has been suggested by circumstantial evidence. For instance, patients with a positive test result for RF in blood have more severe clinical disease and complications than seronegative patients including increased cardiovascular complications.[28] RF can also fix and activate complement by the classic pathway, and there is clear evidence of local complement production and consumption in the rheumatoid joint. Large quantities of IgG RF are produced by rheumatoid synovial tissue and form complexes through self-association. RF-containing immune complexes are readily detected in RA synovial tissue, as well as the surface layers of cartilage. The latter is especially relevant because immobilized complexes can facilitate complement fixation with resultant release of chemotactic peptides. In experiments performed in patients with RA, a marked inflammatory response was elicited when RF from one patient was injected into a joint, but not when normal IgG was given.[29] B cell–targeted therapies such as rituximab can deplete peripheral B lymphocytes and modestly decrease titers of RF. This does not correlate precisely with clinical responses, and synovial RF production is not significantly changed by B cell depletion. Nevertheless, RF levels often decrease in responders and increase again coincident with clinical relapses.

Three-quarters of patients with RA are seropositive using standard tests for RF, although the percentage can be as high as 90% when assayed for IgM RF with enzyme-linked immunosorbent assays. First-degree relatives of seropositive patients with RA are frequently seropositive, suggesting a

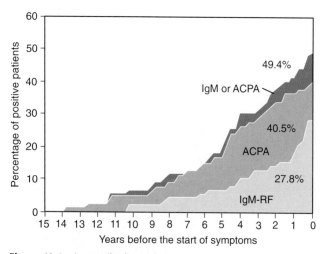

Figure 69-4 Autoantibody production in rheumatoid arthritis. Rheumatoid factors and anticitrullinated protein antibodies (ACPAs) are detected in the blood long before the onset of clinical arthritis in many patients. (*From Nielen MM, van Schaardenburg D, Reesink HW, et al: Specific autoantibodies precede the symptoms of rheumatoid arthritis: a study of serial measurements in blood donors,* Arthritis Rheum 50:380, 2004.)

genetic contribution. Although IgG and IgM RFs are the most abundant in RA, IgE RF has also been demonstrated, especially in patients with extra-articular manifestations. IgE RF can potentially complex with aggregated IgG in synovial tissue, and the subsequent complexes then could degranulate synovial mast cells through activation of Fc receptors in the synovium. IgA RFs are also produced in RA including patients who are seronegative as determined by standard clinical tests that primarily detect IgM RF.

The RFs produced in RA differ from those produced by healthy individuals or from patients with paraproteins. The avidity of RF for the Fc portion of IgG is much greater in RA than in Waldenström's macroglobulinemia or in cryoglobulins. Many RFs expressed by abnormal B cells (such as Waldenström's macroglobulinemia) and by normal B cells in human tonsils are derived from the germline. In contrast, RFs in RA are derived through rearrangements and somatic mutations of the germline genes. RF production can be quite high in rheumatoid synovium; IgM RF represents about 7% of the total IgM and 3% of the total IgG produced by synovial cell cultures.

RFs in RA primarily use the variable heavy 3 (*VH3*) gene and a variety of variable light (VL) genes, whereas natural antibodies with RF activity use *VH1* or *VH4* and the *Vκ3* genes.[30] The kappa light chain repertoire expressed in RF-producing cells isolated from one RA patient was enriched for two specific Vκ genes but contained many somatic mutations and non–germline-encoded nucleotides.[31] Therefore the selection and production of these specific RFs were likely due to antigenic drive rather than derived directly from the germline. Additional RFs have been identified with characteristics similar to an antigen-driven response, although some examples of germline RFs have also been isolated from RA synovium. A crystal structure of one IgM RF bound to IgG showed a key contact residue of the RF with the Fc portion of IgG containing a somatic mutation, supporting the notion that the mutations are related to affinity maturation.

Anticitrullinated Protein Antibodies (ACPAs). One of the most striking recent observations related to autoantibodies is the observation that immunoglobulins that bind to citrullinated proteins are produced by patients with RA and have significant prognostic implications. The discovery originated with reports in the 1970s that antibodies directed against keratin were detected in rheumatoid serum and that the primary target antigen was filament-aggregating protein, filaggrin. These antibodies actually bind to epitopes on filaggrin that contain citrulline, which is derived from post-translational modification of arginine by PADI. Humans have four isoforms of PADI. PADI2 and PADI4 are especially abundant in synovium,[32] and certain SNPs are associated with RA in Asian populations. The function of PADIs in normal immune responses is not certain; citrullination of some chemokines can decrease activity, and modification of histones can regulate gene expression in stressed cells.

Induction of *PADI* expression and citrullination of peptides are not specific to RA and can occur in many inflammatory settings.[33] Not only are other inflammatory arthropathies marked by citrullinated proteins, but other organs such as the lungs in smokers have significant *PADI* activity. The presence of CPs in the lungs of smokers could provide the systemic antigen exposure that can contribute to anti-CP antibody production and begin the long road to developing RA. CPs are present in most animal models of arthritis. Immunohistochemistry demonstrates citrullinated proteins in RA synovial tissue infiltrating cells (Figure 69-5), as well as in extracellular deposits that often colocalize with various isoforms of *PADI*, especially *PADI2* and

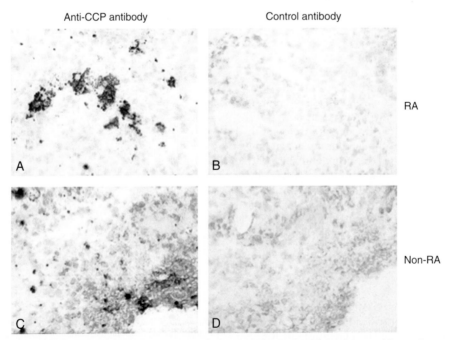

Anti-CCP antibody   Control antibody

RA

Non-RA

Figure 69-5 **A** to **D,** Citrullinated proteins in inflamed synovium. Both rheumatoid arthritis and nonrheumatoid synovium contain citrullinated proteins, detected with an anticyclic citrullinated protein (anti-CCP) antibody (*red-brown* in synovium). Control is an irrelevant antibody. Although citrullinated proteins are not specific, the production of anticitrullinated protein antibodies is more specific to rheumatoid arthritis. *(From Vossenaar ER, Smeets TJ, Kraan MC, et al: The presence of citrullinated proteins is not specific for rheumatoid synovial tissue, Arthritis Rheum 50:3485, 2004.)*

PADI4. Moreover, ACPAs are produced by the rheumatoid synovium, especially tissues with lymphoid aggregates.

The specific proteins that are modified vary widely but include many normal constituents like fibrinogen, vimentin, and fibronectin, as well as xenoproteins like EBV-derived peptides.[34] The pattern of protein citrullination or the specificity of antibodies to particular proteins does not, thus far, have predictive value for developing RA or the severity of disease. One interesting subset involves antibodies that recognize mutant citrullinated vimentin (MCV). These antigens have two modifications that render them more immunogenic: First, there are amino acid changes in the primary sequence such as glycine to arginine. Second, either the new amino acid or another arginine on the protein is citrullinated.[35] The mechanism of amino acid changes has not been defined but could be due to oxidative stress that causes mutations in the genes encoding the protein. These anti-MCV antibodies might be more specific for RA in established disease and also might be more predictive for radiographic progression than standard ACPA tests.[36]

ACPAs are present in the serum of 80% to 90% of RA patients. In some studies, they are also more specific for RA than RF, with specificity approaching 90%. Perhaps most interesting, ACPA, like RF, can appear long before the onset of clinical arthritis and could be a marker for immune hyper-reactivity and subclinical inflammation leading to protein citrullination in a variety of tissues. The more peptides recognized by the repertoire of ACPAs, such as to vimentin, enolase, or various fragments of fibronectin, the greater the likelihood that an individual with arthralgias will develop RA.[37] Of interest, elevated serum cytokines also predicts development of arthritis that meets criteria for RA.[38] A genetic contribution was confirmed in the Native American population, where ACPAs are present in nearly 20% of unaffected first-degree relatives and more than 10% of more distant relatives.[39] ACPAs are also produced by synovial tissue B cells and can be detected in synovial fluid. However, the fact that ACPAs, like RFs, can be detected years before the onset of arthritis and can be found in some normal relatives of RA patients suggests that the autoantibodies alone cannot account for the etiology of the disease.

ACPAs are predictors of more aggressive disease marked by bone and cartilage destruction. In fact, some data suggest that the HLA-DR associations in RA are actually due to an association between the susceptibility epitope and ACPA production. This association extends to accelerated atherosclerosis in RA, where anti-CP positivity is an independent risk factor for ischemic heart disease. In patients with early undifferentiated inflammatory arthritis, ACPAs are also predictive for individuals who will progress to RA.[40]

Despite these caveats, ACPAs do have pathogenic potential. For instance, ACPAs can activate the classical and the alternative complement pathways.[41] In addition, IgE ACPAs from patients with RA can sensitize basophils and mast cells to degranulate. This could enhance increased vascular permeability and influx of inflammatory cells into the synovium.[42] The antibodies have minimal effect when directly injected into mice, and they enhance the arthritogenic potential of anti–type II collagen antibodies in the collagen-induced arthritis model.[43] Mice immunized with

citrullinated fibronectin, but not native fibronectin, can develop inflammatory arthritis.[44] Hence the autoreactivity and autoantibodies are not simply a marker of disease but can participate in the disease process. Citrullination can also increase T cell responses to arthritogenic antigens. For instance, citrullination of albumin leads to the formation of antibodies that also cross-react with the unmodified protein. The citrullinated type II collagen is more immunogenic than the native protein, most likely due to increased affinity in the binding groove of HLA-DR proteins that contain the SE.[45]

Autoimmunity to Cartilage-Specific Antigens

Because synovial tissue inflammation is a hallmark of RA, it is only natural to assume that certain joint-specific antigens might play an etiologic or pathogenic role. The number of potential antigens is extensive, and there is no convincing evidence to date that one specific "rheumatoid" antigen exists. In contrast, the emerging picture of autoimmunity in RA tends to implicate patterns of self-directed responses, rather than a single epitope that encompasses all patients at all times during the disease. It is quite possible that articular autoimmunity could vary with the stage of disease, the clinical manifestations, and treatment.

Type II Collagen. The discoveries that immunization with type II collagen can cause arthritis in rats and mice and that the disease can be passively transferred by IgG fractions containing anticollagen antibodies or by transfer of lymphocytes from affected animals have spawned extensive experiments that illustrate the antigenicity of collagen, the arthrotropic nature of the disease produced, and the dependence on class II MHC genes. T cells are required for initiation of collagen-induced arthritis, and a major immunogenic and arthritogenic epitope on type II collagen resides in a restricted area of the type II collagen chains.

However, type II collagen antibody generation is probably not the initiating event in RA but can amplify the inflammatory response (Table 69-4). Sera from patients with RA contain antibody titers to denatured bovine type II collagen that are significantly higher than those found in control sera[46]; however, there is no difference in antibody titers to native collagen, indicating that the denatured form generated after the breakdown of connective tissue might serve as the immunogen. Anticollagen antibodies purified from the sera of patients with RA can activate complement,

Table 69-4 Examples of Autoantigens in Rheumatoid Arthritis

Cartilage antigens
Type II collagen
gp39
Cartilage link protein
Proteoglycans
Aggrecan
Citrullinated proteins
Glucose-6-phosphoisomerase
HLA-DR (QKRAA)
Heat shock proteins
Heavy-chain binding protein (BiP)
hnRNP-A2
Immunoglobulins (IgG)

generating C5a when they bind to cartilage. In addition, isolated synovial tissue B lymphocytes actively secrete anti–type II collagen antibodies in almost all patients with seropositive RA, whereas articular cells from non-RA patients do not. Synovial fluid T cells also recognize and respond to type II collagen, and 3% to 5% of RA synovial fluid–derived T cell clones are autoreactive to the protein. Of interest, T cell responses to type II collagen, especially a dominant epitope at amino acid 263-270, are much greater if the epitope is glycosylated or if the protein is citrullinated.[47]

gp39 and Other Cartilage-Specific Antigens. Several other cartilage components besides type II collagen have been implicated as potential autoantigens in RA. Among the most provocative is cartilage glycoprotein gp39. Several gp39 peptides can bind to the HLA-DR*0401 molecule and stimulate proliferation of T cells from patients with RA. BALB/c mice, which are often resistant to experimental arthritis, develop polyarticular inflammatory arthritis after immunization with gp39 and complete Freund's adjuvant. Although anti-gp39 antibodies are only detected in a small percentage of patients, it appears to be relatively specific for RA.[48] Other examples of potential cartilage autoantigens include proteoglycans, aggrecan, cartilage-link protein, and other types of collagen. Proteomic analysis of RA serum using peptide arrays to detect multiple autoantibodies also identifies anti-gp39 antibodies in patients with early RA, which may be associated with less aggressive disease.

Autoimmunity to Nonarticular Antigens

Autoimmune responses in RA can also involve antigens that are broadly expressed beyond the joint.[49] These antigen-antibody systems comprise a pattern of autoimmune responses that can potentially lead to synovial inflammation.

Glucose-6-Phosphoisomerase

Spontaneous inflammatory arthritis develops in K/BxN mice due to antigen-specific immunity against a seemingly irrelevant nonarticular antigen.[50] Autoantibodies to the ubiquitous enzyme, glucose-6-phosphate isomerase (GPI) cause the disease, and transient synovitis also develops in normal mice injected with the serum of the affected K/BxN mice. This passive arthritis model serves as a unique tool to study antibody-dependent arthritis and requires the alternate complement pathway, Fc receptors (especially FcRγIII), and mast cells, but not T or B cells. IL-1 is more important than TNF in this model, and the IL-1 knockout mice are almost completely protected from disease. Notably, this effect can be overcome by administration of a TLR ligand like lipopolysaccharide, which shares a downstream signaling pathway with IL-1. Other cytokines, such as IL-6, and signaling pathways, such as p38 MAP kinase and upstream kinases such as MKK3, are also required for full expression of the disease.

Immunohistochemical studies show that the target protein, GPI, adheres to the surface of cartilage, which permits local antibody binding and complement fixation. Initiation of synovial inflammation requires mast cells that increase vascular permeability and provide access to the synovium and cartilage.[51] The initial phase involving mast cell and vascular permeability is augmented by antibody-mediated complement fixation when serum proteins have access to GPI-decorated cartilage.

Although the model appears on first blush to be due to a ubiquitous antigen, articular homing and display of the GPI suggest that it behaves like other arthritis models with "joint-specific" antigens. Although initial data suggested some specificity for RA, anti-GPI antibodies are detected in a relatively small percentage of RA patients and are not specific for the disease. Nevertheless, it might, along with several other antibody systems, contribute to local complement fixation and inflammation.

Heterogeneous Nuclear Ribonuceloprotein-A2 and Heavy-Chain Binding Protein. Several other autoantigens that are expressed in synovium have been characterized in RA, although they are also produced in many other locations. For instance, antibodies directed against the heterogeneous nuclear ribonuceloprotein-A2 (hnRNP-A2), sometimes called RA33, occur in about one-third of RA patients, as well as patients with other systemic autoimmune diseases. However, there may be some specificity for RA when compared with OA and seronegative spondyloarthropathies. Anti-RA33 antibodies are also produced in the TNF transgenic mouse model of rheumatoid arthritis, suggesting that proinflammatory cytokines can independently lead to a breakdown of tolerance for this particular protein.[52] Of interest, RA33-positive patients with early RA tended to have less destructive disease.[53] Although not especially sensitive or specific for RA when used in isolation, an algorithm involving anti-RNP-A2, RF, and anti-CP can be used to predict patients with early synovitis who will progress to erosive RA.[54]

Autoantibodies that bind to stress-protein immunoglobulin heavy-chain binding protein (BiP) have also been observed. About 60% of RA patients have anti-BiP antibodies, and the specificity is reportedly more than 90%. In addition to humoral responses, RA T cells can proliferate in response to this protein. Immunization of mice with BiP does not cause arthritis, but it can cross-tolerize mice and prevent collagen-induced arthritis if administered before immunization with type II collagen. BiP is normally expressed in many tissues but is markedly increased in RA synovium.

Heat Shock Proteins. The heat shock proteins (HSPs) are a family of mainly medium-sized (60 to 90 kD) proteins produced by cells of all species in response to stress. Another smaller HSP (HSP27) can serve as substrates for enzymes such as p38 MAP kinase that regulate stress responses. Immunity against HSPs contributes directly to synovitis and joint destruction in the adjuvant arthritis model in rats in which T lymphocytes recognize an epitope of mycobacterial HSP65 (amino acids 180 through 188). Some of these cells also recognize cartilage proteoglycan epitopes, perhaps explaining the targeting of joints.

Some patients with RA have elevated levels of antibodies to mycobacterial HSPs, especially in synovial fluid. The majority of T cell clones isolated from RA synovial fluid with specificity to mycobacterial components express the γδ–T cell receptor and do not display CD4 or CD8 surface antigens. Freshly isolated synovial fluid T cells from patients with RA briskly proliferate in response to recombinant 65-kD HSP. However, proliferation to other recall antigens such as tetanus toxoid is not increased. Synovial fluid mononuclear cells activated by 60-kD mycobacterial HSP inhibit proteoglycan production by human cartilage explants. Human HSPs including the HSP60 are expressed in the synovium, although the amount expressed per cell appears to be similar in OA, RA, and normal tissue.

SYNOVIAL PATHOLOGY AND BIOLOGY

KEY POINTS

The synovium in RA is marked by intimal lining hyperplasia and sublining infiltration with mononuclear cells, especially CD4+ T cells, macrophages, and B cells.

Intimal lining FLS display unusually aggressive features.

Macrophages in the intimal lining are highly activated and produce many cytokines.

Lymphocytes can either diffusely infiltrate the sublining or form lymphoid aggregates with germinal centers.

Sublining CD4+ T cells mainly display the memory cell phenotype.

Synovial B cells and plasma cells in RA exhibit evidence of antigen-driven maturation and antibody production.

Dendritic cells can potentially present antigens to T cells in synovial germinal centers.

Mast cells produce small molecule mediators of inflammation.

Neutrophils are rarely present in RA synovium but can be abundant in synovial effusions.

The primary inflammatory site in RA is the synovium. Infiltration of synovial tissue with mononuclear cells, especially T cells and macrophages, and synovial intimal lining hyperplasia are hallmarks of the disease (Figure 69-6). In this section, the various cell lineages and histologic patterns of rheumatoid synovium are discussed.

Synovial Intimal Lining Cells: Type A and Type B Synoviocytes

The synovial intimal lining is a loosely organized collection of cells that form an interface between the synovium and the synovial fluid space. The intimal lining cells lack tight junctions and a definite basement membrane. The increase in cell number in RA can be quite substantial. In the normal joint, the lining is only one to two cell layers deep, whereas in RA it is often 4 to 10 cells deep. Two major cell types are found in the lining: a macrophage-like cell known as a type A synoviocyte and a fibroblast-like cell called a type B synoviocyte. The former are derived from the bone marrow and express macrophage surface markers such as CD68, Fc receptors, and CD14, as well as abundant HLA-DR, whereas the latter express little if any class II MHC antigens, are devoid of macrophage markers, and have a scant endoplasmic reticulum. The type B cells, also called FLS, express certain proteins that are unusual for mesenchymal cells including vascular cell adhesion molecule-1 (VCAM-1), CD55 (decay activating factor), cadherin-11, junctional adhesion molecule C (JAM-C), and the proteoglycan-synthesis enzyme, uridine diphosphoglucose dehydrogenase (UDPGD). The relative numbers of type A and B cells are usually similar in normal synovium. There is an absolute increase in both cell types in RA, although the percentage increase in macrophage-like cells is often greater. In addition, the type A synoviocytes tend to accumulate in the more superficial regions of the intimal lining.

Intimal lining synovial macrophages and sublining macrophages are terminally differentiated cells that presumably do not divide in the joint, and the accumulation of cells in RA is likely from the ingress of new bone marrow–derived precursors. Mesenchymally derived type B synoviocytes can divide locally in response to the proliferative factors generated by the activated immune response. Platelet-derived growth factor (PDGF), transforming growth factor-beta (TGF-β), TNF, and IL-1 produced by many different cells combine with products of arachidonic acid metabolism to induce proliferation of these cells. In addition, pluripotential mesenchymal stem cells that arise in the bone marrow and circulate through the blood can migrate into the synovium and differentiate into type B synoviocytes.[55] Retention of macrophages in the intimal lining is probably due to expression of adhesion molecules like VCAM-1 and JAM-C on FLS.

Although local proliferation of cells in the intimal lining likely occurs, rheumatoid synovium rarely shows mitotic figures, and thymidine uptake occurs in only a small percentage of synovial cells. Using a monoclonal antibody that recognizes dividing cells, an even lower rate of cell division

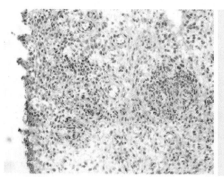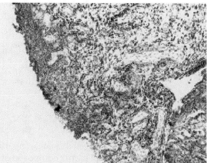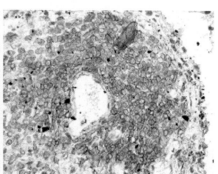

Figure 69-6 Histopathologic appearance of rheumatoid arthritis synovium. Intimal lining hyperplasia, angiogenesis, and a prominent mononuclear cell infiltrate are present. Panels show standard histology *(left panel)*, as well as immunostaining for macrophages *(brown in the intimal lining, middle panel)* and a perivascular T cell aggregate *(right panel)*. *(Courtesy Dr. Paul-Peter Tak.)*

(≈0.05%) is apparent.[56] A somewhat higher percentage of cells that express the cell cycle–specific antigen proliferating cell nuclear antigen (PCNA) is present in RA lining compared with OA. This correlates with the lining cell expression of the proto-oncogene c-myc, a gene that is intimately linked with fibroblast proliferation.

The architecture of the synovial intimal lining is distinct from other lining layers in the body. In contrast to serosal surfaces, the intimal lining does not include epithelial cells, it lacks a basement membrane, and has no tight junctions. Rather than serving as a discrete barrier, it is a loose association of cells that is discontinuous in some locations. Cadherin-11, from a class of adhesion proteins that are ubiquitous in various tissues, serves as the major mediator of homotypic aggregation by FLS.[57] Immunohistochemistry shows abundant expression of this protein in the intimal lining. Its importance in the synovial architecture was confirmed in cadherin-11 knockout mice, in which the intimal lining was virtually nonexistent. Finally, cadherin-11 mediates self-aggregation of FLS in vitro. When the cells are cultured in "micromasses" made of laminin, they migrate to the surface of the particles (Figure 69-7). Macrophages cocultured in the micromasses leads to recruitment of these cells to the surface as well, thereby recapitulating a lining layer with macrophage-like and fibroblast-like cells.[58] Blocking cadherin-11 with antibodies supresses arthritis in the passive K/BxN model. These data suggest that FLS not only

organize the intimal lining formation, but also, like T cells, B cells, and macrophages, play a critical role in the pathogenesis of inflammatory arthritis.

Two major populations of adherent cells can be readily identified when rheumatoid synovium is enzymatically dispersed and cultured in vitro. One type of cell is macrophage-like, which expresses HLA-DR antigens, Fc receptors, and monocyte lineage–differentiation antigens and is capable of phagocytosis. The macrophages, which comprise about 20% of the total cell number in the rheumatoid joint, can be derived either from the intimal lining or the sublining region. These cells are highly activated in the synovium and produce large amounts of inflammatory mediators including cytokines and arachidonic acid metabolites.

A second type is defined by the presence of antigens expressed primarily on fibroblasts and by the absence of phagocytic capability, DR antigens, or antigens of the monocytic lineage. When the enzymatically dispersed cells are cultured for several passages, this latter cell type survives and proliferates, resulting in a relatively homogeneous population of fibroblast-like cells.

Fibroblast-like cells grow slowly, with a doubling time of 5 to 7 days, and can be passaged for several months in vitro. Their doubling rate is rapid at first, perhaps due to the presence of cytokines produced by contaminating macrophages in the culture or a carryover effect from the synovial milieu. Over time, proliferation slows, and after 12 to 15 passages,

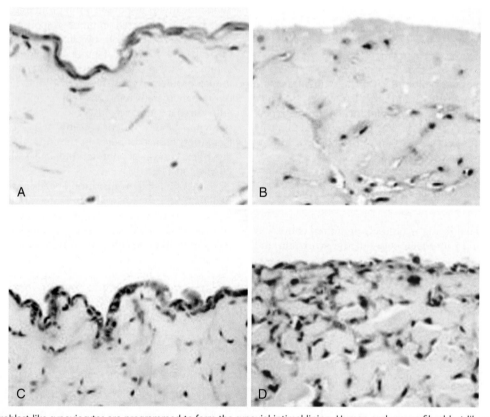

Figure 69-7   Fibroblast-like synoviocytes are programmed to form the synovial intimal lining. Human and mouse fibroblast-like synoviocytes (FLS) spontaneously form lining structures when embedded in a three-dimensional matrix composed of the matrix protein laminin. The cells migrate to the surface of the structure over 3 weeks and resemble an intact synovial lining. The figure shows parallel experiments using human **(A)** and mouse **(C)** fibroblast-like synoviocytes. Of interest, dermal fibroblasts from human **(B)** or mouse **(D)** skin do not migrate to the surface, indicating that the synoviocytes are preprogrammed for this function and that it is not a property of all fibroblasts. *(From Kiener HP, Watts GF, Cui Y, et al: Synovial fibroblasts self-direct multicellular lining architecture and synthetic function in three-dimensional organ culture,* Arthritis Rheum *62:742, 2010.)*

the cells gradually become senescent and ultimately cease to grow. Although it has not been proven that these cells originate solely from the synovial intimal lining, the fact that a significant percentage of cells express VCAM-1 and CD55 suggests that at least some are derived from this region. Synovial fibroblasts from RA have some characteristics reminiscent of tumors or transformed cells (see following).

Experiments examining synovial tissue and FLS gene expression profiles suggest that specific patterns correlate with synovial histopathology.[59] FLS from highly inflamed synovium exhibited a TGF-β gene signature that has also been described in cells with features of both smooth muscle cells and fibroblasts that are found in many mucosal surfaces known as *myofibroblasts*. FLS appear to be involved in wound healing. A second pattern observed in cells derived from relatively noninflammatory RA tissue had increased expression of insulin-like growth factor–regulated genes. Whether the pathogenic processes in the synovium imprint the synoviocytes or vice versa is unknown. Attempts to distinguish RA and OA FLS expression profiles from each other have offered mixed results.

Aggressive Features of RA Fibroblast-like Synoviocytes

Tumor-like Properties. Rheumatoid FLS demonstrate some aggressive properties compared with cells obtained from other synovia or tissues. For instance, adherence to plastic or extracellular matrix is generally required for normal fibroblasts to proliferate and survive in culture. Although FLS typically grow and thrive under conditions that permit adherence, RA synoviocytes can also proliferate in an anchorage-independent manner.[60] In addition, cultured RA synoviocytes can exhibit defective contact inhibition and express a variety of transcription factors, such as c-Myc, that are typically abundant in tumor cells. Poorly regulated cell growth likely occurs in vivo as well, and studies examining X-linked genes demonstrate oligoclonality in the synoviocyte population from RA, but not OA, synovium.[61] This is especially true of cells derived from the invading pannus, which is the most aggressive region of the synovium. Increased telomerase activity, another feature of transformed tissue, is also present in RA synovium and can be observed in FGF-stimulated RA synoviocytes. Epigenetic analysis suggests overexpression of certain microRNAs associated with increased cytokine production.

Matrix Invasion. The most compelling evidence suggesting that RA synoviocytes are permanently altered is derived from studies in a severe combined immunodeficiency (SCID) mouse model where synoviocytes and cartilage are coimplanted. The rheumatoid cells adhere to and invade into the cartilage matrix, whereas osteoarthritis and skin fibroblasts do not[62] (Figure 69-8). Because these synoviocytes are devoid of T cells and macrophages, there is no contribution from an immune response to murine antigens. The invading cells express VCAM-1, which could potentially facilitate adhesion to cartilage or chondrocytes, as well as proteases that digest the cartilage matrix. More recent studies in which explants are introduced into two locations in the SCID mice show that the rheumatoid FLS can migrate from one site to another, presumably via lymphatics and the bloodstream.[63] This raises the intriguing possibility that imprinted, aggressive cells can "metastasize"

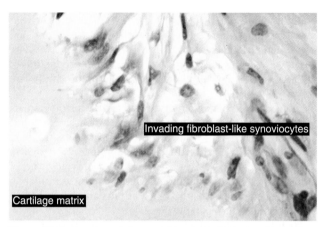

Figure 69-8 Invasion of rheumatoid arthritis (RA) synoviocytes into cartilage explants in severe combined immunodeficiency syndrome (SCID) mice. RA fibroblast-like synoviocytes were coimplanted with normal human cartilage into the renal capsule of SCID mice. Note that the synoviocytes attached to the cartilage and invaded into the matrix. Several chondrocytes in lacunae are also present. *(Courtesy Dr. S. Gay.)*

from joint to joint and contribute to the polyarticular nature of RA.

Blocking IL-1 function in the SCID model with interleukin-1 receptor antagonist (IL-1Ra), a natural antagonist to IL-1, has no effect on synoviocyte invasion but decreases perichondrocyte matrix loss. In contrast, IL-10 or blocking type I metalloproteinase, Ras, or c-Myc expression decreases invasion. Surprisingly, overexpression of soluble TNF receptors has little effect in this model. These studies suggest that excessive production of IL-1 and underexpression of IL-10 contribute to the invasive properties of RA synoviocytes. In another study, transfecting normal synoviocytes with the human papillomavirus gene encoding E6 induced the rheumatoid phenotype. The E6 protein degrades endogenous p53 tumor suppressor protein in synoviocytes. Therefore deficient p53 function can mimic the aggressive phenotype of RA FLS. Overall, these studies paint an interesting picture of RA FLS serving as key effector cells that display unique aggressive properties in inflammatory synovitis.

Synovial T Lymphocytes

Immunohistologic Patterns

In chronic RA, the synovium contains a collection of T lymphocytes that can lead to an organizational structure that resembles a lymph node. The distribution of lymphocytes in the tissue varies from discrete lymphoid aggregates to diffuse sheets of mononuclear cells, with the most prominent location for T cells being the perivascular region. These collections consist of small, CD4+ memory T cells (CD45RO+) with scant cytoplasm. Scattered few CD8+ T cells accumulate in the aggregates, and formation of ectopic germinal centers in RA synovial tissue may depend on them. Peripheral to these foci is a transitional zone with a heterogeneous mixture of cells including lymphocytes, occasional undifferentiated blast cells, plasma cells, and macrophages (see Figure 69-6). Synovial lymphoid aggregates occur in about 15% to 20% of patients; although originally considered specific for RA, it is now clear that they are equally prevalent in psoriatic arthritis and are even seen in some individuals with osteoarthritis.[64] The presence of aggregates correlated with higher production of ACPAs and RF in synovium, but not with clinical disease activity.

Considerable heterogeneity exists in the histologic patterns from patient to patient and within a single joint. Synovial biopsy studies suggest that at least six sites must be evaluated to decrease the risk of sampling error to 10% to 20% or less. In situations where the synovial tissue of more than one joint from an individual patient is available, the same general histopathologic patterns are usually apparent in tissue from separate sites.

Regulation of T Cell Aggregate Formation. T cells often constitute 30% to 50% of cells in RA synovia, and most are CD4[+]. About 5% of cells are B lymphocytes or plasma cells, although in some tissues the percentage can be considerably higher. The B cells are located primarily within reactive lymphoid centers, whereas plasma cells and macrophages are often found outside these centers. This arrangement is consistent with T cell–dependent B lymphocyte activation. Plasma cells, the main immunoglobulin producers, migrate away from the germinal centers after differentiation. CD4 cells in RA synovium are in intimate contact with B lymphocytes, macrophages, and dendritic cells.

Aggregate formation is complex and involves numerous signals to orchestrate the organization of individual cell lineages. In some cases, follicular dendritic cells are present and are involved in forming true germinal centers (see later). The presence or absence of aggregates and germinal centers is a dynamic process. In one study evaluating synovial biopsies, the presence of lymphoid neogenesis was not restricted to patients with autoantibodies. Even though the cytokine and chemokine profile supports the formation of these structures, progression to fully differentiated follicles was uncommon.[65]

Chemokines play a key role in the organization of tissues into lymphoid structures such as aggregates and germinal centers. CXCL13 and CCL21 appear to be especially important, and their expression in rheumatoid synovium correlates with the presence of this microarchitecture.[66] The former, in particular, is produced by synovial follicular dendritic cells. Similarly, plasma cells expressing the chemokine receptor CXCR3 are present in the rheumatoid synovium. The CXCR3 ligand, Mig/CXCL9, is highly expressed by intimal lining synoviocytes and sublining cells and recruits these cells to the T cell aggregates.[67]

The architecture of lymphoid structures in rheumatoid synovium is also regulated by members of the TNF superfamily. Lymphotoxin-α and lymphotoxin-β (LTα and LTβ, respectively), as well as lymphotoxin-related inducible ligand that competes for glycoprotein D binding to herpesvirus entry mediator on T cells (LIGHT) form trimeric molecules in various combinations that can bind to distinct cell surfaces. These three cytokines regulate the function and organization of lymphoid tissues. Deletion of either LTα or LTβ seriously impairs lymphoid development, whereas lymph nodes develop normally in LIGHT-deficient mice. In the SCID mouse model using RA tissue explants, depletion of CD8[+] T cells led to loss of follicular dendritic cells, depletion of LTα1β2, and disintegration of the lymphoid follicles.[68]

Although LTα is difficult to detect in RA, LTβ and LIGHT are present.[69] In addition to regulating lymphoid aggregate and germinal center formation, LT can also directly stimulate FLS to produce chemokines such as CCL2 and CCL5 that attract T cells into the joint. LIGHT also enhances osteoclast differentiation and induces expression of MMP-9, TNF, IL-6, and IL-8 by macrophages. LTβ and LIGHT blockade using soluble receptors decreases the severity of collagen-induced arthritis.[70] However, the inhibitor was not effective in the passive arthritis model in which the pathogenic antibodies were directly administered to mice. Hence the LIGHT axis has a more important role in the early phases of disease when adaptive immunity to joint antigens is developing.

Synovial T Cell Phenotype

Co-stimulatory Molecules. RA synovial T lymphocytes display an activated surface phenotype, with high expression of HLA-DR, CD69, and CD27. The co-stimulatory molecule CD28 is highly expressed by synovial T cells in RA. Its ligands, CD80 and CD86, are also displayed on antigen-presenting cells in the joint, thereby providing an excellent environment for T cell activation. The importance of the CD80/86-CD28 interaction is supported by the observation that abatacept blocks CD80/86 and is effective in RA. Oligoclonal expansion of an unusual T cell population that is CD4[+]CD28[−] is present in RA, especially patients with extra-articular disease.[71] The cells can be cytotoxic and can respond to autoantigens. Other co-stimulatory molecule pairs such as CD40L on T cells and CD40 on antigen-presenting cells are also expressed in RA synovium.

Adhesion Molecules. Synovial lymphocytes also express adhesion molecules of the very late activation antigen (VLA) and lymphocyte function–associated antigen (LFA) superfamily of integrins, as well as help recruit and retain lymphocytes to the synovium. The cytokine milieu of the joint induces adhesion molecules such as intercellular adhesion molecule-1 (ICAM-1), VCAM-1, and connecting segment-1 (CS-1) fibronectin on vascular endothelium. These, in conjunction with chemokines and other chemoattractants, attract cells expressing the correct adhesion molecule counter-receptors on their surface.

Chemokine Receptors. Synovial T cells in RA express characteristic receptors to specific chemokines. The chemokine receptor CCR5 is the ligand for macrophage inhibitory proteins 1α and 1β and is highly expressed in the infiltrating RA T cells. This particular receptor, along with CXCR3, is preferentially found on Th1 cells, an observation that might explain accumulation of this phenotype in the rheumatoid synovium. In fact, expression of nonfunctional CCR5 alleles that protect from HIV infection might diminish the risk of RA. The chemotactic factor stromal cell–derived factor-1 (SDF-1) is also produced by synovial tissue, and its specific receptor, CXCR4, is displayed by rheumatoid synovial T cells. Other T cell phenotypes recruited to the rheumatoid synovium include Th17 cells that express CCR2 or CCR6 and produce IL-17 and CD4[+]CD25[+] Treg cells that can suppress immune responses (see discussion of T cell subsets later). Preferential recruitment of CCR6+ Th17 cells into the rheumatoid joint appears to be due to the local release of the chemokine CCL20.[72]

T Cell Receptor Rearrangements. Numerous groups evaluated T cell receptor gene rearrangements for clues related to antigen-specific expansion. In some patients, a pattern emerged suggesting an increased number of T cells expressing Vβ3, Vβ14, and Vβ17, especially in synovial tissue. These particular Vβ genes are structurally related and are unusually susceptible to activation by superantigens. Most studies have neither found evidence for the restricted clonality of T cells in RA synovial fluid, synovial tissue, and blood nor identified expansion of different Vβ or Vα genes.

Determinants of T Cell Phenotype. The local accumulation of T cells in the joint is not necessarily related to proliferation induced by particular antigen. Instead, antigen-independent processes related to the expression of chemokines and adhesion molecules on vascular endothelium and circulating lymphocytes help determine the mononuclear cell infiltrate. Although local antigen-specific expansion can occur, it is probably responsible for a relatively small percentage of the T cell infiltrate. Cells that encounter their appropriate antigen in the correct cytokine and antigen-presenting cell environment can potentially activate other local cells through direct cell-cell contact or the elaboration of lymphokines. A high level of telomerase activity is also present in synovial lymphocytes in RA, which is a reflection of their proliferative activity and correlates with the severity of synovial inflammation.[73] However, some data suggest that telomerase activity is actually defective in RA T cells and contributes to early senescence of the immune system. An alternative explanation for T cell activation in RA is that antigen presentation mainly occurs in central lymphoid organs. In this scenario, dendritic cells that encounter antigens in the synovium or other sites migrate to lymphatic tissue and then present antigen to naïve T cells. Once activated, these T cells enter the circulation and can home to the joint, where they can produce cytokines and activate resident cells.

Synovial T Cell Immunoreactivity

The histopathologic appearance of RA, with exuberant infiltration of the synovium with T lymphocytes, is characteristic of tissues with chronic antigen-specific responses. However, the synovium can only respond to inflammation in a limited number of ways and many chronic immune-mediated arthropathies have similar histologic patterns. In fact, the appearance of chronic arthritides that are clearly not mediated by T cells (e.g., chronic tophaceous gout) exhibits many of the same features.

The microheterogeneity of the rheumatoid synovial tissue, with different numbers and proportions of cell lineages in each area, suggests that different antigens might be presented at various locations in the synovium. For instance, type II collagen might be presented to T cells one place, proteoglycans elsewhere, and responses to HSPs or viral antigens in yet another region. Although synovial T cells display an activated phenotype, proliferative and cytokine responses are usually less than normal peripheral blood cells

or even autologous peripheral blood T cells from the same patient. Spontaneous and stimulated cytokine production including Th1 factors such as IFN-γ and IL-2 are relatively low. Responses directed toward recall antigens are also deficient, although RA synovial T cells can proliferate briskly to certain HSPs. On the other hand, recent data implicate functional Th17 cells in the synovium, which differentiate in the presence of certain cytokines such as IL-1, IL-6, and/or IL-23 and produce cytokines in the IL-17 family (IL-17A through F).

The mechanisms of decreased responsiveness in the synovial tissue compartment have not been as extensively studied as in synovial fluid or peripheral blood, but they likely include exposure to suppressive factors (e.g., TGF-β or IL-1Ra), abnormal redox potentials that suppress T cell receptor signal transduction, or induction of anergy. Another contributor to local anergy is the relative lack of the co-stimulatory molecule CD80 on HLA-DR+ FLS because coculture of T cells with synoviocytes suppresses subsequent immune responses.

Synovial T cells in RA functionally resemble resting peripheral blood T lymphocytes that have been activated by cytokines rather than antigen.[74] Both synovial and blood T lymphocytes are able to stimulate macrophages to produce TNF in a cell contact–dependent manner. This process is dependent on nuclear factor κB (NFκB) and is mechanistically distinct from T cell activation via the T cell receptor, which is independent of NFκB. Therefore the contribution of T cell to the proinflammatory cytokine milieu may be unrelated to antigen-mediated events and could result from passive activation after exposure to the cytokine environment.

Although increased immune reactivity contributes to the etiology of RA, the search for a specific rheumatoid antigen has not been fruitful. Animal models suggest that breakdown of tolerance can be due to a combination of factors early in development. For instance, mutations in the *ZAP70* gene can lead to spontaneous T cell–dependent inflammatory arthritis in mice.[75] This protein is intimately involved with transducing T cell receptor signals and activating T lymphocytes. An abnormal *ZAP70* gene leads to defective positive and negative selection in the thymus and allows autoreactive T cells to escape. As a result, mice produce autoantibodies (e.g., RF and anti-dsDNA) and develop a severe destructive arthritis. The disease can be transferred by thymocytes or peripheral CD4+ T cells into syngeneic mice with a normal *ZAP70* gene.

The cytokine profile of this model is quite similar to RA, and mice with deficient TNF, IL-1, or IL-6 have reduced synovitis. Of interest, IFN-γ deficiency has no effect, whereas IL-10 deficiency exacerbates disease. These studies demonstrate that minor changes in the T cell receptor complex and signaling can alter T cell selection and induce T cell–dependent arthritis. This is especially relevant in light of the data implicating *PTPN22* in RA because this gene is also involved with T cell receptor signaling. Despite the clear T cell dependence of the model, the cytokines implicated are remarkably similar to autoantibody-dependent models of RA. Therefore the cytokine profile in RA (see later) in many ways represents a final common pathway for a variety of autoimmune mechanisms.

Restoring T Cell Tolerance

Assuming that synovial T cell autoreactivity plays a key role in the pathogenesis of RA, one potential therapeutic approach is to restore tolerance. This concept has been somewhat problematic because the underlying defect has not been defined and could include abnormal thymic selection, poorly defined genetic factors that lead to immune hyper-reactivity, or inadequate regulatory T cell function. The lack of a specific antigen identified as pathogenic also increases the complexity of the problem. What is clear, however, is that current approaches do not "cure" RA because cessation of therapy usually leads to a recurrence of disease.

Aggressive treatment of early RA (within the year of clinical disease) with methotrexate and a TNF inhibitor could lead to long-lasting remissions.[76] In many cases, therapy was withdrawn after 1 year of treatment and patients did not flare for at least an additional year. The mechanism of prolonged remission despite discontinuing therapy in early disease is not defined but appears to differ from clinical experience in chronic RA. Additional individualized therapies that enhance regulatory T cell function, alter costimulation, or delete pathogenic T cells are other ways to restore homeostasis and normal immune function. Examples might include inhibitors of co-stimulatory molecules like CTLA4 or ICOS or to potentially delete subpopulations of T cells that express specific T cell receptor that bind to epitopes critical for autoreactivity. However, the latter strategy based on specific T cell Vβ genes over-represented in RA joints has not been successful.

Synovial B Cells

Synovial B cell and plasma cell hyper-reactivity are viewed increasingly as key participants in the perpetuation and initiation phases of RA. This notion has been fueled by the descriptions of novel spontaneous models of arthritis in mice, such as the K/BxN model, in which loss of tolerance leads to autoantibody production, activation of innate immunity, and chronic synovitis. Furthermore, B cell–directed therapies such as anti-CD20 antibody have demonstrated efficacy in RA.

Cytokine Regulation of Synovial B Cells. Although many rheumatoid synovial tissues exhibit a diffuse infiltration with mononuclear cells, a significant percentage also have discrete lymphoid follicles populated by B cells in the sublining region. Follicular dendritic cells, B cells, plasma cells, and T lymphocytes collect in these aggregates. The germinal centers are highly organized structures in which affinity maturation occurs. B cells are present in the aggregates and express the maturation marker CD20, as well as proliferation antigens such as Ki67. The formation of these structures is dependent on several soluble and membrane-bound cytokines including lymphotoxin. B cells accumulate in lymphoid aggregates in RA synovium under the influence of a variety of chemotactic factors including CCL21 and B cell–attracting chemokine-1 (CXCL13).

A member of the TNF superfamily of cytokines known as B lymphocyte stimulator (BLyS, also called BAFF) has also been identified as a key molecule that regulates B cell differentiation. BLys binds to transmembrane activator and CAML interactor (TACI), which is present on both B and T cells. If this system is blocked using recombinant TACI-Ig to absorb the cytokine and a related B cell differentiation factor called APRIL, then the number of B cells is dramatically reduced and antibody production is decreased. The same construct is effective as a therapeutic agent in collagen-induced arthritis, a model that depends on autoantibody production.[77]

BLyS is produced in RA synovium, especially by macrophages. Synovial lining type B synoviocytes can also release BLyS and can be induced by TNF and IFN-γ in vitro. APRIL is localized mainly to dendritic cells in synovial germinal centers. TACI-Ig, which binds both BLyS and APRIL, disrupts the germinal centers and decreases immunoglobulin receptors in SCID mice implanted with rheumatoid synovium.[78] One clinical trial using an anti-BLyS antibody demonstrated minimal benefit in patients with RA, although a second study showed efficacy. Improved benefit might be possible with a biologic that blocks both APRIL and BLyS, although early studies showed that TACI-Ig significantly decreases serum immunoglobulin concentrations but has limited efficacy in RA.[79]

Synovial B Cell Maturation. B cells isolated directly from germinal centers of RA synovium demonstrate a heterogeneous pattern of V-gene usage and rearrangement. The majority of VH genes are not mutated, suggesting that they are recent immigrants from the peripheral blood and are activated locally. For RF-producing cells, shared mutations containing an identical sequence throughout the variable domain of immunoglobulins have been identified in synovial tissue.[80] Preferential utilization of a limited number of VH and DH gene segments and marked preference for a DH reading frame encoding particular hydrophilic residues have also been observed, consistent with antigen-related selection and maturation. Analysis of expressed heavy-chain variable domains supports the notion that the B cell response in RA synovium is oligoclonal. Similarly, B cell clones isolated from either RA synovium or bone marrow with "nurse-like" cells have limited VH usage.

B cells associated with follicular dendritic cells in the rheumatoid synovium can further differentiate and develop additional mutations, suggesting antigen-driven selection. Plasma cells in other areas of the synovium have distinct rearrangements compared with the B lymphocytes associated with dendritic cells. This raises the question of whether the plasma cells arise locally or migrate from the blood. Although plasma cell rearrangements are not always similar to the B cells, groups of plasma cells use similar genes, albeit with distinct mutations. Therefore the plasma cells could derive from synovial B cell clones that mutated and whose progeny proliferate and differentiate.

What is not certain is whether this process represents an ectopic lymphoid organ performing normal functions or whether it is related to autoimmunity. The presence of abundant autoantibody-producing cells in the synovium supports the latter hypothesis, although normal immune responses might also occur in the joint. Cells that produce RFs, anti–type II collagen antibody, and ACPA populate the RA synovium.

Maturation and survival of B cells depend on stromal cells and cells with nurselike properties that support lymphocyte maturation in the thymus. The synovium of patients with RA also contains nurselike cells, which can increase expression of CD40 and class II MHC proteins on B cells. B cell survival is supported by this population of cells, whereas autoreactive clones evade deletion and produce autoantibodies. A variety of cytokines including GM-CSF, IL-6, and IL-8 are produced by RA nurselike cells, and direct contact with B cells is critical for maximal proliferation and antibody production. Of interest, cultured B cells spontaneously migrate beneath ordinary FLS, which permits them to survive in vitro for prolonged periods of time. The process depends on the interaction of the integrin α4/β1 on B cells with synoviocytes expressing CD106 (VCAM-1). Interference with the B cell–synoviocyte interaction decreases B cell survival and is one potential mechanism by which therapeutic interventions targeted at integrins might suppress autoreactivity and inflammation in RA.

B Cell Depletion in RA. Although the role of T cells and cytokines attracted most of the scientific interest in recent years, clinical trials with an anti-CD20 antibody (rituximab) demonstrating efficacy in RA refocused investigators on B cells and autoantibodies. The precise function of CD20 is not well defined; it is expressed on mature B cells but not plasma cells. Rituximab causes a rapid and profound depletion of peripheral blood B cells. In mice, anti-CD20 antibody depletes B cells in blood, spleen, lymph nodes, and bone marrow. The few remaining B cells in the spleen were of the B1 but not B2 phenotype. Peritoneal B cells are only partially depleted, suggesting that some sites are privileged and protect B cells despite adequate drug penetration.

In RA, serial synovial biopsies demonstrate partial B cell depletion after rituximab therapy despite the virtual absence of peripheral B cells. The clinical responses do not always correlate closely with the extent of synovial depletion, although some patients with the most impressive responses appear to have marked declines in the number of B cells in the post-treatment specimens. Surprisingly, B cell depletion does not consistently decrease autoantibody production or cytokine production in the synovium, nor does a change in ACPA or RF levels predict a clinical response.[81] Longer-term biopsy studies suggest that plasma cells are decreased in synovium 24 weeks after the treatment with rituximab and that this correlates with decreased symptoms.

B Cell Contribution to Synovitis. The simplest explanation for B cell contributions to RA lies in their ability to produce autoantibodies and differentiate into long-lived plasma cells. However, autoantibody titers do not correlate well with disease activity and RA-associated antibodies are detected in individuals without evidence of synovitis. The synovial biopsy data on synovial autoantibody production also suggest that B cells play a more complex and nuanced role in the disease. For example, plasma cells might be a more relevant source of autoantibodies than CD20+ B cells.

Perhaps more important, B cells are potent antigen-presenting cells that could serve this function either in the inflamed synovium or in central lymphoid organs. In an SCID mouse model using rheumatoid synovial explants, T cell activation, lymphoneogenesis, and cytokine production

depended on B cells.[82] In the same model, treatment with TACI-Ig to inhibit APRIL and BLyS decreased synovial inflammation and IFN-γ production in tissues with germinal centers.

B cells can also make a variety of cytokines including LTα, TNF, and IL-6. Although macrophages and synoviocytes might produce greater amounts of proinflammatory factors, production by B cells in strategic locations in the joints and elsewhere might help drive synovitis. A novel subset of regulatory B cells, like regulatory T cells, could decrease inflammatory responses in RA through the production of suppressive cytokines like IL-10 and TGF-β. It is not clear how B cell depletion might select for specific B cell subsets, and it is possible that the regulatory B cells could be relatively enriched.

Dendritic Cells

Dendritic cells (DCs) are potent antigen-presenting cells that populate synovial tissue and synovial effusions of patients with RA. DCs generally sample the environment, especially at mucosal and skin surfaces; process antigens; and then migrate to a central lymphatic site where they present the antigens to T cells. An emerging appreciation of DC function in the etiology of RA led to the concept that the cells could be loaded with local autoantigens and migrate to central lymphoid tissues, where they can participate in the initiation of disease. DCs are also potent producers of type I interferons, which has been implicated in numerous autoimmune diseases such as lupus and RA.

Rheumatoid synovium could function like lymphoid tissues in some circumstances with mature DCs expressing CD86, CD83, and DC-LAMP localized in perivascular lymphocytic infiltrates and aggregates. Ultrastructural analysis of the synovium shows the DCs in contact with lymphocytes, where they can present antigens. The presence of DCs is not unique to RA and has been identified in other inflammatory arthritides including gout and spondyloarthropathies.

DCs are recruited to synovium, like other immunocompetent cells, through the generation of chemotactic factors and expression of the appropriate adhesion molecules. The subsequent localization with the synovium and the formation of microarchitecture such as lymphoid aggregates also depends on production of chemokines in the synovial environment. DCs express the chemokine receptor CCR7, which usually permits them to home to lymphoid tissue and orchestrate organization into the appropriate germinal centers. Synoviocytes in RA express two CCR7 ligands (CCL19 and CCL21), which provide a signal for the DCs to remain in the peripheral tissue. Immature DCs and plasmacytoid DCs are also scattered throughout the synovial sublining region. B cell–enriched lymphoid follicles, which are usually organized around follicular DCs (FDCs), are also found in some RA joint tissues. The source of FDCs is not well defined, but cultured FLS can perform FDC functions in vitro and could contribute in vivo as well. Synoviocytes derived from RA patients can bind to germinal-center B cells and suppress B cell apoptosis.

Follicular DC–containing ectopic lymphoid structures in rheumatoid synovium also express high levels of activation-induced cytosine deaminase, a key gene that participates in immunoglobulin class switching. ACPA-positive plasma cells surround these aggregates, suggesting that the aggregates play a role in autoantibody production. The architecture and ACPA-positive cells persist when tissue is transplanted into SCID mice. Therefore synovial DCs not only help organize the microarchitecture of synovial tissue but also participate in the development of high-affinity IgG autoantibodies.[83]

Cytokines in the rheumatoid synovium such as GM-CSF influence the proliferation and maturation of DCs. Increased numbers are found in the tissue and synovial effusions, where they comprise up to 5% of mononuclear cells. RA synovial tissue DCs do not always behave normally. For example, IL-10 suppresses dendritic cell function, in part by decreasing expression of CD86 and class II MHC molecules. However, RA dendritic cells isolated from the joint are resistant to this effect, possibly because they express lower amounts of the IL-10 receptor.[84] Aside from presenting antigens, DCs also produce cytokines that can influence T cell differentiation in the joint including IL-12 and IL-23, which can enhance the bias toward the Th1 and Th17 (see later) phenotypes; APRIL, which enhances B cell survival; and, as noted earlier, interferons.

Mast Cells, Polymorphonuclear Leukocytes, and Natural Killer Cells

Mast cells are present in the synovial membranes of patients with RA and, in some patients, are located at sites of cartilage erosion. Rheumatoid synovial membranes contain more than 10 times as many mast cells than do control synovial samples from patients undergoing surgery for meniscectomy. Mast cells and histamine are also found in a majority of synovial fluid specimens from inflammatory synovitis. A detailed analysis of several indicators of proliferation and the enumeration of synovial mast cells has demonstrated strong positive correlations between the number of mast cells in synovial tissue and the degree of lymphocyte infiltration.[85] Mast cells from RA synovium express significantly higher amounts of the C5a receptor, compared with OA synovium.

Resident mast cells in synovium respond to cytokines that stimulate mast cell growth and chemotaxis. Extracts of mast cells can induce adherent rheumatoid synovial cells to increase production of PGE_2 and collagenase, and immunostaining of RA synovial mast cells demonstrates tryptase and TNF. Mast cell–derived heparin has significant effects on connective tissue. In particular, it may modulate the effects of hormones on osseous cells and thereby alter the balance of bone synthesis toward degradation.

The role of mast cells in the initiation phase of synovitis was highlighted in the passive K/BxN model in which their absence prevented disease.[86] It is not certain if the cells are required once synovial inflammation has been established and other cell types such as neutrophils supplant the mast cells in some circumstances. For instance, the production of leukotriene B_4 in the same model requires neutrophils but not mast cells in established disease. Treatment of synovial tissue explants cultures with a c-Kit tyrosine kinase inhibitor that blocks stem cell factor signaling and decreased

production of TNF.[87] These data suggest that mast cells might contribute to synovial cytokine production in established disease.

More intriguing, recent data suggest that preformed IL-17A is present in granules of synovial mast cells in RA (Figure 69-9).[88] The conventional view of IL-17 is that it mainly comes from activated T cells. Cultured mast cells released the IL-17 when stimulated with TNF or immune complexes. There is also a correlation between the presence of IgE and FcR1ε and mast cell degranulation in rheumatoid synovium. More direct evidence of mast cell involvement in RA comes from an open label clinical trial using the c-Kit inhibitor masitinib in RA, where evidence of clinical efficacy was observed. c-Kit is a receptor tyrosine kinase that binds to stem cell factor and facilitates mast cell growth and survival.

Despite the abundance of neutrophils in RA synovial effusions, only rare polymorphonuclear leukocytes (PMNs) infiltrate the synovium. NK cells have, however, been identified in RA synovium.[89] Cytotoxic NK cells contain large amounts of granzymes, which are serine proteases. One potentially important immunoregulatory role of NK cells is that they can stimulate B cells to produce RFs. A subset of NK cells that express large amounts of CD56 are unusually abundant in RA synovial tissue and fluid.[90] These cells could potentially produce cytokines or enhance proinflammatory cytokine production by T lymphocytes and macrophages. There is little information on invariant natural killer T cells (iNKT), which respond to lipid antigens. However, blocking CD1d and iNKT function decreases severity of collagen-induced arthritis in mice.

Bone Marrow Cells

Although most attention has been directed at the synovium, cartilage, and cortical bone in RA, the subcortical bone and bone marrow also contribute to synovial inflammatory responses. Primitive bone marrow mesenchymal cells can traverse cortical bone through pores in murine collagen-induced arthritis before the onset of clinical disease, take up residence in the synovium, and produce mediators that enhance synovitis.[91] This process is TNF dependent and is abrogated in mice that lack TNF receptors. CD34+ mesenchymal cells in rheumatoid bone marrow are more highly activated as judged by their NFκB status and their ability to differentiate into fibroblast-like cells that produce MMPs and proangiogenic factors.

Bone marrow can also contribute other relevant cells including macrophage lineage cells that migrate to the synovium and nurselike cells that support the survival of B cells. Just as the bone marrow can influence the synovium, the reverse is also true. Invasive pannus can rupture through cortical bone and invade the marrow space in some patients. When this occurs, B cell aggregates are especially prominent in the marrow and occur in an environment rich in B cell chemoattractants such as CCL21 and B cell survival factors such as BLyS.

The bone marrow changes in RA could be either secondary to synovitis or a primary event (Figure 69-10).[92] The most common explanation for RA is that synovitis occurs first and that it expands into the marrow through

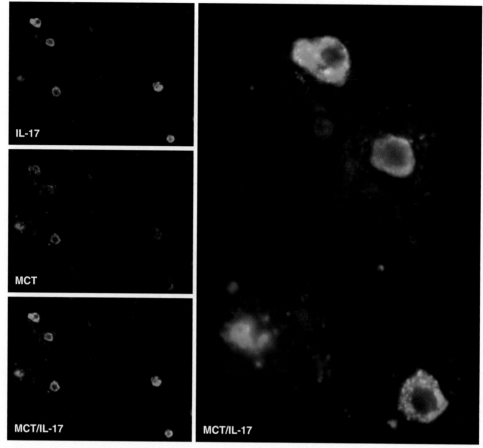

Figure 69-9 Interleukin-17A (IL-17A) in mast cells as a source of IL-17A in rheumatoid arthritis (RA). Traditional paradigms suggest that IL-17 is mainly produced by Th17 cells in the RA synovium. However, mast cells can also produce this cytokine. Immunostaining studies showed that preformed IL-17 could be detected in mast cell granules in RA synovium. Note that the combination image on the right demonstrates IL-17A *(green)* colocalizing with the mast cell marker *(red)*. This suggests a pivotal role of mast cells in the inflammatory response. MCT, mast cell tryptase. *(From Hueber AJ, Asquith DL, Miller AM, et al: Mast cells express IL-17A in rheumatoid arthritis synovium,* J Immunol *184:3336, 2010.)*

soluble factors and direct extension ("outside-in" hypothesis). The notion that bone marrow reactivity might be a primary event and that the activated cells migrate directly to the synovium through cortical bone or via the bloodstream has received increasing attention ("inside-out" hypothesis).

The role of the bone marrow in the pathogenesis of RA is suggested by immunohistologic studies of marrow showing mature B cells and activated T cells forming aggregates, as in the rheumatoid synovium.[93] Functional changes also occur including the ability of marrow mesenchymal cells of RA patients to support B and T cell survival and the production of IL-6 and TNF by marrow cells. Bone marrow mesenchymal cells from RA patients induce B cell growth and support the survival of T cells. Nurselike cells can also be grown from marrow, and marrow monocytes can induce RF production in vitro. There is considerable cross-talk between the synovium and the bone marrow, perhaps via the circulation, diffusion of soluble mediators, or direct migration of cells through cortical pores. The bidirectional interactions between the synovium and the bone marrow suggest that both "inside-out" and "outside-in" mechanisms can participate in RA.

Neural Elements and Rheumatoid Synovium

The synovium in RA is richly innervated with somatic afferent fibers, C-fibers that detect pain, and sympathetic neurons. In addition to providing information to the central nervous system (CNS) on the state of the synovium, peripheral nerves profoundly influence synovial inflammatory responses.[94] For instance, neuropeptides such as substance P and vasoactive intestinal peptide can activate macrophages, increase vascular permeability, and modulate T cell phenotype. Sympathetic fibers can enhance or suppress inflammation depending on the site and timing of stimulation by modulating adrenergic tone. Although vagal branches have not been detected, their primary neurotransmitter acetylcholine is detected in tissues and can suppress synoviocyte cytokine production through the $\alpha7$ nicotinic receptor. Perhaps most interesting, spinal cord circuits can directly modulate synovial inflammation. Activation of adenosine receptors in the spinal cord or inhibition of spinal p38 can markedly decrease synovial inflammation in joint destruction in rat arthritis models. Intrathecal etanercept also blocks peripheral inflammation almost as well as systemic administration of the TNF blocker.[95]

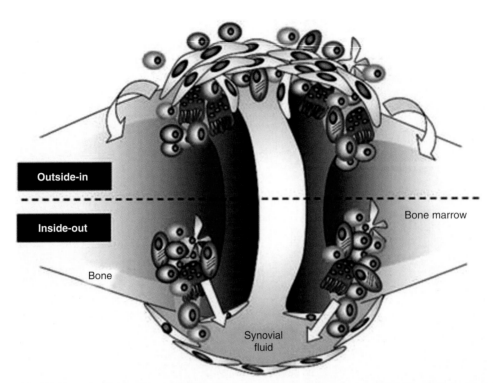

Figure 69-10 Initial synovial lesion in rheumatoid arthritis (RA). Although traditional paradigms suggest that it begins as a synovial disease, the initial insult could be at a distant site. The figure depicts two possible scenarios: (1) RA begins in the synovium and then extends into the bone and bone marrow, and (2) the initial lesion is in the bone marrow, which can extend into the synovium as cells migrate through cortical pores or through the bloodstream. *(From Schett G, Firestein GS: Mr Outside and Mr Inside: classic and alternative views on the pathogenesis of rheumatoid arthritis,* Ann Rheum Dis *69:787, 2010.)*

Synovitis in Early versus Late Rheumatoid Arthritis

Although the synovium during the first few weeks of symptomatic RA occasionally demonstrates a paucity of lymphocyte infiltration, endothelial cell injury, tissue edema, and neutrophil accumulation, in general it has a histologic appearance similar to long-standing disease. The extent of lymphoid aggregation, T cell infiltration, and synovial-lining hyperplasia can resemble chronic disease even when symptoms have been present for a short period of time. The cytokine patterns of these biopsies as determined by immunohistochemical analysis indicated similar levels of T cell (such as IFN-γ) and non–T cell factors (such as IL-1 and TNF). The tumor suppressor gene *p53* is also expressed in early RA, most likely due to intense oxidative stress in the environment.

Biopsies of asymptomatic joints from patients with early or late RA also have lymphocyte infiltration, cytokine production, and *p53* expression. Although IFN-γ, IL-1, and TNF levels are increased compared with normal synovium, they are modestly lower than in clinically active joints. Some cytokines such as IL-8 and the number of macrophages are higher in the painful joints. Macrophage and plasma cell infiltration in early RA might predict more erosive or severe disease. In animal models of arthritis, increased synovial inflammation and expression of proinflammatory transcription factors such as activator protein-1 (AP-1) and NFκB also occur well before clinically evident arthritis.[96]

These studies suggest that patients with "early" RA, as defined by the duration of symptoms, might, in fact, already have chronic disease and that evaluation of truly early disease might require assessment of patients long before the onset of symptoms (if this is even possible). The observation that autoantibodies are produced in RA patients years before the clinical arthritis also supports the notion that a preclinical phase can possibly precede symptomatic synovitis. In addition, profiling cytokine and chemokine levels in stored serum samples of patients who ultimately develop RA show increased levels of chemokines and cytokines, especially in the ACPA-positive population. This reinforces the concept that RA is a continuum that can progress to clinical synovitis. However, the time lines and the environmental stimuli that cause progression are not known.

Animal Models as Surrogates for Rheumatoid Synovitis

Animal models of RA are crucial to understand the biology of synovitis. However, they are an imperfect representation at best for this uniquely human disease. The specific inciting agents are known, the time course is compressed, and disease is induced in genetically pure strains. Despite many differences between various models and human disease, there are many similarities for pathogenic influences such as the presence of autoantibodies and, in many cases, the cytokine profile.[97]

The time course for cytokine and signal transduction activation is an important variable when interpreting therapeutic interventions. For example, IL-6 gene expression is high during a relatively narrow window in collagen-induced arthritis (Figure 69-11).[98] Activation of signaling molecules such as the MAP kinases in the synovium also follows patterns that are similar to, but not identical to, RA. These issues do not invalidate the value of the models, but they do provide context for understanding why so many interventions are effective in preclinical studies but fail in human clinical trials.

SYNOVIAL FLUID AND THE SYNOVIAL FLUID CARTILAGE INTERFACE

KEY POINTS

RA synovial effusions contain neutrophils and mononuclear cells.

Immune complexes that contain autoantibodies such as RFs or anticitrullinated protein antibodies can fix complement, leading to the generation of chemoattractants.

Small molecule mediators of inflammation such as prostaglandins and leukotrienes are present in RA synovial fluid.

Synovial effusions accumulate in the joints of most patients with active RA due to a substantial increase in fluid influx that cannot be removed despite an increase in lymphatic flow. There is an inverse relationship between the molecular weight of proteins and their concentrations in minimally inflamed synovial fluid. High-molecular-weight serum proteins gain access more easily to synovial fluid in inflamed joints, and the relatively high concentration of IgG in RA synovial fluid is good evidence for local synthesis of immunoglobulins. Markedly increased permeance of proteins in rheumatoid patients is also evidence of the severe microvascular lesion in rheumatoid synovitis. Newer techniques evaluating the synovial fluid proteome in RA using mass spectroscopy might provide new insights into the key mediators. More than 400 proteins in RA effusions were identified as potential biomarkers of disease activity including C-reactive protein and six members of the S100 family of calcium granule binding proteins.[99] In general, assays for autoantibodies or assessments of exudate versus transudate in synovial fluid have little value; the concentration of serum proteins in effusions is usually about half to two-thirds the level in the blood.

Polymorphonuclear Leukocytes

Large numbers of PMNs accumulate in rheumatoid synovial effusions and enter via postcapillary venules in the synovium. Neutrophils adhere to activate synovial microvasculature due to their abundant surface expression of selectins and the β_2 integrins. After adherence, chemotactic agents produced by endothelium and resident synovial cells facilitate exit from the intravascular space into the tissue. Thus considering the survival time of PMNs in synovial fluid, an average rheumatoid effusion containing 25,000 PMNs per mm^3 could exceed 1 billion cells each day. The ultimate fate of these cells is usually apoptosis. Neutrophil survival requires expression of the forkhead transcription factor FOXO30.[100] Mice that lack this gene are resistant to inflammatory arthritis due to shortened PMN life span.

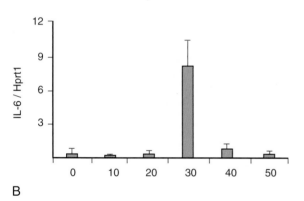

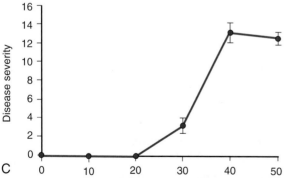

Figure 69-11 Kinetics of synovial activation in collagen-induced arthritis. Although there are many similarities between mouse models and rheumatoid arthritis (RA), the time course of the former is highly compressed and the pathogenic mechanisms might differ. The figure shows the time course for activation of synovial p38 MAP kinase **(A)** and IL-6 gene expression **(B)** in the mouse model. Note that IL-6 expression is high during a relatively limited period of time. The pattern of kinase activation also does not precisely correlate with clinical disease **(C)**. Understanding the time course and pathogenic events of mouse models and how they relate to RA will help with interpretation of the preclinical model. *(From Fukushima A, Boyle DL, Corr M, Firestein GS: Kinetic analysis of synovial signalling and gene expression in animal models of arthritis,* Ann Rheum Dis *69:918, 2010.)*

High concentrations of chemotactic agents in the synovial fluid in RA recruit a large number of cells to the intra-articular cavity. Few PMNs are seen in the synovium itself; once in the tissue they move rapidly to the synovial fluid, drawn by agents such as C5a generated due to complement activation, leukotriene B$_4$ (LTB$_4$), platelet-activating factor, and chemokines. CXC chemokines including ENA-78 and IL-8 is especially abundant in synovial fluid and can attract neutrophils into the intra-articular space. RA PMNs can also release chemokines such as macrophage-inflammatory protein-3α (MIP-3α) into the milieu that promote migration of additional cells into the joint space.

Once in the joint, neutrophils engage immune complexes through Fc receptors, especially FcRγI and FcRγIII, that activate spleen tyrosine kinase (Syk). This process initiates a signaling cascade that includes the MAP kinases and NFκB, cytoskeletal reorganization, release of granule content, generation of reactive oxygen and nitrogen species, and enhanced phagocytosis. Many of the cells contain immune complexes within phagosomes that include IgG and IgM along with RF and complement proteins such as C1q, C3, and C4. PMNs from synovial fluid in RA release de novo synthesized proteins including matrix proteins such as fibronectin, neutral proteinases, and IL-1. Neutrophils also secrete IL-1Ra and oncostatin M, a member of the IL-6 family. Although the amount of IL-1Ra each neutrophil produces is low compared with macrophages, the sheer number of PMNs allows them to produce large amounts in synovial effusions.

Neutrophil cells also release numerous proteases that can adversely affect the lubricating properties of synovial fluid and the integrity of the cartilage including elastase and trypsin. Neutrophil collagenase (MMP-8) can digest native collagen in cartilage, which then makes it susceptible to degradation by other MMPs such as the stromelysins. Although synoviocytes are generally considered major producers of the MMPs, animal models of arthritis suggest that neutrophil-derived proteases play a significant role in cartilage damage.

Although difficult to assess in humans, animal models demonstrate a role for neutrophils in the inflammatory processes. The passive K/BxN and collagen-induced arthritis models, which depend on autoantibodies to bind to the cartilage and fix complement, require neutrophils for full expression of the disease. Depleting neutrophils with antibodies almost completely prevents synovial inflammation in these models. In the K/BxN model, neutrophils also initiate vascular permeability that permits pathogenic antibodies to gain access to the joint space.

Synovial Fluid Lymphocytes

The lymphocyte subsets in synovial fluid differ from that of peripheral blood and synovial tissue. Even though synovial effusions contain an abundance of T cells, the CD4-to-CD8 ratio is actually reversed compared with that of blood or synovial tissue, with an excess of CD8$^+$ cells relative to CD4$^+$ lymphocytes. In addition, synovial tissue is nearly devoid of neutrophils, which often constitute 50% to 75% of synovial fluid cells. The percentage of regulatory T cells (CD4$^+$CD25$^+$) is also higher in synovial fluid than peripheral blood.

Synovial fluid contains T cells, which express high levels of surface HLA-DR antigens. Surface activation antigens are increased on synovial fluid lymphocytes including VLA-1 and CD69. Of CD4$^+$ cells in rheumatoid synovial fluid, most are memory cells and express CD45RO on their surface. Despite the activated phenotype, synovial fluid T cell function is usually deficient compared with peripheral blood cells. For instance, synovial fluid lymphocyte proliferation in response to mitogens or most recall antigens such as tetanus toxoid is significantly less than paired blood T lymphocytes. Mycobacterial antigens and the 60-kD HSP are exceptions because proliferation is actually greater in synovial fluid cells, perhaps because they can also activate TLRs. Cytokine production by synovial fluid T cells in vitro is also low including mitogen-induced expression of IFN-γ and IL-1.

Defective T cell responses by RA synovial fluid mononuclear cells could be due to anti-inflammatory cytokines such as IL-1Ra and TGF-β.[101] Nonspecific components of joint effusions such as hyaluronic acid can be toxic and indirectly suppress T cell activation. The mechanism of diminished T cell activation could also be due to defective TCR signaling. Articular T cells have diminished tyrosine phosphorylation of proteins after stimulation, especially the key signal transduction pathway p38 MAP kinase. Furthermore, tyrosine phosphorylation of the TCR ζ chain, an early event in TCR signaling, is low compared with peripheral blood T cells. The hyporesponsiveness of synovial fluid T cells correlates with a significant decrease in the levels of the intracellular redox-regulating agent glutathione.[102] Restoration of intracellular glutathione increases proliferation of RA synovial fluid T cells. Therefore oxidative stress in the inflamed environment can suppress antigen-specific T cell responses.

Platelets and Platelet Microparticles

Platelets are a rich source of growth factors and cytokines including platelet-derived growth factor (PDGF). They are present in rheumatoid synovial effusions and can form microparticles. This process is dependent on collagen receptor glycoprotein VI. The microparticles activate cultured synoviocytes and, through an IL-1–dependent mechanism, stimulate cytokine secretion. Platelet depletion also suppresses arthritis severity in animal models.

Intra-articular Immune Complexes and Complement Fixation

Synovial Fluid Immune Complexes

Complexes containing immunoglobulins are abundant in the blood and synovial fluid of patients with RA, especially containing IgM. The most prevalent antigens in these aggregates contain IgG complexed with RF due to their ability to bind the Fc portion of immunoglobulin. Using more sensitive techniques, circulating immune complexes in RA contain up to 20 polypeptides including albumin, immunoglobulin, complement, type II collagen, fibrinogen, and acute-phase reactants, as well as DNA. These complexes can potentially fix complement, releasing chemotactic peptides and factors that activate neutrophils and other inflammatory cells.

Immune Complexes Embedded in Cartilage

The aggregates of RF, IgG, and various peptides become embedded into cartilage and other tissues in contact with synovial fluids. Electron microscopic studies demonstrate immunoglobulin complexes with damage to the cartilage matrix in the microenvironment. Immune complexes are absent under areas of cartilage invaded actively by synovial pannus, suggesting that phagocytic cells in the invasive synovium bind to and ingest the immune complexes. This possibility lends credence to the notion that immune complexes deposited in the avascular superficial layers of cartilage in the joint may serve as chemoattractants for the pannus. Immune complexes have been extracted from cartilage of RA and OA patients. Rheumatoid cartilage contains more than 40-fold more IgM and more than 10-fold more IgG than healthy cartilage extracts. IgM RF is found in the majority of RA cartilage extracts but not in OA or healthy control extracts. In addition, more than 60% of the RA cartilage extracts are positive for native and denatured collagen type II antibody.

Synovial Fluid Complement

Biologically active products of complement activation accumulate in synovial fluid during acute inflammation. This observation led to the concept that RA represents an intra-articular immune complex disease. This was the prevailing view of RA until the role of T cells and cytokine networks emerged in the 1980s.

The liver is the major source of complement synthesis in humans, and passive transfer of serum proteins into effusions accounts for many of the complement proteins found there. However, synovial tissue also actively produces complement proteins. Macrophages and fibroblasts produce complement proteins under the influence of cytokines such as IFN-γ, IL-1, and TNF. In situ hybridization shows that C2 is expressed in the synovial intimal lining, whereas C3 appears to be produced by synovial sublining macrophages. Analysis of synovial tissue shows that all complement genes from the classic pathway are expressed in RA, as well as in healthy synovium.

Despite the local production of complement components, the activities of C4, C2, and C3 and total hemolytic complement in rheumatoid synovial effusions are lower than in synovial fluids from patients with other joint diseases. Although the most prominent evidence of activation implicates the classic pathway, cleavage products of the alternate pathway including factor B and properdin have also been documented in RA. IgM RF appears to be a more important determinant of complement activation than IgG RF in serum and synovial fluid. Accelerated catabolism of C4 in RA and the presence of C4 fragments in the plasma correlate with titers of IgM RF.

The interactions between PMNs and the complement system are substantial. Neutrophil lysosomal lysates contain enzymes that cleave complement proteins and generate chemotactic activity such as C5a from serum. C5a, in addition to being a principal chemotactic factor in inflammatory effusions, mediates lysosomal release from human PMNs and induces cytoskeletal rearrangement. The chemotactic anaphylatoxins C3a and C5a are often present in rheumatoid effusions, as are the terminal complement components that comprise the C5b-C9 membrane attack complex. The latter is especially interesting because low levels of the complex can activate synoviocytes in vitro.

Targeting Complement in Rheumatoid Arthritis

Inhibiting complement proteins has obvious therapeutic potential in RA. In addition to theoretic considerations and evidence of complement consumption, a polymorphism in or near the C5 locus has been associated with increased risk of RA. For instance, intra-articular treatment with a soluble complement receptor (sCR1) inhibits joint swelling in rat antigen-induced arthritis. C5-deficient mice have decreased joint inflammation in collagen-induced arthritis and the passive K/BxN model. Absence of C3 or factor B also inhibits collagen-induced arthritis. Unlike the C5 knockout mice, which have normal antibody responses, the C3- and factor B–null animals have lower levels of anti–type II collagen antibodies. The role of C3 convertase has been explored in more detail using transgenic mice that produce the regulatory protein complement receptor 1–related gene/protein y (Crry). These mice have no obvious phenotype and are not more susceptible to infection. However, collagen-induced arthritis is suppressed in the Crry transgenic mice.

These data suggest that classic and alternative complement pathways participate in RA. A humanized anti-C5 antibody has been evaluated in a placebo-controlled study. The antibody inhibits C5 activation and function of the C5b-C9 attack complex. Although the monoclonal antibody was well tolerated, there was only modest evidence of clinical efficacy. Similarly, a C5a receptor antagonist did not decrease inflammation in a short-term placebo-controlled synovial biopsy study even though the compound was effective in preclinical models and blood levels were in the therapeutic range.[103] C5 alone is not sufficient to sustain inflammation in the rheumatoid joint and it probably participates in a redundant inflammatory network. It is not clear whether targeting other complement components such as C3 convertase would be more successful.

Arachidonate Metabolites

Prostaglandins

Arachidonic acid metabolites are produced in the inflamed joint via oxidation by cyclooxygenases (COX) to prostaglandins and thromboxanes or by lipoxygenases to leukotrienes. COX inhibitors are clearly effective in RA, although the effect is modest and is due, in part, to spinal analgesic action. Animal models of arthritis are variably sensitive to prostaglandin; indomethacin almost completely prevents adjuvant arthritis in rats but has minimal benefit in collagen-induced arthritis in mice. This serves as a reminder that results in rodent models do not always correlate with human disease.

Stable prostaglandins, especially PGE_2, produce vasodilation, increase vascular permeability, and are involved centrally in fever. They also display some anti-inflammatory activities that could account for limited efficacy. For example, the drug misoprostol, a prostaglandin analogue, has modest but significant anti-inflammatory or immuno-modulatory effects. Physiologic concentrations of PGE_2 inhibit IFN-γ production by T cells, HLA-DR expression by macrophages, and T cell proliferation.

Production of prostaglandins in RA depends on both COX-1 and COX-2 (see Chapter 24). The former is constitutively expressed and is responsible for the normal endogenous production of prostaglandins in the joint, as well as in other tissues. COX-2, on the other hand, is an inducible enzyme responsible for increased prostaglandin synthesis in inflamed tissue. Cytokines such as IL-1 and TNF induce COX-2 gene expression by cultured synoviocytes and macrophages. COX-2 mRNA and immunoreactive protein are increased in RA synovium.[104] Most nonsteroidal anti-inflammatory drugs including indomethacin and ibuprofen inhibit both enzymes. Much of the anti-inflammatory activity and analgesia in RA results from inhibition of COX-2. Targeting prostaglandin receptors such as E2 or E4 is an alternative approach that might have less deleterious effects on the gastric mucosa and cardiovascular disease. More recent data suggest that EP4 can also act on DCs and T cells to enhance production of Th1 and Th17 cells.[105]

Prostaglandin I_2, like PGE_2, can also contribute to synovial inflammation. For instance, mice lacking the prostaglandin I_2 receptor have significantly decreased arthritis severity in the collagen-induced arthritis model compared with wild type mice even though they make similar amounts of anticollagen antibodies.

Leukotrienes

LTBs are a potent proinflammatory produced by neutrophils and chemotactic for neutrophils, eosinophils, and macrophages. They also promote neutrophil aggregation and adherence to endothelium. Peripheral blood PMNs from rheumatoid patients have an enhanced capacity for LTB_4 production compared with normal individuals.[106] In murine collagen-induced arthritis, LTB_4 antagonists decreased paw swelling and joint destruction, suggesting a pivotal role for this potent chemoattractant. Surprisingly, LTB_4 blockade has minimal efficacy in RA.

Anti-Inflammatory Arachidonic Acid Metabolites

Certain arachidonic acid metabolites such as 15-deoxy-delta(12,14)-PGJ(2) can bind to peroxisome proliferators, activate receptors (PPARs), and inhibit cytokine production and inflammation in animal models of arthritis. Cyclopentenone prostaglandins can also inhibit NFκB by blocking one of the key enzymes that activates this pathway, namely IκB kinase-β (IKKβ). Lipoxins and resolvins represent a unique class of lipid mediators that help resolve inflammatory diseases. Lipoxins (LX) have a trihydroxytetraene structure and are produced from arachidonic acid via the lipoxygenase pathways. LXA_4 binds with high affinity to a G protein–coupled receptor denoted lipoxin A_4 receptor (ALXR). Activation of ALXR inhibits recruitment of neutrophils by attenuating chemotaxis, adhesion, and transmigration into tissues and by diminishing chemokine and cytokine production. LXA_4 significantly decreased cytokine and MMP expression in FLS through an NFκB-dependent mechanism.

PERIPHERAL BLOOD LYMPHOCYTE IMMUNE RESPONSES

Although peripheral lymphocytes are the most accessible, many investigators believe there is greater value studying cells isolated from the primary site of disease. The number of CD4$^+$ helper T cells is mildly increased in the circulation of patients with RA, with a concomitant decrease in CD8$^+$ lymphocytes (and an increased CD4-to-CD8 ratio). The surface phenotype of circulating T cells in RA suggests activation in some studies, but not in others. For instance, an increased percentage of $\alpha\beta$ and $\gamma\delta$ TCR–bearing cells might express HLA-DR and the adhesion protein VLA-4 ($\alpha_4\beta_1$ integrin). The latter is especially critical in that VLA-4 plays an important role in the recruitment of cells to the synovium through interactions with VCAM-1 on endothelial cells. Other markers of activation are not necessarily elevated on RA T cells in the circulation. Therefore peripheral-blood T cells express some, but not all, phenotypic characteristics of activation. It is not clear whether this process occurs in the peripheral or central lymphoid organs or whether cells are activated in the synovium and re-enter the circulation via the synovial lymphatics.

Immunoregulatory dysfunction has been described in RA peripheral lymphocytes. One of the early observations was the inadequate control of EBV-infected B lymphocyte growth due to a defect in T cell function in RA. The abnormal T cell response could be correlated somewhat with disease activity, but it was also noted that the abnormality was present in T cells of some patients with inflammatory arthropathies other than RA.[107] IFN-γ and IL-2 production is significantly suppressed in these RA lymphocyte cultures under certain conditions.

T cell diversity and maturation are abnormal in RA. Whereas thymic output normally decreases with age, this process appears to be accelerated in RA.[108] The presence of T cell receptor rearrangement excision circles (TREC) is a measure of thymic release of mature T cells. Using this parameter, the thymic output in RA may decline prematurely. Similarly, telomere attrition suggests inappropriate "aging" of the T cells. This could be due to a primary defect in peripheral T cell homeostasis or due to impaired thymic function with increased T cell turnover due to chronic immune stimulation. This concept is supported by the observation that telomeric length in RA T cells is shorter than in normal controls and more closely resembles older populations.

Activated B lymphocytes are also present in the peripheral blood of patients with RA. The number of circulating B cells that spontaneously produce RF and other autoantibodies is significantly higher in RA compared with normal individuals. B cells that are enriched in autoantibody production are characterized by a surface determinant CD5. This antigen is normally expressed by T cells, but it is also displayed by fetal B cells and a small number of immature B cells in adults. RA patients with normal circulating numbers of lymphocytes show an abnormal kappa-to-lambda–chain analysis compared with controls, implying oligoclonal B cell proliferation. It is not known whether this reflects expansion of the restricted number of clones capable of producing RF or whether an inciting antigen is something other than IgG and related specifically to RA. On the other hand, normal and RA peripheral blood B cells have equal numbers of B cells that produce IgM anti–type II collagen antibodies. The B cells that accumulate in the synovial fluid, however, produce IgG antibodies that are more likely to be pathogenic.

Attempts to characterize the gene expression profiles in the peripheral blood cells of patients with RA have met with mixed results. In some cases, RNA transcripts can potentially distinguish between RA and psoriatic arthritis and include differential expression of tumor suppressors, MAP kinases, and other proinflammatory proteins. Other limited subsets of genes have been proposed as markers for disease activity or to predict response to targeted therapy. However, additional confirmatory studies are necessary to determine whether these patterns are consistent.

ROLE OF T CELL CYTOKINES

KEY POINTS

Several subsets of T cells have been implicated in the pathogenesis of RA.

Relatively low levels of T cell cytokines are present in RA synovium.

The T cell cytokines that are present, such as IFN-γ and IL-17, can be produced by Th1 cells or Th17 cells.

Regulatory T cell function, which suppresses activation of other T cells, might be low in RA synovium.

The contribution of T cells to synovial inflammation can be through antigen-independent mechanisms such as direct cell-cell contact with macrophages.

The cytokine milieu in RA is rich in factors produced by many cell lineages. Factors produced by T lymphocytes are surprisingly low in RA, whereas those generated by macrophages and by synovial fibroblasts are markedly increased (Table 69-5). The production and contribution of T cell–derived cytokines can be examined based on functional lymphocyte subsets.

T Helper Type 1 Cell Cytokines

Extensive investigation into the cytokine profile of RA suggest a bias toward the Th1 phenotype, which produces cytokines such as IL-2 and IFN-γ and expresses the chemokine receptors CXCR3 and CCR5. Many T cell clones derived from RA synovial tissue produce a Th1 cytokine pattern. Considerable data have accumulated on the relative abundance and function of the prototypic Th1 cytokine, interferon-γ (IFN-γ), which is the most potent inducer of HLA-DR antigens. IFN-γ also induces adhesion molecules on the surface of endothelial cells and can help recruit inflammatory cell accumulation at sites of injury. One of the

Table 69-5 Production of Selected Synovial Cytokines in Rheumatoid Arthritis according to Cellular Source

Cellular Source	Level of Production in Rheumatoid Arthritis Synovium*
T Cells	
Interleukin-2	−
Interleukin-3	−
Interleukin-4	−
Interleukin-6	±
Interleukin-13	±
Interleukin-17A, F	+
Interferon-γ	±
TNF	−
Lymphotoxin-α	−
RANKL	+
GM-CSF	−
Macrophages†/Fibroblasts‡	
Interleukin-1	+++
Interleukin-1Ra	+
Interleukin-6	+++
Interleukin-10	+
Interleukin-12	+
Interleukin-15	++
Interleukin-16	+
Interleukin-18	++
Interleukin-23	+
Interleukin-32	+
Interleukin-33	++
TNF	++
M-CSF	+
GM-CSF	++
BLyS	++
LIGHT	++
RANKL	+
TGF-β	++
Chemokines (e.g., IL-8, MCP-1)	+++
Fibroblast growth factor	++
Interferon-β	++
Dendritic Cells	
Interferon-α	+
Interleukin-12	+
Chemokines (e.g., CXCL13 and CCL21)	+
Mast Cells	
TNF	+
Interleukin-17A	+

*−, absent or very low concentrations; +, present.
†Tissue macrophages or type A synoviocytes.
‡Tissue fibroblasts or type B synoviocytes.
BLyS, B lymphocyte stimulator; GM-CSF, granulocyte-macrophage colony-stimulating factor; MCP-1, monocyte chemoattractant; M-CSF, macrophage colony-stimulating factor; RANKL, receptor activator of NFκB ligand; TGF-β, transforming growth factor-β; TNF, tumor necrosis factor.

most important functions of IFN-γ is its capacity to alter the balance of extracellular matrix synthesis and degradation by decreasing collagen synthesis and inhibiting matrix metalloproteinase (MMP) production by cytokine-stimulated cultured FLS.[109]

Relatively low concentrations of IFN-γ have been detected in RA joints, well below the amounts needed to induce HLA-DR expression on monocytes. The relative lack of IFN-γ in rheumatoid joints has been observed at the level of mRNA using a variety of techniques.

Immunohistochemical analysis clearly demonstrates IFN-γ in small numbers of RA synovial T cells, although the percentage is far less than in chronically inflamed tonsils.

Another major Th1 cytokine, IL-2, is a T cell–derived cytokine that serves as an autocrine or paracrine T cell growth factor. Although it was originally reported to be present in synovial fluid using biologic assay, more specific immunoassays showed that IL-2 is detected in only a small percentage of RA synovial effusions and synovial tissues and, when present, is only found in low concentrations.[110] TNF, GM-CSF, and IL-6 can be expressed by Th1 and Th2 cells. All three are abundant in synovial fluid and produced by RA synovial tissue. However, the primary sources of these cytokines in the rheumatoid joint are macrophages and fibroblasts rather than T cells.

Targeted therapeutics to block Th1 function or recruitment to RA synovium is an attractive concept. Several CCR5 antagonists have been developed because this chemokine receptor serves as a binding protein for HIV and might be used to decrease Th1 cytokine levels in the joint. Some of these have demonstrated efficacy in animal models of arthritis. However, the role of IFN-γ is actually quite complex because administration of the cytokine does not exacerbate disease and, if anything, results in improvement in some patients. IFN-γ knockout mice or IFN-γ receptor deficiency can exacerbate collagen-induced arthritis in mice and serve as a reminder that the effects of cytokines can be highly variable depending on the model and timing of expression.

T Helper Type 2 Cell Cytokines

Although relatively low levels of Th1 cytokines are readily detected, Th2 cytokine levels are exceedingly low in RA. Using immunoassays, IL-4 and LTα are generally not detected in RA synovial fluid. In situ hybridization also shows little or no IL-4 mRNA in RA synovial tissue. When sensitive nested reverse-transcriptase polymerase chain reaction (RT-PCR) techniques are used on synovial biopsies, Th2 cytokines IL-4 and IL-13 are absent in RA, whereas both IFN-γ and IL-12 (a cytokine that induces T cell maturation toward the Th1 phenotype) are usually present. The Th2 cytokine IL-10, which has potent anti-inflammatory activities, is expressed in RA synovium. However, macrophages rather than T cells are the major producers in RA. Some data suggest that synovial fluids in early synovitis have high concentrations of Th2 cytokines such as IL-4 and IL-13 and that this pattern distinguishes patients who progress to RA. As the disease evolves in these patients, the Th2 signature diminishes.[111]

T Helper Type 17 Cytokines

The proinflammatory cytokine produced by Th17 cells, IL-17, exists as six isoforms (IL-17A through F). IL-17A and, to a certain extent, IL-17F mimic many of the activities of IL-1 and TNF with respect to FLS function including induction of collagenase and cytokine production. IL-17A is present in modest, but functionally relevant, concentrations in RA synovial effusions.[112] More important, T cell–derived IL-17A in synovial tissue can synergize with IL-1 and TNF by activating synoviocytes to produce matrix

MMPs and other proinflammatory cytokines. IL-17 receptors IL-17RA and IL-17RC are expressed by synoviocytes and, when engaged, can activate the transcription factor NFκB and initiate an inflammatory cascade. In addition to its effect on mesenchymal cells, IL-17 can participate in bone erosion by enhancing osteoclast activation. Bone resorption in an in vitro model using synovial explants and bone shows that blockade of IL-17, IL-1, and TNF is more effective than blocking the individual factors.

Immunohistochemistry initially suggested that IL-17 is mainly present in sublining T cells, although it could also be derived from mast cells. In some studies, IL-17 is present in the synovium of a minority of RA patients. Because immunoreactive IL-17 can be detected near the erosive front of pannus, it could also participate in extracellular matrix destruction. Animal models of arthritis demonstrate that IL-17 inhibition is anti-inflammatory and protects animals from bone and cartilage destruction.[113] IL-1, IL-23, and/or TGF-β in the joint can potentially enhance Th17 cell differentiation, although the precise cytokine environment for this process in humans and mice can differ. BLyS also has the potential to enhance Th17 cell differentiation and promote inflammatory arthritis. All of these cytokines are present in RA synovium, thereby providing an excellent milieu to enhance the generation of these cells.

The role of the IL-17 family is clear in animal models of arthritis, where blocking IL-17A in particular has dramatic effects on inflammation and matrix destruction. The data in humans are less robust, perhaps because the segregation of human T cells into clear subsets is not as well defined. Early clinical studies with anti-IL-17A antibodies in RA are encouraging, although the benefit is modest compared to TNF inhibitors.[114]

Regulatory T Cells (Tregs)

The role of classically defined inducible regulatory T cells (CD4$^+$CD25$^+$CD127$^+$) in RA remains poorly defined. Deficiency of this subset, which produces IL-10 and TGF-β and regulates other T cells through cell contact, could contribute to autoimmunity. Studies of RA peripheral blood demonstrate normal numbers of Tregs, although the CD4$^+$CD25$^+$ subset appears to accumulate in rheumatoid synovial effusions. However, peripheral blood Treg responses in vitro to stimuli such as anti-CD3 and anti-CD28 antibody displayed an anergic phenotype and were unable to suppress T cell or monocyte cytokine production. Of interest, this abnormality might be reversed when patients are treated with TNF inhibitors.[115] The effect of treatment on synovial Tregs was also observed in a synovial biopsy study. The number of FoxP3$^+$ cells was relatively low in T cell infiltrates identified in rheumatoid synovial biopsies. Interestingly, the number decreased further after intra-articular injection with corticosteroids.[116]

These data suggest that abnormal Treg function could be secondary to cytokine imbalance in RA rather than a primary event. Treatment can have a significant effect on the number and function of Tregs, which makes evaluation of their role in patient samples difficult to interpret. Nevertheless, enhancing or restoring Treg activity as a therapeutic intervention could potentially downregulate other T cells and cytokine production.[117]

Enhancing the number or activity of Tregs has been used to treat animal models of arthritis. Antigen-induced arthritis is exacerbated when CD4+CD25+ cells are depleted and suppressed when they are passively transferred to affected animals. Treg function is low in some inflammation models.[118] Methotrexate also increases Treg function in collagen-induced arthritis. Administration of neuropeptides such as vasoactive intestinal peptide (VIP) appears to suppress collagen-induced arthritis by enhancing the Treg function in synovium and lymph nodes.

T Helper Cell Cytokine Imbalance in RA

The relative abundance of Th1 cells suggests that the synovium resembles a Th1-like delayed-type hypersensitivity reaction and/or a Th17 autoimmune environment. Th2 cytokines and cellular responses that normally suppress Th1 activation are nearly absent, thereby raising the possibility that the lack of T cell activation along the Th2 pathway in RA contributes to disease perpetuation. For example, addition of exogenous IL-10 or IL-4 to cultures of synovial tissue cells or synovial tissue explants suppresses synthesis of proinflammatory cytokines and MMPs by cultured RA synovial tissue explants.[119] The inhibitory action of IL-4 might be mediated by decreased c-Jun and c-Fos expression, which is required for efficient production of MMPs and cytokines. In addition, IL-10 and IL-4 increase the release of other anti-inflammatory cytokines such as IL-1Ra by synovial cells. Although IL-10 protein is present in RA synovial fluid and the gene is expressed by synovial tissue cells,[120] in vitro studies of cultured synovial cells suggest that not enough IL-10 is produced to suppress IFN-γ production.

The notion that Th1 and Th17 cytokines initiate and perpetuate arthritis, whereas Th2 cytokines are suppressive, is supported by studies in animal models. For instance, IL-4 and IL-10 were administered individually or in combination in collagen-induced arthritis.[121] The cytokines had modest or no benefit when used separately, but together the effect was impressive. Clinical improvement correlated with decreased synovial IL-1, TNF, and cartilage destruction. Anti–IL-10 antibody therapy in collagen-induced arthritis accelerates disease. The complexity of cytokine networks in inflammatory arthritis is underscored by studies on the role of IL-12 in collagen-induced arthritis. In early arthritis, IL-12 administration increases the incidence of collagen-induced arthritis, whereas anti–IL-12 is beneficial.[122] However, in late disease, IL-12 administration suppresses arthritis and anti–IL-12 causes an exacerbation. As noted above, administration of anti-IL-17A antibody to block the prototypical Th17 cytokine has only modest benefit. Alternative approaches that inhibit both IL-17A and F, such as soluble receptor constructs, might increase efficacy. The role of Th17 cells is clearer in other inflammatory diseases, most notably psoriasis, where IL-17A blockade demonstrates a robust response.[123]

Although the notion that enhancing Th2 cytokines is attractive, a clinical trial using IL-10 in RA did not demonstrate significant clinical benefit or improvement in histologic evidence of synovial inflammation.[124] It is possible that combinations of Th2 cytokines will be required to coordinate a maximum effect.

Activation of Synovial Cells by Cell-Cell Contact with T Lymphocytes

Even though T cell activation is relatively modest in rheumatoid synovium, direct cell-cell contact permits these cells to participate in synovial cytokine networks and matrix destruction. Membranes prepared from activated T cells can directly stimulate macrophages and FLS to produce cytokines and MMPs.[125] The membrane constituents that regulate this process vary, depending on the particular culture conditions, but include adhesion molecules such as LFA-1 and membrane-bound TNF. Hence a T cell displaying these proteins can potentially contribute to macrophage and fibroblast activation in an antigen-independent fashion. One of the best-characterized consequences of this pathway is the ability of T cells to enhance synovial macrophage TNF production in a contact-dependent manner after exposure to macrophage-derived IL-15.[126]

The concept that lymphocytes can activate cells in the environment through direct contact suggests an unanticipated role for T cells in RA. The traditional paradigm assumes that T cells in the joint respond to a pathogenic stimulus and subsequently drive an antigen-specific response. However, cell-cell contact influences can be antigen-independent and only require colocalization of memory T cells with synoviocytes or macrophages. Because T cells with a memory phenotype accumulate into the joint due to the release of chemoattractants, there is no requirement for a specific arthritogenic antigen to initiate the process. Instead, activation of innate immunity by nonspecific stimuli permits subsequent ingress of the correct T cell phenotype to engage resident synovial lining cells. The combination of adaptive immune responses and antigen-independent stimulation could contribute to the diversity of individual responses to targeted therapy and the relative paucity of complete remissions.

ROLE OF MACROPHAGE AND FIBROBLAST CYTOKINES

KEY POINTS

Macrophage and fibroblast cytokines are abundant in RA synovium.

Cytokine networks involve proinflammatory cytokines such as IL-1, TNF, IL-6, IL-15, IL-18, GM-CSF, and IL-33. These and many other factors help perpetuate synovial inflammation.

Chemokines that recruit inflammatory cells into the joint are commonly produced by macrophages and fibroblasts.

Anti-inflammatory cytokines such as IL-1Ra and IL-10 are produced in rheumatoid synovium, although in amounts insufficient to suppress proinflammatory cyotkine function or production.

Virtually every macrophage and fibroblast proinflammatory mediator investigated in the RA synovium is abundant. In this section, some of the major cytokines and effectors produced in the joint are described, with an emphasis on the prevalence of macrophage and fibroblast products as major forces that perpetuate RA. Macrophages, in particular, are the most vigorous producers of cytokines. The role of macrophage and fibroblast cytokines in the pathogenesis of RA was initially suggested by studies involving patient samples, as well as preclinical experiments in animal models.

Proinflammatory Macrophage and Fibroblast Cytokines

Interleukin-1 Family

The IL-1 family is a ubiquitous group of polypeptides with a wide range of biologic activity; they include IL-1α, IL-1β, IL-18, IL-33, and IL-1Ra, which is a natural inhibitor of IL-1 (see Suppressive Cytokines and Cytokine Antagonists later for a description of IL-1Ra). Abundant animal data indicate that IL-1 can serve as a key regulatory factor in inflammatory arthritis. For instance, recombinant IL-1β induces the accumulation of PMNs and mononuclear leukocytes in the joint space and the loss of proteoglycan from articular cartilage when injected directly into rabbit knee joints. Transgenic mice that overexpress IL-1 also develop inflammatory arthritis, whereas mice that lack the natural IL-1 antagonist IL-1Ra have increased susceptibility to collagen-induced arthritis. In most cases, IL-1 blockade in animal models modestly decreases synovial inflammation while markedly diminishing bone and cartilage destruction.

Interleukin-1. Synovial macrophages are the most prolific source of IL-1 in the joint, and nearly half of all macrophages in the RA synovium express IL-1β.[127] Immunohistologic studies confirm this, with especially abundant IL-1 protein in synovial lining macrophages adjacent to type B synoviocytes and in sublining macrophages near blood vessels. The IL-1 in the lining can subsequently activate type B synoviocytes to proliferate and secrete a variety of mediators. A broad range of stimuli are capable of inducing IL-1 production by macrophages; for example, immunoglobulin Fc fragments and, to a lesser extent, immune complexes, can generate IL-1 production by rheumatoid synovial macrophages. Collagen fragments can induce IL-1 production, and type IX collagen, which has been found only in articular cartilage and localized into intersections of collagen fibrils, is a potent inducer of IL-1 by human monocyte.

Within the rheumatoid joint, IL-1 induces fibroblast proliferation; stimulates the biosynthesis of IL-6, IL-8, and GM-CSF by synovial cells; and enhances collagenase and prostaglandin production. It increases glycosaminoglycan release in human synovial fibroblast cultures, although the effect of IL-1 on the production of intact proteoglycan molecules by intact articular cartilage explants can be the opposite. IL-1 induces a number of adhesion molecules on FLS and endothelial cells including VCAM-1 and ICAM-1 and enhances bone resorption.

IL-1 has been implicated in RA, and inhibition of this mediator using various IL-1 targeted biologic agents has modest anti-inflammatory activity. Even combinations of IL-1 and TNF-directed therapy does not provide benefit beyond TNF blockade alone.[128] In contrast, diseases with a well-defined role for IL-1 such as Still's disease, familial cold autoinflammatory syndrome, Muckle-Wells syndrome, and crystal diseases such as gout have a much better clinical response. These data suggest that IL-1 plays a modest role in the clinical manifestations of RA. Its contributions to cartilage and bone destruction are still uncertain, but preclinical models suggest that the protective effects of TNF blockade are mediated through IL-1.

One explanation for the relatively modest benefit of IL-1 in RA relates to its signaling mechanisms. IL-1 activates NFκB through the kinase MyD88, which is the same pathway as TLRs. When IL-1 signaling is blocked, it is possible that TLR ligands in the synovium including exogenous ones such as peptidoglycan or endogenous ones such as heat shock proteins can provide the stimulus required to overcome IL-1 blockade. This concept was tested in the passive K/BxN model where mice lacking the IL-1 receptor had markedly decreased arthritis severity. When small amounts of the TLR4 ligand lipopolysaccharide were administered, robust synovitis ensued. If a similar system occurs in RA, then IL-1 blockade would be unable to control synovitis as long as TLR signaling remains intact.

Interleukin-18. In addition to IL-1α and IL-1β, a homologous protein in the IL-1 family known as IL-18 has been implicated in RA. This cytokine was originally defined by its ability to bias the immune response toward the Th1 phenotype, especially in the presence of IL-12. In collagen-induced arthritis, IL-18 inhibition significantly attenuates disease.[129] Of particular interest, the same effect was observed in IFN-γ knockout mice, indicating that other non–Th1-related activities of IL-18 might be important. Subsequent studies showed that IL-18 induces GM-CSF, nitric oxide production, and TNF expression by synovial macrophages. IL-18 is expressed by RA synovial tissue, especially by synovial fibroblasts and macrophages, and its production is markedly increased by TNF and IL-1β. A natural inhibitor, the IL-18 binding protein can potentially be used as a therapeutic agent to block both the proinflammatory effects and pro-Th1 effects of IL-18. One potential concern for IL-18 as a target for RA is the fact that the IL-1 convertase inhibitor had only modest benefit. IL-18, like IL-1β, is processed by this enzyme in order to produce biologically active cytokine. Therefore an IL-1 convertase inhibitor theoretically should block both IL-1β and IL-18 release by macrophages.

Interleukin-33. IL-33 is a novel cytokine that signals through the ST2 surface receptor. Like high-mobility-group box 1 (HMGB1), it is an "alarmin" that provides a danger signal due to tissue damage and necrosis with release of intracellular contents. Blocking IL-33 decreases inflammation in several animal models of arthritis including collagen-induced arthritis and antigen-induced arthritis. Mast cells are activated by IL-33 and can subsequently release their content. Thus mast cell–dependent models such as passive K/BxN are less severe in ST2$^{-/-}$ mice.[130] More intriguing, its ability to trigger mast cells could play a role in the release of mast cell products such as TNF and IL-17A in RA synovium. IL-33 can also bias T cells toward the Th2 phenotype, so the fact that it is expressed in RA synovium and synovial effusions raises some questions about its precise function in long-standing disease.

Tumor Necrosis Factor

The TNF superfamily is an extended group of related genes that play a major role in inflammation, immune responses, cell survival, and apoptosis. At least 19 members of the family have been identified, with TNF identified as the eponymous member. Each cytokine has its own preference for cell surface receptor, although there is some promiscuity of receptor binding and functional overlap. The TNF superfamily members exhibit conserved amino acid sequences, suggesting a single ancestral gene. Many include type II membrane protein characteristics and can be released from cell surfaces after proteolytic cleavage. A C-terminal conserved domain called the TNF-homology domain is also shared by several superfamily members. The active forms of the proteins are homotrimers, except for LTα and LTβ, which can form either heterotrimers or homotrimers. Several members have been discussed earlier in the relevant sections. In this section, one of the "founding" members of the superfamily is discussed due to its critical role in synovial inflammation.

TNF is a pleiotropic cytokine that has been implicated as a key proinflammatory cytokine in RA and detected in rheumatoid synovial fluid and serum. It is produced as a membrane-bound protein that is released from the cell surface after proteolytic cleavage by TNF convertase, a membrane MMP. IL-1 and TNF have many similar activities including the ability to enhance cytokine production, adhesion-molecule expression, proliferation, and MMP production by cultured synoviocytes. In some systems, the effects of these two agents are synergistic. Although they share many functions and signal transduction pathways, IL-1 and TNF use distinct surface receptors and intracellular signaling pathways.

The efficacy of TNF inhibitors in RA demonstrates its critical role in the disease; heterogeneity of the rheumatoid process is also apparent because only about one-third of patients have a dramatic response to TNF inhibitors. Efficacy requires continuous therapy because cessation typically leads to a flare of disease. Perhaps more interesting, evidence is beginning to accumulate, suggesting that early aggressive therapy with anti-TNF agents can induce long-term remissions even after therapy is withdrawn. This exciting notion suggests that interventions in the earliest stages of disease could prevent the establishment of chronic synovitis.

TNF, like IL-1, stimulates collagenase and PGE_2 production by human synovial cells, induces bone resorption, inhibits bone formation in vitro, and stimulates resorption of proteoglycan and inhibits its biosynthesis in explants of cartilage. In situ hybridization and immunohistochemical studies show that TNF is primarily produced by synovial macrophages in RA.

Animal models have also supported the general role played by TNF in inflammatory arthritis. For instance, overexpression of TNF in transgenic mice leads to an aggressive and destructive synovitis. In fact, the arthritis also spontaneously occurs in transgenic mice that express only a membrane-bound form of TNF on T cells.[131] TNF blockade is an effective anti-inflammatory agent in many animal models of arthritis,[132] although the effects on bone and cartilage destruction are less prominent than with IL-1

inhibitors and are likely mediated through downstream inhibition of IL-1 production.

TNF inhibition in RA significantly decreases extracellular-matrix destruction as measured by radiographic progression.[133] It is not clear why the bone-protective effects are more prominent in humans than in the animal models. TNF blockade is also more effective in animal models when combined with an IL-1 inhibitor, supporting the additive or synergistic relationship between the two cytokines in animal models. However, this has not been observed in RA.

The mechanism of action for TNF blockers is distinct from other biologic agents. For instance, individuals with an inadequate response to a TNF inhibitor are still likely to respond to either rituximab or abatacept. This supports the notion that multiple independent pathways can contribute to the pathogenesis of RA and the heterogeneous nature of the disease. Surprisingly, clinical responses do not always correlate with protection of the extracellular matrix. Patients with little or no clinical improvement in signs and symptoms of RA still have significant delay or arrest of joint damage. This observation supports the contention that inflammation and destruction could have distinct pathogenic mechanisms such as inhibition of osteoclast maturation, even though synovial inflammation continues unabated.

Interleukin-6 Family

IL-6 is a complex cytokine produced by many cell types including T cells, monocytes, and FLS. Originally defined by its B cell–stimulating properties, it induces immunoglobulin synthesis in B cell lines, is involved in the differentiation of cytotoxic T lymphocytes, and is a major factor in the regulation of acute-phase response proteins like C-reactive protein by the liver. The IL-6 receptor includes a common chain (gp130) that is shared with other cytokines and an IL-6-specific chain (IL-6R). IL-6R can be shed from cell surfaces, bind to IL-6, and deliver it to cells that lack IL-6 receptors by combining with gp130. IL-6 signaling proceeds through the Janus kinases (JAKs), especially JAK1, and phosphorylation of STAT3.

A striking correlation between serum IL-6 activity and serum levels of acute-phase reactants such as C-reactive protein, α_1-antitrypsin, fibrinogen, and haptoglobin occurs in patients with RA. Very high levels of IL-6 are present in RA synovial fluid, and synovial cells in culture from diverse inflammatory arthropathies produce IL-6. In situ hybridization of synovial tissue also shows IL-6 mRNA in the intimal lining, and immunohistochemistry studies show IL-6 protein in the lining and sublining regions. Although many synovial macrophages express the IL-6 gene, the majority of IL-6 appears to be produced by type B synoviocytes.

The pivotal role of IL-6 in RA has been demonstrated by clinical trials using a monoclonal antibody that binds to IL-6R. The clinical responses are similar to TNF inhibitors including protective effects on bone and cartilage damage.[134] Surprisingly, IL-6R antibody is also effective in patients who have not responded to TNF blockade. This observation is surprising considering that TNF is considered upstream of IL-6 in the cytokine cascade and that TNF inhibition markedly decreases IL-6 levels in RA. Neutropenia, increased liver enzymes, and altered blood lipids have been observed with IL-6 inhibition, although the relative importance of these observations is still uncertain. JAK inhibitors have also demonstrated efficacy in RA; this might be due, in part, to the effect on IL-6 signaling.

Cytokines with structural similarity to IL-6 and that share surface-receptor subunits have also been implicated in RA. Several of these, IL-11, leukemia inhibitory factor (LIF), and oncostatin M, are expressed by rheumatoid synovium and can be detected in synovial effusions. The biologic effects of these factors are complex and can be either protective (e.g., by increasing expression of protease inhibitors such as tissue inhibitors of metalloproteinase [TIMP]) or proinflammatory (e.g., by increasing expression of chemokines or MMPs) depending on the culture conditions or the specific model evaluated. This dichotomy among the family members is demonstrated by the fact that IL-11 administration ameliorates collagen-induced arthritis, whereas antibodies to oncostatin M are protective.

Interleukin-12 Family

The IL-12 family includes a group of cytokines that play a key role in the differentiation of T cells and inflammation. IL-12 is a heterodimeric cytokine with two subunits (e.g., p35 and p40) encoded on separate genes and produced by antigen-presenting cells. IL-23 and IL-27 have similar heterodimeric structures to IL-12, with p29/p40 and p28/EB13 components, respectively. In the context of antigen presentation, IL-12, IL-23, and IL-27 can bias T cell responses toward the Th1 phenotype. IL-23 can also play a pivotal role in the production of Th17 cells, along with IL-1 and TGF-β. The IL-12 family of cytokines are generally produced by macrophages in the rheumatoid joint but are also produced by other antigen-presenting cells such as dendritic cells. Although clinical data defining the role of these cytokines are still lacking, there are anecdotal case reports of RA patients with malignancy treated with recombinant IL-12 developing a flare of disease. Animal models including adjuvant arthritis in rats and collagen-induced arthritis in mice are partially ameliorated by neutralization of IL-12, IL-23, or IL-27 depending on the timing of treatment. In some situations, however, IL-27 has anti-inflammatory effects.

Interleukin-15

IL-15 is an IL-2–like cytokine that regulates numerous immunologic functions relevant to RA including T cell chemotaxis and proliferation, production of immunoglobulins by B cells, and the generation of NK cells. Although IL-15 can serve as an IL-2–independent mechanism for activating T cells, its role in RA may be related to its key role in TNF regulation. Macrophages are the primary source of IL-15 in RA, and the cytokine is able to induce a cell-contact mechanism of macrophage TNF production that requires T cells. Although T lymphocytes, or at least their membranes, are required for this process, the macrophages actually produce the TNF. This network provides a potential mechanism whereby local IL-15 production in the synovium can lead to autocrine production of TNF in a T cell–dependent but antigen-independent fashion. IL-15 has

been demonstrated in RA synovial macrophage cells. Soluble IL-15 receptors can function as an IL-15 inhibitor, and when used in vivo can decrease joint inflammation in collagen-induced arthritis. Preliminary clinical trials in RA using an anti-IL-15 antibody had a signal for efficacy, although probably not sufficient to continue developing this particular biologic agent.[135]

Interleukin-32

IL-32 is a novel cytokine that activates NFκB and induces the production of several proinflammatory cytokines and chemokines including TNF, IL-1, IL-6, and IL-8. It has been implicated in Crohn's disease by virtue of its ability to markedly enhance caspase 1 activation and IL-1 production in cells that have been exposed to muramyl dipeptides. More recently, IL-32 was demonstrated by immunohistochemistry in synovial tissues of patients with RA, especially in synovial-lining macrophage-like cells.[136] The level of IL-32 expression correlated with the presence of other cytokines implicated in RA including TNF, IL-1, and IL-18. Injection of IL-32 into the joints of naïve mice causes a robust transient synovitis. The synovial response could be partially abrogated by anti-TNF antibodies, suggesting that IL-32 induces this cytokine in vivo. These data suggest that IL-32 might be upstream from several proinflammatory mediators in RA and could represent a therapeutic target.

Colony-Stimulating Factors

Granulocyte-macrophage colony-stimulating factor (GM-CSF) supports the differentiation of bone marrow precursor cells to mature granulocytes and macrophages. As with other major colony-stimulating factors, GM-CSF also participates in normal immune responses. It is a potent macrophage activator including the induction of HLA-DR expression, IL-1 secretion, intracellular parasite killing, and priming for enhanced release of TNF and PGE_2. Neutrophil function is also regulated by GM-CSF, which enhances antibody-dependent cytotoxicity, phagocytosis, chemotaxis, and the production of oxygen radicals.

RA synovial fluid contains GM-CSF, which is produced by RA synovial tissue cells.[137] The major source in the synovium is macrophages, although IL-1– or TNF-stimulated FLS also express the GM-CSF gene. Its ability to induce HLA-DR gene expression on macrophages might be of particular importance in RA. GM-CSF, not IFN-γ, is the major DR-inducing cytokine in RA synovial effusions. Collagen-induced arthritis in mice is less severe in animals that lack a functional GM-CSF gene or are treated with anti–GM-CSF antibody, which supports the hypothesis that GM-CSF is an important proinflammatory mediator. Anti-GM-CSF antibodies are in clinical development. However, there is some concern that pulmonary alveolar proteinosis might be an adverse event because GM-CSF–deficient mice and autoimmune diseases marked by spontaneous production of anti-GM-CSF antibodies develop this syndrome. A recent phase IIa clinical trial demonstrated potential clinical benefit from an anti-GM-CSF antibody in RA, although long term efficacy and safety still must be evaluated.

Macrophage colony-stimulating factor (M-CSF) is also expressed by RA synovium and is present in synovial effusions. Its primary pathogenic role in RA probably relates to its osteoclast-differentiating capacity. This factor cooperates with RANKL to facilitate bone erosions.

Chemokine Families

Chemokines are a family of related chemoattractant peptides that, with the assistance of adhesion molecules, summon cells into inflammatory sites. They are generally divided into families including CC, CXC, and CX3C based on the position of characteristic cysteine residues.

Many chemokines have been identified in the rheumatoid joint. IL-8, a CXC chemokine that was originally characterized as a potent chemoattractant for neutrophils, along with immune complexes and other chemotactic peptides such as C5a, contributes to the large influx of PMNs into the joint. Immunohistochemical analysis of synovial tissue demonstrates IL-8 protein in sublining perivascular macrophages, as well as in scattered lining cells.[138] Cultured synovial tissue macrophages constitutively produce IL-8, and FLS express the gene if they are stimulated with IL-1 or TNF. IL-8 accounts for about 40% of the neutrophil chemoattractant activity in synovial fluid. In addition, IL-8 activates neutrophils through G protein–coupled receptors and is a potent angiogenesis factor.

Many other chemoattractant proteins are implicated in RA. Macrophage-inhibitory protein-1α, macrophage-inhibitory protein-1β, macrophage chemoattractant protein-1 (MCP-1), and regulated on activation, normally T cell expressed and secreted (RANTES)—members of the CC subfamily—are produced by RA synovium, as are many other CC chemokines.

CXCL16 and epithelial neutrophil-activating peptide-78 (ENA-78) are CXC chemokines and are also abundant along with many others in that family.[139] The former, which binds to CXCR6 on T cells, can contribute to the recruitment of lymphocytes into the synovium. ENA-78 accounts for about 40% of the chemotactic activity for neutrophils in RA synovial fluid. Concentrations of these chemokines are higher in RA synovial effusions compared with noninflammatory arthritides such as OA. Although the chemokines can also be detected in the blood, the levels are considerably lower than in the joint, thereby providing a gradient that signals cells to migrate into the synovium.

As noted earlier, lymphocyte-specific factors might contribute to the germinal center architecture of RA. The CXC factor B cell–activating chemokine-1 (BCA-1; CXCL13) binds to specific CXCR5 receptors on B cells. CXCL13 is expressed in the RA synovial tissues, especially by follicular dendritic cells in germinal centers and likely accounts for B cell migration to these regions.[140] CCL21 and several other factors participate in the anatomic organization of germinal centers, marginal zones, and other regions of lymphoid follicles. Another chemokine, SDF-1, is expressed by synoviocytes and endothelial cells and can play a major role as a chemoattractant for T cells in synovium via its receptor CXCR4. Unlike other chemokine receptors that can bind multiple members of the family, CXCR4 is highly specific for SDF-1 and is expressed by memory CD4+ lymphocytes.

Chemokines have attracted considerable attention as therapeutic targets in order to prevent recruitment of immune cells into the synovium. Numerous preclinical models support the use of chemokine blockers. For instance, antibodies to fractalkine (CXC3L1) suppress murine collagen-induced arthritis, even though anti–type II collagen antibody production was not affected.[141] Anti-CXCL16 antibody also decreases clinical arthritis in the same model. One problem is that the system is highly redundant and several different chemotactic proteins can bind to the same receptor. No clinical improvement was observed in a study using anti-MCP-1 antibody, perhaps because the antibody also altered the kinetics of MCP-1 metabolism. Anti-IL-8 antibodies have met with limited success in psoriasis. More promising results were observed with antibody to IP-10 (CXCL10), which met its primary efficacy end point in a phase II study in RA.

Alternatively, chemokines bind to G protein–coupled receptors and can be targeted to block multiple factors. For instance, CCR1 antagonists, which blocks RANTES and MIP-1α, has been evaluated in clinical trials.[142] Although one compound significantly decreased synovial infiltration by CCR1-expressing cells, no significant improvement was observed. Chemokine receptor blockade has other levels of complexity such as CCR2-deficient mice, which develop more severe arthritis in some models. Several CCR2 antagonists, which block MCP-1, have not demonstrated significant efficacy in RA. These data suggest that the chemokine system including the receptors is both redundant, complex, and, in some cases, perhaps protective in arthritis.

Chemokines and other chemotactic factors (such as C5a and LTB$_4$) can signal through a variety of mechanisms, although many pathways converge on phosphoinositide-3-kinase (PI3K). Of the several PI3K isoforms, PI3Kγ is relatively specific for chemokine signal transduction. This provides an opportunity to block multiple chemokine receptors simultaneously. Proof of concept for this approach was provided by studies in PI3Kγ knockout mice, which have less synovial inflammation in passive and active collagen-induced arthritis than wild-type mice.[143] A small molecule PI3Kγ inhibitor provided similar benefit. Therefore targeting shared intracellular pathways could potentially overcome some of the limitations presented by the complex chemoattractant system.

Platelet-Derived Growth Factor and Fibroblast Growth Factor

PDGF is a potent growth factor that is both chemoattractant and mitogenic for fibroblasts and induces collagenase expression. It is the most potent stimulator of long-term growth of synovial cells in culture. PDGF is expressed in vascular endothelial cells, platelets, and other synovial sublining cells in rheumatoid synovium, compared with healthy tissue. Multiple isoforms of this molecule have been identified (PDGF A through D), all of which have been detected in RA synovial membranes. PDGF D has been identified as an especially potent stimulator of MMP-1 expression in cultured synoviocytes. PDGF is a potent activator of the PI3K pathway, which leads to Akt phosphorylation and supports synoviocyte survival.

Fibroblast growth factors (FGFs) are a family of peptide growth factors with pleiotropic activities. In rheumatoid patients, it is likely that heparin-binding growth factor, the precursor of acidic fibroblast growth factor, is a major mitogen for many cell types and stimulates angiogenesis. Interactions between FGF and proteoglycans is required for biologic activity. It is a potent angiogenic factor, inducing capillary endothelial cells to invade a three-dimensional collagen matrix and form capillaries. Synoviocytes can also be induced to increase expression of RANKL by FGF, thereby enhancing osteoclast activation and bone resorption. FGF is present in RA synovial fluid, and the genes are expressed by synovial cells. Synovial fibroblasts express FGF receptors and proliferate after exposure to the growth factor.

Suppressive Cytokines and Cytokine Antagonists

The proinflammatory cytokine network in RA is offset by a variety of suppressive and anti-inflammatory factors that attempt to reestablish homeostasis. Low production of these suppressive cytokines could potentially contribute to the perpetuation of the synovitis. Many cytokine antagonists or natural immunosuppressives represent potential therapeutic targets for the treatment of inflammatory diseases.

Interleukin-1 Receptor Antagonist

IL-1Ra is a naturally occurring IL-1 inhibitor that binds directly to types I and II IL-1 receptors and competes with IL-1 for the ligand-binding site. Interaction of IL-1Ra with the IL-1 receptors does not result in signal transduction, and, in contrast to IL-1α or -β, the receptor-ligand complex is not internalized after it binds to the IL-1 receptor. Even though IL-1Ra has high affinity for the IL-1 receptor, it is a relatively weak inhibitor because IL-1 can activate cells even if only a small percentage of IL-1 receptors is occupied. Because of this, a substantial excess of the inhibitor is required to saturate the receptor and thereby block IL-1–mediated stimulation (usually 10- to 100-fold excess of IL-1Ra). Recombinant IL-1Ra inhibits a variety of IL-1–mediated events in cultured cells derived from the joint including the induction of MMP and prostaglandin production by chondrocytes and synoviocytes. It can block synovitis in rabbits induced by direct intra-articular injection of recombinant IL-1.

IL-1Ra is present in rheumatoid synovial effusions; much of it is produced by neutrophils and macrophages.[144] Immunohistochemical studies of rheumatoid synovium reveal IL-1Ra protein, especially in perivascular mononuclear cells and the synovial intimal lining. The IL-1Ra protein and mRNA can be detected in synovial macrophages and, to a lesser extent, in type B synoviocytes (Figure 69-12). The presence of IL-1Ra in synovium is not specific to RA because OA synovial tissue also contains IL-1Ra, albeit in lesser amounts. Normal synovium contains little, if any, IL-1Ra protein. Synovial cell culture experiments show that the amount of IL-1Ra is insufficient to antagonize synovial IL-1.

Interleukin-10

IL-10 is an immunosuppressive cytokine that was originally characterized as an inhibitor of T cell cytokine production. Its immunosuppressive actions might be important in pregnancy to suppress an immune response directed against

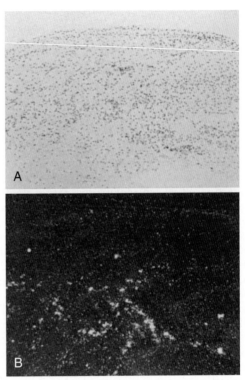

Figure 69-12 Localization of interleukin-1 receptor antagonist (IL-1Ra) messenger RNA in rheumatoid arthritis synovial tissue by in situ hybridization. The specific RNA transcript was detected in perivascular cells, especially macrophages. **A,** Bright field view. **B,** Same area using a dark field filter. Silver grains in the dark field view show the location of IL-1Ra–positive cells.

paternal MHC antigens, and it might regulate susceptibility to some parasitic infections. As noted previously, IL-10 protein is present in RA synovial fluid, and the gene is expressed by synovial tissue macrophages. Serial synovial biopsies in RA patients who were treated with recombinant IL-10 did not show any significant histologic improvement, and clinical responses were not impressive in a limited study.

Transforming Growth Factor-β

TGF-β is a key member of the TGF superfamily, which includes the bone morphogenic proteins that signal through intracellular signaling molecules known as *Smads*. It is widely distributed in different tissues and produced by many cells including T cells, monocytes, and platelets. It suppresses the production of collagenase and induces the expression of TIMP. TGF-β accelerates the healing of incisional wounds and induces both fibrosis and angiogenesis in experimental animal models. Substantial amounts of TGF-β are present in synovial fluid, although it is mainly present in an inactive, latent form, and the mRNA can be detected in RA synovial tissue.[145] Although typically considered an immunosuppressive cytokine with wound-healing properties, the role of TGF-β in RA is complex.

In RA, TGF-β is one of the factors responsible for blunted responses of T cells that have been exposed to synovial fluid. TGF-β also downregulates IL-1 receptor expression on some cell types including chondrocytes. When it is injected directly into the knees of animals, fibrosis and synovial lining hyperplasia develop. In streptococcal cell wall arthritis, parenteral administration or systemic gene therapy with the TGF-β gene ameliorates the disease. However, intra-articular administration of anti–TGF-β antibody decreases arthritis in the injected joint but not in the contralateral joint in the same model. Although mainly considered anti-inflammatory, TGF-β also plays a key role in the development of autoimmunity through the differentiation of T cells into the Th17 phenotype.

Soluble Cytokine Receptors and Binding Proteins

Soluble cytokine receptors and binding proteins can absorb free cytokines and prevent them from engaging functional receptors on cells. Although these obviously could inhibit cytokine action, they also could act as carrier proteins that protect cytokines from proteolytic degradation or deliver them directly to cells such as the IL-6 receptor.

TNF receptors are normally expressed as membrane-bound proteins and can be released from the cell surface after proteolytic cleavage. Soluble p55 and p75 TNF receptors have been detected in RA synovial fluid, sometimes in high concentrations. Soluble TNF receptor levels can be considerably higher than the concentration of TNF in blood or synovial fluid and probably explain why biologically active TNF is difficult to detect in RA synovial fluid despite the presence of immunoreactive protein. Synovial membrane mononuclear cells have increased surface expression and mRNA levels of both TNF receptors compared with OA synovial tissue cells or peripheral blood cells.

Many other soluble receptors and binding proteins are produced in RA, albeit in concentrations too low to effectively suppress the proinflammatory cytokine milieu of the joint. For instance, the IL-1 type II receptor is present in RA synovial fluid, along with lesser amounts of the type I receptor. These soluble receptors can bind to IL-1 or IL-1Ra in synovial effusions. Soluble receptors to IL-15 and IL-17 have been characterized, and an IL-18 binding protein also can inhibit cytokine activity. In some cases, a soluble receptor can protect a cytokine from degradation or transport it to the cells, as with the IL-6 receptor.

Perpetuation of Synovitis by Macrophage-Fibroblast Cytokine Networks

Mapping the cytokine profile in RA led to targeted biologic therapy to inhibit cytokines and supports the concept that cytokine networks play a key role. The network pathway is not autonomous and, except for certain patients with very early disease, discontinuation of anticytokine therapy allows the disease to flare. Nevertheless, paracrine and autocrine cytokine networks in the synovial intimal lining contribute largely to inflammatory arthritis in RA (Figure 69-13).

Several cytokines that have been identified in the synovium or synovial fluid can participate in this system and might explain lining cell hyperplasia, HLA-DR and adhesion-molecule induction, and synovial angiogenesis. The list of potential candidates in this highly redundant system is extensive. Several of these including IL-1, TNF, and IL-6 now have well-defined roles. The first two, along with numerous other factors (e.g., IL-15, IL-18, IL-32) are

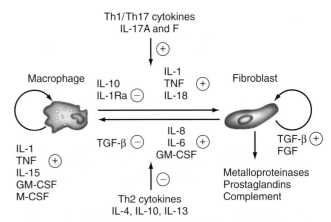

Figure 69-13 Cytokine networks in rheumatoid arthritis (RA). Paracrine and autocrine pathways can lead to activation of fibroblast-like and macrophage-like synoviocytes in the synovial intimal lining. Both positive (+) and negative (–) feedback loops are present, although in RA the former predominate. T helper type 1 (Th1) or Th17 cytokines can potentially enhance the network, whereas Th2 cytokines are suppressive.

produced by synovial macrophages and stimulate synovial fibroblast proliferation and secretion of IL-6, GM-CSF, and chemokines, as well as effector molecules such as MMPs and prostaglandins. GM-CSF, which is produced by both synovial macrophages and IL-1β– or TNF–stimulated synovial fibroblasts, can, in turn, induce IL-1 secretion to form a positive feedback loop. GM-CSF, especially in combination with TNF, also increases HLA-DR expression on macrophages. Macrophage and fibroblast cytokines could also indirectly contribute to the evidence for local T cell and B cell activation including RF production. Newly implicated members of the macrophage-fibroblast cytokine network such as IL-33 can activate other cell lineages such as mast cells that have attracted increased attention in recent years.

The cytokine profile recruits other immune and inflammatory cells into the synovium through the production of chemokines that select specific cell lineages for admission and retention in the synovium. Many of these chemokines including the CXC and CC families are produced by macrophages and fibroblasts and attract neutrophils, macrophages, and specific subpopulations of T and B cells. The sublining chemokine profile including CCL13 and CCL20 helps organize these newly infiltrated cells into organized lymphoid structures in some patients. Other factors such as IL-12 and IL-23 differentiate CD4+ T cells into the Th1 phenotype to produce relatively small amounts of IFN-γ and other relevant cytokines. IL-1 and TGF-β produced mainly by the lining can, along with IL-23, support the production of Th17 cells that release the potent IL-17 family members into the local milieu. All of this occurs in the presence of inhibitor factors, soluble receptors, and binding proteins that are overwhelmed by the inflammatory drive. Other cytokines, such as RANKL and M-CSF, activate osteoclasts that remodel bone.

Even though they do not cause RA, per se, cytokines clearly orchestrate the rheumatoid process. For individual patients, the pivotal cytokine or cytokines that must be blocked could be different, and even this could vary with the stage of disease. Ultimately, understanding the genetic predisposition, the environmental triggers, and the specific patterns of cytokine production could help determine the correct combination of cytokine inhibitors that will be effective.

SIGNAL TRANSDUCTION AND TRANSCRIPTION FACTORS

> **KEY POINTS**
>
> Complex intracellular signaling mechanisms regulate cytokine production and actions in RA synovium.
>
> NFκB, MAP kinases, AP-1, JAK, Syk, and several other pathways are potential therapeutic targets in RA.

Intracellular signal transduction systems transmit information from the environment to the interior of a cell, which can then respond appropriately to stress. The remarkable diversity of signaling pathways and transcription factors provides a selective mechanism for orchestrating activation and repression for appropriate genes. Many of the inflammatory responses observed in RA synovium including the activation of cytokine, proteases, and adhesion-molecule genes can be traced to specific transcription factors and signal transduction pathways.

Nuclear Factor κB

NFκB is a ubiquitous transcription factor that plays a key role in the expression of many genes central to RA including IL-1, TNF, IL-6, and IL-8. NFκB normally resides as an inactive heterodimer or homodimer in the cell cytoplasm associated with an inhibitory protein called IκB that regulates the DNA binding and subcellular localization of NFκB proteins by masking a nuclear localization signal. Extracellular stimuli such as cytokines or TLR agonists initiate a signaling cascade leading to activation of two IκB kinases (IKKα and IKKβ), which phosphorylate IκB at specific NH$_2$-terminal serine residues. Phosphorylated IκB is then selectively ubiquitinated and degraded by the 26S proteasome. This process permits NFκB to migrate to the cell nucleus, where it binds its target genes to initiate transcription.

NFκB is abundant in rheumatoid synovium, and immunohistochemical analysis demonstrates p50 and p65 NFκB proteins in the nuclei of cells in the synovial intimal lining.[146] Although the proteins can also be detected in OA synovium, NFκB activation is much greater in RA because of phosphorylation and degradation of IκB in RA intimal lining cells. Nuclear translocation of NFκB in cultured FLS occurs rapidly after stimulation with many proinflammatory cytokines (e.g., IL-1, TNF, IL-17) or TLR ligands (e.g., peptidoglycan, LPS). NFκB is also a major survival factor for cells and is responsible for resistance to apoptosis in some cell lineages after activation. This is especially important in intestinal inflammation, where IKKβ deficiency can actually increase mucosal damage because the lack of NFκB can increase cell death.

The relevance of NFκB to inflammatory arthritis has been tested in several animal models. Synovial NFκB is rapidly activated, often long before clinical arthritis is evident. Adjuvant arthritis in rats is ameliorated using intra-articular gene therapy with the dominant negative IKKβ construct that blocks the IKK pathway,[147] and streptococcal cell-wall arthritis is blocked with decoy oligonucleotides or a dominant negative IκB adenovirus. NFκB inhibition is associated with decreased synovial cellular infiltration, as well as increased apoptosis. The role of this transcription factor in murine collagen-induced arthritis has been demonstrated using selective IKKβ inhibitors, which suppress arthritis and joint destruction.

Activator Protein-1

Like NFκB, AP-1 regulates many genes implicated in RA including TNF and the MMPs. AP-1 activity can be induced by extracellular signals including cytokines, growth factors, tumor promoters, and the Ras oncoprotein. AP-1 includes members of the Jun and Fos families of transcription factors that form Jun homodimers, Jun-Jun heterodimers, or Jun-Fos heterodimers. Multiple Jun and Fos family members (c-Jun, JunB, JunD, c-Fos, FosB, Fra-1, Fra-2) are expressed in different cell types that mediate the transcription of both unique and overlapping genes. AP-1–driven gene expression is greatly enhanced when one of its components, especially c-Jun, is phosphorylated by the c-Jun N-terminal kinase (JNK).

AP-1 proteins and nuclear binding are elevated in RA synovium, especially in the nuclei of cells in the intimal lining layer.[148] c-Jun and c-Fos proteins are also expressed in the sublining inflammatory infiltrate, albeit to a lesser degree. Localization of AP-1 to the intimal lining correlates with the site where most protease and cytokine genes are overexpressed in RA. AP-1 proteins are usually not detected in normal synovium, although modest amounts have also been detected in OA.

Cytokines such as IL-1 and TNF and TLR ligands probably contribute to the activation of AP-1 in RA synovium. These factors are potent inducers of AP-1 nuclear binding in cultured FLS. The specific Jun family members that constitute AP-1 in synoviocytes have a clear effect on function. For instance, c-Jun increases the production of proinflammatory mediators, whereas JunD suppresses cytokine and MMP production.[149] AP-1 decoy oligonucleotides suppress collagen-induced arthritis and inhibit cytokine production by synovial tissue.

Mitogen-Activated Protein Kinases

MAP kinases, which are signal transduction enzymes activated in response to cellular stress, are composed of parallel protein-kinase cascades that regulate cytokine and MMP gene expression. There are three different families of MAP kinases known as JNK, p38, and extracellular signal-regulated kinase (ERK). MAP kinases phosphorylate selected intracellular proteins, including transcription factors, which subsequently regulate the expression of various genes by transcriptional and post-transcriptional mechanisms. MAP kinases are activated by phosphorylation at conserved threonine and tyrosine residues by a cascade of dual-specificity kinases. These are, in turn, activated by MAP kinase kinase kinases. The relative hierarchy of the individual MAP kinases depends on the cell type and inflammatory stimulus.

The MAP kinases are widely expressed in synovial tissue and are activated in rheumatoid synovium. Phosphorylated ERK, p38, and JNK can be detected by immunohistochemistry or Western blot analysis. All three kinases and their upstream regulators are constitutively expressed by cultured FLS and can be activated within minutes after exposure to cytokines. They regulate production of proinflammatory cytokines and MMPs.

p38 inhibitors are effective anti-inflammatory agents in murine collagen-induced arthritis and rat adjuvant arthritis, possibly by decreasing the production of proinflammatory cytokines. In addition, p38 inhibitors block TNF and IL-6 production by cultured macrophages and synoviocytes, as well as cultured synovial tissue cells. Spinal p38 also plays a major role in pain processing, and inhibitors have potential for analgesic, as well as anti-inflammatory, action. Recent studies suggest that p38 in the central nervous system can regulate peripheral inflammation because intrathecal administration of a p38 inhibitor suppresses inflammation and joint destruction in rat adjuvant arthritis.

Given the putative role of p38 in RA, it is surprising that clinical efficacy of the selective p38 inhibitors is modest, at best.[150] Clinical response rates are rarely greater than 40%, compared with the 60% range for TNF blockers. Perhaps more interesting, an initial decrease in acute-phase reactants is only transient despite adequate drug levels. The explanations for the dissociation among the animal, in vitro, and human data are uncertain, and it is clear that the patterns of kinase and cytokine activation differ. However, p38 regulates several anti-inflammatory pathways in addition to traditional proinflammatory mediators. It is possible that the beneficial effects are mitigated by the loss of these negative feedback loops.

The other two MAP kinases are also potential therapeutic targets. The ERK pathway, which regulates cell growth and some inflammatory mediators, can be blocked by inhibiting its upstream kinases MEK1 and MEK2. One clinical trial with a small molecule inhibitor saw minimal benefit, although the placebo response rate was high. Two of the three JNK isoforms (JNK1 and JNK2) regulate a variety of genes in inflammation including TNF and metalloproteinases. Using a JNK inhibitor, marked protection of bone destruction was observed in the adjuvant arthritis model, along with decreased synovial AP-1 activation and collagenase gene expression.[151] No benefit was observed in the JNK1$^{-/-}$ mice, and only modest cartilage protection was seen in the JNK2$^{-/-}$ animals.

As an alternative to blocking MAP kinases themselves, upstream kinases might be targeted. MKK3 and MKK6, which regulate p38, are activated in the rheumatoid synovial intimal lining. MKK3 knockout and MKK6 knockout mice have markedly decreased joint inflammation in the passive K/BxN model.[152] MKK4 and MKK7 are the main kinases that modulate JNK function and are also activated in the rheumatoid synovium. Only MKK7 is required for cytokine-stimulated JNK activation and MMP expression in cultured synoviocytes.[153] Going even further upstream is also possible, and targeting TAK1, which plays a role in NFκB and JNK activation, could have broader effects.

Janus Activated Kinases and the Signal Transducers and Activators of Transcription

The JAK proteins are key proteins that transduce signals from a wide variety of cytokine and growth factor receptors. Four JAKs have been identified (JAK1, JAK2, JAK3, and TYK1), and they can form heterodimers and homodimers. The specific JAK proteins responsible for individual cytokine responses are not fully elucidated, but some general guidelines are available. JAK3 provides the signaling for many T cell–derived cytokines, and mutations in this gene are responsible for severe immunodeficiency. JAK1/JAK2 is responsible for the IL-6 family and interferons. JAK2/JAK2 signals for growth factors such as erythropoietin. The distribution and expression levels for JAKs in RA are not well defined. However, all four genes are expressed in cultured FLS and immunohistochemistry studies localize JAK3, especially in sublining DCs.[154]

The JAK proteins have become a focus of interest due to the efficacy demonstrated by a JAK inhibitor in RA clinical trials.[155] The benefit observed was similar to biologics, although issues related to adverse events and safety still need to be understood. The best isoform specificity also needs to be defined in order to maximize safety and efficacy. Because IL-6 signals through kinases such as JAK1, one should anticipate that this particular signaling molecule would be especially important for RA. On the other hand, a more T cell–directed approach for indications such as transplantation might focus more on JAK3 and could potentially have longer-term benefits in complex diseases of innate and adaptive immunity.

The JAK proteins phosphorylate the signal transducers and activators of transcription (STATs). The STATS can then translocate to the nuclei, where they can alter gene transcription. STATs have been implicated in the expression of many proinflammatory genes. IFNs signal through STAT1, IL-6 signals through STAT3, and IL-12 signals through STAT4.

Multiple STATs are expressed in rheumatoid synovium. STAT1 activation correlates with disease activity in RA (Figure 69-14), and a STAT1 decoy oligonucleotide suppresses antigen-induced arthritis in mice.[156] In addition, studies of rheumatoid tissue have an expression signature suggesting STAT1-regulated gene expression. STAT3, which is responsible for IL-6 signaling, has also been detected in cells from inflamed joints and can promote survival of cultured FLS. Synovial fluid from RA patients can activate STAT3 due to the presence of IL-6. STAT3 is also strongly phosphorylated in RA synovium, which is consistent with the role of IL-6 in RA and the efficacy of the IL-6 receptor antibody. Surprisingly, activation of the IL-4 pathway (STAT6) has also been demonstrated in RA tissues even though IL-4 expression is low.

Gene signature patterns using microarray technology have been evaluated in RA and correlated to histopathology. These studies can be difficult to interpret because of wide variations in the synovial cell populations, sampling error, and the statistical vagaries of managing large volumes of data. One study suggested that RA patients could be divided into a group with a STAT1 signature and the other with a signature reminiscent of tissue repair and remodeling.[157] With sufficient refinement, one could potentially

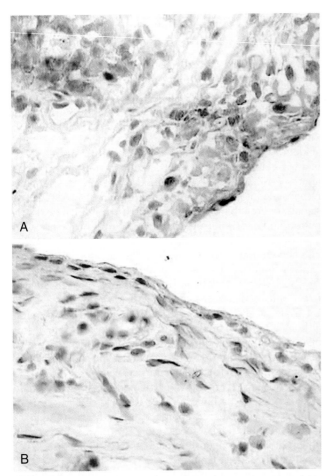

Figure 69-14 Phospho-STAT1 expression in rheumatoid arthritis synovium. Signal transducer and activator of transcription-1 (STAT1) is a transcription factor activated by the Janus kinases that regulates interferon responses. The figure shows expression of STAT1 in the synovial intimal lining using immunohistochemistry **(A). B** shows a synovial biopsy from the same patient after treatment with a traditional disease-modifying antirheumatic drug. Note that expression markedly decreased after therapy. *(From Walker JG, Ahern MJ, Coleman M, et al: Changes in synovial tissue Jak-STAT expression in rheumatoid arthritis in response to successful DMARD treatment,* Ann Rheum Dis 65:1558, 2006.*)*

identify subpopulations of patients that might respond to targeted therapies.

Interferon Regulation: IKK-Related Kinases and Interferon Regulatory Factor-3

Interferon signatures have been noted in several autoimmune diseases including RA. Type I interferons are expressed in RA synovium, especially by synoviocytes in the intimal lining. Regulation of IFN production and the IFN-response genes such as *RANTES, IP-10,* and *MCP-1* involves a pathway that runs parallel to the canonical NFκB pathway and includes two IKK-related kinases, known as IKKε and TANK binding kinase 1 (TBK1). Triggered when TLR3 is ligated by viral dsRNA, IKKε, and TBK1 phosphorylate the transcription factor interferon regulatory factor 3 (IRF3) and induce production of an array of genes that orchestrate this response including RANTES and IFN-β. IKKε and its substrate IRF3 are expressed and highly activated in RA synovium. Using a combination of IKKε$^{-/-}$ mice and genetic constructs that block endogenous IKKε and TBK1 activity, the IKK-related kinases were shown to be a key regulator of

IFN-β, RANTES, and MMP expression in cultured FLS.[158] In contrast to DCs, where IRF7 is the primary IRF that regulates IFN responses, IRF3 is the pivotal factor that is responsible for the IFN signature.[159]

Overexpression of some IRF3-driven genes, most notably IFN-β, could have a beneficial impact in inflammatory arthritis. Mice with collagen-induced arthritis injected with IFN-β or transduced fibroblasts expressing IFN-β have less severe disease compared with controls including decreased bone and cartilage destruction. A clinical trial of IFN-β in RA showed no benefit. An alternative approach might be to inhibit IKK-related kinases to block the chemokines associated with the IFN response and concomitantly treat with low levels of exogenous IFN-β.[160]

Spleen Tyrosine Kinase and Other Signaling Pathways

Several other signaling molecules have been implicated in RA and are potential therapeutic targets. For example, spleen tyrosine kinase (Syk) is involved in immunoreceptor signaling in a variety of cell types. For example, Syk plays a critical role in Fc receptor signaling in macrophages and mast cells. It also participates in B cell activation after ligation of the B cell receptor. A small molecule Syk inhibitor has demonstrated efficacy in patients with RA, although significant benefit was not observed in individuals that did not respond to TNF blockers.[161] c-Kit blockade has also been evaluated in an open-label study that provided a positive signal. PI3 kinases, especially the gamma and delta isoforms, are also attractive therapeutic targets due to their role in innate immunity and cell recruitment. There is no shortage of targets, and many others including upstream MAP kinase regulators, Ras, IL-1 associated kinases (IRAKs), sphingosine kinase-1 (SK-1), and Bruton's tyrosine kinase (BTK) will be evaluated in the future.

CELL SURVIVAL AND DEATH IN RHEUMATOID SYNOVIUM

KEY POINTS

Reactive oxygen and nitrogen in RA joints contribute to a toxic environment that can damage cells and increase inflammation.

Deficient apoptosis, or cell death, can contribute to the accumulation of cells in rheumatoid synovium.

Abnormalities of key regulatory genes such as the p53 tumor suppressor can enhance accumulation of cells in the joint.

Inducing apoptosis can potentially suppress synovial inflammation and joint destruction.

Studies defining the life cycle of cells have opened a new door to understanding the pathogenesis of neoplastic and inflammatory diseases. Although most investigators previously focused on cell proliferation as a mechanism of synovial hyperplasia, increasing attention has been paid to the other side of the equation (i.e., whether insufficient cell death could also contribute to this process). In this section, the role of oxidative damage, programmed cell death, and permanent changes in the genome are discussed because they can alter the natural history of RA.

Reactive Oxygen and Nitrogen

Oxidative stress in the joints of RA patients results from increased pressure in the synovial cavity, reduced capillary density, vascular changes, an increased metabolic rate of synovial tissue, and locally activated leukocytes. The generation of reactive oxygen species can also be facilitated by repetitive ischemia-reperfusion injury in the joint. Tissue injury releases iron and copper ions and heme proteins that are catalytic for free-radical reactions. Electron transport chains are also disrupted in the mitochondria and endoplasmic reticulum, leading to leakage of electrons to form superoxide.

Evidence for increased production of reactive oxygen species in RA patients includes elevated levels of lipid peroxidation products, degradation of hyaluronic acid by free radicals, decreased levels of ascorbic acid in serum and synovial fluid, and increased breath pentane excretion. Moreover, the levels of thioredoxin, a marker of oxidative stress, are significantly higher in synovial fluid from RA patients compared with other forms of arthritis. Peripheral blood lymphocyte DNA from RA patients contains significantly increased levels of the mutagenic 8-oxohydrodeoxyguanosine, which is a product of oxidative damage to DNA, pointing to the genotoxic effects of oxidative stress.

Nitric oxide (NO) production is also high in rheumatoid synovial tissue. Low levels of NO are constitutively produced by endothelial or neuronal synthases, and this is substantially increased by inducible NO synthase after stimulation by cytokines or bacterial products. The nitrite levels in synovial fluid are elevated in RA patients, indicating local NO production. In addition, the urinary nitrate-to-creatinine ratio is increased and inducible NO synthase is present in the synovium.

Apoptosis

Programmed cell death, or apoptosis, removes cells safely from living tissue and permits remodeling, or cell deletion without causing an inflammatory response. Apoptosis is a normal process that is tightly regulated and can be initiated by withdrawal of hormones and growth factors. It is evident in the elimination of autoreactive cells such as thymocytes in the thymus gland and the loss of cells after DNA damage or toxic exposure. It also plays a critical role in immune response by deleting activated T cells and terminating an inflammatory response by rapidly removing neutrophils.

Genes Regulating Apoptosis

The accumulation of cells in RA results from a balance of cell recruitment, cell egress, local proliferation, and local death. Any imbalance can potentially lead to synovial hyperplasia. T cell apoptosis in RA synovial effusions, for instance, is significantly less than lymphocytes from crystal-induced arthropathy. High expression of the antiapoptotic molecule Bcl-2 is found in lymphoid aggregates and protects synovial T cells from programmed cell death. Resistance to apoptosis in vitro increases if RA T cells are cocultured with FLS. The specific adhesion molecules involved are not defined, although the integrin-binding RGD motif

(arginine-glycine-asparagine) blocks the protective effects of synoviocytes.

Fas and its TNF superfamily counter-receptor Fas ligand (FasL) are potent regulators of cell death for many cell types including synovial T cells and synoviocytes. Fas is expressed by rheumatoid synovial fluid T cells, and the number of Fas$^+$ cells in the peripheral blood of RA patients is greater than in healthy controls.[162] Anti-Fas antibody, which cross-links Fas on cell surfaces, rapidly causes apoptosis in synovial fluid B and T lymphocytes in RA, although peripheral-blood T cells are more resistant. Another member of the TNF superfamily, TNF-related apoptosis-inducing ligand (TRAIL) binds to two receptors (DR4 or DR5) to induce caspase-dependent apoptosis. DR5 is expressed in RA FLS but not OA cells, and apoptosis can be induced by either TRAIL or agonistic anti-DR5 antibody.[163]

Studies of apoptosis in RA synovial tissue show only a small number of apoptotic nuclei in the intimal lining and sublining.[164] Electron microscopic studies show rare cells that exhibit the typical findings of programmed cell death. Lymphoid aggregates containing high levels of Bcl-2 have few apoptotic cells. Macrophage apoptosis is also low because they express high levels of the caspase 8 inhibitor FLICE-like inhibitory protein (FLIP), which can inhibit Fas-mediated apoptosis.

The mechanisms for inducing apoptosis in FLS can involve several pathways including induction of JNK and AP-1 activation, inhibition of the kinase Akt, or suppression of NFκB. However, it is comparatively difficult to induce apoptosis in cultured synoviocytes. p53, which typically induces cell-cycle arrest and either DNA repair or apoptosis, is also expressed in the synovial lining and sublining. However, one of the main effectors of p53-mediated apoptosis, p53 upregulated modulator of apoptosis (PUMA), is only present in low concentrations in the synovium and cultured synoviocytes. Synoviocytes are resistant to p53-mediated apoptosis even when cells are forced to overexpress the protein using genetic methods.[165] Fas is constitutively expressed by cultured synoviocytes, and programmed cell death is initiated in a minority of cells when it is cross-linked by anti-Fas antibody. Synoviocyte apoptosis can be initiated by oxidative stress such as hydrogen peroxide or by exposure to nitric oxide.

The relative paucity of apoptosis in RA can also be partially explained by patterns of gene expression that favor cell survival. Sentrin-1, a ubiquitin-like protein, regulates the cell survival by modifying proteins involved in apoptosis. Sentrin-1 is expressed in RA synovium, especially at sites of cartilage invasion, and protects cells from Fas-mediated death. A second protein, phosphatase and tensine homolog on chromosome 10 (PTEN) was originally defined as a key factor that protects from tumorigenesis through antagonism of PI3K, Akt, and many other proliferative pathways. Underexpression of PTEN in RA has been described in rheumatoid synovial intimal lining, as well as cultured FLS.[166]

Therapeutic Interventions That Increase Apoptosis. Fas-induced death has some clinical relevance and has been used successfully in murine collagen-induced arthritis using anti-Fas antibodies and adenovirus encoding for Fas ligand. Anti-Fas antibody also induces synovial cell death in RA synovial tissue explanted in SCID mice. In the SCID mouse model using RA synovial explants, anti-DR5 antibody decreased cartilage erosion. Similarly, adenoviral transfer of TRAIL in a rabbit model of arthritis decreases synovial inflammation.[167] The importance of apoptosis as a regulator of inflammation was confirmed in murine collagen-induced arthritis, where genetic DR5 deficiency exacerbated the disease. Blocking FOXO30 in PMNs is also an effective method of deleting these inflammatory cells and suppressing inflammatory arthritis in mice.

The Bcl2 homology 3 (BH3) domain-only proteins are potent inducers of apoptosis. The challenge is how to get these proteins expressed in the target cell.[168] One of these, Bim, was engineered into a cell membrane permeable protein (TAT-Bim) and evaluated in the passive K/BxN model. The construct decreased arthritis severity in prophylactic and therapeutic treatment protocols and was associated with apoptosis of cells, mainly in the myeloid lineage. Therefore targeted cell death of individual lineages can potentially decrease inflammatory arthritis.

Other molecules that regulate apoptosis have also demonstrated potential utility in animal models. For instance, NFκB blockade in streptococcal cell-wall arthritis induces synovial apoptosis and suppresses arthritis. p53 gene therapy in rabbit antigen-induced arthritis induces synovial apoptosis and decreases inflammation.[169] The pleiotropic activities of p53 were demonstrated in collagen-induced arthritis because p53−/− mice with the disease developed increased inflammation and greater joint destruction in association with decreased apoptosis. Joint damage was mediated by increased expression of collagenase genes in the knockout mice, most likely because p53 directly suppresses MMP gene transcription.[170] However, p53 knockout mice with passive models of arthritis have normal disease severity.[171] This suggests that the protective effects of p53 are partly due to effects on adaptive immunity.

Tumor Suppressor Genes

The p53 tumor suppressor is a key regulator of DNA repair and cell replication. p53 protein expression is significantly greater in the rheumatoid synovium compared with OA and normal tissue.[172] Of interest, p53 protein can also be detected in RA synovium from patients with very early RA. However, its expression is much lower in other inflammatory arthropathies such as reactive arthritis, which might reflect greater DNA damage and oxidative stress in RA.

Somatic mutations in the p53 gene occur in RA synovium could contribute to the unusual phenotype of RA synoviocytes and inadequate apoptosis in synovial tissue.[173] Transition mutations, which are characteristic of damage induced by reactive oxygen or nitric oxide, account for more than 80% of the base changes. Some of the mutant p53 genes exhibit dominant negative characteristics and suppress the function of the wild-type allele. Microdissection studies identified mutant islands with oligoclonal expansion, and the loss of p53 function in a region of RA synovium was associated with increased IL-6 gene expression in the same location. The data suggest that mutations do not cause RA but, instead, are the result of long-standing oxidative stress. The gene alterations can then potentially increase the aggressive nature of the synovium and alter the natural history of RA.

Abnormalities in other genes have also been reported in RA. For instance, synovial T cells in RA have an increased incidence of mutations in the HPRT1 gene. Although not functionally important, these synovial T cells act as a marker for oxidative damage that occurs in the synovial milieu. Some of these abnormal lymphocytes can also be detected in the peripheral blood, suggesting that articular T cells can migrate out of the joint.

Microsatellite instability, which is marked by mutations in mononucleotide and dinucleotide repeat sequences in noncoding DNA, is also significantly greater in RA than OA synovial tissue. Occasional mutations in a coding region microsatellite in the WISP-3 gene, which can regulate type II collagen and aggrecan expression, have been identified in RA synovium. However, similar mutations were observed in OA, suggesting that these are not specific. Mutations in mitochondrial genes have also been described in RA, most likely due to oxidative damage.

Evaluation of DNA mismatch repair (MMR) genes in rheumatoid synovium suggests that the balance of two genes that protect against mutations might contribute to the pattern of DNA damage in RA, with relatively high levels of MSH3 and low levels of MSH6 after reactive nitrogen stress.[174] The former repairs large insertions and deletions, whereas the latter repairs single-base abnormalities. Because most mutations detected in RA involve single bases, the changes in MMR enzyme levels favor these limited mutations rather than more substantial ones.

BLOOD VESSELS IN RHEUMATOID ARTHRITIS

KEY POINTS

Angiogenesis is a dynamic process in RA that provides nutrients to expanding synovium.

Angiogenic factors such as IL-8, FGF, and VEGF can enhance blood vessel proliferation in the synovium.

Microvascular endothelium in the synovium expresses adhesion molecules that guide circulating cells into the joint under the influence of chemoattractants.

Blood vessels play an active role in such inflammatory processes, not only as a means of selecting which cells should enter the tissue but also as a determinant of tissue growth and nutrition through the proliferation of new capillaries. Understanding the structure and function of the microvasculature provides insights into how a highly catabolic tissue such as the rheumatoid synovium can flourish.

Angiogenesis in Rheumatoid Arthritis: Feeding the Starved Synovium

The importance of luxurious new capillary growth early in the development of synovitis has been recognized for many years. The absolute number of blood vessels is increased in RA synovium (Figure 69-15), with a rich network of sublining capillaries and postcapillary venules in histologic sections stained with endothelium-specific antibodies. These blood vessels, however, are not necessarily normal, with a predominance of straight, branching morphology compared

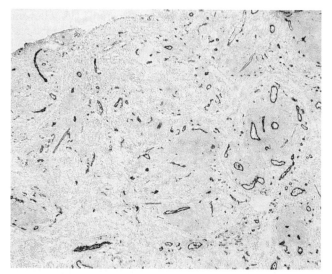

Figure 69-15 Human rheumatoid synovial membrane stained with antibody to von Willebrand factor to delineate blood vessels. Virtually all of these blood vessels formed in response to angiogenic stimuli after the rheumatoid process had been initiated. *(Courtesy Dr. Paul-Peter Tak.)*

with tortuous vessels in psoriatic arthritis synovium. The blood vessels in the inflamed synovium were less mature, probably due to increased DNA damage and decreased recruitment of pericytes. Of interest, the immature vasculature is selectively depleted by TNF blockers in RA.[175]

Hypoxia

The mass of tissue outstrips angiogenesis in RA as determined by the number of blood vessels per unit area and causes local tissue ischemia.[176] Synovial fluid oxygen tensions are remarkably low, lactate measurements are frequently high, and the pH can be as low as 6.8. The mean rheumatoid synovial fluid PO_2 in samples from rheumatoid knees is approximately 30 mm Hg and occasionally less than 15 mm Hg. Another cause of diminished blood flow is increased positive pressure exerted by synovial effusions within the joint, a process that obliterates capillary flow while producing ischemia-reperfusion injury in the joint. Altered vascular flow may not be the only cause of hypoxia in joints; oxygen consumption of the rheumatoid synovium is 20 times normal.

Hypoxia is a potent stimulus for angiogenesis, and many angiogenic factors are regulated by the hypoxia-sensing protein HIF-1α. Low oxygen tension also leads to HIF-1α–induced transcription of VEGF, a specific endothelial cell mitogen that is present in high concentrations in rheumatoid synovial fluid and tissue. Elevated serum concentrations in early disease correlate with subsequent radiographic progress. VEGF also stimulates expression of collagenase, which can degrade the extracellular matrix to make room for the advancing vasculature and pannus. VEGF expression is especially high in the synovial intimal lining, and the angiogenesis factor is also produced by cultured FLS that have been exposed to hypoxia and IL-1. HIF-1α has other functions that regulate inflammation; selective deficiency in myeloid lineage cells suppresses inflammation in the passive K/BxN model of arthritis.[177]

Angiogenic Factors

VEGF can bind to two receptors with tyrosine kinase domains: VEGF-R1/Flt-1 and VEGF-R2. VEGF-R1 regulates inflammatory responses in macrophages such as IL-6 and phagocytosis. VEGF-R1$^{-/-}$ mice are resistant to arthritis in the HTLV1 pX model, which is marked by unregulated proliferation of synovial cells. Small-molecule VEGF-R inhibitors also suppress acute models of inflammation such as carrageenan paw edema and mouse collagen-induced arthritis. Therefore targeting this receptor with a small molecule might suppress the angiogenic and proinflammatory actions of VEGF.

In addition to the hypoxia-driven stimulus for blood vessel growth, the inflammatory cytokine milieu of the joint also encourages angiogenesis. Several proinflammatory factors expressed by the rheumatoid joint including IL-8, FGF, and TNF are angiogenic. Many of these cytokines further enhance angiogenesis by increasing expression of angiopoietins (Ang-1 and Ang-2) by synoviocytes, which can then bind to their tyrosine kinase receptor, Tie-1, on RA capillary endothelial cells. Additional angiogenesis factors derived from activated adhesion molecules on the surface of endothelial cells such as soluble E-selectin and soluble VCAM are released in RA synovium and contribute to vascular proliferation.[178] Limited quantities of some antiangiogenic mediators that inhibit capillary proliferation such as platelet factor-4 and thrombospondin are also produced by the joint.

Vascular remodeling is an active process that involves the continuous creation and resorption of blood vessels. In RA, new capillaries that form under the influence of proangiogenic factors can be identified by the expression of integrins such as $\alpha_v\beta_3$. Endothelial proliferation is especially prominent in synovial tissue regions containing VEGF. Synovial blood vessel involution can also be detected as evidenced by apoptosis of the endothelium in other synovial locations. The ratio of proliferating and involuting blood vessels is significantly higher in RA than OA or normal synovium.

Targeting Angiogenesis

The importance of new blood-vessel formation in inflammatory arthritis was elegantly demonstrated in the collagen-induced arthritis model. The disease was markedly attenuated in animals pretreated with an angiostatic compound similar to fumagillin, which is derived from *Aspergillus*.[179] This compound is cytotoxic to proliferating, but not resting, endothelial cells. In addition, there was regression of established arthritis if treatment was initiated well into the course of the disease. Hence angiogenesis is essential for the establishment and progression of inflammatory arthritis because of the need for blood vessels to either recruit leukocytes or provide nutrients and oxygen to starved tissue.

Targeting HIF-1α with a small molecule inhibitor that blocks nuclear translocation and VEGF induction was effective in adjuvant arthritis.[180] Other small molecules inhibitors of the VEGF-R1 with either antibodies or kinase inhibitors have been successfully tested in preclinical models of arthritis as well. One of these, vatalanib, decreased inflammatory knee arthritis in rabbits.

Several other antiangiogenesis approaches are effective in animal models of arthritis. For instance, thrombospondin 1 overexpression significantly decreased blood vessel density, inflammation, and joint destruction in rat collagen-induced arthritis. Direct intra-articular administration of a cyclic RGD peptide was used in a rabbit model to block $\alpha_v\beta_3$ integrin.[181] As with RA synovium, $\alpha_v\beta_3$ is expressed by proliferating blood vessels in inflamed rabbit synovial tissue. The cyclic peptide decreased joint inflammation, increased endothelial cell apoptosis, and suppressed bone and cartilage destruction.

The ability of RGD to bind selectively to proliferating blood vessels was also used to home a proapoptotic agent to synovial neovasculature in murine collagen-induced arthritis.[182] The cyclic RGD peptide was administered systemically and accumulated in inflamed synovium but not normal joints or other organs. Apoptosis was induced in synovial blood vessels and arthritis regressed. The potent angiogenesis inhibitor endostatin has been tested in the SCID mouse model, and it decreased synovial explant inflammatory cell infiltration and capillary density. Despite the compelling rationale for antiangiogenic therapy, an anti-α_v antibody showed minimal efficacy in a clinical trial, perhaps because other pathways are more important in the synovium.

Adhesion Molecule Regulation

Endothelial cells activated by cytokines and other mediators express adhesion molecules that bind to counter-receptors on mononuclear cells and neutrophils from the circulation and facilitate their recruitment from the blood (see Chapter 25). Several categories of vascular adhesion molecules exist. The selectins (E-, L-, and P-selectin) are a family of adhesion molecules whose primary ligands are carbohydrates, especially sialyl Lewis$_x$, and related oligosaccharides. A second family is integrins, which are heterodimers that include an α- and a β-chain. The counter-receptors depend on the specific combination of these chains and are frequently proteins in the immunoglobulin supergene family or extracellular matrix proteins. Several novel peptides have been described that selectively bind to the blood vessels of human synovial explants in SCID mice and have potential utility as inhibitors of cell adhesion, specifically to joint tissue.

Integrins and Ligands

As one might expect, adhesion molecule expression is increased in the RA synovium due to the rich cytokine milieu. Immunohistochemical techniques localize high levels of ICAM-1 to sublining macrophages, macrophage-like synovial lining cells, and fibroblasts compared with normal tissue.[183] Significant amounts are also present on the majority of vascular endothelial cells. Cultured FLS also constitutively express ICAM-1, which can be markedly increased by TNF, IL-1, and IFN-γ. ICAM-1 and the other ICAM family members can bind to cells expressing the $\beta2$ integrins, especially neutrophils.

Adhesion of $\alpha_4\beta_1$(VLA-4)–expressing mononuclear cells such as memory T cells or monocytes to cytokine-activated endothelial cells can be mediated by VCAM-1 or CS-1 fibronectin. A role for VLA-4 in arthritis has been suggested by a number of experimental observations. In adjuvant arthritis in rats, anti-α_4 antibody decreases lymphocyte accumulation in the joint but not lymph nodes, suggesting that VLA-4 is more important in recruitment to inflamed sites than to noninflamed sites.[184] T lymphocytes isolated from the synovial fluid and synovial membrane of RA patients exhibit increased VLA-4–mediated adherence to VCAM-1, relative to autologous peripheral blood lymphocytes. These studies also suggest that leukocytes expressing functionally activated VLA-4 are selectively recruited to inflammatory sites in RA. Anti-α_4 antibody has potential utility in RA, but enthusiasm is mitigated by effects on host defense observed with natalizumab in multiple sclerosis.

Moderate amounts of VCAM-1 are expressed in RA synovial blood vessels. Surprisingly, the intimal lining is the location of the most intense staining with anti–VCAM-1 antibodies on histologic sections. Even normal synovial tissue expresses VCAM-1 in the lining, albeit less than in RA. Cultured FLS constitutively express small amounts of VCAM-1, and the level is increased by a variety of macrophage and T cell–derived cytokines. VCAM-1 also contributes to T cell adhesion to high endothelial venules in frozen sections of RA synovium.[185] The other VLA-4 counter-receptor, CS-1–containing forms of FN, is restricted to inflamed RA vascular endothelium and the synovial intimal lining.

The integrin $\alpha_4\beta_7$, which also binds to VCAM-1, is a specific adhesion molecule involved in lymphocyte homing to Peyer's patches. Most intraepithelial and lamina propria lymphocytes express $\alpha_4\beta_7$; this molecule is rarely identified in other lymphoid tissues. The expression of $\alpha_4\beta_7$ on peripheral blood lymphocytes from patients with RA is low (similar to normal individuals), but up to a quarter of synovial fluid lymphocytes, mostly CD8$^+$ T lymphocytes, express this adhesion molecule and provide an interesting link between arthritis and the gut.[186]

Selectins

E-selectin expression is also elevated in rheumatoid synovium, although the increase is less dramatic than for the integrins and their counter-receptors. This might be due, in part, to the kinetics of E-selectin expression on endothelial cells, which is transient after stimulation with cytokines.

Therapeutic Potential of Blocking Adhesion Molecules

The therapeutic potential for antiadhesion therapy has been studied in the SCID mouse model. Labeled human peripheral mononuclear cells were injected into engrafted mice, and migration into the tissue was examined.[187] If the mice were treated with TNF, ICAM-1 expression and trafficking into synovium were significantly increased. Anti–ICAM-1 antibody blocked leukocyte migration into the explant under these conditions. In another study, tonsil mononuclear cells also migrated into the RA synovial grafts in SCID mice. RA clinical trials using anti–ICAM-1 therapy have been reported using anti–ICAM-1 antibody or antisense ICAM-1 oligonucleotides, although minimal significant clinical benefit was observed. In addition, mice lacking E- and P-selectin actually had accelerated disease in the collagen-induced arthritis model. This paradoxical result serves as a reminder of the complexity of the inflammatory process.[188]

CARTILAGE AND BONE DESTRUCTION

> ### KEY POINTS
>
> Cartilage degradation and bone destruction in RA are mediated by distinct mechanisms and cell types.
>
> Several classes of proteases including metalloproteinases, serine proteases, cathepsins, and aggrecanases are produced by intimal lining cells in RA, especially FLS.
>
> Synovial lining cells, especially FLS, can invade and damage cartilage in RA.
>
> Bone destruction is mediated by osteoclasts that are activated under the influence of RANKL and other cytokines produced by RA synovium.

Cartilage Destruction and the Pannus-Cartilage Junction

In RA, the cartilage is initially covered by a layer of tissue composed of mesenchymal cells. In the established lesion, macrophage-like and fibroblast-like cells penetrate into cartilage matrix (Figure 69-16). Invasive pannus is more commonly found in metatarsophalangeal joints, compared with hip and knee joints in which a layer of resting fibroblasts appeared to separate pannus from cartilage, perhaps explaining why erosions occur more often around small joints.

FLS from the intimal lining are major effectors of cartilage destruction in RA. They produce prodigious amount of proteases, bind to cartilage, and invade into the extracellular matrix. The pivotal role of synoviocytes in cartilage destruction was demonstrated in arthritis models using cadherin-11 blockade to disrupt the intimal lining.

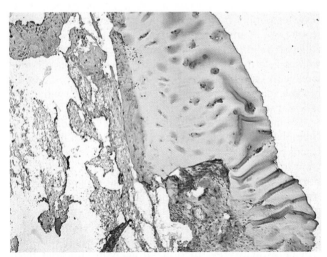

Figure 69-16 Pannus-cartilage junction. The invasive front of pannus burrows into cartilage matrix in rheumatoid arthritis joints. The pannus is primarily composed of macrophages and mesenchymal cells. Immunostaining with anti-CD68 antibody shows the distribution of macrophages in the invasive tissue. *(Courtesy Dr. Paul-Peter Tak.)*

Cartilage destruction is markedly attenuated even though bone erosions progress.[189]

Other cells in the joint, especially neutrophils and cells from the pannus that burrow directly into cartilage, could also be responsible for cartilage, whereas osteoclasts are responsible for bone erosions. More primitive mesenchymal cells isolated directly from the cartilage-pannus junction express phenotypic and functional features of both synoviocytes and chondrocytes and have also been described in the synovium.

Cartilage is destroyed in RA by both enzymatic and mechanical processes. The enzymes induced by factors such as IL-1, IL-17, TNF, phagocytosis of debris by synovial cells, and mechanical trauma degrade the matrix proteins. Early in synovitis, proteoglycans are depleted from the tissue, most likely due to the catabolic effect of cytokines such as IL-1 on chondrocytes with the production of MMPs and aggrecanases, and this leads to mechanical weakening of cartilage. As proteoglycans are depleted, cartilage loses elasticity and becomes susceptible to mechanical fragmentation and fibrillation. Eventually the tissue loses functional integrity concurrent with its dissolution by collagenases and stromelysins. Some of the MMPs responsible for this process are also derived from the chondrocytes themselves. Multiple MMPs, especially stromelysin and collagenase levels, are expressed in RA cartilage, and in situ hybridization studies confirm the presence of the mRNA within chondrocytes.[190] Hence the cartilage is under attack from a multitude of sources: It is bathed in protease-rich synovial fluid, is under extrinsic attack from the invasive pannus, is damaged from within by chondrocytes, and is fragmented by mechanical forces.

Enzymes released by PMNs in synovial fluid including neutrophil collagenase and multiple serine proteases also contribute to cartilage loss. Immune complexes containing RFs are embedded in the superficial layers of cartilage and can attract and activate neutrophils. Electron microscopic examinations of articular cartilage in RA reveal evidence of breakdown of collagen and proteoglycan due to superficial activity of joint fluid enzymes. In a rabbit model of arthritis in which IL-1 was injected directly into the joint, the degree of cartilage damage as measured by proteoglycan levels in synovial fluid correlated best with the stromelysin concentrations in synovial effusions (presumably derived from synoviocytes). Neutrophil depletion of animals did not interfere with subsequent destruction of extracellular matrix, suggesting that MMPs derived from the synovium are more important.

By and large, most animal studies indicate that IL-1 is a key regulator of matrix degradation in arthritis. Although TNF blockade has clear anti-inflammatory effects, chondroprotection is less prominent. The joint destruction observed in TNF-dependent models often requires IL-1. Recent data suggest that IL-17 and TLR ligands can also contribute to joint destruction directly or by synergizing with IL-1 and TNF.

The rate-limiting step in cartilage loss is the cleavage of collagen because proteoglycans are degraded soon after inflammation begins. MMPs, released into the extracellular space and active at neutral pH, are probably responsible for most of the effective proteolysis of articular-cartilage proteins, but other classes of enzymes may contribute to joint destruction. Enzymes such as cathepsins B, D, G, K, L, and H may play a role within and outside cells in degrading noncollagenous matrix proteins. Serine proteinases (e.g., elastase and plasmin) and aggrecanases are doubtless involved as well.

Proteases: Mediators of Joint Destruction

Matrix Metalloproteinases

The MMPs are a family of enzymes that participate in extracellular-matrix degradation and remodeling (see Chapter 8). They are usually secreted as inactive proenzymes, and their proteolytic activity requires limited cleavage or denaturation to reveal a zinc cation at the core. Their activation can be mediated by other proteases including trypsin, plasmin, or tryptase. The substrates for MMPs are varied but quite specific for individual members of the family. Collagenases degrade native collagen types I, II, III, VII, and X, whereas gelatinases are able to degrade denatured or cleaved collagen. Stromelysins have broader specificity and can digest proteoglycans in addition to proteins. They also process procollagenase to the active form, thereby serving as a positive-feedback signal for matrix destruction. Some MMPs such as TNF convertase (TACE) are responsible for the processing and release of cytokines from the cell surface. Many different families of proteinases are found in the joint (Table 69-6), but the MMPs are thought to play a pivotal role in joint destruction.

Regulation of MMP Production. The cytokine milieu has the capacity to induce the biosynthesis of MMPs by synovial cells and alter the balance between extracellular matrix production and degradation. IL-1 and TNF, in particular, induce MMP gene expression by many cells, especially FLS and chondrocytes. The two cytokines are additive or synergistic when used in combination. Many other cytokines and TLR ligands implicated in rheumatoid synovitis can also induce MMP expression including IL-17, LIF, LPS, and peptidoglycans.

MMP induction is mediated by both an increase in gene transcription and mRNA stabilization. Culture medium from rheumatoid synovium stimulates cartilage degradation in vitro, and this is mainly due to IL-1. IL-6 does not induce MMP production by synovial cells but instead increases the production of TIMP-1, a naturally occurring inhibitor of

Table 69-6 Key Proteases and Inhibitors in Rheumatoid Arthritis Synovium

Protease	Inhibitor
Metalloproteinases	TIMP family; α_2-macroglobulin
Collagenase-1	
Collagenase-3	
Stromelysin-1	
92-kD gelatinase	
Serine proteases	SERPINs; α_2-macroglobulin
Trypsin	
Chymotrypsin	
Tryptase	
Cathepsins	α_2-macroglobulin
Cathepsin B	
Cathepsin L	
Cathepsin K	

SERPINs, serine protease inhibitors; TIMP, tissue inhibitor of metalloproteinases.

MMPs. TGF-β inhibits collagenase synthesis and enhances the production of TIMP by fibroblasts and chondrocytes. TGF-β also increases collagen production, shifting the balance from destruction to matrix repair.

Although multiple upstream regulatory sequences are involved in MMP gene transcription, the dominant element in the promoter is AP-1. Other regulatory sites such as an NFκB-like region can also contribute to collagenase expression. AP-1 activity is markedly increased in FLS by proinflammatory cytokines, and its transcriptional activity is mediated by increased expression of components such as c-Jun. The MAP kinases are especially important for this activity, and JNK is the most efficient upstream activator. Glucocorticoids markedly inhibit MMP gene expression by blocking AP-1.

Collagenases and stromelysins have the capacity to degrade virtually all the important structural proteins in the extracellular tissues within joints. Collagenase-1 (MMP-1) cleaves through the triple-helical collagen molecule at a single glycine-isoleucine bond approximately three-quarters of the distance from the NH$_2$-terminus. This enzyme degrades only the interstitial helical collagens (e.g., types I, II, III, and X). It has little or no activity against types IV, V, and IX and other nonhelical collagens or denatured collagen; the degradation of the latter is primarily accomplished by the gelatinases. MMP-1, however, is a relatively inefficient enzyme, whereas collagenase-3 (MMP-13) has more favorable kinetics. Neutrophil collagenase, or MMP-8, is constitutively stored in neutrophil granules and is released into the milieu after degranulation. Of note, rodents lack the collagenase-1 gene, whereas the collagenase-3 gene is preserved. This is especially important to note when evaluating effects of MMP inhibitors in animal models.

MMP Expression in Synovium. The collagenase-1 and collagenase-3 genes are produced by RA synovial tissue, and the latter is highly expressed by chondrocytes in cartilage. In situ hybridization studies show that the primary location of collagenase-1 gene expression in the synovium, like many other MMPs, is the intimal lining, especially in fibroblast-like cells.[191] Subchondral bone is another region in which proteinase expression occurs in RA and could participate in bone resorption. Increased MMP gene expression is an early feature of RA and occurs during the first few weeks of clinically active disease. High expression of collagenase-1, as well as gelatinases such as MMP-2, early in disease correlates with rapidly progressive erosions. Similarly, increased blood levels of the proenzymes are also associated with more severe disease.

Stromelysin-1 (MMP-3) and the other members of the stromelysin family have no activity against most native collagens but effectively degrade type IV collagen, fibronectin, laminin, proteoglycan core protein, and type IX collagen. Stromelysin removes the NH$_2$-terminal propeptides from type I procollagen and is integrally involved in the activation of procollagenase. Like collagenase, stromelysin gene expression occurs mainly in the synovial intimal lining (Figure 69-17). Despite the putative importance of this enzyme in matrix destruction, stromelysin knockout mice are susceptible to collagen-induced arthritis and develop as much joint destruction as mice with functional stromelysin.[192] This observation led to decreased interest in stromelysin inhibitors to treat diseases such as RA.

RA synovium   Stromelysin

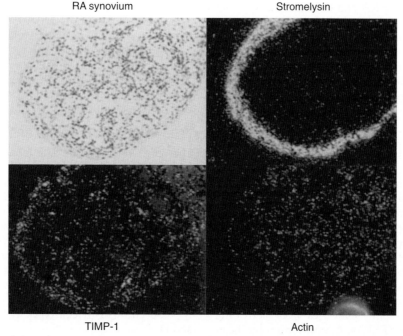

TIMP-1   Actin

Figure 69-17 Localization of stromelysin, tissue inhibitor of metalloproteinases-1 (TIMP-1), and actin mRNA in rheumatoid arthritis (RA) synovial tissue by in situ hybridization. Stromelysin is mainly expressed in the synovial intimal lining, presumably by cytokine-stimulated type B synoviocytes. Bright field and dark field views are shown. *(Courtesy D. Boyle.)*

MMP inhibitors are effective in animal models of rheumatoid arthritis and can suppress bone destruction, as well as the inflammatory synovitis. In models of osteoarthritis, deletion of MMP genes such as stromelysin do not necessarily improve outcomes. Clinical trials in RA using nonselective inhibitors have had minimal success and significant side effects, possibly related to decreased matrix turnover. Inhibitors of TACE (which can also block other MMPs) actually appear to increase disease activity in RA, perhaps due to increased levels of membrane-bound TNF. One of the most consistent side effects experienced by patients treated with MMP inhibitors is increased joint stiffness thought to result from deposition of fibrous tissue without sufficient protease activity to permit removal of matrix proteins. This observation has been replicated in rats, which provides an opportunity to determine if highly selective MMP inhibitors will have a better risk-benefit ratio.

Cysteine Proteases: The Cathepsins

Cathepsins are an extensive family of cysteine proteases that have broad proteolytic activity including activity on types II, IX, and XI collagen and proteoglycans. Like MMPs, the cathepsins are regulated by cytokines and by proto-oncogenes such as Ras. IL-1 and TNF induce cathepsin L expression in cultured FLS.[193] In situ hybridization studies demonstrate expression of cathepsin B and L in RA synovium, especially at sites of erosion. A ribozyme that cleaves cathepsin L decreases FLS invasion and cartilage destruction in the SCID mouse model with implanted cultured synoviocytes.

Cathepsin K has been implicated in bone resorption by osteoclasts. This protease is unique among the cathepsins because it can degrade native type I collagen. It is expressed in RA synovial tissue by both macrophages and fibroblasts and is present in significantly higher concentrations than in OA.[194] Serum levels of cathepsin K correlate with the extent of radiographic damage. A potential role of cathepsins as mediators of bone destruction in arthritis was confirmed in studies in which a cysteine protease inhibitor significantly decreased joint damage in the rat adjuvant arthritis model. In the TNF-transgenic mouse model, lack of the cathepsin K deficiency decreased, but did not eliminate, bone erosions.[195]

Aggrecanases

Aggrecan is a major proteoglycan component of articular cartilage. Because of its large size and negative charge, it contains a considerable amount of water, which increases compressibility. Two proteolytic sites are available on aggrecan in its globular domain. One site is susceptible to MMP cleavage, whereas the other, located 32 amino acids toward the C-terminus, is the site for cleavage by a family of enzymes known as aggrecanases. The two sites can be identified in tissues using monoclonal antibodies after cleavage when specific neoepitopes are revealed.

Normal cartilage contains a surprising amount of aggrecanase neoepitope, suggesting continuous matrix turnover. The level of aggrecanase cleavage product increases with age. Two aggrecanase genes, aggrecanase-1 and aggrecanase-2, have been cloned and are members of the "a disintegrin and metalloproteinase with thrombospondin motif" (ADAMTS) family of proteins (ADAMTS-4 and ADAMTS-5, respectively). They are expressed in OA and RA cartilage, and their proteolytic activity can be detected in synovial fluids. Especially high levels of the neoepitope are present in arthritic cartilage.[196] IL-1 increases aggrecanase expression in cartilage explants, as well as cultures of chondrocytes. Aggrecanase-1 and aggrecanase-2 are constitutively expressed by RA and OA FLS and synovial tissues.[197] Aggrecanase-1 is induced in synoviocytes by cytokines, especially TGF-β, whereas aggrecanase-2 expression remains constant despite TGF-β or IL-1 stimulation. Genetic deletion of aggrecanse-1 has no effect on a murine osteoarthritis model. However, loss of aggrecanase-2 prevents degenerative changes.[198]

Inhibitors of Protease Activity

α_2-Macroglobulin (α_2M) accounts for more than 95% of collagenase inhibitory capacity in serum. The mechanism of inhibition by α_2M involves hydrolysis by the proteinase of a susceptible region in one of the four polypeptide chains of α_2M (sometimes called the "bait"), with subsequent trapping of the proteins within the interstices of the α_2M. Ultimately, the protease is covalently linked to a portion of the α_2M molecule. The serine protease inhibitors (SERPINs) are also abundant in synovial effusions and plasma and can serve a dual purpose of directly blocking serine protease function and indirectly decreasing MMP activity by preventing serine proteases from activating MMP proenzymes. One SERPIN, α_1-antitrypsin, has been well characterized in synovial fluid and is frequently inactivated after oxidation by reactive oxygen species.

A family of proteins that specifically block MMP activity, called TIMPs, has been cloned and characterized. The TIMP proteins block proteinase activity by binding directly to MMPs in a 1:1 molar ratio. TIMP generally binds only to the active enzyme, although exceptions such as TIMP-2 can interact with a progelatinase (MMP-2). The inhibitors bind to MMPs with extremely high avidity. Even though the interaction does not result in new covalent bonds, it is essentially irreversible.

TIMP proteins are present in RA synovial fluid in excess. It is, in fact, difficult to detect free active collagenase and stromelysin because they are usually complexed with the inhibitors. The majority of MMP, however, is in the proenzyme form. Immunohistochemical and in situ hybridization studies have localized the TIMPs in hyperplastic synovial lining cells in rheumatoid synovium, but not in the cells of normal synovium. TIMP gene expression is not significantly altered by IL-1 or TNF but is increased by IL-6, oncostatin M, and TGF-β. TIMP-3 knockout mice have significantly more synovial inflammation and TNF production in antigen-induced arthritis, perhaps because it is not available to inhibit TACE. Similarly, TIMP-1 or TIMP-3 gene transfer limits rheumatoid FLS invasion into cartilage in an SCID mouse model. The function of these genes can extend beyond protease inhibition and include a number of paracrine functions, as well as induction of apoptosis when expressed intracellularly in cultured synoviocytes.

Given the important role of MMPs in tissue destruction, the relative balance between MMPs and TIMPs ultimately determines the fate of the extracellular matrix. The ratio in RA, with its more destructive potential, favors degradation, whereas OA has a lower MMP-to-TIMP ratio. The levels of TIMP gene expression are similar in the two diseases and may well be maximal. The higher ratio in RA results from increased MMP production. This balance between protease and inhibitor can be modified in vivo with drug therapy. For instance, intra-articular corticosteroid injections markedly decrease synovial collagenase, stromelysin, and TIMP gene expression. In contrast, chronic low-dose methotrexate therapy specifically decreases collagenase but not TIMP-1 mRNA.[199] Suppressed collagenase gene expression suggests that a low collagenase-to-TIMP ratio is one mechanism of decreased tissue destruction observed in patients treated with methotrexate.

Regulation of Bone Destruction

Osteoclasts are the major cells responsible for bone degradation. RANKL, which was originally described for its role in T cell–dendritic cell interactions, as well as lymphocyte and lymph node development, is perhaps the single most important factor that modulates bone resorption. Osteoclast development is complex and involves the differentiation of monocytes under the influence of cytokines such as M-CSF in combination with RANKL. Subsequent osteoclast activation can involve several pathways, most of which also depend on the presence of RANKL. Its receptor, known as RANK, is expressed by the osteoclast precursors. RANKL is produced by many cell types including activated T cells and FLS.

Abundant evidence implicates this powerful mechanism in bone destruction caused by inflammatory arthritis. For instance, administration of OPG, a RANKL decoy receptor, to rats with adjuvant arthritis inhibits bone destruction but has almost no effect on inflammation or clinical signs of arthritis.[200] RANKL$^{-/-}$ mice are also protected from bone erosions in the passive K/BxN model of arthritis, although cartilage destruction still occurs. Animal models of arthritis point to IL-17 as a mediator of osteoclast generation. Genetic deficiency of IL-17 or anti-IL-17 antibodies have remarkable bone-sparing effects in these experiments.

RANK, RANKL, and OPG (as well as M-CSF and IL-17) have been detected in the synovium and synovial fluid of patients with RA. The ratio of RANKL to OPG is significantly higher in RA synovial effusions than in either OA or gout, which is consistent with the more destructive nature of RA. Osteoclasts expressing tartrate-resistant acid phosphatase (TRAP), capable of forming resorption lacunae, can be generated from cultured RA synovial cells (Figure 69-18). This activity is blocked by the addition of exogenous OPG. RA synoviocytes and synovial membrane T cells that display RANKL can also induce differentiation of osteoclasts from peripheral blood cells.[201]

The functional relevance of the RANK-RANKL system was confirmed in RA studies in which an anti-RANKL antibody denosumab decreased bone erosions. As predicted from animal model studies, the antibody had no effect on inflammation or clinical signs of synovitis.[202]

A second system that regulates bone remodeling involves the Wingless (Wnt) proteins. Several members of this family bind to receptors that regulate osteoblast differentiation through effects on β-catenin. Wnt signaling is modulated by many other proteins, most notably the Dickkopf (DKK) family. DKK-1 in particular blocks binding of Wnts to its receptors. In TNF-transgenic mice with arthritis, bone erosions are blocked by inhibiting either TNF or DKK-1. With the latter, proliferative bone lesions such as osteophytes formed instead.[203] Therefore DKK-1 is a master switch that determines the fate of bone in inflammatory

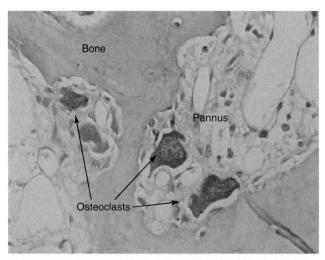

Figure 69-18 Tartrate resistant acid phosphatase–positive osteoclasts are shown invading bone in rheumatoid arthritis (see *arrows* for examples). This process is regulated by RANKL in the presence of other cytokines such as macrophage colony-stimulating factor and tumor necrosis factor. *(Courtesy Dr. Steven Goldring, Dr. Ellen Gravallese, and Dr. Allison Pettit.)*

lesions. When present, bone destruction is favored; when absent, bone formation occurs.

Tissue Repair

Extracellular matrix turnover in RA has been likened to wound healing due to the critical role of collagen production, proteases, and protease inhibitors. Remodeling the matrix by removing damaged proteins is a key element in early repair. Subsequently, the balance shifts to protease inhibition, production of cytokine inhibitors, removal of inflammatory cells through apoptosis, and release of anti-inflammatory eicosanoids such as lipoxins to suppress inflammation. Neutralization of oxidants via glutathione reductase or superoxide dismutase further limits tissue damage.

This process then permits either a return to normal architecture or scar formation. TGF-β, in particular, appears to play a key role in that it increases collagen deposition, suppresses MMP expression, and enhances production of the TIMPs. Although TGF-β levels in the joint are substantial, they are not sufficient to overcome the impressive array of MMPs expressed in synovitis. The repair process is insufficient in RA, perhaps because of persistent T cell activation or autonomous activation of other cell lineages. However, strategies to shift from tissue damage by enhancing endogenous mechanisms might not only suppress symptoms but also enhance appropriate remodeling of the matrix to restore homeostasis

Because the invasive rheumatoid synovium exhibits some properties similar to neoplastic diseases, the possibility that the tissue contains immature cells or embryonic genes that regulate repair has been explored. The embryonic growth factors from the wingless (wnt) and frizzled (fz) gene families have been demonstrated in RA synovium. Normally, these proteins participate in bone marrow progenitor differentiation and limb bud mesenchyme. Wnt5a and Fz5, in particular, are markedly elevated in RA tissues

and cultured synoviocytes. When normal fibroblasts are transfected with the *WNT5A* gene, cytokine expression such as IL-6 increases significantly. Antisense *WNT5A* and dominant negative *WNT5A* vectors diminish cytokine expression by synoviocytes.[204]

These data raise the possibility that immature mesenchymal cells populate the synovium in RA, either as a primary event or as a repair mechanism. Similar primitive mesenchymal cells circulate in the peripheral blood of RA and normal individuals, and in collagen-induced arthritis they infiltrate the synovium before clinically apparent synovial inflammation.

Restoring homeostasis and tissue repair in RA is therefore a complex process that involves the ingress or dedifferentiation of mesenchymal cells that can remodel the matrix. In addition to TGF-β, the function of these cells is modulated by the bone morphogenic proteins (BMPs). The BMPs are members of the TGF-β superfamily and, like TGF-β, signal through the Smad pathway. Several members including BMP-2 and BMP-7 are expressed in the joint and facilitate repair, although inappropriate release can also enhance joint damage or lead to ankylosis or enthesophyte formation.[205] BMP function is also regulated by a family of inhibitors such as Noggin, which can surprisingly limit cartilage damage when overexpressed in murine antigen-induced arthritis. Modulating the relative balance and timing of BMP expression could ultimately be used to either modify the destructive influence of synovitis or regenerate damaged tissues.

SUMMARY

The etiology and pathogenesis of RA remains a complex problem, although the level of understanding has progressed considerably in recent years. Both T cell–dependent and T cell–independent processes contribute to disease initiation and perpetuation. Moreover, disease mechanisms might differ at various stages of the process. These hypotheses have unveiled many novel therapeutic targets and interventions that might lead to significant clinical benefit. Such was the case with the TNF inhibitors, B cell depletion, T cell co-stimulation, and most recently IL-6 inhibition, which have joined the pharmacopoeia for the treatment of RA. Early observations that defined the cytokine profile in arthritis and that delineated the biology of macrophage cytokines led to this breakthrough. Similarly, it is possible that understanding of apoptotic pathways, abnormalities in tumor-suppressor genes, the function of the susceptibility genes, signaling pathways, B cell function, or T cell differentiation will lead to new therapies.

Selected References

1. Firestein GS, Zvaifler NJ: How important are T cells in chronic rheumatoid synovitis?: II. T cell-independent mechanisms from beginning to end, *Arthritis Rheum* 46:298, 2002.
2. Weyand CM, Hicok KC, Conn DL, Goronzy JJ: The influence of HLA-DRB1 genes on disease severity in rheumatoid arthritis, *Ann Intern Med* 117:801, 1992.
3. van der Woude D, Lie BA, Lundström E, et al: Protection against anti-citrullinated protein antibody-positive rheumatoid arthritis is predominantly associated with HLA-DRB1*1301: a meta-analysis of HLA-DRB1 associations with anti-citrullinated protein antibody-positive and anti-citrullinated protein antibody-negative rheumatoid arthritis in four European populations, *Arthritis Rheum* 62:1236, 2010.

4. Rak JM, Maestroni L, Balandraud N, et al: Transfer of the shared epitope through microchimerism in women with rheumatoid arthritis, *Arthritis Rheum* 60:73, 2009.

5. van der Helm-van Mil AH, Verpoort KN, Breedveld FC, et al: The HLA-DRB1 shared epitope alleles are primarily a risk factor for anticyclic citrullinated peptide antibodies and are not an independent risk factor for development of rheumatoid arthritis, *Arthritis Rheum* 54:1117, 2006.

7. Suzuki A, Yamada R, Chang X, et al: Functional haplotypes of PADI4, encoding citrullinating enzyme peptidylarginine deiminase 4, are associated with rheumatoid arthritis, *Nat Genet* 34:395, 2003.

8. Begovich AB, Carlton VE, Honigberg LA, et al: A missense single-nucleotide polymorphism in a gene encoding a protein tyrosine phosphatase (PTPN22) is associated with rheumatoid arthritis, *Am J Hum Genet* 75:330, 2004.

9. Stahl EA, Raychaudhuri S, Remmers EF, et al: Genome-wide association study meta-analysis identifies seven new rheumatoid arthritis risk loci, *Nat Genet* 42:508–514, 2010.

13. Källberg H, Ding B, Padyukov L, et al; EIRA Study Group: Smoking is a major preventable risk factor for rheumatoid arthritis: estimations of risks after various exposures to cigarette smoke, *Ann Rheum Dis* 70:508, 2011.

16. Nelson JL, Hughes KA, Smith AG, et al: Maternal-fetal disparity in HLA class II alloantigens and the pregnancy-induced amelioration of rheumatoid arthritis, *N Engl J Med* 329:466, 1993.

17. Brennan P, Barrett J, Fiddler M, et al: Maternal-fetal HLA incompatibility and the course of inflammatory arthritis during pregnancy, *J Rheumatol* 27:2843, 2000.

18. Karouzakis E, Gay RE, Michel BA, et al: DNA hypomethylation in rheumatoid arthritis synovial fibroblasts, *Arthritis Rheum* 60:3613, 2009.

19. Nile CJ, Read RC, Akil M, et al: Methylation status of a single CpG site in the IL6 promoter is related to IL6 messenger RNA levels and rheumatoid arthritis, *Arthritis Rheum* 58:2686, 2008.

20. Nakamachi Y, Kawano S, Takenokuchi M, et al: MicroRNA-124a is a key regulator of proliferation and monocyte chemoattractant protein 1 secretion in fibroblast-like synoviocytes from patients with rheumatoid arthritis, *Arthritis Rheum* 60:1294, 2009.

21. Stanczyk J, Ospelt C, Karouzakis E, et al: Altered expression of microRNA-203 in rheumatoid arthritis synovial fibroblasts and its role in fibroblast activation, *Arthritis Rheum* 63(2):373–381, 2011.

22. Doran MF, Pond GR, Crowson CS, et al: Trends in incidence and mortality in rheumatoid arthritis in Rochester, Minnesota, over a forty-year period, *Arthritis Rheum* 46:625, 2002.

23. Myasoedova E, Crowson CS, Kremers HM, et al: Is the incidence of rheumatoid arthritis rising? Results from Olmsted County, Minnesota, 1955–2007, *Arthritis Rheum* 62:1572–1582, 2010.

24. Abdollahi-Roodsaz S, Joosten LA, Koenders MI, et al: Local interleukin-1-driven joint pathology is dependent on toll-like receptor 4 activation, *Am J Pathol* 175:2004, 2009.

25. Choe JY, Crain B, Wu SR, Corr M: Interleukin 1 receptor dependence of serum transferred arthritis can be circumvented by toll-like receptor 4 signaling, *J Exp Med* 197:537, 2003.

27. Nielen MM, van Schaardenburg D, Reesink HW, et al: Specific autoantibodies precede the symptoms of rheumatoid arthritis: a study of serial measurements in blood donors, *Arthritis Rheum* 50:38, 2004.

28. Liang KP, Maradit Kremers H, Crowson CS, et al: Autoantibodies and the risk of cardiovascular events, *J Rheumatol* 36(11):2462–2468, 2009.

29. Rawson AJ, Hollander JL, Quismorio FP, Abelson NM: Experimental arthritis in man and rabbit dependent upon serum anti-immunoglobulin factors, *Ann N Y Acad Sci* 168:188, 1969.

31. Lee SK, Bridges SL Jr, Koopman WJ, Schroeder HW Jr: The immunoglobulin kappa light chain repertoire expressed in the synovium of a patient with rheumatoid arthritis, *Arthritis Rheum* 35:905, 1992.

32. De Rycke L, Nicholas AP, Cantaert T, et al: Synovial intracellular citrullinated proteins colocalizing with peptidyl arginine deiminase as pathophysiologically relevant antigenic determinants of rheumatoid arthritis-specific humoral autoimmunity, *Arthritis Rheum* 52:2323, 2005.

33. Vossenaar ER, Smeets TJ, Kraan MC, et al: The presence of citrullinated proteins is not specific for rheumatoid synovial tissue, *Arthritis Rheum* 50:3485, 2004.

35. Damjanovska L, Thabet MM, Levarth EW, et al: Diagnostic value of anti-MCV antibodies in differentiating early inflammatory arthritis, *Ann Rheum Dis* 69:730, 2010.

36. Pruijn GJ, Wiik A, van Venrooij WJ: The use of citrullinated peptides and proteins for the diagnosis of rheumatoid arthritis, *Arthritis Res Ther* 12:203, 2010.

37. van de Stadt LA, van der Horst AR, de Koning MH, et al: The extent of the anti-citrullinated protein antibody repertoire is associated with arthritis development in patients with seropositive arthralgia, *Ann Rheum Dis* 70:128, 2011.

38. Deane KD, O'Donnell CI, Hueber W, et al: The number of elevated cytokines and chemokines in preclinical seropositive rheumatoid arthritis predicts time to diagnosis in an age-dependent manner, *Arthritis Rheum* 62:3161, 2010.

40. López-Longo FJ, Oliver-Miñarro D, de la Torre I, et al: Association between anti-cyclic citrullinated peptide antibodies and ischemic heart disease in patients with rheumatoid arthritis, *Arthritis Rheum* 61:419, 2009.

41. Haisma EM, Levarht EW, van der Woude D, et al: Anti-cyclic citrullinated peptide antibodies from rheumatoid arthritis patients activate complement via both the classical and alternative pathways, *Arthritis Rheum* 60:1923, 2009.

44. Hill JA, Bell DA, Brintnell W, et al: Arthritis induced by posttranslationally modified (citrullinated) fibrinogen in DR4-IE transgenic mice, *J Exp Med* 205:967, 2008.

47. Bäcklund J, Carlsen S, Höger T, et al: Predominant selection of T cells specific for the glycosylated collagen type II epitope (263–270) in humanized transgenic mice and in rheumatoid arthritis, *Proc Natl Acad Sci U S A* 10:1073, 2002.

50. Kouskoff V, Korganow AS, Duchatelle V, et al: Organ-specific disease provoked by systemic autoimmunity, *Cell* 87:811, 1996.

51. Mandik-Nayak L, Allen PM: Initiation of an autoimmune response: insights from a transgenic model of rheumatoid arthritis, *Immunol Res* 32:5, 2005.

53. Nell-Duxneuner V, Machold K, Stamm T, et al: Autoantibody profiling in patients with very early rheumatoid arthritis: a follow-up study, *Ann Rheum Dis* 69:169, 2010.

54. Nell VP, Machold KP, Stamm TA, et al: Autoantibody profiling as early diagnostic and prognostic tool for rheumatoid arthritis, *Ann Rheum Dis* 64:1731, 2005.

55. Corr M, Zvaifler NJ: Mesenchymal precursor cells, *Ann Rheum Dis* 61:3, 2002.

56. Revell PA, Mapp PI, Lalor PA, Hall PA: Proliferative activity of cells in the synovium as demonstrated by a monoclonal antibody, Ki67, *Rheumatol Int* 7:183, 1987.

57. Valencia X, Higgins JM, Kiener HP, et al: Cadherin-11 provides specific cellular adhesion between fibroblast-like synoviocytes, *J Exp Med* 200:1673, 2004.

58. Kiener HP, Watts GF, Cui Y, et al: Synovial fibroblasts self-direct multicellular lining architecture and synthetic function in three-dimensional organ culture, *Arthritis Rheum* 62:742, 2010.

59. van der Pouw Kraan TC, van Gaalen FA, Kasperkovitz PV, et al: Rheumatoid arthritis is a heterogeneous disease: evidence for differences in the activation of the STAT-1 pathway between rheumatoid tissues, *Arthritis Rheum* 48:2132, 2003.

60. Lafyatis R, Remmers EF, Roberts AB, et al: Anchorage-independent growth of synoviocytes from arthritis and normal joints: stimulation by exogenous platelet-derived growth factor and inhibition by transforming growth factor-beta and retinoids, *J Clin Invest* 83:1267, 1989.

61. Imamura F, Aono H, Hasunuma T, et al: Monoclonal expansion of synoviocytes in rheumatoid arthritis, *Arthritis Rheum* 41:1979, 1998.

62. Muller-Ladner L, Kriegsmann J, Franklin BN, et al: Synovial fibroblasts of patients with rheumatoid arthritis attach to and invade normal human cartilage when engrafted into SCID mice, *Am J Pathol* 149:1607, 1996.

64. Cañete JD, Santiago B, Cantaert T, et al: Ectopic lymphoid neogenesis in psoriatic arthritis, *Ann Rheum Dis* 66:720, 2007.

65. Cantaert T, Kolln J, Timmer T, et al: B lymphocyte autoimmunity in rheumatoid synovitis is independent of ectopic lymphoid neogenesis, *J Immunol* 181:785, 2008.

66. Manzo A, Paoletti S, Carulli M, et al: Systematic microanatomical analysis of CXCL13 and CCL21 in situ production and progressive lymphoid organization in rheumatoid synovitis, *Eur J Immunol* 35:1347, 2005.

68. Kang YM, Zhang X, Wagner UG, et al: CD8 T cells are required for the formation of ectopic germinal centers in rheumatoid synovitis, *J Exp Med* 195:1325, 2002.

69. Kim WJ, Kang YJ, Koh EM, et al: LIGHT is involved in the pathogenesis of rheumatoid arthritis by inducing the expression of proinflammatory cytokines and MMP-9 in macrophages, *Immunology* 114:272, 2005.

71. Warrington KJ, Takemura S, Goronzy JJ, Wayland CM: CD4+, CD28− T cells in rheumatoid arthritis patients combine features of the innate and adaptive immune systems, *Arthritis Rheum* 44:13, 2001.

72. Hirota K, Yoshitomi H, Hashimoto M, et al: Preferential recruitment of CCR6-expressing Th17 cells to inflamed joints via CCL20 in rheumatoid arthritis and its animal model, *J Exp Med* 204:2803, 2007.

74. Brennan FM, Hayes AL, Ciesielski CJ, et al: Evidence that rheumatoid arthritis synovial T cells are similar to cytokine-activated T cells: involvement of phosphatidylinositol 3-kinase and nuclear factor kappaB pathways in tumor necrosis factor alpha production in rheumatoid arthritis, *Arthritis Rheum* 46:31, 2002.

78. Seyler TM, Park YW, Takemura S, et al: BLyS and APRIL in rheumatoid arthritis, *J Clin Invest* 115:3083, 2005.

80. Clausen BE, Bridges SL Jr, Lavelle JC, et al: Clonally-related immunoglobulin VH domains and nonrandom use of DH gene segments in rheumatoid arthritis synovium, *Mol Med* 4:240, 1998.

81. Kavanaugh A, Rosengren S, Lee SJ, et al: Assessment of rituximab's immunomodulatory synovial effects (ARISE trial). 1: clinical and synovial biomarker results, *Ann Rheum Dis* 67:402, 2008.

83. Humby F, Bombardieri M, Manzo A, et al: Ectopic lymphoid structures support ongoing production of class-switched autoantibodies in rheumatoid synovium, *PLoS Med* 6:e1, 2009.

86. Lee DM, Friend DS, Gurish MF, et al: Mast cells: a cellular link between autoantibodies and inflammatory arthritis, *Science* 297:1689, 2002.

88. Hueber AJ, Asquith DL, Miller AM, et al: Mast cells express IL-17A in rheumatoid arthritis synovium, *J Immunol* 184:3336, 2010.

90. Dalbeth N, Gundle R, Davies RJ, et al: CD56bright NK cells are enriched at inflammatory sites and can engage with monocytes in a reciprocal program of activation, *J Immunol* 173:6418, 2004.

91. Marinova-Mutafchieva L, Williams RO, Funa K, et al: Inflammation is preceded by tumor necrosis factor-dependent infiltration of mesenchymal cells in experimental arthritis, *Arthritis Rheum* 46:507, 2002.

95. Boyle DL, Jones TL, Hammaker D, et al: Regulation of peripheral inflammation by spinal p38 MAP kinase in rats, *PLoS Med* 3(9):e338, 2006.

96. Han Z, Boyle DL, Manning AM, Firestein GS: AP-1 and NF-κB regulation in rheumatoid arthritis and murine collagen-induced arthritis, *Autoimmunity* 28:197, 1998.

98. Fukushima A, Boyle DL, Corr M, Firestein GS: Kinetic analysis of synovial signalling and gene expression in animal models of arthritis, *Ann Rheum Dis* 69:918, 2010.

100. Jonsson H, Allen P, Peng SL: Inflammatory arthritis requires Foxo3a to prevent Fas ligand-induced neutrophil apoptosis, *Nat Med* 11:666, 2005.

101. Firestein GS, Berger AE, Tracey DE, et al: IL-1 receptor antagonist protein production and gene expression in rheumatoid arthritis and osteoarthritis synovium, *J Immunol* 149:1054, 1992.

102. Maurice MM, Nakamura H, van der Voort EA, et al: Evidence for the role of an altered redox state in hyporesponsiveness of synovial T cells in rheumatoid arthritis, *Immunology* 158:1458, 1997.

103. Vergunst CE, Gerlag DM, Dinant H, et al: Blocking the receptor for C5a in patients with rheumatoid arthritis does not reduce synovial inflammation, *Rheumatology (Oxford)* 46:1773, 2007.

104. Siegle I, Klein T, Backman JT, et al: Expression of cyclooxygenase 1 and cyclooxygenase 2 in human synovial tissue: differential elevation of cyclooxygenase 2 in inflammatory joint diseases, *Arthritis Rheum* 41:122, 1998.

105. Yao C, Sakata D, Esaki Y, et al: Prostaglandin E2-EP4 signaling promotes immune inflammation through Th1 cell differentiation and Th17 cell expansion, *Nat Med* 15:633, 2009.

110. Firestein GS, Xu WD, Townsend K, et al: Cytokines in chronic inflammatory arthritis. I. Failure to detect T cell lymphokines (interleukin 2 and interleukin 3) and presence of macrophage colony-stimulating factor (CSF-1) and a novel mast cell growth factor in rheumatoid synovitis, *J Exp Med* 168:1573, 1988.

111. Raza K, Falciani F, Curnow SJ, et al: Early rheumatoid arthritis is characterized by a distinct and transient synovial fluid cytokine profile of T cell and stromal cell origin, *Arthritis Res Ther* 7:R784, 2005.

112. Chabaud M, Durand JM, Buchs N, et al: Human interleukin-17: A T cell-derived proinflammatory cytokine produced by the rheumatoid synovium, *Arthritis Rheum* 43:963, 1999.

115. Ehrenstein MR, Evans JG, Singh A, Moore S, et al: Compromised function of regulatory T cells in rheumatoid arthritis and reversal by anti-TNFalpha therapy, *J Exp Med* 200:277, 2004.

116. Ruprecht CR, Gattorno M, Ferlito F, et al: Coexpression of CD25 and CD27 identifies FoxP3+ regulatory T cells in inflamed synovia, *J Exp Med* 201:1793, 2005.

118. Morgan ME, Flierman R, van Duivenvoorde LM, et al: Effective treatment of collagen-induced arthritis by adoptive transfer of CD25+ regulatory T cells, *Arthritis Rheum* 52:2212, 2005.

119. Chomarat P, Banchereau J, Miossec P: Differential effects of interleukins 10 and 4 on the production of interleukin-6 by blood and synovium monocytes in rheumatoid arthritis, *Arthritis Rheum* 38:1046, 1995.

123. Hueber W, Patel DD, Dryja T, et al: Effects of AIN457, a fully human antibody to interleukin-17A, on psoriasis, rheumatoid arthritis, and uveitis, *Sci Transl Med* 2:52ra72, 2010.

126. McInnes IB, Leung BP, Sturrock RD, et al: Interleukin-15 mediates T cell-dependent regulation of tumor necrosis factor-alpha production in rheumatoid arthritis, *Nat Med* 3:189–195, 1997.

127. Firestein GS, Alvaro-Gracia JM, Maki R: Quantitative analysis of cytokine gene expression in rheumatoid arthritis, *J Immunol* 144:3347, 1990.

128. Genovese MC, Cohen S, Moreland L, et al: Combination therapy with etanercept and anakinra in the treatment of patients with rheumatoid arthritis who have been treated unsuccessfully with methotrexate, *Arthritis Rheum* 50:1412, 2004.

130. Xu D, Jiang HR, Kewin P, et al: IL-33 exacerbates antigen-induced arthritis by activating mast cells, *Proc Natl Acad Sci U S A* 105:10913, 2008.

131. Georgopoulos S, Plows D, Kollias G: Transmembrane TNF is sufficient to induce localized tissue toxicity and chronic inflammatory arthritis in transgenic mice, *J Inflamm* 46:86,1996.

133. Lipsky PE, van der Heijde DM, St Clair EW, et al: Infliximab and methotrexate in the treatment of rheumatoid arthritis. Anti-tumor necrosis factor trial in rheumatoid arthritis with concomitant therapy study group, *N Engl J Med* 343:1594, 2000.

134. Nishimoto N, Yoshizaki K, Miyasaka N, et al: Treatment of rheumatoid arthritis with humanized anti-interleukin-6 receptor antibody: a multicenter, double-blind, placebo-controlled trial, *Arthritis Rheum* 50:1761, 2004.

136. Joosten LA, Netea MG, Kim SH, et al: IL-32, a proinflammatory cytokine in rheumatoid arthritis, *Proc Natl Acad Sci U S A* 103:3298, 2006.

137. Xu WD, Firestein GS, Taetle R, et al: Cytokines in chronic inflammatory arthritis. II. Granulocyte-macrophage colony-stimulating factor in rheumatoid synovial effusions, *J Clin Invest* 83:876, 1989.

138. Koch AE, Kunkel SL, Burrows JC, et al: Synovial tissue macrophage as a source of the chemotactic cytokine IL-8, *J Immunol* 147:2187, 1991.

140. Schmutz C, Hulme A, Burman A, et al: Chemokine receptors in the rheumatoid synovium: upregulation of CXCR5, *Arthritis Res Ther* 7:R217, 2005.

141. Nanki T, Urasaki Y, Imai T, et al: Inhibition of fractalkine ameliorates murine collagen-induced arthritis, *J Immunol* 173:7010, 2004.

142. Haringman JJ, Smeets TJ, Reinders-Blankert P, Tak PP: Chemokine and chemokine receptor expression in paired peripheral blood mononuclear cells and synovial tissue of patients with rheumatoid arthritis, osteoarthritis, and reactive arthritis, *Ann Rheum Dis* 65:294, 2006.

143. Camps M, Ruckle T, Ji H, et al: Blockade of PI3Kgamma suppresses joint inflammation and damage in mouse models of rheumatoid arthritis, *Nat Med* 11:936, 2005.

147. Tak PP, Gerlag DM, Aupperle KB, et al: Inhibitor of nuclear factor kappaB kinase beta is a key regulator of synovial inflammation, *Arthritis Rheum* 44:1897, 2001.

148. Han Z, Boyle DL, Manning AM, Firestein GS: AP-1 and NF-kB regulation in rheumatoid arthritis and murine collagen-induced arthritis, *Autoimmunity* 28:197, 1998.

151. Han Z, Boyle DL, Chang L, et al: c-Jun N-terminal kinase is required for metalloproteinase expression and joint destruction in inflammatory arthritis, *J Clin Invest* 108:73, 2001.

157. van der Pouw Kraan TC, van Gaalen FA, Kasperkovitz PV, et al: Rheumatoid arthritis is a heterogeneous disease: evidence for differences in the activation of the STAT-1 pathway between rheumatoid tissues, *Arthritis Rheum* 48:2132, 2003.

161. Weinblatt ME, Kavanaugh A, Burgos-Vargas R, et al: Treatment of rheumatoid arthritis with a Syk kinase inhibitor: a twelve-week, randomized, placebo-controlled trial, *Arthritis Rheum* 58:3309, 2008.

166. Pap T, Franz JK, Hummel KM, et al: Activation of synovial fibroblasts in rheumatoid arthritis: lack of expression of the tumour suppressor PTEN at sites of invasive growth and destruction, *Arthritis Res* 2:59, 2000.

168. Scatizzi JC, Hutcheson J, Pope RM, et al: Bim-Bcl-2 homology 3 mimetic therapy is effective at suppressing inflammatory arthritis through the activation of myeloid cell apoptosis, *Arthritis Rheum* 62:441, 2010.

170. Yamanishi Y, Boyle DL, Pinkoski MJ, et al: Regulation of joint destruction and inflammation by p53 in collagen-induced arthritis, *Am J Pathol* 160:123, 2002.

173. Firestein GS, Echeverri F, Yeo M, et al: Somatic mutations in the p53 tumor suppressor gene in rheumatoid arthritis synovium, *Proc Natl Acad Sci U S A* 94:10895, 1997.

175. Izquierdo E, Cañete JD, Celis R, et al: Immature blood vessels in rheumatoid synovium are selectively depleted in response to anti-TNF therapy, *PLoS One* 4:e8131, 2009.

177. Cramer T, Yamanishi Y, Clausen BE, et al: HIF-1alpha is essential for myeloid cell-mediated inflammation, *Cell* 112:645, 2003.

178. Koch AE, Halloran MM, Haskell CJ, et al: Angiogenesis mediated by soluble forms of E-selectin and vascular cell adhesion molecule-1, *Nature* 376:517, 1995.

179. Peacock DJ, Banquerigo ML, Brahn E: Angiogenesis inhibition suppresses collagen arthritis, *J Exp Med* 175:1135, 1992.

181. Storgard CM, Stupack DG, Jonczyk A, et al: Decreased angiogenesis and arthritis in rabbits treated with an αvβ3 antagonist, *J Clin Invest* 103:47, 1998.

184. Issekutz TB, Issekutz AC: T lymphocyte migration to arthritic joints and dermal inflammation in the rat: differing migration patterns and the involvement of VLA-4, *Clin Immunol Immunopathol* 61:436, 1991.

189. Lee DM, Kiener HP, Agarwal SK, et al: Cadherin-11 in synovial lining formation and pathology in arthritis, *Science* 315:1006, 2007.

190. Wolfe GC, MacNaul KL, Buechel FF, et al: Differential in vivo expression of collagenase messenger RNA in synovium and cartilage: quantitative comparison with stromelysin messenger RNA levels in human rheumatoid arthritis and osteoarthritis patients and in two animal models of acute inflammatory arthritis, *Arthritis Rheum* 36:1540, 1993.

192. Mudgett JS, Hutchinson NI, Chartrain NA, et al: Susceptibility of stromelysin 1–deficient mice to collagen-induced arthritis and cartilage destruction, *Arthritis Rheum* 41:110, 1998.

194. Hou WS, Li W, Keyszer G, et al: Comparison of cathepsins K and S expression within the rheumatoid and osteoarthritic synovium, *Arthritis Rheum* 46:663, 2002.

195. Svelander L, Erlandsson-Harris H, Astner L, et al: Inhibition of cathepsin K reduces bone erosion, cartilage degradation and inflammation evoked by collagen-induced arthritis in mice, *Eur J Pharmacol* 613:155, 2009.

196. Lark MW, Bayne EK, Flanagan J, et al: Aggrecan degradation in human cartilage: evidence for both matrix metalloproteinase and aggrecanase activity in normal, osteoarthritic, and rheumatoid joints, *J Clin Invest* 100:93, 1997.

197. Yamanishi Y, Boyle DL, Clark M, et al: Expression and regulation of aggrecanase in arthritis: the role of TGF-beta, *J Immunol* 168:1405, 2002.

198. Stanton H, Rogerson FM, East CJ, et al: ADAMTS5 is the major aggrecanase in mouse cartilage in vivo and in vitro, *Nature* 434:648, 2005.

200. Kong YY, Feige U, Sarosi I, et al: Activated T cells regulate bone loss and joint destruction in adjuvant arthritis through osteoprotegerin ligand, *Nature* 402:304–309, 1999.

201. Kotake S, Udagawa N, Hakoda M, et al: Activated human T cells directly induce osteoclastogenesis from human monocytes: possible role of T cells in bone destruction in rheumatoid arthritis patients, *Arthritis Rheum* 44:1003, 2001.

203. Diarra D, Stolina M, Polzer K, et al: Dickkopf-1 is a master regulator of joint remodeling, *Nat Med* 13:156, 2007.

204. Sen M, Chamorro M, Reifert J, et al: Blockade of Wnt-5A/frizzled 5 signaling inhibits rheumatoid synoviocyte activation, *Arthritis Rheum* 44:772, 2001.

Full references for this chapter can be found on www.expertconsult.com.

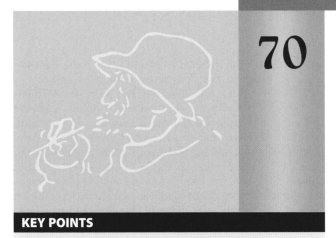

70

Clinical Features of Rheumatoid Arthritis

SUSAN E. SWEENEY •
EDWARD D. HARRIS, Jr. •
GARY S. FIRESTEIN

KEY POINTS

Rheumatoid arthritis is a symmetric inflammatory polyartciular arthritis that mainly affects the small joints of the hands and feet.

Larger joints can be involved, usually later and in a symmetric fashion.

Cartilage destruction and bone erosions are common, especially in rheumatoid factor–positive or anticitrullinated protein antibody–positive patients.

Uncontrolled synovitis can lead to severe deformity, loss of function, and increased mortality due to accelerated atherosclerosis.

Early therapy with aggressive treatment goals improves long-term outcomes in rheumatoid arthritis.

Systemic manifestations include rheumatoid nodules, pulmonary disease, vasculitis, serositis, and eye disease.

EPIDEMIOLOGY AND THE BURDEN OF DISEASE

The prevalence of rheumatoid arthritis (RA) in most populations is around 1% in most populations, with an incidence in women twice that in men. This number was based on many studies of population samples,[1-3] which varied among the surveys from 0.3% to 1.5%. The prevalence of RA in some populations might be changing, however, as suggested by more recent data on incidence rates in different decades. The incidence of RA in Rochester, Minnesota, decreased by 50% between 1950 and 1974. Differences between incidence and prevalence are enhanced by the realization that as the population ages, the prevalence of RA may increase or stay the same, regardless of short term trends in incidence simply because individuals with RA are living longer.

The incidence of RA increases during adulthood, except among men in their 40s through 60s. In Olmsted County, Minnesota, the increased incidence with increasing age continues until age 85, after which the incidence declines.[4] In a 10-year extension of this study, the age-adjusted and sex-adjusted incidence per 100,000 population decreased from 62 in the decade 1955 to 1964 to 32.7 in the decade 1985 to 1994.[5] The decrease was more prominent in women than in men, and the average age at onset of the disease shifted upward. Perhaps more intriguing were cyclic patterns of incidence within decades, suggesting the influence of environmental factors. One explanation for the decline in incidence and the shift toward older age at onset is a birth cohort effect, the greatest impact of which is seen early

in life.[6] A recent update from the Olmsted County, Minnesota, cohort of RA patients from 1955-2007 examined trends in the incidence and prevalence of RA from 1995-2007. During the more recent time period, the incidence of RA in women, but not in men, increased moderately.[7] Causes for this trend reversal in women were not determined but might involve environmental factors. Current incidence rates using this same population-based study of Minnesota patients revealed that the lifetime risk of RA among U.S. adults is 3.6% for women and 1.7% for men.[8]

Throughout the world, pockets of ethnic groups have a much higher incidence of RA. Native Americans constitute one of these groups. In one geographic area between 1986 and 1994, non–Native American populations had an RA prevalence of 1.1% to 0.9%, whereas the prevalence among Algonquian Indians in the same region ranged from 2% to 2.1%, and disease onset was seen 12 years earlier in the Native American population. Among Pima Indians, who bear a very high incidence of RA, a decline in incidence has been correlated with a decrease in seropositivity for rheumatoid factor (RF). The highest likelihood of seropositivity was noted in Pima Indians born at the turn of the 20th century, and seropositivity has decreased ever since that time. This provides additional supportive evidence for a birth cohort effect.[9]

Although newer, more effective therapy for rheumatoid patients has led to reduced morbidity and disability from the disease, dollar costs for RA, which recently surpassed the cost per patient for diabetes, are still substantial. In a panel of individuals with RA in San Francisco followed for 15 years, medical care costs for RA averaged $5,919 per year, and additional costs of $2,582 were incurred for medical but non-RA reasons.[10] More than half of these costs were generated by hospitalization, with some patients bearing costs greater than $85,000/year while their function declined. In another cohort of 4258 patients with RA followed for 17,085 patient-years, lifetime direct medical care costs were estimated to be $93,296.[11]

RISK FACTORS

A predisposition to RA appears to be multifactorial based on the following: (1) Relatively few identical twins have RA (about 15%), even though concordance for the disease is much more likely in twins than in the normal population; (2) despite the powerful influence of the "shared epitope" on HLA-DRB chains in predisposing to the severity of disease, this susceptibility allele is not a risk factor in certain population studies; and (3) the combination of many gene

Supplemental images available on the Expert Consult Premium Edition website.

polymorphisms confers a modestly increased risk for disease. A reasonable hypothesis is that the genetic predisposition to RA involves a propensity to autoimmune responses, but that repeated exposure to environmental agents is ultimately responsible for tipping the balance from subclinical autoimmunity to diseases such as RA. Many of the risk factors for RA are discussed in Chapter 69, especially genetic associations, environmental exposures, and the role of autoantibodies.

CLINICAL PRESENTATIONS OF EARLY RHEUMATOID ARTHRITIS

In the Northern hemisphere, the onset of RA is more frequent in winter than in summer. In several series, onset of RA from October to March in the Northern hemisphere was found to be twice as frequent as in the other 6 months.[12] The appearance of RF or anticitrullinated protein antibodies (ACPAs), also referred to as anticyclic citrullinated protein antibodies (anti-CCPs), often precedes symptoms of arthritis in patients. Approximately half of patients with RA have specific serologic abnormalities several years before the onset of symptoms. A finding of an elevated serum level of immunoglobulin (Ig)M-RF or anti-CCP in a healthy person correlates with increased risk of developing RA.[13] This is especially important in light of the new criteria for RA classification in early RA because symptoms can be minimal for some of those who meet the criteria for diagnosis (see later).

Patterns of Onset

Insidious Onset

RA has an insidious, slow onset over weeks to months in 55% to 65% of cases.[14] The initial symptoms may be systemic or articular. In some people, fatigue, malaise, swollen hands, and diffuse musculoskeletal pain may be the first nonspecific symptoms, with joints becoming involved later. Involvement of tendon sheaths early in the process can focus attention on periarticular structures. In retrospect, the patient often can identify one joint that was involved first, quickly followed by the others. Asymmetric initial presentations (often with increased symmetry developing later in the course of disease) are common. The reason for the symmetry of joint involvement compared with other forms of arthritis, such as the seronegative spondyloarthropathies, is unknown.

Morning stiffness is a cardinal sign of inflammatory arthritis that can appear even before pain and may be related to the accumulation of edema fluid within inflamed tissues during sleep. Morning stiffness dissipates as edema and products of inflammation are absorbed by lymphatics and venules and returned to the circulation by motion accompanying the use of muscles and joints. To be specific for joint inflammation, morning stiffness (e.g., "difficulty moving around") should persist for at least 30 to 45 minutes before disappearing. A similar "gel" phenomenon can occur if a person is inactive during the day.

It is rare for symptoms to remit completely in one set of joints while developing in another. This quality of arthritis

sets RA apart from rheumatic fever or palindromic rheumatism, in which a true migratory pattern of arthritis is common. A subtle, early change in RA is the development of muscle atrophy around affected joints. Muscle efficiency and strength become diminished. As a result, weakness develops that can be out of proportion to pain. Opening doors, climbing stairs, and doing repetitive work rapidly become more demanding. A low-grade fever without chills is rarely present. Depression and anxiety can accentuate symptoms. A small but significant weight loss is common and reflects the catabolic effects of cytokines and associated anorexia.

Acute or Intermediate Onset

Among patients with RA, 8% to 15% have an acute onset of symptoms that peak within a few days. Rarely, a patient can pinpoint the onset of symptoms to a specific time or activity. Symptoms mount, with pain developing in other joints, often in a less symmetric pattern than in patients who have an insidious onset. Acute-onset RA is difficult to diagnose, and sepsis or vasculitis should be ruled out. Fever, suggesting an infectious process, can rarely be a prominent sign. An intermediate type of onset, in which symptoms develop over days or weeks, occurs in 15% to 20% of patients. Systemic complaints are more noticeable than in the insidious type of onset.

Joint Involvement

The joints most commonly involved first in RA are the metacarpophalangeal (MCP) joints, the proximal interphalangeal (PIP) joints, the metatarsophalangeal joints, and the wrists (Table 70-1).[15] Larger joints generally become symptomatic after small joints. Synovitis in large joints is likely to remain asymptomatic for a longer time than in smaller ones, and a biopsy specimen of an asymptomatic knee often shows histologic evidence of synovitis.[16] One anatomic study correlated the area, in square centimeters, of synovial membrane with that of hyaline cartilage in each joint. Joints with the highest ratio of synovium to articular

Table 70-1 Distribution of Joints Involved in Attacks Based on Cumulative Experience with 227 Patients

Joint Involvement	% Patients (Mean)	% Patients (Range)
MCP, PIP	91	74-100
Wrists	78	54-82
Knees	64	41-94
Shoulders	65	33-75
Ankles	50	10-67
Feet	43	15-73
Elbows	38	13-60
Hips	17	0-40
Temporomandibular	8	0-28
Spine	4	0-11
Sternoclavicular	2	0-6
Peri-articular sites	27	20-29

MCP, metacarpophalangeal; PIP, proximal interphalangeal.
Modified from Guerne P-A, Weisman MH: Palindromic rheumatism: part of or apart from the spectrum of rheumatoid arthritis, *Am J Med* 16:451-460, 1992. Copyright 1992, with permission from Excerpta Medica, Inc.

cartilage correlated positively with those most frequently involved in the disease (see Table 70-1).[17]

Early Synovitis: Which Patients Develop Rheumatoid Arthritis?

Distinguishing early RA from other inflammatory arthropathies can be challenging. In its earliest stages, RA might involve only a few joints and may not show the typical symmetric distribution. What diagnostic clues can be used to determine who will progress to classic RA, and who will develop an alternative inflammatory arthritis such as one of the spondyloarthropathies or have a spontaneous remission? The implications for disease management are obvious because early treatment potentially could limit or prevent joint damage and possibly permit long-term remission or even cure. Because 30% to 40% of patients with early inflammatory synovitis have spontaneous remission, accurate identification of patients with RA is essential to avoid undertreatment and overtreatment.

Some of these questions have been addressed by the Leiden Early Arthritis Clinic, which evaluates patients with symptoms of less than 2 years' duration (most patients have symptoms for less than 6 months). In this cohort, only about 20% of patients met criteria for RA when initially evaluated by a rheumatologist.[18] One-third of patients defied categorization and were considered to have "undifferentiated arthritis." When this group of patients was followed for 1 year, 27% ultimately developed RA, and 40% remained undifferentiated. Clinical features that were more commonly seen among patients who developed RA included greater numbers of joints involved (mean of seven joints vs. four joints), longer duration of morning stiffness (90 minutes vs. 60 minutes), and the presence of autoantibodies. These features were insufficient individually to permit early diagnosis of RA, although a composite scoring system has been proposed.[19] The predictive value of this system approaches 90%.

Additional studies from the Leiden Early Arthritis Clinic show that assessment and management of patients with symptoms of less than 12 weeks' duration by a rheumatologist was associated with decreased joint destruction and increased likelihood of disease-modifying antirheumatic drug (DMARD)-free remission.[20] Treatment of early inflammatory synovitis with methotrexate therapy delays progression to RA, but disease ultimately progresses to RA if the medication is discontinued[21] (see Chapter 42).

Among predictive features most likely to be useful in patients, serum autoantibodies might be the most important. ACPAs, in particular, are strongly associated with the evolution of undifferentiated arthritis into RA and progression to erosive disease. In addition, the diversity of citrullinated peptides recognized by ACPAs increased during the period preceding onset of disease in patients who progressed to RA, suggesting that epitope spreading plays a role in the evolution of disease.[22] Other autoantibodies have also been used in a diagnostic algorithm for patients with very early synovitis (symptoms of <3 months' duration), including RFs, anticitrullinated protein, and anti-RA33.[23] Through stepwise analysis of each antibody, RA could be diagnosed in 72% of patients and confirmed by subsequent clinical course and development of RA.

Other Patterns of Disease Onset or Variants of Disease

Palindromic Pattern

Palindromic rheumatism was described by Hench and Rosenberg in 1942. Pain usually begins with pain in one joint or in periarticular tissues; symptoms worsen for several hours to a few days and are associated with swelling and erythema. Then, in reverse sequence, symptoms resolve, leaving no residua. Table 70-2 lists joints involved in a series of 227 patients. An intercritical period, similar to that of gout, is asymptomatic. Half of patients with palindromic rheumatism go on to develop RA, particularly those with HLA-DR4. In a compilation of patients from nine series, only 15% became asymptomatic after at least 5 years with a palindromic syndrome (see Table 70-2).[24] In the remainder, multiple joints became involved, swelling did not subside completely between attacks, and tests for RF became positive. Neither the characteristics of joint fluid nor the pathologic findings of synovial biopsy specimens allow the prediction that RA will evolve from palindromic rheumatism,[25] although it may be worthwhile to measure ACPAs in these people.[26] Those who do not develop RA rarely have constitutional symptoms, and involved joints show no erosion because the synovitis does not become chronic. A more recent study of long-term outcomes in 60 patients diagnosed with palindromic rheumatism revealed that two-thirds of patients developed chronic arthritis, and the risk for chronic arthritis remained for longer than 10 years.[27] Of 51 patients with palindromic rheumatism, 41 experienced marked improvement in frequency and duration of attacks during treatment with antimalarials.[28] The use of antimalarials might reduce the risk of progression to RA.

Table 70-2 Evolution of Patients with Palindromic Rheumatism in Nine Series*

	No. of Cases	Remission or Cure (%)	Persistent PR (%)	RA (%)	Other Diseases (%)
Total or average	653	15 ± 14	48 ± 20	33 ± 17	4 ± 5

*In nine series of patients (653 total), the number undergoing remission or cure, remaining palindromic, evolving toward rheumatoid arthritis (RA), or developing another disease is expressed as an average percentage of the total patient population.

PR, Palindromic rheumatism; RA, rheumatoid arthritis.

Modified from Guerne P-A, Weisman MH: Palindromic rheumatism: part of or apart from the spectrum of rheumatoid arthritis, *Am J Med* 16:451-460, 1992. Copyright 1992, with permission from Excerpta Medica, Inc.

Insidious Onset in Older Individuals

Older individuals (≥65 years old) who develop RA often present with stiffness, limb girdle pain, and diffuse swelling of the hands, wrists, and forearms. Clinical onset that mimics polymyalgia rheumatica or remitting seronegative synovitis with pitting edema (RS3PE) also can occur in the elderly. Individuals with onset at age 60 years or older are less likely to have subcutaneous nodules or RF at the onset of disease, despite the high prevalence of RF in the general population in this age group. Generally, elderly individuals who develop RA tend to have a more benign course than younger people; the frequency of positive tests for RF is lower, but a strong association with HLA-DR4 has been noted. Onset is slow, but stiffness is often incapacitating.

In a study of patients with RA of less than 15 months' duration, older patients had higher scores for joint space narrowing and osteophytes at baseline than patients younger than 55 years. However, no evidence suggested that older patients had more rapid progression of damage, indicating that osteoarthritis was responsible for a significant portion of the damage noted at the onset of disease.[29]

Arthritis Robustus

Arthritis robustus is not so much an unusual presentation of disease as an unusual reaction of patients to the disease.[30] Most patients are men whose disease is characterized by proliferative synovitis, often with deformity, which seems to cause little pain and even less disability. Patients are athletic and invariably keep working (often at physical labor). Periarticular osteopenia is unusual, whereas new bone proliferation at joint margins near significant erosions of bone and cartilage is common. Bulky subcutaneous nodules develop. Subchondral cysts also develop, presumably from excessive pressure caused by synovial fluid within a thick joint capsule during muscular effort.

Rheumatoid Nodulosis

Whether rheumatoid nodulosis is a variant subset of RA or a different entity has not been clarified. The clinical picture includes recurrent pain and swelling in different joints, radiologic subchondral bone cysts, and subcutaneous rheumatoid nodules. In one series of 16 patients followed over 12 years, 6 had an aggressive course indistinguishable from classic erosive polyarticular RA. In 7 patients, cholesterol crystals were found in fluid from the olecranon bursae. Second-line drugs helped articular disease but did not help other components of the process.[31]

COURSE AND COMPLICATIONS OF ESTABLISHED RHEUMATOID ARTHRITIS

Involvement of Specific Joints: Effects of Disease on Form and Function

The effects of rheumatoid synovitis on joints are a complex function of the intensity of the underlying disease, its chronicity, and the stress put on individual joints by the patient. Most well-documented observations of specific joint involvement and complications of the disease were reported in the decades before 1980. Since then, these observations have been refined, but few new data have become available. Despite advances in our understanding of the pathophysiology of RA, including delineation of the cellular and enzymatic pathways that destroy joints, guidelines for the practicing physician—so that the probability that an individual patient would go on to develop erosive disease requiring aggressive treatment can be determined—are only in early stages of development. The spectrum of the clinical course of RA can range from patients who have mild pauciarticular synovitis, with negative serum autoantibodies and few radiographic changes, to those who have unrelenting pain, synovitis, joint damage, and extra-articular manifestations.

Hands and Wrists

The hand and the wrist should be considered together because they form a functional unit. Data have linked disease of the wrist to ulnar deviation of the MCP joints.[32] The hypothesis is that weakening of the extensor carpi ulnaris muscle leads to radial deviation of the wrist as the carpal bones rotate (the proximal row in an ulnar direction and the distal ones in a radial direction). In response to this, ulnar deviation of the fingers (a "zigzag" deformity) keeps the tendons to the phalanges in a normal line with the radius. Other factors, including the tendency for a power grasp to pull the fingers into an ulnar attitude and inappropriate intrinsic muscle action, are also involved (Figure 70-1). Erosion of bone or articular cartilage is not essential for the development of ulnar deviation (Figure 70-2). Significant but reducible ulnar deviation can result from repeated synovitis or muscle weakness in the hands (e.g., in systemic lupus erythematosus, in Parkinson's disease).

Dorsal swelling on the wrist within the tendon sheaths of the extensor muscles is one of the earliest signs of disease. Typically, the extensor carpi ulnaris and extensor digitorum communis sheaths are involved. Rarely, cystic structures resembling ganglia are early findings of RA.

As synovial proliferation develops within the wrist, pressure increases within the relatively nondistensible joint spaces. Proliferative synovium develops enzymatic machinery sufficient to destroy ligaments, tendons, and the articular disk distal to the ulnar head. Pressure and enzymes combine to produce communications among radiocarpal, radioulnar, and midcarpal joints. The integrity of the distal radioulnar joint is lost. The ulnar collateral ligament, stretched by the proliferative synovium of the radioulnar joint, finally ruptures or is destroyed, and the ulnar head springs up into dorsal prominence, where it "floats" and is easily depressed by the examiner's fingers (piano key styloid).

On the volar side of the wrist, synovial protrusion cysts develop; they can be palpated, and their origins can be confirmed by arthrography. The thick transverse carpal ligament provides significant resistance to decompression, however, and the hyperplastic synovium can compress the median nerve, causing carpal tunnel syndrome, often bilaterally.

Progression of disease in the wrist may be characterized by radiographic loss of joint space and bone or by ankylosis (Figure 70-3A). Ultrasound of the wrist correlates with function and classic signs of inflammation and is a

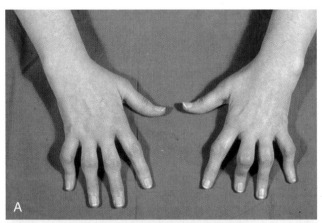

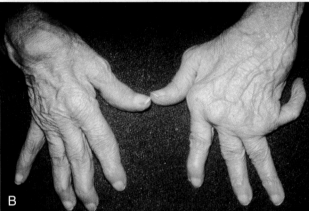

Figure 70-1 **A,** Polyarticular arthritis, especially with fusiform swelling of the proximal interphalangeal joints. Note deformity of wrists with radial deviation. **B,** Complete subluxation with marked ulnar deviation at the metacarpophalangeal joints in a patient with rheumatoid arthritis. The heads of the metacarpals are now in direct contact with the joint capsule instead of the proximal phalanges. *(Courtesy Iain McInnes, MD.)*

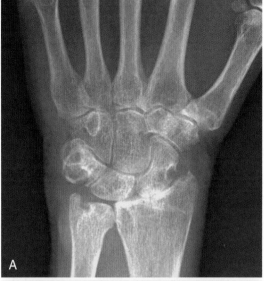

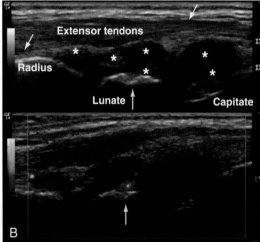

Figure 70-3 **A,** Typical sites of osseous erosion shown on radiographs of a rheumatoid wrist include triquetrum, pisiform, scaphoid, and radius. Erosions are also seen at the ulnar aspect of the distal radius and the distal ulnar styloid process secondary to involvement of the inferior radioulnar compartment. Diffuse cartilage loss is evident in the radiocarpal compartment. **B,** Ultrasound of the rheumatoid wrist dorsal longitudinal view shows synovial proliferation (*), tenosynovial thickening *(white arrows),* synovitis, and synovial hyperemia *(yellow arrows). Upper panel,* grayscale; *lower panel,* power Doppler mode. **(A,** *Courtesy Dr. Barbara Weissman.* **B,** *Courtesy Dr. Arnoldas Ceponis.)*

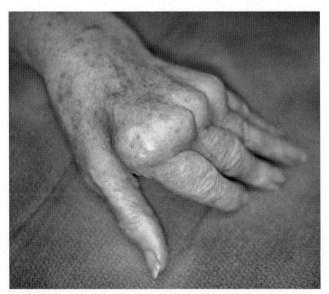

Figure 70-2 Ulnar deviation and subluxation. The hands show typical manifestations of end-stage erosive changes around the metacarpophalangeal joints, with volar dislocation and ulnar drift of the fingers. *(Copyright A.L. Ladd.)*

complementary tool in the evaluation of wrist arthritis in RA (Figure 70-3B). Early detection of carpal bone involvement by RA is also possible with magnetic resonance imaging (MRI), which reveals early synovial proliferation and carpal bone erosions. Bony ankylosis is associated with increased duration and severity of the disease and is found in joints that have been immobilized by pain, inflammation, treatment, or all of these.

The hand may have many joints involved in RA. A sensitive index of hand involvement is grip strength, which simulatneously stresses multiple hand joints. Muscular contraction causes ligamentous tightening around joints, compressing inflamed synovium. The immediate result is weakness, with or without pain; the reflex inhibition of muscular contraction due to pain may be a primary factor in this weakness. Quantitative radiographic scores for joint space narrowing, erosion, and malalignment correlate well with loss of motion but do not correlate with joint count tenderness scores[33]; these data support the concept that inflammatory synovitis and the erosive-destructive potential of proliferative synovitis in RA are not one and the same, but rather reflect different aspects of the same disease.

The swan neck deformity is one of flexion of the distal interphalangeal (DIP) and MCP joints with hyperextension of the PIP joint. The lesion probably begins with shortening of the interosseous muscles and tendons. Shortening of the intrinsic muscles exerts tension on the dorsal tendon sheath, leading to hyperextension of the PIP joint (Figure 70-4A).[34] Deep tendon contracture or, rarely, DIP joint involvement with RA leads to the DIP joint flexion. Marginal erosive changes in DIP joints occur more often in patients with RA who have coexisting osteoarthritis.[35]

If, during chronic inflammation of a PIP joint, the extensor hood stretches or is avulsed, the joint may pop up in flexion, producing a boutonnière deformity (Figure 70-4B). The DIP joint remains in hyperextension.

The most serious result of rheumatoid involvement of the hand is severe resorption of bone that begins at the articular cartilage and spreads along the diaphysis of involved phalanges. Digits appear shortened, excess skin folds are present, and phalanges can be retracted (telescoped) into one another and then pulled out into abnormally long extension, often without pain. With the availability of more effective therapy for RA, this complication has become rare.

Three types of deformity have been described for the thumb:
1. MCP inflammation leads to stretching of the joint capsule and a boutonnière-like deformity.
2. Inflammation of the carpometacarpal joint leads to volar subluxation during contracture of the adductor hallucis.
3. After prolonged disease of both MCP joints, exaggerated adduction of the first metacarpus, flexion of the MCP joint, and hyperextension of the DIP joint result from the patient's need to provide a means to pinch.

One of the most common manifestations of RA in the hands is tenosynovitis in flexor tendon sheaths; this can be a major cause of hand weakness.[36] Tenosynovitis manifests on the volar surfaces of the phalanges as diffuse swelling between joints or as a palpable grating within flexor tendon sheaths in the palm and may occur in half of RA patients.

It is particularly important to diagnose de Quervain's tenosynovitis of the extensors of the thumb because this condition causes severe discomfort and yet is easily treated. Pain originating from these sheaths can be shown by Finkelstein's test, that is, ulnar flexion at the wrist after the thumb is maximally flexed and adducted.

Frequently, rheumatoid nodules develop within tendon sheaths and may "lock" the finger painfully into fixed flexion or cause "trigger" fingers. When they are chronic or recurrent, it may be necessary to inject the tendon sheath or, if that fails, to remove it surgically.

Elbows

RA rarely manifests with severe pain in the elbow, perhaps because the elbow is a stable hinge joint. Nevertheless, involvement of the elbow is common, and if lateral stability at the elbow is lost as the disease progresses, disability can be severe.

The frequency of elbow involvement varies from 20% to 65%, depending on the severity of disease in the patient populations studied. One of the earliest findings, often unnoticed by the patient, is loss of full extension. Because the elbow is principally a connecting joint between the hand and the trunk, the shoulder and the wrists can compensate partially for the loss of elbow motion.

Shoulders

RA of the shoulder not only affects synovium within the glenohumeral joint but also involves the distal third of the clavicle, various bursae and the rotator cuff, and multiple muscles around the neck and chest wall. Severe shoulder pain is often bilateral and can lead to sleep disorders because of difficulty finding a comfortable position. Involvement of the rotator cuff in RA also has been recognized as a principal cause of morbidity. The function of the rotator cuff is to stabilize the humeral head in the glenoid. Weakness of the cuff results in superior subluxation. Rotator cuff tears or insufficiency from other causes can be shown by shoulder arthrography or MRI. In a series of 200 consecutive patients with RA studied by arthrography, 21% had rotator cuff tears, and an additional 24% had evidence of frayed

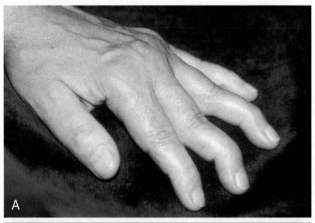
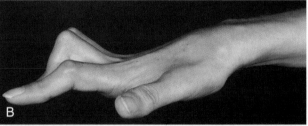

Figure 70-4 **A,** Swan neck deformity. This common deformity leads to hyperextension of the proximal interphalangeal joints and flexion of the distal interphalangeal joints. **B,** Boutonnière deformity. This deformity, which is the opposite of swan neck deformity, is marked by flexion of the proximal interphalangeal joints and extension of the distal interphalangeal joints. *(Courtesy Iain McInnes, MD.)*

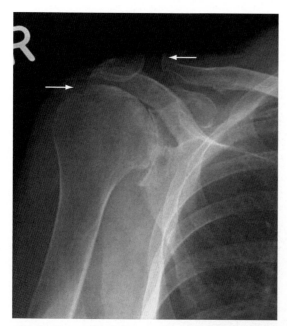

Figure 70-5 Abnormalities of the shoulder in rheumatoid arthritis. The Grashey posterior oblique view of a shoulder shows severe glenohumeral joint space narrowing with marginal erosion and cystic changes of the humeral head adjacent to the greater tuberosity *(lower arrow)*. Elevation of the humeral head with respect to the glenoid indicates chronic rotator cuff tear. Tapering of the distal end of the clavicle is seen, along with widening of the acromioclavicular joint *(upper arrow)*. *(Courtesy Dr. Barbara Weissman.)*

tendons.[37] One likely mechanism behind tears is that the rotator cuff tendon insertion into the greater tuberosity is vulnerable to erosion by the proliferative synovitis that develops there. Previous injury and aging may predispose to the development of tears. Sudden tears may be accompanied by pain and inflammation so great as to suggest infection.

Standard radiographic examinations of the shoulder in RA reveal erosions and superior subluxation (Figure 70-5). Arthrograms, in addition to showing tears of the rotator cuff, can show diffuse nodular filling defects, irregular capsular attachment, bursal filling defects, adhesive capsulitis, and dilation of the biceps tendon sheath (perhaps unique to RA).[38] High-resolution computed tomography (CT) or MRI may provide much of this information without the need for invasive techniques.

Marked soft tissue swelling of the anterolateral aspect of the shoulders in RA may be caused by chronic subacromial bursitis rather than by glenohumeral joint effusions. In contrast to rotator cuff tears, bursal swelling is not associated with decreased range of motion or pain. Synovial proliferation within the subdeltoid bursa might explain the resorption of the undersurface of the distal clavicle seen in this disease. Rarely, the shoulder joint may rupture, with symptoms resembling those of obstruction of venous return from the arm.

Temporomandibular Joints

The temporomandibular joint is commonly involved in RA. Histories reveal that 55% of patients have jaw symptoms at some time during the course of their disease. Radiographic examination reveals structural alterations in 78% of the joints examined. An overbite can develop as the mandibular condyle and the corresponding surface of the temporal bone, the eminentia articularis, are eroded. Physical examination of the rheumatoid patient should include palpation of the temporomandibular joint for tenderness and auscultation for crepitus. Occasionally, patients have acute pain and an inability to close the mouth, necessitating intra-articular glucocorticoid therapy to suppress the acute process.

Temporomandibular joint abnormalities are common in nonrheumatoid populations. The only specific findings for RA in the temporomandibular joint are erosions and cysts of the mandibular condyle detected by CT or MRI. No correlation has been noted between clinical and CT findings of the temporomandibular joint in RA.[39]

Cricoarytenoid Joints

The cricoarytenoid joints are small diarthrodial joints with an important function: They rotate with the vocal cords as the vocal cords abduct and adduct to vary the pitch and tone of the voice. Careful histories may reveal hoarseness in 30% of rheumatoid patients. This hoarseness is not disabling in itself, but the cricoarytenoid joints may become inflamed and immobilized, with the vocal cords adducted to the midline, causing inspiratory stridor. Autopsy examinations have shown cricoarytenoid arthritis in almost half of patients with RA, suggesting that much significant disease of the larynx may be asymptomatic. Although CT scans detected laryngeal abnormalities in 54% of patients with moderately severe RA, no symptoms suggested that these abnormalities would be found.[40] In contrast, findings on indirect laryngoscopy, which detected mucosal and gross functional abnormalities (including rheumatoid nodules), were abnormal in 32% of the same patients and correlated with symptoms of sore throat and difficult inspiration. It follows that the latter examination should be performed in symptomatic rheumatoid patients. Asymptomatic cricoarytenoid synovitis occasionally may lead to aspiration of pharyngeal contents, particularly at night.

Sternoclavicular and Manubriosternal Joints

Sternoclavicular and manubriosternal joints, both possessing synovium and a cartilaginous disk, are often involved in RA. Because of their relative immobility, few symptoms are reported. Patients occasionally describe pain in the sternoclavicular joints, however, while lying on their sides in bed. When symptoms do occur, the physician must be concerned about superimposed sepsis. CT or MRI is useful for careful delineation of the sternoclavicular joint. Manubriosternal involvement is almost never clinically important, although by tomographic criteria, it is common in RA.

Cervical Spine

In contrast to other nonsynovial joints, such as the manubriosternal joint or the symphysis pubis, diskovertebral joints in the cervical spine often manifest osteochondral destruction in RA and on lateral radiographs may be found

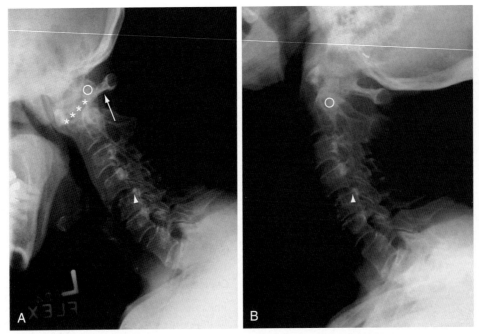

Figure 70-6   Rheumatoid arthritis of the cervical spine. **A,** Lateral radiograph in flexion shows severe anterior atlantoaxial subluxation with a wide anterior atlantodental interval *(asterisks)* and a decreased posterior atlantodental interval *(arrow).* **B,** Almost complete reduction of subluxation is noted on the lateral view in extension. Subaxial subluxation is evident at the level of C4-C5 *(arrowheads)* with erosive changes in various facet joints. O, odontoid. *(Courtesy Dr. Barbara Weissman.)*

to be narrowed (Figure 70-6). Significant pain is reported, but passive range of motion in the absence of muscle spasm may be normal. At least two possible mechanisms have been put forth for this process: (1) extension of the inflammatory process from adjacent neurocentral joints (the joints of Luschka), which are lined by synovium, into the discovertebral area, and (2) chronic cervical instability initiated by apophyseal joint destruction leading to vertebral malalignment or subluxation. This process may produce microfractures of the vertebral end plates, disk herniation, and degeneration of disk cartilage. The atlantoaxial joint is prone to subluxation in several directions and is summarized later.

- The atlas can move anteriorly on the axis (most common). This results from laxity of the ligaments induced by the development of proliferative synovial tissue in adjacent synovial bursae or by fracture or erosion of the odontoid process.
- The atlas can move posteriorly on the axis. This can occur only if the odontoid peg has been fractured from the axis or destroyed.
- The atlas can sublux vertically in relation to the axis (least common). This results from destruction of the lateral atlantoaxial joints or of bone around the foramen magnum. Vertical (superior) migration of the odontoid can develop from unattended anterior or posterior subluxation.

The earliest and most common symptom of cervical subluxation is pain radiating up into the occiput. Two other serious, but less common, clinical patterns include slowly progressive spastic quadriparesis with painless sensory loss in the hands and transient episodes of medullary dysfunction associated with vertical penetration of the dens and probable vertebral artery compression. In the latter, paresthesias may occur in the shoulders or arms during movement of the head.

Physical findings suggestive of atlantoaxial subluxation include loss of occipitocervical lordosis, resistance to passive spine motion, and abnormal protrusion of the axial arch felt by the examining finger on the posterior pharyngeal wall. Radiographic views (lateral, with the neck in flexion) reveal more than 3 mm of separation between the odontoid peg and the axial arch. In symptomatic patients, films in flexion should be taken only after radiographs (including an open-mouth posteroanterior view) have ruled out an odontoid fracture or severe atlantoaxial subluxation. Studies have indicated that CT is useful for showing spinal cord compression by loss of posterior subarachnoid space in patients with C1 to C2 subluxation. MRI has proved particularly valuable in determining pathologic anatomy in this syndrome (Figure 70-7).

Neurologic symptoms often have little relationship to the degree of subluxation and may be related to individual variations in the diameter of the spinal canal. Symptoms of spinal cord compression that demand intervention include altered consciousness, syncope, and loss of sphincter control. Dysphagia, vertigo, convulsions, hemiplegia, dysarthria, nystagmus, and peripheral paresthesias are additional symptoms that require immediate attention.

Some of these symptoms may be related to compression of the vertebral arteries, which must wind through foramina in the transverse processes of C1 and C2, rather than to compression of the spinal cord.

The progression of peripheral joint erosions parallels cervical spine disease in RA. The two coincide in severity and timing; cervical subluxation is more likely to develop

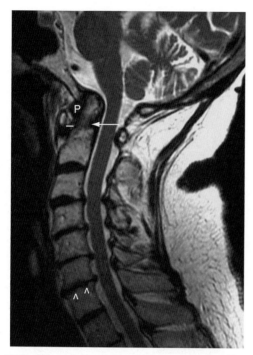

Figure 70-7 Rheumatoid arthritis of the cervical spine. T2-weighted sagittal image shows low signal periodontoid pannus (P). Odontoid process appears irregular secondary to erosion *(arrow)*. The atlantodental distance shows mild widening *(solid line)*. Vertical subluxation can also be seen without signs of cord compression. The anterior subarachnoid space is compromised by disk protrusions at multiple levels. Erosions *(arrowheads)* are seen at the vertebral end plates at the C6-C7 level. *(Courtesy Dr. Barbara Weissman.)*

in patients with erosion of the hands and feet. In a series of patients with RA referred for hip or knee arthroplasty, 61% had radiographic evidence of cervical spine instability.[41]

Is mortality increased in patients with atlantoaxial subluxation? Neurologic signs do not inevitably develop in patients with large subluxations. When signs of cervical cord compression do appear, however, myelopathy progresses rapidly, and 50% of patients die within 1 year.[42] These patients are at risk for these complications if they sustain small falls, whiplash injuries, and general anesthesia with intubation. Cervical collars can be prescribed for symptomatic relief. Operative stabilization may be considered if symptoms are progressive.

Some data support the hypothesis that early C1-to-C2 fusion for atlantoaxial subluxation before the development of superior migration of the odontoid decreases the risk for further progression of cervical spine instability.[43] The incidence of sustained neurologic deterioration related to surgery may be 6%; this emphasizes the importance of a skilled surgical team and of careful assessment of each patient. In many cases, surgical intervention in asymptomatic patients is riskier than conservative management despite the dire appearance of imaging studies.

Vertical atlantoaxial subluxation is important and may follow anterior or posterior subluxation. Symptoms associated with this collapse of the lateral support system of the atlas occur in patients with severe erosive disease. Neurologic findings include decreased sensation in the distribution of cranial nerve V, sensory loss in the C2 area, nystagmus, and pyramidal lesions.

Thoracic, Lumbar, and Sacral Spine

The thoracic, lumbar, and sacral portions of the spine are usually spared in RA. Exceptions include the apophyseal joints; rarely, synovial cysts at the apophyseal joint can impinge as an epidural mass on the spinal cord, causing pain, neurologic deficits, or both.

Hips

The hip is less frequently involved in early RA than in juvenile RA. Hip joint involvement must be ascertained by careful clinical examination; symptoms of hip synovitis include pain in the lower buttock or, more commonly, the groin. Pain on the lateral aspect of the hip is often a manifestation of trochanteric bursitis rather than true hip joint synovitis.

About half of patients with well-established RA have radiographic evidence of hip disease. In contrast to osteoarthritis, in which the femoral head usually migrates superiorly, symmetric thinning of the cartilage in RA leads to axial migration. The femoral head may collapse and be reabsorbed, and the acetabulum is remodeled and pushed medially, leading to protrusio acetabuli (Figure 70-8). Significant protrusion occurs in about 5% of all patients with RA.[44] Loss of internal rotation on physical examination correlates best with radiographic findings. Similar to the situation in other weight-bearing joints, the femoral head may develop cystic lesions that communicate with the joint space.

Knees

In contrast to the hips, synovial inflammation and proliferation in the knees are readily shown on physical examination. Early in knee disease, often within 1 week after the onset of symptoms, noticeable quadriceps atrophy leads to the application of more force than usual through the patella

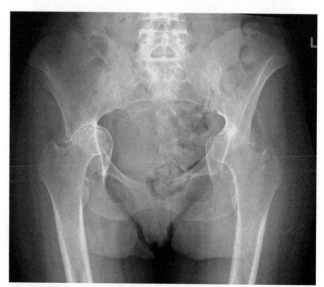

Figure 70-8 Bilateral protrusio acetabuli in rheumatoid arthritis. The medial acetabular margins protrude into the pelvis. Severe accompanying cartilage loss is evident. *(Courtesy Dr. Barbara Weissman.)*

to the femoral surface. Another early manifestation of knee disease in RA is loss of full extension—a functional loss that can become a fixed flexion contracture unless corrective measures are undertaken.

Flexion of a knee with a moderate to large effusion markedly increases intra-articular pressure. The increased intra-articular pressure may cause an outpouching of posterior components of the joint, producing a popliteal or Baker's cyst. This can generate pressures so high in the popliteal space that it may rupture down or dissect into the calf or, less often, superiorly into the posterior thigh. Rupture occurs posteriorly between the medial head of the gastrocnemius and the tendinous insertion of the biceps. Clinically, popliteal cysts and their complications have several manifestations. An intact popliteal cyst may compress superficial venous flow from the lower leg, producing dilation of superficial veins, edema, or both.[45] Rupture of the joint posteriorly with extravasation of joint fluid into the calf may resemble acute thrombophlebitis with swelling and tenderness and may produce systemic signs of fever with leukocytosis. One helpful sign in identifying cyst rupture may be the appearance of a crescentic hematoma beneath one of the malleoli of the ankle.[46] Although arthrography clearly defines the abnormal anatomy of a Baker's cyst, this invasive procedure has been replaced by ultrasonography and, when necessary, MRI (Figure 70-9).

Ankles and Feet

Ankle involvement is usually mild in RA, but damage can occur in severe progressive forms of the disease. Clinical evidence for ankle involvement consists of cystic swelling anterior and posterior to the malleoli. Much of the stability of the ankle depends on the integrity of the ligaments

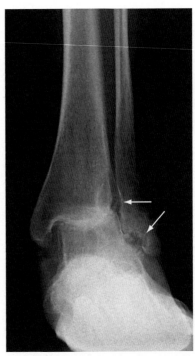

Figure 70-10   Rheumatoid arthritis of the ankle. Diffuse loss of cartilage space can be seen with erosion of the fibula *(arrows)*. Scalloping along the medial border of the distal fibula is designated the fibular notch sign and is a characteristic finding in rheumatoid arthritis. The hindfoot is in valgus alignment.

holding the fibula to the tibia and these two bones to the talus. In RA, inflammatory and proliferative disease may loosen these connections by stretching and eroding the collagenous ligaments, causing erosions (Figure 70-10). The result is incongruity, which progresses to pronation deformities and eversion of the foot.

The Achilles tendon is a major structural component and kinetic force in the foot and ankle. Rheumatoid nodules develop in this collagenous structure, and spontaneous rupture of the tendon has been reported when diffuse granulomatous inflammation is present.[47] The subtalar joint controls eversion and inversion of the foot on the talus; patients with RA invariably have more pain while walking on uneven ground; this is related to the relatively common subtalar joint involvement in RA. Progressive eversion at the subtalar joint, combined with foot pain, leads to a lateral subluxation beginning in the midfoot and the development of a rocker-bottom deformity. Midfoot disease leads to collapse of the arch, which contributes to difficulty walking because of pain.

More than one-third of patients with RA have significant disease in the feet (Figure 70-11). Metatarsophalangeal (MTP) joints are often involved, and gait is altered as pain develops during push-off in striding. Studies have shown that MTPs are the initial site of erosion in many patients. Downward subluxation of the metatarsal heads occurs soon after the MTP joints become involved, producing "cock-up" toe deformities of the PIP joints. Hallux valgus and bunion or callus formation occur if disease continues. Cystic collections representing outpouchings of flexor tendon sheaths often develop under the MTP joints.[48]

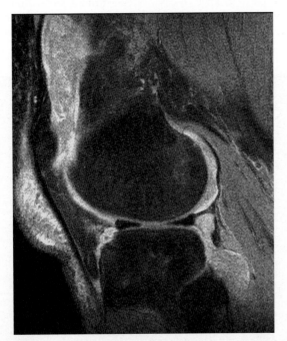

Figure 70-9   Magnetic resonance imaging (MRI) of the knee in rheumatoid arthritis. Sagittal fast spin echo T2-weighted fat-suppressed image allows excellent contrast. Synovial fluid is shown in white as a posterior fluid collection. *(Courtesy Dr. Barbara Weissman.)*

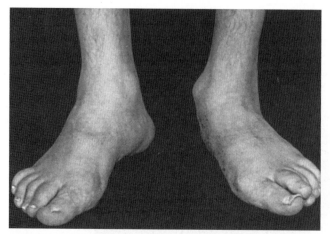

Figure 70-11 Valgus of ankle, pes planus, and forefoot varus deformity of the left foot related to painful synovitis of the ankle, forefoot, and metatarsophalangeal joint in a 24-year-old man with severe rheumatoid arthritis.

Patients with subluxation of metatarsal heads can develop pressure necrosis of the plantar surfaces. Alternatively, those who have subluxation of MTP joints often develop ulceration over the PIP joints that protrude dorsally (hammer toes). The net result is increased pressure on the MTP joints with a sensation described as "walking on marbles" by many patients. Changes caused by the progress of disease and destruction in the foot include intermetatarsal joint ligament stretching in response to inflammation, spreading of the forefoot, anterior migration of the plantar fat pad, and dorsal subluxation of toes followed by plantar subluxation of the metatarsal heads.[49] Concurrently, hallux valgus results in progressive overlap of the second and third toes on top of the great toe.

DIP joints of the foot are rarely affected in RA, but a functional rigid hallux caused by muscle spasm of the great toe intrinsic muscles in an effort to relieve pressure on the lesser metatarsal heads can be extremely painful and may require surgical intervention. Another cause of foot pain in rheumatoid patients is the tarsal tunnel syndrome. In a group of 30 patients with RA, erosions in the feet visible on radiographs and foot pain (4 patients; 13%) were shown by electrodiagnostic techniques to produce slowing of medial or lateral plantar nerve latency, or both.

Extra-articular Complications of Rheumatoid Arthritis

Generally, the number and severity of extra-articular features vary with the duration and severity of the disease. Several of these features may be related to extra-articular foci of an immune response,[50] based on evidence of independent and qualitatively different production of RF in the pleural space, pericardium, muscle, and even meninges. Patients with systemic immune responses have true rheumatoid disease, not just RA. Other unusual proteins and protein complexes in the circulation of patients with active rheumatoid disease include antiphospholipid antibodies, circulating immune complexes, and cryoglobulins. Extra-articular manifestations of RA are associated with excess mortality.[51]

Rheumatoid Nodules

The mature rheumatoid nodule has a central area of necrosis rimmed by a corona of palisading fibroblasts that is surrounded in turn by a collagenous capsule with perivascular collections of chronic inflammatory cells. The earliest nodules, nests of granulation tissue, have been identified measuring less than 4 mm. These nodules grow by accumulating cells that expand centrifugally, leaving behind central necrosis initiated by vasculopathy and compounded by protease destruction of the connective tissue matrix. Nodules occur in 15% to 20% of patients with definite arthritis or RA. They occur most often on extensor surfaces or pressure points, such as the olecranon process and the proximal ulna (Figure 70-12A), as well as on tendons (Figure 70-12B). They are subcutaneous and vary in consistency from a soft, amorphous, entirely mobile mass to a hard, rubbery mass attached firmly to the periosteum.

The appearance of nodules in unusual sites can lead to confusion in diagnosis; they sometimes can appear identical to other types of nodules such as tophi. Sacral nodules may be mistaken for bedsores if the overlying skin breaks down. Occipital nodules also occur in bedridden patients. In the larynx, rheumatoid nodules on the vocal cords may cause progressive hoarseness. Nodules can even be found in the heart and lungs (see later). Nodules on the sclera can produce perforation of this collagenous tissue. Multiple reports describe rheumatoid nodule formation within the central nervous system, involving leptomeninges more frequently than parenchyma.[52] Some patients develop rheumatoid nodules within vertebral bodies, resulting in bone destruction and signs of myelopathy.

Careful histologic study of early lesions[53] suggests that development of the nodule is mediated by affected small arterioles and resulting complement activation and terminal vasculitis. This immunologic response is linked to proliferation of resident histiocytes and fibroblasts and to an influx of macrophages from the circulation. Proliferation of cells and the supporting scaffold of connective tissue are mediated by cytokines expressed in patterns similar to those found in rheumatoid synovium. The cytokine profile of the rheumatoid nodule suggests a T helper-1 (Th1) gene expression pattern similar to that of synovial tissue, including expression of tumor necrosis factor (TNF), interleukin (IL)-1, IL-12, and interferon (IFN)-γ, but not IL-2. More recently, gene expression of IL-17 family members in rheumatoid nodules showed that IL-17A gene expression was minimal in contrast to that of rheumatoid synovial tissue.[54] The absence of IL-17A could be due to decreased IL-23 expression in the nodule. Data from studies using monoclonal antibodies against receptors for complement C3b and C3bi, monocytes, activated macrophages, and HLA-DR molecules suggest that mononuclear phagocytes are constantly being recruited into peripheral layers and subsequently migrate into the palisade to constitute most of the cell population in this area.[55] Other studies using cytochemical markers (nonspecific esterase and CD68 for macrophages, and prolyl hydroxylase for fibroblasts) indicate that a mixture of macrophages and fibroblasts makes up the cellular content of nodules.[56] This evidence fits with data from nodule tissue in organ culture; similar to synovial tissue, cells in the palisading region have

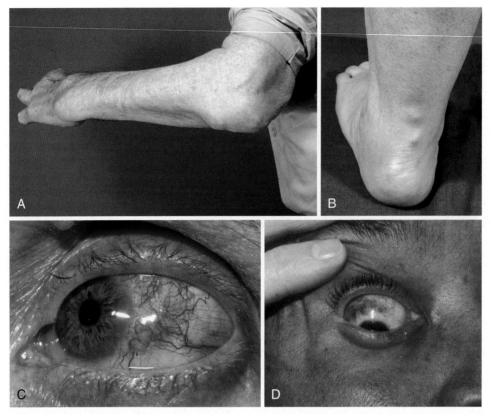

Figure 70-12   Manifestations of increased reactivity of mesenchymal tissue in rheumatoid arthritis include nodules on the elbow **(A)** and on the Achilles tendon **(B)**, as well as episcleritis **(C)** and scleromalacia **(D)**. *(Courtesy Iain McInnes, MD.)*

the capacity to produce collagenase and protease in large quantities.[57]

RF is almost always found in the serum of patients with rheumatoid nodules. Rarely, such nodules are present in the absence of obvious arthritis. A condition called *rheumatoid nodulosis* is characterized by the presence of multiple nodules on the hands, a positive test for RF, episodes of acute intermittent synovitis, and subchondral cystic lesions of small bones of the hands and feet.[58] Many clinicians have noted that during methotrexate therapy, existing nodules may enlarge and new ones may develop, even though symptoms of synovitis regress; the pathophysiology underlying this phenomenon is unknown, although it may relate to the effects of methotrexate on adenosine (see Chapter 61). Discontinuing methotrexate in these patients usually leads to regression of some nodules. Some case reports suggest that TNF inhibitors can be associated with accelerated rheumatoid nodulosis.

The differential diagnosis of rheumatoid nodules includes benign nodules usually found in healthy children that are nontender and appear on the pretibial regions, feet, and scalp. In addition, nodular changes can occur in subcutaneous nodules as rheumatic fever, Gottron's papules in dermatomyositis, and calcinosis in scleroderma. Granuloma annulare consists of intracutaneous nodules that are histologically identical to rheumatoid nodules. Nodules due to xanthomatosis usually have a yellow tinge, and patients have abnormally high plasma lipoprotein and cholesterol levels. Tophi, which are collections of monosodium urate crystals in patients with gout, are associated with small,

punched-out bone lesions and almost always occur in the presence of elevated serum urate concentration. Nodules of multicentric reticulohistiocytosis contain large, lipid-filled macrophages. Numerous proliferative disorders that affect cutaneous tissue, including erythema elevatum diutinum, acrodermatitis chronica atrophicans, bejel, yaws, pinta, and leprosy, can resemble rheumatoid nodules. A rheumatoid nodule, particularly when it occurs on the face, may simulate basal cell carcinoma.

Bone Density

The skeleton has two anatomically and functionally separate components, cortical and trabecular bone, which respond differently to systemic and local diseases and to drugs. RA can be associated with generalized osteopenia and osteoporosis owing to the effects of drugs (especially corticosteroids); cytokine-induced and receptor activator of nuclear factor κB (NFκB) ligand (RANKL)-induced activation of osteoclasts; and the fact that certain groups of patients with the disease, especially postmenopausal women, have other risk factors that enhance the potential for bone loss. Risks for hip fracture and vertebral compression fracture can be high. Bone densitometry should be performed routinely in patients with RA; treatment with bisphosphonates should be considered as an adjunct to therapy.

Because postmenopausal women are at greater risk for osteoporosis, this group should be treated aggressively. Minimizing steroid use is one method that can be used to decrease the risk of osteoporosis in this group and in other patients with RA. Two-phase loss of bone seems to be induced by glucocorticoids: a rapid first phase, when 12% of bone mass disappears in the first 6 to 12 months of therapy, followed by a subsequent chronic phase, which has a slower rate of bone loss.[59] It is encouraging that axial bone loss in patients with RA induced early by glucocorticoids can be reversed.[60] The evaluation, biology, and management of osteoporosis are discussed in Chapter 101. In the relationship between RA and bone, the focus is, appropriately, on osteoporosis; however, diffuse loss of bone in RA, whether or not it is related to glucocorticoid therapy, leads to a high incidence of stress fractures of long bones in RA.[61] The fibula is the most common fracture site. Acute leg pain in a thin, elderly rheumatoid patient, even without a history of trauma, should generate suspicion of a stress fracture. Geodes (i.e., subchondral cysts developed by synovial penetration of the cortex or subchondral plate and subsequent proliferation) weaken bone and can predispose bone to fracture.

Muscle

Clinical weakness is common in RA, but is it caused by muscle involvement in rheumatoid inflammation, or is it a reflex weakness response to pain? Most rheumatoid patients have muscle weakness, but few have muscle tenderness or elevated muscle enzymes in the blood.

In an early autopsy series, focal accumulations of lymphocytes and plasma cells with some contiguous degeneration of muscle fibers were found in all rheumatoid patients—a condition termed *nodular myositis*. More recent studies have pointed to multiple types of muscle disease in RA, although clinically relevant active myositis is uncommon[62]:

- Diminution of muscle bulk with atrophy of type II fibers
- Peripheral neuromyopathy, usually due to a mononeuritis multiplex
- Steroid myopathy
- Active myositis and muscle necrosis with foci of endomysial mononuclear cell infiltration
- Chronic myopathy resembling a dystrophic process, probably the end stage of inflammatory myositis

In biopsy specimens, atrophy of type II fibers is most common. Evidence of myositis and focal necrosis is found occasionally in biopsy specimens of patients with active disease, particularly in a subset with mild synovitis and a disproportionately high erythrocyte sedimentation rate (ESR). In some patients, the lymphocytes in muscle synthesize IgM RF, emphasizing the systemic nature of RA. The patchy "nodules of myositis" contain plasma cells and lymphocytes.

Skin

The most frequently recognized skin lesion in RA is the rheumatoid nodule but several other manifestations may be observed as well. "Senile" purpura resulting from skin atrophy and capillary fragility is especially common in patients treated with glucocorticoids. Palmar erythema is common, but Raynaud's syndrome is rare. Manifestations of vasculitis range from occasional nail fold infarcts to a deep, erosive, scarring pyoderma gangrenosum. Palpable purpura

in rheumatoid patients often occurs as a reaction to a drug that the patient is taking but can be primary and a direct function of the severity of articular disease. Livedo reticularis, the lacy, dusky purple, asymptomatic discoloration seen on the extremities, is believed to signify a deep dermal vasculopathy. It can be present in any or all diffuse connective tissue diseases and often is associated with antiphospholipid antibodies.[63]

Eye

Virtually all ocular manifestations of RA can be considered complications of the disease (see Chapter 44). Keratoconjunctivitis sicca, a component of Sjögren's syndrome, is discussed in Chapter 73. Scleritis and episcleritis are associated with RA. Highly differentiated connective tissues in the eye make rheumatoid manifestations particularly interesting and, when they occur in aggressive form, very serious.

The episclera of the eye is highly vascular compared with the dense sclera. Scleritis, episcleritis, or both occur in less than 1% of rheumatoid patients. In episcleritis, the eye becomes red and, in contrast to conjunctivitis, causes tearing but no discharge. Loss of vision does not occur as a direct result of episcleritis, but a keratitis or a cataract developing secondarily can cause visual loss. Scleritis causes severe ocular pain and dark red discoloration (Figure 70-12C). No discharge is present. Depending on the intensity of the process, scleritis can be localized and superficial or generalized, with or without granulomatous resorption of the sclera down to the uveal layer; when this complication occurs, it is termed *scleromalacia perforans*. In contrast to superficial eye disease, which usually can be treated conservatively with topical steroids, scleritis usually requires systemic or intraocular corticosteroid treatment. In some cases, the sclera can become thin even in the absence of overt inflammation, leading to scleromalacia (Figure 70-12D). Rarely, perilimbic ischemic ulcers can be caused by cryoproteins (RF-IgG complexes) and if untreated can result in perforation of the anterior chamber. Patients with RA who have an associated keratoconjunctivitis sicca secondary to Sjögren's syndrome have pruritic and painful eyes, sometimes leading to chronic blepharitis.

Host Defense and Infection

The incidence of infection as a complication of RA has paralleled the use of glucocorticoids, biologics, and immunosuppressive agents. TNF blockers are especially noteworthy because they have been associated with reactivation of tuberculosis and other opportunistic infections such as histoplasmosis. Pulmonary infections, skin infections, and septic arthritis are the most common infections in RA.[64,65] Difficulty in diagnosis is accentuated by the similarity of aggressive RA to infection, particularly in joints; a "pseudoseptic" arthritis in rheumatoid patients, associated with fever, chills, and grossly purulent synovial fluid, can be part of a severe exacerbation of RA and must be distinguished from infection.[66] Mortality attributable to respiratory infections such as pneumonia and bronchitis is increased in RA patients compared with the general population.[67] A retrospective longitudinal cohort study compared the frequency of infection in a population-based incidence cohort of RA patients versus that in a group of individuals without RA from the same population; this study looked at 7900 to 9100 person-years.[68] A total of 609 RA patients and 609 non-RA patients were studied; 73% were women, and mean patient age was 58 years. Hazard ratios for RA patients versus controls after adjustment for age, sex, smoking status, leukopenia, corticosteroid use, and diabetes mellitus were nearly twofold increased for confirmed infection and for infection requiring hospitalization. Bone, joints, skin, respiratory tract, and soft tissues were the organs with highest hazard ratios. In a subsequent study in this cohort, predictors of infection were identified as increasing age, extra-articular manifestations of RA, leukopenia, and comorbidities such as chronic lung disease, alcoholism, diabetes mellitus, and the use of glucocorticoids.

Traditional DMARD use generally is not associated with a major increased incidence of infection. However, vigilance in using biologic agents is essential because mortality is increased from infection due to immunosuppression.[69] Physicians should always have a low threshold of concern for infection in rheumatoid patients.

Hematologic Abnormalities

Most patients with active RA have a mild normocytic normochromic anemia that correlates with ESR elevation and the activity of the disease. Anemia has mixed causes in RA. One deficiency may mask evidence of others. A useful guide is that three-quarters of rheumatoid patients with anemia have the anemia of chronic disease, whereas one-quarter respond to iron therapy. Patients in both groups may have superimposed vitamin B$_{12}$ or folate deficiency.[70] Hemoglobin of less than 10 is rarely due only to RA. The following guidelines may prove helpful to the clinician in diagnosing the cause of anemia in rheumatoid patients:

- Anemia of chronic disease is associated with a significantly higher serum ferritin concentration than is found in isolated iron deficiency.
- Folate or vitamin B$_{12}$ deficiency or the use of methotrexate can mask iron deficiency, especially in patients taking nonsteroidal anti-inflammatory drugs (NSAIDs) with chronic gastrointestinal blood loss, by increasing the mean cell volume and the mean cell hemoglobin level of erythrocytes.
- The ESR correlates inversely with hemoglobin levels in RA.
- Erythropoietin levels are higher in patients with iron deficiency anemia compared with those with anemia of chronic disease; rheumatoid patients have a diminished response to erythropoietin.[71]

In patients with anemia of chronic disease, the total erythroid heme turnover is slightly reduced, and ineffective erythropoiesis accounts for a much higher than normal percentage of total heme turnover. In contrast to anemia associated with blood loss, ineffective erythropoiesis returns to normal in RA if remission can be induced.[72] Red blood cell aplasia, immunologically mediated, is a rare finding in RA.

Thrombocytosis is often associated with RA. A significant relationship has been noted between thrombocytosis and extra-articular manifestations of rheumatoid disease and disease activity.[73] Eosinophilia (5% of total white blood cell count) has been observed in some patients.

Felty's syndrome comprises an uncommon but severe subset of seropositive, erosive RA symptoms that occur in patients with neutropenia and splenomegaly. Patients with Felty's syndrome have more frequent and robust extra-articular RA manifestations and are at increased risk for infection, skin ulceration, and other complications. Another subset of patients with RA includes those with increased numbers of large granular lymphocytes in the peripheral blood, bone marrow, and liver. These lymphocytes contain many azurophilic granules in the cytoplasm and may account for more than 90% of mononuclear cells in blood. They are increased in certain viral infections. The cells are Fc receptor positive, do not produce IL-2, respond poorly to mitogens, and involve antibody-dependent cell-mediated cytotoxicity activity (expressing CD3, CD8, and CD57) or natural killer cells (expressing CD16 and CD56).[74,75] Among previously described patients with large granular lymphocyte proliferation, almost one-third have had RA.[76] Because the large granular lymphocyte syndrome in patients with RA has the same HLA-DR4 association seen in Felty's syndrome, the proposal has been made that Felty's syndrome and large granular lymphocyte syndrome represent different variants of a broader syndrome comprising RA, neutropenia, large granular lymphocyte expansions, HLA-DR4 positivity, and variable splenomegaly.[77] Neutropenia has been described as an adverse event in more recent drug trials in RA patients, most notably with the humanized anti–IL-6 receptor monoclonal antibody tocilizumab.[78]

Paraproteinemia, typified by monoclonal gammopathies, has a poor prognostic significance when it appears in rheumatoid patients. This evidence for monoclonal B cell proliferation carries with it a high frequency of malignant transformation to lymphoma or myeloma.[79]

Vasculitis

The initial pathologic change in RA is often seen as inflammatory changes in medium and small blood vessels. It is useful to use the term *vasculitis* to group extra-articular complications related not to proliferative granulomas, but rather to inflammatory vascular disease. Systemic rheumatoid vasculitis, one of the most feared complications of RA, has become increasingly uncommon in recent years. This decline in rheumatoid vasculitis, similar to many other extra-articular manifestations, is likely related to marked improvement in therapy resulting from widespread use of methotrexate and new biologic agents. Male gender, long-standing disease, high-titer RF in serum, hypocomplementemia, erosive disease, circulating cryoglobulins, deposition of immune complexes and complement in blood vessels, and extra-articular features such as subcutaneous nodules are variables associated with the development of rheumatoid vasculitis.[80]

Rheumatoid vasculitis affects a very small subset of patients with established, often severe, RA. It can present as the following:

- Distal arteritis (including from splinter hemorrhage, nail fold infarcts, and gangrene) (Figure 70-13)
- Cutaneous ulceration (including pyoderma gangrenosum)
- Peripheral neuropathy (mononeuritis multiplex or sensory stocking-glove neuropathy)

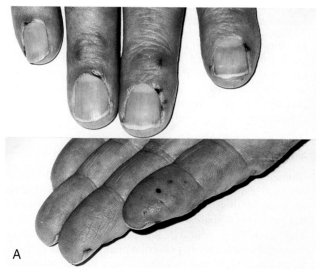

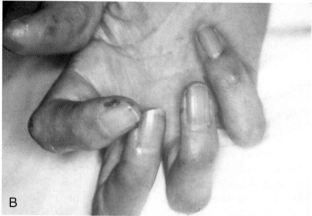

Figure 70-13 **A,** Digital vasculitis in a 65-year-old man with seropositive rheumatoid arthritis. **B,** Nail fold infarcts can occur in patients with rheumatoid arthritis and typically are associated with rheumatoid factor positivity and active joint disease. (**A,** *Courtesy Eileen Moynihan, MD.*)

- Palpable purpura
- Arteritis of viscera, including heart, lungs, bowel, kidney, liver, spleen, pancreas, lymph nodes, or testis

The pathologic finding in rheumatoid vasculitis is a panarteritis. All layers of the vessel wall are infiltrated with mononuclear cells. Fibrinoid necrosis is seen in active lesions. Intimal proliferation may predispose to thrombosis. Obliterative endarteritis of the finger is a common manifestation of vasculitis, and immune complex deposits have been shown in affected vessels.[81] In patients with hypocomplementemia, the cellular infiltrate around the vessels contains neutrophils. In normocomplementemic patients, lymphocytes predominate.

Neurovascular disease may be the only manifestation of vasculitis. The two common clinical patterns include a mild distal sensory neuropathy and a severe sensorimotor neuropathy (mononeuritis multiplex).[82] The latter form is characterized by severe arterial damage on nerve biopsy specimens. Symptoms of the milder form may consist of paresthesias or "burning feet" in association with decreased touch and pin sensation distally. Patients with mononeuritis multiplex have weakness (e.g., footdrop), in addition to sensory abnormalities. Symptoms and signs are identical to those found in polyarteritis nodosa. Rheumatoid pachymeningitis is a rare complication of RA; confined to the dura and pia mater, this process may be limited to certain areas (e.g., lumbar cord, cisternae).[83] Elevated levels of IgG (including IgM and IgG RFs and low-molecular-weight IgM) and immune complexes are found in the cerebrospinal fluid.

Visceral lesions occur generally as claudication or infarction of the organ supplied by the involved arteries. Intestinal involvement with vasculitis manifests as abdominal pain, at first intermittent and progressing often to continuous pain and a tender, quiet abdomen on examination. If infarction develops, resection must be accomplished promptly. Gangrene of digits and extremities, intestinal lesions with bleeding or perforation, cardiac or renal involvement, and mononeuritis multiplex indicate extensive vasculitis and are associated with a poor prognosis.[84]

Other entities in the differential diagnosis for rheumatoid vasculitis include diabetes mellitus, infection, atherosclerosis, and drug reactions. Current practice is to treat organ-specific vasculitis aggressively when it occurs in RA patients, similar to treatment for patients with polyarteritis. This therapeutic approach may be responsible for the small excess mortality in rheumatoid vasculitis patients compared with "controls" with RA alone. In 61 patients with rheumatoid vasculitis, after allowance for general risk factors such as age and sex, the mortality risk was only 1.26 times that of rheumatoid patients without vasculitis.[85]

Renal Disease

The kidney is rarely involved directly in RA but often is compromised indirectly by therapy. Amyloidosis is an unusual complication of chronic RA. AA amyloidosis is one of the most important life-threatening complications of RA. Phenacetin abuse causes renal papillary necrosis; salicylates and other NSAIDs may cause abnormalities as well. Membranous nephropathy is related to therapy with gold salts and penicillamine and was seen when these agents were commonly used to treat RA. Rarely, a focal necrotizing glomerulitis is seen in patients dying with RA and disseminated vasculitis.

Pulmonary Disease

Pleural Disease

Pleuritis is commonly found on autopsy of patients with RA, but clinical disease during life is seen less frequently. In about 20% of patients, pleuritis develops concurrently with the onset of arthritis. Pleuritic pain is not usually a major complaint. Effusions are exudative and can be large enough to cause dyspnea. Characteristics of exudative rheumatoid effusions include a very low glucose concentration in the range of 10 to 50 mg/dL, protein greater than 4 g/dL, mononuclear cells 100 to 3500/mm^3, elevated lactate dehydrogenase, low pH, and depressed total complement activity

(CH_{50}). The low glucose concentrations are of importance because infection (particularly tuberculosis) is the only other condition in which such a low pleural fluid glucose level is seen. Impaired transport of glucose into the pleural space seems to be the cause of this.[86]

Interstitial Pneumonitis and Fibrosis

Pulmonary fibrosis can occur with some regularity in RA and is associated with increased mortality. Similar to findings in scleroderma, physical findings consist of fine, diffuse, dry rales. Radiographs show a diffuse reticular (interstitial) or reticulonodular pattern in both lung fields; this can progress to a honeycomb appearance on plain radiographs and a characteristic lattice network on high-resolution CT scans. Pathologic findings include diffuse fibrosis in the midst of a mononuclear cell infiltrate. The principal functional defect is impairment of alveolocapillary gas exchange with decreased diffusion capacity, best measured using single-breath carbon monoxide diffusion capacities.[87] Interstitial lung disease and RF and ACPA positivity can occur in smokers before articular symptoms develop.[88] This finding has led to the novel hypothesis that RA-specific autoimmunity might be generated in the lung in response to environmental insults such as smoking. Bronchoalveolar lavage may reveal increased numbers of lymphocytes, even in patients with only mildly abnormal chest radiographs and normal pulmonary function test results.[89] In more aggressive disease, a higher proportion of neutrophils can be found in bronchoalveolar lavage. Lymphoid interstitial pneumonitis has been described in patients with RA and Sjögren's syndrome. This relatively indolent disorder is associated with elevated serum globulin levels. Bronchoalveolar lavage shows a primarily lymphocytic response.[90]

Nodular Lung Disease

Pulmonary nodules can appear singly or in clusters that coalesce. Single nodules appear as coin lesions and, when significant peripheral arthritis and nodules are present, can be evaluated by needle biopsy. Caplan's syndrome,[91] in which pneumoconiosis and RA are synergistic, producing a violent fibroblastic reaction with obliterative granulomatous fibrosis, has become a rare occurrence as the respiratory environment in mining operations has improved. Nodules may cavitate, creating a bronchopleural fistula. In several cases, solitary pulmonary nodules in RA patients have proved to be a rheumatoid nodule and a coexistent bronchogenic carcinoma.[92] If the index of suspicion is high for malignancy, the workup should be more aggressive.

Bronchiolitis

An uncommon finding is interstitial pneumonitis that progresses to alveolar involvement and bronchiolitis, respiratory insufficiency, and death. Pathologic studies show a cellular loose fibrosis and a proteinaceous exudate in bronchioles and alveoli; interstitial infiltrations of lymphocytes attest to the immunogenic aspects of the disease. The course and prognosis are similar to those of idiopathic bronchiolitis obliterans with organizing pneumonia.

Pulmonary Hypertension

Pulmonary hypertension is more common in RA than was previously appreciated. Noninvasive echocardiograms have suggested that mild pulmonary hypertension can be detected in more than 30% of patients with RA.[93] Most of these patients are asymptomatic and do not have significant progression.

Small Airways Disease

Defined by a reduced maximal midexpiratory flow rate and maximal expiratory flow rate at 50% of functional vital capacity, small airways disease was observed in 50% of 30 RA patients compared with 22% of a control population.[94] The study was adjusted for pulmonary infection, α1-antitrypsin deficiency, penicillamine treatment, environmental pollution, and smoking. Other investigations have not found small airways dysfunction in RA and have suggested that, if present, it probably is related to factors other than RA.[95] If real, this phenomenon may be part of a generalized exocrinopathic process in the disease, expressed most commonly in Sjögren's syndrome.

Pulmonary Disease due to Treatment of Rheumatoid Arthritis

Many of the drugs used to treat RA are associated with pulmonary toxicity. For instance, methotrexate and leflunomide can cause pulmonary fibrosis in a pattern that resembles RA. Differentiating rheumatoid pulmonary fibrosis from drug-induced fibrosis can be difficult, and this uncertainty might require discontinuing methotrexate therapy in some cases. An idiosyncratic form of methotrexate pulmonary toxicity is less common and usually is accompanied by fever, lung infiltrates, and eosinophilia. Treatment with TNF inhibitors can lead to reactivation of pulmonary or extrapulmonary tuberculosis.

Cardiovascular System

Cardiac disease in RA can take many forms. It has become apparent that increased risk of premature death in RA is due largely to an increased incidence of cardiovascular disease, primarily myocardial infarction and congestive heart failure. Advances in echocardiography have made the diagnosis of pericarditis with endocardial inflammation easier and more specific. Myocardial biopsy through vascular catheters has facilitated diagnosis and classification of myocarditis. In a detailed study of rheumatoid patients using echocardiography, Holter monitors, and electrocardiography, it was reported that 70% of patients with nodular disease and 40% of those with non-nodular RA have some cardiac involvement, including valve thickening or incompetence.[96]

Atherosclerosis

Multiple risk factors for coronary artery disease in RA patients are known, in addition to the risk factors that are relevant in the general population. Patients with prolonged RA have a greater extent of atherosclerosis than patients of the same age with more recent disease onset.[97] Many of the same risk factors noted in RA patients have been implicated in patients without rheumatic diseases, including molecules involved in the immune response, markers of inflammation, and therapeutic agents. It is apparent that, with all else being equal, tobacco smoking is an important factor in augmenting early atherosclerosis in RA patients.[98] In a large, well-studied population of rheumatoid patients at the Mayo Clinic, patients were followed until death, migration from Olmsted County, or 2001. Data show that congestive heart failure was more important than ischemic heart disease as a cause of death.[99] Even in RA patients without clinically evident cardiovascular disease, left ventricular diastolic function and right ventricular diastolic function are reduced.[100]

Pericarditis

Infrequently diagnosed on the basis of history and physical examination in RA, pericarditis is present in 50% of patients at autopsy. In one study, 31% of patients with RA had echocardiographic evidence of pericardial effusion. The same study revealed only rare evidence of impaired left ventricular function in prospectively studied outpatients with RA.[101] Although unusual, cardiac tamponade and/or the more common constrictive pericarditis can develop in RA and may require pericardiectomy. Almost all patients have a positive test for RF, and half have nodules. Preservation of good ventricular function on echocardiography in the face of deteriorating clinical myocardial function should raise a high index of suspicion of constrictive pericarditis.

Myocarditis

Myocarditis is rare but may be due to granulomatous disease or interstitial myocarditis. The granulomatous process resembles subcutaneous nodules and could be considered specific for the disease. Diffuse infiltration of the myocardium by mononuclear cells may involve the entire myocardium and yet may have no clinical manifestations, but it could be suggested by echocardiography.

Endocardial Inflammation

Echocardiographic studies have reported evidence of previously unrecognized mitral valve disease of the anterior leaflet of the mitral valve. Although aortic valve disease and arthritis are more commonly associated with ankylosing spondylitis, numerous patients with granulomatous nodules on the valve have been reported.[102]

Conduction Defects

Atrioventricular block is unusual in RA but is probably related to direct granulomatous involvement. Pathologic examination may reveal proliferative lesions or healed scars. Complete heart block has been described in more than 30 patients with RA. It generally occurs in patients with established erosive nodular disease.[103] Complete heart block usually is permanent and is caused by rheumatoid granulomas in or near the atrioventricular node or bundle of His. Rarely, amyloidosis is responsible for heart block.

Granulomatous Aortitis or Valvular Disease

In severe rheumatoid heart disease, granulomatous disease can spread to involve even the base of the aorta. Occasionally, granulomatous disease associated with RA necessitates urgent valve replacement for aortic regurgitation.[104] With improved therapy for synovitis, these complications (similar to many others) have become rare.

DIAGNOSIS

Criteria to establish the diagnosis of RA are based on an effective clinical history and physical examination, laboratory tests, and exclusion of other diagnoses. No single feature or laboratory test is sufficient for a definitive diagnosis. The 1987 American College of Rheumatology (ACR) criteria for classification usually are not used for diagnosis in individual cases; however, the requirement that objective evidence of synovitis must be present for at least 6 weeks is important, especially because many transient forms of synovitis are observed in primary care settings (Table 70-3). A physician would be less likely to make a premature diagnosis of RA in a patient who might have a self-limited synovitis. To attempt preventing irreversible damage to joints, the diagnosis of RA should be confirmed or ruled out within 2 months after the onset of synovitis.

Classification criteria were revised in 2010 by the ACR and the European League Against Rheumatism (EULAR).[105] The new criteria place greater emphasis on serology and early diagnosis in patients with very few or even no swollen or tender joints (Table 70-4). Symmetric joint disease is not a feature of the new criteria. In addition, classic radiographic changes such as marginal erosions automatically qualify patients for RA classification if they have a single swollen joint. Imaging evidence of synovitis, including ultrasound or MRI, can be used to classify patients even in the absence of symptoms if patients have high titers of RF or ACPA and elevated acute phase reactants. The long-term usefulness and the specificity of the classification of the revised criteria are uncertain, but their use will likely result in earlier diagnosis and treatment. It is important to recognize that these are not diagnostic criteria, and they are used mainly in classifying patients for clinical research.

The characteristic patient with RA reports pain and stiffness in multiple joints, with prominent and prolonged morning stiffness. Joint swelling is boggy and includes soft tissue and synovial fluid. Joints are tender, especially the small joints of the hands and feet, but usually are not painful when the patient is at rest. Palmar erythema and prominent veins on the dorsum of the hand and wrist indicate increased blood flow. DIP joints are rarely involved. The temperature over the involved joints (except the hip) can be elevated, but the joints usually are not red. The range of motion is limited, and muscle strength and function around inflamed joints are diminished. Soft, poorly delineated subcutaneous nodules are often found in the olecranon bursa. Findings on general physical examination are normal except for a possible low-grade fever in a few patients. Soft, small lymph nodes are found occasionally in epitrochlear, axillary, and cervical areas. The history and physical examination are the

Table 70-3 1987 Revised American Rheumatism Association Criteria for Classification of Rheumatoid Arthritis*

Criterion	Definition
Morning stiffness	Morning stiffness in and around the joints lasting at least 1 hour before maximal improvement
Arthritis of ≥3 joint areas	At least 3 joint areas simultaneously having soft tissue swelling or fluid (not bony overgrowth alone) observed by a physician (the 14 possible joint areas are [right or left] PIP, MCP, wrist, elbow, knee, ankle, and MTP joints)
Arthritis of hand joints	At least 1 joint area swollen as above in wrist, MCP, or PIP joint
Symmetric arthritis	Simultaneous involvement of the same joint areas (as in criterion 2) on both sides of the body (bilateral involvement of PIP, MCP, or MTP joints is acceptable without absolute symmetry)
Rheumatoid nodules	Subcutaneous nodules over bony prominences or extensor surfaces, or in juxta-articular regions, as observed by a physician
Serum rheumatoid factor	Demonstration of abnormal amounts of serum rheumatoid factor by any method that has been positive
Radiographic changes	Changes typical of RA on posteroanterior hand and wrist radiographs, which must include erosions or unequivocal bony decalcification localized to or most marked adjacent to involved joints (osteoarthritis changes alone do not qualify)

American College of Rheumatology Criteria	Sensitivity (%)	Specificity (%)
Morning stiffness	68	65
Arthritis in >3 areas	80	43
Arthritis of the hand joints	81	46
Symmetric arthritis	77	37
Rheumatoid nodules	3	100
Rheumatoid factor	59	93
Radiographic change	22	98

Clinical or Laboratory Variable	Persistent Nonerosive Versus Self-Limiting		Persistent Erosive Versus Persistent Nonerosive	
	Odds Ratio	Score	Odds Ratio	Score
Symptom duration at first visit				
>6 weeks, <6 months	2.49	2	0.96	0
>6 months	5.49	3	1.44	0
Morning stiffness >1 hour	1.96	1	1.96	1
Arthritis in ≥3 joints	1.73	1	1.73	1
Bilateral MTP compression pain	1.65	1	3.78	2
Rheumatoid factor positivity	2.99	2	2.99	2
Anticitrullinated protein antibody positivity	4.58	3	4.58	3
Radiographic erosions (hands or feet)	2.75	2	Infinite	Infinite

*For classification purposes, a patient is said to have RA if he or she has satisfied at least four of the seven criteria. Criteria 1 through 4 must be present for at least 6 weeks. Patients with two clinical diagnoses are not excluded. Designation as classic, definite, or probable RA is not to be made.
MCP, metacarpophalangeal; MTP, metatarsophalangeal; PIP, proximal interphalangeal; RA, rheumatoid arthritis.

most sensitive and specific tools for diagnosis of RA. Initial laboratory tests often show the results in the following list (essential tests are indicated with an asterisk [*]):
- Normal white blood cell count and differential*
- Thrombocytosis*
- Mild anemia, normochromic and either normocytic or microcytic*
- Normal urinalysis*
- ESR 30 mm/hr or greater and C-reactive protein level greater than 0.7 pg/mL*
- Normal renal, hepatic, and metabolic tests*
- Normal serum uric acid level
- Positive RF test (about 70% to 80% of patients; occurs in many normal people, in patients with other rheumatic diseases, and in those with chronic infection)*
- ACPA (about 80% to 90% of patients; can be seen in other diseases, including active tuberculosis) (especially useful as diagnostic and prognostic indicator of early synovitis)*

- Other autoantibodies (commonly found but with limited differential diagnosis utility, including antinuclear antibody, SS-A, and SS-B). Although they usually are not clinically indicated, tests for anti–double-stranded DNA and antineutrophil cytoplasmic antibody are usually negative.
- Polyclonal gammopathy as determined by serum protein electrophoresis
- Normal or elevated serum complement level

"Typical" arthrocentesis, when obvious fluid is present, in RA reveals the following:
- Joint fluid is straw-colored, is slightly cloudy, and contains many flecks of fibrin and 5000 to 25,000 white blood cells/mm³; at least 50% of these are polymorphonuclear leukocytes.
- No crystals
- Complement C4 and C2 levels are depressed, but C3 level can be normal.
- Normal synovial fluid glucose level
- Negative cultures and Gram stain

Table 70-4 2010 ACR/EULAR Classification Criteria for Rheumatoid Arthritis (Score-Based Algorithm for Classification in an Eligible Patient [Cutpoint for RA: ≥6/10])

Joint Involvement*	(0-5)
1 medium to large[†] joint	0
2-10 medium to large joints	1
1-3 small[‡] joints (with or without involvement of large joints)	2
4-10 small joints (with or without involvement of large joints)	3
>10 joints[§] (at least one small joint)	5
Serology[‖¶]	**(0-3)**
Negative RF **AND** negative ACPA	0
Low-positive RF **OR** low-positive ACPA	2
High-positive RF **OR** high-positive ACPA	3
Acute Phase Reactants[‖#]	**1**
Normal CRP **AND** normal ESR	0
Abnormal CRP **OR** abnormal ESR	1
Duration of Symptoms**	**(0-1)**
<6 weeks	0
≥6 weeks	1

*Joint involvement refers to any swollen or tender joint on examination, or evidence of synovitis on magnetic resonance imaging or ultrasonography. Distal interphalangeal joints, first carpometacarpal joint, and first metatarsophalangeal joint are excluded from assessment. Categories of joint distribution are classified according to the locations and numbers of involved joints, with placement into the highest category possible based on the pattern of joint involvement.

†Medium to large joints refer to shoulders, elbows, hips, knees, and ankles.

‡Small joints refer to the metacarpophalangeal joints, proximal interphalangeal joints, metatarsophalangeal joints 2 through 5, thumb interphalangeal joints, and wrists.

§In this category, at least one of the involved joints must be a small joint; the other joints can include any combination of large and additional small joints, as well as other joints not specifically listed elsewhere (e.g., temporomandibular, acromioclavicular, sternoclavicular).

‖Individuals should be scored by these criteria only if at least one serologic test and at least one acute phase reactant test result are available. Where a value for a serologic test of acute phase reactant is not available, that test should be considered as negative/normal.

¶Negative refers to international unit (IU) values that are less than or equal to the upper limit of normal (ULN) for the laboratory and assay; low-positive refers to IU values that are greater than the ULN but less than or equal to 3 × ULN for the laboratory and assay; high-positive refers to IU values that are greater than 3 × ULN for the laboratory and assay. Where RF is available only as positive or negative, a positive result should be scored as low-positive for RF.

#Normal/abnormal is determined by local laboratory standards.

**Duration of symptoms refers to patient self-report of the duration or signs or symptoms of synovitis (e.g., pain, swelling, tenderness) of joints that are clinically involved at the time of assessment.

ACPA, anticitrullinated protein/peptide antibody; CRP, C-reactive protein; ESR, erythrocyte sedimentation rate; RF, rheumatoid factor; ULN, upper limit of normal.

Adapted with permission from Aletaha D, Neogi T, Silman AJ, et al: 2010 rheumatoid arthritis classification criteria: an American College of Rheumatology/European League Against Rheumatism collaborative initiative, *Ann Rheum Dis* 69:1580–1588, 2010.

Differential Diagnosis

Other diseases must be excluded before the diagnosis of RA is established.[106] The differential diagnosis of adult polyarthritis is outlined in Table 70-5.[107] The following sections lists various diseases; the relative frequency of each illness is specified as common, uncommon, or rare.

Spondyloarthropathies (Common)

Ankylosing spondylitis, psoriatic arthritis, inflammatory bowel disease–associated arthritis, and reactive arthritis are often referred to as *spondyloarthropathies*. These diseases generally are marked by their respective nonarticular features and the following pattern of joint disease: asymmetric, oligoarticular, lower extremities more than upper extremities, and large joints more than small joints (note that there are

Table 70-5 Discriminating Features in Patients Presenting with Polyarthritis and Fever

Symptom or Sign	Possible Diagnoses
Temperature >40° C	Still's disease
	Bacterial arthritis
	SLE
Fever preceding arthritis	Viral arthritis
	Lyme disease
	Reactive arthritis
	Still's disease
	Bacterial endocarditis
Migratory arthritis	Rheumatic fever
	Gonococcemia
	Meningococcemia
	Viral arthritis
	SLE
	Acute leukemia
	Whipple's disease
Effusion disproportionately greater than pain	Tuberculous arthritis
	Bacterial endocarditis
	Inflammatory bowel disease
	Giant cell arteritis
	Lyme disease
Pain disproportionately greater than effusion	Rheumatic fever
	Familial Mediterranean fever
	Acute leukemia
	Acquired immunodeficiency syndrome
Positive test for rheumatoid factor	Rheumatoid arthritis
	Viral arthritis
	Tuberculous arthritis
	Bacterial endocarditis
	SLE
	Sarcoidosis
	Systemic vasculitis
Morning stiffness	Rheumatoid arthritis
	Polymyalgia rheumatica
	Still's disease
	Some viral and reactive arthritides
Symmetric small joint synovitis	Rheumatoid arthritis
	SLE
	Viral arthritis
Leukocytosis (>15,000/mm³)	Bacterial arthritis
	Bacterial endocarditis
	Still's disease
	Systemic vasculitis
	Acute leukemia
Leukopenia	SLE
	Viral arthritis
Episodic recurrences	Lyme disease
	Crystal-induced arthritis
	Inflammatory bowel disease
	Whipple's disease
	Mediterranean fever
	Still's disease
	SLE

SLE, systemic lupus erythematosus.

From Pinals RS: Polyarthritis and fever, *N Engl J Med* 330:769, 1999. Copyright 1999, Massachusetts Medical Society. All rights reserved.

many exceptions to these general guidelines). The problem in differentiating these diseases from RA arises with a patient (particularly a woman) who has minimal back pain and definite peripheral joint involvement. The presence of low back pain and lumbar involvement helps distinguish these diseases from RA.

In distinguishing patients with reactive arthritis from those with RA, a careful search for heel pain or tenderness and ocular or urethral symptoms is of great importance. Polyarthritis persists chronically in more than 80% of patients with reactive arthritis. The characteristics of enthesopathy in patients with reactive arthritis (i.e., "sausage" digits indicating periarticular soft tissue inflammation, insertional tendinitis, periostitis, and peri-insertional osteoporosis or erosion) may point to the diagnosis.

The differential diagnosis between RA with psoriasis and some forms of psoriatic arthritis may be artificial (see Chapter 43). Some patients with DIP joint involvement and severe skin involvement have a disease that is not RA. Others have a seropositive symmetric polyarthritis that appears to be RA, yet they also have psoriasis. These patients can be treated with the same disease-modifying drugs that are given to patients with progressive RA, including TNF inhibitors.

As a syndrome described extensively in the French literature, synovitis, acne, pustulosis, hyperostosis, osteitis (SAPHO)[108] may resemble psoriatic arthritis and, occasionally, when peripheral arthritis is present, RA. As the name implies, patients variably have severe acne, palmar and plantar pustules, hyperostotic reactions (particularly in the clavicles and sternum), sacroiliitis, and peripheral inflammatory arthritis.

Inflammatory bowel disease (ulcerative colitis and Crohn's disease) is associated with arthritis in 20% of cases (see Chapter 78). Peripheral arthritis occurs more commonly than spondylitis in many series.[109] Ankles, knees, and elbows are the most typically involved peripheral joints, with PIP joints and wrists next in frequency. Simultaneous attacks of arthritis and the development of erythema nodosum are common. Only two or three joints are affected at once. Involvement is usually asymmetric, and erosions are uncommon. The occurrence of peripheral arthritis in inflammatory bowel disease is not related to HLA-B27.

Behçet's syndrome is marked by asymmetric polyarthritis in 50% to 60% of cases (see Chapter 93).[110] It is rare, with a prevalence of less than 1 in 25,000 in the United States. In more than half of cases, the attacks of arthritis are mono-articular. Knees, ankles, and wrists are affected most often; synovial fluid usually contains more than 5000 but less than 30,000 white blood cells/mm³. Joint deformity is unusual. Painful oral and genital ulcers and central nervous system involvement are characteristic. Uveal tract involvement in Behçet's syndrome must be differentiated from the scleritis characteristic of RA in patients with ocular and joint disease.

Enteric infections are complicated occasionally by inflammatory joint disease resembling RA. The joint disease associated with *Yersinia enterocolitica* infection occurs several weeks after the gastrointestinal illness. Knees and ankles are the joints most commonly involved, and most patients

(even patients with peripheral arthritis and no spondylitis) have HLA-B27. Reactive arthritis also has been reported after *Salmonella*, *Shigella*, and *Campylobacter* (*Helicobacter*) *jejuni* infection.

Calcium Pyrophosphate Dihydrate Deposition Disease (Common)

Calcium pyrophosphate dihydrate deposition disease is a crystal-induced synovitis that takes many forms, ranging from a syndrome of indolent osteoarthrosis to that of an acute, hot joint. About 5% of patients have chronic polyarthritis (sometimes referred to as pseudo-RA) associated with proliferative erosion of subchondral bone. Although radiographs are helpful when chondrocalcinosis is present, calcium pyrophosphate dihydrate deposition disease may be present in the absence of calcification on radiographs.[111] Diagnosis then can be made only by arthrocentesis. A radiographic sign of calcium pyrophosphate dihydrate deposition disease that helps to differentiate it from RA is the presence of unicompartmental disease in the wrists (see Chapter 96). On physical examination, the MCPs in calcium pyrophosphate dihydrate deposition disease generally have bony enlargement rather than soft tissue swelling owing to synovial hyperplasia.

Fibromyalgia (Common)

In fibromyalgia, no evidence of synovitis is found (see Chapter 52). Although no specific diagnostic tests define this entity, nonarticular pain and tenderness are common. In an analysis contrasting the pain properties of fibromyalgia versus those of RA,[112] fibromyalgia patients used diverse adjectives to describe their pain, the most common being "pressing," "shooting," "gnawing," "cramping," and "crushing." Most patients in both groups defined the pain as aching and exhausting. Some patients with diffuse connective tissue diseases, including RA, can develop a superimposed fibromyalgia, adding to the difficulty of treating the arthritis.

Gout (Common)

Before a diagnosis of chronic erosive RA is made, chronic tophaceous gout must be ruled out. The reverse applies as well. Features of gouty arthritis that can mimic the features of RA include polyarthritis, symmetric involvement, fusiform swelling of joints, subcutaneous nodules, and a subacute presentation of attacks. Conversely, certain aspects of RA that suggest gouty arthritis include periarticular nodules and seronegative disease (particularly in men). Radiographic findings may be similar, with the appearance of subcortical erosions of RA resembling small osseous tophi in gout. Although large asymmetric erosions with ballooning of the cortex and overhanging edges are more likely to be caused by gout than by RA, this is not always the case. Serologic test results may be misleading as well; RF has been reported in 30% of patients with chronic tophaceous gout who have no clinical or radiographic signs of RA.[113]

Human Immunodeficiency Virus Infection (Common)

Several types of arthropathy have been described in association with human immunodeficiency virus (HIV) infection, including the following[114]:

- Brief, acute arthralgias concurrent with initial HIV viremia
- HIV-associated arthritis, lower extremity noninflammatory oligoarthritis, or a persistent polyarthritis
- Seronegative spondyloarthropathy resembling psoriatic arthritis, or reactive arthritis, often more severe than in patients without HIV infection[115]

It is crucial to rule out HIV in any patient with an acute polyarthritis and fever: HIV-positive patients are at greater risk for toxicity or opportunistic infection when using immunosuppressive drugs (see Chapter 114). HIV-positive patients also can present with syndromes of vasculitis.

Infectious Diseases (Including Viral Causes Such As Hepatitis C) (Common)

Arthritis is commonly associated with viral infection and sometimes can mimic RA. For example, symmetric inflammatory arthritis complicates rubella or rubella vaccination more often in adults than in children and may affect the small joints of the hands. Lymphocytes predominate in synovial effusions of rubella.

Rheumatoid-like arthritis often precedes jaundice in viral hepatitis and is associated with the presence of circulating hepatitis B surface antigen and hypocomplementemia. The surface antigen has been found in synovial tissues with the use of direct immunofluorescence; this supports the concept that this synovitis is mediated by immune complexes.[116] Acute onset of diffuse polyarthritis with small joint effusions and minimal synovial swelling, often accompanied by urticaria, should prompt the physician to request liver function tests in the patient with a history of exposure to hepatitis. With the onset of icterus, arthritis usually resolves without a trace.

Increasing recognition of hepatitis C as a cause of joint problems is related to the availability of specific serologic tests for this virus. About one-third of people infected with hepatitis C virus have arthralgias or arthritis, and in a Korean series, the prevalence of cryoglobulins (mean concentration of 9.8 g/L) was 59%.[117] Patients can present with palmar tenosynovitis, small joint synovitis, carpal tunnel syndrome, and positive tests for RF. The presence of ACPAs can be a useful feature in distinguishing RA from hepatitis C–associated arthritis.[118] Other findings, including mixed cryoglobulinemia syndrome, glomerulonephritis, and cutaneous vasculitis, round out the clinical spectrum of rheumatic complaints associated with this viral infection. Because exacerbation of hepatitis can be associated with the use and the cessation of methotrexate therapy, a good case has been made for testing for hepatitis C every patient with RA scheduled to be started on therapy with this drug.[119]

Fever, sore throat, and cervical adenopathy followed by symmetric polyarthritis are compatible with infection resulting from hepatitis B, rubella, adenovirus type 7, echovirus type 9, *Mycoplasma pneumoniae*, or Epstein-Barr virus and acute rheumatic fever or adult-onset Still's disease. In Japan, many more patients with RA have circulating antibodies against human T-lymphotropic virus type I (HTLV-I), and epidemiologic evidence indicates that HTLV might be associated with an RA-like condition. Multiple nodules within tendon sheaths associated with inflammation resembling rheumatoid tenosynovitis have been described in a patient with HTLV-I arthropathy.[120]

A chronic polyarthritis resembling RA has been described after serologic proof of parvovirus infection. Usually the process is self-limited and does not progress to a destructive synovitis (see Chapter 114). Adults, often those involved in child care, present with a history of a viral-type illness, sometimes with desquamating finger involvement and a diffuse, red facial rash ("slapped cheeks"), followed by arthralgias and synovitis.

Chikungunya is an insect-borne virus found in Africa and Asia that manifests infection as an acute febrile phase with rash followed by prolonged arthralgia or arthritis of multiple joints. Arthritis usually persists for weeks to months but in some cases can last for years.

Polyarthritis after bacterial infection such as poststreptococcal arthritis also can resemble RA. Typically, patients have an antecedent skin or oropharynx group A streptococcal infection in the weeks preceding symptoms. Antistreptolysin O antibody titers are usually elevated. Although the same bacteria can cause glomerulonephritis, it is uncommon to see concomitant arthritis and renal disease.

Lyme Disease (Common in Endemic Areas)

Lyme disease can closely simulate RA in adults or children because of its intermittent course with the development of chronic synovitis. A proliferative, erosive synovitis necessitating synovectomy has evolved in several cases. The histopathologic appearance of the proliferative synovium is not different from that of RA (see Chapter 110), and the Lyme synovial cells produce a similar excess of metalloproteinases. Lyme serologic tests can help distinguish this disease from RA, as can a history of tick bites, characteristic skin rash, or neurologic involvement.

Osteoarthritis (Common)

Although osteoarthritis can begin as a degenerative cartilage disease, and RA begins as synovial inflammation, these diseases can overlap as they progress (Table 70-6). In osteoarthritis, as cartilage deteriorates and joint congruence is altered and stressed, a reactive synovitis often develops. Conversely, because the rheumatoid pannus erodes cartilage, secondary osteoarthritic changes in bone and cartilage occur. In osteoarthritis, involvement of the DIP and first carpometacarpal (CMC) joints is common, but it is rare in RA. Alternatively, MCP and wrist involvement are uncommon in OA. During end stages of degenerative joint disease and RA, involved joints appear the same. In some cases, to differentiate clearly between the two, the physician must delve into the early history and functional abnormalities associated with the disease.

Erosive osteoarthritis occurs frequently in middle-aged women (more frequently than in men) and is characterized

Table 70-6 Factors Useful for Differentiating Early Rheumatoid Arthritis from Osteoarthritis

	Rheumatoid Arthritis	Osteoarthritis
Age at onset	Childhood and adults, peak incidence in 50s	Increases with age
Predisposing factors	Susceptibility epitopes (HLA-DR4, HLA-DR1) PTPN22, PADI4 polymorphisms, and others Smoking	Trauma Congenital abnormalities (e.g., shallow acetabulum)
Early symptoms	Morning stiffness	Pain increases through the day and with use
Joints involved	Metacarpophalangeal joints, wrists, proximal interphalangeal joints most often; distal interphalangeal joints almost never	Distal interphalangeal joints (Heberden's nodes), weight-bearing joints (hips, knees)
Physical findings	Soft tissue swelling, warmth	Bony osteophytes, minimal soft tissue swelling early
Radiologic findings	Periarticular osteopenia, marginal erosions	Subchondral sclerosis, osteophytes
Laboratory findings	Increased C-reactive protein, rheumatoid factor, anticitrullinated protein antibody, anemia, leukocytosis	Normal

by inflammatory changes in PIP joints with destruction and functional ankylosis of the joints. The PIP joints can be red and hot, yet almost no synovial proliferation or effusion occurs; joint swelling involves hard, bony tissue, not synovium. The ESR may be slightly elevated, but RF is not found (see Chapter 99).

Polymyalgia Rheumatica and Giant Cell Arteritis (Common)

Joint radionuclide imaging studies demonstrate increased vascular flow in the synovium of patients with classic polymyalgia rheumatica. Clinical synovitis commonly occurs, but markdly symptomatic arthritis is uncommon. A careful history usually can differentiate shoulder or hip-girdle muscle pain from shoulder or hip joint pain. Examination of synovial biopsy specimens from patients with polymyalgia rheumatica indicates that the synovitis is usually milder than that found in RA.

Several patients have been described whose initial symptom of giant cell arteritis was a peripheral polyarthritis clinically indistinguishable from RA.[121] Among 19 such patients in a group of 522 with biopsy-proven giant cell arteritis, however, only 3 were RF positive. The interval between onsets of each set of symptoms was 3 years or less in 15 of the 19 patients; this suggests a relationship between the two (see Chapter 88). It is known that patients with giant cell arteritis often have HLA-DR4 alleles.

Systemic Lupus Erythematosus (Common)

The distribution of involved joints and deformities in systemic lupus erythematosus (SLE) can be identical to that seen in RA. In contrast to RA, SLE arthritis usually does not cause cartilage destruction or bone erosion. The deformities are often reducible, sometimes leading to normal hand radiographs, owing to the effect of placing the hand firmly on the film cassette. Serologies (antinuclear antibody, anti–double-stranded DNA) and major organ system involvement usually can distinguish RA from SLE. However, RA and SLE can overlap, suggesting a mixed picture of both diseases, sometimes referred to as "rupus." The presence of erosive arthritis in SLE patients is associated with ACPAs.[122] The frequency of erosive arthritis in SLE patients is approximately 10% to 15%, and the subset of SLE patients that are anti-CCP antibody positive are more likely to have erosive

arthritis, suggesting a pathogenic role for the antibody in the formation of erosions.

Musculoskeletal Pain of Thyroid Disease (Common)

In hypothyroidism (see Chapter 121), synovial effusions and synovial thickening can simulate RA.[123] The ESR may be elevated because of hypergammaglobulinemia, but C-reactive protein is normal. The joint fluid is noninflammatory and may have increased viscosity. Knees, wrists, hands, and feet are involved most often, and coexisting calcium pyrophosphate dihydrate deposition disease is frequently found. This syndrome should be distinguished from arthralgias and other nonspecific musculoskeletal problems that often accompany hyperthyroidism and hypothyroidism.

The syndrome of thyroid acropachy complicates less than 1% of cases of hyperthyroidism. This syndrome comprises periosteal new bone formation, which may be associated with a low-grade synovitis similar to hypertrophic osteoarthropathy. Patients with coexisting RA and hyperthyroidism have pain from the arthritis that, although impossible to quantify, seems to exceed the pain expected from the degree of inflammation.

Vasculitis (Uncommon)

Patients with a variety of vasculitides can present with inflammatory arthritis; these syndromes are readily distinguished from RA. Many small vessel vasculitides show palpable purpura and are associated with hepatitis C and cryoglobulinemia. Medium vessel forms of vasculitis, such as granulomatosis with polyangiitis, Churg-Strauss syndrome, or microscopic polyangiitis, include major organ system involvement (e.g., reactive airways disease, glomerulonephritis) and are usually antineutrophil cytoplasmic antibody positive. Polyarteritis nodosa, especially in arthritis associated with hepatitis B, usually is distinguished by renovascular hypertension and other systemic symptoms.

Adult-Onset Still's Disease (Uncommon)

Significant fever at the onset of RA is unusual in adults. Later in the course, if vasculitis or serositis is present, or if intense exacerbations of disease occur, low-grade fever is more common. Adult Still's disease, in contrast, usually manifests with high spiking fevers. Serologic studies (RF and antinuclear antibody) are negative, and patients do not have subcutaneous nodules. Fever patterns in these patients are often quotidian (i.e., reaching normal levels at least once each day). Occasionally, evanescent salmon-colored or pink macules on the trunk and extremities become more prominent when patients are febrile. The cervical spine may be involved, and loss of neck motion may be striking. Approximately 20% of patients with adult-onset Still's disease showed significant functional deterioration from erosive joint disease, similar to RA.[124]

Abnormal liver function tests consistent with hepatitis and severe abdominal pain can be performed and may confound attempts at diagnosis. Liver involvement is observed in most cases and was noted in more than two-thirds of patients in one series[125]; hypergammaglobulinemia is present in more than 60%. Pericarditis and pleural effusions are observed in less than 25% of cases. In contrast to active SLE with nephritis, the serum complement level is normal or high. Serum ferritin levels can be enormously elevated to well beyond levels expected compared with other acute phase reactants in the same individual.[126] When levels are greater than 10,000 ng/mL, physicians should strongly consider adult Still's disease as the diagnosis rather than RA. The glycosylated form of serum ferritin, usually greater than 50% of the total, is reportedly low (mean, 16%) during active phases and in remission.[127]

Yamaguchi and associates[128] developed criteria for establishing the diagnosis of adult Still's disease, which, in numerous series, have greater than 90% sensitivity (Table 70-7). After other diseases have been excluded, adult Still's disease should be considered if five criteria (with more than two being major ones) are met. It is unknown yet whether adding hyperferritinemia would increase the specificity of the diagnosis.

Bacterial Endocarditis (Uncommon)

Arthralgias, arthritis, back pain, and myalgias occur in approximately 30% of patients with subacute bacterial endocarditis.[129] Symptoms typically occur in one or several joints, usually large, proximal ones. This synovitis probably is caused by the deposition of circulating immune complexes. Confusion with RA can occasionally arise because more than half of patients with endocarditis are seropositive for RF. Fever out of proportion to joint findings in the setting of leukocytosis should lead to consideration of infective endocarditis as a diagnostic possibility, even in the absence of a significant heart murmur. Peripheral emboli with digital infarctions may be found, simulating palpable purpura when they occur on the lower legs. Blood cultures

Table 70-7 Criteria for Diagnosis of Still's Disease

Major Criteria	Minor Criteria
Temperature >39° C for >1 week	Sore throat
Leukocytosis >10,000/mm³ with >80% PMNs	Lymph node enlargement
	Splenomegaly
Typical rash	Liver dysfunction (high AST/ALT)
Arthralgias >2 weeks	

ALT, alanine aminotransferase; AST, aspartate aminotransferase; PMNs, polymorphonuclear leukocytes.

should be obtained in all patients with polyarthritis and significant fever. Embolic phenomena with constitutional symptoms, including arthralgias, can be presenting symptoms of atrial myxoma, but this process usually mimics systemic vasculitis or subacute bacterial endocarditis more than RA.

Hemochromatosis (Uncommon)

The characteristic articular feature of hemochromatosis that is almost diagnostic is firm bony enlargement of the MCP joints, particularly the second and third joints, with associated cystic degenerative disease and large hook-like osteophytes on radiographs and, frequently, chondrocalcinosis. Marginal erosions, juxta-articular osteoporosis, synovial proliferation, and ulnar deviation are not seen in the arthropathy of hemochromatosis but are common in RA. Wrists, shoulders, elbows, hips, and knees are involved less often than the MCP joints. Arthritis leads the list of diagnoses provided to patients to explain their symptoms before the diagnosis of hemochromatosis is decided.[131] In the series by McDonnell and colleagues,[131] patients with symptoms received a diagnosis of hemochromatosis only after the symptoms had been present, on average, for an extended period (10 years) and after they had visited an average of 3.5 physicians (see Chapter 118). Other distinguishing features include the fact that hemochromatosis is more common in males, and that patients generally will be RF and ACPA negative and may have other features of iron overload, including CHF, liver abnormalities, adult-onset diabetes, and hyperpigmentation.

Hemophilic Arthropathy (Uncommon)

A deficiency of factor VIII or, less frequently, factor IX, sufficient to produce clinical bleeding, frequently results in hemarthroses. Iron overload at the joint generates a proliferative synovitis that often leads to joint destruction. Because iron stimulates metalloproteinase production by synovial cells, when feasible, large hemarthroses should be aspirated, and the joint should be immobilized and wrapped well. The clotting abnormality is rarely overlooked, however, and it is unlikely that a diagnosis of RA would be made in the setting of hemophilia A or B (see Chapter 119).

Hyperlipoproteinemia (Uncommon)

Achilles tendinitis and tenosynovitis can be presenting symptoms in familial type II hyperlipoproteinemia and may be accompanied by arthritis. Synovial fluid findings may resemble the findings of mild RA, and tendon xanthomas may be mistaken for rheumatoid nodules or gouty tophi. Conversely, bilateral pseudoxanthomatous rheumatoid nodules have been described. Treatment of hyperlipoproteinemia with statins may cause an acute or subacute muscular syndrome that resembles myositis or polymyalgia rheumatica more than it resembles RA (see Chapter 85).

Hypertrophic Osteoarthropathy (Uncommon)

Hypertrophic osteoarthropathy may present as oligoarthritis involving the knees, ankles, or wrists. However, patients generally give a history characteristic of bone pain rather than joint pain. Synovial inflammation accompanies periosteal new bone formation, which is visible on radiographs. Correction of the inciting factor (e.g., cure of pneumonia in a child with cystic fibrosis) is likely to alleviate the synovitis. The synovium is characterized primarily by an increased blood supply and synovial cell proliferation. Little infiltration by mononuclear cells is seen. Pain in the bones that increases when extremities are dependent is characteristic, although it is not always present. If clubbing is not present or is not noticed, this entity may rarely be confused with RA.

Relapsing Seronegative Symmetric Synovitis with Pitting Edema (Uncommon)

Relapsing seronegative symmetric synovitis with pitting edema (RS3PE) is an uncommon syndrome marked by significant pitting edema of the hands with synovial thickening and joint tenderness.[132] It occurs predominantly in elderly men and is characterized by rapid onset of symmetric synovitis and pitting edema over the involved joints. Edema usually occurs in the hands and ankles overlying involved distal joints. Symptoms rapidly respond to short courses of corticosteroids and can lead to residual abnormalities, including flexion contractures of the wrists and fingers. Patients are RF negative, and increased risk of neoplastic disease has been suggested. A poor response to corticosteroid treatment and the presence of constitutional symptoms have been observed in patients with an underlying malignancy. Patients can evolve into other autoimmune diseases, including seronegative RA. In addition, the syndrome might represent a variant of another disease, such as polymyalgia rheumatica or reflex sympathetic dystrophy, rather than a distinct entity.[133]

Rheumatic Fever (Uncommon)

Rheumatic fever is much less common in the developed world than it once was, but it still must be considered in adults with polyarthritis. In adults, arthritis is the most prominent clinical finding of rheumatic fever; carditis is less common than in children; and erythema marginatum, subcutaneous nodules, and chorea are rare. The presentation is often that of an additive, symmetric, large joint polyarthritis (involving lower extremities in 85% of patients), developing within 1 week and associated with a severe tenosynovitis. This extremely painful process is often dramatically responsive to salicylates. In contrast to Still's disease in adults, rheumatic fever generally has no remittent or quotidian fevers and shows evidence of antecedent streptococcal infection. It also has a less protracted course than Still's disease. Many similarities have been noted between rheumatic fever in adults and "reactive" postinfectious synovitis developing from *Shigella*, *Salmonella*, *Brucella*, *Neisseria*, or *Yersinia* infection. As rheumatic fever becomes less common, and because penicillin prophylaxis effectively prevents recurrence of the disease, Jaccoud's arthritis (chronic post–rheumatic fever arthritis) is becoming more rare. This entity, described by Bywaters in 1950,[134] results from severe and repeated bouts of rheumatic fever and synovitis, which stretches joint capsules and produces ulnar deformity of the

hands without erosions. The same deformity can develop in SLE characterized by recurrent synovitis and soft tissue inflammation and in Parkinson's disease. Differentiating rheumatic fever from RA is particularly difficult when subcutaneous nodules are present with rheumatic fever.

Sarcoidosis (Uncommon)

The two most common forms of sarcoid arthritis often can be easily distinguished from RA. In the acute form with erythema nodosum and hilar adenopathy (Löfgren's syndrome), articular problems usually are related to periarthritis affecting large joints of the lower extremities, classically the ankles. Differential diagnosis may be complicated because many of these patients have RF in serum. Joint erosions and proliferative synovitis do not occur in this form of sarcoidosis.

In chronic granulomatous sarcoidosis, cyst-like areas of bone destruction, mottled rarefaction of bone, and a reticular pattern of bone destruction with a lace-like appearance on radiographs may simulate destructive RA. This form of sarcoidosis is often polyarticular, and biopsy of bone or synovium for diagnosis may be essential because often no correlation is noted between joint disease and clinical evidence of sarcoid involvement in other organ systems. Poncet's disease (tuberculous rheumatism) might actually represent granulomatous "idiopathic" arthritis (i.e., sarcoidosis) (see Chapter 117).[135]

Amyloidosis (Uncommon)

Deposits of amyloid can be found in synovial and periarticular tissues and are presumably responsible for the joint problems of some patients. The synovial fluid in amyloid arthropathy is noninflammatory, and particulate material with apple-green fluorescence after Congo red staining may be found in the fluid. Amyloid may cause punched-out bone lesions that rarely can mimic RA erosions. Amyloid formed of β2-microglobulin is found in the joints of patients with chronic renal failure, usually patients who are on dialysis (see Chapter 116).

Malignancy (Uncommon)

Direct involvement by cancer of the synovium usually manifests as a monoarthritis. Non-Hodgkin's lymphoma can manifest as seronegative polyarthritis, without hepatomegaly or lymphadenopathy. Lymphoma can manifest as a symmetric polyarthritis.[136] In children, acute lymphocytic leukemia can manifest as a polyarticular arthritis. Paraneoplastic syndromes and others related to direct involvement with cancer can mimic RA and are described in detail later (see Chapter 122).

Multicentric Reticulohistiocytosis (Rare)

Multicentric reticulohistiocytosis causes severe arthritis mutilans with an opera-glass hand (main en lorgnette).[137] Other causes of arthritis mutilans include RA, psoriatic arthritis, erosive osteoarthritis treated with glucocorticoids, and gout (after tophi are resorbed by treatment with allopurinol). The cell that causes damage to tissues is the multinucleate lipid-laden histiocyte, which apparently releases degradative enzymes sufficient to destroy connective tissue. These cells in aggregate produce multiple small nodules around joints of the hands.

Pigmented Villonodular Synovitis (Rare)

Pigmented villonodular synovitis is a nonmalignant but proliferative disease of synovial tissue that has many functional characteristics similar to those of RA but usually involves only one joint. The histopathologic appearance is characterized by proliferation of histiocytes, multinucleate giant cells, and hemosiderin- and lipid-laden macrophages. Clinically, this is a painless chronic synovitis (most often of the knee) with joint effusions and greatly thickened synovium. Subchondral bone cysts and cartilage erosion may be associated with bulky tissue. It is unclear whether this condition should be classified as an inflammation or as a neoplasm of the synovium (see Chapter 123).

OUTCOMES

Many difficulties are associated with establishing a change in patterns of RA in different time periods or different communities. The best data suggest that clinical manifestations of the disease and the extent of disability are declining. Epidemiologic studies suggest that the disease is not changing, but that earlier, more effective treatment has diminished morbidity.

Criteria for clinical remission were proposed by ACR/EULAR in 2011.[138] Remission can be defined as absence of disease, but its application to RA patients has changed over time. With more effective treatment available, stricter criteria have become more important. Definitions vary widely and can mean absence of clinical and radiologic signs of disease while on treatment, or a disease state with minimal or no activity after therapy is withdrawn. A previous composite system using the Disease Activity Score (DAS) is a mathematical method that includes swollen and tender joints, ESR, and patient assessments of global health.[139] Notably, this criterion does not mean that the patient truly has complete remission with no evidence of synovitis; however, it can be associated with several active joints. ACR criteria from 1981 require absence of joint tenderness, fatigue, joint pain, joint swelling, and morning stiffness, along with a normal ESR. The goal of the ACR/EULAR revised remission criteria was to develop more stringent but achievable criteria for clinical trials. Remission was defined as tender joint count of 1 or less, swollen joint count of 1 or less, C-reactive protein (CRP) of 1 or less, and patient global assessment of 1 or less. In addition, an index-based definition was included as an alternative. Both definitions performed similarly in validation studies. Some controversy still exists regarding whether the goal should be "clinical" or "imaging" remission when ultrasound or MRI evidence of synovitis is considered. The clinical importance of synovitis diagnosed only by imaging in an asymptomatic patient is uncertain.

With increased numbers of effective therapies available, it becomes increasingly important for physicians to be able to determine which patients would be at greatest risk for progressive destructive disease, and which patients would have a more benign illness that is not erosive and is responsive to moderate intervention. In addition to predicting which patients may or may not develop erosion, it is equally important to identify which patients who already have erosions are more likely to progress rapidly to joint destruction. One study of an inception cohort of patients newly presenting with inflammatory polyarthritis confirmed the fact that although the initial radiographic score is, as expected, a powerful predictor of subsequent radiographic damage, high titers of RF and ACPAs continue to be powerful predictors of deteriorating radiographic damage in subjects receiving conventional therapy.[140] ACPAs (e.g., to fibrinogen, to vimentin, to fibronectin) are more specific for RA than for RF, can appear before disease onset, and are predictive of more aggressive and destructive disease.[141] Antimutated citrullinated vimentin antibodies recognize peptides with amino acid substitutions that most likely occur as the result of somatic mutations in the joint and might be more predictive of radiographic progression compared with standard ACPAs.[142]

Joint erosions and deformity may not be the most important aspects of disease for the patients. In several studies, the Health Assessment Questionnaire has been shown to be an excellent predictor of work disability and mortality,[143] and its results can be discrepant from damage measured by radiographs.

Mortality

Infection, renal disease, and respiratory failure traditionally have been the primary factors contributing to excess mortality in RA patients, although congestive heart failure, ischemic heart disease, and peripheral atherosclerosis are more correctly identified as the most common cause of excess mortality in RA (see Chapter 36). In addition, disability develops most rapidly during the first 2 years of RA, supporting the current practice of early aggressive therapy.[144] Persistent premature death and potential widening of the mortality gap in RA patients compared with the general population have been attributed to three potential contributing factors.[145] RA patients are at greater risk for multiple comorbid conditions and poorer outcomes after development of these illnesses. In addition, RA patients often do not receive the best preventive care. Last, systemic inflammation and altered immune responses associated with RA tend to increase and hasten comorbidity and mortality.

Careful epidemiologic studies have indicated that cardiovascular disease is the main cause of increased mortality in RA patients.[146] In the Norfolk Arthritis Register, a primary care–based inception cohort, patients who were seropositive for RF died at an excessive rate within the first 7 years of disease resulting from cardiovascular causes (men, 1.34; women, 2.02) compared with controls.[147] This increased incidence of cardiovascular events in RA patients is independent of traditional risk factors, such as age, sex, smoking status, diabetes mellitus, hypercholesterolemia, systolic blood pressure, and body mass index.[148] The generally accepted explanation is that inflammatory cytokines that are produced in excess in RA (e.g., TNF, platelet-derived growth factor) have the capacity to activate endothelial and subendothelial myofibroblasts, and numerous inflammatory cells are found in atheromatous plaques. Given that nonrheumatoid patients who have higher levels of C-reactive protein than control groups have higher incidences of coronary disease, these data are consistent with hypotheses. Ultrasonography has shown that RA patients have greater thickness of the common carotid and femoral arteries than healthy controls—a finding that was independent of glucocorticoid therapy but was related to the duration and severity of RA.[149] Platelet-derived microparticles, the small vesicles that are released from the plasma membrane when these cells are activated, are elevated in RA in proportion to disease activity.[150] As was noted earlier, the following factors and pathobiologic mechanisms could contribute to atherosclerosis in RA[151]:

- Immune complex–mediated endothelial damage
- Acute phase reactants (C-reactive protein and serum amyloid A, both of which have proinflammatory activity)
- Inflammatory cytokines
- High expression of endothelial cell leukocyte adhesion molecules
- Medications (e.g., steroids)
- Prothrombotic factors (e.g., increased platelets, fibrinogen, and thromboxane)
- Endothelial cell dysfunction induced by inflammation

Therapies considered for rheumatoid patients must consider the effects on atherogenesis. In patients with an unfavorable vascular profile, these considerations might include supplementation with omega-3 fatty acids in the diet, early use of 3-hydroxy-3-methylglutaryl co-enzyme A reductase inhibitors (statins that, in addition to providing lipid-lowering effects, reduce C-reactive protein), attempts to reduce elevated levels of homocysteine induced by methotrexate, avoidance of cyclosporine, and aggressive weight loss disciplines and smoking cessation programs. The IL-6 receptor antibody tocilizumab suppresses several risk factors for mortality, including inflammation, elevated ESR, and elevated C-reactive protein. It also alters the lipid profile by increasing low-density lipoproteins, albeit with a concomitant increase in high-density lipoproteins to maintain a similar ratio. The ultimate effects on cardiovascular risk factors and mortality are still uncertain under these circumstances.

In addition to cardiovascular causes of death associated with RA are causes of death due to complications (articular and extra-articular) of RA and to side effects of therapy. The probability of death varies directly with the severity of complications. Potentially morbid articular complications include the various forms of atlantoaxial subluxation, cricoarytenoid synovitis, and sepsis of involved joints. Unfortunately, mortality from infection in RA has actually increased approximately fourfold to fivefold on average from reports from 1982 to 2004.[65] Extra-articular complications directly causing higher mortality include Felty's syndrome, Sjögren's syndrome, pulmonary complications, and diffuse vasculitis.

One of the largest and best documented studies of survival, prognosis, and causes of death in RA was published by Mitchell and associates.[152] In this prospective trial of 805 patients, which included 12 years of observation, 233 patients died during the course of the study, and survivorship was only 50% of that in population controls. Increased mortality associated with RA is impressive and equals that

seen in all patients with Hodgkin's disease, diabetes mellitus, or stroke (age adjusted).

One prediction suggests that tight control of inflammation might decrease cardiovascular and cerebrovascular events and improve survival. Aggressive use of methotrexate can decrease mortality in patients with cardiovascular or noncardiovascular mortality.[153] Biologic agents such as TNF inhibitors seem to improve survival, especially in women.[154] TNF blockade can potentially exacerbate heart disease, however, and increases mortality in individuals with preexisting congestive heart failure. Longer-term studies are required to assess the impact of new agents such as rituximab and abatacept on mortality (see Chapter 64).

Increased risk for malignancy has been observed in RA, especially with lymphoma. RA patients have a two to three times higher risk of developing Hodgkin's disease, non-Hodgkin's lymphoma, or leukemia compared with the normal population; this is independent of immunosuppressive therapy. Of lymphomas arising in RA, about half are low grade and half are high grade. Most are B cell lymphomas, although it is not clear whether these originate from clonally proliferated lymphocytes associated with RA. Although the relative risk for total cancer in patients with Felty's syndrome is only twofold, the relative risk for non-Hodgkin's lymphoma in this complication of RA is nearly 13-fold[155]—similar to that associated with Sjögren's syndrome.

A meta-analysis of malignancy in adult RA patients indicated that the risk of lung cancer is increased 1.5- to 3.5-fold compared with the general population.[156] Interstitial fibrosis might serve as a risk factor for lung carcinoma, particularly the bronchoalveolar variety.[157] In contrast, risks for colorectal and breast cancer were slightly decreased in RA patients. RA patients have demonstrated a consistently reduced risk for cancer of the gastrointestinal tract.[158] NSAIDs could be responsible for lowering the risk for this form of cancer, as supported by evidence that these drugs can diminish the occurrence and numbers of colonic polyps.

Early clinical trials suggested that solid tumors might be enhanced in patients with RA treated with TNF blockers.[159] Similar data in patients with Wegener's granulomatosis suggest that the combination of etanercept and cyclophosphamide can increase the risk for cancer.[160] However, several large registry studies evaluating the effects of TNF inhibitors on cancer rates in RA patients suggest that the oncogenic effect, if it exists, is small.

Variables Related to Outcome

In attempting to sort out the relative roles of disease manifestations, compared with nondisease factors, in generating disability in RA, investigators have proposed hypothetical models to predict disability in RA using demographic, sociocultural, and clinical characteristics of a consecutive cohort of RA patients.[161] Although their methods could not be used to explain the dynamics of disability in 41% of cases, disease-related factors explained 33% and nondisease factors (e.g., depression and psychologic status, education) accounted for 26% of the disability. Other studies have emphasized the following disease factors, which correlate with a poorer prognosis and a greater likelihood of joint destruction:

Table 70-8 Activities of Daily Living and Visual Analog Questionnaire (see Supplemental Figures 70-1 to 70-12 on www.expertconsult.com)

A. How often is it PAINFUL for you to:	Never	Sometimes	Most of the Time	Always
Dress yourself?	_____	_____	_____	_____
Get into and out of bed?	_____	_____	_____	_____
Lift a cup or glass to your lips?	_____	_____	_____	_____
Walk outdoors on flat ground?	_____	_____	_____	_____
Wash and dry your entire body?	_____	_____	_____	_____
Bend down to pick up clothing from the floor?	_____	_____	_____	_____
Turn faucets on or off?	_____	_____	_____	_____
Get into and out of a car?	_____	_____	_____	_____

B. How much pain have you had in the PAST WEEK? (*mark the scale*)

No pain_____

Pain as bad as it could be

0   **100**

From Callahan LF, Brooks RH, Summey JA, et al: Quantitative pain assessment for routine care of rheumatoid arthritis patients, using a pain scale based on activities of daily living and a visual analog pain scale, *Arthritis Rheum* 30:630, 1987.

- Positive RF in serum[162]
- Positive ACPA in serum
- Rheumatoid nodules[163]
- Elevated Health Assessment Questionnaire level of disability[164]
- Depression[165]
- Persistent ESR elevation (serving as a surrogate for disease control)
- Presence of the shared epitope (QKRAA) on class II major histocompatibility genes

Assessment of the Individual Patient

Assessment of disease activity and its progression is different from prognosis. Prognosis extrapolates from a known set of indices (as noted earlier) and the degree of measured activity of disease to prediction of the outcome. Assessment is the accurate evaluation of disease progression over time. Although the indices listed in the previous section are useful as a way to predict outcomes from one-time measurements, use of three or more assessment measures provides the physician with a graph of progression in an individual patient that he or she can try to flatten out by therapy.[166] Whatever assessment index is used, it should be used early in the patient's disease, so that values are recorded before significant loss of function.

For most patients, a self-report questionnaire based on degrees of difficulty in performing activities of daily living correlates well with joint count, radiographic score, acute phase reactants, grip strength, walking time, functional class estimates, and global self-assessment. One useful self-report includes only eight items from the much longer Stanford Health Assessment Questionnaire (Table 70-8).[167] The limitation of this form—failure to detect clinical improvement in patients with few impairments in activities of daily living—may be offset by its acceptability to patients within busy office practices.

In some situations, more comprehensive joint counts are needed. These include points when large changes in drug therapy are about to be instituted, and when patients are to undergo joint reconstruction by orthopedic or hand surgeons. The Thompson index[168] uses a few joints and weights

data from each joint to reflect the joint surface area, giving a better measure of the "burden of synovitis."

The choice of imaging techniques and measures is important in assessment of the destructive lesions of RA. The inflammatory lesion in RA is reflected reasonably well by heat, pain, swelling, and tenderness. Joint destruction can occur with minimal inflammation, however. MRI and ultrasound provide ways to visualize pannus development and loss of cartilage (see Chapter 58). In each patient, when the diagnosis of RA is reasonably certain, these measures of assessment and estimates of prognosis should be recorded. They should be major determinants of what therapies are instituted (see Chapter 71).

Selected References

1. Wolfe AM: The epidemiology of rheumatoid arthritis: a review. I. Surveys, *Bull Rheum Dis* 19:518–523, 1968.
2. Engel A, Roberts J, Burch TA: Rheumatoid arthritis in adults in the United States, 1960-1962. In *Vital and health statistics*, Series 11, Data from the National Health Survey, Number 17, Washington, DC, 1966, National Center for Health Statistics.
3. Mikkelsen WM, Dodge HJ, Duff IF, et al: Estimates of the prevalence of rheumatic disease in the population of Tecumseh, Michigan, 1959–1960, *J Chronic Dis* 20:351–369, 1967.
4. Linos A, Worthington JW, O'Fallon WM, et al: The epidemiology of rheumatoid arthritis in Rochester, Minnesota: a study of incidence, prevalence and mortality, *Am J Epidemiol* 111:87–98, 1980.
10. Yelin E, Wanke LA: An assessment of the annual and long-term direct costs of rheumatoid arthritis: the impact of poor function and functional decline, *Arthritis Rheum* 42:1209–1218, 1999.
12. Jacoby RK, Jayson MI, Cosh JA: Onset, early stages, and prognosis of rheumatoid arthritis: a clinical study of 100 patients with 11-year follow-up, *BMJ* 2:96–100, 1973.
13. Nielen MM, van Schaardenburg D, Reesink HW, et al: Specific autoantibodies precede the symptoms of rheumatoid arthritis: a study of serial measurements in blood donors, *Arthritis Rheum* 50:380–386, 2004.
14. Fleming A, Crown JM, Corbett M: Early rheumatoid disease. I. Onset, *Ann Rheum Dis* 35:357–360, 1976.
15. Fleming A, Benn RT, Corbett M, et al: Early rheumatoid disease. II. Patterns of joint involvement, *Ann Rheum Dis* 35:361–364, 1976.
17. Mens JM: Correlation of joint involvement in rheumatoid arthritis and in ankylosing spondylitis with the synovial:cartilaginous surface ratio of various joints [letter], *Arthritis Rheum* 30:359–360, 1987.
25. Schumacher HR: Palindromic onset of rheumatoid arthritis: clinical, synovial fluid, and biopsy studies, *Arthritis Rheum* 25:361–369, 1982.

28. Youssef W, Yan A, Russell AS: Palindromic rheumatism: a response to chloroquine, *J Rheumatol* 18:35–37, 1991.

30. De Haas WHD, de Boer W, Griffioen F, et al: Rheumatoid arthritis of the robust reaction type, *Ann Rheum Dis* 33:81–85, 1974.

32. Hastings DE, Evans JA: Rheumatoid wrist deformities and their relation to ulnar drift, *J Bone Joint Surg Am* 57:930–934, 1975.

33. Fuchs HA, Callahan LF, Kaye JJ, et al: Radiographic and joint count findings of the hand in rheumatoid arthritis: related and unrelated findings, *Arthritis Rheum* 31:44–51, 1988.

34. Brewerton DA: Hand deformities in rheumatoid disease, *Ann Rheum Dis* 16:183–197, 1957.

36. Gray RG, Gottlieb NL: Hand flexor tenosynovitis in rheumatoid arthritis: prevalence, distribution, and associated rheumatic features, *Arthritis Rheum* 20:1003–1008, 1977.

37. Ennevaara K: Painful shoulder joint in rheumatoid arthritis: a clinical and radiological study of 200 cases, with special reference to arthrography of the glenohumeral joint, *Acta Rheumatol Scand* 11:1–116, 1967.

38. Huston KA, Nelson AM, Hunder GG: Shoulder swelling in rheumatoid arthritis secondary to subacromial bursitis, *Arthritis Rheum* 21:145–147, 1978.

40. Lawry GV, Finerman ML, Hanafee WN, et al: Laryngeal involvement in rheumatoid arthritis: a clinical, laryngoscopic, and computerized tomographic study, *Arthritis Rheum* 27:873–882, 1984.

41. Smith PH, Benn RT, Sharp J: Natural history of rheumatoid cervical luxations, *Ann Rheum Dis* 31:431–439, 1972.

44. Hastings DE, Parker SM: Protrusio acetabuli in rheumatoid arthritis, *Clin Orthop Relat Res* 108:76–83, 1975.

45. Hench PK, Reid RT, Reames PM: Dissecting popliteal cyst stimulating thrombophlebitis, *Ann Intern Med* 64:1259–1264, 1966.

46. Kraag G, Thevathasan EM, Gordon DA, et al: The hemorrhagic crescent sign of acute synovial rupture [letter], *Ann Intern Med* 85:477–478, 1976.

47. Rask MR: Achilles tendon rupture owing to rheumatoid disease: case report with a nine-year follow-up, *JAMA* 239:435–436, 1978.

48. Bienenstock H: Rheumatoid plantar synovial cysts, *Ann Rheum Dis* 34:98–99, 1975.

49. Calabro JJ: A critical evaluation of the diagnostic features of the feet in rheumatoid arthritis, *Arthritis Rheum* 5:19–29, 1962.

52. Jackson CG, Chess RL, Ward JR: A case of rheumatoid nodule formation within the central nervous system and review of the literature, *J Rheumatol* 11:237–240, 1984.

53. Sokoloff L: The pathophysiology of peripheral blood vessels in collagen diseases. In Orbison JL, Smith DE, editors: *The peripheral blood vessels*, Baltimore, 1963, Williams & Wilkins, p 297.

55. Palmer DG, Hogg N, Highton J, et al: Macrophage migration and maturation within rheumatoid nodules, *Arthritis Rheum* 30:728–736, 1987.

57. Harris ED Jr: A collagenolytic system produced by primary cultures of rheumatoid nodule tissue, *J Clin Invest* 51:2973–2976, 1972.

58. Ginsberg MH, Genant HK, Yu TF, et al: Rheumatoid nodulosis: an unusual variant of rheumatoid disease, *Arthritis Rheum* 18:49–58, 1975.

61. Maddison PJ, Bacon PA: Vitamin D deficiency, spontaneous fractures and osteopenia in rheumatoid arthritis, *BMJ* 4:433–435, 1974.

62. Halla JT, Koopman WJ, Fallahi S, et al: Rheumatoid myositis: clinical and histologic features and possible pathogenesis, *Arthritis Rheum* 27:737–743, 1984.

64. Baum J: Infection in rheumatoid arthritis, *Arthritis Rheum* 14:135–137, 1971.

65. Huskisson EC, Hart FD: Severe, unusual and recurrent infections in rheumatoid arthritis, *Ann Rheum Dis* 31:118–121, 1972.

72. Williams RA, Samson D, Tikerpae J, et al: In-vitro studies of ineffective erythropoiesis in rheumatoid arthritis, *Am J Rheum Dis* 41:502–507, 1982.

73. Farr M, Scott DL, Constable TJ, et al: Thrombocytosis of active rheumatoid disease, *Ann Rheum Dis* 42:545–549, 1983.

81. Fischer M, Mielke H, Glaefke S, et al: Generalized vasculopathy and finger blood flow abnormalities in rheumatoid arthritis, *J Rheumatol* 11:33–37, 1984.

82. Conn DL, McDuffie FC, Dyck PJ: Immunopathologic study of sural nerves in rheumatoid arthritis, *Arthritis Rheum* 15:135–143, 1972.

83. Schmid FR, Cooper NS, Ziff M, et al: Arteritis in rheumatoid arthritis, *Am J Med* 30:56–83, 1961.

84. Geirsson AJ, Sturfelt G, Truedsson L: Clinical and serological features of severe vasculitis in rheumatoid arthritis: prognostic implications, *Ann Rheum Dis* 46:727–733, 1987.

86. Dodson WH, Hollingsworth JW: Pleural effusion in rheumatoid arthritis: impaired transport of glucose, *N Engl J Med* 275:1337–1342, 1966.

89. Tishler M, Grief J, Fireman E, et al: Bronchoalveolar lavage: a sensitive tool for early diagnosis of pulmonary involvement in rheumatoid arthritis, *J Rheumatol* 13:547–550, 1986.

91. Caplan A: Certain unusual radiographic appearances in the chest of coal miners suffering from RA, *Thorax* 8:29, 1953.

95. Sassoon CS, McAlpine SW, Tashkin DP, et al: Small airways function in non-smokers with rheumatoid arthritis, *Arthritis Rheum* 27:1218–1226, 1984.

101. MacDonald WJ Jr, Crawford MH, Klippel JH, et al: Echocardiographic assessment of cardiac structure and function in patients with rheumatoid arthritis, *Am J Med* 63:890–896, 1977.

102. Iveson JM, Thadani U, Ionescu M, et al: Aortic valve incompetence and replacement in rheumatoid arthritis, *Ann Rheum Dis* 34:312–320, 1975.

106. Hoffman GS: Polyarthritis: the differential diagnosis of rheumatoid arthritis, *Semin Arthritis Rheum* 8:115–141, 1978.

109. McEwen C, Lingg C, Kirsner JB: Arthritis accompanying ulcerative colitis, *Am J Med* 33:923, 1962.

110. Zizic TM, Stevens MB: The arthropathy of Behçet's disease, *Johns Hopkins Med J* 136:243–250, 1975.

111. Utsinger PD, Zvaifler NJ, Resnick D: Calcium pyrophosphate dihydrate deposition disease without chondrocalcinosis, *J Rheumatol* 2:258–264, 1975.

113. Kozin F, McCarty DJ: Rheumatoid factor in the serum of gouty patients, *Arthritis Rheum* 20:1559–1560, 1977.

116. Schumacher HR, Gall EP: Arthritis in acute hepatitis and chronic active hepatitis: pathology of the synovial membrane with evidence for the presence of Australia antigen in synovial membranes, *Am J Med* 57:655–664, 1974.

123. Bland JH, Frymoyer JW: Rheumatic syndromes of myxedema, *N Engl J Med* 282:1171–1174, 1970.

125. Appenzeller S, Castro GR, Costallat LT: Adult-onset Still disease in southeast Brazil, *J Clin Rheumatol* 11:76–80, 2005.

129. Churchill MD Jr, Geraci JE, Hunder GG: Musculoskeletal manifestations of bacterial endocarditis, *Ann Intern Med* 87:754–759, 1977.

134. Bywaters EGL: Relation between heart and joint disease including "rheumatoid heart disease" and chronic post-rheumatic arthritis (type Jaccoud), *Br Heart J* 12:101–131, 1950.

135. Poncet A: Address to the Congress Français de Chirurgie, 1897, *Bull Acad Med Paris* 46:194, 1901.

137. Gold RH, Metzger AL, Mirra JM, et al: Multicentric reticulohistiocytosis (lipoid dermatoarthritis): an erosive polyarthritis with distinctive clinical, roentgenographic and pathological features, *AJR Am J Roentgenol* 124:610–624, 1975.

162. Masi AT, Maldonado-Cocco JA, Kaplan SB, et al: Prospective study of the early course of rheumatoid arthritis in young adults: comparison of patients with and without rheumatoid factor positivity at entry and identification of variables correlating with outcome, *Semin Arthritis Rheum* 4:299–326, 1976.

163. Sharp JT, Calkins E, Cohen AS, et al: Observations on the clinical, chemical, and serological manifestations of rheumatoid arthritis, based on the course of 154 cases, *Medicine* 43:41–58, 1964.

Full references for this chapter can be found on www.expertconsult.com.

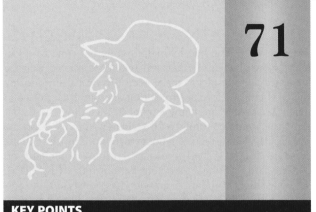

71 Treatment of Rheumatoid Arthritis

JAMES R. O'DELL

KEY POINTS

Diagnose rheumatoid arthritis (RA) early and initiate disease-modifying antirheumatic drug (DMARD) therapy at the time of diagnosis.

Treat all patients to a disease activity target—remission or low disease activity.

It is not important what therapy patients receive as long as they are treated until they reach the target.

For most patients, methotrexate will be the cornerstone of DMARD therapy.

Many patients will require combinations of DMARDs with or without biologics to achieve the target.

Many effective biologic DMARDs are available—all are more effective with methotrexate.

NSAIDS may provide useful symptom control but are rarely indicated without DMARDs.

Glucocorticoids are rapidly effective for most but have side effects. Therefore, use only with other DMARDs and ideally only as a bridge to effective DMARD therapy.

Aggressively address the ubiquitous comorbidities of RA, especially cardiovascular disease.

The treatment of rheumatoid arthritis (RA) has evolved dramatically over the past 30 years, perhaps more so than any of the rheumatic diseases. The majority of patients newly diagnosed with RA in 2013 can expect to have their disease in remission if treated early by a rheumatologist. This remarkable fact has come about because of a tremendous expansion of the number of disease-modifying antirheumatic drugs (DMARDs) available (Table 71-1), the realization that these drugs can and should be used in combinations,[1-3] and the acceptance that all patients should be treated to a target or goal of remission or low disease activity.[1-4] To put the current situation into perspective and to celebrate how far we have come, a look back on the most immediate history of RA treatment as chronicled in the 30 years of the *Textbook of Rheumatology* (TOR) seems appropriate.

When the first edition of TOR was published in 1981, Dr. Ruddy, the author of the RA treatment chapter, discussed intramuscular gold and penicillamine as the mainstay of RA treatment, hydroxychloroquine (HCQ) was mentioned as a possible option, and cyclophosphamide and azathioprine were discussed as experimental therapies. By 1985 and the second edition of TOR, azathioprine was approved for treatment of RA and cyclosporine and

methotrexate (MTX) appeared in experimental sections along with total lymphoid irradiation. By the fourth edition in 1993, Ted Harris, always ahead of his time, championed early DMARD treatment but suggested starting with the least toxic DMARDs—HCQ and sulfasalazine (SSZ). MTX was recommended only after the failure of HCQ, gold, and penicillamine. By 1997 and the fifth edition, early DMARD therapy was firmly established, MTX had moved to the front of the line of DMARD therapy, and combinations of conventional DMARDs were first prominently mentioned. The sixth edition (2001), authored by Mark Genovese, reflected sweeping changes in the landscape: Combination DMARD therapy was firmly established; leflunomide had become an alternative to MTX; and, most importantly, the biologics etanercept (ETAN) and infliximab had forever changed the landscape. In the immediate predecessor to this edition of TOR (2009), the concept of treating to a target was discussed and our armamentarium of biologics had expanded to three anti–tumor necrosis factor (TNF) agents and two biologics with new mechanisms of action: abatacept and rituximab. Critical features of contemporary therapy of RA as discussed in the ninth edition of TOR include the strategy of treating all patients to the goal of remission or low disease activity and emphasizing treating to target and not the drugs used; the rediscovery of conventional combination DMARDs; the introduction of two new TNF inhibitors and a biologic with yet another mechanism of action (anti-IL-6 receptor), tocilizumab; and highlighting the critical role of comorbidities, particularly cardiovascular disease in RA. In this edition, for the first time a section on tapering or discontinuing therapy in patients who are doing well has been added, which illustrates just how far we have come in the past 30 years.

Despite how far we have come, many challenges remain and include first and foremost identifying markers that predict in a differential fashion who will respond to or have side effects from which treatment and developing methods to allow us to measure the amount of immunosuppression that agents are producing. If the current pace of advance continues, the next few editions of TOR may see discussion of RA remissions off all treatments and even treatment of and perhaps cures for "patients" before they develop symptomatic RA.

This chapter attempts to discuss the broad principles of treatment, the goals of RA therapy, the timing of different therapies, and the strategies of employing the plethora of options now available to achieve the best control of each patient. Most of the drugs are not covered in detail here; please refer to other excellent chapters for specifics on the NSAIDs (Chapter 59), glucocorticoids (Chapter 60), traditional DMARDs (Chapter 61), immunoregulatory drugs

Table 71-1 Disease-Modifying Antirheumatic Drugs*

Conventional	Biologics
Methotrexate	Etanercept (Enbrel)
Hydroxychloroquine	Infliximab (Remicade)
Sulfasalazine	Anakinra (Kineret)
Leflunomide	Adalimumab (Humira)
Gold (intramuscular and oral)	Abatacept (Orencia)
Azathioprine	Rituximab (Rituxan)
Minocycline	Certolizumab (Cimzia)
Cyclosporine	Golimumab (Simponi)
Penicillamine	Tocilizumab (Actemra)
Glucocorticoids	

*Currently available drugs that have the ability to slow or halt progression of rheumatoid arthritis including radiographic progression.

(Chapter 62), and anticytokine therapies or biologics (Chapter 63).

GOAL OF RHEUMATOID ARTHRITIS TREATMENT

It is remarkable that rheumatologists now have more than 19 approved conventional or biologic DMARDs to choose from. However, despite all these terrific DMARD options, **the most important paradigm shift for the treatment of RA has been the realization that patients should be treated early and to a target of low disease activity or remission.**[1-4] For those outside the rheumatologic community, this seems like stating the obvious—if you have hypertension, hyperlipidemia, or diabetes, patients are of course treated to get the blood pressure, low-density lipoprotein, or Hb_{A1c}, respectively, down to a defined and easily measured goal. The problem in RA has been having valid reproducible measures of disease activity and remission and then routinely measuring and following those in a clinic. Unfortunately, in RA, there is no single examination finding or laboratory test that satisfactorily measures disease activity.

Many measures have been proposed,[5-10] and all are composite measures that include information derived from some combination of joint examinations, patient and physician assessment of disease activity, patient function, and laboratory measures of inflammation (erythrocyte sedimentation rate [ESR] or C-reactive protein [CRP]). Recently, the American College of Rheumatology (ACR) has endorsed a list of disease activity measures that have been shown to correlate with outcomes. Table 71-2 is a partial list of some of the better known of these measures. Each of these measures have strengths and weaknesses[11]; some rely on only data from the patient, some require complete joint counts by clinicians, and some require laboratory tests to measure

inflammation. The busy clinician rarely has time to document more than 60 tender and swollen joints or wait for laboratory test results to make decisions on patients during their visit. Therefore measures that simplify this process as much as possible are being embraced including those that limit the joints counted to 28 (Disease Activity Score 28 [DAS28]), do not require laboratory tests (Clinical Disease Activity Index [CDAI]), or are entirely dependent on patient data Routine Assessment Patient Index ([RAPID]). There is high correlation among these measures, so currently in the clinic **it is very important that disease activity is measured and less important which measure is used.**

Because none of our therapies cure RA, it seems obvious that the next best goal should be remission. The concept of remission as a goal for RA patients is problematic, however. First, a remission definition that is both relevant and practical has been elusive. To be relevant, remission should be highly predictive of the absence of disease progression over time. To be practical, for clinicians, a remission definition should be easy to apply in real time to patients seen in a clinic as discussed earlier with regard to measures of disease activity. Recently, a new definition of remission for use in clinical trials has been developed by ACR and the European League against Rheumatism (EULAR) (Table 71-3).[12] This definition has been rigorously tested against short-term radiologic outcomes in 1- to 2-year randomized controlled trials (RCTs) follow-up. This definition standardizes remission and is therefore a huge step forward for reporting and comparing results across clinical trials.

However, this definition was designed for clinical trials, not clinical care,[13] where the need to have results of CRPs in real time becomes a problem. Versions of this that do not require laboratory values have been suggested but not fully accepted (e.g., CDAI, Patient Activity Scale). Perhaps more problematic, many believe that remission defined by clinical data alone will always underestimate the amount of low-level disease activity that could be found if synovial biopsies or advanced imaging techniques such as ultrasound (US) or magnetic resonance imaging (MRI) were employed (see Chapter 58). Significant data exists that many and perhaps most RA patients who meet definitions of "remission" have active disease if assessed by US or MRI.[14-16] Indeed, the newly accepted ACR/EULAR definition allows for a swollen joint, which many would argue is not really remission. Another major problem with "remission" is that from currently available data it is not at all clear that remission, regardless of how it is defined, should be the treatment goal for all RA patients. Many patients do well despite low levels of disease activity. This situation may be analogous to the recent studies that show pushing Hb_{A1c} levels below 6.5, which seemed appropriate for diabetic control, was

Table 71-2 Instruments Used to Measure Rheumatoid Arthritis Disease Activity

Instrument	Score Range	Thresholds of Disease Activity			
		Remission	Low	Moderate	High
Disease Activity Score in 28 joints (DAS28)	0-9.4	≤2.6	≤3.2	>3.2 and ≤5.1	>5.1
Simplified Disease Activity Index (SDAI)	0.1-86.0	≤3.3	≤11	>11 and ≤26	>26
Clinical Disease Activity Index (CDAI)	0-76.0	≤2.8	≤10	>10 and ≤22	>22
Rheumatoid Arthritis Disease Activity Index (RADAI)	0-10	≤1.4	<2.2	2.2 and ≤4.9	>4.9
Patient Activity Scale (PAS or PASII)	0-10	≤1.25	<1.9	≥1.9 and ≤5.3	>5.3
Routine Assessment Patient Index Data (RAPID)	0-30	≤1	<6	≥6 and ≤12	>12

Table 71-3 ACR/EULAR Definitions of Remission in Rheumatoid Arthritis Clinical Trials

Boolean-Based Definition
At any time point, patient must satisfy all of the following: Tender joint count ≤1* Swollen joint count ≤1* C-reactive protein ≤1 mg/dL Patient global assessment ≤1 (on a 0-10 scale)

Index-Based Definition
At any time point, patient must have a Simplified Disease Activity Index score of ≤3.3

*Include 28 joints plus feet and ankles.
ACR/EULAR, American College of Rheumatology/European League against Rheumatism.
From Felson DT, Smolen JS, Wells G, et al: American College of Rheumatology/European League against Rheumatism provisional definition of remission in rheumatoid arthritis for clinical trials, *Arthritis Rheum* 63:573–586, 2011.

associated with increased cardiovascular mortality mainly due to hypoglycemia in patients with prior cardiovascular histories.[17]

- When do the risks and considerable expense of some of our RA therapies outweigh the benefits of escalating therapy further?
- Which patient who has improved dramatically but still has two tender or swollen joints needs a third biologic?
- With regard to the previously cited diabetic patients with cardiovascular disease, which RA patients are most at risk if we push too hard for remission?
- Finally, with current therapies, the vast majority of remissions in RA require ongoing treatment with DMARDs, so the concept of a true remission, meaning one where no therapy is required, remains beyond our current reach for the majority of patients.

Despite the problems defining remission or low-disease activity, it is clear that patients do better if clinicians have a goal. The Tight Intensive Control of RA (TICORA) study[18] was the first to convincingly demonstrate this in a randomized fashion. TICORA was a Scottish study in which patients with less than 5 years of disease were randomized to receive either routine care or to receive intensive care. Both groups were treated with an algorithm of conventional DMARDs (Figure 71-1A). The routine care group had regular follow-up and monitoring, while the intensive group was seen monthly and had proscribed escalation of therapy (protocolized) if they had not achieved the goal of low disease activity (defined in this study as DAS ≤ 2.4). Both groups improved significantly, but the group that was treated to a target (intensive group) did significantly better with mean DAS scores (=1.6) in the remission range at 18 months (Figure 71-1B). In the intensive group, 71% achieved an American College of Rheumatology 70% improvement criteria response (ACR70) compared with 18% in the routine care group (P < .0001). Further, this clinical improvement translated to significantly less radiographic progression of erosions compared with the routine group (0.5 vs. 3.0; P = .002). Importantly, this improved disease control was not associated with an increase in treatment-associated adverse events. Finally, despite more frequent visits, intensive therapy resulted in cost savings

even in the short term. These results were particularly remarkable considering they were obtained using conventional DMARDs alone (see Figure 71-1A) without the use of biologics. Findings from other studies have corroborated these findings.[19-21] Further, a meta-analysis of tight control[22] suggested that tight control strategies work best if protocolized, as was done in TICORA.

Although the TICORA investigators selected low disease activity as the target, the target could have been remission as discussed earlier. Most of the previously endorsed measures of disease activity have defined levels that signify "remission" (see Table 71-2). Predictably, the harder we push for remission with increasing numbers and doses of DMARDs, both conventional and biologic, the more toxicity and the expense (Table 71-4) of our treatments become a concern. Both the ACR and EULAR guidelines, as well as recent reviews,[1-4] currently state that low disease activity *or* remission is the goal, and they leave the decision on which one is most appropriate for each unique patient's situation to the clinician. Therefore until further data elucidate this question, clinicians will need to continue to practice the art and science of medicine when selecting the most appropriate target for each patient.

A RANDOMIZED CONTROLLED TRIAL OF TIGHT CONTROL OF RHEUMATOID ARTHRITIS (TICORA)

Intensive therapy: Goal of DAS < 2.4

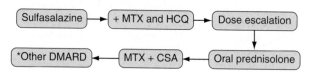

A *Intra-articular steroids were used, but biologics were not.

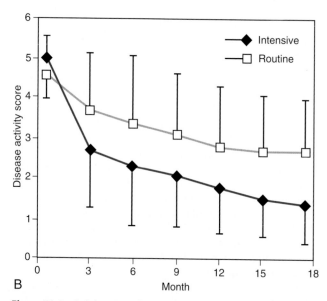

Figure 71-1 A, Schematic of treatment escalation used in TICORA trial. **B,** Comparison of intensive and routine treatment groups. CSA, cyclosporine A; DAS, disease activity score (44 joints); DMARD, disease-modifying antirheumatic drug; HCQ, hydroxychloroquine; MTX, methotrexate. *(Modified with permission from Grigor C, Capell H, Stirling A, et al: Effect of a treatment strategy of tight control for rheumatoid arthritis (the TICORA study): a single-blind randomised controlled trial,* Lancet *364:263–269, 2004.)*

Table 71-4   Average Medication Expense*

Medication	Dosage	Monthly Cost
Methotrexate	20 mg/wk	$26
Hydroxychloroquine	200 mg twice daily	$35
Sulfasalazine	1 g twice daily	$30
Prednisone	10 mg/day	$10
Triple therapy	Above doses	$91
Etanercept	50 mg/wk	$1974
Adalimumab	40 mg every other wk	$1915
Infliximab	300 mg/4 wk	$2264[†]
Rituximab	1500 mg every 6 mo	$1597[‡]
Abatacept	750 mg monthly	$1690[‡]
Tocilizumab	400 mg monthly	$1555[‡]

*U.S. $/month cost to consumer from large national chain pharmacy (Walgreens) in 2011.

[†]Based on average wholesale price as listed by *Redbook* and does not include infusion costs.

[‡]Does not include infusion costs.

CLASSES OF DRUGS

DMARDs: Methotrexate, Sulfasalazine, Hydroxychloroquine, and Leflunomide

The definition of a DMARD is one that has the ability to change (for the better) the course of RA. The most rigorous application of this definition requires RCTs that show not only the ability to change the clinical course of the disease but also the ability to decrease or halt the radiographic progression. By this definition, all of the 10 conventional DMARDs and the 9 biologic DMARDs listed in Table 71-1 qualify with the possible exception of minocycline and HCQ, where only weak evidence exists for radiographic benefits. With the DMARDs listed in Table 71-1 and using these drugs individually or in combinations of two, three, or four as is often done, there are 2569 possible combinations for each individual patient, assuming that biologics are not used in combinations with each other. Obviously, this huge number of choices is both good and bad news for the clinician; it is great to have all the options but impossible to keep them all straight. Therefore to employ these effectively, the clinician must have goals, strategies, and an up-to-date knowledge of the drugs and their interactions and toxicities.

The most widely used conventional DMARDs—MTX, SSZ, HCQ, and leflunomide (LEF)—are discussed in detail in Chapter 61. Together, these four DMARDs along with glucocorticoids (see Chapter 60) currently account for the vast majority of conventional DMARD use. Although less commonly used, gold (both intramuscular [IM] and oral), azathioprine, cyclosporine, and the tetracyclines (minocycline and doxycycline), which are not covered elsewhere in the book, are therefore discussed as follows. Penicillamine is of historical interest[23] but is rarely used and is not discussed in this chapter.

Biologic DMARDs

The biologic DMARDs are discussed in detail in Chapter 63. Within this class of agents we now have the ability to inhibit multiple inflammatory cytokines including TNF (with three monoclonal antibodies (infliximab, adalimumab, and golimumab); the TNF receptor protein (ETAN); and the pegylated Fab fragment certolizumab, interleukin-1 (IL-1) with the IL-1 receptor antagonist (anakinra), IL-6 (monoclonal antibody to the IL-6 receptor tocilizumab) or to kill or inhibit cell lines important in inflammation including B cells (rituximab) and T cells (abatacept). **It is an understatement to say biologics have changed the landscape of RA therapy forever** both in terms of therapeutic expectations and understanding of RA pathogenesis. Because of their often quick onset of action, particularly with the TNF inhibitors, and their ability to retard radiographic progress, they are increasingly used earlier and more often in RA. The challenge for clinicians is to appropriately integrate conventional and biologic therapies and to use biologics when necessary but to make sure the much less expensive conventional therapies have been maximized.

Glucocorticoids

Glucocorticoids, discussed in detail in Chapter 60, have a long and storied history in the treatment of RA. RA was selected as the first disease to be treated with "compound E" at the Mayo Clinic in 1948.[24] Responses were both rapid and dramatic; an analysis of the first 14 patients treated revealed that 100% improved their ESRs by more than 50% within 1 to 3 months, with 80% improving ESRs by at least 70% (an ESR70—a convenient ACR70). Several landmark studies have proven not only clinical efficacy[25-30] but also the significant radiographic efficacy of glucocorticoids.[28,30] The recent COBRA trial[29,30] and the COBRA arm of the BeSt study (discussed later[19,20]) again demonstrated the significant clinical and radiographic benefit that glucocorticoids can provide. Despite the rapid onset and all the other positive benefits of glucocorticoids in RA, their toxicities are also legend. Currently glucocorticoids are most often and most appropriately used along with DMARDs as part of initial "induction" therapy to get RA patients under control rapidly and then aggressively tapered as the slower-acting DMARDs start to kick in. Historically, the belief has been that once an RA patient was on glucocorticoids, he or she would never get off. This is clearly not true with the effective DMARDs now available—successful tapering is the rule.[19,20,31] If a patient cannot be successfully tapered off or at least tapered to an "acceptable" low dose, it is a strong indication that the current DMARD program is not working. Long-term use of doses equivalent to prednisone of greater than 7.5 to 10 mg per day is a clear indication that DMARD therapy needs to be escalated. Importantly, **glucocorticoids should almost never be used in RA without DMARDs.**

Other Conventional DMARDs

Gold Salts

Gold injections have been used in the treatment of RA for close to a century—initially intramuscularly and, more recently, orally. With the advent of newer agents, gold is rarely used in most parts of the world. IM gold is a difficult and cumbersome therapy. It is initiated with weekly IM injections, usually starting with 10 mg the first week, 25 mg the second week, and then 50 mg thereafter, until a response is seen, generally between 3 and 6 months. Once the desired efficacy is seen, the IM injections can eventually be monthly. Frequent monitoring with complete blood counts (CBCs) and urine for protein is necessary. Significant toxicities can occur and include skin rashes, bone marrow depression, and nephrotic syndrome. As problematic as gold treatment is, there is a wealth of evidence that IM gold therapy is beneficial for RA including retarding radiographic progression.[32] Some patients, perhaps 10% to 20% of those started on IM gold, will have essentially complete long-term remissions if maintained on injections every 2 to 4 weeks. Of recent interest was a 48-week RCT in patients with active disease despite MTX; the addition of IM gold to MTX resulted in 61% of patients achieving an ACR20 compared with 30% for the MTX + placebo group (Figure 71-2).[33] Despite the known benefits, there is also ample evidence that the two IM compounds, gold sodium thiomalate and gold sodium thioglucose, are being used less by rheumatologists because of the need for meticulous monitoring for serious toxicity and the inconvenience of administration and monitoring.

Auranofin, the gold oral preparation, has been available for more than 20 years but is rarely used. Auranofin has different and less severe toxicity than the IM gold and reportedly less efficacy. Cytopenia and proteinuria are rare, but an enterocolitis with diarrhea leads to intolerance in many. Auranofin is an effective DMARD,[34] but RCT data show that it is less effective than MTX, IM gold, penicillamine, or SSZ.[35]

Until or unless factors can be found that reliably predict who will get the almost magical clinical response that can be seen with gold, this cumbersome and often difficult-to-manage therapy will continue to disappear. To this end, HLA-DR3 is found in more patients who develop either thrombocytopenia or nephropathy while taking gold injections.[36] These data must be balanced against the evidence that human leukocyte antigen (HLA)-DR3 may be associated with a better response to gold therapy, which corroborates a long-time belief shared by many clinicians that those patients who get rashes on gold are often destined to have excellent clinical responses.

IMMUNOSUPPRESSIVE AGENTS

Azathioprine

Azathioprine (AZA), 50 to 200 mg/day, has been used to treat RA for almost 50 years. Because it has been generic for many years, little recent research has been done. Although clearly not a first-line DMARD in contemporary RA treatment, AZA is most commonly used as a substitute for MTX when there are contraindications or intolerance to MTX. This most commonly arises in patients with the

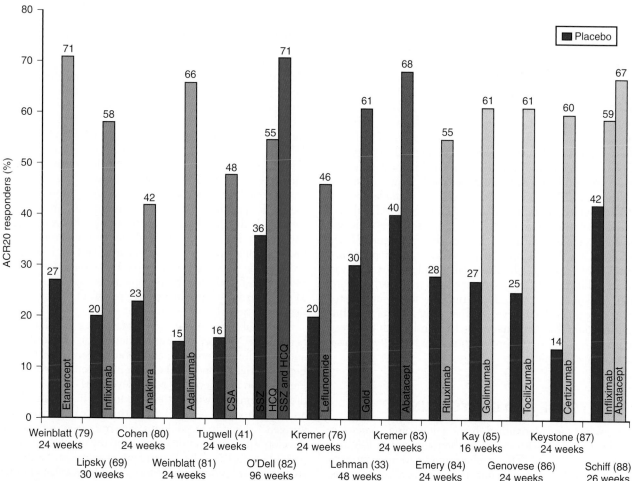

Figure 71-2 Blind trials of therapies in patients with active disease despite methotrexate (MTX). ACR20, American College of Rheumatology 20% composite improvement; CSA, cyclosporine A; HCQ, hydroxychloroquine; SSZ, sulfasalazine.

so-called "MTX flu," but other situations including pregnancy, liver disease, and renal disease may be indications for AZA in RA. Azathioprine is usually used in combination with other conventional or biologic DMARDs. McCarty and co-workers, who was one of the pioneers of combination therapy in RA, has reported on the combination of MTX, AZA, and HCQ in 69 patients treated in an open-label fashion.[37] With this combination, 45% of patients reached remission by the old ACR criteria[38] and this combination was well-tolerated.

Neutropenia is the most common complication of AZA treatment. Neutropenia can be predicted with a genetic test for polymorphisms of the enzyme thiopurine methyltransferase (TMPT). Patients who are homozygous for the mutant polymorphism that is nonfunctional (1 in 300 or 0.3% of patients) are sensitive to bone marrow and other toxicities of AZA. Patients who are heterozygotes (perhaps 10% of the population) may have milder neutropenia.[39] Unfortunately, this test is expensive. In some centers it may cost up to $1000 and is not always reimbursed. Some clinicians elect to start with low doses of 50 mg/day and check CBCs at 2 weeks and then increase the dose as needed if the white blood cell (WBC) count is normal. It has been speculated that the subset of patients with the nonfunctional polymorphisms could be the patients who, when AZA was added to a stable MTX regimen, developed an acute febrile toxic reaction characterized by fever, leukocytosis, and a cutaneous leukocytoclastic vasculitis.[40]

Cyclosporine

In the 1990s, cyclosporine (CSA) gained a foothold in the treatment of RA.[41] Cyclosporine, mostly used in transplantation to prevent allograft rejection, inhibits the activation of $CD4^+$ helper-inducer T lymphocytes by blocking IL-2 and other T helper type 1 cytokine production[42] and by inhibiting CD40 ligand expression in T lymphocytes.[43] The latter effect prevents T cells from delivering CD40 ligand-dependent signals to B cells. Interest in CSA peaked in the mid-1990s when Tugwell and colleagues[44] showed that the addition of CSA (2.5 to 5 mg/kg/day) to a stable dose of MTX provided substantial additive benefit over MTX alone. In the CSA + MTX group, ACR20 responses were achieved by 48% compared with 16% for placebo (see Figure 71-2). Additionally, this therapy seemed to slow radiographic progression of erosions.[45] In this trial, the dose of CSA was decreased if the patient's creatinine level increased to more than 30% of initial values. Unfortunately, follow-up reports on this regimen have revealed that only 22% of patients continued on this combination at 18 months with the most common reasons for discontinuation being hypertension or increasing creatinines.[45]

MINOCYCLINE AND DOXYCYCLINE

Tetracycline and derivatives have a long and somewhat checkered history with regard to the treatment of RA and other arthritides.[46,47] The mechanism of action of tetracyclines in RA is poorly understood. Tetracyclines are, of course, antibiotics, but additionally they inhibit metalloproteinases, modulate immune responses, and have anti-inflammatory effects. No evidence indicates that tetracyclines treat the "infection that causes RA" as was touted by some of the original supporters.[47] However, it is entirely possible that inhibition of nonspecific infections that upregulate the immune response (IL-1, TNF, IL-6) such as periodontitis, bronchitis, and gastritis, to name a few, may be helpful in controlling disease in RA patients. Tetracyclines also have the ability to inhibit biosynthesis and activity of matrix metalloproteinases that have a principal role in degrading articular cartilage in RA. This has been effective in animal models of osteoarthritis (OA) treatment. The presumed mechanism is through chelation of calcium and zinc molecules, which subsequently leads to altered molecular conformations of proenzymes sufficiently to inactive them.[48,49] Minocycline has mild but definite inhibitory effects on synovial T cell proliferation and cytokine production and has been shown to upregulate IL-10 production. Further evidence of its ability to modulate the immune system is the fact that it is known to induce anti-DNA-antibody positive lupus in some patients, especially when used to treat acne.

Given in a dose of 100 mg twice daily, moderate statistically significant improvement in clinical parameters of disease activity was found in patients with established RA treated with minocycline compared with placebo.[50,51] Findings in the treatment of early RA have been more impressive. A study of 46 patients with early rheumatoid factor (RF)-positive RA who had not received previous treatment reported 65% of patients meeting 50% improvement in tender and swollen joints, duration of morning stiffness, and ESR (Paulus criteria), whereas only 13% of the placebo recipients improved similarly over a 6-month period.[52] In 2001 the results of a 2-year trial comparing minocycline with HCQ were published.[31] In this small study of patients with early RF-positive RA, the patients treated with minocycline were more likely to achieve an ACR50 (the primary end point) than the patients treated with HCQ (60% vs. 33%) and were more successful in tapering glucocorticoids. This study reconfirms the potential utility of minocycline, particularly in early RF-positive patients.

Although less studied, there is evidence supporting the use of doxycycline in the treatment of RA. In a trial of patients with early RA, doxycycline plus MTX was compared with the use of MTX alone. Investigators studied low-dose doxycycline (20 mg twice a day) and high-dose doxycycline (100 mg twice a day) in combination with MTX and found that both approaches were superior to MTX alone.[53] Despite the positive results of this study, replication is necessary.

Potential side effects of tetracyclines include lightheadedness, vertigo, rare liver toxicity, drug-induced lupus, and, with longer-term use, cutaneous hyperpigmentation.[54] Elderly patients appear to be at an increased risk of vertigo. Patients on minocycline have developed lupus-like syndromes, complete with autoantibodies including anti-DNA and occasionally perinuclear antineutrophil cytoplasmic antigen.[55] Drug-induced lupus has not been reported to develop with doxycycline or with the use of minocycline in patients with RA. The hyperpigmentation can be impressive and may limit treatment in some.[54] Hyperpigmentation resolves with discontinuation of minocycline and occurs much less commonly if at all with doxycycline.

NONSTEROIDAL ANTI-INFLAMMATORY DRUGS

NSAIDs including salicylates, covered in detail in Chapter 59, have been a ubiquitous part of RA treatment for more than a century. Over the past several decades as toxicities,[56-61] particularly gastrointestinal[56-58] and cardiovascular, have become apparent[58,59] and as DMARDs have become better, the use of NSAIDs has fortunately declined. The somewhat surprising cardiovascular toxicities, now known to be strongly associated with not only the cyclooxygenase-2 (COX-2) specific NSAIDs but essentially all NSAIDs, have been particularly concerning with regard to the RA patient populations in which the main excess mortality is largely due to accelerated cardiovascular disease. Like glucocorticoids, **NSAIDs should rarely be used without DMARDs.** Also like glucocorticoids, the goal should be to taper off as soon as possible to avoid gastrointestinal and cardiovascular toxicities.

Treatment Approaches and Strategies

As detailed earlier, the goal of treatment for all RA patients is remission or at least low disease activity; other than toxicity concerns and affordability issues, **clinicians should not care which drug or combination of drugs are used in an individual patient but should focus on getting patients to target with whatever it takes.** There is no magic or correct DMARD or combination of DMARDs that is right for all patients. Each patient presents a unique challenge and comes with unique expectations, biases, disease activity level, damage burden, comorbidities, and insurance coverage issues. One of the most important areas of investigation in RA is to identify parameters that will predict in a differential fashion which patient will respond to which therapy—so far no clear-cut answers that are applicable to the clinical care of the vast majority of patients have emerged. Some have suggested treatment should be different for RA patients with good prognosis versus poor prognosis. This concept is problematic; separating patients into good versus poor prognosis is difficult. Although data suggest certain features are associated with worse prognosis (Table 71-5), unfortunately no data suggest that stratifying our therapies on the basis of prognosis at the individual patient level yields better outcomes. For example, if we could perfectly score prognosis on a scale of 1 to 10, those patients with intermediate scores would conceivably benefit the most from our most aggressive therapies while those with

THE RA WHEEL OF EMPIRIC THERAPY*

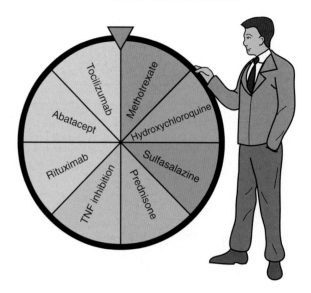

*May need to spin more than once for combination therapy!

Figure 71-3 One approach to selecting therapy for rheumatoid arthritis (RA) patients. *(Courtesy of James R. O'Dell and Robert Wigton, MD.)*

low scores do not need them and those with the highest scores may have an unacceptable benefit-to-toxicity ratio. Most patients who meet criteria for classification of RA in clinic and essentially all of those included in clinical trials have poor-prognosis RA with multiple factors listed in Table 71-5. Regardless of the prognostic factors, the goal for each patient is to achieve at least low disease activity. Until or unless parameters are identified, rheumatologists will of necessity continue to use their clinical judgment at the individual patient level.

Without parameters that predict in a differential way response to medications in terms of efficacy or toxicity, one approach to treatment decisions is illustrated in Figure 71-3. Note that several iterations may be required. This figure indicates that we do not have these much-needed parameters and emphasizes that if we hope to treat RA in a rational, scientific way, it is critical to find these parameters. Figure 71-3 also highlights and reinforces the need to include bio-banks with all of our clinical trials. With regard to individual patients, Figure 71-4 (ACR recommendations[2]) is perhaps a more practical approach. Specific patient populations are discussed as follows.

Treatment of the DMARD-Naïve Patient

The most critically important principle of treating RA effectively is to initiate and rapidly advance DMARD therapy as early as possible. Although this is a universally accepted principle, there is a paucity of rigorous data that directly addresses this point. Few randomized double-blind trials[62-65] in which patients are randomized to early treatment versus late treatment have been conducted, and it is unlikely, not to mention unethical, that any more will be forthcoming. Rather, we accept this foundation principle on the basis of the common and firm belief that treating patients early prevents damage and deformity and preserves

Table 71-5 Factors Associated with Poor Prognosis in Rheumatoid Arthritis

Presence of rheumatoid factor and titer
Presence of antibodies to anticitrullinated protein antibody and titer
Presence of shared epitope (HLA-DR alleles) and number of copies
Presence of erosive disease at presentation
Disease activity at presentation
Magnitude of erythrocyte sedimentation rate or C-reactive protein elevations
Presence of nodules or other extra-articular features
Female gender
Current and past smoking
Obesity

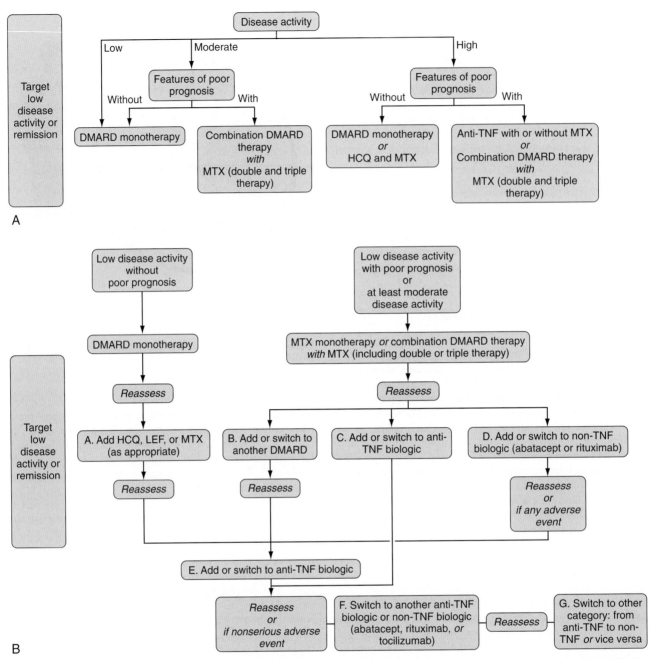

Figure 71-4   American College of Rheumatology recommendations for treatment of rheumatoid arthritis.[2] **A,** Early disease. **B,** Established disease. DMARD, disease-modifying antirheumatic drug; HCQ, hydroxychloroquine; LEF, leflunomide; MTX, methotrexate; TNF, tumor necrosis factor.

function. Many trials and case series provide strong, credible evidence to support this central tenet. Evidence to support this commonsense belief comes from cohort studies of early versus delayed therapy,[66] randomized studies of intensive therapy versus usual care,[18] RCTs of combination versus monotherapy,[19,20,29,67-71] and finally studies of what was previously defined as preclinical RA.[65]

One cohort study of note reported on early RA patients. The first cohort received DMARD therapy early (mean, 123 days after diagnosis), whereas the second cohort received DMARDs very early (mean, 15 days after diagnosis[66]). The first cohort had significantly more radiographic damage at 2 years and, importantly, continued to have radiographic progression while the second did not. The findings of the

TICORA trial (detailed earlier[18]) clearly show the advantages of better control of disease earlier. Multiple studies in early RA have demonstrated that when groups of patients are compared, those that get combinations of therapy fare better than those that get monotherapy.[19,20,29,67-71] COBRA with the combination of MTX, SSZ, and prednisolone versus SSZ alone[29]; FINRACO[67] with the combination of MTX, SSZ, HCQ, and prednisone versus SSZ; BeSt with the multiple combinations compared with step-ups or switches[19,20]; ATTRACT[69] with the combination of infliximab and MTX versus MTX alone and PREMIER with the combination of adalimumab and MTX versus each alone are some examples of these.[70] In all these trials, the combinations outperformed monotherapy.

The PROMPT trial[65] addressed a somewhat different question—patients with inflammatory arthritis who could not yet be classified as RA were randomized to MTX treatment or placebo, and the end point was the development of clinical RA. The MTX-treated group had significantly delayed progression to full-blown RA. Taken together, all these data make a compelling argument for early DMARD therapy in RA.

The new ACR/EULAR RA classification criteria[12] should allow us to classify patients with RA earlier and therefore treat RA patients earlier. The criteria, discussed in detail in Chapter 70, were designed to allow rheumatologists to classify patients in clinical trials with RA as early as possible. Gone is the previous absolute requirement that all patients must have certain features for a minimum of 6 weeks before classification. The 6-week threshold is still acknowledged as important but no longer required, and many patients, particularly those with poor prognostic features, will fulfill criteria before 6 weeks. Importantly, the presence of anticitrullinated protein antibodies (ACPAs), particularly higher-titer antibodies, is weighed heavily in the new criteria (two points). Of note in the previously mentioned PROMPT trial,[65] the benefit of early MTX was seen only in patients who were ACPA positive. Most, if not all, of these patients in PROMPT would fulfill new criteria for classification as RA, so PROMPT can be thought of as a trial to test the very early treatment of RA versus the delayed approach.

The First DMARD

Accepting that DMARD therapy should be started as early as possible, which DMARD should be started? And should we begin with mono or combination DMARD therapies? Although many of the previously cited studies have shown that combinations outperform monotherapy in randomized controlled trials, this does not mean that initial combination therapy should be the standard approach for all patients in the clinic. Most clinicians initially start most patients on mono-DMARD therapy; the evidence to support this is discussed later and is validated by the recent findings of the Treatment of Early Aggressive Rheumatoid (TEAR) trial.[71] The decision of which DMARD to initiate at the individual patient level is complex, and at this time there is clearly no one right answer for all patients and all clinical situations (see Figure 71-3 or 71-4A)—one size, or in this case one drug, clearly does not fit all. Many factors need to be considered including, but not limited to, the patient's disease activity, comorbidities and preference, the relative expense to the patient and to the health care system (weighing the benefits and including direct and indirect costs in our thinking) and importantly where relevant, the patient's desire (both female and male) to conceive. Until or unless parameters that allow selection on the basis of data become available, this complicated decision will still require the best of the clinician's judgment.

With all this said, MTX should be the initial DMARD for the majority of patients. MTX is inexpensive (see Table 71-4), effective, well-tolerated, and, importantly, is the cornerstone of most successful combination therapies (see Figure 71-2). In particular, excellent data exist that anti-TNF therapy with all the currently available agents is much more effective with MTX on board both in terms of clinical and radiographic outcomes[71-74] (see Chapter 61 for specific details on MTX). MTX is usually administered orally at first, although subcutaneous dosing has more predictable bioavailability. In most cases, the dose should be pushed to a minimum of 20 to 25 mg/week if necessary to control disease unless there are contraindications or tolerance problems. Most studies have shown that maximum efficacy may take up to 6 months to achieve but that in most situations, the response at 3 months predicts ultimate success. If MTX is used in this way, approximately 50% of patients will have a good response, and according to consistent data from several trials, approximately 30% will achieve low disease activity status.[18,19,71,74]

Initiating Treatment with a Single DMARD versus Combinations of DMARDs

Although most clinicians still favor starting with monotherapy, combination DMARD therapy has clearly changed the treatment of RA forever. In the early 1990s, the treatment model called for individual DMARDs and then switching to a different DMARD when necessary. At that time, combinations of DMARDs were not used. Studies published in the mid-1990s showing the impressive efficacy and tolerability of various combinations of DMARDs dramatically changed the treatment paradigm.[44,75] Now the majority of RA patients are treated with combinations of two, three, or more DMARDs. The first study that put combination DMARD therapy on the map was the so-called *triple therapy study* by the RAIN group of investigators.[75] This study clearly demonstrated that the triple combination of MTX, HCQ, and SSZ was significantly more effective than MTX alone or the combination of HCQ and SSZ (Figure 71-5). Importantly, this combination of DMARDs did not lead to any increase in toxicity. Multiple publica-

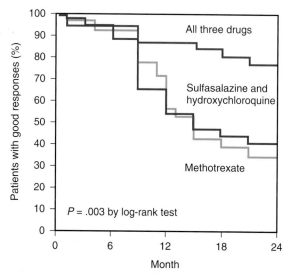

Figure 71-5 Benefits of combination methotrexate/hydroxychloroquine/sulfasalazine (triple) therapy over monotherapy with methotrexate or combination hydroxychloroquine/sulfasalazine. *(Adapted from O'Dell J, Haire C, Erikson N, et al: Treatment of rheumatoid arthritis with methotrexate alone, sulfasalazine and hydroxychloroquine, or a combination of all three medications,* N Engl J Med *334:1287–1291, 1996.)*

tions on other successful combinations of conventional DMARDs soon followed.[29,33,44,67,68,76]

Today, the important question of whether all patients should be started on combinations of DMARDs and then stepped-down or whether started on monotherapy initially and then stepped-up only if patients are not at target is an ongoing debate. Both approaches have their supporters, and data can be presented on both sides of this question. On the one hand, there is no doubt that if short-term responses are looked at in groups of patients, combinations outperform monotherapy. This is true for combinations of conventional DMARDs,[29,67,68] as well as combinations of conventional DMARDs with a biologic.[70] On the other hand, the strategy of initial monotherapy with step-ups only in patients who need it was clearly effective in TICORA (as discussed earlier[18]) and importantly in the BeSt trial[19,20] and TEAR trials (discussed later[71]), and although initial responses were better in both of the latter trials in the clinical parameters of patients initially treated with combinations, all groups in both BeSt and TEAR had identical DAS or DAS28 scores at the end of 2 years. Clinicians do not treat groups of patients but individual patients, and if the results are similar at 2 years or beyond, effective treatment approaches that minimize the number of DMARDs and therefore their potential toxicities and certain expense will be desirable for patients and health care systems alike.

BeSt (Dutch Acronym for Behandel-Strategieen, "Treatment Strategies") Study

BeSt continues to be an important randomized, multicenter trial in which 508 early RA patients were randomized to receive one of four treatment "strategies" in an open-label study.[19,20,77] The four arms of the study were as follows:

- **Group 1:** Sequential DMARD monotherapy; initial MTX 15 mg/week → MTX 25 to 30 mg/week → SSZ → Lef → MTX + infliximab → etc.
- **Group 2:** Step-up combination therapy; initial MTX 15 mg/week → MTX 25 to 30 mg/week → MTX + SSZ → MTX + SSZ + HCQ → + MTX + SSZ + HCQ + prednisone → MTX + infliximab → etc.
- **Group 3:** Initial combination therapy; initial MTX 7.5 mg/week + SSZ 2000 mg/day + prednisone 60 mg/day (tapered to 7.5 mg/day by 7 weeks) → MTX 25 to 30 mg/week + SSZ + prednisone → MTX + CSA + prednisone → MTX + infliximab → etc.
- **Group 4:** Initial MTX and infliximab; initial MTX 25 to 30 mg/week + infliximab 3 mg/kg → infliximab 6 mg/kg every 8 weeks → infliximab 7.5 → infliximab 10 mg/kg every 8 weeks → etc.

Treatment adjustments were made every 3 months with the target of a DAS less than or equal to 2.4 (low disease activity). The DAS is calculated using four variables: Richie Articular Index (66 tender joint count [RAI]), swollen joint count (44 joints [SJC]), the ESR (mm/hour), and the global health assessment score (0 to 100; [GH]); DAS = .53938 × $\sqrt{RAI}$ + .06465 × (SJC) + .33 × ln(ESR) + .00722 × (GH). The major results at 1 and 2 years are shown in Figure 71-6—both combination groups (Groups 3 and 4) improved quicker than Groups 1 and 2, which was expected with high-dose prednisone in Group 3 and high-initial-dose MTX and also infliximab in Group 4. At 1 year, DAS and

other clinical outcomes were similar in all four groups and, importantly, at 2 years they were identical. Health assessment questionnaire (HAQ) scores improved more in the early combination groups (Groups 3 and 4) at 1 year but were not different at 2 years, and radiographic progression at 2 years was greater in Group 1 than in Group 2 and greater in Groups 1 and 2 than in the combination groups (mean modified Sharp van der Heijde Score progression of 9, 5.2, 2.6, and 2.5, respectively). Progression of the joint space narrowing score (importance discussed later), although numerically higher in Group 1, was not statistically different among the four groups (4.3, 2.1, 1.5, 1.2, respectively). Interpretation of these differences is complicated by the fact that despite only 6 months of disease, Group 2 had more radiographic progression at baseline.

Conclusions from BeSt. Treat all patients to a target, and they will all do well, although on many different therapies. It is not so important what patients are on, only that they are at low disease activity or below. Several important caveats apply:

1. The strategy of adding DMARDs as in Group 2 was more effective than the strategy of switching from one DMARD to another, at least for the DMARDs and their order of use in BeSt. Although the clinical outcomes were similar at 2 years for these groups, radiographic progression was greater in Group 1 (mean 9 vs. 5.2), more Group 1 patients required infliximab (26% vs. 6%), and many Group 1 patients ended up on combinations anyway.

2. Initial therapy with combinations of conventional DMARDs (Group 3) or combinations including biologics (Group 4) work more quickly than step-up therapy (Group 2). However, at 2 years, the clinical results were identical. There was a statistical advantage of the combination groups over the step-up group in terms of total radiographic progression (Δ 2.5 points over 2 years); there was no difference in terms of joint space narrowing. This difference in radiographic progression is of no clinical significance unless it continues to grow at similar rates for years. More strategies need to be employed to further change therapies on the basis of radiographic progress in the small group (perhaps 10%) of patients on only conventional therapy where it is relevant.

3. A subset of patients was able to discontinue drug therapy for a period of time. In BeSt, if a DAS score of less than 1.6 was achieved for 6 months, patients were tapered off all medications—this occurred in 115 (23%) of patients. Although many patients relapsed, 59 patients (11.6%) were in remission off all treatment (median follow-up 23 months[77]).

Treatment of Early Aggressive Rheumatoid (TEAR) Trial

The TEAR trial was a landmark study of initial DMARD therapy in patients with early (mean disease duration = 3.6 months), poor-prognosis (all RF positive, CCP positive, or erosive) RA.[71] It is the largest (n = 755) investigator-initiated, randomized, double-blind trial in RA to date. TEAR was a 2-year study and sought to address two critical questions in this early RA population:

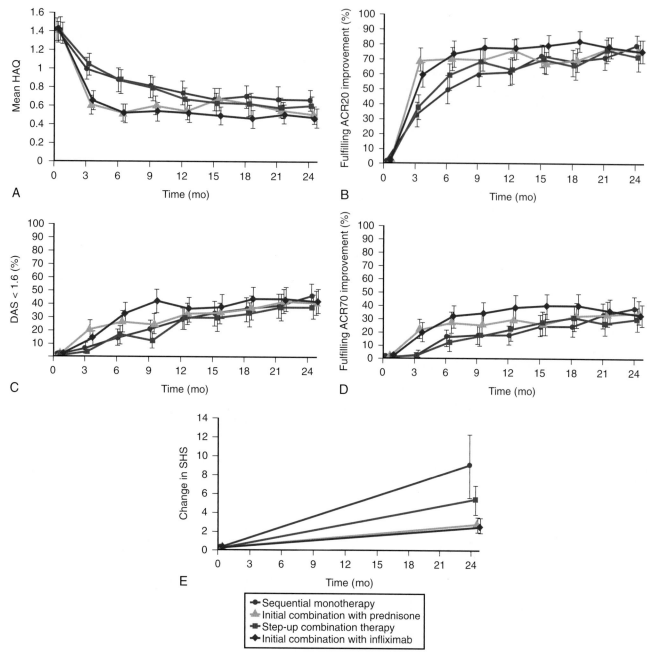

Figure 71-6 A-E, Two-year results of the BeSt study. The error bars indicate 95% confidence intervals. ACR20 indicates American College of Rheumatology 20% composite improvement. DAS, disease activity score; HAQ, health assessment questionnaire; SHS, modified Sharp van der Heijde Score. *(Modified from Goekoop-Ruiterman YP, de Vries-Bouwstra JK, Allaart CF, et al: Comparison of treatment strategies in early rheumatoid arthritis: a randomized trial,* Ann Intern Med *146:406–415, 2007.)*

1. Should patients be initiated on combination therapy or stepped-up to combinations only after a trial of MTX monotherapy?
2. Is combination therapy with MTX-ETAN superior to therapy with MTX-SSZ-HCQ (triple) therapy?

The 755 patients were randomized to the four groups as illustrated in Figure 71-7. Randomization was done in a 2:1 ratio with twice as many patients randomized to the ETAN groups. Patients randomized to the MTX-only groups were stepped-up (72% of patients stepped-up) to their assigned combination at 6 months in a blind fashion unless their DAS28 scores were less than 3.2.

The major clinical findings are nicely illustrated in Figure 71-8. All four groups had excellent improvement—mean change in DAS28 equals 2.8. For the primary end point of the study (mean DAS28 between weeks 48 and 102), all four groups were identical. Patients started on combination therapy (either triple or MTX-ETAN) were better than those started on MTX alone at the 6-month point. However, this difference disappeared within 12 weeks of the step-up point and the step-up group's DAS28s were identical to the other groups for the remainder of the study (see Figure 71-8). Data of functional assessments and quality of life measures closely mirrored the DAS28 results. Radiographics

TEAR STUDY SCHEMA

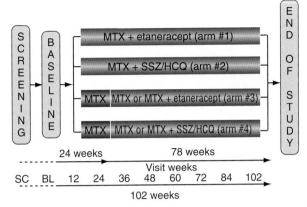

Figure 71-7 Schematic of the four different treatment groups in the TEAR trial.[71] Patients in arms 3 and 4 were treated with methotrexate (MTX) alone and step-up at 24 weeks if DAS28 was greater than 3.2. BL, baseline; HCQ, hydroxychloroquine; SC, screening; SSZ, sulfasalazine.

were done at initiation, at 48 weeks, and at 102 weeks. Radiographic data are presented in Table 71-6, and the cumulative probability plot is shown in Figure 71-9. As shown nicely, the radiographic outcomes of all four groups were superimposable. Table 71-6 shows that there was no difference between the four groups, but if you combine all the ETAN groups and compare them with all the triple therapy groups, the ETAN group had less total modified Sharp score (TSS) progression than the triple therapy group—Δ TSS of 0.51/year ($P = .047$). This small statistical difference was not clinically significant in the 2 years of the

Table 71-6   TEAR Radiographic Results

Treatment Group	N	Δ TSS (over 2 yr)	Standard Deviation
Immediate etanercept	141	0.52	3.24
Immediate triple therapy	74	1.96*	9.48
Step-up etanercept	139	0.76	2.75
Step-up triple therapy	63	1.36	5.00

*One outlier in this group had a Δ TSS of +78.5 points.
  No difference between any of the four treatment groups.
  No difference between combined immediate therapy versus combined step-up.
  Combined etanercept groups had less progression than combined triple therapy ($P = .05$).
  If single outlier is removed from triple therapy group, no difference from etanercept ($P = .07$).
  TEAR, Treatment of Early Aggressive Rheumatoid; TSS, total modified Sharp score.

trial (see later discussion about interpreting radiographic changes in clinical trials). Importantly, extensive data on side effects revealed no differences between the two groups. Many had speculated that serious adverse advents may be more common in the ETAN-treated group, whereas minor toxicities such as gastrointestinal upset and others would be more common in the triple-treated patients—neither was seen in this large, blind, clinical trial.

Conclusions from the TEAR Trial

1. Strategies that initially treat with MTX and step-up to combination therapy only if patients have not achieved target at 6 months are as effective as initial combination therapy in disease control at 1 and 2 years

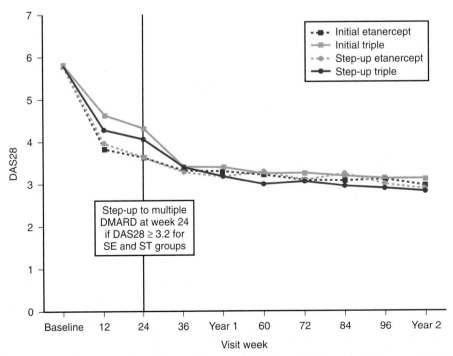

Figure 71-8   Results of treatment in the four groups of the TEAR trial over 102 weeks. DAS28, disease activity score 28; DMARD, disease-modifying antirheumatic drug; SE, Step-up Etanercept; ST, Step-up Triple. (*Modified from Moreland L, O'Dell J, Paulus H, et al: A randomized comparative effectiveness study of oral triple therapy versus etanercept plus methotrexate in early, aggressive rheumatoid arthritis: the TEAR trial,* Arthritis Rheum *2012, doi 10.1002/ art.34498 [Epub ahead of print].*)

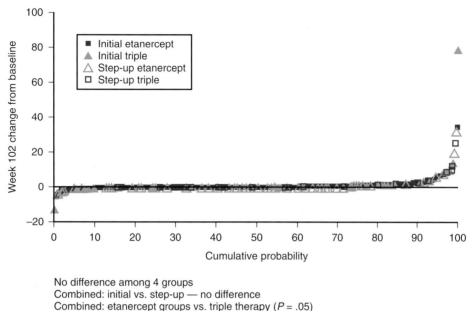

TEAR: PROBABILITY OF RADIOGRAPHIC DAMAGE

No difference among 4 groups
Combined: initial vs. step-up — no difference
Combined: etanercept groups vs. triple therapy ($P = .05$)

Figure 71-9 Percentage of patients with radiographic improvement or progression during the 102 weeks of the TEAR trial[71] by treatment group. Measured by total Sharp score. Marks above the line indicate the amount of radiographic progression, while marks below the line indicate improvement. Thus, in this study, less than 10% of patients in any of the four groups had radiographic progression.

with no difference in clinical or radiographic outcomes. At the core of the debate about initial therapy, single DMARD versus combination, is the question of how soon is soon enough when considering control of RA? Is it important to control synovitis and radiographic progression in days or weeks or is control by 3 to 6 months adequate? No clear long-term data exist to answer this important question. In both the TEAR trial and the BeSt study as discussed earlier, the groups treated with combination therapy early did better quicker, but in both trials the step-up groups looked identical to the early combination groups at 2 years in terms of clinical parameters. However, in both studies the early combination groups had small but statistically significantly less radiographic progression at 2 years. In TEAR, this difference was .5 TSS per year and in BeSt it was 1.3 per year.[20] Therefore central to this issue is the clinical relevance of small degrees of radiographic progression, which is discussed in detail later.

2. The strategy of using triple therapy was as effective as the combination of MTX-ETAN. This is clearly an important observation and should allow clinicians to be comfortable with this conventional therapy combination. Importantly, and somewhat sobering, the mean DAS28s of the four groups between 1 and 2 years of the trial was around 3.0. This means that almost half the patients were not at target (DAS28 < 3.2) regardless of treatment assignment. Therefore in clinical situations, usually after 6 months of therapy these patients should be switched to other therapies to obtain better control of disease. For example, patients on triple therapy are switched to or have ETAN added or MTX-ETAN patients have HCQ and SSZ added. No trial data exist on patients who have failed triple therapy and then are treated with biologics or vice versa.

Treatment of the Patient with Active Disease despite Methotrexate

As discussed earlier, excellent data from clinical trials where patients in general have high disease activity and poor prognostic features show that approximately 30% of patients will achieve a state of low disease activity or better if treated with MTX alone. This figure is consistent across three major trials that documented this response.[19,20,71,74] Of the 70% that have not achieved this level of control, experience suggests that perhaps a third have improved significantly and either the patient or the physician is not willing to escalate therapy. This still leaves approximately 50% of patients who will need something different than MTX monotherapy. The first question to ask is, "Should patients switch to another DMARD or should other DMARDs be added to MTX?" **Data from multiple sources including BeSt, as discussed earlier, strongly support adding conventional DMARDs or biologics to MTX over switching to another DMARD.**[19,20,78] A recent trial has nicely addressed the question of stopping MTX versus continuing MTX in patients with active disease who are started on ETAN. This trial randomized 151 patients to either stopping MTX or continuing MTX while starting ETAN. The group that continued MTX fared much better with ACR20s of 86% versus 64% and experienced significantly less radiographic progression as well.[78]

Excellent data now support the efficacy of 15 different clinically available DMARDs or DMARD combinations when added to MTX in this group of patients (active disease despite MTX). This is true for all of the commonly used DMARDs, conventional and biologics alike. Figure 71-2 highlights the blind clinical trials that have studied currently approved therapies in this patient population.[25,36,69,79-88] The problem for the clinician is that there is a marked paucity of data to compare active therapies with each other in this critically important patient population. Knowing that 15 different treatments are better than a placebo is of limited value because most clinicians do not commonly use placebos to treat patients. Therefore trials that compare active therapies are urgently needed.

Two studies shown in Figure 71-2 provide some insight by comparing active therapies to each other in a limited way. In the study by the RAIN group, the combination of SSZ and HCQ appears to be better than either drug alone when added to MTX.[82] In the study by Schiff and colleagues,[88] abatacept was numerically better than infliximab for efficacy but this difference did not reach statistical significance. This study has been faulted by some because of the low and fixed dose of infliximab (3 mg/kg every 8 weeks). This is a fair criticism with regard to the efficacy comparison, but importantly, even at this "low dose," serious and opportunistic infections were increased in the infliximab group compared with the abatacept group. Serious infections occurred in 1.9% of the abatacept and 8.5% of the infliximab group, and all five opportunistic infections in the trial including both cases of tuberculosis occurred in the infliximab group.

The really critical decision for clinicians is whether to add conventional therapies to MTX or take the leap and add biologics. To date, only two studies have addressed this and, unfortunately, both in an indirect way and with different conclusions. An open-label study (SWEFOT) in this population of patients with active disease despite MTX compared adding SSZ and HCQ (triple) to adding infliximab.[74] At 6 months, both approaches appeared identical with 25% of triple patients and 26% of infliximab and MTX patients responding (EULAR good response); by 1 year, the results were surprisingly different (26% for triple vs. 39% infliximab). It is unclear how these data should be reconciled. One explanation is that infliximab had somehow delayed efficacy with increasing effectiveness between 6 and 12 months. This explanation is problematic because essentially all blind trials have shown that TNF inhibition works quickly and maximum results are achieved by 3 to 6 months. An alternate explanation would be that the open nature of the trial and/or the ability to switch to other therapies affected the perceived responses. Regardless, at 2 years there again was no difference in the number of patients with EULAR good response or the number in remission between these two different approaches.

The second study to address this question, also in an indirect way, was the TEAR trial by Moreland and colleagues as discussed earlier.[71] Although the TEAR trial was designed to look at initial therapy, half of patients initially were treated with MTX alone and are relevant to this discussion. Of these MTX-only patients, 72% or 271 patients did not achieve a DAS28 of less than or equal to 3.2 and were treated with ETAN or the addition of HCQ/SSZ (triple) in a blind fashion. As shown in Figure 71-8, both of these groups looked identical to each other 12 weeks after stepping-up and continued to look identical out to week 102, which was the end of the study. Importantly, with regard to radiographic progression, there was no difference in the radiographic progression of these MTX "failures" in the HCQ/SSZ group versus those in the ETAN group (mean progression of 1.7 vs. 1.1; $P = .57$). Reconciling the findings of the larger blind TEAR trial with the open Swefot trial is difficult, and further data from blind RCTs designed specifically to address this important question are eagerly awaited.

Until further data are available and despite the problems of comparing data across trials, the clinician will have to base the decision of what to add to MTX in this group of patients on the efficacy data presented in Figure 71-2, the economic information presented in Table 71-4, concerns for toxicity in individual patients, and, importantly, patients' wishes. This question of course begs for research, and appropriate clinical trials to address this question are urgently needed. However, addressing this question will take several trials because so many therapies with multiple different mechanisms of action (MOA) have been shown to work in this clinical situation (see Figure 71-2). It would be terrific to be able to select patients on the basis of parameters that suggested which MOA would be most likely to work. Until other data exist, largely because of their long track record, most clinicians favor a TNF inhibitor as the first biologic in this group of patients.

Treatment of "Refractory" Patients or Those with Active Disease despite TNF Inhibition

Despite the effectiveness of conventional DMARD combinations and the TNF inhibitors, a subset of patients will continue to have "unacceptable" levels of disease activity. Estimates of the size of this subset range from 10% to 40% of RA patients. The lack of a universal definition of "refractory" and of "unacceptable" levels of disease activity hampers this discussion. With regard to levels of disease activity, it is clear and probably appropriate that clinicians are willing to tolerate more active disease in this "refractory" group before changing therapy, compared with patients who are naïve to treatment or those treated with active disease despite MTX only. Although clear data are necessary, this approach currently seems prudent as the risk of toxicity and expense of treatment become significant factors.

Increasingly, as our expectations for patients increase, we push to control disease sooner and use biologics earlier and patients are being labeled "refractory" much earlier than ever before. When faced with a "refractory" patient, a close inspection of previous treatments "failed" is in order. It is common for patients to be treated initially with low doses of MTX (≤15 mg orally) for 3 months and then started on a TNF inhibitor with or without MTX. If they still have active disease after a few months, patients get labeled inappropriately as "refractory." It is critical to assess whether MTX therapy has been maximized (see Chapter 61); unless contraindications are present, most patients should have MTX pushed to 25 mg/week and subcutaneous administration should be considered. Data show that triple therapy is as effective as MTX- ETAN,[71] so this combination should be considered when resources are limited before progressing too far down the biologic road.

For patients who are truly refractory, as with the previous section on the patient with active disease despite MTX, we urgently need markers or factors that inform us about the best of many possible approaches. The good news is that we still have multiple options with supportive data even in this difficult patient population, which include switching to another TNF agent,[89-92] starting rituximab,[93] starting abatacept[94] or starting tocilizumab.[95] Currently there are limited data (discussed later) that direct this choice, so until markers or parameters are available, we will make this decision largely empirically (see Figure 71-3).

TNF inhibition has been around the longest, and because of its efficacy and clinicians' comfort level, many would switch to a second TNF inhibitor before switching to a biologic with a different MOA. A number of observational studies and one RCT support this approach.[89-92] From the observational studies, a consistent theme has been that if the first TNF inhibitor was discontinued for toxicity or loss of efficacy, patients have a better chance of efficacy of the second TNF than if the first was discontinued because of primary inefficacy (hazard ratio [HR], 2.7; confidence interval [CI], 2.1 to 3.4[89]). Discontinuation rates, particularly as measured in observational trials, are not the same as efficacy and reflect many things including other treatment options that are available at the time of the study. In the previously cited study published in 2007, golimumab, certolizumab, and tocilizumab were not options.

A single randomized trial has addressed this question of switching to a second TNF inhibitor[92]; golimumab was given after failure of at least one anti-TNF agent, and 43% responded compared with 17% in the placebo-treated group. A special case in this patient population may be patients who have developed antidrug antibodies. Recently, data have been published with regard to antidrug antibodies in patients treated with adalimumab. After 3 years of treatment, 28% of patients developed antidrug antibodies; in 67% of cases, these developed in the first 6 months.[96] Development of antidrug antibodies was associated with lack of or loss of efficacy (HR, 3.0; 95% CI, 1.6 to 5.5), and patients were less likely to achieve remission (HR, 7.1; 95% CI, 2.1 to 23.4). Importantly, 38% of patients with antidrug antibodies compared with 14% of those without discontinued therapy for lack of efficacy (P = .001). Perhaps of more concern was a recent finding that the development of anti–adalimumab antibodies was associated with thromboembolic events (HR, 7.6; 95% CI, 1.3 to 45.1; P = .25[97]). These interesting findings raise the possibility that monitoring patients for development of antidrug antibodies not only to adalimumab but also other biologics may be an important strategy to predict not only lack of efficacy but also to prevent toxicities such as thromboembolic events.

Once a clinician decides to go with a biologic with a different MOA, there are currently three choices (although this will likely increase in coming years): rituximab, abatacept, or tocilizumab. Data to help differentiate among them are scarce. On the basis of strong suggestions in the literature that patients who are seronegative for CCP and RF do less well than seropositive patients when treated with rituximab,[98,99] most clinicians would opt for either abatacept or tocilizumab in the seronegative patient. Randomized trials have shown the efficacy of all three MOAs in this patient population.[93-95] These studies have been similar in design and also in the results of intervention. Patients on MTX with active disease or intolerance to at least one TNF inhibitor have had the TNF inhibitor stopped and are randomized to receive the intervention + MTX or MTX + placebo. Response rates in the three different trials for ACR20 for the active drug versus placebo were rituximab 51% versus 18%,[93] abatacept 50% versus 20%,[94] and tocilizumab 50% versus 10%.[95] All these responses, however, are less robust than in biologic-naïve patients. On the basis of the strikingly similar response rates of 50% across these three trials, there is little to choose from until further predictors of responses or comparison trial data are available. Some have raised concern about treatment with a second biologic after treatment with rituximab, which depresses B cell numbers significantly for at least 6 to 12 months. Limited data from observational studies provide some reassurance as a significant increase in toxicities has not been reported.[100]

What to Do with the Patient in Remission (on DMARDs)

It is a powerful testament of how far therapy for patients with RA has come that it is appropriate to include a new section in this edition on what to do with the patient in remission. It is now common practice for clinicians to ask how to taper DMARDs in patients who are "in remission." Indeed, a recent ACR expert panel acknowledged the importance of this question and included it as one of the top priorities for future investigation.[101] Putting aside the obvious difficulty in defining "remission," be it on clinical grounds, with radiographic evidence or by using advanced imaging, clinicians see an increasing number of patients in "remission" or with low levels of disease activity and are increasingly seeking direction on whom should be tapered off of what medications and when.

Unfortunately, again, little data exist. We do not have laboratory tests, inflammatory parameters, or cytokine profiles that help predict who can be safely tapered. Because of their well-chronicled toxicities, the highest priority should be to get all patients off glucocorticoids and NSAIDs. A number of trials[19,20,31] have shown that with effective DMARD therapy, glucocorticoid tapering is not only possible but should be expected. Perhaps the best example of this is from the BeSt trial in which 92% of Group 3 (the group that got high-dose prednisone up front) was off all prednisone at 2 years.[20] In this trial, prednisone was tapered only if the DAS was at or below 2.4 (low level of disease activity).

Once the patient is off glucocorticoids and perhaps on NSAIDs only as needed but still in remission, it is more difficult to know which drug should be tapered next. A common situation is the patient on combination therapy with MTX and a TNF inhibitor. Because of the expense and concerns for long-term toxicities, it would make sense to taper the TNF inhibitor down to the lowest dose possible. Many of these patients in practice may have been started on this combination initially or had the TNF inhibitor added after only a short course of MTX. These patients may be similar to those in the TEAR trial who were started on the combination of MTX-ETAN.[71] For this group of patients we can infer that approximately 30% of them did not need the ETAN and could have done extremely well on MTX alone just as the 28% of patients who started on MTX alone and did not need to step-up. The MTX-only patients who did not step-up not only had the lowest DAS28 at 2 years (mean, 2.7) but also had the least amount of radiographic progression.[71,102] Unfortunately, we do not know how to select these patients.

If patients have been in remission for 6 months to a year and are being treated with a biologic, it seems prudent to decrease the dose or lengthen the interval between injections. Although most biologics, certainly the subcutaneously administered ones, are dosed in a fixed, one-size-fits-all approach, we know from some of the earlier trials that lower doses than usually clinically prescribed can be effective. As an example, the ERA trial compared doses of ETAN of 10 mg and 25 mg given twice weekly[103]; although the data were slightly better for the higher dose, the low dose clearly had substantial efficacy nearly equal to "full-dose" ETAN, both as measured by clinical (ACR20) and lack of radiographic progression. Therefore a significant percentage of patients may be overdosed, particularly those in remission. In our clinic it is not uncommon to have patients who are in remission taking their 50 mg of ETAN every 2 to 4 weeks or their 40 mg of adalimumab every 3 to 6 weeks.

Although wondering what to do with patients in remission on DMARDs is clearly a wonderful problem to have, further direction is certainly necessary for this emerging and fortunately increasing patient group. Trials to address this question with the collection of biomarkers will be increasingly important as patients continue to do better with current therapies. It is clear that both US and MRI (discussed later) can detect levels of synovitis that are not apparent on clinical examination. As this question is examined further, perhaps we will learn that patients with inflammation by US are not good candidates for discontinuing therapy or, alternatively, US or MRI may provide early warning signs of flares. An interesting recent report indicated that US was able to predict which patients in clinical remission would flare.[104]

Use of Combinations of Biologics

Combinations of conventional DMARDs and combinations of conventional DMARDs (especially MTX) with biologics have played a critical role in the vast improvement in responses to treatments we currently see. However, so far efforts to combine biologic products have not met with success. To date, studies to combine ETAN with anakinra have shown no improvement in disease control with ACR50 of 41% in the ETAN-only arm compared with 31% in the combination arm and have shown an increase in serious infections in the combination arm (7.4% vs. 0%[105]).

Similarly, in patients with active disease despite ETAN (n = 80), patients were randomized to add abatacept or placebo; efficacy showed a nonstatistically significantly trend toward improvement (ACR20 for combination, 48% vs. 31%; P = .07), but again an increased risk of serious adverse events in the combination group (17% vs. 3%) and serious infections (4% vs. 0%).[106] Finally, a recent small trial (n = 51) in which patients with active disease despite MTX and either ETAN or adalimumab were treated with the addition of rituximab or placebo showed modest improvement in efficacy (ACR20 of 30% vs. 17%), and again serious adverse events including infections were numerically greater in the combination-treated group.[107] Despite these less than encouraging results from early biologic combination trials, it is likely that ultimately patients will be treated with combinations of biologics. What is critically needed are good ways to measure the degree of

immune suppression we create with our interventions—a thermostat for TNF, IL-1, or IL-6, if you will.[108] Currently, we are likely inadequately suppressing some patients, therefore not achieving optimal disease control and suppressing others to dangerous levels leading to increased toxicity. When better immune system monitoring techniques are developed, we will be able to better use the biologics we currently have. In addition, it is likely that we will be able to safely and effectively combine biologics to improve outcomes both in terms of efficacy and safety for patients.

Interpreting Radiographic Progression and the Use of Other Imaging Modalities

What is the clinical relevance of radiographic progression? How much progression is significant and over what time period? Are erosions important or should we be concerned only with joint space narrowing? Finally, what role, if any, should US or MRI play in the management of RA?

In clinical trials, treatments of RA are evaluated by clinical parameters (ACR20 responses, DAS, etc.) and radiographic progression (TSS or SHS). This is problematic for a number of reasons. Clinical and radiographic progression is not always parallel. Maybe the most dramatic example of this from an RCT is the PREMIER trial. In the monotherapy arms, MTX alone was significantly better statistically than adalimumab alone, while at the same time, adalimumab alone was better than MTX alone with regard to radiographic progression (Figure 71-10A and B[70]). So which treatment was better? Some would say it is moot because the combination of the two outperformed either monotherapy arm in both measures. However, that misses the point about how to balance radiographic progression versus clinic parameters. Because patients do not come to a clinic complaining of radiographic progression or demanding that it be stopped, the following question is highly relevant: "How is radiographic progression related to things patients do care about—most importantly, physical function?"

Some data relate total Sharp score (TSS) or, similarly, total (SHS) progression to changes on health assessment questionnaires or HAQs (the gold standard for physical function in RA). These data suggest that a change in TSS of 1 equals a change in HAQ of approximately .01.[109] It is well accepted that a clinically significant change in HAQ is approximately .22, so it follows that a change in TSS of 22 is required for a radiographic change to be clinically relevant. This large change is never seen in clinical trials in which active therapies are compared with each other. So although many RCTs have shown statistically significant radiographic progression differences, few if any have shown clinically significant difference within 1 to 2 years of the clinical trial. Additionally, recent data suggest that joint space narrowing correlates well with clinical progression, whereas erosions do not,[110,111] so perhaps we should not be concerned with TSS but only the joint space narrowing component. The next critically important point is over what duration should we be concerned about radiographic progression? If a trial shows Therapy A results in two less TSS points progression per year compared with Therapy B, it follows that if those same therapies are used for 11 years,

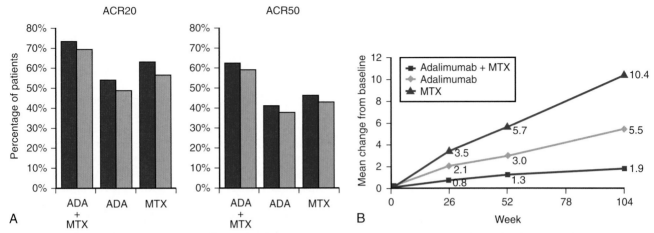

Figure 71-10 Results from the PREMIER trial.[70] **A,** Clinical improvement measured by American College of Rheumatology 20%, 50%, and 70% composite improvement. **B,** Radiographic progression. ADA, adalimumab; MTX, methotrexate. *(Modified from Breedveld FC, Weisman MH, Kavanaugh AF, et al: A multicenter, randomized, double-blind clinical trial of combination therapy with adalimumab plus methotrexate versus methotrexate alone or adalimumab alone in patients with early, aggressive rheumatoid arthritis who had not had previous methotrexate treatment,* Arthritis Rheum *54:26–37, 2006.)*

then patients on Therapy A will have a clinically significant clinical benefit, HAQ .22 less than Therapy B. This is the magnitude of difference (ΔTSS of 1 to 2/year) that has been seen in trials and has led to claims in superiority of one therapy over another. Two problems are readily apparent with this type of extrapolation:

- Within clinical trials patients are often randomized to a therapy and left on it for the duration of the trial regardless of how they are doing. This is not how patients are taken care of in a clinic; if patients are not doing well, therapy is or should be adjusted. Again, the PREMIER trial[70] is an excellent example of this issue—patients were in their assigned groups for 2 years (see Figure 71-10B). Many were not having optimal clinical response, and therapy would have been changed if similar things were happening in a real-life clinical setting. These patients would not still be in the trial demonstrating their predictable radiographic progression, so in any RCT, radiographic progression that occurs after the time the therapy should have had maximum clinical benefit, and therefore patients would have been switched to a new therapy, is not clinically relevant. In the PREMIER trial, the therapies should have had maximal benefit by 6 months, so if the data after that time point include patients who were not at target (at least low disease activity), then it is not relevant to patients seen in a clinic.
- The second point is similar—to extrapolate forward in the example of a change in TSS of 2/year to 11 years of therapy would only be relevant if all patients were doing well clinically. Patients who are not would have their therapies changed before the two TSS progression per year had a chance to become clinically relevant.

Another major reason why radiographic progression is problematic for the clinician is that formal evaluation of radiographic progression is almost never done outside of clinical trials; few, if any, patients in many countries have formal Sharp score assessment of radiographs. In this regard, routine yearly radiographs in RA are not indicated in many

RA patients and only add to the expense of care. This is true for patients who are not doing well clinically—those patients need a change of care regardless of what the radiographs show, and it is also true for patients who are unwilling or unable to change therapies. The small minority of patients who are at target but who are progressing radiographically are the ones we hope to discover important information with serial radiographs. Finally, the way radiographic information is presented in clinical trials is problematic. Most commonly, the mean TSS progression of Group A is compared with Group B and statistics are done. We are told that Therapy A is superior to Therapy B because there is one or two less TSS progression in that group. A much more informative way to look at radiographic outcomes is to look at cumulative probability plots for radiographic changes (Figure 71-11 for the TEMPO trial[72,73] and Figure 71-9 earlier for the TEAR trial[71]). When data are looked at this way, it is readily appreciated that a small number of patients, perhaps 15% to 20% in the TEMPO trial and in many studies even fewer, are driving

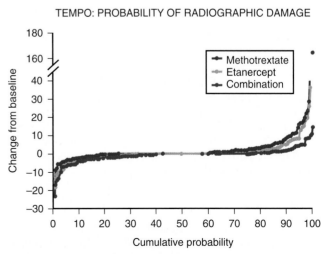

Figure 71-11 Radiographic probability of progression plot from TEMPO.[72,73]

the radiographic outcome. In the TEAR trial, there are no differences across the four groups in the probability plot. With this epiphany, the important questions are who are these patients and how do we focus on this small group that would benefit from a different therapy and not subject the other 80% to 95% to additional risks and expense? Recently, as mentioned earlier, Aletaha and colleagues[110] have called into question the relevance of erosions with regard to clinical correlations and have suggested that joint space narrowing correlates much more strongly with clinical progression. Therefore going forward we need to take this into account.[110]

Finally, what is the place, if any, of "advanced" imaging techniques in evaluating RA patients? Clearly, both US and MRI are powerful techniques to evaluate early erosions and to detect synovitis (see Chapter 58). One potential use of these obviously sensitive techniques, as suggested earlier, is to verify the true absence of synovitis in patients who are felt to be in remission on clinical grounds.[104] Until further research is available, these techniques will remain largely research tools with regard to routine care of RA patients.

ADJUNCTS TO MEDICATIONS

Patient Education

RA is a lifelong disease, so it only makes sense that patients who are educated about their disease do better, and in fact good data exist to show that education leads to better outcomes.[112] Use of the Arthritis Self-Management Program has been shown to lead to less pain, decreased visits to physicians, and economic savings.[113,114] Chronic diseases such as RA affect the whole family, and participation of spouses in educational group sessions leads to additional beneficial effects.[115] Training in stress management is particularly effective in improving measures of helplessness, coping, pain, self-efficacy, and health status.[116] Unfortunately, formal education level, a factor that we cannot modify, is associated with morbidity and mortality rates. Formal educational level is inversely proportional to these outcomes, and this cannot be explained by age, duration of disease, joint count, functional measures, or medications.[117]

Chapter 67 provides an in-depth discussion of many of these important aspects. It is clearly important for patients to take an active role in the management of their chronic disease. The more patients understand their disease and medications, the more control they feel they have over the whole situation. The bond that develops between the patient and physician working together to control this lifelong disease is an important factor in outcome, as well as the satisfaction level of both parties. The stronger the bond is, the less likely that patients will become frustrated and turn to alternative therapies that are not only expensive but may do more harm than good.

Pain Control

If patients with RA are treated early and effectively with DMARDs and therapy is escalated to achieve excellent control of the active components of disease, the need for specific pain medications, particularly narcotics, can be minimized. If pain is a major problem, the clinician should first review the DMARD program and modify it to achieve maximum control of any active synovitis. Unfortunately, some patients will present in the latter course of disease after substantial joint damage has already occurred and will need pain relief. Pain can be the factor that limits effectiveness of physical and occupational therapy, and as pointed out during a special workshop sponsored by the National Advisory Board for Arthritis and Musculoskeletal and Skin Diseases, it is frequently undertreated in patients with arthritis.[118] In addition to inhibiting function, pain is a major cause of depression in patients with polyarthritis. To maximize therapy in patients with early RA or undifferentiated polyarthritis, pain must be controlled without altering consciousness or generating addiction. Treatment strategies favoring education, rest, exercise, and disease-modifying therapies are generally favored as an approach to pain control in arthritis, and strategies that rely on narcotic derivatives may not address control of active RA. In most medical centers, experts in pain management are available for consultation by rheumatologists and primary care physicians (PCPs). There is an excellent discussion of analgesics in rheumatic disease in Chapter 66.

Rest, Exercise, and Activities of Daily Living

Education and supervision of a patient by trained professionals on the importance of finding the best balance of rest and exercise for inflamed joints are essential. This component of therapy can be started well before a definitive diagnosis is made. No matter what the cause, finding this balance should ensure that a patient develops or retains sufficient strength to support joint function without exacerbating inflammation.

Details of physical and occupational therapy are outlined in Chapter 38. A patient with acutely and severely inflamed joints may not be the ideal exercise candidate and may need application of resting splints to immobilize the joint until anti-inflammatory medications, specifically DMARDs, take effect. Even the most painful joints, when splinted, must be moved passively through a full range of motion each day to prevent flexion contractures, particularly in children. For moderately inflamed joints, isometric exercise with muscles contracted in a fixed position (the resting length of the muscle) provides adequate muscle tone without exacerbating joint inflammation and pain. Maximal contractions, held for 6 seconds and repeated 5 to 10 times, performed several times each day, can prevent further loss of muscle mass around arthritic joints.

Patients with well-controlled arthritis will benefit from variable-resistance programs or high-intensity strength training, which has been shown to provide significant improvements in strength, pain, and fatigue levels. Older patients with RA benefit from progressive resistance exercises, similar to younger patients. In a study of older patients given closely regulated workouts on pneumatic resistance equipment, maximal strength of all major exercised muscle groups was increased 75% without exacerbation of clinical disease activity.[119] Prescribed sustained exercise not only increases muscle strength but also helps the ability of patients to perform daily routines, improves global assessments and moods, and can decrease pain.[120]

Most patients with RA should have one or more sessions with a licensed occupational therapist (OT) to learn how to preserve joint function and alignment while carrying out the necessary and enjoyable activities of daily living and to be exposed to the assistive devices that are available. The basic concept is to avoid excessive force applied across non–weight-bearing joints and to avoid unnecessary impact loading on weight-bearing joints. A prospective and controlled Canadian trial demonstrated that home therapy by OTs produced a statistically significant and clinically important improvement in function in RA patients.[121]

Treatment of Comorbidities and Interaction of Rheumatologist with Primary Care Physician

The best possible outcomes for patients with RA can be achieved only with a carefully orchestrated collaboration between PCPs and rheumatologists. On the one hand, the ever-increasing complexity of RA management options, combination therapies, and possible toxicities of therapy have all made it essential that RA patients are seen by rheumatologists. Good evidence indicates that RA patients are more likely to be on DMARDs, are more likely to be on combination DMARDs, and are happier with their care when seen by rheumatologists.[122-124] On the other hand, the realization of the critical nature of the comorbidities associated with RA, especially cardiovascular disease, makes ongoing engagement of a PCP essential[125] to produce optimal outcomes.

Significant data indicate that patients with RA have better outcomes when rheumatologists are the primary manager of the RA. In one series of 561 patients with definite RA followed over 20 years, the patients seen by a rheumatologist during the first 2 years of disease fared significantly better than those who did not.[126] The favorable outcome could be related to an early start of DMARD therapy. Further, data indicate that regular ongoing care by a rheumatologist (mean of 8.6 visits per year) results in less functional disability than for patients who received only intermittent, sporadic care by a rheumatologist.[127] Analysis of these data supported the interpretation that worsening disability was not the reason for intermittent care, but rather a consequence of it. Additionally, evidence supporting care by a rheumatologist showed that patients who had access to a rheumatologist had higher performance scores than patients who saw only a PCP. Access to specialist care resulted in significant improvements in arthritis care, comorbid illness, and health care maintenance overall beyond seeing a PCP alone.[128]

As important as the rheumatologist is, the PCP needs to be closely engaged (Table 71-7). Recently, the

Table 71-7 Role of Primary Care Physicians in Rheumatoid Arthritis

Monitor and aggressively treat cardiovascular risk factors
Monitor and treat/prevent osteoporosis*
Recognize toxicities of rheumatoid arthritis medications and initiate appropriate and timely workup*
Recognize the risks for infections and ensure immunization status is current

*In partnership with a rheumatologist.

comorbidities of RA have been highlighted and include premature atherosclerosis and congestive heart failure, increased risks of osteoporosis and fractures, and increased risks of infections. A recent review by a panel of cardiologists and rheumatologists highlighted RA as a significant risk factor for cardiovascular morbidity and mortality on par with diabetes.[129] In this regard, the PCP needs to aggressively address traditional cardiovascular risk factors such as hypertension and especially hyperlipidemia in RA patients. Statins should be used aggressively because the primary reason for the excess mortality seen in RA is cardiovascular. As an added bonus, statins, probably secondary to their anti-inflammatory effects, have been shown in animal studies of RA models[130] and in at least one RCT in humans[131] to decrease RA activity. Further, there are data that statin use may protect against the development of RA.[132]

Because RA and particularly glucocorticoids are risk factors for osteoporosis, the PCP, in concert with the rheumatologist, needs to address this. Most patients should be receiving calcium and adequate vitamin D_3. Bisphosphonates have been shown to prevent steroid-induced osteoporosis,[133] and their use should be strongly considered in patients on long-term steroids unless there are contraindications (e.g., women of childbearing age).

With the increased infection risk that RA patients have, both because of their disease and therapies, up-to-date immunizations including yearly influenza shots, every 5-year pneumococcal vaccinations, and appropriate zoster vaccinations are critical.[1] The latter is a live-virus vaccination and should be avoided in patients currently receiving biologics. Current recommendations are to give the zoster vaccination 2 weeks before starting any of the biologics. Influenza and pneumococcal vaccinations can be safely given to patients on biologics with reasonable immunologic response,[134] except in patients on rituximab, in whom response is severely impaired.[135,136] The rheumatologist and PCP should push hard for smoking cessation for all the usual reasons plus concern for cardiovascular and pulmonary disease already over-represented in RA; cessation has the added benefit of potentially making patients more responsive to therapies.[137] Finally, because the PCP often sees the patient first during an illness, the PCP needs to be familiar with the common toxicities of RA medications including concerns about MTX in the patient with decreasing renal function, MTX pneumonitis, and the need for heightened concern and aggressive workup of all potential infections including opportunist infections in immunosuppressed patients, particularly those on biologics. Often, the difference between life and death or at least between excellent outcomes and less than optimal results is the rapidity of response to the early warning signs for things as simple as a cellulitis or a pulmonary infiltrate.

Clearly the best care is given by a team: a rheumatologist, a PCP, and an educated patient all working closely together. Timely consultation with physical and occupational therapists and orthopedic surgeons also plays a role in optimal outcomes for RA patients. Although the need for joint replacement surgery is thankfully decreasing, few interventions have been as successful in improving patient mobility and quality of life as having properly timed hip and knee replacements. With the potential of huge changes in health care delivery on the horizon, at least in the United States, it may be an increasing challenge to assure that the right team is always engaged to achieve the best outcomes for each patient.

Evidence That Patients with Rheumatoid Arthritis Are Doing Better

The prognosis for patients with RA has improved dramatically. Every rheumatologist who has been fortunate enough to see the changes over the past quarter of a century is only too happy to witness to this. The days when wheelchairs were commonplace in clinics and many RA patients had symptomatic C1 subluxations, chronic leg ulcers, constrictive pericarditis, and corneal melts are hopefully gone forever. Despite this firmly held perception by clinicians, strong data to support this change have been slow to accumulate.

Recent data from Olmsted County, Minnesota, show that RA patients diagnosed after 1995 lived significantly longer, almost 9 years, than those diagnosed before 1995.[138] In the same cohort of patients in Olmsted County, knee surgery was decreased by 46% and hand surgery by 55%.[139] Data from more than 35,000 U.S. veterans with RA showed a greater than 30% reduction in extra-articular manifestations of RA since the year 2000.[140] Ward, using data from California (years 1983 to 2001), showed that hospitalizations for RA vasculitis or splenectomy for Felty's syndrome decreased by 33% and 71%, respectively.[141] Further, primary knee arthroplasty for RA decreased by 10%. Early unpublished reports from many centers indicate that joint replacement surgery for RA may be reduced by up to 50% to 80%. Data from Sweden and Spain[142] both show that disease activity scores and health assessment scores have significantly improved over the past decade.

Investigators postulate it may take up to 20 years for the results of a change in therapy or approach to fully translate into improvement in long-term outcomes such as joint replacements and mortality. Therefore the encouraging data presented earlier likely reflect our therapies of the early to mid-1990s, and therefore we expect that these early reports are the leading wave of good news as some of the therapeutic principles in use for the past decade began to show their full effect.

Research Agenda: Unmet Needs

As mentioned numerous times, huge gaps remain in our knowledge of how to best use the 19 clinically available DMARDs (see Table 71-1) for optimal patient care. At the top of the list of important clinical questions is the urgent need for factors or parameters that would allow us to differentiate the probability of response to or toxicity from different DMARDs at the level of individual patients. This is important for selection of DMARDs for all the categories of patients discussed earlier—DMARD naïve, those with active disease despite MTX, and those who have failed treatment with MTX plus a TNF inhibitor. With regard to specific trials needed in each of these patient groups, a recent ACR task force was formed to prioritize the clinical research trials needed to most expeditiously advance the knowledge base needed to move RA treatment forward.[101] After making the strong recommendation that all further

trials include biologic samples to aid in our search for factors that differentiate therapeutic responses, they ordered the trial priorities as follows:

- Trials to elucidate the possible role of induction therapy in early disease
- Treatment of active disease despite MTX and the first TNF inhibitor
- Tapering therapy for patients in remission
- Treatment of active disease despite MTX
- Stratifying patients to determine in advance the most appropriate therapy in order to move beyond the current trial and error approach

Except for studies in patients in remission, the task force emphasized the need for trials that compare active therapies with each other. Further trials that demonstrate the superiority of product X over placebo in any of these areas where multiple treatments have already been shown to work will not provide useful information to clinicians trying to make important clinical decisions. True comparative effectiveness research is necessary to address the multiple options available for patients with RA in all of these categories. Further, the task force stressed the importance of innovative trial designs that more closely mirror clinical practice.[101] Examples would include trials that allow escalation or switching of therapies in a blind fashion on the basis of clinical response and not allowing patients with ongoing active disease to continue on fixed therapies after the point of maximal response.

Horizon

It is always difficult to predict the future, particularly in an area where things are changing as rapidly as they are in RA, and certainly the authors of the early editions of TOR could not have predicted we would make the giant strides in RA treatment that we have. As Bill Gates remarked, "We always overestimate the change that will occur in the next 2 years and underestimate the change that will occur in the next 10." By the tenth edition of TOR we will almost certainly have several new biologics and perhaps several new small molecule DMARDs available for treatment. Leading biologic candidates include rilonacept (IL-1 Trap), already approved for cryopyrin-associated periodic syndromes,[143] and potential targets IL-12,[144] IL-17A,[145] IL-23[146] and IL-33.[147] Prime small molecule DMARDs that inhibit signaling molecules, particular Janus kinases (Jak)[148] and spleen tyrosine kinase (Syk),[149] might become available in the next few years and could dramatically change the treatment paradigm yet again.

Regardless of new therapies that expand our portfolio of choices, the two areas where we will need to see the most progress are profiling patients on the basis of parameters that predict differential responses to different therapies and in monitoring the kinds and intensity of immunologic modification that we are producing. If substantial progress can be made in these areas, even without new therapies, we should be able to obtain vastly superior and more expeditious disease control. On a somewhat more pragmatic note, the treatment of RA has become an expensive endeavor and with all the changes in health care and the continuing increases in the cost, it is imperative that we have the appropriate studies to allow us to take the best care of patients for the least cost. If we do not have the appropriate research to justify expensive medications, we may have difficulty justifying their use. Therefore it is critical that trials are designed with this in mind and that long-term costs, both direct and indirect, of suboptimally controlled RA be part of the equation.

It is clear from many observations that the immune response that becomes RA starts [150-152] before most patients present with the classic symptom complex. Studies to elucidate this transition are under way[153] and studies to treat presymptomatic RA are not far behind. Even further, these studies on preclinical disease hold the promise of elucidating the triggers of RA and, if so, the ultimate goal of RA prevention cannot be far behind.

Selected References

1. Saag KG, Teng GG, Patkar NM, et al: American College of Rheumatology 2008 recommendations for the use of nonbiologic and biologic disease-modifying antirheumatic drugs in rheumatoid arthritis, *Arthritis Rheum* 59:762–784, 2008.
2. Singh JA, Furst DE, Bharat A, et al: 2012 update of the 2008 American College of Rheumatology recommendations for the use of disease-modifying antirheumatic drugs and biologic agents in the treatment of rheumatoid arthritis, *Arthritis Care Res (Hoboken)* 64:625–639, 2012.
3. McInnes IB, O'Dell JR: State-of-the-art: rheumatoid arthritis, *Ann Rheum Dis* 69:1898–1906, 2010.
4. Smolen JS, Landewe R, Breedveld FC, et al: EULAR recommendations for the management of rheumatoid arthritis with synthetic and biological disease-modifying antirheumatic drugs, *Ann Rheum Dis* 69:964–975, 2010.
5. van der Heijde DM, van 't Hof M, van Riel PL, et al: Validity of single variables and indices to measure disease activity in rheumatoid arthritis, *J Rheumatol* 20:538–541, 1993.
7. Smolen JS, Breedveld FC, Schiff MHA, et al: A simplified disease activity index for rheumatoid arthritis for use in clinical practice, *Rheumatology (Oxford)* 42:244–257, 2003.
9. Yazici Y, Bergman M, Pincus T: Time to score quantitative rheumatoid arthritis measures: 28-Joint Count, Disease Activity Score, Health Assessment Questionnaire (HAQ), Multidimensional HAQ (MDHAQ), and Routine Assessment of Patient Index Data (RAPID) scores, *J Rheumatol* 35:603–609, 2008.
11. Anderson JK, Caplan L, Yazdany J, et al: Rheumatoid arthritis disease activity measures: American College of Rheumatology recommendations for use in clinical practice, *Arthritis Care Res (Hoboken)* 64:640–647, 2012.
12. Felson DT, Smolen JS, Wells G, et al: American College of Rheumatology/European League Against Rheumatism provisional definition of remission in rheumatoid arthritis for clinical trials, *Arthritis Rheum* 63:573–586, 2011.
13. O'Dell JR, Mikuls TR: To improve outcomes we must define and measure them: toward defining remission in rheumatoid arthritis, *Arthritis Rheum* 63:587–589, 2011.
14. Peluso G, Michelutti A, Bosello S, et al: Clinical and ultrasonographic remission determines different chances of relapse in early and long standing rheumatoid arthritis, *Ann Rheum Dis* 70:172–175, 2011.
15. Saleem B, Brown AK, Keen H, et al: Extended report: should imaging be a component of rheumatoid arthritis remission criteria? A comparison between traditional and modified composite remission scores and imaging assessments, *Ann Rheum Dis* 70:792–798, 2011.
17. The Action to Control Cardiovascular Risk in Diabetes Study Group: Effects of intensive glucose lowering in type 2 diabetes, *N Engl J Med* 358:2545–2559, 2008.
18. Grigor C, Capell H, Stirling A, et al: Effect of a treatment strategy of tight control for rheumatoid arthritis (the TICORA study): a single-blind randomised controlled trial, *Lancet* 364:263–269, 2004.
19. Goekoop-Ruiterman YPM, de Vries-Bouwstra JK, Allaart CF, et al: Clinical and radiographic outcomes of four different treatment strategies in patients with early rheumatoid arthritis (the BeSt study): a randomized, controlled trial, *Arthritis Rheum* 52:3381–3390, 2005.
20. Goekoop-Ruiterman YP, de Vries-Bouwstra JK, Allaart CF, et al: Comparison of treatment strategies in early rheumatoid arthritis: a randomized trial, *Ann Intern Med* 146:406–415, 2007.
22. Schipper LG, van Hulst LT, Grol R, et al: Meta-analysis of tight control strategies in rheumatoid arthritis: protocolized treatment has additional value with respect to the clinical outcome, *Rheumatology (Oxford)* 49:2154–2164, 2010.
24. Hench PS, Kendall EC, Slocumb CH, Polley HF: The effect of a hormone of the adrenal cortex (17-hydroxy-11-dehydrocorticosterone: compound E) and of pituitary adrenocorticotropic hormone on rheumatoid arthritis, *Mayo Clin Proc* 24:181–197, 1949.
25. Joint Committee of the Medical Research Council and Nuffield Foundation on Clinical Trials of Cortisone, ACTH and Other Therapeutic Measures in Chronic Rheumatic Diseases, *Ann Rheum Dis* 18:173, 1959.
27. Kirwan JR and the Arthritis and Rheumatism Council Low-Dose Glucocorticoid Study Group: The effect of glucocorticoids on joint destruction in rheumatoid arthritis, *N Engl J Med* 333:142–146, 1995.
28. Hickling P, Jacoby RK, Kirwan JR and the Arthritis and Rheumatism Council Low Dose Glucocorticoid Study Group: Joint destruction after glucocorticoids are withdrawn in early rheumatoid arthritis, *Br J Rheumatol* 37:930–936, 1998.
29. Boers M, Verhoeven AC, Markusse HM, et al: Randomised comparison of combined step-down prednisolone, methotrexate and sulphasalazine with sulphasalazine alone in early rheumatoid arthritis, *Lancet* 350:309–318, 1997.
31. O'Dell JR, Blakely KW, Mallek JA, et al: Treatment of early seropositive rheumatoid arthritis: a two-year, double-blind comparison of minocycline and hydroxychloroquine, *Arthritis Rheum* 44:2235–2241, 2001.
33. Lehman AJ, Esdaile JM, Klinkhoff AV, et al: METGO Study Group: a 48-week, randomized double-blind, double-observer, placebo-controlled multicenter trial of combination methotrexate and intramuscular gold therapy in rheumatoid arthritis: results of the METGO study, *Arthritis Rheum* 52:1360–1370, 2005.
35. Felson DT, Anderson JJ, Meenan RF: The comparative efficacy and toxicity of second-line drugs in rheumatoid arthritis: results of second-line drugs in rheumatoid arthritis, *Arthritis Rheum* 33:1449, 1990.
36. Sakkas LI, Chikanza IC, Vaughn RW, et al: Gold induced nephropathy in rheumatoid arthritis and HLA class II genes, *Ann Rheum Dis* 52:300, 1993.
37. McCarty DJ, Harman JG, Grassanovich JL, et al: Combination drug therapy of seropositive rheumatoid arthritis, *J Rheumatol* 22:1636–1645, 1995.
39. Black AJ, McLeod HL, Capell HA: Thiopurine methyltransferase genotype predicts therapy limiting severe toxicity from azathioprine, *Ann Intern Med* 129:716, 1998.
40. Blanco R, Martinez-Taboada VM, Gonzalez-Gay MA: Acute febrile toxic reaction in patients with refractory rheumatoid arthritis who are receiving combined therapy with methotrexate and azathioprine, *Arthritis Rheum* 39:1016, 1996.
41. Tugwell P, Bombardier C, Gent M, et al: Low-dose cyclosporine versus placebo in patients with rheumatoid arthritis, *Lancet* 335:1051, 1990.
44. Tugwell P, Pincus T, Yocum D, et al: Combination therapy with cyclosporine and methotrexate in severe rheumatoid arthritis, *N Engl J Med* 333:137, 1995.
45. Stein CM, Pincus T, Yocum D, et al: Combination treatment of severe rheumatoid arthritis with cyclosporine and methotrexate for forty-eight weeks: an open-label extension study. The Methotrexate-Cyclosporine Combination Study Group, *Arthritis Rheum* 40:1843–1851, 1997.
48. Yu LP Jr, Smith GN, Hasty KA, et al: Doxycycline inhibits type XI collagenolytic activity of extracts from human osteoarthritis cartilage and of gelatinase, *J Rheumatol* 18:1450, 1991.
50. Kloppenburg M, Breedveld FC, Terwiel JP, et al: Minocycline in active rheumatoid arthritis: a double-blind, placebo-controlled trial, *Arthritis Rheum* 37:629, 1994.
51. Tilley B, Alarcon G, Heyse S, et al: Minocycline in rheumatoid arthritis: a 48-week, double blind, placebo-controlled trial, *Ann Intern Med* 122:81, 1995.

52. O'Dell JR, Haire CE, Palmer W, et al: Treatment of early rheumatoid arthritis with minocycline or placebo: results of a randomized, double-blind, placebo-controlled trial, *Arthritis Rheum* 40:842, 1997.

53. O'Dell JR, Elliott JR, Mallek JA, et al: Treatment of early seropositive rheumatoid arthritis: doxycycline plus methotrexate versus methotrexate alone, *Arthritis Rheum* 54:621–627, 2006.

54. Fay BT, Whiddon AP, Puumala S, et al: Minocycline-induced hyperpigmentation in rheumatoid arthritis, *J Clin Rheumatol* 14:17–20, 2008.

55. Elkayam O, Levartovsky D, Brautbar C, et al: Clinical and immunological study of 7 patients with minocycline-induced autoimmune phenomena, *Am J Med* 105:484, 1998.

56. Gabriel SE, Jaakkimainen L, Bombardier C: Risk for serious gastrointestinal complications related to use of NSAIDs. A meta-analysis, *Ann Intern Med* 115:787, 1991.

59. Graham DJ, Campen D, Hui R, et al: Risk of myocardial infarction and sudden death in patients treated with cyclo-oxygenase 2 selective and non-selective NSAIDs: nested case-control study, *Lancet* 365:475, 2005.

60. Huerta C, Castellsague J, Varas-Lorenzo C, et al: NSAIDs and risk of ARF in the general population, *Am J Kidney Dis* 45:531, 2005.

62. The HERA Study Group: A randomized trial of hydroxychloroquine in early rheumatoid arthritis: the HERA study, *Am J Med* 98:156–168, 1995.

63. Egsmose C, Lund B, Borg G, et al: Patients with rheumatoid arthritis benefit from early second-line therapy: 5-year follow-up of a prospective double-blind placebo-controlled study, *J Rheumatol* 22:2208–2213, 1995.

65. van Dongen H, van Aken J, Lard LR, et al: Efficacy of methotrexate treatment in patients with probable rheumatoid arthritis. A double-blind, randomized, placebo-controlled trial, *Arthritis Rheum* 56:1424–1432, 2007.

66. Lard LR, Visser H, Speyer I, et al: Early versus delayed treatment in patients with recent-onset rheumatoid arthritis: comparison of two cohorts who received different treatment strategies, *Am J Med* 111(6):446–451, 2001.

67. Möttönen R, Hannonen P, Leirisalo-Repo M, et al: Comparison of combination therapy with single-drug therapy in early rheumatoid arthritis: a randomized trial, *Lancet* 353:1568–1573, 1999.

68. Calguneri M, Pay S, Caliskaner Z, et al: Combination therapy versus monotherapy for the treatment of patients with rheumatoid arthritis, *Clin Exp Rheumatol* 17:699–704, 1999.

69. Lipsky P, et al: Infliximab and methotrexate in the treatment of rheumatoid arthritis, *N Engl J Med* 343(22):1594–1602, 2000.

70. Breedveld FC, Weisman MH, Kavanaugh AF, et al: A multicenter, randomized, double-blind clinical trial of combination therapy with adalimumab plus methotrexate versus methotrexate alone or adalimumab alone in patients with early, aggressive rheumatoid arthritis who had not had previous methotrexate treatment, *Arthritis Rheum* 54:26–37, 2006.

71. Moreland L, O'Dell J, Paulus H, et al: A randomized comparative effectiveness study of oral triple therapy versus etanercept plus methotrexate in early, aggressive rheumatoid arthritis: the TEAR Trial, *Arthritis Rheum* 2012, doi 10.1002/art.34498 (Epub ahead of print).

72. Klareskog L, van der Heijde D, de Jager JP, et al: Therapeutic effect of the combination of etanercept and methotrexate compared with each treatment alone in patients with rheumatoid arthritis: double-blind randomised controlled trial, *Lancet* 363:675–681, 2004.

73. van der Heijde D, Klareskog L, Rodriguez-Valverde V, et al: Comparison of etanercept and methotrexate, alone and combined, in the treatment of rheumatoid arthritis: two-year clinical and radiographic results from the TEMPO study, a double-blind, randomized trial, *Arthritis Rheum* 54:1063–1074, 2006.

74. van Vollenhoven RF, Ernestam S, Geborek P, et al: Addition of infliximab compared with addition of sulfasalazine and hydroxychloroquine to methotrexate in patients with early rheumatoid arthritis (Swefot trial): 1-year results of a randomised trial, *Lancet* 374:459–466, 2009.

75. O'Dell J, Haire C, Erikson N, et al: Treatment of rheumatoid arthritis with methotrexate alone, sulfasalazine and hydroxychloroquine, or a combination of all three medications, *N Engl J Med* 334:1287–1291, 1996.

76. Kremer JM, Genovese MC, Cannon GW, et al: Concomitant leflunomide therapy in patients with active rheumatoid arthritis despite stable doses of methotrexate: a randomized, double-blind, placebo controlled trial, *Ann Intern Med* 137:726–733, 2002.

77. Klarenbeek NB, van der Kooij SM, Güler-Yüksel M, et al: Discontinuing treatment in patients with rheumatoid arthritis in sustained clinical remission: exploratory analyses from the BeSt study, *Ann Rheum Dis* 70:315–319, 2011.

78. Kameda H, Ueki Y, Saito K, et al: Etanercept (ETN) with methotrexate (MTX) is better than ETN monotherapy in patients with active rheumatoid arthritis despite MTX therapy: a randomized trial, *Mod Rheumatol* 20:531–538, 2010.

79. Weinblatt ME, Kremer JM, Bankhurst AD, et al: A trial of etanercept, a recombinant tumor necrosis factor receptor: Fc fusion protein, in patients with rheumatoid arthritis receiving methotrexate, *N Engl J Med* 340:253–259, 1999.

80. Cohen S, Hurd E, Cush J, et al: Treatment of rheumatoid arthritis with anakinra, a recombinant human interleukin-1 receptor antagonist, in combination with methotrexate, *Arthritis Rheum* 46(3):614–624, 2002.

81. Weinblatt ME, Keystone EC, Furst DE, et al: Adalimumab, a fully human anti-tumor necrosis factor alpha monoclonal antibody, for the treatment of rheumatoid arthritis in patients taking concomitant methotrexate: the ARMADA trial, *Arthritis Rheum* 48:35–45, 2003.

82. O'Dell J, Leff R, Paulsen G, et al: Treatment of rheumatoid arthritis with methotrexate and hydroxychloroquine, methotrexate and sulfasalazine, or a combination of the three medications: results of a two-year, randomized, double-blind, placebo-controlled trial, *Arthritis Rheum* 46(5):1164–1170, 2002.

83. Kremer JM, Genant HK, Moreland LW, et al: Effects of abatacept in patients with methotrexate-resistant active rheumatoid arthritis, *Ann Intern Med* 144:865–876, 2006.

84. Emery P, Fleischmann R, Filipowicz-Sosnowska A, et al: The efficacy and safety of rituximab in patients with active rheumatoid arthritis despite methotrexate treatment: results of a phase IIB randomized, double-blind, placebo-controlled, dose-ranging trial, *Arthritis Rheum* 54:1390–1400, 2006.

85. Kay J, Matteson EL, Dasgupta B, et al: Golimumab in patients with active rheumatoid arthritis despite treatment with methotrexate: a randomized, double-blind, placebo-controlled, dose-ranging study, *Arthritis Rheum* 58:964–975, 2008.

86. Genovese MC, McKay JD, Nasonov EL, et al: Interleukin-6 receptor inhibition with tocilizumab reduces disease activity in rheumatoid arthritis with inadequate response to disease-modifying antirheumatic drugs: the tocilizumab in combination with traditional disease-modifying antirheumatic drug therapy study, *Arthritis Rheum* 58:2968–2980, 2008.

87. Keystone E, Heijde D, Mason D Jr, et al: Certolizumab pegol plus methotrexate is significantly more effective than placebo plus methotrexate in active rheumatoid arthritis: findings of a fifty-two-week, phase III, multicenter, randomized, double-blind, placebo-controlled, parallel-group study, *Arthritis Rheum* 58:3319–3329, 2008.

88. Schiff M, Keiserman M, Codding C, et al: Efficacy and safety of abatacept or infliximab vs placebo in ATTEST: a phase III, multicentre, randomized, double-blind, placebo-controlled study in patients with rheumatoid arthritis and an inadequate response to methotrexate, *Ann Rheum Dis* 67:1096–1103, 2008.

89. Hyrich KL, Lunt M, Watson KD, et al: Outcomes after switching from one anti-tumor necrosis factor alpha agent to a second anti-tumor necrosis factor alpha agent in patients with rheumatoid arthritis: results from a large UK national cohort study, *Arthritis Rheum* 56:13–20, 2007.

91. Erickson AR, Mikuls TR: Switching anti-TNF-alpha agents: what is the evidence? *Curr Rheumatol Rep* 9:416–420, 2007.

92. Smolen JS, Kay J, Doyle MK, et al: Golimumab in patients with active rheumatoid arthritis after treatment with tumour necrosis factor alpha inhibitors (GO-AFTER study): a multicentre, randomised, double-blind, placebo-controlled, phase III trial, *Lancet* 374:210–221, 2009.

93. Cohen S, Emery P, Greenwald M, et al: Rituximab for rheumatoid arthritis refractory to anti-tumor necrosis factor therapy, *Arthritis Rheum* 54:2793–2806, 2006.

94. Genovese MC, Becker JC, Schiff M, et al: Abatacept for rheumatoid arthritis refractory to tumor necrosis factor alpha inhibition, *N Engl J Med* 15:1114–1123, 2005.

95. Emery P, Keystone E, Tony HP, et al: IL-6 receptor inhibition with tocilizumab improves treatment outcomes in patients with rheumatoid arthritis refractory to anti-tumour necrosis factor biologicals: results from a 24-week multicentre randomised placebo-controlled trial, *Ann Rheum Dis* 67:1516–1523, 2008.

96. Bartelds GM, Krieckaert CLM, Nurmohamed MT, et al: Development of antidrug antibodies against adalimumab and association with disease activity and treatment failure during long-term follow-up, *JAMA* 305:1460–1468, 2011.

97. Korswagen LA, Bartelds GM, Krieckaert CLM, et al: Venous and arterial thromboembolic events in adalimumab-treated patients with antiadalimumab antibodies, *Arthritis Rheum* 63:877–883, 2011.

98. Mease PJ, Revicki DA, Szechinski J, et al: Improved health-related quality of life for patients with active rheumatoid arthritis receiving rituximab: results of the Dose-Ranging Assessment: International Clinical Evaluation of Rituximab in Rheumatoid Arthritis (DANCER) Trial, *J Rheumatol* 35:20–30, 2008.

100. Genovese MC, Breedveld FC, Emery P, et al: Safety of biological therapies following rituximab treatment in rheumatoid arthritis patients, *Ann Rheum Dis* 68:1894–1897, 2009.

101. American College of Rheumatology Rheumatoid Arthritis Clinical Trial Investigators Ad Hoc Task Force: American College of Rheumatology Clinical Trial Priorities and Design Conference, July 22-23, 2010, *Arthritis Rheum* 63:2151–2156, 2011.

102. O'Dell JR, Curtis RW, Coffield S, et al: Validation of methotrexate first strategy in early rheumatoid arthritis: a randomized, double-blind, 2-year trial, *Arthritis Rheum* 63 Suppl 10:S664, 2011.

103. Bathon JM, Martin RW, Fleischmann RM, et al: A comparison of etanercept and methotrexate in patients with early rheumatoid arthritis, *N Engl J Med* 343(22):1586–1593, 2000.

104. Brown AK, Quinn M, Karim Z, et al: Prediction of flare and long term outcome in DMARD-treated RA patients in remission: the value of imaging and new remission criteria, *Ann Rheum Dis Abstract* OP0061, 2011.

105. Genovese MC, Cohen S, Moreland L, et al: Combination therapy with etanercept and anakinra in the treatment of patients with rheumatoid arthritis who have been treated unsuccessfully with methotrexate, *Arthritis Rheum* 50(5):1412–1419, 2004.

106. Weinblatt M, Schiff M, Goldman A, et al: Selective costimulation modulation using abatacept in patients with active rheumatoid arthritis while receiving etanercept: a randomised clinical trial, *Ann Rheum Dis* 66:228–234, 2007.

107. Greenwald MW, Shergy WJ, Kaine JL, et al: Evaluation of the safety of rituximab in combination with a tumor necrosis factor inhibitor and methotrexate in patients with active rheumatoid arthritis: results from a randomized controlled trial, *Arthritis Rheum* 63:622–632, 2011.

108. O'Dell JR: TNF-α inhibition: The need for a tumor necrosis factor thermostat, *Mayo Clin Proc* 76: 573–575, 2001.

109. Smolen JS, Aletaha D, Grisar JC, et al: Estimation of a numerical value for joint damage-related physical disability in rheumatoid arthritis clinical trials, *Ann Rheum Dis* 69:1058–1064, 2010.

110. Aletaha D, Funovits J, Smolen JS: Physical disability in rheumatoid arthritis is associated with cartilage damage rather than bone destruction, *Ann Rheum Dis* 70:733–739, 2011.

112. Lorig K, Seleznick M, Lubeck D, et al: The beneficial outcomes of the arthritis self-management course are not adequately explained by behavioral change, *Arthritis Rheum* 32:91, 1989.

113. Lorig KR, Mazonson PD, Holman HR: Evidence suggesting that health education for self-management in patients with chronic arthritis has sustained health benefits while reducing health care costs, *Arthritis Rheum* 36:439, 1993.

116. Parker JC, Smarr KL, Buckelew SP, et al: Effects of stress management on clinical outcomes in rheumatoid arthritis, *Arthritis Rheum* 38:1807, 1995.

117. Pincus T, Callahan LF: Formal education as a marker for increased mortality and morbidity in rheumatoid arthritis, *J Chron Dis* 311:552, 1984.

118. Bellamy N, Bradley L: Workshop on chronic pain, pain control, and patient outcomes in rheumatoid arthritis and osteoarthritis, *Arthritis Rheum* 39:357, 1996.

119. Rall LC, Meydani SN, Kehayias JJ, et al: The effect of progressive resistance training in rheumatoid arthritis, *Arthritis Rheum* 39:415, 1996.

121. Helewa A, Goldsmith CH, Lee P, et al: Effects of occupational therapy home service on patients with rheumatoid arthritis, *Lancet* 337:1453, 1991.

122. Criswell LA, Such CL, Yelin EH: Differences in the use of second-line agents and prednisone for treatment of rheumatoid arthritis by rheumatologists and non-rheumatologists, *J Rheumatol* 24:2283, 1997.

124. Solomon DH, Bates DW, Panush RS, et al: Costs, outcomes, and patient satisfaction by provider type for patients with rheumatic and musculoskeletal conditions: a critical review of the literature and proposed methodologic standards, *Ann Intern Med* 127:52, 1997.

125. Rat AC, Henegariu V, Boissier MC: Do primary care physicians have a place in the management of rheumatoid arthritis? *Joint Bone Spine* 71:190, 2004.

126. Wolfe F, Hawley DJ, Cathey MA: Clinical and health status measures over time: prognosis and outcome assessment in rheumatoid arthritis, *J Rheumatol* 18:1290, 1991.

127. Ward MM, Leigh JP, Fries JF: Progression of functional disability in patients with rheumatoid arthritis, *Arch Intern Med* 153:2229, 1993.

128. MacLean CH, Louie R, Leake B, et al: Quality of care for patients with rheumatoid arthritis, *JAMA* 284:984–992, 2000.

129. Friedewald VE, Ganz P, Kremer JM, et al: Rheumatoid arthritis and atherosclerotic cardiovascular disease, *Am J Cardiol* 106: 442–447, 2010.

131. McCarey DW, McInnes IB, Madhok R, et al: Trial of Atorvastatin in Rheumatoid Arthritis (TARA): double-blind, randomised placebo-controlled trial, *Lancet* 363:2015–2021, 2004.

132. Jick SS, Choi H, Li L, et al: Hyperlipidaemia, statin use and the risk of developing rheumatoid arthritis, *Ann Rheum Dis* 68(4):546–551, 2009.

133. Grossman JM, Gordon R, Ranganath VK, et al: American College of Rheumatology 2010 recommendations for the prevention and treatment of glucocorticoid-induced osteoporosis, *Arthritis Care Res (Hoboken)* 62(11):1515–1526, 2010.

134. Fomin I, Caspi D, Levy V, et al: Vaccination against influenza in rheumatoid arthritis: the effect of disease modifying drugs, including TNF alpha blockers, *Ann Rheum Dis* 65(2),191–194, 2006.

136. Bingham CO III, Looney RJ, Deodhar A, et al: Immunization responses in rheumatoid arthritis patients treated with rituximab, *Arthritis Rheum* 62:64–74, 2010.

137. Saevarsdottir S, Wedrén S, Seddighzadeh M, et al: Patients with early rheumatoid arthritis who smoke are less likely to respond to treatment with methotrexate and tumor necrosis factor inhibitors, *Arthritis Rheum* 63:26–36, 2011.

138. Crowson CS, Myasoedova E, Matteson E, et al: Has survival improved in patients recently diagnosed with rheumatoid arthritis? *Arthritis Rheum* 60:S1172, 2009.

139. Shourt CA, Crowson CS, Gabriel SE, et al: Trends in orthopedic surgery utilization among patients with rheumatoid arthritis: a focus on surgery type and gender, *Arthritis Rheum* 62:S652, 2010.

140. Bartels CM, Bell CL, Shinki K, et al: Changing trends in serious extra-articular. manifestations of rheumatoid arthritis among United State veterans over 20 years, *Rheumatology (Oxford)* 49:1670–1675, 2010.

141. Ward M: Decreases in rates of hospitalizations for manifestations of severe rheumatoid arthritis, 1983–2001, *Arthritis Rheum* 50:1122–1131, 2004.

143. Hoffman HM, Throne ML, Amar NJ, et al: Efficacy and safety of rilonacept (interleukin-1 Trap) in patients with cryopyrin-associated periodic syndromes: results from two sequential placebo-controlled studies.

144. Kim W, Min S, Cho M, et al: The role of IL-12 in inflammatory activity of patients with rheumatoid arthritis (RA), *Clin Exp Immunol* 119:175–181, 2000.

148. Kremer JM, Bloom BJ, Breedveld FC, et al: The safety and efficacy of a JAK inhibitor in patients with active rheumatoid arthritis. Results of a double-blind, placebo-controlled phase II a trial of three dosage levels of CP-690,550 versus placebo, *Arthritis Rheum* 60: 1895–1905, 2009.

149. Weinblatt ME, Kavanaugh A, Genovese MC, et al: An oral spleen kinase (Syk) inhibitor for rheumatoid arthritis, *N Engl J Med* 363:1303–1312, 2010.

150. Nielen MM, van Schaardenburg D, Reesink HW, et al: Specific autoantibodies precede the symptoms of rheumatoid arthritis: a study

of serial measurements in blood donors, *Arthritis Rheum* 50:380–386, 2004.

151. Deane KD, O'Donnell CI, Hueber W, et al: The number of elevated cytokines and chemokines in preclinical seropositive rheumatoid arthritis predicts time to diagnosis in an age-dependent manner, *Arthritis Rheum* 62:3161–3172. 2010.

152. Deane KD, Norris JM, Holers VM: Preclinical rheumatoid arthritis: identification, evaluation, and future directions for investigation, *Rheum Dis Clin North Am* 36:213–241, 2010.

153. Kolfenbach JR, Deane KD, Derber LA, et al: A prospective approach to investigating the natural history of preclinical rheumatoid arthritis (RA) using first-degree relatives of probands with RA, *Arthritis Rheum* 61:1735–1742, 2009.

Full references for this chapter can be found on www.expertconsult.com.

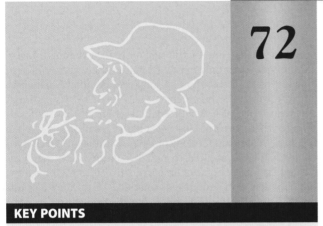

72 Early Synovitis and Early Undifferentiated Arthritis

ANNETTE H.M. VAN DER HELM-VAN MIL • THOMAS W.J. HUIZINGA

KEY POINTS

Early synovitis refers to synovitis that is detected by physical examination; the symptom duration defining *early* has changed over time.

Intervention in arthritis with symptoms less than 12 weeks can be beneficial and can potentially prevent damage later.

Undifferentiated arthritis (UA) is a diagnosis per exclusion. The phenotypic characteristics and outcome change depending on the classification criteria used for rheumatoid arthritis.

Few clinical trials have been performed in UA, and in none of these studies treatment strategies were adjusted to individual patients' chance on spontaneous remission versus progression to rheumatoid arthritis.

WHAT IS EARLY SYNOVITIS?

Recent data suggest that early therapy and achieving low disease activity improve long-term outcomes in inflammatory arthritis.[1,2] These observations have increased awareness among rheumatologists of the importance of early diagnosis and treatment. As a result, considerable pathophysiologic research and clinical trials have focused on identifying early synovitis as soon as possible. Stratifying patients into well-characterized diseases, such as rheumatoid arthritis (RA), is essential so that appropriate therapy can be initiated. Equally important, identifying patients with a high chance for spontaneous remission is needed to avoid overtreating individuals with transient undifferentiated synovitis.

Uniform descriptions of patients and accurate diagnostic criteria for early synovitis are essential for proper interpretation of clinical research. At present, no standardized definition for *early synovitis* is widely accepted. In fact, the definition of *early* has evolved over time. Previously, studies used a cutoff of less than 5 years to define early disease for RA. By the 1990s, duration of symptoms for less than 12 to 24 months was considered early. This duration was chosen because most RA patients incur significant damage when treated conventionally.

The window for modifying disease outcomes might be narrow, and maximum benefit might require interventions even earlier; some evidence suggests that treatment within months might be beneficial. For this reason, several early arthritis cohorts in recent years strictly restrict the inclusion criterion of symptom duration and include only patients with a symptom onset of less than 12 weeks; this is referred

to as *very early synovitis*. Even this definition probably does not capture the earliest phase of disease, as circulating antibodies might appear years before the onset of symptoms in RA, and biomarkers reflecting bone destruction are elevated before arthritis is present.[3,4] Animal models show that histologic evidence of inflammation and activation of signaling pathways can occur well before clinically apparent disease.

Although the term *synovitis* generally refers to a swollen joint detected by physical examination, alternative definitions are also applied. Physical examination might not be sensitive enough, and clinically undetectable synovitis may be present and relevant to identify. Therefore, some studies consider tenderness in the absence of swollen joints as synovitis. For instance, early arthritis clinics might include patients with tenderness but no swollen joints. Others determine synovitis not by physical examination but through the use of imaging modalities such as ultrasound (US) or magnetic resonance imaging (MRI). Different ultrasound techniques are used; of these, traditional B-mode grayscale ultrasonography provides information on synovial thickness, and Doppler imaging measures the synovial blood flow. Ultrasound is easily accessible, rapid, and inexpensive. An important consideration is the reproducibility between readers. Whereas some studies found good or acceptable inter-reader agreement, other studies observed considerable variation between readers. US appears to be valuable, especially in the absence of abnormalities, and the negative predictive value of a normal US result is high. The prognostic implication of abnormal US findings is less clear.[5] More long-term studies are needed to establish which US characteristics have a high positive predictive value for the development of persistent or erosive arthritis.

Until more data become available, the term *early synovitis* generally refers to synovitis that is detected by physical examination. It is important to note that early synovitis refers to a disease symptom but does not reflect any specific diagnosis. The spectrum of final diagnoses in a population of early synovitis patients is presented in Figure 72-1.

EARLY ARTHRITIS CLINICS

Early arthritis clinics are population-based inception cohorts in which patients with synovitis of early onset are included and followed prospectively. These cohorts often contain a wealth of phenotypic information, and the longitudinal design allows the study of factors related to a beneficial or severe course of the disease. Such studies might increase our understanding of the processes involved in arthritis progression. A summary of existing early arthritis cohorts is presented in Table 72-1. Inclusion criteria have changed over

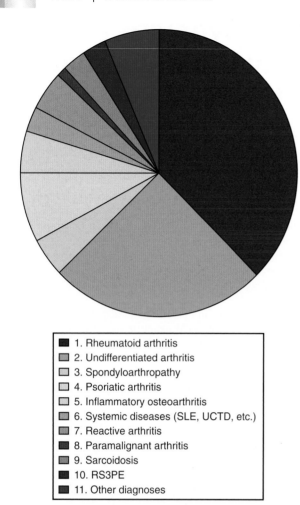

1. Rheumatoid arthritis
2. Undifferentiated arthritis
3. Spondyloarthropathy
4. Psoriatic arthritis
5. Inflammatory osteoarthritis
6. Systemic diseases (SLE, UCTD, etc.)
7. Reactive arthritis
8. Paramalignant arthritis
9. Sarcoidosis
10. RS3PE
11. Other diagnoses

Figure 72-1 Overview of diagnoses of early arthritis patients. (Presented data are based on 2284 early synovitis patients included in the Leiden Early Arthritis Clinic cohort and their diagnosis after 1 year of follow-up.) RS3PE, remitting seronegative symmetrical synovitis with pitting edema; SLE, systemic lupus erythematosus; UCTD, undifferentiated connective tissue disease.

time, in parallel with changing interpretations of the term *early.* Whereas the early arthritis clinics started in or before the 1990s allow inclusion of patients with symptoms up to 2 years, recently started early arthritis clinics focus on very early arthritis and include patients with symptoms less than 12 weeks.

WHAT IS UNDIFFERENTIATED ARTHRITIS?

The term *undifferentiated arthritis* (UA) refers to a subpopulation of early synovitis patients who do not meet criteria for other diseases, including infections, spondyloarthropathies, crystal diseases, and RA. Because it is a diagnosis of exclusion, no classification criteria for UA exist.

European early arthritis cohorts observed that 35% to 54% of the patients included do not meet criteria for other diseases and are considered as UA[6,7]; in the remaining early synovitis patients, a definitive diagnosis could be established at first visits. The frequency of UA is dependent on symptom

duration at the time of the first visit to a rheumatologist. The longer symptoms exist, the more likely that sufficient characteristics are evident to support a definitive diagnosis, and the lower the prevalence of UA will be. In addition, the prevalence of UA will change when classification criteria for rheumatologic diseases change. For example, when the 1987 American College of Rheumatology (ACR) criteria for RA were applied to new-presenting early synovitis patients in the context of an early arthritis clinic in Europe (e.g., Leiden, the Netherlands), about 20% of those patients directly fulfilled the 1987 ACR criteria and thus were classified as RA. At present, few studies evaluating the performance of the 2010 ACR/European League Against Rheumatism (EULAR) criteria are yet available. Initial data from the Leiden clinic suggest that this percentage is increased when the 2010 criteria for RA are applied.[8] The new criteria for RA not only may lead to a lower prevalence of UA, they also may lead to changed patient characteristics in the UA group in that those patients who resembled RA most closely may have departed from the UA population and now are potentially classified as RA.

Characteristics of Undifferentiated Arthritis

Characteristics at first presentation between patients who present with early UA and early RA using the 1987 criteria are somewhat different. Patients with recent-onset UA are younger (mean age, 48 vs. 57 years) and are less frequently female (58% vs. 66%) than early RA patients. UA patients generally have fewer swollen joints and have a greater likelihood of asymmetric synovitis. UA and RA patients do not differ in the acuteness of the start of their complaints, body mass index (BMI), or frequency of a positive family history for RA.[9] UA patients have fewer bone erosions at baseline; in a recent study, erosions were present in 18% of UA patients and 35% of RA patients.[10] Important differences were also noted with regard to autoantibodies. UA patients are RF positive in only 14% and anticitrullinated protein antibody (ACPA) positive in 12% of cases, whereas both of these values are 55% in patients with early RA.[5,6] According to both the 1987 and the 2010 classification criteria for RA, the presence of ACPAs in patients with arthritis is not equal to the classification of RA. Particularly in the case of monoarthritis or oligoarthritis, patients may not fulfill criteria for RA and are labeled as UA. However, early UA patients with ACPAs have a chance of about 70% of classifying under the 1987 ACR criteria 1 year later.

REMISSION RATES IN UNDIFFERENTIATED ARTHRITIS AND RHEUMATOID ARTHRITIS

The natural disease course of UA is variable, depending on the inclusion criteria and the duration of symptoms in several inception cohorts. Spontaneous remission occurs in 40% to 55% of UA patients. In contrast, the remission rate in RA is at most 10% to 15%.[12,13] In these studies, remission was defined as the absence of swollen joints for 1 year or longer after discontinuation of eventual disease-modifying antirheumatic drug (DMARD) therapy and/or discontinuation of participation in the outpatient clinic because the

Table 72-1 Overview of Early Arthritis Cohorts*

Cohort	Inclusion Criteria	Year of Onset	Includes Early Arthritis (Symptoms <2 yr)	Includes Very Early Arthritis (Symptoms <3 mo)
Wichita Arthritis Centre	Undifferentiated polyarthritis syndrome or RA Disease duration <2 yr	1973	X	
Norfolk Arthritis Register	Early inflammatory polyarthritis Age ≥16 yr ≥2 swollen joints Symptom duration ≥4 wk	1989	X	
Leiden EAC	Synovitis of ≥1 joint Symptom duration <2 yr Age >16 yr	1993	X	
Austrian Early Arthritis Registry	Inflammatory arthritis Symptom duration <12 wk	1995		X
Amsterdam	Synovitis of ≥2 joints Symptom duration <3 yr Age >18 yr	1995	X	
Leeds Early Arthritis Centre	Undifferentiated arthritis of the hands Symptom duration <12 mo	1995	X	
Birmingham VEAC	Synovitis of at least one joint Symptom duration ≤3 mo	2000		X
ESPOIR cohort study	Certain RA and UA that may develop into RA Symptom duration <6 mo Age 18-70 yr ≥2 inflammatory joints for the past 6 wk	2002	X	
Toronto Early Arthritis Cohort	Age >16 yr Symptom duration between 6 wk and 12 mo ≥2 swollen joints or 1 swollen MCP or PIP joint with one or more of the following: positive RF, positive ACPA, morning stiffness >45 min, response to NSAIDs, or painful metatarsophalangeal squeeze test	2003	X	
Berlin EAC	≥2 swollen joints Symptom duration between 4 wk and 12 mo	2004	X	
Norwegian Very Early Arthritis (NOR-VEAC)	Synovitis of at least one joint Symptom duration of 16 wk	2004		X
New Castle EAC	Synovitis of at least one joint or inflammatory complaints without a synovitis at physical examination	2006	X	
Rotterdam Early Arthritis CoHort (REACH)	Synovitis ≥1 joint or ≥2 tender joints Symptom duration ≤1 yr	2007	X	

*The presented cohorts include not only early RA patients but also a broader range of early synovitis patients.
ACPA, anticitrullinated protein antibody; MCP, metacarpophalangeal; NSAIDs, nonsteroidal anti-inflammatory drugs; PIP, proximal interphalangeal; RA, rheumatoid arthritis; UA, undifferentiated arthritis.

rheumatologist classified this patient as being in remission. Longer-term follow-up is needed to determine whether symptoms recur many years later. In addition to the difference in frequency of spontaneous remission in UA and RA, the disease duration when spontaneous remission is achieved differs as well. A recent study observed that within UA, the median disease duration until spontaneous remission is 17 months, whereas in RA patients, it takes a median period of 40 months before remission is achieved.[9] Thus, the chance of achieving a natural remission is reduced as the disease process matures. This supports the notion that chronicity might be more easily reversed in the undifferentiated phase of disease.

JOINT DESTRUCTION IN UNDIFFERENTIATED ARTHRITIS AND RHEUMATOID ARTHRITIS

Validated scoring methods are available to measure joint destruction objectively. Most scoring methods assess a limited number of joints. For example, the Sharp-van der Heijde method evaluates metacarpophalangeal (MCP), proximal interphalangeal (PIP), wrist, and metatarsophalangeal (MTP) joints but does not evaluate the distal interphalamgeal or larger joints. Therefore, this method may be less optimal for measuring the level of joint damage in patients who present with predominant synovitis in large joints. In RA, the extent of joint destruction in small joints adequately reflects joint destruction in larger joints. Such data are missing for UA patients.

A recent study evaluated the subgroup of UA patients who developed RA later in time. Radiologic data were compared with those of patients who at first presentation of the disease directly fulfilled the 1987 ACR criteria for RA. Radiographic progression rates between these groups were not different. Health Assessment Questionnaire (HAQ) scores and Disease Activity Score (DAS) measures also were not different between these two groups.[14] Thus, although UA patients as a group have a higher rate of spontaneous remission compared with patients with RA, the subgroup of UA patients who progress to RA have an equally severe course compared with patients classified as RA earlier in the disease. Studies that compare the rate of joint destruction in the total group of early UA patients versus that of patients with early RA have not been performed.

BIOLOGIC MECHANISMS IN UA AND DETERMINANTS OF PROGRESSION TO RA

Our understanding of the processes responsible for progression from UA to RA is far from complete. Risk factors that were identified as independent predictors for RA development may provide clues:

- *Age:* The incidence of RA is clearly age dependent with a rising incidence from 7/100,000 for the age group 18 to 34 years to 107/100,000 for the age group 75 to 84 years.[15] It is unknown why this is so; putative mechanisms include age-related decline in cellular, humoral, and innate immunity.
- *Gender:* Women who present with UA have a twofold greater chance of developing RA compared with men presenting with UA.[15] Sex hormones influence predisposition to autoimmune disease. In general, men are less prone than women. Androgens have anti-inflammatory effects, and estrogens have been reported to suppress arthritis as well.[16,17] Both estrogen and androgen inhibit bone resorption.[18] These results may account for increased progression in postmenopausal females.
- *Number of involved joints and C-reactive protein:* Both markers reflect the level of inflammation and are frequently reported to be associated with progression of synovitis and worse disease outcomes. Although the number of swollen joints and the level of C-reactive protein (CRP) are correlated on a group level, this is often not the case in individual patients, and both markers have their own, independent predictive value. UA patients presenting with CRP levels greater than 50 mg/L have a five times increased risk of being in an early stage of RA. Likewise, patients classified with UA who have polyarthritis have a 1.5 times higher chance of fulfilling the criteria for RA later on compared with patients with monarthritis or oligoarthritis. Moreover, the risk that an early UA patient who has more than 10 swollen joints will develop RA is three times greater than that of patients with monarthritis or oligoarthritis.
- *Autoantibodies:* ACPAs as well as rheumatoid factor (RF) can be present years before the first clinical symptom of synovitis is noted; they are a risk factor for a persistent and destructive course of synovitis. Spontaneous remission is uncommon in ACPA-positive patients. Not only the presence but also the level of ACPAs is of predictive relevance. Despite these strong associations, studies that formally prove that ACPAs themselves are causally related to disease progression are lacking.
- *Environmental factors:* Early UA patients who smoke have a higher risk of development of RA and a destructive disease course. This risk is confined to patients who carry HLA-DRB1 alleles that encode for the so-called shared epitope. Persons who smoke and also carry an HLA-DRB1 shared epitope allele are particularly prone to develop ACPAs, which subsequently are associated with disease persistency and erosiveness.
- *Genetic factors:* Apart from the HLA-DRB1 shared epitope alleles, genetic factors associated with progression from UA to RA are not clearly identified. Most genetic risk factors for RA provide risk for ACPA-positive RA when compared with healthy controls. It is not clear whether these factors are associated with progression from UA to RA as well, and if so, whether such an association is independent of the strong association between ACPAs and development of RA. Identification of new genetic factors has fueled the study of their relevance. In a population of UA patients, information on currently known genetic risk factors for RA does not improve prediction of risk for RA compared with a prediction rule based on common clinical risk factors alone.[19]
- *Additional biomarkers:* The role of biomarkers in the diagnosis of UA is limited. Within RA, it is known that serologic levels of pro–matrix metalloproteinase (MMP)3, receptor activator of nuclear factor κB (NFκB) ligand (RANKL), and osteoprotegerin (OPG) correlate with the rate of joint destruction over time.[20] Biomarkers that specifically reflect or predict disease progression in early UA patients thus far remain unknown.

WINDOW OF OPPORTUNITY

The concept of a window of opportunity suggests that there is a period early in the course of the disease when the disease process can be altered or can even be reversed with a complete return to normality. Treatment during this period might have a greater effect than treatment at a later stage in terms of halting disease progression and achieving remission.[21-23] Several different aspects have been studied, including whether very early UA (<12 weeks) may be an immunopathologically distinct phase compared with later disease.

Studies that focused on synovial tissue did not reveal differences.[24] It is difficult to come to a conclusion from negative studies because one never knows whether the relevant processes have been studied. However, studies that focused on the composition of autoantibody responses have demonstrated that profound maturation of the autoantibody response occurs early during disease.[25]

UA patients who present to an early arthritis clinic within 12 weeks of symptom onset less often progress toward RA compared with UA patients with symptom duration greater than 12 weeks. Similarly, RA patients who at their first visit to a rheumatologist reported symptoms for less than 12 weeks had a lower rate of joint destruction over time and achieved sustained DMARD-free remission more often than RA patients who reported a period greater than 12 weeks before seeing a rheumatologist.[26]

Support for the presence of a window of opportunity is also obtained from trials.[27] An unblinded study of a single dose of corticosteroids in patients with mild early inflammatory arthritis (median, 20 weeks) found that the strongest predictor of disease remission at 6 months (defined as the absence of symptoms and signs in patients without anti-inflammatory treatment) was disease duration less than 12 weeks at the time of therapy.[28] Clinical and radiologic outcomes were significantly better at 3 years in patients who started DMARD therapy within 3 months ("very early") after disease onset compared with a median duration of 12 months at the start of treatment ("early").[22] Remission was achieved in 50% of the very early group compared with 15% of the early group. These data suggest that treatment in very early arthritis might have a greater effect on disease progression and thus underline the relevance of identification and treatment of arthritis in the very early disease phase.

TREATMENT OF UNDIFFERENTIATED ARTHRITIS

Although many rheumatologists have experience treating UA patients, formal data providing information on treatment of UA patients are lacking. Thus far, only a few trials have been performed in UA patients; these are summarized in Table 72-2. One trial observed an effect of steroids in early UA patients—an observation that was not reproduced in another study. Methotrexate is reportedly beneficial in UA patients and is associated with delayed progression to RA and a reduction in the rate of joint destruction. This effect appeared to be predominant among ACPA-positive UA patients but was negligible in ACPA-negative UA patients. However, when methotrexate was discontinued, the rate progression to RA was similar to the placebo arm.

Some biologics have been studied in UA patients. Although surprising lack of efficacy was observed with tumor necrosis factor (TNF) blockers, abatacept was beneficial. The heterogeneous nature of UA patients and the more favorable disease outcome and spontaneous remission rate make it difficult to observe treatment efficacy in the total UA group. Thus the placebo-treated group can have a good remission rate, and differences from the treatment group might be difficult to detect. None of the published randomized trials in UA patients addressed this problem of heterogeneity and stratified patients having a high chance of developing RA or of having a spontaneous remission.

Individualized Treatment of Undifferentiated Arthritis

UA has a variable disease course, ranging between spontaneous remission and severe destruction. Because of this, and because DMARD therapy is potentially toxic, treatment of UA patients should be personalized. The chance for individual patients to progress toward RA or to have a persistent erosive disease course can be estimated using prediction models.[29,30] One of the present prediction rules (Figure 72-2A) is validated using data from early arthritis clinics from Germany, the United Kingdom, Canada, Russia, and Japan; this algorithm is currently used in daily practice in several countries.[29,31-36] The discriminative ability of this model is high. The prediction rule consists of nine variables: age, gender, distribution of involved joints, morning stiffness, numbers of tender and swollen joints, CRP level, and presence of RF and ACPAs. It calculates the risk of developing RA for every UA patient (Figure 72-2B). Such information can facilitate the decision of whether or not to initiate DMARD therapy and might facilitate patient involvement in decision making. In general, a score of 6 or lower is related to a low chance of developing RA (91% chance of not developing RA) and may be a reason to not initiate DMARD therapy. In contrast, patients with a score of 8 or higher have an 84% chance of developing RA; this might be a reason to initiate DMARD therapy in some patients.

Can the 2010 ACR/EULAR criteria[37] be used to identify UA patients who actually have early RA? The presence of new criteria for RA is relevant in that the absence of up-to-date classification criteria had hampered progress with regard to treatment strategies in early RA. The 1987 ACR criteria for RA were not designed to classify RA early and did not include more recent autoantibody tests or imaging modalities. Most randomized clinical trials included patients who fulfilled the 1987 criteria, hence patients with established RA. It is not clear whether the efficacy observed in these trials is the same for patients with early RA or UA.

Table 72-2 Randomized Controlled Trials in Patients with Early Undifferentiated Arthritis

Trial	N	Treatment	Follow-up Duration	Outcome	Effect Compared with Placebo
SAVE trial[38]	389	Single IM injection 120 mg methylprednisolone	52 wk	Drug-free clinical remission	No effect
STIVEA trial[39]	265	3 IM injections 80 mg methylprednisolone	6 and 12 mo	Need to start DMARDs	At 6 mo 61% vs. 76% had started DMARDs; At 12 mo 10% vs. 20% had resolved disease
PROMPT trial[40]	110	Methotrexate therapy during 12 mo	30 mo	Fulfilling the 1987 ACR criteria	40% vs. 53% developed RA; lower radiologic progression
ADJUST trial[41]	56	Abatacept treatment during 6 mo	12 mo	Fulfilling the 1987 ACR criteria	46% vs. 67% developed RA; no effect on radiographic progression
Saleem et al[42]	17	Infliximab at 0, 2, 4, and 16 wk	26 wk	Clinical remission	No effect observed

ACR, American College of Rheumatology; DMARDs, disease-modifying antirheumatic drugs; IM, intramuscular; RA, rheumatoid arthritis.

FORM TO CALCULATE A PATIENT'S PREDICTION SCORE

1. What is the age?   Multiply with 0.02   _____

2. What is the gender?   In case female: 1 point   _____

3. How is the distribution of involved joints?

               In case small joints hands and feet: 0.5 point   _____

               In case symmetric   0.5 point   _____

               In case upper extremities   1 point

       Or: In case upper and lower extremities   1.5 points   _____

4. What is the length of the VAS morning stiffness (range 0-100 mm)?

               In case 26-90 mm   1 point   _____

               In case >90 mm   2 points   _____

5. What is the number of tender joints?

               In case 4-10   0.5 points   _____

               In case 11 or higher   1 point   _____

6. What is the number of swollen joints?

               In case 4-10   0.5 point   _____

               In case 11 or more   1 point   _____

7. What is the C-reactive protein level (mg/L)?

               In case 5-50   0.5 point   _____

               In case 51 or higher   1.5 points   _____

8. Is the rheumatoid factor positive?   If yes   1 point   _____

9. Are the anticitrullinated protein antibodies positive?   If yes   2 points   _____

A   Total score   _____

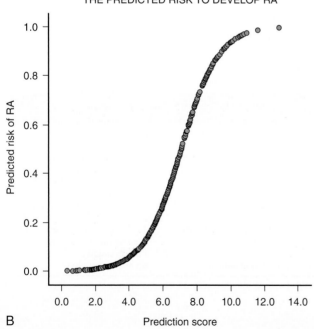

SUBJECTS' PREDICTION SCORES PLOTTED VERSUS THE PREDICTED RISK TO DEVELOP RA

Predicted risk of RA (y-axis: 0.0 to 1.0)

Prediction score (x-axis: 0.0 to 14.0)

B

Figure 72-2 Tool to predict an individual early arthritis patient's probability of developing rheumatoid arthritis (RA). With the calculated prediction score **(A),** the probability can be derived **(B).**[29] VAS, visual analog scale.

The new criteria have mainly been derived for classification and research purposes[37] and require validation for use in clinical practice for early synovitis. The 2010 criteria should not be used as diagnostic criteria until it is demonstrated that patients who fulfill them have a high chance for a persistent or destructive disease course, making 2010 criteria positivity the basis of an argument for starting disease-modifying drugs.

References

1. van Nies JA, de Jong Z, van der Helm-van Mil AH, et al: Improved treatment strategies reduce the increased mortality risk in early RA patients, *Rheumatology (Oxford)* 49:2210–2216, 2010.
2. Puolakka K, Kautiainen H, Pohjolainen T, Virta L: No increased mortality in incident cases of rheumatoid arthritis during the new millennium, *Ann Rheum Dis* 69:2057–2058, 2010.
3. van Schaardenburg D, Nielen MM, Lems WF, et al: Bone metabolism is altered in preclinical rheumatoid arthritis, *Ann Rheum Dis* 70:1173–1174, 2011.
4. Turesson C, Bergström U, Jacobsson LT, et al: Increased cartilage turnover and circulating autoantibodies in different subsets before the clinical onset of rheumatoid arthritis, *Ann Rheum Dis* 70:520–522, 2011.
5. Dougados M, Jousse-Joulin S, Mistretta F, et al: Evaluation of several ultrasonography scoring systems for synovitis and comparison to clinical examination: results from a prospective multicentre study of rheumatoid arthritis, *Ann Rheum Dis* 69:828–833, 2010.
6. van Aken J, van Bilsen JH, Allaart CF, et al:The Leiden Early Arthritis Clinic, *Clin Exp Rheumatol* 21(5 Suppl 31):S100–S105, 2003.
7. Hulsemann JL, Zeidler H: Undifferentiated arthritis in an early synovitis out-patient clinic, *Clin Exp Rheumatol* 13:37–43, 1995.
8. van der Linden MP, Knevel R, Huizinga TW, van der Helm-van Mil AH: Classification of rheumatoid arthritis: comparison of the 1987 ACR and 2010 ACR/EULAR criteria, *Arthritis Rheum* 63:37–42, 2011.
9. de Rooy DP, van der Linden MP, Knevel R, et al: Predicting arthritis outcomes—what can be learned from the Leiden Early Arthritis Clinic? *Rheumatology (Oxford)* 40:93–100, 2011.
10. Verpoort KN, van Gaalen FA, van der Helm-van Mil AH, et al: Association of HLA-DR3 with anti-cyclic citrullinated peptide antibody-negative rheumatoid arthritis, *Arthritis Rheum* 52:3058–3062, 2005.
11. Deleted in proofs.
12. Linn-Rasker SP, Allaart CF, Kloppenburg M, et al: Sustained remission in a cohort of patients with RA: association with absence of IgM-rheumatoid factor and absence of anti-CCP antibodies. *Int J Adv Rheumatol* 2:4–6, 2004.
13. van der Woude D, Young A, Jayakumar K, et al: Prevalence of and predictive factors for sustained disease-modifying antirheumatic drug-free remission in rheumatoid arthritis: results from two large early arthritis cohorts, *Arthritis Rheum* 60:2262–2271, 2009.
14. van Aken J, van Dongen H, le Cessie S, et al: Comparison of long term outcome of patients with rheumatoid arthritis presenting with undifferentiated arthritis or with rheumatoid arthritis: an observational cohort study, *Ann Rheum Dis* 65:20–25, 2006.
15. Doran MF, Pond GR, Crowson CS, et al: Trends in incidence and mortality in rheumatoid arthritis in Rochester, Minnesota, over a forty-year period, *Arthritis Rheum* 46:625–631, 2002.
16. Dunn SE, Ousman SS, Sobel RA, et al: Peroxisome proliferator-activated receptor (PPAR)α expression in T cells mediates gender differences in development of T cell-mediated autoimmunity, *J Exp Med* 204:321–330, 2007.
17. Yoneda T, Ishimaru N, Arakaki R, et al: Estrogen deficiency accelerates murine autoimmune arthritis associated with receptor activator of nuclear factor-kappa B ligand-mediated osteoclastogenesis, *Endocrinology* 145:2384–2391, 2004.
18. Syed F, Khosla S: Mechanisms of sex steroid effects on bone, *Biochem Biophys Res Commun* 328:688–696, 2005.
19. van der Helm-van Mil AH, Toes RE, Huizinga TW: Genetic variants in the prediction of rheumatoid arthritis, *Ann Rheum Dis* 69:1694–1696, 2010.
20. Syversen SW, Landewe R, van der Heijde D, et al: Testing of the OMERACT 8 draft validation criteria for a soluble biomarker reflecting structural damage in rheumatoid arthritis: a systematic literature search on 5 candidate biomarkers, *J Rheumatol* 36:1769–1784, 2009.
21. Finckh A, Liang MH, van Herckenrode CM, de Pablo P: Long-term effect of early treatment on radiographic progression in rheumatoid arthritis; a meta analysis, *Arthritis Rheum* 55:864–872, 2006.
22. Nell VP, Machold KP, Eberl G, et al: Benefit of very early referral and very early therapy with disease modifying anti-rheumatic drugs in patients with early rheumatoid arthritis, *Rheumatology (Oxford)* 43:819–820, 2004.
23. Quinn MA, Emery P: Window of opportunity in early rheumatoid arthritis: possibility of altering the disease process with early intervention, *Clin Exp Rheumatol* 21(5 Suppl 31):S154–S157, 2003.
24. Tak PP, Smeets TJ, Daha MR, et al: Analysis of the synovial cell infiltrate in early rheumatoid synovial tissue in relation to local disease activity, *Arthritis Rheum* 40:217–225, 1997.
25. Willemze A, Ioan-Facsinay A, El-Gabalawy H: Anti-citrullinated protein antibody response associated with synovial immune deposits in a patient with suspected early rheumatoid arthritis, *J Rheumatol* 35:2282–2284, 2008.
26. Van der Linden MP, le Cessie S, Raza K, et al: Long-term impact of delay in assessment of early arthritis patients, *Arthritis Rheum* 62:3537–3546, 2010.
27. Mottonen T, Hannonen P, Korpela M, et al: Delay to institution of therapy and induction of remission using single-drug or combination-disease-modifying antirheumatic drug therapy in early rheumatoid arthritis, *Arthritis Rheum* 46:894–898, 2002.
28. Green M, Marzo-Ortega H, McGonagle D, et al: Persistence of mild, early inflammatory arthritis: the importance of disease duration, rheumatoid factor, and the shared epitope, *Arthritis Rheum* 42:2184–2188, 1999.
29. van der Helm-van Mil AH, le Cessie S, van Dongen H, et al: A prediction rule for disease outcome in patients with recent-onset undifferentiated arthritis: how to guide individual treatment decisions, *Arthritis Rheum* 56:433–440, 2007.
30. Visser H, le Cessie S, Vos K, et al: How to diagnose rheumatoid arthritis early: a prediction model for persistent (erosive) arthritis, *Arthritis Rheum* 46:357–365, 2002.
31. Van der Helm-van Mil AH, Detert J, le Cessie S, et al: Validation of a prediction rule for disease outcome in patients with recent-onset undifferentiated arthritis: moving toward individualized treatment decision-making, *Arthritis Rheum* 58:2241–2247, 2008.
32. Kuriya B, Cheng CK, Chen HM, Bykerk VP: Validation of a prediction rule for development of rheumatoid arthritis in patients with early undifferentiated arthritis, *Ann Rheum Dis* 68:1482–1485, 2009.
33. Tamai M, Kawakami A, Uetani M, et al: A prediction rule for disease outcome in patients with undifferentiated arthritis using magnetic resonance imaging of the wrists and finger joints and serologic autoantibodies, *Arthritis Rheum* 61:772–778, 2009.
34. Bradna P, Soukop T, Bastecj D, Hrncir J: Prediction rule in early and very early arthritis patients, *Ann Rheum Dis* 68(Suppl 3):547, 2009.
35. Luchikhina EL, Karateev DE, Nasonov EL: The use of prediction rule to predict the development of rheumatoid arthritis in Russian patients with early undifferentiated arthritis, *Ann Rheum Dis* 58:2241–2247, 2008.
36. Mjaavatten MD, Van der Helm-van Mil AH, Huizinga TW, et al: Validation of a proposed prediction rule for rheumatoid arthritis in a cohort of 188 patients with undifferentiated arthritis. *Ann Rheum Dis* 167(Suppl II):477, 2008.
37. Aletaha D, Neogi T, Silman AJ, et al; American College of Rheumatology; European League Against Rheumatism: 2010 rheumatoid arthritis classification criteria: an American College of Rheumatology/European League Against Rheumatism collaborative initiative, *Arthritis Rheum* 62:2569–2581, 2010.
38. Machold KP, Landewé R, Smolen JS, et al: The Stop Arthritis Very Early (SAVE) trial, an international multicentre, randomised, double-blind, placebo-controlled trial on glucocorticoids in very early arthritis, *Ann Rheum Dis* 69:495–502, 2010.
39. Verstappen SM, McCoy MJ, Roberts C, et al; STIVEA Investigators: Beneficial effects of a 3-week course of intramuscular glucocorticoid injections in patients with very early inflammatory polyarthritis: results of the STIVEA trial, *Ann Rheum Dis* 69:503–509, 2010.
40. van Dongen H, van Aken J, Lard LR, et al: Efficacy of methotrexate treatment in patients with probable rheumatoid arthritis: a double-

blind, randomized, placebo-controlled trial, *Arthritis Rheum* 56:1424–1432, 2007.

41. Emery P, Durez P, Dougados M, et al: Impact of T-cell costimulation modulation in patients with undifferentiated inflammatory arthritis or very early rheumatoid arthritis: a clinical and imaging study of abatacept (the ADJUST trial), *Ann Rheum Dis* 69:510–516, 2010.

42. Saleem B, Mackie S, Quinn M, et al: Does the use of tumour necrosis factor antagonist therapy in poor prognosis, undifferentiated arthritis prevent progression to rheumatoid arthritis? *Ann Rheum Dis* 67:1178–1180, 2008.

The references for this chapter can also be found on www.expertconsult.com.

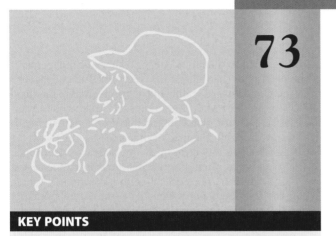

73 Sjögren's Syndrome

E. WILLIAM ST. CLAIR

KEY POINTS

Sjögren's syndrome is divided into primary and secondary forms. The primary form occurs in approximately 0.1% to 0.6% of the general population.

The clinical hallmarks of Sjögren's syndrome are keratoconjunctivitis sicca (dry eyes), xerostomia (dry mouth), and parotid gland swelling.

Extraglandular features of primary Sjögren's syndrome include fatigue, Raynaud's phenomenon, polyarthralgia/arthritis, interstitial lung disease, neuropathy, and purpura.

A chronic mononuclear cell infiltration of the lacrimal and salivary glands is the characteristic histopathologic finding.

A diagnosis of primary Sjögren's syndrome is made by subjective and objective assessment of dry eyes and dry mouth, testing for serum antinuclear antibodies including anti-Ro/SS-A and anti-La/SS-B antibodies, and labial salivary gland biopsy.

Treatment of Sjögren's syndrome aims to provide symptomatic improvement in the symptoms of dry eyes and dry mouth, as well as control of extraglandular manifestations of disease.

HISTORICAL PERSPECTIVE

In 1888 Johann von Mikulicz-Radecki described a case of bilateral painless swelling of the lacrimal, parotid, and submandibular glands,[1] an entity that later bore his name. Reports soon followed showing Mikulicz disease was not a distinct pathologic entity but rather a clinical potpourri of conditions including leukemia, lymphoma, and tuberculosis. Shortly thereafter, salivary gland disease became linked with dryness of the eyes and oral mucosa when Henri Gougerot, a well-known and successful French dermatologist, wrote in 1925 about three cases of salivary gland atrophy with dryness of the eyes, mouth, and vagina. The modern concept of Sjögren's syndrome was firmly rooted in 1933 when Henrik Sjögren, a Swedish ophthalmologist, reported a series of 19 cases of keratoconjunctivitis sicca including two cases with swelling of the major salivary glands.[2] Over the next 2 decades, Sjögren and others published extensively about various facets of the disease that now carries his name (also called Gougerot-Sjögren disease), with most of these contributions coming from European ophthalmologists.

In 1953 Morgan and Castleman[3] published their detailed histopathologic findings from 18 patients with enlarged lacrimal and salivary glands. This pathologic treatise consisted of cases without apparent etiology that had clinical features resembling those of Mikulicz's disease and Sjögren's syndrome. Notably, 15 of the 18 patients were women with lacrimal and salivary gland swelling that developed in the fifth and sixth decades of life. Morgan and Castleman found in the salivary gland tissue a consistent "lymphoid element" accompanied by a striking proliferation of myoepithelial and epithelial cells. The epithelial changes produced a characteristic narrowing or obliteration of the ductal lumen, forming cords of solid cell masses they called *epimyoepithelial islands*. Because of the prominence of these epithelial structures, they advanced the theory that Mikulicz disease had its origins in the ductal epithelium. Morgan and Castleman also recognized that the salivary gland pathology in their cases was similar to that of the patients described by Henrik Sjögren with keratoconjunctivitis sicca. Because Sjögren's patients were mostly middle-aged women, Morgan and Castleman reasoned that Mikulicz disease was a subset of Sjögren's disease but with incomplete clinical manifestations. This now classic paper had the effect of unifying Mikulicz disease and Sjögren's syndrome into a single disease entity, a belief that dominated the field until recently.

When Joseph J. Bunim delivered the Heberden Oration at the Wellcome Foundation in London on December 2, 1960, he enlightened his audience about the latest advances in Sjögren's syndrome.[4] Bunim described in detail the clinical, pathologic, and laboratory findings of the 40 patients with Sjögren's syndrome evaluated by himself, Kurt Bloch, Martin Wohl, Richard Oglesby, and Irwin Ship at the Clinical Center of the National Institutes of Health (NIH). All patients in their series had at least two of the three following features: keratoconjunctivitis sicca, xerostomia (with or without enlargement of the salivary glands), and rheumatoid arthritis. Bunim also knew from the work of others that keratoconjunctivitis sicca and xerostomia, or sicca complex, occurred in some patients with systemic lupus erythematosus, scleroderma, polymyositis, and polyarteritis nodosa. He brought home the point that the exocrinopathy extended beyond the lacrimal and salivary glands to affect the pharynx, larynx, and trachea, as well as the vagina. Many of their patients with Sjögren's syndrome also had extraglandular manifestations such as Raynaud's phenomenon, purpura, pulmonary infiltrates on chest radiograph, and peripheral neuropathy. Talal and Bunim took note of the diagnosis of reticulum cell sarcoma (an older term that includes non-Hodgkin's lymphoma) in three patients and Waldenström's macroglobulinemia in a fourth patient from the NIH cases, drawing attention for the first time to the increased risk of developing lymphoma in this disease.[5] In this report, they speculate that a "chronic state of immunologic hyperactivity and the proliferation of immunologically competent cells producing abnormal tissue antibodies predisposes to the relatively frequent development of malignant lymphoma."[5]

The NIH group also pioneered the characterization of the serologic markers of Sjögren's syndrome. In 1965 they reported that 12 of their 16 patients (75%) with sicca symptoms but no evidence of another connective tissue disease had serum antinuclear antibody (ANA) reactivity by indirect immunofluorescence on rat liver tissue.[6] Applying the Ouchterlony plate method, they further showed that sera from 13 of 16 (81%) of these patients contained precipitating antibodies to SjD and SjT, which were later to be called anti-Ro (SS-A) and anti-La (SS-B) antibodies. Moreover, Bloch and colleagues[7] set the stage for our modern classification schemes by subdividing their patients at the NIH into primary and secondary Sjögren's syndrome. Secondary Sjögren's syndrome was the category reserved for patients with sicca symptoms in the setting of another connective tissue disease such as rheumatoid arthritis, systemic lupus erythematosus, scleroderma, or dermatomyositis, whereas primary Sjögren's syndrome was the designation when the sicca complex occurred in the absence of another connective tissue disease.

In the late 1960s and early 1970s, the investigation of labial salivary gland biopsy for the diagnosis of Sjögren's syndrome led to the development of grading systems for quantifying the intensity of tissue inflammation. In 1968 Chisholm and Mason proposed a grading system for labial salivary gland biopsies that used a simple grading scale (0 to 4) in which grades 0, 1, and 2 represented absent, slight, and moderate mononuclear cell infiltrates, respectively.[8] The higher grades of 3 and 4 corresponded to focal inflammatory cell scores of 1 and greater than 1 per 4 mm² of tissue, where a focus equated to an aggregate of 50 or more mononuclear cells. In this initial study, 9 of the 10 patients with Sjögren's syndrome were classified as grade 3 ($n = 3$) or grade 4 ($n = 6$). By comparison, biopsies had lower grades when they were taken from patients with other chronic inflammatory conditions, as well as controls. For example, among 10 patients with rheumatoid arthritis, the highest biopsy grade was only 3. Twenty other subjects with a variety of other rheumatic diseases (e.g., osteoarthritis, reactive arthritis, psoriatic arthritis, scleroderma) had biopsies with grades of 0 or 1. Although it was a small study by today's standards, this work inspired others to validate and refine these findings. Later, postmortem biopsies from 116 controls without a history of an inflammatory disease were scored with only grade 0, 1, or 2 infiltrates, attesting to the diagnostic specificity of this grading system.[9] However, the Chisholm and Mason grading system had limitations because it was sensitive only at the lower end of the scale and did not discriminate among biopsies with the highest degree of cellular infiltrates or biopsies with two or more foci per 4 mm² of tissue.

To improve on these earlier efforts, Tarpley and coworkers[10] at the NIH developed a grading system that incorporated scales for not only estimating the extent of inflammation but also quantifying the amount of acinar destruction. As expected, they found that labial salivary gland biopsies from patients with the sicca complex alone had higher grades of cellular infiltrates and acinar destruction than those with sicca symptoms and rheumatoid arthritis or rheumatoid arthritis alone. However, grading the acinar destruction did not add diagnostic value independent of the severity of the infiltrates. Greenspan and colleagues[11] from the University of California at San Francisco modified the Chisholm and Mason grading scale when they examined labial salivary gland biopsies from 54 patients with definite or probable Sjögren's syndrome together with 21 controls. Their results reinforced the diagnostic relevance of the focus score, including its relationship to focus size, and highlighted the presence of germinal centers.[11] Grade 4 biopsies (>1 focus per 4 mm² of tissue) were primarily found in the patients with Sjögren's syndrome, with the highest focus scores in patients with the sicca complex in the absence of another connective tissue disease. The range for the focus score was extended from 1 to 12, where a score of 12 was arbitrarily assigned to those specimens with foci so numerous that they were confluent. The focus score was thereafter adopted as the "gold standard" for quantifying chronic inflammation in labial salivary gland biopsies. Because the signs and symptoms of xerostomia were relatively nonspecific indicators of salivary gland involvement in Sjögren's syndrome, other methods such as sialometry, chemical analysis of the saliva, sialography, and scintigraphy were also explored for diagnosing this condition. However, these measures of salivary flow and duct anatomy proved to be diagnostically nonspecific; sialography and scintigraphy had other shortcomings limiting their clinical use.

With a growing interest in Sjögren's syndrome, investigators began to develop classification criteria for comparison of results across studies. In the 1980s, many groups proposed classification criteria for Sjögren's syndrome, aiming to identify patients with a sicca complex caused by a chronic autoimmune disorder. These proposed criteria incorporated a combination of the following items: symptoms of the ocular and oral components; objective measures of lacrimal and salivary gland involvement; a focus score greater than or equal to 1 from a labial salivary gland biopsy; and the presence of serum autoantibodies. Many investigators from Europe, the United States, and Japan contributed to this effort, leading to the general acceptance in 2002 of the revised version of the European criteria proposed by the American-European Consensus group.[12] The International Sjögren's Syndrome Registry, funded in 2003, is collecting data that will inform the natural history of Sjögren's syndrome. It will also support validation of new criteria sets that may be developed from the baseline data of the more than 1200 patients across the world with suspected primary or secondary Sjögren's syndrome.

DEFINITIONS AND CLASSIFICATION CRITERIA

The clinical hallmarks of Sjögren's syndrome are keratoconjunctivitis sicca and xerostomia, or the sicca complex. The term "keratoconjunctivitis sicca" is derived from Latin, and its translation is "dryness of the cornea and conjunctiva." Xerostomia refers to the subjective symptoms of dry mouth. Sjögren's syndrome is subdivided into primary and secondary Sjögren's syndrome. The category of secondary Sjögren's syndrome is reserved for patients with keratoconjunctivitis sicca or xerostomia, or both, in the setting of another connective tissue disease or chronic inflammatory process such as rheumatoid arthritis, systemic lupus erythematosus, polymyositis, systemic sclerosis (scleroderma), or granulomatosis with polyangiitis (formerly Wegener's granulomatosis). Patients are diagnosed with primary Sjögren's syndrome if they manifest signs and symptoms of keratoconjunctivitis sicca and xerostomia in the absence of another connective tissue disease provided they meet serologic or histopathologic criteria. Because primary Sjögren's syndrome is associated with extraglandular features that overlap with those of other connective tissue diseases, it may be difficult in some cases to distinguish from patients with secondary Sjögren's syndrome. The challenge in distinguishing between primary and secondary forms of the disease arises most often in patients with primary Sjögren's syndrome and overlapping features of lupus such as rash, arthritis, and leukopenia. This distinction is often a matter of semantics depending on the preference for "lumping" as opposed to "splitting."

Other terms used to describe Sjögren's syndrome are *autoimmune exocrinopathy*[13] and *autoimmune epithelitis*.[14] In Sjögren's syndrome, the term *exocrinopathy* receives emphasis because of the generalized glandular involvement causing dysfunction of the lacrimal and salivary glands, as well as the apocrine sweat glands of the skin and the submucosal glands of the nose, pharynx, larynx, large airways, and vagina. The term *epithelitis* gains footing from the uniformly activated epithelial cells omnipresent in the lacrimal and salivary glands and other sites of glandular involvement.

International agreement has been reached on the classification of Sjögren's syndrome. By the early 1980s, several criteria sets had been proposed for the classification of Sjögren's syndrome including the Copenhagen criteria,[15] the Japanese criteria,[16] the Greek criteria,[17] and the California criteria.[18] Common to each of these criteria sets was the requirement for objective evidence of keratoconjunctivitis sicca and salivary gland involvement. They differed, however, in their item content and weighting, as well as the methods for assessing salivary gland involvement. For example, some of the criteria relied on whole salivary flow (Copenhagen), whereas other criteria relied on parotid flow rate (Greek, California). Only two of the criteria sets discriminated between primary and secondary Sjögren's syndrome (Copenhagen and Greek).

Movement toward consensus began when the Epidemiology Committee of the European Community conducted a multicenter study involving 26 centers from 12 countries aimed at developing criteria for the classification of Sjögren's syndrome. This group first agreed on the items that should be included in the classification criteria for Sjögren's syndrome and then tested their operational characteristics in a large sample of patients with a clinical diagnosis of primary Sjögren's syndrome (n = 246), secondary Sjögren's syndrome (n = 201), other connective tissues diseases without Sjögren's syndrome (n = 113), and healthy controls (n = 133).[19] Two sets of three questions were selected from a larger body of questions that best correlated with the presence of keratoconjunctivitis sicca and xerostomia, respectively, as judged by clinical experts. The results from objective tests were analyzed by univariate analyses, yielding a tentative list of items based on their sensitivity and specificity for correct classification of the diagnosis. The following six items were chosen for the classification criteria: (I) ocular symptoms; (II) oral symptoms; (III) ocular signs (Schirmer-I-test

≤5 mm/5 min or Rose Bengal score ≥4 by the van Bijsterveld scoring system); (IV) histopathologic features (focus score ≥1 on labial salivary gland biopsy; (V) objective evidence of salivary gland involvement by at least one abnormal test (salivary scintigraphy, parotid sialography, or unstimulated salivary flow rate ≤1.5 mL/15 min); and (VI) at least one of the following serum autoantibodies: anti-Ro/SS-A or anti-La/SS-B antibodies, ANAs, or rheumatoid factor. Exclusion criteria were pre-existing lymphoma, acquired immunodeficiency syndrome, sarcoidosis, and graft-versus-host disease. The presence of four of six criteria (accepting only a positive test for anti-Ro/SS-A or anti-La/SS-B antibodies for item VI had good sensitivity (93.5%) and specificity (94%) for correctly classifying a patient with primary Sjögren's syndrome. It was suggested to be the optimal combination for efficient classification of this condition. For classification of secondary Sjögren's syndrome, the best combination was found to be a positive response for items I or II plus a positive result for any two of items II, IV, and V, resulting in a sensitivity of 85.1% and specificity of 93.9% for this diagnosis. With a positive response to items I or II and only one positive response to items III to V, the sensitivity increased to 95.6% but the specificity dropped to 71.6%.

These preliminary European classification criteria for Sjögren's syndrome were validated in a second study of similar design. Cases of primary Sjögren's syndrome (n = 81), secondary Sjögren's syndrome (n = 76), other connective tissue diseases without Sjögren's syndrome (n = 54), and controls (n = 67) were assembled by expert clinicians at 16 centers from 10 countries to validate the initial results.[20] In this study, it was decided not to use items III (a) (Schirmer-I-test) and V (c) (unstimulated whole salivary flow) to classify patients older than age 60 because the tear and salivary flow by these measures were significantly reduced in the elderly controls from the original study. The results proved to be similar to those of the earlier study, showing a sensitivity of 97.5% and specificity of 94.2% for correctly classifying primary Sjögren's syndrome and a sensitivity of 97.3% and specificity of 91.8% for correctly classifying secondary Sjögren's syndrome. A limitation of this type of study design is the possibility that the sensitivity and specificity of these criteria may be artificially inflated by a "circular bias" deriving from the results of the diagnostic testing on the original selection of patients. These preliminary European classification criteria have also been criticized because a patient may be classified with primary Sjögren's syndrome despite a negative biopsy and the absence of serum anti-Ro/SS-A or anti-La/SS-B antibodies. Thus patients may be classified as having primary Sjögren's syndrome without evidence of an immune basis for their condition.

This conceptual impasse was overcome by the European Study Group on Classification Criteria for Sjögren's Syndrome with a group of American experts. From their previous study, they selected a cohort of 76 patients with primary Sjögren's syndrome, 41 patients with another connective tissue disease but without Sjögren's syndrome, and 63 controls and tested three different combinations of items from the original classification criteria using a receiving operator curve (ROC) analysis. To determine the best possible prediction model, the optimal classifiers were compared with ROC analysis for the three different combinations: C point (positivity for any four of the six items); C* point (positivity of any four of the six items, excluding cases negative for both items IV and VI); and D point (positive for any of the four objective criteria).[12] The C point and the C* point showed the same accuracy (92.7%); however, the C* point had a lower sensitivity than the C point (89.5% vs. 97.4%), but a higher specificity (95.2% vs. 89.4%), and was preferred on the basis of the goal of selecting criteria with a high probability of excluding patients without the disease. The sensitivity and specificity of the D point were 84.2% and 95.2%, respectively, and judged to be comparable with the C* point and acceptable for classification purposes. Therefore patients may now be classified as having primary Sjögren's syndrome if they fulfill four of the six items including either a positive labial salivary gland biopsy or a positive test for serum anti-Ro/SS-A and/or anti-La/SS-B antibodies. This combination avoids the problem of classifying a patient with primary Sjögren's syndrome in the absence of a positive labial salivary gland biopsy or a positive

test for anti-Ro/SS-A and/or anti-La/SS-B antibodies. Alternatively, they may meet the criteria by satisfying any four of the objective items, which was a highly unusual scenario in their data set because nearly all patients with primary Sjögren's syndrome manifested symptoms of dry eyes and/or dry mouth.

The revised classification criteria proposed by the American-European Consensus Group are shown in Table 73-1. It was further specified that the Schirmer-I test be performed with anesthesia and that other ocular dyes such as lissamine green (for conjunctival staining) and fluorescein (for corneal staining) be allowed as replacements for Rose Bengal dye, which was not available in many countries. A positive labial salivary gland biopsy was further defined according to the rules set forth by Daniels and Whitcher.[21] In this case, a positive biopsy must show evidence of focal lymphocytic sialadenitis (FLS), which they defined as dense aggregates of 50 or more lymphocytes in perivascular or periductal locations. These aggregates, or

Table 73-1 Revised International Classification Criteria for Sjögren's Syndrome (SS)

I. Ocular symptoms: a positive response to at least one of the following questions:
   1. Have you had daily, persistent, troublesome dry eyes for more than 3 months?
   2. Do you have a recurrent sensation of sand or gravel in the eyes?
   3. Do you use tear substitutes more than 3 times a day?
II. Oral symptoms: a positive response to at least one of the following questions:
   1. Have you had a daily feeling of dry mouth for more than 3 months?
   2. Have you had recurrently or persistently swollen salivary glands as an adult?
   3. Do you frequently drink liquids to aid in swallowing dry food?
III. Ocular signs—that is, objective evidence of ocular involvement defined as a positive result for at least one of the following two tests:
   1. Schirmer's I test, performed without anaesthesia (≤5 mm in 5 minutes)
   2. Rose bengal score or other ocular dye score (≥4 according to van Bijsterveld's scoring system)
IV. Histopathology: in minor salivary glands (obtained through normal-appearing mucosa), focal lymphocytic sialoadenitis, evaluated by an expert histopathologist, with a focus score greater than 1, defined as a number of lymphocytic foci (which are adjacent to normal-appearing mucous acini and contain more than 50 lymphocytes) per 4 mm² of glandular tissue
V. Salivary gland involvement: objective evidence of salivary gland involvement defined by a positive result for at least one of the following diagnostic tests:
   1. Unstimulated whole salivary flow (≤1.5 mL in 15 minutes)
   2. Parotid sialography showing the presence of diffuse sialectasias (punctate, cavitary or destructive pattern), without evidence of obstruction in the major ducts
   3. Salivary scintigraphy showing delayed uptake, reduced concentration, and/or delayed excretion of tracer
VI. Autoantibodies: presence in the serum of the following autoantibodies:
   1. Antibodies to Ro(SSA) or La(SSB) antigens, or both

Revised Rules for Classification

For Primary SS

In patients without any potentially associated disease, primary SS may be defined as follows:
   a. The presence of any 4 of the 6 items is indicative of primary SS, as long as either item IV (Histopathology) or VI (Serology) is positive.
   b. Any 3 of the 4 objective criteria items (i.e., items III, IV, V, and VI) are present.
   c. The classification tree procedure represents a valid alternative method for classification, although it should be more properly used in clinical-epidemiologic surveys.

For Secondary SS

In patients with a potentially associated disease (for instance, another well-defined connective tissue disease), the presence of item I or item II plus any 2 from among items III, IV, and V may be considered as indicative of secondary SS.

Exclusion Criteria

Past head and neck radiation treatment
Hepatitis C infection
Acquired immunodeficiency syndrome
Pre-existing lymphoma
Sarcoidosis
Graft-versus-host disease
Use of anticholinergic drugs (since a time shorter than fourfold the half-life of the drug)

Reproduced from Classification criteria for Sjögren's syndrome: a revised version of the European criteria proposed by the American-European Consensus Group, Vitali C, Bombardieri S, Jonsson R, et al and the European Study Group on Classification Criteria for Sjögren's Syndrome, *Ann Rheum Dis* 61:554–558, 2002 with permission from BMJ Publishing Group Ltd.

foci, must contain only a small proportion of plasma cells and be located adjacent to normal-appearing acini in lobules without duct dilatation or fibrosis. A minimum threshold for positivity was considered to be greater than or equal to 1 focus per 4 mm^2 of tissue. These rules are important to follow in the interpretation of labial salivary gland biopsies because many specimens, especially from elderly individuals, show patterns of inflammation consistent with chronic sialadenitis, namely mixed lymphocytic and plasma cell infiltrates in association with ductal dilation, acinar atrophy, and fibrosis.

An abnormal parotid sialogram has been clarified in the revised criteria as the presence of diffuse sialectasis according to the scoring system of Rubin and Holt.[22] Positivity by salivary scintigraphy was also further defined as delayed uptake, reduced concentration, or delayed secretion of the tracer, using the method of Schall and colleagues.[23] Parotid sialography and salivary scintigraphy are rarely used clinically in the United States. The revised version also included some modifications to the list of exclusion criteria.

These new revised criteria have also not escaped criticism by some experts because of the possibility that patients may be classified as having primary Sjögren's syndrome without subjective or objective evidence of ocular involvement (satisfying items IV, V, and VI).[24] Others have mentioned the "histologic and immunologic bias" of the revised criteria,[25] but this argument fails if the goal of the classification criteria is to define patients with an immune-mediated condition. Some patients with primary Sjögren's syndrome will test positive for serum ANAs in the absence of anti-Ro/SS-A and anti-La/SS-B antibodies. If such patients have a falsely negative labial salivary gland biopsy, then they will not be classified as having primary Sjögren's syndrome despite a better than average chance otherwise. Another potential shortcoming is the lack of laboratory standardization for the detection of anti-Ro/SS-A and anti-La/SS-B antibodies. Many different methodologies are now available to measure these autoantibodies including the older Ouchterlony plate assay, various commercial enzyme-linked immunosorbent assay (ELISA) kits, and the newer multiplex bead technology. It is unclear if the type of methodology influences the sensitivity or specificity of these criteria. Although these classification criteria have been generally accepted by the medical community, they have not been officially endorsed by the American College of Rheumatology or the European League Against Rheumatism.

Recently, new classification criteria have been published based on data from the International Collaborative Clinical Alliance Cohort.[25a] These criteria have been approved by the American College of Rheumatology. These criteria are derived solely from objective test results and require for classification of primary Sjögren's syndrome at least 2 of the following: (1) a positive test for serum anti-Ro/SS-A and/or anti-La/SS-B antibodies or a positive test for rheumatoid factor and an ANA titer of ≥1 : 320; (2) labial salivary gland biopsy exhibiting focal lymphocytic sialadenitis with a focus score ≥44 mm^2; and (3) keratoconjunctivitis sicca with ocular staining score ≥3. Using an external set of 303 participants, these classification criteria had a sensitivity of 92.5% and a specificity of 95.4%. Further validation of these criteria will be necessary to confirm their performance.

EPIDEMIOLOGY

Primary Sjögren's syndrome ranks among the most common of the autoimmune diseases, with a prevalence rate ranging from 0.1% to 4.6%.[26] However, the epidemiologic data are confounded by variations in the ages of the study populations and differences in the classification criteria used for case identification. For example, the application of the Copenhagen criteria yields a prevalence rate for Sjögren's syndrome 2.7-fold greater than the California criteria, whereas the preliminary European classification criteria captures 2- to 3-fold more patients than the Copenhagen criteria.[27] Bowman and colleagues[28] estimated the prevalence of primary Sjögren's syndrome at 0.1% to 0.6% in a community from the United Kingdom using the revised criteria proposed by the American-European Consensus Group. In a study from Greece employing these same criteria, the age-adjusted mean annual incidence and prevalence rates were 5.3 (confidence interval [CI], 4.5 to 6.1) per 10^5 persons (0.5 for men and 10.1 for women) and 92.8 per 100,000 persons (8.4 for men and 177.4 for women), respectively.[29] The incidence and prevalence rates of primary Sjögren's syndrome are significantly higher in women than men (e.g., approximately 20:1), with a peak incidence in the fifth and sixth decades of life.[29] Primary Sjögren's syndrome occurs infrequently in children with onset as early as 5 years of age.[30] The revised criteria of the American-European Consensus Group may be less sensitive for classifying primary Sjögren's syndrome in children than adults owing to differences between these two age groups in the clinical presentation of this disease.[30]

The prevalence of secondary Sjögren's syndrome associated with rheumatoid arthritis, systemic lupus erythematosus, and systemic sclerosis has been estimated to be 17.1%,[31] 8% to 20%,[32-34] and 14%[35]; respectively. To be classified as secondary Sjögren's syndrome, patients in these studies had at minimum symptoms of keratoconjunctivitis sicca or xerostomia and objective evidence of lacrimal or salivary gland involvement. None of these studies used the preliminary European classification criteria for secondary Sjögren's syndrome.

GENETICS AND PATHOGENESIS

Central to the pathogenesis of primary Sjögren's syndrome is the dysregulation of T cells and B cells, with key contributions from innate pathways of inflammation. Many of these same concepts may apply to the pathogenesis of secondary Sjögren's syndrome; however, most investigation into disease mechanisms has focused on patients with the primary form of the disease, and many of the immunologic features of secondary Sjögren's syndrome are driven by the pathogenic mechanisms underlying the associated disorders.

In primary Sjögren's syndrome, a common theme among models of disease pathogenesis is loss of immunologic tolerance to self-antigens. This failure to recognize self manifests in primary Sjögren's syndrome as the production of serum autoantibodies indicative of the loss of B cell tolerance. Because the appearance of serum autoantibodies may precede the onset of clinical disease, the loss of immune tolerance appears to be permissive but not sufficient to induce clinical disease. T cells reactive with several candidate self-antigens have also been found infiltrating the labial salivary glands of patients with primary Sjögren's syndrome. However, the timing of the evolution of these aberrant T cell responses is unclear with respect to disease onset. Environmental or stochastic factors or both are likely at play in triggering the chronic inflammatory response in the context of a genetically predisposed innate and adaptive immune system.

Because a disproportionately high number of the cases of primary Sjögren's syndrome occur in women, the search for environmental candidates has centered on abnormal regulation of estrogens and androgens. However, no major differences have been found between patients with primary Sjögren's syndrome and healthy controls in serum levels of sex steroid hormones.[36] In addition, treatment with the hormone dehydroepiandrosterone, which acts on the androgen receptor, has shown no clinical efficacy in women with primary Sjögren's syndrome.[37] Among possible viral triggers, Epstein-Barr virus (EBV) and cytomegalovirus (CMV) have received attention in primary Sjögren's syndrome due to their suppressive effects on T cell immunity and their ability to establish persistent infection. In one study, EBV deoxyribonucleic acid (DNA) was found by immunochemical staining in salivary gland biopsies to localize in acinar and ductal epithelial cells[38]; however, the available evidence does not otherwise support a direct role for EBV infection in the pathogenesis of this disease. A 94-bp fragment of cocksackievirus ribonucleic acid (RNA) was also shown to be differentially expressed in salivary gland biopsies from patients with primary Sjögren's syndrome compared with controls,[39] but these results were not replicated in a later study.[40] As yet, the identity of a possible viral trigger remains elusive, if indeed one exists.

It has been difficult to estimate the genetic risk for developing primary Sjögren's syndrome owing to the absence of large twin studies. However, the existence of many large families with two or more members with primary Sjögren's syndrome argues strongly for a genetic component to disease pathogenesis.[41] Primary Sjögren's syndrome is considered to be a complex genetic disorder, similar to the genetic susceptibility of systemic lupus erythematosus and rheumatoid arthritis. It is now clear from genetic studies of human autoimmune diseases that multiple genes contribute to disease risk and that individually each gene confers only modest effects on disease susceptibility.[42] The exception to this rule is the relatively strong signal associated with the human leukocyte antigen (HLA) locus on human chromosome 6p21.3. In populations of European descent, confirmed HLA associations with primary Sjögren's syndrome include DRB1*0301 (DR3), DRB1*1501 (DR2), DQA1*0103, DQA1*0501, DQB1*0201, and DQB1*0601.[43,44] The disease-associated polymorphisms located in the DRB1*0301 and DRB1*1501 loci account for 90% of the HLA genetic contribution. The HLA locus appears to play a major role in the pathogenesis of autoantibody responses associated with primary Sjögren's syndrome. In patients with primary Sjögren's syndrome, higher titers of anti-Ro/SS-A and anti-La/SS-B antibodies have been linked to heterozygosity for the DQA1 and DQB1 alleles.[45]

The genetic susceptibility to primary Sjögren's syndrome will likely include inheritance of genes identified as risk factors in other autoimmune diseases. Familial clustering of cases of primary Sjögren's syndrome with systemic lupus erythematosus, rheumatoid arthritis, and systemic sclerosis, as well as other autoimmune diseases, are consistent with this premise.[46-48] There have been no large-scale genome-wide association studies in primary Sjögren's syndrome. Most efforts to identify disease susceptibility genes in primary Sjögren's syndrome have taken the candidate gene approach. Genes in the type I interferon (IFN) pathway have been the focus of several candidate gene studies because they are highly expressed in the peripheral blood and salivary glands of patients with primary Sjögren's syndrome compared with controls.[49] In a small cohort study, an increased risk of primary Sjögren's syndrome was associated with a single nucleotide polymorphism in the splicing sequence of exon B of the gene encoding IFN regulatory factor 5 (IRF5).[50] IRF5 is among the nine IRFs that signal through Toll-like receptors (TLRs) and is essential for inducing responses through TLR4, 7, and 9.[51] Given the possible inciting roles of viral RNA and DNA, the endosomal TLR7 and TLR9 pathways may be important in primary Sjögren's syndrome for the activation of the type I IFN pathway.[52] A 5-bp insertion/deletion polymorphism (CGGGG insertion/deletion) in the promoter region of the IRF5 transcript has also been linked to primary Sjögren's syndrome.[53] This polymorphism appears to have functional significance because reovirus (double-stranded RNA virus)–infected salivary gland epithelial cells in culture bearing this polymorphism produce higher levels of the IRF5 transcript.[53]

Other susceptibility genes have been identified in primary Sjögren's syndrome, but the findings have not yet been widely replicated. In a case-control study, an increased risk for primary Sjögren's syndrome was associated with a variant haplotype of the transcription factor Signal Transducers and Activator of Transcription 4 (STAT4).[54] This STAT4 polymorphism has also been shown to increase the risk for systemic lupus erythematosus and rheumatoid arthritis. STAT4 is a key intracellular signaling molecule involved in IL-12 and IL-23 signaling and is known to promote the development of T helper 1 (Th1) and T helper 17 (Th17) responses. Polymorphisms in the STAT4 and IRF5 genes appear to be additive in the risk for developing primary Sjögren's syndrome.[55] In other studies, Nordmark and colleagues[56] have identified three gene loci associated with an increased risk of primary Sjögren's syndrome—the early B cell factor (EBF1) gene, the interval encompassing family with sequence similarity 167 member A and B lymphoid tyrosine kinase (FAM167A-BLK), and the tumor necrosis family member 4 (TNFSF4, or the OX40L gene). All three genes are involved in B cell development, which is of particular interest due to the hyperactivated state of B cells in this disease.

The human genome contains conserved noncoding elements with functional sequences including regulatory motifs in promoters and untranslated regions of genes. Some of these conserved noncoding elements encode microRNAs, a novel means for regulation of gene expression. MicroRNAs influence both innate and adaptive immunity and have been shown to play a role in late B cell differentiation and development, as well as the establishment of B cell tolerance. Early studies have shown that microRNA expression patterns in salivary gland tissue can

Table 73-2 Mouse Models of Sjögren's Syndrome*

Mouse Model	Phenotype	Comments
Spontaneous Disease Models		
(NZB)NZW F1 mice	Progressive focal sialadenitis	Glandular involvement F > M
MRL/*lpr*	Lymphocytic infiltration of lacrimal and salivary glands; anti-Ro/SS-A and MR3 antibodies; oligoclonal expansion of T cells and IgA and IgM production in the salivary glands	Normal secretory function; mRNAs for IL-1 and TNF expressed in salivary glands before onset of sialadenitis
NOD and its derivatives NOD.H2h4, NOD.Q, and NOD.P, NOD.E2fl$^{-/-}$, NOD.*scid*	Lymphocytic infiltration of lacrimal and salivary glands; NOD.H2h4 strain (but not parental NOD strain) secretes high levels of anti-Ro/SS-A and anti-La/SS-B antibodies; reduced glandular function	Mice also develop diabetes; exchange of H2 haplotype from H2g7 to H2q (NOD.Q) or H2p (NOD.P) does not affect the frequency of sialadenitis; disruption of ICA69 locus prevents lacrimal gland inflammation and reduces salivary gland inflammation; NOD IFN-$\gamma^{-/-}$ mice do not develop glandular disease; blockade of LT-βR signaling pathway reduces salivary gland infiltrates and improves salivary gland function
NFS/*sld*	Lymphocytic infiltration of lacrimal and salivary glands; anti-α-fodrin antibodies	Aberrant immune responses to α-fodrin; mice develop autoimmune lesions in other organ systems
Experimentally Induced Models		
Carbonic anhydrase (PL/J mice)	Lymphocytic infiltration of salivary glands; antibodies to carbonic anhydrase	
Ro peptides (Balb/c mice)	Lymphocytic infiltration of salivary glands; glandular hypofunction, anti-Ro/SS-A and anti-La/SS-B antibodies	Disease induction requires multiple injections of peptide emulsified in Freund's adjuvant
Transgenic or Knockout Models		
Id3$^{-/-}$	Lymphocytic infiltration of lacrimal and salivary glands; adoptive transfer experiments; anti-Ro/SS-A and anti-La/SS-B antibodies; salivary hyposecretion	Id3 gene involved in TCR-mediated T cell indicate a role for T cells in the development of disease; treatment with anti-CD20 antibodies ameliorates disease
PI3K$^{-/-}$	Lymphocytic infiltration of the lacrimal glands; anti-Ro/SS-A and anti-La/SS-B antibodies	
BAFF transgenic	Lymphocytic infiltration of lacrimal and salivary glands; unique population of marginal zone B cells in salivary glands	No anti-Ro/SS-A or anti-SS-B antibodies; also develop lupus manifestations and anti-DNA antibodies and RF
IL-14α transgenic	Lymphocytic infiltration of lacrimal and salivary glands; hypergammaglobulinemia; <25% of animals develop anti-Ro/SS-A and anti-La/SS-B antibodies; glandular hyposecretion; mild immune complex-mediated renal disease and lymphocytic interstitial pneumonitis	IL-14 is a growth factor for B cells; mice develop large B cell lymphomas later in life; role for LT-α in the salivary gland inflammation; infiltrate primarily B cells with relatively few CD4$^+$ and CD8$^+$ T cells
IL-12 transgenic	Lymphocytic infiltration of lacrimal and salivary glands; anti-La/SS-B antibodies; glandular hyposecretion; increased acinar cell volume	Mice also develop thyroiditis and lung pathology

*See references 58 and 59 for further details.

BAFF, B cell activating factor; F, female; ICA69, islet cell antigen 69; Id3, protein inhibitor of DNA binding 3; IFN-γ, interferon-γ; IL-1, interleukin-1; LT-α, lymphotoxin-α; LT-βR, lymphotoxin β receptor; M, male; MR3, muscarinic receptor subtype 3; NOD, nonobese diabetic; NZB/NZW F1, New Zealand Black × New Zealand White F1 (mouse hybrid); PIK3, phosphoinositide 3-kinase; TNF, tumor necrosis factor.

distinguish patients with Sjögren's syndrome from controls, suggesting a pathologic role for dysregulated microRNA expression in the regulation of the chronic inflammatory response.[57]

Epigenetics refers to the study of inherited changes in gene expression caused by mechanisms other than a change in DNA sequence of that gene. Its principal mechanisms include remodeling of chromatic structure by DNA methylation and histone modification. Thus far, virtually nothing is known about the epigenetics of primary Sjögren's syndrome.

Many insights have been gained about disease mechanisms in primary Sjögren's syndrome from studies of humans with this autoimmune disease, as well as animal models. Experiments in model systems enable hypotheses to be examined in ways not possible in humans and

have contributed to understanding the immunoregulatory disturbances underlying the clinical expression of disease (Table 73-2).[58,59] Whereas these animal models have shed light on disease mechanisms, it has been possible to perform highly significant research in humans with primary Sjögren's syndrome because of the accessibility of labial salivary gland tissue for immunohistopathologic analysis. Studies of labial salivary gland biopsies from patients with this disease have shown approximately 90% of the infiltrating cells are composed of CD4$^+$ T lymphocytes and B lymphocytes, with the remainder an admixture of plasma cells, CD8$^+$ T cells, FoxP3$^+$ T regulatory cells, CD56$^+$ natural killer (NK) cells, and macrophages, as well as myeloid and plasmacytoid dendritic cells (DCs)[60] (Figure 73-1). Most of the infiltrating T cells bear the memory phenotype (CD45RO) and display a restricted T cell receptor (TCR) repertoire representing

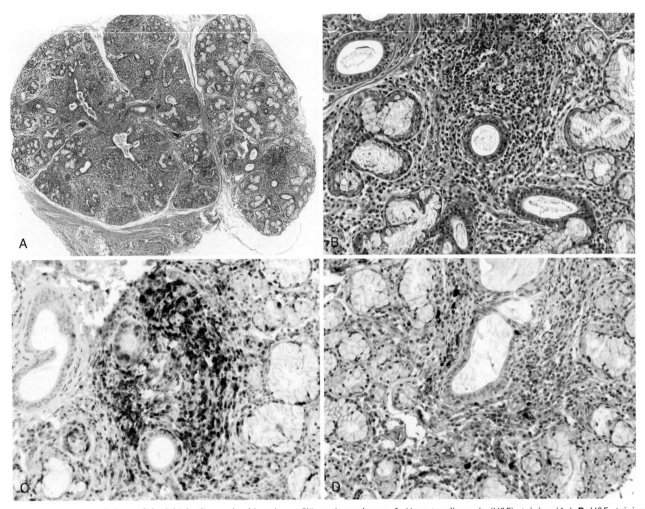

Figure 73-1 Histopathology of the labial salivary gland in primary Sjögren's syndrome. **A,** Hematoxylin-eosin (H&E) staining (4×). **B,** H&E staining (20×). **C,** Anti-CD3 staining of T cells. **D,** Anti-CD21 staining of B cells. Mononuclear cells aggregate in foci throughout the gland in a periductal distribution (**A** and **B**). In this biopsy, most of the mononuclear cells are T cells (**C**) and the minority are B cells (**D**).

several different clonotypes across multiple Vβ families. The proportion of B cells in the infiltrate increases with the severity of the inflammatory lesion.

The infiltrating mononuclear cells tend to coalesce around ducts and blood vessels, and in more severe inflammatory lesions they may form aggregates organized into germinal center (GC)-like structures. The GC-like structures display well-circumscribed mononuclear cell infiltrates with B and T cell components, Ki-67+ proliferating cells, CD21/CD35+ follicular DC networks, and CD31+ high endothelial venules (HEVs).[61] CXCL13 expression by epithelial cells, HEVs, and within germinal center–like structures together with the expression of CXCL12 and CCL21 provides a salivary gland microenvironment capable of attracting and retaining B cells.[62-64] The myeloid DCs and macrophages, the classic antigen-presenting cells, are mostly found in proximity to the ductal epithelium, where they have been shown to secrete tumor necrosis factor (TNF), interleukin-6 (IL-6), IL-10, IL-12, and IL-18. Minor salivary glands also contain a small number of plasmacytoid DCs, the main producers of the type I IFNs.[65] A robust type 1 IFN signature has been detected both in the salivary glands and peripheral blood of patients with primary Sjögren's syndrome.[65,66] The generation of type 1 IFNs by plasmacytoid DCs, among the

first lines of defense against viral infection, is partially dependent on signals through TLR7 and TLR9.

The analysis of T cell cytokines in labial salivary gland biopsies from patients with primary Sjögren's syndrome suggests a predominantly Th1- and Th17-driven response.[67] Studies of the expression of cytokine messenger RNAs (mRNAs) in salivary gland tissue show mainly upregulation of IL-2 and IFN-γ, the Th1-specific cytokines, and lesser quantities of IL-4, IL-5, and IL-13, the Th2-specific cytokines. Th17 cells, so named because they produce IL-17, are also found in the minor salivary glands; the salivary gland microenvironment is also rich in transforming growth factor (TGF)-β, IL-6, and IL-23, which are cytokines known to promote the development of this subset.[68] In addition, the salivary gland infiltrates contain a generous infiltrate of FoxP3+ regulatory T cells.[69] These cells typically show suppressive behavior, but as yet they have an uncertain role in regulating the chronic inflammatory lesion.

Several features of primary Sjögren's syndrome implicate B cells in disease mechanisms. B cells are the source of autoantibodies, but they also activate T cells through their ability to present antigen, are stimulated to secrete proinflammatory and anti-inflammatory cytokines, and facilitate the organization of secondary and tertiary lymphoid tissue.

The frequent presence of hypergammaglobulinemia, circulating immune complexes, mixed monoclonal immunoglobulin M (IgM) cryoglobulinemia, and serum autoantibodies in patients with primary Sjögren's syndrome implies B cells are in a dysregulated state. Most B cells in the salivary gland tissue exhibit a memory phenotype, express somatically hypermutated immunoglobulin V genes, and show preferential changes in V_L gene usage and the length of CDR3 from V_H gene rearrangements, which are findings characteristic of an antigen-driven response.[70] Salivary gland B cells appear to be responding specifically to antigen, although the site of antigen encounter and activation (salivary gland vs. secondary lymphoid tissue) remains uncertain. Germinal center–like structures found in some of the salivary gland biopsies provide an opportune environment for the selection and differentiation of antigen-driven B cell responses. The distribution of peripheral blood B cell subsets in primary Sjögren's syndrome differs from healthy controls, showing increased proportions of $CD27^-$ (naïve) B cells and decreased proportions of $CD27^+$ (memory) B cells.[71] Among several possibilities, these changes in the peripheral blood may result from abnormal trafficking of $CD27^+$ memory B cells to the target tissues, aberrations in B cell development, or both.

Several intrinsic B cell defects have also been found in patients with primary Sjögren's syndrome including abnormal retention of preswitch Ig transcripts in circulating postswitch $CD27^+$ memory B cells[72] and enhanced B cell signaling due to altered kinetics of B cell receptor translocation to lipid rafts.[73] Moreover, studies in patients with primary Sjögren's syndrome have shown increased serum and salivary gland tissue levels of B cell activating factor (BAFF), a B cell prosurvival factor,[74] as well as upregulated salivary gland expression of lymphotoxin (LT)-β mRNA.[75] LT-β is required for the formation of lymph nodes and germinal centers, while the heterodimer LT-α/LT-β can induce the development of ectopic germinal center–like structures. LT-α in soluble form induces the secretion of IFNs and chemokines, which are elevated in the salivary gland tissue from patients with primary Sjögren's syndrome. Levels of IL-14, another B cell growth factor, also appear to be increased in the serum and saliva of patients with primary Sjögren's syndrome.[76] IL-14 transgenic mice have been shown to develop a Sjögren's-like phenotype[77] in which the local tissue response is critically dependent on LT-α.[78] Blocking LT-β receptor signaling in NOD mice ablates the lymphoid organization in the salivary glands and improves their function,[79] further evidence that LTs may play a role in the pathogenesis of Sjögren's syndrome. Finally, abnormal B cell behavior is implied in primary Sjögren's syndrome by the predisposition of this disease toward the development of non-Hodgkin's B cell lymphoma. Interestingly, IL-14 transgenic mice develop large B cell lymphomas later in life.[77]

Anti-Ro/SS-A and anti-La/SS-B antibodies do not appear to have a pathogenic role in disease mechanisms despite their diagnostic and prognostic significance. The stimulating antigen(s) is unknown. An aberrant response to self may be provoked by altered expression of autoantigens. Several models have been proposed to explain the altered expression of autoantigens including differential expression of protein isoforms, post-translational modification, and

abnormal autoantigen presentation via apoptotic blebs, exosomes, or heat shock protein–mediated cross-priming.[80] Ro/SS-A and La/SS-B proteins do in fact show upregulated expression in the vicinity of the immunopathologic lesion in primary Sjögren's syndrome,[80] where they may induce local immune responses. Saliva from patients with this disease has been shown to contain anti-Ro/SS-A and anti-La/SS-B antibodies.[81] Although this finding may be interpreted to reflect local production of autoantibodies, it may also reflect extravasation of proteins from blood vessels into the inflamed tissues.

Among the other autoantibody specificities, those directed against the muscarinic receptor (MR) have attracted the most interest because of their possible role in causing glandular hypofunction. The MR family of receptors is bound by acetylcholine, which mediates the effects of the preganglionic and postganglionic parasympathetic nerve fibers that primarily regulate salivary flow. The muscarinic type 3 receptor (M3R), the target of autoantibodies in primary Sjögren's syndrome, is the subtype that predominately controls salivary flow. Two lines of evidence support the hypothesis that anti-M3R antibodies reduce exocrine gland function. Firstly, serum immunoglobulins from patients with primary Sjögren's syndrome have been shown to bind MR3 receptors on acinar cell membranes; they also have been shown to inhibit acetylcholine-evoked Ca^{2+} responses in a salivary gland cell line.[82] This Ca^{2+}-sensitive response is tightly regulated through intracellular signaling pathways that open the Cl^- channels on the apical membrane, resulting in an osmotic gradient and movement of water into the duct lumen. Secondly, passive transfer of the antibody has been shown to cause glandular hypofunction in NOD mice, an animal model of Sjögren's syndrome.[83] However, the assays for detecting serum anti-M3R antibodies have produced variable results depending on the methodology. For this reason, it has been difficult to determine the diagnostic sensitivity and specificity of serum anti-M3R antibodies in primary Sjögren's syndrome and the possible relationship of these autoantibodies to glandular hypofunction. Other autoantigens have been identified in patients with primary Sjögren's syndrome including α-fodrin, poly(ADP)ribose polymerase, carbonic anhydrase, and ICA69 protein. Despite initial enthusiasm for the possible etiologic role of α-fodrin in primary Sjögren's syndrome, recent studies have shown that serum anti-α-fodrin antibodies are not highly specific for this diagnosis.[84] Autoantibodies to carbonic anhydrase, poly(ADP)ribose polymerase, and ICA69 protein occur in only a minority of patients with primary Sjögren's syndrome and therefore do not appear to be attractive candidates for the initiating autoantigens.

In primary Sjögren's syndrome, the glandular epithelial cell appears to be an active participant in the abnormal immune response. In the salivary gland, the mononuclear cells preferentially congregate around ductal epithelium. The epithelial cells show upregulated expression of HLA class I and II molecules; adhesion molecules such as intercellular adhesion molecule-1 (ICAM-1; CD54), vascular cell adhesion molecule-1 (VCAM-1; CD106) and E-selectin; and co-stimulatory molecules such as CD80 and CD86[85]; they also produce high levels of cytokine mRNAs for IL-1, IL-6, IL-12, IL-18, and TNF,[86-88] as well as BAFF.[74] Ductal epithelial cells have also been shown to express

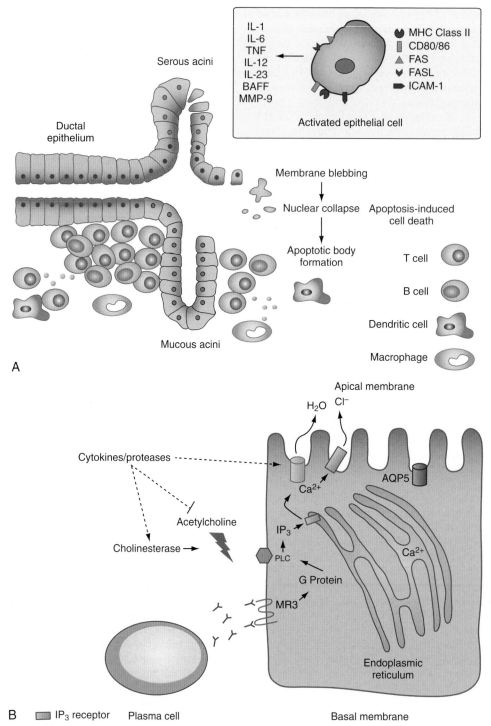

Figure 73-2 Two models for the pathogenesis of salivary gland inflammation in Sjögren's syndrome. **A,** Glandular hypofunction is explained by tissue loss secondary to immune attack, resulting in cytotoxic cell death and apoptosis. Epithelial cells likely play a central role in this process by several mechanisms: antigen-presentation and T cell activation; production of proinflammatory cytokines such as interleukin-1 (IL-1), IL-6, tumor necrosis factor (TNF), IL-12, and IL-23; and secretion of proteases. Epithelial cells also upregulate expression of Fas (FAS) and Fas ligand (FASL), cell surface molecules involved in the activation of apoptotic pathways. Other immune cells such as T cells, B cells, macrophages, and dendritic cells serve to amplify the chronic inflammatory response. In model **B,** glandular hypofunction results from downregulation of receptor-mediated secretion of salivary fluid into the ductal lumen. Acetylcholine binds to muscarinic receptor type 3 (MR3) on the surface of acinar cells, stimulating production of the second messenger inositol 1,4,5-triphosphate (IP$_3$). IP$_3$ in turn diffuses through the cytoplasm until it binds its receptor, IP$_3$R, on the endoplasmic reticulum. This interaction causes calcium to be released into the cytoplasm, which opens Ca^{2+}-sensitive chloride channels on the apical membrane of the cell. Electrochemical neutrality is preserved when Na$^+$ follows chloride across the membrane, while the osmotic gradient propels the water into the ductal lumen. Mechanisms of immune-mediated glandular hypofunction might include inhibition of acetylcholine release by cytokines, increased breakdown of acetylcholine in the epilemmal space by upregulated production of cholinesterases, blockade of M3R by autoantibodies, inhibition of intracellular signaling pathways involved in the fluid secretory process, or altered expression of aquaporin 5 (AQP5), which appears to be primarily responsible for water movement through the apical cell membrane. See reference 96 for more details. BAFF, B cell activating factor; ICAM-1, intercellular adhesion molecule-1; MHC, major histocompatibility complex; MMP-9, matrix metalloproteinase-9; PLC, phospholipase C.

mRNAs for several different proinflammatory chemokines including CXCL13, CCL17, CCL21, and CCL22.[89] Cultured salivary gland epithelial cells also express functional TLR3 and TLR7 molecules,[90,91] endowing a capability to sense pathogens and endogenous molecules produced by injured tissues. Activated epithelial cells are likely driving the aberrant innate and adaptive immune responses not only in the lacrimal and salivary glands but also in the lungs and kidneys, as well as other extraglandular sites.

At least two models exist to explain the glandular hypofunction in Sjögren's syndrome. In one model, it may be hypothesized that the glandular tissue is destroyed by an immune onslaught perpetuated by persistent exposure to self-antigens or other environmental stimulants (e.g., viral infection), leading to apoptosis of acinar epithelial cells and the irreversible loss of salivary gland function[92] (Figure 73-2A). A weakness of this model is that studies suggest epithelial cells rarely undergo apoptosis in the salivary gland tissue despite the fact they upregulate expression of mediators of cell death such as Fas, Fas ligand, and Bax (B cell lymphoma 2–associated X protein).[93] Ligand binding to CD40 expressed on epithelial cells in the salivary gland tissue also leads to Fas-mediated cell death by down-regulating c-FLIP (cellular FLICE-like inhibitor protein), an inhibitor of Fas-mediated cell death.[94] Because no studies have yet shown that an imbalance truly exists between the rates of glandular proliferation and damage, the relevance of this model to glandular hypofunction is uncertain. It also does not explain why many patients with markedly diminished salivary flow retain substantial amounts of normal-appearing acinar tissue in their salivary glands.[95]

A second model[86] assumes apoptosis is not a significant factor in the loss of acinar epithelium and instead posits that glandular function is *inhibited* (and not destroyed) by immune-mediated mechanisms (Figure 73-2B). This model implies a reversibility component to the loss of salivary flow and a pathologic process interrupting M3R activation. Possible mechanisms for such inhibitory effects include a reduction in acetylcholine release, increased breakdown of acetylcholine in the epilemmal space (e.g., acetylcholine must diffuse 100 nm from its release point at the nerve ending to the receptor on the cell), and blockade of M3R by antibodies.[96] Relatively little direct evidence supports any of these mechanisms except for the experiments showing that anti-M3R antibodies may block receptor function. Nevertheless, it is possible that the cytokine milieu in the inflamed glandular tissue interferes with the mechanisms controlling acinar gland function. In the NOD mouse, for example, impairment of salivary gland secretion does not appear to be readily explained by the destruction of acinar glands.[97] Regardless, the "immune destructive" and "immune inhibited" models are not mutually exclusive and may contribute to glandular hypofunction at various stages of the disease.

CLINICAL FEATURES

Keratoconjunctivitis Sicca

Chronic inflammation of the lacrimal glands diminishes secretion of aqueous tears, which if severe, may destroy the conjunctival and bulbar epithelium. Aqueous tear deficiency produces a dry eye, causing symptoms of grittiness or foreign body sensation, burning, photophobia, and eye fatigue. Routine eye examination usually reveals a reduction in the tear flow, as measured by the Schirmer-I-test. Additional findings may include the absence of tears in the conjunctival sac and dilated bulbar conjunctival vessels. Thick mucus may also be seen in the inner canthus of the eye. Slit-lamp examination allows for more detailed visualization of the corneal and conjunctival surface. Following instillation of lissamine green dye or fluoroscein onto the ocular surface, slit-lamp examination may expose devitalized cells or epithelial defects, respectively, signs of corneal and conjunctival damage. Severe dryness may result in corneal abrasion or ulceration.

The anatomy of the tear film informs the differential diagnosis of a dry eye (Table 73-3). The tear film consists

Table 73-3 Differential Diagnosis of Primary Sjögren's Syndrome

Condition	Associated Clinical/Radiologic/Pathophysiologic Features	Immunologic/Histopathologic Profile
Dry Eye (Keratoconjunctivitis Sicca)		
Aqueous Tear Deficiency (Failure of Lacrimal Tear Secretion)		
Sarcoidosis*	Lacrimal and parotid gland enlargement, cervical and hilar adenopathy, ILD, uveitis, arthralgia/arthritis, erythema nodosum	ANA negative or low titer; noncaseating granulomas in multiple organs (e.g., lymph nodes, lungs, spleen, liver, skin, salivary glands)
Chronic hepatitis C infection	Chronic hepatitis	Serum hepatitis C virus antibodies; hepatitis C viremia
Chronic GVHD	Occurs after allogeneic hematopoietic stem cell transplantation; other ocular features include sterile conjunctival inflammation and scarring, with progressive loss of goblet cells and dysfunction of meibomian glands	Lacrimal gland fibrosis, with mild chronic inflammation
Sensory block	Corneal surgery (LASIK), contact lens wear, diabetes	
Motor block	Cranial nerve VII damage	
Age-related	None	
Systemic drugs†		

Continued

Table 73-3   Differential Diagnosis of Primary Sjögren's Syndrome—cont'd

Condition	Associated Clinical/Radiologic/Pathophysiologic Features	Immunologic/Histopathologic Profile
Evaporative (Excessive Water Loss from the Ocular Surface)		
Meibomian gland deficiency	Ocular redness and burning; increased tear break-up time and tear hyperosmolarity; secondary to posterior blepharitis, acne rosacea, seborrheic dermatitis, and drugs (e.g., retinoids)	
Cicatricial pemphigoid[‡]	Scarring of the meibomian orifices, loss of goblet cells	
Poor lid congruity or low blink rate	Proptosis (poor lid congruity), Parkinson's disease (low blink rate)	
Vitamin A deficiency	Impaired goblet cell development	
Dry Mouth (Hyposalivation)		
Amyloidosis	Nephrotic syndrome	ANA negative; monoclonal gammopathy; biopsy often shows amyloid deposits
Hemachromatosis	Cirrhosis	Labial salivary gland biopsy with heavy hemosiderin deposits in the ductal epithelium and loss of acinar glands
Chronic GVHD	Salivary gland dysfunction less common than lacrimal gland dysfunction; may be associated with oral mucosal involvement of chronic GVHD	Periductal inflammation, fibrosis, and glandular atrophy
Chronic hepatitis C infection	See above	Labial salivary gland biopsy shows chronic inflammation similar to that of Sjögren's syndrome
Diabetes mellitus	Type I or type II diabetes	
Radiation therapy	Side effects after radiotherapy for head and neck cancer	Lack of functional acinar cells; damage to ducts, blood vessels, and nerves
Anxiety		
Systemic drugs[†]		
Parotid Gland Enlargement		
Sarcoidosis*	See above	See above
IgG4-related diseases	Multiorgan involvement: lacrimal and salivary gland enlargement, chronic sclerosing sialadenitis, autoimmune pancreatitis, sclerosing cholangitis, lung nodules, interstitial pneumonitis, aortitis, interstitial nephritis, prostatitis, orbital pseudotumor, dacroadenitis, meningitis, hypophysitis	High serum IgG4 levels; lymphoplasmacytic infiltrate and abundance of IgG4[+] plasma cells in tissues
Multicentric Castleman's disease	Lacrimal and salivary gland enlargement (uncommon); fever, lymphadenopathy, hepatomegaly, edema, and ascites (common); increased incidence of non-Hodgkin's lymphoma	Elevated serum IL-6 levels; some patients with increased serum IgG4 levels; lymph node biopsy shows interfollicular plasmacytosis
Diabetes mellitus	More common in type II than type I diabetes	Sialadenosis
Alcoholism		Sialadenosis
HIV lymphoepithelial lesion	Bilateral involvement	Extensive lymphoid infiltrate with reactive germinal centers (CD8 > CD4[+] T cells)
Benign tumors	Painless swelling of the parotid gland; usually unilateral but sometimes bilateral	Pleomorphic adenoma (usually unifocal); Warthin tumor: often multifocal and bilateral; oncocytoma; many other types
Malignant carcinoma	Painless swelling of the parotid gland, facial nerve palsy	Most common: mucoepidermoid carcinoma, acinic cell carcinoma, adenoid cystic
Primary B cell lymphoma	Unilateral or bilateral parotid gland swelling	Marginal zone B cell lymphoma most common subtype (also called *MALT-type*); follicle center and mantle zone lymphomas may also occur in this region; diffuse large B cell lymphoma (rare)
Primary T cell lymphoma	Rarely may present as a parotid gland mass; HTLV-1-associated	Anaplastic large cell or diffuse pleomorphic (medium and large cell)
Calculous duct obstruction	Painful enlargement of salivary glands	Ruptured ducts and obstructive granulomas

*May coexist with primary Sjögren's syndrome.

  †Common offending drugs include: anticholinergics (e.g., antihistamines, tricyclic antidepressants, antispasmodics), clonidine, diuretics, isotretinoin, estrogen replacement therapy, amiodarone.

  ‡May also destroy the lacrimal gland and cause lacrimal duct obstruction late in the clinical course.

  ANA, antinuclear antibodies; GVHD, graft-versus-host disease; HIV, human immunodeficiency virus; HTLV-1, human T lymphotropic virus type 1; IL-6, interleukin-6; ILD, interstitial lung disease; MALT, mucosa-associated lymphoid tissue.

of three major layers: the outer lipid layer, the middle aqueous layer, and the inner mucin layer. In addition to Sjögren's syndrome, conditions associated with infiltration of the lacrimal glands (e.g., sarcoidosis) and diminished tear flow (e.g., medications, aging, and estrogen deficiency) may decrease aqueous tear flow. The lipid layer derives from the meibomian glands and traps the aqueous tear film on the eyeball and protects it from rapid evaporation. Meibomian gland dysfunction, or posterior blepharitis, produces dry eyes from rapid evaporation of tears; it may be present with aqueous tear deficiency and be an aggravating factor in patients with keratoconjuctivitis sicca. Meibomian gland dysfunction is often associated with ocular rosacea and seborrheic dermatitis, two conditions encountered often in clinical practice that lead to symptoms of dry eyes. Lipid degradation resulting from meibomian gland inflammation may produce free fatty acids, which are irritating to the ocular surface and may cause punctate keratopathy. The mucin layer originates from the goblet cells of the conjunctiva and, if deficient, leads to an uneven distribution of the tear film over the surface of the eye. Vitamin A deficiency and Stevens-Johnson syndrome are examples of conditions associated with an abnormal mucin layer.

Xerostomia

The changes in the quality and quantity of the saliva are responsible for the signs and symptoms of xerostomia. Although symptoms of dry mouth are relatively common in the general population, they are usually more severe in Sjögren's syndrome and cause incessant difficulties with chewing and swallowing dry food, altered taste (metallic, salty, or bitter), and prolonged speaking. Patients with xerostomia may have problems wearing dentures. Despite complaints of a dry mouth, many patients will appear to have a normal oral examination owing to residual salivary flow. Others with more severe hypofunction will manifest a dry, sticky, or erythematous oral mucosa.

Two complications of xerostomia are important to the care of patients with xerostomia, expecially those with severe deficits in salivary flow. Xerostomia often results in rampant dental caries, cracked teeth, and loose fillings. Oral candidiasis, the other frequent complication, typically manifests as the atrophic variant, which is characterized by erythema and atrophy of the oral mucosa and filiform papillae on the dorsum of the tongue, with angular cheilitis. Sometimes, a thin, white exudate may appear on the surface of the tongue. The "thrushlike" variant of oral candidiasis is seen much less frequently in patients with xerostomia except in the face of recent antibiotic therapy.

About one-quarter of patients with primary Sjögren's syndrome suffers enlargement of the parotid or submandibular glands during the course of their disease. Chronic swelling is usually painless and may be unilateral or bilateral; it is often diffuse and firm by palpation. Transiently painful episodes of acute swelling and tenderness may also punctuate the clinical course. Acute swelling of the major salivary glands probably results most often from dried mucus obstructing the lumens of the major ducts; it usually subsides within a few days with conservative therapy. Rarely, bacterial infections may cause acute salivary gland swelling and should be considered as a possible etiology if the patient has a fever or other constitutional complaints. Asymmetric gland enlargement with palpable hard nodules that are increasing in size may indicate a neoplasm such as a lymphoma.

Involvement of Other Exocrine Glands

Glandular hypofunction may also affect the nasal passages (meatal obstruction from dried mucus), larynx (hoarseness), trachea (cough), vagina (dyspareunia), and skin (pruritus), producing symptoms of dryness. Virtually any exocrine gland may be involved in this disease.

Extraglandular Manifestations

Nearly three-quarters of patients with primary Sjögren's syndrome manifest signs or symptoms of extraglandular disease. Extraglandular involvement is more likely to occur in patients with serum anti-Ro/SS-A and anti-La/SS-B antibodies, as well as hypergammaglobulinemia, cryoglobulinemia, and hypocomplementemia. However, only about 25% of patients with primary Sjögren's syndrome develop moderate or severe extraglandular disease.

Fatigue, a complex and multifaceted phenomenon, occurs in approximately 70% of patients with primary Sjögren's syndrome.[98] It is also a symptom of depression, chronic anxiety, fibromyalgia, and sleep deficit, as well as a side effect of certain medications. The United Kingdom Sjögren's Interest Group has developed an instrument called the Profile of Fatigue and Discomfort–Sicca Symptoms Inventory (PROFAD-SSI) to specifically measure both somatic (needing rest, poor starting, low stamina, weak muscles) and mental fatigue (poor concentration, poor memory) in this disease.[99] In 547 patients with a confirmed diagnosis of primary Sjögren's syndrome, somatic fatigue was the dominant predictor of physical function and general health.[100] The relative contribution of behavioral and cognitive variables to fatigue was studied in 94 patients with primary Sjögren's syndrome.[101] Although depression was associated with higher levels of fatigue in this study, it was not present in most patients who reported fatigue. The link between fatigue and "biologic disease activity" is not fully understood in primary Sjögren's syndrome. Increased serum cytokines such as IL-6 and type I IFNs, as well as neuroendocrine and autonomic dysfunction are postulated to be contributing factors to the physical and mental aspects of fatigue in this setting.[98]

Raynaud's syndrome has been reported in 13% to 33% of patients with primary Sjögren's syndrome, often preceding the onset of sicca symptoms by several years.[102] Digital ulcers occur only rarely.

Among the dermatologic manifestions, the most common are xerosis, or dry skin; eyelid dermatitis; and angular cheilitis. In addition, many patients develop a variety of other cutaneous manifestations including annular erythema, purpura, and urticarial vasculitis. Annular erythema has been described in several forms: a donut-ring-like erythema with an elevated border (type I); a subacute cutaneous lupus erythematosus (SCLE)-like lesion with marginally scaled polycyclic erythema (type II); and a papular insect bite–like erythema (type III).[103] Histopathologically, these lesions are characterized by a deep perivascular lymphocytic infiltrate without the epidermal changes associated with lupus.[104] In some cases, immunoglobulin and complement deposition is observed along the basement membrane with liquefaction degeneration in the basal layer of the involved skin. The type I lesion appears to be specific for primary Sjögren's syndrome, occurring predominantly in Asian but not Western populations.

Cutaneous vasculitis may be expressed in several different forms including palpable purpura, erythematous papules or macules, and ulcers, with lesions predominantly located in the lower limbs.[105] Such lesions are frequently accompanied by other extraglandular manifestions of disease such as arthritis, peripheral neuropathy, Raynaud's syndrome, anemia, elevated erythrocyte sedimentation rate, hypergammaglobulinemia, serum rheumatoid factor, and serum anti-Ro/SS-A and anti-La/SS-B antibodies. In one study, 27% and 50% of the cases of small vessel, cutaneous vasculitis were present with and without cryoglobulinemia, respectively; 21% of cases were classified as *urticarial vasculitis*.[105] Livedo reticularis has also been described in this setting.

Polyarthalgia occurs frequently in patients with primary Sjögren's syndrome. In a retrospective study, articular symptoms in primary Sjögren's syndrome had a prevalence rate of 45%.[106] Although most patients complain only of polyarthralgia, a subset may develop objective signs of synovitis, which is nonerosive, symmetric, and polyarticular of waxing and waning intensity. Joint symptoms may precede the diagnosis of primary Sjögren's syndrome in up to one-third of cases.[107] In two separate studies, anticyclic citrullinated peptide (anti-CCP) antibodies were detected in serum from 7.5% and 9.9% of patients with primary Sjögren's syndrome.[108,109] However, in only one of these studies was their presence closely associated with synovitis,[109] and in neither study did it appear that serum anti-CCP positivity was associated with radiographic erosions or progression to rheumatoid arthritis.

Involvement of the airways and lung parenchyma in primary Sjögren's syndrome may take several forms including xerotrachea and xerobronchitis; nonspecific interstitial pneumonitis (NSIP); lymphocytic interstitial pneumonitis (LIP), now considered to be a subset of NSIP; usual interstitial pneumonitis (UIP); bronchiolitis; and lymphoma (reviewed in reference 110). The estimated prevalence of pulmonary involvement in primary Sjögren's syndrome varies depending on the thoroughness of the evaluation. In one study involving 123 patients with primary Sjögren's syndrome, 11.4% showed pulmonary signs or symptoms and/or impaired pulmonary function with abnormal chest computed tomography (CT) findings at the time of evaluation.[111]

Evidence of small airways dysfunction is found often in asymptomatic patients with normal radiologic studies. In symptomatic patients, NSIP appears to be the predominant type of lung involvement. The diagnosis can often be made on the basis of clinical presentation, pulmonary function tests (PFTs), and abnormal chest CT findings. PFTs in patients with NSIP show a restrictive pattern with reduced diffusion capacity of lung carbon monoxide (DLCO). Chest CT scans in this condition reveal ground-glass opacities and a reticular nodular pattern. Bronchoalveolar lavage (BAL), which is not usually required for diagnosis, shows evidence of alveolar inflammation, with elevated neutrophil or

lymphocyte counts, or both. LIP is also associated with a restrictive pattern on PFTs. Chest CT findings are ground-glass opacities and thin-walled cysts, with centrilobular nodules, interlobular septal thickening, and bronchovascular bundle thickening (Figure 73-3A). Microscopically, the lung biopsy from patients with LIP shows a diffuse interstitial infiltrate composed of lymphocytes, plasma cells, and histiocytes, which expand the interlobular and alveolar spaces (Figure 73-3B). The PFTs in patients with UIP also show a restrictive pattern like NSIP and LIP, but the chest CT findings of lower lobe fibrosis, honeycombing, and traction bronchiectasis distinguish it from these other two types. Histopathologically, follicular bronchiolitis is

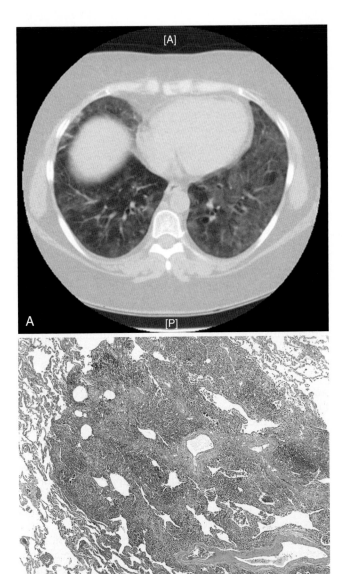

Figure 73-3 Lymphocytic interstitial pneumonitis (LIP) in a 44-year-old woman with primary Sjögren's syndrome. **A,** A slice through the lower lobes of a chest computed tomography scan showing diffuse ground-glass opacities, a scattering of multiple nodules in the periphery, and many thin-walled parenchymal cysts. **B,** Histopathologic examination from a wedge resection of the lower lobe of this patient shows a patchy, nodular interstitial infiltrate composed of mononuclear cells, with widening of the interlobular and alveolar spaces, consistent with LIP. *(Reproduced with permission from ACP Medicine.)*

characterized by nodular lymphocytic infiltrates with germinal center–like structures encircling respiratory bronchioles. PFTs in patients with bronchiolitis may show a restrictive or obstructive functional defect. The chest CT scan usually reveals reticulonodular infiltrates, but it may be normal in mild cases.

Lung biopsy can reveal evidence of not only interstitial lung disease but also other pathologic processes such as low-grade lymphoma or amyloidosis. Ito and colleagues[112] evaluated 33 patients with primary Sjögren's syndrome and biopsy-proven lung disease and found evidence of NSIP in 20 (61%), non-Hodgkin's lymphoma in 4 (12%), diffuse bronchiolitis in 4 (12%), and amyloid in 2 (6%). PFTs revealed restrictive changes in 19 (58%) patients and obstructive changes in 3 (9%) patients. Analysis of BAL fluid from 28 patients from this group was uniformly abnormal, showing elevated lymphocyte counts in 18 (64%) and elevated neutrophil counts in 19 (68%). In 31 patients, chest CT findings revealed an NSIP pattern in 14 (45%) and a UIP pattern in 4 (13%); 3 (10%) showed a pattern of organizing pneumonia. There were no cases of LIP in this series. By comparison, Parambil and colleagues[113] evaluated 18 patients with biopsy-proven lung disease in association with primary Sjögren's syndrome and found a histopathologic pattern of NSIP in 5 (28%) patients, organizing pneumonia in 4 (22%) patients, UIP in 3 (17%) patients, LIP in 3 (17%) patients, lymphoma in 2 (11%) patients, and amyloid in 1 (6%) patient.

Renal disease is infrequently of clinical significance in primary Sjögren's syndrome. Tubular interstitial nephritis, type I renal tubular acidosis (RTA), glomerulonephritis, and nephrogenic diabetes insipidus have been reported in association with this disease. Tubular interstitial nephritis, which is characterized histopathologically by a peritubular lymphocytic infiltrate and fibrosis, rarely progresses to end-stage renal disease.[114,115] A patient with primary Sjögren's syndrome has been described with tubular interstitial nephritis and acquired Gitelman's syndrome and tubular interstitial nephritis, with absence of a sodium-chloride cotransporter in the distal convoluted tubules.[116] Rarely, severe potassium wasting from type I RTA can lead to muscle paralysis.[117] Glomerular disease is exceedingly rare in this setting and may take several forms including membranous, membranoproliferative, mesangial proliferative, and focal crescentic glomerulonephritis.

Patients with primary Sjögren's syndrome have an increased frequency of gastrointestinal symptoms compared with the general population. Dysphagia and heartburn are particularly common complaints that may result from impaired salivary flow or esophageal motility, or both. About one-third of patients with primary Sjögren's syndrome have varying degrees of esophageal dysfunction, although many studies have been unable to correlate symptoms of dysphagia with a functional abnormality.[118] The results of one study suggest that patients with primary Sjögren's syndrome do not have a primary disturbance of esophageal motility, but rather defective clearance of esophageal acid that exposes the esophageal lining to excessive amounts of acid, which in turn, produces morphologic changes and secondary dysmotility.[119] Other results suggest parasympathetic dysfunction might be at the root of the esophageal abnormalities.[118] A case has also been described of a patient with primary Sjögren's syndrome who developed esophageal achalasia in the setting of a sensory ataxic neuropathy, which damaged the myenteric plexus and led to the esophageal abnormality.[120] In addition, chronic atrophic gastritis, which may cause dyspeptic symptoms, has been reported in a small number of cases of primary Sjögren's syndrome.[121]

Patients with primary Sjögren's syndrome may develop liver enzyme abnormalities for a variety of reasons, most often from an associated disorder such as hepatitis C virus infection, autoimmune hepatitis, primary biliary cirrhosis, or a nonspecific hepatitis.[122] Bowel symptoms such as abdominal pain and constipation occur more commonly in patients with primary Sjögren's syndrome than healthy controls, but their etiology is often obscure.[123]

Neurologic abnormalities are protean in primary Sjögren's syndrome, with varied patterns of peripheral and central nervous system involvement. The prevalence of central nervous system involvement that can be directly attributed to primary Sjögren's syndrome is likely to be in the range of 1% to 2%, but much higher rates have been reported with more liberal case definitions. For example, higher prevalence rates are noted when mood disturbances and minor cognitive and affective disturbances are included in the definition of central nervous system (CNS) involvement. Neuropsychiatric symptoms such as depression and minor cognitive disturbances occur in approximately one-third of patients with primary Sjögren's syndrome. However, they are nonspecific clinical disorders that occur frequently in the general population and in patients with other chronic diseases. Rarely, cases have been described in which patients with primary Sjögren's syndrome develop severe cognitive dysfunction. Brain magnetic resonance imaging (MRI) scans in these instances typically show nonspecific T2-weighted, high-intensity signals in the white matter that have an uncertain relationship to the clinical CNS findings. Focal CNS deficits have also been rarely described in patients with primary Sjögren's syndrome and include optic neuropathy, hemiparesis, movement disorders, cerebellar syndromes, recurrent transient ischemic attacks, and motor neuron syndrome.[124] Spinal cord syndromes resembling multiple sclerosis such as transverse myelitis and progressive myelopathy have also been reported in patients with primary Sjögren's syndrome.[125] Patients with primary Sjögren's have been described, too, with neuromyelitis optica in association with serum anti-aquaporin-4 antibodies.[126]

Peripheral nervous system involvement is among the most common of the extraglandular features of primary Sjögren's syndrome. In a cross-sectional study, peripheral neuropathy was diagnosed in 17 (27%) of 62 patients with primary Sjögren's syndrome on the basis of a conventional neurologic examination.[127] However, only 34 (55%) in this group had abnormal nerve conduction velocity studies including 19 (31%) with a motor neuropathy, 8 (13%) with a sensory neuropathy, and 7 (11%) with a sensorimotor neuropathy. Some of the others with normal nerve conduction velocity studies may have had a small fiber neuropathy. Other peripheral neuropathies that have been reported in patients with primary Sjögren's syndrome are cranial neuropathies, autonomic neuropathies, and multiple mononeuropathies.[124] Most cases of peripheral neuropathy are dominated by sensory symptoms and typically do not progress to cause motor weakness.

Beyond lower extremity purpura, systemic vasculitis appears to be a rare manifestation of extraglandular disease. Patients can develop a small vessel vasculitis and cryoglobulinemia in the absence of hepatitis C virus infection and a medium-sized vessel vasculitis with features ranging from multiple mononeuropathies to ischemic bowel.

Lymphoma

Non-Hodgkin's lymphoma (NHL) is a complication of primary Sjögren's syndrome with important prognostic significance. In a recent study, the prevalence of NHL in this disease was 4.3%, with a median time of approximately 7.5 years from the diagnosis of primary Sjögren's syndrome to the development of NHL.[128] Several histopathologic types of NHL have been described in association with primary Sjögren's syndrome including marginal zone B cell lymphoma, follicular cell lymphoma, diffuse large B cell lymphoma, and lymphoplasmacytoid lymphoma. Marginal zone B cell lymphoma, which is a family of low-grade B cell lymphomas, is by far the predominant type of NHL associated with this chronic autoimmune disease.

The mucosa-associated lymphoid tissue (MALT) lymphoma, a type of marginal zone B cell lymphoma, occurs mostly in chronic autoimmune diseases such as primary Sjögren's syndrome. It develops at extranodal sites in relation to mucosae or glandular epithelium such as the lacrimal and salivary glands, lung, gastrointestinal tract, and skin. The earliest histopathologic feature of MALT lymphoma is the finding of monocytoid B cells surrounding the epithelium. Immunochemical staining of these lesions shows their clonality in revealing monotypic infiltrates of either Igκ- or Igλ-light chains.[128] With progression, these lesions show increasing proliferation of neoplastic cells, replacement of reactive follicles, and ductal dilatation. In primary Sjögren's syndrome, MALT lymphomas most often develop in the salivary glands, but they may also develop at other extranodal sites, especially the lung and gastrointestinal tract. In primary Sjögren's syndrome, a fivefold increased risk for lymphoma is conferred by the presence of parotid gland enlargement, splenomegaly, lymphadenopathy, neutropenia, cryoglobulinemia, or low C4.[129]

Associated Diseases

Primary Sjögren's syndrome has been associated with a higher risk for the development of other autoimmune diseases including thyroid disease, autoimmune hepatitis, primary biliary cirrhosis, and celiac disease. Although initial studies found a higher frequency of thyroid disease in patients with primary Sjögren's syndrome than controls, a recent, larger study failed to show a statistically significant difference in the rate of thyroid disease between the two groups.[130] Autoimmune hepatitis and primary biliary cirrhosis occur in less than 5% of patients with primary Sjögren's syndrome, but more precise estimates of their prevalence are not available owing to the absence of well-controlled studies addressing this question. One exception is a Hungarian study showing a 10-fold higher rate of celiac disease in patients with primary Sjögren's syndrome compared with healthy controls.[131]

DIAGNOSIS AND DIAGNOSTIC TESTS

Keratoconjunctivitis Sicca and Xerostomia

A diagnostic suspicion of Sjögren's syndrome is initially raised by complaints of dry eyes and dry mouth. However, many patients do not openly volunteer this information because they do not feel it is important enough to bring to the attention of the physician. Therefore it is essential to inquire about these symptoms if they do not come up during initial history taking. In patients with symptoms of dry eyes and dry mouth, the next step is to confirm the diagnosis by objective testing. An easy method for evaluating aqueous tear flow is the Schirmer's-I test, which is performed by inserting a sterile piece of filter paper in the middle to lateral third of the lower eyelid and measuring the distance tears elute over 5 minutes. A distance of 5 mm or less is the usual cutoff for abnormally low tear production. Although a Schirmer-I test is subject to an approximately 20% rate of false negativity, normal tear flow in the face of ocular foreign body sensations suggests an alternative diagnosis such as blepharitis (see later). Patients with moderate-to-severe symptoms of dry eyes are usually referred to an ophthalmologist for slit-lamp examination. With a slit-lamp, the ophthalmologist can carefully examine the ocular surface, evaluating for any signs of damage. Instillation of lissamine green or fluorescein dye onto the surface of the eye displays the integrity of the conjunctival and corneal surface. Lissamine green dye stains epithelial surfaces lacking mucin (Figure 73-4), whereas the fluorescein dye targets areas of cellular disruption on the ocular surface. Rose Bengal dye, which stains dead or degenerated cells, is no longer preferred for evaluating the ocular surface due to its toxic effects on the cornea.

Several methods may be used for objective assessment of dry mouth, or xerostomia. Only a minority of patients with xerostomia show obvious signs of a dry mucosa on oral examination (e.g., absent sublingual salivary pool, thick and sticky saliva). Sialometry is used to test for functional impairment in salivary flow and refers to the measurement of salivary flow from individual glands (parotid, submandibular, or sublingual) or the mouth as a whole. An unstimulated whole salivary flow rate less than or equal to 1.5 mL/15 min meets the criterion for xerostomia according to the classification criteria developed by the American-European Consensus Group (see Table 73-1). For the collection procedure, the patients should keep their heads tilted forward and swallow once to clear the mouth of excess saliva. At this point, the 15-minute collection period is initiated and then subjects expectorate, as needed, accumulating saliva into a preweighed 50-cm^3 cryovial. Samples are weighed on an analytic balance to determine the volume (1 g = 1 mL) of saliva.

Sialography, another technique for evaluating xerostomia, visualizes radiographic patterns of duct obstruction in the major salivary glands. It is most useful for differentiating an inflammatory process from a neoplasm. This technique calls for injection of radiographic contrast dye into the salivary duct followed by serial radiographs to image the pattern of dye flow. A water-based contrast is strongly preferred to an oil-based contrast because the latter may damage the adjacent salivary gland tissue. Sialography is not routinely

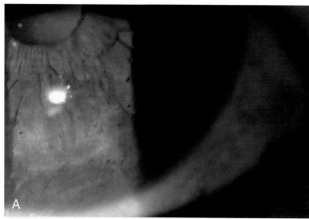

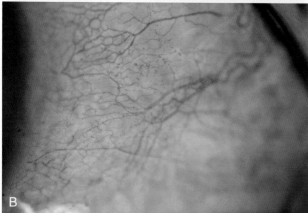

Figure 73-4 Lissamine staining of a dry eye as shown by slit-lamp examination. **A,** Punctate staining of the cornea. **B,** Punctate staining of the conjunctival epithelium. *(A and B, Courtesy W. Craig Fowler, MD, Department of Ophthalmology, University of North Carolina at Chapel Hill.)*

employed in clinical practice because it is an invasive procedure with complications including duct rupture, pain, and infection. Scintigraphy is a radionuclide technique for measuring salivary gland function. After sodium radiolabeled pertechnetate technetium is injected into the blood, it is absorbed into the salivary gland and secreted into the mouth, allowing for determination of the salivary flow rate. The diagnostic sensitivity and specificity of salivary gland scintigraphy for the diagnosis of primary Sjögren's syndrome has been estimated to be 75% and 78%, respectively.[132] Salivary scintigraphy is not widely available for routine testing.

Ultrasonography and MRI have been examined for their ability to detect anatomic abnormalities in the salivary glands of patients with primary Sjögren's syndrome. In comparison with normal individuals, the detection of parenchymal inhomogeneity by ultrasonography in two or more major salivary gland had a sensitivity of 63% and a specificity of 99% for identifying patients with primary Sjögren's syndrome.[133] Although these results are promising, this technique requires further validation and investigation using appropriate disease controls. MRI with sialography may be more sensitive than ultrasonography for detecting glandular structural changes,[134] but further studies are necessary to validate this technique as well.

Labial Salivary Gland Biopsy

Labial salivary gland biopsy has long been considered the gold standard for diagnosing primary Sjögren's syndrome. However, in clinical practice, its use is often reserved for patients in whom the diagnosis remains unclear after a thorough clinical and laboratory evaluation. The biopsy is usually performed by an oral surgeon or otolaryngologist, or other appropriately trained individual. This minor procedure calls for removal of four or more salivary gland lobules through a small incision in the inner lip. A biopsy is considered to be positive if histopathologic analysis shows a focus score of greater than or equal to 1 per 4 mm^2 of tissue, where a focus is defined as a cluster of 50 or more lymphocytes. Using a focus score of greater than or equal to 1 as the cutoff, the sensitivity and specificity of labial salivary gland biopsy for the diagnosis of primary Sjögren's syndrome was reported to be 83.5% and 81.8%, respectively.[19,20] The interpretation of labial salivary gland biopsies is subject to considerable inter-reader variability depending on the experience of the reader. Therefore it is recommended that the biopsy slides be read by an experienced pathologist or other specialist with an appreciation for the nuances of interpretation.

Laboratory Evaluation

Most patients with primary Sjögren's syndrome test positive for serum ANAs. In a large study from Spain, ANAs were detected in sera from 85% of patients with primary Sjögren's syndrome.[135] Approximately one-half and one-third of patients with primary Sjögren's syndrome in this study had anti-Ro/SS-A and anti-La/SS-B antibodies, while about 50% of patients tested positive for rheumatoid factor. There also appears to be a small subset of patients (<5%) with primary Sjögren's syndrome that test negative for serum anti-Ro/SS-A and/or anti-La/SS-B antibodies, but positive for serum anti-centromere antibodies. In one study, such patients with serum anticentromere antibodies had a lower prevalence of dry eyes, hypergammaglobulinemia, and anti-Ro/SS-A and anti-La/SS-B antibodies than other patients with primary Sjögren's syndrome, as well as a higher prevalence of Raynaud's syndrome.[136]

About 5% to 10% of patients with primary Sjögren's syndrome have low blood levels of C3 and C4. For example, 9% of the Spanish cohort referred to earlier had low C3 or C4 levels (13%). About the same proportion of patients with primary Sjögren's syndrome has either type II or III cryoglobulinemia or a monoclonal gammopathy.[135] In type II cryoglobulinemia, the monoclonal gammopathy is usually an IgMκ that has rheumatoid factor activity when the patient resides in a Western or European country; patients of Japanese decent express a higher prevalence of IgA and IgG monoclonal gammopathies.[137] Hematologic abnormalities are observed in about 5% to 15% of patients with primary Sjögren's syndrome and include leukopenia and thrombocytopenia.

Approach to Diagnosis

The clinical diagnosis of primary Sjögren's syndrome is highly likely if a patient with symptoms of dry eyes and dry mouth has objective evidence of keratoconjunctivitis sicca and/or xerostomia in conjunction with a positive test for serum anti-Ro/SS-A and/or anti-La/SS-B antibodies. It may not be necessary to obtain objective evidence of salivary gland involvement if the other clinical and laboratory features are consistent with this diagnosis. In some cases, a clinical diagnosis of primary Sjögren's syndrome may be made in the absence of serum anti-Ro/SS-A and/or anti-La/SS-B antibodies but a moderately or strongly positive test for ANAs. Although accepting a positive ANA alone as the serologic criterion lowers diagnostic specificity, the other clinical and laboratory features can be taken into consideration when making a diagnosis of primary Sjögren's syndromes as opposed to another connective tissue disease or related condition. Because approximately 25% to 50% of patients with primary Sjögren's syndrome test negative for anti-Ro/SS-A and anti-La/SS-B antibodies, a positive test for ANAs may often be the only evidence of an immune-mediated process. Serum ANAs of low titer have relatively little diagnostic value in this setting.

Biopsy of the labial salivary glands may be warranted in cases where signs and symptoms of keratoconjunctivitis sicca and xerostomia are not accompanied by convincing serologic evidence of autoimmunity. The labial salivary gland biopsy is used in this scenario to confirm that glandular hypofunction is associated with a chronic inflammatory process and to explore alternative diagnoses such as sarcoidosis or amyloidosis. In most of these situations, relatively few labial salivary gland biopsies will prove to be positive (focus score ≥1), although a negative result probably reduces the likelihood of primary Sjögren's syndrome to less than 5%.

The diagnosis of primary Sjögren's syndrome in children and adolescents may require special consideration. Compared with adults, children and adolescents present more often with recurrent parotitis, which is not included as a criterion in the recent classification schemes. It has been shown that the inclusion of recurrent parotitis in the classification criteria validated by the American-European Consensus Group increases the sensitivity of diagnosing primary Sjögren's syndrome in children and adolescents from 39% to 76%.[30]

Differential Diagnosis

The differential diagnosis of primary Sjögren's syndrome is broad owing to the variety of conditions that also cause dry eyes and mouth, salivary gland enlargement, and a similar profile of extraglandular manifestations (see Table 73-3). It is important to realize that most patients diagnosed with keratoconjunctivitis sicca by an ophthalmologist do not have primary Sjögren's syndrome, despite a deficiency in aqueous tear flow. The etiology of keratoconjunctivitis in these cases is often obscure and presumably related to aging or hormonal changes or other degenerative processes. Evaporative tear loss secondary to meibomian gland dysfunction is another common cause of dry eyes. Many anticholinergic medications are contributing factors to the sicca complaints. Because approximately 25% of the general population has symptoms of dry mouth, it is not surprising that dry eyes and dry mouth often may coexist in the same patient in the absence of a systemic disease such as Sjögren's syndrome.

Chronic parotitis in association with the sicca complex strongly suggests the diagnosis of Sjögren's syndrome or possibly another systemic disease. Sarcoidosis often comes up in the differential diagnosis of primary Sjögren's syndrome and may even coexist with it. Bilateral diffuse enlargement of the parotid glands from sialadenosis, a noninflammatory process, also may occur in patients with diabetes mellitus who suffer from dry eyes and mouth. In addition, severe hypertriglyceridemia, chronic liver disease, and alcoholism have been associated with sialadenosis and enlargement of the major salivary glands.

A relatively new clinical entity, termed *IgG4-related syndrome* or *IgG4 positive multiorgan lymphoproliferative syndrome,* is emerging as an important consideration in the differential diagnosis of primary Sjögren's syndrome. IgG4-related syndromes are uniquely characterized by high serum levels of IgG4 and tissue biopsies showing a marked infiltration of IgG4+ plasma cells coupled with fibrosis or sclerosis. Compared with primary Sjögren's syndrome, IgG4+-related syndromes do not show the same female predominance and are associated with a lower frequency of dry eyes and mouth, arthralgia, and serum ANA positivity, as well as a higher rate of autoimmune pancreatitis.[138]

TREATMENT

The treatment of primary Sjögren's syndrome aims at reducing the signs and symptoms of dry eyes and dry mouth and ameliorating systemic manifestations (Figure 73-5). Sicca complaints may be lessened in general by withdrawal of medications with drying effects. For the treatment of dry eyes, the patient is advised to avoid central heating and air conditioning, windy environments, and medications that reduce tear and saliva production. Tear supplements are available over the counter in various formulations of different viscosities. Low-viscosity tears are administered more often than high-viscosity tear formulations, which are most useful at bedtime for prolonged lubrication during the sleeping hours. Artificial tears are also available with and without preservatives. Preservative-based tears may worsen dry eyes if they are instilled more than four times per day owing to their toxic effects on the ocular surface. More frequent instillation of tears warrants use of formulations without preservatives.[139]

An ophthalmic preparation of cyclosporine 0.05% (Restasis) has been approved by the U.S. Food and Drug Administration for the treatment of keratoconjunctivitis sicca. In clinical trials, ophthalmic cyclosporine 0.05% has been shown to reduce the signs and symptoms of dry eyes including a statistically significant improvement in tear flow as measured by the Schirmer-I test. Many patients have trouble tolerating ophthalmic cyclosporine because of its burning effects.

Tears may be conserved by blocking the nasolacrimal drainage channels with temporary or permanent occlusion of the punctae, a relatively simple procedure performed by an ophthalmologist. This procedure may be performed in patients with persistent symptoms of dry eyes despite use of artificial tears. Plugs are initially placed in the two inferior punctae because 90% of the tears drain through these channels. Plugs may be later employed to block the two superior

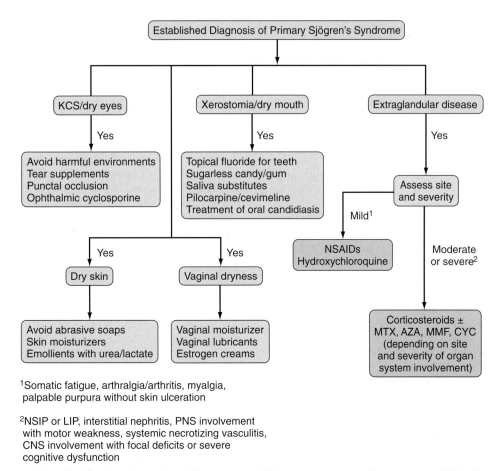

Figure 73-5   Treatment algorithm for Sjögren's syndrome. The treatment of Sjögren's syndrome usually requires a multidisciplinary approach involving rheumatologists, ophthalmologists, dentists/oral surgeons, otolaryngologists, and other subspecialists depending on the extent of extraglandular disease. In all cases, it is prudent to minimize the use of medications that can exacerbate the symptoms of dryness such as antihistamines, antidepressants, muscle relaxers, and other drugs with anticholinergic properties. The treatment of extraglandular disease is individualized according to the site and severity of organ system involvement. The approaches indicated in the algorithm for the treatment of extraglandular disease are not supported by evidence from randomized, controlled trials, but rather from expert opinion based on retrospective case series and clinical experience. AZA, azathioprine; CNS, central nervous system; CYC, cyclophosphamide; KCS, keratoconjunctivitis sicca; LIP, lymphocytic interstitial pneumonitis; MMF, mycophenolate mofetil; MTX, methotrexate; NSAIDs, nonsteroidal anti-inflammatory drugs; NSIP, nonspecific interstitial pneumonitis; PNS, peripheral nervous system.

punctae. Excessive tearing is the most frequent complication of punctual occlusion, which is the rationale for a trial of temporary blockade with dissolvable collagen plugs. Long-term blockage may be achieved using silicone plugs or surgery by cauterization or a laser.

Blepharitis, which commonly occurs in patients with dry eyes, often complicates a dry eye state. Patients with blepharitis may benefit from warm compresses and lid scrubs using an eyelid detergent such as Johnson's Baby Shampoo mixed 1:1 with water. More refractory cases of blepharitis may be managed with chronic doxycycline therapy. Occasionally, the tear film may contain excessive mucous debris that can be dispersed by instillation of a 10% acetylcysteine ophthalmic solution, a mucolytic agent that can be compounded by a pharmacy.

A dry mouth may be managed by replacing existing saliva or stimulating residual salivary flow. Various over-the-counter preparations of artificial saliva are available containing hypromellose or methylcellulose. However, they provide limited relief in most cases because of their short duration of action. Patients may stimulate salivary flow by sucking on sugarless candy or chewing sugarless gum. Two oral secretagogues are available by prescription that stimulate saliva and tear flow. Pilocarpine (Salogen), which acts by stimulating the M3R, is given at a dose of 5 mg three to four times daily and has been shown in controlled clinical trials to improve subjective and objective measures of both dry eyes and dry mouth.[140,141] Cevimeline (Evoxac) also stimulates the M3R and has been similarly shown in trials to improve subjective and objective measures of dry eyes and mouth.[142] Common side effects of these two secretagogues are sweating and flushing, which derive from their mechanism of action. Other possible side effects include visual disturbances, increased urination, nausea, abdominal pain, and diarrhea. Due to their pharmacologic properties, pilocarpine and cevimeline are contraindicated in patients with iritis, narrow angle glaucoma, and moderate-to-severe asthma.

Because xerostomia predisposes to dental carries and broken teeth, daily flossing, frequent dental visits, and regular fluoride applications are recommended for prevention purposes. Oral candidiasis, another complication of xerostimia, may be treated for 10 to 14 days with a nystatin elixir, clotrimazole troches, or fluconazole. Clotrimazole cream is beneficial for the treatment of angular cheilitis, which typically accompanies oral candidiasis.

Patients with primary Sjögren's syndrome also suffer from dryness of the lips, skin, and nasal passages. This problem may be addressed by the frequent application of moisturizers, lip balm, and nasal saline spray. The oily content of vitamin E softgel capsules may be used topically on the skin or the lips for its moisturizing effects. Vaginal dryness with dyspareunia is a frequent complaint of women with primary Sjögren's syndrome. This condition may respond to moisturizers and treatment with a topical estrogen cream. Vaginal lubricants may be necessary for treatment of dyspareunia.

Currently, the therapeutic armamentarium of primary Sjögren's syndrome lacks a proven disease-modifying drug. Clinical experience suggests that symptoms of fatigue, myalgia, and arthralgia/arthritis may respond favorably to treatment with hydroxychloroquine; however, the efficacy of this approach has not been proven in a randomized, controlled clinical trial. Care is taken to avoid doses of hydroxychloroquine exceeding 6.5 mg/kg/day to minimize the risk of retinal toxicity. When this drug is used long term, annual ophthalmologic examinations are recommended to monitor for possible retinal toxicity.

Corticosteroids and other immunosuppressive drugs are often employed for the treatment of organ-threatening extraglandular disease. NSIP and LIP are usually treated with high doses of corticosteroids and other immunosuppressive agents such as azathioprine, mycophenolate mofetil, or cyclophosphamide. Because virtually no controlled data are available supporting the use of these agents for NSIP or LIP, this approach is necessarily empiric and demands judicious monitoring and close follow-up. Bronchiolitis typically improves with high doses of corticosteroids alone, but close follow-up is mandatory for treatment of relapses. Patients who are asymptomatic and have had PFTs showing an isolated mild reduction in DLCO or evidence of small airway disease may be carefully followed without treatment.

Conservative measures may be the only therapy for a sensory peripheral neuropathy where medications such as gabapentin and analgesics may help to control the aggravating and painful neuropathic symptoms. High doses of corticosteroids may produce transient improvement in the symptoms of a peripheral neuropathy, but it is unclear if they provide any long-term benefits and if the benefits outweigh the risks of this treatment. Clinically demonstrable motor loss calls for a more aggressive treatment approach using corticosteroids and other immunosuppressive agents. Some patients with severe motor involvement may benefit from treatment with intravenous immunoglobulin.

A minority of patients with primary Sjögren's syndrome develop recurrent lower extremity purpura. These lesions usually cause burning and stinging and may be associated with lower extremity edema, but they rarely ulcerate. Although moderate to high doses of corticosteroids afford symptomatic relief in most cases, subsequent tapering to low doses and withdrawal usually leads to recurrence of the purpura. Corticosteroid therapy may be avoided in the absence of severe and uncontrollable symptoms or progression to skin ulceration. Support stockings provide symptomatic relief in many cases and can be used in combination with analgesics, antihistamines, or nonsteroidal anti-inflammatory drugs to manage the painful symptoms. The patients are usually left with postinflammatory changes in the skin, which may be an acceptable outcome given the long-term side effects of corticosteroids.

Biologic therapies have been investigated recently for their clinical efficacy and safety in primary Sjögren's syndrome. Infliximab and etanercept, which are TNF inhibitors, have failed in controlled clinical trials to demonstrate therapeutic benefit.[143,144] Preliminary studies of rituximab and epratuzumab have produced mixed results so far,[145-148] and larger studies will be necessary to provide more convincing evidence of clinical efficacy and safety for this indication. Other biologics are on the horizon and will likely be investigated for the treatment of primary Sjögren's syndrome in the near future. The interest in finding a disease-modifying therapy for primary Sjögren's syndrome has led to the initial development of disease activity and damage measures,[149,150] which will require subsequent validation in clinical trials.

OUTCOME

Overall mortality is not increased in patients with primary Sjögren's syndrome compared with the general population, although the subgroup of patients with extraglandular disease has an increased risk of morbidity and death. Compared with the general population, Ioannidis and colleagues[151] showed that mortality was not significantly higher in a cohort of 723 patients with primary Sjögren's syndrome. In this study the patients were subdivided into types I and II according to their risk for complications and death. Approximately 20% of the patients fell into the high-risk, type I group, whereas the remainder in the type II group had no increase in the risk for complications or death. In the type I group, patients presenting with palpable purpura and low C4 levels had a higher risk for long-term complications and death.[151] Similar results were found in another study showing no increase in all-cause mortality among individuals with primary Sjögren's syndrome.[152] Hypocomplementemia has been confirmed as a risk factor for adverse outcomes in another cohort of 336 patients with primary Sjögren's syndrome from Spain.[153]

The disease mechanisms of primary Sjögren's syndrome are being probed with increased interest. The labial salivary gland tissue is readily accessible for biopsy, and the new technologies are dramatically accelerating understanding of the complex pathways intertwining the aberrant innate and adaptive immune responses in this disease. Genetics and genomics are only beginning to permeate the scientific investigation of primary Sjögren's syndrome, and predictably this gap will be filled in the near future. An unanswered question of major import is the cause of the glandular hypofunction. In the earlier stages of disease, it appears that glandular damage does not adequately explain the impaired salivary flow, suggesting that autoantibodies, the cytokine milieu, or both, or other mediators are contributing to these functional abnormalities. Further studies are necessary to address this question owing to the potential reversibility of glandular dysfunction and the nature and timing of therapeutic interventions to be tested in the future.

Although primary Sjögren's syndrome cannot yet claim a disease-modifying therapy, much can be done for patients with this disease by effectively managing the sicca component, ameliorating fatigue and joint pain with hydroxychloroquine therapy, and monitoring for complications. Although biologics such as rituximab may yet prove to be useful for treating Sjögren's syndrome, new therapeutic targets illuminated by translational research will shape the discovery of disease-modifying therapies down the road. Proof of therapeutic efficacy will require instruments that quantify disease activity and damage that are only now under development. Finding that first drug with the properties of disease modification will go a long way toward moving the field forward and expanding the therapeutic options for patients with primary Sjögren's syndrome in the decades to come.

CONCLUSIONS

Primary Sjögren's syndrome occurs nearly as often as rheumatoid arthritis and greater than 10 times more frequently than systemic lupus erythematosus. Therefore it ranks second in prevalence only to rheumatoid arthritis among the autoimmune disorders in the domain of rheumatology. Many patients with mild forms of primary Sjögren's syndrome probably never come to the attention of the rheumatologist, but rather are managed exclusively by primary care physicians, ophthalmologists, otolaryngologists, and dentists. Others may never be referred for a diagnosis because of the frequent misperception that little can be done for patients with Sjögren's syndrome. However, primary Sjögren's syndrome is a systemic autoimmune disease associated with lung, neurologic, and renal involvement; vasculitis; and an increased risk for a low-grade B cell lymphoma, and the rheumatologist is aptly trained to provide an accurate diagnosis and deal effectively with the multisystem complications of this disease.

Selected References

1. Mikulicz J: *Uber eine eigenartige symmetrishe erkankung der tranen und mundspeicheldrusen*, Stuttgart, Germany, 1892, Beitr. Z. Chir. Fesrschr. F. Theodor Billroth, pp 610–630.
2. Sjögren H: Zur kenntnis der keratoconjunctivitis sicca, *Acta Ophthalmol* (Suppl 2):1–151, 1933.
3. Morgan WS, Castleman B: A clinicopathologic study of "Mikulicz's disease", *Am J Pathol* 9:471–503, 1953.
4. Bunim JJ: Heberden Oration. A broader spectrum of Sjögren's syndrome and its pathogenetic implications, *Ann Rheum Dis* 20:1–10, 1961.
5. Talal N, Bunim JJ: The development of malignant lymphoma in the course of Sjögren's syndrome, *Am J Med* 36:529–540, 1964.
6. Beck JS, Anderson JR, Bloch KJ, et al: Antinuclear and precipitating auto-antibodies in Sjögren's syndrome, *Ann Rheum Dis* 24:16–22, 1965.
7. Bloch KJ, Buchanan WW, Wohl MJ, Bunim JJ: Sjögren's syndrome: a clinical, pathological, and serological study of 62 cases, *Medicine* 44:187–231, 1965.
8. Chisholm DM, Mason DK: Labial salivary gland biopsy in Sjögren's disease, *J Clin Pathol* 21:656–660, 1968.
9. Chisholm DM, Waterhouse JP, Mason DK: Lymphocytic sialadenitis in the major and minor salivary gland: a correlation in postmortem subjects, *J Clin Pathol* 23:690–694, 1970.
10. Tarpley TM, Anderson LG, White CL: Minor salivary gland involvement in Sjögren's syndrome, *Oral Surg* 37:64–74, 1974.
11. Greenspan JS, Daniels TE, Talal N, Sylvester RA: The histopathology of Sjögren's syndrome in labial salivary gland biopsies, *Oral Surg* 37:217–229, 1974.
12. Vitali C, Bombardieri S, Jonsson R, et al: Classification criteria for Sjögren's syndrome: a revised version of the European criteria proposed by the American-European consensus group, *Ann Rheum Dis* 61:554–558, 2002.
15. Manthorpe R, Oxholm P, Prause JU, Schiødt M: The Copenhagen criteria for Sjögren's syndrome, *Scand J Rheumatol* (Suppl 61):19–21, 1986.
16. Skopouli FN, Drosos AA, Papaioannou T, Moutsopoulos HM: Preliminary diagnostic criteria for Sjögren's syndrome, *Scand J Rheumatol* (Suppl 61):22–25, 1986.
17. Homma M, Tojo T, Akizuki M, Yamagata H: Criteria for Sjögren's syndrome in Japan, *Scand J Rheumatol* (Suppl 61):26–27, 1986.
18. Fox RI, Robinson CA, Curd JG, et al: Sjögren's syndrome. Proposed criteria for classification, *Arthritis Rheum* 29:577–585, 1986.
19. Vitali C, Bombardieri S, Moutsopoulos HM, et al: Preliminary criteria for the classification of Sjögren's syndrome. Results of a prospective concerted action supported by the European community, *Arthritis Rheum* 36:340–347, 1993.
20. Vitali C, Bombardieri S, Moutsopoulos HM, et al: Assessment of the European classification criteria for Sjögren's syndrome in a series of clinically defined cases: results of a prospective multicentre study, *Ann Rheum Dis* 55:116–121, 1996.
21. Daniels TE, Whitcher JP: Association of patterns of labial salivary gland inflammation with keratoconjunctivitis sicca. Analysis of 618 patients with suspected Sjögren's syndrome, *Arthritis Rheum* 37:869–877, 1994.
22. Rubin H, Holt M: Secretory sialography in diseases of the major salivary glands, *AJR Am J Roentgenol* 77:575–598, 1957.
23. Schall GL, Anderson LG, Wolf RO, et al: Xerostomia in Sjögren's syndrome. Evaluation by sequential salivary scintigraphy, *JAMA* 216:2109–2116, 1971.
26. Gabriel SE, Michaud K: Epidemiological studies in incidence, prevalence, mortality, and comorbidity of the rheumatic diseases, *Arthritis Res Ther* 11:229, 2009.
27. Haugen AJ, Peen E, Hultén B, et al: Estimation of the prevalence of primary Sjögren's syndrome in two age-different community-based populations using two sets of classification criteria: the Horderland Health Study, *Scand J Rheumatol* 37:30–34, 2008.
28. Bowman SJ, Ibrahim GH, Holmes G, et al: Estimating the prevalence among Caucasian women of primary Sjögren's syndrome in two general practices in Birmingham, UK, *Scand J Rheumatol* 33:39–43, 2004.
30. Houghton K, Malleson P, Cabral D, et al: Primary Sjögren's syndrome in children and adolescents: are proposed diagnostic criteria applicable? *J Rheumatol* 32:2225–2232, 2005.
31. Turesson C, O'Fallon WM, Crowson CS, et al: Occurrence of extraarticular disease manifestations is associated with excess mortality in a community based cohort of patients with rheumatoid arthritis, *J Rheumatol* 29:62–67, 2002.
34. Baer AN, Maynard JW, Shaikh F, et al: Secondary Sjögren's syndrome in systemic lupus erythematosus defines a distinct disease subset, *J Rheumatol* 37:1143–1149, 2010.
35. Avouac J, Sordet C, Depinay C, et al: Systemic sclerosis-associated Sjögren's syndrome and relationship to the limited cutaneous subtype: results of a prospective study of sicca syndrome in 133 consecutive patients, *Arthritis Rheum* 54:2243–2249, 2006.
37. Pillemer SR, Brennan MT, Sankar V, et al: Pilot clinical trial of dehydroepiandrosterone (DHEA) versus placebo for Sjögren's syndrome, *Arthritis Care Res* 51:601–604, 2004.
38. Triantafyllopoulou A, Moutsopoulos H: Persistent viral infection in primary Sjögren's syndrome: review and perspectives, *Clin Rev Allergy Immunol* 32:210–214, 2007.
39. Triantafyllopoulou A, Tapinos N, Moutsopoulos HM: Evidence for coxsackievirus infection in primary Sjögren's syndrome, *Arthritis Rheum* 50:2897–2902, 2004.
40. Gottenberg JE, Pallier C, Ittah M, et al: Failure to confirm coxsackievirus infection in primary Sjögren's syndrome, *Arthritis Rheum* 54:2026–2028, 2006.
43. Williams PH, Cobb BL, Namjou B, et al: Horizons in Sjögren's syndrome genetics, *Clinic Rev Allerg Immunol* 32:201–209, 2007.
44. Cobb BL, Lessard CJ, Harley JB, Moser KL: Genes and Sjögren's syndrome, *Rheum Dis Clin N Am* 34:847–868, 2008.
45. Harley JB, Reichlin M, Arnett FC, et al: Gene interaction at HLA-DQ enhances autoantibody production in primary Sjögren's syndrome, *Science* 232:1145–1147, 1986.

49. Mavragani CP, Crow MK: Activation of the type I interferon pathway in primary Sjögren's syndrome, *J Autoimmunity* 35:225–231, 2010.

50. Miceli-Richard C, Comets E, Loiseau P, et al: Association of an IRF5 gene functional polymorphism with Sjogren's syndrome, *Arthritis Rheum* 56:3989–3994, 2007.

51. Takaoka A, Yanai H, Kondo S, et al: Integral role of IRF-5 in the gene induction programme activated by Toll-like receptors, *Nature* 434:243–249, 2005.

53. Miceli-Richard C, Gestermann N, Ittah M, et al: The CGGGG insertion/deletion polymorphism of the IRF5 promoter is a strong risk factor for primary Sjögren's syndrome, *Arthritis Rheum* 60:1991–1997, 2009.

54. Korman BD, Alba MI, Le JM, et al: Variant form of STAT4 is associated with primary Sjögren's syndrome, *Genes Immun* 9:267–270, 2008.

55. Nordmark G, Kristjansdottir G, Theander E, et al: Additive effects of the major risk alleles of IRF5 and STAT4 in primary Sjögren's syndrome, *Genes Immun* 10:68–76, 2009.

56. Nordmark G, Kristjansdottir G, Theander E, et al: Association of EBF1, FAM167A (C8orf13)-BLK and TNFSF4 gene variants with primary Sjögren's syndrome, *Genes Immunity* 12:100–109, 2011.

57. Alevizos I, Alexander S, Turner RJ, Illei GG: MicroRNA expression profiles as biomarkers of minor salivary gland inflammation and dysfunction in Sjögren's syndrome, *Arthritis Rheum* 63:535–544, 2011.

58. Jonsson MV, Delaleu N, Jonsson R: Animal models of Sjögren's syndrome, *Clinic Rev Allerg Immunol* 32:215–224, 2007.

59. Chiorini JA, Cihakova D, Quellette CE, Caturegli P: Sjögren's syndrome: advances in the pathogenesis of animal models, *J Autoimmunity* 33:190–196, 2009.

60. Christodoulou MI, Kapsogeorgou EK, Moutsopoulos HM: Characteristics of the minor salivary gland infiltrates in Sjogren's syndrome, *J Autoimmun* 34:400–407, 2010.

64. Barone F, Bombardieri M, Manzo A, et al: Association of CXCL13 and CCL21 expression with the progressive organization of lymphoid-like structures in Sjögren's syndrome, *Arthritis Rheum* 52:1773–1784, 2005.

65. Gottenberg JE, Cagnard N, Lucchesi C, et al: Activation of IFN pathways and plasmacytoid dendritic cell recruitment in target organs of primary Sjogren's syndrome, *Proc Natl Acad Sci U S A* 103:2770–2775, 2006.

66. Emamian ES, Leon JM, Lessard CJ, et al: Peripheral blood gene expression profiling in Sjögren's syndrome, *Genes Immun* 10:285–296, 2009.

67. Mavragani CP, Moutsopoulos HM: The geoepidemiology of Sjögren's syndrome, *Autoimmunity Rev* 9:A305–A310, 2010.

68. Katsifis GE, Rekka S, Moutsopoulos NM, et al: Systemic and local interleukin-17 and linked cytokines associated with Sjögren's syndrome immunopathogenesis, *Am J Pathol* 175:1167–1177, 2009.

69. Christodoulou MI, Kapsogeorgou EK, Moutsopoulos NM, Moutsopoulos HM: Foxp3+ T-regulatory cells in Sjögren's syndrome: correlation with the grade of the autoimmune lesion and certain adverse prognostic factors, *Am J Pathol* 173:1389–1396, 2008.

71. Bohnhorst J, Bjorgan MB, Thoen JE, et al: Bm1-bm5 classification of peripheral blood B cells reveals circulating germinal center founder cells in healthy individuals and disturbance in the B cell subpopulations in patients with primary Sjögren's syndrome, *J Immunol* 167:3610–3618, 2001.

72. Hansen A, Gosemann M, Pruss A, et al: Abnormalities in peripheral B cell memory of patients with primary Sjögren's syndrome, *Arthritis Rheum* 50:1897–1908, 2004.

73. D'Arbonneau F, Pers JO, Devauchelle V, et al: BAFF-induced changes in B cell receptor-containing lipid rafts in Sjögren's syndrome, *Arthritis Rheum* 54:115–126, 2006.

74. Groom J, Kalled SL, Cutler AH, et al: Association of BAFF/BLyS overexpression and altered B cell differentiation with Sjögren's syndrome, *J Clin Invest* 109:59–68, 2002.

75. Hjelmervik TR, Petersen K, Jonassen I, et al: Gene expression profiling of minor salivary glands clearly distinguishes primary Sjögren's syndrome patients from healthy control subjects, *Arthritis Rheum* 52:1534–1544, 2005.

76. Shen L, Suresh L, Li H, et al: IL-14 alpha, the nexus for primary Sjögren's disease in mice and humans, *Clin Immunol* 130:304–312, 2009.

77. Shen L, Zhang C, Wang T, et al: Development of autoimmunity in interleukin-14alpha transgenic mice, *J Immunol* 177:5676–5686, 2006.

78. Shen L, Suresh L, Wu J, et al: A role for lymphotoxin in primary Sjögren's disease, *J Immunol* 185:6355–6363, 2010.

79. Gatumu MK, Skarstein K, Papandile A, et al: Blockade of lymphotoxin-beta receptor signaling reduces aspects of Sjögren's syndrome in salivary glands of non-obese diabetic mice, *Arthritis Res Ther* 11:R24, 2009.

81. Halse AK, Marthinussen MC, Wahrenherlenius M, Jonsson R: Isotype distribution of anti-Ro/SS-A and anti-La/SS-B antibodies in plasma and saliva of patients with Sjögren's syndrome, *Scand J Rheumatol* 29:13–19, 2000.

82. Li J, Ha Y, Kü N, et al: Inhibitory effects of autoantibodies on the muscarinic receptors in Sjögren's syndrome, *Lab Invest* 84:1430–1438, 2004.

83. Robinson CP, Brayer J, Yamachika S, et al: Transfer of human serum IgG to nonobese diabetic Igµnull mice reveals a role for autoantibodies in the loss of secretory function of exocrine tissues in Sjögren's syndrome, *Proc Natl Acad Sci USA* 95:7538–7543, 1998.

85. Manoussakis MN, Kapsogeorgou EK: The role of epithelial cells in the pathogenesis of Sjögren's syndrome, *Clin Rev Allerg Immunol* 32:225–230, 2007.

86. Fox RI, Kang H, Ando D, et al: Cytokine mRNA expression in salivary gland biopsies of Sjögren's syndrome, *J Immunol* 152:5532–5539, 1994.

89. Xanthou G, Polihronis M, Tzioufas AG, et al: "Lymphoid" chemokine messenger RNA expression by epithelial cells in the chronic inflammatory lesion of the salivary glands of Sjögren's syndrome patients. Possible participation in lymphoid structure formation, *Arthritis Rheum* 44:408–418, 2001.

91. Ittah M, Miceli-Richard C, Gottenberg JE, et al: Viruses induce high expression of BAFF by salivary gland epithelial cells through TLR- and type-I IFN-dependent and -independent pathways, *Eur J Immunol* 38:1058–1064, 2008.

93. Manganelli P, Fietta P: Apoptosis and Sjögren's syndrome, *Semin Arthritis Rheum* 33:49–65, 2003.

94. Ping L, Ogawa N, Sugai S: Novel role of CD40 in Fas-dependent apoptosis of cultured salivary epithelial cells from patients with Sjögren's syndrome, *Arthritis Rheum* 52:573–581, 2005.

96. Dawson LJ, Fox PC, Smith PM: Sjögren's syndrome—the non-apoptotic model of glandular hypofunction, *Rheumatology (Oxford)* 45:792–798, 2006.

97. Jonsson MV, Delaleu N, Brokstad KA, et al: Impaired salivary gland function in NOD mice: association with changes in cytokine profile but not with histopathologic changes in the salivary gland, *Arthritis Rheum* 54:2300–2305, 2006.

98. Ng W, Bowman SJ: Primary Sjögren's syndrome, *Rheumatology (Oxford)* 49:844–853, 2010.

99. Bowman SJ, Booth DA, Platts RG, UK Sjögren's Interest Group: Measurement of fatigue and discomfort in primary Sjögren's syndrome using a new questionnaire tool, *Rheumatology* 43:758–764, 2004.

100. Segal B, Bowman SJ, Fox PC, et al: Primary Sjögren's syndrome: health experiences and predictors of health quality among patients in the United States, *Health Qual Life Outcomes* 7:46, 2009.

101. Segal B, Thomas W, Rogers T, et al: Prevalence, severity, and predictors of fatigue in subjects with primary Sjögren's syndrome, *Arthritis Care Res* 59:1780–1787, 2008.

102. García-Carrasco M, Sisó A, Ramos-Casals M, et al: Raynaud's phenomenon in primary Sjögren's syndrome. Prevalence and clinical characteristics in a series of 320 patients, *J Rheumatol* 29:726–730, 2002.

103. Katayama I, Kotobuki Y, Kiyohara E, Murota H: Annular erythema associated with Sjögren's syndrome: review of the literature on the management and clinical analysis of skin lesions, *Mod Rheumatol* 20:123–129, 2010.

105. Ramos-Casals M, Anaya J, García-Carrasco M, et al: Cutaneous vasculitis in primary Sjögren's syndrome. Classification and clinical significance of 52 patients, *Medicine* 83:96–106, 2004.

106. Fauchais A, Ouattara B, Gondran G, et al: Articular manifestations in primary Sjögren's syndrome: clinical significance and prognosis of 188 patients, *Rheumatology (Oxford)* 49:1164–1172, 2010.

108. Gottenberg J, Mignot S, Nicaise-Rolland P, et al: Prevalence of anti-cyclic citrullinated peptide and anti-keratin antibodies in

patients with primary Sjögren's syndrome, *Ann Rheum Dise* 64:114–117, 2005.

109. Atzeni F, Sarzi-Puttini P, Lama N, et al: Anti-cyclic citrullinated peptide antibodies in primary Sjögren's syndrome may be associated with non-erosive synovitis, *Arthritis Res Ther* 10:R51, 2008.

111. Yazisiz V, Arslan G, Ozbudak IH, et al: Lung involvement in patients with primary Sjögren's syndrome: what are the predictors? *Rheumatol Int* 30:1317–1324, 2010.

112. Ito I, Nagai S, Kitaichi M, et al: Pulmonary manfestations of primary Sjögren's syndrome. A clinical, radiologic, and pathologic study, *Am J Respir Crit Care Med* 171:632–638, 2005.

113. Parambil JG, Myers JL, Lindell RM, et al: Interstitial lung disease in primary Sjögren's syndrome, *Chest* 130:1489–1495, 2006.

115. Maripuri S, Grande JP, Osborn TG, et al: Renal involvement in primary Sjögren's syndrome: a clinicopathologic study, *Clin J Am Soc Nephrol* 4:1423–1431, 2009.

116. Kim YK, Song HC, Kim W, et al: Acquired Gitelman syndrome in a patient with primary Sjögren's syndrome, *Am J Kidney Dis* 52:1163–1167, 2008.

118. Mandl T, Ekberg O, Wollmer P, et al: Dysphagia and dysmotility of the pharynx and oesophagus in patients with primary Sjögren's syndrome, *Scand J Rheumatol* 36:394–401, 2007.

119. Volter F, Fain O, Mathieu E, Thomas M: Esophageal function and Sjögren's syndrome, *Dig Dis Sci* 49:248–253, 2004.

120. Poglio F, Mongini T, Cocito D: Sensory ataxic neuropathy and esophageal achalasia in a patient with Sjögren's syndrome, *Muscle Nerve* 35:532–535, 2007.

122. Matsumoto T, Morizane T, Aoki Y, et al: Autoimmune hepatitis in primary Sjögren's syndrome: pathological study of the livers and labial salivary glands in 17 patients with primary Sjögren's syndrome, *Pathol Int* 55:70–76, 2005.

124. Segal B, Carpenter A, Walk D: Involvement of nervous system pathways in primary Sjögren's syndrome, *Rheum Dis Clin N Am* 34:885–906, 2008.

125. Michel L, Toulgoat F, Desal H, et al: Atypical neurologic complications in patients with primary Sjögren's syndrome, *Semin Arthritis Rheum* 40:338–342, 2011.

126. Kahlenberg JM: Neuromyelitis optica spectrum disorder as an initial presentation of primary Sjögren's syndrome, *Semin Arthritis Rheum* 40:343–348, 2011.

127. Gøransson L, Herigstad A, Tjensvoll AB, et al: Peripheral neuropathy in primary Sjögren's syndrome. A population-based study, *Arch Neurol* 63:1612–1615, 2006.

128. Voulgarelis M, Dafni UG, Isenberg DA, Moutsopoulos HM: Malignant lymphoma in primary Sjögren's syndrome: a multicenter, retrospective, clinical study by the European Concerted Action on Sjögren's Syndrome, *Arthritis Rheum* 42:1765–1772, 1999.

129. Baimpa E, Dahabreh IJ, Voulgarelis M, Moutsopoulos HM: Hematologic manifestations and predictors of lymphoma development in primary Sjögren's syndrome: clinical and pathophysiologic aspects, *Medicine (Baltimore)* 88:284–293, 2009.

130. Ramos-Casals M, García-Carrasco M, Cervera R, et al: Thyroid disease in primary Sjögren's syndrome. Study in a series of 160 patients, *Medicine (Baltimore)* 79:103–108, 2000.

131. Szodoray P, Barta Z, Lakos G, et al: Coeliac disease in Sjögren's syndrome—a study of 111 Hungarian patients, *Rheumatol Int* 24:278–282, 2004.

132. Vinagre F, Santos MJ, Prata A, et al: Assessment of salivary gland function in Sjögren's syndrome: the role of salivary gland scintigraphy, *Autoimmun Rev* 8:672–676, 2009.

133. Wernicke D, Hess H, Gromnica-Ihle E, et al: Ultrasonography of salivary glands—a highly specific imaging procedure for diagnosis of Sjögren's syndrome, *J Rheumatol* 35:285–293, 2008.

134. Niemelä RK, Takalo R, Pääkkö E, et al: Ultrasonography of salivary glands in primary Sjögren's syndrome. A comparison with magnetic resonance imaging and magnetic resonance sialography of parotid glands, *Rheumatology* 43:875–879, 2004.

135. Ramos-Casals M, Solans R, Rosas J, et al: Primary Sjögren's syndrome in Spain. Clinical and immunologic expression in 1010 patients, *Medicine (Baltimore)* 87:210–219, 2008.

136. Vasiliki-Kalliopi KB, Diamanti KD, Vlachoyiannopoulos PG, Moutsopoulos HM: Anticentromere antibody positive Sjögren's syndrome: a retrospective descriptive analysis, *Arthritis Res Ther* 12:R47, 2010.

137. Ramos-Casals M, Cervera R, Yagüe J, et al: Cryoglobulinemia in primary Sjögren's syndrome: prevalence and clinical characteristics in a series of 115 patients, *Semin Arthritis Rheum* 28:200–205, 1998.

138. Masaki Y, Dong L, Kurose N, et al: Proposal for a new clinical entity, IgG$_4$-positive multiorgan lymphproliferative syndrome: analysis of 64 cases of IgG$_4$-related disorders, *Ann Rheum Dis* 68:1310–1315, 2009.

140. Tsifetaki N, Kitsos G, Paschides CA, et al: Oral pilocarpine for the treatment of ocular symptoms in patients with Sjögren's syndrome: a randomised 12 week controlled study, *Ann Rheum Dis* 62:1204–1207, 2003.

141. Vivino FB, Al-Hashimi I, Khan Z, et al: Pilocarpine tablets for the treatment of dry mouth and dry eye symptoms in patients with Sjögren syndrome: a randomized, placebo-controlled, fixed-dose, multicenter trial. P92-01 Study Group, *Arch Intern Med* 159:174–181, 1999.

142. Petrone D, Condemi JJ, Fife R, et al: A double-blind, randomized, placebo-controlled study of cevimeline in Sjögren's syndrome patients with xerostomia and keratoconjunctivitis sicca, *Arthritis Rheum* 46:748–754, 2002.

143. Sankar V, Brennan MT, Kok MR, et al: Etanercept in Sjögren's syndrome: a twelve-week randomized, double-blind, placebo-controlled pilot clinical trial, *Arthritis Rheum* 50:2240–2245, 2004.

144. Mariette X, Ravaud P, Steinfeld S, et al: Inefficacy of infliximab in primary Sjögren's syndrome: results of the randomized, controlled Trial of Remicade in Primary Sjögren's Syndrome (TRIPSS), *Arthritis Rheum* 50:1270–1276, 2004.

145. Steinfeld SD, Tant L, Burmester GR, et al: Epratuzumab (humanised anti-CD22 antibody) in primary Sjogren's syndrome: an open-label phase I/II study, *Arthritis Res Ther* 8:R129, 2006.

146. Dass S, Bowman SJ, Vital EM, et al: Reduction of fatigue in Sjögren syndrome with rituximab: results of a randomised, double-blind, placebo-controlled pilot study, *Ann Rheum Dis* 67:1541–1544, 2008.

147. Devauchelle-Pensec V, Pennec Y, Morvan J, et al: Improvement of Sjögren's syndrome after two infusions of rituximab (anti-CD20), *Arthritis Rheum* 57:310–317, 2007.

148. Pijpe J, van Imhoff GW, Spijkervet FK, et al: Rituximab treatment in patients with primary Sjogren's syndrome: an open-label phase II study, *Arthritis Rheum* 52:2740–2750, 2005.

149. Seror R, Ravaud P, Bowman SJ, et al: EULAR Sjögren's syndrome disease activity index: development of a consensus systemic disease activity index for primary Sjögren's syndrome, *Ann Rheum Dis* 63:1103–1109, 2010.

150. Barry RJ, Sutcliffe N, Isenberg DA, et al: The Sjögren's Syndrome Damage Index—a damage index for use in clinical trials and observational studies in primary Sjögren's syndrome, *Rheumatology (Oxford)* 47:1193–1198, 2008.

151. Ioannidis JP, Vassiliou VA, Moutsopoulos HM: Long-term risk of mortality and lymphoproliferative disease and predictive classification of primary Sjögren's syndrome, *Arthritis Rheum* 46:741–747, 2002.

152. Theander E, Manthorpe R, Jacobsson LT: Mortality and causes of death in primary Sjögren's syndrome: a prospective cohort study, *Arthritis Rheum* 50:1262–1269, 2004.

153. Ramos-Casals M, Brito-Zerón P, Yagüe J, et al: Hypocomplementemia as an immunological marker of morbidity and mortality in patients with primary Sjögren's syndrome, *Rheumatology (Oxford)* 44:89–94, 2005.

Full references for this chapter can be found on www.expertconsult.com.

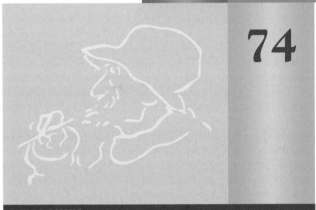

74 Pathogenesis of Ankylosing Spondylitis and Reactive Arthritis

DAVID YU • RIK LORIES •
ROBERT D. INMAN

KEY POINTS

Genetics plays a major role in the etiology of ankylosing spondylitis.

The gene with the greatest contribution to ankylosing spondylitis is HLA-B27.

A major mediator of inflammation is tumor necrosis factor (TNF).

Bone destruction occurs along with pathologic new bone formation in ankylosing spondylitis.

The bone remodeling processes are not necessarily directly linked to the inflammatory processes in ankylosing spondylitis.

Reactive arthritis is initiated by infection outside the joints.

At least in the case of *Chlamydia*-induced arthritis, a modified form of the pathogen can be detected in the joints of some patients.

Ankylosing spondylitis and reactive belong to the family of spondyloarthritis. Reactive arthritis (ReA), is clearly distinct in that it is induced by an episode of acute infection. Accordingly, the pathogenesis of these two diseases will be described in separate sections. For ankylosing spondylitis, it is commonly recognized that two major but "uncoupled" processes coexist inflammation and abnormal bone formation.[1] The process of bone formation in this disease has become a major research frontier.

PATHOGENESIS OF ANKYLOSING SPONDYLITIS

The causes of ankylosing spondylitis are multifactorial and involves a number of interlinking pathways. A considerable number of critical factors have been identified. They can be classified into two groups. One group consists of mediators that are midstream in the pathways leading to inflammation. These mediators are targets of current therapies. The second group of critical factors contributing to ankylosing spondylitis is genetics. How should the degree of contribution of each factor be estimated? For therapeutics, the usefulness of each therapy will be ranked by a statistical value known as *effect size*. In pharmacology, effect size reflects the size of the difference in outcome between groups receiving a drug compared with a group receiving placebo, taking into account the degree of variability within groups. The higher the effect size, the more effective is the therapy. For ranking the genes, we will use the statistical value known as the *population attributable risk*. For each gene, this value represents the incidence of disease in a population that would be eliminated if the gene is absent. The higher the population attributable risk, the greater the contribution to the disease.[2]

Causes of Ankylosing Spondylitis That Are Targets of Therapies

It has been known for more than three decades that most patients with ankylosing spondylitis demonstrate a highly satisfactory response to treatment with nonsteroidal anti-inflammatory drugs (NSAIDs), including the cyclooxygenase-2 (COX-2) inhibitors (coxibs).[3] The effect size for spinal pain is 1.11, which means that there is a 77% probability that a randomly selected NSAID-treated patient will show a better response than a randomly selected placebo-treated patient.[4] This effect size is much greater than in patients with nonspecific chronic low back pain.[5] Because the molecular targets of most NSAIDs are COX-1 and COX-2, and the target of the coxibs is restricted to COX-2, it can be concluded that one of the pathways causing spinal pain in ankylosing spondylitis is the COX-2 pathway.[6] Indeed, the COX-2 pathway generates prostaglandins and thromboxanes, which are strongly proinflammatory. The response of spinal pain in ankylosing spondylitis to NSAIDs is indirect evidence that inflammation is responsible for the pain. In fact, the spinal pain of ankylosing spondylitis is designated as being "inflammatory" rather than "mechanical." The presence of spinal inflammation is validated by magnetic resonance imaging (MRI) observations.[7] Although we know that the COX-2 pathway is responsible in part for the symptoms of ankylosing spondylitis, no information is available as to what triggers this pathway or which downstream mediators are most important.

When responses to NSAIDs are not satisfactory, some patients will be given a trial of a disease-modifying antirheumatic drug (DMARD). Most of the conventional DMARDs useful for rheumatoid arthritis such as methotrexate are much less effective in ankylosing spondylitis.[4] Similar to rheumatoid arthritis, for patients who are resistant to treatment with NSAIDs or conventional DMARDs, there is a very high rate of clinical response to biologically generated agents that target tumor necrosis factor (TNF). Currently, several of these biologics have been approved for the treatment of ankylosing spondylitis in the United States. All are very effective in controlling symptoms. The effect size for etanercept, for example, is 2.25, which means that more than 90% of randomly selected patients will respond better than another randomly selected patient who is treated with placebo.[4] Hence there is little doubt that TNF is a major player in causing the symptoms of ankylosing spondylitis. TNF is a cytokine generated via innate and adaptive immunities by several types of cells, including macrophages, T lymphocytes, and mast cells. TNF is not a factor with a single pathway inducing a single event in a single type of cell. Rather, it is pleiotropic in affecting many cell types, and it induces a network of cytokines and chemokines and other mediators of inflammation.[8] Although it is certain that TNF is a major early upstream mediator in ankylosing spondylitis, no agreement has been reached as to which cell types are specifically responsible for generating TNF, or which processes are disease-specific targets of TNF.

Information derived from the most effective modalities of treatment currently available for ankylosing spondylitis does not provide any concrete clues regarding fundamental causes. As with most chronic diseases, the fundamental causes must be a combination of environmental and genetic factors. What we first need to estimate in ankylosing spondylitis is the degree of contribution of environmental versus genetic factors.

ASSESSMENT OF DEGREE OF CONTRIBUTION BY ENVIRONMENTAL VERSUS GENETIC FACTORS AND IDENTIFICATION OF GENETIC FACTORS

Degrees of contribution of environmental versus genetic factors have been estimated from the degree of concordance among twins. According to those analyses, genetics contributes to more than 90% of the total cause of ankylosing spondylitis. In addition, if there are environmental causes, they are probably ubiquitous, such as enteric bacteria.[9] Indeed, rats carrying the human ankylosing spondylitis–causing transgene HLA-B27 do not develop arthritis when bred in a germ-free environment. However, arthritis will develop once they are transferred to a regular environment.[10] It is thought that the development of arthritis in these rats is related to commensal bacteria, especially in the gastrointestinal tract. In human ankylosing spondylitis, the only enteric bacterium that has been incriminated is *Klebsiella pneumoniae*. As a group, patients with ankylosing spondylitis have higher mean antibody titers to *Klebsiella* compared with control subjects.[11] However, evidence

supporting *Klebsiella* as a cause of ankylosing spondylitis is far less strong than that which supports, for example, that streptococcal infections are a cause of rheumatic fever.

Over the past decade, most of the researchers studying the pathogenesis of ankylosing spondylitis have focused on identification of arthritis-causing genes. According to statistical modeling based on family studies, the disease is caused by up to nine genes with multiplicative interactions among loci.[12] The most important gene, HLA-B27, was discovered in 1973.[13,14] It contributes about 30% of the heritability of the disease. About three decades later, with the development of the technique of genome-wide association study of nonsynonymous single-nucleotide polymorphisms (SNPs), at least four other loci encoding known structural gene sequences have now been reported. In the Wellcome Trust Case Control Consortium and the Australo-Anglo-American Spondylitis Consortium studies, when these genes are ranked according to their degree of contribution, they are listed as follows: HLA-B27, *ERAP1* (endoplasmic reticulum amino peptidase 1, previously known as aminopeptidase-regulating tumor necrosis factor receptor shedding 1, abbreviated as ARTS-1), *IL-23R* (interleukin 23 receptor), *IL-1R2* (interleukin 1 receptor, type II), and *ANTXR2* (anthrax toxin receptor, also known as capillary morphogenesis protein 2, or CMG2). The population attributable risks for the first three are 90%, 26%, and 9%, respectively. Those for *IL-1R2* and *ANTXR2* are probably less than 5%.[15,16] Hence, HLA-B27 is the largest contributor.

How HLA-B27 Induces Ankylosing Spondylitis

The most important gene in ankylosing spondylitis is HLA-B27. In most populations, it is present in more than 90% of patients and in less than 10% of the general population.[17] Rats carrying the HLA-B27 transgene develop arthritis and colitis.[18,19] Using gene terminology from microbiology, it is described as being "essential" for ankylosing spondylitis. Because the association between HLA-B27 and ankylosing spondylitis has been known for more than three decades, the search for how HLA-B27 causes ankylosing spondylitis has been the Holy Grail of many scientists, and an enormous number of publications have been generated. HLA-B27 is an allele of the HLA-B locus of the human leukocyte antigen (HLA) class I antigens. Multiple subtypes of HLA-B27 have been defined.[20] Most experiments attempting to identify the mechanisms of how HLA-B27 mediates arthritis have been carried out with the more common B27*05 and B27*04 subtypes. Multiple hypotheses have been reported regarding how HLA-B27 molecules mediate arthritis. At least three hypotheses are currently under active investigation.

Arthritogenic Peptide Hypothesis

The arthritogenic peptide hypothesis is based on the classic structure and the canonical function of HLA-B alleles. As in all HLA class I molecules, a classic HLA-B27 molecule is a trimolecular complex of a polymorphic HLA class I heavy chain together with a monomorphic light chain ($\beta2$-microglobulin [$\beta2$m]) and a single highly variable peptide (Figure 74-1). Most of the peptides are nanomers that

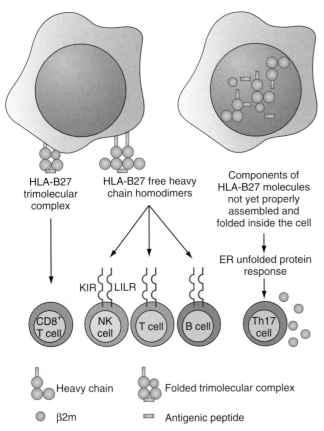

Figure 74-1 Three different structures of HLA-B27 and how they might induce the processes of arthritis. HLA-B27 is first generated as a free heavy chain, which inside the cell becomes associated and folded with β2-microglobulin (β2m) and antigenic peptide, and then becomes expressed on the cell surface as a trimolecular complex. It can also be expressed on the cell surface as homodimers of heavy chains without β2m. ER, endoplasmic reticulum; KIR, killer-cell immunoglobulin-like receptor; LILR, leukocyte immunoglobulin-like receptor; NK, natural killer.

conform to a strict motif, usually with arginine as the second amino acid. The motif of peptides that bind to HLA-B27 is different from that of peptides that bind to other HLA-B alleles or to HLA-A or -C molecules.[21,22] These polymorphisms probably are driven by evolution to survey against ever changing pathogens such as the influenza viruses. The canonical function of HLA-A and -B molecules is to present peptides derived from such intracellular pathogens to CD8+ T lymphocytes to generate a protective adaptive immune response.[23] The reason why this is vulnerable to autoimmunity is that most of the peptides complexed with HLA-A and -B molecules are derived from self-proteins. In health, the hosts are tolerant to all these self-peptides.

The arthritogenic peptide hypothesis postulates that in the case of ankylosing spondylitis, there is a breakdown of tolerance to certain self-peptides, and this breakdown is a consequence of mimicry between the self-peptides and certain pathogen-derived and arthritis-causing peptides.[24] Identification of these arthritogenic peptides demands a great deal of fundamental information concerning the quaternary structures of the HLA-peptide complexes, as well as the dynamics of these structures, the peptide repertoires of candidate pathogens, the repertoires of self-peptides, and last, the repertoires of T cell receptors. At this

point, enormous detail has been generated concerning the structures of HLA-peptide complexes. Reactivity against several self-peptides has also been reported. Many yet untested candidate peptides have recently been identified and will require testing in the future, perhaps with newly developed immunoproteomic techniques.[25,26]

Free Heavy Chain Hypothesis

The free heavy chain hypothesis is based on the observation that HLA-B27 molecules can exist on the cell surface as free heavy chains free of the more usual association with β2m or peptides with the classic HLA-B27 motif (see Figure 74-1). These free heavy chains exist as stable dimers and are capable of engaging allele-specific receptors on natural killer (NK) cells and T lymphocytes. Receptors for HLA-B27 free heavy chain dimers are the *KIR3DL1*001* allele of KIRs (a family of immunoglobulin-like receptors on NK cells and certain subsets of T cells) and the *LILRA1* and *LILRB2* alleles of LILRs (a family of leukocyte immunoglobulin-like receptors on NK cells, T and B cells, and cells of the myeloid lineage).[27] The free heavy chain hypothesis postulates that engagement of these receptors will generate arthritis-causing events. This hypothesis is supported by actual observations of ankylosing spondylitis patients. Such HLA-B27 heavy chain dimers are found on the cell surfaces of mononuclear cells, along with expansion of KIR3DL2-expressing NK and CD4+ T cells responding to such dimers.[28,29]

Unfolded Protein Hypothesis

The unfolded protein hypothesis is different from the previous two in that it is concerned not with activities of HLA-B27 on the cell surface, but with activities inside the cells (see Figure 74-1). Like most surface proteins, the HLA-B27 heavy chains are synthesized linearly into a processing organelle inside the cell by the endoplasmic reticulum (ER). At first, these newly synthesized proteins do not have any conformation and are described as being "unfolded." Then, they are stepwise driven into a series of conformations through sequential complexing with a corresponding series of ER chaperones. These ER chaperones generate conformations in their target proteins by binding to their inappropriately exposed hydrophobic domains, as well as to underglycosylated residues. Through a series of cycles of binding and release with a series of ER chaperones, formation of disulfide bonds, and pairing with the β2m and a peptide, an HLA-B27 molecule will mature into a quaternary and stable form, which then will be transported to the cell surface.[30]

This sequence of events takes place over a period of time. Compared with a few other common HLA alleles, HLA-B27 heavy chains have more prolonged retention times inside the ER. In addition, with HLA-B27, more partially misfolded and unfolded forms are found inside the ER compared with other HLA alleles. Reasons include aberrant disulfide bond formation and multimer formation among the heavy chains, among others. These partially folded or misfolded HLA-B27 proteins remain for a time sequestrated inside the ER, being complexed with chaperones such as the "immunoglobulin heavy chain–binding protein," abbreviated as BiP (GRP78, 78-kD glucose-regulated protein). BiP is a sensor for accumulation of misfolded proteins. It initiates several ER processes, which together are termed *unfolded protein response* (UPR).[31,32] UPR can be cytoprotective or might lead to apoptosis. UPR is associated with a number of diseases, including cancer, diabetes, atherosclerosis, and neurologic disorders. For ankylosing spondylitis, it has been observed in an in vitro system that UPR with HLA-B27 polarizes the cells in response to lipopolysaccharide to cross-talk with the cytokine systems by generating interleukin (IL)-23. The HLA-B27 unfolded protein hypothesis postulates that HLA-B27 induces an unfolded protein response, which, in conjunction with activation by pattern recognition receptors (PRRs) such as those for lipopolysaccharide, would generate proinflammatory cytokines to such a degree as to cause arthritis.[32,33]

How Non–Major Histocompatibility Complex Genes Modify HLA-B27 Physiology

Each of the three hypotheses of how HLA-B27 causes ankylosing spondylitis are based to a large extent on in vitro observations, to a lesser extent on observations in animal models, and even less on patient-derived samples. They are working hypotheses in the sense that they are not yet capable of being translated to the bedside for diagnosis or for development of therapeutics. However, strong support has appeared recently from studies of the biology of ankylosing spondylitis–associated genes identified by the genome-wide association study.

Probably the most important non–major histocompatibility complex (MHC) gene discovered so far is *ERAP1*. The association of *ERAP1* with ankylosing spondylitis has been replicated in multiple populations, including white and nonwhite ethnicities.[34] Equally significant, in one familial study, disease association has been extended to a haplotype of *ERAP1* and *ERAP2*, indicating that the disease association is with a biology common to *ERAP1* and *ERAP2*.[35] *ERAP1* and *ERAP2* are metalloproteinases sharing considerable structural identity with one another. As described earlier, for HLA-B27 to mature into a trimolecular complex inside the endoplasmic reticulum, each heavy chain has to become associated with the monomorphic β2m and a polymorphic peptide. These peptides are derived from proteins that are degraded in the proteasomes outside the endoplasmic reticulum and are transported into the endoplasmic reticulum, often with lengths exceeding the HLA class I peptide motif. *ERAP1* and *ERAP2* are aminopeptidases, which degrade the peptides to suitable lengths to be accommodated into the HLA class I heavy chain–β2m complex.[36,37] It is conceivable that alteration of the expression or the structures of these aminopeptidases can change the peptide repertoire of HLA-B27 or can lead to events postulated by the free heavy chain or the unfolded protein response hypotheses.

How Non–Major Histocompatibility Complex Genes Modify the Cytokine Network

As was described in a previous section, a major mediator of ankylosing spondylitis is TNF. TNF is situated relatively upstream mechanistically in a vast network of arthritis-causing cytokines such as IL-1, -6, and -17.[8] This network is a self-organizing complex kept in balance with self-regulating inhibitors. Three of the non-MHC ankylosing spondylitis genes can potentially perturb such balance in the cytokine network. The activities of two of the ankylosing spondylitis genes—*IL-1R* and *IL-23R*—are self-evident. IL-23R is especially appealing to the pathogenesis of ankylosing spondylitis because it leads to the generation of IL-17, a cytokine that probably holds as pivotal a position as TNF.[38] The other non-MHC ankylosing spondylitis gene, *ERAP1*, apparently has dual biologic activity. Its activities inside the ER have already been described earlier. When present on the cell surface, *ERAP1* aids in release of the receptors for TNF, IL-1, and IL-6.[34,39] It is possible that polymorphisms of *ERAP1* can modify the balance of the cytokine network through this receptor-releasing activity, which favors the development of ankylosing spondylitis.

STRUCTURAL DAMAGE IN ANKYLOSING SPONDYLITIS

Previous sections on research into the pathogenesis of ankylosing spondylitis do not directly address the processes of bone destruction and bone formation. Ankylosing spondylitis (AS) is a disease that typically affects the structures of the spine and the entheses. In the spine, the areas involved are the sacroiliac joints, the vertebral bodies, and the zygapophyseal joints. Enthesitis, on the other hand, is an extra-articular manifestation defined as inflammation at the anatomic zones where ligaments or tendons insert into underlying bone. Examples include the Achilles tendon and the fascia plantaris. Less commonly, peripheral arthritis can also be present in AS patients. Synovitis and enthesitis, joint erosions, bony sclerosis, and progressive bridging of the joint space (ankylosis) characterize sacroiliac joint involvement. In the vertebral bodies, osteitis is associated with loss of trabecular bone, leading to osteoporosis and increased fracture risk.[40] Paradoxically, at the same time, new bone formation can lead to syndesmophyte formation, and eventually ankylosis is found in the same disease and the same patients. In the zygapophyseal joints, inflammation and ankylosis are also recognized. Extra-articular enthesitis is characterized by bone marrow edema and by bony spur formation. A number of features have been proposed as typical for synovitis in AS and related spondyloarthritides, as compared with other rheumatic diseases.[41] These include the presence of specific macrophage subsets, neutrophils, and increased vascularity.

Both inflammation and progressive ankylosis are considered to be separate targets for therapeutic intervention. The two processes are independent of each other, but both can lead to loss of mobility in AS.[42] In the past, most of the research attention has been focused on mechanisms of inflammation. More recently, the process of ankylosis has become a new and high-priority research target. Progressive ankylosis is highly variable between individuals and in most patients shows a fairly slow course.[43] Despite their success in controlling patients' symptoms, anti-TNF strategies have failed to show an inhibitory effect on spinal ankylosis.[44-46] These drugs do have a positive effect on the inflammation-associated osteoporosis that can lead to vertebral fractures.[8]

The link between inflammation and ankylosis, however, remains poorly understood.

Anatomic and Molecular Bases of Ankylosis

Histomorphologic studies of the spine are relatively rare owing to difficulty in accessing the tissues. Based on studies performed decades ago, several different mechanisms of new bone formation have been proposed.[47] Both endochondral and direct bone (also known as membranous) formation appear to play a role. These two different types of bone formation have been best studied during development.[48] The process of endochondral bone formation is critical for the development of the long bones and starts with proliferation and condensation of precursor cells. These cells subsequently differentiate into chondrocytes, which produce an extracellular matrix rich in type II collagen. Articular chondrocytes appear not to further differentiate and have a stable phenotype. Developmental and growth plate chondrocytes, on the other hand, progress into hypertrophic chondrocytes. These cells produce a matrix rich in type X collagen. This matrix gets calcified, is invaded by newly forming vessels, becomes broken down, and is gradually replaced by bone with active osteoblasts as the cellular component. Membranous or direct bone formation is important for the development of the skull and for cortical bone growth.

Unlike endochondral bone formation, in membranous bone formation, progenitor cells directly differentiate into osteoblasts. In ankylosing spondylitis, the shape of the syndesmophytes and their volume suggest that endochondral bone formation is more important than membranous bone formation. However, growth factors that steer endochondral and direct membranous bone formations belong to the same families, and the differentiation process of the progenitor cells is likely determined by the specific localization of the cells and local balances between growth factors. A third process, chondroid metaplasia, has been proposed as an additional mechanism for ankylosing spondylitis. In this process, the chondrocyte matrix is calcified and thus becomes a bone-like tissue. In summary, the temporospatial relationship between inflammation and new bone formation in AS is not clear from these studies. Recent work shows that both classical innate and adaptive immune systems might also participate.[49]

From the molecular perspective, most data concerning ankylosing spondylitis have been derived from mouse models. Based on the view that new bone formation will recapitulate to some extent bone development and growth, a critical role for bone morphogenetic protein (BMP) and Wnt signaling has been proposed (Figure 74-2). In a mouse model of enthesitis, Noggin, a BMP antagonist, inhibits new bone formation originating from the enthesis in peripheral joints.[50] In a human TNF transgenic mouse model of joint destruction, antibodies against DKK1, a Wnt co-receptor antagonist, reversed the arthritis phenotype from erosive to remodeling.[51] Although these animal models have clear limitations, they potentially identify key mechanisms and therapeutic targets.

The specific molecular cascades involved in bone erosion and in osteoporosis in patients with AS have been even less studied. Often it is just assumed that excessive activation of osteoclasts by the receptor activator of nuclear factor κB (NFκB) ligand (RANKL)-RANK system plays a critical role.

Relationship between Inflammation and New Tissue Formation

The specific phenotype of ankylosing spondylitis with progressive spinal ankylosis remains enigmatic. Other diseases such as fibrodysplasia ossificans progressiva, diffuse idiopathic skeletal hyperostosis, and sometimes osteoarthritis, are also characterized by excessive bone formation. These facts and interindividual variability among AS patients suggest that genetic factors may play a role in AS.

Specific localization of new bone formation at entheseal sites suggests that biomechanical factors may play an important role.[52] Bony spurs are found at entheseal sites in degenerative lesions and often are associated with strain. Whether there is a direct relationship between inflammation and new bone formation remains controversial. In most experimental systems, proinflammatory cytokines inhibit chondrogenesis and osteogenesis. In other joint diseases such as rheumatoid arthritis, TNF likely contributes to inhibition of repair by upregulating antagonists of the Wnt signaling pathway such as DKK1.[53] Different and contrasting but not mutually exclusive hypotheses have been put forward to explain the apparent paradox of an inflammatory disease associated with new tissue formation[47,53,54] (see Figure 74-2). Two of these support the concept that inflammation in AS can subside spontaneously, thereby leaving windows of opportunity for tissue repair ultimately leading to ankylosis. The third hypothesis proposes that chronic inflammation and progressive ankylosis are linked, but that they are in molecular terms largely independent processes. In this hypothesis, cell stress and damage at the enthesis are proposed as disease-initiating events.

It remains unclear whether very early treatment of patients with anti-TNF drugs will have an impact on structural progression. It is possible that future therapeutics based on modulation of BMP and Wnt signaling could have an additional effect on ankylosis, but given the critical role of these pathways in the homeostasis of different organs, simple antagonist or agonist approaches may have toxicity issues. The single observation that celecoxib has an effect on structural disease progression indicates that modulation of bone formation is possible.[55] In this case, it is hypothesized that this anti-inflammatory drug has a direct effect on bone formation, and that this particular effect is not linked to symptom control. A major problem in interpreting the results of therapeutic studies so far is that it is not clear which particular patients are prone to new bone formation. Research conducted to identify this specific at-risk patient group will be critical. Moreover, these efforts may lead to better insights into initiating pathophysiologic mechanisms of the disease.

PATHOGENESIS OF REACTIVE ARTHRITIS

Reactive arthritis (ReA)—a sterile synovitis precipitated by an extra-articular infection—has been a challenge for resolving pathogenesis definitively. ReA is the quintessential paradigm of host susceptibility interacting with

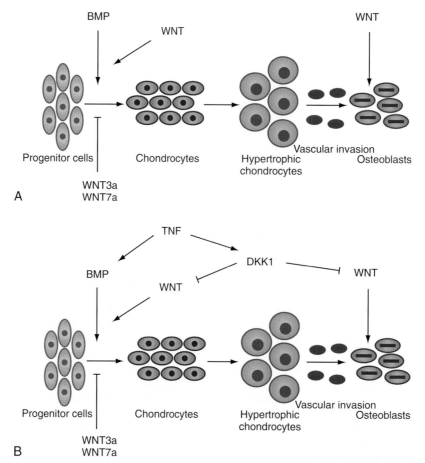

Figure 74-2   Roles of bone morphogenetic proteins (BMPs) and WNTs in endochondral bone formation. **A,** Physiologic endochondral bone formation is stimulated by BMPs. WNTs play a supportive role for BMPs. However, some WNTs have a negative effect on early chondrocyte differentiation. **B,** In the presence of inflammation, tumor necrosis factor (TNF) may stimulate BMP signaling as well as expression of DKK1, which acts as a WNT antagonist. The balance between TNF, BMP, and WNT signaling may determine the onset and progression of ankylosis.

an environmental trigger; as such, it sets a conceptual framework that underlies a broad range of rheumatic diseases. Indeed, ReA occupies an interesting middle ground between autoimmune and autoinflammatory inflammatory diseases.[56] Studies in ReA and undifferentiated oligoarthritis indicate that about 50% of such cases can be attributed to a specific pathogen by a combination of culture and serology, the predominant organisms being *Salmonella, Yersinia,* and *Chlamydia.*[57] Species-specific analysis of serologic responses to pathogens may further enhance this detection rate. A recent population-based study sought to define the epidemiology and clinical spectrum of ReA following culture-confirmed infection with bacterial enteric pathogens in the United States.[58] Telephone interviews were conducted with persons who had culture-confirmed *Campylobacter, Escherichia coli* O157, *Salmonella, Shigella,* or *Yersinia* infection in Minnesota and Oregon between 2002 and 2004. The estimated incidence of ReA following culture-confirmed *Campylobacter, E. coli* O157, *Salmonella, Shigella,* or *Yersinia* infection in Oregon was 0.6 to 3.1 cases per 100,000.

Cytokines in Reactive Arthritis

Analysis of T cell subsets with respect to cytokine profiles is a further method for studying the link between infection

and reactive arthritis. Exposure to different pathogens can stimulate at least two patterns of cytokine production by CD4[+] T cells (T helper [Th]1 and Th2). Th1 cells mediate a protective role against intracellular pathogens. Thus, it would seem appropriate that these cells would be central in clinical complications of such infections. In a study of 11 patients with ReA, it was observed that stimulation of synovial fluid mononuclear cells resulted in secretion of low amounts of interferon (IFN)-γ and TNF but high amounts of IL-10.[59] IL-10 was responsible for suppression of IFN-γ and TNF as judged by the effect of adding IL-10 or anti–IL-10 to cells. Enhanced production of TNF and IFN-γ is observed in chronic ReA when compared with acute ReA or rheumatoid arthritis.[60] TNF dependence of chronic inflammation in the spine draws indirect support from the dramatic changes that follow the institution of anti-TNF therapy in these patients. A study investigated TNF production in healthy subjects with previous *Yersinia*-triggered ReA.[61] The study comprised HLA-B27[+] subjects with ReA (B27[+]ReA[+]), in contrast to B27[+]ReA[-] and B27[-]ReA[-] subjects. It was observed that B27[+]ReA[+] supernatants had higher TNF levels than B27[+]ReA[-] supernatants after stimulation with the phorbol ester, phorbol myristate acetate (PMA), and the calcium ionophore, A23187. Patients who have recovered from *Yersinia* ReA show enhanced TNF production, which may be regulated at the level of monocyte adhesion. A recent study measured levels of several proinflammatory and immunoregulatory cytokines in synovial fluid and sera from patients with ReA and undifferentiated spondyloarthritis, in comparison with rheumatoid arthritis and osteoarthritis.[62] Synovial fluid concentrations of IL-17, IL-6, transforming growth factor (TGF)-β, and IFN-γ were significantly higher in patients with ReA as compared with RA patients. Synovial fluid levels of IL-10 were comparable, but the ratio of IFN-γ/IL-10 was significantly higher in ReA patients than in rheumatoid arthritis patients. IL-17, IL-6, IL-10, and IFN-γ synovial fluid levels were significantly higher than paired serum levels in ReA patients. These findings suggest that Th17 cells, as well as Th1 cells, could be playing a major role in the chronic inflammation seen in ReA.

Innate Immunity and Reactive Arthritis

Recognition that critical host determinants are operational as the first line of defense against pathogens, and that these determinants precede adaptive immunity, represents a major advance in our understanding of host-microbial interactions. ReA represents the paradigm of a dynamic interaction between genetically defined host susceptibility and an environmental trigger. Thus, it is particularly relevant to examine innate immunity of the host because these events, which set the stage for the subsequent development of adaptive immunity, occur early in the course of a challenge by an arthritogenic pathogen. A recent outbreak of salmonellosis was accompanied by ReA and afforded investigators the opportunity to study genetic susceptibility to ReA, which traditionally has been difficult in examining sporadic cases of ReA.[63] Using this cohort and exposed non-ReA individuals as controls, a recent study examined the role of innate immunity in ReA.[64] Genotyping was performed using two TLR2 (*rs5743708* and *rs5743704*) and two TLR4 (*rs4986790* and *rs4986791*) SNPs. No TLR4 exon variants were associated with any clinical events accompanying the *Salmonella* infection. In contrast, one of the rare TLR2 SNPs (*rs5743708*; *R753Q*) was associated with the development of ReA. The TLR2 variant 753Q was not detected in any of the infected individuals with an uncomplicated course. Another TLR2 variant, 631H, was associated with articular symptoms in infected men. This is the first demonstration that genetic variants of TLR2, but not TLR4, are associated with clinical ReA.

The contribution of TLR interactions in *Chlamydia* has also been studied recently.[65] *Chlamydia trachomatis*–inactivated elementary bodies (EBs) and the following antigens were tested for their ability to induce the production of proinflammatory cytokines by human monocytes/macrophages and THP-1 cells: purified lipopolysaccharide, recombinant heat shock protein (rhsp)70, rhsp60, rhsp10, recombinant polypeptide encoded by open reading frame 3 of the plasmid (rpgp3), recombinant macrophage infectivity potentiator (rMip), and recombinant outer membrane protein 2 (rOmp2). Aside from EB, rMip displayed the greatest ability to induce release of IL-1β, TNF, IL-6, and IL-8. Stimulating pathways appeared to involve TLR2/TLR1/TLR6 with the help of CD14 but not TLR4. These data support a role for Mip lipoprotein in the pathogenesis of *C. trachomatis*–induced inflammatory responses and

heighten attention on innate immunity during *Chlamydia* infection.

Response of Reactive Arthritis to Antibiotic Treatment

Recognition that *C. trachomatis* and *C. pneumoniae* species may exist in a persistent metabolically active infective state in the synovium has suggested that persistent chlamydiae may be susceptible to antimicrobial agents. A recent study undertook a 9-month, double-blind prospective trial to assess a 6-month course of combination antibiotics as treatment for *Chlamydia*-induced ReA.[66] Treatment arms consisted of doxycycline and rifampin, azithromycin and rifampin, and placebo. After 6 months of treatment, 17 of 27 subjects (63%) on antibiotics were responders compared with 3 of 15 (20%) on placebo. Antibiotic treatment was associated with significant improvement in the modified swollen joint count and tender joint count. Significantly more subjects became polymerase chain reaction negative at month 6 in the active therapy group than in the placebo group. These data suggest that a 6-month course of combination antibiotics might serve as effective therapy for chronic *Chlamydia*-induced ReA. Further studies will be needed to determine whether this approach is effective in ReA triggered by other pathogens.

References

1. Tam LS, Gu J, Yu D: Pathogenesis of ankylosing spondylitis, *Nat Rev Rheumatol* 6:399–405, 2010.
2. Rowe AK, Powell KE, Flanders WD: Why population attributable fractions can sum to more than one, *Am J Prev Med* 26:243–249, 2004.
3. Goh L, Samanta A: A systematic MEDLINE analysis of therapeutic approaches in ankylosing spondylitis, *Rheumatol Int* 29:1123–1135, 2009.
4. Zochling J, Heijde D, Burgos-Vargas R, et al: ASAS/EULAR recommendationvan ders for the management of ankylosing spondylitis, *Ann Rheum Dis* 65:442–452, 2006.
5. Chou R, Huffman LH: Medications for acute and chronic low back pain: a review of the evidence for an American Pain Society/American College of Physicians clinical practice guideline, *Ann Intern Med* 147:505–514, 2007.
6. Vane JR, Bakhle YS, Botting RM: Cyclooxygenases 1 and 2, *Annu Rev Pharmacol Toxicol* 38:97–120, 1998.
7. Bennett AN, Rehman A, Hensor EM, et al: Evaluation of the diagnostic utility of spinal magnetic resonance imaging in axial spondylarthritis, *Arthritis Rheum* 60:1331–1341, 2009.
8. Tracey D, Klareskog L, Sasso EH, et al: Tumor necrosis factor antagonist mechanisms of action: a comprehensive review, *Pharmacol Ther* 117:244–279, 2008.
9. Brown MA, Kennedy LG, MacGregor AJ, et al: Susceptibility to ankylosing spondylitis in twins: the role of genes, HLA, and the environment, *Arthritis Rheum* 40:1823–1828, 1997.
10. Taurog JD, Maika SD, Satumtira N, et al: Inflammatory disease in HLA-B27 transgenic rats, *Immunol Rev* 169:209–223, 1999.
11. Rashid T, Ebringer A: Ankylosing spondylitis is linked to *Klebsiella*—the evidence, *Clin Rheumatol* 26:858–864, 2007.
12. Brown MA, Laval SH, Brophy S, Calin A: Recurrence risk modelling of the genetic susceptibility to ankylosing spondylitis, *Ann Rheum Dis* 59:883–886, 2000.
13. Brewerton DA, Hart FD, Nicholls A, et al: Ankylosing spondylitis and HL-A 27, *Lancet* 1:904–907, 1993.
14. Schlosstein L, Terasaki PI, Bluestone R, Pearson CM: High association of an HL-A antigen, W27, with ankylosing spondylitis, *N Engl J Med* 288:704–706, 1973.
15. Burton PR, Clayton DG, Cardon LR, et al: Association scan of 14,500 nonsynonymous SNPs in four diseases identifies autoimmunity variants, *Nat Genet* 39:1329–1337, 2007.

16. Reveille JD, Sims AM, Danoy P, et al: Genome-wide association study of ankylosing spondylitis identifies non-MHC susceptibility loci, *Nat Genet* 42:123–127, 2010.

17. Khan MA: Epidemiology of HLA-B27 and arthritis, *Clin Rheumatol* 15(Suppl 1):10–12, 1996.

18. Hammer RE, Maika SD, Richardson JA, et al: Spontaneous inflammatory disease in transgenic rats expressing HLA-B27 and human beta 2m: an animal model of HLA-B27-associated human disorders, *Cell* 63:1099–1112, 1990.

19. Milia AF, Ibba-Manneschi L, Manetti M, et al: HLA-B27 transgenic rat: an animal model mimicking gut and joint involvement in human spondyloarthritides, *Ann N Y Acad Sci* 1173:570–574, 2009.

20. Khan MA: HLA and spondyloarthropathies. In Mehra N, editor: *The HLA complex in biology and medicine*, New Delhi, 2010, Jaypee Brothers Medical Publishers, pp 422–446.

21. Madden DR, Gorga JC, Strominger JL, Wiley DC: The structure of HLA-B27 reveals nonamer self-peptides bound in an extended conformation, *Nature* 353:321–325, 1991.

22. Madden DR, Gorga JC, Strominger JL, Wiley DC: The three-dimensional structure of HLA-B27 at 2.1A resolution suggests a general mechanism for tight peptide binding to MHC, *Cell* 70:1035–1048, 1992.

23. Young AC, Zhang W, Sacchettini JC, Nathenson SG: MHC class I-peptide interactions and TCR recognition, *Cancer Surv* 22:17–36, 1995.

24. Lopez de Castro JA: HLA-B27 and the pathogenesis of spondyloarthropathies, *Immunol Lett* 108:27–33, 2007.

25. Ben Dror L, Barnea E, Beer I, et al: The HLA-B*2705 peptidome, *Arthritis Rheum* 62:420–429, 2010.

26. Lopez de Castro JA: The HLA-B27 peptidome: building on the cornerstone, *Arthritis Rheum* 62:316–319, 2010.

27. Kollnberger S, Bowness P: The role of B27 heavy chain dimer immune receptor interactions in spondyloarthritis, *Adv Exp Med Biol* 649:277–285, 2009.

28. Kollnberger S, Bird LA, Roddis M, et al: HLA-B27 heavy chain homodimers are expressed in HLA-B27 transgenic rodent models of spondyloarthritis and are ligands for paired Ig-like receptors, *J Immunol* 173:1699–1710, 2004.

29. Kollnberger S, Chan A, Sun MY, et al: Interaction of HLA-B27 homodimers with KIR3DL1 and KIR3DL2, unlike HLA-B27 heterotrimers, is independent of the sequence of bound peptide, *Eur J Immunol* 37:1313–1322, 2007.

30. Chapman DC, Williams DB: ER quality control in the biogenesis of MHC class I molecules, *Semin Cell Dev Biol* 21:512–519, 2010.

31. Austin RC: The unfolded protein response in health and disease, *Antioxid Redox Signal* 11:2279–2287, 2009.

32. Turner MJ, Delay ML, Bai S, et al: HLA-B27 up-regulation causes accumulation of misfolded heavy chains and correlates with the magnitude of the unfolded protein response in transgenic rats: implications for the pathogenesis of spondylarthritis-like disease, *Arthritis Rheum* 56:215–223, 2007.

33. Colbert RA, DeLay ML, Layh-Schmitt G, Sowders DP: HLA-B27 misfolding and spondyloarthropathies, *Prion* 3:15–26, 2009.

34. Haroon N, Inman RD: Endoplasmic reticulum aminopeptidases: biology and pathogenic potential, *Nat Rev Rheumatol* 6:461–467, 2010.

35. Tsui FW, Haroon N, Reveille JD, et al: Association of an ERAP1 ERAP2 haplotype with familial ankylosing spondylitis, *Ann Rheum Dis* 69:733–736, 2010.

36. Kanaseki T, Blanchard N, Hammer GE, et al: ERAAP synergizes with MHC class I molecules to make the final cut in the antigenic peptide precursors in the endoplasmic reticulum, *Immunity* 25:795–806, 2006.

37. Yan J, Parekh VV, Mendez-Fernandez Y, et al: In vivo role of ER-associated peptidase activity in tailoring peptides for presentation by MHC class Ia and class Ib molecules, *J Exp Med* 203:647–659, 2006.

38. van den Berg WB, Miossec P: IL-17 as a future therapeutic target for rheumatoid arthritis, *Nat Rev Rheumatol* 5:549–553, 2009.

39. Cui X, Rouhani FN, Hawari F, Levine SJ: An aminopeptidase, ARTS-1, is required for interleukin-6 receptor shedding, *J Biol Chem* 278:28677–28685, 2003.

40. Vosse D, Landewe R, van der Heijde D, et al: Ankylosing spondylitis and the risk of fracture: results from a large primary care-based nested case-control study, *Ann Rheum Dis* 68:1839–1842, 2009.

41. Baeten D, Kruithof E, De Rycke L, et al: Diagnostic classification of spondylarthropathy and rheumatoid arthritis by synovial histopathology: a prospective study in 154 consecutive patients, *Arthritis Rheum* 50:2931–2941, 2004.

42. Machado P, Landewe R, Braun J, et al: Both structural damage and inflammation of the spine contribute to impairment of spinal mobility in patients with ankylosing spondylitis, *Ann Rheum Dis* 69:1465–1470, 2010.

43. Brophy S, Mackay K, Al-Saidi A, et al: The natural history of ankylosing spondylitis as defined by radiological progression, *J Rheumatol* 29:1236–1243, 2002.

44. van der Heijde D, Landewe R, Baraliakos X, et al: Radiographic findings following two years of infliximab therapy in patients with ankylosing spondylitis, *Arthritis Rheum* 58:3063–3070, 2008.

45. van der Heijde D, Landewe R, Einstein S, et al: Radiographic progression of ankylosing spondylitis after up to two years of treatment with etanercept, *Arthritis Rheum* 58:1324–1331, 2008.

46. van der Heijde D, Salonen D, Weissman BN, et al: Assessment of radiographic progression in the spines of patients with ankylosing spondylitis treated with adalimumab for up to 2 years, *Arthritis Res Ther* 11:R127, 2009.

47. Lories RJ, Luyten FP, de Vlam K: Progress in spondylarthritis: mechanisms of new bone formation in spondyloarthritis, *Arthritis Res Ther* 11:221, 2009.

48. Kronenberg HM: Developmental regulation of the growth plate, *Nature* 423:332–336, 2003.

49. Appel H, Kuhne M, Spiekermann S, et al: Immunohistologic analysis of zygapophyseal joints in patients with ankylosing spondylitis, *Arthritis Rheum* 54:2845–2851, 2006.

50. Lories RJ, Derese I, Luyten FP: Modulation of bone morphogenetic protein signaling inhibits the onset and progression of ankylosing enthesitis, *J Clin Invest* 115:1571–1579, 2005.

51. Diarra D, Stolina M, Polzer K, et al: Dickkopf-1 is a master regulator of joint remodeling, *Nat Med* 13:156–163, 2007.

52. McGonagle D, Stockwin L, Isaacs J, Emery P: An enthesitis based model for the pathogenesis of spondyloarthropathy: additive effects of microbial adjuvant and biomechanical factors at disease sites, *J Rheumatol* 28:2155–2159, 2001.

53. Sieper J, Appel H, Braun J, Rudwaleit M: Critical appraisal of assessment of structural damage in ankylosing spondylitis: implications for treatment outcomes, *Arthritis Rheum* 58:649–656, 2008.

54. Maksymowych WP: Disease modification in ankylosing spondylitis, *Nat Rev Rheumatol* 6:75–81, 2010.

55. Wanders A, van der Heijde D, Landewe R, et al: Nonsteroidal anti-inflammatory drugs reduce radiographic progression in patients with ankylosing spondylitis: a randomized clinical trial, *Arthritis Rheum* 52:1756–1765, 2005.

56. Hannu T, Inman R, Granfors K, Leirisalo-Repo M: Reactive arthritis or post-infectious arthritis? *Best Pract Res Clin Rheumatol* 20:419–433, 2006.

57. Fendler C, Laitko S, Sorensen H, et al: Frequency of triggering bacteria in patients with reactive arthritis and undifferentiated oligoarthritis and the relative importance of the tests used for diagnosis, *Ann Rheum Dis* 60:337–343, 2001.

58. Townes JM, Deodhar AA, Laine ES, et al: Reactive arthritis following culture-confirmed infections with bacterial enteric pathogens in Minnesota and Oregon: a population-based study, *Ann Rheum Dis* 67:1689–1696, 2008.

59. Yin Z, Braun J, Neure L, et al: Crucial role of interleukin-10/interleukin-12 balance in the regulation of the type 2 T helper cytokine response in reactive arthritis, *Arthritis Rheum* 40:1788–1797, 1997.

60. Butrimiene I, Jarmalaite S, Ranceva J, et al: Different cytokine profiles in patients with chronic and acute reactive arthritis, *Rheumatology (Oxford)* 43:1300–1304, 2004.

61. Anttonen K, Orpana A, Leirisalo-Repo M, Repo H: Aberrant TNF secretion by whole blood in healthy subjects with a history of reactive arthritis: time course in adherent and non-adherent cultures, *Ann Rheum Dis* 65:372–378, 2006.

62. Singh R, Aggarwal A, Misra R: Th1/Th17 cytokine profiles in patients with reactive arthritis/undifferentiated spondyloarthropathy, *J Rheumatol* 34:2285–2290, 2007.

63. Rohekar S, Tsui FW, Tsui HW, et al: Symptomatic acute reactive arthritis after an outbreak of salmonella, *J Rheumatol* 35:1599–1602, 2008.

64. Tsui FW, Xi N, Rohekar S, et al: Toll-like receptor 2 variants are associated with acute reactive arthritis, *Arthritis Rheum* 58:3436–3438, 2008.

65. Bas S, Neff L, Vuillet M, et al: The proinflammatory cytokine response to *Chlamydia trachomatis* elementary bodies in human macrophages is partly mediated by a lipoprotein, the macrophage infectivity potentiator, through TLR2/TLR1/TLR6 and CD14, *J Immunol* 180:1158–1168, 2008.

66. Carter JD, Espinoza LR, Inman RD, et al: Combination antibiotics as a treatment for chronic *Chlamydia*-induced reactive arthritis: a double-blind, placebo-controlled, prospective trial, *Arthritis Rheum* 62:1298–1307, 2010.

The references for this chapter can also be found on www.expertconsult.com.

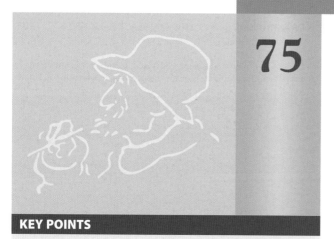

75 Ankylosing Spondylitis

SJEF M. VAN DER LINDEN •
DOMINIQUE BAETEN •
WALTER P. MAKSYMOWYCH

KEY POINTS

The concept of axial spondyloarthritis comprises both nonradiographic axial disease and ankylosing spondylitis (AS) according to the modified New York criteria.

Magnetic resonance imaging of the sacroiliac joints may show inflammation before structural changes appear on conventional radiographs. The modified New York criteria are useful primarily to classify groups of patients (e.g., for clinical or epidemiologic studies). They are not well suited to establish the diagnosis of AS in individual patients.

Nonradiographic axial spondyloarthritic disease occurs about twice as often as AS by modified New York criteria and may show comparable disease activity.

Inflammatory back pain is the usual clue to the early diagnosis of AS and axial spondyloarthritis.

In many populations, AS occurs in 1% to 3% of *HLA-B27*–positive individuals. The disease is more common (about 10%) among first-degree relatives of *HLA-B27*–positive AS patients.

Among patients with chronic inflammatory back pain, *HLA-B27* typing may aid in establishing the diagnosis of AS and axial spondyloarthritis.

Group physiotherapy is more effective than exercises performed at home by the patient.

Expert opinion and BASDAI (Bath ankylosing spondylitis disease activity index) greater than 4 (scale 0 to 10) are important in considering tumor necrosis factor (TNF)-blocking agents if conservative therapy with nonsteroidal anti-inflammatory drugs and physiotherapy fails.

Most AS patients have a normal or marginally elevated erythrocyte sedimentation rate and C-reactive protein level. Patients with normal levels of acute-phase reactants tend to have a somewhat lower response to anti-TNF agents.

Ankylosing spondylitis (AS) belongs to the group of diseases known as the *spondyloarthropathies* or, better, *spondyloarthritides*. This group of disorders constitutes a family of related but heterogeneous conditions rather than a single disease with different clinical manifestations[1] (Tables 75-1 and 75-2).

Radiographic sacroiliitis is considered a hallmark in AS and is found in more than 90% of patients. The inflammation of the sacroiliac (SI) joints and the spine eventually may lead to bony ankylosis. The term *ankylosing spondylitis* is derived from the Greek roots *ankylos*, or "bent" (although it now usually implies fusion or adhesions), and *spondylos*, or "vertebral disk." Ankylosis of the spine tends to appear in late stages of the disease and does not occur in many patients with mild disease.

Many patients with AS have onset of back pain during their third decade of life. It takes, on average, 6 to 8 years between the onset of back pain and establishing a definite diagnosis of AS. This diagnostic delay in the majority of patients results mainly from the relatively late appearance of definite radiographic sacroiliitis on conventional plain radiographs,[2,3] which is a requirement for diagnosis according to the modified New York criteria. Active sacroiliitis on magnetic resonance imaging (MRI) has been shown to predict the later appearance of sacroiliitis on radiographs.[4,5] Thus many patients at an early stage of AS typically present with characteristic clinical symptoms of AS but may not show definite sacroiliitis on radiographs. Therefore they may not be classified as AS cases. In such patients with suspected early AS, sacroiliitis may best be detected on MRI.[3] It has been proposed that a substantial proportion of such patients will develop radiographic sacroiliitis (i.e., structural damage of SI joints) with time and will progress to definite AS, but this hypothesis requires further evaluation in prospective studies. On the other hand, this also implies that a proportion of patients will remain at this (nonradiographic) stage of disease, with inflammation on MRI at some point, but without radiographically detectable damage over the subsequent years.[5] Therefore in order to describe these patients correctly, the term *early AS* has been dropped, with terms such as *preradiographic axial spondyloarthritis*[3] or, more recently, *nonradiographic axial spondyloarthritis*[6] seeming to be more appropriate (Figure 75-1). The term *axial spondyloarthritis* comprises both nonradiographic AS and classic AS (according to the modified New York criteria) and is now considered by ASAS (Assessment of SpondyloArthritis international Society) as the preferred terminology for patients with predominantly spinal disease. The total prevalence of axial spondyloarthritis has been estimated at two to three times that of AS according to the modified New York criteria.[7] In the concept of axial spondyloarthritis, the disease AS represents the tip of the iceberg. Patients with axial spondyloarthritis who have normal SI joints on conventional radiographs often show inflammatory changes on appropriate MRI and may or may not progress to sacroiliitis according to the New York criteria. Such patients may have active disease that needs appropriate treatment. They respond to therapy with biologics. The course and natural history of axial spondyloarthritis without radiographic sacroiliitis is not yet well known. However, although this chapter focuses on radiographic AS, many aspects also apply to patients with axial spondyloarthritis. The interval between the first complaints of the disease and the time of a definite diagnosis may be as long

Table 75-1 Spondyloarthritis

Ankylosing spondylitis
Reactive arthritis
Arthropathy of inflammatory bowel disease (Crohn's disease, ulcerative colitis)
Psoriatic arthritis
Undifferentiated spondyloarthropathies
Juvenile chronic arthritis and juvenile-onset ankylosing spondylitis

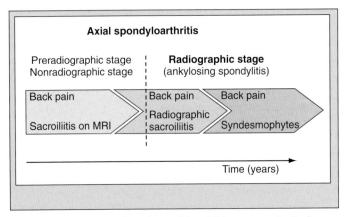

Figure 75-1 Concept of axial spondyloarthritis as an umbrella for patients without radiographic damage and patients with such damage. MRI, magnetic resonance imaging.

as 4 to 9 years.[8] This affects how disease duration is defined. Important components of the definition of disease duration are provided in Table 75-3.[9]

CLASSIFICATION

Criteria for Ankylosing Spondylitis and Axial Spondyloarthritis

The diagnosis of AS is based on clinical features. The disease is "primary" or "idiopathic" if no associated disorder is present; it is "secondary" if the disease is associated with psoriasis or chronic inflammatory bowel disease. In daily practice, a presumptive clinical diagnosis of AS is usually supported by evidence of sacroiliitis on conventional pelvic radiographs; indeed, many think of AS as symptomatic sacroiliitis. The presence of sacroiliitis does not necessarily indicate the presence of AS, however. Moreover, although radiographic sacroiliitis is frequent in AS, it is by no means an early or obligate manifestation of the disease.[10] Contrary to the New York criteria, radiographic evidence of sacroiliitis is not obligatory to fulfill the Rome criteria (Table 75-4). Both sets were primarily intended for use in epidemiologic studies. Lack of either sensitivity or specificity led to a modification of the New York criteria for AS[11] (see Table 75-4). Two criteria—limitation of lumbar spine motion and limitation of chest expansion—appear to reflect disease duration; they are usually not present in early disease.[12] It should be stressed that classification criteria are usually not useful for early diagnosis owing to a lack of sensitivity. In particular, in the early phase of AS, conventional SI radiographs may be normal. MRI is useful to diagnose the disease with predominantly axial manifestations before the presence of radiographic sacroiliitis.[13] To encompass both preradiographic AS and classic AS (according to the modified New York criteria), the Assessment of SpondyloArthritis international Society (ASAS) has proposed classification criteria for axial spondyloarthritis for patients with back pain of at least 3 months' duration and age at onset of complaints before 45 years (Table 75-5). The term *axial spondyloarthritis* has been introduced as an umbrella for the

entire spectrum of spondyloarthritis patients with predominant axial involvement, irrespective of the presence of structural damage on radiographs. Thus axial spondyloarthritis includes nonradiographic axial spondyloarthritis and classical AS (fulfilling the modified New York criteria). According to the ASAS classification criteria for axial spondyloarthritis,[7] a patient with chronic back pain and age at onset before age 45 can be classified as having axial spondyloarthritis if sacroiliitis on imaging (radiographs or MRI) is present plus at least one further spondyloarthritic feature, or, in the absence of sacroiliitis on imaging, if *HLA-B27* plus at least two further spondyloarthritis features are present (see Table 75-5). The sensitivity of the entire set of ASAS criteria for axial spondyloarthritis was 83%, and the specificity was 84%.[7] In the ASAS study on these new criteria, 30% of all patients diagnosed as having axial spondyloarthritis had definite radiographic sacroiliitis and fulfilled the modified New York criteria for AS. Therefore two-thirds were classified as nonradiographic axial spondyloarthritis.[7]

EPIDEMIOLOGY

Prevalence

The prevalence of AS closely parallels the frequency of *HLA-B27*. This holds true for those B27 subtypes that are associated with the disease, but it is not true for populations in which the *HLA-B27*06* subtype that lacks a strong association with AS occurs frequently such as the Indonesian population.[14-16]

Table 75-2 Clinical Characteristics of Spondyloarthritis

Typical pattern of peripheral arthritis—predominantly of lower limb, asymmetric
Absence of rheumatoid factor
Absence of subcutaneous nodules and other extra-articular features of rheumatoid arthritis
Overlapping extra-articular features characteristic of the group (e.g., anterior uveitis)
Significant familial aggregation
Association with *HLA-B27*

Table 75-3 Components of Disease Duration

Onset of axial AS manifestations (inflammatory back pain)
Onset of extra-axial AS manifestations (peripheral arthritis, enthesis)
Onset of associated spondyloarthropathic diseases (acute anterior uveitis, inflammatory bowel disease, psoriasis)
Time since diagnosis of AS by health care provider

AS, ankylosing spondylitis.
From Davis, JC, Dougados M, Braun J, et al: Definition of disease duration in ankylosing spondylitis: reassessing the concept, *Ann Rheum Dis* 65:1518–1520, 2006.

Table 75-4 Criteria for Ankylosing Spondylitis

Rome, 1961

Clinical Criteria

1. Low back pain and stiffness for more than 3 mo, not relieved by rest
2. Pain and stiffness in thoracic region
3. Limited motion in lumbar spine
4. Limited chest expansion
5. History or evidence of iritis or its sequelae

Radiographic Criterion

6. Radiograph showing bilateral sacroiliac changes characteristic of ankylosing spondylitis (this excludes bilateral osteoarthritis of sacroiliac joints)

Definite Ankylosing Spondylitis

Grade 3 or 4 bilateral sacroiliitis with at least one clinical criterion
Or
At least four clinical criteria

New York, 1966

Diagnostic Criteria

1. Limitation of lumbar spine motion in all three planes: anterior flexion, lateral flexion, extension
2. Pain at dorsolumbar junction or in lumbar spine
3. Limitation of chest expansion to 2.5 cm or less measured at level of fourth intercostal space

Grading of Radiographs

Normal, 0; suspicious, 1; minimal sacroiliitis, 2; moderate sacroiliitis, 3; ankylosis, 4

Definite Ankylosing Spondylitis

Grade 3 or 4 bilateral sacroiliitis with at least one diagnostic criterion
Or
Grade 3 or 4 unilateral or grade 2 bilateral sacroiliitis with diagnostic criterion 1 or with criteria 2 and 3

Probable Ankylosing Spondylitis

Grade 3 or 4 bilateral sacroiliitis with no diagnostic criteria

Modified New York, 1984

Criteria

1. Low back pain of at least 3 months' duration improved by exercise and not relieved by rest
2. Limitation of lumbar spine in sagittal and frontal planes
3. Chest expansion decreased relative to normal values for age and sex
4. Bilateral sacroiliitis grade 2 to 4
5. Unilateral sacroiliitis grade 3 or 4

Definite Ankylosing Spondylitis

Unilateral grade 3 or 4, or bilateral grade 2 to 4 sacroiliitis and any clinical criterion

Data from van der Linden SM, Valkenburg HA, Cats A: Evaluation of diagnostic criteria for ankylosing spondylitis: a proposal for modification of the New York criteria, *Arthritis Rheum* 27:361–368, 1984.

Among whites, the estimated prevalence rate of AS as defined by the modified New York criteria ranges from 68 per 100,000 population older than 20 years in the Netherlands to 197 per 100,000 in the United States.[8,17] The prevalence of clinical AS in France is 150 per 100,000 adults, whereas in Norway it is 210 per 100,000 adults.[18,19] The prevalence of the disease in Finland is similar, with a figure of 150 per 100,000 people.[20]

Higher prevalence rates have been reported in central Europe. An epidemiologic study from Berlin reported a prevalence figure of 0.86%.[21] In the general population, AS is likely to develop in about 1% to 2% of *HLA-B27*⁺ adults who have a disease-associated B27 subtype, although there may be regional or geographic differences. For example, in northern Norway, AS may develop in 6.7% of *HLA-B27*⁺ people.[8,22]

The disease is much more common among *HLA-B27*⁺ first-degree relatives of *HLA-B27*⁺ AS patients; roughly 10% to 30% of them have signs or symptoms of AS.[8] In fact, a positive family history of AS is a strong risk factor for the disease.

Incidence

There is no adequate evidence that the incidence of AS has changed in the past few decades. Clinical features, age of onset, and survival time have remained stable.[23] One study revealed an overall age and gender-adjusted incidence of 7.3 per 100,000 person-years. This U.S. figure compares quite well with the Finnish study, which revealed a stable incidence of 8.7 (95% confidence interval [CI], 6.4 to 11.0) per 100,000 people aged 16 or older.[18]

Racial Distribution

AS occurs in all parts of the world, but there are race-related differences in prevalence. This might reflect differences in the distribution of *HLA-B27* among races. Approximately 90% of white patients with AS possess *HLA-B27*, whereas AS and *HLA-B27* are nearly absent (prevalence of B27 < 1%) in African blacks and Japanese. In African-Americans, owing to racial admixture with whites, 2% possess B27, but only about 50% of black patients with AS possess B27. Correspondingly, African-Americans are affected far less frequently than American whites.

Table 75-5 ASAS Classification Criteria for Axial Spondyloarthritis (SpA) (in Patients with Back Pain ≥ 3 Months and Age at Onset < 45 Years)

Sacroiliitis on imaging plus ≥1 SpA feature	OR	**HLA-B27** plus ≥2 other SpA features
SpA Features		**Sacroiliitis on Imaging**
Inflammatory back pain Arthritis Enthesitis (heel) Uveitis Dactylitis Psoriasis Crohn's disease/ulcerative colitis Good response to NSAIDs Family history for SpA *HLA-B27* Elevated CRP*		Active (acute) inflammation on MRI highly suggestive of sacroiliitis associated with SpA OR Definite radiographic sacroiliitis according to modified New York criteria

*Elevated CRP is considered a SpA feature in the context of chronic back pain.

ASAS, Assessment of SpondyloArthritis international Society; CRP, C-reactive protein; HLA-B27, human leukocyte antigen-B27; IBP, inflammatory back pain; MRI, magnetic resonance imaging; NSAIDs, nonsteroidal anti-inflammatory drugs.

From Kollinger S, Bird LA, Roddis M, et al: HLA-B27 heavy chain homodimers are expressed in HLA-B27 transgenic rodent models of spondyloarthritis and are ligands for paired Ig-like receptors, *J Immunol* 173:1699–1710, 2004; and Rudwaleit M: New classification criteria for spondyloarthritis, *Int J Adv Rheumatol* 8:1–7, 2010.

Burden of Disease

AS is associated with a considerable burden to the patient and society. Apart from the axial and articular manifestations, extra-articular manifestations such as enthesitis and acute anterior uveitis and comorbidities such as inflammatory bowel disease and psoriasis contribute to the burden of disease. In addition, a large proportion of patients has spinal osteoporosis, leading to vertebral fractures and thoracic kyphosis. All these features result in a decreased quality of life. Disease status scores for physical functioning and disease activity correlate clearly with psychologic scores for anxiety and depression.[24] The impact of AS can also be seen in various aspects of employment, ranging from requiring assistance at work to increased sick leave and withdrawal from the workforce.[25,26] Apart from the impact on labor force participation, AS patients have an important impact on health care and non–health care resource utilization, resulting in mean total costs (direct and productivity) of about $6700 to $9500 per year per patient when applying the human capital approach to calculate productivity costs.[27-29]

The burden of illness increases with duration of disease. Because the burden due to AS reduces quality of life, and because all types of costs associated with AS result from loss of function and disease activity, early diagnosis and treatment are necessary to prevent or reduce functional decline and improve patient outcome.[30]

PATHOGENESIS

The precise cause of AS is still unclear, but several novel insights are currently emerging. First, several new hypotheses have been proposed to explain the major genetic contribution of HLA-B27. Second, other genetic risk factors have been identified by genome-wide association studies. Third, there is increasing evidence that AS may be driven by abnormal innate immune reactions rather than by autoantigen-specific T and/or B cell reactivity. And finally, the molecular mechanisms of new bone formation and their relationship with inflammation have started to emerge.

HLA-B27

The dominant role of genetic factors is highlighted by data demonstrating disease concordance in 75% of monozygotic twins compared with 13% of nonidentical twins,[31] familial aggregation,[32] and population data demonstrating associations with HLA-B27.[33] About 90% of white AS patients are HLA-B27+. HLA-B27 is the first described and major genetic risk factor for AS but, despite the near-pervasive nature of this association, it has been estimated that B27 contributes only 16% of the total genetic risk. In humans, there appears to be a hierarchy of association of the more than 45 as yet known subtypes of HLA-B27 with AS, ranging from strong association with HLA-B*2705 to weak association with HLA-B*2709. The direct pathogenic role of HLA-B27 is evidenced by the spontaneous spondyloarthritis-like disease in rats overexpressing HLA-B27.[34-36]

The main function of human leukocyte antigen (HLA) class I molecules such as HLA-B27 is to present peptides to CD8+ T cells and, accordingly, the arthritogenic peptide hypothesis proposes that CD8+ T cells are activated by bacterial antigens, for example in the gut, and after recirculation are reactivated in the joint by cartilage or other autoantigens. A number of studies have provided some partial evidence for this concept.[37,38] This hypothesis has been thoroughly questioned by the fact that HLA-B27 transgenic rats develop severe spondyloarthritis-like disease even in the absence of CD8+ T cells.[39,40] Two alternative hypotheses have been proposed more recently, suggesting that HLA-B27 has other specific features independent of antigen presentation that may directly contribute to disease. One theory indicates that HLA-B27 has a special tendency to form heavy chain homodimers that, when present on the cell surface, can trigger direct activation of natural killer (NK) cells through recognition via killer immunoglobulin receptor (KIR)-like receptors.[41,42]

Alternatively, HLA-B27 has a special propensity to misfold in the endoplasmic reticulum and thereby to promote an unfolded protein response, which in turn modulates the functional behavior and cytokine production of myeloid cells.[43-45]

The latter two hypotheses imply a role for altered innate immune responses rather than autoantigen-driven acquired immunity in the pathogenesis of AS.

Population and family studies have shown that HLA-B60 increases susceptibility to AS.[46] This applies to both HLA-B27+ and HLA-B27− persons.

Non–Human Leukocyte Antigen Genes

Two observations clearly suggest a role for non-HLA genetic risk factors. First, there is an increased risk for disease in B27+ first-degree relatives of AS probands (10% to 20%) compared with B27+ individuals in the general population (2% to 5%).[8] Second, disease concordance is 75% in identical twins versus 27% in HLA-B27 concordant dizygotic twins.[31] Genome-wide association studies have now allowed the identification of several of these factors.[47,48] There is a robust association with single-nucleotide polymorphisms (SNPs) in endoplasmic reticulum aminopeptidase-1 (ERAP-1), an enzyme involved in the trimming of peptides for loading in MHC molecules. There is now emerging evidence for a gene-gene interaction between ERAP-1 and HLA-B27, but it remains unknown how the polymorphisms may affect antigen presentation, HLA-B27 homodimer formation, and misfolding. A second strong association is found with SNPs in IL-23R, a genetic feature shared with Crohn's disease and psoriasis. Together with the suggested but not yet confirmed association with STAT3[49] and JAK2 polymorphisms, this suggests the potential involvement of an interleukin (IL)-17 response in AS. Definite association was also found with gene deserts on chromosome 2p15 and 21q22, which warrants further investigation of noncoding ribonucleicacid (RNA) and epigenetic effects in the pathophysiology of this disease. Besides these definite associations, genome-wide association studies have suggested potential associations with tumor necrosis factor (TNF) receptor 1 (TNFR1), the signaling molecule TNFR1-associated death domain protein (TRADD), the TNF superfamily cytokine TNFSF15, IL-1A and the IL-1 receptor 2 (IL-1R2), IL-12B, the vascular morphogenesis protein gene anthrax toxin receptor 2 (ANTXR2), and the innate immune receptor caspase recruitment domain family, member 9 (CARD9).[50]

These associations point toward a potential pathogenic role for altered innate immune responses, TNFR1 signaling, and IL-1.

The importance of TNF to the pathogenesis of AS is highlighted in the phenotype of a transgenic mouse model that overexpresses TNF. These animals develop sacroiliitis characterized by the formation of osteoclasts and granulation tissue.

Autoimmunity versus Autoinflammation

Both the alternative roles for *HLA-B27* besides antigen presentation and the genetic risk factors suggest that AS may not be primarily driven by a canonical autoantigen-specific T and/or B cell reactivity. Indeed, AS does not share genetic risk factors such as PTPN22 or cytotoxic T lymphocyte–associated antigen-4 (CTLA-4) with other autoimmune diseases and lacks disease-specific autoantibodies. On the basis of the predilection of the disease for sites rich in cartilage, it has been proposed that cartilage antigens may be the primary target of an autoimmune response in AS. This hypothesis is supported by several animal models of peripheral and axial arthritis on the basis of the induction of autoimmunity to antigens present in cartilage and fibrous tissue such as aggrecan and versican.[51,52] T cell responses toward the G1 domain of aggrecan have also been observed in human AS, but similar responses were seen in other inflammatory joint disorders, implying a non-specific response to joint damage.[53] Finally, biologic therapies targeting B (such as anti-CD20) or T (such as CTLA4-Ig) cell pathways have limited to no efficacy in AS in proof-of-concept trials.[54,55] Taken together, little strong evidence supports a primary T cell– or B cell–driven autoimmune process in AS.

An alternative hypothesis proposes that AS would be driven by abnormal reactivity of innate immune cells such as macrophages, neutrophils, and mast cells. This hypothesis is supported by several lines of evidence. First, genetic associations with CARD9 and the IL-1 pathway strongly suggest involvement of the inflammasome. Second, histologic studies demonstrated increased infiltration with innate immune cells, but not T, B, or dendritic cells in the peripheral joint and gut of patients with AS.[56-58] Third, human AS and its experimental models have a predilection for sites exposed to either microbial or mechanical stress. The latter aspect has led to the concept that AS and other forms of spondyloarthritis are primarily characterized by inflammation of the so-called synovio-entheseal complex.[59] In this perspective, it is interesting to note that the fibrocartilage protein versican, which could be released during mechanical stress and induces spondylitis in BALB/c mice, is also a ligand for the innate immune receptor TLR2. Formal proof that innate immune alterations may trigger AS remains, however, awaited.

Independently of the exact origin of the inflammation, it is clear that several proinflammatory cytokines are pivotal in the downstream effector mechanisms. TNF plays a crucial role in the disease process as evidenced by the successful introduction of TNF blockade for this disease. Accordingly, transgenic overexpression of TNF in mice leads not only to severe, destructive polyarthritis but also to sacroiliitis.[60] However, it remains incompletely understood which cells are the main producers of TNF in AS, in which form (soluble vs. transmembrane) and through which receptor (TNFR1 or TNFR2) TNF exerts its pathogenic effects, and which are the main target cells. In line with the genetic data, experimental data suggest a role for TNFR1 signaling in stromal cells.[61] Besides TNF, the genetic data and emerging data form functional studies on the unfolded protein response implicate IL-23 and thus possibly IL-17 as important cytokines in the pathogenesis of AS.[62]

Clinical trials targeting the IL-23/IL-17 pathway in AS are currently being performed.

Structural Remodeling and Ankylosis

A crucial and largely unexplained aspect of the pathogenesis of AS is the occurrence of structural remodeling and new bone formation, ultimately leading to ankylosis. Human and experimental studies have revealed three important concepts. First, the remodeling phenotype of AS cannot be explained by the absence of joint destruction because erosive disease is evidenced by histology and radiology and because the cellular and molecular machinery for cartilage and bone destruction is present and operative at the sites of disease.[63,64]

Second, structural remodeling and osteoproliferation are dependent on endochondral bone formation. This process is governed by several molecular pathways including bone morphogenetic protein (BMP) and Wnt signaling.[65,66] There is emerging evidence that several inhibitors of the Wnt pathway are dysfunctional in human spondyloarthritis and that this correlates with new bone formation.[67] Third, osteoproliferation is not critically dependent on inflammation because, despite clinical efficacy on signs and symptoms, TNF blockade fails to halt radiologic progression in AS and both processes can be uncoupled in experimental models.[68,69]

On the other hand, vertebral sites showing signs of inflammation at baseline have a higher risk for subsequent osteoproliferation on follow-up.[70] The exact relationship between inflammation and osteoproliferation needs to be further clarified because it may have important consequences for treatment.

PATHOLOGY

Characteristic pathologic features of AS include inflammation in axial joints, large peripheral joints, and entheses associated with inflammation in subchondral bone marrow. Reparation is also characteristic in terms of the development of chondroid metaplasia, followed by calcification of cartilage and formation of bone, particularly in the axial joints. Fat metaplasia in the axial skeleton at sites of prior inflammation is frequently observed on MRI.

Axial Skeleton

Detailed histopathologic studies of axial involvement in AS are limited owing to the inaccessibility of biopsy material of both SI joints and the spine. A controlled study of SI biopsies from AS patients at various stages of disease and controls showed cellular infiltration with lymphocytes, macrophages, and plasma cells in the synovium and subchondral marrow as the earliest features of disease.[71] Later features include the development of pannus extending from both synovium and subchondral bone marrow, with erosion of articular cartilage and its replacement by granulation tissue. Osteoclast formation and erosion of subchondral bone account for the typical widening of the joint spondyloarthritisce seen on plain radiography. Enthesitis is also evident in later stages of disease at the insertion of the posterior capsule. Reparative changes include cartilage metaplasia at sites of active inflammation, followed by its calcification and then replacement by endochondral bone, leading to obliteration of the joint space by ankylosis. Para-articular changes include bone sclerosis and fat replacement of bone marrow. Regarding the spine, pathologic data are limited except for a number of recent studies of apophyseal joints. Immunohistologic analysis shows subchondral lymphocyte infiltrates with CD4[+] and CD8[+] T cells, together with hypervascularization and foci of CD68[+] osteoclastic cells.[72]

Peripheral Skeleton

Regarding peripheral joint manifestations of AS, histopathologic studies have assessed surgical samples of affected hip joint, synovial biopsies of knee and ankle joint, and enthesitis. Involvement of the hips is characterized by subchondral granulation tissue and osteoclast formation in the femoral heads and acetabulum that is associated with degradation of overlying articular cartilage.[73] Synovial studies have revealed that the type of inflammation is strongly different from that observed in RA, with increased vascularity, increased infiltration with innate immune cells, and absence of specific features of T and B cell autoimmunity.[74-77]

Interestingly, these studies revealed a similar pattern of inflammation in AS in comparison with other subtypes of spondyloarthritis.[78]

Entheseal involvement most frequently occurs at sites rich in fibrocartilage such as the Achilles tendon. Inflammation and chronic cellular infiltration of soft tissues are relatively sparse but may be extensive within the adjacent subchondral bone, particularly in B27[+] individuals.[79] A comparative study of the subchondral marrow from knee and hip joint entheses showed that AS patients clearly differ from those with RA and osteoarthritis with respect to the frequency of marrow inflammation, infiltration with CD8[+] T cells, and presence of hyperosteoclastic erosive lesions.

CLINICAL MANIFESTATIONS

Skeletal Manifestations

Low Back Pain and Stiffness

Back pain is an extremely common symptom, occurring in up to 80% of the general population. Therefore it is important to note that back pain in AS and axial spondyloarthritis has special features that differentiate it from mechanical back pain[80-82] (Table 75-6). In clinical practice inflammatory back pain is often not well recognized.[83] Back pain is the most prevailing diagnostic feature of AS (Table 75-7).

Table 75-6 Aspects of Inflammatory Back Pain in Ankylosing Spondylitis and Axial Spondyloarthritis

Onset of complaints before age 45
Duration of symptoms more than 3 mo (chronic pain)
Located at the lower back
Alternating buttock pain
Awaking due to back pain during the second half of the night
Morning stiffness for at least 30 min
Insidious onset of complaints
Improvement with exercises
No improvement of back pain with rest
Improvement with use of nonsteroidal agents

The pain is initially felt primarily deep in the gluteal region, is dull in character, is difficult to localize, and is insidious in onset. The pain can be severe at this early phase of the disease; it localizes in the SI joints but is occasionally referred toward the iliac crest or greater trochanteric region or down the dorsal thigh. Radiation of buttock pain may suggest root compression of the sciatic nerve. The buttock pain typically alternates from side to side. Coughing, sneezing, or other maneuvers that cause a sudden twist of the back may accentuate pain. Although the pain is often unilateral or intermittent at first, within a few months it usually becomes persistent and bilateral and the lower lumbar area becomes stiff and painful. The pain is associated with a feeling of low back stiffness that is worse in the morning and may awaken the patient from sleep, particularly during the second half of the night. Many patients do not differentiate between low back pain and stiffness. The morning stiffness may last up to 3 hours. Both the stiffness and the pain tend to be eased by a hot shower, an exercise program, or physical activity; they do not improve with rest. Fatigue as a result of chronic back pain and stiffness may be an important problem and can be accentuated by sleep disturbances due to these symptoms.

Chest Pain

With subsequent involvement of the thoracic spine (including costovertebral and costotransverse joints) and the occurrence of enthesitis at the costosternal and manubriosternal joints, patients may experience chest pain accentuated by coughing or sneezing, which is sometimes characterized as "pleuritic." The chest pain is often associated with tenderness over the sternocostal or costosternal junctions. Mild to moderate reduction of chest expansion is often detectable in an early stage of AS. Chest pain occurs relatively often in *HLA-B27*[+] relatives, even in the absence of radiographic evidence of sacroiliitis.[84]

Table 75-7 Diagnostic Features of Ankylosing Spondylitis

Chronic inflammatory spinal pain
Chest pain
Alternate buttock pain
Acute anterior uveitis
Synovitis (predominantly of lower limbs, asymmetric)
Enthesitis (heel, plantar)
Radiographic sacroiliitis
Positive family history of ankylosing spondylitis
Chronic inflammatory bowel disease
Psoriasis

Tenderness

Extra-articular tenderness at certain loci is a prominent complaint in some patients. These lesions are due to enthesitis. Common tender sites are the costosternal junctions, spinous processes, iliac crests, greater trochanters, ischial tuberosities, tibial tubercles, and heels (Achilles tendinitis or plantar fasciitis). Radiographically, bone spurs may develop at these sites.

Joints

The girdle or "root" joints (hips and shoulders) are the most frequently involved extra-axial joints in AS, and pain in these areas is the presenting symptom in up to 15% of patients. Shoulder involvement, but especially hip involvement, may cause considerable physical disability. Coexisting disease in the lumbar spine often contributes significantly to disability of the lower extremities. Hips and shoulders are involved at some stage of disease in up to 35% of patients. Hip disease is more common in Algeria, India, and Mexico. It is relatively more common as a presenting manifestation if the disease starts in childhood (juvenile AS). In boys 8 to 10 years of age, hip disease as a manifestation of juvenile AS is the most frequent type of chronic arthritis. These children with hip disease are mostly HLA-B27+, and they are serologically negative for antinuclear antibodies.

The knee joint may also be affected in AS, often as an intermittent effusion. The temporomandibular joint is involved in about 10% of patients.

Extraskeletal Manifestations

Constitutional symptoms such as fatigue, weight loss, and low-grade fever occur frequently. Other extraskeletal manifestations are more localized.

Eye Disease

Acute anterior uveitis or iridocyclitis is the most common extra-articular manifestation of AS, occurring in 25% to 30% of patients at some time during the course of the disease. There is no clear relationship between activity of the articular disease and this extra-articular manifestation. The onset of eye inflammation is usually acute and typically unilateral, but the attacks may alternate. The eye is red and painful, with visual impairment. Photophobia and increased lacrimation may be present. If the eye remains untreated or if treatment is delayed, posterior synechiae and glaucoma may develop. Most attacks subside in 4 to 8 weeks without sequelae if early treatment is provided. Acute anterior uveitis is more common in B27+ than B27− patients with AS.[85] Relatives who have acute anterior uveitis seem to be at higher risk for AS. The calculated incidence of acute anterior uveitis in a Swiss family study was 89 attacks per 1000 patient-years for AS patients, but only 8 per 1000 person-years among healthy B27+ relatives.[86]

Cardiovascular Disease

Cardiac involvement may be clinically silent or may cause considerable problems. Manifestations of cardiac involvement include ascending aortitis, aortic valve incompetence, conduction abnormalities, cardiomegaly, and pericarditis. In rare situations, aortitis may precede other features of AS. Aortic incompetence was noted in 3.5% of patients who had the disease for 15 years and in 10% after 30 years.[87] Inflammation and dilation of the aorta are the main causes of aortic valve incompetence. Cardiac conduction disturbances are seen with increasing frequency with the passage of time, occurring in 2.7% of those with disease of 15 years' duration and in 8.5% after 30 years.[87] Both aortic incompetence and cardiac conduction defects occur twice as often in patients with peripheral joint involvement. In AS the prevalence of myocardial infarction is increased (4.4% in AS patients compared with 1.2% in the general population in a Dutch study).[88]

Pulmonary Disease

Lung involvement is a rare and late manifestation of AS. It is characterized by slowly progressive fibrosis of the upper lobes of the lungs, appearing, on average, 2 decades after the onset of AS. Patients may complain of cough, dyspnea, and sometimes hemoptysis.[89]

High-resolution computed tomography (CT) may be helpful in detecting interstitial lung disease in patients with respiratory symptoms whose chest radiographs are normal.[90] This imaging technique reveals a high prevalence of lung changes even among AS patients with early disease and without respiratory symptoms. The clinical significance of these findings is unknown. Long-term prospective studies need to be performed.[91]

Pulmonary ventilation is usually well maintained; an increased diaphragmatic contribution helps compensate for chest wall rigidity, which is due to involvement of the thoracic joints in the inflammatory process. Vital capacity and total lung capacity may be moderately reduced as a consequence of the restricted chest wall movement, whereas residual volume and functional residual capacity are usually increased.

Neurologic Involvement

Neurologic complications of AS can be caused by fracture, instability, compression, or inflammation. Traffic accidents or minor trauma can cause spinal fractures. The C5-C6 or C6-C7 level is the most commonly involved site.

As in RA, atlantoaxial joint subluxation, atlantooccipital subluxation, and upward subluxation of the axis may occur in AS as a consequence of instability resulting from the inflammatory process. Spontaneous anterior atlantoaxial subluxation is a well-recognized complication in about 2% of patients and manifests with or without signs of spinal cord compression. It is observed more commonly in patients with spondylitis and peripheral arthritis than in those with exclusively axial involvement.[92]

Causes of neurologic complications due to compression include ossification of the posterior longitudinal ligament (which may lead to compressive myelopathy), destructive intervertebral disk lesions, and spinal stenosis.

The cauda equina syndrome is a rare but serious complication of long-standing AS. The syndrome affects lumbosacral nerve roots. This gives rise to pain and sensory loss, but frequently there are also urinary and bowel symptoms. Gradual onset of urinary and fecal incontinence, impotence, saddle anesthesia, and occasionally loss of ankle jerks occurs. Motor symptoms, if present, are usually mild. CT and MRI allow the accurate noninvasive diagnosis of this complication of AS.[93] No compressive lesions exist. Arachnoiditis and arachnoid adhesions may be important in the pathogenesis.

Renal Involvement

IgA nephropathy has been reported in many patients with AS. These patients often have an elevated immunoglobulin (Ig)A level (93%) and renal impairment (27%) at presentation.[94] Microscopic hematuria and proteinuria may occur in up to 35% of patients. The significance of these findings in terms of subsequent deterioration of renal function is unclear.[95] Amyloidosis (secondary type) is a rare complication. Amyloid deposits detected through abdominal subcutaneous fat aspiration are not invariably associated with a poor renal prognosis.[96]

Osteoporosis

Osteopenia is seen in the early stages of AS.[97] In patients with this disease, osteoporotic deformities of the thoracic spine contribute significantly to abnormal posture, particularly fixed hyperkyphosis.[98] Radiographic damage to the cervical and lumbar spine, thoracic wedging, and disease activity are determinants of hyperkyphosis in AS.[99] An increased occiput-to-wall distance is associated with vertebral fractures. The prevalence of symptomatic osteoporotic spinal fractures is increased in AS.[100] Neurologic complications occur rather frequently, even after minor trauma.[101] Proper assessment of bone density in the spine is difficult in the presence of syndesmophytes because they may give rise to falsely high values. The true fracture risk and complication rate in early and late disease and the relation to disease activity are not yet known. Currently, it is unclear whether any specific antiosteoporotic therapy to prevent spinal fractures is effective.

PHYSICAL FINDINGS

Spinal Mobility

To arrive at an early diagnosis, the physician must perform a thorough physical examination. On examination of the spine, there may be some limitation of motion of the lumbar spine as elicited by forward flexion, hyperextension, or lateral flexion. Early loss of the normal lumbar lordosis is often the first sign and is easily assessed on inspection.

The Schober test (or its modifications) is useful to detect any limitation of forward flexion of the lumbar spine, although it is typically normal in early disease. As the patient stands erect, one mark is placed with a pen on the skin overlying the fifth lumbar spinous process (usually at the level of the posterosuperior iliac spine or the "dimple of Venus," and another mark is placed 10 cm above in the midline. The patient is then asked to bend forward maximally without bending the knees. In healthy people, the distance between the two marks on the skin should increase as the skin stretches. If the distance between both marks does not reach 15 cm, this indicates reduced lumbar spine mobility. Lateral flexion may also be diminished, and spinal rotation may cause pain.

Chest Expansion

Mild to moderate reduction of chest expansion is often detectable in early stages of AS. Normal values are age and sex dependent, and there is considerable overlap between normal values and those obtained from AS patients. Reduction below 5 cm in young persons with an insidious onset of chronic, inflammatory low back pain strongly suggests AS. Chest expansion should be measured on maximal inspiration after forced maximal expiration at the level of the fourth intercostal spondyloarthritisce in males and just below the breasts at the xiphisternal level in females.

Enthesitis

Examination of the ischial tuberosities, greater trochanters, spinous processes, costochondral and manubriosternal junctions, supraspinatus insertion, and iliac crests can determine the presence of enthesitis. Heel pain, especially when getting out of bed, is a characteristic manifestation of Achilles and plantar fasciitis enthesitis.

Sacroiliitis

Direct pressure over the SI joints may elicit pain, as may special testing maneuvers, although the latter lack specificity and sensitivity. These signs may also be negative in early disease or may become negative in late stages as inflammation is replaced by fibrosis or bony ankylosis.

Posture

Over the course of the disease, the patient may lose normal posture. Involvement of the cervical spine is manifested by pain and limitation of neck movement. A forward slope of the neck can be detected by having the patient stand against a wall and try to position his or her occiput against it.

After many years of progression in patients with severe disease, the entire spine may become increasingly stiff, with loss of normal posture from gradual loss of lumbar lordosis and the development of thoracic kyphosis.[98,99] The abdomen becomes protuberant; breathing is primarily by diaphragmatic action. These typical deformities usually evolve after disease duration of 10 years or more.

LABORATORY TESTS

Generally, routine blood tests are not helpful. A normal erythrocyte sedimentation rate (ESR) or normal C-reactive protein (CRP) level does not exclude active disease. An elevated ESR or CRP is reported in up to 75% of patients, but it may not correlate with clinical disease activity.[102] In an unselected patient population, an elevated ESR and CRP was present in 45% and 38%, respectively, of patients with spinal disease only, compared with 62% and 61%, respectively, of patients with peripheral arthritis with or without inflammatory bowel disease. Neither ESR nor CRP is superior in assessing disease activity.[103] A mild normochromic anemia may be present in 15% of patients. Elevation of serum alkaline phosphatase (derived primarily from bone) is seen in some patients but is unrelated to disease activity or duration. Some elevation of serum IgA is frequent in AS. Its level correlates with acute-phase reactants. Active disease is associated with decreased lipid levels, particularly high-density lipoprotein cholesterol, resulting in a more atherogenic lipid profile.[104]

IMAGING STUDIES

Conventional Radiography

The typical radiographic changes of AS are seen primarily in the axial skeleton, especially in the SI, discovertebral, apophyseal, costovertebral, and costotransverse joints. They evolve over many years, with the earliest, most consistent, and most characteristic findings seen in the SI joints. However, otherwise typical AS has been described in the absence of radiographic evidence of sacroiliitis.[8] The radiographic findings of sacroiliitis are usually symmetric and consist of blurring of the subchondral bone plate, followed by erosions and sclerosis of the adjacent bone. The changes in the synovial portion of the joint (i.e., the lower two-thirds of the joint) result from inflammatory synovitis and osteitis of the adjacent subchondral bone.[105] The cartilage covering the iliac side of the joint is much thinner than that covering the sacral side. Therefore the erosions and subchondral sclerosis are typically seen first and tend to be more prominent on the iliac side.

In the upper one-third of the SI joint, where strong intraarticular ligaments hold the bones together, the inflammatory process may lead to similar radiographic abnormalities. Progression of the subchondral bone erosions can lead to pseudowidening of the SI joint space. Over time, gradual fibrosis, calcification, interosseous bridging, and ossification occur. Erosions become less obvious, but the subchondral sclerosis persists, becoming the most prominent radiographic feature.

Ultimately, usually after several years, there may be complete bony ankylosis of the SI joints, with resolution of bony sclerosis. It is practical to grade radiographic sacroiliitis according to the New York criteria (Table 75-8).

Bony erosions and osteitis ("whiskering") at sites of osseous attachment of tendons and ligaments are frequently seen, particularly at the calcaneus, ischial tuberosities, iliac crest, femoral trochanters, supraspinatus insertion, and spinous processes of the vertebrae. In the early stages of the evolution of syndesmophytes, there is inflammation of the superficial layers of the annulus fibrosus, with subsequent reactive sclerosis and erosions of the adjacent corners of the

Table 75-8 Grading of Sacroiliitis: New York Criteria

Grade 0, normal
Grade 1, suspicious
Grade 2, minimal sacroiliitis
Grade 3, moderate sacroiliitis
Grade 4, ankylosis

vertebral bodies. This combination of destructive osteitis and repair leads to "squaring" of the vertebral bodies. This squaring is associated with gradual ossification of the annulus fibrosus and eventual "bridging" between vertebrae by syndesmophytes.[106] There are often concomitant inflammatory changes, ankylosis in the apophyseal joints, and ossification of the adjacent ligaments. In a number of patients, this may ultimately result in a virtually complete fusion of the vertebral column ("bamboo spine").

Hip involvement may lead to symmetric, concentric joint spondyloarthritisce narrowing, irregularity of the subchondral bone with subchondral sclerosis, osteophyte formation at the outer margin of the articular surface, and, ultimately, bony ankylosis of these joints.

Several validated scoring methods are available to quantify structural damage in AS: the Bath AS radiology index (BASRI), the Stoke AS spondylitis score (SASSS), and the modified SASSS.[107-109] The BASRI includes scores for the cervical and lumbar spine, as well as the SI joints. A similar score for the hips is also available. The SASSS evaluates the lumbar spine only; the modified SASSS assesses the anterior, cervical, and lumbar spine. These scoring methods are most suited for use in clinical trials and observational studies.

Computed Tomography and Magnetic Resonance Imaging

The conventional plain pelvic radiograph is still the initial tool for the evaluation of SI joints in patients with inflammatory low back pain. This technique, however, lacks sensitivity in early sacroiliitis because it only detects structural abnormalities that are the consequence of inflammation. CT may detect bone abnormalities such as sclerosis and erosion sooner than plain radiography, but its use is limited by radiation exposure and it does not detect changes in soft tissues or bone marrow where early features of sacroiliitis develop. MRI sequences that are used in routine practice to image the SI joint can detect sacroiliitis in 50% of patients with preradiographic SpA.[110] These sequences include fat-saturating techniques, such as short tau inversion recovery (STIR), that are very sensitive in the detection of bone marrow edema, which is a frequent finding in AS-related inflammation of the musculoskeletal system (Figure 75-2). The T1-weighted sequence allows detection of erosions and fat infiltration, which may occur early in disease and is associated with resolution of inflammation. Diagnostic MRI should include both sequences, while the role of contrast enhancement with gadolinium is still unclear due to its substantial cost and prolonged time for imaging, which patients may find difficult to endure.

Similarly, plain spinal radiographs only show abnormalities once disease is well established, and it plays a minor role in diagnostic or ongoing routine evaluation except to detect other causes of back pain, such as spinal fractures. Characteristic abnormalities include square vertebrae, shiny corners (the Romanus lesion), spondylodiscitis (the Anderson lesion), and syndesmophytes with partial and complete fusion. Spinal inflammation can only be visualized by MRI, where it is typically seen as bone marrow edema in the vertebrae at both anterior and posterior vertebral corners as well as around the intervertebral disk. Lateral and posterior

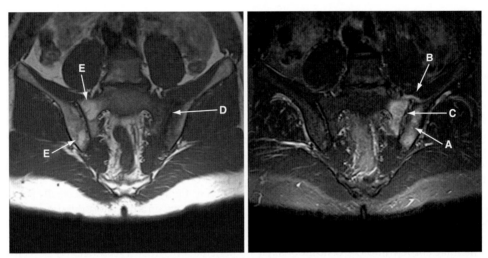

Figure 75-2   T1-weighted *(left)* and short-tau inversion recovery sequence magnetic resonance *(right)* images of 23-year-old male with inflammatory back pain and equivocal pelvic radiograph demonstrating the following features: *A,* Bone marrow edema in left iliac and sacral bones. *B,* Capsular inflammation. *C,* Joint space inflammation. *D,* Diffuse erosion of left iliac bone with widening of joint space. *E,* Fat infiltration in right sacrum and ilium.

elements such as the costovertebral and costotransverse joints, facet joints, pedicles, and spinal ligaments can also show inflammatory lesions.[111] MRI and ultrasonography can be very useful to assess enthesitic problems such as Achilles tendinitis and heel pain.

Quantification of spinal inflammation using MRI is highly sensitive to change and is increasingly recognized as an essential component of clinical trials. MRI scores for inflammation correlate with CRP but not with symptoms. Increasing evidence supports an association between MRI inflammation and the future development of structural changes on radiography.[112,113]

DIAGNOSIS

Clinical manifestations of AS usually begin in late adolescence or early adulthood; only rarely do they begin after age 40 years.[8] The diagnosis of AS at an early stage of disease depends primarily on a careful history and physical examination. Two features of the history are critical: (1) the presence of inflammatory low back pain and stiffness and (2) a positive family history for AS.

Low back pain is common in the general population and is frequently due to noninflammatory, nonspecific mechanical causes. However, the low back pain in AS has typical "inflammatory" features (see Table 75-6). A history of inflammatory low back pain can be used as a diagnostic tool. A reassessment of the clinical history for diagnostic purposes among young to middle-aged adults (younger than 50 years) with chronic back pain and an established diagnosis of either AS or mechanical back pain revealed a sensitivity of 37% (95% CI, 28 to 46), a specificity of 84% (95% CI, 76 to 90), a positive likelihood ratio of 2.3 (95% CI, 1.4 to 3.7), and a post-test probability of AS of 11% (given a pretest probability of 5%) if two of the four parameters listed in Table 75-9 were present. If three or four of these items were present, the sensitivity was 34% (95% CI, 25 to 43), the specificity was 97% (95% CI, 92 to 99), the positive likelihood ratio was 12.4 (95% CI, 4.0 to 40), and the post-test probability of AS was 39%.[81] Because the prevalence of AS in many white populations is as low as approximately

0.1% to 0.3%, applying the clinical history as a test for the disease in such low-probability settings provides rather low post-test probability values. However, a positive family history increases the pretest probability of AS from 0.1% for a person belonging to the general population to about 10% for any first-degree relative of an AS proband.[8] The probability of having AS for a first-degree relative with a positive family history of AS increases from 10% to nearly 50% if this relative has inflammatory low back pain. In contrast, the likelihood of having AS increases from 0.1% to only 1% for a person who has inflammatory back pain (without any other inflammatory indications listed in Table 75-9) but has a negative family history for AS.

A definite diagnosis of AS is usually established by radiographic evidence of bilateral sacroiliitis. The plain anteroposterior view of the pelvis is usually adequate for diagnostic purposes. There is, however, considerable intraobserver and interobserver variation in the radiographic diagnosis of sacroiliitis for both conventional pelvic films and CT of the SI joints. Training in reading these films has limited value. Improvement in sensitivity tends to be associated with a decrease in specificity.[117]

In most adult patients, AS can be diagnosed clinically without the *HLA-B27* test. This assessment has no additional value in established disease or as a pure screening tool.[118] However, in young patients with inflammatory chronic back pain, a positive *HLA-B27* test increases the likelihood of having AS, particularly if imaging of the SI

Table 75-9   Proposed Criteria for Inflammatory Back Pain in Young to Middle-aged Adults* with Chronic Back Pain

Morning stiffness of at least 30 min duration
Improvement of back pain with exercise but not with rest
Awakening because of back pain during second half of night only
Alternating buttock pain

*Younger than 50 yr.
From Rudwaleit M, Metter A, Listing J, et al: Inflammatory back pain in ankylosing spondylitis: a reassessment of the clinical history for application as classification and diagnostic criteria, *Arthritis Rheum* 65:569–578, 2006.

joints does not provide conclusive results. Usually, however, the contribution of *HLA-B27* typing to purely clinical factors in diagnosing axial manifestations of AS among patients with inflammatory back pain of short duration is rather limited, whereas MRI may help in classifying patients as having spondyloarthritis or nonspondyloarthritis.[119]

Physicians are reluctant to make the diagnosis of AS when radiographic evidence of sacroiliitis is not present. Relatives of AS patients in particular may have signs and symptoms of AS including inflammatory back pain but sometimes do not show radiographic sacroiliitis even after lengthy follow-up. Radiographic sacroiliitis is frequent in AS but is by no means an early or obligate manifestation of the disease. In patients with a clinical diagnosis of possible AS, radiographic sacroiliitis may never become manifest or only after appropriate follow-up. Therefore diagnosing this type of disease, which fits entirely into the concept of axial spondyloarthritis, early, before (conventional) radiographic evidence of sacroiliitis is manifest, constitutes a challenge to the clinician. This is especially true as more effective treatments become increasingly available. In this context, the term (nonradiographic) axial spondyloarthritis is often used. An approach based on pretest probabilities and likelihood ratios has been proposed to diagnose early disease with predominantly axial manifestations before convincing evidence of radiographic sacroiliitis is present.[81] The majority of patients diagnosed clinically with preradiographic axial spondyloarthritis have MRI evidence of spondyloarthritis,[120] and the severity of bone edema on MRI has been shown to predict the development of radiographic sacroiliitis on follow-up.[121] Consequently, MRI is now an acceptable imaging criterion for the diagnosis of spondyloarthritis and is especially useful when the history points to inflammatory back pain, the pelvic radiograph is normal or equivocal, and the patient is positive for B27.

AS rarely develops after age 40; however, late-onset AS does occur. In this case, there may be little or no clinical involvement of the axial skeleton initially, but patients may show moderate oligoarthritis with low cell counts in the synovial fluid and pitting edema of the lower limbs.[122]

At the other end of the age scale, juvenile-onset AS is not uncommon among young patients with spondyloarthritis. Such patients tend to have enthesitis and peripheral arthritis, which may be severe and disabling.

ANKYLOSING SPONDYLITS IN MALES AND FEMALES

Clinically, AS is more common in males, with a reported male-to-female ratio of about 2:1 to 3:1. However, extrapolation of studies employing the genetic marker *HLA-B27* suggests that, on the basis of radiographs of the SI joints, prevalence rates are about equal in both sexes.[8]

Disease expression is thought to be different in males and females. A case-control study comparing 35 female patients with 70 male patients as controls showed no differences in spinal symptoms, chest expansion, peripheral arthritis, extra-articular manifestations, or functional outcome. The males with AS more often had radiographic spinal changes and hip joint involvement than their female counterparts. There is still some controversy, but overall, there are no

significant clinical or radiographic differences between women and men with AS. However, on average, the disease seems to be more severe in men.[123,124]

Fertility among female patients with AS is normal.[125] Most patients (50% to 60%) do not experience major changes in disease activity during pregnancy, but an increase in morning stiffness and low back pain, particularly at night, may occur at about the 20th week of gestation and last for a few days to weeks.[126] In about 50% of patients, an exacerbation of symptoms is seen within the first half year after delivery. Sacroiliitis including complete ankylosis of the SI joints does not constitute a contraindication for vaginal delivery. Epidural anesthesia is usually possible because most patients have a rather short duration of disease and do not have extensive spinal syndesmophytes. The fetal outcome is not impaired in patients with AS. Every pregnancy in patients with this disease should be considered potential high risk, however, and such pregnancies require close collaboration between rheumatologists and obstetricians.

An uncontrolled study among 612 AS patients (mean age, 50.8 years; 71.6% males) reported a substantial impact on sexual relationships (response rate, 38%). Poor function, depression, disease activity, unemployment, and poor self-efficacy were independently associated with greater impact on patients' sexual relationships.[127]

OUTCOME

The course of AS is highly variable, characterized by spontaneous remissions and exacerbations. Its prognosis has generally been considered rather favorable. The disease may run a relatively mild or self-limited course. However, the disease may also remain active over many years. Life expectancy is somewhat reduced, particularly after 10 years of disease.[128] A study from Finland indicates that the risk of dying for patients with AS is increased by 50% compared with controls matched for age and gender. Causes of death include complications of the disease such as amyloidosis and spinal fractures, as well as cardiovascular, gastrointestinal, and renal disease.[129] There is no convincing evidence that the natural history of the disease has essentially changed over the past few decades.[130,131] No differences exist between familial and sporadic AS in terms of age at onset, age at diagnosis, or prevalence of peripheral arthritis and acute anterior uveitis.[132]

Functional limitations increase with disease duration. Although structural damage seen on radiographs is clearly associated with physical function and spinal mobility at the group level, individual patients with normal radiographs might exhibit a major reduction in spinal mobility, whereas those with severe radiographic abnormalities might function quite well in everyday tasks.[133]

Recent data show that the functional prognosis of AS is less favorable than was previously thought. Withdrawal from work in those with paid jobs varies from 10% after 20 years of disease duration to 30% after 10 years, depending on the characteristics of the patients included and the social security system considered.[134-137] The age- and sex-adjusted withdrawal rate from labor-force participation was 3.1 times higher among Dutch patients compared with the general population.[137] Older age at disease onset, manual work, lower educational level, and coping strategies characterized by the limitation and pacing of activities were associated with a higher risk for work disability.[135-137] Vocational counseling, job training, easy access to the workplace, and support of colleagues and management may reduce the probability of withdrawal from work.[134,138] Sick leave in those with paid jobs was linked to disease activity and presence of extraspinal disease manifestations.[134,137,139] Patients with peripheral joint involvement are more likely to take sick leave than are AS patients with axial manifestations only.

Overall, the first 10 years of disease are particularly important with respect to subsequent outcome. Most of the loss of function among patients with AS occurs within this period and is associated with the presence of peripheral arthritis, spinal radiographic changes, and development of a so-called bamboo spine.[140] In a retrospective study of patients with spondyloarthropathies including AS, of at least 10 years' duration, seven variables were associated with disease severity if these factors occurred within the first 2 years of follow-up. These factors, expressed as an odds ratio together with its 95% CI, are as follows: arthritis of hip joints (22.9; 4.4 to 118), ESR more than 30 mm/hr (7; 4.8 to 9.5), poor efficacy of nonsteroidal anti-inflammatory drugs (NSAIDs) (8.3; 2.6 to 27.1), limitation of lumbar spine (7; 2 to 25), sausage-like digits (8.5; 1.5 to 9.0), oligoarthritis (4.3; 1.4 to 13.1), and onset before age 16 years (3.5; 1.1 to 12.8).[141] Although radiographic progression is highly variable among patients, radiographic evidence of spinal involvement, especially the presence of syndesmophytes, appears to be the primary factor that independently predicts further radiographic progression.[142] The long-term results of total hip replacement in AS are satisfactory. The outcome of 138 total hip replacements and 12 revisions was good or very good in 86%, and 63% of patients had no pain. Mobility was good or very good in 44%. The mean follow-up was 7.5 years (range, 1 to 34 years). Altogether, 69% of the male hip recipients younger than 60 years were at work at the time of the survey.[143]

ASSESSMENT AND MONITORING

Signs and symptoms such as spinal pain and limitation of motion might be due to current disease activity or to damage. A plethora of tools is available to assess these dimensions. For example, there are many ways to measure limitation of motion of the lumbar spine. New instruments have been developed to assess various aspects of the disease including the Bath and Edmonton AS metrology indices, Bath AS global index, BASRI, Bath AS disease activity index, and Dougados functional index.[144-149] However, standardization and validation of many of these instruments are lacking or incomplete. An international Assessment in Ankylosing Spondylitis (ASAS) working group was formed with the aim of selecting, proposing, and testing core sets of measures for different settings.[150] It was thought that a certain set of variables should be targeted to a specific task. For example, when assessing the efficacy of physical therapy, it would not be realistic to include measures of radiographic changes of the spine. Clearly, the set of measures for a drug's disease-modifying capabilities will differ from a set that measures analgesic effectiveness only. Four settings have been defined: disease-controlling

Table 75-10 World Health Organization–International League of Associations for Rheumatology Core Sets for Ankylosing Spondylitis

Domain	Instrument
Function	BASFI or Functional Index Dougados
Pain	VAS: last week, spine pain at night due to AS
	VAS: last week, spine pain due to AS
Spinal mobility	Chest expansion and modified Schober and occiput to wall distance (lateral spinal flexion or BASMI)
Patient global assessment	VAS: last week
Stiffness	Duration of morning spine stiffness, last week
Peripheral joints and entheses	Number of swollen joints (44 joint count); validated enthesis index
Acute-phase reactants	Erythrocyte sedimentation rate
Spine radiographs	Lateral view of lumbar spine and lateral view of cervical spine
Hip radiographs	Pelvic radiograph including sacroiliac joints and hips
Fatigue	VAS on fatigue from BASDAI

Disease-controlling antirheumatic therapy domains: 1-10; symptom-modifying antirheumatic drug domains: 1-5, 10; physical therapy domains: 1-5, 10; clinical record-keeping domains: 1-7.

AS, ankylosing spondylitis; BASDAI, Bath ankylosing spondylitis disease activity index; BASFI, Bath ankylosing spondylitis functional index; BASMI, Bath ankylosing spondylitis metrology index; VAS, visual analogue scale.

From van der Heijde D, Calin A, Dougados M, et al: Selection of instruments in the core set for DC-ART, SMARD, physical therapy, and clinical record keeping in ankylosing spondylitis: progress report of ASAS Working Group—assessments in ankylosing spondylitis, *J Rheumatol* 26:951–954, 1999.

antirheumatic therapy; symptom-modifying antirheumatic drugs such as NSAIDs; physical therapy; and clinical record keeping in daily practice (Table 75-10).[150] Also, criteria to assess the response of individual patients have been developed and validated. These ASAS-20 improvement criteria are frequently used in clinical trials.[151] In addition, more stringent improvement criteria—ASAS-40 and ASAS-5/6—have been proposed,[152] as well as criteria to define partial remission. The three sets of improvement criteria and the partial remission criteria are presented in Table 75-11.[151,152] The recently developed Ankylosing Spondylitis Disease Activity Score (ASDAS) enables defining disease activity states and demonstrating improvement by applying cutoff values.[153]

A needs-based quality-of-life instrument specific for AS has been developed. It is well accepted and easy to perform and, in terms of assessing the impact of interventions, has shown good scaling and psychometric properties and sensitivity to change.[154,155]

MANAGEMENT

A systematic review of the literature on the management of AS culminated in a series of treatment propositions developed by ASAS/European League Against Rheumatism (EULAR) that emphasize the key evidence-based components of disease management (Table 75-12; Figure 75-3).[156,157] For most patients, AS is a relatively mild disease with a good functional prognosis. Most do not experience significant extraskeletal manifestations except for acute anterior

Table 75-11 Assessment in Ankylosing Spondylitis (ASAS) International Working Group Improvement Criteria and Partial Remission Criteria

ASAS-20 Improvement Criteria

At least 20% improvement and 10 units improvement in 3 of the 4 following domains, without 20% or more worsening and 10 units worsening in the remaining domain:
  BASFI
  Morning stiffness
  Patient global assessment
  Pain

ASAS-40 Improvement Criteria

At least 40% improvement and 20 units improvement in 3 of the 4 following domains, without any worsening in the remaining domain:
  BASFI
  Morning stiffness
  Patient global assessment
  Pain

ASAS-5/6 Improvement Criteria

At least 20% improvement in 5 of the 6 following domains:
  BASFI
  Morning stiffness
  Patient global assessment
  Pain
  Acute-phase reactants
  Spinal mobility

ASAS Partial Remission Criteria

A value below 20 units in all 4 domains of the ASAS-20 improvement criteria

BASFI, Bath ankylosing spondylitis functional index.
From Anderson J.J, Baron G, van der Heijde D, et al: Ankylosing spondylitis assessment group preliminary definition of short-term improvement in ankylosing spondylitis, *Arthritis Rheum* 44:1876–1886, 2001; and Brandt J, Listing J, Sieper J, et al: Development and preselection of criteria for short term improvement after anti-TNFα treatment in ankylosing spondylitis, *Ann Rheum Dis* 63:1438–1444, 2004.

uveitis, which occurs in about 30% of patients. Usually, this eye disease can be well managed with eye drops containing corticosteroids to reduce inflammation and with pupil-dilating, atropine-like agents to prevent or diminish synechiae. At the outset, patients should be warned that acute

ASAS/EULAR recommendations for the management of AS

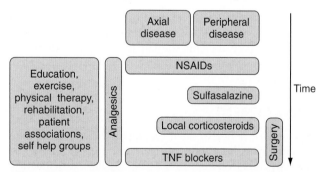

Figure 75-3 Recommended management of ankylosing spondylitis (AS), based on clinical expertise and research evidence. The disease progression with time moves vertically from top to bottom. ASAS/EULAR, Assessment in Ankylosing Spondylitis/European League Against Rheumatism; NSAIDs, nonsteroidal anti-inflammatory drugs; TNF, tumor necrosis factor.

anterior uveitis may occur at any time during the course of the disease.

The treatment objectives in AS are to relieve pain, stiffness, and fatigue and to maintain good posture and good physical and psychosocial functioning.[158] No drug is currently available that significantly influences the course of spinal disease and retards the process of ossification in particular. Similarly, evidence is lacking that any of the conventional disease-modifying antirheumatic drugs including sulfasalazine and methotrexate alter or inhibit the inflammation seen in the spine and entheses in AS.

A full explanation of the disease, its course, possible complications (e.g., acute anterior uveitis), and its prognosis is essential to achieve compliance by the patient. Self-help groups provide important information and social support. In addition, patient organizations often provide access to hydrotherapy and group physiotherapy. Exercises are the mainstay of treatment. Preferably, they should be started after a hot shower or a hot bath. Swimming and extension-promoting exercises or sporting activities such as volleyball or cross-country skiing are appropriate. These activities counteract the kyphotic effects of pain and fatigue on posture and reduce stiffness. Patients should avoid vigorous or contact sports if the spine has become fused or osteoporotic because such a spine is susceptible to fracture.

Appliances such as driving mirrors may improve comfort and safety, especially if there is considerable involvement of the cervical spine. In that case, appropriate neck support is also required to reduce the risk of fracturing the vulnerable osteoporotic cervical spine as a consequence of traffic accidents. For the same reason, automobile air bags are strongly recommended.

Physiotherapy

Evidence indicates that physiotherapy in the form of exercises is effective, at least in the short term (up to 1 year). In a randomized, controlled trial, a program of supervised physiotherapy in groups was superior to individualized programs in improving thoracolumbar mobility and fitness. The program, which consisted of hydrotherapy, exercises, and sporting activities twice weekly for 3 hours per session, resulted in improved overall health and less stiffness, as reported by the patient.[159] An intensive 3-week spondyloarthritis exercise therapy program resulted in marked improvement in both subjective and objective assessments that lasted for up to 9 months. Health resource utilization, in particular NSAID use and sick leave, was significantly reduced during this 9-month follow-up period. The clinical benefits of such treatments can be achieved at acceptable costs.[160,161] A Cochrane review concluded that a home exercise program is better than no intervention, supervised group physiotherapy is better than home exercises, and that combined inpatient spa-exercise therapy followed by supervised outpatient weekly group physiotherapy is better than weekly group physiotherapy alone (level A evidence) (Table 75-13).[162] The tendency toward positive effects of physiotherapy in the management of AS calls for further research in this field. New trials should also address other physiotherapy interventions commonly used in clinical practice. Moreover, the impact on physical functioning of physiotherapy in patients who respond well to biologics needs

Table 75-12 First Update of the ASAS/EULAR Recommendations for the Management of Ankylosing Spondylitis (AS)

The overreaching principles of the management of patients with AS are:
  AS is a potentially severe disease with diverse manifestations, usually requiring multidisciplinary treatment coordinated by the rheumatologist
  The primary goal of treating the patient with AS is to maximize long term health-related quality of life through control of symptoms and inflammation, prevention of progressive structural damage, preservation/normalization of function, and social participation
  Treatment of AS should aim at the best care and must be based on a shared decision between the patient and the rheumatologist
The optimal management of patients with AS requires a combination of nonpharmacologic and pharmacologic treatment modalities

1. General Treatment

The treatment of patients with AS should be tailored according to:
  The current manifestations of the disease (axial, peripheral, entheseal, extra-articular symptoms and signs)
  The level of current symptoms, clinical findings, and prognostic indicators
  The general clinical status (age, gender, comorbidity, concomitant medications, psychosocial factors)

2. Disease Monitoring

The disease monitoring of patients with AS should include:
  Patient history (e.g., questionnaires)
  Clinical parameters
  Laboratory tests
  Imaging
    All according to the clinical presentation as well as the ASAS core set
The frequency of monitoring should be decided on an individual basis depending on:
  Course of symptoms
  Severity
  Treatment

3. Nonpharmacologic Treatment

The cornerstone of nonpharmacologic treatment of patients with AS is patient education and regular exercise
Home exercises are effective. Physical therapy with supervised exercises, land or water based, individually or in a group, should be preferred as these are more effective than home exercises
Patient associations and self-help groups may be useful

4. Extra-articular Manifestations and Comorbidities

The frequently observed extra-articular manifestations (e.g., psoriasis, uveitis, and inflammatory bowel disease) should be managed in collaboration with the respective specialists
Rheumatologists should be aware of the increased risk of cardiovascular disease and osteoporosis

5. Nonsteroidal Anti-inflammatory Drugs (NSAIDs)

NSAIDs, including coxibs, are recommended as first-line drug treatment for AS patients with pain and stiffness
Continuous treatment with NSAIDs is preferred for patients with persistently active, symptomatic disease
Cardiovascular, gastrointestinal, and renal risks should be taken into account when prescribing NSAIDs

6. Analgesics

Analgesics, such as paracetamol and opioid (like) drugs, might be considered for residual pain after previously recommended treatments have failed, are contraindicated, and/or are poorly tolerated

7. Glucocorticoids

Corticosteroid injections directed to the local site of musculoskeletal inflammation may be considered
The use of systemic glucocorticoids for axial disease is not supported by evidence

8. Disease-modifying Antirheumatic Drugs (DMARDs)

There is no evidence for the efficacy of DMARDs, including sulfasalazine and methotrexate, for the treatment of axial disease
Sulfasalazine may be considered in patients with peripheral arthritis

9. Anti–Tumor Necrosis Factor (TNF) Therapy

Anti-TNF therapy should be given to patients with persistently high disease activity despite conventional treatments according to the ASAS recommendations
There is no evidence to support the obligatory use of DMARDs before or concomitant with anti-TNF therapy in patients with axial disease
There is no evidence to support a difference in efficacy of the various TNF inhibitors on the axial and articular/entheseal disease manifestations, but in the presence of inflammatory bowel disease a difference in gastrointestinal efficacy needs to be taken into account
Switching to a second TNF blocker might be beneficial, especially in patients with loss of response
There is no evidence to support the use of biologic agents other than TNF inhibitors in AS

10. Surgery

Total hip arthroplasty should be considered in patients with refractory pain or disability and radiographic evidence of structural damage, independent of age
Spinal corrective osteotomy may be considered in patients with severe disabling deformity
In patients with AS and an acute vertebral fracture, a spinal surgeon should be consulted

11. Changes in the Disease Course

If a significant change in the course of the disease occurs, causes other than inflammation, such as a spinal fracture, should be considered and appropriate evaluation, including imaging, should be performed

ASAS, Assessment in Ankylosing Spondylitis; EULAR, European League Against Rheumatism.
From van der Heijde D, Sieper J, Maksymowych WP, et al: 2010 update of the international ASAS recommendations for the use of anti-TNF agents in patients with axial spondyloarthritis, *Ann Rheum Dis* 70:905–908, 2010.

Table 75-13   Cochrane Review of Physiotherapeutic Interventions and Spondyloarthritis Therapy for Patients with Ankylosing Spondylitis: Conclusions

Home exercise programs are better than no intervention
Supervised group physiotherapy is better than home exercise
Combined inpatient spondyloarthritis and exercise therapy followed by supervised outpatient weekly group physiotherapy is better than weekly group physiotherapy alone

From Dagfinrud H, Kvien TK, Hagen KB: Physiotherapy interventions for ankylosing spondylitis, *Cochrane Database Syst Rev* (4):CD002822, 2004.

to be assessed. Although these patients may experience relief of symptoms, the formation and progression of syndesmophytes may not be influenced by TNF-blocking agents.[68] This reinforces the ongoing need for supplementary therapeutic modalities such as physiotherapy in some patients with AS.

Lying prone for 15 to 30 minutes once or several times a day is useful to reverse the tendency toward kyphosis, which is aggravated by pain and fatigue, as well as flexion contractures of the hip joints. Patients should sleep fully supine on a firm mattress with only a small neck-support pillow.

Medication

Nonsteroidal Anti-inflammatory Drugs

The efficacy and effectiveness of NSAID therapy for the alleviation of symptoms have been well established (level A evidence). When given for prolonged periods of up to a year, there may be improvement in spinal mobility and acute-phase reactants.[163] Many NSAIDs are effective in patients with AS, and no NSAID has documented superiority in terms of efficacy. Selective cyclooxygenase-2 (COX-2) inhibitors have similar efficacy to conventional NSAIDs (level A evidence).[164] A nonselective NSAID is appropriate for most patients with AS, who tend to be relatively young and without comorbidity. A COX-2–selective agent may be used in the presence of risk factors for peptic ulceration, although both categories of NSAIDs may exacerbate inflammatory bowel disease. Once-daily drug regimens may improve patient compliance. Up to 2 weeks may be required to demonstrate maximal symptomatic benefit from an NSAID. If symptomatic relief is inadequate, a switch to another NSAID may be worthwhile; failure of two NSAIDs should prompt an exploration of other management strategies.

Given the gastrointestinal and cardiovascular risks of taking NSAIDs or coxibs, one must address whether this treatment should be on a daily or an "on-demand" basis. A 2-year randomized, prospective, controlled trial in AS patients compared the efficacy of continuous NSAID therapy with that of intermittent on-demand use. The results suggest that continuous therapy retards radiographic disease progression.[165] This study is in line with an older study that also suggested a possible disease-controlling effect of continuous therapy.[166] However, these findings require confirmation by studies less liable to bias.[167]

Second-Line Drugs

Borrowing well-established concepts in the treatment of RA, disease-controlling therapy for AS has been defined as an agent that decreases inflammatory manifestations of disease, sustains or improves function, and prevents or decreases the rate of progression of structural damage. Although most of the second-line agents developed primarily for RA have been studied in AS, none can be considered disease controlling in AS. The greatest amount of data is available for sulfasalazine, which was first proposed as a therapy for AS in 1984, based on the common association between inflammatory bowel disease and spondyloarthritis, the description of inflammatory lesions in the ileum of patients with spondyloarthritis, and its success in the treatment of intestinal inflammation.[168] A total of 11 double-blind, placebo-controlled trials have been published, as well as two meta-analyses. The results of the two largest trials were consistent, demonstrating no significant benefit for sulfasalazine in AS, although subgroup analysis showed that patients with (peripheral) polyarthritis—mostly those with psoriatic arthritis, but also AS patients with peripheral joint involvement—had a significant but modest response.[169,170] An important limitation in most of these studies was the long disease duration (>10 years) of recruited patients, and it has been suggested that early disease may be more responsive to therapy. However, a 24-week placebo-controlled trial that recruited 230 patients meeting European Spondyloarthropathy Study Group (ESSG) criteria for spondyloarthritis and with symptom duration of less than 5 years confirmed that sulfasalazine was ineffective.[171] The most recent meta-analysis, based on 11 trials, concluded that this agent has a significant impact only on the ESR and the severity of spinal stiffness (level A evidence).[172] The primary indication for the use of sulfasalazine in routine practice is a patient who has concomitant peripheral arthritis and has had an inadequate response to NSAIDs and physical modalities.

The evaluation of methotrexate in AS has been limited to case reports and open analyses, mostly reported in abstract form. These studies have included limited numbers of patients for periods of 6 months to 3 years, at doses from 7.5 to 15 mg weekly. The results have been mixed, with some benefit noted in patients with concomitant peripheral arthritis. Two small placebo-controlled trials assessed methotrexate in doses of 10 and 7.5 mg weekly for 24 weeks, with contradictory findings.[173,174] A meta-analysis concluded that there was no evidence of efficacy and that higher-quality trials, larger sample sizes, longer durations of treatment, and higher dosages of methotrexate were necessary before any definitive conclusions could be drawn (level B evidence).[175]

Corticosteroids may be effective for local intra-articular treatment in AS including the SI joints, if given under fluoroscopic guidance (level B evidence). Systemic steroids are of unproven benefit and are thought to be less effective than in RA (level C evidence). Leflunomide has been studied in AS, and although an open-label study suggested a benefit in patients with peripheral arthritis, a small placebo-controlled study reported no benefit (level B evidence).[176,177] A controlled dose-response (60 mg vs. 10 mg) evaluation of a bisphosphonate, pamidronate, given intravenously on a monthly basis for 6 months showed evidence of symptomatic efficacy, primarily in patients with only axial disease (level B evidence).[178] However, this finding needs to be confirmed.

Thalidomide has been used in two open-label studies in AS because it enhances the degradation of TNF messenger RNA. In a Chinese study, improvement was reported in 80% of patients, with deterioration 3 months after treatment discontinuation. Frequent side effects are drowsiness, constipation, and dizziness (level B evidence).[179]

Biologic Therapies

A milestone in the treatment of AS is the development of anti-TNF therapies. The rationale is based on the finding of TNF expression in SI joint biopsies of AS patients, the observation that overexpression of TNF leads to sacroiliitis in animal models, and earlier clinical trial data demonstrating the efficacy of one anti-TNF agent, infliximab, in Crohn's disease. Four anti-TNF agents are of proven benefit in AS according to pivotal phase III trials (level A evidence): infliximab, etanercept, adalimumab, and golimumab. Infliximab is an IgG1 chimeric monoclonal antibody with the Fab portion derived from the mouse. It is given in a dose of 3 to 5 mg/kg every 6 to 8 weeks after loading at 0, 2, and 6 weeks. Etanercept is a recombinant 75-kD TNF receptor IgG1 fusion protein that is self-administered by subcutaneous injection either once (50 mg) or twice (25 mg) weekly. Adalimumab and golimumab are human monoclonal antibodies that are self-administered by subcutaneous injection on alternate weeks (40 mg) or monthly (50 mg), respectively. None require concomitant therapy with methotrexate.

All these agents demonstrate ASAS-20 response rates of 55% to 60% and ASAS-40 response rates of 45% to 50% in phase III trials.[180-184] Even higher response rates have been observed in patients with preradiographic axial spondyloarthritis and short disease duration who received adalimumab or infliximab in placebo-controlled trials.[185,186] Improvement is evident by 2 to 4 weeks and is sustained as long as the patient remains on treatment; virtually all patients relapse by 4 months after discontinuation of treatment.[183] Significant improvement is also observed in function, spinal mobility, peripheral synovitis, enthesitis score, and quality of life. Sick leave and work disability are reduced. The number of patients who must be treated to achieve one patient who experiences at least 50% improvement in disease activity is just two (95% CI, 1 to 6). Objective parameters of disease activity that show improvement include acute-phase reactants, synovial histopathology, and MRI features of inflammation in the spine and SI joints.[187] As of now, no evidence indicates that these agents are disease controlling with respect to the prevention of structural damage on plain radiography.[68] Response to treatment appears to be increased in those with high disease activity and worse in those with a long disease duration, impaired function, and no discernible evidence of inflammation on MRI.[188] However, patients with complete spinal ankylosis may benefit from these treatments.[182] Adverse events in AS patients are no different from those reported in RA, and infusion reactions in patients receiving infliximab have been no more frequent than in RA patients on concomitant methotrexate. All anti-TNF agents are effective for psoriasis, and the monoclonal anti-TNF antibodies, infliximab and adalimumab, also have demonstrated efficacy in both uveitis and colitis. Patients who fail to respond to one anti-TNF agent may respond to an alternative anti-TNF agent.

Recommendations for the use of anti-TNF therapies have been developed (Table 75-14).[189-191] These new therapeutic modalities identify important clinical questions to be answered by further research. All the anti-TNF agents examined to date have symptom-modifying properties, but their long-term safety and disease-controlling effects in terms of preventing structural damage have yet to be demonstrated.

Surgery

Involvement of the hip joint may cause serious disability. Ectopic bone formation may occur, but the outcome of total hip replacement is generally favorable.[143]

Vertebral osteotomy may be required in selected cases to correct marked flexion deformity when forward vision is severely impaired. Diaphragmatic herniation may result from the procedure.

SUMMARY

Although understanding of AS genetics has improved greatly, knowledge about its cause and pathogenesis is far from complete. Much has been accomplished in terms of classification and assessment of the disease. Treatment with biologics such as anti-TNF is effective, but such therapy has not yet been shown to inhibit radiographic progression of spinal syndesmophytes. The challenge now is to determine how to predict and improve outcomes at the level of individual patients, in particular for those patients who will develop important structural changes and functional decline.

Future Directions

The long interval (on average) between the first symptoms of AS and the clinical diagnosis must be shortened.

Research into factors that accurately predict final outcome at the time of diagnosis is essential.

Study of which factors predict response to biologic therapy for individual AS patients is highly desirable. In addition, the long-term effects of treatment with biologics are not yet fully known.

Evidence of the effectiveness of preventing damage in terms of the development of syndesmophytes is still contradictory. It is largely unknown what triggers the process of ankylosing.

A few studies suggest that continuous (versus intermittent) use of NSAIDs or coxibs may slow the progression of axial radiographic manifestations of AS. These findings, however, are controversial. Therefore further studies on this issue are required.

Table 75-14 2010 Update of Recommendations for the Use of Anti–Tumor Necrosis Factor (TNF) Agents in Patients with Axial Spondyloarthritis (SpA)

	Recommendation
Patient Selection	
Diagnosis	Patients fulfilling modified New York Criteria for definitive AS* or the ASAS criteria for axial SpA
Active disease	Active disease for ≥4 wk
	BASDAI ≥ 4 (0-10)† and a positive expert opinion‡
Treatment failure	**All patients** should have had adequate therapeutic trials of at least two NSAIDs. An adequate therapeutic trial is defined as at least two NSAIDs over a 4-wk period in total at maximum recommended or tolerated anti-inflammatory dose unless contraindicated
	Patients with predominantly axial manifestations do not have to take DMARDs before anti-TNF treatment can be started
	Patients with symptomatic peripheral arthritis should have an insufficient response to at least one local steroid injection if appropriate and should normally have had an adequate therapeutic trial of a DMARD, preferably sulfasalazine
	Patients with symptomatic enthesitis must have failed appropriate local treatment
Assessment of Disease	
ASAS Core Set of Daily Practice	
Physical function (BASFI or Dougados functional index)	
Pain (VAS for spine at night from AS in the past week and VAS for spine from AS in the past week)	
Spinal mobility (chest expansion, modified Schober and occiput to wall distance, and lateral lumbar flexion)	
Patient's global assessment (VAS for the past week)	
Stiffness (duration of morning spine stiffness in the past week)	
Peripheral joints and entheses (number of swollen joints [44 total], enthesitis score such as developed in Maastricht, Berlin, or San Francisco)	
Acute-phase reactants (erythrocyte sedimentation rate or C-reactive protein)	
Fatigue (VAS)	
BASDAI	
VAS for overall level of fatigue or tiredness in the past week	
VAS for overall level of AS neck, back, or hip pain in the past week	
VAS for overall level of pain or swelling in joints other than neck, back, or hips in the past week	
VAS for overall discomfort from any areas tender to touch or pressure in the past week	
VAS for overall level of morning stiffness from time of awakening in the past week	
Duration and intensity (VAS) of morning stiffness from time of awakening (up to 120 min)	
Assessment of Response	
Responder criteria	BASDAI: 50% relative change or absolute change of 2 (on 0-10 scale) *and* expert opinion in favor of continuation
Time of evaluation	After at least 12 wk

*Modified New York criteria (van der Linden et al, 1984): radiologic criterion (sacroiliitis, grade ≥II bilaterally or grade III to IV unilaterally) and at least two out of three clinical criteria (low back pain and stiffness for more than 3 mo that improves with exercise but is not relieved by rest; limitation of motion of the lumbar spine in both the sagittal and frontal planes; limitation of chest expansion relative to normal values correlated for age and sex).

†BASDAI assessed on a 0-10 VAS or NRS.

‡The expert is a doctor, usually a rheumatologist, with expertise in inflammatory back pain and the use of biologic agents. Experts should be locally defined. An expert opinion should consider clinical features (history and examination) as well as either serum acute-phase reactant levels or imaging results, such as radiographs demonstration rapid progression or magnetic resonance imaging scans indicting inflammation.

ASAS core set for daily practice: physical function (BASFI); pain (VAS/NRS, last week, spine at night, due to AS and VAS/NRS, last week, spine due to AS); spinal mobility (chest expansion, cervical rotation, occiput-to-wall distance, modified Schober, and lateral lumbar flexion or BASMI); patient's global assessment (VAS/NRS, last week); stiffness (duration of morning stiffness, spine, VAS/NRS, last week); peripheral joints and entheses (number of swollen joints [44 joints count], enthesitis score such as developed in Maastricht, Berlin, or San Francisco); acute-phase reactants (preferably C-reactive protein); fatigue (VAS/NRS).

AS, ankylosing spondylitis; ASAS, Assessment in SpondyloArthritis international Society; BASDAI, Bath Ankylosing Spondylitis Disease Activity Index; BASFI, Bath Ankylosing Spondylitis Functional Index; BASMI, Bath Ankylosing Spondylitis Metrology Index; DMARD, disease-modifying antirheumatic drug; NRS, numeric rate scale; NSAIDs, nonsteroidal anti-inflammatory drugs; VAS, visual analogue scale.

From van der Heijde D, Sieper J, Maksymowych WP, et al: 2010 update of the international ASAS recommendations for the use of anti-TNF agents in patients with axial spondyloarthritis, *Ann Rheum Dis* 70:905–908, 2010.

Selected References

2. Mau W, Zeidler H, Mau R, et al: Clinical features and prognosis of patients with possible ankylosing spondylitis. Results of a 10-year follow-up, *J Rheumatol* 15:1109–1114, 1988.

5. Oostveen J, Prevo R, den Boer J, et al: Early detection of sacroiliitis on magnetic resonance imaging and subsequent development of sacroiliitis on plain radiography. A prospective, longitudinal study, *J Rheumatol* 26:1953–1958, 1999.

6. Bennett AN, McGonagle D, O'Connor P, et al: Severity of baseline magnetic resonance imaging-evident sacroiliitis and *HLA-B27* status in early inflammatory back pain predict radiographically evident ankylosing spondylitis at eight years, *Arthritis Rheum* 58:3413–3418, 2008.

14. D'Amato M, Fiorillo MT, Carcassi C, et al: Relevance of residue 116 of *HLA-B27* in determining susceptibility to ankylosing spondylitis, *Eur J Immunol* 25:3199–3201, 1995.

15. Lopez-Larrea C, Sujirachato K, Mehra NK, et al: *HLA-B27* subtypes in Asian patients with ankylosing spondylitis, *Tissue Antigens* 45:169–176, 1995.

16. Nasution AR, Marjuadi A, Kunmartini S, et al: *HLA-B27* subtypes positively and negatively associated with spondylarthropathy, *J Rheumatol* 24:1111–1114, 1997.

19. Saraux A, Guillemin F, Guggenbuhl F, et al: Prevalence of spondyloarthropathies in France: 2001, *Ann Rheum Dis* 64:1431–1435, 2005.

20. Kaipiainen-Seppanen O, Aho K, Heliovaara M: Incidence and prevalence of ankylosing spondylitis in Finland, *J Rheumatol* 24:496–499, 1997.

21. Braun J, Bollow M, Remlinger G, et al: Prevalence of spondyloarthropathies in *HLA-B27* positive and negative blood donors, *Arthritis Rheum* 41:58–67, 1998.

23. Carbone LD, Cooper C, Michet CJ, et al: Ankylosing spondylitis in Rochester, Minnesota, 1935-1989, *Arthritis Rheum* 35:1476–1482, 1992.

24. Martindale J, Smith J, Sutton CJ, et al: Disease and psychological status in ankylosing spondylitis, *Rheumatology (Oxford)* 45:1288–1293, 2006.

33. Gonzalez-Roces S, Alvarez MV, Gonzalez S, et al: *HLA-B27* and worldwide susceptibility to ankylosing spondylitis, *Tissue Antigens* 49:116–123, 1997.

34. Hammer RE, Maika SD, Richardson JA, et al: Spontaneous inflammatory disease in transgenic rats expressing *HLA-B27* and human beta 2m: An animal model of *HLA-B27*-associated human disorders, *Cell* 63:1099–1112, 1990.

35. Taurog JD, Richardson JA, Croft JT, et al: The germfree state prevents development of gut and joint inflammatory disease in *HLA-B27* transgenic rats, *J Exp Med* 180:2359–2364, 1994.

36. Tran TM, Dorris ML, Satumtira N, et al: Additional human beta-2 microglobulin curbs *HLA-B27* misfolding and promotes arthritis and spondylitis without colitis in male *HLA-B27*-transgenicrats, *Arthritis Rheum* 54:1317–1327, 2006.

43. Mear JP, Schreiber KL, Münz C, et al: Misfolding of *HLA-B27* as a result of its B pocket suggests a novel mechanism for its role in susceptibility to spondyloarthropathies, *J Immunol* 163:6665–6670, 1999.

45. Turner MJ, Sowders DP, DeLay ML, et al: *HLA-B27* misfolding in transgenic rats is associated with activation of the unfolded protein response, *J Immunol* 175:2438–2448, 2005.

51. Glant T, Mikecz K, Arzoumanian A, et al: Proteoglycan-induced arthritis in Balb/c mice, *Arthritis Rheum* 30:201–212, 1987.

53. Zou J, Zhang Y, Thiel A, et al: Predominant cellular immune response to the cartilage autoantigenic G1 aggrecan in ankylosing spondylitis and rheumatoid arthritis, *Rheumatology (Oxford)* 42:846–855, 2003.

68. van der Heijde D, Landewé R, Baraliakos X, et al: Radiographic findings following two years of infliximab therapy in patients with ankylosing spondylitis, *Arthritis Rheum* 58:3063–3070, 2008.

71. Francois RJ, Gardner DL, Degrave EJ, Bywaters EGL: Histopathologic evidence that sacroiliitis in ankylosing spondylitis is not merely enthesitis, *Arthritis Rheum* 43:2011–2024, 2000.

80. Calin A, Porta J, Fries JF, Schurman DJ: Clinical history as a screening test for ankylosing spondylitis, *JAMA* 237:2613–2614, 1977.

85. Khan MA, Kushner I, Braun WE: Comparison of clinical features in *HLA-B27* positive and negative patients with ankylosing spondylitis, *Arthritis Rheum* 20:909–912, 1977.

87. Graham DC, Smythe HA: The carditis and aortitis of ankylosing spondylitis, *Bull Rheum Dis* 9:171–174, 1958.

89. Strobel ES, Fritschka E: Case report and review of the literature: fatal pulmonary complications in ankylosing spondylitis, *Clin Rheumatol* 16:617–622, 1997.

90. Casserly IP, Fenlon HM, Breatnach E, et al: Lung findings on high-resolution computed tomography in idiopathic ankylosing spondylitis: correlation with clinical findings, pulmonary function testing and plain radiography, *Br J Rheumatol* 36:677–682, 1997.

92. Ramos-Remus C, Gomez-Vargas A, Hernandez-Chavez A, et al: Two year follow-up of anterior and vertical atlantoaxial subluxation in ankylosing spondylitis, *J Rheumatol* 24:507–510, 1997.

93. Tyrrell PNM, Davies AM, Evans N: Neurological disturbances in ankylosing spondylitis, *Ann Rheum Dis* 53:714–717, 1994.

94. Lai KN, Li PKT, Hawkins B, et al: IgA nephropathy associated with ankylosing spondylitis: occurrence in women as well as in men, *Ann Rheum Dis* 48:435–437, 1989.

95. Vilar MJ, Cury SE, Ferraz MB, et al: Renal abnormalities in ankylosing spondylitis, *Scand J Rheumatol* 26:19–23, 1997.

96. Gratacos J, Orellana C, Sanmarti R, et al: Secondary amyloidosis in ankylosing spondylitis: a systematic review of 137 patients using abdominal fat aspiration, *J Rheumatol* 24:912–915, 1997.

97. Lee YS, Schlotzhauer T, Ott SM, et al: Skeletal status of men with early and late ankylosing spondylitis, *Am J Med* 103:233–241, 1997.

100. Cooper C, Carbone L, Michet CJ, et al: Fracture risk in patients with ankylosing spondylitis: a population based study, *J Rheumatol* 21:1877–1882, 1994.

102. Khan MA, Kushner I: Diagnosis of ankylosing spondylitis. In Cohen AS, editor: Progress in clinical rheumatology, vol 1, Orlando, 1984, Grune & Stratton, pp 145–178.

105. Schichikawa K, Tsujimoto M, Nishioka J, et al: Histopathology of early sacroiliitis and enthesitis in ankylosing spondylitis. In Ziff M, Cohen SB, editors: The spondyloarthropathies: advances in inflammation research, vol 9, New York, 1985, Raven Press.

106. Aufdermaur M: Pathogenesis of square bodies in ankylosing spondylitis, *Ann Rheum Dis* 48:628–631, 1989.

107. Calin A, Mackay K, Santos H, Brophy S: A new dimension to outcome: application of the Bath ankylosing spondylitis radiology index, *J Rheumatol* 26:988–992, 1999.

108. Dawes PT: Stoke ankylosing spondylitis spine score, *J Rheumatol* 26:993–996, 1999.

110. Weber U, Lambert RGW, Ostergaard M, et al: The diagnostic utility of magnetic resonance imaging in spondylarthritis: an international multicenter evaluation of one hundred eighty-seven subjects, *Arthritis Rheum* 62:3048–3058, 2010.

112. Bennett AN, McGonagle D, O'Connor P, et al: Severity of baseline magnetic resonance imaging—evident sacroiliitis and HLA-B27 status in early inflammatory back pain predict radiographically evident ankylosing spondylitis at eight years, *Arthritis Rheum* 58: 3413–3418, 2008.

118. Khan MA, Khan MK: Diagnostic value of *HLA-B27* testing in ankylosing spondylitis and Reiter's syndrome, *Ann Intern Med* 96:70–76, 1982.

122. Dubost JJ, Sauvezie B: Late onset peripheral spondyloarthropathy, *J Rheumatol* 16:1214–1217, 1989.

123. Kidd B, Mullee M, Frank A, et al: Disease expression of ankylosing spondylitis in males and females, *J Rheumatol* 15:1407–1409, 1988.

124. Jimenez-Balderas FJ, Mintz G: AS: clinical course in women and men, *J Rheumatol* 20:2069–2072, 1993.

128. Khan MA, Khan MK: Survival among patients with ankylosing spondylitis: a lifetable analysis, *J Rheumatol* 8:86–90, 1981.

129. Lehtinen K: Mortality and causes of death in 398 patients admitted to hospital with ankylosing spondylitis, *Ann Rheum Dis* 52:174–176, 1993.

130. Calin A, Elswood J, Rigg S, et al: Ankylosing spondylitis: an analytical review of 1500 patients—the changing pattern of disease, *J Rheumatol* 15:1234–1238, 1988.

131. Fries JF, Singh G, Bloch DA, et al: The natural history of ankylosing spondylitis: is the disease really changing? *J Rheumatol* 16:860–863, 1989.

134. Guillemin F, Briancon S, Pourel J, Gaucher A: Long-term disability and prolonged sick leaves as outcome measurements in ankylosing spondylitis: possible predictive factors, *Arthritis Rheum* 33:1001–1006, 1990.

135. Ramos-Remus C, Prieto-Parra RE, Michel-Diaz J, et al: A five-year cumulative analysis of labor-status and lost working days in patients with ankylosing spondylitis (AS), *Arthritis Rheum* 41(Suppl):1136, 1998.

140. Gran JT, Skomsvolly JF: The outcome of ankylosing spondylitis: a study of 100 patients, *Br J Rheumatol* 36:766–771, 1997.

141. Amor B, Silva-Santos R, Nahal R, et al: Predictive factors for the long-term outcome of spondyloarthropathies, *J Rheumatol* 21:1883–1887, 1994.

143. Calin A, Elswood J: The outcome of 138 total hip replacements and 12 revisions in ankylosing spondylitis: high success rate after a mean followup of 7.5 years, *J Rheumatol* 16:955–958, 1989.

145. Jenkinson TR, Mallorie PA, Whitelock H, et al: Defining spinal mobility in ankylosing spondylitis (AS): the Bath AS Metrology Index (BASMI), *J Rheumatol* 21:1694–1698, 1994.

147. Calin A, Garrett S, Whitelock H, et al: A new approach to defining functional ability in ankylosing spondylitis: the development of the Bath ankylosing spondylitis functional index (BASFI), *J Rheumatol* 21:2281–2285, 1994.

148. Dougados M, Gueguen A, Nakache JP, et al: Evaluation of a functional index and an articular index in ankylosing spondylitis, *J Rheumatol* 15:302–307, 1988.

149. Garrett S, Jenkinson T, Whitelock H, et al: A new approach to defining disease status in AS: the Bath ankylosing spondylitis disease activity index (BASDAI), *J Rheumatol* 21:2286–2291, 1994.

151. Anderson JJ, Baron G, van der Heijde D, et al: Ankylosing spondylitis assessment group preliminary definition of short-term improvement in ankylosing spondylitis, *Arthritis Rheum* 44:1876–1886, 2001.

158. Khan MA, Skosey JL: Ankylosing spondylitis and related spondylo-arthropathies. In Samter M, editor: *Immunological diseases*, Boston, 1988, Little, Brown, pp 1509–1538.

163. Dougados M, Gueguen A, Nakache JP, et al: Ankylosing spondylitis: what is the optimum duration of a clinical study? A one year versus 6 weeks non-steroidal anti-inflammatory drug trial, *Rheumatology (Oxford)* 38:235–244, 1999.

165. Wanders A, van der Heijde D, Landewe R, et al: Nonsteroidal anti-inflammatory drugs reduce radiographic progression in patients with ankylosing spondylitis: a randomized controlled trial, *Arthritis Rheum* 52:1756–1765, 2005.

166. Boersma JW: Retardation of ossification of the lumbar vertebral column in ankylosing spondylitis by means of phenylbutazone, *Scand J Rheumatol* 5:60–64, 1976.

167. Akkoc N, van der Linden S, Khan MA: Ankylosing spondylitis and symptom-modifying vs disease-modifying therapy, *Clin Rheumatol* 20:539–557, 2006.

168. Amor B, Kahan A, Dougados M, Delrieu F: Sulphasalazine in anky-losing spondylitis, *Ann Intern Med* 101:878, 1984.

169. Dougados M, van der Linden S, Leirisalo-Repo M, et al: Sulfasalazine in the treatment of spondyloarthropathy, *Arthritis Rheum* 38:618–627, 1995.

170. Clegg DO, Reda DJ, Weisman MH, et al: Comparison of sulfasalazine and placebo in the treatment of ankylosing spondylitis, *Arthritis Rheum* 39:2004–2012, 1996.

173. Roychowdhury B, Bintley-Bagot S, Hunt J, Tunn EJ: Methotrexate in severe ankylosing spondylitis: a randomised placebo controlled, double-blind observer study, *Rheumatology* 40(Suppl 1):43, 2001.

174. Gonzalez-Lopez L, Garcia-Gonzalez A, Vazquez-del-Mercado M, et al: Efficacy of methotrexate in ankylosing spondylitis: a random-ized, double-blind, placebo-controlled trial, *J Rheumatol* 31:1568–1574, 2004.

176. Haibel H, Rudwaleit M, Braun J, et al: Six month open label trial of leflunomide in ankylosing spondylitis, *Ann Rheum Dis* 64:124–126, 2005.

177. Van Denderen JC, Van der Paardt M, Nurmohamed MT, et al: Double-blind study of leflunomide in the treatment of active ankylos-ing spondylitis, *Ann Rheum Dis* 63(Suppl 1):SAT0033, 2004.

178. Maksymowych WP, Jhangri GS, Fitzgerald AA, et al: A six-month randomized, controlled, double-blind, dose response comparison of intravenous pamidronate (60 mg versus 10 mg) in the treatment of nonsteroidal antiinflammatory drug-refractory ankylosing spondyli-tis, *Arthritis Rheum* 46:766–773, 2002.

179. Huang F, Gu J, Zhao W, et al: One-year open-label trial of thalido-mide in ankylosing spondylitis, *Arthritis Rheum* 47:249–254, 2002.

Full references for this chapter can be found on www.expertconsult.com.

76 Reactive Arthritis and Undifferentiated Spondyloarthritis

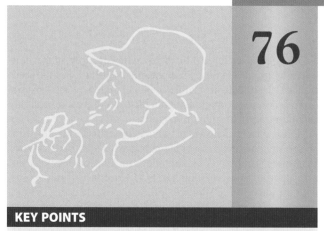

J.S. HILL GASTON

KEY POINTS

Reactive arthritis is a form of spondyloarthritis triggered by particular infections.

Undifferentiated spondyloarthritis can have both peripheral and axial features.

Undifferentiated spondyloarthritis is a provisional diagnosis—many cases will evolve into other forms of spondyloarthritis.

Diagnosis of reactive arthritis rests on symptoms and signs of spondyloarthritis, including extra-articular disease, and evidence of preceding infection.

Reactive arthritis is often self-limited, but chronic forms require disease-modifying antirheumatic drugs (DMARDs) and even biologics.

Treatment of undifferentiated spondyloarthritis depends on whether axial or peripheral disease is predominant.

Two forms of spondyloarthritis will be reviewed in this chapter: reactive arthritis and undifferentiated spondyloarthritis. The other members of the spondyloarthritis group—ankylosing spondylitis, psoriatic arthritis, and arthritis associated with inflammatory bowel disease—are described elsewhere, and current thinking on common features that operate in the pathogenesis of all forms of spondyloarthritis can be found in Chapter 74.

DEFINITIONS AND TERMINOLOGY

Reactive Arthritis

The term **reactive arthritis** is sometimes used loosely, and unhelpfully, to mean "any arthritis that comes on after some kind of infection," that is, as a "reaction" to infection. In this way, diseases such as Lyme disease and rheumatic fever are sometimes termed "reactive," as are postviral forms of arthritis. However, this is potentially confusing; it is better to have a broad category of **postinfectious arthritis** and to reserve the term **reactive arthritis** for the arthritis that follows infection *and* shares features with other forms of spondyloarthritis.[1,2] These include clinical features such as frequent evidence of enthesitis, in addition to arthritis, extra-articular features, particularly those involving eyes and skin, and, as required for a spondyloarthritis family member, a clear association with HLA-B27.[3] Using this definition, a relatively small list of bacteria (and no viruses) are common triggers of reactive arthritis (Table 76-1), and a longer "tail" of infections have occasionally been reported

as causes. These organisms principally infect the gastrointestinal and genitourinary tracts, although *Chlamydia pneumoniae* (now sometimes termed *Chlamydophila pneumoniae*) is an exception[4-6] because it causes respiratory infection.

Another unhelpful term is **Reiter's syndrome** or Reiter's triad—consisting of urethritis, conjunctivitis, and arthritis. There are four main reasons for consigning this term to the dustbin of history. First, Hans Reiter was by no means the first to describe reactive arthritis—on this basis, reactive arthritis would be Leroy-Fiessinger-Reiter syndrome, a term that obviously lacks utility. Second, Reiter erroneously attributed the postdysenteric cases he described to spirochetal infection. Third, Reiter had an association with the Third Reich.[7,8] Fourth, the inclusion of urethritis in Reiter's triad leads to the mistaken assumption that cases of reactive arthritis with urethritis are likely to be due to sexually acquired infection.[9] This is not the case because urethritis is not uncommon in patients whose reactive arthritis is triggered by enteric infection, especially HLA-B27+ patients,[10] and the cases Reiter described in World War I had arthritis associated with dysentery. Therefore, Reiter's syndrome is at best a synonym for reactive arthritis and is neither useful nor required, but the "triad" does not distinguish a clinically important subgroup of reactive arthritis.

Reactive arthritis secondary to gastrointestinal infection is sometimes bracketed with spondyloarthritis associated with inflammatory bowel disease as **enteropathic arthritis.**[11] However, although links between the gut and arthritis are very important pathologically, particularly in spondyloarthritis, enteropathic arthritis is really an ill-defined overlap term, which often includes other forms of arthritis that do not have classic features of spondyloarthritis but occur in relation to gastrointestinal disorders. Examples include Whipple's disease and celiac disease.

Undifferentiated Spondyloarthritis

Obvious overlap has been noted between different members of the spondyloarthritis family. By definition, patients with undifferentiated spondyloarthritis have arthritis that fails to satisfy diagnostic or classification criteria for one of the other forms. Thus, it may not be legitimate to regard undifferentiated spondyloarthritis as a separate "disease" because over time, patients often develop new features, which means that their disease is no longer "undifferentiated." The commonest of these is development of radiographic changes in the sacroiliac joints that allow the patient to satisfy criteria for ankylosing spondylitis. This occurs in approximately 60% of patients in many series,[12] and all ankylosing spondylitis patients will pass through an "undifferentiated" phase

Table 76-1   Organisms Associated with Reactive Arthritis

Common
Gastrointestinal Pathogens
Salmonella species
Campylobacter jejuni and *Campylobacter coli*
Yersinia enterocolitica and *Yersinia pseudotuberculosis*
Shigella flexneri; less commonly, *Shigella sonnei* or *Shigella dysenteriae*
Clostridium difficile
Genitourinary Pathogens
Chlamydia trachomatis
?*Mycoplasma* species
Respiratory Pathogens
Chlamydia pneumoniae
Reported
Mycobacterium bovis bacillus Calmette-Guérin
Enterotoxigenic *Escherichia coli* and many others in small numbers of case reports

(often termed *axial spondyloarthritis*) if seen before developing structural changes on radiographs. Likewise, patients may develop psoriasis at some point after the onset of their spondyloarthritis. In cases where there is a family history of psoriasis or features such as dactylitis, which is very common in psoriatic arthritis, the term *psoriatic arthritis sine psoriasis* is sometimes used, but if patients fail to meet diagnostic criteria for psoriatic arthritis (such as the recently devised Classification Criteria for Psoriatic Arthritis [CASPAR][13]), they should be classified as having undifferentiated spondyloarthritis. Note that in the absence of a personal or family history of skin or nail psoriasis, patients fulfill the CASPAR criteria for psoriatic arthritis only if they have dactylitis *and* juxta-articular new bone formation on hand or foot radiographs, *and* lack rheumatoid factor. In addition, underlying inflammatory bowel disease may declare itself clinically only at some point after the onset of undifferentiated spondyloarthritis.

Finally, as discussed in the following section, it may be difficult to make a certain diagnosis of reactive arthritis, particularly when evidence of a triggering infection is absent or incomplete, resulting in significant overlap between reactive arthritis and undifferentiated spondyloarthritis—hence their being considered together in this chapter.

CLASSIFICATION CRITERIA FOR REACTIVE ARTHRITIS AND UNDIFFERENTIATED SPONDYLOARTHRITIS

Because both reactive arthritis and undifferentiated spondyloarthritis are members of the spondyloarthritis group, patients can first be identified as having spondyloarthritis by means of rather wide classification criteria. It must be recognized that classification criteria are devised to allow homogeneous sets of patients with particular features to be defined. This is critical for research studies, ensuring that different investigators report on the same set of patients. Thus classification criteria are not, and should not be used

as, diagnostic criteria; clinicians will certainly make confident clinical diagnoses for patients who fail to fulfill particular classification criteria. Nevertheless, such criteria often serve as a convenient checklist of the features that are usually present in a given disease.

The two best known classification criteria for all forms of spondyloarthritis considered together are those devised by Amor[14] (Table 76-2) and the later European Spondyloarthropathy Study Group (ESSG) criteria[15] (Table 76-3). The Amor criteria allocate "points" to 12 features characteristic of spondyloarthritis, and classification is based on reaching a specified total score of 6 points. The ESSG criteria are applied to patients with inflammatory back pain or oligoarthritis, with the presence of additional features required for classification. The sensitivity and specificity achieved by the Amor and ESSG criteria vary in different series and inevitably depend on the population to which they are applied, but these values are usually around 80% and 90%, respectively. A more recent development in the classification of spondyloarthritis has been the separation of axial (spine and sacroiliac) inflammation from peripheral arthritis, with recognition that in different forms of spondyloarthritis, one or another of these may predominate, although with time many patients will develop both. To aid classification of axial spondyloarthritis, which traditionally requires radiographic sacroiliitis, as exemplified by the modified New York criteria for ankylosing spondylitis (AS),[16] magnetic resonance imaging (MRI) changes of sacroiliitis have been included in the recently published Assessment of SpondyloArthritis international Society [ASAS] criteria[17]) (Table 76-4). MRI sacroiliitis is carefully defined as bone marrow edema on short tau inversion recovery (STIR) sequences, or as osteitis on T1 images with contrast medium, localized to subchondral or periarticular bone marrow. The

Table 76-2   Amor Criteria for Spondyloarthritis

Clinical Symptoms or Past History of:	Points
Lumbar or dorsal pain during the night, or morning stiffness of lumbar or dorsal spine	1
Asymmetric oligoarthritis	2
Buttock pain	1
Alternating buttock pain	2
Dactylitis of finger or toe	2
Heel pain or other well-defined enthesopathy	2
Iritis	2
Nongonococcal urethritis or cervicitis within 1 mo of arthritis onset	1
Acute diarrhea within 1 mo of arthritis onset	1
Psoriasis, balanitis, or inflammatory bowel disease	2
Radiology	
Sacroiliitis (grade ≥2 if bilateral; grade ≥3 if unilateral)	3
Genetic Background	
HLA-B27+ or family history of ankylosing spondylitis, reactive arthritis, uveitis, psoriasis, or inflammatory bowel disease	2
Response to Treatment	
Good response to NSAIDs within 48 hr, or relapse within 48 hr if NSAIDs withdrawn	2

For a definitive diagnosis of spondylarthritis, ≥6 points is required; 5 points indicates probable spondyloarthritis.
NSAIDs, nonsteroidal anti-inflammatory drugs.

Table 76-3 European Spondyloarthropathy Study Group Criteria for Spondyloarthritis

For patients with:
    Inflammatory spinal pain
    or
    Synovitis that is asymmetric or is present predominantly in the lower limbs
+ ≥1 if:
    Family history of spondyloarthropathy
    Psoriasis
    Inflammatory bowel disease
    Urethritis, cervicitis, or acute diarrhea within 1 mo of onset of arthritis
    Alternating buttock pain
    Enthesitis
    Sacroiliitis

changes are also required to be multiple or present in at least two consecutive slices. Therefore, patients younger than 45 years of age, with at least 3 months' history of back pain or sacroiliitis on MRI (or on radiographs), plus at least one feature from the list of spondyloarthritis-associated signs and symptoms shown in Table 76-4, fulfill the criteria. In the absence of sacroiliitis, HLA-B27⁺ individuals can still be classified as having axial spondyloarthritis when two or more of these features are present. These ASAS criteria represent a recent and welcome development, but it remains to be determined what the specificity and sensitivity of MRI changes in sacroiliac joints will be when used in routine practice in nonresearch settings.

The main driver for developing the ASAS criteria for axial spondyloarthritis has been the need to define early ankylosing spondylitis without requiring radiologic changes in the sacroiliac joints. Because these often take years to develop, new criteria were required to identify, investigate, and treat patients with early ankylosing spondylitis. Nevertheless, not all patients who fulfill the criteria for axial spondyloarthritis go on to develop ankylosing spondylitis, that is, early ankylosing spondylitis is a subset of axial

Table 76-4 Assessment of SpondyloArthritis international Society Classification Criteria for Axial Spondyloarthritis (SpA)

For patients with back pain for ≥3 mo and aged <45 yr:
Sacroiliitis on imaging   +   ≥1 SpA feature
or
HLA-B27   +   ≥2 other SpA features
Sacroiliitis on imaging defined as:
    Active acute inflammation on magnetic resonance imaging highly suggestive of sacroiliitis associated with SpA
    or
    Definitive radiographic sacroiliitis according to the modified New York criteria
SpA features comprising:
    Arthritis
    Enthesitis (heel)
    Inflammatory back pain
    Dactylitis
    Uveitis
    Psoriasis
    Inflammatory bowel disease
    Good response to nonsteroidal anti-inflammatory drugs
    Family history of SpA
    HLA-B27
    Elevated C-reactive protein

spondyloarthritis. Patients who do not progress to radiographic changes or other clinical features of ankylosing spondylitis will continue to be classified as having undifferentiated spondyloarthritis.

The new ASAS criteria for axial disease are clearly useful for identifying patients with undifferentiated spondyloarthritis. In reactive arthritis, acute inflammatory back pain is common, but no studies have established the frequency of MRI-defined sacroiliitis in this disease, or of MRI-defined changes in the spine, although the latter are not used in the ASAS classification. Thus the ASAS criteria for axial spondyloarthritis are not likely to be very useful in reactive arthritis.

More relevant to reactive arthritis are the ASAS criteria for classification of peripheral spondyloarthritis, which have also been published and discussed recently[18,19] (Table 76-5). These are applied to patients who present with arthritis, particularly asymmetric oligoarticular lower limb arthritis OR enthesitis OR dactylitis. These patients are classified as having peripheral spondyloarthritis if they have **one** additional feature from the list shown in Table 76-5. In the absence of any of these features, **two** features from an additional list are required: arthritis, enthesitis, dactylitis, inflammatory back pain, or family history of spondyloarthritis. Note that because these criteria are applied to patients who present with arthritis or enthesitis or dactylitis, this second list gives weight to the occurrence of these symptoms in combination. These criteria achieved a sensitivity of 78% and a specificity of 83%, representing a compromise between lower sensitivity and greater specificity of the Amor or ESSG criteria. How the ASAS criteria will fare in more general use remains to be seen; they were developed in a population in whom 85% were younger than age 45, and 30% had radiographic changes in sacroiliac joints that met modified New York criteria for ankylosing spondylitis, even though they did not have back pain at recruitment.

Used together, ASAS criteria for axial and peripheral spondyloarthritis should classify all those patients who have some form of spondyloarthritis (again recalling that some patients will be *diagnosed* with spondyloarthritis even though

Table 76-5 Assessment of SpondyloArthritis international Society Classification Criteria for Peripheral Spondyloarthritis

For patients with:
    Peripheral arthritis (usually asymmetric, lower limb)
    or
    Enthesitis
    or
    Dactylitis
+ 1 of:
    HLA-B27
    Genitourinary or gastrointestinal infection
    Psoriasis
    Inflammatory bowel disease
    Magnetic resonance imaging sacroiliitis
    or
+ 2 of:
    Arthritis
    Enthesitis
    Dactylitis
    Inflammatory back pain
    Family history of spondyloarthritis

Table 76-6 Proposed Definition of the Diagnosis of Reactive Arthritis

Patients can be confidently diagnosed with reactive arthritis if they have:
1. **Classic clinical features:**
Asymmetric oligoarthritis, predominantly lower limbs
Enthesitis
Extra-articular signs
and
Proven infection by *Salmonella, Campylobacter, Yersinia, Shigella,* or *Chlamydia* (whether symptomatic or not)
or
Proven infection by other organisms previously reported to be associated with reactive arthritis (e.g., *Clostridium difficile, Mycobacterium bovis* bacillus Calmette-Guérin)
2. **Any acute inflammatory arthritis, including monoarthritis and/or axial inflammation**
and
Proven infection by reactive arthritis–associated bacteria
3. **Classic clinical features (as listed in No. 1)**
and
Diarrhea or urethritis/cervicitis within the previous 6 wk, infection not proven

they do not meet these *classification* criteria). Of those who meet ASAS criteria, some will have documented psoriasis or inflammatory bowel disease, or radiologic sacroiliitis, and therefore can be classified as having a particular form of spondyloarthritis. The remainder will have undifferentiated spondyloarthritis or reactive arthritis. In relation to diagnosis, checking the features included in the classification criteria will allow the clinician to identify patients in whom some form of spondyloarthritis is likely, and will prompt additional clinical examination and investigations that may clarify the diagnosis or even elicit additional criteria.

In relation to reactive arthritis, there is no wholly satisfactory definition of the disease.[20] One practical proposal is shown in Table 76-6. In the setting of an outbreak of food poisoning, when all those known to have been infected with *Salmonella* or *Campylobacter* can be followed up, all who develop new joint symptoms can be regarded as having reactive arthritis, but inevitably this also includes patients with only arthralgias.[21,22] Joint symptoms have a high background prevalence in the community, and it is difficult to be certain that those reported by patients following infection are genuinely related to the infection and not to preexisting conditions that assume new prominence in the context of an infection, or to questionnaires seeking such symptoms.

In practice therefore it is best to regard only patients with new definite joint swelling, enthesitis, or inflammatory back pain as having reactive arthritis—most of these will fulfill the ASAS criteria for peripheral spondyloarthritis. In specialist rheumatology practice, as compared with community surveys, reactive arthritis patients will have clear evidence of joint inflammation and commonly enthesitis. What is often less certain is the nature of any triggering infection; the degree of certainty runs from patients with culture-proven infection with an organism previously known to cause reactive arthritis, to those who may have only a history suggesting a preceding infection or serologic evidence of infection without clinical history. A "gold standard" for reactive arthritis, requiring spondyloarthritis and unequivocal demonstration of preceding infection by

culture (or polymerase chain reaction [PCR]), would allow diagnosis of only a minority of cases, but less strict criteria inevitably result in an overlap with undifferentiated spondyloarthritis. Some surveys of patients given the latter diagnosis have produced immunologic evidence, particularly when synovial fluid T cell responses to reactive arthritis–associated organisms are measured, which suggests that a significant proportion (up to 50%) may actually have reactive arthritis.[23]

INCIDENCE OF REACTIVE ARTHRITIS AND UNDIFFERENTIATED SPONDYLOARTHRITIS

Several community studies have examined reactive arthritis, mainly in Scandinavia, where HLA-B27 prevalence is high. A study in Oslo suggested an incidence of 4 to 5 per 100,000 for both *Chlamydia*-induced and enteric infection–related disease,[24] and similar results were reported in Finland.[25] Reactive arthritis following gastroenteritis has been systematically investigated by Leirisalo-Repo and colleagues, who studied populations known to have been infected with *Salmonella, Campylobacter, Yersinia,* and *Shigella* and provided follow-up by questionnaire and clinical examination to determine the incidence of new inflammatory symptoms in the joints and back, and of clinical reactive arthritis.[21,22,26,27] Together these studies suggest that 7% to 12% of those infected develop reactive arthritis, and other studies agree with this.[28-30] An incidence of 4.3 per 100,000 and 0.13 per 100,000, respectively, for *Campylobacter* and *Shigella* was reported in population studies in Finland; the low figure for *Shigella* reflected the finding that this organism was always contracted outside Finland. In other reports of outbreaks of gastroenteritis, widely differing incidences of reactive arthritis have been reported from 0 to 55%.[31] The reasons for this are not clear but may reflect the particular serotype involved, the dose of bacteria to which subjects were exposed, and the severity of the gastroenteritis. One curious feature is the declining incidence of reactive arthritis due to *Chlamydia* infection set against a large increase in chlamydial infection generally. The explanation is unclear but may relate to the younger age group of those infected and their lack of previous exposure to related organisms.[32]

The prevalence of undifferentiated spondyloarthritis has been estimated at 0.7% in one study, which identified all those meeting ESSG criteria and then removed those (≈60%) with defined forms of spondyloarthritis.[33] Because the proportion of those with undifferentiated disease who will eventually proceed to ankylosing spondylitis is approximately 60%, the prevalence of persistent undifferentiated disease is approximately 0.3%; an unknown proportion of these may have undiagnosed reactive arthritis.

CLINICAL FEATURES AND DIAGNOSIS OF REACTIVE ARTHRITIS

History

The arthritis is usually acute in onset and is normally oligoarticular, with a predilection for the lower, weight-bearing, limbs. Mild cases picked up in surveys of populations following outbreaks of infection often have polyarthritis or polyarthralgia, but those who present clinically usually have marked synovitis with large effusions, such that septic or crystal-induced arthritis enters the differential diagnosis. A definitive diagnosis of reactive arthritis is greatly aided by two additional aspects of history: extra-articular features and preceding infection. Conjunctivitis is often transient and painless and therefore is discovered only by careful history—sometimes the red eye is noticed only by relatives. Inflammatory back symptoms or enthesitis (heel or plantar fascia pain) may be regarded as minor in comparison with the presenting joint, and a history of these features has to be specifically sought. Specific questioning is needed to elicit a history of preceding infection—the patient will not necessarily spontaneously assume a link between infection and subsequent arthritis, particularly if there is a gap of several weeks between events, although the onset of joint symptoms is rarely more than 4 weeks after infection. Gastrointestinal upset may be minor in some cases (especially with *Yersinia* infection[34]), and a sexual history will rarely be volunteered spontaneously.

Signs

- *Joints:* Careful examination for mild involvement of joints other than the presenting ones is important, particularly in apparent monoarthritis; discovery of even mild synovitis of a proximal interphalangeal (PIP) or wrist joint, in addition to a grossly swollen knee, greatly decreases the likelihood of septic arthritis.
- *Entheses:* Major entheses should be examined for signs of inflammation (Figure 76-1); loss of weight bearing due to ankle or knee arthritis may mean that the patient is unaware of significant Achilles tendinitis or plantar fasciitis. The Maastricht Ankylosing Spondylitis Enthesitis Score (MASES) provides a helpful list of 13 major entheses: first and fourth costochondral joints, L + R; anterior and posterior iliac spines, L + R; iliac crest, L + R; fifth lumbar spinous process; and Achilles tendon insertion, L + R, which should be checked.[35] Missing from this list but readily examined is the calcaneal plantar fascia insertion. Alternatively,

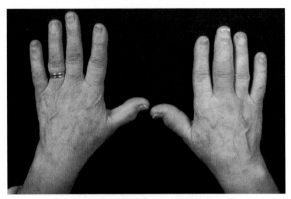

Figure 76-2 Dactylitis of the right middle finger.

the Mander index may be used.[36] Tendinitis may combine with arthritis to produce characteristic dactylitis in fingers or toes (Figure 76-2).

- *Extra-articular disease:* The characteristic skin rash associated with reactive arthritis, keratoderma blenorrhagica (Figure 76-3), should be sought on soles and palms—again, the former may not be evident to the patient. Histologically, the rash is identical to psoriasis, but skin biopsy is rarely required to establish the nature of the rash. The other typical associated rash is circinate balanitis on the glans penis (Figure 76-4); this also needs to be specifically sought, particularly in uncircumcised males. Erythema nodosum is seen in *Yersinia* infection but rarely in other reactive arthritis–associated infections. Mouth or palatal ulcers are often painless and may not be reported by the patient. Conjunctivitis sometimes is still present when the patient is first seen by a rheumatologist, but ongoing pain or visual disturbance raises the possibility of uveitis and requires full ophthalmologic assessment.

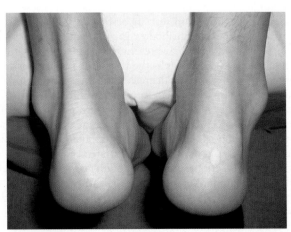

Figure 76-1 Enthesitis of right Achilles tendon.

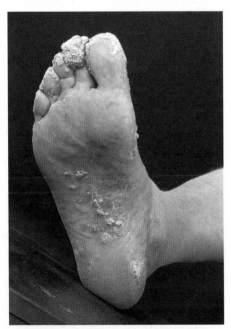

Figure 76-3 Keratoderma blenorrhagica.

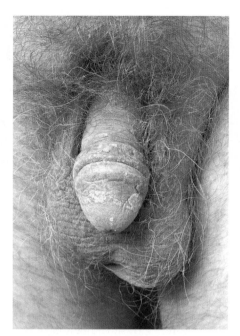

Figure 76-4 Circinate balanitis.

Investigations

Blood Tests

Inflammatory markers (erythrocyte sedimentation rate [ESR], C-reactive protein [CRP]) will be raised, often impressively so, with CRP greater than 100 mg/L; white cell count and differential will usually show neutrophilia; serum urate is useful in relation to an alternative diagnosis, and glucose should be measured to allow interpretation of synovial fluid glucose.

Tests on Synovial Fluid

Because the differential diagnosis of reactive arthritis very commonly includes septic arthritis or crystal-induced disease, synovial fluid should be aspirated whenever possible. Cell count, bacteriologic culture, glucose levels, and examination under polarizing microscope for crystals are needed to exclude septic and crystal arthritis.

In a research setting, measurement of synovial T cell recognition of triggering organisms or specific bacterial antigens as proliferation (usually uptake of ^{3}H-thymidine) or cytokine production has been informative. It is also possible to examine cells in synovial fluid using flow cytometry[37-40] for surface phenotype and intracellular cytokine staining. Recently, increased numbers of CD4[+] T lymphocytes producing interleukin (IL)-17 have been described in reactive arthritis synovial fluid.[41] However, currently, none of these research tests can be used diagnostically. They are unlikely to ever achieve high specificity because production of proinflammatory cytokines such as IL-17 or interferon-γ is common to various forms of inflammatory arthritis. In addition, memory T cells are recruited to inflamed joints so that, for example, a patient with active RA and an incidental Chlamydia infection is likely to have Chlamydia-specific T cells in the synovial fluid and tissue. Nevertheless, when there is a high pretest probability of reactive arthritis (i.e.,

the patient has signs and symptoms consistent with this diagnosis), the finding of marked responses to one particular reactive arthritis–associated organism is likely to be relevant diagnostically and may lead to confirmation of the nature of the triggering infection by other means.

Microbiology

Culture and Other Means of Detecting Bacteria. The aim is to gather evidence to implicate a reactive arthritis–associated organism. For gastrointestinal infection, stool culture should be carried out; organisms such as Salmonella and Yersinia may persist in the gut for several weeks after gastroenteritis has resolved. Yersinia has the unusual property of growing at 4° C, which allows improved detection of the organism by maintaining the stool sample at 4° C for 24 to 48 hours prior to culture; microbiology laboratories should be informed that Yersinia infection is being considered to allow them to do this. Stool culture for Yersinia is also appropriate in patients without gastrointestinal symptoms because symptoms are often mild in infection with this organism. For genitourinary infection, swabs should be obtained from the urethra or vagina for culture of Chlamydia trachomatis and, if indicated, from the throat and rectum. However, in view of the difficulty involved in culturing chlamydiae, nucleic acid amplification techniques (ligase chain reaction [LCR], PCR) are generally preferred and can be performed on urine samples or by self-administered swabs, both of which are acceptable to patients. Use of PCR to identify Chlamydia in synovial fluid has not yet been developed sufficiently.[42] PCR is also helpful in establishing a diagnosis of Chlamydia pneumoniae infection when arthritis is seen in association with respiratory tract infection. The presence of chlamydiae can be detected in urine or sputum by means of an enzyme-linked immunosorbent assay (ELISA) to detect chlamydial lipopolysaccharide (LPS).

Serology. Although culture or direct demonstration of the organism is preferred, in some circumstances serology can provide reliable evidence of a preceding infection. Its effectiveness depends very much on the frequency of infection in the community and therefore on the proportion of subjects with pre-existing antibodies. For Salmonella species, and increasingly for Campylobacter, antibodies are commonly detected in healthy subjects because of a high level of community exposure to these organisms. In these cases therefore, diagnosis will rest, at best, on an increased titer of pathogen-specific antibodies in acute and convalescent sera. Because patients may present to rheumatologists in the convalescent phase, as far as the triggering infection is concerned, this substantially decreases the utility of serology in diagnosing these infections. In contrast, infection with Yersinia or Shigella is not prevalent in Western societies, so that detection of specific antibodies carries greater significance even if immunoglobulin (Ig)M antibodies or a fourfold increase in titer cannot be demonstrated. For detection of chlamydial infection, serology generally has not proved reliable. Micro-immunfluorescence tests can be carried out, in which dilutions of sera are applied to multi-well slides containing organisms; this is regarded as the "gold standard" for Chlamydia serology. However, again the prevalence of antibodies in the population is high, particularly for

C. pneumoniae in older subjects. Individual recombinant chlamydial antigens have been used to devise additional serologic tests, but none has yet been established for general use.

HLA-B27 Testing

Testing for HLA-B27 generally is not required to make the *diagnosis* of reactive arthritis. Although more severe cases such as those seen in secondary care are strongly associated with HLA-B27 (70% to 80% of cases are positive), the percentage of positivity is much less in milder cases and is highly variable in different published series. However, HLA-B27 testing is worthwhile because it may identify patients with an increased likelihood of persistent disease, in whom early introduction of disease-modifying antirheumatic drugs (DMARDs) would be indicated (see later).

Imaging

Radiographs of affected joints are unlikely to be useful diagnostically when reactive arthritis presents, but baseline films are useful for future management. Imaging techniques that can identify inflammation of affected joints or entheses are what is required; the choice lies between ultrasound (particularly power Doppler studies), scintigraphy, and MRI. As noted previously, MRI may reveal sacroiliitis or other evidence of axial involvement but is not required for joints with clinically obvious synovitis—the norm in reactive arthritis. Power Doppler ultrasonography appears promising for detecting enthesitis but is not without difficulties in interpretation.[43-45] This technique may also reveal enthesitis in rheumatoid arthritis, thereby producing difficulties for the ASAS classification criteria, but this enthesitis is usually noted in relation to nearby synovitis rather than as the predominant inflammatory lesion. Likewise, scintigraphy did not perform particularly well in detecting sacroiliitis in a population with chronic back pain[46]; it might perform better in young patients with sacroiliitis due to reactive arthritis, because the background prevalence of abnormalities in healthy young controls is likely to be much lower.

TREATMENT OF REACTIVE ARTHRITIS

Control of Symptoms

Most patients (80% to 90%) will have self-limiting disease, which does not require disease-modifying drugs. Symptomatic measures include full-dose nonsteroidal anti-inflammatory drugs (NSAIDs), preferably long-acting, with the choice between selective and nonselective drugs dependent on the patient's risk of gastrointestinal bleeding versus cardiovascular disease; in young patients, the former predominate, so there is a preference for agents such as etoricoxib.[47] Additional analgesics may be required. Intra-articular corticosteroids are very useful when infection has been confidently excluded, and injection of enthesitis may also be required with avoidance of the Achilles tendon insertion, in view of the tendency of this tendon to rupture. In patients with severe disease and systemic features, parenteral or short-course oral steroids may be used. Patients require physiotherapy to maintain muscle bulk and range of movement. Informal psychologic support is often crucial because, although the disease is self-limiting, it commonly takes 6 to 12 months to remit. In a young, previously fit patient, this is perceived as a major medical event, curtailing many sporting and leisure activities, and sometimes interfering with employment.

Disease-Modifying Drugs

Few controlled trials have examined the use of DMARDs in reactive arthritis. Such patients were included in a trial of sulfasalazine in spondyloarthritis,[48] and sulfasalazine was also tested in reactive arthritis.[49] The natural tendency of spontaneous remission makes it difficult for investigators to conduct trials to determine the effectiveness of DMARDs, but sulfasalazine showed effectiveness in 62% of reactive arthritis patients as compared with 48% in placebo. In undifferentiated spondyloarthritis, sulfasalazine was reported not to be effective, although an unexpected effect on axial symptoms, but not peripheral arthritis, was recorded.[50] This result is at variance with other findings.[51,52] When should DMARDs be introduced in reactive arthritis? Patients who have severe, persistent disease or recurrent disease, particularly those who are HLA-B27+, are candidates for the early introduction of DMARDs. However, even patients with very severe presentation can settle rapidly with NSAIDs and intra-articular steroids, so only those who are responding slowly or whose disease flares significantly after an initial response would justify introduction of DMARDs within the first 3 months of disease. Those who relapse after having responded well initially are also likely to require DMARDs. The risk-benefit ratio of sulfasalazine is favorable, and the drug is a logical choice in cases triggered by enteric infection. Patients who fail sulfasalazine can progress to methotrexate or leflunomide, or a combination of the two. Note however, that none of these recommendations on the use of DMARDs has been properly tested in controlled trials. In view of the favorable course in most patients, there is reluctance to test early use of drugs such as methotrexate in the way that is now commonplace in rheumatoid arthritis (RA).

Biologics

Only in rare cases have biologics such as tumor necrosis factor (TNF)-blocking agents[53-55] or tocilizumab[56] been used in reactive arthritis, although they appear to be effective. They have not been reported to be associated with recrudescence of infection—an important consideration in view of evidence for persistence of triggering organisms such as *Chlamydia*[57,58] or *Yersinia*.[59] In light of reports of increased numbers of T helper (Th)17 cells in reactive arthritis joints and genetic evidence implicating the IL-17 axis in spondyloarthritis, rational future use of biologics might suggest the use of inhibitors of IL-23—ustekinumab, which recognizes the shared IL-12/23 p40 subunit and is effective in psoriasis,[60,61] or a IL-23–specific antibody targeting the p19 unit, currently in trial, or IL-17 itself. IL-6 and IL-1 are also implicated in generating Th17 cells,[62] and the efficacy of tocilizumab (in a single case report) may reflect an effect on the generation of Th17 cells.

Antibiotics

By definition, the joint in reactive arthritis is sterile, so there is no prima facie case for treatment of arthritis with antibiotics. Obviously, chlamydial infection in the genitourinary tract requires conventional treatment to avoid damage and scarring, particularly in females; *Chlamydia pneumoniae* respiratory tract infection also needs treatment. In general, food poisoning does not require antibiotics, although ciprofloxacin is often used to reduce symptom duration.[63]

In relation to arthritis, the use of prolonged courses of antibiotics has been advocated in view of increasing evidence of persistence of the organism, within the joint and elsewhere, despite adequate antibiotic treatment of the primary infection; this applies particularly to chlamydia infection. Several placebo-controlled trials have examined the effects of prolonged courses of antibiotics (3 to 6 months), which are effective with reactive arthritis–associated bacteria (tetracycline, ciprofloxacin, and azithromycin) and with outcome in reactive arthritis.[64-68]. For disease due to enteric infection, the results are uniformly negative. In an early trial, post hoc subgroup analysis suggested a beneficial effect of prolonged lymecycline in *Chlamydia*-induced disease[64]; an effect of prolonged antibiotics on *Chlamydia*-induced arthritis was not confirmed in subsequent trials,[68,69] although some studies may not have had sufficient *Chlamydia*-induced cases. A recent and controversial study used a combination of antibiotics, rifampicin with doxycycline, and azithromycin, which were chosen to be effective against persistent, slowly dividing organisms; investigators reported effectiveness in *Chlamydia*-induced reactive arthritis, including in patients with long-standing disease (mean duration, 10 to 14 years).[70,71] Seventeen of 27 antibiotic-treated patients achieved the trial end point compared with 3 of 15 receiving placebo, and treatment was associated with clearance of chlamydiae as detected by PCR. The trial involved relatively small numbers, and the findings require confirmation.

OUTCOME IN REACTIVE ARTHRITIS

A vast majority of patients with reactive arthritis make a full recovery with no chronic joint damage, although in more severe cases, 12 to 18 months may be required for complete resolution of symptoms. Remaining patients have progressive spondyloarthritis with relapses and involvement of new joints and entheses in the absence of any evidence of re-infection, and often increasing prominence of axial symptoms and radiographic changes of ankylosing spondylitis.[72] HLA-B27 is the main factor predisposing to chronicity or recurrence in reactive arthritis and is worth testing for this reason. It is possible that polymorphisms in other genes,[73] including those that influence susceptibility to AS,[74] will also affect outcome in reactive arthritis, but this remains to be tested. Of course it may be argued that HLA-B27+ patients are predisposed to both reactive arthritis and other forms of spondyloarthritis, and therefore might develop two diseases rather than reactive arthritis evolving into ankylosing spondylitis, but the clinical impression suggests evolution rather than development of a new disease.

Severe arthritis (large effusions, multiple joints, and very high levels of CRP and ESR) does not necessarily correlate with persistent disease, but complete recovery will usually take longer (6 to 12 months) compared with milder disease. Young active patients require counseling to prepare them for this.

DIAGNOSIS AND TREATMENT OF UNDIFFERENTIATED SPONDYLOARTHRITIS

Because, as discussed previously, undifferentiated spondyloarthritis by definition is not a "specific" disease, a detailed account of its diagnosis and treatment is somewhat redundant.

Diagnosis

Briefly, patients present rheumatologically with arthritis or enthesitis, or dactylitis, which is itself a combination of these conditions. In such cases, the diagnosis will be based on additional features of spondyloarthritis, as detailed in the ASAS classification criteria for axial or peripheral arthritis. An algorithm for diagnosing axial disease on this basis has been published.[75] Every attempt should be made to rescue the patient from the undifferentiated diagnosis to a more distinct form of spondyloarthritis, but this will not always be possible, especially in those with early disease and in a percentage of those with long-standing disease.

Investigations

These have already been detailed in relation to reactive arthritis. In cases with predominantly axial disease, inflammatory markers may not be elevated.

Treatment

Patients with undifferentiated spondyloarthritis will have different combinations of axial and peripheral disease. Where axial disease predominates, management will most resemble that for ankylosing spondylitis. Patients usually will require full-dose NSAIDs (a good response to these reinforces the diagnosis), axial symptoms are generally refractory to conventional DMARDs, and a proportion of patients will require treatment with biologics, particularly anti-TNF, when symptom control with NSAIDs proves inadequate.[76,77] An important research question is whether early intervention with anti-TNF will prevent progression of undifferentiated spondyloarthritis to ankylosing spondylitis, that is, whether the "window of opportunity" concept leading to early aggressive treatment of rheumatoid arthritis might also apply to ankylosing spondylitis. Peripheral disease is managed in a similar fashion to psoriatic arthritis, or reactive arthritis in its more chronic, established form, with the use of DMARDs—sulfasalazine, methotrexate, and leflunomide, given individually or in combination. In the absence of psoriasis or a family history of psoriasis, hydroxchloroquine can be used, often as an add-on to another more powerful DMARD. Finally, the antibiotic regimen recently reported to be effective in *Chlamydia*-induced reactive arthritis was first tested in undifferentiated arthritis on the assumption that it might be related to *Chlamydia*[78]; findings showed some efficacy.[79]

UNANSWERED QUESTIONS AND FUTURE RESEARCH

1. How Many Patients Currently Classified as Undifferentiated Spondyloarthritis Actually Have Reactive Arthritis?

Answering this question requires better diagnostic techniques. For *Chlamydia*-induced reactive arthritis, detection of bacteria-specific mRNA has been reported, even in late disease. However, the problems of using PCR with high levels of amplification while avoiding contamination have not been fully resolved. Given that chlamydiae might traffic to any inflamed joint, and therefore may be identified by PCR in, for example, RA joints, it may be that a specific transcript or set of transcripts will be associated with bacterial persistence in the joint, which drives reactive arthritis. Equally, a synovial tissue or fluid gene expression "signature" characteristic of reactive arthritis may exist (better still, a peripheral blood signature) and may be used for diagnosis. This would be particularly useful in reactive arthritis triggered by enteric organisms because bacteria-specific mRNA in the joints of these patients has only occasionally been reported.

2. Do Antibiotics Have Any Role in the Treatment of Established Reactive Arthritis?

This question has been re-opened, at least for *Chlamydia*-induced arthritis, by recent data reporting successful treatment with combinations of azithromycin or tetracycline and rifampicin. These observations need to be repeated and expanded. A positive result would lead to exploration of the same combinations in other forms of reactive arthritis.

3. What Is the Role of HLA-B27 in Inducing Susceptibility to Reactive Arthritis, and What Other Genes Influence Susceptibility?

These questions are generic for our understanding of the pathogenesis of spondyloarthritis. They have rightly been addressed initially in ankylosing spondylitis, where the incidence of HLA-B27 is very high and case definitions can be well controlled. Mechanisms for the mode of action of HLA-B27, which emerge from these studies, can be re-examined in reactive arthritis, where an interaction with the consequences of intracellular infection might be expected. Although this was initially seen in terms of HLA-B27 presenting "spondylitogenic" peptides from reactive arthritis–associated bacteria, other mechanisms involving homodimeric B27 heavy chains or induction of the unfolded protein response may present opportunities for interactions with bacteria. As other genes associated with ankylosing spondylitis are identified, they need to be tested in reactive arthritis. There is a need therefore to establish cohorts of reactive arthritis patients in which the diagnosis is certain so that accurate genetic work can be done.

References

1. Ahvonen P, Sievers K, Aho K: Arthritis associated with *Yersinia enterocolitica* infection, *Acta Rheumatol Scand* 15:232–253, 1969.
2. Keat A: Reiter's syndrome and reactive arthritis in perspective, *N Engl J Med* 309:1606–1615, 1983.
3. Aho K, Ahvonen P, Lassus A, et al: HL-A antigen 27 and reactive arthritis, *Lancet* ii:157–159, 1973.
4. Saario R, Toivanen A: *Chlamydia pneumoniae* as a cause of reactive arthritis, *Br J Rheumatol* 32:1112, 1993.
5. Braun J, Laitko S, Treharne J, et al: *Chlamydia pneumoniae*—a new causative agent of reactive arthritis and undifferentiated oligoarthritis, *Ann Rheum Dis* 53:100–105, 1994.
6. Hannu T, Puolakkainen M, Leirisalo-Repo M: *Chlamydia pneumoniae* as a triggering infection in reactive arthritis, *Rheumatology (Oxford)* 38:411–414, 1999.
7. Wallace D, Weisman M: Should a war criminal be rewarded with eponymous distinction? The double life of Hans Reiter. *J Clin Rheumatol* 6:49–54, 2000.
8. Keynan Y, Rimar D: Reactive arthritis—the appropriate name, *Isr Med Assoc J* 10:256–258, 2008.
9. Ford D: Prevention of a false diagnosis of sexually acquired reactive arthritis by synovial lymphocyte responses, *J Rheumatol* 17:1335–1336, 1990.
10. Laitinen O, Leirisalo M, Skylv G: Relation between HLA-B27 and clinical features in patients with yersinia arthritis, *Arthritis Rheum* 20:1121–1124, 1977.
11. Gaston JSH, Lillicrap MS: Arthritis associated with enteric infection, *Best Pract Res Clin Rheumatol* 17:219–239, 2003.
12. Zochling J, Brandt J, Braun J: The current concept of spondyloarthritis with special emphasis on undifferentiated spondyloarthritis, *Rheumatology (Oxford)* 44:1483–1491, 2005.
13. Taylor W, Gladman D, Helliwell P, et al: Classification criteria for psoriatic arthritis: development of new criteria from a large international study, *Arthritis Rheum* 54:2665–2673, 2006.
14. Amor B, Dougados M, Mijiyawa M: Criteres de classification des spondylarthropathies, *Rev Rhum Mal Osteoartic* 57:85–89, 1990.
15. Dougados M, van der Linden S, Juhlin R, et al: The European Spondylarthropathy Study Group preliminary criteria for the classification of spondylarthropathy, *Arthritis Rheum* 34:1218–1227, 1991.
16. van der Linden S, Valkenburg HA, Cats A: Evaluation of diagnostic criteria for ankylosing spondylitis: a proposal for modification of the New York criteria, *Arthritis Rheum* 27:361–368, 1984.
17. Rudwaleit M, Landewe R, van der Heijde D, et al: The development of Assessment of SpondyloArthritis international Society classification criteria for axial spondyloarthritis (part I): classification of paper patients by expert opinion including uncertainty appraisal, *Ann Rheum Dis* 68:770–776, 2009.
18. Rudwaleit M, van der Heijde D, Landewe R, et al: The Assessment of SpondyloArthritis international Society classification criteria for peripheral spondyloarthritis and for spondyloarthritis in general, *Ann Rheum Dis* 70:25–31, 2011.
19. Zeidler H, Amor B: The Assessment in Spondyloarthritis International Society (ASAS) classification criteria for peripheral spondyloarthritis and for spondyloarthritis in general: the spondyloarthritis concept in progress, *Ann Rheum Dis* 70:1–3, 2011.
20. Pachecotena C, Burgosvargas R, Vazquezmellado J, et al: A proposal for the classification of patients for clinical and experimental studies on reactive arthritis, *J Rheumatol* 26:1338–1346, 1999.
21. Hannu T, Mattila L, Rautelin H, et al: *Campylobacter*-triggered reactive arthritis: a population-based study, *Rheumatology (Oxford)* 41:312–318, 2002.
22. Hannu T, Mattila L, Siitonen A, Leirisalo-Repo M: Reactive arthritis attributable to *Shigella* infection: a clinical and epidemiological nationwide study, *Ann Rheum Dis* 64:594–598, 2005.
23. Fendler C, Laitko S, Sorensen H, et al: Frequency of triggering bacteria in patients with reactive arthritis and undifferentiated oligoarthritis and the relative importance of the tests used for diagnosis, *Ann Rheum Dis* 60:337–343, 2001.
24. Kvien TK, Glennas A, Melby K, et al: Reactive arthritis: incidence, triggering agents and clinical presentation, *J Rheumatol* 21:115–122, 1994.
25. Savolainen E, Kaipiainen-Seppanen O, Kroger L, Luosujarvi R: Total incidence and distribution of inflammatory joint diseases in a defined population: results from the Kuopio 2000 arthritis survey, *J Rheumatol* 30:2460–2468, 2003.

26. Hannu T, Mattila L, Siitonen A, Leirisalo-Repo M: Reactive arthritis following an outbreak of *Salmonella typhimurium* phage type 193 infection, *Ann Rheum Dis* 61:264–266, 2002.

27. Hannu T, Mattila L, Nuorti JP, et al: Reactive arthritis after an outbreak of *Yersinia pseudotuberculosis* serotype O:3 infection, *Ann Rheum Dis* 62:866–869, 2003.

28. Inman RD, Johnston ME, Hodge M, et al: Postdysenteric reactive arthritis: a clinical and immunogenetic study following an outbreak of salmonellosis, *Arthritis Rheum* 31:1377–1383, 1988.

29. Pope JE, Krizova A, Garg AX, et al: *Campylobacter* reactive arthritis: a systematic review, *Semin Arthritis Rheum* 37:48–55, 2007.

30. Townes JM, Deodhar AA, Laine ES, et al: Reactive arthritis following culture-confirmed infections with bacterial enteric pathogens in Minnesota and Oregon: a population-based study, *Ann Rheum Dis* 67:1689–1696, 2008.

31. Toivanen A, Toivanen P: *Reactive arthritis*, Boca Raton, Fla, 1988, CRC Press, Inc.

32. Telyatnikova N, Gaston JSH: Prior exposure to infection with *Chlamydia pneumoniae* can influence the T-cell-mediated response to *Chlamydia trachomatis*, *FEMS Immunol Med Microbiol* 47:190–198, 2006.

33. Braun J, Bollow M, Remlinger G, et al: Prevalence of spondylarthropathies in HLA-B27 positive and negative blood donors, *Arthritis Rheum* 41:58–67, 1998.

34. Kihlstrom E, Foberg U, Bengtsson A, et al: Intestinal symptoms and serological response in patients with complicated and uncomplicated *Yersinia enterocolitica* infections, *Scand J Infect Dis* 24:57–63, 1992.

35. Heuft-Dorenbosch L, Spoorenberg A, van Tubergen A, et al: Assessment of enthesitis in ankylosing spondylitis, *Ann Rheum Dis* 62:127–132, 2003.

36. Mander M, Simpson JM, McLellan A, et al: Studies with an enthesis index as a method of clinical assessment in ankylosing spondylitis, *Ann Rheum Dis* 46:197–202, 1987.

37. Gaston JSH, Life PF, Merilahti Palo R, et al: Synovial T lymphocyte recognition of organisms that trigger reactive arthritis, *Clin Exp Immunol* 76:348–353, 1989.

38. Life PF, Bassey EOE, Gaston JSH: T-cell recognition of bacterial heat-shock proteins in inflammatory arthritis, *Immunol Rev* 121:113–135, 1991.

39. Thiel A, Wu PH, Lauster R, et al: Analysis of the antigen-specific T cell response in reactive arthritis by flow cytometry, *Arthritis Rheum* 43:2834–2842, 2000.

40. Thiel A, Wu P, Lanowska M, et al: Identification of immunodominant CD4$^+$ T cell epitopes in patients with *Yersinia*-induced reactive arthritis by cytometric cytokine secretion assay, *Arthritis Rheum* 54:3583–3590, 2006.

41. Shen H, Goodall JC, Gaston JS: Frequency and phenotype of T helper 17 cells in peripheral blood and synovial fluid of patients with reactive arthritis, *J Rheumatol* 37:2096–2099, 2010.

42. Kuipers JG, Sibilia J, Bas S, et al: Reactive and undifferentiated arthritis in North Africa: use of PCR for detection of *Chlamydia trachomatis*, *Clin Rheumatol* 28:11–16, 2009.

43. Kiris A, Kaya A, Ozgocmen S, Kocakoc E: Assessment of enthesitis in ankylosing spondylitis by power Doppler ultrasonography, *Skeletal Radiol* 35:522–528, 2006.

44. D'Agostino MA, Aegerter P, Jousse-Joulin S, et al: How to evaluate and improve the reliability of power Doppler ultrasonography for assessing enthesitis in spondylarthritis, *Arthritis Rheum* 61:61–69, 2009.

45. D'Agostino MA, Said-Nahal R, Hacquard-Bouder C, et al: Assessment of peripheral enthesitis in the spondylarthropathies by ultrasonography combined with power Doppler: a cross-sectional study, *Arthritis Rheum* 48:523–533, 2003.

46. Song IH, Brandt H, Rudwaleit M, Sieper J: Limited diagnostic value of unilateral sacroiliitis in scintigraphy in assessing axial spondyloarthritis, *J Rheumatol* 37:1200–1202, 2010.

47. van der Heijde D, Baraf HSB, Ramos-Remus C, et al: Evaluation of the efficacy of etoricoxib in ankylosing spondylitis: results of a fifty-two-week, randomized, controlled study, *Arthritis Rheum* 52:1205–1215, 2005.

48. Dougados M, Vanderlinden S, Leirisalo-Repo M, et al: Sulfasalazine in the treatment of spondylarthropathy: a randomized, multicenter, double-blind, placebo-controlled study, *Arthritis Rheum* 38:618–627, 1995.

49. Clegg DO, Reda DJ, Weisman MH, et al: Comparison of sulfasalazine and placebo in the treatment of reactive arthritis (Reiter's syndrome): a Department of Veterans Affairs Cooperative Study, *Arthritis Rheum* 39:2021–2027, 1996.

50. Braun J, Zochling J, Baraliakos X, et al: Efficacy of sulfasalazine in patients with inflammatory back pain due to undifferentiated spondyloarthritis and early ankylosing spondylitis: a multicentre randomised controlled trial, *Ann Rheum Dis* 65:1147–1153, 2006.

51. Clegg DO, Reda DJ, Weisman MH, et al: Comparison of sulfasalazine and placebo in the treatment of ankylosing spondylitis: a Department of Veterans Affairs Cooperative Study, *Arthritis Rheum* 39:2004–2012, 1996.

52. Chen J, Liu C: Is sulfasalazine effective in ankylosing spondylitis? A systematic review of randomized controlled trials, *J Rheumatol* 33:722–731, 2006.

53. Meador R, Hsia E, Kitumnuaypong T, Schumacher HR: TNF involvement and anti-TNF therapy of reactive and unclassified arthritis, *Clin Exp Rheumatol* 20(6 Suppl 28):S130–S134, 2002.

54. Schafranski MD: Infliximab for reactive arthritis secondary to *Chlamydia trachomatis* infection, *Rheumatol Int* 30:679–680, 2010.

55. Wechalekar MD, Rischmueller M, Whittle S, et al: Prolonged remission of chronic reactive arthritis treated with three infusions of infliximab, *J Clin Rheumatol* 16:79–80, 2010.

56. Tanaka T, Kuwahara Y, Shima Y, et al: Successful treatment of reactive arthritis with a humanized anti-interleukin-6 receptor antibody, tocilizumab, *Arthritis Rheum* 61:1762–1764, 2009.

57. Schumacher H, Arayssi T, Branigan P, et al: Surveying for evidence of synovial *Chlamydia trachomatis* by polymerase chain reaction (PCR): a study of 411 synovial biopsies and synovial fluids, *Arthritis Rheum* 40:S270, 1997.

58. Carter JD, Hudson AP: Reactive arthritis: clinical aspects and medical management, *Rheum Dis Clin North Am* 35:21–44, 2009.

59. Gaston JSH, Cox C, Granfors K: Clinical and experimental evidence for persistent *Yersinia* infection in reactive arthritis, *Arthritis Rheum* 42:2239–2242, 1999.

60. Papp KA, Langley RG, Lebwohl M, et al: Efficacy and safety of ustekinumab, a human interleukin-12/23 monoclonal antibody, in patients with psoriasis: 52-week results from a randomised, double-blind, placebo-controlled trial (PHOENIX 2), *Lancet* 371:1675–1684, 2008.

61. Leonardi CL, Kimball AB, Papp KA, et al: Efficacy and safety of ustekinumab, a human interleukin-12/23 monoclonal antibody, in patients with psoriasis: 76-week results from a randomised, double-blind, placebo-controlled trial (PHOENIX 1), *Lancet* 371:1665–1674, 2008.

62. Ghoreschi K, Laurence A, Yang XP, et al: Generation of pathogenic T(H)17 cells in the absence of TGF-beta signalling, *Nature* 467:967–971, 2010.

63. Pichler HE, Diridl G, Stickler K, Wolf D: Clinical efficacy of ciprofloxacin compared with placebo in bacterial diarrhea, *Am J Med* 82:329–332, 1987.

64. Lauhio A, Leirisalo Repo M, Lahdevirta J, et al: Double-blind, placebo-controlled study of three-month treatment with lymecycline in reactive arthritis with special reference to *Chlamydia* arthritis, *Arthritis Rheum* 34:6–14, 1991.

65. Toivanen A, Yli-Kertulla J, Luukainen R, et al: Effect of antimicrobial treatment on chronic reactive arthritis, *Clin Exp Rheumatol* 11:301–307, 1993.

66. Sieper J, Fendler C, Laitko S, et al: No benefit of long-term ciprofloxacin treatment in patients with reactive arthritis and undifferentiated oligoarthritis: a three-month, multicenter, double-blind, randomized, placebo-controlled study, *Arthritis Rheum* 42:1386–1396, 1999.

67. Yli-Kertulla T, Luukkainen R, Yli-Kertulla U, et al: Effect of a three month course of ciprofloxacin on the outcome of reactive arthritis, *Ann Rheum Dis* 59:565–570, 2000.

68. Kvien TK, Gaston JS, Bardin T, et al: Three month treatment of reactive arthritis with azithromycin: a EULAR double blind, placebo controlled study, *Ann Rheum Dis* 63:1113–1119, 2004.

69. Putschky N, Pott HG, Kuipers JG, et al: Comparing 10-day and 4-month doxycycline courses for treatment of *Chlamydia trachomatis*-reactive arthritis: a prospective, double-blind trial, *Ann Rheum Dis* 65:1521–1524, 2006.

70. Carter JD, Hudson AP: The evolving story of *Chlamydia*-induced reactive arthritis, *Curr Opin Rheumatol* 22:424–430, 2010.

71. Carter JD, Espinoza LR, Inman RD, et al: Combination antibiotics as a treatment for chronic *Chlamydia*-induced reactive arthritis: a double-

blind, placebo-controlled, prospective trial, *Arthritis Rheum* 62:1298–1307, 2010.

72. Kaarela K, Jantti JK, Kotaniemi KM: Similarity between chronic reactive arthritis and ankylosing spondylitis: a 32-35-year follow-up study, *Clin Exp Rheumatol* 27:325–328, 2009.

73. Tsui FW, Xi N, Rohekar S, et al: Toll-like receptor 2 variants are associated with acute reactive arthritis, *Arthritis Rheum* 58:3436–3438, 2008.

74. Reveille JD, Sims AM, Danoy P, et al: Genome-wide association study of ankylosing spondylitis identifies non-MHC susceptibility loci, *Nat Genet* 42:123–127, 2010.

75. Rudwaleit M, van der Heijde D, Khan MA, et al: How to diagnose axial spondyloarthritis early, *Ann Rheum Dis* 63:535–543, 2004.

76. Brandt J, Haibel H, Reddig J, et al: Successful short term treatment of severe undifferentiated spondyloarthropathy with the anti-tumor necrosis factor-alpha monoclonal antibody infliximab, *J Rheumatol* 29:118–122, 2002.

77. Brandt J, Khariouzov A, Listing J, et al: Successful short term treatment of patients with severe undifferentiated spondyloarthritis with the anti-tumor necrosis factor-alpha fusion receptor protein etanercept, *J Rheumatol* 31:531–538, 2004.

78. Savolainen E, Kettunen A, Narvanen A, et al: Prevalence of antibodies against *Chlamydia trachomatis* and incidence of *C. trachomatis*-induced reactive arthritis in an early arthritis series in Finland in 2000, *Scand J Rheumatol* 38:353–356, 2009.

79. Carter JD, Valeriano J, Vasey FB: Doxycycline versus doxycycline and rifampin in undifferentiated spondyloarthropathy, with special reference to *Chlamydia*-induced arthritis: a prospective, randomized 9-month comparison, *J Rheumatol* 31:1973–1980, 2004.

The references for this chapter can also be found on www.expertconsult.com.

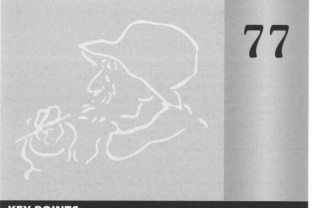

77

Psoriatic Arthritis

OLIVER FITZGERALD

KEY POINTS

Psoriatic arthritis should be suspected in a patient with an asymmetric joint distribution pattern who may have additional clinical features, such as dactylitis, enthesitis, or inflammatory-type back pain, and who is negative for rheumatoid factor.

New classification criteria, the Classification of Psoriatic Arthritis (CASPAR) criteria, have been validated.

Psoriatic arthritis is a progressive disease, with 47% of patients developing erosions within 2 years of diagnosis. Polyarticular disease and an elevated erythrocyte sedimentation rate are markers of poor outcome.

An essential core set of domains and instruments is now agreed as being necessary for inclusion in clinical trials.

Studies of synovial tissue have highlighted an increase in vascularity and the presence of neutrophils as helping to distinguish spondyloarthropathy from rheumatoid arthritis. Change in synovial CD3+ T cell infiltration might correlate with clinical response to treatment.

Prominent entheseal involvement with bone marrow edema at entheseal insertions on magnetic resonance imaging has prompted the hypothesis that psoriatic arthritis may originate at the enthesis.

A role for CD8+ T cells and the innate immune response has been proposed.

Although there is a paucity of evidence for efficacy of disease-modifying antirheumatic drugs in psoriatic arthritis, tumor necrosis factor inhibitors have proved effective for skin and joint disease.

Psoriatic arthritis is a member of the spondyloarthropathy family and may be defined as an inflammatory arthropathy associated with psoriasis and usually negative for rheumatoid factor. Until the 1950s, an inflammatory arthritis occurring in the presence of psoriasis was thought to represent rheumatoid arthritis (RA) occurring coincidentally with psoriasis. Based primarily on clinical and radiologic grounds and using the rheumatoid factor, the distinction between RA and psoriatic arthritis became gradually accepted. Wright described the classic clinical features in 1959, and together with his colleague Moll, he published his classification criteria in 1973.[1,2] These criteria have remained until recently the simplest and the most frequently used in clinical studies. The American Association of Rheumatism included psoriatic arthritis as a distinct clinical entity in the classification of rheumatic diseases for the first time in 1964.[3]

EPIDEMIOLOGY

Epidemiologic studies have supported the concept that psoriatic arthritis is a unique disease entity separate from RA. The prevalence of inflammatory arthritis is increased among patients with psoriasis, ranging from 7% to 25% compared with a general population estimate of 2% to 3%. The prevalence of psoriasis among subjects with arthritis also is increased at 2.6% to 7% compared with a general population estimate of 0.1% to 2.8%.[4]

Psoriasis affects about 2% of the population. The prevalence varies, with 5% to 10% of Russians and Norwegians affected, and only 0% to 0.3% of West Africans or Native Americans affected.[5] Onset of psoriasis may occur at any age, but it most frequently peaks in the 20s. Although no gender predilection has been reported, a genetic predisposition has been noted.

Among patients with psoriasis, 7% to 42% develop arthritis. This figure varies so widely in part because of a lack of widely accepted diagnostic criteria; it also varies according to which population is being studied. The exact prevalence and incidence of psoriatic arthritis are unknown. The reported prevalence of psoriatic arthritis ranged from 0.056% to 0.28% in a large population-based study in the United States.[6] Cases were defined as patients who reported a "physician diagnosis" of psoriasis and psoriatic arthritis. Prevalence was calculated at 0.25% (95% confidence interval, 0.18% to 0.31%). Kay and colleagues[7] did a prevalence study in northeast England to evaluate records from six general practices; 81 of 772 psoriasis subjects had an inflammatory arthritis with a prevalence of 0.28%. The reported incidence of psoriatic arthritis has varied from 3 to 23 cases per 100,000. Data from Rochester, New York, have shown an incidence rate of 6.59 per 100,000, whereas in Finland, 16 new cases of psoriatic arthritis were identified in a population of 87,000, yielding a mean incidence rate of 23 per 100,000.[8,9] Using the Icelandic genealogy database, risk ratios (RRs) for developing psoriatic arthritis spanning five generations were estimated.[10] Results confirmed a strong and complex genetic component with a significant risk ratio up to the fourth-degree relatives of psoriatic arthritis patients, as well as an important environmental contribution.

CLINICAL FEATURES

Plaque psoriasis or psoriasis vulgaris is the most common skin phenotype in patients with psoriatic arthritis. Other patterns of skin involvement may be seen (Figure 77-1). Although arthritis usually develops in a setting of an established diagnosis of psoriasis, some patients may be unaware that they have psoriasis, or psoriasis may develop after the onset of arthritis in approximately 15% of cases.[11] In a clinical study, the incidence of development of arthritis in patients with psoriasis remained constant (74 per 1000 person-years), while the prevalence increased with time since diagnosis of psoriasis, reaching 20.5% after 30 years.[12] If a patient presents with the classic articular manifestations of psoriatic arthritis but does not volunteer psoriasis or the presence of a rash, it is incumbent on the physician to examine the patient's skin carefully, including the scalp and nails, because psoriasis frequently lurks in such areas. Examples of nail dystrophic changes are shown in Figure 77-2.

Although a more recent U.S. study suggests that the prevalence of psoriatic arthritis among psoriasis patients increases with psoriasis severity,[6] in clinical practice, little relationship has been observed between severity of skin

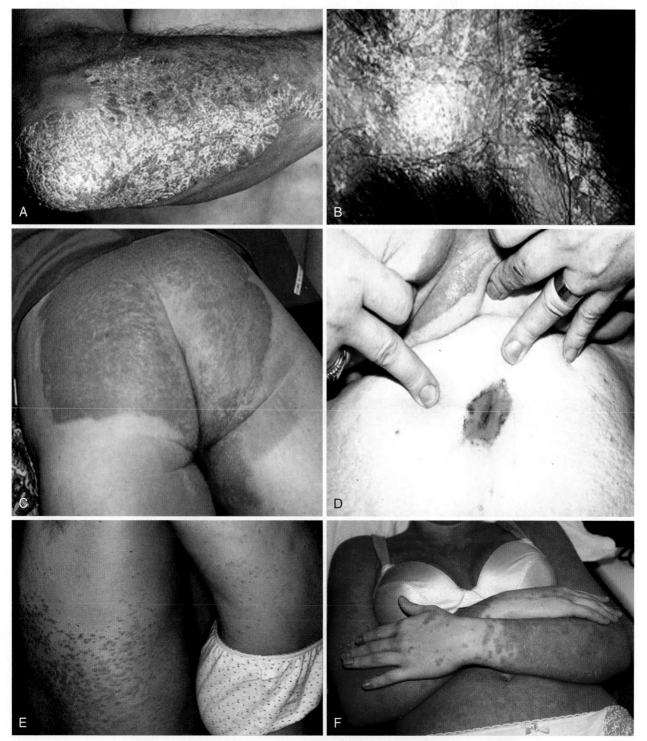

Figure 77-1 Clinical phenotypes in psoriasis: plaque psoriasis (psoriasis vulgaris). **A,** At extensor surface of elbow and on scalp **(B).** Genital psoriasis **(C).** Inframammary and umbilical flexural psoriasis **(D).** Guttate psoriasis in a father and child **(E).** Erythrodermic psoriasis on the trunk and upper limbs **(F).**

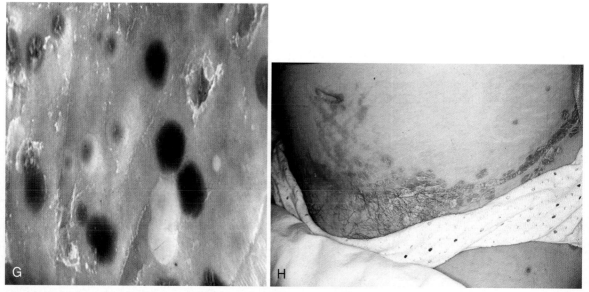

Figure 77-1, cont'd **G,** Pustular psoriasis on the foot. **H,** The Koebner phenomenon on a surgical abdominal wound.

involvement and severity of arthritis. In one prospective study, only 35% of patients reported that their skin and joint components flared at the same time.[11] Other systemic features of joint inflammation are common in patients with psoriatic arthritis, including stiffness after rest and fatigue. In one study of fatigue, a number of factors, including disease activity, physical disability, pain, and psychologic distress, contributed to fatigue, with comorbid fibromyalgia and hypertension further adding to the challenge.[13] Compared with other core outcome measures, fatigue has been found to be an independent outcome measure that is sensitive to change.[14]

Patients with psoriatic arthritis present with symptoms and signs of joint, entheseal, or spinal inflammation. The joints involved at presentation in 129 early psoriatic arthritis patients are shown in Figure 77-3. In one of their seminal papers on psoriatic arthritis, Wright and Moll[15] described five clinical patterns of psoriatic arthritis (Figure 77-4):

1. Asymmetric oligoarthritis
2. Symmetric polyarthritis

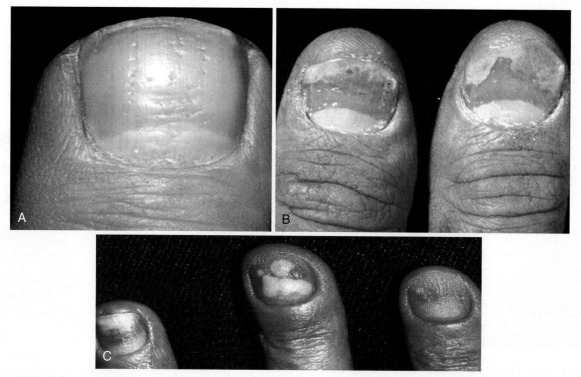

Figure 77-2 Nail dystrophic changes. **A,** Nail pitting; **B,** onycholysis; and **C,** severe destructive change with nail loss and pustule formation.

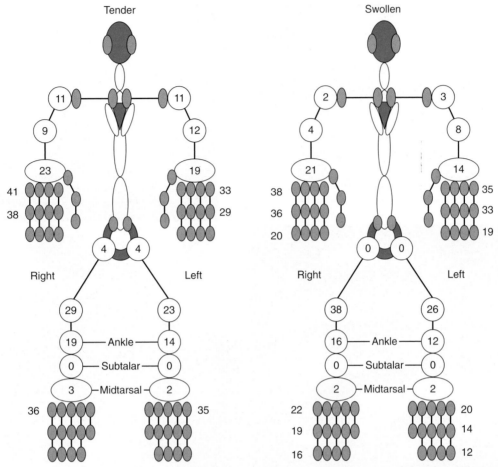

Figure 77-3 Frequency (%) of peripheral limb joint involvement in 129 patients with early psoriatic arthritis as assessed by joint tenderness and swelling (distal interphalangeal joints of hand and proximal and distal interphalangeal joints of feet not assessed for tenderness as part of Ritchie Articular Index).

3. Predominant distal interphalangeal (DIP) joint involvement
4. Predominant spondyloarthritis
5. Destructive (mutilans) arthritis

These classification criteria are the most commonly quoted, although many alternative criteria have been proposed. Variability in the definition of terms has led to differences in the reported frequency of psoriatic arthritis in subsets among the different studies. The pattern of joint involvement is not fixed; the patient's disease may fluctuate and may be influenced by treatment. In a study of 129 patients with early psoriatic arthritis, 53 of 77 initially classified as polyarticular were reassessed at 2 years; 26 of 53 (49%) patients were subsequently classified as oligoarticular, 19 of 53 (36%) remained classified as polyarticular, and 12 of 53 (23%) were in remission.[16]

The Classification of Psoriatic Arthritis (CASPAR) study has included in the analysis a breakdown of disease pattern subtypes.[17] This multicenter study included data on 588 psoriatic arthritis cases and 536 controls. In contrast to the original Moll and Wright paper, but similar to many subsequent publications, approximately 63% of patients had polyarticular joint involvement compared with 13% with oligoarticular disease. The other patterns of joint involvement described by Moll and Wright occurred much less

commonly. Predominant DIP disease was found in less than 5%, but DIP involvement can occur in any of the subtypes. Predominant spondyloarthritis is uncommon, although spinal involvement may be found in 40% to 70% of psoriatic arthritis cases, depending on whether or not radiographs are taken.[18] Risk factors for spinal involvement include severe peripheral arthritis and HLA-B27.[19] Finally, arthritis mutilans, a destructive form of arthritis associated with flail joints, is rare, although more patients may develop this form of joint involvement with time if their disease is not properly controlled.

Features that are typical of psoriatic arthritis, including dactylitis and enthesitis, are helpful in diagnosis. Dactylitis, which is characterized by a sausage-shaped swelling of the fingers or toes (see Figure 77-4B), may be found in 29% to 33.5% of psoriatic arthritis patients at first presentation, and 48% may have an episode of dactylitis during follow-up.[16,20] Ultrasound and magnetic resonance imaging (MRI) studies have shown that joint and tenosynovial inflammation are prominent in involved digits.[21,22] Enthesitis, inflammation at tendon and ligament insertion into bone, is a feature of all of the spondyloarthropathies and may be a presenting feature in psoriatic arthritis. Overall, enthesitis is found in 38% of patients at presentation.[16] The most common entheseal sites involved are the Achilles and plantar fascia

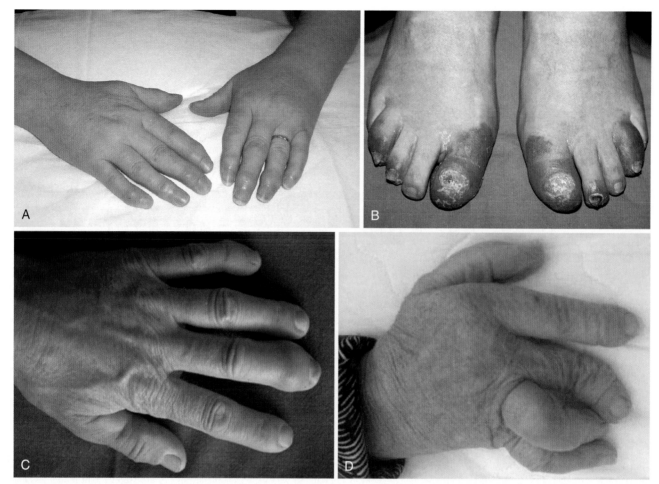

Figure 77-4 Patterns of peripheral joint disease: asymmetric polyarticular disease. **A,** Distal interphalangeal joint involvement and forearm lymphedema. **B,** Toe dactylitis with skin and nail change. **C,** Predominant distal interphalangeal joint involvement. **D,** Arthritis mutilans.

insertions. Other sites include the insertions of the quadriceps and patellar tendons, the iliac crest, the rotator cuff, and the epicondyles at the elbow. Patients have reported pain at these sites, with tenderness and sometimes swelling noted on examination. Entheseal involvement may be asymptomatic, and ultrasound is more sensitive than clinical palpation. Often spurs are detected on x-ray, although spurs are not always associated with symptoms.

With the obvious exception of psoriasis and nail dystrophic change, extra-articular disease is less common in psoriatic arthritis than in RA. Iritis or uveitis occurs in 7% to 18%, more bilateral than in ankylosing spondylitis, but is usually found in patients with spinal involvement.[11,23] Numerous studies have suggested that psoriatic arthritis patients have a higher prevalence of inflammatory bowel disease, sometimes asymptomatic and detected only on biopsy specimen.[24,25] Whether this inflammatory bowel disease is coincidental or is possibly related to medication effects remains to be clarified. Distal limb edema or lymphedema may occur more commonly in psoriatic arthritis; one case-control study found it in 21% of psoriatic arthritis patients compared with 4.9% of controls (see Figure 77-4A).[26] Finally, amyloid is rare but is described in psoriatic arthritis.

DIFFERENTIAL DIAGNOSIS

Certain articular features if present are useful in distinguishing psoriatic arthritis from RA, including dactylitis, DIP involvement, and inflammation at entheseal sites (Table 77-1; see Figure 77-4). In addition, inflammatory-type back pain or sacroiliitis on plain x-ray or MRI should raise the suspicion of psoriatic arthritis because spinal involvement is uncommon in RA. The absence of rheumatoid nodules

Table 77-1 Clinical Features That Distinguish Psoriatic Arthritis from Rheumatoid Arthritis

	Psoriatic Arthritis	Rheumatoid Arthritis
Psoriasis	+	−
Symmetric	+	++
Asymmetric	++	+
Enthesopathy	+	−
Dactylitis	+	−
Nail dystrophy	+	−
Human immunodeficiency virus association	+	−

or other systemic features common to RA can be another useful differentiating feature.

Distinguishing psoriatic arthritis from other spondyloarthropathies is also important. Dactylitis may be a feature in reactive arthritis, where a palmoplantar pustular rash (keratoderma blennorrhagicum) may be clinically and histologically indistinguishable from pustular psoriasis (see Figure 77-1G). In relation to spinal involvement, sacroiliitis may be unilateral more frequently, and the spinal changes on plain radiography may be more asymmetric in psoriatic arthritis than with classic ankylosing spondylitis. Finally, crystal-associated arthropathies occasionally can confuse, especially with monoarticular disease, and are best distinguished by synovial fluid crystal analysis. Serum urate levels may be increased in patients with psoriatic arthritis, adding to the confusion. To aid dermatologists and general physicians in identifying those with psoriatic arthritis, a number of screening tools for arthritis in patients with psoriasis have been proposed and are the subject of a current head-to-head comparative study.

LABORATORY FEATURES

No diagnostic laboratory test for psoriatic arthritis is known. Although the absence of rheumatoid factor is considered an important distinguishing feature from RA, low levels of rheumatoid factor may be found in patients (5% to 16%) with typical psoriatic arthritis features. Until a more definitive diagnostic test becomes available, it is difficult to be categorical about diagnosis in these patients. Cyclic citrullinated peptide antibodies initially were thought to be specific to RA, but it is now recognized that cyclic citrullinated peptide antibodies are found in approximately 5% of psoriatic arthritis patients as well.[27] Acute phase markers, such as erythrocyte sedimentation rate, C-reactive protein, and serum amyloid A, may be elevated in psoriatic arthritis patients, but less commonly and to a lesser degree than in RA patients. These markers are elevated in particular in patients with polyarticular disease and act as a marker of poor prognosis.[28] Finally, as was mentioned previously, hyperuricemia may be found in association with metabolic abnormalities in psoriatic arthritis patients and may not reflect the extent of skin involvement.

RADIOGRAPHIC FEATURES

Although substantial advances have been made in the application, in particular, of musculoskeletal ultrasound (MSUS) and of MRI in patients with arthritis, including psoriatic arthritis, plain radiographic imaging remains the "gold standard" for assessing bony changes in peripheral joints in psoriatic arthritis.

Plain Radiography

Sixty-seven percent of patients with established psoriatic arthritis have radiographic abnormalities,[11] and 47% of patients with recent-onset psoriatic arthritis will have developed erosions within 2 years of disease onset.[16] Distinctive radiographic features reflect in some cases the clinical phenotype (Figure 77-5). These features include asymmetric joint involvement; involvement of the interphalangeal joints of the fingers and toes, with features of bony erosion and resorption sometimes seen together and resulting in the classic "pencil-in-cup" deformity; joint space narrowing or involvement of entheseal sites, often with bony spurs or periostitis developing; and spinal involvement, frequently less severe and asymmetric than in classic ankylosing spondylitis.

Radiographic progression in psoriatic arthritis is slow in early stages of the disorder, with the mean modified Sharp (to include DIP joints in the hands) erosion score at presentation increasing from 1.2 to 3 at 2 years.[16] Larson and Sharp scoring systems have been used in psoriatic arthritis, but neither the Larson nor the Sharp score has been developed specifically for psoriatic arthritis or has been extensively validated.

Musculoskeletal Ultrasound

Many MSUS applications are useful in psoriatic arthritis; these applications are likely to develop further as the technology (in particular, power Doppler) that can be used to allow identification of blood flow is further advanced (Figure 77-6). Already it has been shown that MSUS is more sensitive than clinical examination in detecting knee synovitis in patients with various arthritides, including psoriatic arthritis.[29] One study has suggested further that this increased sensitivity may result in reclassification of some patients as polyarticular when they were previously diagnosed as oligoarticular on clinical grounds.[30] This reclassification may result in significant changes in prognosis and therapy. Finally, MSUS has been used in objective monitoring of the response of synovitis to therapy.[31]

MSUS features at the enthesis include entheseal thickening, hypoechoic change, increased vascularity as shown on power Doppler, tenosynovitis, and bony erosions or enthesophyte formation.[32,33] MSUS has been shown to be more sensitive than clinical examination in detecting lower limb enthesopathy.[33,34] MSUS has been used in studies of dactylitic digits. Together with MRI, MSUS has shown dactylitis to be due to a combination of synovial and tenosynovial inflammation.[21,22] Finally, MSUS guidance for small joint or entheseal aspiration or injection may have particular application in patients with psoriatic arthritis.

Magnetic Resonance Imaging

MRI studies have been particularly useful in offering new insights into disease pathogenesis in psoriatic arthritis. Based on the prominent entheseal-related bone marrow edema seen on MRI, McGonagle and colleagues[35] have proposed that psoriatic arthritis, in contrast to RA, is an entheseal-based disease. MRI can be used to study all aspects of joint involvement, including the enthesis, but use of MRI as a routine clinical tool in psoriatic arthritis has not been clarified. Application of MRI to the spine or sacroiliac joints in psoriatic arthritis may prove especially helpful, as has been shown in ankylosing spondylitis, but studies in psoriatic arthritis patients are awaited. Preliminary studies have suggested that MRI can be useful as an outcome measure in the detection of synovitis or of vascularity in patients with psoriatic arthritis undergoing biologic therapies (Figure 77-7). More detailed studies are required. A new MRI

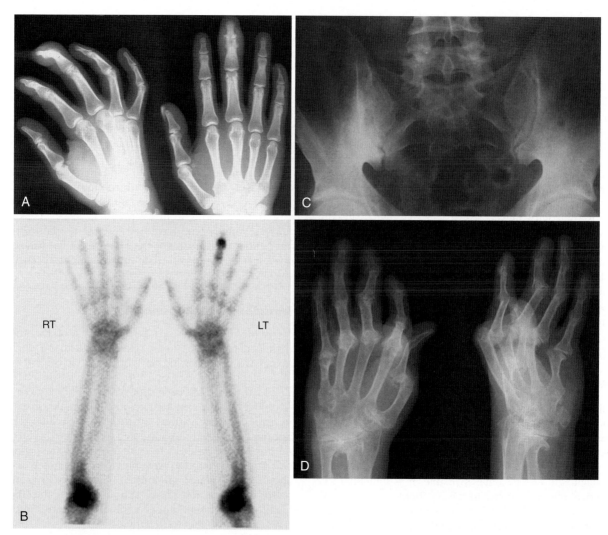

Figure 77-5　Radiologic features in psoriatic arthritis. **A,** Third left distal interphalangeal joint monoarthritis with prominent new bone formation. **B,** Bone scan from same patient as in **A. C,** Asymmetric right-sided sacroiliitis. **D,** Severe destructive changes (arthritis mutilans) with multiple erosions and "pencil-in-cup" deformities. *(Courtesy Dr. Robin Gibney.)*

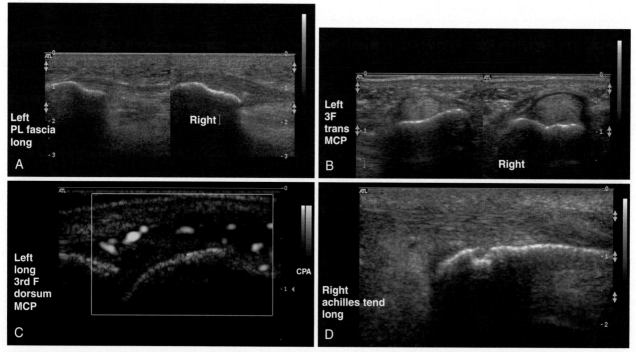

Figure 77-6　Musculoskeletal ultrasound features in psoriatic arthritis. **A,** Right plantar fascia thickening compared with the left. **B,** Transverse section through left third finger at the metacarpophalangeal joint showing right tenosynovitis. **C,** Power Doppler ultrasound through left third finger at the metacarpophalangeal joint confirming increased vascularity (synovitis). **D,** Right Achilles tendinitis with calcaneal erosion. *(Courtesy Dr. Robin Gibney.)*

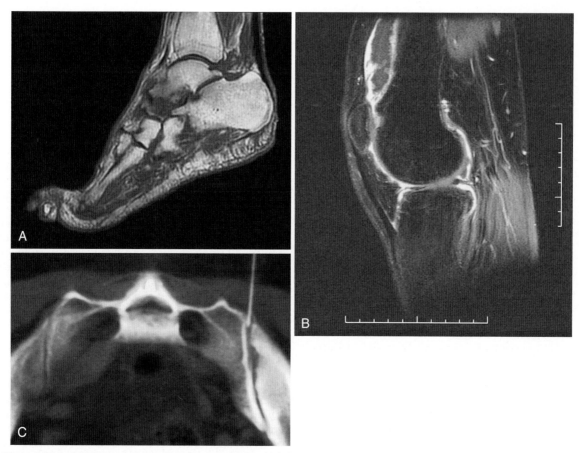

Figure 77-7 A, T1-weighted magnetic resonance imaging (MRI) of left foot confirming severe talonavicular disease with bone edema. **B,** Contrast-enhanced MRI of an inflamed knee joint in psoriatic arthritis showing synovial enhancement and large suprapatellar effusion. **C,** Computed tomography scan of sacroiliac joint showing sclerosis, erosion, and needle in place just before corticosteroid injection. *(Courtesy Dr. Robin Gibney.)*

scoring system has been proposed to measure articular inflammation and damage in patients with psoriatic arthritis (PsAMRIS).[36]

Other Imaging Modalities

The use of other imaging modalities, such as computed tomography (CT) or scintigraphy, has largely been superseded by MRI. CT is now reserved mainly for patients for whom MRI is contraindicated, or for whom MRI is unavailable. Positron emission tomography has been found to be comparable with MSUS and MRI in RA knees; this work needs to be extended to psoriatic arthritis. In a study using high-resolution CT imaging, structural bone changes were compared between RA and psoriatic arthritis. Smaller Ω-shaped and tubule-shaped erosions, as well as large sometimes corona-shaped osteophytes, are typical of psoriatic arthritis.[37]

DIAGNOSIS

A diagnostic test for psoriatic arthritis is currently unavailable. Nevertheless, in its simplest form, psoriatic arthritis can be considered as an arthritis occurring in the presence of psoriasis, but in the absence of rheumatoid factor. Most psoriatic arthritis patients meet this simple definition. The arthritis can be predominantly spinal, it may involve only

entheseal sites, psoriasis may present after arthritis in 15% of cases, and low-titer positive rheumatoid factor may be found. Recognizing these difficulties, the CASPAR group published new classification criteria based on an analysis of 588 psoriatic arthritis cases and 536 controls (Table 77-2).[38] These criteria have yet to be validated in other large patient cohorts, and they should not be used in individual patient diagnosis. In the setting of clinical research, the CASPAR criteria have a specificity of 0.987 and a sensitivity of 0.914. For the individual patient, an algorithm for diagnosis is suggested in Figure 77-8.

CLINICAL COURSE AND OUTCOME

Five early psoriatic arthritis cohorts have been studied.[16,39-42] The mean disease duration in these cohorts was 6 to 12 months, the median age at onset of psoriasis was 27 to 31 years, and the median age at onset of arthritis was 38 to 52 years. Overall, little relationship was noted between skin disease severity and onset of psoriatic arthritis; the small joints of hands and feet were most commonly involved; the DIP joints were involved in one-third of patients, usually in association with nail disease, which was present in two-thirds; dactylitis and enthesitis were present in one-third; and spinal involvement only was found in 2% to 4%, but was present in 20% overall. At follow-up, disease had continued to progress in most patients, with 47% developing

Table 77-2   CASPAR Classification Criteria for
Psoriatic Arthritis

Inflammatory articular disease (joint, spine, or entheseal) with ≥3
points from the following:
1. Evidence of psoriasis (one of a, b, or c)
   a. Current psoriasis*: psoriatic skin or scalp disease present
      today as judged by a rheumatologist or dermatologist
   b. Personal history of psoriasis: history of psoriasis that may be
      obtained from patient, family physician, dermatologist,
      rheumatologist, or other qualified health care provider
   c. Family history of psoriasis: history of psoriasis in a first-
      degree or second-degree relative according to patient report
2. Psoriatic nail dystrophy: typical psoriatic nail dystrophy,
   including onycholysis, pitting, and hyperkeratosis observed on
   current physical examination
3. Negative test for rheumatoid factor: by any method except
   latex, but preferably by ELISA or nephelometry, according to the
   local laboratory reference range
4. Dactylitis (one of a or b)
   a. Current swelling of an entire digit
   b. History: history of dactylitis recorded by a rheumatologist
5. Radiologic evidence of juxta-articular new bone formation:
   ill-defined ossification near joint margins (but excluding
   osteophyte formation) on plain x-rays of hand or foot

*Current psoriasis scores 2, whereas all other items score 1.
   Specificity 0.987, sensitivity 0.914.
   CASPAR, Classification of Psoriatic Arthritis; ELISA, enzyme-linked immu-
nosorbent assay.

erosive disease within 2 years.[16] Markers for progression included polyarticular disease and an elevated erythrocyte sedimentation rate. Long-term follow-up studies have shown significant morbidity and increased mortality in psoriatic arthritis: 17% of patients have five or more deformed joints, 40% to 57% have a deforming arthritis, 20% to 40% have spinal involvement, 11% to 19% are disabled, and mortality is increased compared with the general population.[11,43,44] In one study, carotid intimal medial thickness was increased in psoriatic arthritis patients compared with

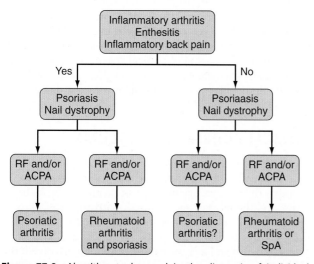

Figure 77-8 Algorithm to be used in the diagnosis of individual patients presenting with possible psoriatic arthritis. Some patients may present with typical articular manifestations of psoriatic arthritis, but in the absence of skin or nail disease. They can be diagnosed as having definite psoriatic arthritis only when psoriasis subsequently develops. ACPA, anticitrullinated protein antibody; RF, rheumatoid factor; SpA, spondyloarthropathy.

controls (but was significantly reduced compared with an RA cohort of similar disease duration [unpublished observations]).

COMORBIDITIES IN PSORIATIC ARTHRITIS

Similar to the recent emphasis on the importance of comorbidities in psoriasis,[45] a number of studies have highlighted cardiovascular risk factors and the metabolic syndrome in psoriatic arthritis. In one study of 109 psoriatic arthritis patients compared with 699 RA and 122 ankylosing spondylitis controls, the adjusted odds ratio for the metabolic syndrome was 2.44 (1.48 to 4.01; $P < .001$) with adjusted odds ratios significantly increased for central obesity, impaired fasting glucose, and low high-density lipoprotein (HDL) cholesterol.[46] The European League Against Rheumatism (EULAR) has published evidence-based guidelines for cardiovascular risk management in patients with inflammatory arthritis.[47]

OUTCOME DOMAINS AND INSTRUMENTS

Measuring response to treatment of psoriatic arthritis in clinical trials has been the subject of much interest for members of the Group for Research and Assessment of Psoriasis and Psoriatic Arthritis (GRAPPA) and Outcome Measures in Rheumatoid Arthritis Clinical Trials (OMERACT). Many of the data that have been used to date in clinical trials have been adapted from RA and have not been validated. Controversial issues have included the number of joints to count, the usefulness of the acute phase response in psoriatic arthritis, and how important is it to include a measure of function or quality of life. An essential core set of domains that must be included in clinical trials has now been agreed on, with other domains necessary but not mandatory, and yet others requiring considerably more research (Figure 77-9). Instruments for many of these domains have yet to be developed and validated, and some instruments, such as the Psoriasis Assessment Severity Index (PASI), have acknowledged limitations. Table 77-3 lists the currently available instruments for the core domains. Instruments for dactylitis and enthesitis have been proposed and validated.[48,49]

In the setting of clinical trials, numerous composite scores (e.g., American College of Rheumatology [ACR]20, ACR50, ACR70; EULAR Disease Activity Score [DAS] response criteria) have been used in psoriatic arthritis, most again adapted from RA and not extensively validated in psoriatic arthritis. One scoring system was developed for psoriatic arthritis—the PsARC; although it has been used in numerous studies, it too has not been extensively validated and is considered perhaps insufficiently responsive and discriminant.[50] Much work is required to develop a validated and responsive composite instrument for psoriatic arthritis. More recently, minimal disease activity criteria were developed and validated,[51] and two disease activity indices have been proposed. The Disease Activity index for Psoriatic Arthritis (DAPSA) appears to work well for

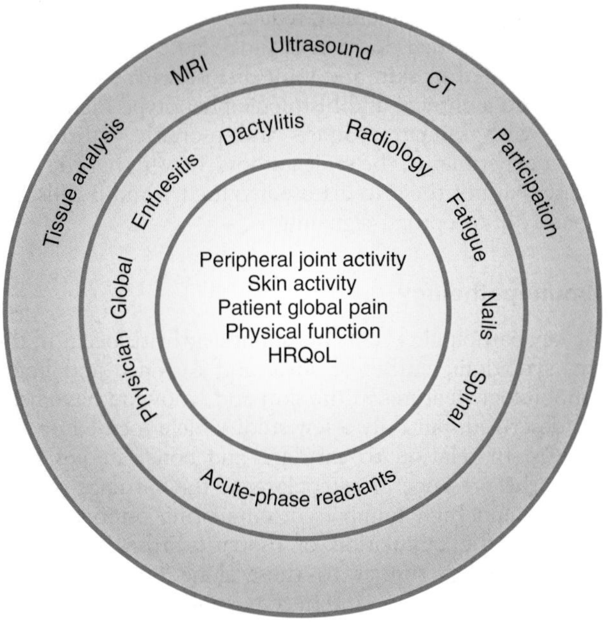

Figure 77-9 Outcome domains in psoriatic arthritis. The central core domains are considered essential for inclusion in clinical trials. The middle circle contains domains that are considered important but not essential. The outer circle contains domains that all require further research and validation. CT, computed tomography; HRQoL, health-related quality of life; MRI, magnetic resonance imaging.

joint-related disease and is easy to apply.[52] The Composite Psoriatic Disease Activity Index (CPDAI) better reflects all of the domains potentially involved in psoriatic arthritis[53]; thus unlike the DAPSA, this instrument could distinguish treatment responses between two doses of etanercept in the PRESTA trial dataset (FitzGerald, personal communication). Finally, Gladman and colleagues used data from placebo-controlled trials.[54]

Table 77-3 Core Set Instruments Proposed for Use in Clinical Trials

Domain	Instrument
Peripheral joint inflammation	Tender/swollen joint count 68/66
Patient global assessment	Instrument under study proposed*
Skin assessment	Psoriasis Assessment Severity Index (if body surface area ≥3%)
	Lesion score (erythema, induration, scale)
	Body surface area
Pain	Visual analogue scale or numeric rating scale
Physical function	HAQ/SF-36 physical function composite
Health-related quality of life	Generic
	Disease specific (e.g., DLQI, PsAQoL)

*Cauli A, Gladman DD, Mathiew A, et al: Patient global assessment in psoriatic arthritis: a multicenter GRAPPA and OMERACT study, *J Rheumatol* 38:898–903, 2011.

DLQI, Dermatology Life Quality Index; HAQ, health assessment questionnaire; PsAQoL Psoriatic Arthritis Quality of Life; SF-36, Short Form health survey.

PATHOGENESIS

Many studies have explored key components of disease pathogenesis, including the contribution of genetic factors, the role of infection or trauma, studies of animal models or involved sites of disease, and the importance of components of the immune system such as cytokines.

Genetic Factors

Familial clustering of psoriasis and psoriatic arthritis is well described. Twin studies in psoriasis have shown a high rate of concordance in monozygotic twins.[55] The genetic basis for this clustering has been the subject of extensive investigations in psoriasis, but has been much less well studied in psoriatic arthritis. Studies of psoriatic arthritis have often included patients as a subset of larger psoriasis cohorts, and the diversity of clinical phenotypes has not often been recognized.

A strong association between psoriasis and the human leukocyte (HLA)-C region of the major histocompatibility complex (MHC) has long been recognized. Whether this was HLA-Cw6 itself, found in approximately 60% of psoriasis cohorts, or a region telomeric to this has been the subject of much controversy. Elder[56] definitively showed that the HLA susceptibility region for psoriasis is HLA-Cw6, which is often in linkage disequilibrium with other HLA-B alleles such as HLA-B57, HLA-B37, and HLA-B13. The presence of HLA-Cw6 is associated with an earlier age of onset of psoriasis (type 1 disease, <40 years old) and with more extensive and severe disease. In individuals with psoriatic arthritis, the association with HLA-Cw6 is slightly weaker, whereas additional associations have been found with HLA-B27, chiefly in patients with predominant spinal disease, and with HLA-B38 and HLA-B39.[57]

These findings have been interpreted to suggest that the MHC association with psoriasis lies close to the HLA-C region, whereas the association with the articular manifestations more likely lies in or close to the HLA-B region. A study of a large cohort of psoriatic arthritis patients in the United Kingdom has found HLA-Cw6 to be in linkage disequilibrium with HLA-DRBI*07, and that possession of both alleles was associated with fewer involved or damaged joints (Pauline Ho, personal communication, 2007).[58]

Other genes within the MHC region have been explored in psoriasis and psoriatic arthritis. Tumor necrosis factor (TNF) promoter polymorphisms or a gene in linkage disequilibrium with TNF may predispose the patient to or increase susceptibility to psoriasis and to psoriatic arthritis. One study has found further an association between the TNF-308 A allele and disease progression in early psoriatic arthritis.[59] Whole-genome scans in psoriasis have identified additional non-MHC susceptibility regions, known as the PSORS regions on chromosomes 4, 6, and 17. To date, no candidate genes have been identified.

Increasing evidence suggests that an additional or distinct genetic contribution is responsible for the development of psoriatic arthritis. Investigators have pointed to an MHC class I chain-related A (MICA)-A9 polymorphism, which confers additional relative risk, in particular for polyarticular disease, in psoriasis patients who carry Cw*0602.[60] MICA-A9 polymorphism was found in linkage disequilibrium with HLA-B alleles (B*5701, B*3801). These results suggest that the *MICA* gene or other nearby genes may be involved in the development of psoriatic arthritis. Additionally, a genome scan identified a paternally influenced locus on chromosome 16—a region not known to be implicated in psoriasis susceptibility.[61]

Finally, two genome-wide association studies in psoriatic arthritis have been reported.[62,63] These studies have confirmed associations with HLA-C and interleukin (IL)-12B, and they have identified a new susceptibility region TRAF3IP2 on chromosome 6p, which encodes a protein involved in IL-17 signaling, and which interacts with members of the Rel/ nuclear factor κB (NFκB) transcription factor family.

Environmental Factors

The role of environmental factors in triggering skin or joint disease in patients with psoriasis or psoriatic arthritis has been supported largely by clinical observations, although the mechanism is poorly understood. It has long been recognized that there is a strong association between guttate psoriasis and preceding streptococcal infections in children.[64] That this association might be related to a streptococcal superantigen has been proposed. Some authors have found bacterial antigens in synovial tissue samples from psoriatic arthritis patients, but this may be no different from those in noninflammatory control subjects.[65]

The Koebner phenomenon (see Figure 77-1H) has been reported to occur in 52% of patients with psoriasis. The Koebner phenomenon is the development of psoriasis along the site of skin trauma. It has been proposed that trauma may play a role in triggering episodes of joint inflammation, and the term *deep Koebner phenomenon* has been coined. Although the role of trauma has not been proved, in one study, 24.6% of patients reported a traumatic event before the onset of arthritis.[66]

Finally, a link between stress and exacerbation of psoriasis has been proposed, supported largely by clinical observational studies. A similar association may exist in psoriatic arthritis, but this has not been systematically examined.

Animal Models

Although spondyloarthropathy has been detected in a variety of primates, rodent models have proved helpful in deciphering pathogenic pathways. In rodents transgenic for HLA-B27 class I molecules, skin, nail, and joint features have been described that mimic some of the features of the human phenotype.[67] When HLA-B27 transgenic rats were raised in a germ-free environment, they seemed to be protected from joint disease. Mice genetically lacking MHC class II have developed skin and joint disease, but confined to the distal phalanges with skin and nail disease also on the affected digits.[68] Involvement of the distal phalanges and nails was reported in aging male DBA/1 mice from different litters that were caged together from 12 weeks.[69] In these animals, dactylitis, periostitis, and ankylosing enthesitis were observed.

Finally, JunB protein was shown to be expressed in normal and in clinically uninvolved psoriatic skin, but expression was considerably reduced in involved psoriatic lesions.[70] Epidermal deletion of JunB and c-Jun in a mouse model resulted in skin and joint disease with 100% penetrance and a clinical and histologic phenotype highly consistent with human psoriasis and psoriatic arthritis. In further experiments, the same authors showed that the joint disease, but not the skin disease, required T and B cells and intact TNF receptor 1 signaling.

Immunopathology

The key pathologic events in psoriatic arthritis occur in the skin, synovium, entheseal sites, and cartilage and bone. Pathobiologic features in the skin and synovium have been well described, but only a few studies have focused on the enthesis. In relation to cartilage and bone, studies have shown the presence of osteoclasts at the cartilage-pannus junction and high numbers of circulating osteoclast precursors in the circulation of psoriatic arthritis patients. Detailed studies similar to those done on RA on the synovial-cartilage-bone interface possibly could yield valuable information regarding joint destruction in psoriatic arthritis.

Psoriasis Skin

Involved psoriasis skin is characterized by epidermal hyperplasia, mononuclear leukocytes in the papillary dermis, neutrophils in the stratum corneum, and an increase in various subsets of dendritic cells.[71] CD8+ T cells are the predominant T cell subset chiefly found in the epidermis, whereas dermal T cells contain a mixture of CD4+ and CD8+. Most T cells in skin lesions express addressin, a cutaneous lymphocyte antigen, in contrast to circulating T cells and T cells found in the inflamed synovium in psoriatic arthritis.[72] Finally, vascular changes are prominent in psoriasis with impressive growth and dilation of superficial blood vessels.

Psoriatic Synovium

Many early studies of synovial pathology in psoriatic arthritis highlighted the presence of prominent and striking vascular changes. In the first study that compared psoriatic arthritis and RA synovial tissue, quantitative immunopathologic analysis confirmed these prominent vascular changes and found that vessel number was significantly increased in psoriatic arthritis.[73] Lining layer hyperplasia was less marked in psoriatic arthritis, and fewer macrophages were seen trafficking into the synovium and out to the lining layer. The numbers of T lymphocytes and their subsets and the number of B cells were similar to the frequency found in RA. Although neutrophil infiltration was not assessed, this study examined adhesion molecule expression further in the two patient subgroups and found E-selectin expression to be considerably reduced in psoriatic arthritis. Many of these observations have been confirmed by other authors.

In a study by Kruithof and co-workers,[74] the synovial immunopathologic features in patients with spondyloarthropathy, including psoriatic arthritis, were compared with the features seen in RA.[74] Using a semi-quantitative scoring system, the authors identified many features characteristic of the spondyloarthropathy group as a whole and in the psoriatic arthritis subgroup alone. Increased vascularity, higher neutrophil numbers (also seen in involved psoriasis skin), and a higher number of infiltrating CD163[+] macrophages, a marker of mature tissue macrophages, reliably distinguished spondyloarthropathy from RA. No significant differences were seen between oligoarticular versus polyarticular psoriatic arthritis.

The important role of the vasculature in psoriatic arthritis pathogenesis is perhaps most elegantly shown by the large numbers of tortuous and dilated blood vessels observed through an arthroscopic view of psoriatic joints.[75] An interaction of key growth factors is thought to regulate closely the new vessel formation or angiogenic process. Growth factors, including TNF, transforming growth factor (TGF)-β, platelet-derived growth factor (PDGF), angiopoietins (ANG-1, ANG-2), and vascular endothelial growth factor (VEGF), have been described in skin and synovial tissue.[76,77] Because this expression is found at an early stage of inflammation, it may represent a primary event in psoriatic arthritis as opposed to a reaction or response to hypoxia. One possibility is that there is a genetic predisposition to endothelial activation, which results in new vessel formation and increased cellular trafficking.

Of interest, two studies have identified a change in synovial CD3[+] T cell infiltration as correlating with clinical response in patients commencing biologic therapies[78] (Pontifex, personal communication). Changes in CD3 infiltration also correlated with changes in MRI assessment of synovitis (Pontifex). Changes in CD3 infiltration may well prove to be a useful tissue biomarker of treatment response.

Entheseal Sites

Laloux and associates[79] described the immunopathologic features of the enthesis in patients undergoing joint replacement surgery with spondyloarthropathy, including psoriatic arthritis, and compared them with RA. The number of patients was small in this study, but a consistent increase in CD8[+] T cell expression was observed at the enthesis in patients with psoriatic arthritis compared with RA patients. Ultrasound-guided biopsy of five sites of acute enthesitis in early spondyloarthropathy confirmed an inflammatory response with increased vascularity and cellular, predominantly macrophage, infiltration.[80] These findings are consistent with the well-described association of psoriatic arthritis with HLA class I antigens. They also are consistent with the previously described dominance of activated and mature CD8[+] T cells in psoriatic arthritis synovial fluid samples compared with RA.[81] It is attractive to suggest that entheseally derived antigens might trigger an immune response in adjacent synovial tissue. To date, evidence for this hypothesis has not been found, although this is clearly an area for future study. A search for candidate antigens common to the enthesis and the skin might be informative.

Cytokines

Synovial explant tissues obtained from psoriatic arthritis joints have been shown to produce higher levels of the T helper type 1 (Th1) cytokines interleukin (IL)-2 and interferon-γ protein than explants similarly cultured from osteoarthritis and RA patients.[82] This Th1 lymphocyte profile also has been observed in psoriasis plaques.[83] The cytokines IL-1β and TNF were released by psoriasis synovial explants in high concentrations. In contrast, IL-4 and IL-5 were not identified, but IL-10 was highly expressed in psoriatic synovium, although not in skin. A similar pattern of cytokine production in psoriatic arthritis synovium was shown using immunohistochemical and gene expression techniques.[84,85] Other innate cytokines, such as IL-18 and IL-15, are present in psoriatic arthritis synovial tissue and are downregulated by methotrexate therapy.

The role of Th17 cells has been explored, and an important immunomodulatory role has been better established in psoriasis than in psoriatic arthritis. Comparison of lesional skin gene expression in responders versus nonresponders to etanercept revealed rapid downmodulation of innate IL-1β and IL-8 sepsis cascade cytokines in both groups, but only responders downregulated IL-17 pathway genes to baseline levels.[86] An increase in circulating Th17 cells has been found in psoriatic arthritis,[87] and an increase in IL-17 has been found in skin, synovial tissue, and synovial fluid of psoriatic arthritis patients.[88] Further supporting a key role for the Th17 pathway, genetic polymorphisms in key cytokines involved in differentiation of T cells to Th1 and Th17 subtypes, IL-12 and IL-23, have been found to be associated with susceptibility to both psoriasis and psoriatic arthritis,[89] and inhibition of the common p40 subunit of IL-12/IL-23 has led to clinical improvement in both skin and joint manifestations.[90]

TNF levels are elevated in psoriatic skin, synovium, and joint fluid of patients with psoriatic arthritis.[82,91] Several lines of evidence support the concept that TNF is an important cytokine in the psoriatic joint. TNF transgenic mice exhibit extensive bone destruction similar to that observed in some psoriatic arthritis patients. In a study of 129 patients with early psoriatic arthritis, patients with erosions were significantly more likely to have the TNF-308 A allele, an allele associated with high TNF production.[59] As was mentioned earlier, immunohistochemical and gene expression studies have shown marked upregulation of TNF in the psoriatic synovial membrane. Histopathologic analysis of synovial specimens from eight spondyloarthropathy patients, four of whom had psoriatic arthritis, treated with the anti-TNF monoclonal antibody infliximab revealed decreased vascularity, synovial lining thickness, and mononuclear cell infiltration after therapy.[92,93] In another study, a significant reduction in the quantity of infiltrating macrophages, the CD31[+] vascular area, αvβ3-positive neovessels/*Ulex europaeus* agglutinin–positive vessels, VEGF and its receptor KDR/flk-1 (VEGFR-2), and SDF-1–positive vessels in psoriatic arthritis synovium was noted after 8 weeks (three infusions) of infliximab treatment.[94]

Matrix Metalloproteinases and Cartilage Destruction

Radiographs of psoriatic joints often reveal cartilage loss manifested as joint space narrowing. Similar to RA, matrix metalloproteinases (MMPs) and tissue inhibitors of MMPs (TIMPs) were identified in psoriatic arthritis synovial lining and sublining layers.[95,96] In particular, immunohistochemical studies revealed that MMP-9 localized to blood vessel walls, whereas MMP-1, MMP-2, MMP-3, TIMP-1, and TIMP-2 showed a cellular and interstitial staining pattern in the synovial lining. Serum levels of MMP-3 exhibited a marked and rapid decrease after successful anti-TNF therapy, raising the possibility that this molecule may serve as a biomarker. In another study, similar levels of MMP-1 and MMP-3 mRNA were detected in RA and psoriatic arthritis synovial tissue despite the fact that RA patients exhibited more erosions on plain radiographs.[97] The elevated ratio of MMPs to TIMP-1 in synovial tissue favored cartilage degradation, although expression of MMPs was not significantly elevated at the cartilage-pannus junction compared with other sites. These reports indicate that MMPs are upregulated in psoriatic arthritis synovium, but their precise functions remain to be defined.

Bone Remodeling

Radiographs of psoriatic arthritis joints can reveal markedly altered bone remodeling in the form of bone resorption (tuft resorption or osteolysis, large eccentric erosions, and pencil-in-cup deformities) and new bone formation (periostitis, spur or enthesophyte formation, bony ankylosis). Important in bone resorption, psoriatic joint biopsy specimens show large multinucleated osteoclasts in deep resorption pits at the bone-pannus junction.[98] Osteoclastogenesis (differentiation of monocytes into osteoclasts) is a contact-dependent process directed by osteoblasts and stromal cells in the bone marrow. These cells release signals necessary for differentiation of an osteoclast precursor derived from the CD14+ monocyte population into an osteoclast.

One of these signals is the receptor activator of nuclear factor κB ligand (RANKL), a member of the TNF superfamily that binds to receptor activator of nuclear factor κB (RANK) on the surface of osteoclast precursors and osteoclasts. This ligand-receptor interaction stimulates proliferation and differentiation of osteoclast precursors and activation of osteoclasts. It has been proposed that the relative expression of RANKL and of its natural antagonist osteoprotegerin (OPG) ultimately controls osteoclastogenesis. In psoriatic arthritis synovial tissues, marked upregulation of RANKL protein and low expression of osteoprotegerin were detected in the adjacent synovial lining.[98] Osteoclasts also were noted in cutting cones traversing the subchondral bone, supporting a bidirectional attack on the bone in psoriatic joints. In addition, osteoclast precursors, derived from circulating CD14+ monocytes, were markedly elevated in the peripheral blood of patients with psoriatic arthritis compared with healthy controls. Treatment of patients with psoriatic arthritis with anti-TNF agents significantly decreased the level of circulating osteoclast precursor, supporting a central role for TNF in the generation of this precursor population. Although abundantly expressed, there appeared to be little relationship between expression of RANKL, OPG, and RANK and both systemic and local inflammation,[99] and also little relationship between the decline in osteoclast precursor numbers and bone marrow edema following etanercept treatment.[100]

The mechanisms responsible for new bone formation in the psoriatic joint are poorly understood. Higher circulating levels of bone formation markers, in particular bone alkaline phosphatase, in psoriatic arthritis patients as compared with RA patients both before and after anti-TNF therapy commenced has been demonstrated (Szentepetery, personal communication). TGF-β and VEGF may be pivotal in this process of new bone formation, given that TGF-β is strongly expressed in synovial tissues isolated from patients with ankylosing spondylitis and synergizes with VEGF to induce bone formation in animal models.[101] De Klerck and colleagues[102] showed that the bone morphogenetic proteins (BMPs) BMP-2 and BMP-7 are upregulated in regions of pathologic new bone formation. The same investigators showed that expression of phosphorylated Smad-1 and Smad-5, important signaling molecules downstream of BMP, was markedly increased in regions of new bone formation taken from the calcaneus in a patient with Achilles tendinitis and periostitis. These studies provide evidence that potential mediators of ankylosis and periostitis in the psoriatic enthesis and joint include BMP molecules and possibly VEGF and TGF-β. Finally, the Wnt pathway and the balance between Wnt and the Wnt antagonist dickkopf-1 (DKK-1), which binds to the Wnt receptor complex on the surfaces of osteoblast lineage cells, may well be of considerable importance in the disordered bone remodeling found in psoriatic arthritis.

Summary

In considering a model for disease pathogenesis in psoriatic arthritis, we have to try to take into account genetic susceptibility; the role of the environment; cellular immunologic mechanisms; and secreted cytokines, chemokines, and other proteins. For some time, the primary hypothesis has been that psoriatic arthritis is an HLA class I–restricted, antigen-driven immune process (Figure 77-10). Considerable evidence has been presented to support this hypothesis; however, despite careful analysis of T cell receptor phenotype, no antigen-driven process other than that driven by Epstein-Barr virus has been identified.[103] The potential role of components of the innate immune response, such as Toll-like receptors or cells bearing natural killer receptors, is currently under active investigation. It is possible that the interaction of environmental factors, such as those derived from pathogens or expressed after trauma, with Toll-like receptors in a genetically susceptible individual may set in train intracellular signaling events leading to cytokine release, immune activation, and release of destructive enzymes such as MMPs (Figure 77-11).

TREATMENT

In considering treatment strategies for psoriatic arthritis, the diverse nature of the clinical phenotype (peripheral arthritis, skin and nail disease, axial disease, dactylitis, and enthesitis) may complicate therapeutic decisions because not all treatments are effective for all features, and patients often display a mixture of all of the features simultaneously. GRAPPA published a systematic review of the evidence for treatment strategies in psoriatic arthritis; this review provided treatment guidelines that are currently being revised. The reader is referred to this GRAPPA publication for a detailed review of the evidence; Figure 77-12 is a proposed preliminary algorithm for treatment choices.[104] Treatment

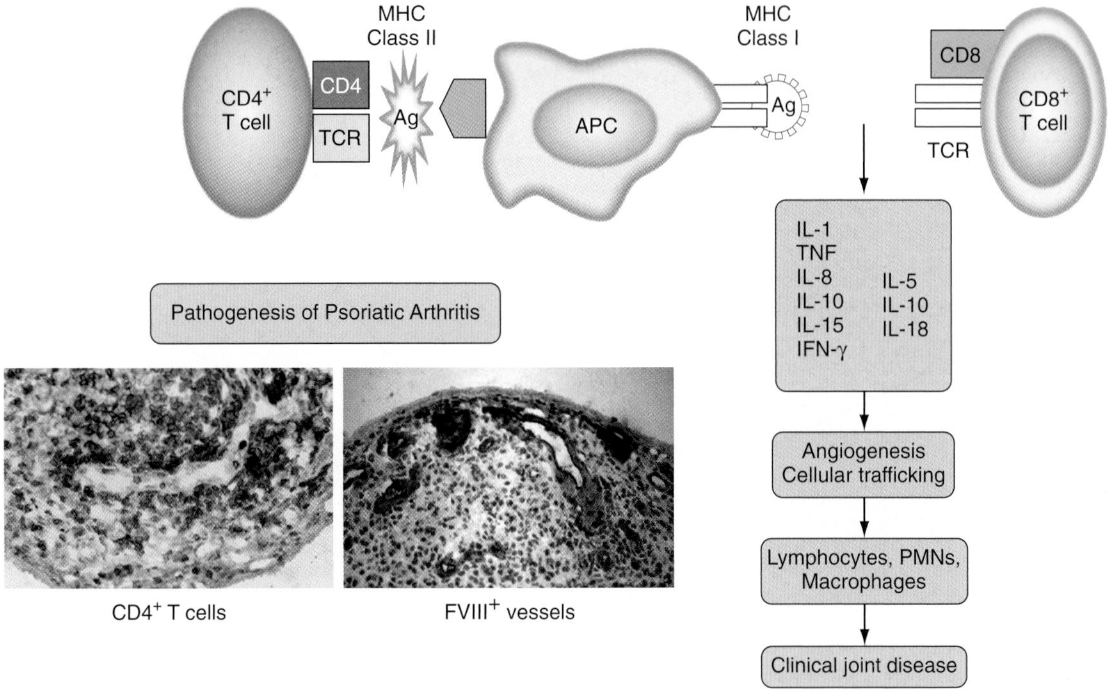

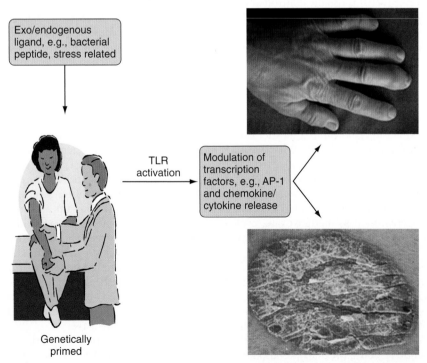

Figure 77-10 Traditional disease pathogenesis model in psoriatic arthritis. APC, antigen-presenting cell; IFN, interferon; IL, interleukin; MHC, major histocompatibility complex; PMNs, polymorphonuclear neutrophils; TCR, T cell receptor; TNF, tumor necrosis factor.

choices may be driven by the disease feature considered most severe at the time of evaluation. Finally, in reviewing the evidence for therapeutic effect presented in the following section, recommendations from the Agency for Health Care Policy and Research were used, whereby interventions are scored by categories of evidence (level 1 through 4) and strength of recommendation (grade A through D).[105]

Traditional Agents

Although there is little published evidence of a favorable therapeutic effect in psoriatic arthritis, nonsteroidal anti-inflammatory drugs are most often the agents first used in psoriatic arthritis, whatever the clinical phenotype (level 1b, grade A).[106] Expert opinion supports the use of

Figure 77-11 Alternative model incorporating new disease pathogenesis concepts. TLR, Toll-like receptor.

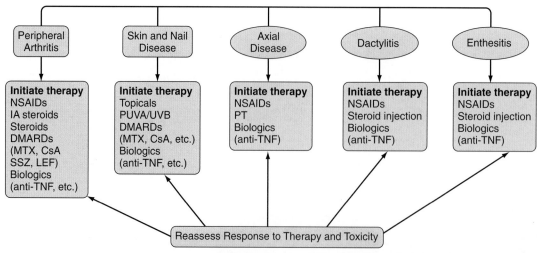

Figure 77-12 Preliminary treatment algorithm for the various clinical manifestations in psoriatic arthritis. CsA, cyclosporin A; DMARDs, disease-modifying antirheumatic drugs; IA, intra-articular; LEF, leflunomide; MTX, methotrexate; NSAIDs, nonsteroidal anti-inflammatory drugs; PT, physical therapy; PUVA, psoralen plus ultraviolet A; SSZ, sulfasalazine; TNF, tumor necrosis factor; UVB, ultraviolet B. *(From Kavanaugh AF, Ritchlin CT: Systematic review of treatments for psoriatic arthritis: an evidence based approach and basis for treatment guidelines,* J Rheumatol *33:1417–1421, 2006.)*

nonsteroidal anti-inflammatory drugs, although occasional exacerbations of psoriasis have been reported. The use of systemic corticosteroids is not evidence based (level 4, grade D), although 24% of patients in one study were taking prednisolone.[107] Concerns have arisen suggesting that exacerbations of psoriasis may follow corticosteroid withdrawal. No randomized controlled trials have examined intra-articular steroids in psoriatic arthritis or the use of local entheseal or dactylitis injections. Expert opinion indicates that intra-articular steroids can be quite effective, especially in oligoarticular disease, or where localized entheseal involvement is present, as in plantar fasciitis (level 4, grade D). Mild skin disease (PASI <10) is usually controlled with topical steroids or vitamin D derivatives; the latter are best used for maintenance therapy.[108]

Systemic therapy is considered in patients with three or more inflamed joints despite conventional therapy, as described previously; persistent or treatment-resistant axial, entheseal, or dactylitic disease, especially where multiple sites are involved; or moderate or severe psoriasis (PASI >10). Randomized controlled trials of disease-modifying antirheumatic drugs (DMARDs) are few and limited by size. Based on evidence and expert opinion, nearly all DMARDs may have small to moderate beneficial effects on peripheral joints, enthesitis, and dactylitis.[106,109,110] Axial features and nail disease do not seem to respond.[111] Good or moderate improvements in skin disease have been reported with some of the older systemic agents, such as methotrexate, cyclosporine, sulfasalazine, leflunomide, and acetretin (all level 1b, grade A).[108]

The best evidence for DMARD use comes from studies of peripheral joint disease and of psoriasis. Six randomized controlled trials have studied the use of sulfasalazine in psoriatic arthritis (level 1a, grade A); the largest included 221 patients. Fifty-nine percent of patients achieved a therapeutic response (PsARC), but consistent with other studies, a high therapeutic response (42.7%) was also noted in placebo-treated patients.[50]

Methotrexate remains for many rheumatologists the DMARD of first choice for patients with psoriatic arthritis, but evidence for its use is limited (level 3, grade B). A small, prospective randomized controlled trial concluded that methotrexate was as effective as cyclosporine; another study of 72 patients with active psoriatic arthritis and an incomplete response to methotrexate, in which cyclosporine was added in, showed significant differences only in synovitis as detected by MSUS and PASI score in favor of the combination therapy.[31,112] Although evidence for methotrexate is lacking, an open study reported significant reductions in synovial cellular infiltration and in cytokine gene expression after 3 months of therapy.[85] Although evidence suggests that cyclosporine may be as effective as methotrexate, its use is limited because its toxicity profile is considered to be high (level 1b, grade B).[113]

Perhaps the best randomized controlled trial in psoriatic arthritis of a DMARD examined the use of leflunomide (level 1b, grade A).[114] This trial included 190 patients who received leflunomide or placebo for 24 weeks. Fifty-nine percent of patients treated with leflunomide compared with 30% of patients given placebo met the primary response criteria (PsARC), with significant, although small, improvements in other individual parameters, including joint scores, health assessment questionnaire results, PASI, and Dermatology Life Quality Index scores. Regarding some older DMARDs, such as gold salts and antimalarials, no evidence of treatment benefit has been found; exacerbation of psoriasis has been reported, and these agents cannot be recommended. One small, randomized controlled trial with azathioprine suggested benefit with a reduction in Ritchie score (level 2b, grade B). Finally, apart from the cyclosporine/methotrexate study referred to earlier, little or no evidence suggests that DMARD combination therapy is beneficial or safe in psoriatic arthritis.

With the exception of psoriasis, there is a paucity of evidence that DMARDs are beneficial for the other features of psoriatic arthritis, including dactylitis, axial disease, or enthesitis. Absence of evidence does not mean absence of an effect, however. Further randomized controlled trials specifically examining these features in psoriatic arthritis are required. In psoriasis, methotrexate and cyclosporine have been shown to be highly and probably equally effective (level 1b, grade A).[108] Adverse effects, in particular with cyclosporine, may limit usage in some patients.

Biologics

The approach to treatment in psoriatic arthritis has changed considerably with the introduction of biologic therapies. As a result of numerous large, well-conducted, randomized controlled trials, accumulating evidence indicates that anti-TNF treatments are effective in controlling peripheral arthritis symptoms and signs, improving quality of life, and preventing radiologic progression (overall level 1b, grade A).[106] Indeed higher rates of Disease Activity Score (DAS)28 remission are found in psoriatic arthritis patients as compared with RA patients after 1 year of anti-TNF therapy.[115] Patients receiving 25 mg subcutaneously twice weekly of etanercept showed significant improvement in American College of Rheumatology (ACR)20 responses (59% vs. 15%) at 12 weeks compared with placebo.[116] At 12 months, radiographic disease progression (modified total Sharp score) was inhibited in the etanercept group (−0.03 unit) compared with worsening of +1.00 unit in the placebo group.

Although the anti-TNF therapies have not been compared in any study, their effect on peripheral arthritis seems to be similar. Evidence indicates that anti-TNF therapies are also effective for other disease features, such as nail disease, enthesitis, and dactylitis.[109,110,117] These studies are limited by the absence of a validated instrument to measure these features. With psoriasis, the effects of anti-TNF therapies can be quite dramatic.[118] In particular with antibody therapy, highly significant improvements in PASI scores were achieved (e.g., PASI = 75 in 59% of adalimumab-treated patients vs. 1% in placebo-treated patients after 24 weeks; PASI = 90 in 50%).[119] Better skin but not articular responses have been demonstrated in etanercept patients treated with 50 mg twice weekly as compared with once weekly.[120]

Alefacept is a fusion protein of soluble lymphocyte function antigen 3 with Fc fragments of immunoglobulin (Ig) G1. Alefacept was the first biologic agent approved for the treatment of moderate to severe psoriasis (level 1b, grade A). Efficacy was dose dependent and slow, but PASI = 75 was achieved in 33% of patients at some point.[121] Alefacept in combination with methotrexate was evaluated in 185 patients with active psoriatic arthritis.[122] At 6 months, 54% of alefacept-treated patients versus 23% of placebo-treated patients achieved an ACR20 response. Finally, efalizumab, a humanized monoclonal antibody targeting the CD11a component of lymphocyte function antigen 1, has been approved for the treatment of psoriasis, with PASI = 75 achieved in 22% to 39% in randomized controlled trials,[118] but this agent has since been withdrawn owing to safety issues. To date, no evidence for a beneficial effect of efalizumab in other psoriatic arthritis joint manifestations has been observed. Finally, inhibition of the common p40 subunit of IL-12/IL-23 has demonstrated good efficacy in psoriasis,[123] and ustekinumab has now been approved for treatment. A phase II clinical trial in psoriatic arthritis suggests reasonable efficacy for joint disease,[90] but additional studies are required.

References

1. Wright V: Rheumatism and psoriasis: a re-evaluation, *Am J Med* 27:454–462, 1959.
2. Moll JMH, Wright V: Psoriatic arthritis, *Semin Arthritis Rheum* 3:55–78, 1973.
3. Blumberg BS, Bunim JJ, Calkins E, et al: ARA nomenclature and classification of arthritis and rheumatism (tentative), *Arthritis Rheum* 7:93–97, 1964.
4. Gladman DD, Antoni C, Mease P, et al: Psoriatic arthritis: epidemiology, clinical features, course, and outcome, *Ann Rheum Dis* 64(Suppl 2):ii14–ii17, 2005.
5. Krueger G, Ellis CN: Psoriasis—recent advances in understanding its pathogenesis and treatment, *J Am Acad Dermatol* 53(Suppl 1):S94–S100, 2005.
6. Gelfand JM, Gladman DD, Mease PJ, et al: Epidemiology of psoriatic arthritis in the population of the United States, *J Am Acad Dermatol* 53:573, 2005.
7. Kay L, Perry-James J, Walker D: The prevalence and impact of psoriasis in the primary care population in northeast England, *Arthritis Rheum* 42:S299, 1999.
8. Shbeeb M, Uramoto KM, Gibson LE, et al: The epidemiology of psoriatic arthritis in Olmsted County, Minnesota, USA, 1982-1991, *J Rheumatol* 27:1247–1250, 2000.
9. Savolainen E, Kaipiainen-Seppanen O, Kroger L, et al: Total incidence and distribution of inflammatory joint diseases in a defined population: results from the Kuopio 2000 arthritis survey, *J Rheumatol* 30:2460–2468, 2003.
10. Karason A, Love TJ, Gudbjornsson B: A strong heritability of psoriatic arthritis over four generations—the Reykjavik Psoriatic Arthritis Study, *Rheumatology (Oxford)* 48:1424–1428, 2009.
11. Gladman DD, Shuckett R, Russell ML, et al: Psoriatic arthritis (PSA)—an analysis of 220 patients, *Q J Med* 62:127–141, 1987.
12. Christophers E, Barker JN, Griffiths CE, et al: The risk of psoriatic arthritis remains constant following initial diagnosis of psoriasis among patients seen in European dermatology clinics, *J Eur Acad Dermatol Venereol* 24:548–554, 2010.
13. Husted JA, Tom BD, Farewell VT, Gladman DD: Longitudinal analysis of fatigue in psoriatic arthritis, *J Rheumatol* 37:1878–1884, 2010.
14. Minnock P, Kirwan J, Veale D, et al: Fatigue is an independent outcome measure and is sensitive to change in patients with psoriatic arthritis, *Clin Exp Rheumatol* 28:401–404, 2010.
15. Moll JMH, Wright V: Familial occurrence of psoriatic arthritis, *Ann Rheum Dis* 22:181–195, 1973.
16. Kane D, Stafford L, Bresnihan B, et al: A prospective, clinical and radiological study of early psoriatic arthritis: an early synovitis clinic experience, *Rheumatology* 42:1460–1468, 2003.
17. Helliwell PS, Porter G, Taylor WJ: Polyarticular psoriatic arthritis is more like oligoarticular psoriatic arthritis, than rheumatoid arthritis, *Ann Rheum Dis* 66:113–117, 2007.
18. Battistone MJ, Manaster BJ, Reda DJ, et al: The prevalence of sacroiliitis in psoriatic arthritis: new perspectives from a large, multicenter cohort. A Department of Veterans Affairs Cooperative Study, *Skeletal Radiol* 28:196–201, 1999.
19. Chandran V, Tolusso DC, Cook RJ, Gladman DD: Risk factors for axial inflammatory arthritis in patients with psoriatic arthritis, *J Rheumatol* 37:809–815, 2010.
20. Brockbank JE, Stein M, Schentag CT, et al: Dactylitis in psoriatic arthritis: a marker for disease severity? *Ann Rheum Dis* 64:188–190, 2005.
21. Kane D, Greaney T, Bresnihan B, et al: Ultrasonography in the diagnosis and management of psoriatic dactylitis, *J Rheumatol* 26:1746–1751, 1999.
22. Olivieri I, Barozzi L, Pierro A, et al: Toe dactylitis in patients with spondyloarthropathy: assessment by magnetic resonance imaging, *J Rheumatol* 24:926–930, 1997.
23. Queiro R, Torre JC, Belzunegui J, et al: Clinical features and predictive factors in psoriatic arthritis-related uveitis, *Semin Arthritis Rheum* 31:264–270, 2002.

24. Schatteman L, Mielants H, Veys EM, et al: Gut inflammation in psoriatic arthritis: a prospective ileocolonoscopic study, *J Rheumatol* 22:680–683, 1995.

25. Williamson L, Dockerty JL, Dalbeth N, et al: Gastrointestinal disease and psoriatic arthritis, *J Rheumatol* 31:1469–1470, 2004.

26. Cantini F, Salvarani C, Olivieri I, et al: Distal extremity swelling with pitting edema in psoriatic arthritis: a case-control study, *Clin Exp Rheumatol* 19:291–296, 2001.

27. Korendowych E, Owen P, Ravindran J, et al: The clinical and genetic associations of anti-cyclic citrullinated peptide antibodies in psoriatic arthritis, *Rheumatology (Oxford)* 44:1056–1060, 2005.

28. Gladman DD, Farewell VT, Nadeau C: Clinical indicators of progression in psoriatic arthritis: multivariate relative risk model, *J Rheumatol* 22:675–679, 1995.

29. Karim Z, Wakefield RJ, Quinn M, et al: Validation and reproducibility of ultrasonography in the detection of synovitis in the knee: a comparison with arthroscopy and clinical examination, *Arthritis Rheum* 50:387–394, 2004.

30. Wakefield RJ, Green MJ, Marzo-Ortega H, et al: Should oligoarthritis be reclassified? Ultrasound reveals a high prevalence of subclinical disease, *Ann Rheum Dis* 63:382–385, 2004.

31. Fraser AD, van Kuijk AW, Westhovens R, et al: A randomised, double blind, placebo controlled, multicentre trial of combination therapy with methotrexate plus cyclosporine in patients with active psoriatic arthritis, *Ann Rheum Dis* 64:859–864, 2005.

32. Balint PV, Sturrock RD: Inflamed retrocalcaneal bursa and Achilles tendonitis in psoriatic arthritis demonstrated by ultrasonography, *Ann Rheum Dis* 59:931–933, 2000.

33. D'Agostino MA, Said-Nahal R, Hacquard-Bouder C, et al: Assessment of peripheral enthesitis in the spondylarthropathies by ultrasonography combined with power Doppler: a cross-sectional study, *Arthritis Rheum* 48:523–533, 2003.

34. Balint PV, Kane D, Wilson H, et al: Ultrasonography of entheseal insertions in the lower limb in spondyloarthropathy, *Ann Rheum Dis* 61:905–910, 2002.

35. McGonagle D, Conaghan PG, Emery P: Psoriatic arthritis: a unified concept twenty years on, *Arthritis Rheum* 42:1080–1086, 1999.

36. Ostergaard M, McQueen F, Wiell C, et al: The OMERACT psoriatic arthritis magnetic resonance imaging scoring system (PsAMRIS): definitions of key pathologies, suggested MRI sequences, and preliminary scoring system for PsA hands, *J Rheumatol* 36:1816–1824, 2009.

37. Finzel S, Englbrecht M, Engelke K, et al: A comparative study of periarticular bone lesions in rheumatoid arthritis and psoriatic arthritis, *Ann Rheum Dis* 70:122–127, 2011.

38. Taylor W, Gladman D, Helliwell P, et al: Classification criteria for psoriatic arthritis: development of new criteria from a large international study, *Arthritis Rheum* 54:2665–2673, 2006.

39. Harrison BJ, Silman AJ, Barrett EM, et al: Presence of psoriasis does not influence the presentation or short-term outcome of patients with early inflammatory polyarthritis, *J Rheumatol* 24:1744–1749, 1997.

40. Jones SM, Armas JB, Cohen MG, et al: Psoriatic arthritis: outcome of disease subsets and relationship of joint disease to nail and skin disease, *Br J Rheumatol* 33:834–839, 1994.

41. Punzi L, Pianon M, Rossini P, et al: Clinical and laboratory manifestations of elderly onset psoriatic arthritis: a comparison with younger onset disease, *Ann Rheum Dis* 58:226–229, 1999.

42. Khan M, Schentag C, Gladman DD: Clinical and radiological changes during psoriatic arthritis disease progression, *J Rheumatol* 30:1022–1026, 2003.

43. Torre Alonso JC, Rodriguez Perez A, Arribas Castrillo JM, et al: Psoriatic arthritis (PA): a clinical, immunological and radiological study of 180 patients, *Br J Rheumatol* 30:245–250, 1991.

44. Hanly JG, Russell ML, Gladman DD: Psoriatic spondyloarthropathy: a long term prospective study, *Ann Rheum Dis* 47:386–393, 1988.

45. Tobin AM, Veale DJ, Fitzgerald O, et al: Cardiovascular disease and risk factors in patients with psoriasis and psoriatic arthritis, *J Rheumatol* 37:1386–1394, 2010.

46. Mok C, Ko G, Ho L, et al: Prevalence of atherosclerotic risk factors and the metabolic syndrome in patients with chronic inflammatory arthritis, *Arthritis Care Res* 62:195–202, 2011.

47. Peters MJ, Symmons DP, McCarey D, et al: EULAR evidence-based recommendations for cardiovascular risk management in patients with rheumatoid arthritis and other forms of inflammatory arthritis, *Ann Rheum Dis* 69:325–331, 2010.

48. Helliwell PS, Firth J, Ibrahim GH, et al: Development of an assessment tool for dactylitis in patients with psoriatic arthritis, *J Rheumatol* 32:1745–1750, 2005.

49. Healy PJ, Helliwell PS: Measuring clinical enthesitis in psoriatic arthritis: assessment of existing measures and development of an instrument specific to psoriatic arthritis, *Arthritis Rheum* 59:686–691, 2008.

50. Clegg DO, Reda DJ, Mejias E, et al: Comparison of sulfasalazine and placebo in the treatment of psoriatic arthritis. A Department of Veterans Affairs Cooperative Study, *Arthritis Rheum* 39:2013–2020, 1996.

51. Coates LC, Helliwell PS: Validation of minimal disease activity criteria for psoriatic arthritis using interventional trial data, *Arthritis Care Res* 62:965–969, 2010.

52. Schoels M, Aletaha D, Funovits J, et al: Application of the DAREA/DAPSA score for assessment of disease activity in psoriatic arthritis, *Ann Rheum Dis* 69:1441–1447, 2010.

53. Mumtaz A, Gallagher P, Kirby B, et al: Development of a preliminary composite disease activity index in psoriatic arthritis, *Ann Rheum Dis* 70:272–277, 2011.

54. Gladman DD, Tom BD, Mease PJ, Farewell VT: Informing response criteria for psoriatic arthritis (PsA). II. Further considerations and a proposal—the PsA joint activity index, *J Rheumatol* 37:2559–2565, 2010.

55. Eastmond CJ: Psoriatic arthritis: genetics and HLA antigens, *Baillieres Clin Rheumatol* 8:263–276, 1994.

56. Elder JT: PSORS1: linking genetics and immunology, *J Invest Dermatol* 126:1205–1206, 2006.

57. Gladman DD, Farewell VT: The role of HLA antigens as indicators of disease progression in psoriatic arthritis: multivariate relative risk model, *Arthritis Rheum* 38:845–850, 1995.

58. Ho PY, Barton A, Worthington J, et al: Investigating the role of the HLA-Cw*06 and HLA-DRB1 genes in susceptibility to psoriatic arthritis: comparison with psoriasis and undifferentiated inflammatory arthritis, *Ann Rheum Dis* 67:677–682, 2008.

59. Balding J, Kane D, Livingstone W, et al: Cytokine gene polymorphisms: association with psoriatic arthritis susceptibility and severity, *Arthritis Rheum* 48:1408–1413, 2003.

60. Gonzalez S, Martinez-Borra J, Lopez-Vazquez A, et al: MICA rather than MICB, TNFA, or HLA-DRB1 is associated with susceptibility to psoriatic arthritis, *J Rheumatol* 29:973–978, 2002.

61. Karason A, Gudjonsson JE, Upmanyu R, et al: A susceptibility gene for psoriatic arthritis maps to chromosome 16q: evidence for imprinting, *Am J Hum Genet* 72:125–131, 2003.

62. Hüffmeier U, Uebe S, Ekici AB, et al: Common variants at TRAF3IP2 are associated with susceptibility to psoriatic arthritis and psoriasis, *Nat Genet* 42:996–999, 2010.

63. Ellinghaus E, Ellinghaus D, Stuart PE, et al: Genome-wide association study identifies a psoriasis susceptibility locus at TRAF3IP2, *Nat Genet* 42:991–995, 2010.

64. Rasmussen JE: The relationship between infection with group A beta hemolytic streptococci and the development of psoriasis, *Pediatr Infect Dis J* 19:153–154, 2000.

65. Wilbrink B, van der Heijden IM, Schouls LM, et al: Detection of bacterial DNA in joint samples from patients with undifferentiated arthritis and reactive arthritis, using polymerase chain reaction with universal 16S ribosomal RNA primers, *Arthritis Rheum* 41:535–543, 1998.

66. Langevitz P, Buskila D, Gladman DD: Psoriatic arthritis precipitated by physical trauma, *J Rheumatol* 17:695–697, 1990.

67. Yanagisawa H, Richardson JA, Taurog JD, et al: Characterization of psoriasiform and alopecic skin lesions in HLA-B27 transgenic rats, *Am J Pathol* 147:955–964, 1995.

68. Bardos T, Zhang J, Mikecz K, et al: Mice lacking endogenous major histocompatibility complex class II develop arthritis resembling psoriatic arthritis at an advanced age, *Arthritis Rheum* 46:2465–2475, 2002.

69. Lories RJ, Matthys P, de Vlam K, et al: Ankylosing enthesitis, dactylitis, and onychoperiostitis in male DBA/1 mice: a model of psoriatic arthritis, *Ann Rheum Dis* 63:595–598, 2004.

70. Zenz R, Eferl R, Kenner L, et al: Psoriasis-like skin disease and arthritis caused by inducible epidermal deletion of Jun proteins, *Nature* 437:369–375, 2005.

71. Bos JD, de Rie MA, Teunissen MB, et al: Psoriasis: dysregulation of innate immunity, *Br J Dermatol* 152:1098–1107, 2005.

72. Pitzalis C, Cauli A, Pipitone N, et al: Cutaneous lymphocyte antigen-positive T lymphocytes preferentially migrate to the skin but not to the joint in psoriatic arthritis, *Arthritis Rheum* 39:137–145, 1996.

73. Veale D, Yanni G, Rogers S, et al: Reduced synovial membrane macrophage numbers, ELAM-1 expression, and lining layer hyperplasia in psoriatic arthritis as compared with rheumatoid arthritis, *Arthritis Rheum* 36:893–900, 1993.

74. Kruithof E, Baeten D, De Rycke L, et al: Synovial histopathology of psoriatic arthritis, both oligo- and polyarticular, resembles spondyloarthropathy more than it does rheumatoid arthritis, *Arthritis Res Ther* 7:R569–R580, 2005.

75. Reece RJ, Canete JD, Parsons WJ, et al: Distinct vascular patterns of early synovitis in psoriatic, reactive, and rheumatoid arthritis, *Arthritis Rheum* 42:1481–1484, 1999.

76. Fearon U, Griosios K, Fraser A, et al: Angiopoietins, growth factors, and vascular morphology in early arthritis, *J Rheumatol* 30:260–268, 2003.

77. Leong TT, Fearon U, Veale DJ: Angiogenesis in psoriasis and psoriatic arthritis: clues to disease pathogenesis, *Curr Rheumatol Rep* 7:325–329, 2005.

78. van Kuijk AW, Gerlag DM, Vos K, et al: A prospective, randomized, placebo-controlled study to identify biomarkers associated with active treatment in psoriatic arthritis: effects of adalimumab treatment on synovial tissue, *Ann Rheum Dis* 68:1303–1309, 2009.

79. Laloux L, Voisin MC, Allain J, et al: Immunohistological study of entheses in spondyloarthropathies: comparison in rheumatoid arthritis and osteoarthritis, *Ann Rheum Dis* 60:316–321, 2001.

80. McGonagle D, Marzo-Ortega H, O'Connor P, et al: Histological assessment of the early enthesitis lesion in spondyloarthropathy, *Ann Rheum Dis* 61:534–537, 2002.

81. Costello P, Bresnihan B, O'Farrelly C, et al: Predominance of CD8+ T lymphocytes in psoriatic arthritis, *J Rheumatol* 26:1117–1124, 1999.

82. Ritchlin C, Haas-Smith SA, Hicks D, et al: Patterns of cytokine production in psoriatic synovium, *J Rheumatol* 25:1544–1552, 1998.

83. Austin LM, Ozawa M, Kikuchi T, et al: The majority of epidermal T cells in psoriasis vulgaris lesions can produce type 1 cytokines, interferon-gamma, interleukin-2, and tumor necrosis factor-alpha, defining TC1 (cytotoxic T lymphocyte) and TH1 effector populations: a type 1 differentiation bias is also measured in circulating blood T cells in psoriatic patients, *J Invest Dermatol* 113:752–759, 1999.

84. Danning CL, Illei GG, Hitchon C, et al: Macrophage-derived cytokine and nuclear factor kappaB p65 expression in synovial membrane and skin of patients with psoriatic arthritis, *Arthritis Rheum* 43:1244–1256, 2000.

85. Kane D, Gogarty M, O'Leary J, et al: Reduction of synovial sublining layer inflammation and proinflammatory cytokine expression in psoriatic arthritis treated with methotrexate, *Arthritis Rheum* 50:3286–3295, 2004.

86. Zaba LC, Suárez-Fariñas M, Fuentes-Duculan J, et al: Effective treatment of psoriasis with etanercept is linked to suppression of IL-17 signaling, not immediate response TNF genes, *J Allergy Clin Immunol* 124:1022–1010.e1-395, 2009.

87. Jandus C, Bioley G, Rivals JP, et al: Increased numbers of circulating polyfunctional Th17 memory cells in patients with seronegative spondylarthritides, *Arthritis Rheum* 58:2307–2317, 2008.

88. Raychaudhuri SK, Raychaudhuri SP: Scid mouse model of psoriasis: a unique tool for drug development of autoreactive T-cell and Th-17 cell-mediated autoimmune diseases, *Indian J Dermatol* 55:157–160, 2010.

89. Filer C, Ho P, Smith RL, et al: Investigation of association of the IL12B and IL23R genes with psoriatic arthritis, *Arthritis Rheum* 58:3705–3709, 2008.

90. Gottlieb A, Menter A, Mendelsohn A, et al: Ustekinumab, a human interleukin 12/23 monoclonal antibody, for psoriatic arthritis: randomised, double-blind, placebo-controlled, crossover trial, *Lancet* 373:633–640, 2009. Erratum in: *Lancet* 376:1542, 2010; *Lancet* 373:1340, 2009.

91. Partsch G, Steiner G, Leeb BF, et al: Highly increased levels of tumor necrosis factor-alpha and other proinflammatory cytokines in psoriatic arthritis synovial fluid, *J Rheumatol* 24:518–523, 1997.

92. Baeten D, Kruithof E, Van den Bosch F, et al: Immunomodulatory effects of anti-tumor necrosis factor alpha therapy on synovium in spondyloarthropathy: histologic findings in eight patients from an open-label pilot study, *Arthritis Rheum* 44:186–195, 2001.

93. Kruithof E, De Rycke L, Roth J, et al: Immunomodulatory effects of etanercept on peripheral joint synovitis in the spondylarthropathies, *Arthritis Rheum* 52:3898–3909, 2005.

94. Canete JD, Pablos JL, Sanmarti R, et al: Antiangiogenic effects of anti-tumor necrosis factor alpha therapy with infliximab in psoriatic arthritis, *Arthritis Rheum* 50:1636–1641, 2004.

95. Ribbens C, Martin y Porras M, Franchimont N, et al: Increased matrix metalloproteinase-3 serum levels in rheumatic diseases: relationship with synovitis and steroid treatment, *Ann Rheum Dis* 61:161–166, 2002.

96. Vandooren B, Kruithof E, Yu DT, et al: Involvement of matrix metalloproteinases and their inhibitors in peripheral synovitis and down-regulation by tumor necrosis factor alpha blockade in spondylarthropathy, *Arthritis Rheum* 50:2942–2953, 2004.

97. Kane D, Jensen LE, Grehan S, et al: Quantitation of metalloproteinase gene expression in rheumatoid and psoriatic arthritis synovial tissue distal and proximal to the cartilage-pannus junction, *J Rheumatol* 31:1274–1280, 2004.

98. Ritchlin CT, Haas-Smith SA, Li P, et al: Mechanisms of TNF-alpha- and RANKL-mediated osteoclastogenesis and bone resorption in psoriatic arthritis, *J Clin Invest* 111:821–831, 2003.

99. Vandooren B, Cantaert T, Noordenbos T, et al: The abundant synovial expression of the RANK/RANKL/osteoprotegerin system in peripheral spondylarthritis is partially disconnected from inflammation, *Arthritis Rheum* 58:718–729, 2008.

100. Anandarajah AP, Schwarz EM, Totterman S, et al: The effect of etanercept on osteoclast precursor frequency and enhancing bone marrow oedema in patients with psoriatic arthritis, *Ann Rheum Dis* 67:296–301, 2008.

101. Peng H, Wright V, Usas A, et al: Synergistic enhancement of bone formation and healing by stem cell-expressed VEGF and bone morphogenetic protein-4, *J Clin Invest* 110:751–759, 2002.

102. De Klerck B, Carpentier I, Lories RJ, et al: Enhanced osteoclast development in collagen-induced arthritis in interferon-gamma receptor knock-out mice as related to increased splenic CD11b+ myelopoiesis, *Arthritis Res Ther* 6:R220–R231, 2004.

103. Curran SA, Fitzgerald OM, Costello PJ, et al: Nucleotide sequencing of psoriatic arthritis tissue before and during methotrexate administration reveals a complex inflammatory T cell infiltrate with very few clones exhibiting features that suggest they drive the inflammatory process by recognizing autoantigens, *J Immunol* 172:1935–1944, 2004.

104. Kavanaugh AF, Ritchlin CT: Systematic review of treatments for psoriatic arthritis: an evidence based approach and basis for treatment guidelines, *J Rheumatol* 33:1417–1421, 2006.

105. Shiffman RN, Shekelle P, Overhage JM, et al: Standardized reporting of clinical practice guidelines: a proposal from the Conference on Guideline Standardization, *Ann Intern Med* 139:493–498, 2003.

106. Soriano ER, McHugh NJ: Therapies for peripheral joint disease in psoriatic arthritis: a systematic review, *J Rheumatol* 33:1422–1430, 2006.

107. Grassi W, De Angelis R, Cervini C: Corticosteroid prescribing in rheumatoid arthritis and psoriatic arthritis, *Clin Rheumatol* 17:223–226, 1998.

108. Strober BE, Siu K, Menon K: Conventional systemic agents for psoriasis: a systematic review, *J Rheumatol* 33:1442–1446, 2006.

109. Ritchlin CT: Therapies for psoriatic enthesopathy: a systematic review, *J Rheumatol* 33:1435–1438, 2006.

110. Helliwell PS: Therapies for dactylitis in psoriatic arthritis: a systematic review, *J Rheumatol* 33:1439–1441, 2006.

111. Nash P: Therapies for axial disease in psoriatic arthritis: a systematic review, *J Rheumatol* 33:1431–1434, 2006.

112. Spadaro A, Riccieri V, Sili-Scavalli A, et al: Comparison of cyclosporin A and methotrexate in the treatment of psoriatic arthritis: a one-year prospective study, *Clin Exp Rheumatol* 13:589–593, 1995.

113. Mihatsch MJ, Wolff K: Consensus conference on cyclosporin A for psoriasis, February 1992, *Br J Dermatol* 126:621–623, 1992.

114. Kaltwasser JP, Nash P, Gladman D, et al: Efficacy and safety of leflunomide in the treatment of psoriatic arthritis and psoriasis: a multinational, double-blind, randomized, placebo-controlled clinical trial, *Arthritis Rheum* 50:1939–1950, 2004.

115. Saber TP, Ng CT, Renard G, et al: Remission in psoriatic arthritis: is it possible and how can it be predicted? *Arthritis Res Ther* 12:R94, 2010.

116. Mease PJ, Kivitz AJ, Burch FX, et al: Etanercept treatment of psoriatic arthritis: safety, efficacy, and effect on disease progression, *Arthritis Rheum* 50:2264–2272, 2004.

117. Cassell S, Kavanaugh AF: Therapies for psoriatic nail disease: a systematic review, *J Rheumatol* 33:1452–1456, 2006.

118. Boehncke WH, Prinz J, Gottlieb AB: Biologic therapies for psoriasis: a systematic review, *J Rheumatol* 33:1447–1451, 2006.

119. Mease PJ, Gladman DD, Ritchlin CT, et al: Adalimumab for the treatment of patients with moderately to severely active psoriatic arthritis: results of a double-blind, randomized, placebo-controlled trial, *Arthritis Rheum* 52:3279–3289, 2005.

120. Sterry W, Ortonne JP, Kirkham B, et al: Comparison of two etanercept regimens for treatment of psoriasis and psoriatic arthritis: PRESTA randomised double blind multicentre trial, *BMJ* 340:c147, 2010.

121. Lebwohl M, Christophers E, Langley R, et al: An international, randomized, double-blind, placebo-controlled phase 3 trial of intramuscular alefacept in patients with chronic plaque psoriasis, *Arch Dermatol* 139:719–727, 2003.

122. Mease PJ, Gladman DD, Keystone EC: Alefacept in combination with methotrexate for the treatment of psoriatic arthritis: results of a randomized, double-blind, placebo-controlled study, *Arthritis Rheum* 54:1638–1645, 2006.

123. Krueger GG, Langley RG, Leonardi C, et al; CNTO 1275 Psoriasis Study Group: A human interleukin-12/23 monoclonal antibody for the treatment of psoriasis, *N Engl J Med* 356:580–592, 2007.

The references for this chapter can also be found on www.expertconsult.com.

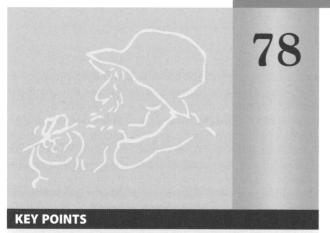

78 | Enteropathic Arthritis

FRANK A. WOLLHEIM •
MONIKA RONNEBERGER

KEY POINTS

The gut wall is a leaky barrier exposed to commensal and pathogenic microorganisms.

Microbiota are essential for maturation and regulation of the immune system.

Gastrointestinal lymphoid tissue–microbiota interaction balances between inflammatory defense and tolerance.

Genetic polymorphisms in Crohn's disease can result in relative immune deficiency.

Some types of joint disease in inflammatory bowel disease are genetically determined.

HLA-B27 interacts with non–major histocompatibility complex genes.

Celiac disease is common in adults, 25% of whom have joint manifestations.

Patients with Whipple's disease often present with joint symptoms.

Microscopic colitis is accompanied by extraenteric autoimmune manifestations.

This chapter deals with rheumatic conditions associated with gut pathology, which are commonly designated as *enteropathic arthritis*. People realized centuries ago that dysentery was sometimes followed by arthritis, a condition now known as *reactive arthritis*. Although it is a well-established example of enteropathic arthritis, reactive arthritis is covered in Chapter 76. This chapter covers musculoskeletal problems associated with inflammatory bowel disease (IBD), celiac disease (CeD), and other less common conditions. New insight into gut physiology, its barrier function, regulation of immune responses, and trophic functions is emerging. Knowledge regarding detailed interactions implicated in the generation of joint disease, however, remains incomplete. The fine-tuning of permeability, interactions between gut contents and gut mucosa, the nature of the gastrointestinal-associated lymphoid tissue, and how gastrointestinal-associated lymphoid tissue generates arthritis are at the core of this chapter.

GUT BIOLOGY AND THE MICROBIOTA

KEY POINTS

The gut mucosa is a leaky barrier and is covered by an "unstirred" layer.

Eighty percent of the gut wall consists of immune cells.

Gut permeability is delicately regulated and is disturbed in disease.

The gastrointestinal tract has three major biologic functions: serving as a barrier against hostile environmental factors; affecting fluid and food absorption and excretion of waste products; and producing major trophic host functions. The gut mucosa has an estimated surface area of 300 to 400 m^2, which is 200 times the body's skin surface area. This mucosa is constantly exposed to potentially harmful environmental agents against which defense is essential, but at the same time tolerance toward a normal microflora must be maintained. In order to fulfill these diverse functions, the gut is an immunologically privileged organ. Disturbances can lead to food allergy or inflammatory bowel disease (Figure 78-1).

The gut epithelium constitutes a so-called leaky barrier. It consists of intestinal epithelial cells including Paneth cells in deep crypts, mucus-secreting goblet cells, M cells, and lymphocytes. It is covered by a thin layer of fluid separated from luminal flow and peristalsis of the intestine, the so-called unstirred layer, which slows down the diffusion of solutes and prevents loss of digestive enzymes. An increased thickness of the unstirred layer may contribute to malabsorption in CeD. Underneath the basal membrane is the lamina propria, which contains immune cells including lymphocytes, dendritic cells, and macrophages (Figure 78-2).[1] The plasma membrane of the epithelial cells is impermeable to most hydrophilic solutes in the absence of specific transporters. The structure of the interepithelial paracellular space consists of the tight junction, the adherens junction, and the desmosome (see Figure 78-2B). The tight junction is considered rate limiting for permeability. A perijunctional actomyosin ring condensation is regulated by myosin light chain kinase (MLCK), which has been shown to have a central role in regulating tight junction transport and in tumor necrosis factor (TNF)-induced permeability increase.[2] TNF inhibition will influence permeability via inhibition of MLCK transcription. Overexpression of MLCK, on the other hand, results in increased permeability and activation of immune cells in transgenic mice.[3] Although initially healthy, these mice were prone to accelerated colitis if challenged.

Na$^+$ solutes smaller than 5000 daltons can pass through the epithelium freely, whereas bacterial products and dietary antigens are dependent on active transport mechanisms. Altered gut permeability can be observed in several diseases, among them nonalcoholic fatty liver disease.[4] In this condition alterations in the zona occludens 1 (ZO1) expression result in perturbation of permeability. Genetic and exogenous factors such as drugs, nicotine, microorganisms,[5] and cytokines are potential triggers of pathology by influencing paracellular functions in the gut epithelium.

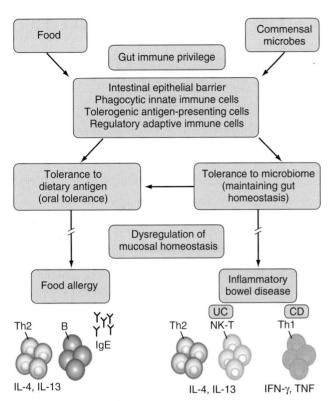

Figure 78-1   Immune privilege in the gut. CD, Crohn's disease; IFN, interferon; IL, interleukin; NK-T, natural killer T cell; TNF, tumor necrosis factor; UC, ulcerative colitis. *(From Iweala OI, Nagler CR: Immune privilege in the gut: the establishment and maintenance of non-responsiveness to dietary antigens and commensal flora,* Immunol Rev *213:82–100, 2006.)*

Assessment of mucosal permeability and transport can be achieved by oral feeding of lactalbumin, lactoglobulin, polyethylene glycol particles, ^{51}Cr-labeled ethylenediamine tetraacetic acid (EDTA), and sugars such as lactulose and mannitol, followed by urinalysis. In addition, intestinal permeability and function can be studied by regional perfusion with the help of endoscopic techniques that close off segments of the gut with inflatable balloons.[6] A study applying enzyme-linked immunosorbent assays to fluid collected by this technique showed marked local immunity to a number of food-related antigens in patients with rheumatoid arthritis.[7] Ethnic differences in gut permeability have also been described.[8]

The healthy gut harbors a mixture of native bacteria acquired at birth or shortly thereafter that retains a relatively constant composition; it also has a smaller population of transient bacteria of varying composition. The former are essential for health and live in symbiosis; the latter contain potential pathogens. Whereas the stomach and duodenum normally contain less than 10^3 mucosa-adhering bacteria, the number of bacteria increases to 10^4 in the jejunum and 10^7 in the ileum. Most of the latter group comprises gram-negative aerobic species. In the colon, the bacterial density is 10^{12} or more, consisting mostly of anaerobic bacteria. Transit time is fast in the upper gut and slow in the distal gut, but the immunologic impact of the microflora is higher in the proximal parts of the gut.[9] In other words, the total number of bacterial cells called the *human microbiota* is 10 times that of cells in the body.[10]

Analysis of the 16S bacterial ribosomal RNA gene sequence has revealed the presence of a bewildering number of phylotypes in the human gastrointestinal tract, and the number of genes in the microbiome is estimated to be 100 times that of the human genome.[11] There is also a high degree of diversity among healthy individuals and some correlation with obesity and other conditions. Most phylotypes have not been cultured, and their functions remain unknown. The potential pathogenicity of individual commensal microbes is demonstrated in a recent paper showing that a single species of segmental filamentous bacteria can trigger autoimmune arthritis in germ-free K/BxN mice by activating Th17 cells in lamina propria.[12]

The normal trophic functions of the gut require this microflora, as demonstrated by host defects in germ-free animals. Bacteria digest food carbohydrates into short-chain fatty acids, which facilitate the absorption of Ca^{2+}, Mg^{2+}, and Fe^{2+} ions; synthesize amino acids and vitamins; and secrete antibacterial protective substances. Some 300 to 500 different species are represented, and the composition is unique for each individual. Figure 78-3 shows some of the common colonic species and their functions.[9]

Gastrointestinal-Associated Lymphoid Tissue and Its Interactions

KEY POINTS
Microbiota are the major regulators of gastrointestinal-associated lymphoid tissue.
Retinoic acid promotes IgA and lymphocyte homing.
Flagellin stimulates dendritic cells to induce Th17 cells.
Vascular adhesion protein-1 is expressed in gut and synovium and is a putative therapeutic target.
Gut lymphocytes express α4β7, αEβ7, and CCR9, which are important for homing.

Gastrointestinal-associated lymphoid tissue (GALT) is a part of the mucosal immune system, a prominent feature of which is the dominating output of secretory immunoglobulin (Ig)A. This was discovered analyzing tears and saliva in the early 1960s.[13] GALT is the largest lymphoid organ of the body, constituting 25% of the mucosal mass. Cellular components of GALT are localized in Peyer's plaques, gut lymphoid follicles, lamina propria, and intraepithelial T cells. GALT is part of a complex defense and tolerance regulating system involving specialized dendritic cells (DCs) and intestinal epithelial cells (IECs) (Figure 78-4). Commensal bacteria interact with IECs, which send signals to DCs mediated by anti-inflammatory substances (e.g., thymic stromal lymphopoietin [TSLP]) and to lamina propria DCs. Bacteria also interact directly with DCs by means of their polysaccharide A. A subset of lamina propria DCs expresses CD11b^{hi}, CD11c^{hi}, and Toll-like receptor (TLR5). When exposed to bacterial flagellin, these DCs promote the differentiation of T helper 17 (Th17) cells. These DCs also produce retinoic acid. IEPs also produce retinoic acid from dietary vitamin A, APRIL (*a proliferation-inducing*

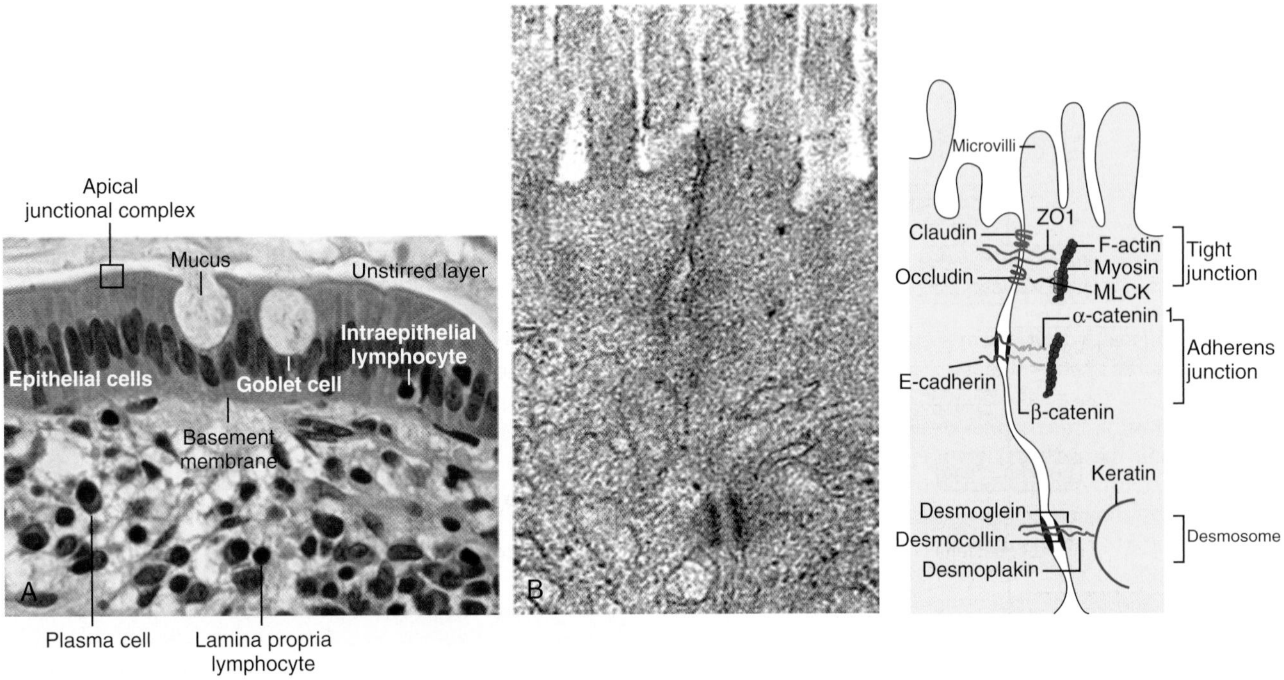

Figure 78-2 Anatomy of the mucosal barrier. **A,** The human intestinal mucosa is composed of a simple layer of columnar epithelial cells, as well as the underlying lamina propria and muscular mucosa. Goblet cells, which synthesize and release mucin, as well as other differentiated epithelial cell types, are present. The unstirred layer, which cannot be seen histologically, is located immediately above the epithelial cells. The tight junction, a component of the apical junctional complex, seals the paracellular space between epithelial cells. Intraepithelial lymphocytes are located above the basement membrane but are subjacent to the tight junction. The lamina propria is located beneath the basement membrane and contains immune cells including macrophages, dendritic cells, plasma cells, lamina propria lymphocytes, and, in some cases, neutrophils. **B,** An electron micrograph and corresponding line drawing of the junctional complex of an intestinal epithelial cell. Just below the base of the microvilli, the plasma membranes of adjacent cells seem to fuse at the tight junction, where claudins, zonula occludens 1 (ZO1), occludin, and F⁻ actin interact. E⁻ cadherin, α⁻ catenin 1, β⁻ catenin, catenin δ1 (also known as *p120 catenin;* not shown), and F⁻ actin interact to form the adherens junction. Myosin light chain kinase (MLCK) is associated with the perijunctional actomyosin ring. Desmosomes, which are located beneath the apical junctional complex, are formed by interactions among desmoglein, desmocollin, desmoplakin, and keratin filaments. *(From Turner JR: Intestinal mucosal barrier function in health and disease,* Nat Rev Immunol *9:799–809, 2009.)*

ligand), and BAFF. Retinoic acid stimulates the expression of the integrin α4β7 and CCR9, thereby influencing gut-homing lymphocytes.[14] It was recently shown that Wnt–β-catenin signaling is required for the stimulation of expression of anti-inflammatory mediators by intestinal DCs.[15] Bacteria can also penetrate into Peyer's patches (PPs) and create a symbiotic environment with host cells.[16] Cytokines such as interleukin (IL)-10 and transforming growth factor (TGF)-β serve anti-inflammatory functions. Retinoic acid, APRIL, and BAFF contribute to the dominating IgA production in local lymphoid cells. Gut enterochromaffin cells produce 5-hydroxytryptamine, which has anti-inflammatory effects and chromogranins with both proinflammatory and anti-inflammatory effects.[17] Some of these not yet fully understood interactions are depicted in Figure 78-5. Plasma cells in the lamina propria become programmed to produce IgA, but the production is also skewed to formation of dimeric IgA, pIgA, in which the monomers are connected by joint, or J, chains.[18] Intestinal epithelial glycoprotein pIgR, a polymeric immunoglobulin receptor that is also called *secretory component* (SC), is produced in IECs. It is a 100-kD transmembrane receptor for polymeric immunoglobulin, pIgA, and IgM. SC/pIgR is abundantly present in Peyer's patches in the distal ileum. The pIgR in IECs combines with pIgA and to a lesser extent with IgM to form secretory IgA, SIgA, and SIgM, respectively, which are exported into the lumen and constitute a

noninflammatory, non–complement-binding first line of defense. It is estimated that a healthy adult secretes 3 to 5 g of SIgA into the gut daily (Figures 78-6 and 78-7).[18] Breast-feeding provides the newborn with abundant SIgA and SIgM, which confers passive protection and also regulates much of the child's immune system[19] (Figure 78-8).

From the Peyer's patches, primed B lymphocytes disseminate throughout the body's mucous membranes, notably to other parts of the alimentary tract. Primed T lymphocytes also disseminate into the circulation and lymph nodes and home into target organs such as salivary glands (in Sjögren's disease), lungs, and synovium.[19] Vascular adhesion protein-1 (VAP-1) expressed on synovial epithelial cells is involved in lymphocyte homing, and P-selectin is a part of macrophage recruitment. VAP-1 is a bifunctional glycoprotein with both adhesive and amino-oxidative properties.[20] Inhibition of this molecule is in development in oncology. A monoclonal antibody is protective against collagen-induced arthritis, and VAP-1 may become a target in the treatment of enteropathic arthritis. Most T lymphocytes in the mucosal lamina propria are CD4⁺, whereas intraepithelial T cells are mostly CD8⁺. Gut-associated lymphocytes preferentially express the integrins α4β7 and αEβ7 and the integrin receptor CCR9 on stimulation by intestinal dendritic cells.[20]

Induction of oral tolerance to type II collagen has demonstrated how GALT activation may ameliorate

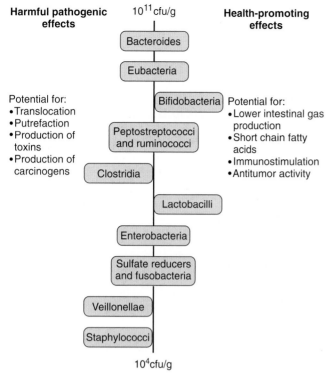

Figure 78-3 Physiologic roles of the intestinal microflora. *(From Salminen S, Bouley C, Boutron-Ruault MC, et al: Functional food science and gastrointestinal physiology and function,* Br J Nutr *80(Suppl 1):S147–S171, 1998.)*

inflammatory joint disease (see Figure 78-7).[21] A chain of events in the pathogenesis of enteropathic arthritis can begin with gastrointestinal infection with the appropriate microorganism in a genetically predisposed patient. This causes local inflammation in the gut mucosa, formation of secretory IgA, increased permeability, absorption of foreign material, and triggering of T lymphocytes. Circulating immune complexes and memory T cells localize to joints and cause synovitis (Figure 78-9). Figure 78-10 summarizes recent understanding of how colonization by segmented filamentous bacteria triggers arthritis in mice.

In conclusion, the gut wall is a highly diversified immunologic, endocrine, and digestive organ. Its interaction with the microbiota potentially mediates both protective and harmful signals (e.g., triggering enteropathic arthritis).

INFLAMMATORY BOWEL DISEASE

Epidemiology

KEY POINTS
The incidence and prevalence of inflammatory bowel disease are higher in developed societies.
Smoking increases the risk in both CD and ulcerative colitis.
Smokeless nicotine (snuff) may be inert or protective.
Ethnic influences are present.

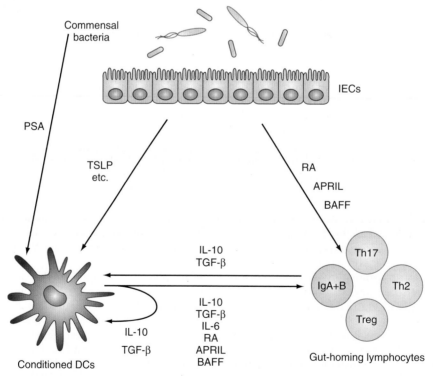

Figure 78-4 Tolerance induction machinery in the gut. Under the influence of commensal bacteria and their products, conditioned intestinal epithelial cells (IECs) constitutively produce anti-inflammatory molecules such as thymic stromal lymphopoietin (TSLP) to limit the inflammation-induced signals, leading to the development of tolerogenic dendritic cells (DCs). Tolerogenic DCs might also be induced by direct stimulation with *Bacteroides fragilis*–derived polysaccharide A (PSA). Once the tolerogenic DCs are developed, they preferentially produce critical factors for the induction of Th2 cells, Tregs, Th17 cells, and IgA⁺ B cells. IECs also produce retinoic acid (RA), a proliferation-inducing ligand (APRIL), and B cell activating factor belonging to the tumor necrosis factor family (BAFF), which probably affect the development of these lymphocyte subsets. Communication among the commensal flora, IECs, and gut immune system is bidirectional, but only a part of the bidirectional communication is shown in this figure. IL, interleukin; TGF-β, transforming growth factor-β. *(From Tezuka H, Ohteki T: Regulation of intestinal homeostasis by dendritic cells,* Immunol Rev *234:247–258, 2010.)*

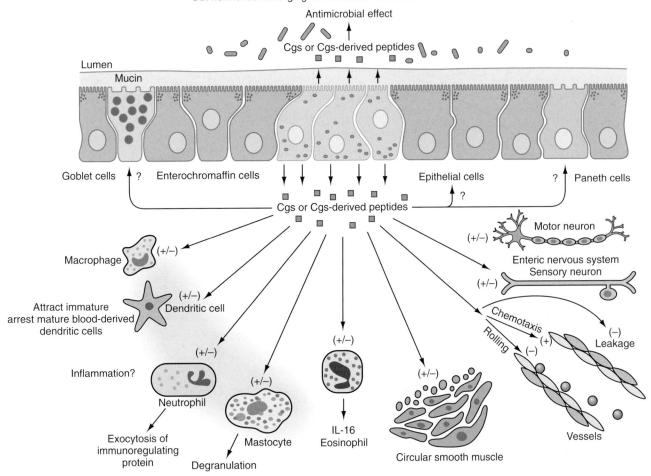

Figure 78-5 Putative role of chromogranins (Cgs) in immune activation and inflammation. Luminal or internal inflammatory stimuli causes alteration in Cgs or Cgs-derived peptides release. They may act locally on Paneth, goblet, and epithelial cells, as well as on immune cells such as macrophages, dendritic cells, neutrophils, mastocytes, and eosinophils. Endothelial permeability, chemotaxis, rolling, smooth muscle contractility, and the enteric nervous system can also be modulated. IL-16, interleukin-16; (−) inhibition; (+) activation. *(From Khan WI, Ghia JE: Gut hormones: emerging role in immune activation and inflammation,* Clin Exp Immunol *161:19–27, 2010.)*

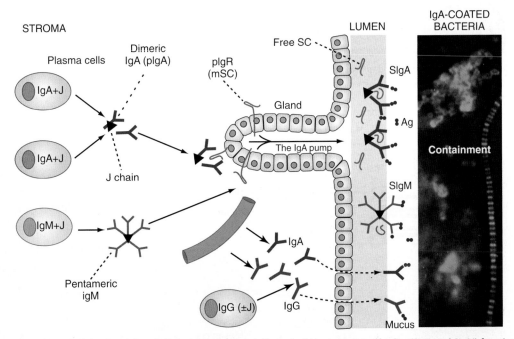

Figure 78-6 Receptor-mediated export of dimeric IgA and pentameric IgM to provide secretory antibodies (SIgA and SIgM) functioning in immune exclusion of antigen (Ag) at the mucosal surface. Polymeric Ig receptor (pIgR) is expressed basolaterally as membrane secretory component (mSC) on secretory epithelial cells and mediates transcytosis of dimeric IgA and pentameric IgM, which are produced with incorporated J chain (IgA + J and IgM + J) by mucosal plasma cells. Although J chain is often produced by mucosal IgG plasma cells (70% to 90%), it does not combine with this isotype and is therefore degraded intracellularly as denoted (±J). Locally produced (and serum-derived) IgG is therefore not subject to pIgR-mediated transport but can be transmitted paracellularly to the lumen together with monomeric IgA as indicated. Free SC (depicted in mucus) is generated when pIgR in its unoccupied state *(top basolateral symbol)* is cleaved at the apical face of the epithelium-like bound SC in SIgA and SIgM. Commensal bacteria in the *right-hand panel* are coated in vivo with SIgA, which aids their containment and thereby promotes host-microbial mutualism. *(From Brandtzaeg P: Mucosal immunity: induction, dissemination, and effector functions,* Scand J Immunol *70:505–515, 2009.)*

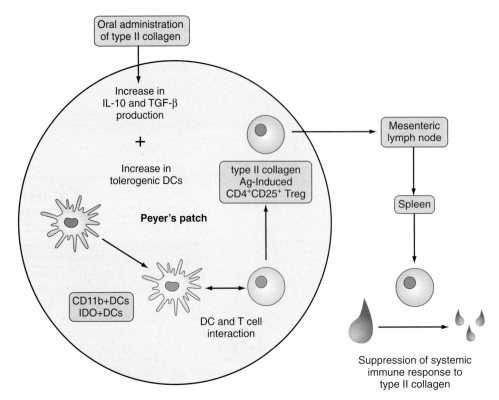

Figure 78-7 Role of Peyer's patch (PP) dendritic cells (DCs) in type II collagen oral tolerance. As a result of repeated oral administration of type II collagen, the production of anti-inflammatory cytokines such as interleukin-10 (IL-10) and transforming growth factor-β (TGF-β) by PP cells is enhanced and the populations of CD11c⁺CD11b⁺DCs and IDO⁺DCs are increased in PP. Then, through DC–T cell interaction, type II collagen inducible CD4⁺CD25⁺Foxp3⁺ and regulatory T cells are generated in the PP. Regulatory T cells generated in the PP move to the mesenteric lymph node and then enter the systemic circulation, where they suppress the systemic immune response to CII. *(From Park KS, Park MJ, Cho ML, et al: Type II collagen oral tolerance; mechanism and role in collagen-induced arthritis and rheumatoid arthritis,* Mod Rheumatol *19(6):581–589, 2009.)*

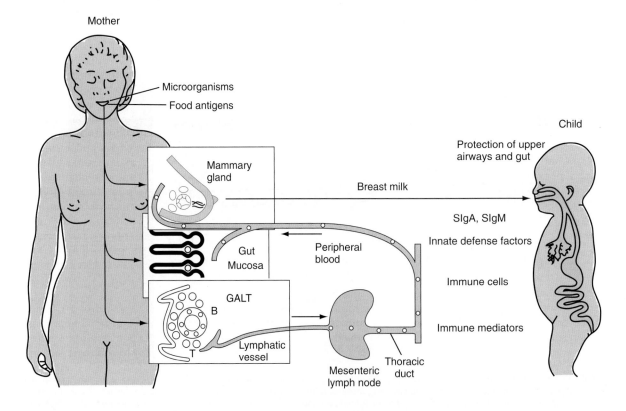

Figure 78-8 Integration of mucosal immunity between mother and newborn. Primed B (and probably T) cells from Peyer's patch migrate via lymph and peripheral blood to the lactating mammary gland, resulting in the presence in breast milk of secretory antibodies (SIgA and SIgM) specific for enteric antigens. GALT, gastrointestinal-associated lymphoid tissue. *(From Brandtzaeg P: Mucosal immunity: integration between mother and the breast-fed infant,* Vaccine *21:3382–3388, 2003.)*

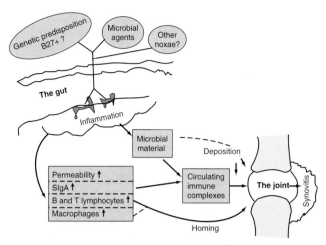

Figure 78-9 Immune pathogenesis of enteropathic arthritis.

The prevalence and incidence of IBD are higher in developed countries. Demographics in developing countries, however, show an increase of IBD. Prevalence of Crohn's disease (CD) is not decreasing, although immigration from minor developed countries is accelerating.[22] The prevalence of CD and ulcerative colitis (UC) is about equal, and in the United States one observes between 50 and 100 cases per 100,000 population.[5] In recent years, the incidence of UC has decreased in Western countries, whereas the previously low incidence of IBD in Eastern Europe, South America, and the Pacific has increased.[22,23] This may be due in part to better reporting. Ethnic affiliation has an influence on the prevalence, although it is still unknown to what extent this is due to genetic or environmental factors. For example, the Jewish population has a higher susceptibility in general but prevalence approaches that of the background population. Romanies have a remarkably lower risk of developing IBD compared with the average Hungarian population.[24,25] However, ethnic differences in the prevalence of extraintestinal manifestation have not been reported so far.

The incidence of CD and UC in a large Swedish population–based study was 11 per 100,000 and 18 per 100,000 person-years, respectively.[26] In this study it was also shown that "ever smokers" had a relative risk of 1.5 (95% confidence interval [CI], 1.2 to 1.8) and 1.3 (1.1 to 1.5), respectively. It was also shown that "ever users" of moist snuff were not at increased risk of developing IBD. Therefore the nicotine component probably does not contribute to susceptibility. On the basis of the immunosuppressive signal mediated by nicotinic acetylcholine α receptors, smokeless nicotine may be innocent or indeed protective.[27] The overall concordance in monozygotic twins is 36%, but it is only 16% in UC.[28] The onset of disease is highest

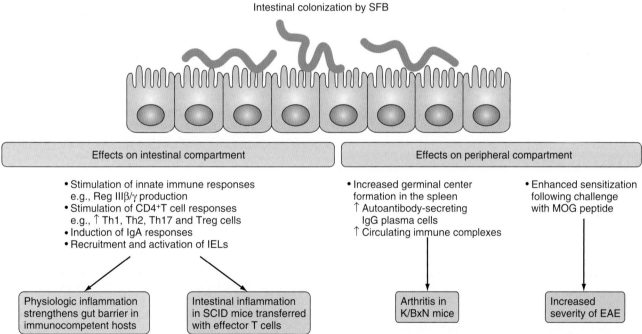

Figure 78-10 Effects of colonization of the gut immune system. Segmented filamentous bacteria (SFB) are spore-forming bacteria that are related to the genus *Clostridium*.[51] Inherited from the mother microbiota, SFB develop strong interactions with the ileal mucosa and in immunocompetent mice, the bacteria can largely recapitulate the inducing effects of the whole microbiota on the postnatal maturation of the gut immune system. SFB induce the production of Reg IIIβ/γ microbicidal peptides,[23,45] which protect against colonizing pathogens.[46] Additionally, SFB simultaneously activate strong secretory IgA responses,[44] induce the recruitment and activation of cytotoxic intraepithelial lymphocytes (IELs), and drive various T cell responses including a robust T helper 17 (Th17) cell response.[28,45] In immunocompetent mice, SFB-induced proinflammatory and regulatory responses balance each other, which results in physiologic inflammation that strengthens the gut barrier. By contrast, colonization by SFB promotes the development of colitis in severe combined immunodeficient (SCID) mice that have been reconstituted with effector T cells.[52] Intestinal colonization by SFB can also promote the development of inflammatory diseases outside of the gut. SFB promote arthritis in autoimmune nonobese diabetic (NOD) mice that express a transgenic T cell receptor (TCR) that is specific for a self-peptide (known as K/BxN mice), an effect ascribed to the induction of Th17 cells.[54] SFB also enhance the severity of myelin oligodendrocyte glycoprotein (MOG)-induced experimental autoimmune encephalomyelitis (EAE). These aggravating effects may reflect the strong adjuvant properties of SFB. *(From Cerf-Bensussan N, Gaboriau-Routhiau V: The immune system and the gut microbiota: friends or foes? Nat Rev Immunol 10(10):735–744, 2010.)*

Table 78-1 Extraintestinal Manifestations of Inflammatory Bowel Disease

Feature or Disease	Crohn's	Ulcerative Colitis
Peripheral arthritis	≈15%	≈10%
Axial or sacroiliac arthritis	≈15%-20%	≈10%-15%
Septic arthritis	Rare	Not reported
Skin		
Erythema nodosum	Up to 15%	<15%
Erythema multiforme	Rare	?
Pyoderma gangrenosum	0.5%-2%	0.3%-0.4% in severe disease
Aphthous ulcers	Rare	1%-8%
Nephrolithiasis (oxalate)	<15%	?
Amyloidosis	Very rare	Not reported
Liver disease	3%-5%	7%
Uveitis	13%	4%
Vasculitis	Takayasu's	<5%
Clubbing of fingers	Yes	1%-5%
Increased prevalence of asthma	Yes	Yes
Increased prevalence of multiple sclerosis	No	Yes

between 15 and 30 years of age, but IBD can start at any age. CD has a second peak later in life. There are no marked sex differences of IBD. Joint involvement has been reported in up to 25% of patients.[6] Lower figures were reported from a large population-based Canadian study,[29] but the study excluded peripheral arthritis, which may explain why less than 10% of patients had "arthritis." Interestingly, asthma and multiple sclerosis were overrepresented in two studies of extraintestinal autoimmune manifestations of IBD (Table 78-1).[30]

Genetics

> **KEY POINTS**
>
> At least 30 genetic associations have been identified in CD, and several occur in UC.
>
> *NOD2* (previously known as *CARD15*), *IRGM*, and *ATG16L1* are associated with DCs.
>
> *IL23R* and *MDR1* are associated with both CD and UC.
>
> *IL23R* deletion protects against colitis in mice.
>
> CD has features of defective intracellular microbial handling.

Etiopathogenic research regarding IBD is in an active stage of development. New technology including genome-wide association studies (GWAS) has identified at least 31 genes showing replicated associations with CD[31] and a similar number for UC.[32] Approximately half of these associations are shared by both diseases. The strongest associations apart from human leukocyte antigen (HLA) are with the *NOD2* (formerly known as *CARD15*) gene on chromosome 16 and the *IL23R* on chromosome 1. *NOD2* and *NOD1* are cytosolic sensors for the bacterial peptidoglycan muramyl dipeptide and trigger the synthesis of antibacterial α-defensins.[33,34] Reduced mucosal expression of these defensins is found in

patients with CD.[35] IL23 signaling can result in activation of Th17 cells in the gut. The importance of IL23 is supported by the finding that *IL23R* −/− mice are resistant to induction of colitis.[36] Also, IL23 is upregulated in patients with CD.[37] Another association is found with the transcription factor STAT3, which is involved in Th17 activation. STAT3 is present on innate and reactive immune cells and is present in increased amounts in the gut mucosa.[38] Another confirmed genetic association is that with *ERAP1*, an endoplasmic reticulum aminopeptidase previously known as *ARTS1*.[39] *ERAP1* functions by trimming the length of peptides before loading into the grove of HLA, and therefore it could play a role in the triggering of immune reactions in various locations such as gut and joint. A recent Spanish study looked at the Fc receptor gene FcRL-3, which is associated with susceptibility to RA, and found an association with peripheral arthritis in CD. Although this needs replication in other studies, it may indicate an example of a gene combination influencing disease phenotype.[40] However, it is clear that no single gene or combination of genes alone can account for manifest IBD and clearly the intestinal microflora remains a major suspect as contributor to the cause of IBD, although final proof is lacking. Experimental models of IBD require presence of gut bacteria. Postoperative therapy with metronidazole has prolonged the time to relapse.[14] Whereas *CARD15* mutations were present in 43% of patients in the initial French study,[41] later population studies found a much lower prevalence in northern European populations and no correlation in Asians. *CARD15* mutations are not related to susceptibility in the United States. High expression of *CARD15* messenger RNA has been found in the small intestine, and it is believed to be a regulator of nuclear factor κB (NFκB) signaling after the engagement of TLRs. *IBD3* on chromosome 6 has shown the most constant association with IBD, and *HLA-DRB1*0103* has been linked to severe UC in several studies.[20] Further, a TNF microsatellite gene factor was associated with CD but not with UC. HLA-DR2 and DR3 associations have been linked to UC but not to CD.

Mutations of the detoxifying ATP-binding cassette, subfamily B, member 1 gene (*ABCB1*), also known as multidrug resistance 1 gene (*MDR1*), are strongly downregulated in unaffected colonic tissue of both CD and UC. *TLR4* and *TLR5* associations have been identified in several populations; this may be of special interest because they act in synergy with *CARD15* and *CARD4* in the induction of proinflammatory cytokines. TLR inhibitors are being investigated for therapeutic efficacy. Recently, researchers found a role for a virus as the contributing trigger in gene-manipulated mice, when mice with a disrupted autophagy gene, *ATG16L1*, were infected with a specific strain of murine norovirus and developed CD-like disease.[37]

Pathogenesis

CD and UC are clinically distinct entities with a different pathogenesis, but genetic evidence also shows common features. Both are familial, but hereditary factors are more important in CD, according to twin studies. Whereas the entire gut wall is involved in a patchy way in CD, diffuse mucosal pathology is typical of UC. T lymphocyte proliferation and cytokine generation are also different. In CD, a

Th1 response dominates,[42] but no such dominance has been documented for UC. Increased amounts of proinflammatory cytokines, TNF, interleukin (IL)-1β, IL-6, IL-17, and IL-8, are released locally in both diseases (see Figure 78-1).[43]

The interplay between the intestinal microflora and genetic host factors is disturbed in IBD. The microbial contribution is still largely unclear, but animal work indicates that parts of the normal gut flora may be involved. In addition, pathogenic organisms such as *Clostridium difficile* have been linked to exacerbations of IBD.[44] As discussed earlier, genetic factors related to both innate and adaptive immunity are involved in susceptibility to IBD. Experimental work with transgenic animals transfected with human *HLA-B27* and β₂-microglobulin has shown that certain strains of conventional mice and rats develop spondyloarthropathies, whereas identical animals in a germ-free environment are protected.[45,46] In human IBD, *HLA-B27* remains a strong predisposing factor, but only in those individuals with spinal joint involvement. Jejunal fluid from patients with ankylosing spondylitis (AS) and rheumatoid arthritis collected with the closed-segment endoscopic technique contained antibodies against *Klebsiella pneumoniae*, *Escherichia coli*, and *Proteus mirabilis*.[5] A disturbed and augmented local immune response in parts of the gut against a variety of microorganisms is emerging as a prevalent feature of several chronic joint diseases, but it has not been examined in IBD with this endoscopic technique. The viral contribution cited earlier indicates an important role for Paneth cells and disturbed autophagy in the pathogenesis.[47]

Gene manipulation in mice indicates that IL-2, IL-10, and transforming growth factor (TGF)-β may be protective factors and that *HLA-B27* may influence cytokine expression.[48] Altered cytokine balance in the gut mucosa may be an important contributing pathogenic factor.

Increased gut permeability has already been alluded to as an important factor in pathogenesis.[6] Bacteria recovered from the gut lumen in IBD are covered by immunoglobulin, part of which is circulatory IgG.[49] Increased leakage of tissue fluid from the inflamed mucosa allows the egress of complement-binding IgG, which may contribute to inflammation and further augment permeability. The altered immune response to bacteria differs between CD and UC.[50] Increased gut permeability in IBD is under genetic influence. Basal permeability was normal in a study of relatives of patients with CD, but it became abnormally increased after the ingestion of acetylsalicylic acid.[51] Environmental influences on permeability may be partly mediated by bacterial endotoxin. An in vitro perfusion study on rat gut showed that serosal rather than mucosal application of endotoxin impairs the barrier.[52] Absorbed bacterial material could therefore add to an already damaged barrier.

Clinical Features

KEY POINTS

Peripheral arthritis in CD and UC occurs in two distinct forms.

Enthesitis pain is more pronounced than in AS.

Sclerosing cholangitis develops in 5% of IBD.

Table 78-2 Distinct Features of Inflammatory Bowel Disease

Feature	Crohn's	Ulcerative Colitis
Replicated non-HLA genetic associations	CARD15/NOD2, IRGM, ATG16L1, IL23R	IL23R
Concordance in monozygotic twins	36%	19%
Non-*HLA* genes	Several	Several
Gut permeability sensitive to acetylsalicylic acid on genetic base	Yes	?
T lymphocyte response in gut	Th1, Th17 (interferon-γ↑)	No Th1-Th2 imbalance, Th17
Fas ligand expression	No	Yes
Effect of smoking	Negative	Negative
Correlation of gut activity to arthritis symptoms	No	Yes
Intercellular adhesion molecule-1 antisense therapy	Beneficial	No response (?)
Response to anti–tumor necrosis factor therapy	Well established	Probably effective

Although CD and UC are clinically distinct entities, they share many features (Table 78-2). Spinal involvement occurs in 10% to 20% of cases and may be the only articular manifestation or accompany oligoarthritis.[53] Spinal involvement is often silent, so its prevalence is underestimated; it may precede the onset of IBD or appear later.[6] In contrast to AS, there is an equal sex distribution. In general, the involvement is similar to or identical with that in classic AS, although small differences have been found.[54] Changes in enteropathic disease tended to be milder, squaring was more prevalent, and Romanus lesions were rare. The majority of radiographic features were similar. As noted, spinal symptoms may be mild or absent, but when present, they do not correlate with intestinal symptoms. The issue is complicated by the association of AS with silent CD, as diagnosed by biopsy.[55] In full-blown IBD-related AS, the prevalence of B27 is between 50% and 70%, which is lower than in AS not associated with IBD.[6]

Between 5% and 15% of patients in most studies develop peripheral arthritis, slightly more often in CD than in UC (Table 78-3). CD patients with large bowel disease (≈70%)

Table 78-3 Peripheral Joint Disease in Inflammatory Bowel Disease

Feature	Type II (>5 Joints)	Type I (<5 Joints)
Ulcerative colitis	3% of all UC; 3% of all CD	2% of all UC; 5% of all CD
Crohn's disease	6% of all UC; 0% of all CD	4% of all UC; 6% of all CD
Clinical course	Self-limited arthritis	Persistent arthritis
Course of IBD	Relapsing in < 85%	Relapsing in 30%-40%
MHC association	HLA-B27, B35, DRB1*0103	HLA-B44

CD, Crohn's disease; HLA, human leukocyte antigen; IBD, inflammatory bowel disease; MHC, major histocompatibility complex; UC, ulcerative colitis.

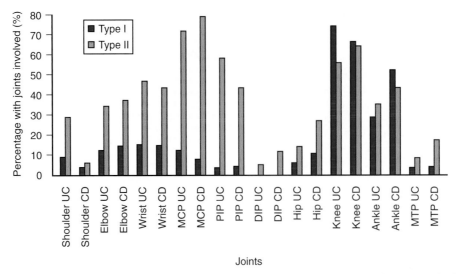

Figure 78-11 Articular distribution of peripheral arthropathies in inflammatory bowel disease. CD, Crohn's disease; DIP, distal interphalangeal joint; MCP, metacarpophalangeal joint; MTP, metatarsophalangeal joint; PIP, proximal interphalangeal joint; UC, ulcerative colitis. *(From Orchard TR, Wordsworth BP, Jewell DP: Peripheral arthropathies in inflammatory bowel disease: their articular distribution and natural history,* Gut *42:387, 1998.)*

and intestinal complications, such as fistulas or abscesses, are more likely to develop peripheral arthritis than patients with disease limited to the ileum.

IBD arthritis is often nondestructive and reversible, but erosive changes may also occur. Limited histopathologic evidence indicates the presence of granulomas in CD and nonspecific synovitis in UC.[6] In CD patients, rapidly destructive septic arthritis has been reported in the hip. Joint symptoms tend to coincide with gut activity in UC but not in CD. Total colectomy is associated with remission of arthritis in half the patients with UC, but paradoxically, arthritis may also begin after surgery.[56] This may represent a form of bypass arthritis and is related to altered gut microbiology in a blind loop.

On the basis of examination of about 1500 patients with IBD, an important distinction was made between two forms of peripheral arthritis[57] (Figure 78-11). Oligoarthritis, or type I, affects fewer than five joints, whereas polyarthritis, or type II, involves more than five joints. The highest prevalence was found in metacarpophalangeal, proximal interphalangeal, knee, and ankle joints. Shoulder involvement was more common in UC, but joint involvement was otherwise strikingly similar. The majority of type I arthritis cases were acute and resolved within 6 weeks, whereas the type II cases persisted.[58] Type I arthritis was 12 times more prevalent in carriers of the rare *HLA-DRB1*0103* allele, type II arthritis was associated with HLA-B44, and sacroiliitis in CD was associated with *CARD15* polymorphisms.[59] This is an example of genetic influence on disease phenotype and may be a clue to pathogenesis.

Clubbing of fingers, uveitis, and skin manifestations are other extraintestinal manifestations of IBD, with a higher frequency in CD. Erythema nodosum, which is usually self-limited, is most frequent in young female patients with UC. Pyoderma gangrenosum is a more severe, painful, ulcerating skin reaction that is frequently associated with systemic disease[60] (Figure 78-12). In a series of 86 patients with pyoderma gangrenosum seen at the Mayo Clinic between 1970 and 1983, 31 had IBD.[6] Erythema nodosum, uveitis, and

peripheral arthritis commonly occur together in IBD and have been linked to *HLA-DRB1*0103* and TNF gene polymorphism.[61] Uveitis is also a feature of other spondyloarthropathies such as AS and reactive arthritis. In IBD, however, uveitis is more often bilateral, and the tendency toward chronicity is more pronounced.[62,63] Up to 5% of the patients with UC and CD can develop primary sclerosing cholangitis (PSC), a progressive liver disease that can lead to end-stage liver fibrosis.[64,65] The risk of developing colorectal cancer is increased in IBD and related to the extent of the colonic involvement and disease duration. Colorectal cancer mortality has decreased significantly in the past few decades, however, due to better surveillance and earlier diagnosis.[66,67]

Diagnosis

Because of the lack of specific tests to confirm a suspicion of IBD-related arthritis, a careful history and clinical examination, supplemented by imaging, are the principal

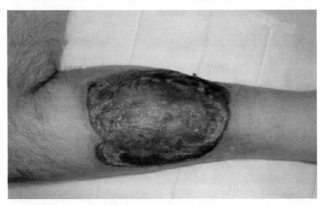

Figure 78-12 Pyoderma gangrenosum in a case of Crohn's disease. *(From Rothfuss KS, Stange EF, Herrlinger KR: Extraintestinal manifestations and complications in inflammatory bowel diseases,* World J Gastroenterol *12:4819–4831, 2006.)*

diagnostic tools. Arthropathy can precede intestinal symptoms in a subgroup of patients, and thus colonoscopy with histologic exploration can be informative regarding the origin of occurring joint symptoms. Fecal calprotectin has emerged as a sensitive screening test for IBD and helps to select cases for endoscopic exploration.[64] As mentioned earlier, genetic mapping has shown interesting clinical correlates, but genotyping is not part of the routine clinical workup at present, except perhaps for *HLA-B27*. Stool cultures should be performed when infection with special pathogens is suspected. In patients with apparent IBD and monoarthritis, joint aspiration is important to exclude septic arthritis, especially before starting immunosuppressive therapy.

Treatment

> ### KEY POINTS
>
> Symptomatic treatment of joint disease in IBD is often adequate.
>
> In disease-modifying antirheumatic drug–unresponsive disease, TNF inhibitors may work.
>
> Interferon-γ, IL-23, and IL-6 are potential new targets.
>
> Probiotic efficacy is unproved.

Joint manifestations are considered secondary to active IBD. Current dogma states that treating the latter will benefit the former, but there is no rigorous proof. Placebo effects account for perhaps 20% of the treatment response in IBD; therefore only placebo-controlled evidence can be trusted. To bring into focus the arthritic discomforts, symptomatic relief is still the main target because in general, IBD-associated arthritis is nondestructive. Pain control with nonsteroidal anti-inflammatory drugs (NSAIDs) is a possible problem owing to their potential induction of flares. However, they are widely used, often well tolerated, and remain an important tool, especially in patients with primary involvement of the spine or enthesitis. Experience with the selective cyclooxygenase-2 inhibitor celecoxib, although limited, has failed to show improved gastrointestinal tolerance in comparison with other NSAIDs.[67]

Sulfasalazine and its derivative 5-acetylsalicylic acid (5-ASA) inhibit the function of NFκB, and several studies have shown the efficacy of these drugs compared with placebo in UC but not in CD.[5] Glucocorticoids are effective in both forms of IBD, although the response of uveitis to topical therapy with glucocorticoids may be less prompt than in other forms of uveitis.[6] In patients with oligoarthritis, intra-articular glucocorticoid injection can be effective and safer than oral administration. Azathioprine has been widely used to maintain remission in IBD. It has proven long-term efficacy in both UC colitis and CD, according to a large European study.[68] It should not be combined with 5-ASA owing to a pharmacokinetic interaction.[69] If azathioprine is not tolerated, methotrexate is recommended under frequent monitoring for signs of hepatotoxicity.

TNF inhibition with infliximab results in remission of gastrointestinal manifestations in close to 60% of patients

Table 78-4 Approved Biologics for Crohn's Disease (as of 2012)

United States	European Union	Switzerland
Infliximab	Infliximab	Infliximab
Adalimumab	Adalimumab	Adalimumab
Certolizumab pegol		Certolizumab pegol
Natalizumab (limited)		

with CD, as confirmed in several placebo-controlled studies.[70] Similar data are available for adalimumab, even in patients with previous infliximab exposure[71] and certolizumab pegol.[72] Interestingly, etanercept, which is not beneficial for intestinal manifestation, seems to be effective for spinal and peripheral involvement. An overview of approved anti-TNF therapy in CD is given in Table 78-4.

Infliximab was found to be superior to placebo in UC patients resistant to conventional drug therapy, although the evidence is less robust if compared with glucocorticoid therapy.[73] However, for UC, infliximab remains the only currently approved TNF-inhibiting treatment. A recent Swedish study shows higher survival on drug therapy among patients of male sex and with peripheral arthritis.[74]

Natalizumab, targeting α4 integrin, has shown promising effects in both multiple sclerosis and CD. However, enthusiasm was reduced after the occurrence of three cases of lethal progressive leukoencephalitis.[75] The drug is still in limited use. ABT-874/J695, an anti-interleukin 12/23 antibody and ustekinumab, directed against the shared subunit p40, are more effective compared with placebo in first studies with patients suffering from CD.[76,77]

Currently anti–interferon (IFN)-γ antibodies such as fontolizumab are being investigated for their efficacy in CD, and early data suggest a significant response compared with placebo.[78] In a pilot study, tocilizumab, an anti-interleukin-6 receptor monoclonal antibody, showed significant but not complete response in patients with active CD.[79] Probiotics, although commercially promoted, have not been proved effective in IBD.[80] Metronidazole, ciprofloxacin, and other poorly absorbed broad-spectrum antibiotics have been widely tested in controlled studies, but there is no convincing evidence that they are better than placebo and they are usually inferior to glucocorticoids.[81]

Outcome

No prospective studies have addressed the outcome of arthritis complicating IBD. Central and peripheral arthritis shares most features with spondyloarthropathies not associated with or with silent IBD.

BRUCELLA ARTHRITIS

Epidemiology

Brucellosis has been eradicated in Western Europe and North America but is still a major zoonosis in areas of South America, the Middle East, India, and other places where goat and sheep farming is practiced and poverty is prevalent. With increased global travel, sporadic cases can be expected in Europe and the United States. In endemic areas, the reported incidence is between 1 and 200 cases per 100,000.[82]

Cause and Pathogenesis

Brucella are small gram-negative bacteria that infect macrophages and are harbored in the liver, spleen, and bone marrow; from there, they can spread to joints. The four species causing human disease are *Brucella melitensis*, *Brucella abortus*, *Brucella suis*, and *Brucella canis*. *Brucella* arthritis is thought to be reactive on the basis of the failure to grow microorganisms from joint fluid and the poor response to antibiotic therapy, but this has never been proved.[6]

Clinical Features and Diagnosis

Brucellosis causes arthritis in about one-third of cases. The main locations are the spine in adults and the peripheral joints in children and adolescents. Knees, hips, and ankles are the dominant peripheral locations. Sacroiliitis can be extremely acute and painful. Rising titers of serum antibodies and a confirmatory culture solidify the diagnosis. Case reports describe septic prepatellar bursitis[83] and olecranon bursitis[84] and indicate that fluid from these lesions can be diagnostic.

Treatment and Outcome

Rifampicin 600 to 900 mg and doxycycline 200 mg daily for at least 6 weeks are recommended by the World Health Organization, but other combinations have been tried.[82] The arthritis can become destructive unless treated early. Spinal stenosis may be a complication.

BYPASS ARTHRITIS-DERMATITIS SYNDROME

Epidemiology

Improved surgical techniques for overweight treatment have eliminated a major cause of bypass arthritis-dermatitis syndrome. It may occur as a rare complication in gastrointestinal diseases with defective peristalsis, systemic sclerosis, and IBD, particularly after colorectal surgery.[6]

Cause and Pathogenesis

Bacterial overgrowth in a blind loop is the likely cause. The formation and absorption of complement-binding immune complexes with increased gut permeability are contributing factors in pathogenesis.

Clinical Features and Diagnosis

The main features seen in patients in the 1970s were an intensely painful oligoarthritis of the large and small joints and the spine, without structural changes, and a recurrent papulopustular rash (Figure 78-13). Today, gastrointestinal dysfunction in combination with painful, nondestructive oligoarthritis and intermittent papular skin rash may be encountered.

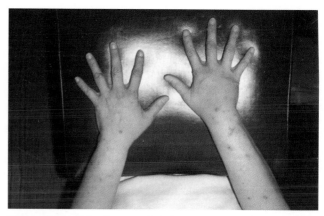

Figure 78-13 Relapsing pustulosis in a patient with bypass arthritis-dermatitis.

Treatment and Outcome

Correction of gastrointestinal function, administration of nonresorbed antibiotics such as neomycin, and symptomatic pain relief are the principal therapeutic options. Prolonged complaints have been reported, but cure is the rule.

CELIAC DISEASE

Epidemiology

CeD is a common condition with a global distribution. It used to be considered most prevalent in children, but new evidence shows that it is even more common in adults. Intestinal symptoms may be minimal or absent; consequently, published prevalence figures of 1% may be too low.[6,85,86] In juvenile idiopathic arthritis CeD has been found in 6% to 7% of cases.[86]

Cause and Pathogenesis

CeD is caused by an immune reaction to partly digested wheat gluten by T lymphocytes in the gut of genetically HLA-DQ2–positive or HLA-DQ8–positive individuals. A seminal observation was the finding that tissue transglutaminase is the major autoantigen in CeD.[85] It was shown in 2002 that dietary gluten is partly digested by gastric enzymes to generate a stable 33–amino acid peptide that is deamidated by tissue transglutaminase.[87] The peptide is then presented in the context of HLA-DQ2 or HLA-DQ8 to CD4+ T cells, resulting in IFN-γ release and inflammation, altered gut permeability, and eventually villus atrophy. Autoantibodies against tissue transglutaminase are also formed.[85] CeD can now be considered as a systemic disease that may involve GI-related pathology, as well as endocrine, skin, locomotor, and neural abnormalities (Figure 78-14).[86]

Clinical Features and Diagnosis

Only two-thirds of patients present with diarrhea or irritated bowel symptoms. Nonspecific signs such as fatigue, headache, and arthralgias may occur and delay a correct

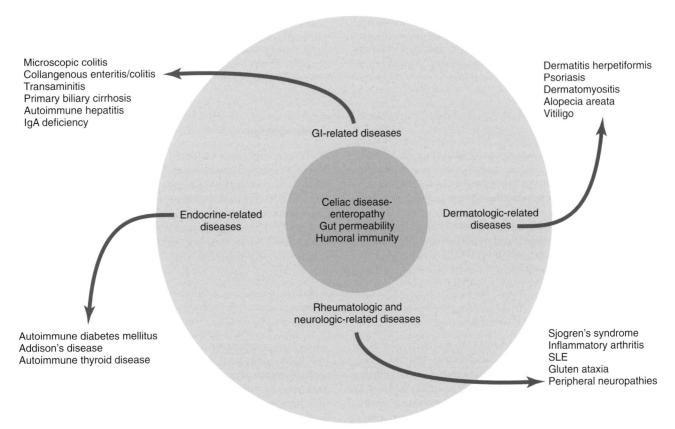

Microscopic colitis
Collangenous enteritis/colitis
Transaminitis
Primary biliary cirrhosis
Autoimmune hepatitis
IgA deficiency

Dermatitis herpetiformis
Psoriasis
Dermatomyositis
Alopecia areata
Vitiligo

GI-related diseases

Endocrine-related
diseases

Celiac disease-
enteropathy
Gut permeability
Humoral immunity

Dermatologic-related
diseases

Autoimmune diabetes mellitus
Addison's disease
Autoimmune thyroid disease

Rheumatologic and
neurologic-related diseases

Sjogren's syndrome
Inflammatory arthritis
SLE
Gluten ataxia
Peripheral neuropathies

Figure 78-14   Celiac disease as a multiorgan systemic condition. GI, gastrointestinal; SLE, systemic lupus erythematosus. *(From Barton SH, Murray JA: Celiac disease and autoimmunity in the gut and elsewhere, Gastroenterol Clin North Am 37(2):411–428, 2008.)*

diagnosis.[86] CeD is a systemic disease that can involve type I diabetes, anemia, osteoporosis, neuropathies, and joint symptoms in up to 25% of patients.[88] This can be an asymmetric oligoarthritis or polyarthritis, and axial involvement is common. Arthritis may be the presenting symptom of the disease.[89]

In addition to small bowel biopsy, the diagnosis can be established by assaying for the presence of serum for IgA antitissue transglutaminase antibodies and IgA antiendomysial antibodies.[90]

Treatment and Outcome

Elimination of gluten from the diet is the rational therapy and is often the only one required. In addition, various experimental approaches have been discussed but are not yet supported by data. These include the administration of IL-10 to boost regulatory T cells, the induction of tolerance by nasal application of gluten peptides, and gene therapy. No specific therapy has been established for the joint problems.

Children with verified CeD still have abnormal mucosa in adulthood and must continue the dietary restriction. There are no outcome reports dealing with joint involvement.

WHIPPLE'S DISEASE

Epidemiology

Whipple's disease is a rare condition. Incidence and prevalence figures are unknown. A retrospective French study identified 52 patients, 73% of whom were men.[6]

Genetics and Pathogenesis

Whipple's disease, or intestinal lipodystrophy, as it was initially called in 1907,[6] is an intestinal infection with a unique microorganism called *Tropheryma whipplei*, belonging to the Actinomycetes family. The organism has been found in sewage, but the source of infection in humans is not known. Six different genotypes have been confirmed in culture from diseased tissue.[91]

The organism lives in macrophages, and these elicit a skewed lymphocyte response, with suppressed Th1 dominating Th2 cells. Expression of the cytokine IL-16 stimulates growth of the pathogen.[92] In vitro monocytes from patients with Whipple's disease express CD163, possibly explaining a reduced oxidative impact against *T. whipplei*.[93] A correlation between different clinical manifestations and variable genotypes of the bacterium has not been identified, and host factors seem to be crucial for the kind of manifestation.[94] Altered gut permeability may be implicated in joint involvement. In a cohort of 122 European patients, an association between HLA alleles *DRB1*13* and *DQB1*06* and Whipple's disease was found, supporting a genetic contribution to susceptibility.[95]

Clinical Features

The disease can have many faces and may remain undiagnosed for many years. Recurrent fever; malaise; hematologic, pulmonary, and cardiac disturbances; and neurologic and ophthalmic symptoms are sometimes present and misinterpreted. Articular symptoms, however, are the presenting feature in 67% of cases, compared with intestinal symptoms in only 15%. Eventually, 83% of patients develop diarrhea, abdominal pain, and malnutrition. Arthralgias and arthritis are most commonly seen in knee joints but can localize in any peripheral joint, as well as in spinal joints and disks. Sacroiliitis has been described.

Diagnosis

The diagnostic test of choice rests on immune histology, with the occurrence of periodic acid–Schiff–positive material, an abundance of CD68+ macrophages, and staining with antisera specific for *T. whipplei*. Quantitative PCR of saliva and stool has been suggested as a noninvasive screening method.[96] PCR of cerebrospinal fluid can detect central nervous system involvement.[97] The organism can grow out in culture, which takes an average of 30 days. In one study, only 2 of 10 small bowel specimens were culture positive; the yield is higher using sterile cardiac or nerve tissue.[91] Culture therefore remains a research tool.

Treatment

No randomized, controlled studies are available. Initial treatment should be ceftriaxone for 2 weeks to ensure entrance into the central nervous system. Then oral trimethoprim-sulfamethoxazole is administered for a prolonged or indefinite period. In case of intolerance or lack of efficacy, tetracycline can be used. A prospective comparison between ceftriaxone and meropenem treatment for 2 weeks followed by trimethoprim-sulfamethoxazole for 1 year showed good 3-year remission in both groups.[98] However, immune histology still shows some evidence of remaining pathology,[99] indicating that recurrence could be anticipated after discontinued therapy.

Use of penicillin, streptomycin, and chloramphenicol has been abandoned.[99]

Outcome

Without treatment, Whipple's disease is chronic or relapsing, usually progressive, and ultimately fatal. With adequate antibiotic therapy, clinical remission is usually complete or near complete.

MICROSCOPIC COLITIS

Microscopic colitis (MC) is a name given to two conditions presenting with profuse diarrhea. The first, collagenous colitis (CC), was described in 1976, and the second, lymphocytic colitis (LC), was published in 1989.[100] They are now joined by a rare third condition called collagenous gastritis (CG).[101] Apart from gastrointestinal symptoms, they all may be associated with extraintestinal autoimmune manifestations.

Epidemiology

Although initially considered rare, it is now evident that MC is a common cause of watery diarrhea in several populations. The minimal overall annual incidence is 1 to 5 cases per 100,000. It is 5 to 10 times more common in individuals older than the age of 65 and distinctly more common in women.[100] The female-to-male ratio is 7:1 in collagenous colitis and 2:1 in lymphocytic colitis. The peak incidence is seen among those 60 to 80 years old. For some years the incidence seemed to be increasing, but this has now leveled off.[102]

Cause

The cause is unknown. Although no strong genetic factor has been identified, an association with HLA-DQ2 and with a polymorphism in the *TNF* gene has been described.[100] Exposure to antirheumatic therapy has been suspected in MC patients with rheumatoid arthritis on the basis of the observation that arthritis usually precedes the onset of CC. Reaction against some luminal factor is deduced from the observation that histology is normalized when ileostomy is performed but recurs after closure. Drugs that are prime suspects include NSAIDs and acetylsalicylic acid, lansoprazole, ranitidine, sertraline, and ticlopidine.[102] CC, LC, and CG all seem to be associated with CeD, autoimmune thyroid disease, and arthritis, but no causal relationship is established.

Pathogenesis

Infection is suspected, but no agent has been identified. Luminal factors are strongly suggested by almost complete histologic normalization after performing ileostomy and recurrence of pathology and symptoms after its closure.[102] Connective tissue growth factor was markedly increased in the subepithelial zone of biopsies from CC patients analyzed by reverse transcription PCR, indicating a pathogenic role for connective tissue growth factor (CTGF).[103] If confirmed, this may lead to targeted therapy of CC.

Clinical Features

Chronic, intermittent (or sometimes chronic, persistent) painful watery stools, weight loss, and fatigue are the cardinal intestinal symptoms. There is no difference between collagenous and lymphocytic colitis in this regard. The course is acute or chronic but usually benign.

CC and LC are associated with a variety of rheumatic syndromes in 10% to 20% of cases. These include Sjögren's syndrome, nondestructive oligoarthritis, migratory arthralgias, sacroiliitis, and rheumatoid arthritis. A survey of 63 consecutive cases in one Swedish center identified 8 cases of rheumatoid arthritis and 3 cases of AS, clearly

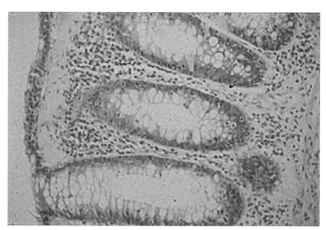

Figure 78-15 Collagenous colitis. Note the intact epithelium and massive subepithelial collagen layer. *(Courtesy Dr. Claes Lindström.)*

suggesting a correlation between colitis and chronic joint disease.[102]

Diagnosis

The diagnosis can be made only by histology obtained at colonoscopy. Endoscopic examination is essentially normal. Lindström found a characteristic thickening of the collagen layer under the gut epithelium. This layer is normally 3 μm, but in CC, it is more than 10 μm and may reach 50 to 100 μm (Figure 78-15). In addition, one can see inflammation and an increased number of lymphocytes. The histology of LC shows an abundance of epithelial lymphocytes (Figure 78-16). In both conditions, the gut epithelium remains intact, although colonic mucosal tears are occasionally present.

Treatment and Outcome

Nonspecific antidiarrheal therapy with 2 to 16 mg loperamide is often effective. Open studies have indicated efficacy of mesalamine 800 mg three times daily either as

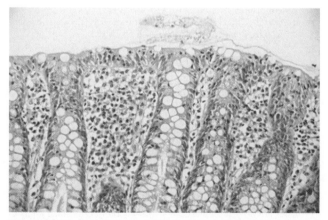

Figure 78-16 Lymphocytic colitis. Note the epithelial lesions with intraepithelial lymphocytosis and inflammation of the lamina propria. *(From Wollheim FA: Collagenous colitis and rheumatology,* Curr Rheumatol Rep *2:183–184, 2000.)*

monotherapy or in combination with cholestyramine 4 g/day. Budesonide 9 mg/day has good immediate effect but gut relapse is common.[100]

PONCET'S DISEASE AND BACILLE CALMETTE-GUÉRIN–INDUCED ARTHRITIS

Tuberculous arthritis, or Poncet's disease, is a rare aseptic form of insidious fever, weakness, and arthritis described mostly in young adults suffering from extrapulmonary tuberculosis.[14] It responds slowly to antituberculous therapy, and in the absence of pulmonary changes, the intestine is assumed to be the port of entry. The attenuated *Mycobacterium* strain bacille Calmette-Guérin (BCG) is used intradermally as an adjuvant in cancer therapy to stimulate T cell–mediated immunity; it is also instilled into the urinary bladder to treat superficial cancer.

Epidemiology

No epidemiologic data are available. A recent review identified 50 bona fide cases of Poncet's disease.[104] Aseptic arthritis occurs in 0.4% to 0.8% of patients treated with the instillation of BCG for bladder malignancy,[6] and anecdotal evidence indicates an increased prevalence of *HLA-B27* among them.[105] This finding was associated with sacroiliitis in 20% and oligoarthritis with predominant localization to the lower limbs; it occurred more often in men. In cases of reactive arthritis occurring after the intradermal administration of BCG, 6 of 10 patients were women and symmetric hand arthritis dominated. In view of the global increase of tuberculosis incidence, one should exercise vigilance regarding possible new cases of Poncet's arthritis.

Cause and Pathogenesis

An aseptic complication of active tuberculosis or the administration of BCG precipitates the process. By definition, it is a reactive arthritis, which means that the infectious agent triggers an immune reaction; however, the enteropathic nature is not firmly established. *HLA-B27* may be a susceptibility factor in post-BCG arthritis.[6]

Mycobacterium heat shock protein 65 has been incriminated in both these sterile forms of arthritis, as well as in others.[106] Mycobacterial and human heat shock proteins are 50% homologous, and one hypothesis is that both the therapeutic efficacy and the arthritis are caused by cross-reactive T lymphocytes. Heat shock protein also has homologies with proteoglycan and HLA-DR. The pathogenesis of arthritis after intravesical instillation of BCG might be different and related to antigen persistence, setting the stage for a kind of reactive arthritis.

Clinical Features and Diagnosis

Insidious fever, weakness, and arthritis are described mostly in young adults suffering from extrapulmonary tuberculosis.[6] The arthritis consists of oligoarthritis or polyarthritis of large or small joints, or both. The onset is not as acute as in regular enteric reactive arthritis. Most peripheral joints can be affected.[6] An interesting case was identified in Finland with the help of a sensitive ELISPOT IFN-γ release test. The patient was a female 55-year-old hospital attendant presenting migratory arthritides of an ankle and toes.[107]

Arthritis developing in the presence of active tuberculosis or after recent exposure to BCG and proven to be aseptic is sufficient for diagnosis.

Treatment and Outcome

There is no established treatment. Post-BCG cases usually heal within 3 months. However, despite negative culture results, 4 to 6 months of conventional antituberculous therapy is often practiced.[107]

ENTEROVIRAL AND HEPATITIS VIRUS–ASSOCIATED ARTHRITIS

Epidemiology

Enterovirus infections, like other common virus infections, often give rise to arthralgias. The precise prevalence is not known. Hepatitis B and hepatitis C disease cause joint manifestations in 10% to 25% of cases.

Genetics and Pathogenesis

No genetic factors have been identified. *Enterovirus* species can invade joints and may rarely be isolated from joint fluid.[108] Immune complex–mediated activation may result in viral hepatitis. A preferential deposition of such immune complexes in joints results in arthralgias and arthritis.[109] In hepatitis C disease, precipitation of cryoglobulins is often observed. Molecular mimicry has been proposed but not proved.[110] Viral persistence in host cells with continuous production of viral protein expressed on cell surfaces has been observed.[111] Immunosuppressive therapy may reactivate latent virus growth and may be misinterpreted as increased disease activity in patients with other rheumatologic conditions.

Clinical Features

Hepatitis B may be associated with a variety of general symptoms including fever, abdominal pain, nausea, and vomiting after a prodromal period of up to 6 months. Among these patients, 10% to 25% also develop articular symptoms, which may present during the prodromal phase. Preferentially, locations are hands and knees. In addition to morning stiffness, migratory arthritis is common. Interestingly, a coincident appearance of urticaria-like rash, predominantly of the legs, is common. The arthritis characteristically disappears with the onset of jaundice.[112-114]

Less than 5% of hepatitis B–infected individuals develop a chronic disease with persistent or remitting articular manifestations. The disease is self-limited and only requires symptomatic treatment.[110,115]

Hepatitis C virus is associated with joint symptoms in 20% of cases. Other frequent symptoms are myalgia, glomerulonephritis, and vasculitis or essential mixed cryoglobulinemia, which may become severe. Oligoarthritis occurs in one-third of the cases, whereas two-thirds develop polyarticular disease.[109,116]

Enteroviruses, coxsackieviruses, and echoviruses are only associated with arthropathy in less than 1% of cases, but due to the high prevalence of the primary disease the number of arthritis cases is not trivial.[116-118] After an incubation period of 3 to 5 days the patients develop fever, fatigue, headache, pharyngitis, myalgia, rash, pleuritic pain, and conjunctivitis or, alternatively, nausea, abdominal pain, enteric cramps, vomiting, and diarrhea. Joint symptoms are self-limited and disappear within days, although recurrence can occur. Any peripheral joint may be affected.[119]

References

1. Turner JR: Intestinal mucosal barrier function in health and disease, *Nat Rev Immunol* 9(11):799–809, 2009.
2. Wang F, Graham WV, Wang Y, et al: Interferon-gamma and tumor necrosis factor-alpha synergize to induce intestinal epithelial barrier dysfunction by up-regulating myosin light chain kinase expression, *Am J Pathol* 166(2):409–419, 2005.
3. Su L, Shen L, Clayburgh DR, et al: Targeted epithelial tight junction dysfunction causes immune activation and contributes to development of experimental colitis, *Gastroenterology* 136(2):551–563, 2009.
4. Miele L, Valenza V, La Torre G, et al: Increased intestinal permeability and tight junction alterations in nonalcoholic fatty liver disease, *Hepatology* 49(6):1877–1887, 2009.
5. Wollheim FA: Enteropathic arthritis. In Kelley WN, Harris ED Jr, Ruddy S, Sledge CB, editors: *Textbook of rheumatology*, ed 5, Philadelphia, 1997, WB Saunders, p 1006.
6. Wollheim FA: Enteropathic arthritis. In Kelley WN, Harris ED Jr, Ruddy S, Sledge CB, editors: *Textbook of rheumatology*, ed 7, Philadelphia, 2005, WB Saunders, p 1165.
7. Hvatum M, Kanerud L, Hällgren R, Brandtzaeg P: The gut-joint axis: cross reactive food antibodies in rheumatoid arthritis, *Gut* 55:1240–1247, 2006.
8. Iqbal TH, Lewis KO, Gearty JC, Cooper BT: Small intestinal permeability to mannitol and lactulose in the three ethnic groups resident in west Birmingham, *Gut* 39:199, 1996.
9. Guarner F: Enteric flora in health and disease, *Digestion* 73(Suppl 1):5–12, 2006.
10. Hattori M, Taylor TD: The human intestinal microbiome: a new frontier of human biology, *DNA Res* 16(1):1–12, 2009.
11. Eckburg PB, Bik EM, Bernstein CN, et al: Diversity of the human intestinal microbial flora, *Science* 308(5728):1635–1638, 2005.
12. Wu HJ, Ivanov II, Darce J, et al: Gut-residing segmented filamentous bacteria drive autoimmune arthritis via T helper 17 cells, *Immunity* 32(6):815–827, 2010.
13. Tomasi TB: The discovery of secretory IgA and the mucosal immune system, *Immunol Today* 13(10):416–418, 1992.
14. Tezuka H, Ohteki T: Regulation of intestinal homeostasis by dendritic cells, *Immunol Rev* 234(1):247–258, 2010.
15. Manicassamy S, Reizis B, Ravindran R, et al: Activation of beta-catenin in dendritic cells regulates immunity versus tolerance in the intestine, *Science* 329(5993):849–853, 2010.
16. Obata T, Goto Y, Kunisawa J, et al: Indigenous opportunistic bacteria inhabit mammalian gut-associated lymphoid tissues and share a mucosal antibody-mediated symbiosis, *Proc Natl Acad Sci U S A* 107:7419–7424, 2010.
17. Khan WI, Ghia JE: Gut hormones: emerging role in immune activation and inflammation, *Clin Exp Immunol* 161(1):19–27, 2010.
18. Brandtzaeg P: Mucosal immunity: induction, dissemination, and effector functions, *Scand J Immunol* 70:505–515, 2009.
19. Brandtzaeg P: Mucosal immunity: Integration between mother and the breast-fed infant, *Vaccine* 21:3382–3388, 2003.
20. Marttila-Ichihara F, Smith DJ, Stolen C, et al: Vascular amine oxidases are needed for leukocyte extravasation into inflamed joints in vivo, *Arthritis Rheum* 54:2852–2862, 2006.
21. Jalkanen S, Salmi M: VAP-1 and CD73, endothelial cell surface enzymes in leukocyte extravasation, *Arterioscler Thromb Vasc Biol* 28(1):18–26, 2008.

22. Logan I, Bowlus CL: The geoepidemiology of autoimmune intestinal diseases, *Autoimmun Rev* 9(5):A372–A378, 2010.

23. Lakatos PL: Recent trends in the epidemiology of inflammatory bowel diseases: up or down? *World J Gastroenterol* 12:6102–6108, 2006.

24. Karlinger K, Györke T, Makö E, et al: The epidemiology and pathogenesis of inflammatory bowel disease, *Eur J Radiol* 35:154–167, 2000.

25. Roth MP, Petterson FM, McElree C, et al: Geographic origins of Jewish patients with inflammatory bowel disease, *Gastroenterology* 97:900, 1989.

26. Carlens C, Hergens MP, Grunewald J, et al: Smoking, use of moist snuff, and risk of chronic inflammatory diseases, *Am J Respir Crit Care Med* 181(11):1217–1222, 2010.

27. Andersson J: The inflammatory reflex–introduction, *J Intern Med* 257(2):122–125, 2005.

28. Tysk C, Lindberg E, Jarnerot G, Floderus-Myrhed B: Ulcerative colitis and Crohn's disease in an unselected population of monozygotic and dizygotic twins: a study of heritability and the influence of smoking, *Gut* 29:990, 1988.

29. Bernstein CN, Wajda A, Blanchard JF: The clustering of other chronic inflammatory diseases in inflammatory bowel disease: a population-based study, *Gastroenterology* 129:827–836, 2005.

30. Loftus EV Jr: Inflammatory bowel disease extending its reach, *Gastroenterology* 129:1117–1120, 2005.

31. Barrett JC, Hansoul S, Nicolae DL, et al: Genome-wide association defines more than 30 distinct susceptibility loci for Crohn's disease, *Nat Genet* 40(8):955–962, 2008.

32. McGovern DP, Gardet A, Törkvist L: *Nat Genet* 42(4):332–337, 2010.

33. Vermeire S: Review article: Genetic susceptibility and application of genetic testing in clinical management of inflammatory bowel disease, *Aliment Pharmacol Ther* 24(Suppl 3):2–10, 2006.

34. Voss E, Wehkamp J, Wehkamp K, et al: NOD2/CARD15 mediates induction of the antimicrobial peptide human beta-defensin-2, *J Biol Chem* 281:2005–2011, 2006.

35. Hugot JP, Laurent-Puig P, Gower-Rousseau C, et al: Mapping of a susceptibility locus for Crohn's disease on chromosome 16, *Nature* 379:821–823, 1996.

36. Ahern PP, Schiering C, Buonocore S, et al: Interleukin-23 drives intestinal inflammation through direct activity on T cells, *Immunity* 33(2):279–288, 2010.

37. Neurath M: IL-23: A master regulator in Crohn disease, *Nature Med* 13:26–28, 2007.

38. Cénit MC, Alcina A, Márquez A, et al: STAT3 locus in inflammatory bowel disease and multiple sclerosis susceptibility, *Genes Immun* 11(3):264–268, 2010.

39. Brown MA: Genetics of ankylosing spondylitis, *Curr Opin Rheumatol* 22(2):126–132, 2010.

40. Mendoza JL, Lana R, Martin MC, et al: FcRL3 gene promoter variant is associated with peripheral arthritis in Crohn's disease, *Inflamm Bowel Dis* 15(9):1351–1357, 2009.

41. Fuss IJ, Neurath M, Boirivant M, et al: Disparate CD4⁺ lamina propria (LP) lymphokine secretion profiles in inflammatory bowel disease: Crohn's disease LP cells manifest increased secretion of IFN-γ, whereas ulcerative colitis LP cells manifest increased secretion of IL-5, *J Immunol* 157:1261, 1996.

42. Camoglio L, Te Velde AA, Tigges AJ, et al: Altered expression of interferon-γ and interleukin-4 in inflammatory bowel disease, *Inflamm Bowel Dis* 4:285, 1998.

43. Guimbaud R, Bertrand V, Chauvelot-Moachon L, et al: Network of inflammatory cytokines and correlation with disease activity in ulcerative colitis, *Am J Gastroenterol* 93:2397, 1998.

44. Mylonaki M, Langmead L, Pantes A, et al: Enteric infection in relapse of inflammatory bowel disease: importance of microbiological examination of stool, *Eur J Gastroenterol Hepatol* 16:775–778, 2004.

45. Hammer RE, Maika SD, Richardson JA, et al: Spontaneous inflammatory disease in transgenic rats expressing HLA-B27 and human β₂ m: an animal model of *HLA-B27*-associated human disorders, *Cell* 63:1099, 1990.

46. Taurog JD, Richardson JA, Croft JT, et al: The germfree state prevents development of gut and joint inflammatory disease in HLA-B27 transgenic rats, *J Exp Med* 180:2359, 1994.

47. Cadwell K, Patel KK, Maloney NS, et al: Virus-plus-susceptibility gene interaction determines Crohn's disease gene *ATG16L1* phenotypes in intestine, *Cell* 141(7):1135–1145, 2010.

48. Rath HC, Herfarth HH, Ikeda JS, et al: Normal luminal bacteria, especially *Bacteroides* species, mediate chronic colitis, gastritis, and arthritis in HLA-B27/human β₂-microglobulin transgenic rats, *J Clin Invest* 98:945, 1996.

49. van der Waaij LA, Kroese FG, Visser A, et al: Immunoglobulin coating of faecal bacteria in inflammatory bowel disease, *Eur J Gastroenterol Hepatol* 16:669–674, 2004.

50. Macpherson A, Khoo UY, Forgacs I, et al: Mucosal antibodies in inflammatory bowel disease are directed against intestinal bacteria, *Gut* 38:365, 1996.

51. Söderholm JD, Olaison G, Lindberg E, et al: Different intestinal permeability patterns in relatives and spouses of patients with Crohn's disease: an inherited defect in mucosal defence? *Gut* 44:96, 1999.

52. Osman NE, Waström B, Karlsson B: Serosal but not mucosal endotoxin exposure increases intestinal permeability in vitro in the rat, *Scand J Gastroenterol* 33:1170, 1998.

53. Wordsworth P: Arthritis and inflammatory bowel disease, *Curr Rheumatol Rep* 2:87, 2000.

54. Helliwell PS, Hickling P, Wright V: Do the radiological changes of classical ankylosing spondylitis differ from the changes found in the spondylitis associated with inflammatory bowel disease, psoriasis, and reactive arthritis? *Ann Rheum Dis* 57:135, 1998.

55. Mielants H, Veys EM, Goemaere S, et al: A prospective study of patients with spondyloarthropathy with special reference to HLA-B27 and to gut histology, *J Rheumatol* 20:1353, 1993.

56. Andreyev HJ, Kamm MA, Forbes A, Nicholls RJ: Joint symptoms after restorative proctocolectomy in ulcerative colitis and familial polyposis coli, *J Clin Gastroenterol* 23:35, 1996.

57. Orchard TR, Wordsworth BP, Jewell DP: Peripheral arthropathies in inflammatory bowel disease: their articular distribution and natural history, *Gut* 42:387, 1998.

58. Orchard TR, Thiyagaraja S, Welsh KI, et al: Clinical phenotype is related to HLA genotype in the peripheral arthropathies of inflammatory bowel disease, *Gastroenterology* 118:274, 2000.

59. Peeters H, Vander Cruyssen B, Laukens D, et al: Radiological sacroiliitis, a hallmark of spondylitis, is linked with *CARD15* gene polymorphisms in patients with Crohn's disease, *Ann Rheum Dis* 63:1131, 2004.

60. Rothfuss KS, Stange EF, Herrlinger KR: Extraintestinal manifestations and complications in inflammatory bowel diseases, *World J Gastroenterol* 12:4819–4831, 2006.

61. von den Driesch P: Pyoderma gangrenosum: a report of 44 cases with follow-up, *Br J Dermatol* 137:1000, 1997.

62. Orchard TR, Chua CN, Ahmad T, et al: Uveitis and erythema nodosum in inflammatory bowel disease: clinical features and the role of HLA genes, *Gastroenterology* 123:714, 2002.

63. Banares A, Hernandez-Garcia C, Fernandez-Guitierrez B, Jover JA: Eye involvement in the spondyloarthropathies, *Rheum Dis Clin North Am* 24:771, 1998.

64. Lee YM, Kaplan MM: Primary sclerosing cholangitis, *N Engl J Med* 332:924, 1995.

65. Kaplan GG, Laupland KB, Butzner D, et al: Incidence, clinical spectrum, and outcomes of primary sclerosing cholangitis in adults and children: a population based analysis, *Am J Gastroenterol* 102:1042, 2007.

66. Ekbom A, Helmick C, Zack M, et al: Ulcerative colitis and colorectal cancer: a population-based study, *N Engl J Med* 323:1228, 1990.

67. Ekbom A, Helmick C, Zack M, Adami HO: Increased risk of large-bowel cancer in Crohn's disease with colonic involvement, *Lancet* 336:357, 1990.

68. Holtmann MH, Krummenauer F, Claas C, et al: Long-term effectiveness of azathioprine in IBD beyond 4 years: a European multicenter study in 1176 patients, *Dig Dis Sci* 51:1516–1524, 2006.

69. Hande S, Wilson-Rich N, Bousvaros A, et al: 5-Aminosalicylate therapy is associated with higher 6-thioguanine levels in adults and children with inflammatory bowel disease in remission on 6-mercaptopurine or azathioprine, *Inflamm Bowel Dis* 12:251–257, 2006.

70. Akobeng AK, Zachos M: Tumor necrosis factor-alpha antibody for induction of remission in Crohn's disease, *Cochrane Database Syst Rev* (1):CD003574, 2004.

71. Swoger JM, Loftus EV Jr, Tremaine WJ, et al: Adalimumab for Crohn's disease in clinical practice at Mayo clinic: the first 118 patients, *Inflamm Bowel Dis* 16(11):1912–1921, 2010.

72. Sandborn WJ, Abreu MT, D'Haens G, et al: Certolizumab pegol in patients with moderate to severe Crohn's disease and secondary failure to infliximab, *Clin Gastroenterol Hepatol* 8(8):688–695, e2, 2010.

73. Lawson MM, Thomas AG, Akobeng AK: Tumour necrosis factor alpha blocking agents for induction of remission in ulcerative colitis, *Cochrane Database Syst Rev* (3):CD005112, 2006.

74. Kristensen LE, Karlsson JA, Englund M, et al: Presence of peripheral arthritis and male sex predicting continuation of anti-tumor necrosis factor therapy in ankylosing spondylitis: an observational prospective cohort study from the South Swedish Arthritis Treatment Group Register, *Arthritis Care Res (Hoboken)* 62(10):1362–1369, 2010.

75. Berger JR: Natalizumab and progressive multifocal leucoencephalopathy, *Ann Rheum Dis* 65(Suppl 3):iii48–iii53, 2006.

76. Mannon PJ, Fuss IJ, Mayer L, et al: Anti-interleukin-12 antibody for active Crohn's disease, *N Engl J Med* 351:2069, 2004.

77. Sandborn WJ, Feagan BG, Fedorak RN, et al: A randomized trial of ustekinumab, a human interleukin-12/23 moniclonal antibody, in patients with moderate-to-severe Crohn's disease, *Gastroenterology* 135:1130, 2008.

78. Reinisch W, Hommes DW, Van Assche G, et al: A dose escalating, placebo controlled, double blind, single dose and multidose, safety and tolerability study of fontolizumab, a humanised anti-interferon gamma antibody, in patients with moderate to severe Crohn's disease, *Gut* 55(8):1138–1144, 2006.

79. Ito H, Takazoe M, Fukuda Y, et al: A pilot randomized trial of a human anti-interleukin-6 receptor monoclonal antibody in active Crohn's disease, *Gastroenterology* 126:989, 2004.

80. Rolfe V, Fortun P, Hawkey C, Bath-Hextall F: Probiotics for maintenance of remission in Crohn's disease, *Cochrane Database Syst Rev* (4):CD004826, 2006.

81. Perencevich M, Burakoff R: Use of antibiotics in the treatment of inflammatory bowel disease, *Inflamm Bowel Dis* 12:651–664, 2006.

82. McGill PE: Geographically specific infections and arthritis, including rheumatic syndromes associated with certain fungi and parasites, *Brucella* species and *Mycobacterium leprae*, *Best Pract Res Clin Rheumatol* 17:289–307, 2003.

83. Wallach JC, Delpino MV, Scian R, et al: Prepatellar bursitis due to *Brucella abortus*: case report and analysis of the local immune response, *J Med Microbiol* 59:1514–1518, 2010.

84. Turan H, Serefhanoglu K, Karadeli E, et al: A case of brucellosis with abscess of the iliacus muscle, olecranon bursitis, and sacroiliitis, *Int J Infect Dis* 13(6):e485–487, 2009.

85. Lee SK, Green PH: Celiac sprue (the great modern-day imposter), *Curr Opin Rheumatol* 18:101–107, 2006.

86. Barton SH, Murray JA: Celiac disease and autoimmunity in the gut and elsewhere, *Gastroenterol Clin North Am* 37(2):411–428, 2008.

87. Shan L, Molberg O, Parrot I, et al: Structural basis for gluten intolerance in celiac sprue, *Science* 297:2275–2279, 2002.

88. Lubrano E, Ciacci C, Ames PR, et al: The arthritis of coeliac disease: prevalence and pattern in 200 adult patients, *Br J Rheumatol* 35:1314, 1996.

89. Slot O, Locht H: Arthritis as presenting symptom in adult coeliac disease: two cases and review of the literature, *Scand J Rheumatol* 29:260, 2000.

90. van der Windt DA, Jellema P, Mulder CJ, et al: Diagnostic testing for celiac disease among patients with abdominal symptoms: a systematic review, *JAMA* 303(17):1738–1746, 2010.

91. Fenollar F, Birg ML, Gauduchon V, Raoult D: Culture of *Tropheryma whippelii* from human samples: a 3-year experience (1999 to 2002), *J Clin Microbiol* 41:3816–3822, 2003.

92. Moos V, Kunkel D, Marth T, et al: Reduced peripheral and mucosal *Tropheryma whippeli*-specific Th1 response in patients with Whipple's disease, *J Immunol* 177:2015–2022, 2006.

93. Moos V, Schmidt C, Geelhaar A, et al: Impaired immune functions of monocytes and macrophages in Whipple's disease, *Gastroenterology* 138:210, 2010.

94. Martinetti M, Biagi F, Badulli C, et al: The HLA alleles DRB1*13 and DQB1*06 are associated to Whipple's disease, *Gastroenterology* 136:2289, 2009.

95. Li w, Fenollar F, Rolain JM, et al: Genotyping reveals a wide heterogeneity of *Tropheryma whipplei*, *Microbiology* 154:521, 2008.

96. Fenollar F, Laouira S, Lepidi H, et al: Value of *Tropheryma whipplei* quantitative polymerase chain reaction assay for the diagnosis of Whipple disease: usefulness of saliva and stool specimens for first line screening, *Clin Infect Dis* 47:659, 2008.

97. von Herbay A, Ditton HJ, Schuhmacher F, Maiwald M: Whipple's disease: staging and monitoring by cytology and polymerase chain reaction analysis of cerebrospinal fluid, *Gastroenterology* 113:434, 1997.

98. Feurle G, Junga N, Marth T: Efficacy of ceftriaxone or meropenem as initial therapies in Whipple's disease, *Gastroenterology* 138:478, 2010.

99. Mahnel R, Marth T: Progress, problems, and perspectives in diagnosis and treatment of Whipple's disease, *Clin Exp Med* 4:39–43, 2004.

100. Williams JJ, Beck PL, Andrews CN, et al: Microscopic colitis—a common cause of diarrhoea in older adults, *Age Ageing* 39(2):162–867, 2010.

101. Leung ST, Chandan VS, Murray JA, Wu TT: Collagenous gastritis: histopathologic features and association with other gastrointestinal diseases, *Am J Surg Pathol* 33(5):788–798, 2009.

102. Tysk C, Bohr J, Nyhlin N, Wickbom A, Eriksson S: Diagnosis and management of microscopic colitis, *World J Gastroenterol* 14(48):7280–7288, 2008.

103. Günther U, Bateman AC, Beattie RM, et al: Connective tissue growth factor expression is increased in collagenous colitis and coeliac disease, *Histopathology* 57(3):427–435, 2010.

104. Kroot EJ, Hazes JM, Colin EM, Dolhain RJ: Poncet's disease: reactive arthritis accompanying tuberculosis. Two case reports and a review of the literature, *Rheumatology (Oxford)* 46:484–489, 2007.

105. Lugo-Zamudio GE, Yamamoto-Furusho JK, Delgado-Ochoa D, et al: Human leukocyte antigen typing in tuberculous rheumatism: Poncet's disease, *Int J Tuberc Lung Dis* 14:916–920, 2010.

106. Macía Villa C, Sifuentes Giraldo W, Boteanu A, et al: Reactive arthritis after the intravesical instillation of BCG, *Reumatol Clin* 2012 Feb 27. [Epub ahead of print]

107. Valleala H, Tuuminen T, Repo H, et al: A case of Poncet disease diagnosed with interferon-gamma-release assays, *Nat Rev Rheumatol* 5:643–647, 2009.

108. Pawlotsky JM, Roudot-Thoraval F, Simmonds P, et al: Extrahepatic immunological manifestations in chronic hepatitis C and hepatitis C virus serotypes, *Ann Intern Med* 122:169, 1995.

109. Rivera J, Garcia-Monforte A, Pineda A, Millan Nunez-Cortes J: Arthritis in patients with chronic hepatitis C virus infection, *J Rheumatol* 26:420, 1999.

110. Wands JR, Mann E, Alpert E, et al: The pathogenesis of arthritis associated with acute hepatitis B surface antigen-positive hepatitis, *J Clin Invest* 55:930, 1975.

111. Soderlund M, von Essen R, Haapasaari J, et al: Persistence of parvovirus B 19 DANN in synovial membranes, *Lancet* 349:1063, 1997.

112. Ganem D, Prince AM: Hepatitis B virus infection—natural history and clinical consequences, *N Engl J Med* 350:1118, 2004.

113. Hsu HH, Feinstone SM, Houfnagle JH: Acute viral hepatitis. In Mandell GL, Bennett JE, Dolin R, editors: *Mandell, Douglas and Bennett's principles and practices of infectious diseases*, ed 4, New York, 1995, Churchill Livingstone.

114. Alarcon GS, Townes AS: Arthritis in viral hepatitis. Report of two cases and review of the literature, *Johns Hopkins Med J* 132:1, 1973.

115. Shumaker JB, Goldfinger SE, Alpert E, et al: Arthritis and rash, *Arch Intern Med* 133:483, 1974.

116. Rosner I, Rozenbaum M, Toubi E, et al: The case for hepatitis C arthritis, *Semin Arthritis Rheum* 33:375, 2004.

117. Blotzer JW, Myers AR: Echovirus-associated polyarthritis. Report of a case with synovial fluid and synovial histological characterization, *Arthritis Rheum* 21:978, 1978.

118. Hurst NP, Martynoga AG, Nuki G, et al: Coxsackie B infection and arthritis, *Br Med J (Clin Res Ed)* 286:605, 1983.

119. Zeichhardt H, Grunert H-P: Enteroviruses. In Armstrong D, Cohen J, editors: *Infectious disease textbook*, ed 1, London, 1999, Mosby.

The references for this chapter can also be found on www.expertconsult.com.

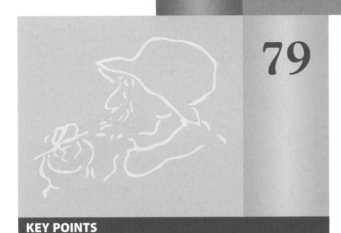

79

Etiology and Pathogenesis of Systemic Lupus Erythematosus

MARY K. CROW

KEY POINTS

Systemic lupus erythematosus (SLE) results from chronic and recurrent activation of the immune system, with production of antibodies and other protein products contributing to inflammation and tissue damage.

SLE is a disease with typical onset in the childbearing years and most common in females, suggesting a role for both hormones and as yet uncharacterized sex-related factors in disease pathogenesis.

Progress in genetic analysis has resulted in identification of genetic variants associated with SLE, with most related to innate and adaptive immune system function. Complement deficiencies confer the highest risk of disease, and mutations in *TREX1* point to impaired regulation of endogenous nucleic acids as an important pathogenic mechanism.

Environmental factors contribute to initiation of lupus and lupus flares.

The discovery of the Toll-like receptor family of innate immune receptors has led to important advances that point to a significant role for innate immune system activation in SLE pathogenesis.

A contribution of nucleic acid–containing immune complexes as stimuli for endosomal Toll-like receptors has added an important new role for immune complexes in the pathogenesis of SLE.

Production of type I interferon (IFN), broad expression of type I IFN–inducible genes, and the effects of IFN on immune system activation and function have emerged as central mechanisms of lupus pathogenesis.

Impaired regulation of the adaptive immune response contributes to autoantibody production and has informed development of new therapies.

Platelets and neutrophils, along with neutrophil extracellular material, have gained new attention as important pathogenic effectors. Complement remains an important mediator of inflammation.

Systemic lupus erythematosus (SLE) represents one of the most significant diseases in all of medicine. Predominantly targeting young women in their childbearing years and with

the potential to cause significant physical disfigurement, morbidity, and occasionally mortality, lupus is the focus of strong advocacy to support research that will generate insights into disease pathogenesis. In fact, characterization of the immunologic contributors to lupus, the prototype systemic autoimmune disease, has been the focus of particularly intense study since the flowering of the discipline of immunology in the 1950s and 1960s. Recent efforts to define the genetic variations that underlie susceptibility to lupus have supported the central role of the immune system in disease pathogenesis but have extended the view of lupus pathology beyond the important role of autoantibodies to include a significant contribution of the innate immune system to disease. An underlying role for the vasculature as a target of the immune system and its products is gaining renewed interest as an important component of lupus pathogenesis. Together, these recent advances provide important insights into how the intersection of genetic variations with environmental triggers amplifies immune system activation and target organ vulnerability to generate the classic manifestations of lupus and its clinically significant comorbidities. Figure 79-1 provides a schematic overview of many of the contributors to SLE and how they interact to drive autoimmunity and tissue damage.

HISTORICAL VIEW OF LUPUS PATHOGENESIS

Insights into the immunopathogenic mechanisms that account for development of autoimmunity in patients with SLE and the tissue damage that results in disease have come in fits and starts over many decades. Progress has been informed by the scientific tools available at the time along with the acute observations of clinicians and research scientists. Descriptions of the clinical manifestations of disease suggested a multisystem disease that typically involves skin and joints, with renal, cardiac, and neurologic pathology suspected and then documented once histologic studies were performed. Alterations of blood vessels in many organs were recognized as an important component of the disease process in early studies, with the pathognomonic "onion

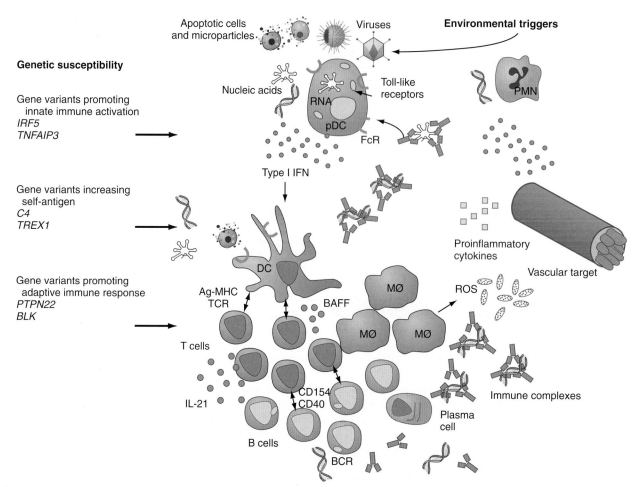

Figure 79-1 Contributors to systemic lupus erythematosus (SLE) pathogenesis. Mechanisms that promote development of SLE are related to the underlying genetic profile of the individual. Many of the disease-associated genetic variants (examples are illustrated) contribute to excessive production or impaired clearance of stimulatory nucleic acids; increased generation of products of the innate immune response, particularly type I interferon (IFN); or an altered threshold for activation or efficiency of signaling of cells of the adaptive immune response. In most cases multiple genetic risk variants are required to establish a state of immune activation that is receptive to environmental triggers that promote development of autoimmunity. In rare cases, a mutation of a critical regulator of immune activation might be sufficient to initiate the altered immune state that can lead to disease. Type I interferon is a product of plasmacytoid dendritic cells (pDCs), and activation of those cells by intracellular nucleic acids or exogenous triggers such as a virus or debris derived from damaged or dying cells might represent mechanisms of initiation of disease. Once IFN-α is produced, it mediates numerous effects on immune system cells that mimic the response to a viral infection. The antigen-presenting capacity of myeloid dendritic cells can be augmented, promoting activation of self-reactive T cells and differentiation of B cells toward production of pathogenic antibodies. Activated T cells express CD154 (CD40 ligand) and produce interleukin-21 (IL-21), providing effective help for B cells to generate antibody-producing plasma cells. IFN-α also supports the production of B cell activating factor (BAFF), a survival and differentiation factor for B cells. Once autoantibodies are produced, immune complexes amplify immune activation by accessing endosomal Toll-like receptors in pDCs and B cells and deposit directly in the vicinity of blood vessels, inducing complement activation, inflammation, and tissue damage. Reactive oxygen species (ROS) and proinflammatory cytokines produced by monocytes and macrophages contribute to tissue damage, as does IFN-α, which stimulates endothelial cells and is associated with poor vascular repair and sclerosis. BCR, B cell receptor; DC, dendritic cell; MHC, major histocompatibility complex; MØ, macrophage; PMN, polymorphonuclear neutrophil; RNA, ribonucleic acid; TCR, T cell receptor.

skinning" of splenic arterioles, cellular infiltration and damage to renal glomeruli, and vasculopathy in skin and brain demonstrated clinically by manifestations such as nephritis, livedo reticularis, and stroke. The lupus erythematosus (LE) cell, described by Hargraves in 1948, suggested that engulfment of cellular debris, a mechanism that remains an important concept in considerations of lupus pathogenesis, was active at sites of inflammation.

The recognition that antibodies directed at cellular components, particularly cell nuclei, were present in the sera of patients with SLE directed the attention of the investigator community toward the immune system and the conclusion that lupus reflected an autoimmune process. Together with pathologic studies of kidneys from lupus nephritis that showed deposition of immunoglobulin and complement components in kidney glomeruli, the elution of anti-deoxyribonucleic acid (DNA) autoantibodies from lupus kidneys contributed to the concept that autoantibodies, particularly anti-DNA antibodies, were pathogenic. Isolation from lupus sera of complexes of antibody with DNA or DNA-binding proteins such as histones was an important factor in classifying SLE as predominantly an immune complex–mediated autoimmune disease. Although lupus pathogenesis does depend on those immune complexes and the inflammatory responses that they induce, subsequent investigation identified virtually all cell components and many soluble immune system products as contributors to the immune system dysfunction that ultimately accounts for disease in SLE.

The development of the field of cellular immunology in the 1970s and the later identification of the T cell antigen receptor, along with families of co-stimulatory molecules mediating interactions between T cells and antigen-presenting cells or B cells, led to the implication of self-reactive T cells as important regulators of immune responses, as well as helpers for B cell differentiation to autoantibody-producing cells in the case of patients with SLE. Numerous deficiencies in T cell function including altered production of typical T cell cytokines such as interleukin-2 (IL-2) were described, and studies of murine lupus models strongly supported the essential role that T cells play in lupus pathogenesis.

The discovery of Toll-like receptors (TLR) in the 1990s, the recognition that those receptors recognize common determinants expressed by microbes, and the demonstration that TLRs mediate immune system activation was a major advance, perhaps the most significant milestone in many decades, that has led to gains in understanding of lupus pathogenesis. Characterization of the typical exogenous ligands of each of the TLRs has been followed by identification of endogenous ligands for their receptors, with nucleic acids being the most relevant for amplification of immune system activation and autoimmunity in SLE. It is not yet clear if the TLRs act to augment immunologic activity that is initiated by other molecular pathways or if they are also essential as sensors for the primary initiators of autoimmune disease.

In spite of these considerable gains in elucidating the pathogenesis of SLE, the environmental triggers and genetic susceptibility factors that lead to the initiation of autoimmunity in some individuals but not in others remain largely undefined. Regarding triggers of disease, clinical observations have pointed to exposure to sunlight, microbial infection, and certain drugs as factors that can lead to initiation or exacerbation of lupus. Whether there is a common thread among these environmental triggers is not clear, but ultraviolet light–mediated DNA damage and modification of DNA methylation are among the processes that might render self–nucleic acid stimulatory to the immune system.

Significant technologic advances in recent years, together with development of consortia of investigators who have cooperated to share biologic samples from patient cohorts and control subjects, have supported important progress in defining the genetic variants that show a statistical association with a diagnosis of SLE. These recent genome-wide association studies (GWASs) have built on long-standing observations of the high risk of disease in patients with complement deficiencies to identify lupus-associated genes that encode important components of molecular pathways that promote production of type I interferon (IFN), alter the threshold for activation of lymphocytes, or generate immune stimuli.

Together, these scientific advances have led to the recent, long-awaited activity in drug development programs targeting mechanisms likely to impact lupus disease activity or clinical progression. This chapter reviews those recent studies that have illuminated the immunopathogenesis of SLE.

GENETIC CONTRIBUTIONS TO LUPUS PATHOGENESIS

Current concepts in genetic studies of complex human diseases including SLE identify both common variants with a small impact on risk of disease, as well as low-frequency mutations that can have a great impact on the risk of developing lupus or a lupus-like syndrome.

Observations of several individuals with SLE within a family, along with a high frequency of concordance of SLE in identical twins, have pointed to a strong genetic contribution to SLE. Data suggest that concordance of clinical lupus disease in twins is 10 times more frequent in monozygotic than in dizygotic twins, although the highest reported concordance rate is still only 57%. Moreover, the suggestion that multiple autoimmune diseases are associated with common genetic susceptibility factors is supported by the aggregation of several distinct autoimmune diseases within a family. The pace of discovery of common genetic variants, typically identified by statistical analysis of single nucleotide polymorphisms (SNPs) in relation to a diagnosis of SLE, has markedly accelerated in recent years, as the cost of genotyping thousands of patient and control samples has become feasible. Publication of two important collaborative genome-wide association studies, one by the SLE Genetics (SLEGEN) consortium and the other organized by Genentech, identified at least nine new genes or genomic loci associated with SLE.[1,2] Since presentation of those studies, additional lupus-associated genetic variants have been confirmed or at least strongly supported.[3] The common theme among the lupus-associated genes is that the vast majority encode proteins implicated in immune system function. Although this result is not surprising, it confirms the essential contribution of the immune system to the autoimmunity, inflammation, and tissue damage that characterize lupus disease and points to the most significant molecular pathways that mediate altered immune function.

The lupus-associated genes that play likely roles in lupus pathogenesis can be grouped on the basis of their roles in immune function (Table 79-1). In parallel to the requirements for immune system activation stimulated by foreign antigens, SLE-associated genes are involved in generation of self-antigen, activation of the innate immune response, and activation of the adaptive immune response. Although the specific functional alterations that are conferred by the lupus-associated variant compared with the more common variant have yet to be defined in detail, in most cases there is sufficient information regarding function to allow formulation of hypotheses that can be tested in functional genetic studies.

The rare but high-risk deficiencies in complement pathway gene products, including C2, C4, and C1q, are thought to contribute to lupus pathogenesis by impairing clearance of cellular debris, a function that is typically supported by those complement components. Increased availability of nuclear debris can provide sufficient self-antigen for induction of self-reactive T cells or serve as an

Table 79-1 Genetic Variants Associated with Systemic Lupus Erythematosus (SLE)

Major Histocompatibility Complex (MHC) Genes Associated with SLE
Homozygous deficiencies of early complement components (C2, C4A, C4B) (increase risk 5- to 10-fold)
HLA-DR2 (increases relative risk twofold to threefold)
HLA-DR3 (increases relative risk twofold to threefold)
DR2/DRX associated with anti-Sm antibodies
DR3/DRX associated with anti-Ro and anti-La antibodies
DR2/DR3 associated with anti-Ro, anti-La, and/or anti-Sm and also associated with anti-dsDNA antibodies
DR3/DR3 associated with anti-Sm antibodies

Non-MHC Genes Associated with SLE
Homozygous deficiency of C1q (increases risk 5- to 10-fold)

Associations Based on Linkage Studies
Fc gamma receptor IIa *(FCGR2A)*
Fc gamma receptor IIIa *(FCGR3A)*
Programmed cell death 1 *(PDCD1)*

Associations Based on Candidate Gene Studies
C-reactive protein *(CRP)*
Interferon regulatory factor 5 *(IRF5)* (supported by GWAS)
Interleukin-10 *(IL-10)*
Protein tyrosine phosphatase 22 *(PTPN22)* (supported by GWAS)

Associations Based on or Confirmed by Genome-Wide Association Studies
B cell scaffold protein with ankyrin repeats *(BANK1)*
B lymphocyte specific tyrosine kinase *(BLK)*
V-ETS avian erythroblastosis virus E26 oncogene homolog 1 *(ETS1)*
Ubiquitin-conjugating enzyme E2L *(UBE2L3)*
Ikaros family zinc finger 1 *(IKZF1)*
Interleukin-1 receptor associated kinase/methyl-CpG-binding protein 2 *(IRAK1/MECP2)*
Integrin αM *(ITGAM)*
Juxtaposed with another zinc finger gene *(JAZF1)*
PHD and ring finger domains 1 *(KIAA1542/PHRF1)*
WD repeat- and FYVE domain-containing protein 4 *(WDFY4)*
V-yes Yamaguchi sarcoma viral related oncogene homolog *(LYN)*
Nicotinamide nucleotide adenylyltransferase 2 *(NMNAT2)*
PR domain-containing protein 1 (BLIMP1) *(PRDM1)*
PXK domain-containing serine/threonine kinase *(PXK)*
RAS guanyl nucleotide-releasing protein 3 *(RASGRP3)*
Solute carrier family 15, member 4 *(SLC15A4)*
Signal transducer and activator of transcription 4 *(STAT4)*
Tumor necrosis factor–induced protein 3 *(TNFAIP3)*
Tumor necrosis factor ligand superfamily, member 4 (OX40L) *(TNFSF4)*
TNFAIP3-interacting protein 1 *(TNIP1)*
3-prime repair exonuclease 1 *(TREX1)*
XK, Kell blood group complex subunit-related family, member 6 *(XKR6)*

Rare Genetic Mutations Associated with Lupus
3-prime repair exonuclease 1 *(TREX1)*
Ribonuclease H2, subunit A-C *(RNASEH2A-C)*
SAM domain- and HD domain-containing protein 1 *(SAMHD1)*

GWAS, genome-wide association study.

endogenous adjuvant for activation of the innate immune response. The ancestral major histocompatibility complex (MHC) 8.1 haplotype block, HLA-B8/DR3/DQw2/C4AQO, that is associated with lupus susceptibility, encodes the alleles B8 and DR3 and bears a short *C4B* gene and no *C4A* gene, whereas other nonrisk haplotypes carry either a longer *C4B* segment and/or one or more copies of *C4A*. In fact, the relative risk related to the C4A null allele

is twice that of either HLA-B8 or DR3, pointing to the significance of the C4 genes in disease risk.[4] It should be noted that this risk haplotype is also associated with accelerated disease in patients infected with human immunodeficiency virus (HIV), insulin-dependent diabetes mellitus, and several other autoimmune diseases. Deficiency of C1q, the recognition protein for the classical complement pathway, might contribute to disease on the basis of its important role in promoting clearance of apoptotic cell debris by mononuclear phagocytes.[5] C1q plays an additional role in inhibition of IFN-α production by directing stimulatory immune complexes to monocytes rather than IFN-producing plasmacytoid dendritic cells. Through this mechanism C1q deficiency can augment IFN-α and promote broad immune dysregulation.[6] C-reactive protein (CRP), a member of the pentraxin family, also contributes to clearance of apoptotic debris. Polymorphisms in *CRP* have been associated with SLE and with decreased levels of CRP, but it remains unclear how much of the genetic contribution to basal CRP levels is due to variations within the gene itself versus variations in other genes.

Recent studies of families with a lupus-like disease, the Aicardi-Goutières syndrome, suggest that mutations in genes encoding nucleases that cleave either DNA or ribonucleic acid (RNA) might result in excess stimulatory nucleic acid and innate immune system activation.[7,8] Aicardi-Goutières and several related conditions are characterized by skin lesions, autoantibodies, central nervous system disease, and high levels of type I IFN. Mutations in the *TREX1* gene, encoding DNase III, a 3′-5′ exonuclease, as well as two additional genes, *RNASEH2* and *SAMHD1*, are associated with this syndrome.[9] A functional connection between *TREX1* and control of type I IFN production was demonstrated in a murine model in which *TREX1* deficiency resulted in increased levels of IFN-β.[10] A recent analysis of more than 8000 lupus patients found *TREX1* mutations in approximately 0.5% of patients. In addition, a common variant in the *TREX1* gene conferred an odds ratio for diagnosis of lupus of 1.73 compared with healthy controls.[11] Taken together, these recent demonstrations of association of rare genetic variants of enzymes that regulate degradation of nucleic acids with SLE point to the central role of those nucleic acids as triggers for immune system activation and disease.

A large number of lupus-associated single nucleotide polymorphisms (SNPs) are found in genes that encode proteins involved in induction of type I IFN or response to that family of cytokines.[12-14] IFN regulatory factor 5 (IRF5) and IRF7 are cytoplasmic proteins that translocate to the nucleus after effective activation of the endosomal TLRs by DNA or RNA. IRF5 and IRF7 then act as transcription factors to initiate transcription of IFN-α and other proinflammatory mediators. *TNFAIP3* encodes A20, a protein that regulates several proinflammatory cellular mechanisms including signaling through endosomal TLRs and activation of nuclear factor κB (NFκB).[15] Genetic variants in *IRF5*, *IRF7*, *TNFAIP3*, and numerous other lupus-associated genetic variants can be mapped to molecular pathways responsible for induction of innate immune system activation or responsiveness to its products, particularly IFN-α.

A third set of lupus-associated gene variants contributes to altered thresholds for lymphocyte activation or efficiency of cell activation. The ancestral MHC 8.1 haplotype that has been shown to be strongly associated with a diagnosis of SLE, along with other autoimmune diseases, appears to influence the early stages of immune system activation. Although more efficient presentation of self-antigens by disease-associated MHC class II alleles would seem to be the most likely mechanism by which the MHC risk haplotype confers predisposition to autoimmunity, available data point to a number of immune alterations, many focused on the T cell, in healthy individuals bearing the ancestral haplotype.[4] The impact of those alleles is best defined clinically as determining immune responses that generate particular autoantibody specificities, and the alleles seem to be important in determining whether anti-DNA autoantibodies, antibodies specific for RNA-associated proteins, or both types of autoantibodies can be induced and produced through T cell–dependent B cell differentiation.[16] Additional lupus-associated variants that alter adaptive immune system activation are involved in cytokine signaling such as STAT4 or efficiency of signaling downstream of the T and B cell surface antigen receptors such as PTPN22 in the case of both T and B cells and LYN, BANK, BLK, TNFAIP3, and others in the case of B cells.

A fourth category of lupus-associated genetic variants defines determinants of target organ damage. The understanding of genetic determinants of target organ vulnerability to immune mediated or oxidative damage is less well developed than is the role of genetic variants in altered immune system function in SLE, but identification of polymorphisms in members of the kallikrein gene family are associated with SLE and suggest areas for future investigation.[17] Table 79-1 lists many of the genetic variants documented to have a statistical association with a diagnosis of SLE.

Although impressive progress based on GWAS has identified statistical association of sequence variations in genes or genetic loci with a diagnosis of SLE, the functional consequences of those variations have not been extensively characterized. The best developed insights regarding the impact of lupus-associated variants on immune function have derived from studies of gene products involved in production of type I IFN. The risk alleles for IRF5 and IRF7 are associated with increased serum type I IFN activity in those patients who demonstrate autoantibodies targeting DNA or RNA-associated proteins.[12,18] Those studies support the hypothesis that nucleic acid–containing immune complexes are important stimuli that act through endosomal TLRs such as TLR7 and TLR9, those TLRs that mediate cell signals through the IRF5 and IRF7 transcription factors.

The impressive collaborative efforts that have successfully collected sufficient patient and control samples and performed the required genotyping and statistical analyses have defined or at least confirmed those molecular pathways that are central to the immunopathogenesis of SLE. The strong support for activation and altered regulation of the TLR pathway, along with variations in lymphocyte signaling, point to potential therapeutic targets for future study. In addition, the recent identification of less common mutations in enzymes required for degradation of intracellular nucleic acids suggests that further study of the TLR-independent pathways of innate immune system activation, mediated by nucleic acid sensors and their associated kinases

and adaptor molecules, might be another fruitful area for further investigation.

Subphenotype analysis will continue to amplify the information that can be gleaned from patient and control genotyping. A recent study of anti-dsDNA+ and anti-dsDNA− SLE patients, along with healthy controls, identified HLA-DR3, STAT4, and ITGAM as significantly associated with the presence of anti-dsDNA antibodies.[19] A case-only analysis additionally associated PTPN22, IRF5, and PTTG1 with anti-dsDNA antibodies. In contrast, a distinct group of lupus-associated genes showed comparable association between anti-dsDNA positive and negative patients, including FCGR2A, OX40L, IL10, PXK, UHRF1BP1, PRDM1, BLK, and IRAK1. Although it is possible that some of these variants are associated with distinct autoantibody specificities, it is more likely that they represent risks for other aspects of lupus pathogenesis, perhaps contributing to inflammation and tissue damage.

Whether the insights regarding specific genetic susceptibility factors can be used to predict development of lupus or particular manifestations of disease is as yet unclear. Recent studies have attempted to determine the predictive value of accumulated genetic risk variants. Although increased numbers of lupus-associated alleles are associated with some increased risk of disease and the number of lupus-associated genetic alleles is significantly higher in patients with anti-dsDNA antibodies than in those without those autoantibodies, at this time, it would not appear that genotyping for lupus risk is sufficiently informative to warrant practical application in patient management.[20]

FEMALE PREDOMINANCE OF SYSTEMIC LUPUS ERYTHEMATOSUS

A discussion of genetic contributions to SLE pathogenesis cannot ignore the dramatic 9:1 female predominance of the disease. Of all of the characteristic clinical features of lupus, it is the extreme sex skewing that remains least understood. Hormonal contributions to immune system activation are likely to represent a component of the female predominance of the disease; estrogen can modulate lymphocyte activation, and prolactin has been shown to be expressed at increased levels in lupus serum.[21]

Granting a contribution of hormones to increased immune activation, it would appear that additional concepts should be entertained to understand why 9 or 10 females are diagnosed with SLE for every male lupus patient. It is intriguing that Klinefelter's syndrome, characterized by a 47,XXY genotype, is increased 14-fold among men with SLE compared with men without SLE.[22] These data are proposed to support an X chromosome gene dose effect as an important contributor to SLE pathogenesis. Identifying the X chromosome as a possible risk factor for SLE provides a basis for new hypotheses regarding disease susceptibility, but the nature of that risk remains undefined. A possible role for altered regulation of epigenetic processes such as DNA methylation has been raised, and murine studies have supported the impact of duplications of portions of the X chromosome that encode the TLR7 gene in activation of the innate immune system, production of type I IFN, and generation of autoimmunity.[23] Investigation of altered gene dosage in human patients has not confirmed a similar duplication of the *TLR7* gene, and studies of DNA methylation are most suggestive of altered DNA methylation reflecting generalized immune activation rather than a primary etiologic event.[24] Further studies of epigenetic regulation of X chromosome structure and gene expression are warranted.

A potential pathogenic role for the distinct events that occur in the ovary compared with those in the testes also deserves further study. Onset of SLE most typically occurs in the childbearing years, after menarche and before menopause. A positive association between early menarche and SLE has been observed, and breastfeeding confers a protective effect.[25] Both observations might be consistent with molecular and cellular events related to ovulation as factors contributing to lupus pathogenesis. It is intriguing to consider that the biology of germ cell maturation, with female germ cells undergoing a second meiotic division before ovulation each month, might involve mechanisms and mediators that affect immune recognition. Although not yet fully understood, the carefully orchestrated demethylation and remethylation of DNA, along with the production of regulatory RNAs and RNA-associated proteins such as so-called PIWI proteins, in the germ cells and associated somatic cells might provide a source of stimulatory nucleic acid–containing complexes that could access TLR-dependent or TLR-independent pathways and result in immune activation.[26] The challenge in pursuing such concepts is the obvious limitation on access to ovarian tissue for study, although murine models might be helpful in that regard.

ENVIRONMENTAL TRIGGERS OF LUPUS

Concordance rates for development of SLE in identical twins range from 24% to 57%, and it is understood that both environmental factors and stochastic events (i.e., chance) contribute to development of SLE in an individual. Although some environmental triggers of disease have been identified on the basis of clinical observation and epidemiologic studies (Table 79-2), in general there is incomplete understanding of the range of factors that can induce disease and the mechanisms by which they do so. Socioeconomic factors have been demonstrated to contribute to poor outcomes in lupus patients, likely related to poor access to care.[27] The distinct contributions of low socioeconomic status versus genetic factors that impact disease severity in certain ethnic groups are difficult to dissect.

Clinical manifestations that are often present at the time of diagnosis including fatigue and arthralgias have suggested that a virus might initiate the disease. In fact, epidemiologic studies demonstrating higher prevalence of antibodies specific for Epstein-Barr virus (EBV) antigen in children with SLE compared with the general population, as well as higher frequency of anti-EBV antibodies in a military cohort before diagnosis of lupus, support a possible role for that virus in disease pathogenesis.[28] In addition, SLE patients demonstrate increased EBV DNA in blood.

Several potential mechanisms might account for a pathogenic role for EBV in SLE including production of EBV-encoded RNAs that induce type I IFN, utilization of B cell signaling pathways to promote B cell activation and differentiation, and generation of autoantibodies reactive

Table 79-2 Environmental Factors That Might Play a Role in the Pathogenesis of Systemic Lupus Erythematosus (SLE)

Definite
Ultraviolet B light

Probable
Estrogen and prolactin—in humans, female-to-male ratio is 9:1 between menarche and menopause, 3:1 in young and old
EBV
Lupus-inducing medications*
Hydralazine
Procainamide
Isoniazid
Hydantoins
Chlorpromazine
Methyldopa
Penicillamine
Minocycline
Tumor necrosis factor inhibitors
Interferon-α

Possible
Dietary factors
Alfalfa sprouts and related sprouting foods containing canavanine
Pristane and other hydrocarbons
Infectious agents other than EBV
Bacterial DNA
Smoking
Human retroviruses or endogenous retroelements
Endotoxins, bacterial lipopolysaccharides
Vitamin D deficiency

*Although each drug listed and many others can induce lupus-like symptoms in predisposed individuals, there is little evidence that they can induce true SLE or even activate disease in individuals with spontaneous, established SLE. If the clinical care of a patient with SLE would benefit from the use of one of these drugs, the drug should not be withheld.

DNA, deoxyribonucleic acid; EBV, Epstein-Barr virus.

with DNA or RNA-binding proteins through a molecular mimicry mechanism.[29] EBV-encoded small RNAs or EBERs are expressed in cells latently infected with EBV. EBERs induce expression of type I IFN after binding to the dsRNA-dependent protein kinase (PKR) and activating signaling through a TLR-independent pathway. Latent membrane protein 1, encoded by EBV, can act as a mimic of CD40 and promote B cell dysfunction and autoimmunity in lupus-susceptible mice.[30] A recent study demonstrates that antibodies specific for the virus-encoded EBNA-1 protein can also react with dsDNA.[31] The molecular basis of this apparent cross-reactivity is not known, although DNA can associate with EBNA-1 and might account for the described antibody reactivity. T cell responses specific for EBV have been studied in patients with lupus and found to be deficient, perhaps contributing to the increased numbers of EBV-infected mononuclear cells and increased copy number of EBV DNA found in SLE patients.[32]

Environmental toxins are of interest, yet their potential role in lupus pathogenesis has not been comprehensively explored. Data support current smoking as a risk factor for SLE, with a dose response relating pack years of smoking to risk. As is currently proposed with regard to pathogenesis of rheumatoid arthritis, smoking might provide an inflammatory stimulus to epithelial or mononuclear cells in the lungs, promoting protein modification or nonspecific inflammation. Silica has also been proposed as a potential pathogenic factor in SLE on the basis of its known capacity to serve as an adjuvant.[33]

Two well-described triggers of lupus, ultraviolet light and certain drugs, are likely to promote lupus pathogenesis through their effects on DNA. Ultraviolet (UV) light has many effects on skin cells including induction of DNA breaks that might alter gene expression or lead to apoptotic or necrotic cell death. Even in the absence of cell death, DNA breaks or prolonged maintenance of DNA-protein cross-links might provide either an adjuvant or antigenic stimulus to the immune system. Altered DNA methylation has been proposed as a likely mechanism of drug-induced lupus.[34] In the case of hydralazine, the drug inhibits extracellular signal-regulated kinase (ERK) pathway signaling, resulting in decreased expression of DNA methyltransferase 1 (DNMT1) and DNMT3a, two enzymes that mediate DNA methylation. Altered DNA methylation modifies gene expression and might also expose potential ligands for TLR-mediated immune system activation.

INNATE IMMUNE SYSTEM ACTIVATION IN SYSTEMIC LUPUS ERYTHEMATOSUS

Arguably the most significant recent advance that has improved understanding of the pathogenesis of SLE and other autoimmune and inflammatory diseases is the discovery of the TLRs and, more generally, the elucidation of the central role of innate immune system activation in regulation of the adaptive immune response, inflammation, and tissue repair. The TLRs are composed of an ectodomain with leucine-rich repeats, a transmembrane domain, and a cytoplasmic domain that associates with adaptor molecules that initiate signaling, resulting in activation of members of the IFN-regulatory factor family, NFκB, and members of the MAP kinase family. TLR-independent innate immune activation is initiated by intracytoplasmic nucleic acid sensors such as RIG-I and MDA5, which use distinct adaptors to trigger signal transduction through IRFs and the NFκB pathway. Over the past decade studies of nucleic acid–responsive TLRs and TLR-independent nucleic acid sensors that result in production of type I IFNs and other proinflammatory mediators have identified a direct pathogenic role for nucleic acids and nucleic acid–containing immune complexes as mediators of immune dysfunction in lupus. These studies complement the demonstration of broad expression of type I IFN-inducible genes in peripheral blood cells of lupus patients, referred to as the "IFN signature."[35-37] Together, the data point to the innate immune response and its products as significant factors in lupus pathogenesis. Table 79-3 describes many of the key components of the TLR-dependent and TLR-independent immune system pathways that are important in activation and control of lupus immune responses.

The endosomal TLRs, particularly TLR7, reactive with single-stranded RNA, and TLR9, reactive with unmethylated CpG-rich DNA, have been associated with lupus pathogenesis on the basis of in vitro studies that demonstrate activation of those TLRs by immune complexes that gain access to their intracytoplasmic compartment with the help of Fc receptors that bind the Fc fragment of

Table 79-3 Key Components of TLR-dependent and TLR-independent Innate Immune Response Pathways Relevant to the Pathogenesis of SLE

TLR-dependent Pathway
Receptors
Endosomal TLRs (TLR7 and TLR9) TLR4 TLR3?
Adaptors
Myeloid differentiation primary response gene 88 (MyD88) Toll/IL-1 receptor (TIR)-domain-containing adaptor protein (TIRAP) TIR-domain-containing adaptor protein inducing interferon-β (TRIF) TRIF-related adaptor molecule (TRAM) TNF receptor-associated factor 6 (TRAF6)
Kinases
Interleukin-1 receptor associated kinase-1 (IRAK1) IRAK4 Mitogen-activated protein kinase kinase kinase 7 (MAP3K7/TAK1) I-kappa B kinase alpha and beta (IKKα/β) I-kappa B kinase gamma (NEMO)
Transcription Factors
Interferon regulatory factor 3 (IRF3) IRF5 IRF7 Nuclear factor κB (NFκB)
Regulators
MyD88 short (MyD88s) Toll-interacting protein (TOLLIP) A20 (encoded by *TNFAIP3*)
TLR-independent Pathway
Receptors
Retinoic acid–inducible gene 1 (RIG-I) Melanoma differentiation-associated gene 5 (MDA5) DEXH box polypeptide 58 (DHX58/LGP2) Eukaryotic translation initiation factor 1-alpha kinase 2 (EIF2AK2/PKR) Z-DNA binding protein 1 (ZBP1/DAI)
Adaptors
Mitochondrial antiviral signaling protein (MAVS/IPS-1/VISA/CARDIF) Fas-associated via death domain (FADD) TRAF3
Kinases
Receptor-interacting serine threonine kinase 1 (RIP1) IKKε TANK-binding kinase 1 (TBK1)
Transcription Factors
IRF3 NFκB
Regulators
Tripartite motif-containing protein 25 (TRIM25) Ring finger protein 135 (RNF135) RNF125 Cyclindromatosis (CYLD) Heat shock protein 90 (HSP90)

SLE, systemic lupus erythematosus; TLR, Toll-like receptor.

immunoglobulin in the complex.[38-40] Clinical data demonstrating association of autoantibodies with specificity for RNA-binding proteins (such as Ro, La, Sm, and RNP) with high expression of IFN-induced genes in patient peripheral blood cells point to a significant role for RNA-containing immune complexes in innate immune activation and IFN production.[41] Associated neutrophil-derived proteins including high mobility group box 1 (HMGB1) and the cathelicidin protein LL37 can facilitate access of those immune complexes to the TLR-containing endosome. Lupus mice made deficient in one or another TLR have supported the role of TLR7 in generating type I IFN, autoantibodies specific for RNA-binding proteins and disease.[42] TLR9 activation can also generate IFN-α, but the findings from *TLR9*-deficient MRL/*lpr* mice have been somewhat confusing because those mice show more severe disease, suggesting that the activation of TLR9 might actually be protective. It appears that TLR9 activation can regulate the *TLR7* pathway, resulting in reduced production of RNA-related autoantibodies.[43] In addition to demonstrating

the important role of the endosomal TLRs in lupus pathogenesis, the data link TLR pathway activation with production of particular autoantibody specificities. These significant advances in characterization of the role of TLRs and the innate immune response in lupus disease have suggested new therapeutic approaches that are currently being pursued (Figure 79-2).

The elucidation of the mechanisms of induction of type I IFN, with plasmacytoid dendritic cells (pDCs) the major producers, have promoted studies that identified roles for additional cell types in amplification of this pathway. Platelets, largely ignored in studies of SLE pathogenesis, were shown to promote IFN production by pDCs through signals mediated by CD40 ligand (CD154) on activated platelets and CD40 on the pDCs.[44] One of the

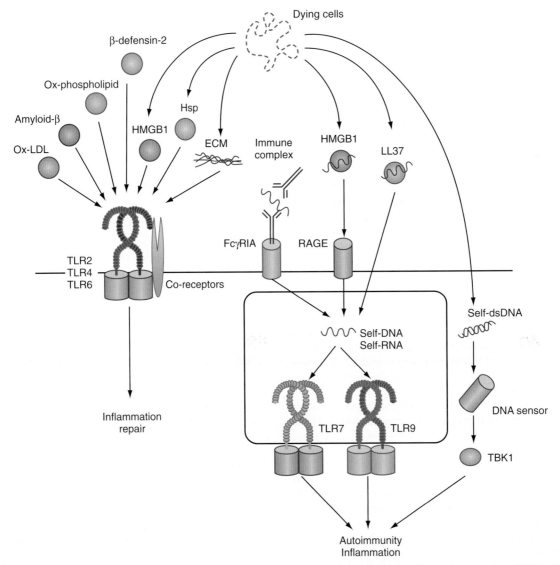

Figure 79-2 Endogenous stimuli for innate immune system activation. Endogenous molecules released by dying cells such as high mobility group box 1 (HMGB1) and β-defensins are recognized by cell surface Toll-like receptors (TLRs) and induce production of inflammatory mediators. Self-DNA or self-RNA, either in association with HMGB1 or LL37 or in the form of immune complexes that bind Fc receptors, is internalized into endosomal TLRs and transducer signals that result in transcription of type I interferon or proinflammatory cytokines. Self-nucleic acids can also be recognized by cytoplasmic sensors and trigger gene expression that contributes to immune activation, autoimmunity, and inflammation. DNA, deoxyribonucleic acid; ECM, extracellular matrix; Hsp, heat shock protein; LDL, low-density lipoprotein; RAGE, receptor for advanced glycation end products; RNA, ribonucleic acid; TBK1, TANK-binding kinase 1. *(From Kawai T, Akira S: The role of pattern-recognition receptors in innate immunity: update on Toll-like receptors, Nat Immunol 11:373–384, 2010.)*

initial microarray data sets demonstrating an IFN gene expression signature in peripheral blood cells of pediatric lupus patients also detected expression of genes that are typically expressed in granulocytes.[35] Recent studies from several groups have extended this observation and have documented low-density granulocytes in the circulation of lupus patients.[45]

Neutrophil extracellular traps (NETs) have gained attention as potential mediators of innate immune system activation. The NETs derive from a discrete cellular process, termed *NETosis*, in which aggregates of chromatin including DNA and its associated histones, HMGB1, LL37, elastase, and myeloperoxidase, are systematically extruded from nuclei into the extracellular environment. Generation of the NETs can be induced by interaction of neutrophils with vascular endothelial cells, activated platelets, or various cytokines. Recent data also implicate nucleosomes and RNA-containing immune complexes in the induction of NETosis.[46-48] Although NETs have only recently been linked to SLE, they present an intriguing and possibly significant mechanism that might account for observed alterations in immune function. They have the capacity to induce production of type I IFN by pDCs, serve as a source of relevant self-antigens for presentation to T lymphocytes, and mediate vascular damage and thrombosis.[49]

As described earlier, the elucidation of a significant role for the nucleic acid–sensing TLRs in recent years has drawn attention to the important role of autoantigen in driving disease in lupus. The contribution of apoptotic debris, either through increased apoptosis and/or impaired clearance of apoptotic cells, has been assumed for a number of years to be at least one likely mechanism that drives immune system activation and focuses its specificity on nucleic acids and their associated proteins. Apoptotic blebs are enriched in the typical targets of autoantibodies such as Ro and Sm. Recent attention on so-called *microparticles*, small membrane-enclosed particles released by activated and dying cells, has generated data demonstrating binding of those particles by some autoantibodies in lupus plasma.[50] A combination of increased generation of nuclear material, perhaps modified, and impaired clearance may be important mechanisms of lupus immunopathogenesis. The role of C1q and complement components in the clearance of apoptotic debris has been suggested as an explanation for the strong association of C1q, C2, and C4 deficiencies with SLE.[51] A second role for complement components that likely reduces the pathogenicity of immune complexes is the capacity of complement to solubilize immune complexes, reducing the likelihood that those complexes would deposit in tissue and cause damage.[52]

ADAPTIVE IMMUNE SYSTEM ALTERATIONS IN SYSTEMIC LUPUS ERYTHEMATOSUS

T cell function has been carefully studied in SLE patients for several decades, and deficiencies or alterations in signaling pathways, production of cytokines, cell proliferation, and regulatory functions have been documented.[53] CD4+ T cells are viewed as a requirement for development of lupus on the basis of their essential role in providing helper signals that drive differentiation of B cells to autoantibody-producing cells. Although some in vitro experiments have supported the capacity of cytokines such as IL-21 and B cell activating factor (BAFF)/B lymphocyte stimulator (BLyS) and TLR ligands to mediate antibody production by B cells, T cells are recognized as the most efficient drivers of B cell differentiation.[54]

The activation status and signaling mechanisms of lupus T cells are distinct from those of T cells from healthy individuals. Among the alterations in function is decreased proliferation in response to self-non–T cells or allogeneic-non–T cells or in response to presentation of soluble antigens. In contrast, T cell proliferation induced by direct activation of the T cell antigen receptor is at least as strong as observed in control cells. Lupus T cells readily express CD40 ligand (CD154) after activation and maintain expression of that important co-stimulatory molecule longer than control T cells, leading to augmented help for activation and differentiation of B cells exposed to those T cells. Another long-standing observation is that lupus T cells produce less IL-2 than control T cells, perhaps one factor that contributes to impaired generation of IL-2-dependent T regulatory cells. The molecular basis of the altered T cell activation in lupus patients is complex, but at least one factor might be the observed substitution of the T cell receptor zeta chain with the common gamma chain that is a component of the Fc receptor signaling machinery. Correction of this defect can normalize T cell signaling and IL-2 production.[55] Augmented calcium responses following T cell receptor ligation have been observed, and hyperpolarization of mitochondria in T cells has been associated with altered T cell activation and function.[56]

An interesting observation from studies of lupus T cells might reflect more global epigenetic alterations to the lupus genome that impact autoimmunity. Treatment of mouse and human T cells with 5-azacytidine resulted in increased expression of the lymphocyte function antigen-1 (LFA1; CD11a) adhesion molecule and increased proliferative responses to self-non–T cells.[57] Lupus T cells studied ex vivo show hypomethylation of CG-rich areas of the genome, and a recent report of genome methylation in identical twins discordant for lupus demonstrated relatively less methylation of the twin with active lupus.[24] Multiple mechanisms have been postulated to contribute to DNA demethylation in lupus lymphocytes including increased expression of growth arrest and DNA damage-induced 45alpha (GADD45alpha), a protein that removes methyl groups from DNA, decreased expression of DNAMT1, and ERK pathway signaling.[34]

Generalized lymphopenia is typical of SLE, but expansions of specific T cell populations have been described. The recently documented T follicular helper population, characterized by expression of ICOS, CXCR5, and Bcl6 and by production of IL-21, mediates important signals that promote differentiation of autoantigen-specific B cells.[58,59] A population of CD8+ cells with a memory phenotype is associated with poor prognosis, possibly based on tissue damage mediated by those cells.[60]

The regulation and function of T regulatory cells (Tregs), with capacity to suppress immune responses, and Th17 cells, which promote inflammation by production of IL-17, have been intensively studied in recent years. Some studies of lupus patients do show a relative depletion of Tregs and increased Th17 cells and IL-17.[61] The functional impact of those alterations in human lupus is still not clear.

Cytokine production is altered in SLE, with decreased production of IL-2 a characteristic feature of patient T cells, as it is of individuals carrying the HLA 8.1 haplotype.[4] Athough this deficiency in IL-2 was initially linked to the often poor proliferative responses of lupus T cells stimulated with autologous or allogeneic T cells or soluble antigen, the recognition that IL-2 is important for maintenance of T regulatory cells suggests another mechanism through which impaired production of IL-2 might contribute to immune system activation and autoimmunity.[62]

B cell regulation is also impaired in SLE, contributing to differentiation to production of autoantibodies and cytokines. The activated phenotype of SLE B cells has the potential to promote efficient presentation of specific self-antigens to T cells. It has not been entirely clear whether altered B cell function is strictly secondary to increased availability of T cell help, B cell survival, proliferation and differentiation factors, and signaling through TLRs or whether primary B cell dysfunction also contributes to autoimmunity. Recent studies characterizing the B cell repertoire using single-cell polymerase chain reaction and cloning of individual immunoglobulin transcripts will permit improved understanding of the role of altered B cell tolerance mechanisms in the bone marrow versus secondary effects of T cell and cytokine help in generating self-reactive antibody specificities. BAFF/BLyS, IL-10, and IL-21 are among the candidate therapeutic targets that could modify the B cell differentiation program, a suggestion supported by clinical studies of BAFF/BLyS blockade. An additional approach toward improved regulation of B cell function is suggested by recent data demonstrating an association between vitamin D deficiency and presence of antinuclear antibodies in healthy individuals and increased B cell activation and serum type I IFN activity in vitamin D–deficient SLE patients.[63]

The baseline activation status of lupus B cells, as well as their response to antigen stimulation, is altered when compared with B cells from healthy individuals, and current studies are exploring the functional implications of lupus-associated genetic variants in several kinases, phosphatases, and adaptor molecules such as BLK, BANK, and PTPN22 for B cell function. Studies of the risk variant of *PTPN22* in B cells from healthy subjects point to the influence of that lupus-associated variant on impaired counterselection of self-reactive B cells.[64] *LYN* deficiency in mice is associated with a lupus-like phenotype, and similar deficiencies in the LYN kinase have been described in lupus B cells.[65] Polymorphisms in the gene encoding Lyn studied in European-descent individuals could potentially impact B cell signaling and autoimmunity.[66] The gene encoding the inhibitory Fc receptor, *FCGR2B*, is polymorphic, and several variants have been associated with SLE.[67,68] SLE B cells show decreased expression of this FcR and altered cytokine production when engaged by immune complexes. Interestingly, the inhibitory capacity of FcγRIIb can be exploited using an engineered bifunctional antibody that coligates CD19 and FcγRIIb.[69] This antibody suppressed B cell functions in a mouse engrafted with human B cells.

Current investigations of antibody-producing cells are defining several categories of B lineage cells that contribute to autoimmunity and disease. Long-lived plasma cells that are maintained by chemokines and stromal cell products in protective niches in the bone marrow are proposed as sources of those lupus autoantibodies such as anti-Sm and anti-Ro that are chronically maintained at fairly constant levels. Those antibodies have been refractory to modulation by immunosuppressive or B cell depletion therapy.[70] In contrast, circulating preplasma cells or plasmablasts are sources of anti-dsDNA antibodies that fluctuate in some patients in association with variations in disease activity and might be more amenable to anti–B cell therapy.[71]

The T and B cell alterations that have been described in studies of lupus immune function are undoubtedly a reflection of multiple genetic variations that play out in altering threshold for cell activation and efficiency of cell signaling. They are also the result of interactions among those lymphocytes, along with antigen-presenting cells and their products, that over time amplify the overall level of immune activation. Increased production of type I IFN and presence of antinuclear antibodies in healthy family members of lupus patients likely reflect the consequences of genetic variations that are among the factors that predispose to SLE. When the circuits of immune activation are amplified by environmental triggers, conditions are in place to generate the characteristic T and B cell autoimmunity that is required for tissue damage and disease.

AUTOIMMUNITY IN SYSTEMIC LUPUS ERYTHEMATOSUS

Autoantibodies are traditionally viewed as essential mediators of pathology in SLE, particularly when they are in the form of immune complexes. Virtually all lupus patients demonstrate a positive antinuclear antibody test, and the majority of patients have one or more of the characteristic autoantibody specificities that have been associated with lupus (see also Chapter 55). Among those, anti-dsDNA and anti-Smith (Sm) are most specific for SLE. Interestingly, those specificities have been linked functionally in murine studies that demonstrate that dsDNA can bind to a peptide comprising amino acids 83-119 of the SmD1 protein, and T cells specific for that peptide provide help for production of anti-dsDNA antibody.[72,73] Anti-Ro, anti-La, and anti-RNP antibodies are characteristic of SLE but are also seen in other systemic autoimmune diseases. These characteristic autoantibodies in SLE can be categorized in relation to their targets including DNA and DNA-binding proteins, typically aggregated in nucleosomes that contain histones; RNA and RNA-associated proteins, typically aggregated in cytoplasmic or nuclear ribonucleoprotein particles; phospholipids exposed in plasma membranes and associated proteins such as β_2-glycoprotein I; and cell membrane proteins, typically those expressed on blood cells. Some of these self-antigens typically targeted by lupus autoantibodies are most likely accessed by antigen-presenting cells in the form of cell membrane–enclosed blebs derived from apoptotic cells or microparticles, small aggregates of cellular material derived from cells and generated after flipping of phosphatidylserine to the outer aspect of the cell membrane in the setting of cell activation or apoptosis. Although some patients who present with a clinical picture characteristic of SLE do not have significant titers of those autoantibodies, it is likely that those patients have undefined autoimmunity targeted at unspecified antigens.

The pathogenic antibodies in SLE tend to be those produced by cells that are far along in the B cell differentiation process, either preplasma cells or plasma cells, and have undergone immunoglobulin class switching, a process that is driven by CD4+ T helper cells and in some cases by TLR ligands together with B cell differentiation factors such as IL-21 and BLyS/BAFF.[54] It is not possible to define the earliest step in the generation of pathogenic autoantibodies, and in fact it is probable that the generation of autoimmunity can begin in any number of ways. Presentation of self-antigen by an excessively activated antigen-presenting cell, stochastic activation of low-avidity self-reactive T cells that are present in healthy individuals but have the potential to expand and drive differentiation of B cells with broad specificity for self-antigens, or direct activation of self-reactive B cells in the presence of activating TLR ligands such as those provided by demethylated CpG-rich DNA from bacteria or viruses or self-derived nuclear debris might all be starting points for development of pathogenic autoimmunity. The process might begin with production of type I IFN by a virus-infected cell or a cell with impaired degradation of intracellular nucleic acids, altering the threshold for activation of the immune system by subsequent exposures to self-antigens. Less important than the precise starting point is the observation that autoimmunity develops and builds over time, with presence of autoantibodies observed more than 5 years before clinical manifestations of disease appear and the range of specificities of antigens targeted expanding over time.[74] The data from analysis of prevalence of several lupus autoantibodies among sera collected from members of the military who later developed SLE demonstrate an intriguing sequence, with anti-Ro antibodies typically presenting earliest, anti-dsDNA antibodies appearing several years later, and anti-Sm, the antibody specificity most specific for a diagnosis of SLE, appearing approximately at the time of clinical diagnosis. This pattern, along with studies from murine models demonstrating determinant spreading of autoantibody specificities not only to distinct proteins within a nucleic acid–protein particle but also to other self-antigen targets, provides clues to lupus pathogenesis that are not yet understood but hold promise for future breakthroughs in elucidating important pathogenic mechanisms.[75] Additional autoantibody specificities that are associated with lupus activity and with proliferative lupus nephritis and are thought to be pathogenic include those reactive with C1q. Anti-C1q antibodies appear to recognize neoepitopes of C1q when it is bound to early apoptotic cells.[76]

A shift from a predominant polyclonal IgM picture toward polyclonal IgG, driven by T cell help and cytokines, occurs over time in most patients with lupus and with development of tissue pathology and damage. In fact, some IgM antibodies that have self-reactivity are viewed as protective, with the switch from IgM to IgG or IgA representing an important point of altered immune regulation that contributes to the immunopathogenesis of SLE. Some of these IgM natural antibodies react with apoptotic cells and actually inhibit their activation through TLRs.[77]

In addition to immunoglobulin class, with class-switched antibodies better able to access extravascular spaces compared with IgM antibodies, amino acid sequence and charge of the antigen-binding site can influence pathogenicity. Arginines in the CDR3 region of anti-dsDNA antibodies are characteristic and influence binding to their DNA target. Molecular mimicry is a concept that has been applied to reactivity of antibodies specific for a microbial protein that also react with self-antigens, but the concept can also be applied to those antibodies that unexpectedly bind to two distinct self-antigens. For example, some anti-dsDNA antibodies were found to bind to a peptide that is a feature of glutamate receptors on central nervous system neurons.[78] Beyond features of Ig class and antigen-binding site that influence access to tissue and affinity of binding, glycosylation and complement-fixing capacity are important determinants of the antibody's capacity to bind to Fc receptors and promote complement activation, resulting in target cell death or inflammation.

The role of SLE autoantibodies in the pathogenesis of the disease has traditionally focused on the deposition of immune complexes in skin, renal glomerulus, and other sites of tissue injury, along with a potential contribution of direct targeting of antibodies to local or "planted" antigens. But in recent years, with the recognition that nucleic acid–containing immune complexes can directly induce cell signaling and new gene transcription after accessing endosomal TLRs, an additional important pathogenic role for autoantibodies as immune modulators has been defined.

Particular lupus autoantibody specificities have been associated with specific clinical manifestations of disease (Table 79-4). Perhaps the best developed characterization of the mechanisms by which an autoantibody mediates disease is the role of maternal-derived anti-Ro antibody in the neonatal lupus syndrome. After transplacental transfer of anti-Ro antibody, RNA-containing immune complexes are proposed to form, activating the production of cytokines that contribute to fibrosis of the cardiac conduction system.[79] This scenario, similar to that which mediates production of type I IFN by pDCs, identifies nucleic acid–autoantibody immune complexes as regulators of cytokine production that results in tissue damage. Anti-Ro and anti-La antibodies, although common to several autoimmune diseases, are also characteristic in association with sicca symptoms, subacute cutaneous lupus, and, as noted, in neonatal lupus. Anti-RNP antibodies are seen in both SLE and mixed connective tissue disease.

Antiphospholipid antibodies, with lupus anticoagulant the most informative antibody profile, contribute to placental damage and vascular thrombosis, as well as thrombocytopenia in the antiphospholipid syndrome and in some patients with lupus. Recent studies in a murine model indicate that tissue damage and thrombosis depend on activation of the complement system by the antiphospholipid antibodies.[80] Similar mechanisms might be relevant in forms of lupus renal disease characterized by microangiopathy.

Table 79-4 Correlation among Clinical Manifestations of Systemic Lupus Erythematosus and Autoantibodies, Immune Complexes, and T Cells

Manifestation	Autoantibodies	Immune Complexes	T Cells
Nephritis	Anti-dsDNA	+	+
	Anti-Ro		
	Anti-C1q		
	Ids 16/6, 3I and GN2		
Arthritis	?	+	+
Dermatitis	Anti-Ro		+
	Anti-dsDNA		
	Id 16/6		
Vasculitis	Anti-Ro	+	+
Central nervous system	Antiribosomal P	+	
	Antineuronal		
	Anti-NR2		
Hematologic:			
Lymphopenia	Antilymphocyte		
Hemolysis	Antierythrocyte		
Thrombocytopenia	Antiplatelet	+	
Clotting	Antiphospholipid		
Fetal loss	Antiphospholipid		
Neonatal lupus	Anti-Ro		
Sicca syndrome	Anti-Ro		+
Mild disease	Anti-RNP without		
	other autoantibody		
	except antinuclear antibody		

MECHANISMS OF TARGET ORGAN DAMAGE

Clinical disease is ultimately a reflection of tissue damage mediated by the inflammatory sequelae of the described autoimmunity and immune system activation, along with an exaggerated or aberrant repair response. The classic view of the mechanisms that result in tissue damage involves activation of the complement system by immune complexes deposited in tissue, as well as release of products of phagocytes including enzymes released from neutrophil granules and reactive oxygen intermediates from macrophages. Recent studies in mouse and human systems involving extensive analysis of renal infiltrating cells at various points in the disease process have identified a monocyte population that has undergone differentiation to generate a functional phenotype that mediates what is apparently uncontrolled tissue repair, contributing to sclerosis and organ dysfunction.[81] Studies in a murine model have shown that IFN-α can also contribute to development of crescents in lupus kidneys.[82]

The role of the vasculature as a significant target organ contributing to disease in lupus has once again come to the fore, after several decades that have focused predominantly on the immune system and the contributions of autoantibodies to pathology.[83] Altered structure and function of both venous and arterial vessels have been noted for many years including the periarteriolar concentric onion skinning seen in spleen, microangiopathy and associated microthrombi seen in some organs, and the endothelial dysfunction that has been associated with premature atherosclerosis in lupus patients. Recent studies have focused on the potential role of type I IFN on endothelial cells and endothelial cell progenitor cells and have postulated that increased production of IFN is at least one contributor to impaired vascular repair.[84] A role for granulocytes and proinflammatory lipids has also been proposed.[49,85] Characterization of the micropathology of the vasculature in Degos disease, a syndrome with some common pathologic features with SLE, has drawn attention to the association of activation of the IFN pathway with vascular sclerosis and endothelial damage.[86] A possible direct contribution of type I IFN to vascular injury supplements the previously described role of complement activation products C3a and C5a and expression of endothelial cell surface adhesion molecules E-selectin, vascular cell adhesion molecule 1 (VCAM-1), and intercellular adhesion molecule 1 (ICAM-1) in lupus flares.

SUMMARY

Considerable gains in understanding mechanisms of lupus pathogenesis have established the knowledge base that will underlie future advances in development of targeted therapies that will improve patient outcomes. The recognition of a central role for innate immune system activation including the role of type I IFN in lupus pathogenesis has been a major advance in recent years. Rapid progress in characterizing the genetic variants that are associated with a diagnosis of lupus has provided strong support for alterations in molecular pathways that regulate nucleic acid degradation, TLR signaling and lymphocyte activation thresholds, and signaling efficiency as important mechanisms that determine disease susceptibility. The products of the immune system including autoantibodies and their immune complexes, cytokines, and complement components, along with proinflammatory mediators and reactive oxygen products released from neutrophils and macrophages, remain key mediators of tissue damage. But an additional pathogenic role for nucleic acid–containing immune complexes as immune modulators through their important capacity to access and activate endosomal TLRs is an important new concept that can guide future therapeutic approaches. Targeting the components of innate immune system activation that affect the TLR pathway along with modulation of T cell help for B cell differentiation to autoantibody-producing cells would appear to be a rational therapeutic strategy in light of our current understanding of pathogenic mechanisms.

References

1. Harley JB, Alarcon-Riquelme ME, Criswell LA, et al: Genome-wide association scan in women with systemic lupus erythematosus identifies susceptibility variants in ITGAM, PXK, KIAA1542 and other loci, *Nat Genet* 40(2):204–210, 2008.
2. Hom G, Graham RR, Modrek B, et al: Association of systemic lupus erythematosus with C8orf13-BLK and ITGAM-ITGAX, *N Engl J Med* 358(9):900–909, 2008.
3. Deng Y, Tsao BP: Genetic susceptibility to systemic lupus erythematosus in the genomic era, *Nat Rev Rheumatol* 6(12):683–692, 2010.
4. Price P, Witt C, Allcock R, et al: The genetic basis for the association of the 8.1 ancestral haplotype (A1, B8, DR3) with multiple immunopathological diseases, *Immunol Rev* 167:257–274, 1999.
5. Mevorach D: Clearance of dying cells and systemic lupus erythematosus: the role of C1q and the complement system, *Apoptosis* 15(9):1114–1123, 2010.
6. Santer DM, Hall BE, George TC, et al: C1q deficiency leads to the defective suppression of IFN-alpha in response to nucleoprotein containing immune complexes, *J Immunol* 185(8):4738–4749, 2010.
7. Rice G, Newman WG, Dean J, et al: Heterozygous mutations in *TREX1* cause familial chilblain lupus and dominant Aicardi-Goutieres syndrome, *Am J Hum Genet* 80(4):811–815, 2007.
8. Lee-Kirsch MA, Gong M, Chowdhury D, et al: Mutations in the gene encoding the 3′-5′ DNA exonuclease TREX1 are associated with systemic lupus erythematosus, *Nat Genet* 39(9):1065–1067, 2007.
9. Rice GI, Bond J, Asipu A, et al: Mutations involved in Aicardi-Goutieres syndrome implicate SAMHD1 as regulator of the innate immune response, *Nat Genet* 41(7):829–832, 2009.
10. Stetson DB, Ko JS, Heidmann T, Medzhitov R: Trex1 prevents cell-intrinsic initiation of autoimmunity, *Cell* 134(4):587–598, 2008.
11. Namjou B, Kothari PH, Kelly JA, et al: Evaluation of the *TREX1* gene in a large multi-ancestral lupus cohort, *Genes Immun* 12(4):270–279, 2011.
12. Niewold TB, Kelly JA, Flesch MH, et al: Association of the IRF5 risk haplotype with high serum interferon-alpha activity in systemic lupus erythematosus patients, *Arthritis Rheum* 58(8):2481–2487, 2008.
13. Kariuki SN, Franek BS, Kumar AA, et al: Trait-stratified genome-wide association study identifies novel and diverse genetic associations with serologic and cytokine phenotypes in systemic lupus erythematosus, *Arthritis Res Ther* 12(4):R151, 2010.
14. Ramos PS, Williams AH, Ziegler JT, et al: Genetic analyses of interferon pathway-related genes reveals multiple new loci associated with systemic lupus erythematosus (SLE), *Arthritis Rheum* 63:2049–2057, 2011.
15. Boone DL, Turer EE, Lee EG, et al: The ubiquitin-modifying enzyme A20 is required for termination of Toll-like receptor responses, *Nat Immunol* 5(10):1052–1060, 2004.
16. Graham RR, Ortmann W, Rodine P, et al: Specific combinations of HLA-DR2 and DR3 class II haplotypes contribute graded risk for disease susceptibility and autoantibodies in human SLE, *Eur J Hum Genet* 15(8):823–830, 2007.
17. Liu K, Li QZ, Delgado-Vega AM, et al: Kallikrein genes are associated with lupus and glomerular basement membrane-specific antibody-induced nephritis in mice and humans, *J Clin Invest* 119(4):911–923, 2009.
18. Salloum R, Franek BS, Kariuki SN, et al: Genetic variation at the IRF7/PHRF1 locus is associated with autoantibody profile and serum interferon-alpha activity in lupus patients, *Arthritis Rheum* 62(2):553–561, 2010.
19. Chung SA, Taylor KE, Graham RR, et al: Differential genetic associations for systemic lupus erythematosus based on anti-dsDNA autoantibody production, *PLoS Genet* 7(3):e1001323, 2011.
20. Taylor KE, Chung SA, Graham RR, et al: Risk alleles for systemic lupus erythematosus in a large case-control collection and associations with clinical subphenotypes, *PLoS Genet* 7(2):e1001311, 2011.
21. Cohen-Solal JF, Jeganathan V, Hill L, et al: Hormonal regulation of B-cell function and systemic lupus erythematosus, *Lupus* 17(6):528–532, 2008.
22. Scofield RH, Bruner GR, Namjou B, et al: Klinefelter's syndrome (47,XXY) in male systemic lupus erythematosus patients: support for the notion of a gene-dose effect from the X chromosome, *Arthritis Rheum* 58(8):2511–2517, 2008.
23. Deane JA, Pisitkun P, Barrett RS, et al: Control of Toll-like receptor 7 expression is essential to restrict autoimmunity and dendritic cell proliferation, *Immunity* 27(5):801–810, 2007.
24. Javierre BM, Fernandez AF, Richter J, et al: Changes in the pattern of DNA methylation associate with twin discordance in systemic lupus erythematosus, *Genome Res* 20(2):170–179, 2010.
25. Costenbader KH, Feskanich D, Stampfer MJ, Karlson EW: Reproductive and menopausal factors and risk of systemic lupus erythematosus in women, *Arthritis Rheum* 56(4):1251–1262, 2007.
26. Castañeda J, Genzor P, Bortvin A: piRNAs, transposon silencing, and germline genome integrity, *Mutat Res* 714:95–104, 2011.
27. Alarcon GS, Calvo-Alen J, McGwin G Jr, et al: Systemic lupus erythematosus in a multiethnic cohort: LUMINA XXXV. Predictive factors of high disease activity over time, *Ann Rheum Dis* 65(9):1168–1174, 2006.
28. Moon UY, Park SJ, Oh ST, et al: Patients with systemic lupus erythematosus have abnormally elevated Epstein-Barr virus load in blood, *Arthritis Res Ther* 6(4):R295–302, 2004.
29. Poole BD, Templeton AK, Guthridge JM, et al: Aberrant Epstein-Barr viral infection in systemic lupus erythematosus, *Autoimmun Rev* 8(4):337–342, 2009.
30. Peters AL, Stunz LL, Meyerholz DK, et al: Latent membrane protein 1, the EBV-encoded oncogenic mimic of CD40, accelerates autoimmunity in B6.Sle1 mice, *J Immunol* 185(7):4053–4062, 2010.
31. Yadav P, Tran H, Ebegbe R, et al: Antibodies elicited in response to EBNA-1 may cross-react with dsDNA, *PLoS One* 6(1):e14488, 2011.
32. Kang I, Quan T, Nolasco H, et al: Defective control of latent Epstein-Barr virus infection in systemic lupus erythematosus, *J Immunol* 172(2):1287–1294, 2004.
33. Costenbader KH, Kim DJ, Peerzada J, et al: Cigarette smoking and the risk of systemic lupus erythematosus: a meta-analysis, *Arthritis Rheum* 50(3):849–857, 2004.
34. Gorelik G, Fang JY, Wu A, et al: Impaired T cell protein kinase C delta activation decreases ERK pathway signaling in idiopathic and hydralazine-induced lupus, *J Immunol* 179(8):5553–5563, 2007.
35. Bennett L, Palucka AK, Arce E, et al: Interferon and granulopoiesis signatures in systemic lupus erythematosus blood, *J Exp Med* 197(6):711–723, 2003.
36. Baechler EC, Batliwalla FM, Karypis G, et al: Interferon-inducible gene expression signature in peripheral blood cells of patients with severe lupus, *Proc Natl Acad Sci U S A* 100(5):2610–2615, 2003.
37. Crow MK, Kirou KA, Wohlgemuth J: Microarray analysis of interferon-regulated genes in SLE, *Autoimmunity* 36(8):481–490, 2003.
38. Lovgren T, Eloranta ML, Bave U, et al: Induction of interferon-alpha production in plasmacytoid dendritic cells by immune complexes containing nucleic acid released by necrotic or late apoptotic cells and lupus IgG, *Arthritis Rheum* 50(6):1861–1872, 2004.
39. Bave U, Magnusson M, Eloranta ML, et al: Fc gamma RIIa is expressed on natural IFN-alpha-producing cells (plasmacytoid dendritic cells) and is required for the IFN-alpha production induced by apoptotic cells combined with lupus IgG, *J Immunol* 171(6):3296–3302, 2003.
40. Barrat FJ, Meeker T, Gregorio J, et al: Nucleic acids of mammalian origin can act as endogenous ligands for Toll-like receptors and may promote systemic lupus erythematosus, *J Exp Med* 202(8):1131–1139, 2005.
41. Kirou KA, Lee C, George S, et al: Activation of the interferon-alpha pathway identifies a subgroup of systemic lupus erythematosus patients with distinct serologic features and active disease, *Arthritis Rheum* 52(5):1491–1503, 2005.
42. Christensen SR, Shupe J, Nickerson K, et al: Toll-like receptor 7 and TLR9 dictate autoantibody specificity and have opposing inflammatory and regulatory roles in a murine model of lupus, *Immunity* 25(3):417–428, 2006.
43. Nickerson KM, Christensen SR, Shupe J, et al: TLR9 regulates TLR7- and MyD88-dependent autoantibody production and disease in a murine model of lupus, *J Immunol* 184(4):1840–1848, 2010.

44. Duffau P, Seneschal J, Nicco C, et al: Platelet CD154 potentiates interferon-alpha secretion by plasmacytoid dendritic cells in systemic lupus erythematosus, *Sci Transl Med* 2(47):47ra63, 2010.

45. Denny MF, Yalavarthi S, Zhao W, et al: A distinct subset of proinflammatory neutrophils isolated from patients with systemic lupus erythematosus induces vascular damage and synthesizes type I IFNs, *J Immunol* 184(6):3284–3297, 2010.

46. Lindau D, Ronnefarth V, Erbacher A, et al: Nucleosome-induced neutrophil activation occurs independently of TLR9 and endosomal acidification: implications for systemic lupus erythematosus, *Eur J Immunol* 41(3):669–681, 2011.

47. Garcia-Romo GS, Caielli S, Vega B, et al: Netting neutrophils are major inducers of type I IFN production in pediatric systemic lupus erythematosus, *Sci Transl Med* 3(73):73ra20, 2011.

48. Lande R, Ganguly D, Facchinetti V, et al: Neutrophils activate plasmacytoid dendritic cells by releasing self-DNA-peptide complexes in systemic lupus erythematosus, *Sci Transl Med* 3(73):73ra19, 2011.

49. Villanueva E, Yalavarthi S, Berthier CC, et al: Netting neutrophils induce endothelial damage, infiltrate tissues, and expose immunostimulatory molecules in systemic lupus erythematosus, *J Immunol* 187(1):538–552, 2011.

50. Ullal AJ, Reich CF 3rd, Clowse M, et al: Microparticles as antigenic targets of antibodies to DNA and nucleosomes in systemic lupus erythematosus, *J Autoimmun* 36(3-4):173–180, 2011.

51. Gullstrand B, Martensson U, Sturfelt G, et al: Complement classical pathway components are all important in clearance of apoptotic and secondary necrotic cells, *Clin Exp Immunol* 156(2):303–311, 2009.

52. Johnston A, Auda GR, Kerr MA, et al: Dissociation of primary antigen-antibody bonds is essential for complement mediated solubilization of immune precipitates, *Mol Immunol* 29(5):659–665, 1992.

53. Crispin JC, Kyttaris VC, Terhorst C, Tsokos GC: T cells as therapeutic targets in SLE, *Nat Rev Rheumatol* 6(6):317–325, 2010.

54. Ettinger R, Sims GP, Robbins R, et al: IL-21 and BAFF/BLyS synergize in stimulating plasma cell differentiation from a unique population of human splenic memory B cells, *J Immunol* 178(5):2872–2882, 2007.

55. Nambiar MP, Fisher CU, Warke VG, et al: Reconstitution of deficient T cell receptor zeta chain restores T cell signaling and augments T cell receptor/CD3-induced interleukin-2 production in patients with systemic lupus erythematosus, *Arthritis Rheum* 48(7):1948–1955, 2003.

56. Fernandez D, Bonilla E, Mirza N, et al: Rapamycin reduces disease activity and normalizes T cell activation-induced calcium fluxing in patients with systemic lupus erythematosus, *Arthritis Rheum* 54(9):2983–2988, 2006.

57. Richardson B: DNA methylation and autoimmune disease, *Clin Immunol* 109(1):72–79, 2003.

58. Simpson N, Gatenby PA, Wilson A, et al: Expansion of circulating T cells resembling follicular helper T cells is a fixed phenotype that identifies a subset of severe systemic lupus erythematosus, *Arthritis Rheum* 62(1):234–244, 2010.

59. Choi YS, Kageyama R, Eto D, et al: ICOS receptor instructs T follicular helper cell versus effector cell differentiation via induction of the transcriptional repressor Bcl6, *Immunity* 34(6):932–946, 2011.

60. McKinney EF, Lyons PA, Carr EJ, et al: A CD8+ T cell transcription signature predicts prognosis in autoimmune disease, *Nat Med* 16(5):586–591, 2010.

61. Xing Q, Wang B, Su H, et al: Elevated Th17 cells are accompanied by FoxP3+ Treg cells decrease in patients with lupus nephritis, *Rheumatol Int* 32(4):949–958, 2012.

62. Lieberman LA, Tsokos GC: The IL-2 defect in systemic lupus erythematosus disease has an expansive effect on host immunity, *J Biomed Biotechnol* 2010:740619, 2010.

63. Ritterhouse LL, Crowe SR, Niewold TB, et al: Vitamin D deficiency is associated with an increased autoimmune response in healthy individuals and in patients with systemic lupus erythematosus, *Ann Rheum Dis* 70:1569–1574, 2011.

64. Menard L, Saadoun D, Isnardi I, et al: The *PTPN22* allele encoding an R620W variant interferes with the removal of developing autoreactive B cells in humans, *J Clin Invest* 121:3635–3644, 2011.

65. Flores-Borja F, Kabouridis PS, Jury EC, et al: Decreased LYN expression and translocation to lipid raft signaling domains in B lymphocytes from patients with systemic lupus erythematosus, *Arthritis Rheum* 52(12):3955–3965, 2005.

66. Lu R, Vidal GS, Kelly JA, Delgado-Vega AM, et al: Genetic associations of LYN with systemic lupus erythematosus, *Genes Immun* 10(5):397–403, 2009.

67. Li X, Wu J, Carter RH, Edberg JC, et al: A novel polymorphism in the Fcgamma receptor IIB (CD32B) transmembrane region alters receptor signaling, *Arthritis Rheum* 48(11):3242–3252, 2003.

68. Blank MC, Stefanescu RN, Masuda E, et al: Decreased transcription of the human FCGR2B gene mediated by the -343 G/C promoter polymorphism and association with systemic lupus erythematosus, *Hum Genet* 117(2-3):220–227, 2005.

69. Horton HM, Chu SY, Ortiz EC, et al: Antibody-mediated coengagement of FcgammaRIIb and B cell receptor complex suppresses humoral immunity in systemic lupus erythematosus, *J Immunol* 186(7):4223–4233, 2011.

70. Hiepe F, Dorner T, Hauser AE, et al: Long-lived autoreactive plasma cells drive persistent autoimmune inflammation, *Nat Rev Rheumatol* 7(3):170–178, 2011.

71. Jacobi AM, Mei H, Hoyer BF, et al: HLA-DRhigh/CD27high plasmablasts indicate active disease in patients with systemic lupus erythematosus, *Ann Rheum Dis* 69(1):305–308, 2010.

72. Dieker JW, Van Bavel CC, Riemekasten G, et al: The binding of lupus-derived autoantibodies to the C-terminal peptide (83–119) of the major SmD1 autoantigen can be mediated by double-stranded DNA and nucleosomes, *Ann Rheum Dis* 65(11):1525–1528, 2006.

73. Langer S, Langnickel D, Enghard P, et al: The systemic and SmD183–119-autoantigen-specific cytokine memory of Th cells in SLE patients, *Rheumatology (Oxford)* 46(2):238–245, 2007.

74. Arbuckle MR, McClain MT, Rubertone MV, et al: Development of autoantibodies before the clinical onset of systemic lupus erythematosus, *N Engl J Med* 349(16):1526–1533, 2003.

75. Jiang C, Deshmukh US, Gaskin F, et al: Differential responses to Smith D autoantigen by mice with HLA-DR and HLA-DQ transgenes: dominant responses by HLA-DR3 transgenic mice with diversification of autoantibodies to small nuclear ribonucleoprotein, double-stranded DNA, and nuclear antigens, *J Immunol* 184(2):1085–1091, 2010.

76. Bigler C, Schaller M, Perahud I, et al: Autoantibodies against complement C1q specifically target C1q bound on early apoptotic cells, *J Immunol* 183(5):3512–3521, 2009.

77. Chen Y, Khanna S, Goodyear CS, et al: Regulation of dendritic cells and macrophages by an anti-apoptotic cell natural antibody that suppresses TLR responses and inhibits inflammatory arthritis, *J Immunol* 183(2):1346–1359, 2009.

78. DeGiorgio LA, Konstantinov KN, Lee SC, et al: A subset of lupus anti-DNA antibodies cross-reacts with the NR2 glutamate receptor in systemic lupus erythematosus, *Nat Med* 7(11):1189–1193, 2001.

79. Reed JH, Clancy RM, Purcell AW, et al. β2-Glycoprotein I and protection from anti-SSA/Ro60-associated cardiac manifestations of neonatal lupus, *J Immunol* 187(1):520–526, 2011.

80. Girardi G, Berman J, Redecha P, et al: Complement C5a receptors and neutrophils mediate fetal injury in the antiphospholipid syndrome, *J Clin Invest* 112(11):1644–1654, 2003.

81. Bethunaickan R, Berthier CC, Ramanujam M, et al: A unique hybrid renal mononuclear phagocyte activation phenotype in murine systemic lupus erythematosus nephritis, *J Immunol* 186(8):4994–5003, 2011.

82. Triantafyllopoulou A, Franzke CW, Seshan SV, et al: Proliferative lesions and metalloproteinase activity in murine lupus nephritis mediated by type I interferons and macrophages, *Proc Natl Acad Sci U S A* 107(7):3012–3017, 2010.

83. Hopkins P, Belmont HM, Buyon J, et al: Increased levels of plasma anaphylatoxins in systemic lupus erythematosus predict flares of the disease and may elicit vascular injury in lupus cerebritis, *Arthritis Rheum* 31(5):632–641, 1988.

84. Kaplan MJ: Premature vascular damage in systemic lupus erythematosus, *Autoimmunity* 42(7):580–586, 2009.

85. McMahon M, Grossman J, Skaggs B, et al: Dysfunctional proinflammatory high-density lipoproteins confer increased risk of atherosclerosis in women with systemic lupus erythematosus, *Arthritis Rheum* 60(8):2428–2437, 2009.

86. Magro CM, Poe JC, Kim C, et al: Degos disease: a C5b-9/interferon-alpha-mediated endotheliopathy syndrome, *Am J Clin Pathol* 135(4):599–610, 2011.

The references for this chapter can also be found on www.expertconsult.com.

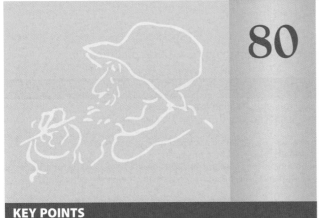

80

Clinical Features of Systemic Lupus Erythematosus

MARIA DALL'ERA • DAVID WOFSY

CLASSIFICATION CRITERIA

Systemic lupus erythematosus (SLE) is the prototypic systemic autoimmune disease characterized by diverse multisystem involvement and the production of an array of autoantibodies. Clinical features in individual patients can be quite variable, ranging from mild joint and skin involvement to severe life-threatening internal organ disease. Criteria for the classification of SLE were initially developed by the American College of Rheumatology (ACR) in 1971, revised in 1982, and revised for a second time in 1997[1,2] (Table 80-1). A person must fulfill 4 of 11 criteria to be classified as SLE, all other reasonable diagnoses having been excluded. A patient does not have to manifest all 4 criteria simultaneously; the required 4 of 11 criteria can be fulfilled over a period of weeks or years. The ACR criteria were developed as a means of classifying patients with SLE for the purpose of inclusion in clinical and epidemiologic studies. In clinical practice, these criteria are often cited to support a diagnosis of SLE. However, it should be emphasized that fulfillment of these classification criteria is not an absolute requirement for diagnosis. Rather, diagnosis typically rests on the judgment of an experienced clinician who recognizes a characteristic constellation of symptoms and signs in the setting of supportive serologic studies, after exclusion of alternative differential diagnostic possibilities. Recently, a concerted effort has been made to further revise the classification criteria, for example, to make lupus nephritis a "stand-alone" criterion, to increase the weight of neurologic manifestations, and/or to add a low-complement criterion. These proposed changes to the classification criteria are currently in development.

EPIDEMIOLOGY

Prevalence and incidence rates of SLE vary widely in the literature. Reported prevalence frequencies range from 20 to 240 per 100,000 persons, and reported incidence rates range from 1 to 10 per 100,000 person-years.[3] This variation is partly due to methodological differences between studies (e.g., different case definitions of SLE and methods of case ascertainment). One study from Rochester, Minnesota, determined that the incidence of SLE increased almost fourfold between the time periods of 1950 to 1979 and 1980 to 1992.[4] This increase in reported incidence may reflect a combination of factors, including an actual increase in disease, changes in population demographics, more widespread case-finding efforts, and detection of milder cases.

Prevalence and incidence of SLE vary across gender, geographic regions, and racial/ethnic groups. SLE demonstrates a striking female predominance with a peak incidence during reproductive years. The degree of female predominance varies with age. The female-to-male ratio is 10 to 15:1 in adults, 3:1 in older-onset SLE, and 8:1 in children.[5] The prevalence of SLE is believed to be approximately three- to fourfold higher in African-American, Asian, and Hispanic populations compared with white populations.[6] SLE is rare among blacks in Africa.

Most SLE patients present with their disease between 15 and 64 years of age.[7] Patients with pediatric-onset SLE (<16 years old) are more likely to be African-American than those with later-onset SLE.[7] SLE tends to be more severe in men and in pediatric patients. Late-onset SLE (>50 years old) is characterized by a more insidious onset with a higher occurrence of serositis and pulmonary involvement and a lower incidence of malar rash, photosensitivity, alopecia, Raynaud's phenomenon, neuropsychiatric disease, and nephritis.[7]

CLINICAL FEATURES

Systemic lupus erythematosus has protean clinical manifestations that may differ dramatically from patient to patient. Just as the signs and symptoms of SLE vary widely among patients, so too does the severity of disease. Some patients with lupus will have relatively mild disease that never threatens a life-sustaining organ; other patients will progress rapidly to life-threatening disease.

The great variability in the expression and severity of SLE constitutes a major challenge to accurate diagnosis.

Table 80-1   1997 Update of the 1982 Revised American College of Rheumatology Classification Criteria for Systemic Lupus Erythematosus*

Criterion	Definition
Malar rash	Fixed erythema, flat or raised, over the malar eminences, sparing the nasolabial folds
Discoid rash	Erythematous raised patches with adherent keratotic scale and follicular plugging; atrophic scarring may occur in older lesions
Photosensitivity	Skin rash as a result of unusual reaction to sunlight, by patient history or physician observation
Oral ulcers	Oral or nasopharyngeal ulceration, usually painless, observed by a physician
Arthritis	Nonerosive arthritis involving two or more peripheral joints, characterized by tenderness, swelling, or effusion
Serositis	a. Pleuritis-convincing history of pleuritic chest pain or rub heard by a physician or evidence of pleural effusions *or* b. Pericarditis-documented by electrocardiogram or rub or evidence of pericardial effusion
Renal disorder	a. Persistent proteinuria >0.5 g/day, >3+ if quantification not performed *or* b. Cellular casts: may be red blood cell, hemoglobin, granular tubular, or mixed
Neurologic disorder	a. Seizures: in the absence of offending drugs or known metabolic derangements (e.g., uremia, acidosis, electrolyte imbalance) *or* b. Psychosis: in the absence of offending drugs or known metabolic derangements (e.g., uremia, acidosis, electrolyte imbalance)
Hematologic disorder	a. Hemolytic anemia with reticulocytosis *or* b. Leukopenia <4000/mm^3 *or* c. Lymphopenia <1500/mm^3 *or* d. Thrombocytopenia <100,000/mm^3 in the absence of offending drugs
Immunologic disorder	a. Anti-DNA: antibody to native DNA in abnormal titer *or* b. Anti-Smith: presence of antibody to Sm nuclear antigen *or* c. Positive finding of antiphospholipid antibodies based on (1) abnormal serum concentration of IgG or IgM anticardiolipin antibodies, (2) positive test result for lupus anticoagulant using a standard method, or (3) false-positive serologic test for syphilis known to be positive for at least 6 mo and confirmed by *Treponema pallidum* immobilization or fluorescent treponemal antibody absorption test
Positive antinuclear antibody	An abnormal titer of antinuclear antibody by immunofluorescence or an equivalent assay at any point in time and in the absence of drugs known to be associated with drug-induced lupus syndromes

*The presence of four or more criteria is required for systemic lupus erythematosus classification. Exclude all other reasonable diagnoses.

Although it is difficult to pinpoint their precise frequencies, it is clear that the most common presenting manifestations are constitutional symptoms (fever, fatigue, and/or weight loss), cutaneous manifestations (e.g., malar rash), and articular manifestations (arthritis and/or arthralgia). Each of these manifestations appears to be present in at least 50% of lupus patients at the time of diagnosis. The other clinical features of SLE are much less likely to be presenting manifestations, although virtually any of them might be the first clue to the correct diagnosis. More commonly, these manifestations appear over time as the disease evolves. Taken together, various descriptive studies in the literature[1,8-12] support a cumulative frequency of symptoms and signs that is summarized in Table 80-2.

Table 80-2   Frequencies of Various Manifestations of Systemic Lupus Erythematosus*

Manifestation	Frequency
Constitutional symptoms (fatigue, fever, weight loss)	90%-95%
Mucocutaneous involvement (malar rash, alopecia, mucosal ulcers, discoid lesions, etc.)	80%-90%
Musculoskeletal involvement (arthritis/arthralgia, avascular necrosis, myositis, etc.)	80%-90%
Serositis (pleuritis, pericarditis, peritonitis)	50%-70%
Glomerulonephritis	40%-60%
Neuropsychiatric involvement (cognitive impairment, depression, psychosis, seizures, stroke, demyelinating syndromes, peripheral neuropathy, etc.)	40%-60%
Autoimmune cytopenia (anemia, thrombocytopenia)	20%-30%

*Systemic lupus erythematosus is a heterogeneous disease that can affect virtually any organ system in variable ways.

Mucocutaneous Involvement

Mucocutaneous involvement is very common in SLE. Gilliam and colleagues have categorized cutaneous lupus erythematosus (LE) lesions as "lupus specific" or "lupus nonspecific" based on the histopathologic finding of interface dermatitis[13,14] (Table 80-3). The presence of lupus-specific lesions confirms the diagnosis of cutaneous LE; lupus nonspecific lesions can occur in diseases other than lupus. Lupus-specific lesions are further subdivided into acute lupus erythematosus (ACLE), subacute lupus erythematosus (SCLE), and chronic cutaneous lupus erythematosus (CCLE) lesions, based on additional clinical and histopathologic information. Discoid lupus is the most common subtype of CCLE. SCLE and CCLE can occur as distinct isolated entities or as one of several manifestations of SLE. The risk of SLE varies with each cutaneous subset. One study of 161 patients with lupus-specific lesions showed that the classification criteria for SLE were present in 72% of patients with ACLE, 58% with SCLE, 28% with any form of discoid lupus, and 6% with localized discoid lupus confined to head and neck. Patients commonly displayed more than one type of cutaneous lesion.[15]

Acute Cutaneous Lupus Erythematosus

Acute cutaneous lupus erythematosus (ACLE) lesions can be localized or generalized. The hallmark feature of ACLE is localized to the malar region ("butterfly rash") and is characterized by confluent, macular or papular erythema lasting days to weeks that occurs symmetrically on the cheeks and bridge of the nose, sparing the nasolabial folds (Figure 80-1). Induration and scaling may occur. The malar rash of SLE can be mimicked by a variety of other facial

Table 80-3 Gilliam Classification of Skin Lesions Associated with Lupus

A. Lupus erythematosus (LE)-specific skin lesions
1. Acute cutaneous LE (ACLE)
   Localized ACLE
   Generalized ACLE
2. Subacute cutaneous LE (SCLE)
   Annular SCLE
   Papulosquamous SCLE
3. Chronic cutaneous LE (CCLE)
   Classical discoid LE (DLE): (a) localized; (b) generalized
   Hypertrophic DLE/verrucous DLE
   Lupus panniculitis/profundus
   Mucosal DLE
   LE tumidus
   Chilblain LE
   Lichenoid DLE (DLE-lichen planus overlap)
B. LE-nonspecific skin lesions
1. Cutaneous vascular disease
   Vasculitis
      Leukocytoclastic vasculitis
      Polyarteritis nodosa–like
   Vasculopathy
      Degos disease–like
      Atrophe blanche–like
      Periungal telangiectasia
      Livedo reticularis
      Thrombophlebitis
      Raynaud's phenomenon
      Erythromelalgia
2. Nonscarring alopecia
   "Lupus hair"
   Telogen effluvium
   Alopecia areata
3. Sclerodactyly
4. Rheumatoid nodules
5. Calcinosis cutis
6. LE-nonspecific bullous lesions
7. Urticaria
8. Papulonodular mucinosis
9. Cutis laxa/anetoderma
10. Acanthosis nigricans (type B insulin resistance)
11. Erythema multiforme (Rowell's syndrome)
12. Leg ulcers
13. Lichen planus

rashes, including acne, rosacea, seborrheic dermatitis, perioral dermatitis, atopic dermatitis, and erysipelas. If the diagnosis remains uncertain after an extensive clinical and serologic evaluation, biopsy of the rash can aid in distinguishing cutaneous lupus from other dermatologic conditions. It is important to remember that other forms of lupus-specific skin lesions such as discoid lupus can also occur in the malar distribution.

The generalized form of ACLE refers to widespread macular or maculopapular erythema occurring in a photosensitive distribution on any area of the body. The palmar surfaces, dorsa of the hands, and extensor surfaces of the fingers are commonly involved. In contrast to Gottron's papules of dermatomyositis, the erythema of ACLE spares the metacarpalphalangeal joints and typically is located between the interphalangeal joints. In severe forms of ACLE, a widespread bullous eruption similar to toxic epidermal necrolysis (TEN) can occur. ACLE lesions heal without scarring, although temporary postinflammatory hyperpigmentation may be observed.

Subacute Cutaneous Lupus Erythematosus

Subacute cutaneous lupus erythematosus (SCLE) is characterized by the presence of nonscarring, photosensitive lesions that can take one of two distinct forms: (1) papulosquamous lesions that resemble psoriasis, or (2) annular-polycyclic lesions with peripheral scale and central clearing (Figure 80-2). These two forms can occur concurrently in the same patient. SCLE has a predilection for the back, neck, shoulders, and extensor surfaces of the arms and usually spares the face. The lesions typically last for weeks to months and heal without scarring. Uncommonly, a severe TEN-like eruption can evolve from SCLE lesions after sun exposure.[16] SCLE, particularly the annular subtype, is strongly associated with the presence of anti-SSA/Ro antibody.[17] Several drugs are known to induce SCLE; angiotensin-converting enzyme inhibitors, terbinafine, hydrochlorothiazide, and calcium channel blockers are common culprits. Finally, SCLE has been implicated as a paraneoplastic syndrome.[18]

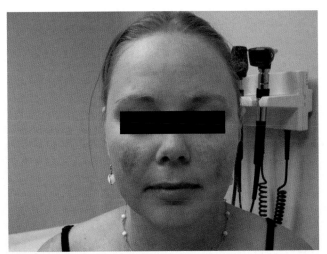

Figure 80-1 Localized acute cutaneous lupus erythematosus (malar rash, butterfly rash). This lesion is characterized by macular or papular erythema in a malar distribution, sparing the nasolabial folds.

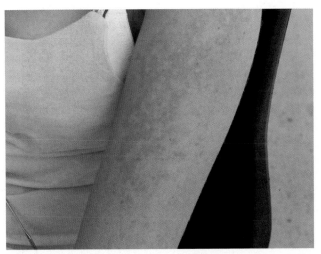

Figure 80-2 Subacute cutaneous lupus (papulosquamous variant). Lesions typically involve the back, neck, shoulders, and extensor surfaces of the arms and usually spare the central area of the face. Lesions heal without scar.

Chronic Cutaneous Lupus Erythematosus

Chronic cutaneous lupus erythematosus (CCLE) refers to a variety of subtypes of photosensitive lesions that can lead to skin atrophy and scar and that may persist for several months. Discoid lupus (DLE) is the most common subtype of CCLE and is subdivided into localized discoid lupus (limited to head and neck) and generalized discoid (occurring above and below the neck) (Figures 80-3 and 80-4). The term "discoid" refers to the sharply demarcated disk-shaped appearance of the lesions. The lesions are raised, erythematosus plaques with adherent scale that commonly occur on the scalp, face, and neck. The cheeks, nose, ears, and upper lip are classic locations. Typically, a raised, erythematous border denotes the actively expanding component. Follicular plugging is a characteristic finding. Left untreated, DLE can result in permanent alopecia and disfigurement. Squamous cell carcinoma has been described as a sequela of long-standing DLE; thus, active surveillance of known lesions and evaluation of changing lesions are critical.[19] Other subtypes of DLE include mucosal DLE (described later) and hypertrophic LE. Hypertrophic LE consists of chronic, indurated lesions that are covered by hyperkeratotic, multilayered scales. These lesions can be a source of diagnostic confusion because they may visually and histologically resemble squamous cell carcinoma.[20]

Other forms of CCLE include lupus panniculitis/profundus and chilblain lupus. Lupus panniculitis is a lobular panniculitis that has a predilection for the scalp, face, arms, buttocks, and thighs. When a cutaneous discoid lesion

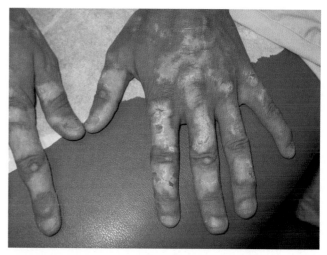

Figure 80-4 Discoid lupus erythematosus involving the dorsa of the hands. The lesions spare the proximal interphalangeal joints, a characteristic feature of lupus-specific rashes.

overlies the panniculitis, the entity is referred to as *lupus profundus*.[21] Biopsy is often necessary to secure the diagnosis because reports have described T cell lymphoma mimicking panniculitis. However, biopsy should be performed carefully because the lesions have a tendency to break down. Lupus panniculitis is one of the few panniculitides that can occur above the waist. Lupus panniculitis is associated with low risk of concomitant SLE. Chilblain lupus manifests as tender, erythematous, or violaceous papules occurring on acral areas, especially fingers, toes, heels, nose, and ears. The lesions are brought on by cold, damp air.

Other Systemic Lupus Erythematosus Skin Lesions

SLE patients can develop lupus-nonspecific skin lesions such as cutaneous leukocytoclastic vasculitis, bullous lesions, periungal erythema, and livedo reticularis. Cutaneous leukocytoclastic vasculitis most commonly presents as palpable purpura on the lower extremities. Bullous lupus erythematosus is a rare cutaneous manifestation characterized by subepidermal vesiculobullous skin changes. It is manifested by a nonscarring bullous eruption[22] (Figure 80-5). SLE may be associated with other bullous disorders such as bullous pemphigoid and dermatitis herpetiformis. The physical examination finding of periungal erythema represents dilation of the capillaries at the base of the nail. These capillaries can be visualized at the bedside with a dermatoscope or ophthalmoscope. Other disorders associated with periungal erythema include scleroderma and mixed connective tissue disease (MCTD). Unlike scleroderma and MCTD, SLE is not associated with capillary dropout. Livedo reticularis is characterized by an erythematous to violaceous reticular or net-like pattern of the skin. It is highly associated with the antiphospholipid antibody syndrome.

Photosensitivity

Photosensitivity occurs frequently in SLE. In one study, photoprovocation testing caused an abnormal skin reaction to ultraviolet A, ultraviolet B, or visible light in greater than 90% of lupus patients.[23] Most abnormal skin reactions

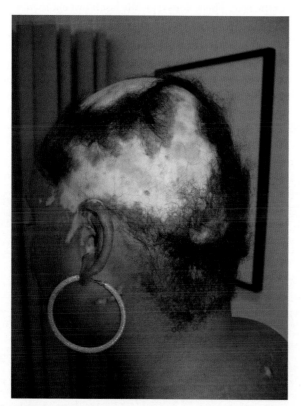

Figure 80-3 Discoid lupus erythematosus involving the face and scalp. Discoid lesions are a form of chronic cutaneous lupus and are commonly found on the scalp, face, and external ears. If untreated, these lesions can lead to permanent alopecia and disfigurement.

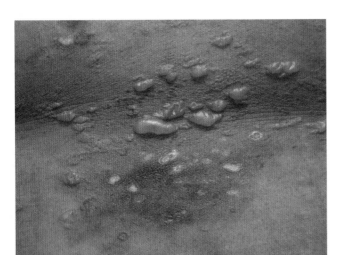

Figure 80-5 Bullous lupus erythematosus. These lesions are a rare manifestation of lupus and are characterized by nonscarring bullous lesions.

occurred 1 to 2 weeks after exposure to light and persisted for weeks to months. Photosensitive patients may report worsening of their systemic disease symptoms such as fatigue and joint pain following sun exposure. During evaluation of a photosensitive patient, polymorphous light eruption (PMLE) and phototoxic medications are important diagnostic considerations.[24] Accurate differentiation between PMLE and lupus is essential because PMLE is treated by ultraviolet radiation phototherapy, but lupus is worsened by it. PMLE can occur concomitantly in patients with known SLE.

Alopecia

Scarring alopecia is a common complication of discoid lupus. Scalp discoid lesions most frequently develop on the vertex and parietal areas.[25] Nonscarring alopecia in SLE patients can take several forms. "Lupus hair" is characterized by short, irregularly sized hair at the frontal hairline and is associated with active systemic disease.[26] Telogen effluvium manifests as diffuse hair thinning. Lastly, the incidence of alopecia areata (discrete areas of hair loss) is believed to be increased in SLE.[27]

Mucosal Ulcers

SLE patients commonly develop nasal or oral lesions that represent the mucosal counterparts of cutaneous lupus.[28] Acute oral lupus lesions present as red macules, palatal erythema or petechiae, erosions, or ulcerations. These lesions are usually painless. Subacute oral lesions are rare, and are characterized by well-demaracted, round, red patches. Oral discoid lesions present as painful, well-demarcated, round, red lesions with white radiating hyperkeratotic striae. When the lesions evolve, they may take on a honeycomb appearance. Oral discoid lupus frequently involves the lip and spreads from the vermilion border to the skin of the lip. Lupus oral ulcers have a gradual onset and can occur anywhere on the oral mucosa, the most common locations being the hard palate, buccal musosa, and vermilion border.[29] These lesions are most commonly unilateral or asymmetric. The relationship between the presence of oral lesions and systemic disease activity remains unclear. Note that oral candidiasis and oral lichen planus can take on a similar appearance to SLE oral ulcers. The histopathology and immunopathology of musosal lesions are similar to the alterations seen in the skin. Vasculitis is absent.

DERMATOPATHOLOGY AND IMMUNOPATHOLOGY

A skin biopsy is useful in the diagnosis of cutaneous lupus in the setting of an atypical clinical presentation. Immunofluorescence should always be performed along with conventional histology. "Lupus-specific" skin lesions are characterized by an interface dermatitis consisting of a mononuclear cell infiltrate at the dermal-epidermal junction. Other pathologic findings present in lupus skin lesions include basal layer vasculopathic degeneration of keratinocytes, perivascular and periadnexal inflammation, follicular plugging, mucin deposition, and hyperkeratosis. These findings occur to different degrees in various lupus-specific skin lesions, with discoid lesions showing the most profound changes.[30] In contrast, early ACLE lesions may have minimal histopathologic findings and only a sparse lymphocytic infiltrate.

Immunofluorescence demonstrates granular deposition of immunoglobulin and complement components along the dermal-epidermal junction. Immunoglobulin (Ig)G and IgM are the most common immunoglobulin subtypes deposited. Various complement components including C3, C1q, and the membrane attack complex have also been identified. Direct immunofluorescence (DIF) of nonlesional, sun-exposed skin is called the *lupus band test*. Although a positive lupus band test is often seen in patients with SLE, this may also be seen in patients with other rheumatic diseases, as well as in healthy people. In one study, 20% of healthy young adults had a positive DIF in sun-exposed skin.[31] It is important to note that serologic testing with antinuclear antibody (ANA), anti–double-stranded DNA (anti-dsDNA), and anti-Smith (anti-SM) has largely supplanted use of the lupus band test in confirming the diagnosis of SLE. DIF of nonlesional, sun-protected skin is believed to be more specific for SLE.

MUSCULOSKELETAL

Arthritis

Arthritis and arthralgias are very common manifestations of SLE, present in up to 90% of patients at some point during the course of their disease.[32] Severity of involvement can range from mild joint pain to deforming arthritis. Although any joint can be involved, lupus arthritis is characterized by a symmetric, inflammatory arthritis predominantly affecting the knees, wrists, and small joints of the hands.[33] Synovial effusions are typically small and not as inflammatory as those present in rheumatoid arthritis. Hand deformities can occur as a result of ligamental and/or joint capsule laxity and joint subluxation. This manifestation is called "Jaccoud's-like arthropathy" because it resembles the arthropathy that develops in patients with a history of rheumatic fever (Figure 80-6). Lupus hand deformities are reducible.

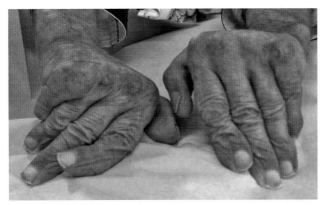

Figure 80-6 Jaccoud's-like arthropathy. These hand deformities resemble those that develop in patients with a history of rheumatic fever and are caused by ligamentous and/or joint capsule laxity. Deformities in the hands, such as ulnar drift at the metacarpophalangeal joints, swan neck and boutonnière deformities, and hyperextension at the interphalangeal joint of the thumb, closely resemble the deformities seen in rheumatoid arthritis. Absence of erosions on radiographs and their reducibility distinguish this condition from the deforming arthritis of rheumatoid arthritis. *(Courtesy Dr. D. Vassilopoulos.)*

Jaccoud's-like arthropathy sometimes occurs in the foot as well.[34]

Although lupus arthritis is not classically associated with erosions on plain radiography, erosive disease has been described in a small subset of patients.[35] In addition, MRI studies have shown occasional erosions in some patients with lupus arthritis.[36] Erosive arthritis is more commonly a feature of MCTD. Some studies have demonstrated an association between lupus erosive arthritis and the presence of anticyclic citrullinated protein (anti-CCP) antibodies.[35] In addition to arthritis, tendinitis or tenosynovitis is frequently observed in SLE patients.[37] Tendon rupture is a very uncommon occurrence.

Synovial biopsies from lupus arthritis patients have shown a variety of abnormalities, including deposition of fibrin-like material, focal or diffuse synovial lining cell proliferation, vascular congestion, perivascular mononuclear cell infiltration, vasculitis, and obliteration of vessel lumina.[38] Radiographic studies of patients with SLE have revealed changes such as cystic bone lesions, periarticular soft tissue swelling, demineralization, acral sclerosis, joint subluxations, and erosions.[39,40]

Avascular Necrosis

Avascular necrosis (AVN), also referred to as aseptic necrosis and ischemic necrosis, is a painful and disabling condition that occurs in some SLE patients.[41] AVN is the end result of interruption of the blood supply to bone, leading to reactive hyperemia of adjacent bone, demineralization, and then collapse. The most commonly affected sites include the femoral heads, tibial plateaus, and femoral condyles, but smaller joints can be involved as well. AVN is often bilateral, and joint effusions may occur. AVN of the femoral head should be suspected in an SLE patient with groin pain that is worsened with weight bearing and movement of the hip. The pain may radiate down the side of the thigh, and a limp might be evident. Although both plain radiographs and magnetic resonance imaging (MRI) can be helpful in

the diagnosis of AVN, MRI is the more sensitive test. One prospective MRI study of 45 SLE patients on glucocorticoid therapy demonstrated that 34% of patients developed silent osteonecrosis of the femoral head.[42] However, MRI studies may be too sensitive an indicator, in that some lupus patients with suggestive MRI findings never progress to clinical symptoms of AVN. Therefore, MRI findings should always be interpreted in the context of the clinical setting. The use of high doses of glucocorticoids is a well-known risk factor for the development of AVN, but AVN has also been described in SLE patients who have never used glucocorticoids. An MRI study of 72 newly diagnosed SLE patients demonstrated that AVN typically developed within the first 3 months of initiation of high-dose glucocorticoids.[43] Epidemiologic studies have shown that high disease activity as measured by the Systemic Lupus Erythematosus Disease Activity Index (SLEDAI) and the use of cytotoxic medications are also associated with AVN.[44,45]

Myositis

Although myalgias occur commonly in SLE, true myositis is relatively rare. One study of SLE patients at the National Institutes of Health (NIH) found a prevalence of myositis of 8%.[46] In most of those patients, myositis was one of the presenting features of SLE. Myositis usually involves the proximal upper and lower extremities. Histologic findings in SLE myositis are often less pronounced than those observed in polymyositis.

A biopsy study of 55 unselected SLE patients demonstrated that several pathologic changes, including type II fiber atrophy, lymphocytic vasculitis, and myositis, were increased in SLE patients compared with control patients.[47]

It is important to distinguish myositis secondary to SLE from myopathy caused by glucocorticoids, antimalarial agents, or statins because the treatment is very different. Muscle enzymes such as creatine phosphokinase (CPK) and aldolase are typically normal in patients with both glucocorticoid- and hydroxychloroquine-induced myopathy. Biopsy specimens usually reveal characteristic findings, including vacuolar changes in hydroxychloroquine myopathy and type II fiber atrophy in glucocorticoid myopathy in the absence of inflammation. Finally, it is important to think broadly about other potential causes of myopathy and myositis in SLE patients, including thyroid disease, electrolyte abnormalities, and infectious myositis. One must also consider the possibility of MCTD because myositis can be a prominent feature of that disorder.

RENAL INVOLVEMENT

General Considerations

Renal involvement is common in SLE and is a significant cause of morbidity and mortality.[48] It is estimated that up to 90% of SLE patients will have pathologic evidence of renal involvement on biopsy, but only 50% will develop clinically significant nephritis. The clinical presentation of lupus nephritis is highly variable, ranging from asymptomatic hematuria and/or proteinuria to frank nephrotic syndrome to rapidly progressive glomerulonephritis with loss of renal function. Lupus nephritis typically develops within the first

36 months of the disease, although there are exceptions. Thus, periodic screening for the presence of nephritis is a critical component of the ongoing evaluation and management of SLE patients. Routine screening procedures include inquiring about new-onset polyuria, nocturia, or foamy urine and looking for the presence of hypertension or lower extremity edema. It is important to screen at regular intervals for the presence of proteinuria and/or hematuria and a change in serum creatinine; in active SLE patients, screening at 3-month intervals is prudent.

Types of Renal Involvement in Systemic Lupus Erythematosus

Several forms of renal involvement have been noted in SLE, including immune complex–mediated glomerulonephritis (most common form), tubulointerstitial disease, and vascular disease. Glomerulonephritis is characterized by immune complex deposition and inflammatory cell infiltration into the glomerulus. The pattern of glomerular injury is primarily related to the site of immune complex deposition. Tubulointerstitial and vascular disease can occur with or without immune complex–mediated glomerulonephritis. Tubulointerstitial disease has been observed in up to 66% of SLE renal biopsy specimens[49] and is characterized by inflammatory cell infiltrates, tubular damage, and interstitial fibrosis. The presence of tubulointerstitial disease is a strong predictor of poor long-term renal outcome.[50]

Renal vascular lesions in SLE include "lupus vasculopathy," thrombotic microangiopathy (TMA), vasculitis, and nonspecific vascular sclerosis.[51,52] Lupus vasculopathy is defined as the presence of immunoglobulin and complement-containing hyaline thrombi within the glomerular capillary or arteriolar lumina. Inflammatory changes to the vascular wall are absent. TMA is characterized by the presence of fibrin thrombi within the glomerular capillary or arteriolar lumina and may be associated with the presence of antiphospholipid antibodies. The finding of TMA should prompt consideration of antiphospholipid antibody syndrome nephropathy (APSN). Although exceedingly rare, true vasculitis characterized by leukocyte infiltration and fibrinoid necrosis of arterial walls can occur. Nonspecific sclerotic vascular lesions characterized by fibrous intimal thickening are commonly observed. The presence of such vascular lesions is associated with decreased renal survival.[53] In addition to the lupus-related renal lesions described previously, SLE patients may develop renal abnormalities that are unrelated to their underlying SLE. Such pathologic lesions include focal segmental glomerulosclerosis (FSGS), hypertensive nephrosclerosis, and thin basement membrane disease.[54] In an SLE patient in whom renal disease is suspected, renal biopsy is critical in distinguishing between these potential causes and in guiding appropriate management decisions.

Laboratory Evaluation

Urinalysis

Performance of a urinalysis with microscopy is essential in the screening and monitoring of lupus nephritis.[55] Hematuria, pyuria, dysmorphic red blood cells, red blood cell casts,

and white blood cell casts may all be present. Red blood cell casts are very specific, but not sensitive, for the diagnosis of glomerulonephritis. Early morning urine specimens, which tend to be concentrated and acidic, are ideal for the detection of red blood cell casts. White blood cells, red blood cells, and white blood cell casts may indicate the presence of tubulointerstitial involvement. Hematuria in the absence of proteinuria might be due to urolithiasis, menstrual contamination, or bladder pathology, particularly transitional cell carcinoma in a patient with previous cyclophosphamide exposure.

Accurate measurement of proteinuria is critical because proteinuria is a very sensitive indicator of glomerular damage. In addition, studies of chronic kidney disease have shown that the magnitude of proteinuria is a strong predictor of glomerular filtration rate decline.[56] Normal daily protein excretion is less than 150 mg. Although the gold standard tool is an accurately collected 24-hour urine protein, this test can be cumbersome for patients and is prone to errors in undercollection and overcollection. Thus, many clinicians are currently using the random spot urine protein-to-creatinine ratio out of convenience. Use of the spot ratio is controversial because data suggest that the spot ratio often is not representative of the findings in a timed collection, especially in the range of 0.5 to 3.0 (the range of most lupus nephritis flares).[57] However, a spot ratio can be a helpful screening test for the presence of proteinuria and is useful in differentiating nephrotic from nonnephrotic range proteinuria.[58] Urine dipstick should not be used for the quantification of proteinuria because it reflects protein concentrations and varies depending on the volume of the sample. Many experts currently recommend calculation of the protein:creatinine ratio from a 12- or 24-hour urine collection as the gold standard of proteinuria assessment.[59]

Measurement of Renal Function

Although easy to measure, serum creatinine is a fairly insensitive indicator of early decline in glomerular filtration rate (GFR). Creatinine is freely filtered across the glomerulus and is also secreted by the proximal tubule. As GFR falls, the rise in serum creatinine is counteracted by increased tubular creatinine secretion. In addition, hemodynamic changes such as those caused by treatment with angiotensin-converting enzyme inhibitors or nonsteroidal anti-inflammatory drugs are a common cause of changes in serum creatinine levels in the absence of progression of underlying renal disease. However, trending serum creatinine over time is a reasonable method by which to follow a patient's renal function. Some clinicians prefer to utilize equations that estimate GFR, such as the Cockcroft-Gault and Modification of Diet in Renal Disease (MDRD) study equations. Whichever method is chosen, the detection of changes in renal function over time is more important than the absolute level when following lupus nephritis patients in clinical practice.

Renal Biopsy

When an SLE patient has clinical or laboratory features that suggest the presence of nephritis, a renal biopsy should be performed to confirm the diagnosis, evaluate the degree of disease activity, and determine an appropriate course of treatment.

Before renal biopsy, ultrasonography is recommended to assess kidney size and structure and to rule out renal vein thrombosis. Kidney size of less than 75% of normal is a relative contraindication to biopsy.[60] SLE glomerulonephritis is classified by the International Society of Nephrology/Renal Pathology Society (ISN/RPS) into six categories based on light microscopic, immunofluorescent, and electron micrographic findings[61] (Table 80-4 and Figure 80-7).

An individual biopsy might exhibit just one of the ISN/RPS pathologic classes or a combination of classes. Class I is characterized by normal appearing glomeruli on light microscopy and mesangial immune deposits on immunofluorescence. Class II is characterized by mesangial proliferation on light microscopy and mesangial deposits on immunofluorescence. Class III and IV lupus nephritis lesions are highly inflammatory and are characterized by immune complex deposition in the subendothelial space. They have traditionally been described as "proliferative" because of the presence of proliferating endocapillary cells within the glomeruli. They are believed to be interrelated lesions that differ in the distribution of endocapillary immune complex deposition. Class III denotes that less than 50% of glomeruli are involved, and class IV denotes that 50% or more of glomeruli are involved. Class IV lesions are subcategorized according to whether most glomeruli show focal (<50% of the glomerular tuft) or global (≥50% of the glomerular tuft) involvement. These lesions are further described as active

(A), chronic (C), or a mixture of the two (A/C). Thick subendothelial immune deposits form classic "wire loop" lesions. Class V lupus nephritis is characterized by immune complex deposition in the subepithelial space, resulting in widespread thickened capillary loops. These findings are similar to those observed in idiopathic membranous nephritis. However, the presence of concomitant mesangial deposits plus or minus tubuloreticular inclusion bodies would favor the diagnosis of lupus. This lesion is commonly manifested clinically as nephrotic range proteinuria. Class V nephritis may occur in a pure histopathologic form or in combination with features of class III or class IV nephritis. Class VI nephritis is defined by the presence of more than 90% globally sclerotic glomeruli. In addition to the type of glomerular pathology, the ISN/RPS classification system dictates that tubulointerstitial disease and/or vascular disease should be noted on the diagnostic line.

Immunofluorescence studies are an important supplement to the findings on light microscopy. Immunofluorescence reveals the type and pattern of immune complex deposition. Lupus nephritis is characterized by a granular pattern of immunofluorescence along the glomerular basement membrane, mesangium, and/or tubular basement membranes. The characteristic findings of lupus nephritis are sometimes referred to as the "full-house" pattern, because IgG, IgM, IgA, C3, and C1q are all found in the deposits. Electron microscopy is useful in more precisely localizing the sites of immune complex deposition. The finding of tubuloreticular inclusion bodies within endothelial cells is strongly suggestive of the diagnosis of lupus nephritis. However, because tubuloreticular inclusion bodies are

Table 80-4 International Society of Nephrology/Renal Pathology Society Classification of Lupus Nephritis

WHO Type	
Class I	**Minimal Mesangial Lupus Nephritis**
	Normal glomeruli by light microscopy, but mesangial immune deposits by immunofluorescence
Class II	**Mesangial Proliferative Nephritis**
	Purely mesangial hypercellularity of any degree or mesangial matrix expansion by light microscopy, with mesangial immune deposits.
	Few isolated subepithelial or subendothelial deposits may be visible by immunofluorescence or electron microscopy, but not by light microscopy
Class III	**Focal Lupus Nephritis**
	Active or inactive focal, segmental, or global endocapillary or extracapillary glomerulonephritis involving <50% of all glomeruli, typically with focal subendothelial immune deposits, with or without mesangial alterations
Class IV	**Diffuse Lupus Nephritis**
	Active or inactive diffuse, segmental, or global endocapillary or extracapillary glomerulonephritis involving ≥50% of all glomeruli, typically with diffuse subendothelial immune deposits, with or without mesangial alterations. This class is subdivided into diffuse segmental (IV-S) lupus nephritis when ≥50% of the involved glomeruli have segmental lesions, and diffuse global (IV-G) lupus nephritis when ≥50% of the involved glomeruli have global lesions. Segmental is defined as a glomerular lesion that involves less than half of the glomerular tuft. This class includes cases with diffuse wire loop deposits, but with little or no glomerular proliferation
Class V	**Membranous Lupus Nephritis**
	Global or segmental subepithelial immune deposits or their morphologic sequelae by light microscopy and by immunofluorescence or electron microscopy, with or without mesangial alterations
	Class V nephritis may occur in combination with class III or class IV, in which case both are diagnosed
	Class V nephritis may show advanced sclerotic lesions
Class VI	**Advanced Sclerotic Lupus Nephritis**
	≥90% of glomeruli globally sclerosed without residual activity

WHO, World Health Organization.

Adapted from Weening JJ, et al: The classification of glomerulonephritis in systemic lupus erythematosus revisited, *J Am Soc Nephrol* 15:241, 2004.

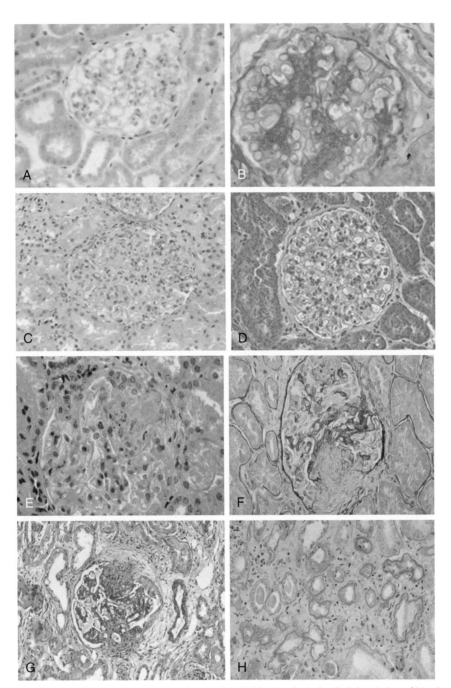

Figure 80-7 **A** through **D,** World Health Organization types of lupus. (See Table 80-4 for a detailed description of histologic findings.) **A,** Normal glomerulus (type I). **B,** Mesangial proliferative (type II). **C,** Proliferative nephritis. Dramatic increase in mesangial and endocapillary cellularity produces a lobular appearance of the glomerular tufts and compromises the patency of most capillary loops. When less than 50% of glomeruli are involved, nephritis is denoted as focal (type III). When more than 50% of glomeruli are involved, nephritis is denoted as diffuse (type IV). **D,** Membranous nephropathy (type V). In membranous lupus nephropathy, the capillary walls of the glomerular tuft are prominent and widely patent, resembling "stiff" structures with decreased compliance. **E** through **H,** High-risk histologic features suggesting severe nephritis. **E,** Fibrinoid necrosis with karyorrhexis in a patient with focal proliferative glomerulonephritis. **F** and **G,** Cellular crescents with layers of proliferative endothelial cells and monocytes lining Bowman's capsule along with a predominantly mononuclear interstitial infiltrate. **H,** Severe interstitial fibrosis and tubular atrophy. Note the thickening of the tubular basement membranes and tubular epithelial degeneration with separation of residual tubules caused by deposition of collagenous connective tissue among tubules.

associated with increased levels of interferon alpha, chronic viral infections such as hepatitis B/C and the human immunodeficiency virus (HIV) must be ruled out.

Renal biopsy is especially important because urinary parameters such as hematuria and the degree of proteinuria imperfectly predict the underlying renal pathology.[62,63]

Hematuria might be absent in patients with severe class IV nephritis, and proteinuria can be modest in patients with class V nephritis. A repeat renal biopsy may be indicated in certain clinical settings (e.g., if a patient is not responding appropriately to therapy, if a patient unexpectedly worsens after having achieved a good response to therapy). Repeat renal biopsy can be useful in detecting class transformation that occurs in 15% to 50% of lupus nephritis patients during the course of their disease. Class transformation can occur spontaneously or as a result of treatment.

Outcome

Each ISN/RPS histopathologic class portends a distinct renal prognosis. Patients with class I and class II nephritis have an excellent renal prognosis and do not require any specific therapy. In contrast, the long-term renal prognosis of class III or class IV nephritis is believed to be poor in the absence of immunosuppressive therapy. Although the long-term renal prognosis of class V nephritis is more favorable than that of class III or class IV nephritis, class V patients are more likely to suffer from morbid complications of the nephrotic syndrome, including cardiovascular disease, thromboembolic disease, and hyperlipidemia. Several epidemiologic studies have defined demographic, clinical, and histopathologic factors associated with renal outcome in patients with lupus nephritis. Studies have shown that African-Americans and Hispanics/Latinos generally experience a worse renal prognosis than white and Chinese populations. The reasons for this disparity most likely involve a combination of genetic and socioeconomic factors. A retrospective analysis of 65 patients at the NIH suggested that age greater than 30 years, African-American race, low hematocrit, elevated serum creatinine, and low C3 complement were associated with increased probability of renal failure. The histologic features of cellular crescents and interstitial fibrosis were also associated with worse renal prognosis.[50]

PLEUROPULMONARY INVOLVEMENT

Pleuropulmonary manifestations of SLE are diverse and can involve any aspect of the lung (Table 80-5).

Pleuritis

Up to 50% of SLE patients will develop pleuritis. Clinically apparent pleural effusions are typically small, bilateral, and exudative.[64] Pleuritis is commonly manifested by pleuritic chest pain, but pleural effusions may be asymptomatic and detected on routine chest radiography performed for another purpose. Massive pleural effusions requiring pleurocentesis and/or pleurodesis are uncommon but have been reported.[65] The presence of pleuritis usually corresponds to active SLE in other organ systems.[66] Thoracoscopic evaluation has demonstrated nodules on the visceral pleura with immunoglobulin deposits detected on immunfluorescence. The differential diagnosis of pleural effusions in an SLE patient includes infection, malignancy, and heart failure. In addition, pleural effusions are a common feature of drug-induced lupus. In the absence of infection, high levels of serum C-reactive protein (CRP) have been found to correlate well with the presence of pleuritis and other forms of serositis in SLE.[66,67] Thus, serum CRP may be a useful clue to the presence of pleuritis.

Lupus Pneumonitis

Acute lupus pneumonitis is a rare manifestation of SLE that presents as a severe, acute respiratory illness with fever, cough, pulmonary infiltrates, and hypoxemia. Chest radiography usually reveals bilateral, lower lobe, acinar infiltrates that often occur in conjunction with a pleural effusion. Histopathologic findings are nonspecific and include diffuse alveolar damage, inflammatory cell infiltrates, hyaline membranes, and alveolar hemorrhage.[68] Immunofluorescence studies have demonstrated granular deposits of IgG and C3 within the alveolar septa.[69] Because clinical and pathologic features of acute lupus pneumonitis are nonspecific, careful evaluation is critical to exclude other potential pulmonary processes such as infection. If routine blood and sputum cultures are nondiagnostic, bronchoscopy with

Table 80-5   Pleuropulmonary Manifestations of Systemic Lupus Erythematosus

Manifestation	Key Features
Pleuritis	May occur with or without effusion
	May correlate with elevated serum C-reactive protein
Pleural effusion	May be asymptomatic
	Usually small, bilateral, exudative
	Common feature of drug-induced lupus
	Must exclude infection, malignancy, heart failure
Acute pneumonitis	Severe respiratory illness with fever, cough, pulmonary infiltrates, hypoxemia
	Pleural effusion may be present
	High mortality rate
	Bronchoscopy with bronchoalveolar lavage might be necessary to exclude infection
Chronic interstitial lung disease	May develop after acute pneumonitis or in a more insidious fashion
	Presents as dyspnea on exertion, pleuritic chest pain, nonproductive cough
	High-resolution computed tomography more sensitive than chest x-ray in detecting disease
	Must exclude infection, pulmonary edema, malignancy
Diffuse alveolar hemorrhage	Presents as dyspnea and cough, alveolar infiltrates, fall in blood hemoglobin level
	Hemoptysis may not be present
	Diffusion capacity of carbon monoxide typically increased
	Bronchoscopy with bronchoalveolar lavage confirms the diagnosis and excludes infection
	High mortality rate
Pulmonary arterial hypertension	Presents as dyspnea on exertion, fatigue, chest pain, nonproductive cough
	Diagnosis should be confirmed with right heart catheterization
	Exclude secondary causes of pulmonary hypertension, including thromboembolic disease
Shrinking lung syndrome	Dyspnea, low lung volumes, elevation of hemi-diaphragms in absence of lung parenchymal involvement

bronchoalveolar lavage can be useful in detecting pulmonary pathogens. A "tree and bud" pattern on high-resolution computed tomography (HRCT) may suggest the presence of an atypical pneumonia. Acute lupus pneumonitis is associated with significant morbidity and mortality. One series of 12 patients reported a mortality rate of 50% with deaths from respiratory failure, opportunistic infection, and thromboembolic events. Three of the surviving patients progressed to chronic interstitial pneumonitis.[70]

Chronic Interstitial Lung Disease

Chronic interstitial lung disease is a rare manifestation of SLE. It occurs more commonly in other connective tissue diseases such as systemic sclerosis, rheumatoid arthritis, and polymyositis/dermatomyositis. Interstitial lung disease in the setting of SLE can develop after one or more episodes of acute pneumonitis but can also occur in an insidious fashion.[70] Symptoms are similar to those seen in patients with idiopathic interstitial lung disease and include dyspnea on exertion, pleuritic chest pain, and chronic, nonproductive cough. The diagnosis of interstitial lung disease is often made on the basis of clinical-radiologic findings; lung biopsy is not routinely performed. Chest radiography might be normal early in the disease but can show reticular opacities. Pulmonary function studies show a restrictive pattern with reduction in total lung capacity and reduction in the diffusion capacity of carbon monoxide (DLCO). HRCT is more sensitive than chest radiography in detecting interstitial lung disease and in distinguishing reversible lesions (ground glass opacities) from irreversible fibrotic lesions. Nonspecific interstitial pneumonia (NSIP) and usual interstitial pneumonia (UIP) are the most common patterns detected on histopathology and HRCT. Before making the diagnosis of interstitial lung disease, it is important to exclude infection, pulmonary edema, and malignancy.

Diffuse Alveolar Hemorrhage

Diffuse alveolar hemorrhage (DAH) is a life-threatening manifestation of SLE that occurs in less than 2% of patients. It is characterized by acute or subacute onset of dyspnea and cough in the setting of new alveolar infiltrates on chest radiography and a fall in blood hemoglobin level. Similar to other causes of DAH, hemoptysis is not universally present. Although most patients are too ill to receive this test, the DLCO is typically increased in the setting of DAH owing to the presence of extravascular hemoglobin within the alveoli. Bronchoscopy with bronchoalveolar lavage (BAL) is important in ruling out infection and confirming the diagnosis. Characteristic findings include visualization of blood in the airways and serosanguineous BAL fluid that does not clear with continued lavage. Hemosiderin-laden macrophages may be seen in the BAL fluid. Various histopathologic patterns have been described in lupus DAH, including bland pulmonary hemorrhage, capillaritis, diffuse alveolar damage, and vasculitis of small arterioles and small muscular pulmonary arteries. DAH usually occurs in the setting of serologically and clinically active SLE, and lupus nephritis is the most common concurrent SLE manifestation. However, DAH occasionally may be the initial manifestation of SLE. Mechanical ventilation is often required,[71]

and infectious complications are common. Despite aggressive therapy, mortality from DAH continues to be 50%.

Pulmonary Arterial Hypertension

Pulmonary arterial hypertension (PAH) is a rare, devastating complication of SLE that is defined as a mean pulmonary artery pressure greater than 25 mm Hg at rest on right heart catheterization. Other key findings on heart catheterization include a normal pulmonary capillary wedge pressure and elevated pulmonary capillary resistance. Symptoms of PAH include dyspnea on exertion, fatigue, chest pain, and nonproductive cough. Physical examination findings may include a pronounced second pulmonary heart sound, a left parasternal lift, and signs of a volume-overloaded state. Chest radiography and HRCT are important in excluding lupus pneumonitis. Chest radiography may show cardiomegaly and a prominent pulmonary artery segment. The electrocardiogram often shows right axis deviation. Pulmonary function studies demonstrate a reduction in DLCO. Although transthoracic Doppler echocardiography is a decent screening test for PAH, the diagnosis should be confirmed by right heart catheterization. Similar to interstitial lung disease, PAH more commonly occurs in association with scleroderma and mixed connective tissue disease.

In an SLE patient who has been diagnosed with PAH, an evaluation must be performed for secondary causes of pulmonary hypertension. Ventilation and perfusion (V/Q) lung scan and/or helical computed tomography are useful in excluding chronic thromboembolic disease. Echocardiography can rule out left heart failure and intracardiac shunting. A sleep study can be useful in ruling out obstructive sleep apnea. An evaluation for interstitial lung disease is necessary. Some studies suggest that PAH occurs more commonly in patients with Raynaud's phenomenon.

Other

Shrinking lung syndrome occurs in a small subset of SLE patients and should be considered when evaluating an SLE patient with unexplained dyspnea and pleuritic chest pain.[72,73] The cause of the disorder remains controversial. Diaphragmatic myopathy, abnormal chest wall expansion, phrenic neuropathy, and pleural inflammation/fibrosis have been reported as possible factors. The prognosis of this syndrome seems to be good, and progressive respiratory failure is uncommon.

Although symptomatic bronchiolar disease is uncommon in SLE, abnormalities in pulmonary function studies have been reported in up to two-thirds of SLE patients.[74] One study of nonsmoking SLE patients found that 24% of patients had pulmonary function studies consistent with small airway disease. Rare case reports of bronchiolitis obliterans organizing pneumonia (BOOP) in the setting of SLE have been described.[75]

CARDIOVASCULAR INVOLVEMENT

Cardiovascular disease is a frequent complication of SLE and may involve the pericardium, myocardium, valves, and coronary arteries.

Pericarditis

Pericarditis, with or without an effusion, is the most common cardiac manifestation of SLE, occurring in more than 50% of SLE patients at some point during the course of their disease.[76] Pericardial effusions are usually small and asymptomatic and typically are detected on echocardiography performed for another indication. Consistent with this observation, necropsy studies have shown that histopathologic evidence of pericarditis is much more common than clinically symptomatic disease during life.[77] Symptomatic pericarditis classically presents as sharp, precordial chest pain that is improved in the upright position. A pericardial rub and tachycardia may be detected on cardiac auscultation. The electrocardiogram demonstrates diffuse ST segment elevation. Similar to pleuritis, pericarditis usually occurs in the setting of active SLE in other organ systems. Although rare, SLE pericarditis complicated by large effusions and tamponade physiology have been reported. Purulent effusions necessitating pericardiocentesis have also been described, but rarely. The differential diagnosis of precordial chest pain in an SLE patient includes costochondritis, gastroesophageal reflux disease, pulmonary embolism, myocardial ischemia, pleuritis, pneumonitis, and pulmonary hypertension.

Myocarditis

Myocarditis, an uncommon manifestation of SLE, should be suspected in a patient presenting with various combinations of the following clinical features: unexplained heart failure or cardiomegaly, unexplained tachycardia, and unexplained electrocardiographic abnormalities. Echocardiography can confirm the presence of systolic or diastolic dysfunction and/or global hypokinesis. If myocarditis is suspected, an endomyocardial biopsy may be helpful in confirming the diagnosis and excluding other causes of cardiomyopathy such as hydroxychloroquine toxicity. The distinguishing pathologic finding of hydroxychloroquine toxicity is myocyte vacuolization in the absence of active myocarditis. Histopathologic findings of SLE myocarditis include perivascular and interstitial mononuclear cell infiltration and sometimes fibrosis and scar.[77]

Valvular Abnormalities

Several valvular abnormalities have been described in patients with SLE, including Libman-Sacks endocarditis (also known as atypical verrucous endocarditis), valvular thickening, valvular regurgitation, and valvular stenosis. One transesophageal echocardiographic (TEE) study demonstrated a prevalence of valvular abnormalities of 61% in SLE patients compared with 9% of controls, with vegetations present in 43% of SLE patients compared with none of the controls.[78] Valvular thickening with a predilection for the mitral and aortic valves was the most common abnormality, occurring in 50% of SLE patients. Valvular regurgitation and stenosis were detected in 25% and 4% of patients, respectively.[78] In this study, the presence and progression of valvular disease were not associated with SLE disease activity or treatment. Over a follow-up period of up to 5 years, some valvular abnormalities resolved and some

new lesions occurred. The combined incidence of stroke, peripheral embolism, congestive heart failure, infective endocarditis, need for valve replacement, and death was 22% among patients with valvular disease compared with 15% in those without valvular disease.[78]

Libman-Sacks endocarditis has been recognized in multiple pathologic studies as a characteristic valvular abnormality in SLE. Libman-Sacks verrucae typically appear as pea-sized, flat or raised, granular lesions that occur most commonly on the ventricular aspects of the mitral valve posterior leaflet.[77] The verrucae often extend onto the adjacent left ventricular mural endocardium and may lead to adherence of the leaflet and chordae tendineae to the ventricular mural endocardium, resulting in valvular regurgitation. All four valves may be involved, but recent studies suggest a predominance of left-sided lesions. The lesions are frequently clinically silent because they are typically found on the undersurface of valve leaflets, surrounded by fibrous tissue. Histologically, two types of verrucae have been described: (1) active lesions consisting of fibrin clumps with infiltrating lymphocytes and plasma cells, and (2) healed lesions consisting of dense vascularized fibrous tissue with or without calcification.[77] Combinations of active and healed lesions also occur. Verrucae typically do not contain polymorphonuclear cells; thus, the presence of such cells should prompt consideration of infectious endocarditis. Immunopathologic studies have demonstrated immunoglobulin and complement deposition in a granular pattern at the base of the valve, along the valve leaflet, and within the verruca itself.[79] Cardiac murmurs are frequently heard in patients with SLE. They may simply result from high-flow states such as fever and anemia, or they may reflect cardiac pathology such as mitral valve prolapse or infective endocarditis. When a new murmur is evaluated, a transthoracic echocardiogram (TTE) is an appropriate first test. However, TEE should be utilized in the event of a nondiagnostic TTE or in a patient with suspected thromboembolic events. TEE has been shown to be superior to TTE for detection of Libman-Sacks endocarditis.[80] Although thromboembolic events are believed to be rare complications of Libman-Sacks endocarditis, one study showed that valvular heart disease detected on TTE was associated with the presence of cerebral infarcts on MRI.[81] It remains uncertain whether the incidence of valvular disease is increased in SLE patients who also have circulating antiphospholipid antibodies.

Coronary Artery Disease

Both intramural and extramural coronary artery disease is increased in patients with SLE. Necropsy studies have demonstrated fibrous intimal proliferation of small intramural coronary arteries and obstruction of these arteries with hyaline material.[77] These lesions are similar to those observed in pathologic studies of renal and central nervous system tissue in SLE patients. The large epicardial coronary arteries may be obstructed owing to arterial emboli, in situ thrombosis, vasculitis, or atherosclerotic disease. True coronary artery vasculitis is exceedingly rare. In contrast, atherosclerotic disease is a well-recognized complication of long-standing SLE.[82] Autopsy studies have demonstrated atherosclerosis in 25% to 40% of SLE patients.[77,83] One epidemiologic study demonstrated that young women with

SLE have a 50-fold higher risk of myocardial infarction compared with age-matched controls.[84] A multicenter inception cohort determined that male sex and older age at SLE diagnosis were significantly associated with the presence of atherosclerotic disease.[85] Although patients with SLE are more likely to have classic atherosclerotic risk factors such as hypertension and exposure to corticosteroids, these risk factors alone do not fully account for the increased risk of atherosclerosis seen in SLE patients.[86] Thus, SLE itself is believed to be an independent risk factor.

The possibility of coronary artery disease must be considered in any SLE patient presenting with chest pain and/or shortness of breath, and one should have a low threshold for a functional evaluation with a cardiac stress test. Cardiac catheterization might also be necessary for diagnosis and therapeutic intervention. It is important to evaluate these patients for the presence of antiphospholipid antibodies because coronary artery thrombosis may be a manifestation of the antiphospholipid antibody syndrome. Evaluation for and treatment of modifiable risk factors such as obesity, smoking, hypertension, and hyperlipidemia are important in mitigating the development and progression of atherosclerotic disease.

NEUROPSYCHIATRIC INVOLVEMENT

General Considerations

Neuropsychiatric lupus (NPSLE) consists of a broad range of neurologic and psychiatric manifestations that can involve any aspect of the central or peripheral nervous system. With the intention of improving the terminology and classification of NPSLE, an American College of Rheumatology (ACR) subcommittee categorized NPSLE into 19 distinct syndromes encompassing the central (CNS) and peripheral (PNS) nervous system[87] (Table 80-6). The extent of this classification system underscores the complexity of NPSLE. CNS disorders range from diffuse processes such as acute confusional state, headache, psychosis, and mood disorders to more focal processes such as seizures, myelopathy, and chorea. It is notable that the ACR classification system has removed the cryptic term "lupus cerebritis" from the vernacular. Although the ACR case definitions are very helpful in providing a framework in which to think about

Table 80-6 American College of Rheumatology Classification of Neuropsychiatric Syndromes in Systemic Lupus Erythematosus

Central Nervous System	Peripheral Nervous System
Aseptic meningitis	Guillain-Barré syndrome
Cerebrovascular disease	Autonomic disorder
Demyelinating syndrome	Mononeuropathy, single/multiplex
Headache	Myasthenia gravis
Movement disorder	Cranial neuropathy
Myelopathy	Plexopathy
Seizure	Polyneuropathy
Acute confusional state	
Anxiety disorder	
Cognitive dysfunction	
Mood disorder	
Psychosis	

and study NPSLE, accurate attribution of neuropsychiatric manifestations remains challenging. It is often difficult to distinguish whether neuropsychiatric symptoms are due to active SLE or to other factors such as infection, metabolic abnormalities, severe hypertension, adverse effects of medications, or independent neurologic or psychiatric problems. No laboratory or imaging study is sufficiently sensitive or specific to confirm the diagnosis of neuropsychiatric SLE. Instead, the diagnosis is based on a thorough clinical evaluation that is corroborated by findings (or lack thereof) on brain imaging, serologic testing, lumbar puncture, and neuropsychiatric assessment.

Pathogenesis

Multiple pathogenic mechanisms are undoubtedly involved in the various NPSLE syndromes, but in most cases the precise pathogenesis is unknown. Many of the manifestations can be grouped into two broad categories: primary vascular injury and primary inflammatory injury. A combination of the two categories can also occur. Vascular injury includes damage to both large and small vessels via thromboembolic events, often as a consequence of antiphospholipid syndrome. In some patients, vasculopathy of small vessels may be due to vascular hyalinization, perivascular inflammation, and endothelial proliferation. In contrast, inflammatory-mediated injury might result from increased permeability of the blood-brain barrier, intrathecal production of inflammatory cytokines, and damage from antineuronal antibodies. Histopathologic studies have demonstrated multiple CNS abnormalities, including large and small multifocal infarctions, hemorrhage, bland small vessel vasculopathy, cortical atrophy, brain edema, and demyelination. True vasculitis of cerebral vessels is rare. Several autoantibodies have been implicated in the pathogenesis of some neuropsychiatric manifestations, particularly psychosis, but they lack sufficient sensitivity or specificity to guide diagnosis.[88]

Approach to Diagnosis

The diagnostic evaluation of a patient with potential NPSLE is tailored to the presenting neuropsychiatric manifestation. Depending on the manifestation, consultation with a neurologist and/or a psychiatrist is advised. The most important first step is exclusion of an alternative explanation for the neuropsychiatric symptoms/signs. Lumbar puncture with cerebrospinal fluid (CSF) examination is useful for exclusion of an infectious origin. Mild lymphocytic pleocytosis and elevated CSF protein are sometimes observed but are not uniformly present. CSF findings are not sensitive or specific enough to confirm a diagnosis of neuropsychiatric SLE. It is important to recognize that infection is a common cause of CNS symptoms in SLE patients who are hospitalized with altered mental status,[89] and must be rigorously ruled out. Progressive multifocal leukoencephalopathy (PML) is a rare infection that also merits consideration in an SLE patient presenting with symptoms of CNS dysfunction. PML occurs more frequently in SLE patients than in patients with other rheumatic diseases, even in the absence of significant immunosuppressive therapy.[90] Thus, in an SLE patient with unexplained new neurologic symptoms, polymerase chain reaction (PCR) of the CSF for the presence of John Cunningham (JC) virus should be considered. In situations where PCR is negative, brain biopsy might be needed to confirm the diagnosis. Electromyography and nerve conduction studies are important in the setting of suspected peripheral neuropathy. Electroencephalogram (EEG) is necessary in the evaluation of seizure. Neuropsychological testing may be helpful in the setting of suspected cognitive dysfunction.

MRI is the preferred imaging modality in patients with suspected NPSLE. The most common noted abnormalities are small, hyperintense, T2-weighted, focal white matter lesions located in the periventricular and subcortical white matter of the frontoparietal region of the brain. However, these findings are nonspecific and can be observed in other disease processes such as atherosclerotic vascular disease and multiple sclerosis. Other common MRI findings include cortical atrophy, ventricular dilation, cerebral edema, diffuse white matter abnormalities, focal atrophy, infarction, leukoencephalopathy, and hemorrhage.[91] MRI is especially useful in detecting the presence of infarcts, hemorrhage, and myelopathy and sometimes can help to exclude infectious conditions such as brain abscess.[91] MRI is most likely to show abnormalities in the setting of focal neurologic deficits, seizures, chronic cognitive dysfunction, and antiphospholipid antibody–mediated disease and is less likely to show abnormalities in the setting of headache, acute confusional state, and psychiatric syndromes.

Estimates of the prevalence of NPSLE have varied widely in the literature, largely depending on the extent to which headache and/or mild cognitive abnormalities have been included in the analysis. However, the preponderance of these studies suggests that CNS manifestations predominate over PNS manifestations. Several of the more common syndromes and associated differential diagnoses are described in the following paragraphs.

Selected Neuropsychiatric Lupus Syndromes

Headaches are reported in more than 50% of SLE patients, but attribution of the headache to SLE is extremely difficult. Both migrainous and tension-type headaches have been described. One meta-analysis[92] determined that the prevalence of primary headache syndromes was not different between SLE and control patients, and that headache was not related to SLE disease activity. The evaluation of headache in an SLE patient should be similar to that in a non-SLE patient and should be directed by the presence or absence of worrisome features such as fever, meningismus, altered mental status, and focal neurologic signs.

Cognitive dysfunction, manifested primarily by deficits in thinking, memory, and concentration, is being increasingly recognized in SLE patients. Some have estimated a prevalence of up to 80%, although serious cognitive impairment is much less common. Some studies suggest that cognitive dysfunction may be associated with the presence of antiphospholipid antibodies, but a causal relationship has not been definitively established. Documentation of the presence and extent of cognitive dysfunction via neuropsychiatric testing can be useful in establishing a baseline in a particular patient that can be followed over time, particularly when a therapeutic intervention is being considered.

Psychiatric disorders such as psychosis, depression, and anxiety can occur in SLE, and consultation with a psychiatrist is highly recommended in the evaluation of patients with these symptoms. An SLE patient presenting with psychosis represents a distinct diagnostic and therapeutic challenge. The differential diagnosis includes CNS infection, primary schizophrenia, systemic metabolic abnormalities, and psychosis occurring as a side effect of corticosteroid therapy or illicit drugs. Steroid-induced psychosis is dose dependent and typically occurs within the first 2 weeks of treatment initiation.

Although rare, demyelinating syndromes such as optic neuritis and myelitis can occur as part of the spectrum of NPSLE. Optic neuritis is characterized by pain with eye movement, central visual field loss, and a waxing and waning course.[93] Optic neuritis should be differentiated from ischemic optic neuropathy, which typically presents with acute, painless loss of vision and lack of significant improvement in vision over time.[94] Myelitis is characterized by the onset of bilateral lower extremity paresthesia, numbness, and weakness that can rapidly progress to involve the upper limbs and the muscles of respiration. A sensory level is usually noted, and autonomic involvement of the bowel and bladder is common. Band-like pain or discomfort around the abdomen is a characteristic symptom. It is important to differentiate myelitis from other causes of myelopathy, including infection, structural spinal cord abnormalities, and vascular insult to the spinal cord. Spinal cord MRI is the critical first test. CSF examination is important to rule out infection.

The combination of optic neuritis and myelitis presents a special clinical challenge because this combination of features can occur in the setting of SLE, multiple sclerosis (MS), or neuromyelitis optica (NMO).[95] Complicating matters, the clinical presentation of antiphospholipid antibody syndrome can mimic demyelinating disease. A thorough clinical history, MRI, CSF analysis, and serologic testing are helpful in distinguishing these entities. NPSLE and MS can have identical white matter lesions on brain MRI. Spinal cord lesions may differ in that MS spinal cord lesions usually span an area measuring less than two spinal segments, but SLE lesions are often longitudinally extensive with involvement of more than three spinal cord segments. Although oligoclonal bands may be present in the CSF of both SLE and MS patients, the absence of oligoclonal bands and the presence of a pleocytosis significantly lessen the likelihood of MS. Although a positive ANA has been described in up to 27% of patients with MS,[95] more specific subserologies such as anti-dsDNA and anti-Sm favor the diagnosis of SLE. NMO is defined as manifested by two of the following three features: presence of the NMO IgG antibody (antibody to aquaporin 4), absence of brain lesions diagnostic of MS, and longitudinally extensive myelitis on MRI.[96] The NMO antibody has a specificity of greater than 90% for the diagnosis of NMO. However, SLE and NMO may occur concurrently in a given patient.

Patients with SLE are at increased risk of stroke, with ischemic stroke being more common than intracerebral hemorrhage.[97] Studies have demonstrated an association between the presence of antiphospholipid antibodies (aPL) and/or valvular heart disease and the risk of stroke.[81] Brain MRI is a critical test in the diagnosis of ischemic or hemorrhagic stroke, and magnetic resonance angiography (MRA) can detect vessel aneurysms. Echocardiography, carotid ultrasound, and electrocardiography are important diagnostic tests in the setting of suspected thromboembolic cerebrovascular disease.

Peripheral neuropathy has been observed in up to 20% of SLE patients and typically is characterized by a symmetric, length-dependent sensory or sensorimotor polyneuropathy. Vasculitis of the vasa nervorum and demyelination are two well-recognized pathogenic mechanisms. When the results of nerve conduction studies (NCS) are normal, small-diameter nerve fibers are likely involved. Small-fiber involvement frequently presents as fluctuating numbness and tingling of the upper extremities and hands. A devastating, large-fiber vasculitic neuropathy can also develop in patients with SLE. Autonomic neuropathies, cranial neuropathies, and abnormalities of the neuromuscular junction resembling myasthenia gravis have also been described.

GASTROINTESTINAL INVOLVEMENT

SLE can involve any part of the gastrointestinal system. Dysphagia is noted in up to 13% of patients, and manometric studies have detected abnormalities of esophageal motility.[98] Decreased peristalsis is most commonly observed in the upper one-third of the esophagus. In contrast to scleroderma, involvement of the lower esophageal sphincter is rare in SLE.[99] A variety of potential pathogenic mechanisms have been described, including muscle atrophy, inflammation of esophageal muscle, and ischemic or vasculitic damage to the Auerbach plexus.

Abdominal pain, sometimes accompanied by nausea and vomiting, has been reported in up to 40% of SLE patients and can be due to SLE-related causes, medication side effects, and non–SLE-related causes such as infection.[98] When evaluating an SLE patient with abdominal pain, it is critical to rule out non-SLE conditions. It is important to note that when patients are treated with corticosteroids and/or other immunosuppressives, clinical signs of an acute abdomen such as rebound tenderness can be masked. Thus, delay in diagnosis is common. SLE-related causes of abdominal pain may include peritonitis, pancreatitis, mesenteric vasculitis, and intestinal pseudo-obstruction. Although autopsy studies have revealed evidence of peritoneal inflammation in up to 72% of SLE patients,[100] the presence of ascites is rare. If an SLE patient presents with abdominal pain and ascites, paracentesis is warranted to rule out infection. Peritonitis can also occur in the setting of mesenteric ischemia, bowel infarction, and pancreatitis. Thus, abdominal imaging is an important part of the initial evaluation.

Pancreatitis due to SLE is uncommon and usually is associated with active SLE in other organs. When considering the possible diagnosis of pancreatitis, it is important to note that elevated serum amylase may be misleading in that it has been observed in SLE patients in the absence of pancreatitis.[101] Although corticosteroids and azathioprine have been associated with the development of pancreatitis in non-SLE patients, these medications do not seem to play a major role in the development of pancreatitis in SLE patients.[102] It is important to rule out non-SLE causes of pancreatitis such as biliary disease, alcohol consumption, and hypertriglyceridemia.

Mesenteric vasculitis is a very rare manifestation of SLE that can present with a range of symptoms from cramping, bloating, and anorexia to an acute abdomen with diarrhea and gastrointestinal hemorrhage. Accurate diagnosis and prompt treatment are essential to prevent the potential catastrophic complications of necrotic bowel, perforation, and sepsis. Abdominal radiography may show distention of bowel loops, thickening and thumbprinting of the bowel wall, and/or free air in the abdomen. Ultrasonography may be useful in demonstrating bowel wall edema and thickening. Abdominal CT is thought to be the most useful imaging modality for the early diagnosis of mesenteric ischemia and can demonstrate prominence of mesenteric vessels with a palisade pattern supplying dilated bowel loops, ascites, and bowel wall thickening with a double halo sign.[103] Gastroscopy and colonoscopy can sometimes reveal findings of ischemia and ulceration. Because lupus mesenteric vasculitis typically involves the small vessels (arterioles and venules) of the bowel submucosa, mesenteric angiography is usually nondiagnostic. However, angiography can be helpful in ruling out larger vessel causes of mesenteric ischemia, such as polyarteritis nodosa, atherosclerotic disease, or thrombosis resulting from antiphospholipid antibody disease.

Liver test abnormalities have been described in up to 60% of SLE patients at some point during the course of their illness, but clinically significant liver disease is rarely a direct manifestation of SLE.[104] For this reason, the presence of liver disease should prompt a search for non-SLE causes, including medications such as nonsteroidal anti-inflammatory drugs, methotrexate, and azathioprine. Abnormal liver enzymes may be caused by hepatic steatosis as a result of obesity, concomitant diabetes mellitus, or treatment with corticosteroids. Infections such as viral hepatitis, cytomegalovirus (CMV), and Epstein-Barr virus (EBV) must also be excluded. Once medications and infections have been ruled out as possible culprits, persistent liver test abnormalities should prompt an investigation with an abdominal ultrasound and possibly a liver biopsy. Lupus hepatitis is believed to be a distinct entity from autoimmune hepatitis.[105] Lupus hepatitis is typically characterized by the presence of lobular inflammation with a paucity of lymphoid infiltrates. These findings contrast with those of autoimmune hepatitis, in which periportal (interface) inflammation and dense lymphoid infiltrates dominate. Although ANA is frequently seen in these disorders, anti–smooth muscle and anti-LKM antibodies are more frequently noted in autoimmune hepatitis than in lupus hepatitis. Rarely, nodular regenerative hyperplasia complicates SLE. This disorder causes diffuse nodularity of the liver with little fibrosis and can result in portal hypertension. Nodular regenerative hyperplasia is also associated with the presence of antiphospholipid antibodies in some patients.[106] Vascular disorders of the liver such as Budd-Chiari syndrome, hepatic veno-occlusive disease, and hepatic infarction have been described, especially in the setting of antiphospholipid antibodies.

Other rare gastrointestinal manifestations of SLE include intestinal pseudo-obstruction and protein-losing enteropathy. Intestinal pseudo-obstruction is characterized by decreased intestinal motility caused by dysfunction of the visceral smooth muscle or enteric nervous system.[107] The small bowel is more frequently involved than the large bowel. Presenting symptoms include abdominal pain, nausea, vomiting, and abdominal distention. Patients with protein-losing enteropathy experience abdominal pain, profound pitting edema, and diarrhea and are noted to have a hypoalbuminemia. Other causes of hypoalbuminemia, such as nephrotic syndrome from renal disease, must be excluded.

OPHTHALMOLOGIC

SLE can affect the eye in a variety of ways. The most common ocular manifestation is keratoconjunctivitis sicca (KCS), which can occur in the presence or absence of secondary Sjögren's syndrome.[108] Retinal abnormalities can be detected on ophthalmoscopic examination as retinal hemorrhages, vasculitic-appearing lesions, cotton wool spots, and hard exudates. SLE retinopathy is believed to be an immune complex–mediated vasculopathy and/or the result of microthrombotic events. The presence of retinal abnormalities has been shown to correlate with lupus nephritis, CNS lupus, and the presence of antiphosholipid antibodies.[109] Episcleritis and scleritis can occur in SLE. Uveitis is extremely rare. Discoid lupus can involve the lower eyelid and conjunctiva. Glucocorticoids and antimalarial agents, two medications commonly used for the treatment of SLE, can affect the eye. Posterior subcapsular cataracts and elevated intraocular pressure are well-described complications of glucocorticoid therapy, and maculopathy is a rare but serious complication of the use of hydroxychloroquine and chloroquine. The risk of retinal toxicity is low if the daily dose of chloroquine is kept below 3 mg/kg of ideal body weight and the daily dose of hydroxychloroquine is kept at or below 6.5 mg/kg of ideal body weight..

HEMATOLOGIC

Hematologic involvement is common in SLE; all three blood cell lines can be affected. When evaluating a patient with the hematologic abnormalities as described later, it is always necessary to consider the potential of myelosuppression from medications such as methotrexate, azathioprine, mycophenolate mofetil, and cyclophosphamide. In addition, corticosteroids are a common cause of lymphopenia and leukocytosis secondary to neutrophilia.

Anemia

Anemia of chronic disease (ACD) is the most common anemia in SLE. It is a normochromic, normocytic anemia characterized by the presence of low serum iron, low transferrin, and normal to increased serum ferritin. ACD can coexist with anemias resulting from other processes. Autoimmune hemolytic anemia (AIHA) should be suspected in the setting of the following laboratory abnormalities: increased serum unconjugated bilirubin, increased lactate dehydrogenase (LDH), increased reticulocyte count, and reduced serum haptoglobin. The direct Coombs' test is typically positive and usually is mediated by warm-reacting IgG anti-erythrocyte antibodies. The peripheral blood smear demonstrates spherocytosis. Some reports have suggested an association between AIHA and the presence of anticardiolipin antibodies.[110,111] A positive direct Coombs' test can

occur without hemolysis. AIHA may be the presenting manifestation of SLE, or it may predate full-blown SLE by many years.

Microangiopathic hemolytic anemia (MAHA), characterized by the presence of schistocytes on peripheral blood smear, should prompt consideration of thrombotic thrombocytopenic purpura–hemolytic uremic syndrome (TTP-HUS). TTP is a syndrome consisting of MAHA, thrombocytopenia, fever, neurologic symptoms, and renal involvement, and may be associated with SLE. Because MAHA, thrombocytopenia, neurologic symptoms, and renal involvement can also occur in catastrophic antiphospholipid antibody syndrome (CAPS), antiphospholipid antibodies should always be measured as part of the evaluation. Blood loss, renal insufficiency, pure red cell aplasia, and medication-induced myelotoxicity are additional potential causes of anemia in SLE patients.

Leukopenia

Leukopenia occurs in approximately 50% of SLE patients and can occur secondary to lymphopenia and/or neutropenia. One study of 158 newly diagnosed, clinically active SLE patients demonstrated that 75% of patients had lymphocyte counts lower than 1500 cells/μL, and that lymphopenia eventually developed in 93% of patients.[112] The presence of lymphocytoxic antibodies in some SLE patients correlates with lymphopenia and with disease exacerbation.[113] Lymphopenia may be a side effect of treatment with glucocorticoids or other immunosuppressive agents. Neutropenia due to SLE can result from immune-mediated destruction or marrow suppression.

Thrombocytopenia

Mild thrombocytopenia is noted in up to 50% of SLE patients, but severe thrombocytopenia can also occur. Thrombocytopenia can be the result of immune-mediated platelet destruction similar to immune thrombocytopenic purpura (ITP). The platelet IIb/IIIa antigen is the primary target. Thrombocytopenia can also be caused by a consumptive process such as TTP or splenomegaly. Antithrombopoietin antibodies have been found in the sera of some SLE patients and have been correlated with lower platelet counts.[114] Chronic, low-level thrombocytopenia is a characteristic feature of the antiphospholipid antibody syndrome. Similar to AIHA, isolated ITP may pre-date the development of complete SLE by several years.[115]

LYMPHADENOPATHY AND SPLENOMEGALY

Lymphadenopathy commonly occurs in association with active SLE and is characterized by the presence of enlarged, soft, nontender lymph nodes. Lymphadenopathy can be focal or generalized; the cervical, axillary, and inguinal regions are typically involved. Lymph node histopathology demonstrates reactive hyperplasia and varying degrees of coagulative necrosis. The presence of hematoxylin bodies is specific for SLE. Histologic features of Castleman's disease have been reported.[116] The differential diagnosis of lymphadenopathy in an SLE patient includes infection and/or a lymphoproliferative process; lymph node biopsy is sometimes required for diagnosis. Splenomegaly can be observed in patients with SLE and may be associated with hepatomegaly. Histopathologic studies demonstrate periarterial fibrosis (onion-skin lesions). Splenic atrophy and functional asplenism have also been reported.[117]

DIAGNOSIS

Establishing the diagnosis of SLE can be challenging because of its heterogeneous disease manifestations and waxing and waning clinical course. No clinical manifestation or laboratory test can serve as a definitive diagnostic test. Instead, SLE is diagnosed on the basis of a constellation of characteristic symptoms, signs, and laboratory findings in the appropriate clinical context. Although the ACR classification criteria (see Table 80-1) cannot always be relied upon for diagnostic purposes in individual patients, they serve as useful reminders of the wide variety of clinical features that can be seen in SLE.

Serologic Tests

Serologic tests play an important role in the diagnosis of SLE. SLE is the prototypic systemic humoral autoimmune disease. As such, it is characterized by production of a wide variety of autoantibodies, which often provide important diagnostic information[118] (Table 80-7). The hallmark serologic feature is the presence of ANAs, as reflected by a positive ANA test. The gold standard method for detecting ANA is indirect immunofluorescence using a human epithelial cell tumor line (HEp2 cell line). With this method, the ANA test is highly sensitive in that it is positive in more than 95% of people with SLE. Because of a desire for automation and cost savings, some laboratories are utilizing the enzyme-linked immunosorbent assay (ELISA) as the method of testing for ANA. However, the ELISA method is less accurate than the immunofluorescence method, resulting in a higher false-negative rate. Positive ANA tests also occur in many other autoimmune diseases, including rheumatoid arthritis, scleroderma, polymyositis, and autoimmune thyroiditis, among others. ANAs are also detectable in low titers (<1:80) in many people without autoimmune disease, especially in the elderly.[119] Therefore, a positive test is not sufficient to establish the diagnosis of SLE. On the other hand, a negative test can be helpful in ruling out SLE. Although "ANA-negative" SLE has been reported, it is very rare with the immunofluorescence method of testing. In those rare instances, other tests (e.g., anti-Ro/SSA) confirm the presence of lupus-associated autoantibodies.[120]

Once it has been established that ANAs are present, it is important to determine which particular nuclear antigens may be the target of the autoantibodies, because some of these antigen-specific responses provide great diagnostic specificity. The most important of these tests is the test for antibodies to double-stranded DNA (anti-dsDNA). Anti-dsDNA antibodies are present in no more than 50% to 60% of patients with lupus, so their absence does not exclude the possibility of SLE. However, the presence of these antibodies is highly specific for SLE and therefore can be very helpful in establishing a definitive diagnosis. Similarly, antibodies to the Sm antigen have great specificity for SLE, but these antibodies are present in even fewer SLE patients ($\approx$30%). The Sm antigen is a component of extractable nuclear antigens (ENAs), a term that refers to a heterogeneous mixture of non-DNA nuclear antigens that can be "extracted" from cells in the laboratory. These antigens are primarily ribonucleoproteins that can be divided into two major subsets based on their susceptibility to digestion by ribonuclease. The ribonuclease-sensitive antigens are designated RNP. Ribonuclease-resistant antigens are designated Sm (because these antibodies were first detected in a patient named Smith). Unlike anti-Sm, anti-RNP is not specific for SLE. However, high titers of anti-RNP antibodies can be helpful in supporting the diagnosis of MCTD.[121]

Numerous other autoantibodies can be found in patients with SLE. Antibodies to cytoplasmic antigens, such as Ro and La (SSA and SSB), can be found in some patients with SLE. Although these autoantibodies lack both sensitivity and specificity for SLE, they sometimes are associated with distinct clinical syndromes. The best example of such a relationship involves the presence of anti-Ro antibodies in more than 90% of cases of neonatal lupus.[122,123] Anti-Ro antibodies are also seen with increased frequency in patients with SCLE.[124] Other autoantibodies may be directed against cell surface molecules or against circulating proteins. For example, antibodies to blood components can be responsible for hemolytic anemia, neutropenia, or thrombocytopenia, and antibodies to phospholipids can be detected in some SLE patients with or without antiphospholipid syndrome (see Chapter 82). It should be noted that rheumatoid

Table 80-7 Autoantibodies and Clinical Significance in Systemic Lupus Erythematosus (SLE)

Autoantibody	Prevalence in SLE	Clinical Significance
Antinuclear Antibody		
Anti-dsDNA	60%	95% specificity for SLE; fluctuates with disease activity; associated with glomerulonephritis
Anti-Smith	20%-30%	99% specificity for SLE; associated with anti-U1RNP antibodies
Anti-U1RNP	30%	Antibody associated with mixed connective tissue disease and lower frequency of glomerulonephritis
Anti-Ro/SSA	30%	Associated with Sjögren's syndrome, photosensitivity, SCLE, neonatal lupus, congenital heart block
Anti-La/SSB	20%	Associated with Sjögren's syndrome, SCLE, neonatal lupus, congenital heart block, anti-Ro/SSA
Antihistone	70%	Also associated with drug-induced lupus
Antiphospholipid	30%	Associated with arterial and venous thrombosis, pregnancy morbidity

SCLE, subacute cutaneous lupus erythematosus.

factor (anti-IgG) can be found in 15% to 20% of people with SLE, whether or not joint disease is present.[125] Anti-CCP antibodies can also be present.

Complement consumption arising from immune complex disease may lead to hypocomplementemia in patients with SLE.[126,127] Because hypocomplementemia is rare in other diseases, its presence in a patient with SLE can provide valuable supportive evidence for the diagnosis. Moreover, because hypocomplementemia most likely reflects complement activation by immune complexes, its presence is often a sign of active disease. However, hereditary complement deficiencies may be found in patients with SLE (C1q, C2, C4), so absence of a particular complement component does not always reflect consumption.[128-130] For this reason, it is often necessary to measure more than one complement component (e.g., C3 and C4) before concluding that hypocomplementemia is due to active disease.

The utility of serologic tests in assessing disease activity and predicting disease flares remains a topic of controversy. In the absence of a hereditary complement deficiency, hypocomplementemia is a reliable indicator that the disease is active, but normal complement levels do not rule out active disease. Titers of anti-dsDNA antibodies correlate with disease activity in some patients, but not in others. One recent study attempted to resolve the long-standing debate about the prognostic value of changes in lupus serology.[131] In this study, patients with clinically quiescent lupus underwent monthly monitoring for levels of anti-dsDNA, C3a, C3, C4, and CH50 to identify patients with serologically active, clinically quiescent disease. These patients were then randomized to treatment with corticosteroids or placebo to determine whether treatment of serologically active disease could prevent impending clinical flares. The results were equivocal. Some patients with serologically active disease flared, and some flares were apparently prevented. However, in most control subjects, serologic deterioration was not followed by a clinical flare, and most of the flares that occurred in the original patient population that had been monitored were not preceded by serologic deterioration. Thus, there remains no substitute for knowledge of a particular patient's pattern or whether there is an association between clinical and serologic manifestations in that patient.

DIFFERENTIAL DIAGNOSIS

Because of the involvement of multiple organ systems and the lack of specificity of symptoms and/or signs, many systemic diseases can mimic SLE. Thus, before a diagnosis of SLE is established, a comprehensive search for infectious, malignant, and other autoimmune diseases must be undertaken.

Several viral infections can produce symptoms and signs that are present in SLE. In addition, many viral illnesses are associated with the production of autoantibodies. A careful patient history with serologic testing for the potential pathogen should help to secure the correct diagnosis. Parvovirus B19 classically presents with fever, rash, symmetric inflammatory polyarthritis, and cytopenias. Furthermore, the presence of ANA, anti-dsDNA, and hypocomplementemia has been observed in a few cases. Cytomegalovirus and Epstein-Barr virus can mimic SLE in that patients often present with fatigue, cytopenias, abdominal pain, and liver test abnormalities. Acute HIV infection typically presents with fever, diffuse lymphadenopathy, and oral ulcers. Patients with hepatitis B and C can develop inflammatory arthritis and positive autoantibodies.

Malignancy, particularly non-Hodgkin's lymphoma, can manifest with constitutional symptoms, joint pain, cytopenias, lymphadenopathy, rash, and a positive ANA. One must be particularly alert to the possibility of malignancy in an older patient presenting with a new lupus-like syndrome. It is important to ensure that patients undergo appropriate malignancy screening tests.

Other autoimmune diseases such as RA, dermatomyositis, and Still's disease often share similar clinical features with SLE. Differentiating between these disorders might be difficult in early phases of the disease. Patients with RA and SLE may develop a symmetric inflammatory arthritis with a predilection for the wrists and small joints of the hands. ANA and rheumatoid factor (RF) may be elevated in both disorders, although anti-CCP antibody suggests RA, and anti-dsDNA or anti-Sm suggests SLE. The photosensitive, erythematous rashes of dermatomyositis and SLE can appear clinically and histopathologically identical. A careful patient history and supporting serologies will aid in making the correct diagnosis. Mixed connective tissue disease (MCTD) must also be considered when evaluating a patient for possible SLE. MCTD is a syndrome characterized by a high-titer anti-RNP antibody in conjunction with clinical features that are often present in SLE, scleroderma, and/or polymyositis. Patients frequently present with puffy, swollen hands and Raynaud's phenomenon. In contrast to SLE, patients with MCTD can develop an erosive arthritis that looks very similar to RA.

Careful evaluation for drug-induced lupus should be undertaken in every new patient in whom the diagnosis of SLE is suspected. This is especially important in an older person presenting with a lupus-like syndrome. Arthralgia, myalgia, fever, and serositis are common manifestations. A wide variety of drugs have been implicated in the development of drug-induced lupus; minocycline, procainamide, hydralazine, isoniazid, interferon alpha, and anti-TNF agents are well-known culprits. Hydrochlorothiazide is associated with SCLE. All of these drugs may cause a positive ANA. Minocycline is occasionally associated with anti-dsDNA antibodies and perinuclear-staining antineutrophil cytoplasmic antibodies (P-ANCA), and anti-TNF agents can cause positive anti-dsDNA antibodies. Antihistone antibodies are present in more than 95% of cases of drug-induced lupus, with the exception of those cases caused by minocycline However, antihistone antibodies cannot be used to confirm a diagnosis of drug-induced lupus because up to 80% of idiopathic SLE patients will also produce antihistone antibodies.

NEONATAL LUPUS

Neonatal lupus is a passively acquired autoimmune disease of neonates that results from transplacental passage of maternal anti-SSA and/or anti-SSB antibodies.[132] It can occur in mothers with SLE, in those with Sjögren's syndrome, or in patients in whom an autoimmune disease has not been diagnosed. Neonatal lupus can involve multiple organ systems, including heart, skin, liver, and the hematologic system; the most severe complications are congenital complete heart block and cardiomyopathy.[133] The term *neonatal lupus* stems from early observations that the skin lesions in affected newborns were similar to the lesions of SCLE.

Congenital complete heart block is associated with a neonatal mortality rate as high as 20%, and most patients will eventually require a permanent pacemaker. This complication occurs in up to 2% of babies born to mothers who are positive for anti-Ro/SSA and/or anti-LA/SSB antibodies. Once a woman has given birth to a baby with complete heart block, the risk for recurrence in a subsequent pregnancy is approximately 15%. Evidence from in vitro studies suggests that during fetal development, fetal cardiocytes undergo apoptosis that results in expression of Ro/SSA and La/SSB on the cell surface. Binding of anti-Ro/SSA and/or anti-La/SSB to fetal cardiocytes leads to inflammatory injury and subsequently to fibrosis of the atrioventricular (AV) node and surrounding tissue. The sinoatrial (SA) node may also be involved. Prospective studies have shown that the vulnerable period for the fetal heart is between 16 and 24 weeks of gestation. Thus, it is recommended that mothers with anti-Ro/SSA and/or anti-La/SSB antibodies undergo monitoring with fetal echocardiography beginning at 16 weeks' gestation. The hope has been that detection of early stages of heart block (first-degree and second-degree block) might allow for treatment that would prevent progression to third-degree heart block. Currently, the treatment of choice is maternal administration of a fluorinated glucocorticoid such as dexamethasone. Fluorinated glucocorticoids are preferred because of their ability to cross the placenta and enter the fetal circulation. However, treatment of incomplete fetal heart block remains controversial because the benefits have not been clearly delineated, and glucocorticoids have been associated with several fetal side effects such as intrauterine growth retardation, oligohydramnios, and adrenal suppression. Complete heart block is irreversible even with treatment, and first- or second-degree heart block may or may not reverse with treatment. Complicating matters, complete heart block can occur in the absence of preceding first- or second-degree block. In addition to conduction blocks, structural cardiac abnormalities have been observed in the setting of neonatal lupus, including, but not limited to, patent ductus arteriosus, ventricular septal defect, atrial septal defect, and patent foramen ovale. Myocarditis and pericarditis have also been described.

Rash, a common manifestation of neonatal lupus, consists of erythematous, annular lesions that resemble the annular subtype of SCLE. The rash typically occurs on the scalp, face, trunk, and extremities with a predilection for the periorbital area; it often develops after exposure of the newborn to ultraviolet light. Lesions typically occur within the first 4 to 6 weeks of life but may be present at birth. The rash is self-limiting and does not necessitate treatment. Lesions tend to resolve by 6 months of age, at which time maternal anti-Ro/SSA and/or anti-La/SSB antibodies are no longer present in the baby's circulation. Less common manifestations of neonatal lupus include hepatic, hematologic, and neurologic involvement.[134] Hepatic manifestations include asymptomatic elevation of liver function tests, hepatitis, hepatomegaly, cholestasis, and cirrhosis.

Hematologic manifestations include thrombocytopenia, autoimmune hemolytic anemia, and leukopenia. Neurologic complications, including myelopathy, seizures, and aseptic meningitis, have been reported.

Selected References

1. Tan EM, Cohen AS, Fries JF, et al: The 1982 revised classification of systemic lupus erythematosus, *Arthritis Rheum* 11:1271–1277, 1982.
2. Hochberg MC: Updating the American College of Rheumatology revised criteria for the classification of systemic lupus erythematosus, *Arthritis Rheum* 40:1725, 1997.
3. Pons-Estel GJ, Alarcon GS, Scofield L, et al: Understanding the epidemiology and progession of systemic lupus erythematosus, *Semin Arthritis Rheum* 39:257–268, 2010.
4. Uramoto KM, Michet CJ, Thumboo J, et al: Trends in the incidence and mortality of systemic lupus erythematosus, 1950–1992, *Arthritis Rheum* 42:46–50, 1999.
5. Ballou SP, Khan MA, Kushner I: Clinical features of systemic lupus erythematosus, *Arthritis Rheum* 25:55–60, 1982.
6. Chakravarty EF, Bush TM, Manzi S, et al: Prevalence of adult systemic lupus erythematosus in California and Pennsylvania in 2000: estimates obtained using hospitalization data, *Arthritis Rheum* 56:2092–2094, 2007.
7. Boddaert J, Huong DL, Amoura Z, et al: Late-onset systemic lupus erythematosus: a personal series of 47 patients and pooled analysis of 714 cases in the literature, *Medicine* 83:348–359, 2004.
8. Dubois EL, Tuffanelli DL: Clinical manifestations of systemic lupus erythematosus: computer analysis of 520 cases, *JAMA* 190:104–111, 1964.
9. Estes D, Christian CL: The natural history of systemic lupus erythematosus by prospective analysis, *Medicine* 50:85–95, 1971.
10. Hochberg MC, Boyd RE, Ahearn JM, et al: Systemic lupus erythematosus: a review of the clinico-laboratory features and immunopathogenetic markers in 150 patients with emphasis on demographic subsets, *Medicine* 64:285–295, 1985.
11. Pistiner M, Wallace DJ, Nessim S, et al: Lupus erythematosus in the 1980s: a survey of 570 patients, *Semin Arthritis Rheum* 21:55–64, 1991.
12. Vitali C, Bencivelli W, Isenberg DA, et al;: European Consensus Study Group for Disease Activity in SLE: Disease activity in systemic lupus erythematosus: report of the Consensus Study Group of the European Workshop for Rheumatology Research. I. A descriptive analysis of 704 European lupus patients, *Clin Exp Rheumatol* 10:527–539, 1992.
13. Gilliam JN, Sontheimer RD: Distinctive cutaneous subsets in the spectrum of lupus erythematosus, *J Am Acad Dermatol* 4:471–475, 1981.
14. Sontheimer RD: The lexicon of cutaneous lupus erythematosus: a review and personal perspective on the nomenclature and classification of the cutaneous manifestations of lupus erythematosus, *Lupus* 6:84–95, 1997.
15. Watanabe T, Tsuchida T: Classification of lupus erythematosus based upon cutaneous manifestations: dermatologic, systemic, and laboratory features in 191 patients, *Dermatology* 190:277–283, 1995.
17. Gilliam JN, Sontheimer RD: Skin manifestations of SLE, *Clin Rheum Dis* 8:207–218, 1982.
18. Chaudhry SI, Murphy LA, White IR: Subacute cutaneous lupus erythematosus: a paraneoplastic dermatosis? *Clin Exp Dermatol* 30:655–658, 2005.
19. Parikh N, Choi J, Li M, et al: Squamous cell carcinoma arising in a recent plaque of discoid lupus erythematosus, in a sun-protected area, *Lupus* 19:210–212, 2010.
20. Perniciaro C, Randle HW, Perry HO: Hypertrophic discoid lupus erythematosus resembling squamous cell carcinoma, *Dermatol Surg* 21:255–257, 1995.
21. Walling HW, Sontheimer RD: Cutaneous lupus erythematosus: issues in diagnosis and treatment, *Am J Clin Dermatol* 10:365–381, 2009.
22. Vassileva S: Bullous systemic lupus erythematosus, *Clin Dermatol* 22:129–138, 2004.
23. Sanders CJ, Van Weelden H, Kazzaz GA, et al: Photosensitivity in patients with lupus erythematosus: a clinical and photobiological study of 100 patients using a prolonged phototest protocol, *Br J Dermatol* 131:131–137, 2003.
24. Tutrone WD, Spann CT, Scheinfeld N, Deleo VA: Polymorphic light eruption, *Dermatol Ther* 16:28–39, 2003.

25. Fabbri P, Amato L, Chiarini C, et al: Scarring alopecia in discoid lupus erythematosus: a clinical, histopathologic and immunopathologic study, *Lupus* 13:455–462, 2004.

26. Alarcon-Segovia D, Cetina JA: Lupus hair, *Am J Med Sci* 267:241–242, 1974.

28. Nico MM, Vilela MA, Rivitti EA, Lourenço SV: Oral lesions in lupus erythematosus: correlation with cutaneous lesions, *Eur J Dermatol* 18:376–381, 2008.

29. Jonsson R, Heyden G, Westberg NG, Nyberg G: Oral mucosal lesions in systemic lupus erythematosus—a clinical, histopathological and immunopathological study, *J Rheumatol* 11:38–42, 1984.

30. David-Bajar KM, Davis BM: Pathology, immunopathology, and immunohistochemistry in cutaneous lupus erythematosus, *Lupus* 6:145–157, 1997.

32. Grossman JM: Lupus arthritis, *Best Pract Res Clin Rheumatol* 23:495–506, 2009.

33. Labowitz R, Schumacher HR: Articular manifestations of systemic lupus erythematosus, *Ann Intern Med* 74:911–921, 1971.

34. Morley KD, Leung A, Rynes RI: Lupus foot, *Br Med J* 284:557–558, 1982.

35. Chan MT, Owen P, Dunphy J, et al: Associations of erosive arthritis with anti-cyclic citrullinated peptide antibodies and MHC Class II alleles in systemic lupus erythematosus, *J Rheumatol* 35:77–83, 2008.

36. Ostendorf B, Scherer A, Specker C, et al: Jaccoud's arthropathy in systemic lupus erythematosus: differentiation of deforming and erosive patterns by magnetic resonance imaging, *Arthritis Rheum* 48:157–165, 2003.

37. Boutry N, Hachulla E, Flipo RM, et al: MR imaging findings in hands in early rheumatoid arthritis: comparison with those in systemic lupus erythematosus and primary Sjögren syndrome, *Radiology* 236:593–600, 2005.

39. Weissman BN, Rappoport AS, Sosman JL, Schur PH: Radiographic findings in the hands in patients with systemic lupus erythematosus, *Radiology* 126:313–317, 1978.

40. Leskinen RH, Skrifvars BV, Laasonen LS, Edgren KJ: Bone lesions in systemic lupus erythematosus, *Radiology* 153:349–352, 1984.

41. Dubois EL, Cozen L: Avascular (aseptic) bone necrosis associated with systemic lupus erythematosus, *JAMA* 174:966–971, 1960.

42. Nagasawa K, Tada Y, Koarada S, et al: Very early development of steroid-associated osteonecrosis of femoral head in systemic lupus erythematosus: prospective study by MRI, *Lupus* 14:385–390, 2005.

43. Oinuma K, Harada Y, Nawata Y, et al: Osteonecrosis in patients with systemic lupus erythematosus develops early after starting high dose corticosteroid treatment, *Ann Rheum Dis* 60:1145–1148, 2001.

44. Fialho SC, Bonfa E, Vitule LF, et al: Disease activity as a major risk factor for osteonecrosis in early systemic lupus erythematosus, *Lupus* 16:239–244, 2007.

45. Calvo-Alén J, McGwin G, Toloza S, et al; LUMINA Study Group: Systemic lupus erythematosus in a multiethnic US cohort (LUMINA): XXIV. Cytotoxic treatment is an additional risk factor for the development of symptomatic osteonecrosis in lupus patients: results of a nested matched case-control study, *Ann Rheum Dis* 65:785–790, 2006.

46. Tsokos GC, Moutsopoulos HM, Steinberg AD: Muscle involvement in systemic lupus erythematosus, *JAMA* 246:766–768, 1981.

47. Lim KL, Abdul-Wahab R, Lowe J, Powell RJ: Muscle biopsy abnormalities in systemic lupus erythematosus: correlation with clinical and laboratory parameters, *Ann Rheum Dis* 53:178–182, 1994.

48. Danila MI, Pons-Estel GJ, Zhang J, et al: Renal damage is the most important predictor of mortality within the damage index: data from LUMINA LXIV, a multiethnic US cohort, *Rheumatology (Oxford)* 48:542–545, 2009.

50. Austin HA 3rd, Boumpas DT, Vaughan EM, Balow JE: Predicting renal outcomes in severe lupus nephritis: contributions of clinical and histologic data, *Kidney Int* 45:544–550, 1994.

51. Descombes E, Droz D, Drouet L, et al: Renal vascular lesions in lupus nephritis, *Medicine* 76:355–368, 1997.

52. Appel GB, Pirani CL, D'Agati V: Renal vascular complications of systemic lupus erythematosus, *J Am Soc Nephrol* 4:1499–1515, 1994.

53. Banfi G, Bertani T, Boeri V, et al: Renal vascular lesions as a marker of poor prognosis in patients with lupus nephritis. Gruppo Italiano per lo Studio della Nefrite Lupica (GISNEL), *Am J Kidney Dis* 18:240–248, 1991.

54. Baranowska-Daca E, Choi YJ, Barrios R, et al: Nonlupus nephritides in patients with systemic lupus erythematosus: a comprehensive clinicopathologic study and review of the literature, *Hum Pathol* 32:1125–1135, 2001.

55. Austin HA: Clinical evaluation and monitoring of lupus kidney disease, *Lupus* 7:618–621, 1998.

56. Keane WF: Proteinuria: its clinical importance and role in progressive renal disease, *Am J Kidney Dis* 35(4 Suppl 1):S97–S105, 2005.

57. Birmingham DJ, Rovin BH, Shidham G, et al: Spot urine protein/creatinine ratios are unreliable estimates of 24 h proteinuria in most systemic lupus erythematosus nephritis flares, *Kidney Int* 72:865–870, 2007.

58. Ginsberg JM, Chang BS, Matarese RA, Garella S: Use of single voided urine samples to estimate quantitative proteinuria, *N Engl J Med* 309:1543–1546, 1983.

59. Fine DM, Ziegenbein M, Petri M, et al: A prospective study of protein excretion using short-interval timed urine collections in patients with lupus nephritis, *Kidney Int* 76:1284–1288, 2009.

60. Grande JP, Balow JE: Renal biopsy in lupus nephritis, *Lupus* 7:611–617, 1998.

61. Weening JJ, D'Agati VD, Schwartz MM, et al: The classification of glomerulonephritis in systemic lupus erythematosus revisited, *J Am Soc Nephrol* 15:241–250, 2004.

62. Eiser AR, Katz SM, Swartz C: Clinically occult diffuse proliferative lupus nephritis: an age-related phenomenon, *Arch Intern Med* 139:1022–1025, 1979.

63. Jacobsen S, Starklint H, Petersen J, et al: Prognostic value of renal biopsy and clinical variables in patients with lupus nephritis and normal serum creatinine, *Scand J Rheumatol* 28:288–299, 1999.

64. Good JT Jr, King TE, Antony VB, Sahn SA: Lupus pleuritis: clinical features and pleural fluid characteristics with special reference to pleural fluid antinuclear antibodies, *Chest* 84:714–718, 1983.

65. Breuer GS, Deeb M, Fisher D, Nesher G: Therapeutic options for refractory massive pleural effusion in systemic lupus erythematosus: a case study and review of the literature, *Semin Arthritis Rheum* 34:744–749, 2005.

66. Man BL, Mok CC: Serositis related to systemic lupus erythematosus: prevalence and outcome, *Lupus* 14:822–826, 2005.

67. ter Borg EJ, Horst G, Limburg PC, et al: C-reactive protein levels during disease exacerbations and infections in systemic lupus erythematosus: a prospective longitudinal study, *J Rheumatol* 17:1642–1648, 1990.

68. Haupt HM, Moore GW, Hutchins GM: The lung in systemic lupus erythematosus: analysis of the pathologic changes in 120 patients, *Am J Med* 71:791–798, 1981.

70. Matthay RA, Schwarz MI, Petty TL, et al: Pulmonary manifestations of systemic lupus erythematosus: review of twelve cases of acute lupus pneumonitis, *Medicine* 54:397–409, 1975.

71. Todd DJ, Costenbader KH: Dyspnea in a young woman with active systemic lupus erythematosus, *Lupus* 18:777–784, 2009.

72. Hoffbrand BI, Beck ER: Unexplained dyspnea and shrinking lungs in systemic lupus erythematosus, *Br Med J* 1:1273–1277, 1965.

74. Andonopoulos AP, Constantopoulos SH, Galanopoulou V, et al: Pulmonary function of nonsmoking patients with systemic lupus erythematosus, *Chest* 94:312–315, 1988.

76. Crozier IG, Li E, Milne MJ, Nicholls MG: Cardiac involvement in systemic lupus erythematosus detected by echocardiography, *Am J Cardiol* 65:1145–1148, 1990.

77. Bulkley BH, Roberts WC: The heart in systemic lupus erythematosus and the changes induced in it by corticosteroid therapy: a study of 36 necropsy patients, *Am J Med* 58:243–264, 1975.

78. Roldan CA, Shively BK, Crawford MH: An echocardiographic study of valvular heart disease associated with systemic lupus erythematosus, *N Engl J Med* 335:1424–1430, 1996.

79. Bidani AK, Roberts JL, Schwartz MM, Lewis EJ: Immunopathology of cardiac lesions in fatal systemic lupus erythematosus, *Am J Med* 69:849–858, 1980.

80. Roldan CA, Qualls CR, Sopko KS, Sibbitt WL Jr: Transthoracic versus transesophageal echocardiography for detection of Libman-Sacks endocarditis: a randomized controlled study, *J Rheumatol* 35:224–229, 2008.

81. Roldan CA, Gelgand EA, Qualls CR, Sibbitt WL Jr: Valvular heart disease by transthoracic echocardiography is associated with focal brain injury and central neuropsychiatric systemic lupus erythematosus, *Cardiology* 108:331–337, 2007.

82. Urowitz MB, Bookman AA, Koehler BE, et al: The bimodal mortality pattern of systemic lupus erythematosus, *Am J Med* 60:221–225, 1976.

83. Haider YS, Roberts WC: Coronary arterial disease in systemic lupus erythematosus: quantification of degrees of narrowing in 22 necropsy patients (21 women) aged 16 to 37 years, *Am J Med* 70:775–781, 1981.

84. Manzi S, Meilahn EN, Rairie JE, et al: Age-specific incidence rates of myocardial infarction and angina in women with systemic lupus erythematosus: comparison with the Framingham study, *Am J Epidemiol* 145:408–415, 1997.

85. Urowitz MB, Gladman D, Ibanez D, et al;: Systemic Lupus International Collaborating Clinics: Atherosclerotic vascular events in a multinational inception cohort of systemic lupus erythematosus, *Arthritis Care Res* 62:881–887, 1995.

86. Esdaile JM, Abrahamowicz M, Grodzicky T, et al: Traditional Framingham risk factors fail to fully account for accelerated atherosclerosis in systemic lupus erythematosus, *Arthritis Rheum* 44:2331–2337, 1991.

87. The American College of Rheumatology nomenclature and case definitions for neuropsychiatric lupus syndromes, *Arthritis Rheum* 42:599–608, 1999.

88. Karassa FB, Afeltra A, Ambrozic A, et al: Accuracy of anti-ribosomal P protein antibody testing for the diagnosis of neuropsychiatric systemic lupus erythematosus: an international meta-analysis, *Arthritis Rheum* 54:312–324, 2006.

89. Futrell N, Schultz LR, Millikan C: Central nervous system disease in patients with systemic lupus erythematosus, *Neurology* 42:1649–1657, 1992.

90. Molloy ES, Calabrese LH: Progressive multifocal leukoencephalopathy: a national estimate of frequency in systemic lupus erythematosus and other rheumatic diseases, *Arthritis Rheum* 60:3761–3765, 2009.

91. Sibbitt WL Jr, Brooks WM, Kornfeld M, et al: Magnetic resonance imaging and brain histopathology in neuropsychiatric systemic lupus erythematosus, *Semin Arthritis Rheum* 40:32–52, 2010.

92. Mitsikostas DD, Sfikakis PP, Goadsby PJ: A meta-analysis for headache in systemic lupus erythematosus: the evidence and the myth, *Brain* 127(Pt 5):1200–1209, 2004.

93. Lin YC, Wang AG, Yen MY: Systemic lupus erythematosus-associated optic neuritis: clinical experience and literature review, *Acta Ophthalmol* 87:204–210, 2009.

95. Ferreira S, D'Cruz DP, Hughes GR: Multiple sclerosis, neuropsychiatric lupus and antiphospholipid syndrome: where do we stand? *Rheumatology (Oxford)* 44:434–439, 2005.

97. Krishnan E: Stroke subtypes among young patients with systemic lupus erythematosus, *Am J Med* 118:1415.e1–e7, 2005.

98. Sultan SM, Ioannou Y, Isenberg DA: A review of gastrointestinal manifestations of systemic lupus erythematosus, *Rheumatology* 38:917–932, 1999.

100. Hoffman BI, Katz WA: The gastrointestinal manifestations of systemic lupus erythematosus: a review of the literature, *Semin Arthritis Rheum* 9:237–247, 1980.

101. Reynolds JC, Inman RD, Kimberly RP, et al: Acute pancreatitis in systemic lupus erythematosus: report of twenty cases and a review of the literature, *Medicine* 61:25–32, 1982.

102. Nesher G, Breuer GS, Temprano K, et al: Lupus-associated pancreatitis, *Semin Arthritis Rheum* 35:260–267, 2006.

103. Ko SF, Lee TY, Cheng TT, et al: CT findings at lupus mesenteric vasculitis, *Acta Radiol* 38:115–120, 1997.

104. Runyon BA, LaBrecque DR, Anuras S: The spectrum of liver disease in systemic lupus erythematosus: report of 33 histologically-proved cases and review of the literature, *Am J Med* 69:187–194, 1980.

105. Youssef WI, Tavill AS: Connective tissue diseases and the liver, *J Clin Gastroenterol* 35:345–349, 2002.

108. Davies JB, Rao PK: Ocular manifestations of systemic lupus erythematosus, *Curr Opin Ophthalmol* 19:512–518, 2008.

109. Ushiyama O, Ushiyama K, Koarada S, et al: Retinal disease in patients with systemic lupus erythematosus, *Ann Rheum Dis* 59:705–708, 2000.

110. Fong KY, Loizou S, Boey ML, Walport MJ: Anticardiolipin antibodies, haemolytic anaemia and thrombocytopenia in systemic lupus erythematosus, *Br J Rheumatol* 31:453–455, 1992.

111. Delezé M, Alarcón-Segovia D, Oria CV, et al: Hemocytopenia in systemic lupus erythematosus: relationship to antiphospholipid antibodies, *J Rheumatol* 16:926–930, 1989.

112. Rivero SJ, Díaz-Jouanen E, Alarcón-Segovia D: Lymphopenia in systemic lupus erythematosus: clinical, diagnostic, and prognostic significance, *Arthritis Rheum* 21:295–305, 1978.

113. Winfield JB, Winchester RJ, Kunkel HG: Association of cold-reactive antilymphocyte antibodies with lymphopenia in systemic lupus erythematosus, *Arthritis Rheum* 18:587–594, 1975.

115. Rabinowitz Y, Dameshek W: Systemic lupus erythematosus after "idiopathic" thrombocytopenic purpura: a review, *Ann Intern Med* 52:1–28, 1960.

116. Kojima M, Nakamura S, Morishita Y, et al: Reactive follicular hyperplasia in the lymph node lesions from systemic lupus erythematosus patients: a clinicopathological and immunohistological study of 21 cases, *Pathol Int* 50:304–312, 2000.

118. Kavanaugh A, Tomar R, Reveille J, et al: Guidelines for clinical use of the antinuclear antibody test and tests for specific autoantibodies to nuclear antigens, *Arch Pathol Lab Med* 124:71–81, 2000.

119. Tan EM, Feltkamp TE, Smolen JS, et al: Range of antinuclear antibodies in "healthy" individuals, *Arthritis Rheum* 40:1601–1611, 1997.

120. Maddison PJ, Provost TT, Reichlin M: Serologic findings in patients with "ANA-negative" systemic lupus erythematosus, *Medicine* 60:87–94, 1981.

121. Sharp GC, Irvin WS, Tan EM, et al: Mixed connective tissue disease: an apparently distinct rheumatic disease syndrome associated with a specific antibody to an extractable nuclear antigen (ENA), *Am J Med* 52:148–159, 1972.

122. Watson RM, Lane AT, Barnett NK, et al: Neonatal lupus erythematosus: a clinical, serological and immunogenetic study with review of the literature, *Medicine* 63:362–378, 1984.

123. McCauliffe DP: Neonatal lupus erythematosus: a transplacentally acquired autoimmune disorder, *Semin Dermatol* 14:47–53, 1995.

124. David-Bajar KM, Bennion SD, DeSpain JD, et al: Clinical, histologic, and immunofluorescent distinctions between subacute cutaneous lupus erythematosus and discoid lupus erythematosus, *J Invest Dermatol* 99:251–257, 1992.

125. Singer JM: The latex fixation test in rheumatic diseases, *Am J Med* 31:766–779, 1961.

126. Lloyd W, Schur PH: Immune complexes, complement, and anti-DNA in exacerbations of systemic lupus erythematosus (SLE), *Medicine* 60:208–217, 1981.

127. Swaak AJG, Gorenwold J, Bronsveld W: Predictive value of complement profiles and anti-dsDNA in systemic lupus erythematosus, *Ann Rheum Dis* 45:359–366, 1986.

128. Kirschfink M, Petry F, Khirwadkar K, et al: Complete functional C1q deficiency associated with systemic lupus erythematosus (SLE), *Clin Exp Immunol* 94:267–272, 1993.

129. Agnello V: Complement deficiency states, *Medicine* 57:1–24, 1978.

130. Sturfelt G, Truedsson L, Johansen H, et al: Homozygous C4A deficiency in systemic lupus erythematosus: analysis of patients from a defined population, *Clin Genet* 38:427–433, 1990.

131. Tseng C-E, Buyon JP, Kim M, et al: The effect of moderate-dose corticosteroids in preventing severe flares in patients with serologically active, but clinically stable, systemic lupus erythematosus: findings of a prospective, randomized, double-blind, placebo-controlled trial, *Arthritis Rheum* 54:3623–3632, 2006.

132. Izmirly PM, Rivera TL, Buyon JP: Neonatal lupus syndromes, *Rheum Dis Clin N Am* 33:267–285, 2007.

133. Cimaz R, Spence DL, Hornberger L, Silverman ED: Incidence and spectrum of neonatal lupus erythematosus: a prospective study of infants born to mothers with anti-Ro autoantibodies, *J Pediatr* 142:678–683, 2003.

134. Silverman E, Jaeggi E: Non-cardiac manifestations of neonatal lupus erythematosus, *Scand J Immunol* 72:223–225, 2010.

Full references for this chapter can be found on www.expertconsult.com.

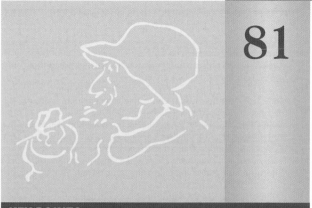

81

Treatment of Systemic Lupus Erythematosus

GEORGE BERTSIAS •
ANTONIOS FANOURIAKIS •
DIMITRIOS T. BOUMPAS

KEY POINTS

The standard of care for SLE with severe, major organ involvement involves the combination of high-dose glucocorticoids with pulses of intravenous cyclophosphamide CYC. However, this regimen is associated with significant toxicity including gonadal failure in young women. Mycophenolate mofetil (MMF) is at least equally effective and has a better toxicity profile than CYC in the treatment of moderately severe proliferative lupus nephritis (PLN). Maintenance of renal remission in moderate to severe PLN may be achieved with both azathioprine and MMF.

In lupus nephritis refractory to standard immunosuppressive therapy, calcineurin inhibitors (cyclosporin A, tacrolimus) have demonstrated some efficacy exerting significant antiproteinuric effects.

SLE pregnancies are considered high risk for maternal and fetal complications, underscoring the importance of family counseling and planning before pregnancy is sought. Common effective means of contraception are generally safe in SLE patients.

Pediatric-onset SLE is associated with high disease severity and rapid damage accrual. Treatment is guided by experience obtained in adult patients and involves the combination of glucocorticoids and immunosuppressive agents for severe manifestations.

Infections contribute to significant morbidity in SLE. Strategies to decrease their impact include (1) education aimed at both patients and physicians; (2) immunizations similar to those available to the general population; (3) minimization of exposure to glucocorticoids; and (4) prompt initiation of antimicrobial therapy in suspected infection.

The realization that a significant proportion of SLE patients features disease- and treatment-related comorbidities has shifted attention to adjunct therapies and primary prevention strategies such as renoprotective and cardiovascular disease risk reduction measures.

CLINICAL COURSE AND GENERAL TREATMENT STRATEGY

KEY POINTS

Treatment of moderate or severe systemic lupus erythematosus (SLE) requires an initial period of intensive immunosuppressive therapy (induction therapy) to control aberrant immunologic activity, recover function, and halt tissue injury, followed by a longer period of less intense and less toxic therapy (maintenance therapy) to consolidate remission and prevent future flares.

SLE patients experience poor quality of life, which is only in part associated with disease activity and organ damage.

The management of systemic lupus erythematosus (SLE) is challenging due to the clinical heterogeneity and the unpredictable course of the disease.[1] SLE activity usually follows the flare pattern, which is characterized by a relapsing-remitting course. However, an equal number of patients have continuously active disease, and only a few have long periods of disease quiescence.[2,3] Despite improvements in overall survival (85% to 90% during the first 10 years), some SLE patients are still at risk for premature death.[4,5] Persistent inflammation inevitably results in irreversible major organ damage, which is linked to decreased quality of life and increased mortality.[6] Accordingly, therapeutic strategies should aim at reducing overall burden of systemic inflammation. Achieving these goals requires (1) accurate assessment of disease activity and flares, (2) stratification according to severity of target organ involvement, (3) use of safe and effective drugs to induce remission promptly and prevent flares, and (4) prevention and management of disease and treatment-related comorbidities.[7]

In general, patients with mild lupus manifestations (skin, joint, and mucosal involvement) are treated with antimalarials or disease-modifying antirheumatic drugs (DMARDs), alone or in combination with low-dose oral glucocorticoids (GCs). Severe SLE with major organ involvement requires an initial period of intensive immunosuppressive therapy (*induction therapy*) to control aberrant immunologic activity and halt tissue injury, followed by a longer period of less intensive and less toxic *maintenance therapy*, to consolidate remission and prevent flares.[8] Immunosuppressive therapy enables for the use of lower GC doses, thus reducing its deleterious effects.

SLE patients experience poor quality of life, which is only in part associated with disease activity and organ damage. Important contributors include fatigue, fibromyalgia, depression, and cognitive dysfunction.[9,10] Treating physicians should regularly address these issues and engage symptomatic or remedial therapies as indicated. The realization that a significant proportion of patients features disease- and treatment-related comorbidities has shifted attention to adjunct therapies and primary prevention strategies such as renoprotective and cardiovascular disease risk reduction measures.

PATIENT AND PHYSICIAN PREFERENCES

KEY POINTS

Patients have a preference for full disclosure of medication risks and treatment alternatives. They also favor an active or collaborative role in decision making involving their health care.

Health professionals are increasingly encouraged to involve patients in treatment decisions, recognizing them as experts with a unique knowledge of their own health and their preferences for treatments, health states, and outcomes.[11] This approach may be particularly challenging in patients with severe lupus who may benefit from cytotoxic therapy, which is, however, associated with significant toxicity. This was demonstrated in a study of 93 well-educated women with mild lupus and good health status who were presented with descriptions of cyclophosphamide (CYC) and azathioprine (AZA) and were then asked to indicate their preferred choice of hypothetical treatment.[12] The study patients had a strong preference for full disclosure of medication risks and treatment alternatives, and they preferred a collaborative role in decision making involving their health care. Nearly all (98%) participants chose AZA over CYC when both drugs conferred an equal probability of renal survival. Although most subjects switched preferences to CYC for better renal survival, a significant proportion (15% to 31%) were unwilling to switch to CYC for improved short- or long-term renal survival. Preference for the long-term benefits of CYC was greater among college than high school graduates, which could reflect a better understanding of the probabilities presented in the study among those with a higher education level. This underscores the importance of providing patients with tailored information to ensure that all patients accurately perceive the risks and benefits related to prescribed medications.

On the other hand, the relative paucity of high-quality evidence to guide therapeutic decisions for various disease manifestations has been a cause for practice pattern variation among lupus experts. Many opinions about the treatment of lupus are based on personal perception rather than valid observation. To facilitate physicians who are in the care of these patients, the European League Against Rheumatism (EULAR) Task Force on SLE has developed management recommendations based on evidence and expert opinion (see Evidence and Expert-based Recommendations in SLE later).

DRUGS USED IN THE TREATMENT OF SYSTEMIC LUPUS ERYTHEMATOSUS

KEY POINTS

The target dose of glucocorticoids should be 0.25 mg/kg every other day for 2 to 3 months, which is acceptable for long-term use. Concomitant use of immunosuppressive agents facilitates tapering and decreases cumulative toxicity.

Antimalarials are effective for skin and mucocutaneous manifestations. Their use has been associated with reduced organ damage accrual.

Azathioprine (AZA) is effective as an induction and a maintenance regimen in mild to moderate SLE including nephritis.

The combination of high-dose glucocorticoids with pulses of intravenous CYC remains the standard of care for severe SLE with major organ involvement.

MMF is at least equally efficacious and has a better toxicity profile than CYC in the treatment of moderately severe PLN.

Calcineurin inhibitors (cyclosporin A, tacrolimus), used alone or in combination with other immunosuppressive agents, have demonstrated efficacy in refractory to cytotoxic therapy lupus nephritis.

Based on evidence from uncontrolled studies, the American College of Rheumatology and the European League Against Rheumatism–European Renal Association have included rituximab (anti-CD20 mAb) as a therapeutic option for selected cases of lupus nephritis refractory to conventional immunosuppressive treatment.

There is an unprecedented array of promising biologic therapies currently in development in SLE.

Glucocorticoids

GCs exert broad inhibitory effects on immune responses mediated by T and B cells, as well as on the effector functions of monocytes and neutrophils. On the basis of these effects and their rapid onset of action, GCs have been remarkably efficacious in managing acute SLE manifestations. However, only two small randomized controlled trials (RCTs) have been conducted to demonstrate their efficacy in lupus.[13,14]

Low-dose GC therapy (≤ 7.5 mg prednisone equivalent per day) is generally used when other initial therapies (antimalarials) are not tolerated or are inadequate to control disease activity. In moderate to severe disease, GCs are used as either single or background therapy in combination with immunosuppressive agents, at doses 0.5 to 1 mg/kg prednisone equivalent in a single dose usually in the morning. When combined with immunosuppressive agents, the GC dose should rarely exceed 0.5 to 0.6 mg/kg prednisone due to concerns for infections and other toxicities. Tapering of GC dose starts after the first 4 to 6 weeks of therapy, targeting a dose of 0.25 mg/kg every other day at 2 to 3 months, which is acceptable for long-term use. Concomitant use of immunosuppressive agents facilitates tapering and decreases cumulative GC toxicity.

Tseng and colleagues[15] examined the effect of a short course of moderate-dose GC in preventing flares in clinically stable but serologically active SLE. Severe flares, requiring increase in prednisone dose or addition of an immunosuppressive agent, or both, occurred in 6 out of 20 patients on placebo, as compared with none of the 21 patients who took prednisone (30 mg for 2 weeks, 20 mg for 1 week, and 10 mg for 1 week). The results agree with those of Bootsma and colleagues[13] and suggest that in clinically stable but serologically active SLE patients, short-term GC therapy may avert a severe flare. This effect must be balanced against risks for overtreating patients with higher cumulative GC doses.

In severe, rapidly progressing disease or when doses greater than 0.6 mg/kg/day prednisone equivalent are required to control disease activity, GC pulse therapy may be introduced.[16,17] Intravenous (IV) pulses of methylprednisolone (MP) (250 to 1000 mg daily for 1 to 3 consecutive days) are used, although there is no strong evidence to support a survival advantage. In addition to expediting remission, IV-MP pulses may allow for the use of lower GC doses during the induction period. In a trial from the National Institutes of Health (NIH), 82 patients with moderate to severe proliferative lupus nephritis (PLN) were randomized to receive sequential induction-maintenance therapy with IV-MP alone, IV-MP plus IV-CYC, or IV-CYC alone.[18] Renal remission was significantly more common in both IV-CYC groups regardless of whether or not they received IV-MP. In the extended follow-up of the trial cohort, an analysis of protocol completers found that doubling of serum creatinine (SCr) was significantly lower in the combination group than in the IV-CYC group (relative risk [RR] 0.095).[19] These findings indicate that combining IV-CYC with IV-MP in the treatment of lupus nephritis (LN) may confer an advantage in long-term renal outcomes without added toxicity.

GC toxicity may involve early (mood effects, acne, myalgias, infections); later (metabolic); and late-onset (osteoporosis, avascular bone necrosis, cataract, cardiovascular disease) adverse events. Although confounded by increased systemic disease activity, most effects are considered to be dependent on the cumulative dose and duration and, to a lesser extent, route of administration. Tailoring GC use on the basis of individual patient profile (disease activity, risk for toxicity) and prompt initiation of primary prevention measures (antiosteoporotic treatment) is of paramount importance.

Antimalarials and DMARD Therapy

Hydroxychloroquine

Antimalarial drugs, mainly chloroquine and hydroxychloroquine (HCQ), are commonly prescribed to SLE patients with skin and joint manifestations but are increasingly identified as an adjuvant treatment for achieving remission in severe lupus. A systematic review concluded that use of antimalarials resulted in a greater than 50% reduction in general SLE disease activity and to a moderate reduction in severe flares and GC dose.[20] Beneficial effects on the lipid profile and subclinical atherosclerosis markers have also been described. Intriguingly, prospective observational studies have reported an inverse association between use of HCQ and accrual of irreversible organ damage, as measured using the Systemic Lupus International Collaborating Clinics–American College of Rheumatology Damage Index (SDI) (adjusted hazard ratio [HR], 0.73), and overall mortality rates (adjusted HR, 0.14 to 0.32).[20] Although these findings may be confounded by milder forms of disease usually present in SLE patients who are prescribed antimalarials, the presumptive mode of action of antimalarials by inhibition of innate immunity pathways provides a plausible explanation for their multifold beneficial effects.[21] HCQ is well tolerated with low rates of mild gastrointestinal and skin adverse events. Retinal toxicity is uncommon (estimated at 0.1% in patients who received HCQ for more than 10 years[20]), but routine ophthalmologic evaluation is recommended (annual screening during the first 5 years of usage is recommended for individuals who are treated with high HCQ dose [>6.5 mg/kg], for those treated more than 5 years, or for those who have other complicating factors).[22]

Methotrexate

Methotrexate (MTX), an antifolate agent commonly prescribed for rheumatoid arthritis (RA), has been used as steroid-sparing treatment for articular and cutaneous manifestations of SLE.[23] MTX is administered weekly either orally or parenterally. Concomitant administration of folic acid (2.5 to 5 mg/week, not until 24 hours after the intake of MTX) is recommended to minimize toxicity (Table 81-1). Fortin and colleagues[24] evaluated the efficacy of MTX in a 12-month placebo-controlled RCT in 86 SLE patients. Patients had mild to moderate disease, with musculoskeletal (93%), cardiovascular (74%), and hematologic (69%) manifestations. Approximately half of the patients in each group were on oral prednisone, whereas 41 patients in the placebo group versus 27 in the MTX group were on antimalarials. Among participants with comparable baseline prednisone dose, those on MTX received on average 1.33 mg/day less prednisone during the trial period compared with those in the placebo group. Fewer patients in the MTX group were also started on GCs (5% vs. 26% in the placebo group). MTX use was associated with a reduction in the mean during-trial Systemic Lupus Activity Measure (SLAM) score of 0.86 units. Together, these data suggest that MTX could be a reasonable alternative steroid-sparing agent in mild to moderate SLE.

Leflunomide

Leflunomide, currently used in RA, has been used in LN refractory or intolerant to standard immunosuppressive therapy. Leflunomide requires a loading dose of 100 mg/day for 3 days followed by 20 mg/day thereafter. In a multicenter observational study, 110 patients with biopsy-proven PLN were assigned to either oral leflunomide or IV-CYC (monthly pulses 0.5 g/m²), both in combination with oral prednisone (0.8 mg/kg/day for 4 weeks, then tapered).[25] After 6 months, complete and partial remission rates were 21% and 52% in the leflunomide group and 18% and 55% in the IV-CYC group, respectively. Repeat kidney biopsies showed significant reduction in activity index and pathologic transformation of 10 cases of diffuse to focal PLN. Similar rates of adverse events were observed in the two study groups and included mostly herpes zoster infection, alopecia, and hypertension. Better-designed RCTs are necessary to establish the efficacy, if any, of leflunomide in PLN. The drug is teratogenic and is contraindicated in patients who are trying to become or are pregnant.

Cytotoxic Therapy

Cyclophosphamide

Pharmacology and Route of Administration. CYC is an alkylating agent that depletes both T and B cells and reduces the production of autoantibodies in lupus. Both oral and IV administration of CYC result in similar plasma concentrations, and the serum half-life is approximately 6 hours. CYC is metabolized to various active metabolites by cytochrome P-450 in the liver or other tissues such as transitional epithelial cells of the bladder or lymphocytes. Drugs that induce hepatic microsomal enzymes (barbiturates,

Table 81-1 Recommended Therapeutic Drug Monitoring in Systemic Lupus Erythematosus

Drug	Dosage	Dose Adjustment	Toxicities Requiring Monitoring	Baseline Evaluation	Laboratory Monitoring
Azathioprine	50-100 mg/day in 1-3 doses with food	↓ 25% if eGFR 10-30 mL/min; ↓ 50% if eGFR < 10 mL/min	Myelosuppression, hepatotoxicity, lymphoproliferative diseases	CBC, platelets, SCr, AST or ALT	CBC and platelets every 2 wk with changes in dosage; baseline tests every 1-3 mo
Mycophenolate mofetil	1-3 g/day in 2 divided doses with food	Maximum 1 g/day if eGFR < 25 mL/min	Myelosuppression, hematotoxicity, infection	CBC, platelet, SCr, AST or ALT	CBCs and platelets every 1-2 wk with changes in dosage; baseline tests every 1-3 mo
Cyclophosphamide	50-150 mg/day in a single dose with breakfast. Lots of fluids (at least 3 L water/day), empty bladder before bedtime	↓ 25% if eGFR 25-50 mL/min; ↓ 30-50% if eGFR < 25 mL/min; ↓ 25% if serum Bil 3.1-5 mg/dL or transaminases >3 times ULN	Myelosuppression, hemorrhagic cystitis, myeloproliferative disease, malignancies	CBC, platelet, SCr, AST or ALT, urinalysis	CBC with differential every 1-2 wk, with changes in dosage and then every 1-3 mo; keep WBC > 4000/mm³ with dose adjustment; urinalysis, AST or ALT every 3 mo; urinalysis every 6-12 mo following cessation
Methotrexate	7.5-15 mg/wk in 1-3 doses with food or milk/water	↓ 50% if eGFR 10-50 mL/min; avoid use if eGFR < 10 mL/min; avoid use in hepatic dysfunction (serum Bil 3.1-5 mg/dL or transaminases >3 times ULN)	Myelosuppression, hepatic fibrosis, pneumonitis	CxR, hepatitis B/C serology in high-risk patients, AST or ALT, SAlb, ALP, SCr	CBC with platelet, AST, SAlb, SCr every 1-3 mo
Cyclosporin A	100-400 mg/day in 2 doses at the same time every day with meal or between meals	Avoid in impaired renal function	Renal insufficiency, anemia, hypertension	CBC, SCr, uric acid, AST or ALT, SAlb, ALP, blood pressure	SCr every 2 wk until dose is stable, then monthly; CBC, potassium, AST or ALT, SAlb, and ALP every 1-3 mo; drug levels only with doses > 3 mg/kg/day
Tacrolimus	1-3 mg/day in 2 doses at the same time every day	Cautious use in liver or renal insufficiency	Renal insufficiency, neurotoxicity, malignancy, infections, hyperkalemia	SCr, potassium, AST or ALT, glucose, blood pressure	Baseline tests once a week for the first 3-4 wk, then every 1-3 mo; monitor drug trough levels
Leflunomide	100 mg/day in a single dose for 3 days, then 10-20 mg/day	Avoid in hepatic dysfunction (serum Bil 3.1-5 mg/dL or transaminases >3 times ULN)	Myelosuppression, hepatotoxicity, fetal toxicity	CBC, SCr, AST or ALT, SAlb, ALP	CBC, AST or ALT, SAlb, and ALP monthly for 6 mo, then every 1-3 mo; monthly monitoring if MTX coadministered
Rituximab	1000 mg on day 1 and 15	None	HBV reactivation (rare)	CBC, SCr, AST or ALT, HBV serology (high-risk patients), TST	CBC and platelets

ALP, alkaline phosphatase; ALT, alanine transaminase; AST, aspartate transaminase; Bil, bilirubin; CBC, complete blood cell count; CxR, chest x-ray; eGFR, estimated glomerular filtration rate; HBV, hepatitis B; LFTs, liver function tests; MTX, methotrexate; SAlb, serum albumin; SCr, serum creatinine; TST, tuberculin skin testing; ULN, upper limit of normal; WBC, white blood cell count.

alcohol, phenytoin, rifampin) may accelerate the metabolism of CYC into its active metabolites and thus increase its pharmacologic and toxic effects. Conversely, drugs that inhibit the hepatic microsomal enzymes (antimalarials, tricyclic antidepressants, and allopurinol) may slow the conversion of CYC to active metabolites. Approximately 20% of the drug is excreted by the kidney, whereas 80% is

processed by the liver. Dose modification is necessary for patients with renal impairment but not in liver disease.

The NIH trials demonstrated equivalent efficacy yet lower toxicity with monthly IV (0.5 to 1 g/m²) versus oral regimens, which led to the predominant use of IV-CYC in clinical practice (Table 81-4). Reversible myelotoxicity is common and dose related. After pulse therapy, the nadir of lymphocyte count occurs on days 7 to 10 and that of granulocyte count on days 10 to 14. The risk of infection increases with a white blood cell count less than 3000 cells/mm^3, so the dose should be adjusted to keep it above this level (see Table 81-1). A prompt recovery from granulocytopenia usually occurs after 21 to 28 days. Thrombocytopenia is rare in CYC monotherapy. Reversible alopecia and nausea are common, whereas infections (especially herpes zoster), gonadal toxicity, and malignancy (including bladder toxicity and carcinoma) are less frequent though much more serious adverse events (see Comorbidities in Systemic Lupus Erythematosus and Women's Health Issues later).

Use in Lupus Nephritis. RCTs with long-term follow-up have shown that intermittent pulse IV-CYC therapy is effective for moderate to severe PLN.[33] CYC may retard progressive renal scarring, preserve renal function, and reduce the risk for the development of end-stage renal disease (ESRD) requiring dialysis or renal transplantation. Following induction therapy, a maintenance regimen is necessary to decrease the risk of flares.[34] NIH studies have demonstrated that combination pulse therapy with IV-CYC and IV-MP improves renal outcomes without increasing toxicity.[18,19] On the basis of these studies, the authors propose 7 monthly pulses of IV-CYC (0.5 to 1 g/m^2) followed by quarterly pulses for at least 1 year beyond remission. For patients with moderate to severe disease, monthly pulses of IV-MP are given during the induction period.

Because of toxicity concerns and the appreciation that the disease may be less severe in whites, European investigators sought alternative IV-CYC protocols. In the Euro-Lupus Nephritis Trial involving mostly patients with milder forms of disease (mean SCr, 1.2 mg/dL; mean proteinuria, 3 g/day), less intensive regimens of IV-CYC (6 fortnightly pulses at a fixed dose of 500 mg each in combination with three daily doses of 750 mg of IV-MP) followed with AZA as maintenance had comparable efficacy and less toxicity than high-dose IV-CYC (8 pulses).[35] Mean survival rate at 10 years was 92% for both groups; ESRD and doubling of SCr rates did not differ between the two groups.[36] Therefore low-dose IV-CYC may be an alternative option for white patients with moderately severe LN.

Austin and colleagues[37] compared cyclosporin A (5 mg/kg/day, then adjusted according to changes in SCr), IV-CYC (0.5 to 1 g/m^2 × 6 monthly doses), and GC alone in an RCT in 42 patients with lupus membranous nephropathy (LMN) (median GFR, 83 mL/min/1.73 m^2; median proteinuria, 5.4 g/day). All patients received alternate-day oral prednisone (1 mg/kg every other day for 8 weeks, then tapered to 0.25 mg/kg every other day). At 1 year, the cumulative probability of remission was 27% with prednisone, 60% with IV-CYC, and 83% with CsA. Rates of nephrotic syndrome relapse per 100 patient-months were 2.0 with CsA versus 0.2 with IV-CYC. Thus although IV-CYC and CsA are equally effective as induction therapy in LMN, CsA may require maintenance therapy (with lower doses of CsA, or AZA, or MMF) to prevent relapses.

Use in Extrarenal Disease. CYC has demonstrated efficacy in life-threatening extrarenal lupus manifestations such as severe thrombocytopenia (platelet count <20,000/mm^3), neurologic disease, abdominal vasculitis, acute pneumonitis/alveolar hemorrhage, and extensive skin disease.[38,39] Barile-Fabris and colleagues[40] have reported

superiority of IV-CYC against IV-MP for severe nonthrombotic neurologic SLE. In this trial, 32 patients were randomized to receive 3 pulses of 1 g of IV-MP followed by one of the following two treatments: pulses of 1 g IV-MP (monthly for 4 months, then every 2 to 3 months for 1 year) or IV-CYC (0.75 g/m^2 monthly for 1 year and then every 3 months for another year). Seizures were the most common syndrome; other manifestations included peripheral neuropathy, optic neuritis, transverse myelitis, brain stem disease, coma, and internuclear ophthalmoplegia. Clinical response was observed in 18 of 19 patients who received IV-CYC as compared with 7 of 13 who received IV-MP. Thus the combination of pulses of IV-MP with IV-CYC is considered as treatment of choice for severe inflammatory neurologic SLE.

Other Agents

Chlorambucil. Chlorambucil (CAB) is an aromatic alkylating agent with substitution of the N-methyl group of mechlorethamine with phenylbutyric acid. The drug is given orally (0.1 to 0.2 mg/kg/day) with good absorption. The effects on immune functions are comparable with those described for CYC. Adverse events are also similar to those of CYC, except for bladder toxicity. More prolonged and less predictable bone marrow suppression can be observed. CAB has been associated with increased risk for leukemia. There is limited experience with the use of CAB in SLE, yet favorable outcomes in renal and extrarenal manifestations such as neuropsychiatric, vasculitis, and multiorgan involvement have been reported. In a retrospective study of 19 patients with predominantly LMN, Moroni and colleagues[56] showed that CAB combined with alternate-month cycles of IV-MP was more effective than IV-MP alone in inducing remission of nephrotic syndrome (64% vs. 38%) and preserving renal function over a period of 83 months. However, the use of CAB for LMN or other lupus manifestations is limited.

Fludarabine. Fludarabine induces profound immunosuppression by depleting T and B lymphocytes and is used in the treatment of hematologic malignancies. A single pilot study in patients with active PLN was terminated prematurely due to severe hematologic toxicity.[57] It is unlikely that fludarabine will be used in SLE.

Antimetabolites Calcineurin Inhibitors

Azathioprine

AZA interferes with the de novo synthesis of inosinic acid and inhibits the conversion of purine bases such as inosine to adenine and guanine ribonucleotides. AZA in doses of 2 to 2.5 mg/kg/day has been remarkably safe in the long term without significantly increasing the risk for infection, whereas it is associated with a marginally increased risk for malignancy. Gastrointestinal complaints are frequent, leading 15% to 30% of patients to discontinue the drug within 6 months. Mild liver enzyme elevation may occur, but severe liver injury is rare. Reversible, dose-related bone marrow toxicity is also common; leukopenia is encountered in approximately 4.5% and thrombocytopenia in 2% of patients receiving low-dose AZA (see Table 81-1). Notably,

AZA toxicity is idiosyncratic and has been associated with genetic polymorphisms resulting in decreased thiopurine methyltransferase (TPMT) activity and impaired ability to detoxify intermediate metabolites.[26] Concomitant use of allopurinol substantially increases AZA toxicity and should be avoided.

In lupus, manifestations such as mild PLN, thrombocytopenia with platelet count in the range of 20 to $50 \times 10^3/mm^3$, and serositis may respond to AZA, usually in combination with moderate to high GC doses (Tables 81-2 and 81-3). Its efficacy as an induction-maintenance regimen has been tested in low-risk European patients with PLN who were randomized to receive pulse IV-CYC plus prednisone versus IV-MP plus AZA plus a tapering dose of prednisone.[27] After 2 years, both groups received maintenance therapy with AZA plus prednisone. The two groups did not differ in terms of induction of remission, mean SCr and proteinuria levels during the first 2 years. However, after a median follow-up duration of 5.7 years, rates of doubling of baseline SCr and of renal relapses were higher in the AZA group. Thus the authors believe that AZA may be used in mild LN and in patients strongly opposed to CYC.

AZA has also been considered a safe and efficacious option for maintenance of remission in SLE including cases of moderately severe PLN.[28,29] Two RCTs have compared AZA versus mycophenolate mofetil (MMF) as maintenance regimens in PLN. In the MAINTAIN trial, which included only European patients, both agents were equally efficacious in terms of time-to-renal flare, number of severe flares, renal remission, and doubling of SCr.[30] In contrast, the ALMS trial, which included a larger number of patients with multiethnic backgrounds, reported increased renal flares in the AZA versus the MMF group (see Mycophenolate Mofetil later).[31] To this end, both agents can be used as maintenance therapy on the basis of availability, clinical experience, and potential for pregnancy because MMF is associated with an increased risk of spontaneous abortion and fetal malformation. On the basis of their significant difference in cost, patients with mild to moderate LN, especially white individuals, could first be treated with AZA.[32]

Mycophenolate Mofetil

Pharmacology. MMF is a prodrug of mycophenolic acid, a potent inhibitor of inosine monophosphate dehydrogenase that is indispensable for the de novo synthesis of guanosine nucleotides. The lack of any salvage nucleotide synthesis pathway in lymphocytes renders them a selective target for MMF. Conversely, other tissues with high proliferative activity (skin, intestine, neutrophils) that have an intrinsic salvage guanosine synthesis pathway can escape the antiproliferative effects, which explains its more favorable toxicity profile compared with CYC. MMF has excellent oral bioavailability with peak levels occurring within 1 to 2 hours after administration and half-life of 17 hours. Although therapeutic drug monitoring to guide MMF dosing has been proposed in renal transplantation, validation of therapeutic MPA monitoring in LN is still required.[41] Antacids and cholestyramine decrease the bioavailability

Table 81-2 Indications for Immunosuppressive Therapy in Systemic Lupus Erythematosus

General Indications
Involvement of major organs or extensive involvement of nonmajor organs (skin) refractory to other agents, or both
Failure to respond to or inability to taper corticosteroids to acceptable doses for long-term use

Specific Organ Involvement
Renal
Proliferative or membranous nephritis (nephritic or nephritic syndrome), or both
Hematologic
Severe thrombocytopenia (platelets <20,000/mm³)
Thrombotic thrombocytopenic purpura–like syndrome
Severe hemolytic or aplastic anemia, or immune neutropenia not responding to glucocorticoids
Pulmonary
Lupus pneumonitis or alveolar hemorrhage, or both
Cardiac
Myocarditis with depressed left ventricular function, pericarditis with impending tamponade
Gastrointestinal
Abdominal vasculitis
Nervous System
Transverse myelitis, cerebritis, optic neuritis, psychosis refractory to corticosteroids, mononeuritis multiplex, severe peripheral neuropathy

Table 81-3 Recommended Immunosuppressive Therapy for Major Organ Involvement in Systemic Lupus Erythematosus

Disease Severity	Induction Therapy	Maintenance Therapy
Mild	High-dose GC (0.5-1 mg/kg/day prednisone ×4-6 wk, tapered to 0.125 mg/kg every other day within 3 mo) alone or in combination with AZA (1-2 mg/kg/day)	Low-dose GC (prednisone ≤0.125 mg/kg on alternative days) alone or with AZA (1-2 mg/kg/day)
	If no remission within 3 mo, treat as moderately severe	Consider further gradual tapering at the end of each year of remission
Moderate	MMF (2 g/day) (or AZA) with GC as above; if no remission after the first 6-12 mo, treat as severe	MMF tapered to 1.5 g/day for 6-12 mo and then to 1 g/day; consider further tapering at the end of each year in remission
		Alternative: AZA (1-2 mg/kg/day)
Severe	Pulse IV-CYC alone or in combination with pulse IV-MP for the first 6 mo (background GC 0.5 mg/kg/day for 4 wk, then taper)	Quarterly pulses of IV-CYC for at least 1 year beyond remission
	If no response, consider adding RTX or switch to MMF	Alternative: AZA (1-2 mg/kg/day), MMF (1-2 g/day)

AZA, azathioprine; CYC, cyclophosphamide; GC, glucocorticoid; IV, intravenous; MMF, mycophenolate mofetil; MP, methylprednisolone; RTX, rituximab.

Table 81-4 National Institutes of Health Protocol for Administration and Monitoring of Pulse Intravenous Cyclophosphamide Therapy

Estimate GFR by standard methods (Cockcroft-Gault or the Modification of Diet in Renal Disease formula)

Calculate body surface area (m^2): BSA = √Height (cm) × Weight (kg)/3600

Cyclophosphamide (Cytoxan) (CYC) dosing and administration:

  Initial dose 0.75 g/m^2 (0.5 g/m^2 if GFR less than one-third of expected normal)

  Administer CYC in 150 mL normal saline IV over 30-60 min (alternative: equivalent dose of pulse CYC may be taken orally in highly motivated and compliant patients)

  Determine WBC at days 10 and 14 after each CYC pulse (patient should delay prednisone until after blood tests drawn to avoid transient steroid-induced leukocytosis)

  Adjust subsequent doses of CYC to maximum dose of 1 g/m^2 to keep nadir WBC >1500/mm^3. If WBC nadir falls <1500/mm^3, decrease next dose by 25%

Repeat IV-CYC pulses monthly (every 3 wk in extremely aggressive disease) for another 6 mo (total 7 pulses), then quarterly for 1 year after remission is achieved (inactive urine sediment, proteinuria <1 g/day, normalization of complement (and ideally anti-dsDNA), and minimal or no extrarenal lupus activity)

Protection of urine bladder against CYC-induced hemorrhagic cystitis

  Diuresis with 5% dextrose and 0.45% saline (2 L at 250 mL/hr). Frequent voiding; continue high-dose oral fluids for 24 hr. Patients return to clinic if they cannot sustain an adequate fluid intake

  Consider mesna (each dose 20% of total CYC dose) intravenously or orally at 0, 2, 4, and 6 hr after CYC dosing. Mesna is especially important to use when sustained diuresis may be difficult to achieve or if pulse CYC is administered in an outpatient setting

  If anticipating difficulty with sustaining diuresis (e.g., severe nephrotic syndrome) or with voiding (e.g., neurogenic bladder), insert a 3-way urinary catheter with continuous bladder flushing with standard antibiotic irrigating solution (e.g., 3 L) or normal saline for 24 hr to minimize risk of hemorrhagic cystitis

Antiemetics (usually administered orally)

  Dexamethasone (10 mg single dose) *plus*

  Serotonin receptor antagonists: granisetron 1 mg with CYC dose (usually repeat dose in 12 hr); ondansetron 8 mg three times daily for 1-2 days

Monitor fluid balance during hydration. Use diuresis if patient develops progressive fluid accumulation

Complications of pulse CYC

  Expected: nausea and vomiting (central effect of CYC) mostly controlled by serotonin receptor antagonists; transient hair thinning (rarely severe at CYC doses ≤1 g/m^2)

  Common: significant infection diathesis only if leukopenia not carefully controlled; modest increase in herpes zoster (very low risk of dissemination); infertility (male and female); amenorrhea proportional to age of the patient during treatment and to the cumulative dose of CYC. In females at high risk for persistent amenorrhea, consider using leuprolide 3.75 mg subcutaneously 2 wk before each dose of CYC

CYC, cyclophosphamide; GFR, glomerular filtration rate; IV, intravenous; WBC, white blood cell count.

of MMF, and the coadministration with AZA should be avoided. MMF may be teratogenic and should not be administered during pregnancy.

Use in Lupus Nephritis

Induction Therapy. Initial RCTs indicated equal or even superior efficacy of MMF over CYC in inducing remission in PLN, but their findings were limited by flaws in the design such as the low number of patients, the underrepresentation of severe forms of LN, and the short follow-up.[28,42-44] The Aspreva Lupus Management Study (ALMS), one of the largest and most racially diverse RCT in LN that included a total of 370 patients, 27% of whom had estimated GFR less than 60 mL/min/1.73 m^2, failed to demonstrate superiority of MMF (2 to 3 g/day) over monthly pulses of IV-CYC (0.5 to 1 g/m^2).[45] Both groups received oral prednisone, with a defined taper from a maximum starting dose of 60 mg/day. At 6 months, response rates were similar for both groups (56% for MMF, 53% for IV-CYC) and there were no differences in adverse events. Subsequently, three meta-analyses of RCTs have concluded that MMF is as effective as CYC (pooled relative risk [RR] for complete remission ranging 1.49 to 1.61) and has a better safety profile (pooled RR, 0.15 to 0.17 for amenorrhea; 0.41 to 0.78 for leukopenia; 0.77 to 0.83 for infections) as induction therapy for PLN.[46-48] MMF may therefore be considered as induction therapy in moderately severe PLN, especially when gonadal toxicity is an issue.

MMF has demonstrated antiproteinuric effects in LMN,[49] but there is lack of large RCTs to formally test its efficacy.

A pooled analysis of 84 patients with pure LMN who participated in the ALMS trial[45] and in the study by Ginzler and colleagues[44] demonstrated comparable remission rates (percentage change of proteinuria and SCr were the primary end points) in MMF- and IV-CYC-treated patients.[50] A trial testing MMF monotherapy in idiopathic membranous nephropathy failed to demonstrate efficacy.[51] More data are necessary to delineate the role of MMF in the management of LMN.

Maintenance Therapy. Contreras and colleagues[28] compared MMF versus AZA or quarterly pulses of IV-CYC as maintenance therapy in PLN following remission with 7 IV-CYC pulses. In this trial of 59 patients, 95% were black or Hispanic, 78% had diffuse PLN, with average SCr 1.6 mg/dL and serum albumin 2.7 mg/dL. After a follow-up of 72 months, MMF and AZA were superior to IV-CYC in terms of relapse-free survival (78% for MMF, 58% for AZA, 4% for IV-CYC), mortality, infections, and amenorrhea. This study was criticized for the insufficient number of patients to demonstrate superiority, the use of lower doses of IV-CYC, and the use of higher doses of GC, which may have decreased efficacy and increased the risk for infections. Two large multicenter RCTs have compared MMF versus AZA as maintenance regimen in PLN. The MAINTAIN Nephritis Trial included 105 European patients with moderately severe class III to IV PLN (10% had baseline SCr >1.4 mg/dL, 39% had proteinuria ≥3 g/day) who received induction therapy with 3 daily 750-mg IV-MP pulses followed by oral GC and 6 fortnightly IV-CYC pulses (500 mg per pulse).[30]

On the basis of randomization performed at baseline, AZA (target dose: 2 mg/kg/day) or MMF (target dose: 2 g/day) was given at week 12 to all patients. Over a 3-year period, the two groups did not differ in terms of time-to-renal flare, number of severe flares, renal remission, or doubling of SCr. Adverse events did not differ between the groups except for blood cytopenias, which were more frequent in the AZA group. These results are different from those reported for the ALMS maintenance part.[31] This study included 227 patients (44% nonwhites) and showed a failure rate of 32% in the AZA group versus 16% in the MMF group at 3 years after successful induction therapy during the first part of the study with either MMF or IV-CYC. Differences in the study design and the induction protocol, the number and ethnicity of the included patients, and the outcome measures may account for the discrepant results. Of note, an RCT in ANCA-positive vasculitis found that MMF was less effective than AZA for maintaining disease remission following induction therapy with IV-CYC and GC.[52] To this end, both MMF and AZA may be used for maintenance of remission in PLN on the basis of availability and potential for pregnancy.

Use in Extrarenal Lupus. A systematic review of open-label trials concluded that MMF may be effective for refractory skin and blood manifestations in SLE.[53] A posthoc analysis of the ALMS trial data in LN patients showed that MMF was equally efficacious with IV-CYC pulse therapy (both in combination with tapered prednisone) on general disease activity.[54] At week 24, BILAG-defined remission was achieved in the general (100% in MMF vs. 94% in IV-CYC), mucocutaneous (84% vs. 93%), musculoskeletal (91% vs. 96%), and hematologic (60% vs. 67%) domains. Normalization of C3/C4 and anti-dsDNA titers also occurred at a similar rate. Conversely, MMF showed no efficacy in preventing extrarenal flares in 75 patients who were followed at a single center for 5 years for renal (71%) or nonrenal disease.[55] A substantial number of patients experienced flares during the second and third years of treatment, particularly in hematologic, mucocutaneous, and musculoskeletal domains. While awaiting additional data to define the efficacy of MMF in extrarenal lupus, the drug may be used in patients with moderately severe lupus who are intolerant or have not adequately responded to AZA.

Cyclosporin A

Pharmacology. Cyclosporin A (CsA), a fungus-derived calcineurin inhibitor that deactivates T cells, also reduces antigen presentation and autoantibody production by lupus B cells. Following oral administration, peak serum concentration occurs within 1 to 8 hours. Drug concentration is measured in whole blood, but this is rarely necessary in autoimmune diseases, unless CsA is used in doses greater than or equal to 3 mg/kg/day. Clinical response occurs 1 to 2 months after treatment initiation. Several drugs interact with CsA, leading to reduced (rifampin, phenytoin, phenobarbital, nafcillin) or increased (erythromycin, clarithromycin, azoles, calcium channel blockers, amiodarone, allopurinol, colchicine) drug concentrations. The drugs may also augment CsA nephrotoxic effects (NSAIDs, aminoglycosides, quinolones, angiotensin-converting enzyme [ACE] inhibitors, amphotericin B). Common adverse events include mild gastrointestinal complaints, hirsutism, gingival hyperplasia, and mild elevation in serum alkaline phosphatase levels. Tremor, paresthesias, electrolyte disturbances (hyperkalemia and hypomagnesemia), and hyperuricemia may also occur. Hypertension occurs in nearly 20% of patients receiving CsA and is controlled by either reduction of the dose or antihypertensive treatment. A major adverse effect is nephrotoxicity, which is reversible after adjustment of the dose or drug discontinuation, and CsA should be avoided in patients with impaired renal function (see Table 81-1).

Use in Proliferative Lupus Nephritis. Uncontrolled studies have demonstrated efficacy of CsA when used in combination with GC or in between quarterly doses of IV-CYC in refractory-to-conventional treatment PLN. Beneficial effects include reduction in proteinuria, stabilization of renal function, improvement in overall disease activity, and a modest steroid-sparring effect. Rihova and colleagues[58] prospectively studied 31 LN patients (n = 24 with class III/IV nephritis) who were treated with CsA (5 mg/kg/day in two equal doses and then adjusted to trough level 80 to 120 ng/mL) and low-dose prednisone. After a mean of 7 months, all but two patients achieved complete response, defined as proteinuria less than 1 g/day and improved or stabilized renal function. About half of these patients, however, experienced a renal flare after CsA withdrawal.

Moroni and colleagues[29] compared AZA with CsA as maintenance therapies in 69 patients with diffuse PLN and preserved renal function. All patients received induction therapy with 3 daily pulses of 1 g IV-MP, followed by prednisone and oral CYC for 3 months. They were then assigned to receive either CsA (4 mg/kg/day for 1 month and then tapered to 2.5 to 3 mg/kg/day) or AZA (1.5 to 2 mg/kg/day) for 2 to 4 years. The two groups did not differ in flare-ups, proteinuria, and blood pressure levels. Both agents were well tolerated. In another study, 40 patients with newly diagnosed PLN and mild renal insufficiency were randomly assigned to sequential induction and maintenance therapy with either CYC or CsA.[59] The CYC regimen included 8 pulses IV-CYC (10 mg/kg) administered within 9 months, followed by 4 to 5 oral CYC boluses; CsA was given orally 4 to 5 mg/kg/day for 9 months and then tapered to 3.75 to 1.25 mg/kg/day within the next 9 months. Both groups received oral MP (0.8 mg/kg/day, then tapered). In the intention-to-treat analysis, 16 patients in the CYC group (76%) and 13 patients in the CsA group (68%) achieved complete or partial response at 9 months (induction phase). At the end of maintenance phase (18 months), the respective percentages were 52% for CYC and 95% for CsA. The trend for more favorable response in the CsA group was due to a higher proportion of patients achieving a 50% or greater decrease in proteinuria (38% in CYC group vs. 74% in CsA group). Despite its methodology flaws, this trial provides evidence for efficacy of CsA in mild to moderate proteinuric PLN with preserved renal function.

Use in Membranous Lupus Nephropathy. Balow and Austin[37] performed an RCT in 42 patients with MLN to compare prednisone alone or in combination with CsA or monthly pulses of IV-CYC. Remission rates at 1 year were 27% for prednisone, 60% for IV-CYC, and 83% for CsA. During follow-up, however, rates of nephrotic syndrome relapse were 10-fold higher in the CsA than the IV-CYC group, suggesting that despite its effectiveness as induction therapy, CsA may require maintenance therapy to prevent relapses in MLN.

Use in Extrarenal Lupus. Uncontrolled studies of short duration have shown improvement in disease activity, anti-dsDNA titers, and cytopenias with modest GC reduction in SLE patients who received low-dose CsA.[60,61] The BILAG group performed a multicenter, nonblinded RCT to compare the steroid-sparing effect of CsA (titrated to 2.5 to 3.5 mg/kg/day in two divided doses and adjusted to changes in SCr) versus AZA (2 to 2.5 mg/kg/day) in severe lupus requiring 15 or greater mg/day prednisone.[62] Eighty-nine patients (66% whites) were randomized; 66% had active disease (defined as a BILAG A or B in any systems), and 34% entered the study because a different steroid-sparing agent was required. At 12 months, the unadjusted mean reduction in prednisolone dose was 9.5 ± 8.1 mg in the CsA group and 10.2 ± 6.2 mg in the AZA group. These improvements, however, were deemed as suboptimal for both drugs because almost 50% of patients with active disease at baseline failed to respond. The two groups did not differ in any of the secondary end points, namely disease activity, response to treatment, flares, damage accrual, and quality-of-life measures. In terms of safety, 23 patients (49%) who received CsA developed hypertension and another 6 patients (13%) showed a rise in SCr, both successfully managed by CsA dose reduction or addition of antihypertensive treatment. Thus CsA may be used as an alternative steroid-sparing agent to AZA in SLE patients, but with monitoring of the renal function and blood pressure.

Tacrolimus

Tacrolimus is a 10 to 100 times more potent calcineurin inhibitor than CsA. Systemic administration has been associated with dose-dependent reversible nephrotoxicity and blood pressure elevation, albeit less often than CsA. Other reported adverse effects include cardiomyopathy in children, anxiety, seizures, delirium and tremor, diabetes, and hyperlipidemia. In a pilot study of 10 SLE patients with skin and musculoskeletal disease, tacrolimus administered at doses of 1 to 3 mg/day for 1 year resulted in a significant reduction in SLE Disease Activity Index (SLEDAI) score and the dose of GC.[63] Tacrolimus has also demonstrated beneficial effects in refractory-to-conventional therapy PLN and LMN.[64-66] Miyasaka and colleagues[67] conducted a placebo-controlled, double-blind trial in 63 patients with active mild-to-moderate nephritis requiring 10 or greater mg/day prednisone. They were randomized to receive a 28-week course of either tacrolimus (3 mg/day) or placebo in combination with GC (≤10 mg/day). In intention-to-treat analysis, only tacrolimus-treated patients had significant improvement in the author-defined nephritis disease activity index; 4 out of 27 patients in the tacrolimus group as compared with 1 out of 33 in the placebo group achieved proteinuria less than 0.3 g/day. Higher rates of GI toxicity and hyperglycemia were observed in the tacrolimus group.

Tacrolimus has been used in combination with MMF in severe or resistant LN. Cortés-Hernandez and colleagues[68] prospectively studied 70 patients with moderately severe PLN who received induction therapy with 3 daily pulses of IV-MP (1 g/dose) and oral MMF (2 g/day), in conjunction with oral prednisone (1 mg/kg/day for 4 weeks, then tapered). In case of renal flare or treatment failure despite an increase in MMF dose, oral tacrolimus (0.075 mg/kg/day, adjusted to trough level 5 to 10 ng/mL) was added. At the end of the 65-month follow-up, tacrolimus had been started in 17 patients (24%), with 12 of them achieving complete or partial response after an average of 24 months. Tacrolimus/MMF combination therapy (tacrolimus 4 mg/day, MMF 2 g/day) has also been compared against IV-CYC (6 to 9 pulses of 1 g/m²) in patients with mixed class IV + V LN.[69] In this study, patients had mean estimated GFR of 98 mL/min, proteinuria 4.4 g/day, and most had previously been treated with MMF or CYC. Both groups received 3 daily pulses of IV-MP (0.5 g/day) and then switched to oral prednisone. After 6 months, 10 patients in the "multitarget" group versus 1 patient in the IV-CYC group achieved complete remission. Combination therapy was well tolerated, and no major effects were observed. This is in contrast, however, with the significant toxicity reported in other patients with LN who received the same combination therapy.[70] Therefore additional studies with a larger number of patients and longer follow-up are necessary to establish the efficacy, safety, and specific indications of such a multidrug approach in LN.

Biologic Therapies

B Cell–Depleting Therapies

B cells play a key role in lupus pathogenesis by several means. First, they produce pathogenic autoantibodies that cause tissue damage by immune complex formation, complement activation, and direct cytotoxicity. They also function as antigen-presenting cells and secrete inflammatory cytokines that activate T cells.

Rituximab. Rituximab (RTX) is a chimeric mouse-human monoclonal antibody targeting the cell membrane protein CD20, which is expressed in all developmental stages of B cells, except for the hematopoietic stem cell and the plasma cell. Its mechanism of action involves cytotoxicity through complement activation, antibody-dependent cell-mediated cytotoxicity, and induction of apoptosis. RTX has been used in more than 450 SLE patients with refractory-to-cytotoxic therapy SLE, mainly as add-on therapy to GCs or other immunosuppressive agents, or both.[71,72] Clinical response was noted in more than 80%, with manifestations such as neuropsychiatric disease,[73] PLN, and autoimmune cytopenias, showing higher response rates. Data from a French lupus registry including a total of 136 patients also indicated response rates of at least 70% for various manifestations, with autoimmune cytopenias exhibiting the most favorable outcomes (85% for hemolytic anemia, 92% for thrombocytopenia). A clinically significant decrease in SLEDAI by 3 or more units was observed in 71%.[74] With regard to LN, a meta-analysis of observational studies found an overall complete and partial response rate with RTX therapy of 69%, with lower rates observed in LMN.[75] Two European cohorts, however, have reported comparable response rates in patients with PLN and LMN who received RTX in combination with steroids and IV-CYC.[76]

Unexpectedly, two RCTs failed to demonstrate efficacy of RTX in SLE. The EXPLORER trial assessed the effects of RTX over 52 weeks in patients with active moderate to severe extrarenal SLE.[77] A total of 257 patients were randomized to receive RTX or placebo (two biweekly infusions of 1000 mg at baseline and at 6 months), in combination with background immunosuppression (AZA, MMF, MTX) and prednisone at a dose of 0.5 to 1 mg/kg/day, not tapered until day 16 after the first RTX infusion. At week 52, no difference was observed between RTX and placebo in the primary (BILAG-defined major or partial clinical response) or any of the secondary end points. The LUNAR trial evaluated the efficacy of RTX versus placebo, both in combination with MMF (3 g/day), in 144 patients with active PLN.[78] By week 52, there was no significant difference between the two groups in terms of complete or partial renal response. Both studies were criticized for suboptimal design, mainly due to background therapies with high doses of oral GC and immunosuppressive drugs, which could have masked RTX effects. Alternatively, RTX may be more efficacious in patients with aggressive disease refractory to conventional treatment, as were most patients included in open-label trials.

RTX is generally well tolerated with mild infusion reactions being the most common adverse event, usually prevented by premedication with antihistamines and GCs. Mild infections are common (up to 20%), but the overall risk for serious or opportunistic infections is not significantly increased.[79] Following the report of a few cases of progressive multifocal leukoencephalopathy (PML) in RTX-treated patients with RA and SLE, the U.S. Food and Drug Administration (FDA) has issued an alert about possible RTX and PML links. More data are necessary to evaluate whether RTX indeed increases the inherent risk for PML in SLE. Together, although RTX cannot be considered first-line therapy for mild to moderate SLE, its use may be justified in severe refractory cases on the basis of mounting evidence from open-label trials. Accordingly, the American College of Rheumatology (ACR) and the EULAR–European Renal Association have included rituximab (anti-CD20 mAb) as a therapeutic option for selected cases of LN refractory to conventional immunosuppressive treatment.[80a,80b]

Ocrelizumab. The BELONG trial evaluated the efficacy and safety of ocrelizumab (humanized anti-CD20 monoclonal antibody) versus placebo, both in combination with either MMF (up to 3 g/day) or IV-CYC (Euro-Lupus protocol) in 378 patients with PLN.[80] The study was prematurely terminated due to increased rates of serious and opportunistic infections in ocrelizumab-treated patients, both when combined with MMF and IV-CYC.

B Cell Inhibitors

Epratuzumab. Epratuzumab is a recombinant anti-CD22 monoclonal antibody that modulates lupus B cell function.[81] CD22 is a membrane co-receptor for the B cell receptor mediating inhibitory signaling through attenuation of calcium efflux. In 14 SLE patients with moderately active disease, epratuzumab therapy resulted in reduction in BILAG scores by greater than or equal to 50% in more than 70% of patients at 6 weeks and in nearly 40% of patients at 18 weeks.[82] Drug tolerability was acceptable, and mild infections occurred in a minority of participants. Positive results have been announced for a phase IIb placebo-controlled, dose-defining trial in moderate to severe SLE. Using a composite BILAG-based response index, patients who received epratuzumab 600 mg weekly or 1200 mg biweekly achieved almost twofold higher response rates than the placebo group at the end of the 12-week treatment cycle. A similar rate of adverse events was recorded in the two groups.[83] Phase III trials in moderate and severe SLE are under way.

Belimumab. The B lymphocyte stimulator protein (BLyS, also known as B cell activation factor [BAFF]) and the proliferation-inducing ligand (APRIL) are growth factors important for B cell survival and maturation. BLyS binds to three different B cell receptors, namely the transmembrane activator and calcium-modulating cyclophilin ligand interactor (TACI), the B cell maturation antigen (BCMA), and the BAFF receptor (BAFF-R), whereas APRIL signals through TACI and BCMA.[84]

Belimumab is a fully human anti-BLyS monoclonal antibody. An initial phase II trial of belimumab in combination with GCs and/or immunosuppressive agents in 449 active SLE patients did not meet its primary end points.[85] In a posthoc analysis, however, serologically active patients (ANA titer ≥1:80 or anti-dsDNA positive) had a significantly higher response by week 52 in terms of SLEDAI and physician's global assessment. These two parameters were combined with BILAG to define a novel activity index, the SLE responder index (SRI), which revealed favorable response rates for belimumab.[86]

Two subsequent phase III placebo-controlled RCTs (BLISS-52, BLISS-76) evaluated two different doses of belimumab (1 mg/kg, 10 mg/kg; dosed IV on days 0, 14, 28, and then every 28 days) on top of standard therapy in more than 1500 serologically positive SLE patients, using the SRI as the primary end point. Belimumab treatment resulted in a modest albeit significant reduction in disease activity and needs for additional GC, coupled with an increase in time-to-first flare.[87] In BLISS-52, 58% achieved the primary end point in the high-dose belimumab arm versus 44% in the placebo group; the respective figures in BLISS-76 were 43% for belimumab and 34% for placebo. There were no significant differences in infectious adverse events between the two drugs. These data opened the way for approval of this agent for the treatment of SLE.

Atacicept. Atacicept (TACI-Ig) is a recombinant fusion protein of the extracellular domain of TACI and the human IgG1.Fc domain. TACI mediates signals from both BLyS and APRIL, thus affecting memory B cells, plasma cells, and immunoglobulin production. This was illustrated in two phase Ib placebo-controlled trials in patients with mild to moderate SLE.[88,89] Both studies found no difference in adverse events between the two study groups, with the exception of mild injection-site reactions in patients receiving atacicept. However, a phase II/III trial of atacicept in combination with MMF in LN was prematurely terminated due to increased infection rates.

Co-stimulation Blockade

CD40-Ligand Blockade. CD40-ligand (CD40L) is expressed on activated T cells and stimulates antigen-presenting cells including B cells through engagement with CD40. Anti-CD40L treatment resulted in improvement of renal disease and increased survival in NZB/W F1 lupus mice.[90] Two fully humanized monoclonal anti-CD40L antibodies have been developed for therapeutic trials in humans: BG9588 and IDEC-1310. The latter showed no efficacy in mild to moderate SLE.[91] The encouraging results by the use of BG9588 (improvement in serologic activity and decrease in hematuria in 28 patients with PLN) were overpowered by the occurrence of serious thromboembolic events.[92]

Abatacept. Abatacept (CTLA4-Ig) is a recombinant protein that comprises the extracellular domain of human CTLA-4 fused to the Fc portion of human IgG1 and antagonizes CD28-mediated T cells. It is approved for the treatment of moderate to severe RA and juvenile idiopathic arthritis. CTLA4-Ig delayed disease progression in lupus-prone mice, especially when combined with CYC.[93] A placebo-controlled, phase IIb trial of abatacept in combination with GC and background immunosuppressive therapy in 175 SLE patients with skin, joint, cardiovascular, and respiratory manifestations failed to meet its primary end point.[94] After 1 year, the proportion of patients with new BILAG A/B flare after steroid taper did not differ between the two groups. However, the trial design may have undermined potential efficacy of abatacept because patients were started on high doses of GC (30 mg/day) and tapering began on day 29 or 57. Posthoc analysis showed that patients with polyarthritis benefited more from abatacept treatment. Serious adverse events were significantly more frequent in the abatacept group (20% vs. 7% in placebo) including bronchitis, diverticulitis, and gastroenteritis. Two RCTs are currently under way to evaluate abatacept in combination with MMF or IV-CYC in LN.

Anticytokine Therapy

Tumor Necrosis Factor Inhibitors. Tumor necrosis factor (TNF) has divergent effects on the immune systemic in lupus. In an open-label study, seven SLE patients with moderately active disease received four doses of 300 mg infliximab on day 0 and at weeks 2, 6, and 10, in combination with AZA or MTX. Anti-dsDNA and other autoantibodies increased in most patients, peaking 4 to 10 weeks after the last infliximab infusion but returning to baseline levels thereafter.[95] In the prospective follow-up of 13 patients, 6 out of 9 patients with LN had a long-term (up to 5 years) response after four infusions of infliximab in combination with AZA.[96] All five patients with severe arthritis responded, but only for 2 months after the last infusion. Long-term therapy was associated with high rates of serious adverse events. In another small open-label study in resistant proliferative or membranous LN, treatment with infliximab in combination with oral prednisone and CsA resulted in transient reduction of proteinuria and stabilization of renal function.[97] Together, it is unlikely that TNF inhibition will be used routinely in SLE treatment.

Interferon Inhibition. Type I interferon (IFN-α) has been implicated in lupus pathogenesis through breakdown of immune tolerance. Serum IFN levels are increased and correlate with disease activity, and gene expression studies have identified an "interferon signature" in a subset of SLE patients.[98] A phase I trial evaluated the effects of a single dose of anti-IFN-α monoclonal antibody (MEDI-545) in SLE.[99] It was noted to downregulate IFN-inducible genes and other signaling pathways such as GM-CSF, TNF, IL-10, IL-1β, and BAFF. Two phase II trials are ongoing to assess safety and efficacy of anti-IFN therapy in lupus.

Anti-IL-6 Therapy. In lupus-prone mice, blockade of IL-6 or its receptor reduced anti-dsDNA levels, ameliorated proteinuria, and increased survival.[100] Tocilizumab, a humanized monoclonal antibody against the α-chain of the IL-6 receptor, has shown efficacy in RA. Illei and colleagues[101] tested tocilizumab in 16 patients with moderately active SLE, in combination with low-dose GC. Patients received tocilizumab (2, 4, 8 mg/kg) biweekly for 12 weeks and were monitored for an additional 8 weeks. Results revealed a correlation between clinical and serologic efficacy, evidenced by reduction in SLAM and SLEDAI indices, acute-phase reactants, and anti-dsDNA levels. Dose-dependent neutropenia (median decrease in neutrophil count by 56% in the 8 mg/kg group) and frequent infections (upper respiratory and urinary tract) were observed. To resolve issues on efficacy and safety, a larger trial is necessary.

Anti-IL-10 Therapy. IL-10 is upregulated in SLE and correlates with disease activity, although its exact pathogenic role has not been elucidated. An open-label trial in six steroid-dependent SLE patients showed improvement in disease activity reported up to 6 months after the administration of an anti-IL-10 murine monoclonal antibody (BN10) for 21 days.[102] However, all patients developed antibodies against BN10, and new trials are awaited with a human anti-IL-10 monoclonal antibody.

Other Therapies

Intravenous Immunoglobulin

Intravenous immunoglobulin (IVIG) exerts immunosuppressive effects by interaction with anti-idiotypic antibodies, interference with the complement and cytokines, cytolysis of target cells, induction of apoptosis through Fc receptors, and modulation of co-stimulatory molecules.[103] In an RCT of 14 patients, IVIG (400 mg/kg for 5 consecutive days monthly for 18 months) was as effective as pulse IV-CYC (1 g/m^2 every 2 months for 6 months, then every 3 months for 1 year) as maintenance therapy of PLN.[104] In another study, high-dose IVIG (2 g/kg divided over 5 days) in 1 to 8 monthly courses was administered in 20 SLE patients with cytopenias, massive proteinuria, arthritis, fever, arthralgia, mood changes, and psychosis. IVIG therapy resulted in improvement in SLEDAI and dose of GC.[105] Common adverse events include fever, myalgia, headache, and arthralgia; less common are aseptic meningitis, nephropathy in patients who receive sucrose-containing preparations, and thromboembolic complications in older patients with atherosclerotic risk factors. The drug is contraindicated in IgA deficiency.

Synthetic Tolerogens

Tolerogenic peptides aim at restoring immune tolerance in lupus. Abetimus sodium (LJP-394) contains four identical dsDNA strands covalently linked to a small molecule platform. It is thought to reduce anti-dsDNA antibodies by binding and clearance of soluble anti-dsDNA antibodies and B cell receptor cross-linking on dsDNA-specific B cells. Initial studies showed decrease of anti-dsDNA levels, prolongation of the time-to-renal flare, and reduced renal flares, especially in patients with high-affinity anti-dsDNA antibodies.[106-108] However, a phase III placebo-controlled trial in 317 LN patients failed to meet its primary end point (prolongation of time to renal flare), although abetimus-treated patients had 21% fewer flares, reduced proteinuria, and improved SLEDAI scores.[109] The drug was well tolerated, and a 900-mg dosage was introduced in another trial, with no additional benefit.[110] The spliceosomal peptide P140 is another tolerogen that has demonstrated benefit in early SLE trials. In a dose-escalation study in 20 patients with moderate SLE, the drug significantly decreased anti-dsDNA levels and slightly reduced SLEDAI.[111] The results of an ongoing phase IIb trial using SRI as efficacy index are awaited.

Dehydroepiandrosterone

Dehydroepiandrosterone (DHEA) is a naturally occurring inactive steroid in adrenal glands, testes, and ovaries. Seven RCTs including a total of 842 patients have been performed to assess efficacy and safety of DHEA in SLE. Their meta-analysis showed that the drug had modest clinical effect only in mild to moderate disease.[112] DHEA treatment also resulted in improvement in health-related quality of life measurements.

Clofazimine

Clofazimine (CFZ) (100 mg/day), an antimicrobial used in the treatment of leprosy, has shown efficacy in the treatment of skin involvement in lupus.[113] However, it should be reserved for patients with exclusively cutaneous disease because it may provoke severe lupus flares.

MANAGEMENT OF SPECIFIC SYSTEMIC LUPUS ERYTHEMATOSUS MANIFESTATIONS AND TREATMENT ALGORITHMS

KEY POINTS

Skin manifestations in SLE usually respond to sun exposure prophylaxis, topical glucocorticoids, and systemic antimalarials.

Risk stratification based on renal pathology, demographic, and clinical and laboratory characteristics enables the identification of LN patients at high risk for renal dysfunction who may benefit from aggressive cytotoxic therapy.

In moderately severe PLN, mycophenolate mofetil may be preferred as induction regimen, especially when gonadal toxicity is a concern. Failure to achieve response after the initial 6 months of therapy should evoke decisions about intensifying or altering immunosuppressive therapy.

Combination of monthly pulses of intravenous CYC and pulse intravenous methylprednisolone is the treatment of choice for severe LN. If substantial improvement occurs after the first 6 months, maintenance therapy with azathioprine or mycophenolate mofetil may be started.

Glucocorticoids alone or in combination with immunosuppressive agents are recommended for neuropsychiatric events felt to reflect an immune/inflammatory process; antiplatelet and/or anticoagulation therapy is recommended for events related to antiphospholipid antibodies.

Antiplatelet or anticoagulation therapies, or both, are necessary in patients with antiphospholipid syndrome to prevent recurrent events, but the intensity of such therapies remains controversial.

Mucocutaneous and Joint Disease

No single therapeutic agent has been officially approved for cutaneous lupus erythematosus (CLE). Mild malar rash and other photosensitive rashes usually respond to prophylaxis from sun exposure, but the use of sunscreens with high sun protection factor cannot be overemphasized. Topical GCs reduce redness and scaling. In an RCT of 78 patients with discoid lupus erythematosus (DLE), high-potency topical fluocinonide 0.05% was more effective than low-potency hydrocortisone 1% (response rates 27% vs. 10%, respectively).[114] Calcineurin inhibitors (tacrolimus, pimecrolimus) are a useful alternative, especially for the face, because they cause less atrophic and rosacea-like effects than topical steroids.

In refractory to topical therapy skin disease, systemic antimalarials may be used alone or in combination with oral GCs (up to 20 mg/day). HCQ was equally effective and had more favorable safety profile than the oral retinoid acitretin in an RCT of 58 DLE patients.[115] Other systemic treatment remains largely empiric. MTX has shown efficacy in refractory subacute CLE and DLE.[116] Alternative choices include retinoids, dapsone, MMF, and IV-CYC.[39] Thalidomide and IVIG should be reserved for patients with severe recalcitrant CLE due to potential serious neurotoxicity and high cost, respectively (Figure 81-1).[117,118]

Lupus arthritis follows the pattern of nonerosive symmetric polyarthritis primarily affecting the small joints of the hands and feet. In mild arthritis, initial therapy should be based on antimalarials. In persistent or aggressive disease, utilization of DMARDs is advocated. In a prospective controlled study, SLEDAI scores, need for steroids, and articular involvement were significantly improved in SLE patients receiving MTX for 6 months.[119] Leflunomide is used less often. Anti-TNF agents have been implicated for anti-dsDNA antibody development or even drug-induced lupus. RTX may be used in severe lupus arthritis refractory to DMARDs.

Lupus Nephritis

Induction Therapy

Current therapeutic strategies in LN include an initial *induction* phase aimed at substantially improving disease

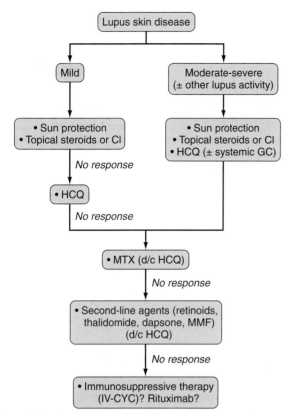

Figure 81-1 Suggested algorithm for the management of cutaneous manifestations in SLE. (See text for details.) CI, calcineurin inhibitors; d/c, discontinue; GC, glucocorticoids; HCQ, hydroxychloroquine; IV-CYC, pulse intravenous cyclophosphamide; MMF, mycophenolate mofetil; MTX, methotrexate. (Modified from Kuhn A, Ruland V, Bonsmann G: Cutaneous lupus erythematosus: update of therapeutic options: Part II, J Am Acad Dermatol 65:e195–213, 2010; and Kuhn A, Ruland V, Bonsmann G: Cutaneous lupus erythematosus: update of therapeutic options: Part I, J Am Acad Dermatol 65:e179–193, 2010.)

Table 81-5 Severity of Lupus Nephritis

Proliferative Nephritis	
Mild	Class III nephritis without severe histologic features (crescents, fibrinoid necrosis)*; low chronicity index (≤3); normal renal function; non-nephrotic range proteinuria
Moderately severe	Mild disease as defined above with partial or no response after the initial induction therapy, or delayed remission (>12 mo), or
	Focal proliferative nephritis with adverse histologic features or reproducible SCr increase ≥30%, or
	Class IV nephritis without adverse histologic features
Severe	Moderately severe as defined above but not remitting after 6-12 mo of therapy, or
	Proliferative disease with impaired renal function and fibrinoid necrosis or crescents in >25% of glomeruli, or
	Mixed membranous and proliferative nephritis, or
	Proliferative nephritis with high chronicity alone (chronicity index >4) or in combination with high activity (chronicity index >3 and activity index >10), or
	Rapidly progressive glomerulonephritis (doubling of SCr within 2-3 mo)
Membranous Nephropathy	
Mild	Non-nephrotic range proteinuria with normal renal function
Moderate	Nephrotic range proteinuria with normal renal function at presentation
Severe	Nephrotic range proteinuria with impaired renal function at presentation (≥30% increase in SCr)

*Concomitant therapy with corticosteroids or immunosuppressive drugs, or both, may modify urinary sediment and histologic findings and should be taken into consideration.

SCr, serum creatinine.

activity (or even attaining remission), followed by a *maintenance* phase, in which the goal is to maximize the therapeutic effect and consolidate the response. Risk stratification, according to renal pathology[120] and patient demographic, clinical and laboratory characteristics, enables the identification of patients at risk for renal dysfunction or ESRD, or both, who may benefit from aggressive cytotoxic therapy (Table 81-5).[8,121]

For *mild* class I/II disease, a limited trial of prednisone (0.5 to 1 mg/kg/day for 4 to 6 weeks and then tapered to alternate day 0.125 to 0.25 mg/kg if remission occurs) is indicated. The use of three consecutive daily pulses of IV-MP may expedite remission and allow for the use of lower GC doses (0.5 mg/kg/day). Addition of immunosuppressive therapy (AZA 1 to 2 mg/kg/day) either from the beginning or during GC tapering may decrease cumulative steroid dose. If the patient does not achieve complete remission (clearing of cellular casts and proteinuria, normalization of complement, minimal lupus activity) within 3 months or if nephritis worsens, therapy with MMF or monthly pulse IV-CYC should be initiated. Delay in immunosuppressive therapy because of a partial response beyond the 3 to 4 months may have an adverse impact on response to therapy, thus increasing the risk for flare.

In *moderately severe* PLN, meta-analyses of RCTs comparing MMF with CYC confirmed the efficacy of the former for induction therapy; claims of superiority toward CYC were not substantiated. MMF is increasingly used as a first-line treatment for most PLN cases due to its favorable toxicity profile, whereas CYC is reserved for the most severe ones. For whites, the low-dose (Euro-Lupus) IV-CYC regimen may be equally efficacious and less toxic than the high-dose (NIH) regimen. Both earlier[122] and recent[36,123,124] studies underscore the significance of early response to therapy at 6 months (defined as a decrease in SCr level and proteinuria <1 g/day) as a strong predictor of good long-term renal outcome. Thus failure to achieve response after the initial 6 months of therapy should precipitate decisions about switching from MMF to pulse IV-CYC.

In *severe* LN, the authors recommend induction therapy with 7 monthly pulses of IV-CYC in combination with 3 initial pulses of IV-MP at the start, followed by pulses of IV-MP in combination with IV-CYC at monthly intervals (1 pulse/month) for the first 6 to 12 months (see Table 81-3). High doses of prednisone (0.5 to 1 mg/kg/day tapered after 4 weeks) should be continued during the induction period. Addition of plasma exchange is of no benefit in terms of survival. For patients strongly opposing pulses of IV-CYC, alternative induction regimens include (1) daily oral MMF (1 g twice a day for 12 months with increase to 3 g/day if no response in 6 to 8 weeks) or (2) monthly pulses of IV-MP (1 g/m^2 daily) for three doses and then at monthly

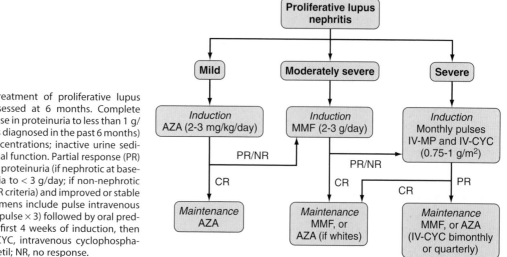

Figure 81-2 Recommended treatment of proliferative lupus nephritis. Renal response is assessed at 6 months. Complete response (CR) is defined as decrease in proteinuria to less than 1 g/day (or < 0.3 g/day if nephritis was diagnosed in the past 6 months) with normal serum albumin concentrations; inactive urine sediment; and improved or stable renal function. Partial response (PR) is defined as significant change in proteinuria (if nephrotic at baseline ≥ 50% decrease in proteinuria to < 3 g/day; if non-nephrotic at baseline but not meeting the CR criteria) and improved or stable renal function. All induction regimens include pulse intravenous methylprednisolone (IV-MP) (1 g/pulse × 3) followed by oral prednisone (0.5 to 0.6 mg/kg for the first 4 weeks of induction, then tapered). AZA, azathioprine; IV-CYC, intravenous cyclophosphamide; MMF, mycophenolate mofetil; NR, no response.

intervals for 6 to 12 months if there is steady progress to remission. Adherence to the National Kidney Foundation–Kidney Disease Outcomes Quality Initiative (NKF-KDOQI) guidelines for the management of renal diseases is of utmost importance. Figure 81-2 summarizes the treatment recommendations for PLN.[125]

Maintenance Therapy

Following induction of remission, patients with mild to moderate disease may be treated with low-dose GC (7.5 to 15 mg prednisone on alternate day) or AZA, with CsA being an alternative agent. For maintenance therapy in moderately severe disease, MMF or AZA could be used on the basis of availability and potential for pregnancy because MMF is associated with an increased risk of spontaneous abortion and fetal malformation. Because of the significant difference in the cost between the two drugs, patients with less severe LN could first be treated with AZA, especially white individuals.

In severe disease, our preferred approach is quarterly pulse IV-CYC until 1 year beyond remission. If substantial improvement occurs, this could be followed by AZA or MMF after the first 6 months. Microscopic hematuria or non-nephrotic proteinuria may not clear for several months, even when most other clinical parameters have remitted. Remission may occur at an average of 1.5 to 2 years after therapy. Thus discontinuing pulse IV-CYC therapy because of lack of achieving remission before completing at least 2 years of treatment is not justified unless there is definite disease worsening (reproducible increase in SCr and/or >50% increase in proteinuria at the nephrotic range). In selected patients with severe disease who have achieved remission, MMF may be used as a maintenance regimen (see Figure 81-2).[126]

Lupus Membranous Nephropathy

LMN with mesangial expansion (pure membranous) and low-grade proteinuria (<2 g/day) carries a low risk for progression to ESRD (20% at 10 years) and may require renin-angiotensin axis blockade and low-dose GC. Persistent nephrotic-range proteinuria, abnormal renal function, and black race have been implicated as high-risk features and are indications for immunosuppressive therapy.[127] Uncontrolled studies indicate beneficial effects of the combination of GC with AZA or calcineurin inhibitors in mild to moderate LMN.[65,128] In the RCT of Austin and colleagues[37] oral CsA and pulse IV-CYC were equally successful in inducing remission. Nephrotic syndrome relapses were more common in the CsA group, suggesting that these patients should receive maintenance therapy with lower CsA doses or other immunosuppressive agent. MMF has emerged as an efficacious regimen with more favorable safety profile for both induction and maintenance therapy of class V LN on the basis of the pooled data from two RCTs comparing MMF versus IV-CYC in moderately severe LN.[50] However, this will have to be proven in larger trials with longer follow-up. Mixed membranous and proliferative histology (especially when diffuse proliferation is present) has a worse prognosis, even from pure proliferative disease. These patients should be aggressively treated as those with PLN. Bao and colleagues[69] have reported interesting results using the combination of prednisone, MMF, and tacrolimus as induction therapy for mixed class IV+V LN. In this trial, multitarget therapy was associated with higher rates of complete response compared with pulse IV-CYC. These results need to be confirmed before adopting this regimen.

Treatment of Renal Flares

Approximately 30% to 50% of patients with moderate to severe PLN will relapse after achieving partial or complete remission.[129-131] *Nephritic* flares are characterized by active urine sediment and reproducible increase of SCr (≥30% increase) and may adversely affect renal prognosis; *proteinuric* flares without significant changes in renal function have a more benign prognosis.[131,132] Risk factors for progression to ESRD after a nephritic flare are patients with marked loss of renal function (SCr >2 mg/dL) at the time of response, partial response to therapy, and high chronicity and activity indices at renal biopsy. Flares are more common in African-American patients and patients with undetectable serum C3/C4 levels. However, pre-emptive treatment in the face of abnormal serology (rising anti-dsDNA or reduced C3/C4 titers, or both) may result in overtreating a large number of patients. Mild to moderate flares (stable SCr, subnephrotic proteinuria) may be treated with GC in combination with AZA or MMF. Calcineurin inhibitors (alone or added to existing immunosuppressive therapy) have also demonstrated efficacy. For severe nephritic flares, reinstitution of cytotoxic therapy with monthly pulses of IV-CYC and IV-MP is the authors' preferred approach, with MMF considered as an alternative agent. RTX has also been successfully used in a small case series.

Central Nervous System Disease

Less than 40% of neuropsychiatric events in SLE patients can be attributed to lupus, whereas the remaining cases represent complications of the disease or its therapy, or they may be caused by infections, metabolic abnormalities, and drug adverse effects. Neuropsychiatric SLE (NPSLE) is a clinical challenge, and difficulties include the correct attribution of neuropsychiatric syndromes to SLE, the selection of proper diagnostic examinations, and optimal treatment. To facilitate the management of these patients, EULAR has published recommendations using an evidence-based approach followed by expert consensus (Table 81-6).[133] All nonlupus contributing factors should be identified and treated, and symptomatic therapy should be considered if appropriate. Moderate to high doses of GCs alone or in combination with immunosuppressive therapy (AZA for mild to moderate cases, IV-CYC for severe ones) may be used for neuropsychiatric events felt to reflect an immune/inflammatory process (particularly acute confusional state, aseptic meningitis, myelitis, optic neuritis, refractory seizure disorder, peripheral neuropathies, psychosis) or when they occur in the context of active generalized lupus, following exclusion of non-SLE-related causes.[40] Although a placebo-controlled trial reported improved cognition in five out of eight SLE patients with inactive disease and mild cognitive dysfunction who were treated with low-dose prednisone (0.5 mg/kg/day for 21 days, then tapered), GCs should not be routinely administered in these patients unless to control concurrent SLE or other overt NPSLE activity. In severe NPSLE refractory to cytotoxic therapy, the use of plasma exchange, IVIG, and RTX has been reported in uncontrolled studies, with varying rates of success. Antiplatelet or anticoagulation therapy are recommended for NPSLE related to aPL antibodies, especially for thrombotic cerebrovascular disease (see Antiphospholipid Syndrome later).

Hematologic Disease

Peripheral cytopenias are common but usually mild in SLE. A thorough clinical and laboratory evaluation is necessary to exclude offending drugs or other secondary causes. Mild

Table 81-6 Approach to Systemic Lupus Erythematosus (SLE) Patients with Neuropsychiatric Manifestations

What Are the Risk Factors for NPSLE?
Generalized (non-CNS) lupus activity or damage, previous or other concurrent major NPSLE manifestation(s), persistently positive moderate-to-high titers of aPL antibodies
When to Suspect NPSLE
Any SLE patient at risk who presents with new-onset neurologic or psychiatric manifestations without an apparent cause In patients with subtle or mild signs or symptoms, a high index of suspicion is required to exclude underlying overt NPSLE
Is It NPSLE?
Mild manifestations (headache, mood disorders, anxiety, mild cognitive dysfunction, polyneuropathy without electrophysiologic confirmation) are common (up to 40%) but are not usually related to lupus Non–SLE-related causes (infections, metabolic disturbances, drug adverse effects) must be excluded Most (40%-50%) lupus-related events occur at onset or during the first 2-4 yr after SLE diagnosis, common (50%-60%) in the presence of generalized lupus activity Attribution to lupus more likely when NPSLE risk factors are present
What Diagnostic Workup Is Indicated?

Magnetic resonance imaging is the preferred neuroimaging test and may help to identify:
  Ischemic/thrombotic, demyelinating, or infectious processes
  T2-weighted white matter lesions: in the absence of other confounding factors (increased age, long-standing SLE, atherosclerotic risk factors, heart valve disease) may reflect underlying CNS lupus activity (especially when ≥5 in number, ≥6-8 mm in size, bihemispheric)
Cerebrospinal fluid analysis should be performed when CNS infection is suspected; mild abnormalities common in active NPSLE
Other tests as indicated: electroencephalogram to diagnose seizure disorder, neuropsychologic tests to assess cognitive dysfunction, nerve conduction studies for peripheral neuropathy

What Is the Treatment of NPSLE?

Control aggravating factors (infection, dehydration, metabolic abnormalities, hypertension)
Control symptoms (anticonvulsants, antidepressants, antipsychotics)
Glucocorticoids and/or immunosuppressive therapy in cases of:
  Acute confusional state, aseptic meningitis, myelitis, optic neuritis, refractory seizure disorder, peripheral neuropathies, severe psychosis
  Control generalized (non-CNS) lupus activity
Antithrombotic or antiplatelet therapy
  aPL-associated NPSLE (particularly cerebrovascular disease, ischemic optic neuropathy, chorea) or when antiphospholipid syndrome–associated thrombotic events are present

CNS, central nervous system; NPSLE, neuropsychiatric systemic lupus erythematosus.

cytopenias require no specific therapy other than regular monitoring. In more severe cases (platelet count $< 50 \times 10^3/$ mm^3 or active bleeding, neutrophil count $<1000/mm^3$), GCs (1 mg/kg/day with gradual tapering) are the mainstay of treatment.[134] Pulses of IV-MP followed by lower doses of prednisone (0.6 mg/kg/day) may be used alternatively. Steroid-sparing agents (AZA, CsA) can be added during steroid tapering.[61] Patients with steroid-resistant thrombocytopenia may be candidates for splenectomy, especially when there is no significant lupus activity in other organs. Early reports from the 1980s have shown a satisfactory response to splenectomy with progressive rise in platelet counts. Prophylactic measures for avoidance of infectious complications in patients undergoing splenectomy are mandatory. These include immunization against encapsulated bacteria (*Streptococcus pneumoniae*, *Neisseria meningitidis*, *Haemophilus influenzae*) and influenza virus, as well as prophylactic antibiotic coverage when necessary.

Resistant life-threatening cytopenias may require potent immunosuppressive therapy. Monthly pulses of IV-CYC have been shown to reverse severe refractory autoimmune thrombocytopenia.[135] In severe neutropenia, however, the risk for potential leukocyte toxicity of CYC should be considered. The use of lower-dose IV-CYC (Euro-Lupus protocol) is associated with a better safety profile and is advocated by some centers. RTX may be considered in patients with refractory neutropenias, especially when the use of IV-CYC is hampered by its potential myelotoxicity.[72,74] Of note, RTX may also be associated with both early- and late-onset neutropenia, which is usually self-limited.[136]

Treatment of immune thrombocytopenia may sail into a new era with the development of novel thrombopoietin mimetic agents that enhance platelet production. Two such agents, romiplostim and eltrombopag, were shown to be superior than standard of care in large RCTs and have been approved for the treatment of immune thrombocytopenia.[137,138] They resulted in a greater incidence of sustained platelet response, less bleeding, fewer transfusions, reduced requirement for other treatments (including splenectomy), and greater improvement in quality of life. Adverse events were minimal. The ultimate place these remedies will take in the armamentarium against immune thrombocytopenia (before or after splenectomy) will depend on their long-term efficacy/safety profile and their cost compared with the potentially curative and relatively safe choice of splenectomy.

Supportive treatment may be necessary for severe cytopenias or associated complications. Febrile neutropenia should be treated with broad-spectrum antibiotics and, if neutrophil counts are less than $500/mm^3$, with human G-CSF. Serious hemolytic anemia (Hb <7 g/dL) may require red blood cell transfusions, whereas platelet transfusions are best avoided unless invasive procedures are planned.

Antiphospholipid Syndrome

aPL antibodies (anticardiolipin [aCL], anti–β_2-glycoprotein I [anti-β_2GPI], and lupus anticoagulant [LAC]) are encountered in 30% to 40% of SLE and are associated with increased risk for thrombo-occlusive incidents. The combination of vascular thrombosis or obstetric morbidity, or both, and persistently positive aPL antibodies measured at least 12 weeks apart, defines antiphospholipid syndrome (APS).[139,140]

Thrombotic Antiphospholipid Syndrome

APS-associated thrombosis requires antiplatelet and/or anticoagulation therapy to prevent recurrent events, but the intensity of such therapies remains controversial. On the basis of the results of two systematic reviews,[141,142] patients with definite APS and first venous or arterial noncerebral/noncoronary thrombosis should receive oral anticoagulation (warfarin) at a target international normalized ratio (INR) 2 to 3, although some experts recommend higher-intensity anticoagulation following arterial thrombotic events.[139] Data from the Antiphospholipid Antibodies and Stroke Study (APASS) and large RCTs in the general population suggest that antithrombotic therapy is not superior to antiplatelet therapy for secondary thromboprophylaxis after noncardioembolic stroke or transient ischemic attack.[143] Because many patients studied were elderly and had low titers of aPL antibodies, determined at a single time point, the conclusions may be limited to these populations. Acute coronary artery syndromes should be treated according to the evidence base for the general population. For patients with recurrent thrombotic events, anticoagulation should target INR 3 to 4, especially if they have high-risk aPL profile (LAC or aCL IgG at higher titers, or anti-β_2GPI plus LAC or aCL).[144] Additional atherothrombotic risk factors should be aggressively controlled. The role of newer classes of anticoagulants (direct thrombin inhibitors, oral direct factor Xa inhibitors)—currently licensed for the management of venous thromboembolism in the general population—for secondary APS thromboprophylaxis remains to be determined.

HCQ, in addition to its anti-inflammatory effects, has been proposed to exert antithrombotic properties through inhibiting platelet aggregation and arachidonic acid release from stimulated platelets. Use of HCQ has been associated with reduced rates of thrombosis in both aPL-positive and aPL-negative patients.[145] A systematic review of epidemiologic studies found evidence for antithrombotic effect of HCQ in SLE patients, especially in studies accounting for exposure previous to the event.[20] These results have not been confirmed in large prospective cohort studies,[146] and controlled studies are necessary to determine the effectiveness of HCQ for primary thromboprophylaxis. RCTs have also shown a protective effect of rosuvastatin (20 mg/day) against thrombosis (including cardiovascular events and venous thromboembolism) in healthy adults with normal low-density lipoprotein levels and elevated C-reactive protein (>2 mg/dL).[147,148] These findings justify the conduction of clinical trials of statins in aPL-positive patients. In small case series, RTX has demonstrated beneficial effects in severe APS cases including resolution of symptoms (especially thrombocytopenia) and reduction in aPL antibody titers.[149]

Pregnancy in Antiphospholipid Syndrome

Pregnant SLE-APS patients are at increased risk for complications including maternal thrombosis, recurrent spontaneous abortions before 10 weeks' gestation, and late adverse pregnancy outcomes such as fetal death, pre-eclampsia, fetal growth restriction, and preterm birth.[150,151] For women with APS and a history of pregnancy complications or thrombosis, or both, a meta-analysis of three RCTs concluded that the combination of unfractionated heparin and aspirin confers a significant benefit in live births (odds ratio [OR] for first trimester loss, 0.26; number needed to treat [NNT], 4).[152] The pooled effect of low-molecular-weight heparin was also favorable (OR 0.70) but not statistically significant. Conversely, combination therapy of either unfractionated or low-molecular-weight heparin with aspirin had no effect in prevention of late-pregnancy losses. Results from RCTs do not specifically define optimum treatment for women with fetal death (>10 weeks' gestation) or previous early delivery (<34 weeks' gestation) because of severe pre-eclampsia or placental insufficiency. Nonetheless, most experts recommend low-dose aspirin and either prophylactic or intermediate-dose heparin. A beneficial effect of low-dose aspirin in primary prevention of thrombotic events and miscarriage in SLE with persistently positive moderate to high titers of aPL antibodies has been suggested by some,[145,153] but not all,[154] studies. Neither aspirin combined with low-molecular-weight heparin nor aspirin alone improved the live birth rate, as compared with placebo, among women with unexplained recurrent miscarriage.[155]

Vitamin K antagonists are teratogenic and should be avoided between 6 and 12 weeks of gestation; even after 12 weeks of gestation they should be used cautiously due to increased risk for fatal bleeding. Antithrombotic coverage of the postpartum period is recommended for all APS patients irrespective of their thrombotic history. Women with previous thrombosis will need long-term anticoagulation, and treatment is generally switched to warfarin as soon as the patient is clinically stable after delivery.[139,156] In patients with no previous thrombosis, the recommendation is prophylactic-dose heparin or low-molecular-weight heparin therapy for 4 to 6 weeks after delivery, although warfarin is an option. Both heparin and warfarin are safe during breastfeeding.

Other Antiphospholipid Syndrome Manifestations

A distinct type of small-vessel vaso-occlusive nephropathy with histologic features of thrombotic microangiopathy and chronic vascular lesions, termed *APS nephropathy*, should be suspected in aPL-positive patients with hypertension, proteinuria (usually mild to moderate), hematuria, and renal impairment.[157,158] These patients may benefit from aggressive immunosuppressive therapy along with anticoagulation, but development of ESRD is common.[159] A minority of patients (<1%) can suffer from a potentially life-threatening variant of APS, catastrophic APS (CAPS), which is characterized by multiple small-vessel thromboses resulting in multiorgan failure.[160] Approximately 70% of patients manifest renal involvement, usually resulting in severe hypertension, proteinuria, hematuria, and renal impairment. The condition is associated with 50% mortality rate and may be treated with combination of anticoagulation and immunosuppressive therapy (high-dose GC alone or in combination with CYC) plus attempts to reduce aPL titers (plasma exchange, IVIG).

ADDITIONAL ISSUES

KEY POINTS

Pregnancy outcome in SLE is optimal when disease is clinically quiescent for at least 6 months.

The risks of treatment during pregnancy must be weighed against the risks of an untreated SLE flare, with potential deleterious effects on the mother and the fetus.

The treatment of pediatric-onset SLE is similar to that in adult SLE patients.

Treatment of Refractory Systemic Lupus Erythematosus

IV-CYC in combination with IV-MP has long been considered the treatment of choice for most patients with severe, life-threatening lupus. Mounting evidence from uncontrolled studies supports the beneficial effects of RTX (alone or in combination with IV-CYC) in refractory SLE.[161-163] Higher response rates have been reported for skin, blood, central nervous system (CNS), and renal manifestations.[74] Advantages from the use of RTX include its favorable toxicity profile and the rapid onset of action.[73] MMF may rescue a few refractory SLE patients including LN cases with inadequate response to CYC. However, its efficacy in critically ill patients requires further documentation. Calcineurin inhibitors have also shown efficacy in resistant-to-standard immunosuppressive therapy lupus,[164] particularly LN,[165] and benefits of combination therapy with MMF were reported in a small RCT.[69] For selected patients with CNS involvement, autoimmune thrombocytopenia, or APS, IVIG may be considered as an adjunct therapy. Synchronized therapy with plasmapheresis and pulse IV-CYC has been used in severe PLN cases.[166]

High-dose chemotherapy with autologous hematopoietic stem cell transplantation (HSCT) has been used in SLE.[167] The rationale is to maximally suppress the immune system with an immunoablative regimen (usually high-dose CYC combined with equine antithymocyte globulin and pulse IV-MP) and then rescue the patient from prolonged cytopenias by the infusion of mobilized CD34-enriched stem cells. A few patients who received HSCT experienced improvement in disease activity, but relapses were common.[168] In a pilot study, 15 patients refractory to conventional treatment (n = 14 with nephritis) received a small dose of allogeneic bone marrow–derived mesenchymal stem cells (1×10^6/kg by IV injection).[169] Prednisolone was tapered from week 2 onwards, and IV-CYC was continued with larger intervals. Rapid and sustained improvements in autoantibody levels, proteinuria, and nonrenal manifestations were reported, with no significant acute toxicity. Until more data are available, stem cell transplantation remains an experimental procedure that needs to be considered in critically ill lupus patients, ideally in experienced centers.

Treatment of Lupus in Pregnancy

Pregnancy may increase disease activity and precipitate the appearance of flares (13% to 74%), which are usually mild.

Lupus pregnancies are considered high risk for maternal and fetal complications. A recent meta-analysis reviewing 2571 pregnancies in SLE patients reported unsuccessful pregnancy and preterm birth rates of 23% and 39%, respectively, while maternal complications included nephritis (16%), hypertension (16%), and pre-eclampsia (7%).[151] A history of LN and the presence of aPL antibodies were associated with development of hypertension and premature birth.

The management of a pregnant woman with an SLE flare is challenging and should be dealt with on a multidisciplinary basis (Table 81-7). The risks of treatment with potential deleterious effects on the mother and the fetus must be balanced against the risks of untreated disease. Mild flares involving the skin, joints, and blood are usually treated with GC. The latter are relatively safe, although they carry a small risk of harm (increased risk of cleft palate in children, intrauterine growth retardation, maternal hypertension, diabetes) and thus should be used in the lowest enough doses to control disease activity. HCQ has a good safety record despite crossing the placenta. AZA, although listed as FDA category D, can be used with caution as a steroid-sparing agent. The same holds true for CsA (category C). In contrast, CYC is a major teratogen and should not be used unless there is no available alternative for organ-threatening disease in the mother, preferentially in the late second or third trimester. Fetal loss due to CYC toxicity may occur. MMF and MTX are listed as category D and X, respectively, and should be avoided. For biologic agents, data regarding safety during pregnancy are lacking and their use is generally discouraged. Pregnant SLE patients with a severe renal flare (active urinary sediment, increase in SCr) can be treated with high-dose GC and antihypertensives, *excluding* ACE inhibitors, whereas AZA can be used cautiously to allow steroid tapering. Prompt delivery of the fetus at the earliest safe time point possible is warranted.

Neonatal lupus occurs in some babies born by mothers with anti-SSA/Ro or anti-SSB/La antibodies, or both. The most serious complication is neonatal complete heart block (CHB), which occurs in up to 2% of such pregnancies and carries a 20% to 30% mortality risk. The risk of recurrence in a mother having already borne a child with CHB ranges from 14% to 19%.[170] Therefore all women with SLE should be evaluated for the presence of anti-Ro/La antibodies. The most vulnerable period for the development of conduction disturbances is between week 18 and 26 of gestation, during which anti-Ro/La–positive patients should be evaluated with weekly fetal Doppler echocardiography for the prompt identification of conduction anomalies, mainly PR interval prolongation. If CHB develops, no modality has been shown to reverse it. In contrast, a large observational study in 118 pregnant women with anti-Ro antibodies showed that first-degree block may be reversed by fluorinated GCs such as dexamethazone (4 mg/day) initiated at the time of diagnosis and continued throughout pregnancy.[171] Two trials found no beneficial effect of IVIG on prevention of recurrence of congenital heart block in Ro/SSA-positive mothers.[172,173]

Regarding breastfeeding, the American Academy of Pediatrics (AAP) states that nursing is permissible for women receiving GC but the interval between dose and nursing should be at least 4 hours if the prednisone dosage is greater than 20 mg/day. Antimalarials may be continued during lactation, whereas AZA is not recommended due to possible risk for immunosuppression, carcinogenicity, and growth restriction of the child. MTX, MMF, CsA, leflunomide, and CYC are also contraindicated.

The high-risk features of SLE pregnancy and the possible risk for adverse outcomes highlight the importance of family counseling and planning before pregnancy is sought. It is generally accepted that pregnancy outcome is optimal when disease is clinically quiescent for at least 6 months and, in cases of kidney involvement, if renal function is normal or near normal. Until this desired goal is reached, common effective means of contraception should be taken to avoid unplanned pregnancies (see Women's Health Issues).

Table 81-7 Approach to the Management of Pregnancy in Systemic Lupus Erythematosus

Planning of pregnancy
Ensure that lupus is inactive for at least 6 mo
Reassure patient: small risk for major flare
Discourage pregnancy if SCr >2 mg/dL
Determine aPL antibodies and other antibodies that may be of relevance (anti-SSA, anti-SSB)
Obtain baseline serology and chemistry labs (SCr, SAlb, uric acid, anti-dsDNA, C3/C4)
Be aware of the small risk for CHB, especially in women with both anti-SSA and anti-SSB antibodies or with a prior episode of CHB. In such cases, may monitor for CHB between 16 and 24 wk of gestation
Monitor closely blood pressure and proteinuria. Should this develop, differentiate between active nephritis and pre-eclampsia
Presence of generalized lupus activity, active urine sediment, and low serum complement are in favor of lupus nephritis
For patients with antiphospholipid syndrome, consider combined heparin and aspirin to reduce risk for pregnancy loss and thrombosis. Patients with aPL antibodies may be treated with aspirin, although there are no adequate data to support its use

CHB, congenital heart block.

Treatment of Pediatric Systemic Lupus Erythematosus

Pediatric-onset SLE (pSLE) represents 15% to 20% of all SLE cases and is associated with higher disease severity and more rapid damage accrual than adult-onset SLE. The use of antimalarials (HCQ 4 to 6 mg/kg/day) is helpful in children with skin disease and arthritis. In mild nephritis (class II or mild class III LN), normal renal function, normal blood pressure, and non-nephrotic proteinuria, oral GCs (≤1 mg/kg/day) may suffice to control disease. Initial pulses of IV-MP (30 mg/kg/day up to a maximum dose of 1 g/day for 3 consecutive days) may allow for lower oral prednisone dose (0.5 mg/kg/day). In patients with class III nephritis and high activity index or class IV disease, pulse therapy with IV-MP and IV-CYC (0.75 to 1 g/m^2) should be considered. Lehman and colleagues[174,175] studied clinical and histologic progression of class III/IV nephritis in 16 children who completed at least 3 years of continuous treatment with IV-CYC. Significant improvements in disease activity, renal function, and renal activity index were observed. In a retrospective study of 28 patients with class IV LN who received IV-CYC and oral GC, repeat biopsy showed histologic improvement in 20 out of 25 children. At last follow-up, 3.5 ± 2.3 years after second biopsy, 26 patients retained normal renal function.[176] In PLN with preserved renal function and non-nephrotic proteinuria, MMF could be used.[177] A single study has reported good outcomes with the combination of MMF and CsA in severe class III/IV LN patients who responded inadequately to initial induction therapy with MMF and GC.[178]

Both AZA and MMF are efficacious maintenance regimens in pediatric PLN.[179,180] Baskin and colleagues[181] studied 20 pSLE patients with severe PLN who received 6-month induction therapy with pulse IV-MP (30 mg/kg, followed by oral prednisone 0.5 to 1.0 mg/kg/day) and IV-CYC (500 mg/m²). AZA (2 mg/kg/day) was commenced as a remission-maintaining regimen in all patients; in 10 patients, treatment subsequently switched to oral MMF (1200 mg/m²/day) because of intolerance or lack of efficacy. Following this approach, 14 patients (70%) achieved complete remission and another 3 (15%) had partial remission. An alternate-day regimen of 10 to 15 mg oral prednisone should be aimed at during the maintenance phase.

Renal flares remain an important issue that has not been adequately addressed. Alternative to a second course of IV-CYC and GC, which may be associated with significant long-term toxicity, is the combination of IV MTX and CYC administered for 9 months.[175] Although data for RTX are limited, it may be used (600 mg/m², maximum dose of 1 g/m² on days 1 and 15) in refractory renal and extrarenal disease.[182,183] RTX can be used as monotherapy or in combination with CYC, under the following dosage scheme: 500 to 750 mg/m² on days 2 and 16.

Significant CNS involvement usually warrants combination of high-dose steroids with an immunosuppressive agent such as CYC or AZA.[147] To date, there is no study documenting an increased rate of serious adverse effects such as life-threatening infections or secondary neoplasia in children with SLE receiving cytotoxic therapy compared with adults. All children with LN should be regularly reviewed to treat accompanying hypertension, proteinuria, and renal dysfunction. Monitoring for normal growth, physical and pubertal development, and bone density is important, especially for patients on long-term treatment with GC.

COMORBIDITIES IN SYSTEMIC LUPUS ERYTHEMATOSUS

KEY POINTS

The diagnostic approach and management of an SLE patient with possible infection should consider: (1) the dominant clinical syndrome, (2) the history of epidemiologic exposures, and (3) the "net-state" of immunosuppression.

Immunizations are safe and effective in SLE patients but must be avoided in active disease. Inactivated live vaccines are contraindicated in patients taking immunosuppressive drugs or high-dose glucocorticoids.

In SLE patients with end-stage renal disease, hemodialysis may be preferred over chronic ambulatory peritoneal dialysis. Renal transplantation is a potential alternative.

SLE patients are at increased risk for cardiovascular disease, and strict adherence to general population guidelines for primary prevention is recommended.

Cervical dysplasia is increased in women with lupus. HPV vaccination should be considered until the age of 25 years, similarly to the general population.

Infections and Immunizations

Risk Factors and General Management

Infections account for 20% to 55% of all deaths in SLE patients. Susceptibility to infections may be due to underlying immune dysregulation and therapeutic factors, particularly high-dose GCs and immunosuppressive drugs. A broad spectrum of infections have been reported in SLE including bacterial, mycobacterial, viral, fungal and parasitic infections, with the respiratory, urinary tract, and CNS as the most commonly involved sites.[184] Risk factors for infections include increased clinical or serologic lupus activity, or both, at baseline[185,186]; major organ involvement (especially renal[187] and lung involvement[188]); lymphopenia; persistent neutropenia (<1000/mm³)[189]; hypoalbuminemia (especially for severe CNS infections[190]); high dose of GC (each increase of 10 mg/day prednisone is associated with 11-fold increased risk for serious infection[188]); and prior (within the last 6 months) use of immunosuppressive drugs (especially AZA and CYC).[186,191,192]

The evaluation of a lupus patient who receives immunosuppressive therapy and presents with symptoms or signs suggestive of infection possesses diagnostic and therapeutic challenges (Figure 81-3). This is complicated by the fact that active SLE per se is associated with increased risk for infection, and on the other hand, viral infections can mimic a lupus flare. Findings that favor the diagnosis of infection include the presence of shaking chills, leukocytosis and/or neutrophilia (especially in the absence of steroid therapy), increased numbers of band forms or metamyelocytes on peripheral blood smear, and concomitant immunosuppressive therapy.[192-195] The diagnosis of SLE fever is favored by the presence of leukopenia (not explained by cytotoxic therapy), normal or only slightly increased C-reactive protein, low C3/C4, and elevated anti-DNA antibodies. If fever fails to resolve in a patient receiving prednisone 20 to 40 mg daily, it is likely that that fever is due to infection, not SLE. Elevated serum procalcitonin (PCT) levels have been reported to be predictive of bacterial or mycotic infections,[196] although their diagnostic utility in patients with systemic autoimmune diseases has been questioned.[197] Pending microbiology results, adequate antimicrobial therapy (including broad-spectrum antibiotics in suspected nosocomial infection) is recommended to reduce adverse outcomes.[198,199]

Specific and Opportunistic Infections

Tuberculosis Infection. Tuberculosis (TB) infection rates are 6- to 60-fold higher in SLE patients than the general population[200] and may be caused by both *Mycobacterium tuberculosis* (MTB) and nontuberculous mycobacterium (NTM).[201] Extrapulmonary involvement is

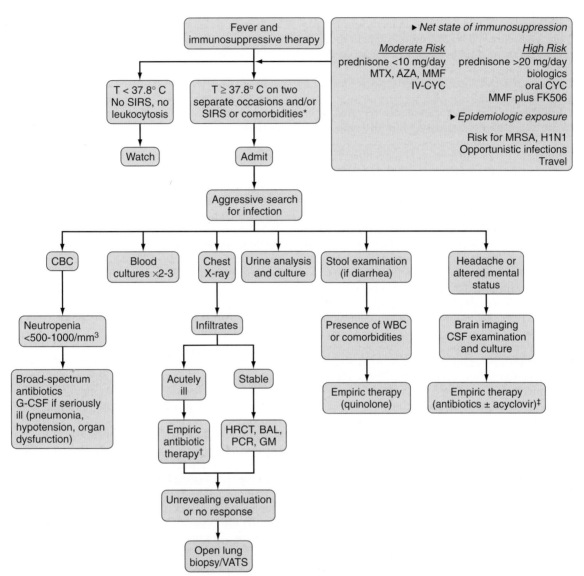

Figure 81-3 Initial assessment and management of systemic lupus erythematosus patients who receive immunosuppressive therapy and present with fever or other symptoms and signs suggestive of infection. *, Systemic inflammatory response syndrome (SIRS): T ≥38° C or <36° C, tachycardia (heart rate >90/min), tachypnea (respiratory rate >20/min), white blood cells (WBC) >12,000/mm³; comorbidities: age older than 65 years, diabetes, chronic cardiopulmonary disease. †, Consider empirical therapy for *Pneumocystis* pneumonia in severe hypoxemia or diffuse pulmonary infiltrates. ‡, Consider tuberculosis and other opportunistic central nervous system (CNS) infections. AZA, azathioprine; BAL, bronchoalveolar lavage; CBC, complete blood count; CSF, cerebrospinal fluid; G-CSF, granulocyte colony-stimulating factor; GM, galactomannane; H1N1, influenza H1N1; HRCT, high-resolution chest tomography; IV-CYC, intravenous cyclophosphamide; MMF, mycophenolate mofetil; MRSA, methicillin-resistant *Staphylococcus aureus*; MTX, methotrexate; PCR, polymerase chain reaction; T, temperature; VATS, video-assisted thoracoscopy. *(Modified from Papadimitraki ED, Bertsias K, Chamilos MD, Boumpas DT: Systemic lupus erythematosus: cytotoxic drugs. In Tsokos G, Buyon JP, Koike T, Lahita RG, editors: Systemic lupus erythematosus, ed 5, St Louis, 2010, Elsevier, pp 1083–1108.)*

common and ranges from 52% to 74% of TB infections. Tuberculin skin testing (TST) is recommended for patients who are candidates for treatment with long-term prednisone greater than or equal to 15 mg/day or immunosuppressive drugs. Because of the isoniazid age-related hepatotoxicity (4.6% in individuals older than 65 years of age vs. 0.3% in 20- to 30-year-old individuals), TST is advocated only for moderate-risk patients younger than 65 years of age. TB diagnosis can be established by conventional methods including the presence of a suggestive clinical presentation, a positive TST, and microbiologic confirmation (by the identification of bacilli in the smear or positive cultures). In selected patients, when these measures are nondiagnostic, typical histologic abnormalities such as granulomas may help in the diagnosis. The advent of the T cell IFN-γ release assays, a more specific test than the tuberculin skin test, may improve the detection of latent TB infection.

Pneumocystis jiroveci Infection. The incidence of *Pneumocystis* pneumonia in SLE patients on CYC approximates 0.15%. Risk factors include lymphopenia (≤750/mm³) during lupus treatment, high disease activity, renal involvement, interstitial pulmonary fibrosis, and high prednisone dosage.[202] Some authors recommend *Pneumocystis* pneumonia prophylaxis (one double-strength tablet of trimethoprim-sulfamethoxazole three times a week or dapsone 100 mg/day if allergic to sulfamethoxazole) for patients on high-dose GC (≥20 mg/day prednisone or equivalent) alone or in combination with cytotoxic drugs, especially if CD4 count is less than 300 cells/mm³. Of note, risk of allergic reactions to sulfamethoxazole may be increased in SLE patients.

Viral Infections. The most commonly reported viral infections in SLE patients are parvovirus B19 and cytomegalovirus (CMV) (predominantly in severely immunosuppressed patients). The latter may mimic a lupus flare or present with specific organ involvement such as hepatitis, gastrointestinal bleeding, or pulmonary infiltrates. Renal insufficiency, lymphopenia, APS manifestations, treatment with CYC, multiorgan involvement at presentation, and a lower frequency of antiviral treatment have been related to fatal viral infection in SLE cohorts.[203,204] The introduction of direct antigenic (CMV pp65 antigenemia) and molecular (quantitative polymerase chain reaction [PCR]) testing has revolutionized the diagnosis of CMV infection in the setting of immune suppression. Viral load has proven useful for diagnosis of infection, prediction of disease, and monitoring response to therapy. However, detection of small amounts of viral DNA in peripheral blood by PCR is not necessarily indicative of clinically significant CMV infection, and correct interpretation of test results may require consultation with an infectious diseases specialist. Further confirmatory diagnosis of organ-specific involvement can be made by histologic detection of characteristic inclusion bodies. Increased age (≥60 years), symptomatic infection, and lymphopenia (all three correlating with CMV antigenemia above 5.6/10⁵ PMNs) have been associated with fatal outcome, and their presence may therefore prompt initiation of antiviral therapy.[204]

Varicella-zoster virus (VZV) reactivation is an important issue in SLE patients. Risk factors include history of CYC or AZA exposure, the presence of concurrent or previous malignancy, and LN. Shingles dissemination and bacterial superinfection are mostly linked to high-dose GC treatment.[205] SLE patients do not display increased risk for HIV infection, and screening should be based on individualized risk factors. Due to risks of occurrence and reactivation of the infection following immunosuppressive therapy, particularly when steroids are administered, screening for hepatitis C and B virus is prudent before starting such therapies.

Immunizations

Although vaccination may hypothetically induce polyclonal cell activation in lupus precipitating a flare, it is felt to be safe.[206] Vaccines, however, should not be given to patients with active disease. Inactivated live vaccines (measles, mumps, rubella, polio, VZV, and vaccinia [smallpox]) are contraindicated in patients taking immunosuppressive drugs or prednisone, or both, at a dose greater than 20 mg/day. Influenza vaccine is safe and effective, although seroprotection and seroconversion rates are lower than those in healthy controls[207,208]; booster vaccination does not increase antibody titers in annually vaccinated patients.[209] Pneumococcal vaccine is also safe, but the resultant antibody titers may be decreased in SLE patients; use of GC may contribute to blunted antibody responses. Protective immune response can be achieved safely in SLE patients

with both tetanus toxoid and *H. influenzae* type B in addition to pneumococcus.

According to the Advisory Committee on Immunization Practices (ACIP) guidelines and EULAR guidelines,[210] individuals older than 60 years of age should be vaccinated with a single dose of VZV vaccine. This is a live-attenuated vaccine and should be administered at least 14 days before initiation, or it should be deferred for at least 1 month after discontinuation of high-dose GC or immunosuppressive therapy. Therapy with low-dose MTX (<0.4 mg/kg/week) or AZA (<3 mg/kg/day) is not considered sufficiently immunosuppressive to create vaccine safety concerns. Kuruma and colleagues[211] reported on hepatitis B vaccination in inactive SLE patients treated with low-dose GC and not receiving immunosuppressive drugs, negative for anti-dsDNA and aCL antibodies. Patients were administered a recombinant vaccine. All patients developed protective antibodies, and there were no SLE flares.

Chronic Kidney Disease and End-Stage Renal Disease

Risk Factors and Dialysis

Approximately 10% to 20% of SLE patients will develop ESRD. Clinical predictors are abnormal SCr values at presentation, delay in treatment initiation, failure to achieve remission, and systolic hypertension.[212-215] Progression of LN to the point of dialysis does not necessarily indicate ESRD because 5% to 10% of patients will recover sufficient renal function to interrupt dialysis at least temporarily. Patients with rapid deterioration of renal function are more likely to have a reversible physiologic (dehydration, infection, acute tubular necrosis) or pathologic (crescentic glomerulonephritis) component accounting for their renal insufficiency. In these patients, immunosuppressive therapy (pulse of IV-MP and IV-CYC 0.4 to 0.5 g/m², administered 8 to 10 hours before dialysis) may continue during dialysis.

The 5-year survival rate of SLE patients on dialysis approximates 80% to 90%, comparable with that in non-SLE dialysis patients.[216] Hemodialysis may be the first choice of renal replacement therapy, especially for patients who are still on immunosuppressive therapy, due to increased rates of infectious complications (most commonly peritonitis) and hospital admissions in patients on chronic ambulatory peritoneal dialysis (CAPD).[216,217] Irrespective of the dialysis mode, most patients with advanced renal disease experience a decline in lupus activity. Discontinuation of cytotoxic therapy may be considered in patients with steadily rising SCr to greater than or equal to 5 mg/dL with inactive urine sediment, renal biopsy showing exclusively scarring and atrophy, or contracted renal size. Judicious use of GCs and immunosuppressive drugs is essential to minimize the risk for septic complications. Cardiovascular morbidity and mortality are also increased in patients with ESRD, underscoring the need for tight control of atherosclerotic risk factors.[218]

Renal Transplantation

Renal transplantation is a viable alternative for lupus patients with ESRD. Graft and patient survival rates are comparable with those in other patient groups, although this is not confirmed in all studies.[216] Results are superior with living than cadaveric donor transplantation (5-year graft survival rates 77% to 89% vs. 41% to 58%). If a living donor is available, the possibility for pre-emptive transplantation can be considered because this approach is associated with superior graft and patient outcomes in other kidney diseases.[219] Nevertheless, a period of at least 3 months on dialysis may allow some patients to recover adequate renal function for significant time periods.

There are no prospective studies comparing various immunosuppressive regimens after renal transplantation in SLE. Calcineurin inhibitors should generally be included in the induction phase (6 to 12 months) on the basis of observations of improved graft survival rates since their introduction in lupus transplantation.[220] Due to potential nephrotoxicity and adverse effects on cardiovascular disease (CVD) risk factors, their use should be minimized during the maintenance phase and other immunosuppressive agents (MMF, AZA) should be preferentially employed. Recurrence of LN (usually mild mesangial proliferative disease) in the renal allograft is a rare event (2% to 3%) and not an important cause of graft loss. Risk factors for recurrent LN include non-Hispanic black race, female gender, age younger than 33 years, and living donor transplantation.[221-223] APS has been associated with post-transplant renal thrombosis and poor graft outcome and warrants anticoagulation therapy.[224]

Cardiovascular Morbidity

SLE patients have a 2.3 to 7.5 increased risk for developing coronary heart disease compared with age-matched controls, after adjusting for traditional CVD risk factors.[225] In lupus, traditional CVD risk factors are reinforced by disease-related risk factors such as circulating prothrombotic aPL antibodies, antibodies against high-density lipoprotein cholesterol (HDL-C) interfering with its function, a typical lupus-pattern of dyslipidemia (low HDL-C, high triglycerides, normal or slightly elevated low-density lipoprotein cholesterol (LDL-C), and abnormal serum homocysteine levels), and the proatherogenic effect of systemic inflammation.[226]

Tight control of CVD risk factors is recommended for SLE patients, according to risk stratification and the presence of comorbidities. Hypertension requires diligent monitoring and treatment because it has been associated with worse outcomes in LN. For patients with nephritis and proteinuria greater than 1 g/day, target blood pressure should be less than 110/70 mm Hg. For most cases, ACE inhibitors or angiotensin receptor blockers (ARBs), or both, are the initial treatments of choice. For dyslipidemia, Wajed and colleagues[227] advocated for the institution of dietary or lipid-lowering therapy toward a target LDL-C less than 101 mg/dL in all SLE patients without stratifying for presence of other risk factors. Similarly, many clinicians follow the National Cholesterol Education Program Adult Treatment Panel III guidelines for the use of statins in primary CVD prevention, considering SLE as a coronary heart disease risk factor equivalent to diabetes. However, this approach is not universally accepted because it may lead to overtreatment of LDL-C levels.[228] Nonetheless, aggressive

treatment of dyslipidemia (target LDL-C <100 mg/dL and triglycerides <150 mg/dL) is recommended for patients with multiple risk factors, especially those with moderate or severe lupus. Although CVD is the leading cause of death among women and it carries a higher mortality than men (44% vs. 27%), a large survey revealed that only 13% of the women recognized the magnitude of the problem.[229] This, coupled with the greater challenge the diagnosis of coronary disease poses in women compared with men owing to its often atypical presentation, emphasizes the importance of sensitization of lupus women regarding their increased probability to develop CVD.[230]

Osteoporosis

Ongoing disease activity, premature menopause caused by use of immunosuppressive drugs, relative vitamin D deficiency due to avoidance of sun exposure, and the use of systematic GCs all contribute to reduced bone mineral density (BMD) in SLE patients.[231] Vertebral compression fractures are common, especially as the age of patients increases.[232] Quality indicators regarding osteoporosis prevention and therapy suggest that (1) all SLE patients receiving prednisone greater than or equal to 7.5 mg/day for 3 or more months should undergo BMD testing unless already on antiresorptive or anabolic therapy and receive osteoporosis prophylaxis with calcium and vitamin D supplements and (2) patients receiving prednisone greater than or equal to 7.5 mg/day for 1 or more months and having a central T score of −2.5 or less or a history of fragility fracture should be treated with an antiresorptive or anabolic agent unless contraindications exist.[233] This daily prednisone dosage is higher than the guidelineproposed by the ACR for prevention of steroid-induced osteoporosis (5 mg/day) in the general patient population. The authors recommend osteoporosis prophylaxis with daily prednisone doses of greater than or equal to 5 mg for postmenopausal women and greater than or equal to 7.5 mg for premenopausal women.

Malignancy in Lupus

Hematologic malignancies (particularly non-Hodgkin's lymphoma [NHL]) and cervical and lung cancer occur more commonly in SLE compared with the general population, followed by rare forms of malignancy affecting the hepatobiliary tract and the vulva/vagina. Immunosuppressive therapy (with the potential for mutagenesis and the impairment of antitumor immune surveillance) and intrinsic SLE-related mechanisms (chronic antigenic stimulation, impaired surveillance) may account for this risk.

NHL is associated with SLE (standardized incidence ratio [SIR], 3.6),[234,235] with the most commonly identified histologic subtype being diffuse large B cell lymphoma, which usually runs an aggressive course. Hodgkin's lymphoma (HL) is also more frequent in SLE (SIR, 3.2).[236] The risk for hematologic malignancies may increase after exposure to immunosuppressive medications, particularly after a period of 5 years following cessation of therapy. Because SLE and lymphomas share clinical manifestations (fever, lymphadenopathy, splenomegaly, cytopenias, and monoclonal expansion of B cells), a high index of suspicion is necessary for early detection of the latter. In such cases, an aggressive investigation is warranted with appropriate imaging studies and potentially lymph node biopsy.

Cervical dysplasia is increased in women with lupus[237,238] as a result of impaired clearance of human papillomavirus (HPV) due to exposure to immunosuppressive agents, particularly CYC (increase by 1 g of IV-CYC exposure corresponding to 13% increased risk of cervical intraepithelial neoplasia [CIN]). Therefore SLE should be regarded as a risk factor for cervical malignancy and high-risk HPV infection. The authors would recommend cervical cytology for cancer screening once (EULAR) or twice (U.S. Preventive Services Task Force) in the first year and then annually, adding HPV testing to the first-year-obtained cervical smears and then modifying subsequent screening on the basis of these results (cervical cytology screening every 6 months for women with detectable HPV DNA and annually for others). Although the efficacy of HPV vaccine has not been investigated in patients with autoimmune diseases, EULAR guidelines concluded that HPV vaccination should be considered for women with SLE until the age of 25 years, similar to the general population.[210]

SLE patients have a moderately increased risk for lung cancer (SIR, 1.4), mostly adenocarcinomas,[235] yet this risk is higher in SLE patients who smoke.[239] While waiting for the final verdict on the use of chest computed tomography as a screening test in the smoking population, smoking and nonsmoking patients should be evaluated similarly to the general population. With regard to breast cancer, there is no evidence for increased risk in SLE and thus no particular recommendation should be applied beyond screening guidelines used in the general population.

Emergencies in Patients with Lupus

SLE patients may visit the emergency department (ED) for complications related to lupus itself, lupus treatment, or unrelated reasons. Critical questions confronting the clinician are (1) whether the event is related to lupus and (2) whether in the presence of lupus the management should differ. In general, lupus-related emergencies frequently occur when disease is active. For example, approximately 60% of primary NPSLE events occur in the presence of generalized lupus activity. Common symptoms bringing lupus patients to the ED are fever, shortness of breath, and chest pain. Poor compliance, low education level, severity of the underlying disease, and higher damage scores are risk factors for hospitalization.

SLE patients might also develop life-threatening organ dysfunction, related to disease activity or immunosuppressive therapy, severe enough to require admission to the intensive care unit (ICU). Infections are the leading cause of admission (45% to 61%). Hsu and colleagues[240] studied 51 SLE patients admitted to the ICU and identified intracranial hemorrhage, gastrointestinal hemorrhage, and septic shock as poor outcome predictors. High APACHE II scores and use of vasopressors have been associated with patient mortality.[241] Overall mortality in SLE patients admitted to the ICU is high, although it has declined during the past decade (from 47% to 24%).[241,242] An aggressive search for infection together with recommended empiric antimicrobial therapy is crucial. When it is not clear whether the underlying process is related to infection or active disease,

empiric antimicrobial therapy together with high-dose GC (0.5 to 1 mg/kg/day) may suffice. Once infection has been ruled out, pulse steroids or CYC, or both, may be used. Agents such as IVIG, plasmapheresis, and RTX may be considered as adjuvant therapy in life-threatening disease or in cases of deterioration or inadequate response following 1 to 2 weeks of therapy.

WOMEN'S HEALTH ISSUES

> **KEY POINTS**
>
> Synthetic gonadotropin releasing hormone analogues significantly decreased rates of gonadal failure in young women with severe SLE treated with CYC.
>
> Contraceptive methods including hormone agents are generally safe for most SLE patients.

Premature ovarian failure is an age- and dose-dependent adverse effect of CYC therapy, whereas male gonadal toxicity may be observed with as little as 7 g cumulative CYC dose. Strategies to preserve fertility in postpubertal SLE women include hormonal contraceptives, gonadotropin releasing hormone (GnRH) antagonists, and embryo and oocyte cryopreservation. Ovarian tissue banking for future tissue transplantation has been suggested for prepubertal girls. Individual patient preferences should be considered when deciding about fertility preservation. Some authors have suggested that coadministration of GnRH antagonists confers protection against premature ovarian failure and therefore recommend a GnRH antagonist–based protocol in CYC-treated female patients. In men receiving CYC for malignancies, frequency of azoospermia ranges from 30% to 90%. Administration of testosterone and sperm banking represent valid strategies for preservation of testicular function and fertility (see Table 81-4).[243]

Contraceptive methods are generally safe for most SLE patients. Previous research had suggested that hormonal agents might increase the risk of disease flares. However, two RCTs found no increase in flares in those without severe disease activity at study entry, and a systematic review concluded that benefits of use outweigh potential risks for most contraceptive methods.[244] However, women with positive aPL antibodies should avoid combined hormonal methods because of an increased risk for thrombosis. Coexisting conditions such as severe thrombocytopenia, atherosclerosis, hypertension, and venous thrombosis could also make certain contraceptives less advisable.

Women with SLE may experience lower urinary tract symptoms, often accompanied by voiding dysfunction (small bladder capacity, low urinary flow rate).[245] Urinary bladder involvement is thought to contribute to recurrent urinary tract infections in some SLE patients.[246] The approach to investigation and management of recurrent urinary tract infections is similar to that in the general population; control of disease activity may prevent bladder dysfunction. Lupus mastitis represents a rare form of lupus panniculitis occurring in 2% of women with SLE and may clinically mimic breast carcinoma.[247] GC treatment is generally effective, but refractory forms may necessitate surgical excision.

EVIDENCE AND EXPERT-BASED RECOMMENDATIONS IN SYSTEMIC LUPUS ERYTHEMATOSUS

Due to the systemic nature of SLE, multiple medical subspecialties are involved in the care of these patients, dictating an integrated approach to their care. To this end, EULAR has developed recommendations covering the most important aspects in the diagnosis, management, and monitoring.[125,133,210,248] These recommendations—developed not only for the specialists but for all internists and primary care physicians—are based on a combined research-based evidence approach and expert opinion consensus.

Future Directions

This past decade has witnessed major advances in defining risk factors and phenotypes, elucidating pathogenesis, and optimizing treatment. Recognition of adjuvant-like factors that promote the production of type I interferon via Toll-like receptors offers new targets for therapy in addition to those targeting B and T cells. Exploration of the genetic and environmental factors that determine susceptibility to disease may eventually lead to the identification of individuals at risk and elucidate the primary events that cause autoimmunity. In contrast to monogenic diseases, the expansion of personalized medicine in lupus awaits a more complete description of predisposition. Genome-wide, next-generation sequencing efforts now under way will provide within the next few years a more comprehensive description of the relations between genome sequence variation and clinical phenotypes.

Meanwhile, new drugs have been added to the armamentarium against the disease and new therapeutic strategies are aimed at inducing prompt remission with more intense therapy and prevention of flares with less toxic therapies. The introduction of MMF has added a useful new drug while providing additional valuable insights in trial design in lupus. Despite past efforts devoted to arguing on the choice of specific agents, there is finally a consensus that what is more important is a strategy aiming at remission and its maintenance with the treatment that best fits the patient. With the approval of the first biologic agent in March 2011, the disease is finally showing signs of yielding to more targeted therapy and unraveling its heterogeneity and complexity. Most importantly, it has become clearer than ever that optimal long-term outcome requires not only treatment of the disease flares but also management of its comorbidities. To this end, lupus highlights the need for a multidisciplinary approach and superb internal medicine skills.

Selected References

2. Nikpour M, Urowitz MB, Ibanez D, Gladman DD: Frequency and determinants of flare and persistently active disease in systemic lupus erythematosus, *Arthritis Rheum* 61:1152–1158, 2009.
4. Doria A, Iaccarino L, Ghirardello A, et al: Long-term prognosis and causes of death in systemic lupus erythematosus, *Am J Med* 119:700–706, 2006.
5. Ippolito A, Petri M: An update on mortality in systemic lupus erythematosus, *Clin Exp Rheumatol* 26:S72–S79, 2008.
6. Chambers SA, Allen E, Rahman A, Isenberg D: Damage and mortality in a group of British patients with systemic lupus erythematosus followed up for over 10 years, *Rheumatology (Oxford)* 48:673–675, 2009.
7. Bertsias GK, Salmon JE, Boumpas DT: Therapeutic opportunities in systemic lupus erythematosus: state of the art and prospects for the new decade, *Ann Rheum Dis* 69:1603–1611, 2010.
8. Bertsias G, Boumpas DT: Update on the management of lupus nephritis: let the treatment fit the patient, *Nat Clin Pract Rheumatol* 4:464–472, 2008.
10. Kiani AN, Petri M: Quality-of-life measurements versus disease activity in systemic lupus erythematosus, *Curr Rheumatol Rep* 12:250–258, 2010.
12. Fraenkel L, Bogardus S, Concato J: Patient preferences for treatment of lupus nephritis, *Arthritis Rheum* 47:421–428, 2002.
13. Bootsma H, Spronk P, Derksen R, et al: Prevention of relapses in systemic lupus erythematosus, *Lancet* 345:1595–1599, 1995.
14. Denburg SD, Carbotte RM, Denburg JA: Corticosteroids and neuropsychological functioning in patients with systemic lupus erythematosus, *Arthritis Rheum* 37:1311–1320, 1994.
15. Tseng CE, Buyon JP, Kim M, et al: The effect of moderate-dose corticosteroids in preventing severe flares in patients with serologically active, but clinically stable, systemic lupus erythematosus: findings of a prospective, randomized, double-blind, placebo-controlled trial, *Arthritis Rheum* 54:3623–3632, 2006.
18. Gourley MF, Austin HA 3rd, Scott D, et al: Methylprednisolone and cyclophosphamide, alone or in combination, in patients with lupus nephritis. A randomized, controlled trial, *Ann Intern Med* 125:549–557, 1996.
19. Illei GG, Austin HA, Crane M, et al: Combination therapy with pulse cyclophosphamide plus pulse methylprednisolone improves long-term renal outcome without adding toxicity in patients with lupus nephritis, *Ann Intern Med* 135:248–257, 2001.
20. Ruiz-Irastorza G, Ramos-Casals M, Brito-Zeron P, Khamashta MA: Clinical efficacy and side effects of antimalarials in systemic lupus erythematosus: a systematic review, *Ann Rheum Dis* 69:20–28, 2010.
22. Marmor MF, Carr RE, Easterbrook M, et al: Recommendations on screening for chloroquine and hydroxychloroquine retinopathy: a report by the American Academy of Ophthalmology, *Ophthalmology* 109:1377–1382, 2002.
23. Carneiro JR, Sato EI: Double blind, randomized, placebo controlled clinical trial of methotrexate in systemic lupus erythematosus, *J Rheumatol* 26:1275–1279, 1999.
24. Fortin PR, Abrahamowicz M, Ferland D, et al: Steroid-sparing effects of methotrexate in systemic lupus erythematosus: a double-blind, randomized, placebo-controlled trial, *Arthritis Rheum* 59:1796–1804, 2008.
27. Grootscholten C, Ligtenberg G, Hagen EC, et al: Azathioprine/methylprednisolone versus cyclophosphamide in proliferative lupus nephritis. A randomized controlled trial, *Kidney Int* 70:732–742, 2006.
28. Contreras G, Pardo V, Leclercq B, et al: Sequential therapies for proliferative lupus nephritis, *N Engl J Med* 350:971–980, 2004.
29. Moroni G, Doria A, Mosca M, et al: A randomized pilot trial comparing cyclosporine and azathioprine for mainentance therapy in diffuse lupus nephritis over four years, *Clin J Am Soc Nephrol* 1:925–932, 2006.
30. Houssiau FA, D'Cruz D, Sangle S, et al: Azathioprine versus mycophenolate mofetil for long-term immunosuppression in lupus nephritis: results from the MAINTAIN Nephritis Trial, *Ann Rheum Dis* 69:2083–2089, 2010.
31. Wofsy D, Appel GB, Dooley MA, et al: Aspreva Lupus Management Study maintenance results, *Lupus* 19:S27, 2010.
32. Boumpas DT, Bertsias GK, Balow JE: A decade of mycophenolate mofetil for lupus nephritis: is the glass half-empty or half-full? *Ann Rheum Dis* 69:2059–2061, 2010.
33. Austin HA 3rd, Klippel JH, Balow JE, et al: Therapy of lupus nephritis. Controlled trial of prednisone and cytotoxic drugs, *N Engl J Med* 314:614–619, 1986.
34. Boumpas DT, Austin HA 3rd, Vaughn EM, et al: Controlled trial of pulse methylprednisolone versus two regimens of pulse cyclophosphamide in severe lupus nephritis, *Lancet* 340:741–745, 1992.

35. Houssiau FA, Vasconcelos C, D'Cruz D, et al: Immunosuppressive therapy in lupus nephritis: the Euro-Lupus Nephritis Trial, a randomized trial of low-dose versus high-dose intravenous cyclophosphamide, *Arthritis Rheum* 46:2121–2131, 2002.

36. Houssiau FA, Vasconcelos C, D'Cruz D, et al: The 10-year follow-up data of the Euro-Lupus Nephritis Trial comparing low-dose and high-dose intravenous cyclophosphamide, *Ann Rheum Dis* 69:61–64, 2010.

37. Austin HA 3rd, Illei GG, Braun MJ, Balow JE: Randomized, controlled trial of prednisone, cyclophosphamide, and cyclosporine in lupus membranous nephropathy, *J Am Soc Nephrol* 20:901–911, 2009.

40. Barile-Fabris L, Ariza-Andraca R, Olguin-Ortega L, et al: Controlled clinical trial of IV cyclophosphamide versus IV methylprednisolone in severe neurological manifestations in systemic lupus erythematosus, *Ann Rheum Dis* 64:620–625, 2005.

42. Chan TM, Li FK, Tang CS, et al: Efficacy of mycophenolate mofetil in patients with diffuse proliferative lupus nephritis. Hong Kong-Guangzhou Nephrology Study Group, *N Engl J Med* 343:1156–1162, 2000.

43. Chan TM, Tse KC, Tang CS, et al: Long-term study of mycophenolate mofetil as continuous induction and maintenance treatment for diffuse proliferative lupus nephritis, *J Am Soc Nephrol* 16:1076–1084, 2005.

44. Ginzler EM, Dooley MA, Aranow C, et al: Mycophenolate mofetil or intravenous cyclophosphamide for lupus nephritis, *N Engl J Med* 353:2219–2228, 2005.

45. Appel GB, Contreras G, Dooley MA, et al: Mycophenolate mofetil versus cyclophosphamide for induction treatment of lupus nephritis, *J Am Soc Nephrol* 20:1103–1112, 2009.

46. Kamanamool N, McEvoy M, Attia J, Ingsathit A, et al: Efficacy and adverse events of mycophenolate mofetil versus cyclophosphamide for induction therapy of lupus nephritis: systematic review and meta-analysis, *Medicine (Baltimore)* 89:227–235, 2010.

50. Radhakrishnan J, Moutzouris DA, Ginzler EM, et al: Mycophenolate mofetil and intravenous cyclophosphamide are similar as induction therapy for class V lupus nephritis, *Kidney Int* 77:152–160, 2010.

51. Dussol B, Morange S, Burtey S, et al: Mycophenolate mofetil monotherapy in membranous nephropathy: a 1-year randomized controlled trial, *Am J Kidney Dis* 52:699–705, 2008.

52. Hiemstra TF, Walsh M, Mahr A, et al: Mycophenolate mofetil vs azathioprine for remission maintenance in antineutrophil cytoplasmic antibody-associated vasculitis: a randomized controlled trial, *JAMA* 304:2381–2388, 2010.

54. Ginzler EM, Wofsy D, Isenberg D, et al: Nonrenal disease activity following mycophenolate mofetil or intravenous cyclophosphamide as induction treatment for lupus nephritis: findings in a multicenter, prospective, randomized, open-label, parallel-group clinical trial, *Arthritis Rheum* 62:211–221, 2010.

55. Posalski JD, Ishimori M, Wallace DJ, Weisman MH: Does mycophenolate mofetil prevent extra-renal flares in systemic lupus erythematosus? Results from an observational study of patients in a single practice treated for up to 5 years, *Lupus* 18:516–521, 2009.

56. Moroni G, Maccario M, Banfi G, et al: Treatment of membranous lupus nephritis, *Am J Kidney Dis* 31:681–686, 1998.

57. Illei GG, Yarboro CH, Kuroiwa T, et al: Long-term effects of combination treatment with fludarabine and low-dose pulse cyclophosphamide in patients with lupus nephritis, *Rheumatology (Oxford)* 46:952–956, 2007.

58. Rihova Z, Vankova Z, Maixnerova D, et al: Treatment of lupus nephritis with cyclosporine—an outcome analysis, *Kidney Blood Press Res* 30:124–128, 2007.

59. Zavada J, Pesickova S, Rysava R, et al: Cyclosporine A or intravenous cyclophosphamide for lupus nephritis: the Cyclofa-Lune study, *Lupus* 19:1281–1289, 2010.

62. Griffiths B, Emery P, Ryan V, et al: The BILAG multi-centre open randomized controlled trial comparing cyclosporine vs azathioprine in patients with severe SLE, *Rheumatology (Oxford)* 49:723–732, 2010.

67. Miyasaka N, Kawai S, Hashimoto H: Efficacy and safety of tacrolimus for lupus nephritis: a placebo-controlled double-blind multicenter study, *Mod Rheumatol* 19:606–615, 2009.

68. Cortés-Hernandez J, Torres-Salido MT, Medrano AS, et al: Long-term outcomes—mycophenolate mofetil treatment for lupus nephritis with addition of tacrolimus for resistant cases, *Nephrol Dial Transplant* 25:3939–3943, 2010.

69. Bao H, Liu ZH, Xie HL, et al: Successful treatment of class V+IV lupus nephritis with multitarget therapy, *J Am Soc Nephrol* 19:2001–2010, 2008.

71. Murray E, Perry M: Off-label use of rituximab in systemic lupus erythematosus: a systematic review, *Clin Rheumatol* 29:707–716, 2010.

72. Ramos-Casals M, Garcia-Hernandez FJ, de Ramon E, et al: Off-label use of rituximab in 196 patients with severe, refractory systemic autoimmune diseases, *Clin Exp Rheumatol* 28:468–476, 2010.

73. Tokunaga M, Saito K, Kawabata D, et al: Efficacy of rituximab (anti-CD20) for refractory systemic lupus erythematosus involving the central nervous system, *Ann Rheum Dis* 66:470–475, 2007.

74. Terrier B, Amoura Z, Ravaud P, et al: Safety and efficacy of rituximab in systemic lupus erythematosus: results from 136 patients from the French AutoImmunity and Rituximab registry, *Arthritis Rheum* 62:2458–2466, 2010.

76. Jonsdottir T, Gunnarsson I, Mourao AF, et al: Clinical improvements in proliferative vs membranous lupus nephritis following B-cell depletion: pooled data from two cohorts, *Rheumatology (Oxford)* 49:1502–1504, 2010.

77. Merrill JT, Neuwelt CM, Wallace DJ, et al: Efficacy and safety of rituximab in moderately-to-severely active systemic lupus erythematosus: the randomized, double-blind, phase II/III systemic lupus erythematosus evaluation of rituximab trial, *Arthritis Rheum* 62:222–233, 2010.

78. Rovin BH, Furie R, Latinis K, et al: Efficacy and safety of rituximab in patients with active proliferative lupus nephritis: The Lupus Nephritis Assessment with Rituximab study, *Arthritis Rheum* 64:1215–1226, 2012.

86. Furie RA, Petri MA, Wallace DJ, et al: Novel evidence-based systemic lupus erythematosus responder index, *Arthritis Rheum* 61:1143–1151, 2009.

92. Boumpas DT, Furie R, Manzi S, et al: A short course of BG9588 (anti-CD40 ligand antibody) improves serologic activity and decreases hematuria in patients with proliferative lupus glomerulonephritis, *Arthritis Rheum* 48:719–727, 2003.

94. Merrill JT, Burgos-Vargas R, Westhovens R, et al: The efficacy and safety of abatacept in patients with non-life-threatening manifestations of systemic lupus erythematosus: results of a twelve-month, multicenter, exploratory, phase IIb, randomized, double-blind, placebo-controlled trial, *Arthritis Rheum* 62:3077–3087, 2010.

96. Aringer M, Houssiau F, Gordon C, et al: Adverse events and efficacy of TNF-alpha blockade with infliximab in patients with systemic lupus erythematosus: long-term follow-up of 13 patients, *Rheumatology (Oxford)* 48:1451–1454, 2009.

99. Yao Y, Richman L, Higgs BW, et al: Neutralization of interferon-alpha/beta-inducible genes and downstream effect in a phase I trial of an anti-interferon-alpha monoclonal antibody in systemic lupus erythematosus, *Arthritis Rheum* 60:1785–1796, 2009.

101. Illei GG, Shirota Y, Yarboro CH, et al: Tocilizumab in systemic lupus erythematosus: data on safety, preliminary efficacy, and impact on circulating plasma cells from an open-label phase I dosage-escalation study, *Arthritis Rheum* 62:542–552, 2010.

103. Zandman-Goddard G, Blank M, Shoenfeld Y: Intravenous immunoglobulins in systemic lupus erythematosus: from the bench to the bedside, *Lupus* 18:884–888, 2009.

109. Cardiel MH, Tumlin JA, Furie RA, et al: Abetimus sodium for renal flare in systemic lupus erythematosus: results of a randomized, controlled phase III trial, *Arthritis Rheum* 58:2470–2480, 2008.

111. Muller S, Monneaux F, Schall N, et al: Spliceosomal peptide P140 for immunotherapy of systemic lupus erythematosus: results of an early phase II clinical trial, *Arthritis Rheum* 58:3873–3883, 2008.

112. Crosbie D, Black C, McIntyre L, et al: Dehydroepiandrosterone for systemic lupus erythematosus, *Cochrane Database Syst Rev* (4):CD005114, 2007.

117. Kuhn A, Ruland V, Bonsmann G: Cutaneous lupus erythematosus: update of therapeutic options Part II, *J Am Acad Dermatol* 65:e195–213, 2011.

118. Kuhn A, Ruland V, Bonsmann G: Cutaneous lupus erythematosus: update of therapeutic options: Part I, *J Am Acad Dermatol* 65:e179–193, 2010.

120. Weening JJ, D'Agati VD, Schwartz MM, et al: The classification of glomerulonephritis in systemic lupus erythematosus revisited, *J Am Soc Nephrol* 15:241–250, 2004.

123. Chen YE, Korbet SM, Katz RS, et al: Value of a complete or partial remission in severe lupus nephritis, *Clin J Am Soc Nephrol* 3:46–53, 2008.

124. Houssiau FA, Vasconcelos C, D'Cruz D, et al: Early response to immunosuppressive therapy predicts good renal outcome in lupus nephritis: lessons from long-term followup of patients in the Euro-Lupus Nephritis Trial, *Arthritis Rheum* 50:3934–3940, 2004.

125. Bertsias G, Ioannidis JP, Boletis J, et al: EULAR recommendations for the management of systemic lupus erythematosus. Report of a Task Force of the EULAR Standing Committee for International Clinical Studies Including Therapeutics, *Ann Rheum Dis* 67:195–205, 2008.

128. Mok CC, Ying KY, Yim CW, et al: Very long-term outcome of pure lupus membranous nephropathy treated with glucocorticoid and azathioprine, *Lupus* 18:1091–1095, 2009.

129. Illei GG, Takada K, Parkin D, et al: Renal flares are common in patients with severe proliferative lupus nephritis treated with pulse immunosuppressive therapy: long-term followup of a cohort of 145 patients participating in randomized controlled studies, *Arthritis Rheum* 46:995–1002, 2002.

130. Mok CC, Ying KY, Ng WL, et al: Long-term outcome of diffuse proliferative lupus glomerulonephritis treated with cyclophosphamide, *Am J Med* 119:355 e25-33, 2006.

131. Mok CC, Ying KY, Tang S, et al: Predictors and outcome of renal flares after successful cyclophosphamide treatment for diffuse proliferative lupus glomerulonephritis, *Arthritis Rheum* 50:2559–2568, 2004.

133. Bertsias GK, Ioannidis JP, Aringer M, et al: EULAR recommendations for the management of systemic lupus erythematosus with neuropsychiatric manifestations: report of a task force of the EULAR standing committee for clinical affairs, *Ann Rheum Dis* 69:2074–2082, 2010.

134. Hepburn AL, Narat S, Mason JC: The management of peripheral blood cytopenias in systemic lupus erythematosus, *Rheumatology (Oxford)* 49:2243–2254, 2010.

139. Ruiz-Irastorza G, Crowther M, Branch W, Khamashta MA: Antiphospholipid syndrome, *Lancet* 376:1498–1509, 2010.

140. Cohen D, Berger SP, Steup-Beekman GM, et al: Diagnosis and management of the antiphospholipid syndrome, *BMJ* 340:c2541, 2010.

142. Ruiz-Irastorza G, Hunt BJ, Khamashta MA: A systematic review of secondary thromboprophylaxis in patients with antiphospholipid antibodies, *Arthritis Rheum* 57:1487–1495, 2007.

145. Tektonidou MG, Laskari K, Panagiotakos DB, Moutsopoulos HM: Risk factors for thrombosis and primary thrombosis prevention in patients with systemic lupus erythematosus with or without antiphospholipid antibodies, *Arthritis Rheum* 61:29–36, 2009.

147. Ridker PM, Danielson E, Fonseca FA, et al: Reduction in C-reactive protein and LDL cholesterol and cardiovascular event rates after initiation of rosuvastatin: a prospective study of the JUPITER trial, *Lancet* 373:1175–1182, 2009.

150. Tincani A, Bazzani C, Zingarelli S, Lojacono A: Lupus and the antiphospholipid syndrome in pregnancy and obstetrics: clinical characteristics, diagnosis, pathogenesis, and treatment, *Semin Thromb Hemost* 34:267–273, 2008.

151. Smyth A, Oliveira GH, Lahr BD, et al: A systematic review and meta-analysis of pregnancy outcomes in patients with systemic lupus erythematosus and lupus nephritis, *Clin J Am Soc Nephrol* 5:2060–2068, 2010.

152. Ziakas PD, Pavlou M, Voulgarelis M: Heparin treatment in antiphospholipid syndrome with recurrent pregnancy loss: a systematic review and meta-analysis, *Obstet Gynecol* 115:1256–1262, 2010.

154. Erkan D, Harrison MJ, Levy R, et al: Aspirin for primary thrombosis prevention in the antiphospholipid syndrome. A randomized, double-blind, placebo-controlled trial in asymptomatic antiphospholipid antibody–positive individuals, *Arthritis Rheum* 56:2382–2391, 2007.

155. Kaandorp SP, Goddijn M, van der Post JA, et al: Aspirin plus heparin or aspirin alone in women with recurrent miscarriage, *N Engl J Med* 362:1586–1596, 2010.

160. Cervera R, Bucciarelli S, Plasin MA, et al: Catastrophic antiphospholipid syndrome (CAPS): descriptive analysis of a series of 280 patients from the "CAPS Registry," *J Autoimmun* 32:240–245, 2009.

161. Gunnarsson I, Sundelin B, Jonsdottir T, et al: Histopathologic and clinical outcome of rituximab treatment in patients with cyclophosphamide-resistant proliferative lupus nephritis, *Arthritis Rheum* 56:1263–1272, 2007.

162. Jonsdottir T, Gunnarsson I, Risselada A, et al: Treatment of refractory SLE with rituximab plus cyclophosphamide: clinical effects, serological changes, and predictors of response, *Ann Rheum Dis* 67:330–334, 2008.

165. Moroni G, Doria A, Ponticelli C: Cyclosporine (CsA) in lupus nephritis: assessing the evidence, *Nephrol Dial Transplant* 24:15–20, 2009.

167. Traynor AE, Schroeder J, Rosa RM, et al: Treatment of severe systemic lupus erythematosus with high-dose chemotherapy and haemopoietic stem-cell transplantation: a phase I study, *Lancet* 356:701–707, 2000.

169. Liang J, Zhang H, Hua B, et al: Allogenic mesenchymal stem cells transplantation in refractory systemic lupus erythematosus: a pilot clinical study, *Ann Rheum Dis* 69:1423–1429, 2010.

171. Friedman DM, Kim MY, Copel JA, et al: Prospective evaluation of fetuses with autoimmune-associated congenital heart block followed in the PR Interval and Dexamethasone Evaluation (PRIDE) Study, *Am J Cardiol* 103:1102–1106, 2009.

172. Pisoni CN, Brucato A, Ruffatti A, et al: Failure of intravenous immunoglobulin to prevent congenital heart block: findings of a multicenter, prospective, observational study, *Arthritis Rheum* 62:1147–1152, 2010.

173. Friedman DM, Llanos C, Izmirly PM, et al: Evaluation of fetuses in a study of intravenous immunoglobulin as preventive therapy for congenital heart block: results of a multicenter, prospective, open-label clinical trial, *Arthritis Rheum* 62:1138–1146, 2010.

175. Lehman TJ, Edelheit BS, Onel KB: Combined intravenous methotrexate and cyclophosphamide for refractory childhood lupus nephritis, *Ann Rheum Dis* 63:321–323, 2004.

176. Askenazi D, Myones B, Kamdar A, et al: Outcomes of children with proliferative lupus nephritis: the role of protocol renal biopsy, *Pediatr Nephrol* 22:981–986, 2007.

180. Benseler SM, Bargman JM, Feldman BM, et al: Acute renal failure in paediatric systemic lupus erythematosus: treatment and outcome, *Rheumatology (Oxford)* 48:176–182, 2009.

181. Baskin E, Ozen S, Cakar N, et al: The use of low-dose cyclophosphamide followed by AZA/MMF treatment in childhood lupus nephritis, *Pediatr Nephrol* 25:111–117, 2010.

184. Navarra SV, Leynes MS: Infections in systemic lupus erythematosus, *Lupus* 19:1419–1424, 2010.

188. Ruiz-Irastorza G, Olivares N, Ruiz-Arruza I, et al: Predictors of major infections in systemic lupus erythematosus, *Arthritis Res Ther* 11:R109, 2009.

191. Bosch X, Guilabert A, Pallares L, et al: Infections in systemic lupus erythematosus: a prospective and controlled study of 110 patients, *Lupus* 15:584–589, 2006.

201. Mok MY, Wong SS, Chan TM, et al: Non-tuberculous mycobacterial infection in patients with systemic lupus erythematosus, *Rheumatology (Oxford)* 46:280–284, 2007.

203. Ramos-Casals M, Cuadrado MJ, Alba P, et al: Acute viral infections in patients with systemic lupus erythematosus: description of 23 cases and review of the literature, *Medicine (Baltimore)* 87:311–318, 2008.

206. Abu-Shakra M: Safety of vaccination of patients with systemic lupus erythematosus, *Lupus* 18:1205–1208, 2009.

210. van Assen S, Agmon-Levin N, Elkayam O, et al: EULAR recommendations for vaccination in adult patients with autoimmune inflammatory rheumatic diseases, *Ann Rheum Dis* 70:414–422, 2010.

211. Kuruma KA, Borba EF, Lopes MH, et al: Safety and efficacy of hepatitis B vaccine in systemic lupus erythematosus, *Lupus* 16:350–354, 2007.

212. Chrysochou C, Randhawa H, Reeve R, et al: Determinants of renal functional outcome in lupus nephritis: a single centre retrospective study, *QJM* 101:313–316, 2008.

216. Rietveld A, Berden JH: Renal replacement therapy in lupus nephritis, *Nephrol Dial Transplant* 23:3056–3060, 2008.

220. Chelamcharla M, Javaid B, Baird BC, Goldfarb-Rumyantzev AS: The outcome of renal transplantation among systemic lupus erythematosus patients, *Nephrol Dial Transplant* 22:3623–3630, 2007.

222. Contreras G, Mattiazzi A, Guerra G, et al: Recurrence of lupus nephritis after kidney transplantation, *J Am Soc Nephrol* 21:1200–1207, 2010.

227. Wajed J, Ahmad Y, Durrington PN, Bruce IN: Prevention of cardiovascular disease in systemic lupus erythematosus–proposed guidelines for risk factor management, *Rheumatology (Oxford)* 43:7–12, 2004.

233. Yazdany J, Panopalis P, Gillis JZ, et al: A quality indicator set for systemic lupus erythematosus, *Arthritis Rheum* 61:370–377, 2009.

234. Bernatsky S, Ramsey-Goldman R, Rajan R, et al: Non-Hodgkin's lymphoma in systemic lupus erythematosus, *Ann Rheum Dis* 64:1507–1509, 2005.

235. Bernatsky S, Boivin JF, Joseph L, et al: An international cohort study of cancer in systemic lupus erythematosus, *Arthritis Rheum* 52:1481–1490, 2005.

238. Tam LS, Chan AY, Chan PK, et al: Increased prevalence of squamous intraepithelial lesions in systemic lupus erythematosus: association with human papillomavirus infection, *Arthritis Rheum* 50:3619–3625, 2004.

242. Ansell SM, Bedhesi S, Ruff B, et al: Study of critically ill patients with systemic lupus erythematosus, *Crit Care Med* 24:981–984, 1996.

243. Silva CA, Bonfa E, Ostensen M: Maintenance of fertility in patients with rheumatic diseases needing antiinflammatory and immunosuppressive drugs, *Arthritis Care Res (Hoboken)* 62:1682–1690, 2010.

244. Culwell KR, Curtis KM, del Carmen Cravioto M: Safety of contraceptive method use among women with systemic lupus erythematosus: a systematic review, *Obstet Gynecol* 114:341–353, 2009.

248. Mosca M, Tani C, Aringer M, et al: European League Against Rheumatism recommendations for monitoring patients with systemic lupus erythematosus in clinical practice and in observational studies, *Ann Rheum Dis* 69:1269–1274, 2010.

Full references for this chapter can be found on www.expertconsult.com.

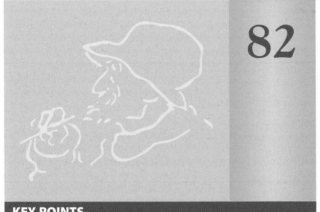

82 Antiphospholipid Syndrome

DORUK ERKAN • JANE E. SALMON • MICHAEL D. LOCKSHIN

KEY POINTS

Antiphospholipid antibodies (aPLs) are a family of autoantibodies directed against phospholipid-binding plasma proteins, most commonly β_2-glycoprotein I.

The clinical manifestations range from asymptomatic to catastrophic antiphospholipid syndrome (APS).

Stroke is the most common presentation of arterial thrombosis; deep vein thrombosis is the most common venous manifestation.

Pregnancy losses typically occur after 10 weeks' gestation (fetal loss), but earlier losses also occur.

Catastrophic APS is a rare form of APS that consists of multiple thromboses of medium and small arteries occurring over days.

Diagnosis should be made in the presence of characteristic clinical manifestations and persistently positive aPLs (measured at least 12 weeks apart).

Prevention of secondary thrombosis lacks a risk-stratified approach; the effectiveness of high-intensity anticoagulation in APS patients with vascular events is not supported by prospective controlled studies.

A common strategy to prevent fetal loss in aPL-positive patients with a history of pregnancy morbidities is low-dose aspirin and heparin.

Primary thrombosis prevention in persistently aPL-positive individuals requires a risk-stratified approach; elimination of reversible thrombosis risk factors and prophylaxis during high-risk periods are crucial. The effectiveness of aspirin in persistently aPL-positive patients without vascular events is not supported by prospective controlled studies.

Currently, no evidence indicates that anticoagulation is effective for nonthrombotic manifestations of aPLs, such as thrombocytopenia or heart valve disease.

Catastrophic APS patients usually receive a combination of anticoagulation, corticosteroids, intravenous immunoglobulin (IVIG), and plasma exchange.

Diagnosis of the antiphospholipid syndrome (APS) requires that a patient have both a clinical event (thrombosis or pregnancy morbidity) and the persistent presence of antiphospholipid antibody (aPL), documented by a solid phase serum assay (anticardiolipin or anti–β_2-glycoprotein I [anti-β_2GPI] immunoglobulin [Ig]G or IgM), a coagulation assay (inhibitor of phospholipid-dependent clotting—the lupus anticoagulant test), or both. Preliminary (Sapporo) classification criteria for APS,[1] revised in 2004,[2] are listed in Table 82-1.

Certain factors are not included as criteria but may be helpful in the diagnosis of individual patients. These include IgA anticardiolipin or anti-β_2GPI, valvular heart disease, thrombocytopenia, early preeclampsia, and livedo reticularis (Table 82-2). These factors are rare, nonstandardized, or nonspecific phenomena that are too unreliable for use in clinical studies, but they occur in a sufficient number of patients to support a suspected diagnosis.

APS can occur as an isolated diagnosis, or it can be associated with systemic lupus erythematosus (SLE) or another rheumatic disease. Transient aPL, but probably not the syndrome, can be induced by drugs and infection.[3]

EPIDEMIOLOGY

Low-titer, usually transient, anticardiolipin occurs in up to 10% of normal blood donors,[4,5] and moderate- to high-titer anticardiolipin or a positive lupus anticoagulant test occurs in less than 1%. The prevalence of positive aPL tests increases with age. Ten percent to 40% of SLE patients[5] and approximately 20% of rheumatoid arthritis patients[6] have positive aPL tests.

Based on a limited number of uncontrolled and non–risk-stratified studies, asymptomatic (no history of vascular or pregnancy events) aPL-positive patients have a 0% to 4% annual risk of thrombosis; patients with other autoimmune diseases such as SLE are at the higher end of the range.[7,8] The aPL profile (low vs. high risk for thrombosis) and patients' clinical characteristics (presence or absence of other acquired or genetic thrombosis risk factors) influence the individual risk of thrombosis.[9] Ten percent of first-stroke victims have aPLs,[10] especially those who are young (up to 29%),[5,11] as do up to 20% of women who have suffered three or more consecutive fetal losses.[12] Fourteen percent of patients with recurrent venous thromboembolic disease have aPLs.[13]

CAUSE

The main antigen to which aPLs bind is not a phospholipid but rather a phospholipid-binding plasma protein, namely, β_2GPI (apolipoprotein H). β_2GPI is normally present in serum at a concentration of 200 mg/mL, is a member of the complement control protein family, and has five repeating domains and several alleles. An octapeptide in the fifth domain and critical cysteine bonds are necessary for both phospholipid binding and antigenicity[14]; a first-domain site activates platelets.[15,16] In vivo, β_2GPI binds to phosphatidylserine on activated or apoptotic cell membranes, including those of trophoblasts, platelets, and endothelial cells. Under physiologic conditions, β_2GPI may function

Table 82-1 Revised Sapporo Classification Criteria for Antiphospholipid Syndrome

Clinical Criteria

1. Vascular thrombosis*
   One or more clinical episodes[†] of arterial, venous, or small vessel thrombosis[‡] in any tissue or organ
2. Pregnancy morbidity
   (a) One or more unexplained deaths of a morphologically normal fetus at or beyond the 10th wk of gestation, *or*
   (b) One or more premature births of a morphologically normal neonate before the 34th wk of gestation because of eclampsia, severe preeclampsia, or recognized features of placental insufficiency[§], *or*
   (c) Three or more unexplained consecutive spontaneous abortions before the 10th wk of gestation, with maternal anatomic or hormonal abnormalities and paternal and maternal chromosomal causes excluded

Laboratory Criteria

1. Lupus anticoagulant present in plasma on two or more occasions at least 12 wk apart, detected according to the guidelines of the International Society on Thrombosis and Hemostasis
2. Anticardiolipin antibody of immunoglobulin (Ig)G or IgM isotype in serum or plasma, present in medium or high titer (>40 GPL or MPL, or >99th percentile), on two or more occasions at least 12 wk apart, measured by a standardized ELISA
3. Anti–β_2-glycoprotein I antibody of IgG or IgM isotype in serum or plasma (in titer >99th percentile) present on two or more occasions at least 12 wk apart, measured by a standardized ELISA

Definite APS is present if at least one of the clinical criteria and one of the laboratory criteria are met. Classification of APS should be avoided if less than 12 wk or more than 5 yr separate the positive antiphospholipid antibody test and the clinical manifestation. In studies of populations of patients who have more than one type of pregnancy morbidity, investigators are strongly encouraged to stratify groups of subjects according to a, b, or c above.

*Coexisting inherited or acquired factors for thrombosis are not reasons to exclude patients from APS trials. However, two subgroups of APS patients should be recognized by the presence and absence of additional risk factors for thrombosis. Indicative (but not exhaustive) cases include age (>55 yr in men and >65 yr in women), the presence of any of the established risk factors for cardiovascular disease (hypertension, diabetes mellitus, elevated low-density lipoprotein or low high-density lipoprotein cholesterol, cigarette smoking, family history of premature cardiovascular disease, body mass index >30 kg/m², microalbuminuria, estimated glomerular filtration rate <60 mL/min), inherited thrombophilias, oral contraceptive use, nephritic syndrome, malignancy, immobilization, and surgery. Thus, patients who fulfill these criteria should be stratified according to contributing causes of thrombosis.
[†]A thrombotic episode in the past can be considered a clinical criterion, provided that thrombosis is proved by appropriate diagnostic means, and that no alternative diagnosis or cause of thrombosis is found.
[‡]Superficial venous thrombosis is not included in the clinical criteria.
[§]Generally accepted features of placental insufficiency include an abnormal or nonreassuring fetal surveillance test (e.g., nonreactive nonstress test) suggestive of fetal hypoxemia, an abnormal Doppler flow velocimetry waveform analysis suggestive of fetal hypoxemia (e.g., absent end-diastolic flow in the umbilical artery), oligohydramnios (e.g., amniotic fluid index ≤5 cm), or a postnatal birth weight less than the 10th percentile for gestational age.
Investigators are strongly advised to classify APS patients participating in studies into one of the following categories: I, more than one laboratory criteria present (any combination); IIa, only lupus anticoagulant present; IIb, only anticardiolipin antibody present; IIc, only anti–β_2-glycoprotein I antibody present. APS, antiphospholipid syndrome; ELISA, enzyme-linked immunosorbent assay.
From Miyakis S, Lockshin MD, Atsumi T, et al: International consensus statement on an update of the classification criteria for definite antiphospholipid syndrome, *J Thromb Haemost* 4:295–306, 2006.

in the elimination of apoptotic cells[17] and as a natural anticoagulant.[18]

Other, less relevant antigens targeted by aPLs are prothrombin, annexin V, protein C, protein S, high- and low-molecular-weight kininogens, tissue plasminogen activator, factor VII, factor XI, factor XII, complement component C4, and complement factor H.[19]

In experimental animal models, passive or active immunization with viral peptides,[20] bacterial peptides,[21] and heterologous β_2GPI[22] induces polyclonal aPLs and clinical events associated with APS. These data suggest that pathologic autoimmune aPL is induced in susceptible humans by infection via molecular mimicry.

Table 82-2 Other Features Suggesting the Presence of Antiphospholipid Antibodies

Clinical
Livedo reticularis
Thrombocytopenia (usually 50,000-100,000 platelets/mm³)
Autoimmune hemolytic anemia
Cardiac valve disease (vegetations or thickening)
Multiple sclerosis–like syndrome, chorea, or other myelopathy

Laboratory
IgA anticardiolipin antibody
IgA anti–β_2-glycoprotein I

However, infection-induced aPLs (syphilitic and nonsyphilitic *Treponema*, *Borrelia burgdorferi*, human immunodeficiency virus, *Leptospira*, or parasites) are usually β_2GPI independent and bind phospholipids directly.[23] Drugs (chlorpromazine, procainamide, quinidine, and phenytoin) and malignancies (lymphoproliferative disorders) can also induce β_2GPI-independent aPLs. Conversely, autoimmune aPLs bind β_2GPI or other phospholipid-binding plasma proteins, which in turn bind negatively charged phospholipids such as cardiolipin (β_2GPI-dependent aPLs).

Low levels of aPLs may be present normally; one of the functions of normal aPLs may be to participate in the physiologic removal of oxidized lipids.

PATHOGENESIS

Antiphospholipid antibody is most likely related to thrombosis through multiple mechanisms; a proposed pathogenesis is illustrated in Figure 82-1. The process begins with activation or apoptosis of platelets, endothelial cells, or trophoblasts, during which phosphatidylserine (a negatively charged phospholipid) migrates from the inner to the normally electrically neutral outer cell membrane. Circulating β_2GPI binds to phosphatidylserine, and then aPL binds to a β_2GPI dimer.[24]

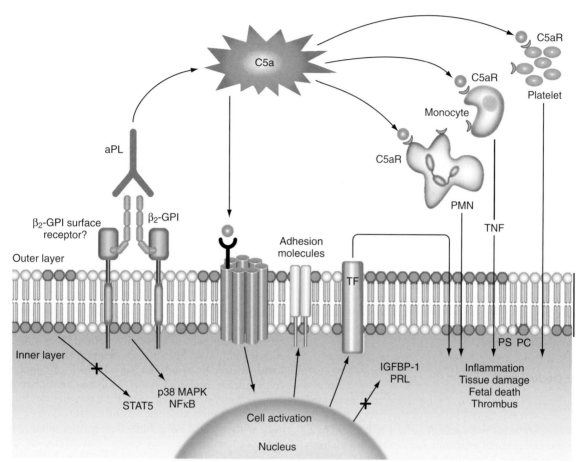

Figure 82-1 Proposed mechanism of antiphospholipid antibody (aPL)-related thrombosis and placental injury. The negatively charged phospholipid phosphatidylserine (PS, *yellow circles*) migrates from the inner to the outer cell membrane during activation or apoptosis of platelets and endothelial cells, and it is normally present on trophoblasts. The neutral phospholipid phosphatidylcholine (PC, *red circles*) is the major constituent of the outer layer of unactivated cells. Dimeric β₂-glycoprotein I (β₂GPI) then binds to PS (probably via β₂GPI surface receptors such as apoER2′, annexin A2, or a Toll-like receptor), and aPL binds to β₂GPI, activating the classic complement pathway and leading to the generation of C5a, which induces (1) expression of adhesion molecules (e.g., intracellular adhesion molecule-1) and tissue factor [TF]), and (2) activation of monocytes, polymorphonuclear (PMN) cells, and platelets, resulting in the release of proinflammatory mediators (e.g., tumor necrosis factor [TNF], vascular endothelial growth factor receptor-1) and initiation of the prothrombotic stage. Both nuclear factor κB (NFκB) and p38 mitogen-activated protein kinase (p38 MAPK) may play a role in the intracellular signaling cascade. Antiphospholipid antibodies also downregulate the expression of trophoblast signal transducer and activator of transcription 5 (STAT5), reducing the endometrial stromal cell production of prolactin (PRL) and insulin growth factor binding protein-1 (IGFBP-1).

Antiphospholipid antibody–β₂GPI dimer binding activates the complement cascade extracellularly; initiates an intracellular signaling cascade, probably through the C5a and β₂GPI surface receptors; and recruits and activates inflammatory effector cells, including monocytes, neutrophils, and platelets, leading to the release of proinflammatory products (e.g., tumor necrosis factor [TNF], oxidants, proteases) and the induction of a prothrombotic phenotype.[25-27] The putative receptor of β₂GPI binding protein that transduces signals from the cell membrane to the nucleus is not yet identified and may vary among cells. The following candidates have been suggested: apoER2 (a member of the low-density lipoprotein receptor superfamily), annexin A2, and a Toll-like receptor.[28-30] Both nuclear factor κB and p38 mitogen-activated protein kinase may play a role in the intracellular signaling cascade.[31,32]

In addition, through downregulation of the signal transducer and activator of transcription 5 (STAT5), aPLs inhibit the production of placental prolactin and insulin growth factor–binding protein-1,[33] and they adversely affect the formation of a trophoblast syncytium, placental apoptosis,

and trophoblast invasion—all processes that are required for the normal establishment of placental function.

Other possible contributory mechanisms of aPL-mediated thrombosis include inhibition of coagulation cascade reactions catalyzed by phospholipids (e.g., activation of circulating procoagulant proteins, inhibition of protein C and S activation), induction of tissue factor (a physiologic initiator of coagulation) expression on monocytes, reduction of fibrinolysis, and interaction with the annexin V anticoagulant shield in the placenta.[29]

In experimental animal models, aPLs cause fetal resorption and increase the size and duration of trauma-induced venous and arterial thrombi.[34,35] Inhibiting complement activation prevents experimental aPL-induced fetal death and angiogenic dysregulation–associated abnormal placental development and preeclampsia; C5 knockout mice carry pregnancies normally despite aPL,[36] implying that a complement-mediated effector mechanism is an absolute requirement for fetal death to occur. Complement activation is also required for experimental thrombosis.[37,38] In addition, aPL-induced reduction of heparin-binding epidermal growth factor–like growth factor leads to defective placentation.[39]

Because high-level aPLs may persist for years in asymptomatic persons, it is likely that vascular injury, endothelial cell activation, or both immediately precede the occurrence of thrombosis in those bearing the antibody (second-hit hypothesis). Of note, at least 50% of APS patients with vascular factors possess other acquired thrombosis risk factors at the time of their events.[40,41]

Persons congenitally lacking β_2GPI[42] and β_2GPI knockout mice appear normal.[43] β_2GPI polymorphisms influence the generation of aPLs in individuals, but they have only a weak relationship to the occurrence of APS.[44] A cluster of 50 upregulated genes may have an effect on the occurrence of thrombosis in aPL-positive individuals.[45]

CLINICAL FEATURES

Clinical manifestations range from asymptomatic aPL positivity (no history of vascular or pregnancy events) to catastrophic APS (multiple thromboses occurring over days). Thus patients should not be evaluated and managed as if they have a single disease.

Vascular Occlusion

APS affects all organ systems. Its principal manifestations are venous or arterial thromboses and pregnancy loss (see Table 82-1). Except for their severity, the youth of affected patients, and the unusual anatomic locations (Budd-Chiari syndrome; sagittal sinus and upper extremity thromboses), venous thromboses in APS do not differ clinically from thromboses attributable to other causes. Similarly, arterial thromboses differ from non–aPL-associated thromboses only by their recurrent nature, unusual locations, and occurrence in young patients. Deep vein thrombosis and stroke are the most common clinical manifestations of APS. Renal thrombotic microangiopathy, glomerular capillary endothelial cell injury, and thrombosis of renal vessels cause proteinuria without cells in the urine or hypocomplementemia and may lead to severe hypertension, renal failure, or both.[46]

Pregnancy Morbidity

Pregnancy losses in patients with aPLs typically occur after 10 weeks' gestation (fetal loss), although earlier losses also occur. These pre-embryonic or embryonic pregnancy losses (<10 weeks' gestation) are commonly due to chromosomal and other genetic defects. Pregnancy in those with APS is often normal until the second trimester, when fetal growth slows and amniotic fluid volume decreases. APS patients may develop severe, early preeclampsia or HELLP (hemolysis, elevated liver enzymes, low platelets) syndrome. Placental infarction is a cause of fetal growth restriction or death; nonthrombotic mechanisms of placental dysfunction also may occur.[47] Prior late pregnancy losses predict future losses, independent of the aPL profile.

Miscellaneous and Noncriteria Manifestations

Many patients have livedo reticularis or thrombocytopenia (Figure 82-2), although these conditions are not specific for

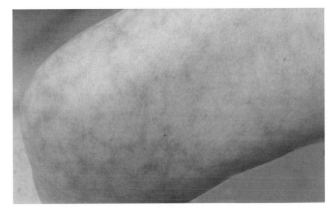

Figure 82-2 Livedo reticularis in antiphospholipid syndrome.

APS. Cardiac valve disease (vegetations, thickening, or both), a late manifestation, may necessitate valve replacement. Its pathogenesis in APS is unknown. Recent studies suggest that APS does not add to the risk of atherosclerosis imparted by SLE.[48] Pulmonary hypertension may develop owing to recurrent pulmonary embolism or small vessel thrombosis; rarely, aPL-positive patients may present with diffuse pulmonary hemorrhage. Some patients develop nonfocal neurologic symptoms such as lack of concentration, forgetfulness, and dizzy spells. Multiple small, hyperintense lesions seen on magnetic resonance imaging (MRI), primarily in the periventricular white matter, do not correlate well with clinical symptoms. Rarely, high-affinity antiprothrombin antibodies may cause hemorrhage by depleting prothrombin (lupus anticoagulant hypoprothrombinemia syndrome).[49]

Catastrophic Antiphospholipid Syndrome

Catastrophic APS is a rare, abrupt, life-threatening complication. It consists of multiple thromboses of medium and small arteries occurring (despite apparently adequate anticoagulation) over a period of days and causing stroke; cardiac, hepatic, adrenal, renal, and intestinal infarction; and peripheral gangrene.[4,50] In a review of 220 patients with catastrophic APS, the main clinical manifestations included renal involvement in 154 patients (70%), pulmonary in 146 (66%), cerebral in 133 (60%), cardiac in 115 (52%), and cutaneous in 104 (47%).[51] Acute adrenal failure may be the initial clinical event. Proposed formal criteria for this syndrome are shown in Table 82-3.[52] Patients often have moderate thrombocytopenia; erythrocytes are less fragmented than in the hemolytic uremic syndrome or thrombotic thrombocytopenic purpura, and fibrin split products are not strikingly elevated. Renal failure and pulmonary hemorrhage may occur. Tissue biopsies show noninflammatory vascular occlusion.

DIAGNOSIS AND DIAGNOSTIC TESTS

Laboratory Studies

The diagnosis of APS requires a positive lupus anticoagulant test or a moderate- to high-titer anticardiolipin or anti-β_2GPI IgG or IgM test in patients with characteristic clinical manifestations. Patients with negative lupus anticoagulant

Table 82-3 Preliminary Criteria for the Classification of Catastrophic Antiphospholipid Syndrome (APS)

1. Evidence of involvement of three or more organs, systems, or tissues*
2. Development of manifestations simultaneously or in less than 1 wk
3. Confirmation by histopathology of small vessel occlusion in at least one organ or tissue†
4. Laboratory confirmation of the presence of antiphospholipid antibody (lupus anticoagulant or anticardiolipin or anti–β₂-glycoprotein I antibodies)‡

Definite Catastrophic APS

All four criteria

Probable Catastrophic APS

Criteria 2 through 4 and two organs, systems, or tissues involved
Criteria 1 through 3, except no confirmation 6 wk apart owing to early death of patient not tested before catastrophic episode
Criteria 1, 2, and 4
Criteria 1, 3, and 4 and development of a third event more than 1 wk but less than 1 mo after the first, despite anticoagulation

*Usually, clinical evidence of vessel occlusions, confirmed by imaging techniques when appropriate. Renal involvement is defined by a 50% rise in serum creatinine, severe systemic hypertension, proteinuria, or some combination of these.

†For histopathologic confirmation, significant evidence of thrombosis must be present, although vasculitis may coexist occasionally.

‡If the patient has not been diagnosed previously with APS, laboratory confirmation requires that the presence of antiphospholipid antibody be detected on two or more occasions at least 6 wk apart (not necessarily at the time of the event), according to proposed preliminary criteria for the classification of APS.

From Asherson RA, Cervera R, de Groot PG, et al: Catastrophic antiphospholipid syndrome: international consensus statement on classification criteria and treatment guidelines, *Lupus* 12:530–534, 2003.

and anticardiolipin tests should be tested for IgA anticardiolipin and IgG, IgM, or IgA anti-β₂GPI when there is a high suspicion for APS. Positive aPL results require a repeat test after 12 or more weeks to exclude a transient, clinically unimportant antibody. The diagnosis of APS should be questioned if less than 12 weeks or more than 5 years separate the positive aPL test from the clinical manifestation.[2]

The lupus anticoagulant test is a more specific but less sensitive predictor of thromboses than is anticardiolipin test; it correlates better with aPL-related clinical events.[53] However, both false-positive and false-negative lupus anticoagulant test results may occur in anticoagulated patients. Documentation of a lupus anticoagulant requires a four-step process: (1) demonstration of a prolonged phospholipid-dependent coagulation screening test, such as activated partial thromboplastin time or dilute Russell viper venom time (however, low-level abnormalities are not clearly linked to APS); (2) failure to correct the prolonged screening test by mixing the patient's plasma with normal platelet-poor plasma, demonstrating the presence of an inhibitor; (3) shortening or correction of the prolonged screening test by the addition of excess phospholipid, demonstrating phospholipid dependency; and (4) exclusion of other inhibitors.[54] Approximately 80% of patients with lupus anticoagulant have anticardiolipin, and 20% of patients positive for anticardiolipin have lupus anticoagulant.[55]

The anticardiolipin enzyme-linked immunosorbent assay (ELISA) is sensitive but not specific for the diagnosis of APS.[56] Although the widely available ELISA test for IgG and IgM anticardiolipin is standardized, considerable variability exists among commercial laboratories that perform the test, especially for the IgA isotype.[57] Low-titer anticardiolipin or anti-β₂GPI, transient aPLs, and antibody to noncardiolipin phospholipids (phosphatidylserine, phosphatidylethanolamine) have no or less proven relationship to APS. ELISA tests other than anticardiolipin and anti-β₂GPI are neither standardized nor widely accepted as predictors of clinical illness.

A false-positive test for syphilis does not fulfill the laboratory criteria, but it should alert physicians to order the aPL tests previously described, especially in patients with a history of aPL-related clinical manifestations.

Whether to test persons with venous occlusive disease or recurrent fetal loss simultaneously for protein C, protein S, and antithrombin III deficiency or for the factor V Leiden and prothrombin mutations is a matter of economics and clinical likelihood; such testing is advisable when feasible. It is useful to test persons with arterial occlusive disease for hyperhomocysteinemia.

Antinuclear and anti-DNA antibodies occur in approximately 45% of patients clinically diagnosed as having primary APS without an accompanying illness[58]; these antibodies do not mandate the additional diagnosis of SLE if the patient has no clinical indicators of SLE. Thrombocytopenia in APS is usually modest (>50,000/mm³); proteinuria and renal insufficiency occur in patients with thrombotic microangiopathy. Pathologic examination demonstrates small artery and glomerular thrombi and recanalization (Figure 82-3). Hypocomplementemia, erythrocyte casts, and pyuria are not characteristic of thrombotic microangiopathy and, when present, imply lupus glomerulonephritis. Erythrocyte sedimentation rate, hemoglobin, and leukocyte count are usually normal in patients with uncomplicated primary APS, except during acute thrombosis. Prothrombin fragment 1 + 2 and other markers of coagulation activation do not predict impending thrombosis.

Imaging Studies

MRI shows vascular occlusion and infarction consistent with clinical symptoms, with no special characteristics (other than multiple, otherwise unexplained cerebral infarctions in a young person). Multiple small, hyperintense white matter lesions are common and do not unequivocally imply brain infarction. Occlusions usually occur in vessels below the resolution limits of angiography; hence, angiography or magnetic resonance angiography is not indicated unless clinical findings suggest medium- or large-vessel disease. Echocardiography or cardiac MRI may show severe Libman-Sacks endocarditis and intracardiac thrombi.[59]

Pathology

Skin, renal, and other tissues show thrombotic occlusion of all caliber arteries and veins, acute and chronic endothelial injury and its sequelae, and recanalization in late lesions. Uteroplacental insufficiency was once thought to be due to thrombosis or spiral artery vasculopathy (atherosis, intimal thickening, fibrinoid necrosis, and absence of physiologic changes in the spiral arteries).[60] Consistent with the importance of inflammation in murine models of APS, recent

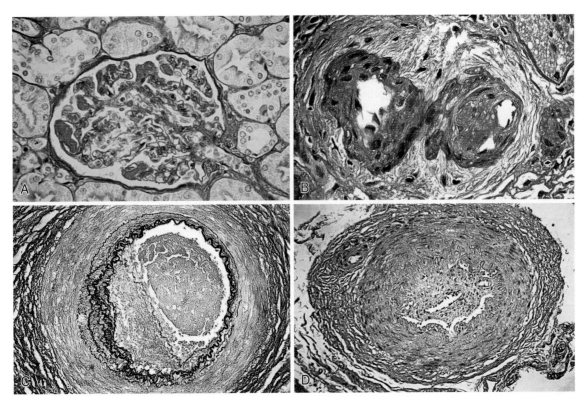

Figure 82-3　Renal thrombotic microangiopathy in antiphospholipid syndrome (APS). **A,** Kidney biopsy from a 35-year-old woman with primary APS, microhematuria, and non-nephrotic proteinuria. The glomerulus contains microthrombi and occluding capillary lumina, and endothelial swelling is evident. **B,** The same patient's small renal artery contains organized thrombus, with recanalization and arteriosclerosis (periodic acid–Schiff, ×100). **C,** Autopsy specimen from a 45-year-old man with primary APS. Note the thrombus in various stages of organization, intact elastic lamina with focal reduplication, and medial thickening (elastic Verhoeff stain, ×100). **D,** The same patient's medium-sized peripheral artery. Note the organized thrombus with recanalization, severe fibrointimal thickening, medial hypertrophy, and extreme stenosis of the lumen (hematoxylin and eosin, ×75). *(Courtesy Dr. Surya V. Seshan.)*

findings demonstrate inflammatory infiltrates, particularly macrophages, and suggest that inflammation contributes to placental injury in patients.[61] The finding of necrotizing vasculitis suggests concomitant lupus or other connective tissue disease. No other diagnostic immunofluorescence or electron microscopic findings have been reported.

Differential Diagnosis

Infection-induced anticardiolipin is usually transient and is more commonly IgM than IgG.[62] Transient aPLs or low-titer anticardiolipin is inconclusive for diagnosis. Research laboratories can distinguish autoimmune from infection-induced aPLs by determining the antibody's β_2GPI dependence. In a patient who has lupus or lupus-like disease, livedo reticularis, or long-standing thrombocytopenia and who has a persistently positive aPL test in addition to APS-related symptoms, it is usually unnecessary to exclude other diagnoses.

Because the prevalence of aPL-positive ELISA tests increases with age, and because the differential diagnosis of vascular occlusion is broader than it is in young adults, particular care is necessary in diagnosing APS in patients older than 60 years. Sustained high-titer anticardiolipin IgG, livedo reticularis, thrombocytopenia, coexisting rheumatic disease, and absence of other causes support a diagnosis of APS.

Five percent to 21% of women with recurrent pregnancy losses, and 0.5% to 2% of normal pregnant women, have

aPLs. Heritable deficiency of protein C, protein S, and antithrombin III and the presence of the factor V Leiden (A506G), prothrombin (G20210A), and methylene tetrahydrofolate reductase (MTHFR, C677T) mutations are less common causes of fetal loss.[63] Attribution of pregnancy loss to APS is most certain when no coexisting plausible explanation is known, when the loss occurs after demonstration of a fetal heartbeat (10 weeks), when a significant aPL profile is repeatedly positive before and after pregnancy, and when the placenta shows vasculopathy and infarction. A single pregnancy loss before 10 weeks' gestation in a patient with a low-positive anticardiolipin test is more likely to be attributable to fetal chromosomal abnormalities, infection, or maternal hormonal or anatomic abnormalities.

Independent coagulopathies may further increase thrombotic risk in patients with aPLs. These and other acquired thrombotic risk factors (hypertension, diabetes, nephrotic syndrome, venous insufficiency, immobility) are alternative causes of thromboembolic disease. Arterial occlusion occurs in patients with thrombotic thrombocytopenic purpura, infected or sterile emboli of cardiac or vascular origin, septicemia, hyperhomocysteinemia, myxoma, Takayasu's arteritis, polyarteritis nodosa, and severe Raynaud's disease. The relationship of Sneddon's syndrome (stroke and livedo reticularis, with or without aPLs) to APS is uncertain.

Catastrophic APS has few mimics. Among them are sepsis, disseminated intravascular coagulation, thrombotic thrombocytopenic purpura, hemolytic uremic syndrome, polyarteritis nodosa, and disseminated embolization from myxoma, atrial thrombus, or atherosclerotic plaque. Small vessel occlusions occurring in rapid succession suggest disseminated intravascular coagulation. Severe cerebral and renal disease suggests thrombotic thrombocytopenic purpura; renal failure and hemolysis suggest hemolytic uremic syndrome. Antiphospholipid antibodies are rarely present in patients with the alternative diagnoses. Acute adrenal insufficiency is characteristic of APS and Waterhouse-Friderichsen syndrome.

TREATMENT

Thrombosis

Treatment recommendations are summarized in Table 82-4. Anticoagulation with heparin is the treatment for acute thrombosis in APS patients. Warfarin, occasionally in association with low-dose aspirin, is used for secondary thrombosis prophylaxis. Two randomized, controlled trials demonstrated that moderate warfarin (international normalized ratio [INR], 2 to 3) and high-intensity warfarin (INR, 3 to 4) are equally protective against recurrence in APS patients after the first thrombosis.[64,65] The intensity of anticoagulation for aPL-related arterial thrombosis is still a matter for debate because in both studies, patients with arterial events constituted less than half of the study

Table 82-4 Treatment Recommendations for Persistently Antiphospholipid Antibody–Positive Individuals

Clinical Circumstance	Recommendation
Asymptomatic	No treatment*
Venous thrombosis	Warfarin INR 2.5 indefinitely
Arterial thrombosis	Warfarin INR 2.5 indefinitely
Recurrent thrombosis	Warfarin INR 3-4 ± low-dose aspirin
Pregnancy:	
First pregnancy	No treatment†
Single pregnancy loss at <10 wk	No treatment†
≥1 Fetal or ≥3 (pre)-embryonic losses, no thrombosis	Prophylactic heparin‡ + low-dose aspirin throughout pregnancy, discontinue 6-12 wk postpartum
Thrombosis regardless of pregnancy history	Therapeutic heparin§ or low-dose aspirin throughout pregnancy, warfarin postpartum
Valve nodules or deformity	No known effective treatment; full anticoagulation if emboli or intracardiac thrombi demonstrated
Thrombocytopenia >50,000/mm³	No treatment
Thrombocytopenia <50,000/mm³	Prednisone, IVIG
Catastrophic antiphospholipid syndrome	Anticoagulation + corticosteroids + IVIG or plasmapheresis

*Aspirin (81 mg/day) may be considered in high-risk patients with multiple non-aPL cardiovascular risk factors.
†Aspirin (81 mg/day) may be considered.
‡Enoxaparin 0.5 mg/kg subcutaneously once daily.
§Enoxaparin 1 mg/kg subcutaneously twice daily or 1.5 mg/kg subcutaneously once daily.
INR, international normalized ratio; IVIG, intravenous immunoglobulin.

population. Although APS patients with arterial thrombosis who are at high risk for recurrence may require high-intensity anticoagulation, in the absence of risk-stratified studies, *high risk* has no consensus definition and currently is based solely on clinical judgment.

Aspirin is the standard of care after an ischemic stroke or a transient ischemic attack to prevent a recurrence in aPL-negative patients. Although most aPL-positive patients with ischemic strokes receive warfarin, the Antiphospholipid Antibody in Stroke Study (APASS) concluded that for selected aPL-positive patients who do not have atrial fibrillation or high-grade stenosis, aspirin and warfarin (target INR, 2.2) are equivalent in terms of both efficacy and major bleeding complications.[66] The APASS results probably do not apply to conventionally defined APS because the average age of study participants was much higher than that of the average APS population; in addition, the aPL determination was performed only once at study entry, and the titer cutoff for assigning a patient to the positive anticardiolipin group was very low. However, aspirin is an option for older aPL-positive patients who have a single low-titer anticardiolipin test, and whose presentation is one stroke.

Some patients require larger than expected doses of both heparin and warfarin to achieve therapeutic anticoagulation. Uncommonly, positive lupus anticoagulant tests cause the INR to be unreliable.[67] Patients with constantly fluctuating INR levels and/or recurrent events despite therapeutic INR may be monitored by the measurement of anti–factor Xa activity or another appropriate assay.

For well-anticoagulated patients who continue to have thromboses, the addition of aspirin (81 to 325 mg/day) can be considered. Experimental (in vitro and/or animal models) and clinical evidence (in lupus patients) suggests that hydroxychloroquine may decrease the incidence of thrombosis; similarly, experimental evidence indicates that statins can interfere with aPL-mediated thrombosis.[68] However, controlled studies are needed to determine the effectiveness of hydroxychloroquine and statins in aPL-positive patients. Corticosteroids have no established role in the treatment of APS but are used for rheumatic symptoms in patients with accompanying systemic autoimmune illness. However, high doses of corticosteroids usually are given empirically to patients with severe thrombocytopenia, hemolytic anemia, and catastrophic APS.

No controlled studies in APS patients have been published for clopidogrel, pentoxifylline, aspirin-dipyridamole, argatroban, hirudin, and other new anticoagulant agents. Neither hirudin nor fondaparinux inactivates complement, and neither drug protects mice with experimental APS against pregnancy loss, so they may be ineffective in human disease. Clinical experience suggests that thrombolytic agents for acute thrombosis are unhelpful because reocclusion occurs rapidly.

Currently available data, although retrospective and not risk-stratified, indicate that lifelong anticoagulation of APS patients who have had vascular events is appropriate.[69] However, recent recognition that some patients have full remission of antibody, and that most thrombotic events have recognizable triggers, raises the possibility of discontinuing anticoagulation in highly selected patients when the triggers are eliminated.

Pregnancy Morbidity

Heparin is indicated at the diagnosis of pregnancy in an aPL-positive woman who has had prior pregnancy losses attributable to APS. Because warfarin is teratogenic, only unfractionated or low-molecular-weight heparin is used for the treatment of affected pregnancies in the United States; in other countries, converting to warfarin after the first trimester may be considered acceptable.[70] Most physicians with a special interest in this field now use low-molecular-weight heparin owing to decreased risk of thrombocytopenia and osteoporosis.

Patients with prior fetal losses later than 10 gestational weeks should be treated with prophylactic heparin (enoxaparin 30 to 40 mg subcutaneously once daily), together with low-dose aspirin; this regimen increases the fetal survival rate from 50% (untreated) to 80%.[71,72] Women who have had prior thromboses must be fully anticoagulated (enoxaparin 1 mg/kg subcutaneously twice daily or 1.5 mg/kg subcutaneously once daily) throughout pregnancy because the risk of new thrombosis markedly increases both during pregnancy and during the postpartum period. Even with treatment, prematurity and fetal growth restriction may occur. Clopidogrel and newer antithrombotic agents have not been cleared for use in pregnancy but, together with intravenous immunoglobulin (IVIG) and hydroxychloroquine, they may be considered in patients who are unable to use heparin, or who fail heparin treatment.

In aPL-positive women with prior thrombosis, warfarin is changed to heparin or low-molecular-weight heparin before conception, if possible, or at the first missed menstrual period. In aPL-positive women without prior thrombosis, if heparin is indicated during pregnancy, treatment begins after confirmation of pregnancy, continues until 48 hours before anticipated delivery (to allow epidural anesthesia), and resumes for 8 to 12 weeks during the postpartum period. Some physicians recommend the initiation of heparin before conception; no clinical trial supports this recommendation, however, and the risk associated with longer-duration heparin therapy is considerable. Patients in most published series received low-dose aspirin as well as heparin, but the benefit of adding aspirin is unknown.

Because of the risk of postpartum thrombosis, it is prudent to continue anticoagulation for 8 to 12 weeks during the postpartum period and then to discontinue it by tapering the doses. If desired, conversion from heparin to warfarin may be accomplished after the first or second postpartum week. Breastfeeding is permissible with both heparin and warfarin.

No studies unequivocally justify the treatment of women with aPLs during a first pregnancy, women with only very early losses, or women whose aPL titers are low or transient. Nonetheless, it is common to offer such patients low-dose aspirin.

Asymptomatic Antiphospholipid Antibody–Positive Individuals

Persistence of aPLs for decades without clinical events is well documented. The probability that an asymptomatic person incidentally found to have aPLs will eventually develop the syndrome is likely low.[7] Anticoagulation is not indicated for the prophylactic treatment of asymptomatic aPL-positive individuals. For those with moderate- to high-titer anticardiolipin and persistent aPLs, education about the meaning of abnormal tests is appropriate, as is a discussion of warning signs to be reported. Elimination of reversible thrombosis risk factors and prophylaxis during high-risk periods, such as surgical procedures, are crucial. The necessity for and the effectiveness of aspirin are not supported by the current literature; in a recent randomized, double-blind, placebo-controlled trial, low-dose aspirin (81 mg) appeared to be no better than placebo in preventing first thrombotic episodes in persistently asymptomatic aPL-positive patients; the incidence rate of first thrombosis was relatively low.[9]

Although drugs that induce lupus (hydralazine, phenytoin) may also induce aPLs, they may be prescribed for patients with aPLs if no alternatives are available. Drugs that promote thrombosis (estrogen and estrogen-containing oral contraceptives) are not currently deemed safe, even for asymptomatic women serendipitously known to have high-titer antibodies. This advice does not translate to a recommendation to test all normal women before prescribing such medications, but it does suggest that special attention and further evaluation should be provided to those with family histories or clinical suggestions of rheumatic disease, livedo reticularis, biologic false-positive tests for syphilis, or borderline thrombocytopenia. No reliable information is available regarding the safety of progestin-only contraception, "morning after" contraception, or the use of raloxifene, bromocriptine, or leuprolide in APS patients. A small retrospective review of women undergoing artificial reproductive technology (in vitro fertilization) procedures demonstrated no thrombotic events.[73]

Antiphospholipid Antibody–Positive Individuals with Ambiguous Events

Some patients with positive aPL tests have clinical events of ambiguous meaning (dizzy or confusional episodes, nonspecific visual disturbances, very early pregnancy loss). No consensus has been reached regarding the treatment of such persons. Because full anticoagulation carries high risk, many physicians prescribe low-dose (81 mg) aspirin, hydroxychloroquine, or both daily. No published data support or repudiate this recommendation. Based on the presumed pathogenesis, some physicians prescribe anticoagulation for patients with livedo reticularis, thrombocytopenia, leg ulcers, thrombotic microangiopathy, or valvulopathy. The efficacy of anticoagulation is unknown in these conditions. One small, descriptive, cross-sectional study provides evidence that B cell depletion with rituximab is well tolerated and can be effective for refractory thrombocytopenia and skin ulcers in aPL-positive patients.[74] An open-label phase IIa descriptive pilot study assessing the effectiveness and safety of rituximab in patients with noncriteria and/or anticoagulation-resistant manifestations of aPL is in progress (Clinical Trials.gov Identifier: NCT00537290).

Catastrophic Antiphospholipid Syndrome

The onset of catastrophic APS is usually sudden and immediately life threatening. Early diagnosis can be a challenge, especially in patients with no history of APS. However, early diagnosis is critical because, in contrast to other causes of multiple organ dysfunction syndrome, appropriate therapy includes anticoagulation and corticosteroids in combination with repeated plasma exchange, IVIG, and, in desperate situations, other modalities such as cyclophosphamide or rituximab. However, mortality remains as high as 48% despite all attempts at effective therapy.[75] No systematic studies have examined the treatment of catastrophic APS owing to the rarity of the condition.

Antiphospholipid Antibody–Negative Individuals with a Clinical Event

In patients clinically suspected of having APS but with normal anticardiolipin, lupus anticoagulant, and anti-β$_2$GPI tests, alternative causes of clotting must be sought. Even among patients with concomitant rheumatic disease, APS may not be the cause of recurrent thromboembolism or pregnancy loss. Patients with SLE develop emboli from SLE-related cardiac valvular disease, vasculitis, or atheroma. Other patients have factor V Leiden or some other procoagulant mutation. Recurrent pregnancy losses may be caused by chromosomal abnormalities, uterine infection, diabetes, hypertension, or non-aPL coagulopathy. The concept of "seronegative" APS is not recognized.

OUTCOME

Pulmonary hypertension, neurologic involvement, myocardial ischemia, nephropathy, gangrene of extremities, and catastrophic APS are associated with a worse prognosis. During long-term follow-up, serious morbidity and disability occur in an unpredictable proportion of primary APS patients who experience major vascular events and in those who have delays in diagnosis and treatment. Thus, the long-term functional outcome of primary APS patients is poor; at 10 years, one-third of patients develop permanent organ damage, and one-fifth are unable to perform everyday activities.[76]

In a retrospective study of obstetric APS patients without thrombosis, 35% developed aPL-related clinical events during 8 years of follow-up[77]. The studied populations were highly selected referral populations that may have been biased toward severe disease, but follow-up studies of obstetric patients with autoantibodies show similar results.[78]

Long-term outcomes of children born of APS pregnancies are not known. In many patients with long-standing APS, the development of severe cardiac valvular disease necessitates valve replacement, and rare patients develop renal failure due to thrombotic microangiopathy. Immediate thrombosis may cause loss of a transplanted kidney or other organ; aPL positivity correlates with poor graft survival after renal transplantation in SLE patients.[79]

Serious perioperative complications may occur despite prophylaxis in aPL-positive patients because they are at additional risk for thrombosis when undergoing surgical procedures. Thus perioperative strategies should be clearly identified before any surgical procedure is performed; in addition, pharmacologic and physical antithrombosis interventions should be vigorously employed, periods without anticoagulation should be kept to an absolute minimum, intravascular manipulation for access and monitoring

should be minimized, and any deviation from a normal course should be considered a potential disease-related event.[80]

References

1. Wilson WA, Gharavi AE, Koike T, et al: International consensus statement on preliminary classification criteria for antiphospholipid syndrome: report of an international workshop, *Arthritis Rheum* 42:1309–1311, 1999.
2. Miyakis S, Lockshin MD, Atsumi T, et al: International consensus statement on an update of the classification criteria for definite antiphospholipid syndrome, *J Thromb Haemost* 4:295–306, 2006.
3. Gharavi AE, Sammaritano LR, Wen J, et al: Characteristics of human immunodeficiency virus and chlorpromazine-induced antiphospholipid antibodies: effect of beta 2 glycoprotein I on binding to phospholipid, *J Rheumatol* 21:94–99, 1994.
4. Vila P, Hernandez MC, Lopez-Fernandez MF, et al: Prevalence, follow-up and clinical significance of the aCL in normal subjects, *Thromb Haemost* 72:209–213, 1994.
5. Petri M: Epidemiology of the antiphospholipid antibody syndrome, *J Autoimmun* 15:145–151, 2000.
6. Olech E, Merrill JT: The prevalence and clinical significance of antiphospholipid antibodies in rheumatoid arthritis, *Curr Rheumatol Rep* 8:100–108, 2006.
7. Giron-Gonzalez JA, Garcia del Rio E, Rodriguez C, et al: Antiphospholipid syndrome and asymptomatic carriers of antiphospholipid antibody: prospective analysis of 404 individuals, *J Rheumatol* 31:1560–1567, 2004.
8. Somers E, Magder LS, Petri ML: Antiphospholipid antibodies and incidence of venous thrombosis in a cohort of patients with systemic lupus erythematosus, *J Rheumatol* 29:2531–2536, 2002.
9. Erkan D, Harrison MJ, Levy R, et al: Aspirin for primary thrombosis prevention in the antiphospholipid syndrome: a randomized, double-blind, placebo-controlled trial in asymptomatic antiphospholipid antibody-positive individuals, *Arthritis Rheum* 56:2382–2391, 2007.
10. The Antiphospholipid Antibody Stroke Study (APASS) Group: Anticardiolipin antibodies are an independent risk factor for first ischemic stroke, *Neurology* 43:2069–2073, 1993.
11. Levine SR, Brey RL, Sawaya KL, et al: Recurrent stroke and thrombo-occlusive events in the antiphospholipid syndrome, *Ann Neurol* 38:119–124, 1995.
12. Stephenson MD: Frequency of factors associated with habitual abortion in 197 couples, *Fertil Steril* 66:24–29, 1996.
13. Ginsberg JS, Wells PS, Brill-Edwards P, et al: Antiphospholipid antibodies and venous thromboembolism, *Blood* 86:3685–3691, 1995.
14. Koike T, Ichikawa K, Kasahara H: Epitopes on beta2-GPI recognized by anticardiolipin antibodies, *Lupus* 7(Suppl 2):S14, 1998.
15. Shi T, Giannakopoulos B, Yan X, et al: Anti-beta2-glycoprotein I antibodies in complex with beta2-glycoprotein I can activate platelets in a dysregulated manner via glycoprotein Ib-IX-V, *Arthritis Rheum* 54:2558–2567, 2006.
16. Reddel SW, Wang YX, Sheng YH, et al: Epitope studies with anti-beta 2-glycoprotein I antibodies from autoantibody and immunized sources, *J Autoimmun* 15:91–96, 2000.
17. Casciola-Rosen L, Rosen A, Petri M, et al: Surface blebs on apoptotic cells are sites of enhanced procoagulant activity: implications for coagulation events and antigenic spread in systemic lupus erythematosus, *Proc Natl Acad Sci U S A* 93:1624–1629, 1996.
18. Mori T, Takeya H, Nishioka J, et al: Beta 2-glycoprotein I modulates the anticoagulant activity of activated protein C on the phospholipid surface, *Thromb Haemost* 75:49–55, 1996.
19. Bertolaccini ML, Hughes GR: Antiphospholipid antibody testing: which are most useful for diagnosis? *Rheum Dis Clin North Am* 32:455–463, 2006.
20. Gharavi AE, Pierangeli SS, Harris EN: Origin of antiphospholipid antibodies, *Rheum Dis Clin North Am* 27:551–563, 2001.
21. Blank M, Krause I, Fridkin M, et al: Bacterial induction of autoantibodies to beta2-glycoprotein-I accounts for the infectious etiology of antiphospholipid syndrome, *J Clin Invest* 109:797–804, 2002.
22. Gharavi AE, Sammaritano LR, Wen J, et al: Induction of antiphospholipid antibodies by immunization with beta 2 glycoprotein I (apolipoprotein H), *J Clin Invest* 90:1105–1109, 1992.

23. Arvieux J, Renaudineau Y, Mane I, et al: Distinguishing features of anti-beta2 glycoprotein I antibodies between patients with leprosy and the antiphospholipid syndrome, *Thromb Haemost* 87:599–605, 2002.

24. Lutters BC, Derksen RH, Tekelenburg WL, et al: Dimers of beta 2-glycoprotein 1 increase platelet deposition to collagen via interaction with phospholipids and the apolipoprotein E receptor 2', *J Biol Chem* 278:33831–33838, 2003.

25. Bordron A, Dueymes MY, Levy Y, et al: Anti-endothelial cell antibody binding makes negatively charged phospholipids accessible to antiphospholipid antibodies, *Arthritis Rheum* 41:1738–1747, 1998.

26. Simantov R, LaSala J, Lo SK, et al: Activation of cultured vascular endothelial cells by antiphospholipid antibodies, *J Clin Invest* 96:2211–2219, 1996.

27. Font J, Espinosa G, Tassies D, et al: Effects of β2-glycoprotein I and monoclonal anticardiolipin antibodies in platelet interaction with subendothelium under flow conditions, *Arthritis Rheum* 46:3283–3289, 2002.

28. van Lummel M, Pennings MT, Derksen RH, et al: The binding site in β2-glycoprotein I for ApoER2 on platelets is located in domain V, *J Biol Chem* 280:36729–36736, 2005.

29. Erkan D, Lockshin MD: What is antiphospholipid syndrome? *Curr Rheumatol Rep* 6:451–457, 2004.

30. Romay-Penabad Z, Montiel-Manzano MG, Shilagard T: Annexin A2 is involved in antiphospholipid antibody-mediated pathogenic effects in vitro and in vivo, *Blood* 114:3074–3083, 2009.

31. Dunoyer-Geindre S, de Moerloose P, Galve-de Rochemonteix B, et al: NFkappaB is an essential intermediate in the activation of endothelial cells by anti-beta2-glycoprotein 1 antibodies, *Thromb Haemost* 88:851–857, 2002.

32. Pierangeli SS, Vega-Ostertag M, Harris EN: Intracellular signaling triggered by antiphospholipid antibodies in platelets and endothelial cells: a pathway to targeted therapies, *Thromb Res* 114:467–476, 2004.

33. Mak IYH, Brosens JJ, Christian M, et al: Regulated expression of signal transducer and activator of transcription, Stat5, and its enhancement of PRL expression in human endometrial stromal cells in vitro, *J Clin Endocrinol Metab* 87:2581–2587, 2002.

34. Pierangeli SS, Liu XW, Barker JH, et al: Induction of thrombosis in a mouse model by IgG, IgM, and IgA immunoglobulins from patients with the antiphospholipid syndrome, *Thromb Haemost* 74:1361–1367, 1995.

35. Jankowski M, Vreys I, Wittevrongel C, et al: Thrombogenicity of β2-glycoprotein I-dependent antiphospholipid antibodies in a photochemically-induced thrombosis model in the hamster, *Blood* 101:157–162, 2003.

36. Girardi G, Bulla R, Salmon JE, et al: The complement system in the pathophysiology of pregnancy, *Mol Immunol* 43:68–77, 2006.

37. Fleming SD, Egan RP, Chai C, et al: Anti-phospholipid antibodies restore mesenteric ischemia/reperfusion-induced injury in complement receptor 2/complement receptor 1-deficient mice, *J Immunol* 173:7055–7061, 2004.

38. Girardi G, Yarilin D, Thurman JM, et al: Complement activation induces dysregulation of angiogenic factors and causes fetal rejection and growth restriction, *J Exp Med* 203:2165–2175, 2006.

39. Di Simone N, Marana R, Castellani R: Decreased expression of heparin-binding epidermal growth factor-like growth factor as a newly identified pathogenic mechanism of antiphospholipid-mediated defective placentation, *Arthritis Rheum* 62:1504–1512, 2010.

40. Kaul M, Erkan D, Sammaritano L, et al: Assessment of the 2006 revised antiphospholipid syndrome (APS) classification criteria (abstract), *Arthritis Rheum* 54:S796, 2006.

41. Erkan D, Yazici Y, Peterson MG, et al: A cross-sectional study of clinical thrombotic risk factors and preventive treatments in antiphospholipid syndrome, *Rheumatology* 41:924–929, 2002.

42. Bancsi LF, van der Linden IK, Bertina RM: Beta 2-glycoprotein I deficiency and the risk of thrombosis, *Thromb Haemost* 67:649–653, 1992.

43. Sheng Y, Reddel SW, Herzog H, et al: Impaired thrombin generation in beta 2-glycoprotein I null mice, *J Biol Chem* 276:13817–13821, 2001.

44. Kamboh MI, Manzi S, Mehdi H, et al: Genetic variation in apolipoprotein H (beta2-glycoprotein I) affects the occurrence of antiphospholipid antibodies and apolipoprotein H concentrations in systemic lupus erythematosus, *Lupus* 8:742–750, 1999.

45. Potti A, Bild A, Dressman HK, et al: Gene-expression patterns predict phenotypes of immune-mediated thrombosis, *Blood* 107:1391–1396, 2006.

46. Bhandari S, Harnden P, Brownjohn AM, et al: Association of anticardiolipin antibodies with intraglomerular thrombi and renal dysfunction in lupus nephritis, *Q J Med* 91:401–409, 1998.

47. Rand JH, Wu X, Andree HAM, et al: Pregnancy loss in the antiphospholipid-antibody syndrome: a possible thrombogenic mechanism, *N Engl J Med* 337:154–160, 1997.

48. Roman MJ, Shanker BA, Davis A, et al: Prevalence and correlates of accelerated atherosclerosis in systemic lupus erythematosus, *N Engl J Med* 349:2399–2406, 2003.

49. Erkan D, Bateman H, Lockshin MD: Lupus-anticoagulant-hypoprothrombinemia syndrome associated with systemic lupus erythematosus: report of 2 cases and review of literature, *Lupus* 8:560–564, 1999.

50. Erkan D, Cervera R, Asherson RA: Catastrophic antiphospholipid syndrome: where do we stand? *Arthritis Rheum* 48:3320–3327, 2003.

51. Cervera R, Font J, Gomez-Puerta JA, et al: Validation of the preliminary criteria for the classification of catastrophic antiphospholipid syndrome, *Ann Rheum Dis* 64:1205–1209, 2005.

52. Asherson RA, Cervera R, de Groot PG, et al: Catastrophic antiphospholipid syndrome: international consensus statement on classification criteria and treatment guidelines, *Lupus* 12:530–534, 2003.

53. Galli M, Luciani D, Bertolini G, et al: Lupus anticoagulants are stronger risk factors for thrombosis than anticardiolipin antibodies in the antiphospholipid syndrome: a systematic review of the literature, *Blood* 101:1827–1832, 2003.

54. Brandt JT, Triplett DA, Alving B, et al: Criteria for the diagnosis of lupus anticoagulants: an update, *Thromb Haemost* 74:1185–1190, 1995.

55. Cervera R, Piette JC, Font J, et al: Antiphospholipid syndrome: clinical and immunologic manifestations and patterns of disease expression in a cohort of 1000 patients, *Arthritis Rheum* 46:1019–1027, 2002.

56. Day HM, Thiagarajan P, Ahn C, et al: Autoantibodies to β2-glycoprotein I in systemic lupus erythematosus and primary antiphospholipid syndrome: clinical correlations in comparison with other antiphospholipid antibody tests, *J Rheumatol* 25:667–674, 1998.

57. Erkan D, Derksen WJ, Kaplan V, et al: Real world experience with antiphospholipid antibody tests: how stable are results over time? *Ann Rheum Dis* 64:1321–1325, 2005.

58. Lockshin MD, Sammaritano LR, Schwartzman S: Brief report: validation of the Sapporo criteria for antiphospholipid antibody syndrome, *Arthritis Rheum* 43:440–443, 2000.

59. Erel H, Erkan D, Lehman TJ, et al: Diagnostic usefulness of 3 dimensional gadolinium enhanced magnetic resonance venography in antiphospholipid syndrome, *J Rheumatol* 29:1338–1339, 2002.

60. Khong TY, De Wolf F, Robertson WB, et al: Inadequate maternal vascular response to placentation in pregnancies complicated by preeclampsia and by small-for-gestational-age infants, *Br J Obstet Gynaecol* 93:1049–1059, 1986.

61. Stone S, Pijnenborg R, Vercruysse L, et al: The placental bed in pregnancies complicated by primary antiphospholipid syndrome, *Placenta* 27:457–467, 2006.

62. Levy RA, Gharavi AE, Sammaritano LR, et al: Characteristics of IgG antiphospholipid antibodies in patients with systemic lupus erythematosus and syphilis, *J Rheumatol* 17:1036–1041, 1990.

63. Kupferminc MJ, Eldo A, Steinman N, et al: Increased frequency of genetic thrombophilia in women with complications of pregnancy, *N Engl J Med* 340:9–13, 1999.

64. Crowther MA, Ginsberg JS, Julian J, et al: Comparison of two intensities of warfarin for the prevention of recurrent thrombosis in patients with the antiphospholipid antibody syndrome, *N Engl J Med* 349:1133–1138, 2003.

65. Finazzi G, Marchioli R, Brancaccio V, et al: A randomized clinical trial of high-intensity warfarin vs conventional antithrombotic therapy for the prevention of recurrent thrombosis in patients with the antiphospholipid syndrome (WAPS), *J Thromb Haemost* 3:848–853, 2005.

66. Levine SR, Brey RL, Tilley BC, et al: Antiphospholipid antibodies and subsequent thrombo-occlusive events in patients with ischemic stroke, *JAMA* 291:576–584, 2004.

67. Ortel TL, Moll S: Monitoring warfarin therapy in patients with lupus anticoagulants, *Ann Intern Med* 127:177–185, 1997.

68. Erkan D, Lockshin MD: New approaches for managing antiphospholipid syndrome, *Nat Clin Pract Rheumatol* 5:160–170, 2009.

69. Brunner HI, Chan WS, Ginsberg JS, et al: Long term anticoagulation is preferable for patients with antiphospholipid antibody syndrome: result of a decision analysis, *J Rheumatol* 29:490–501, 2002.
70. Vilela VS, de Jesus NR, Levy RA: Prevention of thrombosis during pregnancy, *Isr Med Assoc J* 4:794–797, 2002.
71. Kutteh WH: Antiphospholipid antibody-associated recurrent pregnancy loss: treatment with heparin and low-dose aspirin is superior to low-dose aspirin alone, *Am J Obstet Gynecol* 174:1584–1589, 1996.
72. Rai R, Cohen H, Dave M, et al: Randomised controlled trial of aspirin and aspirin plus heparin in pregnant women with recurrent miscarriage associated with phospholipid antibodies (or antiphospholipid antibodies), *BMJ* 314:253–257, 1997.
73. Guballa N, Sammaritano L, Schwartzman S, et al: Ovulation induction and in vitro fertilization in systemic lupus erythematosus and antiphospholipid syndrome, *Arthritis Rheum* 43:550–556, 2000.
74. Tenedios F, Erkan D, Lockshin MD: Rituximab in the primary antiphospholipid syndrome (PAPS) (abstract), *Arthritis Rheum* 52:4078, 2005.
75. Vero S, Asherson RA, Erkan D: Critical care review: catastrophic antiphospholipid syndrome, *J Intensive Care Med* 21:144–159, 2006.
76. Erkan D, Yazici Y, Sobel R, et al: Primary antiphospholipid syndrome: functional outcome after 10 years, *J Rheumatol* 27:2817–2821, 2000.
77. Erkan D, Merrill JT, Yazici Y, et al: High thrombosis rate after fetal loss in antiphospholipid syndrome: effective prophylaxis with aspirin, *Arthritis Rheum* 44:1466–1467, 2001.
78. Gris JC, Bouvier S, Molinari N, et al: Comparative incidence of a first thrombotic event in purely obstetric antiphospholipid syndrome with pregnancy loss: the NOH-APS observational study, *Blood* 119:2624–2632, 2012.
79. Raklyar I, DeMarco PJ, Wu J, et al: Anticardiolipin antibody correlates with poor graft survival in renal transplantation for systemic lupus erythematosus, *Arthritis Rheum* 52:S384, 2005.
80. Erkan D, Leibowitz E, Berman J, Lockshin MD: Perioperative medical management of antiphospholipid syndrome: Hospital for Special Surgery experience, review of the literature and recommendations, *J Rheumatol* 29:843–849, 2002.

The references for this chapter can also be found on www.expertconsult.com.

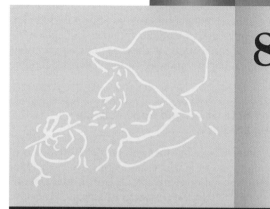

83 Etiology and Pathogenesis of Scleroderma

JOHN VARGA

KEY POINTS

Scleroderma/systemic sclerosis (SSc) has a complex pathogenesis and protean clinical manifestations reflecting the underlying early immune dysregulation and microangiopathy, as well as subsequent systemic fibrosis.

There is marked patient-to-patient variability in clinical and laboratory manifestations, disease course, and molecular signatures, suggesting the existence of distinct disease subsets.

Vascular lesions in small blood vessels occur early and progress to obliterative vasculopathy that causes tissue hypoxia, oxidative stress, and vascular complications.

Immune dysregulation manifested by autoantibodies, evidence of innate immune activation, and the "interferon signature" is prominent in SSc, but its role as a primary factor in pathogenesis has not been established. Genetic association studies implicate the human leukocyte antigen (HLA) and other immunoregulatory genes that are also associated with systemic lupus erythematosus.

Fibrosis is associated with sustained mesenchymal cell activation by growth factors, cytokines, chemokines, hypoxia and reactive oxygen species, and aberrant reactivation of developmental pathways.

Scleroderma or systemic sclerosis (SSc) is an uncommon disease of unknown cause and complex pathogenesis. The hallmarks of SSc are (1) autoimmunity, (2) inflammation, (3) functional and structural alterations in small blood vessels, and (4) interstitial and vascular fibrosis in the skin and internal organs. This unique constellation of distinct but related pathophysiologic features, illustrated in Figure 83-1, accounts for the characteristic clinical manifestations of SSc. Early-stage disease may be dominated by inflammation and vascular injury, whereas in advanced disease fibrosis and vascular insufficiency are most prominent. However, there is enormous patient-to-patient variability in these features. Recent advances in cell and molecular biology, mouse genetic engineering, functional genomics, and genetic association studies reveal the involvement of a large number of molecules, pathways, and cell types in SSc, yielding an increasing nuanced picture of the pathogenesis. Environmental triggers in a genetically susceptible individual are thought to induce a cascade of events with early vascular injury, immune cell activation, the generation of autoimmunity, and subsequent fibroblast activation and matrix accumulation that results in chronic and progressive tissue damage. Over time, vascular insufficiency and widespread fibrosis cause disruption of vital organs, accounting for the substantial morbidity and mortality of SSc.

ETIOLOGY

Neither the cause of SSc nor the precise contribution of genetic factors is fully understood. Evidence indicates that infectious agents, environmental toxins, and drugs, as well as microchimerism, are potential triggers.

Genetic Risk: Family Studies

Familial clustering of a disease is considered as evidence of inherited disease susceptibility, but such clustering might be explained by shared environmental exposures, shared genetic background, or the interaction between genes and environment.[1] The risk of SSc is increased among first-degree relatives of SSc cases compared with the general population. In one U.S. study, the relative risk of SSc among first-degree relatives of cases was 13, with a rate of 1.6% compared with 0.026% in the general population, identifying a family history of SSc as the strongest known risk factor.[2] The only twin study of SSc to date reported a relatively small disease concordance rate (4.7%), although the concordance rate for positive antinuclear antibody (ANA) was 90% for monozygotic (identical) twins and 40% for dizygotic (fraternal) twins.[3] Raynaud disease and pulmonary fibrosis show increased prevalence in pedigrees of SSc patients.[4] Moreover, autoimmune diseases among first-degree family members of SSc patients have been reported in up to 36% of cases, with hypothyroidism, hyperthyroidism, rheumatoid arthritis, and systemic lupus erythematosus (SLE) most common.

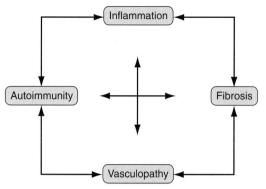

Figure 83-1 The pathophysiologic quartet underlying systemic sclerosis. Patients with systemic sclerosis display evidence of inflammation, autoimmunity, vasculopathy, and fibrosis. Autoimmunity and vasculopathy generally precede the onset and contribute to the progression of fibrosis. Vascular obliteration and interstitial fibrosis perpetuate and further exacerbate chronic autoimmunity and inflammation. *(Courtesy Kathleen Kelley.)*

Genetic Association Studies: Immune Susceptibility Genes for Scleroderma

The past decade has witnessed rapid progress in delineating genetic susceptibility factors in SSc. Genetic association studies using candidate gene approaches and, more recently, genome-wide association (GWA) studies have been performed in large multinational patient cohorts. The major histocompatibility complex (MHC) is the dominant genetic region implicated in autoimmune disease, although the role of specific human leukocyte antigen (HLA) alleles in pathogenesis remains unknown. The interpretation of HLA associations is complicated by the extensive linkage disequilibrium of risk haplotypes. Specific HLA alleles have long been known to be associated with SSc and specific autoantibodies. For instance, a case-contol study of SSc revealed strong associations with HLA DRB1*1104, DQA1*0501, and DQB1*0301 haplotypes.[5] Candidate gene approaches typically look for changes in single nucleotides (single nucleotide polymorphisms [SNPs]), the most common form of deoxyribonucleic acid (DNA) variation. Non-HLA susceptibility genes associated with SSc include the protein tyrosine phosphatase nonreceptor 22 (PTPN22), which has been associated with SLE, myasthenia gravis, vitiligo, and Addison's disease; interleukin (IL)-1β and NLRP1, an inflammasome scaffold that promotes pro-IL-1β maturation and processing; and interferon regulatory factor 5 (IRF5), a transcription factor in the Toll-like receptor

(TLR) pathway that mediates type I interferon (IFN) induction and is associated with SLE, as well as SSc and interstitial lung disease. The association of IRF5 with SSc is particularly interesting, in light of the role of IFN type I in immune responses. Table 83-1 summarizes SSc susceptibility genes identified to date. In addition to classic SNPs, informative genetic polymorphisms in SSc include variations of copy numbers, rare allelic variants, and epigenetic changes. The identification of these genetic associations will require in-depth analysis using deep-sequencing technologies.

Other Candidate Genes and Genome-wide Association Studies

Candidate gene approaches focusing on genes involved in vascular homeostasis or matrix remodeling have to date not yielded robust associations with SSc. A British study identified a functional SNP in the connective tissue growth factor (CTGF) promoter region associated with SSc. However, in another study an apparent association with SPARC could not be validated in an independent cohort. Potential explanations for discrepancies among genetic association studies include ethnic differences in the study populations and disease heterogeneity.

Several GWA studies in large and ethnically diverse populations are currently under way. These unbiased approaches have the advantage over candidate gene studies in that they are driven by discovery rather than a priori hypotheses. The first large-scale SSc GWA study analyzed 300,000 SNPs in a cohort of 2296 white cases and 5014 healthy controls.[6] Statistically significant associations were found with SNPs in the HLA region, as well as *IRF5*, *TNFAIP3*, and *CD247*, a gene implicated in T cell signaling and also associated with susceptibility to SLE. Although genetic association studies represent a rapidly evolving area of research, the results to date can be summed up as follows: (1) Genetic variants associated with SSc susceptibility are involved in innate and adaptive immune responses, and (2) they are shared with SLE and other autoimmune diseases. It is worth noting that important associations can be missed by GWA studies using current technologies. Moreover, despite the wealth of emerging information, the genetic associations discovered to date are of relatively modest magnitude, with odds ratios that are generally less than 1.5. This finding points to the potential importance of gene-gene interactions (epistasis), particularly for genes within the same molecular pathways, and gene-environment

Table 83-1 Systemic Sclerosis (SSc) Susceptibility Genes

Locus	Chromosome	Associated SSc Subset	Potential Pathogenic Mechanism
HLA	6	Various	Antigen presentation
PTPN22	1p3.2	Topo1+ positive	T and B cell activation
NLRP1	17p13.2	dcSSc, pulmonary fibrosis	Inflammasome component, IL-1β processing
IRF5	7q32	dcSSc	Transcription factor required for induction of type I interferon
STAT4	2q32.3	lcSSc, ACA	Transcription factor for IL-12 and IL-23
BANK1	4q24	dcSSc	Adaptor involved in B cell signaling
TNFSF4	1q25	SSc	T cell co-stimulation
T-bet	17.q21.32	SSc	Transcription factor for Th1 T cell polarization

Based on published candidate gene studies and genome-wide association studies as of 2011.
ACA, anticentromere antibody; dcSSc, diffuse cutaneous SSc; IL, interleukin; lcSSc, limited cutaneous SSc; SSc, systemic sclerosis.

interactions. A current challenge in SSc research is how to handle the large volume of new information emerging from GWA studies. Moreover, it will be important to delineate how genes shared among diverse autoimmune conditions contribute to disease-specific phenotypes. Shedding light on this important problem will require large collaborative studies involving phenotypically well-characterized populations of varied ethnic background and meta-analyses.

INFECTIOUS AGENTS: VIRUSES

Along with exposure to certain environmental and occupational agents and drugs, viruses such as human cytomegalovirus (hCMV) and parvovirus B19 have been implicated as potential triggers for SSc. Patients with SSc have anti-hCMV antibodies directed against the UL83 and UL94 protein epitopes on hCMV. Anti-UL94 antibodies can induce endothelial cell apoptosis and fibroblast activation, suggesting a direct role for antiviral antibodies in tissue damage. Antitopoisomerase-I can cross-react with hCMV-derived proteins, implicating molecular mimicry as a mechanism linking hCMV infection and SSc.[7] Cytomegalovirus is implicated in the pathogenesis of allograft vasculopathy, a complication of organ transplantation characterized by vascular neointima formation and smooth muscle cell proliferation strikingly reminiscent of the obliterative proliferative vasculopathy seen in SSc. In dermal fibroblasts, hCMV stimulates synthesis of the profibrotic growth factor connective tissue growth factor (CTGF, CCN2) in vitro.[8] Evidence of human parvovirus B19 infection has also been reported in patients with SSc.

ENVIRONMENTAL EXPOSURES, DIETARY SUPPLEMENTS, DRUGS AND RADIATION

Although reports of putative geographic clustering suggest a role for shared environmental exposures, careful investigations have generally failed to substantiate apparent clusters of SSc. On the other hand, well-documented epidemic outbreaks of SSc-like illnesses with acute onset and chronic course have been reported. One such illness, called the *toxic oil syndrome*, occurred in Spain and was linked to the ingestion of contaminated rapeseed cooking oils.[9] In the United States, dietary supplements containing L-tryptophan were implicated in an explosive outbreak of the eosinophilia-myalgia syndrome (EMS) in 1989.[10] The EMS epidemic subsided following the ban on L-tryptophan, but sporadic cases of EMS following ingestion of L-tryptophan and other food supplements continue to be reported. Although scleroderma-like skin fibrosis was a prominent manifestation of these apparently de novo toxicoepidemic syndromes, along with multisystem involvement, chronic course, and autoimmunity, the associated clinical, histopathologic, and laboratory features clearly differentiate them from SSc.[11] The frequency of SSc appears to be increased among men with occupational exposure to silica dust. This was recently confirmed by a meta-analysis of 16 observational studies, with risk estimates as high as 15.[12] Other exposures linked with SSc include polyvinyl chloride, toluene, xylene, trichloroethylene, and organic solvents. Additional reports

Table 83-2 Environmental Agents and Drugs Implicated in Scleroderma-like Syndromes

Chemicals
Silica
Heavy metals
Mercury
Organic chemicals
Vinyl chloride
Benzene
Toluene
Trichloroethylene
Drugs
Bleomycin
Pentazocine
Taxol
Cocaine
Dietary Supplement/Appetite Suppressants
L-tryptophan (contamination)
Mazindol
Fenfluramine
Diethylpropion

alleged an association between SSc and environmental exposures to pesticides, hair dyes, and industrial fumes. Although exposure to cigarette smoke is known to increase the risk of multiple autoimmune diseases, there is no evidence to date implicating it as a risk factor for SSc.

Certain drugs have been implicated in SSc-like illnesses. The best studied is the anticancer drug bleomycin, which induces skin and lung fibrosis in the mouse (see later). Other potentially implicated drugs include pentazocine, the taxenes docetaxel and paclitaxel, and cocaine. The use of appetite suppressants has been linked to the development of pulmonary arterial hypertension (PAH). The occurrence of SSc in women following cosmetic breast augmentation with silicone implants raised significant concern regarding a possible causal association.[13] Subsequent large-scale epidemiologic surveys and a meta-analysis, however, failed to confirm an increased risk of SSc or of other connective tissue diseases among women with silicone breast implants.[14] Radiation treatment for malignant neoplasms has been linked with the onset of de novo SSc, as well as exacerbation of tissue fibrosis in patients with pre-existing SSc.[15] Some of the environmental agents and drugs that have been linked with the development of SSc are listed in Table 83-2.

MICROCHIMERISM

Healthy women harbor immunologic stem cells of fetal origin that persist for many years following pregnancy, a condition called *microchimerism*. Some studies found that the number of circulating fetal cells is elevated in women with SSc compared with healthy women.[16,17] Moreover, cells with a male chromosome, presumably from a prior pregnancy with a male fetus, have been detected in affected organs from women with SSc. It has been speculated that persistence of fetal cells in SSc may be linked to the development of the disease through a graft-versus-host response triggered by the fetal cells or through a maternal (auto) immune response against the fetal cells.

PATHOLOGY

General Features

The pathologic hallmarks of SSc are a noninflammatory proliferative/obliterative vasculopathy affecting small arteries and arterioles in multiple vascular beds and interstitial and vascular fibrosis, most prominent in the skin, lungs, and heart.[18] Inflammation is generally absent in long-standing SSc, but in early-stage disease inflammatory cell infiltrates in many organs may be prominent. In the skin, the infiltrates are located predominantly around blood vessels and in the reticular dermis and are composed primarily of CD4+ T lymphocytes and monocytes, whereas in the lungs, cellular infiltrates consist predominantly of CD8+ T lymphocytes.

Vascular Pathology

Vascular injury and activation are the earliest and possibly primary events in SSc. Histopathologic evidence of vascular damage is present before fibrosis and can be detected in involved and uninvolved skin, indicating a generalized process.[19] Raynaud phenomenon and other vascular manifestations typically precede other manifestations of SSc. Additional signs of vasculopathy include cutaneous telangiectasia; nailfold capillary changes (giant capillaries, hemorrhages, and avascular areas); PAH; digital tip pitting; gastric antral vascular ectasia (also called *watermelon stomach*); and scleroderma renal crisis. The most characteristic histopathologic finding in the small and medium-sized arteries is bland intimal proliferation (Figure 83-2). Intimal hypertrophy, a finding that SSc shares with chronic allograft arteriopathy, is thought to result from proliferation and migration of myointimal cells and local accumulation

of collagen.[20] The vascular basement membranes are thickened and reduplicated. These changes are most prominent in blood vessels of the heart, lungs, kidneys, and gastrointestinal tract. A systematic survey of SSc skin biopsies revealed a marked reduction in the number of capillaries (rarefaction) and loss of vascular endothelial cadherin, a molecule required for vascular tube formation.[21] Remarkably, this study showed that clinical improvement following high-dose immunosuppressive therapy was accompanied by capillary regeneration in the skin.

Impaired fibrinolysis, increased levels of von Willebrand factor, and ongoing platelet aggregation are prominent. Endothelial cell injury itself causes further platelet aggregation, release of platelet-derived growth factor (PDGF) and endothelin-1 (ET-1), and endothelial cell apoptosis.[22] Vasculitic lesions and immune complex deposition in the vessel walls are uncommon. In late stages of the disease, extensive fibrin deposition and perivascular fibrosis cause progressive luminal occlusion, and eventually there is striking paucity of small blood vessels and capillaries in lesional tissue.[23] Loss of vascular supply leads to chronic tissue hypoxia. Widespread proliferative/obliterative vasculopathy of small and medium-sized arteries and capillary rarefaction are the pathologic hallmarks of all forms of SSc. In patients with SSc-associated PAH, pulmonary arteriolar intimal proliferation and evidence of veno-occlusive disease are prominent, whereas in contrast to idiopathic PAH, plexogenic arteriopathy does not occur.[24]

Tissue Fibrosis

Fibrosis is characterized by excessive accumulation of fibrillar collagens, fibronectin, elastin, proteoglycans, cartilage oligomeric matrix protein (COMP), and many other structural extracellular matrix (ECM) molecules. The process causes disruption and, ultimately, complete obliteration of tissue architecture. Most prominently affected are the lungs, gastrointestinal tract, heart, tendon sheath, and perifascicular tissue surrounding skeletal muscle. Histopathologic examination of these organs shows homogeneous and relatively acellular connective tissue with thick hyalinized collagen bundles.

ORGAN-SPECIFIC PATHOLOGIC FINDINGS

Skin

Fibrosis of the skin, the hallmark of SSc, is accompanied by marked expansion of the dermis with obliteration of the hair follicles, sweat glands, and sebaceous glands and other skin appendages. Collagen fiber accumulation is most prominent in the reticular (deep) dermis and progressively invades the subjacent adipose layer with entrapment of fat cells. Early-stage SSc skin biopsies reveal dermal edema and perivascular infiltrates composed of T lymphocytes and monocytes (Figure 83-3). Less commonly, mast cells and eosinophils may also be detected.[25,26] The proportion of α–smooth muscle actin–positive myofibroblasts, a mesenchymal cell type that is intermediate between fibroblasts and contractile smooth muscle cells and plays a major role in fibrogenesis, is increased in the lesional skin.[27] With

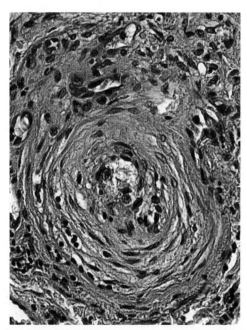

Figure 83-2 Histologic appearance of systemic sclerosis vasculopathy. A pulmonary arteriole showing extensive medial hypertrophy and intimal thickening, leading to narrowing of the vascular lumen.

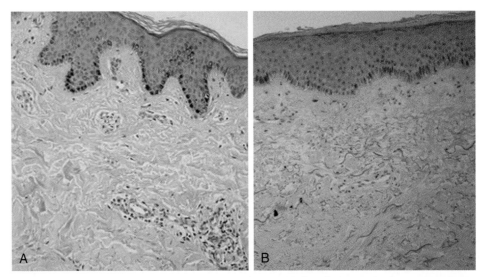

Figure 83-3 Histology of skin in diffuse cutaneous systemic sclerosis. There is perivascular infiltration in the dermis with inflammatory cells of multiple lineages. Microvascular endothelial cell activation and increased extracellular matrix deposition are also seen **(A).** Later there is regression of the inflammatory features. Secondary structures within the skin such as hair follicles and sebaceous and sweat glands are reduced, and rete pegs are flattened **(B).** H&E stain, original magnification ×40.

disease progression, the skin undergoes atrophy with loss of epidermal-dermal ridges and effacement of the rete pegs reminiscent of the changes seen in aging skin. The fibrotic dermis is largely acellular and contains dense accumulation of compact hyalinized collagen bundles, fibronectin, hyaluronic acid, and other structural proteins. Sweat glands and eccrine glands atrophy with loss of periglandular adipose tissue. The subcutaneous adipose layer is obliterated. In a double-blind study of 45 SSc skin biopsies, the histologic grade of skin fibrosis was found to closely correlate with the extent of clinical skin involvement.[28] Reduction in the number of dermal lymphatic vessels, which can be marked, contributes to interstitial fluid accumulation and edema.[29] Paucity of dermal capillaries (rarefaction) is associated with chronic tissue hypoxia that induces angiogenic factors such as vascular endothelial growth factor (VEGF). Evidence of tissue hypoxia can even be found in clinically uninvolved, apparently "normal" skin.[30]

Biochemical analysis shows that the collagens in the fibrotic dermis are normal, and relative proportions of the main fibrillar collagens (type I and type III) are comparable with those of normal skin.[31] In contrast, the minor nonfibrillar type VII collagen, normally restricted to the dermal-epidermal basement membrane zone, is abundant throughout the lesional dermis. The enzymes mediating post-translational collagen modification such as lysyl hydroxylase (PLOD2) are elevated, resulting in an increase in aldehyde-derived collagen cross-links, which may account for the dense sclerotic nature of the fibrotic dermis.[32]

Genome-wide expression profiling of lesional skin using DNA microarray technology provides an increasingly clearer understanding of the activation events that underlie fibrosis. Results from several studies reveal strikingly altered gene expression patterns in SSc skin biopsies compared with healthy controls. Remarkably, clinically involved and uninvolved skin appear to be indistinguishable in terms of their gene expression profiles. Many genes involved in ECM homeostasis and in transforming growth factor-β (TGF-β),

CCN2, IL-13, and Wnt signaling pathways show elevated expression.[33,34] Furthermore, a number of genes reflecting a bone/cartilage phenotype are elevated in the skin. A particularly intriguing finding from these studies is that skin biopsies from different individuals show marked heterogeneity at the level of their "molecular signature," with at least five distinct and reproducible patterns identified to date.[35]

Lungs

In early-stage SSc, the lungs show patchy infiltration of the alveolar walls with lymphocytes, plasma cells, macrophages, and eosinophils (Figure 83-4). At this stage, bronchoalveolar lavage fluid contains elevated proportions of inflammatory leukocytes. With progression, interstitial lung fibrosis

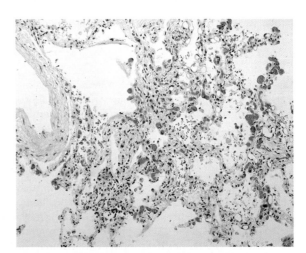

Figure 83-4 Histologic appearance of the lung. Evidence of intersitial lung disease is common in systemic sclerosis. Although there is substantial variation in the appearance of lung histology, consistent features include reduction in air spaces and thickening of alveolar walls with matrix deposition. Inflammatory cell infiltrates may be prominent. Lung biopsy is rarely required for diagnosis.

and vascular damage predominate, often coexisting within the same lesions. Intimal thickening of the pulmonary arteries, best seen with elastin stain, underlies PAH and at autopsy is often associated with multiple pulmonary emboli and myocardial fibrosis.

Lung fibrosis in SSc is characterized by expansion of the alveolar interstitium due to accumulation of collagens and other connective tissue proteins. The typical histologic pattern is nonspecific interstitial pneumonitis (NSIP), a form of interstitial lung disease characterized by mild to moderate interstitial inflammation, type II pneumocyte hyperplasia, and fairly uniform distribution of fibrosis. Less commonly, SSc is associated with the usual interstitial pneumonia (UIP) pattern that is characterized by scattered fibroblastic foci and patchy distribution of fibrosis and has a worse prognosis.[36] Progressive alveolar septal thickening ultimately results in obliteration of the air spaces and honeycombing, as well as consequent loss of pulmonary blood vessels. This process impairs gas exchange and contributes to worsening of pulmonary hypertension. Extensive pulmonary fibrosis may also predispose to primary lung carcinoma.

Gastrointestinal Tract

Prominent pathologic changes can occur at any level from the mouth to the rectum. The esophagus is virtually always affected, with fibrosis in the lamina propria, submucosa, and muscular layers and characteristic vascular lesions.[37] Replacement of the normal intestinal architecture results in disordered peristaltic activity, gastroesophageal reflux and small bowel dysmotility, pseudo-obstruction, and bacterial overgrowth. Chronic gastroesophageal reflux is complicated by esophageal inflammation, ulcerations, and stricture formation. Up to one-third of SSc patients with severe gastroesophageal reflux develop Barrett's esophagus, characterized by metaplasia of the normal squamous lining of the esophagus into columnar epithelium.[38] Because Barrett's metaplasia is a premalignant lesion associated with a greater than 30-fold increased risk of adenocarcinoma, patients with Barrett's esophagus need ongoing monitoring for dysplasia and adenocarcinoma.

Kidneys

In the kidneys vascular lesions predominate, and glomerulonephritis is rare except in overlap syndromes. Chronic renal ischemia is associated with shrunken glomeruli and other ischemic changes. Patients with acute scleroderma renal crisis show a thrombotic microangiopathy that is indistinguishable from other forms of malignant hypertension.[39] Histopathologic changes are most prominent in the small interlobular and arcuate renal arteries, which show reduplication of elastic lamina, marked intimal proliferation (onion skinning), and fibrinoid necrosis of the arteriolar walls.[40] Similar pathologic changes have also been reported in SSc patients who do not have renal crisis. Intimal thickening leads to severe narrowing and total obliteration of the lumen, often with microangiopathic hemolysis. Tubular changes such as flattening and degeneration of tubular cells occur secondary to vascular insufficiency. The clinical picture of scleroderma renal crisis may resemble thrombotic thrombocytopenic purpura (TTP). However, reduced to absent levels or activity of von Willebrand factor cleaving protease (ADAMTS13) has not been reported in scleroderma renal crisis. Figure 83-5 shows the characteristic histologic features associated with scleroderma renal crisis.

Heart

At autopsy, evidence of cardiac involvement is found in up to 80% of patients with SSc.[41] Modest pericardial effusions are common; occasionally fibrosis and constrictive pericarditis may occur. A characteristic pathologic finding is myocardial contraction band necrosis, which is thought to reflect repeated episodes of ischemia-reperfusion due to "myocardial Raynaud phenomenon."[42] Significant interstitial and perivascular fibrosis in the heart may occur in the absence of clinically evident heart involvement. Skeletal muscle myositis in SSc is occasionally accompanied by acute myocarditis.[43]

PATHOLOGIC FINDINGS IN OTHER ORGANS

Fibrosis of the thyroid glands is common. Broad bands of fibrous tissue are seen in the thyroid gland, with atrophy and obliteration of the follicles, in the absence of inflammation. Abnormal thyroid function tests and antithyroid antibodies are common. Erectile dysfunction is frequent and may be a presenting manifestation of the disease in men. Pathologic examination shows extensive proliferative/obliterative changes in the penile blood vessels.[44] Fibrosis of the salivary and lacrimal glands in the absence of inflammation can occur and may be associated with Sjögren's syndrome. Synovial biopsies show fibrosis and characteristic vascular changes in the small arterioles.[45]

ANIMAL MODELS OF SCLERODERMA

Animal models of human disease are indispensible research tools to facilitate the understanding of complex disease states. Such models are used to identify the cellular and molecular components of pathologic process, discover potential therapeutic targets, and develop and evaluate novel treatment strategies. A large number of putative SSc models have been reported, but to date none fully reproduce each of the four cardinal features of the disease: obliterative and proliferative microangiopathy, autoimmunity, inflammation, and fibrosis.[46] However, as illustrated in Figure 83-6, particular animal models recapitulate selected disease features. Broadly speaking, current mouse models can be divided into four types: (1) naturally occurring disease models, in which spontaneous mutations are associated with a genetically transmitted scleroderma-like phenotype such as tight skin (Tsk1/+ mouse); (2) induced models in which the scleroderma phenotype is elicited by chemical exposures or by manipulation of the immune system (bleomycin-induced skin and lung fibrosis); (3) transplantation of HLA-mismatched bone marrow cells resulting in chronic sclerodermatous graft-versus-host disease; and (4) genetic manipulations giving rise to engineered mouse strains with heritable scleroderma-like traits.

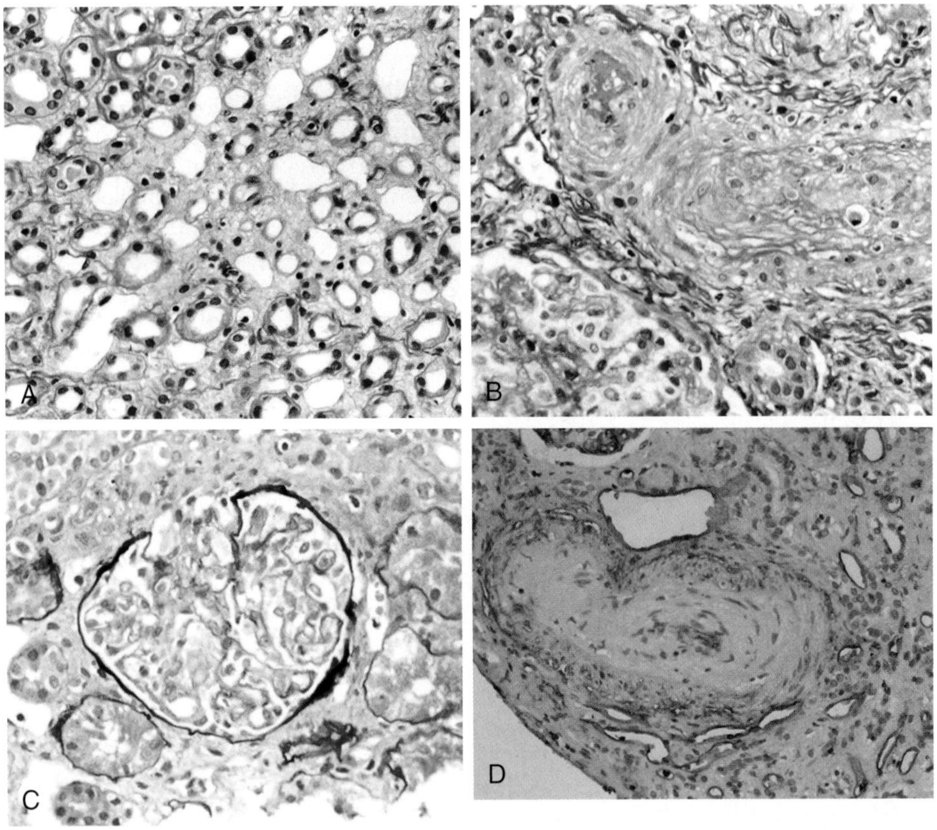

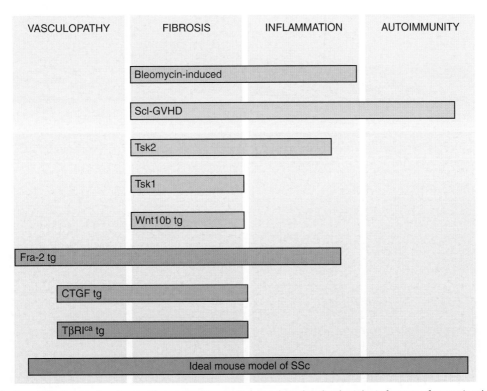

Figure 83-5 Histologic appearance of scleroderma renal crisis. Characteristic histologic findings include interstitial fibrosis **(A)** and occlusion of intrarenal arteries with neointima formation, fibrinoid necrosis of the vessel wall, and reduplication of the internal elastic lamina **(B)**. The glomeruli are shrunken and lack inflammatory cells or proliferative changes **(C)**. Intravascular thrombosis resembling the changes of thrombotic thrombocytopenic pupura may be present **(D)**.

Figure 83-6 Animal models of systemic sclerosis. Mouse models recapitulate selected pathophysiologic features of systemic sclerosis (SSc). Shown are the principal disease processes of SSc (inflammation, autoimmunity, microangiopathy, and fibrosis) and the extent to which they are represented in commonly used mouse models. CTGF, connective tissue growth factor; GVHD, graft-versus-host disease; tg, transgenic. *(Modified from Distler JH, Distler O, Beyer C, Schett G: Animal models of systemic sclerosis: prospects and limitations,* Arthritis Rheum *62(10):2831–2844, 2010.)*

Heritable Animal Models of Scleroderma

The Tsk1/+ mouse is characterized by diffuse skin thickening and tethering to the underlying subcutaneous tissue. Mice homozygous for the Tsk1 mutation die in utero at 8 to 10 days of gestation. However, heterozygous mice (Tsk1/+) survive and develop tight skin. In contrast to SSc, Tsk1/+ mice show prominent subcutaneous hyperplasia but relatively unremarkable dermis.[47] Furthermore, the lungs of Tsk1/+ mice show emphysematous changes rather than fibrosis, and microangiopathy has not been reported. Although inflammation is uncommon, Tsk1/+ mice develop autoantibodies directed against topoisomerase-I. The Tsk1 mutation is now known to be an intragenic tandem duplication fibrillin-1 gene.[48] Fibrillin-1 is a large ECM protein that is widely distributed in microfibrils, and in addition to its structural role also modulates the latency and activation of TGF-β.[49] Fibrillin-1 gene mutations are associated with Marfan's disease with multiple tissues showing activation of TGF-β. The fibrillin-1 duplication mutation in Tsk1/+ mice gives rise to an abnormally large 450-kD protein. No corresponding fibrillin-1 mutations have been demonstrated in patients with SSc. Although it has been hypothesized that accumulation of the abnormally large mutant fibrillin-1 destabilizes the matrix[50] or perturbs the homeostatic control of TGF-β latency, the precise mechanisms linking the Tsk1/+ mutation in fibrillin-1 to the development of cutaneous hyperplasia are unknown.

Another animal model of scleroderma is the Tsk2 mouse that spontaneously develops scleroderma-like skin changes by 3 to 4 weeks of age.[51] In contrast to Tsk1/+ mice, Tsk2/+ mice have fibrotic dermis with extensive infiltration with mononuclear inflammatory cells and show evidence of autoimmunity. The Tsk2 mutation, originally induced in normal mice by exposure to ethylnitrosourea, is located on chromosome 1 and is inherited as an autosomal dominant trait, although the underlying molecular defect has not yet been identified.

Inducible Animal Models of Scleroderma

Chronic skin and lung fibrosis (Figure 83-7) can be induced in BALB/c or C57 mice by subcutaneous injections of bleomycin or oxidative agents. Bleomycin is an antitumor

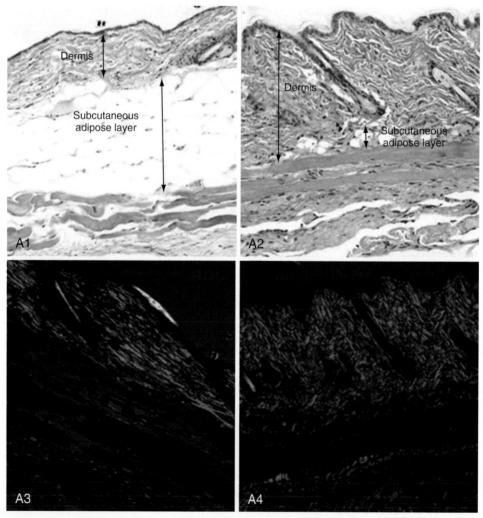

Figure 83-7 Bleomycin-induced mouse model of systemic sclerosis. Mice received subcutaneous injection of PBS (**A1, A3**) or bleomycin (**A2, A4**) for 28 days. **A1-A4,** Skin changes. **A1** and **A2,** H&E stain; **A3** and **A4,** Sirius red stain. Note dermal fibrosis and loss of subcutaneous adipose layer (**A2**), and increased collagen accumulation (**A4**).

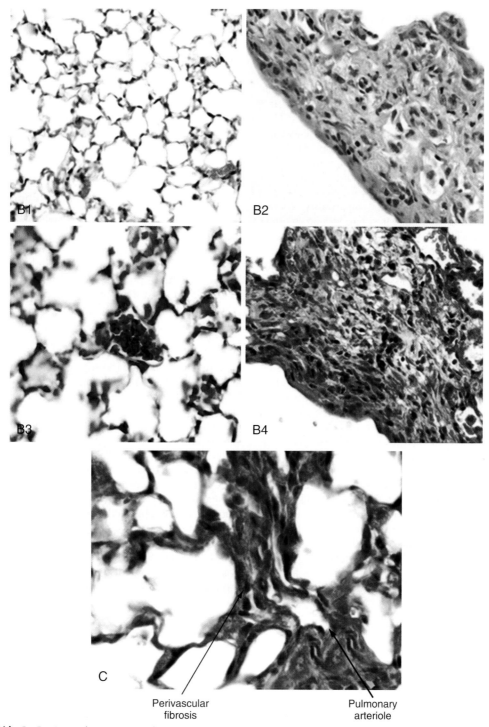

Figure 83-7, cont'd   B1-B4, Lung changes. **B1** and **B2,** H&E stain; **B3** and **B4,** Trichrome stain. Note dense lung fibrosis obliterating the alveolar parenchyma **(B2, B4). C,** Perivascular fibrosis in pulmonary arteriole. *(Courtesy D. Melichian.)*

chemotherapy drug that has long been recognized to be complicated by pulmonary fibrosis. The sequence of bleomycin-induced histopathologic changes in mice closely resembles those seen in SSc: early and self-limited mononuclear cell infiltration and increased expression of cytokines such as TGF-β, IL-4, IL-6, IL-13, and monocyte chemotactic protein-1 (MCP-1), followed by the appearance of dermal fibrosis with excessive collagen deposition and accumulation of α–smooth muscle actin–positive myofibroblasts.[52] Bleomycin-induced fibrosis may be linked to reactive oxygen species (ROS) generation, as well as direct activation of innate immunity via TLR2. In contrast to SSc, bleomycin-induced mouse scleroderma is not associated with either microangiopathic changes or autoantibodies and skin fibrosis is limited in extent and duration. Nevertheless, in light of its reproducibility, relative strain independence, and ease of induction, this mouse model is widely used for investigating specific molecules and pathways in the development and treatment of fibrosis. Injection of oxidative agents (such as hydroxyl radicals or hypochlorite) into the skin in BALB/c mice induces skin and lung fibrosis, as well as the appearance of SSc-specific autoantibodies.[53] The pathologic changes are linked to the generation of hydrogen peroxide and other ROS. Subcutaneous injection of TGF-β induces granulation tissue and only transient fibrosis, but simultaneous injection of CTGF along with TGF-β results in persistent fibrosis, suggesting that CTGF is required for sustaining the fibrotic response. However, adenovirus-mediated delivery of constitutively active TGF-β receptor I is sufficient to induce local dermal fibrosis. Transplantation of bone marrow or spleen cells into sublethally irradiated minor histocompatibility locus–mismatched recipient mice results in sclerodermatous graft-versus-host disease. This mouse model displays interstitial and perivascular fibrosis in the skin and lung and autoimmunity.[54] Skin fibrosis is preceded by mononuclear cell infiltration with elevated TGF-β and chemokine expression.

Genetic Manipulations in Mice Giving Rise to Scleroderma-like Phenotypes

Mouse strains with genetic gain-of-function or loss-of-function modifications resulting in spontaneous scleroderma-like phenotypes have been created. These transgenic, knockin, and knockout mice provide robust novel experimental tools in scleroderma research. Mouse strains with constitutive or inducible expression of TGF-β signaling in fibroblasts recapitulate key clinical, histologic, and biochemical features of SSc and provide support for the role of perturbed TGF-β signaling in pathogenesis.[55,56] Other promising transgenic models of SSc include mice overexpressing CTGF, PDGF receptor (PDGFR)-α, Wnt10b, and Fra-2 and mice null for caveolin-1, relaxin, Fli-1, and fetuin A.[57] Scleroderma-like fibrotic, vascular, and calcific changes in the skin, as well as in some cases the lungs, develop spontaneously in these mice. Other genetically engineered mice show increased sensitivity to the induction of fibrosis. Examples include T-bet null and VEGF null mice. These emerging mouse models provide new exciting research opportunities for the discovery of molecules and pathways underlying the pathogenetic features of SSc.

PATHOGENESIS

Integrated Overview

The pathogenesis of SSc is complex, and existing animal models capture only some of its diverse pathologic and clinical attributes. An integrated view of pathogenesis must integrate the cardinal features of SSc: vascular injury and damage, inflammation with activation of the innate and adaptive arms of the immune system, and fibroblast activation resulting in generalized interstitial and vascular fibrosis. Although evidence for each can be found in each SSc patient, the relative individual contribution of these processes to the clinical manifestations varies from one patient to another. As illustrated in Figure 83-1, complex and dynamic interplay between these distinct processes is thought to be responsible for initiating, amplifying, and sustaining tissue damage in SSc.[58]

Vasculopathy

Vascular injury is likely to be the initiating and proximal event in SSc (see Figure 83-5). Evidence of vascular involvement is early and widespread, and its progression over time is associated with significant clinical sequelae. The presence of nailfold microvascular changes, detected by capillaroscopy, in an individual with isolated Raynaud phenomenon identifies an elevated risk of progression to SSc, indicating that microvasculopathy precedes other clinical manifestations of the disease.

Vascular Injury and the Activated Endothelium

The initial vascular insult is triggered by circulating factors such as (unidentified) cytotoxic molecules or T cell–derived proteolytic granzymes.[59] Other potential causes of vascular injury include antiendothelial cell autoantibodies, vasculotropic viruses, inflammatory cytokines, ROS, and other forms of environmental stress. Vascular injury causes endothelial cell activation, with increased expression of vascular endothelial cell adhesion molecule-1 and E-selectin, altered secretion of vasoactive mediators, platelet activation, and activation of the thrombotic and fibrinolytic cascades.[60] In the injured arterioles and capillaries, activated endothelial cells may undergo transdifferentiation to mesenchymal cells via a process termed *endothelial-mesenchymal transition*. This process driven by TGF-β and Notch is associated with loss of endothelial markers such as CD31 and progressive acquisition of mesenchymal markers such as α–smooth muscle actin. Although endothelial-mesenchymal transition has been documented in cancer, recent studies identify endothelial cell-derived fibroblasts in cardiac and pulmonary fibrosis, suggesting that this form of endothelial cell plasticity may also play a role in SSc. Platelet activation is a prominent early feature of vascular injury in SSc and is associated with the release of thromboxane A_2, PDGF, and TGF-β, which potentiate vasoconstriction and also contribute to fibroblast activation and myofibroblast transdifferentiation. Pericytes, which are smooth muscle–like structural cells found in the walls of small blood vessels, show marked hyperplasia in lesional skin from patients with early-stage SSc and express the surface marker Thy-1 (CD90) and receptors for PDGF.[61,62]

Functional abnormalities of the vascular endothelium include impaired production of and responsiveness to endothelium-derived vasodilatory factors such as nitric oxide (NO), thrombomodulin, calcitonin gene-related peptide, and prostacyclins. The ensuing imbalance of vasodilators and vasoconstrictors impairs blood flow responses. Recurrent episodes of ischemia-reperfusion create oxidative stress with the generation of H_2O_2 and other ROS. Damaged microvessels show increased vascular permeability and enhanced transendothelial leukocyte migration. Platelets are exposed to subendothelial structures, which further aggravates platelet aggregation. Activated endothelial cells release the extremely potent vasoconstrictor ET-1, which promotes leukocyte adhesion, vascular smooth muscle cell proliferation, and fibroblast activation (Figure 83-8). Levels of ET-1 are elevated in the blood and in bronchoalveolar lavage fluids from patients with SSc.[63] Ultimately

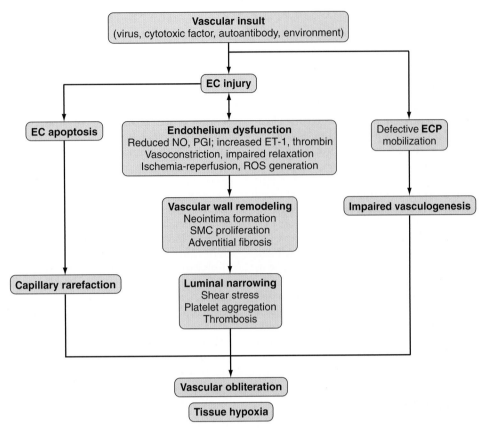

Figure 83-8 Pathogenesis of vasculopathy. Initial vascular insult results in endothelial cell (EC) injury and activation, with reversible functional changes, increased expression of adhesion molecules, and enhanced leukocyte diapedesis resulting in perivascular inflammation. Damaged endothelium promotes platelet aggregation and thrombin release and shows impaired production of vasodilators such as nitric oxide (NO), increased production of vasoconstrictors such as endothelin-1 (ET-1), and release of reactive oxygen species (ROS). Consequent vasoconstriction and defective vasodilation aggravate vascular damage, leading to irreversible and progressive vascular wall remodeling, luminal occlusion, platelet aggregation, in situ thrombosis, and tissue hypoxia. Loss of blood vessels may be further compounded by insufficient vasculogenesis. ECP, endothelial cell progenitor; PGI, prostaglandin I; SMC, smooth muscle cell.

fibrinolytic and coagulation cascades are activated, culminating in intravascular fibrin deposition and thrombosis.

Vascular Damage and Vasculogenesis

In the medium-sized and larger vessels a combination of hypertrophy of the intimal and medial layers and adventitial fibrosis causes progressive luminal narrowing. Together with endothelial cell apoptosis, the process culminates in obliterative vasculopathy and vascular rarefaction, with the characteristic striking decrease of blood vessels seen angiographically in late-stage SSc. Loss of microvasculature results in reduced blood flow and chronic tissue hypoxia, which induces hypoxia-inducible factor-1 (HIF-1) α-dependent genes such as VEGF and its receptors. There is substantial controversy regarding the balance of proangiogenic and antiangiogenic factors in SSc. In some studies, the plasma levels of the angiogenesis inhibitor endostatin, a degradation product of type XVIII collagen, were reported to be increased.[64] Other studies, however, found elevated levels of the proangiogenic factors VEGF, fibroblast growth factor, and PDGF. Furthermore, the expression of VEGF and its receptors was also elevated in lesional tissue.[65,66] It is currently unclear why, in the face of tissue hypoxia and elevated angiogenic factors, SSc is associated with progressive loss of blood vessels. Recent studies implicate defective vasculogenesis as a potential explanation. A reduction in the number of bone marrow-derived circulating endothelial progenitor cells and their impaired differentiation into mature endothelial cells has been described in SSc patients.[67-69] Because CD34+ circulating endothelial progenitor cells are required for physiologic vasculogenesis in ischemic tissues, defective progenitor cell mobilization or function compromises the vascular repair. Whether the reduction in circulating endothelial progenitor cells in SSc is due to "exhaustion" of the bone marrow, destruction in the peripheral circulation or some other process, remains unresolved.

Hypoxia

The widespread microangiopathy and resultant capillary loss in affected tissues leads to decreased blood flow and consequent hypoxia. With the onset of fibrosis, excessive ECM accumulation increases diffusion distance from blood vessels to cells, further aggravating tissue hypoxia.[70] Hypoxia is a potent inducer of the basic helix-loop-helix transcription factors HIF-1α and HIF-1β. Under normoxic conditions, cellular HIF-1α is undetectable due to its rapid and efficient proteasomal degradation mediated by the tumor suppressor von Hippel-Lindau (vHL) protein. Because in hypoxic cells pVHL is unable to bind to its target, HIF-1α

is protected from degradation and translocates into the nucleus, binds to hypoxia-responsive DNA regulatory sequences, and induces the transcription of hypoxia-regulated genes involved in erythropoiesis, angiogenesis, and glucose metabolism. Hypoxia is also a potent in vitro and in vivo stimulus for ECM remodeling genes such as collagens, prolyl hydroxylases, and lysyl oxidase and promotes epithelial cell differentiation into activated myofibroblasts.[71,72] These and other hypoxia-induced profibrogenic responses are partially mediated by autocrine TGF-β. A recent paper provides compelling experimental support for the role of hypoxia in exacerbating fibrosis.[73] In this study, mice with myeloid-cell-specific deletion of VEGF showed markedly increased tissue hypoxia and activated Wnt–β-catenin signaling upon bleomycin-induced lung injury, culminating in striking exacerbation of fibrosis.

The presence of severe tissue hypoxia in SSc has been documented noninvasively, and oxygen levels in the skin were shown to inversely correlate with skin thickness. In another study using a needle electrode inserted into the dermis, SSc patients exhibited significantly reduced levels of PO_2 (23.7 mm Hg vs. 33.6 mm Hg in controls). Interestingly, HIF-1α in the lesional skin was undetectable, rather than elevated, as is the case with the hypoxia-inducible VEGF.

Oxidative Stress and Reactive Oxygen Species

Oxidative stress and elevated levels of ROS are implicated in the pathogenesis of SSc.[74] ROS might be generated from the endothelium in response to repeated episodes of ischemia reperfusion. Normal fibroblasts exposed to TGF-β or to stimulatory PDGFR autoantibodies generate ROS, whereas explanted SSc skin fibroblasts spontaneously produce excessive amounts of ROS via the membrane NADPH oxidase Nox4.[75] Hydrogen peroxide and other oxygen free radicals in turn stimulate collagen synthesis, TGF-β secretion, and other fibrotic responses in fibroblasts. A role for ROS in pathogenesis is further supported by a

mouse model of scleroderma induced by subcutaneous injections of peroxynitrite or hypochlorite.[53]

IMMUNE DYSREGULATION

Introduction

A resurgence of interest in understanding the role of immune dysregulation in the pathogenesis of SSc is occurring. Both the innate and adaptive arms of the immune system are activated in early SSc, and autoimmunity manifested by highly specific and mutually exclusive autoantibodies is prominent throughout the course of the disease. Lesional tissues show prominent perivascular accumulation of mononuclear inflammatory cells, whereas circulating leukocytes (including T cells, B cells, monocytes, and dendritic cells) show evidence of activation and polarization and display the "type I interferon signature" associated with SLE and other autoimmune diseases (Figure 83-9). The strong genetic associations between SSc and HLA Class II locus polymorphisms provide support for the immunologic basis of SSc. Nevertheless, whether immune dysregulation is a primary or significant factor in SSc pathogenesis still remains to be established. Current clinical trials are evaluating the efficacy of myeloablative therapy followed by hematopoietic reconstitution as a therapeutic strategy to "reset the immune system" in SSc.

Cellular Effectors of Immune Dysregulation in Scleroderma: T Cells, B Cells, and Monocytes/Macrophages

T Cell Activation

Activation of T cells is evident in lesional tissues, as well as in peripheral blood, and appears to play a direct role in tissue injury. In early SSc, activated CD4 and CD8 T lymphocytes and monocytes/macrophages, and less commonly B cells, eosinophils, mast cells and NK cells, are observed

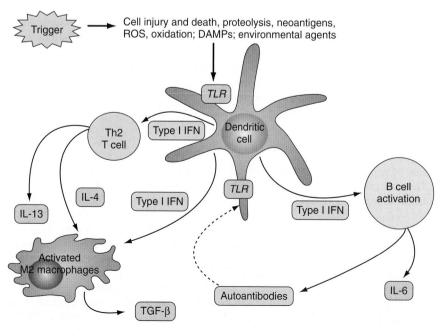

Figure 83-9 Complex immune dysregulation in scleroderma. An inciting event such as infection, oxidative damage, necrotic/apoptotic cell debris, or environmental toxins causes activation of dendritic cells, possibly via Toll-like receptors (TLRs). Activated dendritic cells produce type I interferon (IFN), which causes Th2 T cell polarization, monocyte differentiation to an alternately activated (M2) phenotype, and B cell activation with plasma cell maturation and production of autoantibodies. Autoantibodies form immune complexes that in turn further induce type I IFN production via TLR signaling. Th2-polarized T cells and M2 macrophages secrete profibrotic chemokines and cytokines, inducing fibroblast activation. Additional T cell subsets such as Tregs and Th17 may also be involved. DAMPs, damage-associated molecular patterns; IL, interleukin; ROS, reactive oxygen species; TGF-β, transforming growth factor-β.

in perivascular regions in the lesional skin, lungs, and other affected organs; these inflammatory cell infiltrates are detectable before the appearance of fibrosis.[76] In situ hybridization studies show prominent procollagen gene expression in early-stage SSc skin in fibroblasts that are adjacent to inflammatory cells, suggesting a role for the inflammatory cells or their soluble products in inducing fibroblast activation.[77] The extent of lymphocytic tissue infiltration correlates with the severity and progression of skin fibrosis.

Tissue-infiltrating T cells are predominantly CD3+ and CD4+ and express activation markers CD69, CD45, HLA-DR, and the IL-2 receptor. These T cells display restricted T cell receptor signatures indicative of oligoclonal T cell expansion in response to an as-yet unidentified antigen.[78] In the lungs, a predominance of CD8+ and γ/δ T cells is observed.[79] It is not known whether T cells in lesional tissue are activated nonspecifically (by cytokines or chemokines) or specifically in response to an antigen. Evidence of T cell activation in SSc is also detected in the peripheral blood, with elevated serum levels of IL-2 and IL-2 receptor expression, and spontaneous cytokine secretion. Peripheral blood lymphocytes show the "IFN signature" defined by the upregulation of type I IFN-inducible genes.[80-82] Increased expression of LFA-1 and α1 integrins may enable T cells to adhere directly to endothelium and fibroblasts. Circulating CD4+ T cells also express elevated chemokine receptors. At the same time, vascular endothelial cells express ICAM-1, E-selectin, and other adhesion molecules that facilitate leukocyte diapedesis.

Th1/Th2 Cytokine Balance and Polarized Immune Responses

Evidence implicates an altered balance between T helper (Th)1 and Th2 cytokines in fibrosis. T cells polarized to a Th2 pattern secrete abundant IL-4, IL-5, and IL-13, with only low levels of the hallmark Th1 cytokine IFN-γ. The Th2 cytokines are considered to be profibrogenic because they can directly stimulate collagen synthesis and myofibroblast transdifferentiation, as well as induce TGF-β, a powerful modulator of immune regulation and ECM accumulation. In contrast, IFN-γ blocks these responses and exerts antifibrotic effects. Thus skewing of the immune response toward a Th2 pattern could create a profibrotic environment.

Animal studies support the significance of a Th2-polarized immune response in fibrosis. For example, T cells that have been Th2 polarized in vitro induce fibrosis when passively transferred in mice. Moreover, mice lacking the transcription factor T-bet, which directs T cell differentiation of T cells toward a Th1-predominant phenotype, spontaneously show a Th2-polarized immune response and develop exaggerated skin fibrosis in response to bleomycin.[83,84]

Patients with SSc display an altered Th1/Th2 cytokine balance with a predominant Th2 profile. For example, both the serum levels of IFN-γ and in vitro IFN-γ production by peripheral blood monocytes are reduced. Microarray analysis of SSc peripheral blood leukocytes showed elevated expression of GATA3, a transcription factor controlling Th2 polarization. Cloned CD4+ T cells from SSc skin biopsies secrete IL-4 but not IFN-γ.[85] T cell lines generated from SSc skin biopsies show prominent CD8 expression and produce high levels of IL-4. Similarly, alveolar CD8+ T cells

show elevated Th2 cytokine production, and the Th2 predominance predicts accelerated decline in lung function.[86] By analyzing the ratio of chemokine receptors associated with Th1 versus Th2 responses, peripheral blood T cells in SSc were shown to have a Th2-predominant pattern that predicted the presence and progression of interstitial lung disease.[87] Proteomic and DNA microarray analysis demonstrated a Th2 cytokine predominance in SSc bronchoalveolar lavage fluids and CD8+ lymphocytes. A longitudinal study of SSc patients showed that skin improvement over time was associated with a decline in serum levels of Th2 cytokines and a concomitant increase in IL-12, a Th1 cytokine.[88]

Other T Cell Subsets

The Th17 subset of T lymphocytes is implicated in the pathogenesis of rheumatoid arthritis and other inflammatory diseases. SSc patients have increased numbers of IL-17 producing CD4+ T cells in both the peripheral blood and bronchoalveolar lavage fluid.[89] Patterns of Th1, Th2, and Th17 predominant immune responses might be useful in identifying specific clinical phenotypes in SSc.

Suppressor regulatory T cells (Tregs) are important in controlling autoimmunity. Interestingly, although the frequency of peripheral blood Treg cells was increased in SSc patients, they showed impaired suppressive activity and secretion of TGF-β and IL-10.[90] Other studies failed to replicate these findings but demonstrated reduced numbers of Foxp3+ CD4+ T cells in the lesional skin compared with other inflammatory skin diseases.

Monocytes and Macrophages

Phagocytic monocytes and macrophages regulate innate immunity and tissue repair. Monocytes are a major source of cytokines and chemokines including IL-1, tumor necrosis factor (TNF), MCP-1, PDGF, and TGF-β, all of which are important in inflammatory and fibroproliferative responses. In addition, monocytes produce collagenases and other matrix-degrading enzymes that mediate tissue remodeling. Macrophages are prominent among the mononuclear cells infiltrating the lesional skin in early SSc and express Siglec-1 and AIF-1, markers of IFN-induced activation. Macrophages exhibit discrete phenotypes in response to specific stimuli, with alternatively activated (M2) macrophages induced in response to IL-4 and TGF-β secreting profibrotic mediators. M2 macrophages accumulate in various organs in animal models of fibrosis, and may be important in pathogenesis. In SSc patients with active lung disease, alveolar macrophages show an M2 phenotype characterized by secretion of profibrotic mediators TGF-β, PDGF, and IL-13. Evidence of local mast cell and eosinophil activation and degranulation is sometimes prominent in lesional skin.

Dendritic Cells

These potent antigen-presenting cells found in the skin and circulation bridge innate and adaptive immunity, and by modulating T cell, B cell, and monocyte/macrophage function shape the immune response (see Figure 83-9).

Dendritic cells are the major source of type I IFN and can also secrete fibrogenic cytokines including TGF-β. Recent studies show that CD11c+ dendritic cells accumulate in fibrotic tissue in animal models and in patients with SSc. Activated dendritic cells in the lesional tissue might directly or indirectly modulate resident fibroblast activation. Moreover, monocyte-derived dendritic cells from the peripheral blood in SSc show altered in vitro responses to TLR2/3 ligands and increased secretion of IL-6 and IL-10, which favors a Th2 skewing of the immune response.[91]

AUTOIMMUNITY

Autoantibodies in Scleroderma: Pathogenetic Considerations

Humoral autoimmunity, manifested by the presence of autoantibodies with multiple antigenic specificities, can be detected in the serum in virtually all patients. The presence of SSc autoantibodies has significant utility in diagnosis and classification, as well as in predicting organ-specific complications and clinical course. In contrast, a direct role of autoantibodies in tissue damage has not been conclusively established. Autoantibodies in SSc tend to be highly specific and mutually exclusive, and they show strong association with individual disease phenotypes and immunogenetic backgrounds. The levels of autoantibodies, particularly antitopoisomerase I, may correlate with the extent of skin and lung fibrosis and fluctuate with disease activity.

Various hypotheses exist to explain the generation of autoantibodies in SSc. According to one hypothesis, self-antigens such as topoisomerase I undergo proteolytic cleavage in the presence of ROS, resulting in exposure of normally cryptic epitopes and break in immune tolerance.[92] Other potential mechanisms include molecular mimicry as a consequence of viral infection, chronic B cell hyperreactivity, and increased expression or altered subcellular localization of potential autoantigenic peptides. Alternately, SSc autoantibodies might be generated from B cells activated by endogenous TLR7 ligands such as nucleic acid–containing cellular debris.

Several reports describe biologically active autoantibodies directed against ECM components, cell membrane PDGF receptors, fibroblasts, and endothelial cells in SSc patients. Stimulatory autoantibodies can induce target cell activation or apoptosis in vitro.[93,94] In one study, autoantibodies against the PDGF receptor were detected in each of the SSc patients evaluated in one study and shown to induce ROS generation and multiple signaling cascades in normal skin fibroblasts, resulting in myofibroblast differentiation. It is not yet known whether these autoantibodies precede, or are a consequence of, fibrosis, and their direct pathogenetic role in SSc remains to be established.

B Cells in Scleroderma

Recent studies provide evidence for a potential direct role for B lymphocytes in the pathogenesis of SSc. B cells have multiple immune regulatory functions in addition to the generation of antibodies including antigen presentation, cytokine production, lymphoid organogenesis, and T cell differentiation. Although B cells are not generally prominent in microscopic sections of lesional tissue, DNA microarray analyses demonstrated a molecular signature indicative of activated B cells with increased expression of immunoglobulin genes in some SSc skin biopsies. B cells were also prominent in SSc lung biopsies.[95] Patients with SSc display intrinsic abnormalities of B cells, with elevated numbers of naïve B cells, and reduced numbers of plasma cells.[96] Memory B cells are chronically activated and display increased CD95 and CD86, as well as CD19, a signaling cell surface receptor that regulates intrinsic and antigen receptor–induced B cell responses. Transgenic mice overexpressing CD19 develop spontaneous autoimmunity and high titers of antitopoisomerase I antibodies. Altered B cell function and chronic B cell activation in SSc may not only account for autoantibody production but also contribute to fibrosis because activated B cells secrete IL-6, which directly stimulates fibroblast activation and collagen synthesis. Patients with SSc also have elevated levels of the potent B cell survival factor B cell activating factor belonging to the TNF family (BAFF) in the serum and in lesional skin, as well as increased BAFF receptor expression on B cells. In light of the emerging role of B cells in the pathogenesis of SSc, therapies targeting B cells are under consideration.

Type I Interferon Signature and Innate Immune Signaling: Similarities to Systemic Lupus Erythematosus

Stimulation of denditic cells and other cell types by ligands of TLR3 results in robust secretion of type I IFN. Accordingly, the presence of IFN or IFN-induced cellular responses suggests TLR-mediated innate immune signaling. Type I IFNs (α and β) are themselves potent modulators of innate immunity. Elevated expression of IFN-regulated genes (the "IFN signature") was first described in SLE patients.[97] Circulating immune complexes containing antinucleic acid autoantibodies serve as endogenous TLR3 ligands that stimulate type I IFN secretion by dendritic cells and macrophages. Similar to SLE, an IFN signature has been detected in circulating leukocytes from SSc patients. Indeed, a recent study reported that the most highly expressed genes in SSc peripheral blood leukocytes were IFN regulated and similar to those detected in SLE.[81] Moreover, incubation of normal leukocytes with SSc sera induced the secretion of IFN, indicative of TLR3 activation by nucleic acid–containing immune complexes in the serum.[98] Interestingly, serum levels of IFN are only inconsistently elevated in SSc. These observations identify an important role for TLR-mediated innate immune signaling and type I IFNs in SSc and highlight immunopathogenic similarities between SLE and SSc, but they fail to explain why these two related autoimmune diseases display largely nonoverlapping clinical phenotypes. The direct pathogenetic role of type I IFN in the development of microangiopathy and fibrosis in SSc remains to be established.

FIBROSIS

Overview

Fibrosis, characterized by replacement of normal tissue architecture with stiff paucicellular connective tissue, is

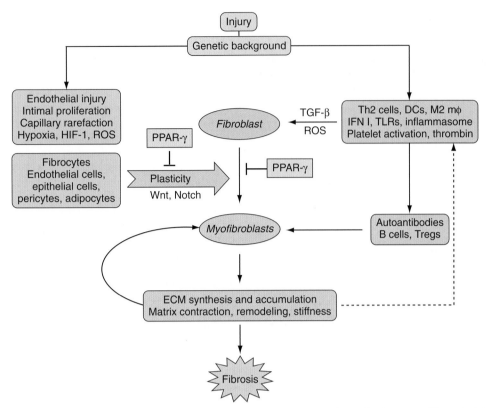

Figure 83-10 Pathogenesis of fibrosis. Fibrosis is the end result of immune dysregulation and vascular damage and hypoxia. Injury causes vascular damage, perivascular inflammation, and innate immune signaling, with oxidative stress, secretion of inflammatory and fibrogenic cytokines and chemokines, autoantibodies, fibroblast activation, and myofibroblast accumulation. Circulating mesenchymal progenitor cells traffic to and accumulate within the lesional tissue and transdifferentiate into fibrotic fibroblasts, accelerating matrix accumulation. Tissue hypoxia, matrix remodeling, and stiffness further contribute to fibroblast activation, which causes disruption of tissue architecture and organ failure. DCs, dendritic cells; ECM, extracellular matrix; HIF-1, hypoxia-inducible factor-1; IFN, interferon; PPAR-γ, peroxisome proliferator-activated receptor-γ; ROS, reactive oxygen species; TGF-β, transforming growth factor-β; TLRs, Toll-like receptors.

the pathologic hallmark of SSc and can be viewed as a form of aberrant wound healing. Fibrosis represents the end result of a complex series of vascular and immune-mediated responses to injury in a genetically predisposed individual. As illustrated in Figure 83-10, injured or activated vascular and immune cells produce soluble mediators, autoantibodies, and ROS that induce the activation and differentiation of mesenchymal effector cells, culminating in excessive and ultimately irreversible ECM accumulation and remodeling.

Extracellular Matrix

The ECM consists of a cellular compartment of resident fibroblasts and myofibroblasts and infiltrating cells, as well as connective tissue composed of large structural proteins such as collagens, proteoglycans, fibrillins, and adhesion molecules. The ECM also serves as a reservoir for sequestering growth factors and matricellular proteins that, together with the connective tissue compartment, control the differentiation, function, and survival of mesenchymal cells. Excessive connective tissue accumulation results from overproduction by fibroblasts activated by soluble factors, hypoxia, and ROS; signals from the surrounding ECM; or via cell-cell interactions. Impaired matrix degradation and turnover, as well as expansion of the pool of ECM-producing mesenchymal cells, also play roles.

Regulation of Collagen Synthesis

The family of collagens is composed of more than two dozen structural proteins with critical roles in organ development, growth, and differentiation. The ECM of the skin, bones, and tendons is composed largely of type I collagen, with smaller amounts of associated type III collagen. Type II collagen is found mainly in articular cartilage. The fibrillar collagens consist of three α chains wound into a characteristic triple helix, a structure made possible by the presence of a glycine at every third residue of repeating Gly-X-Y sequence, where X is frequently a proline and Y is frequently a hydroxyproline. During their biosynthesis, fibrillar collagens undergo extensive enzymatic modifications inside the cell and additional processing following their secretion. Covalent cross-linking stabilizes the collagen fiber network in the extracellular space.

Type I collagen synthesis is regulated by cytokines and other soluble extracellular factors, ROS, hypoxia, and cell-cell and cell-matrix contact (Table 83-3). Environmental cues allow fibroblasts to respond to dynamic tissue requirements during development and tissue repair. The genes encoding the various collagens harbor cis-acting regulatory elements that are specifically recognized by DNA-binding transcription factors. Sp1, Ets1, Smad2/3, Egr-1, and CCAAT-binding factor (CBF) stimulate, and Sp3, C/EBP, YB1, c-Krox, and Fli-1 suppress transcription.[99] These

Table 83-3 Extracellular Factors Potentially Contributing to the Pathogenesis of Fibrosis in Systemic Sclerosis

Signal	Cellular Source
TGF-β	Inflammatory cells (macrophages, T cells), platelets, fibroblasts
PDGF	Platelets, macrophages, fibroblasts, endothelial cells
CTGF/CCN2	Fibroblasts
IGF-1	Fibroblasts
IL-1α	Keratinocytes
IL-4, IL-13	Th2 lymphocytes, mast cells
IL-6	Macrophages, B cells, T cells, fibroblasts
Chemokines (MCP-1, MCP-3)	Neutrophils, epithelial cells, endothelial cells, fibroblasts
Fibroblast growth factor	Fibroblasts
ET-1	Endothelial cells
Wnt ligands	Developmental pathway aberrantly reactivated
Notch/Jagged	Developmental pathway aberrantly reactivated
Hypoxia	Hypoxic underperfused tissue
ROS	Generated from ischemia reperfusion

CTGF, connective tissue growth factor; ET-1, endothelin-1; IGF-1, insulin-like growth factor-1; IL, interleukin; MCP, monocyte chemotactic protein; PDGF, platelet-derived growth factor; ROS, reactive oxygen species; SSc, systemic sclerosis; TGF-β, transforming growth factor-β.

transcription factors interact with one another and with non-DNA-binding cofactors, scaffold proteins, and chromatin-modifying enzymes such as p300/CBP, PCAF, and histone deacetylases. The activities and interactions of transcription factors and cofactors are controlled by extracellular cues. Enzymes that modify chromatin structure, causing it to unwind, enhance DNA-binding factor access to cognate cis-acting regulatory sequences and facilitate transcription.[100] Alterations in the levels, activities, or interactions among the various transcription factors, co-factors, and chromatin-modifying enzymes contribute to persistent fibroblast activation in SSc.

Effector Cells of Fibrosis: Fibroblasts

Fibroblasts are versatile spindle-shaped cells that are capable of both synthesis and degradation of ECM. Although unstimulated fibroblasts are biosynthetically quiescent, under the influence of appropriate extracellular signals they secrete ECM macromolecules and growth factors, cytokines and growth factors; adhere to and contract connective tissue; and transdifferentiate into myofibroblasts. Together, these biosynthetic, proinflammatory, contractile, and adhesive functions enable fibroblasts to execute effective wound healing. Whereas under physiologic conditions the fibroblast repair program is self-limited, pathologic fibrosis is characterized by uncontrolled fibroblast activation that results in exaggerated ECM accumulation and remodeling.[101] Recent DNA microarray studies reveal that fibroblasts explanted from different anatomic locations differ markedly in their pattern of gene expression, suggesting that fibroblasts in different sites in the body could be considered distinct differentiated cell types.[102] The apparent "positional memory" of fibroblasts is governed by genetic imprinting by the homeobox (HOX) family transcription factors.

Effector Cells of Fibrosis: Myofibroblasts, Pericytes, Endothelial Cells, and Cellular Plasticity

In fibrosis, the tissue pool of activated mesenchymal cells is expanded by not only proliferation of resident fibroblasts but also transdifferentiation of other cell types, as well as the influx of bone marrow–derived mesenchymal progenitor cells. Myofibroblasts characterized by the cytoskeletal protein α–smooth muscle actin are specialized cells that arise from resident fibroblasts, as well as epithelial and endothelial cells and fibrocytes in response to TGF-β. Myofibroblasts synthesize collagens, tissue inhibitor of metalloproteinases (TIMPs), and other ECM components and are a major source of TGF-β during the fibrotic response. During normal wound healing, myofibroblasts are detected transiently in the early granulation tissue and then disappear via apoptosis. The removal of fibroblasts is a crucial step in wound resolution. In pathologic fibrogenesis myofibroblasts persist in lesional tissue, resulting in excessively contracted ECM that is characteristic of chronic scar.

Pericytes are mesenchymal cells in the walls of small blood vessels that are normally in intimate contact with the underlying endothelium and regulate vascular homeostasis. In SSc patients, a marked increase in microvascular pericyte compartment and increased expression of PDGF receptors has been reported. Activated pericytes can transdifferentiate into collagen-producing fibroblasts and myofibroblasts, thus linking microvascular injury and fibrosis.

Under certain conditions, epithelial cells can also undergo transformation to fibroblasts. Epithelial-mesenchymal transition (EMT) plays a vital role during vertebrate embryonic development. On stimulation, epithelial cells lose characteristic markers and cell-cell adhesion and acquire fibroblast markers such as α–smooth muscle actin. Pathologic EMT occurs prominently in cancer and is increasingly implicated in renal fibrosis and idiopathic pulmonary fibrosis.[103] Similar to epithelial cells, vascular endothelial cells can, on injury, undergo a transition to fibroblasts. This process, called *EndMT*, has been demonstrated in various forms of experimentally induced fibrosis. Both EMT and EndMT are stimulated by TGF-β and Notch, and both processes might be implicated in tissue fibrosis in SSc.

Fibrocytes and Monocyte-Derived Mesenchymal Progenitor Cells

Fibrocytes are bone marrow–derived CD34+ mesenchymal progenitor cells normally present in small numbers in the peripheral blood that can present antigen and also synthesize collagen.[104] These bone marrow–derived cells express CD14+ (a monocyte marker), as well as chemokine receptors (CCR3, CCR5, and CXCR4), which allows them to accumulate in specific tissues. The role for circulating fibrocytes and their trafficking into lesional tissue in the pathogenesis of fibrosis was established in animal models using neutralizing antibodies and in CXCR4-deficient mice. Mice with accelerated senescence have an increased number of circulating fibrocytes and show increased sensitivity to bleomycin-induced fibrosis. It is thought that in lesional tissue, fibrocytes undergo differentiation into activated myofibroblasts, losing the CD14 and CD34 markers in the process, and contribute to the progression of fibrosis. Other studies have identified multipotent monocyte-derived mesenchymal progenitor cells in peripheral blood. However, the role of fibrocytes and other bone marrow–derived progenitor cells in SSc-associated fibrosis remains speculative.

MOLECULAR DETERMINANTS OF FIBROSIS: TRANSFORMING GROWTH FACTOR-β

The expression of ECM genes is normally tightly regulated by paracrine/autocrine mediators, cell-cell contact, hypoxia, and contact with the surrounding ECM. Multiple cytokines are implicated in SSc (see Table 83-3). Of these, TGF-β is considered to be the master regulator of both physiologic fibrogenesis (wound healing and tissue repair) and pathologic fibrosis. TGF-β plays essential roles in normal tissue repair, angiogenesis, and immune regulation and is implicated in cancer, fibrosis, and autoimmunity. Most cell types secrete TGF-β as a latent complex that is sequestered within the ECM. Under appropriate conditions, latent TGF-β is converted to its biologically active form that is capable of triggering cellular responses. The activation of latent TGF-β is controlled in part by fibrillin-1 and is mediated by integrins, thrombospondins, αvβ6 integrin, and proteolytic enzymes. Because of its fundamental role in orchestrating fibrotic responses, TGF-β is considered as a potential therapeutic target in SSc. Blocking TGF-β activity via biologic approaches using neutralizing antibodies and blocking intracellular TGF-β signaling using small molecular kinase inhibitors such as the c-Abl blocker imatinib mesylate (Gleevec) are undergoing evaluation. To date, small clinical trials of such interventions have not shown signficant efficacy in modifying the course of fibrosis.

Cellular Signaling by Transforming Growth Factor-β: Canonical Smad Pathways

A member of a large cytokine superfamily that also includes activin and bone morphogenetic proteins, TGF-β is secreted by platelets, monocytes/macrophages, dendritic cells, and fibroblasts, and most cell types express surface receptors for TGF-β. The type of response elicited by TGF-β is specific for the target cell lineage and is context dependent. In mesenchymal cells, TGF-β acts as a potent inducer of fibrillar collagen synthesis; stimulates fibroblast proliferation, migration, adhesion, and transdifferentiation into myofibroblasts; and suppresses the production of matrix-degrading metalloproteinases (Table 83-4). In endothelial and epithelial cells, TGF-β drives transdifferentiation into fibroblasts. Activated TGF-β binds to the type II TGF-β receptor, triggering an intracellular signal transduction cascade that leads to the induction of target genes. The evolutionarily conserved canonical TGF-β signal transduction pathway involves phosphorylation of the type I TGF-β receptor, a serine-threonine kinase that in turn phosphorylates cytosolic Smads. Ligand-induced phosphorylation of Smad2/3 allows them to form heterocomplexes with Smad4 and translocate into the nucleus, where they bind to a consensus Smad-binding element (SBE) and recruit

Table 83-4 Fibrogenic Activities of Transforming Growth Factor-β (TGF-β) Relevant to Systemic Sclerosis

Recruits monocytes
Stimulates synthesis of collagens, fibronectin, proteoglycans, elastin, tissue inhibitor of metalloproteinases; inhibits matrix metalloproteinases
Stimulates fibroblast proliferation, chemotaxis
Induces fibrogenic cytokine production: connective tissue growth factor; autoinduction; blocks type II interferon synthesis and activity
Stimulates production of endothelin-1
Stimulates generation of reactive oxygen species
Stimulates expression of surface receptors for TGF-β, PDGF
Induces fibroblast mitogenic responses to PDGF-AA
Promotes fibroblast-myofibroblast differentiation, monocyte-fibrocyte differentiation
Promotes epithelial-mesenchymal transition, endothelial mesenchymal transition
Inhibits fibroblast and myofibroblast apoptosis

PDGF, platelet-derived growth factor.

transcriptional cofactors such as the histone acetylase p300/CBP, resulting in gene transcription. Conserved SBE sequences are found in many TGF-β-inducible genes including type I collagens, PAI-1, α–smooth muscle actin, and CTGF. Ligand-induced signal transduction through the Smad pathway is tightly controlled by endogenous inhibitors such as Smad7 and BAMBI.

Noncanonical Transforming Growth Factor-β Signaling

Although the Smad pathway is the central mediator of signals from the TGF-β receptors, recent evidence indicates the existence of alternative non-Smad pathways. Non-Smad signaling molecules activated by TGF-β include protein kinases (c-Abl, p38 and JNK, integrin-associated focal adhesion kinase FAK, and TGF-β activated kinase TAK1); lipid kinases such as PI3 kinase and its downstream target Akt; and the calcium-dependent phosphatase, calcineurin. Signaling via c-Abl is particularly relevant to SSc because this nonreceptor tyrosine kinase implicated in chronic myelogenous leukemia (CML) mediates profibrotic signals induced by TGF-β and PDGF and is activated in SSc fibroblasts.[105] Imatinib is an effective small molecule inhibitor of c-Abl that is highly effective for the treatment of CML. In scleroderma skin fibroblasts in culture imatinib reversed the abnormal ECM gene expression, and in mouse models of scleroderma, imatinib treatment prevented the development of skin fibrosis.[106]

CYTOKINES, GROWTH FACTORS, CHEMOKINES, AND LIPID MEDIATORS

Multiple cytokines, growth factors, chemokines, and eicosanoids that regulate ECM accumulation and mesenchymal cell function show aberrant expression or activity in SSc. Soluble mediators such as CTGF, PDGF, IL-4, IL-6, IL-13, adenosine, prostaglandin F2α, and lysophosphatidic acid (LPA1) each contribute to the pathogenesis of fibrosis and therefore represent potential therapeutic targets.

Connective Tissue Growth Factor/CCN2

CTGF is a cysteine-rich 40-kD member of the CCN early-response gene family. This matricellular growth factor is implicated in angiogenesis, wound healing, and development. In normal adults, CTGF is undetectable, but its expression is markedly elevated in fibrotic conditions. Serum levels of CTGF correlate with the extent of skin and pulmonary fibrosis in SSc patients. The expression of CTGF can be induced in normal fibroblasts by TGF-β, IL-4, and VEGF, whereas TNF and iloprost block stimulation. Transgenic mice overexpressing CTGF develop scleroderma-like diffuse skin fibrosis and microvascular pathology.[107] In vitro, CTGF exerts multiple profibrotic effects in normal fibroblasts. Because many of these CTGF effects parallel those induced by TGF-β, it has been suggested that TGF-β responses are mediated through endogenous CTGF. The identity of the cellular CTGF receptors and the mechanism of action underlying CTGF profibrotic responses remain incompletely characterized.

Platelet-Derived Growth Factor

PDGFs are disulfide-bonded heterodimeric proteins that act mainly on stromal cells and regulate the wound healing process. Originally isolated from platelets, PDGF isoforms are also secreted from macrophages, endothelial cells, and fibroblasts. PDGF, signaling via the α and β transmembrane receptors, acts as a potent mitogen and chemoattractant for fibroblasts. Moreover, PDGF induces ROS generation and stimulates the synthesis of collagen, fibronectin, and proteoglycans, as well as the secretion of TGF-β1; MCP-1, and IL-6. Transgenic mice expressing a constitutively active PDGF-α receptor develop progressive fibrosis in the skin and multiple organs.[108] Lesional skin fibroblasts from SSc patients show elevated PDGF and PDGF-β receptor expression,[109] and PDGF levels are increased in the bronchoalveolar lavage fluid. In SSc patients, serum antibodies to the PDGF receptor induce fibroblast activation and ROS generation in vitro; however, these antibodies are not specific for SSc and have also been detected in patients with graft-versus-host disease.

Developmental Pathways: Wnt and Notch

Wnt and Notch developmental pathways required for embryogenesis appear to be deregulated in fibrosis and SSc. The Wnts comprise a family of poorly soluble glycoproteins with dual roles in cell-cell adhesion and transcriptional regulation. Although Wnts have essential roles in morphogenesis, stem cell homeostasis, and cell fate determination, abnormal Wnt signaling is implicated in colorectal cancer, as well as rheumatoid and osteoarthritis, osteoporosis, PAH, and aging. Intracellular Wnt signaling is mediated via canonical (β-catenin) and noncanonical pathways, and there is extensive cross-talk with TGF-β signaling. Transcription of a large number of genes with diverse biologic functions including multiple genes associated with tissue remodeling and pathologic fibrosis are induced by Wnts through β-catenin. Transgenic mice overexpressing Wnt10b or a constitutively-active mutant β-catenin develop exuberant wound healing, dermal fibrosis, and increased collagen synthesis in the skin.[110] Lungs from patients with idiopathic pulmonary fibrosis show increased nuclear β-catenin accumulation at fibrotic foci. Expression profiling analysis of SSc skin biopsies shows elevated expression of Wnt ligands, Wnt receptors, and Wnt targets. Notch is a transmembrane receptor activated by its ligand, Jagged, which has a fundamental role in embryonic development, wound healing, and tissue repair. Notch signaling regulates endothelial cell and fibroblast responses including myofibroblast differentiation. A mouse model of scleroderma showed markedly activated Notch signaling in the skin and lungs, and the activity of ADAM-17, a proteinase induced by TGF-β and ROS that initiates Notch signal transduction, was elevated in SSc skin biopsies.[111]

Interleukins

IL-1 is secreted by multiple cell types. A recent study showed that SSc epidermal keratinocytes are activated and secreted IL-1α. Co-culture of SSc keratinocytes with normal skin fibroblasts resulted in fibroblast activation and myofibroblast differentiation that was mediated by IL-1α secreted by keratinocytes. The Th2 cytokine IL-4 stimulates fibroblast proliferation, chemotaxis, collagen synthesis, and production of TGF-β, CTGF, and TIMP. Serum levels of IL-4 are elevated in SSc, and the number of IL-4-producing T lymphocytes is increased in peripheral blood and skin. IL-6, produced by monocytes and T lymphocytes, fibroblasts, and endothelial cells, stimulates collagen and TIMP-1 synthesis and promotes a Th2-polarized immune response. The biologic activities of IL-6 are mediated via the JAK-STAT intracellular signaling pathway shared with other cytokines. Serum levels of IL-6 are elevated in SSc and correlated with the severity of skin involvement. IL-13 is implicated in asthma and other fibrotic conditions. The profibrotic effects of IL-13 involve both indirect mechanisms due to stimulation of TGF-β production by macrophages and direct stimulation of fibroblast proliferation and collagen synthesis. Serum levels of IL-13 are elevated in SSc.

Chemokines

Chemokines represent a superfamily of more than 40 low-molecular-weight soluble mediators originally characterized by their chemotactic effects on leukocytes but now recognized to have a broad range of cellular targets and biologic activities. They play important roles in angiogenesis, wound healing, and fibrosis. The CC chemokine MCP-1 stimulates collagen production directly, as well as through induction of endogenous TGF-β production. Serum levels of MCP-1, along with those of MIP-1α, IL-8, CXCL8, and CCL18, are elevated in SSc and correlate with the severity of skin fibrosis. Mononuclear cells and dermal fibroblasts from SSc patients spontaneously produce these chemokines, and lesional SSc fibroblasts show constitutive upregulation of the MCP-1 receptor CCR2. Because MCP-1 drives a Th2 response, the MCP-1–CCR2 axis is thought to play a major role in the pathogenesis of SSc by amplifying collagen stimulation and promoting Th2 cytokine production. Significantly, MCP-1 null mice are resistant to the development of fibrosis induced by bleomycin.[112] Enhanced MCP-1 and MCP-3 expression was noted in lesional skin in SSc, particularly in early disease. These chemokines promote transendothelial migration of mononuclear cells in vitro. The levels of MIP-1α, CXCL8, and CCL18 are also elevated in SSc bronchoalveolar lavage fluid. One study showed that elevated CCL18 levels identified SSc patients who had pulmonary fibrosis, and changes in CCL18 serum levels showed a strong negative correlation with changes in lung function in this cohort. Additional chemokines overexpressed in lesional tissue or serum in patients with SSc or in animal models of scleroderma include RANTES and PARC (CC chemokines), as well as IL-8, MIP-2, and fractalkine (CXC chemokines). The insulin-like growth factor binding protein-1 (IGFBP-1) stimulates collagen synthesis and fibroblast proliferation and induces TGF-β. Patients with SSc have elevated levels of IGF-1 in bronchoalveolar lavage fluids. Expression of IGFBP-3 is markedly elevated in SSc fibroblasts. Adenovirally mediated overexpression of IGFBP-5 resulted in the induction of chronic scleroderma-like fibrosis in mice.[113]

Bioactive Lipids

A variety of bioactive lipids are potent modulators of fibroblast function. Although some prostanoids inhibit fibrotic responses through a variety of mechanisms, prostaglandin F ($PGF_2^α$) was shown to be elevated in patients with pulmonary fibrosis and can stimulate collagen production and fibroblast proliferation.[114] Mice with targeted deletion of the PGF receptor are protected from bleomycin-induced pulmonary fibrosis. Lysophosphatidic acid (LPA), generated via the hydrolysis of membrane phospholipids, exerts multiple biologic activities via G protein–coupled transmembrane receptors. Recently LPA was shown to induce fibroblast chemotaxis and CTGF production. The levels of LPA are elevated in the lungs of patients with pulmonary fibrosis. Moreover, LPA1 knockout mice are protected from bleomycin-induced skin and lung fibrosis. A recent study indicates that LPA induces αvβ6 integrin-mediated TGF-β activation in epithelial cells, contributing to sustained autocrine TGF-β signaling.[115]

Regulation of Fibroblast Function via Innate Immune Signaling: Toll-like Receptors and the Inflammasome

The IFN signature observed in SSc leukocytes and genetic association with mediators of innate immunity support the role of TLR-mediated innate immune responses in SSc. All cell membrane and endosomal TLRs are expressed on normal fibroblasts. Activation of TLR4 by lipopolysaccharide (LPS) plays a critical role in liver fibrosis, with sensitization to TGF-β as the underlying mechanism. In addition, TLR4 also induced the expression of the profibrotic transcription factors Egr-1 and Egr-2. In SSc, fibroblast TLRs might be activated by endogenous TLR ligands called *damage-associated molecular patterns* generated by tissue injury, autoimmunity, and oxidative stress. Endogenous TLR ligands that could play a role in SSc belong to three categories: ECM-derived molecules such as hyaluronan and

its small-molecular-weight degradation products, tenascin C, alternatively spliced extra domain A (EDA) of fibronectin and biglycan; cellular stress proteins such as HMGB1 and Hsp60; and nucleic acids and immune complexes released from damaged or necrotic cells. The expression of both TLR3 and TLR4 is elevated in SSc skin and lung biopsies and is accompanied by substantial increases in hyaluronan, tenascin C, and alternately spliced fibronectin levels. The TLR3 ligand poly(I:C) causes dramatic induction of type I IFN, IL-6, and other inflammatory cytokines, as well as ECM molecules, in normal fibroblasts. These observations suggest that fibroblasts exposed to endogenous TLR ligands during tissue injury switch to an activated phenotype. In this way, fibroblast TLR signaling initiated by damage-associated endogenous TLR ligands in SSc might convert a self-limited regenerative tissue repair into an aberrant and intractable fibrotic scar.

Recently identified innate immune sensors in addition to TLRs include NOD-like receptors (NLRs), RIG-I, and Nalp3. These intracellular receptors respond to cytosolic nucleic acids, damage-associated endogenous molecules, and environmental signals such as silica, bleomycin, and gadolinium. Once activated, these receptors facilitate inflammasome assembly with activation of caspase-1 and secretion of proIL-1β and IL-18. *NLRP1* is a susceptibility gene for SSc and associated pulmonary fibrosis. Inflammasome activation and IL-1β play an important role in experimental mouse fibrosis and appear to be important in fibroblast activation of SSc as well.[116]

Negative Regulation of Extracellular Matrix Accumulation

To prevent excessive matrix accumulation and scarring in response to injury, redundant biologic mechanisms have evolved. Fibroblasts are equipped with endogenous molecules that repress ECM gene expression and TGF-β stimulation. For example, Smad7 is an inhibitory Smad that blocks TGF-β signal transduction by accelerating ubiquitin-mediated TGF-β receptor degradation. Functional impairment of Smad7 was demonstrated in SSc fibroblasts. Other cell-intrinsic endogenous repressors of collagen synthesis include the transcription factors Sp3, Fli-1, p53, Ras, Nrf2, and the nuclear hormone receptor, peroxisome proliferator-activated receptor-γ (PPAR-γ). Impaired expression, induction, or function of these endogenous inhibitors may be responsible for failure to limit fibroblast activation in SSc.

Interferon-γ

IFN-γ, produced primarily by Th1 lymphocytes, is a major negative regulator of collagen gene expression and fibroblast activation. IFN-γ represses collagen gene expression and abrogates stimulation induced by TGF-β.[117] IFN-γ is also a potent inhibitor of fibroblast proliferation, fibroblast-mediated matrix contraction, and myofibroblast transdifferentiation. Significantly, some studies have shown that fibroblasts from patients with SSc are relatively resistant to the inhibitory effects of IFN-γ. Clinical trials of IFN-γ in SSc have demonstrated a modest and inconsistent improvement in skin fibrosis.

Peroxisome Proliferator-Activated Receptor-γ

PPAR-γ is an intracellular molecule that modulates TGF-β signaling and mesenchymal cell plasticity and is functionally associated with fibrosis. Originally identified in adipocytes as a key regulator of adipogenesis and lipid metabolism, PPAR-γ is a dual function molecule acting as both a nuclear hormone receptor and ligand-inducible transcription factor. Multiple lipid moieties and electrophilic prostanoids such as 15d-prostaglandin J$_2$ (15d-PGJ$_2$) serve as endogenous ligands for PPAR-γ. Insulin-sensitizing drugs such as rosiglitazone and pioglitazone are potent pharmacologic PPAR-γ agonists. PPAR-γ modulates vascular and immune processes, and abnormal PPAR-γ function is implicated in lipodystrophy, atherosclerosis, PAH, and inflammatory diseases. Activation of fibroblasts with 15d-PGJ$_2$ or pharmacologic PPAR-γ ligands resulted in a virtual abrogation of TGF-β-induced collagen production, myofibroblast transdifferentiation, EMT, and other Smad3-dependent transcriptional responses. The expression and activity of PPAR-γ are impaired in patients with diffuse cutaneous SSc (dcSSc).[118] Furthermore, PPAR-γ expression shows an inverse relationship with enhanced TGF-β signaling in lesional tissue. Of note, multiple factors implicated in SSc pathogenesis including TGF-β, Wnt ligands, IL-13, hypoxia, LPA, and CTGF potently inhibit PPAR-γ expression, which might account for impaired PPAR-γ expression in SSc. Together, these findings implicate altered PPAR-γ expression and function in SSc.

SCLERODERMA FIBROBLAST

Fibroblasts explanted from lesional skin or fibrotic lungs of patients with SSc display an abnormal activated phenotype that persists during their serial passage in vitro, indicating autonomous alteration in cell function. The "SSc phenotype" is characterized by the following: enhanced ECM synthesis, secretion of profibrotic cytokines and chemokines, and resistance to IFN-γ and other inhibitory signals. Moreover, SSc fibroblasts show features of myofibroblast transdifferentiation, in part because of constitutive activation of the FAK focal adhesion kinase. It remains unsettled whether the activated SSc fibroblast phenotype represents an intrinsic abnormality or activation in response to exogenous stimuli in the fibrotic milieu.

Numerous molecules of signal transduction and transcriptional regulation have been reported to be abnormally expressed or constitutively activated in SSc fibroblasts. The list includes protein kinase C, Smad3, Egr-1, p300, and c-Abl. Elevated expression of the prosurvival factors Bcl-2 and Akt in SSc fibroblasts may play a role in their relative resistance to apoptosis. Because most of the SSc fibroblast characteristics can be induced in normal fibroblasts by treatment with TGF-β, it has been suggested that the SSc phenotype is due to autocrine TGF-β signaling. The levels of TGF-β receptors are elevated on SSc fibroblasts, which might enable these cells to mount a robust response to endogenously produced TGF-β or to low levels of environmental TGF-β. Furthermore, SSc fibroblasts have elevated levels of thrombospondin and αvβ3 integrins, which mediate latent TGF-β activation at the cell surface. Consistent with the autocrine TGF-β hypothesis, SSc fibroblasts

show constitutive TGF-β signaling, with elevated Smad3 activation, and constitutive interaction with the histone acetyltransferase p300/CBP. Other studies demonstrate defective expression or function of endogenous suppressors of TGF-β signaling and ECM production, suggesting that failure to terminate fibroblast activation may represent a fundamental defect in SSc. Endogenous molecules that negatively regulate fibroblast activation include Fli-1, PTEN, PPAR-γ, and Smad7. Autocrine TGF-β activation of fibroblasts cannot fully account for all of the phenotypic hallmarks of SSc fibroblasts such as constitutive CTGF production, indicating that both Smad-independent TGF-β signaling mechanisms, as well as non-TGF-β–mediated activation events, are involved in the induction or maintenance of the SSc phenotype. The autonomous SSc phenotype could also result from abnormal integrin-mediated signaling from the surrounding ECM. Moreover, epigenetic alterations in SSc fibroblasts are associated with persistent and heritable fibroblast dysfunction. For example, silencing the *FLI-1* gene, an important endogenous negative regulator of collagen gene expression, by DNA methylation or chromatin histone deacetylation suppresses its expression in fibroblasts from lesional skin, which increases collagen synthesis.

References

1. Dieudé P, Boileau C, Allanore Y: Immunogenetics of systemic sclerosis, *Autoimmun Rev* 10(5):282–290, 2011.
2. Arnett FC, Howard RF, Tan F, et al: Increased prevalence of systemic sclerosis in a Native American tribe in Oklahoma, *Arthritis Rheum* 39(8):1362–1370, 1996.
3. Feghali-Bostwick C, Medsger TA Jr, Wright TM: Analysis of systemic sclerosis in twins reveals low concordance for disease and high concordance for the presence of antinuclear antibodies, *Arthritis Rheum* 48(7):1956–1963, 2003.
4. Frech T, Khanna D, Markewitz B, et al: Heritability of vasculopathy, autoimmune disease, and fibrosis in systemic sclerosis: a population-based study, *Arthritis Rheum* 62(7):2109–2116, 2010.
5. Arnett FC, Gourh P, Shete S, et al: Major histocompatibility complex (MHC) class II alleles, haplotypes and epitopes which confer susceptibility or protection in systemic sclerosis: analyses in 1300 Caucasian, African-American and Hispanic cases and 1000 controls, *Ann Rheum Dis* 69(5):822–827, 2010.
6. Radstake TR, Gorlova O, Rueda B, et al: Genome-wide association study of systemic sclerosis identifies CD247 as a new susceptibility locus, *Nat Genet* 42(5):426–429, 2010.
7. Muryoi T, Kasturi KN, Kafina MJ, et al: Antitopoisomerase I monoclonal autoantibodies from scleroderma patients and tight skin mouse interact with similar epitopes, *J Exp Med* 175(4):1103–1109, 1992.
8. Markiewicz M, Smith EA, Rubinchik S, et al: The 72-kilodalton IE-1 protein of human cytomegalovirus (HCMV) is a potent inducer of connective tissue growth factor (CTGF) in human dermal fibroblasts, *Clin Exp Rheumatol* 22(3 Suppl 33):S31–S34, 2004.
9. Tabuenca JM: Toxic-allergic syndrome caused by ingestion of rapeseed oil denatured with aniline, *Lancet* 2(8246):567–568, 1981.
10. Hertzman PA, Blevins WL, Mayer J, et al: Association of the eosinophilia-myalgia syndrome with the ingestion of tryptophan. *N Engl J Med* 322(13):869–873, 1990.
11. Mori Y, Kahari VM, Varga J: Scleroderma-like cutaneous syndromes, *Curr Rheumatol Rep* 4(2):113–122, 2002.
12. McCormic ZD, Khuder SS, Aryal BK, et al: Occupational silica exposure as a risk factor for scleroderma: a meta-analysis, *Int Arch Occup Environ Health* 83(7):763–769, 2010.
13. Varga J, Schumacher HR, Jimenez SA: Systemic sclerosis after augmentation mammoplasty with silicone implants, *Ann Intern Med* 111(5):377–383, 1989.
14. Janowsky EC, Kupper LL, Hulka BS: Meta-analyses of the relation between silicone breast implants and the risk of connective-tissue diseases, *N Engl J Med* 342(11):781–790, 2000.

15. Varga J, Haustein UF, Creech RH, et al: Exaggerated radiation-induced fibrosis in patients with systemic sclerosis, *JAMA* 265(24):3292–3295, 1991.
16. Artlett CM, Smith JB, Jimenez SA: Identification of fetal DNA and cells in skin lesions from women with systemic sclerosis, *N Engl J Med* 338(17):1186–1191, 1998.
17. Nelson JL, Furst DE, Maloney S, et al: Microchimerism and HLA-compatible relationships of pregnancy in scleroderma, *Lancet* 351(9102):559–562, 1998.
18. D'Angelo WA, Fries JF, Masi AT, Shulman LE: Pathologic observations in systemic sclerosis (scleroderma). A study of fifty-eight autopsy cases and fifty-eight matched controls, *Am J Med* 46(3):428–440, 1969.
19. Freemont AJ, Hoyland J, Fielding P, et al: Studies of the microvascular endothelium in uninvolved skin of patients with systemic sclerosis: direct evidence for a generalized microangiopathy, *Br J Dermatol* 126(6):561–568, 1992.
20. Prescott RJ, Freemont AJ, Jones CJ, et al: Sequential dermal microvascular and perivascular changes in the development of scleroderma, *J Pathol* 166(3):255–263, 1992.
21. Fleming JN, Nash RA, McLeod DO, et al: Capillary regeneration in scleroderma: stem cell therapy reverses phenotype? *PLoS One* 3(1):e1452, 2008.
22. Kahaleh MB: Endothelin, an endothelial-dependent vasoconstrictor in scleroderma. Enhanced production and profibrotic action, *Arthritis Rheum* 34(8):978–983, 1991.
23. Yousem SA: The pulmonary pathologic manifestations of the CREST syndrome, *Hum Pathol* 21(5):467–474, 1990.
24. Overbeek MJ, Vonk MC, Boonstra A, et al: Pulmonary arterial hypertension in limited cutaneous systemic sclerosis: a distinctive vasculopathy, *Eur Respir J* 34(2):371–379, 2009.
25. Hawkins RA, Claman HN, Clark RA, Steigerwald JC: Increased dermal mast cell populations in progressive systemic sclerosis: a link in chronic fibrosis? *Ann Intern Med* 102(2):182–186, 1985.
26. Cox D, Earle L, Jimenez SA, et al: Elevated levels of eosinophil major basic protein in the sera of patients with systemic sclerosis, *Arthritis Rheum* 38(7):939–945, 1995.
27. Jelaska A, Korn JH: Role of apoptosis and transforming growth factor beta1 in fibroblast selection and activation in systemic sclerosis, *Arthritis Rheum* 43(10):2230–2239, 2000.
28. Verrecchia F, Laboureau J, Verola O, et al: Skin involvement in scleroderma—where histological and clinical scores meet, *Rheumatology (Oxford)* 46(5):833–841, 2007.
29. Rossi A, Sozio F, Sestini P, et al: Lymphatic and blood vessels in scleroderma skin, a morphometric analysis, *Hum Pathol* 41(3):366–374, 2010.
30. Davies CA, Jeziorska M, Freemont AJ, Herrick AL: The differential expression of VEGF, VEGFR-2, and GLUT-1 proteins in disease subtypes of systemic sclerosis, *Hum Pathol* 37(2):190–197, 2006.
31. Varga J, Bashey RI: Regulation of connective tissue synthesis in systemic sclerosis, *Int Rev Immunol* 12(2-4):187–199, 1995.
32. van der Slot AJ, Zuurmond AM, Bardoel AF, et al: Identification of PLOD2 as telopeptide lysyl hydroxylase, an important enzyme in fibrosis, *J Biol Chem* 278(42):40967–40972, 2003.
33. Whitfield ML, Finlay DR, Murray JI, et al: Systemic and cell type-specific gene expression patterns in scleroderma skin, *Proc Natl Acad Sci U S A* 100(21):12319–12324, 2003.
34. Gardner H, Shearstone JR, Bandaru R, et al: Gene profiling of scleroderma skin reveals robust signatures of disease that are imperfectly reflected in the transcript profiles of explanted fibroblasts, *Arthritis Rheum* 54(6):1961–1973, 2006.
35. Milano A, Pendergrass SA, Sargent JL, et al: Molecular subsets in the gene expression signatures of scleroderma skin, *PLoS One* 3(7):e2696, 2008.
36. Bouros D, Wells AU, Nicholson AG, et al: Histopathologic subsets of fibrosing alveolitis in patients with systemic sclerosis and their relationship to outcome, *Am J Respir Crit Care Med* 165(12):1581–1586, 2002.
37. Roberts CG, Hummers LK, Ravich WJ, et al: A case-controlled study of the pathology of oesophageal disease in systemic sclerosis (scleroderma), *Gut* 55(12):1697–1703, 2006.
38. Wipff J, Allanore Y, Soussi F, et al: Prevalence of Barrett's esophagus in systemic sclerosis, *Arthritis Rheum* 52(9):2882–2888, 2005.
39. Fisher ER, Rodnan GP: Pathologic observations concerning the kidney in progressive systemic sclerosis, *AMA Arch Pathol* 65(1):29–39, 1958.
40. Trostle DC, Bedetti CD, Steen VD, et al: Renal vascular histology and morphometry in systemic sclerosis. A case-control autopsy study, *Arthritis Rheum* 31(3):393–400, 1988.
41. Follansbee WP, Zerbe TR, Medsger TA Jr: Cardiac and skeletal muscle disease in systemic sclerosis (scleroderma): a high risk association, *Am Heart J* 125(1):194–203, 1993.
42. Fernandes F, Ramires FJ, Arteaga E, et al: Cardiac remodeling in patients with systemic sclerosis with no signs or symptoms of heart failure: an endomyocardial biopsy study, *J Card Fail* 9(4):311–317, 2003.
43. Follansbee WP, Zerbe TR, Medsger TA Jr: Cardiac and skeletal muscle disease in systemic sclerosis (scleroderma): a high risk association, *Am Heart J* 125(1):194–203, 1993.
44. Nehra A, Hall SJ, Basile G, et al: Systemic sclerosis and impotence: a clinicopathological correlation, *J Urol* 153(4):1140–1146, 1995.
45. Schumacher HR Jr: Joint involvement in progressive systemic sclerosis (scleroderma): a light and electron microscopic study of synovial membrane and fluid, *Am J Clin Pathol* 60(5):593–600, 1973.
46. Distler JH, Distler O, Beyer C, Schett G: Animal models of systemic sclerosis: prospects and limitations, *Arthritis Rheum* 62(10):2831–2844, 2010.
47. Baxter RM, Crowell TP, McCrann ME, et al: Analysis of the tight skin (Tsk1/+) mouse as a model for testing antifibrotic agents, *Lab Invest* 85(10):1199–1209, 2005.
48. Siracusa LD, McGrath R, Ma Q, et al: A tandem duplication within the fibrillin 1 gene is associated with the mouse tight skin mutation, *Genome Res* 6(4):300–313, 1996.
49. Neptune ER, Frischmeyer PA, Arking DE, et al: Dysregulation of TGF-beta activation contributes to pathogenesis in Marfan syndrome, *Nat Genet* 33(3):407–411, 2003.
50. Lemaire R, Farina G, Kissin E, et al: Mutant fibrillin 1 from tight skin mice increases extracellular matrix incorporation of microfibril-associated glycoprotein 2 and type I collagen, *Arthritis Rheum* 50(3):915–926, 2004.
51. Christner PJ, Peters J, Hawkins D, et al: The tight skin 2 mouse. An animal model of scleroderma displaying cutaneous fibrosis and mononuclear cell infiltration, *Arthritis Rheum* 38(12):1791–1798, 1995.
52. Takagawa S, Lakos G, Mori Y, et al: Sustained activation of fibroblast transforming growth factor-beta/Smad signaling in a murine model of SSc, *J Invest Dermatol* 121(1):41–50, 2003.
53. Servettaz A, Goulvestre C, Kavian N, et al: Selective oxidation of DNA topoisomerase 1 induces systemic sclerosis in the mouse, *J Immunol* 182(9):5855–5864, 2009.
54. Zhang Y, McCormick LL, Desai SR, et al: Murine sclerodermatous graft-versus-host disease, a model for human scleroderma: cutaneous cytokines, chemokines, and immune cell activation, *J Immunol* 168(6):3088–3098, 2002.
55. Sonnylal S, Denton CP, Zheng B, et al: Postnatal induction of transforming growth factor beta signaling in fibroblasts of mice recapitulates clinical, histologic, and biochemical features of scleroderma, *Arthritis Rheum* 56:334–344, 2007.
56. Denton CP, Lindahl GE, Khan K, et al: Activation of key profibrotic mechanisms in transgenic fibroblasts expressing kinase-deficient type II Transforming growth factor-β receptor (TβRIIδk), *J Biol Chem* 280(16):16053–16065, 2005.
57. Lakos G, Takagawa S, Varga J: Animal models of SSc, *Methods Mol Med* 102:377–393, 2004.
58. Varga J, Abraham DJ, Systemic sclerosis: paradigm multisystem fibrosing disorder, *J Clin Invest* 117(3):557–567, 2007.
59. Kahaleh MB, Sherer GK, LeRoy EC: Endothelial injury in scleroderma, *J Exp Med* 149(6):1326–1335, 1979.
60. Cerinic MM, Valentini G, Sorano GG, et al: Blood coagulation, fibrinolysis, and markers of endothelial dysfunction in systemic sclerosis, *Semin Arthritis Rheum* 32(5):285–295, 2003.
61. Rajkumar VS, Sundberg C, Abraham DJ, et al: Activation of microvascular pericytes in autoimmune Raynaud's phenomenon and systemic sclerosis, *Arthritis Rheum* 42(5):930–941, 1999.
62. Rajkumar VS, Howell K, Csiszar K, et al: Shared expression of phenotypic markers in systemic sclerosis indicates a convergence of pericytes and fibroblasts to a myofibroblast lineage in fibrosis, *Arthritis Res Ther* 7(5):R1113–1123, 2005.
63. Cambrey AD, Harrison NK, Dawes KE, et al: Increased levels of endothelin-1 in bronchoalveolar lavage fluid from patients with systemic sclerosis contribute to fibroblast mitogenic activity in vitro, *Am J Respir Cell Mol Biol* 11(4):439–445, 1994.

64. Hebbar M, Peyrat JP, Hornez L, et al: Increased concentrations of the circulating angiogenesis inhibitor endostatin in patients with systemic sclerosis, *Arthritis Rheum* 43(4):889–893, 2000.

65. Distler O, Distler JH, Scheid A, et al: Uncontrolled expression of vascular endothelial growth factor and its receptors leads to insufficient skin angiogenesis in patients with systemic sclerosis, *Circ Res* 95(1):109–116, 2004.

66. Distler O, Del Rosso A, Giacomelli R, et al: Angiogenic and angiostatic factors in systemic sclerosis: increased levels of vascular endothelial growth factor are a feature of the earliest disease stages and are associated with the absence of fingertip ulcers, *Arthritis Res* 4(6):R11, 2002.

67. Kuwana M, Okazaki Y, Yasuoka H, et al: Defective vasculogenesis in systemic sclerosis, *Lancet* 364(9434):603–610, 2004.

68. Kuwana M, Kaburaki J, Okazaki Y, et al: Increase in circulating endothelial precursors by atorvastatin in patients with systemic sclerosis, *Arthritis Rheum* 54(6):1946–1951, 2006.

69. Del Papa ND, Quirici N, Soligo D, et al: Bone marrow endothelial progenitors are defective in systemic sclerosis, *Arthritis Rheum* 54(8):2605–2615, 2006.

70. Beyer C, Schett G, Gay S, et al: Hypoxia in the pathogenesis of systemic sclerosis, *Arthritis Res Ther* 11(2):220, 2009.

71. Distler JH, Jüngel A, Pileckyte M, et al: Hypoxia-induced increase in the production of extracellular matrix proteins in systemic sclerosis, *Arthritis Rheum* 56(12):4203–4215, 2007.

72. Zhou D, Dada LA, Wu M, et al: Hypoxia-induced alveolar epithelial-mesenchymal transition requires mitochondrial ROS and hypoxia-inducible factor 1, *Am J Physiol Lung Cell Mol Physiol* 297(6): L1120–1130, 2009.

73. Stockmann C, Kerdiles Y, Nomaksteinsky M, et al: Loss of myeloid cell-derived vascular endothelial growth factor accelerates fibrosis, *Proc Natl Acad Sci U S A* 107(9):4329–4334, 2010.

74. Gabrielli A, Avvedimento EV, Krieg T: Scleroderma, *N Engl J Med* 360(19):1989–2003, 2009.

75. Svegliati S, Cancello R, Sambo P, et al: Platelet-derived growth factor and reactive oxygen species (ROS) regulate Ras protein levels in primary human fibroblasts via ERK1/2. Amplification of ROS and Ras in systemic sclerosis fibroblasts, *J Biol Chem* 280(43):36474–36482, 2005.

76. Roumm AD, Whiteside TL, Medsger TA Jr, Rodnan GP: Lymphocytes in the skin of patients with progressive systemic sclerosis. Quantification, subtyping, and clinical correlations, *Arthritis Rheum* 27(6):645–653, 1984.

77. Kahari VM, Sandberg M, Kalimo H, et al: Identification of fibroblasts responsible for increased collagen production in localized scleroderma by in situ hybridization, *J Invest Dermatol* 90(5):664–670, 1988.

78. Sakkas LI, Xu B, Artlett CM, et al: Oligoclonal T cell expansion in the skin of patients with systemic sclerosis, *J Immunol* 168(7):3649–3659, 2002.

79. Yurovsky VV, Wigley FM, Wise RA, White B: Skewing of the CD8+ T-cell repertoire in the lungs of patients with systemic sclerosis, *Hum Immunol* 48(1-2):84–97, 1996.

80. York MR, Nagai T, Mangini AJ, et al: A macrophage marker, Siglec-1, is increased on circulating monocytes in patients with systemic sclerosis and induced by type I interferons and Toll-like receptor agonists, *Arthritis Rheum* 56(3):1010–1020, 2007.

81. Assassi S, Mayes MD, Arnett FC, et al: Systemic sclerosis and lupus: points in an interferon-mediated continuum, *Arthritis Rheum* 62(2):589–598, 2010.

82. Duan H, Fleming J, Pritchard DK, et al: Combined analysis of monocyte and lymphocyte messenger RNA expression with serum protein profiles in patients with scleroderma, *Arthritis Rheum* 58(5):1465–1474, 2008.

83. Lakos G, Melichian D, Wu M, Varga J: Increased bleomycin-induced skin fibrosis in mice lacking the Th1-specific transcription factor T-bet, *Pathobiology* 73(5):224–237, 2006.

84. Aliprantis AO, Wang J, Fathman JW, et al: Transcription factor T-bet regulates skin sclerosis through its function in innate immunity and via IL-13, *Proc Natl Acad Sci U S A* 104(8):2827–2830, 2007.

85. Mavalia C, Scaletti C, Romagnani P, et al: Type 2 helper T-cell predominance and high CD30 expression in systemic sclerosis, *Am J Pathol* 151(6):1751–1758, 1997.

86. Parel Y, Aurrand-Lions M, Scheja A, et al: Presence of CD4+ CD8+ double-positive T cells with very high interleukin-4 production

potential in lesional skin of patients with systemic sclerosis, *Arthritis Rheum* 56(10):3459–3467, 2007.

87. Boin F, De Fanis U, Bartlett SJ, et al: T cell polarization identifies distinct clinical phenotypes in scleroderma lung disease, *Arthritis Rheum* 58(4):1165–1174, 2008.

88. Matsushita T, Hasegawa M, Hamaguchi Y, et al: Longitudinal analysis of serum cytokine concentrations in systemic sclerosis: association of interleukin 12 elevation with spontaneous regression of skin sclerosis, *J Rheumatol* 33(2):275–284, 2006.

89. Radstake TR, van Bon L, Broen J, et al: The pronounced Th17 profile in systemic sclerosis (SSc) together with intracellular expression of TGFbeta and IFNgamma distinguishes SSc phenotypes, *PLoS One* 4(6):e5903, 2009.

90. Radstake TR, van Bon L, Broen J, et al: Increased frequency and compromised function of T regulatory cells in systemic sclerosis (SSc) is related to a diminished CD69 and TGFbeta expression, *PLoS One* 4(6):e5981, 2009.

91. van Bon L, Popa C, Huijbens R, et al: Distinct evolution of TLR-mediated dendritic cell cytokine secretion in patients with limited and diffuse cutaneous systemic sclerosis, *Ann Rheum Dis* 69(8):1539–1547, 2010.

92. Casciola-Rosen L, Wigley F, Rosen A: Scleroderma autoantigens are uniquely fragmented by metal-catalyzed oxidation reactions: implications for pathogenesis, *J Exp Med* 185(1):71–79, 1997.

93. Baroni SS, Santillo M, Bevilacqua F, et al: Stimulatory autoantibodies to the PDGF receptor in systemic sclerosis, *N Engl J Med* 354(25):2667–2676, 2006.

94. Henault J, Robitaille G, Senecal JL, Raymond Y: DNA topoisomerase I binding to fibroblasts induces monocyte adhesion and activation in the presence of anti-topoisomerase I autoantibodies from systemic sclerosis patients, *Arthritis Rheum* 54(3):963–973, 2006.

95. Lafyatis R, O'Hara C, Feghali-Bostwick CA, Matteson E: B cell infiltration in systemic sclerosis-associated interstitial lung disease, *Arthritis Rheum* 56(9):3167–3168, 2007.

96. Sato S, Hasegawa M, Fujimoto M, et al: Quantitative genetic variation in CD19 expression correlates with autoimmunity, *J Immunol* 165(11):6635–6643, 2000.

97. Baechler EC, Batliwalla FM, Karypis G, et al: Interferon-inducible gene expression signature in peripheral blood cells of patients with severe lupus, *Proc Natl Acad Sci U S A* 100(5):2610–2615, 2003.

98. Kim D, Peck A, Santer D, et al: Induction of interferon-alpha by scleroderma sera containing autoantibodies to topoisomerase I: association of higher interferon-alpha activity with lung fibrosis, *Arthritis Rheum* 58(7):2163–2173, 2008.

99. Ramirez F, Tanaka S, Bou-Gharios G: Transcriptional regulation of the human alpha 2(I) collagen gene (COL1A2), an informative model system to study fibrotic diseases, *Matrix Biol* 25(6):365–372, 2006.

100. Ghosh AK, Varga J: Transcriptional coactivators p300/CBP and type I collagen gene expression, *Current Sci* 85:155–161, 2003.

101. Varga J, Abraham DJ: Systemic sclerosis: paradigm multisystem fibrosing disorder, *J Clin Invest* 117(3):557–567, 2007.

102. Chang HY, Chi JT, Dudoit S, et al: Diversity, topographic differentiation, and positional memory in human fibroblasts, *Proc Natl Acad Sci U S A* 99:12877–12882, 2002.

103. Kalluri R, Neilson EG: Epithelial-mesenchymal transition and its implications for fibrosis, *J Clin Invest* 112(12):1776–1784, 2003.

104. Abe R, Donnelly SC, Peng T, et al: Peripheral blood fibrocytes: differentiation pathway and migration to wound sites, *J Immunol* 166(12):7556–7562, 2001.

105. Bhattacharyya S, Ishida W, Wu M, et al: A non-Smad mechanism of fibroblast activation by transforming growth factor-beta via c-Abl and Egr-1: selective modulation by imatinib mesylate, *Oncogene* 28(10):1285–1297, 2009.

106. Distler JH, Jüngel A, Huber LC, et al: Imatinib mesylate reduces production of extracellular matrix and prevents development of experimental dermal fibrosis, *Arthritis Rheum* 56(1):311–322, 2007.

107. Sonnylal S, Shi-Wen X, Leoni P, et al: Selective expression of connective tissue growth factor in fibroblasts in vivo promotes systemic tissue fibrosis, *Arthritis Rheum* 62(5):1523–1532, 2010.

108. Olson LE, Soriano P: Increased PDGFRalpha activation disrupts connective tissue development and drives systemic fibrosis, *Dev Cell* 16(2):303–313, 2009.

109. Klareskog L, Gustafsson R, Scheynius A, Hallgren R: Increased expression of platelet-derived growth factor type B receptors in the

skin of patients with systemic sclerosis, *Arthritis Rheum* 33:1534–1541, 1990.

110. Wei J, Melichian D, Komura J, et al: Canonical Wnt signaling induces skin fibrosis and subcutaneous lipoatrophy: a novel mouse model for scleroderma? *Arthritis Rheum* 63:1707–1717, 2011.

111. Kavian N, Servettaz A, Mongaret C, et al: Targeting ADAM-17/notch signaling abrogates the development of systemic sclerosis in a murine model, *Arthritis Rheum* 62(11):3477–3487, 2010.

112. Ferreira AM, Takagawa S, Fresco R, et al: Diminished induction of skin fibrosis in mice with MCP-1 deficiency, *J Invest Dermatol* 126(8):1900–1908, 2006.

113. Yasuoka H, Hsu E, Ruiz XD, et al: The fibrotic phenotype induced by IGFBP-5 is regulated by MAPK activation and egr-1-dependent and -independent mechanisms, *Am J Pathol* 175(2):605–615, 2009.

114. Oga T, Matsuoka T, Yao C, et al: Prostaglandin F(2alpha) receptor signaling facilitates bleomycin-induced pulmonary fibrosis independently of transforming growth factor-beta, *Nat Med* 15(12):1426–1430, 2009.

115. Tager AM, LaCamera P, Shea BS, et al: The lysophosphatidic acid receptor LPA1 links pulmonary fibrosis to lung injury by mediating fibroblast recruitment and vascular leak, *Nat Med* 14(1):45–54, 2008.

116. Gasse P, Mary C, Guenon I, et al: IL-1R1/MyD88 signaling and the inflammasome are essential in pulmonary inflammation and fibrosis in mice, *J Clin Invest* 117(12):3786–3799, 2007.

117. Varga J, Olsen A, Herhal J, et al: Interferon-gamma reverses the stimulation of collagen but not fibronectin gene expression by transforming growth factor-beta in normal human fibroblasts, *Eur J Clin Invest* 20(5):487–493, 1990.

118. Wei J, Ghosh AK, Sargent JL, et al: PPARγ downregulation by TGFβ in fibroblast and impaired expression and function in systemic sclerosis: a novel mechanism for progressive fibrogenesis, *PLoS One* 5(11):e13778, 2010.

The references for this chapter can also be found on www.expertconsult.com.

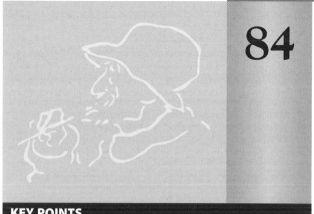

84

Clinical Features and Treatment of Scleroderma

FRANCESCO BOIN • FREDRICK M. WIGLEY

HISTORICAL PERSPECTIVE

Some consider that the first description of systemic sclerosis (scleroderma) was put forth in 1753 by Cario Curzio (Naples, Italy).[1] However, a careful review of the reported case suggests that the diagnosis was really *scleroedema* because of the distribution of the skin changes and the fact that the 17-year-old female improved with bloodletting, warm milk, and small doses of quicksilver. In 1836, Fantonetti (1791-1877), a Milanese physician, became the first to use the word *scleroderma* to designate a skin disease in an adult. However, it is likely that this patient also had scleroedema. The first convincing case of scleroderma was reported in 1842; then several acceptable cases were published before 1847, when Gintrac used the term *sclerodermie*, establishing this condition as a specific clinical entity.[2] By 1860, numerous cases had been reported, and articles reviewing the disease were published. Maurice Raynaud (1834-1881) described a patient with *sclerodermie* and cold-induced "asphyxie locale"—this was the first description of Raynaud's phenomenon in scleroderma. Sir William Osler described scleroderma while at Johns Hopkins Hospital between 1891 and 1897.[3] Osler recognized the systemic nature of the disease and was so impressed with the severity of scleroderma that he wrote:

> In its more aggravated forms, diffuse scleroderma is one of the most terrible of all human ills. Like Tithonous, to "whither slowly," and like him to be "beaten down and marred and wasted" until one is literally a mummy, encased in an ever-shrinking, slowly contracting skin of steel, is a fate not pictured in any tragedy, ancient or modern.

Matsui (Japan, 1924) emphasized the importance of visceral involvement as part of scleroderma based on several autopsies. Goetz (Capetown, 1945) further confirmed the multisystem involvement and suggested that the disease be named *progressive systemic sclerosis*.[4]

The concept of subtypes of scleroderma began in 1964, when Winterbauer reported cases with the CRST (calcinosis, *Raynaud's* phenomenon, sclerodactyly, and *telangiectasia*) syndrome.[5] A similar group of patients was reported in 1920 and was named after the authors—the Thiberge-Weissenbach syndrome. Velayos and colleagues recognized that esophageal dysmotility was common in these patients, so it is now called the CREST syndrome.[6] In 1969, 58 autopsy cases of scleroderma were compared with matched controls.[7] The organs found to be frequently and significantly involved by this disease were the skin, gastrointestinal tract, lungs, kidneys, skeletal muscle, and pericardium. This report first described the systemic nature of scleroderma vascular disease with findings of both kidney and lung arterial changes. In 1979, Rodnan introduced a clinical method to evaluate the extent of skin disease.[8] Steen and Medsger with others conducted extensive surveys of large populations of scleroderma patients, defining the clinical course and specific subtypes of disease. In the 1970s, an expert subcommittee established diagnostic criteria, and Leroy and colleagues suggested the classification of two major subsets of disease defined by skin involvement: *limited* and *diffuse*. Later, work by several investigators recognized that scleroderma has an autoimmune basis with occurrence of specific autoantibodies associated with subtypes of disease and useful in predicting disease course.

Scientific work in the modern era has revealed details regarding the pathogenesis of the disease and has led to the recognition that scleroderma is a complex polygenetic autoimmune disease associated with a unique disease process involving tissue fibrosis. Although no drug has yet been discovered with clear disease-modifying properties and ability to fully control the underlying disease process, major progress has been made in managing specific organ disease. The discovery that an angiotensin-converting enzyme inhibitor could reverse the scleroderma renal crisis in the 1970s has changed the course of kidney disease in scleroderma and has improved the survival of patients. Current therapies for gastrointestinal, cardiac, pulmonary, vascular, and interstitial lung disease have improved quality of life and survival.

EPIDEMIOLOGY

Incidence and Prevalence

Scleroderma is a rare disease with an estimated incidence of approximately 18 to 20 cases per million population per year, and a prevalence of 100 to 300 cases per million population. Reported rates vary by method of ascertainment, population under study, and definition of disease. Scleroderma is found in all races and in various geographic areas, but the prevalence and severity of disease vary among different racial and ethnic groups. The prevalence of scleroderma appears to be greater in the United States, where it has been estimated at 24.2 per 100,000, than in Europe, where recent studies in Iceland, England, France, and Greece have estimated rates ranging from 7.1 to 15.8 per 100,000.[9] In Australia, estimates are similar to those in the United States, and Japan has a lower reported prevalence— similar to that in Europe.[10] The highest scleroderma prevalence is reported among Choctaw Native Americans, in whom the disease appears to be more severe.[11] Several surveys in the United States show that African-Americans have a higher age-specific incidence rate and experience more severe disease than whites.[12] Occurrence is not different from urban to rural areas. Occasional reports have described unusually large numbers of cases of scleroderma observed in restricted geographic regions, suggesting nonrandom distribution of the disease. For example, in a rural area in the province of Rome, a geographic cluster of scleroderma and disease with related features was reported, suggesting prevalence 1000 times greater than expected.[13] Likewise, a study in the United Kingdom reported a higher prevalence of scleroderma in three geographic areas clustered near airports compared with other areas of the United Kingdom.[14]

The average age at onset is between 35 and 50 years, and the disease is more common among women (3 to 7:1 female-to-male ratio). Disease onset in the elderly is well described; it is uncommon for the disease to become manifest before the age of 25 years. Older age at onset is associated with increased risk for multisystem disease and, in particular, pulmonary arterial hypertension (PAH). A progressive increase in the incidence of scleroderma has been noted with increasing age. Over the period from 1963 to 1982, in Pittsburgh, Pennsylvania, the highest rates of scleroderma were observed between the ages of 45 and 54 years in black women, and between the ages of 55 and 64 years in white women.[15] Younger age at disease diagnosis among black women compared with white women was reported from Detroit, Michigan.[9]

Survival

Mortality among scleroderma patients is high, and most deaths are attributed directly to the disease manifestations.[16] In fact, the prognosis in scleroderma is highly variable, and survival is influenced by disease subtype, degree of internal organ involvement, and comorbid conditions. Factors associated with poor prognosis include diffuse skin disease, the presence of pulmonary disease (particularly PAH), renal involvement, multisystem disease, evidence of heart disease, older age at disease onset, and the presence of anemia. The standardized mortality rate (SMR) is the measure used to assess the relative mortality of a disease in comparison with the general population. Surveys of scleroderma patients report an SMR from 1.46 to 7.1. A survey found that among 284 scleroderma patients who died, the median disease duration as estimated from the onset of Raynaud's

phenomenon until death was 7.1 years for patients with diffuse skin disease, and 15.0 years for those with limited skin disease. Among non–scleroderma-related causes of death are, as expected, infection, malignancy, and cardiovascular events. Although premature atherosclerosis has been implicated as the cause of early death in other inflammatory autoimmune diseases, an increased prevalence of macroscopic coronary artery or cerebrovascular involvement beyond that expected in the general population has not yet been demonstrated in scleroderma.

Several studies suggest that the main cause of death has changed over time. Improved survival in recent years is thought to be secondary to more effective treatments for specific organ-based complications. It seems clear that the natural history of scleroderma renal complications has changed secondary to the use of angiotensin-converting enzyme (ACE) inhibitors for renal crisis. Historically, patients with scleroderma renal crisis had 1-year survival less than 15%.[17] Recent case-control studies conducted after the introduction of ACE inhibitors suggest greater than 85% 1-year survival. Pharmacologic prevention and treatment of interstitial lung disease and PAH are thought to have an impact. Cohort studies have demonstrated improved overall survival among scleroderma patients. At one scleroderma center, 10-year survival from disease diagnosis improved from 54% in the 1972-1981 group to 66% in the 1982-1991 group.[18] Another survey found that 5-year survival among diffuse cutaneous scleroderma patients improved from 69% in 1990-1993 to 84% in 2000-2003 (P = .018), whereas 5-year survival among limited cutaneous scleroderma patients remained unchanged at 93% and 91%, respectively.[19]

Environmental Exposures

Geographic clustering of scleroderma cases suggests that environmental exposure may be responsible for the disease, but definitive proof is still lacking. Epidemics of scleroderma-like illness following exposure to dietary (L-tryptophan or adulterated rapeseed oil), occupational (silica), or pharmacologic toxins (e.g., bleomycin, gadolinium-based contrast media) support the idea that environmental exposure can trigger a fibrotic disease. Typical scleroderma is found among coal miners and workers exposed to silica, particularly male workers. A meta-analysis of the risk of silica exposure found that the combined estimator of relative risk (CERR) was 1.03 (95% confidence interval [CI], 0.74 to 1.44) in females and 3.02 (95% CI, 1.24 to 7.35) in males.[20] Although occupational exposure to solvents (paint thinner or removers, mineral spirits, trichloroethylene, trichloroethane, perchloroethane, gasoline, aliphatic hydrocarbons, halogenated hydrocarbons, and BTX solvents containing benzene, toluene, or xylene) or polyvinyl chloride is reported to be associated with scleroderma, the role of these agents in causing disease is controversial and remains unproven. Likewise, case reports have suggested that silicone present in breast implants has triggered scleroderma, but large epidemiologic surveys have not found a greater incidence of scleroderma than expected in women with breast implants or exposure to silicone. Drugs implicated as potentially causative for systemic sclerosis (SSc)-like illnesses include bleomycin, pentazocine, and cocaine.

Genetic Factors

Although the absolute risk for family clustering remains low (1%), studies from Australia and the United States suggest that a family history of scleroderma increases the risk of disease, with a relative risk of first-degree relatives around 14 and of siblings in the range of 15 to 19.[21] Genetic factors were investigated by a survey of 42 twin pairs among which at least one twin had scleroderma.[22] The overall concordance rate was low at 4.7%, and was similar between monozygotic and dizygotic twin pairs. Although an association between major histocompatibility complex (MHC) alleles and scleroderma has been reported, this has not been confirmed consistently.[23] This finding argues against strong genetic susceptibility and favors a role for environmental and/or epigenetic events.

OVERVIEW OF CLINICAL FEATURES

Diagnostic Criteria

A subcommittee of the American College of Rheumatology (ACR) established diagnostic criteria based on a consensus of experts who evaluated a multicenter survey of scleroderma patients compared with other patient groups (Table 84-1).[24] The purpose of these criteria was to provide diagnostic certainty and consistency for research and other documentary exercises. The single finding of thickening of the skin typical of scleroderma proximal to the metacarpophalangeal (MCP) joints of the hands is considered a major criterion confirming the diagnosis. This includes changes on the face, arms, legs, or trunk. If skin thickening is found only distal to the MCP joints, then two of three minor criteria (digital pits, sclerodactyly, and pulmonary fibrosis on chest radiograph) must be present to confirm the diagnosis. These criteria are very specific (98%) for making the diagnosis of scleroderma but are considered too restricted in that they exclude patients with early or mild expression of the disease. Many patients with skin thickening limited to the fingers and some with no skin changes are recognized

Table 84-1 Establishing Diagnosis of Scleroderma

ACR Criteria Must have (a) or two of (b), (c), or (d)	a. Proximal SSc (proximal to MCPs/MTPs) b. Digital pits c. Sclerodactyly d. Pulmonary fibrosis (CXR; HRCT)
CREST Criteria Must have three of the five features	Calcinosis Raynaud's phenomenon Esophageal dysmotility Sclerodactyly Telangiectasias
Minor Criteria*† Must have all three	Definite Raynaud's phenomenon Abnormal capillary loops Specific scleroderma autoantibody

*Some experts continue to classify patients with minor criteria only as undifferentiated connective disease with scleroderma features.

†Proximal areas include the face. Autoantibody includes anticentromere, antitopoisomerase (Scl-70), and anti-RNA polymerase III.

ACR, American College of Rheumatology; CREST, calcinosis, Raynaud's phenomenon, esophageal dysfunction, sclerodactyly, telangiectasias; CXR, chest x-ray; HRCT, high-resolution computed tomography; MCPs, metacarpophalangeal joints; MTPs, metatarsophalangeal joints; SSc, systemic sclerosis.

to have systemic disease and yet do not meet the ACR criteria. Large longitudinal surveys confirm that a high percentage of patients with definitive Raynaud's phenomenon and typical scleroderma nail-fold capillary changes, along with scleroderma-specific autoantibodies, develop scleroderma within a 2- to 4-year period of follow-up.[25] Therefore, although the ACR criteria have a definite role in defining cases for research purposes, the clinician needs to take into account subtle features of the disease to make an early diagnosis for management purposes. Most experts would accept the finding of three of the five features of the CREST syndrome (calcinosis, Raynaud's phenomenon, esophageal dysfunction, sclerodactyly, telangiectasias) to make a clinical diagnosis of scleroderma. In clinical practice, one needs to recognize that some patients will not develop skin changes and yet they do have systemic disease (systemic sclerosis sine scleroderma), and many patients will present with partial expression of the disease (e.g., Raynaud's with nail-fold changes only) and later will develop well-defined disease. Experts argue that patients with partial expression, especially when a specific scleroderma-related autoantibody is present, should be considered to have a diagnosis of scleroderma and should be treated accordingly.

Classification and Clinical Subsets

The scleroderma disease process is complex, and its clinical expression is very heterogeneous such that the disease is expressed in several distinct clinical phenotypes. Classifying patients into subtypes is useful both for investigative purposes and for clinical practice. A specific subtype can define increased risk for internal organ involvement and overall prognosis. The traditional way to classify patients is by the degree of skin thickening as determined by physical examination. The skin is scored by pinching a fold and deciding whether it is abnormally thickened because of the scleroderma process. A committee of experts decided by consensus that two major groups of patients can be identified based on the distribution of skin changes and associated clinical and laboratory outcomes as observed (Figure 84-1).[26] Patients are considered to have *diffuse skin disease* if skin changes are found proximal to the elbows and/or knees or on the trunk, excluding the face. These patients tend to have higher risk of multisystem disease and poor survival. Patients are considered to have *limited disease* if skin changes occur distal to the elbows and/or knees and not on the trunk. Facial skin thickening can be present in the limited group. Some argue that the term *CREST syndrome* should be eliminated, and that these patients should be classified in the limited skin group. Others feel that the CREST syndrome is a unique subtype within the broader group of limited skin diseases with a distinct disease course.

Another less popular classification system divides patients into three groups based on skin changes: limited (fingers only), intermediate (skin to the elbows or knees), and diffuse (skin above the elbows and/or knees and/or trunk). Studies using this classification have found that the intermediate group had distinct clinical outcomes, including an intermediate survival statistic between limited (best) and diffuse (worse).[27] A subtype of disease with absence of skin fibrosis has been recognized and is referred to as *scleroderma sine scleroderma*. Serologic studies have shown that the

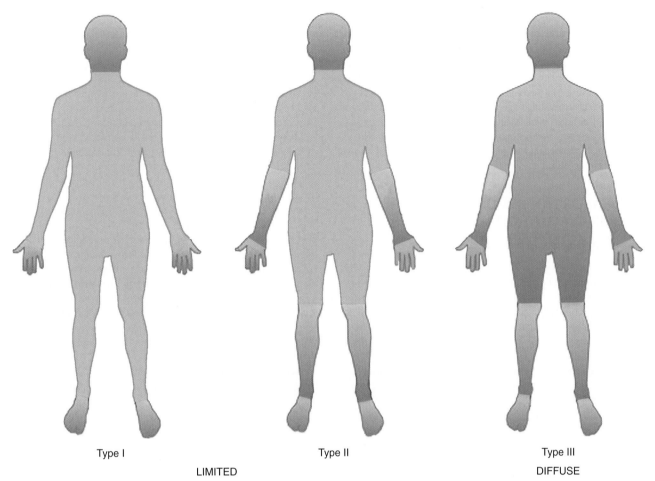

Type I   Type II   Type III

LIMITED   DIFFUSE

Figure 84-1 Classification of scleroderma and clinical subsets. Most experts classify scleroderma into two major groups: limited and diffuse. Limited includes patients with no skin changes (systemic sclerosis "sine" scleroderma), and type I or II, who do not have more proximal limb or truncal involvement.

presence of specific autoantibodies predicts clinical features of the disease, suggesting that the classification might be based on the autoantibody type (see "Natural History"). Patients with early or partial expression of the disease (e.g., Raynaud's phenomenon alone with nail-fold capillary loop abnormalities) are often diagnosed as having undifferentiated connective tissue disease (UCTD). About 20% of these patients will develop clear features of scleroderma, usually within 2 to 4 years of follow-up.[25]

Scleroderma patients often have features of another rheumatic or autoimmune disease. These patients are considered to have an *overlap syndrome*. The most common overlap syndromes are polyarthritis, myositis, sicca complex, and hypothyroidism. Less common are primary biliary cirrhosis, autoimmune hepatitis, vasculitis, rheumatoid arthritis, and antineutrophil cytoplasm antibody (ANCA)-associated pauci-immune glomerulonephritis. Mixed connective tissue disease (MCTD) is an overlap syndrome, with features of scleroderma, polymyositis, lupus-like rashes, and rheumatoid-like polyarthritis.

Natural History of Disease

The natural history of scleroderma varies a great deal depending on the specific subtype of disease established in

a patient. Scleroderma tends to be a chronic monophasic illness, unlike systemic lupus erythematosus, which is characterized by quiescence interrupted by sudden disease flares. The pattern of the disease and the degree or type of internal organ involvement are variable but generally can be predicted by the extent of skin affected. Internal organ disease is more severe in patients with the diffuse skin type than in those with limited scleroderma. The disease course is usually indolent in patients with sclerodactyly alone. In these patients, years pass from onset of Raynaud's phenomenon before obvious organ dysfunction manifests, although explosive multisystem disease can emerge rapidly over several months in patients with widespread skin changes. Likewise, when patients with diffuse skin disease experience skin improvement, new internal organ disease is generally uncommon. The degree of skin thickening varies in extent and progression over time, with some cases stopping after several months with relatively mild disease, and others progressing over years to involve most of the body surface (see "Skin Involvement").

Patients classified in the *limited scleroderma* group may have intermediate skin involvement, with skin extending over the hands and forearms or lower legs but not over the trunk. These patients appear to have an intermediate disease course that is not as severe as that of patients with widespread skin disease. The intermediate group has decreased survival compared with patients with only sclerodactyly. Although the degree of skin disease provides a rough guide by which to predict disease course, many exceptions have been noted. Variability is associated with other clinically defined factors, including age, gender, and racial/ethnic background. Late age at onset increases the risks for PAH and poor survival. Males may have a more aggressive disease course than females. African-American or Native American race predicts a worse disease course and worse multisystem disease.[9]

GENERAL PRINCIPLES OF DISEASE EVALUATION

Measuring Disease Activity and Severity

One of the challenges in studying or caring for patients with scleroderma consists of determining and measuring disease activity, severity, and damage. These measures are not independent of each other and thus cannot be considered in isolation. Activity is a measure of ongoing disease that is dynamic and reversible; it is a direct reflection of ongoing biologic processes such as autoimmune-mediated inflammation or progressive tissue fibrosis. Severity is a measure of the impact of damage on the whole person or a specific organ at any given time. In the extreme, severity is a measure of irreversible end-stage damage. It is important to distinguish reversible disease activity from irreversible damage in that both can cause clinical distress, yet intervention differs for the two. Patients with scleroderma accumulate irreversible damage over time, thus the measure of activity is best done in early disease, when disease has the potential of being reversed.

Measurement of changes in skin thickness (modified Rodnan skin score) is used as a surrogate measure of disease severity and a predictor of extent of organ involvement and overall prognosis (see skin manifestation section).[28] It is also used as a quantifiable, easily obtainable, and valid score, changing over time in response to therapy. Thus, the skin score is now used as a measure of disease activity and is employed in clinical trials as a primary outcome measure. In patients with diffuse skin disease, improvement in skin score is associated with better clinical outcome. A core set of items covering 11 domains (skin, musculoskeletal, cardiac, pulmonary, renal, gastrointestinal, health-related quality of life measures, global health, Raynaud's phenomenon, digital ulcers, and the biomarkers erythrocyte sedimentation rate and C-reactive protein) is now considered to provide the minimum clinically relevant treatment effect values, as defined by consensus of experts in the field.[29] More detailed scales for specific organs are also in use. For example, a skin assessment tool combines the modified Rodnan skin score with a visual analogue score (VAS) of the patient's assessment of skin activity, a VAS score of the physician's assessment of skin activity, and measures obtained by a durometer.[30] A gastrointestinal scale has been developed to define mild to severe gastrointestinal disease.[31] Experts who reviewed current outcome measures in assessing PAH as related to scleroderma decided that lung vascular and pulmonary arterial pressures and cardiac function as measured by right heart catheterization and echocardiography;

exercise testing as measured by 6-minute walk and oxygen saturation with exercise, New York Heart Association functional class, severity of dyspnea on a VAS, and measures of quality of life and function obtained by Short Form 36 and the Health Assessment Questionnaire and Disability Index (HAQ-DI); and physician global scale as measured by survival are all important measures. Other outcome measures that are considered valid include Raynaud's condition score for Raynaud's severity, forced vital capacity, and Mahler's dyspnea index to follow interstitial lung disease, serum creatinine, blood pressure, and complete blood count during a scleroderma renal crisis, as well as serum creatine phosphokinase to follow muscle disease.

A scleroderma severity scale has been developed by Medsger to assess disease severity status in individual patients both at a given time and longitudinally (Table 84-2).[32] This scale is based on scoring that ranges from 0 (normal) to 4 (end-stage) for each organ system involved in scleroderma, including a general measure, along with measures of the peripheral vascular system, skin, joints and tendons, gastrointestinal tract, lung, heart, and kidney. This severity scale is now used by many experts to define the status of a patient in clinical trials and in research investigating risk for clinical outcomes.

The Health Assessment Questionnaire and Disability Index (HAQ-DI) is a self-administered tool initially developed for rheumatoid arthritis to measure functional impairment; it has been validated and used in scleroderma as well, where it correlates with objective physical signs and reflects the disease course. Higher degrees of impairment are found by HAQ scores in scleroderma patients with diffuse skin disease, higher skin scores, abnormal hand function, presence of myopathy or friction rubs, and joint pain.[33] Change in the HAQ score occurs with changes in skin involvement and progressive organ disease.[34] The HAQ is useful in evaluating patients with Raynaud's and correlates with the severity and presence of digital ulcers. VAS instruments that assess disease in various domains specific for scleroderma are added to the HAQ to focus on scleroderma-specific issues, including measures of Raynaud's and digital ulcers. In addition, the Short Form 36 survey, a simple self-report tool composed of 36 items in 8 domains, is used to assess health-related quality of life.

Developing an activity scale is much more challenging than establishing severity measures. Attempts include evaluating changes in skin score and evidence of active lung disease and documenting congestive heart failure or a scleroderma renal crisis. A composite score generated as a physician global assessment has been used to measure disease activity. This simple global score has merit but is influenced, besides activity, by organ severity and irreversible damage.[35] A European study group developed the Valentini disease activity index, which currently is used in clinical studies.[36] This index provides more of an organ-specific assessment than a measure of global activity. The Medsger disease severity scale has the potential to measure activity if used in studies with serial observations, when individual organ scales can be combined into a composite score. Intermediate clinical and serologic biomarkers are under investigation as candidates to define and predict disease activity and prognosis, but none has proved reliable or valid. Measures of acute phase factors (e.g., erythrocyte

Table 84-2 Medsger Systemic Sclerosis Severity Scale*

Organ System	0 (Normal)	1 (Mild)	2 (Moderate)	3 (Severe)	4 (End Stage)
General	Wt loss <5%; Ht 37%+; Hb 12.3+ g/dL	Wt loss 5%-10%; Ht 33%-37%; Hb 11.0-12.2 g/dL	Wt loss 10%-15%; Ht 29%-33%; Hb 9.7-10.9 g/dL	Wt loss 15%-20%; Ht 25%-29%; Hb 8.3-9.6 g/dL	Wt loss 20+%; Ht 25%; Hb <8.3 g/dL
Peripheral vascular	No Raynaud's; Raynaud's not requiring vasodilators	Raynaud's requiring vasodilators	Digital pitting scars	Digital tip ulcerations	Digital gangrene
Skin	TSS 0	TSS 1-14	TSS 15-29	TSS 30-39	TSS 40+
Joint/tendon	FTP 0-0.9 cm	FTP 1.0-1.9 cm	FTP 2.0-3.9 cm	FTP 4.0-4.9 cm	FTP 5.0+ cm
Muscle	Normal proximal muscle strength	Proximal weakness, mild	Proximal weakness, moderate	Proximal weakness, severe	Ambulation aids required
Gastrointestinal tract	Normal esophagogram; normal small bowel series	Distal esophageal hypoperistalsis; small bowel series abnormal	Antibiotics required for bacterial overgrowth	Malabsorption syndrome; episodes of pseudo-obstruction	Hyperalimentation required
Lung	DLCO 80+%; FVC 80+%; no fibrosis on radiograph; sPAP <35 mm Hg	DLCO 70%-79%; FVC 70%-79%; basilar rales; fibrosis on radiograph; sPAP 35-49 mm Hg	DLCO 50%-69%; FVC 50%-69%; sPAP 50-64 mm Hg	DLCO <50%; FVC <50%; sPAP 65+ mm Hg	Oxygen required
Heart	ECG normal; LVEF 50+%	ECG conduction defect; LVEF 45%-49%	ECG arrhythmia; LVEF 40%-44%	ECG arrhythmia requiring therapy; LVEF 30%-40%	CHF; LVEF <30%
Kidney	No history of SRC with serum creatinine <1.3 mg/dL	History of SRC with serum creatinine <1.5 mg/dL	History of SRC with serum creatinine 1.5-2.4 mg/dL	History of SRC with serum creatinine 2.5-5.0 mg/dL	History of SRC with serum creatinine >5.0 mg/dL or dialysis required

*If two items are included for a severity grade, only one is required for the patient to be scored as having disease of that severity level.

CHF, congestive heart failure; DLCO, diffusing capacity for carbon monoxide, % predicted; ECG, electrocardiogram; FTP, fingertip-to-palm distance in flexion; FVC, forced vital capacity, % predicted; Hb, hemoglobin; Ht, hematocrit; LVEF, left ventricular ejection fraction; sPAP, estimated pulmonary artery pressure by Doppler echo; SRC, scleroderma renal crisis; TSS, total skin score; Wt, weight.

Adapted from Medsger TA Jr, Bombardieri S, Czirjak L, et al: Assessment of disease severity and prognosis, *Clin Exp Rheumatol* 21(3 Suppl 29):S51, 2003.

sedimentation rate, C-reactive protein) are nonspecific but are included by expert consensus in some systems designed to measure disease activity. Currently, no "gold standard" is available to measure disease activity in scleroderma, and defining biomarkers or other measures of disease activity remains a major challenge.

Autoantibodies

Measurement of the autoantibodies present in scleroderma can be helpful in determining the clinical features and prognosis of the disease, in that specific scleroderma-related autoantibodies have been established as strong predictors of disease outcome and the pattern of organ complications

(Table 84-3).[37] The three most frequently observed types of scleroderma-specific autoantibodies are anticentromere, antitopoisomerase I, and anti-RNA polymerase III antibodies.

Anticentromere patients tend to be older white women. Skin disease usually is limited and most often involves just the fingers. The disease course is indolent, and often the diagnosis is delayed until anticentromere antibodies are discovered or late organ disease becomes evident. Patients frequently develop features of the CREST syndrome. Subcutaneous calcinosis is a late manifestation, appearing in areas such as small clusters on the fingers and along the forearm and anterior lower leg. Raynaud's phenomenon can become severe and is associated with increased risk for

Table 84-3 Autoantibodies and Associated Phenotypes in Scleroderma

Antigen	Subtype	Clinical Phenotype
Topoisomerase 1 (Scl70)	Diffuse	Pulmonary fibrosis, cardiac involvement
Centromere (protein B, C)	Limited	Severe digital ischemia, PAH, sicca syndrome, calcinosis
RNA polymerase III	Diffuse	Severe skin disease, tendon rubs, renal crisis (±sine scleroderma)
U3-RNP (fibrillarin)	Diffuse or limited	Primary PAH; esophageal, cardiac, and renal involvement; muscular disease
Th/To	Limited	Pulmonary fibrosis, rare renal crisis, lower GI dysfunction
B23	Diffuse or limited	PAH, lung disease
Cardiolipin, β_2GPI	Limited	PAH, digital loss
PM/Scl	Overlap	Myositis, pulmonary fibrosis, acro-osteolysis
U1-RNP	Overlap	SLE, inflammatory arthritis, pulmonary fibrosis

GI, gastrointestinal; GPI, glycoprotein I; PAH, pulmonary arterial hypertension; RNA, ribonucleic acid; RNP, ribonucleoprotein particle; SLE, systemic lupus erythematosus.

Adapted from Boin F, Rosen A: Autoimmunity in systemic sclerosis: current concepts, *Curr Rheumatol Rep* 9:165–172, 2007.

macrovascular disease. Higher risk for digital gangrene and amputation is noted in the anticentromere–positive group. Interstitial lung disease is less common and is isolated and progressive; pulmonary vascular disease with PAH and right heart failure occur in a significant proportion of patients. Overall, however, anticentromere antibodies generally are predictors of a favorable prognosis. The presence of anticentromere antibodies can also be seen in patients with primary Sjögren's syndrome who do not have scleroderma.

Antitopoisomerase I antibodies are seen in 30% of African-American patients and are correlated with a poor prognosis and higher scleroderma-related mortality. Interstitial lung disease (ILD) is highly associated with anti-topoisomerase, independent of the degree of skin disease. Patients usually have diffuse skin disease and are at risk for rapid skin changes and renal crisis, usually in the first few years from disease onset. Raynaud's phenomenon may be the first symptom, followed in the first years of disease by skin changes and joint-tendon involvement leading to contractures, particularly in the fingers and elbows. The degree of skin thickening varies a great deal in these patients, but usually the level of severity of skin involvement is established in the first 1 to 3 years of disease.

Anti-RNA polymerase III antibodies are associated with rapid and aggressive diffuse skin disease and renal involvement. These patients have the worst cutaneous involvement with rapid widespread skin disease associated with signs and symptoms of deep tissue fibrosis involving joints, tendons, and muscles. Flexion contractures of fingers, wrist, elbows, shoulders, hips, knees, and ankles are complications that can occur within a few months of onset of disease activity. Friction rubs are common. A "fibrosing" myopathy without inflammation, along with skin and joint disease, leads to loss of strength and flexibility. Significant disability occurs in early disease. Anti-RNA polymerase III–positive patients are not likely to have severe gastrointestinal disease and are relatively protected from developing ILD or pulmonary vascular disease. However, they are at high risk (approximately 25% to 40% of patents) for developing scleroderma renal disease with hypertensive crisis. Risk is greatest in the early years, when skin is rapidly changing. Heart disease can be a late complication, but major disability from skin and deep tissue disease is the most worrisome long-term problem in this subtype of scleroderma.

Other antinucleolar antibodies are found among subgroups of patients with scleroderma and are associated with specific clinical phenotypes and clinical outcomes. Of these, anti-Th/To antibodies and anti-PM/Scl antibodies are associated with limited skin disease, whereas anti-U3-RNP (fibrillarin) antibodies are associated with diffuse disease. Anti-Th/To is at increased risk for development of severe ILD and pulmonary hypertension. Anti-U3-RNP is another predictor of a less favorable prognosis with a higher frequency of internal organ involvement, including interstitial lung disease, PAH, and renal crisis. It is frequently present in African-Americans and is associated with diffuse skin disease and poor prognosis. Hyperpigmented and hypopigmented skin changes are common, and contractures of large joints associated with inflammatory or fibrotic muscle disease lead to significant morbidity. Cardiac disease is often

subclinical until late-stage disease, when both right and left heart failure can occur.

Anti-PM/Scl, anti-Ku, and anti-U1-RNP antibodies are seen mainly in patients with overlap syndromes. The presence of anti-Pm/Scl is associated with acute onset of weakness due to inflammatory muscle disease and higher risk for interstitial lung disease. Anti-Ku positivity has been demonstrated to be strongly associated with muscle and joint involvement. Anti-U1-RNP is seen in patients with mixed connective tissue disease and is common among African-Americans with limited scleroderma. Polyarthritis, myositis, and lupus with skin or renal involvement are common complications. A subset can develop diffuse skin disease, and risk for late onset of PAH is increased overall. Although an uncommon anti-B23 autoantibody is associated with pulmonary arterial hypertension, up to 11% of patients with scleroderma can test negative for antinuclear antibodies.

CLINICAL MANIFESTATIONS AND TREATMENT

General Principles of Management

Several basic principles can be of help in managing patients with scleroderma. The first is that scleroderma encompasses subsets of disease, each with a unique clinical phenotype; thus carefully determining the specific subtype of the patient sets the scene for deciding therapy. Clinical problems and disease activity in scleroderma are highly variable in expression, even within a given subtype. This variability is thought to be secondary to different susceptibility to, or risk for, systemic complications. It is also due to the presence of a dynamic biologic process unique to scleroderma. Therefore, patients move through stages of the disease process with disease activity that varies with time and can shift in nature. Signs of classic inflammatory events are often present during the initial phase of the disease, but later, an indolent subclinical fibrotic process is dominant and gradually causes organ damage. Although the skin may be the site of the most dramatic physical findings, scleroderma is a multisystem disease, and the physician must search for early organ-based complications, including cardiopulmonary, gastrointestinal, renal, or musculoskeletal involvement. Understanding the shortcomings of current investigations, not getting locked into "traditional" therapy, focusing on an organ-specific approach, and defining the disease subtype and level of disease activity are most important in establishing optimal management. Although no good studies have been conducted to prove the effectiveness of this approach, it seems reasonable to use combination therapy with rapid control of the inflammatory immune process early on, followed by maintenance immunosuppression for an extended time. The anti-inflammatory program is then coupled with organ-specific therapy (see later sections). The missing component in this comprehensive approach is the availability of a direct antifibrotic agent able to prevent the progression of fibrosis once the inflammatory phase is under control. Obviously, early intervention is most important for success; once irreversible tissue or organ damage is noted, supportive care becomes the main and often the only option.

RAYNAUD'S PHENOMENON

Raynaud's phenomenon (RP) is an exaggerated vascular response of the digital arterial circulation triggered by cold ambient temperature and emotional stress. The diagnosis of RP is based on a history of excessive cold sensitivity and recurrent events of sharply demarcated pallor and/or cyanosis of the skin of the digits (Figure 84-2). Blanching reflects digital arterial vasospasm, and cyanosis occurs secondary to the deoxygenation of sluggish venous blood flow. Some skin blushing (redness) may follow owing to reactive hyperemia after regular blood flow has been restored. Raynaud's phenomenon occurs in 3% to 15% of the general population. It is more common among females (3 to 4:1) and is likely to begin before 20 years of age. During cold exposure (particularly during shifting temperatures and winter months), Raynaud's attacks increase in frequency and intensity. Raynaud's phenomenon can be categorized clinically into primary and secondary forms (Figure 84-3). Primary RP occurs when no disease process is associated with recurrent vasospastic events. Distinguishing primary RP from that associated with an underlying disorder is frequently challenging. Young age at onset (<20 years), symmetric manifestations of symptoms, mild to moderate severity, no association with digital ulceration or tissue gangrene, normal nail-fold capillary examination, and a negative antinuclear antibody (ANA) titer are all indicative of primary RP.[38] Secondary RP occurs in a variety of settings, including connective tissues disorders and other rheumatic conditions, occupational trauma (e.g., hypothenar hammer syndrome), the use of certain drugs (e.g., antimigraine agents, ergotamine derivatives, bleomycin), increased blood viscosity, and compressive or obstructive vascular disease (e.g., thoracic outlet syndrome, atherosclerosis, thromboangiitis obliterans).

Nail-fold capillaroscopy is the tool most commonly used at the bedside to distinguish patients with primary RP from those with scleroderma or another rheumatic disease. Maricq and associates first described the abnormal pattern of nail-fold capillary vessels seen in scleroderma.[39] The simplest method of detection is to coat the skin of the nail fold with immersion oil and then view the area using a bifocal dissecting microscope or a hand-held device such as an ophthalmoscope set at 20 or 40 diopters. A computerized nail-fold videocapillaroscopy technique is used in specialty centers. This technique provides enhanced digital images that can assess local blood flow and follow the disease course.[40] Although patients with primary RP may have normal, thin, palisading nail-fold capillary loops (Figure 84-4), in secondary RP, capillary loop dilation/enlargements and dropouts represent the salient features. Patterns of capillary abnormalities appear to correlate with the course of systemic disease manifestations. Capillary dilation (giant capillaries), microhemorrhages, and some disorganization of the capillary network are typical of early disease; dropouts, avascular areas, and signs of neoangiogenesis with bizarre architectural distortion manifest at later stages of scleroderma.[41,42] Approximately 20% to 30% of patients with RP and abnormal nail-fold capillary changes will develop clinical features of scleroderma, usually within a 2- to 3-year period.[25] Patients presenting with RP, nail-fold capillary changes, and the presence of a scleroderma-related autoantibody have a 70% to 80% chance of developing scleroderma within 2 to 3 years from presentation. Therefore, capillaroscopy represents an important standard tool that can be used to examine patients presenting with RP.

In scleroderma, RP and digital ischemia are the clinical manifestations of both fixed structural vascular disease and abnormal regulation of local vasomotor control. Cold-induced vasoconstriction of peripheral blood vessels normally occurs via sympathetic stimulation. Abnormal thermoregulation is associated with a nonvasculitic vasculopathy characterized by endothelial dysfunction and a fibrotic proliferation, which produces an increase in collagen content of the intima of small and medium vessels and causes loss of vessel flexibility and obliteration of their lumina. Digital pitting with loss of fingertip tissue and small, painful, superficial ulcerations are very common and usually are noted secondary to disease affecting the small arteries and arterioles of the skin (Figure 84-5). Large, deep ulceration of the distal portion of the finger is a consequence of larger-vessel (e.g., digital artery) occlusion associated with severe vasospasm. The latter event usually presents as a sharp demarcation of the distal digit with intense, localized pain secondary to ischemia. Failure to reverse these events may lead to loss of the whole digit or limb secondary to deep tissue infarction.

Although a number of methods may be used to objectively score attacks of RP, no test is considered practical or reproducible enough to replace the clinical criteria for diagnosis and management. Patients with an active RP attack

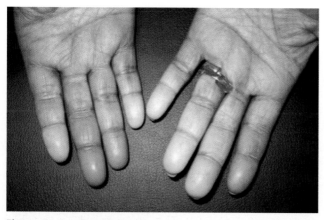

Figure 84-2 Active Raynaud's phenomenon with well-demarcated pallor at the fingertips in a scleroderma patient.

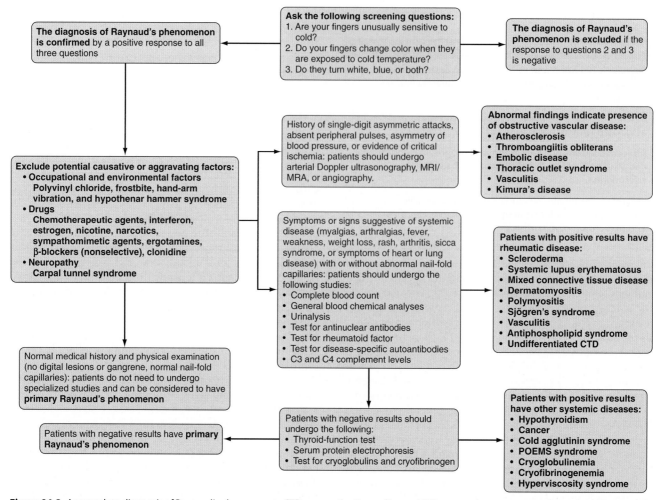

Figure 84-3 Approach to diagnosis of Raynaud's phenomenon. CTD, connective tissue disease; MRA, magnetic resonance angiography; MRI, magnetic resonance imaging; POEMS, polyneuropathy, organomegaly, endocrinopathy, monoclonal gammopathy, and skin changes.

will present with coolness of the involved distal fingertips and/or toes, which can be associated with a line of demarcation of skin pallor or cyanosis. In later stages of severe RP, if left untreated, one may find signs of critical digital ischemia resulting in painful and unremitting digital ulcerations. Such findings warrant immediate medical treatment. Several methods may be used to assess the severity of RP. Traditionally, the patient is asked to use a diary to record the frequency and duration of attacks during days of usual activity. Raynaud's condition score (RCS) is a patient-based measure that takes into account the impact of RP on the patient, including pain, discomfort, and effect on daily function. Other laboratory-based measures, including laser Doppler, thermography, and plethysmography methods, are used in an attempt to obtain objective data.

Treatment of Raynaud's Phenomenon and Digital Ischemia

The primary goal in the management of RP is prevention of digital ischemia through the use of nonpharmacologic and pharmacologic measures (Figure 84-6). In the setting of acute digital ischemia, rapid intervention using both treatment modalities is required. The primary and most important nonpharmacologic therapy for prevention is avoidance

of cold ambient temperatures, particularly transitioning from a warm or hot environment to a cold one. A warm ambient temperature reduces the frequency and severity of RP. All patients with RP should understand that clothing should be layered and loose-fitting, with the goal of maintaining a warm core body temperature, not just warmth of the affected extremities. Patients who have an acute ischemic event are best treated with rest in a warm environment (home or hospital), insulated from cold temperatures. Other potential therapies include minimizing emotional distress (reducing sympathetic tone) and avoiding aggravating factors such as smoking, sympathomimetic drugs (e.g., preparations for the common cold), migraine headache medications (e.g., serotonin agonists), and nonselective β-blockers (e.g., propranolol). Although behavioral therapies (biofeedback, autogenic training, and classical conditioning) are reported to be helpful, their benefit is controversial, and they play no role in the management of acute ischemia related to scleroderma.[43] In fact, biofeedback alone is not helpful for primary RP.

Drug therapy for RP in scleroderma includes the use of a variety of oral or systemic vasodilators. Calcium channel blockers are considered to be first-line therapeutic agents in the treatment of RP. This class of medication works primarily by inducing arterial vasodilation through direct

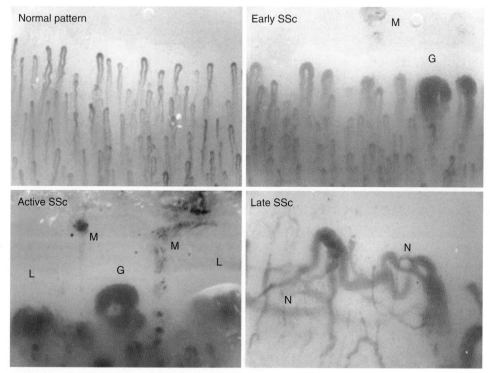

Figure 84-4 Patterns of nail-fold capillary abnormalities assessed by videocapillaroscopy in scleroderma patients. *Top right,* "Early pattern" shows the presence of few enlarged/giant capillaries, few capillary hemorrhages, and no evident loss or distortion of capillaries. *Bottom left,* "Active pattern" presents with frequent dilated capillary loops, frequent microhemorrhages, moderate loss of capillaries, and mild disorganization of the capillary architecture. *Bottom right,* "Late pattern" is characterized by severe loss of capillaries with avascular areas, ramified/bushy capillaries (neovascularization), and disorganization of the normal capillary architecture. G, giant capillaries; L, loss of capillaries; M, microhemorrhages; N, neoangiogenesis; SSc, systemic sclerosis. *(Courtesy Professor Maurizio Cutolo.)*

inhibition of contraction of vessel smooth muscle cells; however, these agents provide additional benefits by reducing oxidative and inhibiting platelet activation.[44,45] Most published studies evaluating the efficacy of calcium channel blockers in RP have employed dihydropyridines (e.g., nifedipine, amlodipine, nisoldipine, isradipine, felodipine), and few have looked at nondihydropyridines, which appear to be more efficacious in primary than in secondary RP.[46,47] A meta-analysis of 17 studies evaluating the efficacy of short- and long-acting formulations of calcium channel blockers reported a 33% reduction in attack severity and a near 50% reduction in the number of attacks per week.[48] The current recommendation is to use an extended-release formulation of a calcium channel blocker for treatment of nonurgent RP. The dose should be titrated to clinical efficacy, but common side effects (hypotension, headache, pedal edema) should be monitored. For urgent cases of RP, a short-acting formulation of the medication is preferred, but titration should be carefully monitored. Although calcium channel blockers are the agents most likely to be effective, a host of other vasodilators are used, including nitrates, phosphodiesterase-5 inhibitors (e.g., sildenafil), intravenous prostaglandins, and sympatholytic agents (e.g., prazosin).

Among other agents being tested in the treatment of RP are drugs that enhance nitric oxide availability—serotonin uptake blockers (e.g., fluoxetine), Rho-kinase inhibitors, local injection of botulinum toxin (Botox), antioxidants (acetylcysteine), angiotensin receptor blockers, and selective α2-adrenergic receptor antagonists. A combination of

these agents, if tolerated, can be used in refractory cases. Various formulations of topical and oral nitroglycerin are employed.[49,50] Although some degree of efficacy is obtained, use of nitroglycerin is limited by substantial side effects, including headache, dizziness, and local skin irritation. The cyclic guanine monophosphate phosphodiesterase-5 inhibitors are thought to be effective in the treatment of RP by sustaining the vasodilatory effect of nitric oxide.[51,52] Studies using phosphodiesterase inhibitors have reported variable effects, and the ideal drug and dosing have not yet been defined. Despite the theoretical advantage of angiotensin-converting enzyme (ACE) inhibitors, a study of quinapril showed that these medications did not affect the occurrence of digital ulcers or the frequency or severity of RP episodes.[53] Thus, although ACEs are critical for the treatment of a scleroderma renal crisis (see renal section), they do not have a major role in the management of RP.

New emphasis is being placed on prevention of scleroderma vascular disease through the use of immunosuppressive and vasoprotective drugs. HMG-CoA (3-hydroxy-3-methylglutaryl-coenzyme A) reductase inhibitors (statins) can modify progression of vascular injury and can prevent vascular ischemia through different pleiotropic functions, as by improvement of endothelial dysfunction, reduction of clotting, and introduction of some anti-inflammatory effects.[54,55] Data suggest that statins may increase the number of endothelial progenitor cells and may improve vascular remodeling after injury.[56,57] In a randomized, placebo-controlled study of scleroderma patients with secondary RP,

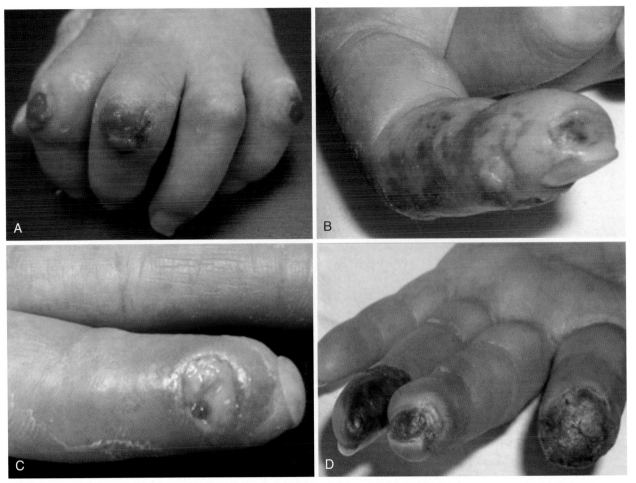

Figure 84-5 Scleroderma and Raynaud's phenomenon can be associated with digital ulcerations and severe digital ischemia. **A,** Traumatic ulcers over the proximal interphalangeal joints. **B** and **C,** Ischemic digital ulcerations secondary to small arterial disease. **D,** Digital gangrene secondary to macrovascular disease.

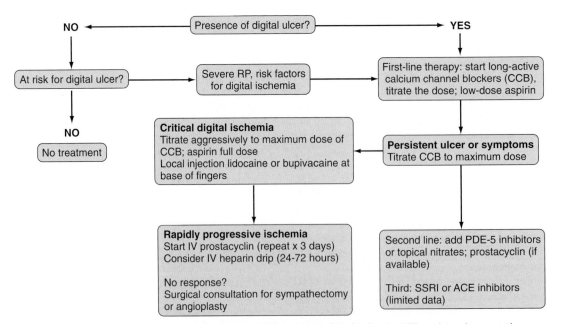

Figure 84-6 Approach to drug treatment of Raynaud's phenomenon (RP) and acute digital ischemia. ACE, angiotensin-converting enzyme; IV, intravenous; PDE-5, phosphodiesterase-5; SSRI, selective serotonin reuptake inhibitor.

statin use significantly decreased the number of digital ulcers formed.[58]

Intravenous infusions of vasodilating prostaglandins (alprostadil, epoprostenol, iloprost, treprostinil) reduce the severity and frequency of Raynaud's attacks and are most helpful during periods of sustained critical ischemia. These prostaglandins are efficacious in the treatment of RP because of their strong vasodilating effect, inhibition of platelet aggregation, and enhancement of vascular function through other mechanisms. Intravenous prostacyclins can be given intermittently to patients with scleroderma during winter months or throughout the year, or they can be used acutely during a vascular crisis. Oral prostaglandins have variable absorption and are not yet available.

Endothelin-1 is strongly implicated in the pathogenesis of RP and the vascular disease of scleroderma.[59] Bosentan, an endothelin-1 receptor blocker, was studied in a randomized, placebo-controlled, double-blind multicenter study that showed efficacy in preventing new digital ulcers, along with improved hand function, but it did not improve healing of existing ulcers compared with placebo.[60]

Sympathectomy is a viable option for patients with RP who are unresponsive to medical therapy; it should be considered as acute intervention during a critical ischemic event. Localized digital sympathectomy with lysis of fibrosis around the vessel is effective for acute ischemia and has mostly replaced cervical sympathectomy.[61,62] Responses to sympathectomies suggest that the long-term benefit derived from these interventions is limited. In fact, Raynaud's attacks eventually recur, and medical therapy is needed to prevent new events.

Careful assessment for correctable macrovascular disease should be done when confronted with acute digital ischemia, particularly when the whole finger is demarcated, or when the event involves a lower extremity. In this setting, appropriate studies such as arterial Doppler ultrasound or angiographic imaging are warranted. If macrovascular disease is present, vascular surgery may help to alleviate the occlusive process. Preferential involvement of the ulnar artery has been reported in scleroderma patients.[63]

Patients with critical digital ischemia should be hospitalized to reduce vasospastic activity, maintain warmth, and permit rapid initiation of vasodilator therapy. Intravenous vasodilating prostaglandins can be infused to maximize vasodilation. Antiplatelet therapy with low-dose aspirin may be useful, but its benefit is unproven in the acute setting. Heparinization may be considered during acute ischemic crises of the digits, but chronic anticoagulation in scleroderma is not recommended. Chemical sympathectomy of the affected digit, performed by local infiltration with lidocaine or bupivacaine, may provide immediate relief. For refractory cases, a surgical approach to digital sympathectomy is used.

Ischemic digital lesions should be treated with topical antibiotics and daily cleansing with soap and water. Débridement procedures should be performed very cautiously because tissue trauma may extend the injury owing to the avascular nature of the digital tissue. Digital lesions that progress to dry gangrene should be permitted to undergo autoamputation. Surgical amputation is best offered only for intractable pain or deep tissue infection.

SKIN INVOLVEMENT

The most overt clinical manifestation of scleroderma is skin disease. The degree of involvement can vary among patients, and involvement can change in severity and distribution over time in the same individual. Almost every scleroderma patient presents with skin thickening and hardening due to increased collagen and extracellular matrix deposition in the dermis. The distribution of skin changes is characteristic, with more frequent and intense involvement of fingers, hands, forearms, distal legs, feet, and face, and, to a lesser degree, the proximal limbs and anterior trunk. Sparing of the midback is typical. Scleroderma is classically subdivided into *limited* and *diffuse* cutaneous forms (Figure 84-7). Limited scleroderma is defined by skin thickening restricted to the face and limbs distally to the elbows and knees. Commonly, in this form of the disease, only the fingers and the face are involved. In contrast, diffuse cutaneous involvement is characterized by widespread skin thickening, including proximal limbs and truncal areas. Proximal skin involvement defines the diffuse cutaneous subset but may be absent in early stages of disease. Signs of skin thickening are not apparent in the setting of other disease manifestations (e.g., Raynaud's phenomenon, nail-fold capillary abnormalities), nor is evidence of internal organ involvement. This clinical presentation is referred to as *systemic sclerosis sine scleroderma*. Traditionally, patients are clustered into limited and diffuse skin subsets, but evidence suggests the existence of an intermediate group of patients. Each subset of disease defined by the degree of skin thickening has a unique pattern of disease manifestation and risk for specific clinical outcomes. Therefore, expression of skin disease can be used as a predictor or a "clinical biomarker" of the disease course. The variable degree of skin involvement can be quantified by physical examination. The most widely accepted scoring system (modified Rodnan skin score) is applied by pinching the skin in 17 different body areas and subjectively averaging the thickness of each specific site from 0 = normal to 3 = very thick (Figure 84-8). The skin score (maximum, 51) is a useful clinical measurement tool that can be used to quantify the severity of skin disease.[28] Although the overall extent of skin involvement as measured by the skin score can predict certain clinical outcomes, it does not define the quality of the skin process nor the level of disease activity at any single point in time. Therefore, it is important to follow the skin score over time and to measure changes sequentially to monitor disease progression.

Cutaneous involvement in scleroderma begins with clinical signs of inflammation. This is called the *edematous phase* because it is characterized by nonpitting edema of affected body areas. In limited scleroderma, this event is mild and is restricted to the digits; however, in the diffuse form of the disease, cutaneous swelling and edema can be widespread and so impressive in the limbs as to mimic a fluid overload state such as congestive heart failure. Edema can also cause local tissue compression. For example, upon involvement of the wrist area, scleroderma patients are not infrequently diagnosed with carpal tunnel syndrome (especially at disease onset) to explain hand and wrist discomfort. In association with edema, signs and symptoms of inflammation are

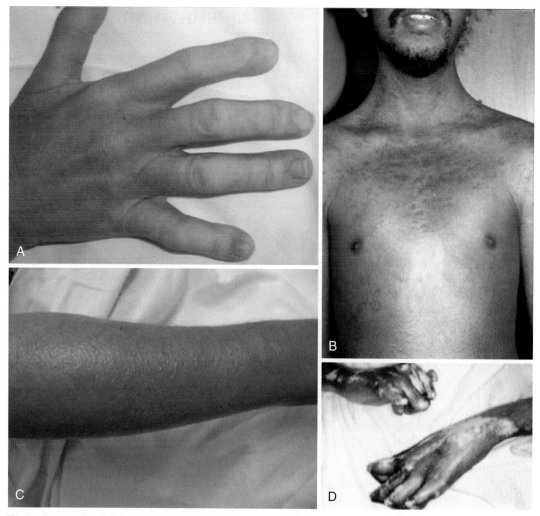

Figure 84-7 Skin involvement in scleroderma is subdivided into "limited" and "diffuse" cutaneous forms. **A,** Sclerodactyly in limited cutaneous disease. **B,** Truncal changes in diffuse cutaneous disease. **C,** Inflammatory signs in early active skin disease. **D,** Finger contracture in the chronic fibrotic phase of skin involvement in scleroderma.

common. Erythema of the skin and intense pruritus and pain (see Figure 84-7C) are characteristic of advancing active diffuse skin disease. This pain has a neuropathic quality with a reported "pins and needles" sensation. The disease process leads to loss of skin appendages, as well as decreased hair growth and loss of sweat and exocrine glands; thus the skin surface becomes dry and uncomfortable. Small papules can be seen in areas of trauma as the result of scratching, giving the surface a cobblestone texture. The

edematous phase continues for several weeks but eventually gives way to a fibrotic stage, with protracted activity that may last months or years.

During the fibrotic phase, acute inflammation is clinically less obvious, and deposition in the dermis of excessive collagen and other extracellular material thickens the skin, making it inflexible and causing further loss of skin appendages. Fibrosis extends beyond the dermis into the deeper layers with loss of subcutaneous adipose tissue

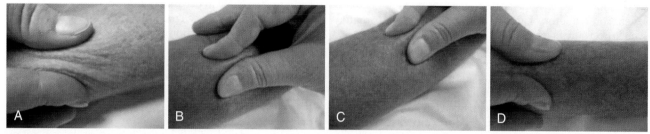

Figure 84-8 Method used to semi-quantify skin thickness in scleroderma. The modified Rodnan skin score is obtained by clinical palpation of 17 different body areas (fingers, hands, forearms, upper arms, chest, abdomen, thighs, lower legs, and feet) and subjective averaging of the thickness of each specific site: 0 = normal (**A**); 1 = mild (**B**); 2 = moderate (**C**); and 3 = severe (**D**). The maximum score is 51.

(lipodystrophy). In late stages of the disease, skin actually thins with atrophy and has a noninflammatory bound-down appearance. Deeper tissue fibrosis causes permanent contractures around joints or may involve underlying muscle, causing a myopathy (see Figure 84-7D). Patients with diffuse cutaneous scleroderma develop the most dramatic widespread skin changes; those with limited skin disease may note only puffy fingers and digital thickening typical of sclerodactyly. A masked facies, small oral and orbital apertures, and vertical furrowing of the perioral skin are consequences of skin and soft tissue fibrosis. In some patients, gum atrophy and facial skin tightening make the front teeth appear more prominent. Flexion contractures of fingers, wrists, and elbows often appear secondary to dermal sclerosis and fibrosis with atrophy of underlying tissues. Skin ulcers can develop as a complication of avascular fibrotic or damaged thinned skin and are very common at sites of trauma, such as over the digital metacarpophalangeal or proximal interphalangeal joints or at the tip of the elbows, particularly when joint contractures are present at these sites (see Figure 84-5). Ulcerations may be noted secondary to underlying vascular disease and tissue ischemia (see vascular disease section). Ankle or lower extremity ulcers occur rarely secondary to macrovascular occlusive disease or comorbid conditions (venous disease). Hypopigmentation (vitiligo-like) and/or hyperpigmentation of the skin ("salt-and-pepper" appearance) can develop typically on the face, arms, and trunk (Figure 84-9A). General tanning of the skin may be seen, even in the absence of sun exposure.

Active skin involvement might persist for the first 12 to 18 months of the disease, with no further clinical signs of inflammation or progressive skin fibrosis seen after this interval. During this later stage, the skin begins to repair and can return to normal texture or, in areas most severely affected (e.g., fingers, hands), can become thin and atrophic. During this recovery phase, new robust hair growth is seen, particularly on the forearms, and itching and pain disappear, consistent with spontaneous resolution of disease activity. After years from disease onset, the skin rarely relapses again into an active phase and gradually can recover normal texture and color. Patients who established over time their phenotype as limited to the fingers (plus or minus facial changes) do not convert to the diffuse form of the disease.

Telangiectasias are erythematous matted skin lesions of vascular origin; for this reason, they blanch on local pressure. They are composed of vasodilated postcapillary venules without evidence of inflammation and resemble the type of lesions seen in Osler-Weber-Rendu disease (hereditary hemorrhagic telangiectasia). Telangiectasias develop primarily on the fingers, hands, face, and mucous membranes, but they may also be found on the limbs and trunk (Figure 84-9B). They tend to become more numerous over time in both limited and diffuse types of skin disease, and are more obvious in white patients with limited scleroderma. The biologic mechanism leading to the development of telangiectasias in scleroderma is thought to be related to the underlying chronic tissue hypoxia that stimulates abnormal secretion of vascular growth factors (e.g., vascular endothelial growth factor [VEGF]). Thus, the development of telangiectasias may indicate ongoing vascular injury and abnormal vascular repair or angiogenesis. The total burden

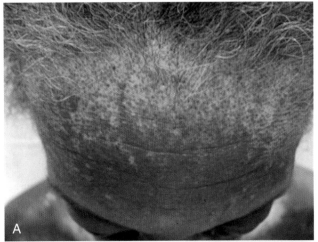

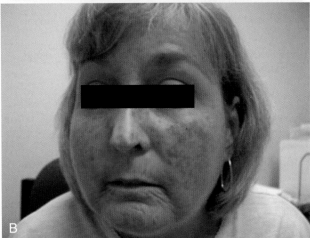

Figure 84-9 Skin manifestations in scleroderma patients. **A,** Vitiligo-like ("salt and pepper") discoloration of the forehead. **B,** Large facial telangiectasias.

of telangiectasias is associated with increased risk of pulmonary hypertension, suggesting that they are clinical biomarkers of systemic vascular disease. Nail-fold capillary abnormalities can be observed after immersion oil is applied to the skin surface at the base of the fingernails, and direct visualization is performed using an ophthalmoscope or by videocapillaroscopy. In early scleroderma, dilated capillary loops (giant capillaries) and microhemorrhages may be seen. At later stages, the nail-fold capillaries are attenuated and disorganized (see section on vascular changes).

Despite evidence of active inflammation during the early edematous phase of scleroderma skin involvement, systemic corticosteroids do not appear to be effective in stopping disease progression. A variety of other immunomodulatory drugs and newer agents with potential "disease-modifying properties" (i.e., antifibrotic) have been used to control the skin disease, but to date, none has proved uniformly successful (see treatment section). In the early active stage of diffuse scleroderma, pruritus can be one of the most distressing symptoms. Antihistamines, analgesics, or tricyclic antidepressants (e.g., doxepin) are often used but usually provide only partial benefit. Dryness of the skin surface results from damage to the exocrine structures caused by decreased or absent natural oil (sebum) production. This can worsen pruritus, leading to skin trauma due to repetitive scratching. Ulceration and secondary tissue infection may also result. The best approach to treatment is characterized by frequent topical application of an emollient preparation, periodic cleansing with soap and water, and use of topical antibiotics for any traumatic skin ulceration. Physical therapy is most important to prevent severe skin and joint contractures, and to help patients with activities of daily living.

GASTROINTESTINAL INVOLVEMENT

KEY POINTS

Manifestations of gut dysmotility are universally present in scleroderma and can affect any segment of the gastrointestinal tract.

Involvement of the upper GI tract is more common and can present with severe symptoms.

Dysfunction and failure of the lower GI tract are associated with poor prognosis.

Almost every scleroderma patient has symptoms of gastrointestinal disease, ranging from mild gastroesophageal reflux disease (GERD) to severe bowel dysfunction, which can be life threatening. Virtually any segment of the gastrointestinal tract can be affected (Table 84-4).

Oropharynx

Patients may report that chewing is difficult because of decreased facial flexibility caused by skin and deeper tissue fibrosis. Perioral skin tightening can result in a decreased oral aperture and inability to open the mouth wide enough

for proper dental care or to bite into large solid foods such as an apple (Figure 84-10). Dry membranes resulting from decreased saliva production can lead to difficult mastication. In some patients, periodontal disease and gum regression cause loosening of teeth, which further affects chewing capacity.

Upper pharyngeal function is usually normal, but a subset of patients may develop a myopathy that causes weakness of pharyngeal muscles, mimicking a neuromuscular disease.[64] This manifestation is characterized by pharyngeal dysfunction with problems initiating swallowing and frequent coughing due to laryngeal penetration and can be associated with increased risk for aspiration of foods or liquids. Although limited pathologic studies of the upper pharyngeal structures have examined scleroderma, both myositis and fibrosis are known to occur.

Esophagus

Dysphagia resulting from esophageal disease is the most common gastrointestinal symptom, occurring in approximately 90% of patients. Heartburn, regurgitation, and dysphagia for pills and solids (more than liquids) are the most common symptoms, but atypical retrosternal pain (particularly at night), periodic cough, a sense of food "sticking" in the esophagus, and nausea can result from esophageal dysfunction. Esophageal involvement in scleroderma is characterized by loss of normal smooth muscle function, especially in the lower two-thirds of the esophagus, and hypotonia of the lower esophageal sphincter (Figure 84-11A). Functional studies of esophageal motility suggest that neural dysfunction is common in patients with scleroderma, and that this may precede myopathic dysfunction and histologic changes in smooth muscle layers.[65] Manometric evaluation has identified the presence of esophageal hypomotility in areas that later did not show any histologic

Table 84-4 Gastrointestinal Manifestations of Scleroderma

Site	Manifestation	Management
Oropharynx	Perioral tight skin	Regular dental and periodontal care
	Decreased oral aperture	Artificial saliva
	Periodontitis, gum disease	
	Dry mouth	
	Swallowing difficulties	Targeted swallowing exercises and rehabilitation
	Coughing, aspiration	
Esophagus	Acid reflux (heartburn)	Lifestyle modifications
	Dysphagia	Proton pump inhibitors
		Prokinetics
	Strictures	Upper gastrointestinal endoscopy
	Barrett's esophagus	
Stomach	Gastroparesis, dyspepsia	Prokinetics
	Gastric antral vascular ectasia	Proton pump inhibitors, iron replacement
		Endoscopic laser or cryotherapy
		Transfusions
		Surgery
Small and large intestine	Hypomotility, constipation	Mild laxatives
		Promotility agents
	Bacterial overgrowth, diarrhea	Rotational antibiotics
	Pseudo-obstruction	Octreotide
	Pneumatosis intestinalis	Avoidance of surgery
	Malabsorption	Enteral or parenteral nutrition support
	Colonic pseudodiverticula	
Anorectum	Sphincter incompetence	Biofeedback, sacral nerve stimulation, surgery

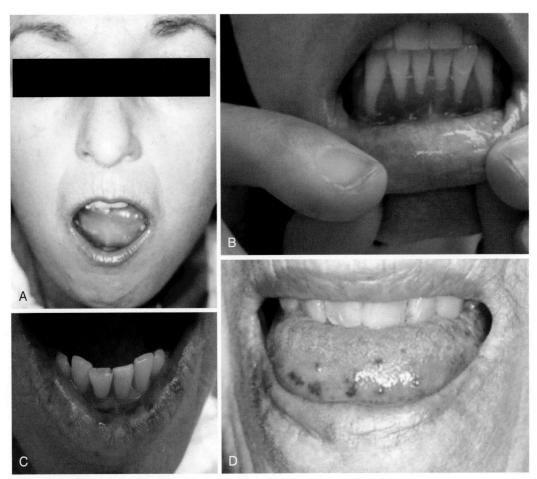

Figure 84-10 Oral manifestations. **A,** Perioral skin tightening with decreased oral aperature, furrowing around the lips, and dry membranes. **B,** Periodontal disease with regression of gum and loosening of teeth. **C** and **D,** Telangiectasias on lips and tongue.

abnormality of the smooth muscle. Other studies have shown esophageal smooth muscle activity in response to pharmacologic stimulation (methacholine challenge) early in the disease, but not in patients with more advanced scleroderma. The cause of these abnormalities is unknown, but clear evidence indicates that neural dysfunction precedes muscle disease.

Tissue fibrosis is often evoked as the cause of esophageal disease in scleroderma. However, pathologic studies demonstrate atrophy of the smooth muscle layers of the distal esophagus in the absence of significant fibrosis. Ischemia of the esophagus in scleroderma is suggested by functional studies that show impaired esophageal blood flow following cold exposure and rewarming protocols. Noninflammatory intimal layer hyperplasia in arterioles of the gastrointestinal tract has been described. Inflammatory infiltrates usually are not present in the smooth muscle unless severe transmural esophagitis is present. This suggests that inflammation is not a cardinal feature of the pathogenesis of esophageal smooth muscle lesions in scleroderma.

The severity of esophageal symptoms may not accurately reflect the seriousness of the underlying disease. Therefore, every patient with scleroderma should be fully evaluated for esophageal involvement. If untreated, gastrointestinal reflux may lead to esophagitis, bleeding, esophageal strictures, or precancerous lesions such as Barrett's esophagus. The asymptomatic patient without abnormal laboratory testing

(anemia, positive evidence of gastrointestinal bleeding) does not require specific interventions. Patients with mild GERD can be treated empirically with proton pump inhibitors and then can be followed clinically if they become symptom free with normal laboratory data. When more severe symptoms are present (e.g., GERD with dysphagia), or when treatment with proton pump inhibitors fails, an upper gastrointestinal endoscopy is necessary to fully assess the anatomy of the esophagus and the extent of related disease. Direct endoscopy is appropriate to rule out Barrett's esophagus, stricture, or a site of uncontrolled esophagitis or bleeding. Barium swallow and cine-esophagography are sensitive tests for esophageal strictures. However, direct measurement of esophageal motility via esophageal manometry may be needed if the cause of symptoms such as atypical chest pain is unclear. Although complications from Barrett's esophagus (e.g., esophageal cancer) are uncommon, periodic re-endoscopy to reassess status is recommended, even if symptoms are under therapeutic control.

It is critical that patients alter eating behavior to complement medication therapy. Patients often do better by eating more frequent smaller meals, avoiding food intake for several hours before bedtime, moving the main meal toward mid-day, taking a walk after meals to help gastroesophageal emptying, and eliminating foods that aggravate symptoms (e.g., spicy sauces, caffeinated or carbonated beverages). Bedtime is often the time of severe reflux. This can be

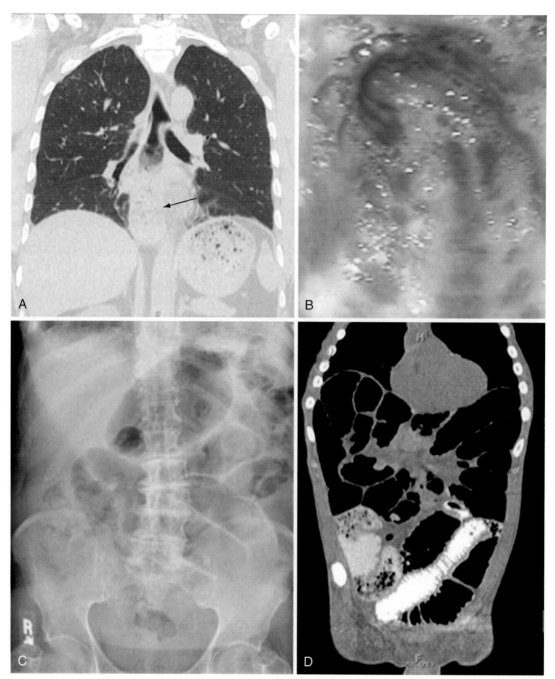

Figure 84-11 Gastrointestinal manifestations in scleroderma. **A**, Chest computed tomography (CT) (sagittal view) showing severe esophageal dysmotility with dilation and *(arrow)* retention of gastric content. **B**, Upper endoscopy: gastric antral vascular ectasias presenting as "watermelon" stomach. **C** and **D**, Plain abdominal x-ray and abdominal CT: small intestinal dysmotility with pseudo-obstruction, pneumatosis cystoides intestinalis.

improved by avoiding filling the stomach at least 2 to 3 hours before bedtime and by elevating the head and trunk during sleep. Treatment of reflux by suppression of gastric acid with antacids or histamine-2 (H_2)- is helpful but overall disappointing in scleroderma. Conversely, proton pump inhibitors (e.g., omeprazole, lansoprazole) can be very effective. Usually, long-term daily use is required. Higher doses may be used periodically for breakthrough symptoms. If symptoms are not controlled with recommended medication dosages, then a formal 24-hour ambulatory pH study may be necessary to determine whether persistent symptoms are due to uncontrolled acid reflux. A prokinetic drug (e.g.,

metoclopramide, domperidone, erythromycin) should be added when symptoms of dysphagia or endoscopic findings of esophagitis are present despite the use of effective acid suppression. These medications tend to be effective during early disease but are less likely to help later on, with advanced esophageal dysfunction. Long-term use of prokinetics may be needed. Many patients respond to relatively low doses, for example, at bedtime alone. Given the increased risk of neurologic complications with the use of metoclopramide, many recommend domperidone as a relatively safer alternative when long-term prokinetic treatment is needed.

Stomach

The degree of delayed gastric emptying (gastroparesis) is underappreciated in scleroderma, and gastroparesis often causes early satiety, aggravation of GERD symptoms, anorexia, abdominal pain, a sensation of bloating, or nausea. Frequently, weight loss in scleroderma patients is a consequence of poor caloric intake due to lack of appetite from poor gastric function. Prokinetics are used to improve gastric emptying and related symptoms. Gastritis or gastric ulcer can occur. Dilation of the microvasculature in the gastric mucosa is found in a subset of patients. This manifestation, also called *gastric antral vascular ectasia* (GAVE), is thought to be caused by an abnormal angiogenesis, leading to bizarre dilation of microvessels and arterial-venous (A-V) malformations similar to the telangiectasias seen in the skin, lips, and oral mucous membranes. In general, these lesions are asymptomatic, but they can be responsible for occult gastrointestinal bleeding. Extensive clusters of A-V malformations lead to the presence of longitudinal red stripes in the inner lining of the stomach, converging to the pylorus and described on endoscopy as "watermelon stomach," based on their appearance (Figure 84-11B). Endoscopic therapy with laser photocoagulation or cryotherapy can be used to ablate bleeding vessels. Rarely, bleeding associated with GAVE is refractory and requires multiple transfusions, repeated laser or cryotherapy, or even gastric surgery (e.g., antral or gastric resection).

Lower Gastrointestinal Tract

Bloating, abdominal distention, diarrhea, and constipation are common complaints caused by dysmotility of the small and large bowel. Functional and pathologic studies again suggest that microvascular disease, neural dysfunction, smooth muscle atrophy, and tissue fibrosis similar to those seen in the esophagus are causing the bowel disease. Most cases present in similar fashion to irritable bowel syndrome (IBS). Constipation due to sluggish or atonic bowel function can result in repeated bouts of diarrhea with malabsorption, progressive loss of weight, and severe malnutrition. Diarrhea is thought to be caused by bacterial overgrowth as a consequence of bowel dysfunction, but other causes have been considered, including decreased mesenteric blood flow or pancreatic insufficiency. Recurrent episodes of pseudo-obstruction constitute one of the most serious intestinal problems in scleroderma. These episodes are sometimes mistaken for surgical emergencies. Pseudo-obstruction is a manifestation of profound loss of bowel smooth muscle function, causing severe dysmotility and segments of luminal dilation. Pneumatosis cystoides intestinalis sometimes complicates scleroderma of the bowel when gas leaks into the diseased intestinal wall and tracks into the mesentery of the gut or the peritoneal cavity, mimicking a bowel perforation (Figure 84-11C and D). Asymptomatic wide-mouthed diverticula, also resulting from fibrosis and atrophy of the bowel wall, are pathognomonic of scleroderma. Volvulus, stricture, and perforation are uncommon complications of severe bowel involvement.

Management of the lower gastrointestinal tract includes avoiding a constipation-diarrhea cycle through adequate fiber ingestion, use of stool softener (docusate), or, if constipation is severe, periodic doses of osmotic laxatives (polyethylene glycol). Lubiprostone is helpful if chronic constipation predominates. Other prokinetic drugs are less effective for treatment of the lower gastrointestinal tract. Octreotide is reported to help patients with severe lower GI hypomotility and pseudo-obstruction. In cases with bloating, recurrent bouts of diarrhea, or episodes of pseudo-obstruction, the use of cyclic antibiotics and/or probiotics is helpful. Total parenteral nutrition may become necessary in patients with severe scleroderma-related bowel disease without response to other medical therapy. The presence of intestinal failure is a poor prognostic complication. Fecal incontinence can result in scleroderma caused by dysfunction of both internal (atrophy and fibrosis) and external (weakness) anal sphincters. Successful treatment includes firming stool texture, performing exercises to strengthen the pelvic muscles, providing biofeedback methods, and conducting surgical repair of aggravating factors such as rectal prolapse or severe hemorrhoids.

PULMONARY INVOLVEMENT

Pulmonary involvement is found in most scleroderma patients. Interstitial lung disease and pulmonary hypertension are recognized as the most common lung complications and now are regarded as the major cause of death in scleroderma. In combination, it is estimated that they are responsible for 60% of scleroderma-related deaths.[18] They are present in many patients at the same time, but one process may dominate over the other. Lung disease can occur without symptoms, or it can cause progressive respiratory failure and severe limitation of the quality of life. Additional pulmonary complications such as chronic aspiration, pleural disease, spontaneous pneumothorax, neuromuscular weakness, drug-induced pneumonitis, and lung cancer need to be considered in the differential diagnosis of a scleroderma patient presenting with respiratory symptoms.

Interstitial Lung Disease

> **KEY POINTS**
>
> Lung disease is a major cause of morbidity and mortality in scleroderma patients.
>
> Pulmonary fibrosis occurs in both limited and diffuse subsets of scleroderma, with a variable disease course in terms of severity and outcome.
>
> Nonwhite and antitopoisomerase 1–positive patients generally have the worst prognosis.
>
> Pulmonary function testing (spirometry and diffusing capacity) is helpful for screening and monitoring of interstitial lung disease (ILD). The degree of lung fibrosis on high-resolution computed tomography (HRCT) predicts outcome.
>
> Treatment for scleroderma-related ILD is limited to immunosuppression.
>
> Risk factors for pulmonary arterial hypertension include late onset of scleroderma, limited phenotype, presence of numerous telangiectasias, and positive anticentromere antibodies.

Interstitial lung disease (ILD) is the most common lung manifestation, occurring to some degree in about 80% of patients with diffuse cutaneous scleroderma and in 20% of patients with limited skin disease. Higher risk to develop severe progressive ILD has been observed in patients with diffuse skin involvement, African-Americans, Native Americans, and those positive for antitopoisomerase 1 (Scl-70), anti-U3-RNP, or anti-Th/To antibodies. Data from a recent study of patients with active lung disease show that patients with limited and those with diffuse scleroderma were indistinguishable with regard to their baseline pulmonary functions, although patients with limited skin disease presented with more extensive pulmonary fibrosis, perhaps reflecting a delay in diagnosis and more advanced progression of lung disease before study entry.[66]

ILD typically manifests with declining lung volumes and increased parenchymal fibrosis with reticular interstitial thickening that is greatest at the lung bases. Pathologic studies have shown that the most common histologic pattern of fibrosing alveolitis in scleroderma is nonspecific interstitial pneumonia (NSIP), as opposed to usual interstitial pneumonia (UIP), which is instead the common presentation of idiopathic pulmonary fibrosis. A mixed pattern of NSIP and UIP can also be found. The histopathologic classification does not appear to predict outcome, which is more related to baseline disease severity and functional respiratory measures.[67] For this reason, a surgical lung biopsy is not required in the setting of scleroderma patients who are following a typical disease course. Although ILD is

usually characterized by a functional restrictive ventilatory defect with reduced gas exchange, at later stages of the disease some degree of airway obstruction can be found in association with honeycombing of lung parenchyma and bronchiectasis. Pleural reactions are not common in scleroderma. Rare cases of spontaneous pneumothorax, adult respiratory distress syndrome, and pulmonary hemorrhage have been reported. Aspiration secondary to gastroesophageal reflux disease (GERD), secondary infection, and heart failure can complicate the course of scleroderma lung disease. Some authors consider GERD associated with chronic aspiration a potential inciting factor for the development of ILD in scleroderma.[68]

During earlier stages of ILD, the underlying active fibrosing alveolitis may be totally asymptomatic and may not be detected by conventional chest radiographs. The most common symptoms of scleroderma lung disease are dyspnea (initially on exertion) and fatigue. Chest pain is not typical, and nonproductive cough is usually a late complication, particularly in association with the presence of traction bronchiectasis. Coughing in scleroderma often is not a primary lung problem but rather is a manifestation of GERD with associated laryngeal irritation. The most characteristic finding of ILD on physical examination is bilateral fine inspiratory crackles (i.e., "velcro" rales) at the lung bases. Pulmonary function testing (PFT) is the method most commonly used to detect interstitial lung disease (Figure 84-12). The earliest functional abnormality is a reduction in the single breath diffusion capacity of carbon monoxide

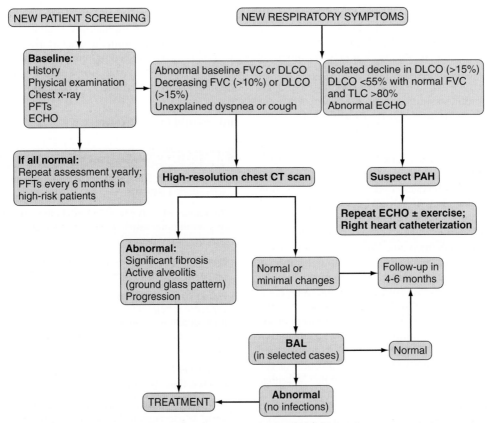

Figure 84-12 Approach to lung disease in scleroderma. This approach is recommended for all patients with scleroderma with both new-onset and long-standing disease. BAL, bronchoalveolar lavage; CT, computed tomography; DLCO, diffusing capacity; ECHO, echocardiography; FVC, forced vital capacity; PAH, pulmonary arterial hypertension; PFT, pulmonary function test; TLC, total lung capacity.

(DLCO). Although a decline in DLCO correlates with the severity of pulmonary fibrosis as measured by HRCT and predicts worse outcome, it is not a very specific measure and can be abnormal also in the context of pulmonary vascular disease and underlying chronic obstructive disease/emphysema. A restrictive ventilatory defect is identified by a depression of the forced vital capacity (FVC) and the total lung capacity (TLC). Serial measurements of FVC are the most reliable tool with which to follow ILD. A decline in FVC of more than 10% from baseline is often indicative of disease activity and is associated with increased mortality. Lung function may remain stable after an initial decline at disease onset, or it can progress at 4- to 6-month intervals until severe disease develops after a few years. Patients presenting with a normal FVC during early stages of scleroderma have a better lung prognosis, and an early reduction in FVC is likely to be associated with further progression of lung involvement, usually within the first 2 to 3 years from disease onset. The presence of ILD predicts increased mortality. One study found that patients with severe ILD have a 9-year survival rate of approximately 30%, whereas patients with no severe organ involvement have a 72% survival rate.[18] The most rapid decline in FVC is thought to occur within the initial 3 years from disease onset, but progression of ILD can occur in later years, so it is recommended that respiratory status be monitored on a regular basis, and that pulmonary function be tested yearly.

High-resolution computed tomography (HRCT) is more accurate than chest radiography in evaluating diffuse lung disease; it is a well-established, sensitive, and noninvasive method of detecting and characterizing ILD in scleroderma. The extent of pulmonary fibrosis on HRCT correlates closely with PFT abnormalities and can be used to predict prognosis.[69] Recent evidence shows that the degree of HRCT changes coupled with the level of lung function deficit can be used to generate a simple staging system (limited vs. extensive disease) with good prognostic value.[70] An FVC of less than 70% or a disease extent on HRCT greater than 20% predicts ILD progression and higher mortality. HRCT features of fibrosis are present in 55% to 65% of all patients with scleroderma and in almost every patient with abnormal pulmonary function tests. The earliest and most common abnormality on HRCT is usually found in the posterior and basilar portion of the lungs in the form of increased subpleural lung attenuations in the absence of distinct architectural distortion. With progression of the disease, increased "ground glass" opacities (GGO) are seen, but it has been well established that these changes alone are not always indicative of active inflammation, nor can they predict progression itself. Subsequent detection of a fine reticular pattern often precedes overt pulmonary fibrosis manifested by parenchymal distortion, reticular intralobular interstitial thickening, traction bronchiectasis and bronchiolectasis, and, in the late stages, honeycomb and cystic air spaces (Figure 84-13). When reticular interstitial abnormalities are present on HRCT, regression of disease rarely, if ever, occurs.

Pathologic studies on scleroderma patients with early lung disease have shown that lung fibrosis is preceded by the presence of a mixed interstitial inflammatory infiltrate spilling into the alveolar spaces (alveolitis). It has been assumed that measuring abnormal levels of inflammatory cells in the bronchoalveolar lavage (BAL) would have allowed identification of patients with active lung disease at risk for progression and with potential benefit from immunosuppressive therapy. Published data have shown that an abnormal BAL cell count, in particular with increased granulocytes (neutrophils and eosinophils), is associated with more severe lung disease and mortality in patients with scleroderma ILD.[71] However, the value of BAL cytology in predicting lung disease progression or response to treatment has not been uniformly confirmed. Few observational studies have indicated that the presence of BAL granulocytic alveolitis was associated with significant deterioration of lung function tests over time in patients not receiving immunosuppressive therapy.[72] In contrast, other studies did not find a clear association between BAL cellular abnormalities and clinical outcomes.[73] At present, evidence to recommend routine clinical use of BAL cytology to predict outcome in patients with scleroderma and ILD is still insufficient.

Early detection and prompt therapeutic intervention remain essential in preventing progression of lung disease. Current treatment of scleroderma-related ILD is most often directed against the immune response and the inflammatory process mediating lung injury and tissue fibrosis. A randomized placebo-controlled study comparing 1 year of oral cyclophosphamide versus placebo suggests some modest benefit of the active drug (improvement in FVC).[66] This benefit was sustained at 18 months but was completely lost after 2 years' follow-up, suggesting that a sequential or maintenance immunosuppressive approach may be indicated to retain the clinical response. Other studies suggest benefit using intravenous monthly cyclophosphamide followed by azathioprine as maintenance therapy. Several small retrospective studies have shown moderate benefit from mycophenolate mofetil (MMF) with improvement in or stabilization of lung function, suggesting that this drug may prove to be a safe and effective treatment in scleroderma patients, and a possible alternative to cyclophosphamide. Although more studies are needed to confirm the benefit of immunosuppressive therapy in scleroderma-associated ILD, newer drugs are under investigation, including targeted biologic immunotherapies and antifibrotic molecules (see general therapy section). More aggressive immunosuppressive protocols such as autologous or allogeneic hematopoietic stem cell transplantation, preceded by myeloablative or immunoablative conditioning regimens, are under investigation, but their treatment toxicity remains a concern.

It remains very important to pursue careful selection of patients and to treat only those with evidence of active lung disease. In fact, in most cases, no or minimal progression to severe disease is seen despite some evidence of underlying pulmonary fibrosis. This is best done with serial studies and careful assessment of both pulmonary function tests and HRCT scans.

Lung transplantation is an option in patients with severe ILD not responsive to medical therapy. Carefully selected scleroderma patients undergoing lung transplantation have similar morbidity and mortality as patients undergoing transplantation for idiopathic lung disease.[74] A retrospective survey of 47 scleroderma patients who underwent lung transplantation found that 1- and 3-year survival rates were 68% and 46%, respectively.

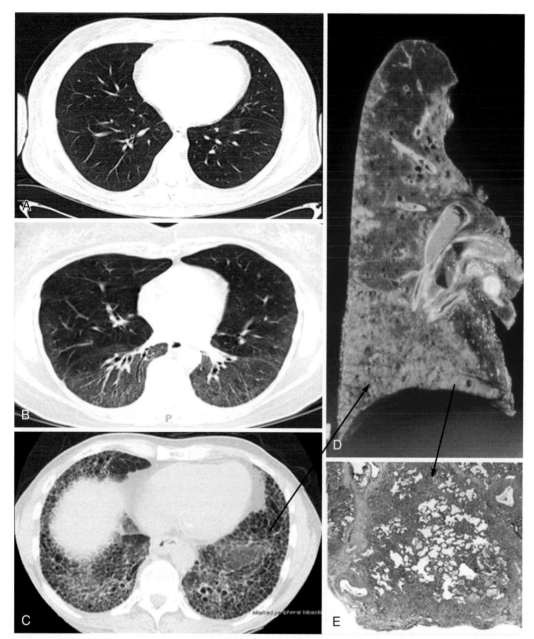

Figure 84-13 Scleroderma-related interstitial lung disease: high-resolution chest computed tomography scan showing **(A)** normal lung, **(B)** active alveolar inflammation ("ground glass" opacification), and **(C)** end-stage lung disease with honeycombing. **D**, Gross pathology. **E**, Histology showing fibrosing alveolitis.

Pulmonary Hypertension

Pulmonary arterial vascular disease is a common manifestation of scleroderma; when associated with pulmonary arterial hypertension (PAH), it represents a difficult clinical challenge with life-threatening consequences. The pulmonary vascular process can be indolent and remain clinically silent, or it may lead to respiratory distress secondary to severe PAH and associated right heart failure. Typical symptoms associated with clinically manifested PAH include dyspnea on exertion, fatigue, and, less commonly, chest pain or syncope. Physical examination may be normal during early stages of PAH, but as the disease progresses, a systolic murmur of tricuspid regurgitation, a loud pulmonic component, the S2, an S3 gallop, and signs of right heart failure

(right-sided parasternal heave, prominent and elevated jugular venous pulse, hepatomegaly, signs of fluid overload with peripheral edema) are seen. Later in the disease, patients become dyspneic with little activity, have a resting tachycardia, and may appear cyanotic. Sudden syncope or death can occur owing to hypoxia and congestive heart failure.

PAH is usually a late complication of scleroderma, typically manifesting after 10 years from disease onset, particularly in patients with limited cutaneous involvement. Considering the potentially devastating consequences of PAH, early diagnosis is very important. Simple bedside examination is not very sensitive, particularly during early stages; thus it is recommended to screen every scleroderma patient using objective testing such as electrocardiography

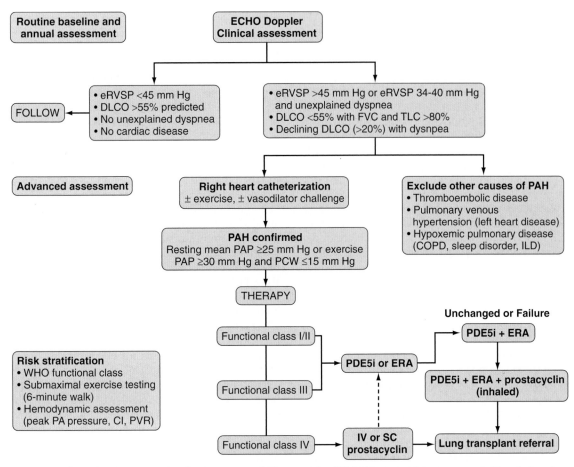

Figure 84-14 Approach to scleroderma-associated pulmonary arterial hypertension (PAH). This approach is recommended for all scleroderma patients with new-onset disease or especially long-standing disease with limited scleroderma. CI, cardiac index; COPD, chronic obstructive pulmonary disease; DLCO, diffusing capacity; ECHO, echocardiography; ERA, endothelin receptor antagonist; eRVSP, estimated right ventricular systolic pressure; FVC, forced vital capacity; ILD, interstitial lung disease; IV, intravenous; PA, pulmonary artery systolic pressure; PAP, pulmonary artery pressure; PCW, capillary wedge pressure; PDE5i, phosphodiesterase-5 inhibitor; PVR, pulmonary vascular resistance; SC, subcutaneous; TLC, total lung capacity on pulmonary function testing. Functional class: World Health Organization (WHO) functional classification of disease severity in PAH according to level of function and associated symptoms. Increasing WHO functional class reflects more severe symptoms and greater restriction in activity.

(ECG), echocardiography (ECHO), and pulmonary function testing (Figure 84-14). The ECG can be normal, but as disease progresses, signs of right-sided heart strain with right ventricular hypertrophy and right axis deviation can be observed. Detection by ECHO of increased right ventricular systolic pressure (RVSP) is useful, but values need to be confirmed by right heart catheterization (RHC), given the possibility of false-positive or false-negative results. When the ECHO estimates an RVSP greater than 45 mm Hg, about 95% of the time this will be confirmed by RHC.[75] Some use the tricuspid gradient (TG) as a measure of pulmonary artery pressure. Additional noninvasive screening includes pulmonary function testing. A low diffusing capacity (DLCO) without evidence of obstructive or restrictive lung disease (low forced vital capacity, or FVC) suggests a defect in gas exchange secondary to pulmonary vascular disease or PAH. DLCO may progressively decline for years before the diagnosis of PAH is established.[76] Increased serum N-terminal pro-brain natriuretic peptide (NT-proBNP) may indicate the presence of PAH and right heart strain, even when levels are modestly elevated (>395 pg/mL).[77] The diagnosis of PAH should be confirmed by RHC, providing direct measurement of pulmonary

hemodynamics. PAH is defined as resting mean pulmonary arterial pressure equal to or greater than 25 mm Hg, with normal pulmonary capillary wedge pressure equal to or less than 15 mm Hg. In addition to confirming abnormal hemodynamic values, the RHC can help in differentiating true PAH from pulmonary venous hypertension secondary to left heart failure or pulmonary occlusive disease. The 6-minute walk test can provide baseline functional information but cannot accurately assess the severity of PAH. Because in scleroderma patients, baseline hemodynamic parameters do not correlate well with the clinical course of PAH, new cardiopulmonary dynamic testing such as exercise stress ECHO and exercise during RHC have been introduced, but their role in diagnosing or monitoring PAH has not yet been fully established.

Based on the definition and the tools used to obtain measurements, the prevalence of PAH in scleroderma has been reported with variability. Using ECHO as a diagnostic tool, the prevalence of PAH has been estimated at between 30% and 50% of all studied patients, and investigations using confirmatory RHC have detected a prevalence of 8% to 12%.[78,79] Clinically, scleroderma-related pulmonary vascular disease can present in three different ways. In some patients, it manifests and progresses as severe isolated PAH in the absence of other significant lung disease. In others, it can be associated with mild or severe pulmonary fibrosis that is believed to drive vascular disease and PAH by causing chronic hypoxia coupled with destruction of lung parenchyma and underlying vasculature. Association of ILD and PAH usually entails a worse prognosis. In a third group of patients, pulmonary vascular disease presents with dyspnea on exertion, isolated decline of the DLCO with no significant signs of ILD (i.e., low lung volumes), and a normal resting ECHO and/or RHC. These patients are considered to have microvascular lung disease and may be at high risk to develop overt PAH. Increased risk of developing PAH has been associated with limited skin disease, late age at onset of scleroderma, presence of numerous telangiectasias, low DLCO, and presence of anti-U3-RNP antibody. Some studies suggest that the presence of anticentromere, anti-B23, and anti-β_2-glycoprotein I antibodies also increases the risk for PAH.

PAH has a major impact on quality of life and survival of affected patients. The natural course of the disease is characterized by progression of hemodynamic impairment, resulting in right heart failure and leading to a poor outcome. Despite the availability of newer targeted therapies, the median survival in scleroderma patients with PAH ranges between 1 and 3 years.[80,81] A progressive rapid increase in pulmonary pressure is more likely to occur in patients with limited skin disease and late age at onset of scleroderma.[82] This more aggressive course is associated with high mortality. Survival in patients with ILD-associated PAH is significantly worse (3-year survival, 46%) than in those with PAH alone (3-year survival, 64%).[83] This difference is possibly explained by the presence in scleroderma of underlying comorbidities, and in particular of biventricular heart (myocardial) involvement. A 10-fold increase in NT-proBNP blood levels is associated with higher mortality.[84,85] ECHO findings can help predict prognosis. For example, the degree of tricuspid annular plane systolic excursion (TAPSE) reflects right ventricular function. A TAPSE of less than 1.8 cm is associated with decreased survival in patients with PAH.[86] A recent survey identified that pulmonary vascular resistance, stroke volume index, and pulmonary arterial capacitance were strong predictors of survival.[87] This suggests that right ventricular dysfunction is associated with poorer outcome. Male gender and higher New York Heart Association functional class also impact prognosis negatively. It is suggested that survival has improved with current modes of therapy. One survey found 47% 2-year survival in historical controls as opposed with 71% among patients treated with modern therapy.[88]

All patients with PAH are encouraged to continue an active lifestyle as tolerated. Formal educational and exercise programs can improve their quality of life. Conventional therapy includes diuretic therapy (loop and potassium-sparing diuretics) and supplemental oxygen therapy if needed. Anticoagulation is used if there is no defined risk for bleeding. Although calcium channel blockers may help patients with evidence of acute vasodilative response during hemodynamic testing, this is an uncommon finding in scleroderma. In recent years, a number of targeted agents have become available for the treatment of PAH. Many clinical trials testing these drugs in primary PAH have

included about 20% of patients with connective tissue disease, primarily scleroderma. Specific therapies include prostaglandin derivatives (epoprostenol, treprostinil, beraprost, iloprost), endothelin receptor antagonists (bosentan, sitaxsentan, ambrisentan), and phosphodiesterase-5 inhibitors (sildenafil, tadalafil, vardenafil). These interventions can improve hemodynamics, exercise tolerance, and quality of life. No evidence from clinical trials suggests that any one of these agents is superior to another. Most believe that early intervention is most important, and that combination therapy may be helpful (see Figure 84-14). Decisions regarding the preferred agents to use and how to deliver them are based mostly on personal preferences and the clinical status of the individual patient. For patients with mild to moderate disease (functional class I or II), a single oral agent is usually started (i.e., sildenafil, bosentan, ambrisentan). Our preference is to use sildenafil, given its favorable side effect profile. Patients presenting with more severe disease (class III or IV) and those failing monotherapy are usually treated with intravenous or inhaled prostaglandins alone or in combination with one or two oral agents. Sildenafil and bosentan can be used in combination, even if concern arises about their interaction and increased hepatotoxicity.[89,90] Lung or heart-lung transplantation for PAH remains the treatment of last resort when medical therapy fails. Patients with scleroderma who are carefully selected for transplantation have an outcome that is similar to those with other causes of lung disease. PAH in scleroderma is a progressive disease for which no specific or single therapy may suffice. Therefore, careful longitudinal monitoring is important. Noninvasive testing with periodic clinical assessment with 6-minute walk time, repeat pulmonary function testing, and ECHO studies are helpful. When a major therapeutic decision is needed, such as switching or adding a new therapy, a repeat RHC may be indicated. Further improvement in survival of scleroderma patients with PAH may result from future therapeutic interventions targeting the underlying inflammatory process and the dysregulated endothelial proliferation mediating pulmonary vascular remodeling and consequent failure of the right heart.

CARDIAC INVOLVEMENT

The clinical manifestations of heart disease in scleroderma are highly variable, ranging from clinically silent cardiac involvement to frank heart failure. The reported prevalence of heart disease varies from 10% to more than 50%, depending on the diagnostic method used, but in general it tends to be underestimated. Symptoms such as dyspnea, chest pain, or palpitations are commonly thought to be secondary to more obvious organ involvement such as the lungs or the upper gastrointestinal tract, and the contribution of heart disease often is not appreciated until later stages. Cardiac disease can occur in both diffuse and limited subtypes of scleroderma and can manifest as a primary heart problem or in association with other organ failure. When clinically evident, heart disease entails an overall poor prognosis and predicts shortened survival.[91] Along with pulmonary fibrosis and PAH, cardiac disease accounts for the majority of deaths in scleroderma. One study found that 25% of deaths could be directly related to heart disease (mostly heart failure and arrhythmias).[16] In a large meta-analysis, cardiac involvement was associated with increased mortality (hazard ratio, 2.8; 95% confidence interval [CI], 2.1 to 3.8) after adjustments for age and gender.[92] A survey comparing 129 scleroderma patients with a left ventricle ejection fraction (LVEF) of less than 55% with 256 subjects with normal LVEF demonstrated that male gender, age, digital ulcerations, myositis, and no use of calcium channel blockers were independent factors associated with left ventricular dysfunction.[93]

Cardiac disease in scleroderma can be characterized by involvement of the endocardium, myocardium, and pericardium, separately or concomitantly. As a consequence, pericardial effusion, auricular and/or ventricular arrhythmias, conduction disease, valvular regurgitation, myocardial ischemia, myocardial hypertrophy, and heart failure are all reported. Clinically overt pericarditis is uncommon, but asymptomatic and hemodynamically benign pericardial effusions are frequently detected by ECHO. In a controlled study, significant pericardial effusion was found in about 15% of patients compared with 4% of controls.[94] Pathologic studies have shown that some degree of pericardial involvement is detectable in 33% to 77% of scleroderma patients, usually with evidence of a fibrinous pericarditis with adhesions and chronic inflammatory cell infiltrates.[95] Hemodynamic compromise secondary to tamponade physiology is rare but may require acute intervention with anti-inflammatory medication, pericardiocentesis, or creation of a pericardial window for slow decompression. The presence of a large pericardial effusion even if asymptomatic is a poor prognostic sign, particularly if associated with PAH or renal disease.

Focal myocardial fibrosis is the hallmark of established primary heart involvement in SSc and usually is not secondary to atherosclerotic coronary artery disease. In fact, pathologic studies and a survey of coronary angiograms have found little involvement of coronary arteries in scleroderma patients.[7,96] Unlike other rheumatic diseases such as rheumatoid arthritis or SLE, scleroderma does not exhibit unequivocally an increased risk for coronary artery disease independent from usual risk factors. Nevertheless, typical angina symptoms should make one consider atherosclerosis of the coronary vessels or another process. Atypical chest pain can also be caused by musculoskeletal problems, esophageal reflux disease, or PAH mimicking cardiac disease. The fibrotic lesions in the heart of scleroderma patients are patchy, involve the myocardium of both ventricles, and usually are accompanied by evidence of microvascular disease with concentric intimal hypertrophy associated with fibrinoid necrosis of the intramural coronary arteries and arterioles.[97] This results in reduced coronary flow reserve even with normal epicardial coronary arteries and in the absence of clinically manifested cardiac dysfunction.[98] Vasospasm and associated myocardial perfusion defects are demonstrated to occur at rest, with exercise, and following cold exposure.[99] These findings suggest that myocardial fibrosis may be associated with reversible vasospasm of the microvascular coronary circulation, and that vasodilating agents such as calcium channel blockers may have the capacity to improve coronary flow and prevent further cardiac damage.[100] Patients with angina-like chest pain may need to undergo angiographic studies because nuclear perfusion studies are likely to be abnormal as a result of microvascular disease.

Electrocardiography (ECG) and Holter monitoring will often show some heart conduction defect or asymptomatic arrhythmia; these are thought to be consequences of myocardial fibrosis. Premature ventricular contractions are the most common abnormality, but sinus node dysfunction, first-degree heart block, supraventricular arrhythmias (supraventricular tachycardia, atrial fibrillation), and ventricular arrhythmias (ventricular tachycardia) are also observed. Complete heart block is uncommon. Scleroderma-related syncope is an ominous manifestation of late-stage PAH or an important arrhythmia. When an arrhythmia is suspected, a Holter monitoring study should be ordered promptly. More extensive evaluation with electrophysiologic studies is indicated in serious cases because a pacemaker or ablative therapy can help in management of these life-threatening complications.

Transthoracic echocardiography (TTE) is a widely used type of noninvasive cardiac testing; it represents a sensitive tool to detect the presence of cardiac disease. TTE can provide estimates of elevated right ventricular (RV) and pulmonary artery pressures, as well as evidence of right heart dysfunction such as atrial and ventricular dilation or septal wall motion abnormalities. A depressed left ventricular (LV) contractility is not frequently detected in scleroderma patients with the use of conventional TTE, but relaxation abnormalities can be found in up to 40% of cases.[101] Left ventricular diastolic dysfunction is detected especially in patients with diffuse scleroderma, and may occur in the absence of systemic hypertension (independent of renal disease) and in association with pulmonary vascular disease. Although TTE is very helpful in monitoring underlying cardiac abnormalities later in the disease process, it lacks some sensitivity during preclinical stages of heart involvement. Novel diagnostic methods such as tissue Doppler echocardiography (TDE), with or without strain imaging, and magnetic resonance imaging (MRI) have been applied more recently to study myocardial disease in scleroderma, showing the ability to detect abnormalities earlier than conventional echocardiography and with greater accuracy.[102,103] Provocative exercise testing during echocardiography can be used to detect underlying diastolic dysfunction and pulmonary hypertension not previously recognized by resting studies.

Cardiac evaluation has been improved by the systematic measurement of brain natriuretic peptide (BNP) or its prohormone N-terminal pro-BNP (NT-proBNP). Blood levels of NT-proBNP reflect both RV and LV volume or pressure overload. It can be a useful test and a prognostic marker for following right or left heart failure in scleroderma patients.[85,104]

Patients with diffuse cutaneous scleroderma and skeletal muscle inflammation (polymyositis) are particularly prone to develop severe cardiomyopathy and to have a particularly poor prognosis. Acute myocarditis can also occur in association with inflammatory muscle disease and can present as sudden-onset heart failure. Prompt institution of immunosuppressive treatment is indicated in these cases. An endomyocardial biopsy may be helpful in differentiating overt myocarditis from the myocardial fibrosis commonly present in scleroderma patients.

RENAL INVOLVEMENT

KEY POINTS

Scleroderma renal crisis (SRC) is a life-threatening condition that occurs in 5% to 10% of scleroderma patients.

Risk factors for SRC include early diffuse skin disease, use of corticosteroids, and the presence of anti-RNA polymerase III antibodies.

Early pharmacologic intervention with angiotensin-converting enzyme inhibitors is crucial to control and possibly reverse the disease process.

Renal involvement in scleroderma is classically characterized by the abrupt onset of very high blood pressure (malignant hypertension), elevated plasma renin, and rising serum creatinine reflective of acute renal failure, along with a constellation of symptoms and clinical manifestations such as headaches, malaise, hypertensive retinopathy, encephalopathy, and pulmonary edema, usually referred to as *scleroderma renal crisis* (SRC). Renal disease in scleroderma can also be asymptomatic, and despite the high prevalence of histopathologic renovascular lesions typical of scleroderma vasculopathy, clinically important renal dysfunction, independent of scleroderma renal crisis, is seen in only a minority of patients.[105] Although SRC is the most recognized renal complication, abnormal renal function can be explained by factors other than intrinsic scleroderma renal disease such as medication side effects, comorbid conditions, or associated heart, gastrointestinal, or lung disease. One survey suggested that mild unexplained proteinuria without loss of renal function or evidence of glomerular disease is a common sign of renal disease in scleroderma.[106] A superimposed inflammatory kidney disease can also occur in scleroderma. Several cases of pauci-immune necrotizing crescentic glomerulonephritis associated with myeloperoxidase (MPO)-specific antineutrophilic cytoplasmic antibodies (ANCAs) have been reported in scleroderma patients with a presentation mimicking SRC.[107]

SRC needs to be considered in scleroderma patients with sudden and severe elevation of blood pressure, with or without renal failure; in patients with sudden renal failure, with or without hypertension; and in patients with sudden-onset microangiopathic hemolytic anemia, with or without hypertension or renal failure. Nonmalignant hypertension alone without signs of renal dysfunction or mild urine abnormalities is unlikely to be due to SRC. Scleroderma renal crisis occurs in 5% to 10% of patients and mostly in those with diffuse scleroderma. It usually is encountered within the first 2 to 4 years from disease onset. The estimated median duration of scleroderma at the time of SRC diagnosis is 8 months.[108,109] Occurrence in later disease is uncommon.[108] Patients at greatest risk of developing SRC are those with diffuse cutaneous scleroderma, particularly those with the rapidly progressive skin disease. SRC is a rare complication in patients with limited scleroderma (approximately 1% to 2%). African-Americans and patients with diffuse skin disease who are treated with a high dose of corticosteroid (>40 mg/day of prednisone) or low-dose cyclosporine are at increased risk of developing an SRC. A long-term low dose of prednisone may also be a risk factor for SRC. For this reason, it is recommended to avoid corticosteroids or to use doses less than 10 mg daily if necessary. Renal crisis is also associated with a positive ANA (speckled pattern) anti-U3-RNP and usually is not seen in patients with anticentromere antibodies. Antibodies to RNA polymerase III have been found in about 60% of patients with SRC in one survey.[108] Although antitopoisomerase I antibodies are prevalent in patients with diffuse skin disease, no association between their presence and SRC has been reported. Nonmalignant hypertension, abnormal urinalysis, and isolated increases in plasma renin activity are not predictors of an SRC.[110]

Patients experiencing SRC present with typical signs of malignant hypertension, including headache, altered vision, signs of congestive heart failure, florid pulmonary edema, confusion, or neurologic signs secondary to hypertensive encephalopathy in the setting of an abnormally high blood pressure, usually above 150/90 mm Hg. Hypertensive encephalopathy is characterized by acute or subacute onset of lethargy, fatigue, confusion, headaches, visual disturbances (including blindness from hypertensive retinopathy), seizures, or cerebral hemorrhage. In about 10% of cases, SRC occurs with normal blood pressure. New-onset anemia, asymptomatic pericardial effusion, and cardiac disease may precede an SRC. Laboratory testing at onset may show normal or high creatinine, modest to absent proteinuria, and/or microscopic hematuria. Renal insufficiency usually is not the presenting problem in an SRC but rather is a late complication of untreated disease. However, a rapid rise in serum creatinine can occur over several days with a fairly benign urinalysis—less than 2 g of protein excretion in 24 hours—and a mild hematuria with some granular casts. A microangiopathic hemolytic anemia and thrombocytopenia can accompany or precede an SRC and may be the only finding in a normotensive patient. This presentation with normotensive SRC usually entails a worse prognosis. Distinguishing SRC-associated thrombotic microangiopathy from idiopathic thrombotic thrombocytopenic purpura may be difficult but is important because treatments differ. Accurate assays for ADAMTS (a disintegrin and metalloproteinase [ADAM family] with thrombospondin-1 domains)-13 activity can be helpful because its level should be normal in scleroderma.

Poorer outcome is more frequent among males and among patients presenting with creatinine greater than 3 mg/dL (265 mmol/L). Approximately two-thirds of patients with SRC will require renal support with dialysis, but about half will recover function and be able to discontinue therapy, usually within several weeks, most before 6 months.[108] However, cases of recovery from up to 24 months of dialysis support have been reported, distinguishing SRC from other causes of renal failure. The renal crisis truly mimics malignant hypertension, with rapidly progressive renal failure secondary to microvascular disease, vasospasm, and tissue ischemia. The characteristic lesion of vascular disease such as intimal hyperplasia or luminal narrowing involving in particular the renal arcuate arteries is detected even in patients without SRC. Although the renal pathology is now well described, the pathogenesis of the renal crisis remains poorly understood. It is assumed that intrinsic renal vessel disease is complicated by an intense vasospasm triggering high levels of plasma renin, which results in malignant hypertension.

Before the discovery of angiotensin-converting enzyme (ACE) inhibitors, hypertensive renal crisis had almost uniformly a fatal outcome. In contrast, patients treated with ACE inhibitors have a good outcome 60% of the time, and death or end-stage renal disease is now much less common. The mortality rate at 1 year associated with SRC has decreased from 76% to less than 15%. However, despite aggressive antihypertensive therapy, the 5-year survival of patients with SRC remains only 65%. Although ACE inhibitors are standard therapy in SRC, it remains unclear whether other related drugs such as angiotensin receptor blockers (ARBs) can be effective in treating or preventing a crisis. Endothelin and other mediators of vascular disease are implicated in the pathogenesis of SRC; thus interference with endothelin function by a specific inhibitor may offer a novel therapeutic approach. A vasodilating prostaglandin (prostacyclin) may also provide rapid control of blood pressure while improving renal blood flow. The overall outcome in SRC remains unsatisfactory in terms of acute disease outcome, morbidity, and need for renal transplantation or long-term renal support with dialysis. Data suggest that use of an ACE inhibitor before a crisis does not prevent an SRC.[108]

Any newly developed hypertension in a scleroderma patient should be urgently evaluated because the key to successful therapy is early detection and rapid intervention (Figure 84-15). Patients with SRC should be hospitalized and immediately started on an ACE inhibitor. Captopril, a rapid-acting ACE inhibitor, should be started, to allow dose increases until systolic blood pressure is down by 20 mm Hg/24 hr while avoiding hypotension. Treatment continues with an ACE inhibitor even if creatinine continues to rise. When full doses of an ACE inhibitor are not controlling blood pressure, other antihypertensive medications may be added, including calcium channel blockers, endothelin inhibitors, and prostacyclin or an ARB (which is infused). Some patients continue to have progressive renal failure despite attaining control of blood pressure. Other causes of renal disease always need to be considered, especially in patients with limited scleroderma, and in those with a high level of proteinuria or abnormal urinalysis such as red cell casts. Renal biopsy should be done to confirm the diagnosis and to gain insight into the prognosis by determining the degree of renal damage. Detection on kidney biopsy of other forms of glomerular inflammation is important in that it will dictate a different specific treatment approach.

Successful renal transplantation has been performed in scleroderma patients, providing an overall survival benefit over long-term dialysis. Renal allograft survival at 3 years is about 60%, which is comparable with the rate observed in systemic lupus erythematosus. It is not recommended to pursue renal transplantation until it is clear that recovery will not spontaneously occur. This can be determined in part by assessing the degree of damage on renal biopsy and by waiting at least 6 months (some suggest 2 years) after recovery from the acute crisis. Recurrence of SRC is uncommon (5%) after renal transplant.

MUSCULOSKELETAL INVOLVEMENT

Musculoskeletal symptoms are almost always present in scleroderma, usually are multifactorial in origin, and often are the initial symptoms of the disease. The most common

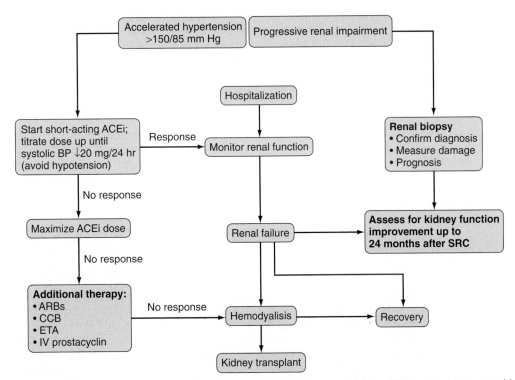

Figure 84-15 Management of scleroderma renal crisis. ACEi, angiotensin-converting enzyme inhibitor; ARB, angiotensin receptor blocker; BP, blood pressure; CCB, calcium channel blocker; ETA, endothelin receptor antagonist; IV, intravenous; SRC, scleroderma renal crisis.

symptoms are nonspecific pain, stiffness, and diffuse muscular discomfort that mimics a flu-like syndrome. Impaired hand function, characterized by decreased hand mobility, reduced dexterity, and decreased grip force, is in particular a major source of difficulty in performing activities of daily living. The degree and type of musculoskeletal disease vary a great deal and are influenced by the duration of disease, the level of overall disease activity, and the subtype of skin involvement. For example, in early diffuse scleroderma, pain is often widespread in areas of skin inflammation and advancing fibrosis that can involve joint structures, tendons, subcutaneous tissue, and underlying muscle. In later-stage diffuse disease, joint contractures and muscle atrophy are often associated with pain and loss of function, causing significant disability. In limited scleroderma patients, puffy fingers and loss of hand function and grip may be the only musculoskeletal symptoms throughout the disease course. Although histologic evidence suggests that synovitis occurs, arthralgias, pain, and stiffness without signs of frank arthritis constitute the usual clinical picture. However, overlap syndromes of rheumatoid-like polyarthritis or inflammatory muscle disease can dominate the clinical picture in an individual patient.

In the early edematous phase of diffuse scleroderma, patients often are diagnosed with a carpal tunnel syndrome due to soft tissue swelling and inflammation in the hand and wrist area. Erosive arthritis with joint space narrowing can be seen, but soft tissue swelling, periarticular osteopenia, and contractures of the joint are more common. Distal bone resorption, osteolysis, and periarticular calcinosis are found in the fingers of patients with later-stage diffuse scleroderma. Contractures of the proximal interphalangeal (PIP) and metacarpophalangeal (MCP) joints are most common, and rarely of the distal interphalangeal (DIP) joint. Patients with diffuse skin disease develop contractures of large joints, including wrist, elbows, shoulders, hips, knees, and ankles. These contractures are the hallmark of severe scleroderma and are associated with fibrosis and ankylosis of the joint, resulting from disease in the overlying skin, fascia, joint capsule, and tendons.

Tendon friction rubs can be felt as a coarse crepitus over joints or over the forearm or lower leg with adjacent joint movement. These rubs are thought to be secondary to low-grade tenosynovitis, local edema, and fibrosis of the tendon sheath, fascia, and joint structures. Friction rubs are seen primarily in patients with diffuse skin disease; when present, they are an indicator of a poor overall prognosis. They are found in about 15% to 30% of patients and are more common in those with diffuse skin disease and in patients with antitoposiomerase, anti-RNA polymerase, or anti-U3-RNP antibodies.[111]

The prevalence of signs of joint inflammation in scleroderma is estimated in relatively small observational studies to be about two-thirds of patients.[112,113] A large multicenter survey reported the frequencies of synovitis, tendon friction rubs, and joint contractures to be 16%, 11%, and 31%, respectively.[114] Synovitis, tendon friction rubs, and joint contractures are more likely to occur together and are more prevalent in patients with the diffuse cutaneous subset. These manifestations also tend to be associated with severe vascular, muscular, renal, and interstitial lung involvement. Synovitis, joint contracture, and tendon friction rubs are associated with more severe disease and with systemic inflammation.

Erosive arthritis is commonly associated with periarticular calcinosis (Figure 84-16A) and can be seen with significant bone loss or osteolysis. A radiologic survey of 120 patients found abnormalities including erosion (21%), joint space narrowing (28%), arthritis (defined by concomitant erosion and joint space narrowing) (18%), radiologic demineralization (23%), acro-osteolysis (22%), flexion contracture (27%), and calcinosis (23%).[114] Radiologic studies using ultrasonography and MRI confirm that hand involvement is striking, with articular, bone, and soft tissue changes.[115,116] Resorption of distal phalanges was significantly associated with digital ulcers and extra-articular calcification; flexion contracture was associated with the diffuse cutaneous form and with high Health Assessment Questionnaire (HAQ) disability scores.[117] Calcinosis is most often seen in patients with digital ulcers but was similarly observed in patients with the diffuse or limited cutaneous subtype. Calcinosis is often seen in the subcutaneous tissue in areas of trauma such as the extensor surfaces of the forearms, elbows, or patellae. Unlike the more diffuse calcinosis seen in myositis patients, calcium deposits in scleroderma tend to be found in clusters around joints and sites of trauma. These deposits can restrict joint motion and may be associated with acute inflammation similar to a gouty arthritis, or the deposits can rupture through the skin, weeping a thick white material. Once the skin is broken, secondary infection can occur.

Erosive polyarthritis, seemingly specific for scleroderma, or seropositive rheumatoid arthritis can occur in patients with limited or diffuse skin disease. However, the prevalence of scleroderma with rheumatoid arthritis overlap is unusual (1% to 2%) with an estimated incidence of 5%.[114,118,119] This is confirmed by the low frequency of anticyclic citrullinated protein antibodies found in patients with scleroderma and arthritis. When an inflammatory arthritis is present, traditional medications used in rheumatoid arthritis can be helpful. One case series demonstrated that the tumor necrosis factor (TNF) inhibitor etanercept appeared to be efficacious in improving active inflammatory joint disease in a subset of scleroderma patients, and it was generally safe and well tolerated.

A sense of weakness in the muscles of the hands, arms, and legs is very common (80%) and can be subtle or profound. One study found measurable weakness in 30% of patients with proximal more than distal strength compromised. Myopathy in an individual scleroderma is often multifactorial, but patients with myopathy are at increased risk for poor outcome and decreased survival.[120] Weakness is often caused by muscle atrophy secondary to the inflexibility due to joint disease and fibrotic skin with lack of usual mobility and exercise. It can also occur because of malnutrition resulting from scleroderma bowel disease. Muscle weakness in scleroderma may be secondary to direct muscle disease. In diffuse scleroderma, fibrosis can extend into the striated muscle, causing muscle atrophy and clinical weakness. This has been called a *fibrosing myopathy*. It presents in the setting of severe diffuse skin disease with joint contractures and mild elevation of creatine phosphokinase (CPK). Electromyography (EMG) demonstrates nonirritable myopathy, and muscle biopsy shows little inflammation,

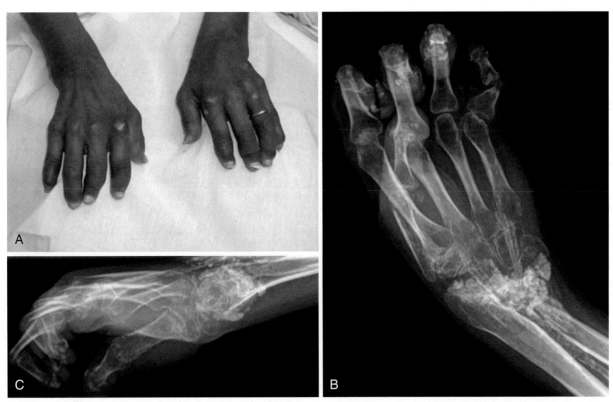

Figure 84-16 A, Hands of a scleroderma patient showing reabsorption of distal phalanges corresponding to radiographic evidence of (**B** and **C**) acroosteolysis, calcinosis, and joint erosions.

fibrosis, and type 2 muscle atrophy. The fibrosing myopathy does not respond to traditional anti-inflammatory medications, including corticosteroids. This type of muscle disease is associated with cardiomyopathy, heart failure, and arrhythmia that can be severe and irreversible.[120]

Approximately 5% to 10% of scleroderma patients have an inflammatory muscle disease that can follow the same course as polymyositis and other forms of idiopathic inflammatory myopathy. Patients present with rapid proximal muscle weakness associated with high CPK. EMG shows irritable myopathy, and muscle biopsy is typical of an inflammatory myositis. In some cases with severe polymyositis, myocarditis can occur with heart failure. High levels of anti-PM/Scl-100 antibodies are found in about 4% of patients with SSc, and these patients often present with acute inflammatory muscle disease. Patients with muscle weakness should be fully evaluated for underlying causes with the use of laboratory measures of muscle enzymes, electromyographic studies, magnetic resonance imaging, and muscle biopsy. These studies will help differentiate inflammatory muscle disease form other forms of myopathy.

ENDROCRINE INVOLVEMENT

Endocrine dysfunction can complicate the course and management of scleroderma patients. The most common endocrine problem associated with scleroderma is thyroid disease, and the frequency of other endocrinopathies is similar to that of the general population. Thyroid disease is reported in 10% to 15% of patients with scleroderma.[121,122] A case-control study found a 10 to 14 times increased risk of hypothyroidism in scleroderma.[123] Evidence for both fibrosis of

the thyroid and autoimmune injury exists. Patients with features of the CREST syndrome (subcutaneous calcinosis, Raynaud's phenomenon, esophageal hypomotility, sclerodactyly, and telangiectasias) are more likely to have hypothyroidism than those with diffuse skin disease. An autoimmune basis for thyroid disease is suggested by one series, which found Hashimoto's thyroiditis in 6% and Graves' disease in 3% of patients.[124] A survey of 719 scleroderma patients found that 273 (38%) had at least one other autoimmune condition; the most frequent was autoimmune thyroid disease.[125] Thyroid autoantibodies are commonly found in scleroderma patients with hypothyroidism. In addition, the association of CREST syndrome with autoimmune hypothyroidism and primary biliary cirrhosis has been reported, suggesting multiple autoimmune targets in these patients. Thyroid disease may not be recognized in patients with subclinical disease or with symptoms associated with chronic multisystem disease. It is recommended that thyroid function should be monitored periodically, especially in patients with limited scleroderma with the CREST syndrome and in those with long-standing disease.

OTHER ASSOCIATED MANIFESTATIONS

It must be recognized that in patients who have scleroderma, several less common and often forgotten complications of this disease may require attention. Awareness of these associated problems can improve quality of life and prevent undue distress. Bone disease can occur for a variety of reasons. Most patients with scleroderma are women who are near or in menopause, and therefore are at risk for osteoporosis and its complications. This risk is increased by the chronic inflammatory nature of the disease, disuse, and several commonly used medications. Malabsorption and lack of sun exposure may lead to vitamin D deficiency, and bowel dysfunction can limit calcium intake. Avascular necrosis of carpal bones of the wrist is reported and is thought to be secondary to scleroderma peripheral vascular disease. In addition, osteolysis or bony resorption of the tips or tufts of the fingers, middle phalanges, distal radius, and ulna bones (less commonly, the distal clavicle, ribs, mandible, and distal toes) may occur (Figure 84-16B and C). Acro-osteolysis is fairly common, presenting with shortening of the finger or pain of the fingertip. Osteolysis is thought to be a manifestation of peripheral vascular disease and poor nutritional blood flow on affected bones. Neurologic complications can be a significant unrecognized problem. The central nervous system is generally spared in scleroderma, but unilateral or bilateral trigeminal neuralgia is known to occur in a subset of patients. Peripheral neuropathy occurs in a higher percentage of patients than expected owing to multiple causes, including nutritional deficiency from gastrointestinal disease, entrapment neuropathy, vasculitis, or vasculopathy of small vessels typical of scleroderma vascular disease. Carpal tunnel syndrome can complicate diffuse scleroderma and may occur in patients with associated inflammatory joint disease.

Muscle weakness is very common, and the presence of a myopathy is associated with a poor prognosis. Multiple factors, including inflammatory polymyositis, disuse atrophy, malnutrition, medications, and a fibrosing myopathy associated with diffuse scleroderma skin disease, can cause muscle dysfunction. Autoimmune hepatitis and biliary cirrhosis are reported in patients with the CREST syndrome. It is recommended that all patients with scleroderma be screened for associated autoimmune-mediated liver disease because it usually responds to immunosuppressive therapy.

Dry eyes (keratoconjunctivitis sicca) and/or mucous membranes (xerostomia) occur in about 25% of patients. Dry eyes may occur as the result of severe facial periorbital skin fibrosis inhibiting full closure of the eyelids. Topical artificial tears should be used frequently in these cases. Facial changes alter oral aperture and decrease facial flexibility. Vertical lines around the lips and thinning of the lips along with pinching of the nose affect self-esteem, especially in younger women. A decreased oral aperture prevents easy daily oral hygiene and dental procedures. Loosening of the teeth happens because of loss of normal periodontal ligament attaching the tooth to the alveolar bone. Decreased saliva and difficulty performing usual dental hygiene can lead to significant periodontal disease. Treatment of oral manifestations requires early referral for experienced dental care and frequent cleaning with fluoride treatment. Pilocarpine and cevimeline are agonists for the muscarinic cholinergic receptors that can increase saliva and improve symptoms of xerostomia.

Most data suggest normal fertility in scleroderma, but during pregnancy, risk for hypertension, scleroderma renal crisis, or premature fetal loss is increased. Sexual performance is often affected, particularly in women with diffuse disease. Decreased sexual satisfaction is associated with painful inflexible joints, dry vaginal membranes, and general fatigue. Erectile dysfunction and associated impotence among male scleroderma patients have been reported in more than 80% of men with scleroderma. This results from local fibrosis of the corporeal smooth muscle and scleroderma microvascular disease. Psychogenic and medication-induced sexual dysfunction must be considered.

Several causes of lower extremity lesions can occur, including skin fibrosis, stasis dermatitis, lipodermatosclerosis, panniculitis, subcutaneous calcinosis, and leg ulcers. Leg ulcers may result from traumatic breakdown of atrophic fibrotic skin, ischemic ulcers secondary to scleroderma vascular disease, vaculitis, and occlusive vascular events resulting from an associated hypercoagulable state. Livedoid vasculopathy is a rare complication causing skin ulcerations on the lower leg and foot as the result of small vessel vasculitis or small vessel thrombosis.

PSYCHOSOCIAL ASPECTS

Scleroderma is a disease that can alter virtually every aspect of the patient's life. Although scleroderma is often mild in its expression, the patient is now faced with a life crisis and must deal with a rare chronic disease that is complex and is not completely understood by the medical community. Patients learn that scleroderma is potentially a life-threatening disease that alters physical capacity and can be disfiguring. At the onset of the disease, patients are often confused, anxious, and frightened. Fear and misunderstanding become a major source of distress. Studies of psychosocial adjustment support the conclusion that a substantial proportion of patients with scleroderma have difficulty adapting to the disease and have reduced quality of life measures. Although little evidence suggests that scleroderma directly affects the central nervous system with a direct organic cause for altered mental status, a complex array of medications used to treat the disease and its complications may have some influence on mood and sense of well-being.

Psychosocial aspects of the disease do not appear to be consistently influenced by age, gender, ethnicity, education, or marital status. However, some data suggest that being disabled with low financial income leads to higher psychological distress. Evidence suggests that depression in scleroderma patients is common and is related more to the patient's personality, the degree of pain, and the level of social support than to actual disease severity. Disease-related disability, as measured by the Health Assessment Questionnaire Disability Index (HAQ-DI), is a more important predictor of adjustment problems than are disease symptoms related to severity. Pain and fatigue are common in scleroderma. Together with depressive symptoms, they are the most significant determinants of physical functioning and social adjustment—two important components of health-related quality of life—in patients with limited and diffuse disease subtypes.

Personality traits influence the degree of psychological adjustment. Patients with scleroderma who describe themselves as anxious, worried, tense, or detail-oriented are more likely to be depressed than patients who describe themselves as agreeable or extraverted and outgoing. Disease unpredictability and lack of control cause increased distress. High self-reported uncertainty is related to poor adjustment. Thus, increasing the patient's understanding of the disease and expectations through education may reduce uncertainty and improve quality of life. Body image dissatisfaction is a significant concern. Patients are distressed by disease-related changes in visible parts of their body, especially the fingers and hands. A survey found that tight skin and facial changes were not as distressful as hand deformity with finger contractions and hand dysfunction. Sexual function is affected in both men and women with scleroderma. A significant proportion of men experience erectile dysfunction. Women with scleroderma, particularly those with diffuse skin disease, have high levels of sexual impairment compared with women with other chronic diseases for which sexual function has received greater attention. Both may have a decreased sexual drive during the disease course. The impact of sexual function on quality of life is not well studied, but it exists as a problem and should be appropriately addressed as part of comprehensive care.

Psychological factors with demonstrated relevance to scleroderma include pain, depression, and distress about disfigurement, physical function, and social function. Although these dimensions of quality of life are interrelated, pain, depression, and distress about disfigurement are common and may respond to psychological intervention. This begins with providing compassionate support beyond just ordering medications. It is important to spend time in a comfortable setting educating patients about scleroderma, providing a clear understanding of the degree of their disease and explaining to them what they need to do and what can be done for relief. Having insight into social support and life circumstances, including financial distress, work environment, and family structure, provides a framework for helping to decrease external distress. For example, a family conference held to explain the reality of the health situation or the needs of the patient can reduce home tension and can clarify the patient's capacity in their family role. An adjustment in the work environment (e.g., permission for a space heater) can make a difference. Clearly, effective social support improves quality of life. Follow-up visits that provide time to discuss issues of coping and social support are most important. Recognizing the personality of patients while addressing their specific concepts is helpful. Treating underlying depression and especially providing effective management of disease-related pain help to improve quality of life and reduce social and psychological distress. Body image dissatisfaction is a significant concern in women with scleroderma and should be assessed routinely. Early identification and treatment of body image dissatisfaction may help to prevent depression and psychosocial impairment in this population. The possibility of premature death from the disease is a major cause of fear and needs to be addressed with the patient and the family. Most often, life expectancy is not influenced by the disease, yet patients fear death because they have scleroderma. When a patient is facing death from severe disease, appropriate honest and sensitive support must be provided.

THERAPEUTIC APPROACH FOR DISEASE MODIFICATION

Immunotherapy

Scleroderma is thought to be an inflammatory connective tissue disorder triggered by an autoimmune process.[66]

Nonselective immunosuppressive treatments are usually employed in scleroderma to treat specific organ manifestations such as early progressing skin disease, active interstitial lung disease, and underlying inflammatory joint or muscle disease (Table 84-5). Cyclophosphamide (CYC) has shown some modest efficacy in scleroderma-related ILD in a randomized placebo-controlled trial. Current therapeutic protocols use CYC as a daily oral regimen or as monthly intravenous (IV) therapy, until control of disease is achieved. The CYC is often followed by maintenance treatment with azathioprine (AZA) or mycophenolate mofetil (MMF), agents that have antiproliferative effects on inflammatory cells and in particular on activated T and B lymphocytes.[126] Uncontrolled studies suggest benefit of MMF in both ILD

Table 84-5 Immunotherapeutic Treatments in Scleroderma

Therapeutic Category	Drug	Clinical Studies (Reference)
Nonselective immunotherapy	Cyclophosphamide	Tashkin 2006[66] Hoyles 2006[126] Nadashkevich 2006[157] Tashkin 2007[158]
	Mycophenolate mofetil	Liossis 2006[128] Nihtyanova 2007[129] Gerbino 2008[159] Zamora 2008[160] Derk 2009[127]
	Azathioprine	Dheda 2004[161] Nadashkevich 2006[157] Paone 2007[162] Berezne 2008[132]
	Methotrexate	van den Hoogen 1996[133] Pope 2001[134]
T cell–targeted immunotherapy	Cyclosporin A	Clements 1993[136] Filaci 1999[163] Morton 2000[135]
	Antithymocyte globulin	Matteson 1996[164] Stratton 2001[165]
	Extracorporeal photopheresis	Rook 1993[166] Krasagakis 1998[167] Knobler 2006[137]
	Sirolimus (rapamycin)	Su 2009[168]
B cell–targeted immunotherapy	Rituximab	Lafyatis 2009[139] Smith 2010[138] Daoussis 2010[169]
Intravenous immunoglobulins	IVIG	Levy 2000[170] Amital 2003[171] Levy 2004[172] Ihn 2007[173] Nacci 2007[174]
Biologic immunotherapy	TNF inhibitors Etanercept Infliximab	Lam 2007[175] Denton 2009[176]
Antifibrotic therapy	CAT-192 (anti–TGF-β ab)	Denton 2007[146] Gordon 2009[177]
	Imatinib mesylate	Pope 2009[178]
Cell-based immunotherapy	Autologous HSCT	Binks 2001[140] McSweeney 2002[179] Farge 2004[141] Nash 2007[180] Oyama 2007[142]

HSCT, hematopoietic stem cell transplantation; IVIG, intravenous immunoglobulin; TGF-β, transforming growth factor-beta; TNF, tumor necrosis factor.

and active scleroderma skin disease.[127-129] Evidence supporting the use of AZA as a primary agent to treat scleroderma-related ILD is weak and remains limited to small retrospective studies. Two open-label trials support its role as maintenance therapy after primary CYC immunosuppression.[130-132]

Methotrexate (MTX) is frequently used in scleroderma to treat associated inflammatory arthritis and myositis. MTX efficacy in skin disease and lung function has been investigated in two randomized placebo-controlled trials showing only a small benefit on skin scores after 6 months (weekly intramuscular injections) or 12 months (weekly oral therapy), respectively.[133,134] Based on the findings of these studies, many experts use MTX for active skin disease.

Selective immunotherapy has also been used in scleroderma (see Table 84-5). T lymphocyte–directed treatments such as cyclosporin A, sirolimus (rapamycin), and antithymocyte globulin (ATG) have shown some benefit.[135,136] However, these studies generally were small and were limited by drug toxicity. The use of extracorporeal photoimmunotherapy or photopheresis (ECP) has been reported with modest improvement in skin disease but lack of any efficacy on internal organ manifestations.[137] This approach is not currently supported. Preliminary studies of rituximab, a chimeric immunoglobulin (Ig)G1 monoclonal antibody directed against CD20, a surface molecule expressed on early pre-B and mature B cells, have not yet demonstrated solid evidence of clinical benefit.[138,139] However, therapeutic strategies based on B cell depletion remain an active area of research. Administration of intravenous immunoglobulins (IVIG) to scleroderma patients has been reported in uncontrolled studies with some evidence that it can improve skin fibrosis or joint disease.

Studies of cell-based immunotherapy using autologous hematopoietic stem cell transplantation (HSCT) preceded by myeloablative conditioning regimens are under way for severe cases of scleroderma. Overall, preliminary data suggest that this approach is effective in improving skin fibrosis and providing stabilization of the lung and other organ function.[140,141] However, significant concern regarding toxicity and treatment-related mortality exists such that this approach is still considered investigational and is used only in patients with life-threatening diffuse scleroderma. Nonmyeloablative (immunoablative) conditioning regimens with or without HSCT have demonstrated similar results.[142,143]

Treatment of Fibrosis

To date, no drugs have proved able to reverse the fibrotic disease process in scleroderma, but several potential agents are being used off-label or are under investigation. Their use is still based on in vitro data, animal studies, or case series because formal well-designed controlled trials are still missing.

D-Penicillamine is a chelating agent that blocks collagen cross-linking and thus has the potential to have an antifibrotic effect. Several case reports and retrospective reviews have suggested that D-penicillamine is beneficial.[144] A double-blind, randomized clinical trial comparing the efficacy of low-dose versus high-dose D-penicillamine in early diffuse scleroderma found no significant difference between skin scores of the two groups at 24 months.[145] Given the potential toxicity of D-penicillamine, its lack of effectiveness in the only controlled trial, and the long duration before benefit was achieved in several uncontrolled surveys, the drug has fallen out of favor and generally is not used.

Transforming growth factor-beta (TGF-β) is a cytokine known to promote fibroblast proliferation and differentiation, in addition to upregulation of collagen and extracellular matrix synthesis. Therefore, it represents an appealing target to specifically control progression of collagen and extracellular deposition in tissues. A human recombinant neutralizing TGF-β antibody was studied versus placebo in a relatively small phase I/II trial in patients with early diffuse scleroderma.[146] No clinical benefit was observed when skin score or lung function testing parameters were evaluated. Although the results of this study were negative, it does not negate the idea that another more potent neutralizing antibody might be helpful.

Imatinib, dasatinib, and nilotinib are small molecules that inhibit the tyrosine kinase activity of the abl-kinases and platelet-derived growth factor (PDGF) receptors, thus interfering with important profibrotic pathways activated in scleroderma. In addition, dasatinib inhibits Src kinases, which are also involved in fibroblast differentiation and secretory function.[147] Several uncontrolled trials with tyrosine kinase inhibitors are currently under way, with early data analysis reporting conflicting results. Adverse events were common, including fluid retention, nausea, fatigue, and elevation of creatine kinase. Therefore, although a potent antifibrotic effect has been shown by tyrosine kinase inhibitors in vitro or in animal models, clinical studies to date have not provided solid evidence for their use in treating skin and systemic fibrosis in scleroderma. Formal clinical trials are needed.

Halofuginone, a plant-derived alkaloid with antifibrotic properties via inhibition of TGF-β and T cell activation, is known to reduce collagen production in animal models. Only limited use of topical halofuginone therapy in scleroderma skin disease is reported with some encouraging results.[148] Rosiglitazone is an agonist of peroxisome proliferative-activator receptor gamma (PPAR-γ) and has been shown to suppress in vitro fibroblast production of collagen and to alleviate fibrosis in the bleomycin-induced scleroderma mouse model.[149] Pirfenidone (5-methyl-1-phenylpyridin-2[1H]-one) is a novel antifibrotic agent with evidence of benefit in patients with idiopathic pulmonary fibrosis (IPF).[150] Clinical trials in scleroderma have not been performed. Neutralizing antibodies against connective tissue growth factor (CTGF) can effectively suppress the development of skin fibrosis in animal models, and anti-CTGF therapy is now under consideration to treat scleroderma.[151]

Treatment of Vascular Disease

Although scleroderma is generally considered a fibrosing disorder, it is well recognized that underlying vasculopathy plays a fundamental role in its pathogenesis and associated tissue injury. In RP, small and medium-sized peripheral blood vessels involved in tissue nutrition and body thermoregulation are affected. The pathologic and clinical consequences of scleroderma vascular disease are not limited to the skin but are widespread and are found in all involved organs. Currently, no guidelines have been put forth for the treatment of scleroderma vascular disease. Therefore, pharmacologic therapies are focused on the treatment of organ-specific disease such as scleroderma renal crisis, PAH, and RP. Conventional treatment strategies have been limited to the use of nonspecific vasodilator agents (see Raynaud's phenomenon section). More recently, it has been appreciated that agents targeting specific biologic processes involved in vascular disease (i.e., prostacyclin, endothelin antagonists, and phosphodiesterase inhibitors) may have a broader beneficial effect on scleroderma (see Raynaud's phenomenon and pulmonary hypertension section).

SUMMARY OF CURRENT PRACTICAL RECOMMENDATIONS FOR TREATMENT

The key to current management of scleroderma is to not isolate treatment to one problem that seems to be dominant, but to appreciate the complexity and dynamics of this multisystem disease (Table 84-6). It is clear that use of just one drug is not effective in managing scleroderma, and that long-term therapy is required with possible adjustments based on specific clinical circumstances. A combination therapy approach that attempts to treat the immune response, the vascular disease, and the underlying tissue fibrosis is recommended.

Patients with severe RP should be on vasodilators and antiplatelet therapy with aspirin. Vasodilator treatment should start with a calcium channel blocker, with a second agent added if needed. This can be a phosphodiesterase inhibitor or intermittent intravenous prostacyclin (it is hoped that oral prostacyclin will be available soon). If digital ulcers are recurring, then the addition of an endothelin inhibitor or a statin is suggested.

Patients with hypertensive renal disease should be treated urgently with an ACE inhibitor or, if needed, with additional ARBs or antihypertensives, including calcium channel blockers or a prostacyclin analogue. The use of ACE inhibitors to prevent a scleroderma renal crisis is not recommended.

All patients need periodic professional dental care, and if loss of saliva is noted, the use of pilocarpine or cevimeline is recommended. Patients with upper gastrointestinal disease should be treated with lifestyle changes such as improving their eating habits with proton pump inhibitors, in case of unremitting symptoms with a prokinetic drug (metoclopramide, domperidone). If the lower intestinal tract is involved, then rotating antibiotics can improve episodes of pseudo-obstruction, diarrhea, or malabsorption.

First-line therapy for active skin disease has not yet been established, but we recommend immunosuppressive therapy based on severity and level of disease activity. Although most recommend methotrexate, we prefer mycophenolate for mild disease and cyclophosphamide for severe aggressive disease (daily oral, monthly IV). More innovative therapies are needed and may include antithymocyte globulin, immunoablation or myeloablation with or without hematopoietic stem cell rescue, and intravenous gamma globulin given alone or in combination with other immunosuppressive agents. Participation of patients in new clinical trials should be pursued.

Active interstitial lung disease should be treated with immunosuppressive therapy. Induction therapy with cyclophosphamide (6 to 12 months; daily oral or monthly IV therapy) followed by maintenance (several years) with mycophenolate or azathioprine is recommended. Mycophenolate or azathioprine alone is a reasonable alternative.

Pulmonary vascular disease and PAH are best treated with vasoactive drugs, including endothelin-1 inhibitors, phosphodiesterase inhibitors, or prostacyclin analogues, given alone or in combination. The role of anticoagulation or immunosuppressive agents is not yet defined. Treatment of associated heart failure is most important.

Cardiac disease should be treated with vasoactive drugs such as calcium channel blockers, other antihypertensive agents, diuretics, and antiarrhythmic medications.

Table 84-6 Current Recommendations for Treatment of Scleroderma

Manifestation	Primary Therapy	Alternative/Second-Line Therapy
Raynaud's phenomenon	Vasodilators (CCB) Antiplatelet	PDE5 inhibitors, prostacyclin, endothelin antagonists
Hypertensive renal disease	ACE inhibitors	ARBs, CCB, prostacyclin, renal transplant (wait at least 24 mo)
GI involvement	**Upper GI** Dental/periodontal care, lifestyle modifications, proton pump inhibitors, prokinetics	EGD to treat stenosis and/or GAVE
	Lower GI Probiotics, rotational antibiotics	Total parenteral nutrition
Skin	Mycophenolate mofetil, cyclophosphamide	IVIG, ATG, research trial (severe cases)
Interstitial lung disease	Cyclophosphamide, mycophenolate mofetil, azathioprine	Research trial
Pulmonary arterial hypertension	PDE5 inhibitors, endothelin antagonists, prostacyclin	Combination therapy, atrioseptostomy, lung transplant, research trial
Cardiac involvement	Heart failure therapy, diuretics, CCB	Immunosuppression (myocardial inflammation)
Joints	Prednisone, methotrexate, TNF inhibitors	IVIG (if contractures and rubs are present), PT/OT
Muscles	Prednisone, methotrexate, azathioprine	IVIG
Psychosocial	Antidepressants, pain control, sleep control	Support group

ACE, angiotensin-converting enzyme; ARBs, angiotensin receptor blockers; ATG, antithymocyte globulin; CCB, calcium channel blockers; EGD, esophagogastroduodenoscopy; GAVE, gastric antral vascular ectasia; GI, gastrointestinal; HSCT, hematopoietic stem cell transplantation; IVIG, intravenous immunoglobulin; PDE5, phosphodiesterase-5 inhibitor; PT/OT, physical therapy/occupational therapy; TNF, tumor necrosis factor.

Immunosuppression should be used if inflammatory muscle or pericardial disease is present.

Inflammatory arthritis should be treated in a similar fashion to the approach used in treating rheumatoid arthritis. However, a fibrosing process causing a nonerosive arthropathy with friction rubs and joint contractures is best treated with the same medications used for active scleroderma skin disease.

Treatment for muscle disease will vary depending on the presence of inflammatory myositis or a nonirritable fibrosing myopathy. The former is treated with corticosteroids, methotrexate, or other immunosuppressive agents effective in immune-mediated polymyositis. The fibrosing process is best treated with the same approach used for scleroderma skin disease.

All patients need emotional and physical support. Scleroderma is a painful disease, and managing pain is essential for reducing depression and improving quality of life. This may require the use of sleep aids (e.g., lorazepam, zolpidem) and/or intermittent use of narcotics. Physical and occupational therapy is most important early in the course of the disease to reduce pain and improve activities of daily living. Family counseling helps the patient cope by providing a clear understanding of what is needed at home. Adjustment of the work environment (e.g., limiting time at work, adjusting room temperature, changing work

assignment) or helping to obtain disability support is also important. Open communication between the physician and the patient provides an essential element of care.

LOCALIZED SCLERODERMA

Localized scleroderma is a nonsystemic skin disease that is seen primarily in children.[152] It can be divided into five major types: plaque morphea, generalized morphea, bullous morphea, linear morphea, and deep morphea. Mixed forms with different types of localized scleroderma occurring at the same time are observed in about 15% of patients. The most common form of localized scleroderma is an isolated circular patch of thickened skin called *plaque morphea* (Figure 84-17A and B). The histology is characterized by mononuclear cellular infiltrates (particularly during active phases) and deposition of thick bundles of collagen. It is usually confined to the dermis, but occasionally it can present with local panniculitis or deeper fibrosis. Multiple morphea lesions *(generalized morphea)* can involve extensive areas of the skin surface and occasionally can coalesce, mimicking the skin changes of systemic sclerosis (Figure 84-17D). In some cases, the morphea lesions may appear nodular and resemble keloids *(keloid morphea)* or, rarely, may form subepidermal bullae *(bullous morphea)* (Figure 84-17C). Inactive morphea may appear as flat areas of hyperpigmented

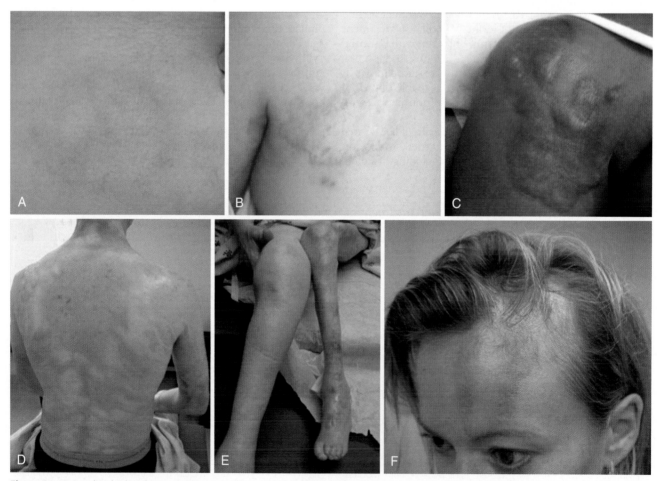

Figure 84-17 Localized scleroderma. **A**, Plaque morphea active and **(B)** inactive. **C**, Keloid morphea. **D**, Generalized morphea. **E**, Linear scleroderma affecting a lower limb and **(F)** the face (en coup de sabre).

skin. Active plaque morphea lesions present as enlarging geographic lesions with raised violaceous borders and ivory-white sclerotic centers. Localized scleroderma can also present as a linear streak (*linear scleroderma*) that crosses dermatomes and is associated with tracking of fibrosis from the skin into deeper tissues, including muscle and fascia (Figure 84-17E). In severe cases, linear scleroderma causes dramatic growth deformities of bone and supporting tissues in the affected regions. Linear scleroderma that affects the face and/or scalp associated with atrophy of muscle, underlying bone, and, rarely, brain tissue is called *en coup de sabre* ("sword stroke") lesion (Figure 84-17F). Progressive hemifacial atrophy (Parry-Romberg syndrome) presents with atrophy of subcutaneous tissue, muscle, and bone without skin fibrosis. A close relationship among seizures, central nervous system (CNS) abnormalities, and ocular malfunction has been noted among these subtypes. Fasciitis with deep subcutaneous sclerosis can be seen in association with morphea lesions. *Pansclerotic morphea* is an uncommon but aggressive and disabling type of localized scleroderma that follows a progressive course despite treatment. It involves skin and deep tissues mimicking systemic sclerosis, but typically it spares the distal portion of the extremities, and the distribution of fibrosis acquires a "tank top" pattern on the trunk.

Although localized scleroderma may be disfiguring and disabling, it is generally a self-limited process that is not associated with a systemic illness. Patients with localized scleroderma have antinuclear antibodies most often directed against histones, chromatin, or nucleosomes, suggesting the presence of a specific underlying autoimmune process. Recent studies suggest that a combination of systemic corticosteroids and methotrexate can be effective treatment for localized scleroderma. Uncontrolled trials of topical therapy with ultraviolet (UV)A-1 phototherapy suggest that this treatment can be helpful for morphea lesions.

MIMICS OF SCLERODERMA

Several conditions that present with various degrees of skin fibrosis can be potentially confused with scleroderma (Table 84-7).[153] These disorders have different origins and exhibit distinct clinical characteristics, skin pathology, and disease associations. They often are detected in the primary care setting, and patients are referred to rheumatologists for further evaluation.

In the early 19th century, many cases of *scleredema* were mistakenly thought to be scleroderma. Scleredema is characterized by thick, indurated skin secondary to collagen and mucin deposition that normally begins on the trunk, especially over the upper back and shoulders, and can spread to arms, legs, and face. Scleredema occurs in the setting of three associated conditions: It can be a transient clinical manifestation following infection; a more persistent disorder associated with insulin-dependent diabetes; or an idiopathic process associated with a monoclonal gammopathy. It is seen in 2% to 15% of diabetic patients, particularly among those with poorly controlled disease. The course of scleredema varies with the underlying associated condition. It tends to resolve in several months when secondary to an infection, and it is improved with control of the diabetic state. No therapy has proved effective, but

Table 84-7 Spectrum of Scleroderma-like Fibrosing Skin Disorders

Immune-Mediated/Inflammatory
Eosinophilic fasciitis
Graft-versus-host disease
Lichen sclerosus et atrophicus
POEMS syndrome
Overlap (systemic lupus erythematosus, dermatomyositis)
Metabolic
Phenylketonuria
Porphyria cutanea tarda
Hypothyroidism (myxedema)
Deposition
Scleromyxedema
Systemic amyloidosis
Nephrogenic systemic fibrosis (or nephrogenic fibrosing dermopathy)
Scleredema adultorum
Lipodermatosclerosis
Occupational
Polyvinyl chloride
Organic solvents
Silica
Epoxy resins
Genetic
Progeroid disorders (progeria, acrogeria, Werner's syndrome)
Stiff skin syndrome (or congenital fascial dystrophy)
Toxic or Iatrogenic
Bleomycin
Pentazocine
Carbidopa
Eosinophilia-myalgia syndrome (L-tryptophan)
Toxic oil syndrome (aniline denatured rapeseed oil)
Postradiation fibrosis

POEMS, polyneuropathy, organomegaly, endocrinopathy, monoclonal gammopathy, and skin changes.
Adapted from Boin F, Hummers LK: Scleroderma-like fibrosing disorders, *Rheum Dis Clin North Am* 34:199–220, 2008.

UVA-1 treatment or PUVA (phototherapy) is reported to be of benefit.

Eosinophilic fasciitis (EF), also called diffuse fasciitis with eosinophilia or Shulman's syndrome or fasciitis-panniculitis syndrome, can also mimic scleroderma. Eosinophilic fasciitis is more common in males and presents as rapid and progressive stiffening of the arms, legs, and trunk. Inflammation and fibrosis within fascia create puckering of the skin and deep venous tracks (the "groove sign"). Because the inflammatory process is deep to cutaneous tissues, the superficial layers of the skin may be pinched readily in EF, in contrast to the thickened dermis involved in scleroderma. EF spares the fingers, is not associated with RP or nail-fold capillary abnormalities, and is not associated with systemic manifestations.[154] Peripheral eosinophilia is present in about 80% of cases but is not required to make a diagnosis. EF associates with a number of hematologic disorders, including immune-mediated anemia or thrombocytopenia, pure red-cell aplasia, myelodysplastic syndromes, and lymphoproliferative processes (T or B cell lymphoma, multiple myeloma). A diagnosis is made by clinical examination and by full-thickness biopsy that includes the fasciae. EF generally responds to corticosteroid therapy and can completely resolve over several months. However, a small percentage of patients will have progressive, nonresponsive disease.

Scleromyxedema (papular mucinosis) closely mimics the cutaneous manifestations of scleroderma. The skin has a flesh-colored papular eruption, giving it a cobblestone feel to light palpation. Distribution is typical with particular involvement of the glabellum, posterior auricular area, and neck. The skin of the trunk and limbs also can become involved. Patients usually are between 30 and 70 years old and have an associated monoclonal gammopathy that usually is of the IgG type with lambda light chains. The presence of RP, sclerodactyly, esophageal dysmotility, pulmonary hypertension, and a myopathy can mimic features of scleroderma. Nail-fold capillary changes do not occur, and neurologic complications with encephalopathy, seizures, coma, and psychosis are reported. Scleromyxedema responds rapidly to treatment with intravenous immunoglobulin, but maintenance therapy must be continued to prevent relapse.[155]

Nephrogenic systemic fibrosis (NSF) is a fibrosing disorder that occurs in patients with end-stage renal failure usually on chronic dialysis or following recent renal transplantation.[156] NSF usually develops over a short time (days to weeks) and then follows a chronic progressive course. This disorder is characterized by thickened, hardened skin with brawny hyperpigmentation and raised plaques, and then loss of limb function due to contractures secondary to subacute and chronic fibrosis of the skin, fasciae, and muscles. The face is usually spared. Deep fibrosis leads to flexion contractions and skin ulcerations. It is now clear that exposure to gadolinium-containing contrast agents in the setting of renal impairment triggers the disease process. Gadolinium deposits are found in involved tissues. By routine microscopy, findings range from a very subtle proliferation of dermal fibroblasts in early lesions to a florid proliferation of fibroblasts and dendritic cells in fully developed cases. Although it has been suggested that improvement can occur with improved renal function, no effective therapy has been confirmed. Reports of benefit with the use of imatinib mesylate are encouraging, but aggressive physical therapy, care to prevent skin ulcerations, pain control, and emotional support are the mainstay of therapy.

Scleroderma-like skin changes have been reported in a number of other disorders, including the carcinoid syndrome, chronic graft-versus-host disease, porphyria cutanea tarda, POEMS syndrome (*polyneuropathy, organomegaly, endocrinopathy, monoclonal gammopathy, and scleroderma-like skin changes*), bleomycin exposure, Werner's syndrome, and phenylketonuria. Eosinophilia-myalgia syndrome and toxic oil syndrome are conditions of historic interest resulting from ingestion of toxic contaminants and presenting with scleroderma-like features.

Selected References

1. Rodnan GP, Benedek TG: An historical account of the study of progressive systemic sclerosis (diffuse scleroderma), *Ann Intern Med* 57:305–319, 1962.
6. Velayos EE, Masi AT, Stevens MB, et al: The 'CREST' syndrome: comparison with systemic sclerosis (scleroderma), *Arch Intern Med* 139:1240–1244, 1979.
7. D'Angelo WA, Fries JF, Masi AT, et al: Pathologic observations in systemic sclerosis (scleroderma): a study of fifty-eight autopsy cases and fifty-eight matched controls, *Am J Med* 46:428–440, 1969.
8. Rodnan GP, Lipinski E, Luksick J: Skin thickness and collagen content in progressive systemic sclerosis and localized scleroderma, *Arthritis Rheum* 22:130–140, 1979.
9. Mayes MD, Lacey JVJ, Beebe-Dimmer J, et al: Prevalence, incidence, survival, and disease characteristics of systemic sclerosis in a large US population, *Arthritis Rheum* 48:2246–2255, 2003.
11. Arnett FC, Howard RF, Tan F, et al: Increased prevalence of systemic sclerosis in a Native American tribe in Oklahoma: association with an Amerindian HLA haplotype, *Arthritis Rheum* 39:1362–1370, 1996.
15. Steen VD, Oddis CV, Conte CG, et al: Incidence of systemic sclerosis in Allegheny County, Pennsylvania: a twenty-year study of hospital-diagnosed cases, 1963-1982, *Arthritis Rheum* 40:441–445, 1997.
16. Tyndall AJ, Bannert B, Vonk M, et al: Causes and risk factors for death in systemic sclerosis: a study from the EULAR Scleroderma Trials and Research (EUSTAR) database, *Ann Rheum Dis* 69:1809–1815, 2010.
17. Steen VD, Medsger TA Jr: Long-term outcomes of scleroderma renal crisis, *Ann Intern Med* 133:600–603, 2000.
18. Steen VD, Medsger TA: Changes in causes of death in systemic sclerosis, 1972-2002, *Ann Rheum Dis* 66:940–954, 2007.
19. Nihtyanova SI, Tang EC, Coghlan JG, et al: Improved survival in systemic sclerosis is associated with better ascertainment of internal organ disease: a retrospective cohort study, *Q J Med* 103:109–115, 2010.
21. Arnett FC, Cho M, Chatterjee S, et al: Familial occurrence frequencies and relative risks for systemic sclerosis (scleroderma) in three United States cohorts, *Arthritis Rheum* 44:1359–1362, 2001.
24. Preliminary criteria for the classification of systemic sclerosis (scleroderma). Subcommittee for scleroderma criteria of the American Rheumatism Association Diagnostic and Therapeutic Criteria Committee, *Arthritis Rheum* 23:581–590, 1980.
25. Kallenberg CG, Wouda AA, Hoet MH, et al: Development of connective tissue disease in patients presenting with Raynaud's phenomenon: a six year follow up with emphasis on the predictive value of antinuclear antibodies as detected by immunoblotting, *Ann Rheum Dis* 47:634–641, 1988.
26. LeRoy EC, Medsger TA Jr: Criteria for the classification of early systemic sclerosis, *J Rheumatol* 28:1573–1576, 2001.
27. Barnett AJ, Miller M, Littlejohn GO: The diagnosis and classification of scleroderma (systemic sclerosis), *Postgrad Med J* 64:121–125, 1988.
28. Clements PJ, Lachenbruch PA, Ng SC, et al: Skin score: a semiquantitative measure of cutaneous involvement that improves prediction of prognosis in systemic sclerosis, *Arthritis Rheum* 33:1256–1263, 1990.
31. Khanna D, Hays RD, Maranian P, et al: Reliability and validity of the University of California, Los Angeles Scleroderma Clinical Trial Consortium Gastrointestinal Tract Instrument, *Arthritis Rheum* 61:1257–1263, 2009.
32. Medsger TA Jr, Silman AJ, Steen VD, et al: A disease severity scale for systemic sclerosis: development and testing, *J Rheumatol* 26:2159–2167, 1999.
34. Steen VD, Medsger TA Jr: The value of the Health Assessment Questionnaire and special patient-generated scales to demonstrate change in systemic sclerosis patients over time, *Arthritis Rheum* 40:1984–1991, 1997.
36. Valentini G, Della Rossa A, Bombardieri S, et al: European multicentre study to define disease activity criteria for systemic sclerosis. II. Identification of disease activity variables and development of preliminary activity indexes, *Ann Rheum Dis* 60:592–598, 2001.
37. Steen VD, Powell DL, Medsger TA Jr: Clinical correlations and prognosis based on serum autoantibodies in patients with systemic sclerosis, *Arthritis Rheum* 31:196–203, 1988.
38. LeRoy EC: Raynaud's phenomenon, scleroderma, overlap syndromes, and other fibrosing syndromes, *Curr Opin Rheumatol* 4:821–824, 1992.
39. Maricq HR, LeRoy EC: Patterns of finger capillary abnormalities in connective tissue disease by "wide-field" microscopy, *Arthritis Rheum* 16:619–628, 1973.

41. Herrick AL, Cutolo M: Clinical implications from capillaroscopic analysis in patients with Raynaud's phenomenon and systemic sclerosis, *Arthritis Rheum* 62:2595–2604, 2010.

42. Cutolo M, Sulli A, Pizzorni C, et al: Nailfold videocapillaroscopy assessment of microvascular damage in systemic sclerosis, *J Rheumatol* 27:155–160, 2000.

46. Comparison of sustained-release nifedipine and temperature biofeedback for treatment of primary Raynaud phenomenon: results from a randomized clinical trial with 1-year follow-up, *Arch Intern Med* 160:1101–1108, 2000.

47. Kahan A, Amor B, Menkes CJ: A randomised double-blind trial of diltiazem in the treatment of Raynaud's phenomenon, *Ann Rheum Dis* 44:30–33, 1985.

48. Thompson AE, Pope JE: Calcium channel blockers for primary Raynaud's phenomenon: a meta-analysis, *Rheumatology (Oxford)* 44:145–150, 2005.

49. Anderson ME, Moore TL, Hollis S, et al: Digital vascular response to topical glyceryl trinitrate, as measured by laser Doppler imaging, in primary Raynaud's phenomenon and systemic sclerosis, *Rheumatology* 41:324–328, 2002.

51. Fries R, Shariat K, von Wilmowsky H, et al: Sildenafil in the treatment of Raynaud's phenomenon resistant to vasodilatory therapy, *Circulation* 112:2980–2985, 2005.

52. Gore J, Silver R: Oral sildenafil for the treatment of Raynaud's phenomenon and digital ulcers secondary to systemic sclerosis, *Ann Rheum Dis* 64:1387, 2005.

57. Kuwana M, Kaburaki J, Okazaki Y, et al: Increase in circulating endothelial precursors by atorvastatin in patients with systemic sclerosis, *Arthritis Rheum* 54:1946–1951, 2006.

58. Abou-Raya A, Abou-Raya S, Helmii M: Statins: potentially useful in therapy of systemic sclerosis-related Raynaud's phenomenon and digital ulcers, *J Rheumatol* 35:1801–1808, 2008.

59. Mayes MD: Endothelin and endothelin receptor antagonists in systemic rheumatic disease, *Arthritis Rheum* 48:1190–1199, 2003.

60. Korn JH, Mayes M, Matucci Cerinic M, et al: Digital ulcers in systemic sclerosis: prevention by treatment with bosentan, an oral endothelin receptor antagonist, *Arthritis Rheum* 50:3985–3993, 2004.

62. Kotsis SV, Chung KC: A systematic review of the outcomes of digital sympathectomy for treatment of chronic digital ischemia, *J Rheumatol* 30:1788–1792, 2003.

64. Yarze JC, Varga J, Stampfl D, et al: Esophageal function in systemic sclerosis: a prospective evaluation of motility and acid reflux in 36 patients, *Am J Gastroenterol* 88:870–876, 1993.

65. Lock G, Straub RH, Zeuner M, et al: Association of autonomic nervous dysfunction and esophageal dysmotility in systemic sclerosis, *J Rheumatol* 25:1330–1335, 1998.

66. Tashkin DP, Elashoff R, Clements PJ, et al: Cyclophosphamide versus placebo in scleroderma lung disease, *N Engl J Med* 354:2655–2666, 2006.

67. Bouros D, Wells AU, Nicholson AG, et al: Histopathologic subsets of fibrosing alveolitis in patients with systemic sclerosis and their relationship to outcome, *Am J Respir Crit Care Med* 165:1581–1586, 2002.

68. Christmann RB, Wells AU, Capelozzi VL, et al: Gastroesophageal reflux incites interstitial lung disease in systemic sclerosis: clinical, radiologic, histopathologic, and treatment evidence, *Semin Arthritis Rheum* 40:241–249, 2010.

69. Goldin JG, Lynch DA, Strollo DC, et al: High-resolution CT scan findings in patients with symptomatic scleroderma-related interstitial lung disease, *Chest* 134:358–367, 2008.

70. Goh NS, Desai SR, Veeraraghavan S, et al: Interstitial lung disease in systemic sclerosis: a simple staging system, *Am J Respir Crit Care Med* 177:1248–1254, 2008.

71. Silver RM, Metcalf JF, Stanley JH, et al: Interstitial lung disease in scleroderma: analysis by bronchoalveolar lavage, *Arthritis Rheum* 27:1254–1262, 1984.

72. Silver RM, Wells AU: Histopathology and bronchoalveolar lavage, *Rheumatology (Oxford)* 47(Suppl 5):v62–v64, 2008.

73. Mittoo S, Wigley FM, Wise R, et al: Persistence of abnormal bronchoalveolar lavage findings after cyclophosphamide treatment in scleroderma patients with interstitial lung disease, *Arthritis Rheum* 56:4195–4202, 2007.

74. Schachna L, Medsger TA Jr, Dauber JH, et al: Lung transplantation in scleroderma compared with idiopathic pulmonary fibrosis and idiopathic pulmonary arterial hypertension, *Arthritis Rheum* 54:3954–3961, 2006.

75. Hsu VM, Moreyra AE, Wilson AC, et al: Assessment of pulmonary arterial hypertension in patients with systemic sclerosis: comparison of noninvasive tests with results of right-heart catheterization, *J Rheumatol* 35:458–465, 2008.

76. Steen V, Medsger TA Jr: Predictors of isolated pulmonary hypertension in patients with systemic sclerosis and limited cutaneous involvement, *Arthritis Rheum* 48:516–522, 2003.

77. Allanore Y, Borderie D, Avouac J, et al: High N-terminal pro-brain natriuretic peptide levels and low diffusing capacity for carbon monoxide as independent predictors of the occurrence of precapillary pulmonary arterial hypertension in patients with systemic sclerosis, *Arthritis Rheum* 58:284–291, 2008.

79. Hachulla E, Gressin V, Guillevin L, et al: Early detection of pulmonary arterial hypertension in systemic sclerosis: a French nationwide prospective multicenter study, *Arthritis Rheum* 52:3792–3800, 2005.

80. Fisher MR, Mathai SC, Champion HC, et al: Clinical differences between idiopathic and scleroderma-related pulmonary hypertension, *Arthritis Rheum* 54:3043–3050, 2006.

81. Kawut SM, Taichman DB, Archer-Chicko CL, et al: Hemodynamics and survival in patients with pulmonary arterial hypertension related to systemic sclerosis, *Chest* 123:344–350, 2003.

82. Chang B, Wigley FM, White B, et al: Scleroderma patients with combined pulmonary hypertension and interstitial lung disease, *J Rheumatol* 30:2398–2405, 2003.

83. Mathai SC, Hummers LK, Champion HC, et al: Survival in pulmonary hypertension associated with the scleroderma spectrum of diseases: impact of interstitial lung disease, *Arthritis Rheum* 60:569–577, 2009.

84. Williams MH, Handler CE, Akram R, et al: Role of N-terminal brain natriuretic peptide (N-TproBNP) in scleroderma-associated pulmonary arterial hypertension, *Eur Heart J* 27:1485–1494, 2006.

86. Forfia PR, Fisher MR, Mathai SC, et al: Tricuspid annular displacement predicts survival in pulmonary hypertension, *Am J Respir Crit Care Med* 174:1034–1041, 2006.

87. Campo A, Mathai SC, Le Pavec J, et al: Hemodynamic predictors of survival in scleroderma-related pulmonary arterial hypertension, *Am J Respir Crit Care Med* 182:252–260, 2010.

88. Williams MH, Das C, Handler CE, et al: Systemic sclerosis associated pulmonary hypertension: improved survival in the current era, *Heart* 92:926–932, 2006.

89. Hoeper MM, Faulenbach C, Golpon H, et al: Combination therapy with bosentan and sildenafil in idiopathic pulmonary arterial hypertension, *Eur Respir J* 24:1007–1010, 2004.

92. Ioannidis JP, Vlachoyiannopoulos PG, Haidich AB, et al: Mortality in systemic sclerosis: an international meta-analysis of individual patient data, *Am J Med* 118:2–10, 2005.

94. Allanore Y, Meune C, Kahan A: Outcome measures for heart involvement in systemic sclerosis, *Rheumatology* 47(Suppl 5):v51–v53, 2008.

95. Byers RJ, Marshall DA, Freemont AJ: Pericardial involvement in systemic sclerosis, *Ann Rheum Dis* 56:393–394, 1997.

97. James TN: De subitaneis mortibus. VIII. Coronary arteries and conduction system in scleroderma heart disease, *Circulation* 50:844–856, 1974.

99. Alexander EL, Firestein GS, Weiss JL, et al: Reversible cold-induced abnormalities in myocardial perfusion and function in systemic sclerosis, *Ann Intern Med* 105:661–668, 1986.

101. Kahan A, Allanore Y: Primary myocardial involvement in systemic sclerosis, *Rheumatology (Oxford)* 45(Suppl 4):iv14–iv17, 2006.

102. Meune C, Avouac J, Wahbi K, et al: Cardiac involvement in systemic sclerosis assessed by tissue-doppler echocardiography during routine care: a controlled study of 100 consecutive patients, *Arthritis Rheum* 58:1803–1809, 2008.

104. Fijalkowska A, Kurzyna M, Torbicki A, et al: Serum N-terminal brain natriuretic peptide as a prognostic parameter in patients with pulmonary hypertension, *Chest* 129:1313–1321, 2006.

106. Steen VD, Syzd A, Johnson JP, et al: Kidney disease other than renal crisis in patients with diffuse scleroderma, *J Rheumatol* 32:649–655, 2005.

108. Penn H, Howie AJ, Kingdon EJ, et al: Scleroderma renal crisis: patient characteristics and long-term outcomes, *Q J Med* 100:485–494, 2007.

109. Teixeira L, Mouthon L, Mahr A, et al: Mortality and risk factors of scleroderma renal crisis: a French retrospective study of 50 patients, *Ann Rheum Dis* 67:110–116, 2008.

110. Clements PJ, Lachenbruch PA, Furst DE, et al: Abnormalities of renal physiology in systemic sclerosis: a prospective study with 10-year followup, *Arthritis Rheum* 37:67–74, 1994.

111. Steen VD: Autoantibodies in systemic sclerosis, *Semin Arthritis Rheum* 35:35–42, 2005.

113. Baron M, Lee P, Keystone EC: The articular manifestations of progressive systemic sclerosis (scleroderma), *Ann Rheum Dis* 41:147–152, 1982.

114. Avouac J, Walker U, Tyndall A, et al: Characteristics of joint involvement and relationships with systemic inflammation in systemic sclerosis: results from the EULAR Scleroderma Trial and Research Group (EUSTAR) database, *J Rheumatol* 37:1488–1501, 2010.

117. Avouac J, Guerini H, Wipff J, et al: Radiological hand involvement in systemic sclerosis, *Ann Rheum Dis* 65:1088–1092, 2006.

118. Szucs G, Szekanecz Z, Zilahi E, et al: Systemic sclerosis-rheumatoid arthritis overlap syndrome: a unique combination of features suggests a distinct genetic, serological and clinical entity, *Rheumatology (Oxford)* 46:989–993, 2007.

122. Kahl LE, Medsger TA Jr, Klein I: Prospective evaluation of thyroid function in patients with systemic sclerosis (scleroderma), *J Rheumatol* 13:103–107, 1986.

123. Antonelli A, Ferri C, Fallahi P, et al: Clinical and subclinical autoimmune thyroid disorders in systemic sclerosis, *Eur J Endocrinol* 156:431–437, 2007.

126. Hoyles RK, Ellis RW, Wellsbury J, et al: A multicenter, prospective, randomized, double-blind, placebo-controlled trial of corticosteroids and intravenous cyclophosphamide followed by oral azathioprine for the treatment of pulmonary fibrosis in scleroderma, *Arthritis Rheum* 54:3962–3970, 2006.

127. Derk CT, Grace E, Shenin M, et al: A prospective open-label study of mycophenolate mofetil for the treatment of diffuse systemic sclerosis, *Rheumatology (Oxford)* 48:1595–1599, 2009.

128. Liossis SN, Bounas A, Andonopoulos AP: Mycophenolate mofetil as first-line treatment improves clinically evident early scleroderma lung disease, *Rheumatology (Oxford)* 45:1005–1008, 2006.

129. Nihtyanova SI, Brough GM, Black CM, et al: Mycophenolate mofetil in diffuse cutaneous systemic sclerosis—a retrospective analysis, *Rheumatology (Oxford)* 46:442–445, 2007.

130. Paone C, Chiarolanza I, Cuomo G, et al: Twelve-month azathioprine as maintenance therapy in early diffuse systemic sclerosis patients treated for 1-year with low dose cyclophosphamide pulse therapy, *Clin Exp Rheumatol* 25:613–616, 2007.

132. Berezne A, Ranque B, Valeyre D, et al: Therapeutic strategy combining intravenous cyclophosphamide followed by oral azathioprine to treat worsening interstitial lung disease associated with systemic sclerosis: a retrospective multicenter open-label study, *J Rheumatol* 35:1064–1072, 2008.

133. van den Hoogen FH, Boerbooms AM, Swaak AJ, et al: Comparison of methotrexate with placebo in the treatment of systemic sclerosis: a 24 week randomized double-blind trial, followed by a 24 week observational trial, *Br J Rheumatol* 35:364–372, 1996.

134. Pope JE, Bellamy N, Seibold JR, et al: A randomized, controlled trial of methotrexate versus placebo in early diffuse scleroderma, *Arthritis Rheum* 44:1351–1358, 2001.

136. Clements PJ, Lachenbruch PA, Sterz M, et al: Cyclosporine in systemic sclerosis: results of a forty-eight-week open safety study in ten patients, *Arthritis Rheum* 36:75–83, 1993.

137. Knobler RM, French LE, Kim Y, et al: A randomized, double-blind, placebo-controlled trial of photopheresis in systemic sclerosis, *J Am Acad Dermatol* 54:793–799, 2006.

138. Smith V, Van Praet JT, Vandooren B, et al: Rituximab in diffuse cutaneous systemic sclerosis: an open-label clinical and histopathological study, *Ann Rheum Dis* 69:193–197, 2010.

139. Lafyatis R, Kissin E, York M, et al: B cell depletion with rituximab in patients with diffuse cutaneous systemic sclerosis, *Arthritis Rheum* 60:578–583, 2009.

140. Binks M, Passweg JR, Furst D, et al: Phase I/II trial of autologous stem cell transplantation in systemic sclerosis: procedure related mortality and impact on skin disease, *Ann Rheum Dis* 60:577–584, 2001.

141. Farge D, Passweg J, van Laar JM, et al: Autologous stem cell transplantation in the treatment of systemic sclerosis: report from the EBMT/EULAR Registry, *Ann Rheum Dis* 63:974–981, 2004.

142. Oyama Y, Barr WG, Statkute L, et al: Autologous non-myeloablative hematopoietic stem cell transplantation in patients with systemic sclerosis, *Bone Marrow Transplant* 40:549–555, 2007.

143. Tehlirian CV, Hummers LK, White B, et al: High-dose cyclophosphamide without stem cell rescue in scleroderma, *Ann Rheum Dis* 67:775–781, 2008.

144. Derk CT, Huaman G, Jimenez SA: A retrospective randomly selected cohort study of D-penicillamine treatment in rapidly progressive diffuse cutaneous systemic sclerosis of recent onset, *Br J Dermatol* 158:1063–1068, 2008.

145. Clements PJ, Furst DE, Wong WK, et al: High-dose versus low-dose D-penicillamine in early diffuse systemic sclerosis: analysis of a two-year, double-blind, randomized, controlled clinical trial, *Arthritis Rheum* 42:1194–1203, 1999.

146. Denton CP, Merkel PA, Furst DE, et al: Recombinant human anti-transforming growth factor beta1 antibody therapy in systemic sclerosis: a multicenter, randomized, placebo-controlled phase I/II trial of CAT-192, *Arthritis Rheum* 56:323–333, 2007.

147. Skhirtladze C, Distler O, Dees C, et al: Src kinases in systemic sclerosis: central roles in fibroblast activation and in skin fibrosis, *Arthritis Rheum* 58:1475–1484, 2008.

148. Pines M, Snyder D, Yarkoni S, et al: Halofuginone to treat fibrosis in chronic graft-versus-host disease and scleroderma, *Biol Blood Marrow Transplant* 9:417–425, 2003.

149. Wu M, Melichian DS, Chang E, et al: Rosiglitazone abrogates bleomycin-induced scleroderma and blocks profibrotic responses through peroxisome proliferator-activated receptor-gamma, *Am J Pathol* 174:519–533, 2009.

152. Laxer RM, Zulian F: Localized scleroderma, *Curr Opin Rheumatol* 18:606–613, 2006.

153. Boin F, Hummers LK: Scleroderma-like fibrosing disorders, *Rheum Dis Clin North Am* 34:199–220, 2008.

154. Lakhanpal S, Ginsburg WW, Michet CJ, et al: Eosinophilic fasciitis: clinical spectrum and therapeutic response in 52 cases, *Semin Arthritis Rheum* 17:221–231, 1988.

155. Blum M, Wigley FM, Hummers LK: Scleromyxedema: a case series highlighting long-term outcomes of treatment with intravenous immunoglobulin (IVIG), *Medicine* 87:10–20, 2008.

156. Kribben A, Witzke O, Hillen U, et al: Nephrogenic systemic fibrosis: pathogenesis, diagnosis, and therapy, *J Am Coll Cardiol* 53:1621–1628, 2009.

157. Nadashkevich O, Davis P, Fritzler M, et al: A randomized unblinded trial of cyclophosphamide versus azathioprine in the treatment of systemic sclerosis, *Clin Rheumatol* 25:205–212, 2006.

158. Tashkin DP, Elashoff R, Clements PJ, et al: Effects of 1-year treatment with cyclophosphamide on outcomes at 2 years in scleroderma lung disease, *Am J Respir Crit Care Med* 176:1026–1034, 2007.

159. Gerbino AJ, Goss CH, Molitor JA: Effect of mycophenolate mofetil on pulmonary function in scleroderma-associated interstitial lung disease, *Chest* 133:455–460, 2008.

160. Zamora AC, Wolters PJ, Collard HR, et al: Use of mycophenolate mofetil to treat scleroderma-associated interstitial lung disease, *Respir Med* 102:150–155, 2008.

162. Paone C, Chiarolanza I, Cuomo G, et al: Twelve-month azathioprine as maintenance therapy in early diffuse systemic sclerosis patients treated for 1-year with low dose cyclophosphamide pulse therapy, *Clin Exp Rheumatol* 25:613–616, 2007.

165. Stratton RJ, Wilson H, Black CM: Pilot study of anti-thymocyte globulin plus mycophenolate mofetil in recent-onset diffuse scleroderma, *Rheumatology (Oxford)* 40:84–88, 2001.

168. Su TI, Khanna D, Furst DE, et al: Rapamycin versus methotrexate in early diffuse systemic sclerosis: results from a randomized, single-blind pilot study, *Arthritis Rheum* 60:3821–3830, 2009.

169. Daoussis D, Liossis SN, Tsamandas AC, et al: Experience with rituximab in scleroderma: results from a 1-year, proof-of-principle study, *Rheumatology (Oxford)* 49:271–280, 2010.

172. Levy Y, Amital H, Langevitz P, et al: Intravenous immunoglobulin modulates cutaneous involvement and reduces skin fibrosis in systemic sclerosis: an open-label study, *Arthritis Rheum* 50:1005–1007, 2004.

174. Nacci F, Righi A, Conforti ML, et al: Intravenous immunoglobulins improve the function and ameliorate joint involvement in systemic sclerosis: a pilot study, *Ann Rheum Dis* 66:977–979, 2007.

175. Lam GK, Hummers LK, Woods A, et al: Efficacy and safety of etanercept in the treatment of scleroderma-associated joint disease, *J Rheumatol* 34:1636–1637, 2007.

176. Denton CP, Engelhart M, Tvede N, et al: An open-label pilot study of infliximab therapy in diffuse cutaneous systemic sclerosis, *Ann Rheum Dis* 68:1433–1439, 2009.

179. McSweeney PA, Nash RA, Sullivan KM, et al: High-dose immunosuppressive therapy for severe systemic sclerosis: initial outcomes, *Blood* 100:1602–1610, 2002.

180. Nash RA, McSweeney PA, Crofford LJ, et al: High-dose immunosuppressive therapy and autologous hematopoietic cell transplantation for severe systemic sclerosis: long-term follow-up of the US multicenter pilot study, *Blood* 110:1388–1396, 2007.

Full references for this chapter can be found on www.expertconsult.com.

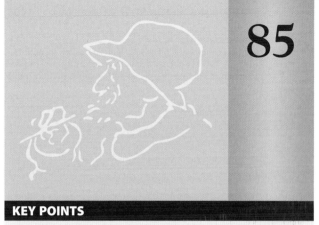

85 Inflammatory Diseases of Muscle and Other Myopathies

KANNEBOYINA NAGARAJU •
INGRID E. LUNDBERG

KEY POINTS

Myopathies are a heterogeneous group of muscle diseases characterized by symmetric proximal muscle weakness and frequent involvement of other organs.

Myopathies are often accompanied by elevated levels of serum muscle enzymes and abnormal electromyograms.

Histology shows varying degrees of inflammation and muscle fiber degeneration and regeneration.

Some patients have autoantibodies that bind to molecules involved in protein synthesis, and these antibodies are often associated with distinct clinical phenotypes.

Corticosteroids and cytotoxic drugs are common therapies.

HISTORY OF INFLAMMATORY MUSCLE DISEASES

Inflammatory muscle diseases are a heterogeneous group of systemic autoimmune rheumatic disorders characterized by chronic muscle weakness, muscle fatigue, and mononuclear cell infiltration into skeletal muscle. These disorders were described in the literature more than a century ago as generalized muscle disorders affecting principally the trunk and proximal limb muscles, with or without skin involvement.[1-5] It was also recognized that these diseases can range from acute and even fatal to slow, progressive, chronic, insidious conditions, with patterns of relapse and remission. Steiner's[6] summary of myositis cases in 1903 made a clear distinction between idiopathic polymyositis (PM) and other forms of myositis caused by bacteria and parasites,[6] and Stertz[7] in 1916 first reported an association between dermatomyositis (DM) and internal malignancy.[7] At about the same time, Batten[8] described the first case of DM with classic histologic features in a child.

Since the 1940s, it has been recognized that PM may occur in the absence of cutaneous lesions, muscle pain, or constitutional symptoms. It may present in an acute, subacute, or chronic insidious form, with some fraction of cases showing systemic features or involvement of organs and tissues.[9] The differential diagnosis has been described independently by several investigators, and the most chronic form was differentiated from an adult variety of muscular dystrophy.[10-12] Banker and Victor[13] noted that DM in children was different and involved a greater degree of vascular inflammation and thrombosis (systemic angiopathy). The first, and still widely used, classification scheme and set of diagnostic criteria for myositis were proposed by Bohan and Peter in 1975.[14,15] They include PM and DM but not the later-described subset known as inclusion body myositis

(IBM). IBM was later defined by the presence of distinct histopathologic changes including vacuoles and nuclear and cytoplasmic inclusions, as well as by distinct clinical features including resistance to glucocorticoids.[16,17] Debate continues whether IBM should be considered an idiopathic inflammatory myopathy (IIM). We have chosen to include information on IBM in this chapter because it is clinically relevant to the differential diagnosis of PM.

EPIDEMIOLOGY

The actual annual incidence of inflammatory myopathy is currently unknown. Because these diseases are so rare, no large-scale epidemiologic studies have been reported; however, several retrospective studies have reported an annual incidence of less than 10 per million individuals[18-22] (Table 85-1). This may be an overestimate, given that the Peter and Bohan diagnostic criteria used in these studies did not distinguish IBM as a separate disease entity. The prevalence of IBM has been estimated to be 10.7 per million in the United States, 9.3 per million in Australia, and 4.9 per million in the Netherlands.[23-25] The age-adjusted prevalence of IBM for those older than 50 years was reported as 16 to 35 per million.[24,25] In some geographic areas, IBM appears to be the most common acquired progressive myopathy, representing 16% to 28% of all inflammatory myopathies.[25] There may be referral biases in these studies. The incidence-prevalence studies need to be interpreted cautiously, given that most have not reported confidence intervals for their rates.

The incidence of the various myopathies varies according to ethnicity, age, and gender. Some studies have reported that the incidence of PM is higher in black patients than in white patients.[18] IIMs can occur in any age group, from early childhood to late in adult life. The onset of PM is usually in the late teens or older, with the mean age at onset being 50 to 60 years; DM shows two peaks—5 to 15 years and 45 to 65 years. IBM is commonly seen in individuals older than 50 years and is rare in younger adults. Some studies have reported gender-specific incidence rates. For example, in the case of PM and DM, females are more commonly affected than males (ratio > 2 : 1), whereas in IBM, the converse is true (again, >2 : 1 ratio).

Inflammatory myopathies can occur in association with other autoimmune connective tissue diseases such as scleroderma, systemic lupus erythematosus (SLE), rheumatoid arthritis, Sjögren's syndrome, polyarteritis nodosa, and sarcoidosis. Significant proportions of all myositis patients (11% to 40%) have an associated connective tissue disease.[23,26,27] Several studies have also confirmed an association between malignancies and inflammatory myopathies.

Table 85-1 Incidence of Inflammatory Myopathies by Country

Country	Study Dates	Incidence (million/yr)	Reference
United States	1963-1982	5.5	18
United States	1947-1968	5.0	20
Australia	1989-1991	7.4	21
Sweden	1984-1993	7.6	22
Israel	1960-1976	2.1	205

A 2-decade-long retrospective study of myositis patients revealed about 12% (37/309) of the patients are associated with malignant diseases. A majority (81%) (30/37) of these patients had DM, and the remainder (19%) had PM. In about 68% of these cases malignancy and myositis appeared within 1 year. The most frequent malignancies associated with myositis were breast tumors and adenocarcinomas, and successful treatment of the underlying malignant disease improved the clinical disease course of myositis. Overall survival rate was considerably worse for DM compared with other forms of myositis.[28] Similar observations were made in a nationwide cohort study in Taiwan that indicated although the general risk of cancer was increased in IIM patients, cancers of the nasopharynx, lung, and breast tissue were the most likely to be diagnosed in both PM and DM patients. Detection of malignancies most frequently occurred within 1 year of being diagnosed with an IIM, with the likelihood of developing a malignancy decreasing over time.[29] Overall, the frequency of malignancies varies widely (4% to 42%) in different studies,[19,30] but in general the incidence of malignancy is higher in DM patients than in IBM or PM patients.[31] It is difficult to determine the relative risks for a particular malignancy because a variety of malignancies are associated with myositis, and only small numbers of individual malignancies have been reported in any one study.

ETIOLOGY OF MYOSITIS

Genetic Risk Factors

An association with immune response genes and occasional reports of familial clustering of myositis support the role of genetic factors in these diseases.[32-37] Polymorphisms in human leukocyte antigen (HLA) class I and II genes are known genetic risk factors for several autoimmune diseases including myositis, but the mechanisms for these associations remain unclear. One possibility is that because the gene products influence T cell repertoire development, tolerance, and immune responses to foreign agents, certain polymorphisms may be selected on the basis of environmental triggers. It appears that haplotypes HLA-DRB1*0301 and HLA-DQA1*0501 are the strongest known genetic risk factors for all forms of myositis in whites; however, different phenotypes have additional HLA risk and protective factors.[37,38] It has been shown that in African-American patients neither DRB1*0301 nor DQA1*0501 is strongly associated with myositis. Instead, the HLA-DRB1*08 allele shows the highest general risk for developing myositis, whereas the HLA-DRB1*14 allele is strongly protective in African-American patients.[39] The HLA-B8/DR3/DR52/

DQ2 haplotype is found in a significant proportion of IBM patients.[40] The risk and protection conferred by HLA associations differ significantly among different ethnic and serologic groups. For example, in some populations (e.g., Koreans, Mesoamericans), there is no association with HLA genes.[35] Further, HLA-DRB1*0301, which is a risk factor in whites, is a protective factor in the Japanese population.[41] The HLA-DRB1*0301, HLA-DQA1*0501, and HLA-DQB1*0201 alleles are strongly associated with myositis-specific antibodies in PM patients.[42] Mechanistic data supporting the role of HLA molecules in disease pathogenesis are, unfortunately, lacking at present. Some studies have reported that maternally derived chimeric cells are present in the peripheral blood and muscle tissues of juvenile DM patients, suggesting that HLA alleles control the occurrence of chimerism and explain the HLA association found in these disorders.[43,44] Like other autoimmune disease conditions, myositis is a complex multigenic disorder involving other non-HLA immune response genes (e.g., cytokines and receptors including tumor necrosis factor [TNF], interleukin [IL]-1, and tumor necrosis factor receptor [TNFR]-1); complement components (e.g., C4, C2); immunoglobulin heavy-chain allotypes, and T cell receptors.[45] The exact contribution of the genetic component in these disorders is currently unknown, in part because of their rarity, the small number of subjects in any single cohort, and the heterogeneity in disease phenotype. International collaborative efforts are currently under way to address these issues and to identify potential genetic and environmental risk factors in myositis.

Environmental Risk Factors

The temporal association of myositis onset and environmental agents in certain individuals suggests that specific exposures in the context of certain genetic backgrounds can initiate muscle inflammation. Common environmental agents implicated in myositis include infectious organisms such as viruses and bacteria and noninfectious agents such as drugs and food supplements (Table 85-2). For example, enteroviruses (influenza, coxsackievirus, echoviruses) and retroviruses (human T-lymphotropic virus-I) are known to induce muscle inflammation. The myositis associated with enteroviruses usually occurs in children and is generally self-limited. A viral cause is strengthened by the presence of high-titer antiviral antibodies and viral particles in patients' serum and tissue samples,[46,47] as well as the induction of muscle inflammation by enteroviruses in animal models. Attempts to identify virus in the tissues of IIM patients by sensitive techniques such as polymerase chain reaction have failed, leading to doubts about the viral cause of these diseases[48] and ruling out continual viral infection as a cause of the ongoing muscle inflammation in these patients. However, it is possible that viruses initially trigger the disease process before being eliminated by the host's immune response, thus explaining the absence of viral genomes in the myositis muscle tissue. Similarly, some microorganisms such as staphylococci, clostridia, and mycobacteria are known to affect skeletal muscle and cause acute muscle inflammation, but there is no evidence that these organisms actually cause chronic, self-sustaining muscle inflammation.

Table 85-2 Possible Environmental Risk Factors

Infectious Agents
Viruses
Picornavirus family, enteroviruses
Polio, coxsackievirus types A and B, echoviruses
Retroviruses
HIV-1, HTLV-I
Parvovirus B19
Hepatitis C virus
Hepatitis B virus
Bacteria
Staphylococci
Clostridia
Mycobacteria
Parasites
Toxoplasma gondii
Trypanosoma cruzi
Borrelia burgdorferi

Noninfectious Agents
Drugs
D-Penicillamine
Corticosteroids
Chloroquine
Statins (atorvastatin, lovastatin, pravastatin, simvastatin)
Lipid-lowering fibrates (bezafibrate, clofibrate, gemfibrozil)
L-Tryptophan
Biologic agents (e.g., growth hormone, interferon-α, interleukin-2)
Vaccination for tetanus, BCG, diphtheria, hepatitis B, hepatitis A
Miscellaneous drugs (e.g., local anesthesia, hydroxyurea, leuprolide acetate)
Ultraviolet radiation exposure
Miscellaneous agents (e.g., silicone breast implants, chronic graft-versus-host disease associated with bone marrow transplantation, collagen injection, silica exposure)

BCG, bacille Calmette-Guérin; HIV, human immunodeficiency virus; HTLV-I, human T-lymphotropic virus I.

Parasites such as *Toxoplasma gondii*, *Trypanosoma cruzi*, and *Borrelia burgdorferi* have been implicated in the triggering of IIMs. The evidence in support of a parasitic cause includes the recovery of parasites from some myositis patients and their serologic response to the parasites; improvement in myositis symptoms after treatment with antiparasitic drugs; a histologic picture of inflammation including infiltration of macrophages and CD4 T cells; and induction of myositis after parasitic infection in animal models.[49-55] Despite these observations, it is difficult to establish a direct link between any parasitic infections and myositis in human patients because there is often no history of antecedent parasitic infection.

Ultraviolet (UV) light irradiation is likely to be a risk factor for the development of DM because epidemiologic data have demonstrated a latitude gradient of PM and DM, with the latter being more frequent closer to the equator and the former being more frequent in northern countries. The ratio between PM and DM is associated with a latitude gradient and is directly correlated with UV light irradiation. This observed correlation is particularly strong in a subset of DM patients with anti–Mi-2 autoantibodies, indicating that UV light may be an environmental risk factor for its development. The association between UV light exposure and subtype of myositis suggests that UV light is an exogenous modifier that can influence the clinical phenotype in PM and DM.[56]

It appears that malignancy is an additional risk factor for the development of myositis, and there is a strong association between DM and malignancies. This early clinical observation has been confirmed in epidemiologic studies.[30,57] With regard to PM and IBM, the association with malignancy is less convincing. The increased risk of malignancy associated with DM has been established both at the time of DM diagnosis and more than 10 years after diagnosis. The pathophysiologic mechanism for the association between malignancy and DM has not been clarified, but there could be several explanations. The strong association between malignancy and the onset of DM indicates that the latter could be a paramalignant phenomenon; that is, the development of myositis is a consequence of the malignancy (related to autoantigens), or the malignancy and DM share disease mechanisms. Thus the molecular mechanisms underlying this unique association are currently unclear. However, there is some evidence that removal of a tumor sometimes results in amelioration of muscle weakness, and tumor reappearance sometimes coincides with muscle weakness, suggesting that these two are linked.[28] A recent report has shed some light on this connection by showing that myositis-specific antigens are highly expressed in cancer tissues, as well as in regenerating muscle cells of myositis patients.[58,59] The authors propose that in cancer-associated myositis, an autoimmune response directed against cancer cross-reacts with regenerating muscle cells, enabling a feed-forward loop of tissue damage and antigen selection.[60] This association must be explored further because cancer-associated myositis patients almost never develop myositis-specific autoantibodies, which are protective for the development of cancer. For malignancies that develop during established disease, the potential explanations include the presence of chronic inflammation or prolonged immunosuppressive treatment, which could contribute to the development of malignancy.

A recent report noted a novel association of myositis with hypertension, diabetes, and ischemic heart disease. The prevalence of hypertension and diabetes in this population was 62% and 29%, respectively, considerably higher than the background prevalence of 9.4% and 4%. These authors suggest that hypertension and ischemic heart disease were more likely to be present before the diagnosis of myositis, whereas hypertension and diabetes occurred more frequently following the diagnosis of myositis in DM patients in comparison with PM or IBM patients, suggesting that it is essential to perform a comprehensive assessment of vascular risk factors in these patients.[61] The same group also reported that patients with IIM are at 75% increased risk for mortality, and cardiovascular diseases followed by infection and malignancy account for the commonest causes of death.[62]

Mimics of Myositis

A variety of insults induce the clinical and pathologic spectrum that mimics myositis in some individuals (see Table 85-2). A number of drugs are known to cause a myopathy that closely mimics myositis. For example, D-penicillamine causes clinically and histologically indistinguishable IIM.[63] Likewise, commonly used lipid-lowering drugs such as statins (e.g., atorvastatin, lovastatin) can cause a myopathy that resembles inflammatory myositis. These agents inhibit 3-hydroxy-3-methylglutaryl-coenzyme A (HMG-CoA) reductase, a rate-limiting enzyme involved in the conversion of HMG-CoA to mevalonic acid, thereby preventing the synthesis of bioactive sterol and nonsterol metabolic intermediates in the cholesterol synthetic pathway. The mechanism by which these drugs cause myopathy is not clear yet.[64-66] However, a recent study showed anti-HMGCR antibodies in patients with statin-induced autoimmune myopathy. It has been suggested that statins upregulate HMG-CoA autoantigen in regenerating muscle cells that in turn sustain an autoimmune response even after statin withdrawal, providing a mechanism for statin-induced immune-mediated necrotizing myopathy.[67] Other drugs such as hydroxyurea can cause skin rashes that resemble DM.[68] TNF inhibitors have been associated with the onset of autoimmune diseases such as vasculitis and a lupus-like syndrome. Recent reports implicate that TNF inhibitors in inflammatory arthritis patients may either induce or exacerbate DM or anti-Jo-1 positive PM.[69,70] Some other reports point to the vaccine adjuvant aluminum hydroxide as a cause of macrophagic myofasciitis. The histology shows infiltration by macrophages and some CD8+ T cells into the endomysium, perimysium, and epimysium, together with clinically elevated creatine kinase (CK) levels, muscle weakness, myalgias, fatigue, and arthralgias.[71] Despite some reports of vaccine-induced myositis, systematic investigation has failed to link any vaccine to myositis.[72]

PATHOGENESIS

Significant advances have been made in our understanding of the pathogenesis of the human inflammatory myopathies.[73-78] It is generally thought that IIMs are autoimmune in origin because they are frequently associated with other autoimmune diseases (e.g., Hashimoto's thyroiditis) and collagen vascular diseases (e.g., scleroderma); many patients exhibit an autoantibody response including the presence of myositis-specific autoantibodies; some studies provide evidence for lymphocyte-mediated muscle fiber injury; and a favorable response to immunosuppressive therapies in some patients supports an autoimmune cause of these disorders.

Humoral Immune Response

More than 50% of all IIM patients have uniquely defined autoantibodies—some of which are specific to myositis, and some of which are merely associated with myositis. These are generally referred to as myositis-specific autoantibodies (MSAs) and myositis-associated autoantibodies (MAAs), respectively. MAAs include autoantibodies to various nuclear and cytoplasmic antigens. Antinuclear antibodies (ANAs) present in myositis are not particularly associated with any disease subgroup, whereas MSAs that are directed against antigens of the protein synthesis pathway (e.g., aminoacyl–transfer RNA [tRNA] synthetases and signal recognition particles) and nuclear components (e.g., nuclear helicase [Mi-2]) are often associated with distinct clinical disease groups and subgroups (e.g., tRNA synthetases with interstitial lung disease, Mi-2 with DM) (Table 85-3).

Table 85-3 Myositis-Specific Antibodies

Autoantibodies	Clinical Disease/Features
Antisynthetase autoantibodies*	More common in polymyositis than dermatomyositis; interstitial lung disease, arthritis, Raynaud's phenomenon, fevers, mechanic's hands
Signal recognition particle (SRP)†	Polymyositis; possible severe disease and cardiac involvement
Chromodomain helicase DNA binding proteins 3 and 4 (Mi-2α and β)‡	Dermatomyositis

*Common antisynthetase antibodies found in myositis are targeted to histidyl-tRNA synthetase (Jo-1), threonyl-tRNA synthetase (PL-7), alanyl-tRNA synthetase (PL-12), isoleucyl-tRNA synthetase (OJ), glycyl-tRNA synthetase (EJ), and asparaginyl-tRNA synthetase (KS).
†Autoantibodies commonly bind to a 54-kD SRP protein in the U.S. patient population and 72-, 54-, and 9-kD proteins in the Japanese population.
‡Targets a 240-kD helicase protein that is part of the nucleosome remodeling deacetylase complex.

Anti–histidyl-tRNA synthetase antibodies are the most frequent and are present in about 16% to 20% of myositis patients.[79-81] Antibodies against other aminoacyl-tRNA synthetases such as threonyl-tRNA synthetase (PL-7), alanyl-tRNA synthetase (PL-12), isoleucyl-tRNA synthetase (OJ), glycyl-tRNA synthetase (EJ), and asparaginyl-tRNA synthetase (KS) are found less frequently (1% to 3%). Anti–Mi-2 antibodies are strongly associated with DM,[82,83] with prominent features such as Gottron's papules, heliotrope rash, the V sign, and the shawl sign. An individual usually has only one MSA because MSAs are often mutually exclusive. The MSAs are most common in patients with other autoimmune diseases and are infrequent or absent in IBM patients and those with malignancies, muscular dystrophies, or other myopathies. These antibodies are sometimes present before the onset of clinical disease.[84]

MAAs such as PM-Scl are frequently associated with a characteristic overlap syndrome that includes features of scleroderma.[85,86] This syndrome is characterized by mild muscle disease, prominent arthritis, and limited skin involvement; it frequently responds to therapy.[87] Some myositis patients also have other MAAs such as anti-snRNP, anti-Ro/SSA, anti-Ku, and anti-PMS1. Antibodies recognizing an uncharacterized 56-kD large nuclear ribonucleoprotein have been found in a majority of myositis patients (86%), and the antibody titer appears to vary with disease activity, suggesting its importance in our understanding of disease pathogenesis and its potential usefulness as a clinical disease marker.[88] Some of the MSAs show strong immunogenetic associations; for example, antibodies against aminoacyl-tRNA synthetases are associated with HLA-DQA1*0501, anti-SRP with DR5, anti–Mi-2 with DR7, and anti–PM-Scl with DR3.[37] Neither the molecular mechanisms that initiate and perpetuate the autoimmune response nor the precise role of these autoantibodies in the pathogenesis of myositis is currently known. However, these antibodies serve as excellent clinical markers and can help diagnose and categorize these heterogeneous disorders into homogeneous subgroups.

Cell-Mediated Immune Response

At the cellular level, there are distinct differences in the distribution and location of the various lymphocyte subsets in the muscle tissues in different IIMs. Two major patterns of inflammatory cell infiltrates are seen in muscle tissue. The first has a predominantly perivascular distribution (Figure 85-1A), often in perimysial areas (Figure 85-1C), and is largely made up of CD4+ T cells, macrophages, and dendritic cells. Occasionally, B cells are present in some patients. This pattern is seen mainly in DM patients with skin rash but occasionally in patients without a rash. The second pattern has a predominantly endomysial distribution (Figure 85-1B), with mononuclear inflammatory cells often surrounding and sometimes invading non-necrotic muscle fibers. These inflammatory cellular infiltrates are comprised primarily of CD8+ T cells and macrophages, but CD4+ T cells and dendritic cells are also present. This pattern is generally seen in patients without skin rashes and often in those classified as having PM or IBM. In some patients, the two patterns of inflammation are seen in the same biopsy. The two distinct locations and the varying compositions of the inflammatory cell populations in the two areas suggest two different pathogenic mechanisms—one that targets the blood vessels and one that targets the muscle fibers. Notable inflammation is also seen in other organs.

The vascular involvement in patients with DM is also manifested in the skin and can be seen clinically in the form of nail-fold changes and changes in the gastrointestinal (GI) tract. The capillaries show clear hyperplasia, vacuolization, and necrosis, contributing to an ischemia that could cause fiber damage.[89,90] One of the earliest events in the pathogenesis of DM appears to be activation of the complement cascade. This leads to the subsequent deposition of complement components, which in turn results in the deposition of lytic membrane attack complexes in the endothelial cells and the eventual loss of capillaries due to complement-mediated damage. The capillaries are abnormally thickened and enlarged and look like high endothelial venules, which are characteristics of vessels that facilitate lymphocyte trafficking (Figure 85-2). The capillaries also show signs of neovascularization.[91] This loss of capillaries results in some of the histopathologic features characteristic of this disease: capillary necrosis and loss, perivascular inflammation and ischemia (rarely seen), and perifascicular atrophy (a late feature; see Figure 85-1C and D). Recent studies also point out a role for type I interferon (IFN)-inducible genes in the pathogenesis of DM. It has been shown that plasmacytoid dendritic cells produce type I IFN and induce expression of IFN-inducible proteins such as MxA and IFN-inducible gene 15 (ISG15) at perifascicular myofibers and capillaries of DM biopsies, suggesting that injury to muscle fibers and capillaries occurs due to the intracellular overproduction of one or more type I IFN-inducible proteins in DM[92,93]-induced genes Although no direct comparison has been reported, the pathologic changes in juvenile and adult DM appear to be similar, except that all the basic pathologic features are more prominent in the childhood form (see later). The factors that initiate complement activation in this disease are poorly understood; however, the consequences of complement-mediated damage are clearly visible in DM.[94]

The endomysial inflammatory aggregates contain a high percentage of T cells, particularly activated CD8+ T cells, macrophages, and CD4+ T cells and few natural killer cells. Immunoelectron microscopic studies have provided evidence of the invasion, replacement, and probable destruction of non-necrotic muscle fibers by T cells and macrophages.[95] It is suggested that CD8+ cytotoxic T lymphocytes (CTLs) recognize major histocompatibility

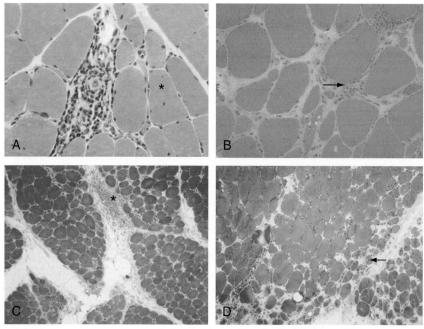

Figure 85-1 Hematoxylin and eosin staining of muscle biopsy showing perivascular inflammation. **A,** Variation in fiber size and central nucleation *(asterisk)*. **B,** Endomysial inflammation and increased fibrosis *(arrow)*. **C,** Perimysial inflammation *(asterisk)*. **D,** Perifascicular atrophy *(arrow)*. *(B, Courtesy Dr. Inger Nemmesmo. D, Courtesy Dr. Paul Plotz.)*

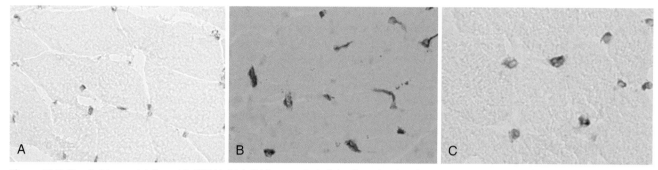

Figure 85-2 Muscle biopsy staining with CD146 (Mel-CAM), an endothelial cell marker. Results are shown in normal **(A)**, dermatomyositis **(B)**, and polymyositis **(C)** subjects. Note the abnormal capillary size in both dermatomyositis and polymyositis.

complex (MHC) class I on muscle fibers and may mediate muscle fiber damage. Infiltrating CTLs express perforin-containing granules, which are characteristically oriented toward the target muscle fiber, indicating that muscle fiber injury may be partially mediated by perforin-dependent cytotoxic mechanisms (Figure 85-3B and C).[96] In PM and IBM, there is evidence of clonal proliferation of CD8+ T cells, both within the muscle and in the peripheral circulation.[97,98] T cell lines from patients demonstrate cytotoxicity against autologous myotubes,[99] suggesting that the muscle fiber injury in PM and IBM is mediated by CTLs. CTLs are known to mediate target cell damage by both perforin–granzyme B and Fas-FasL pathways. The overexpression of antiapoptotic molecules such as Bcl-2, Fas-associated death domain–like IL-1 converting enzyme inhibitory protein (FLIP), and human inhibitor of apoptosis protein–like protein in skeletal muscle of myositis patients suggests that perforin–granzyme B–mediated CTL damage may play a predominant role in muscle fiber injury and dysfunction in myositis.[100-102]

In contrast to previous concepts, recent studies also show accumulations of B cells, plasma cells, myeloid dendritic cells, late-activated macrophages expressing 25F9 marker, as well as CD8+ CD28− and CD4+ CD28− T cells (TCR V[β]-expanded T cells) in the skeletal muscle and in the peripheral circulation of PM, DM, and IBM patients. These CD28− cells and late-activated macrophages expressing 25F9 marker are hypothesized to exhibit cytotoxic potential and produce proinflammatory cytokines in IIM skeletal muscle.[103,104] Another study also explored the potential role of FOXP3+ Treg cells in the pathology of myositis. These authors reported that the number of Treg cells correlated with the degree of inflammation in IIMs and suggested that these cells might serve to counterbalance activity of cytotoxic T cells in myositis.[105]

On the basis of the data described, two different pathways have been proposed as major mediators of muscle damage and inflammation: one mediated through T lymphocytes (CTLs) directed against muscle fibers, predominating in PM and IBM, and the other directed against

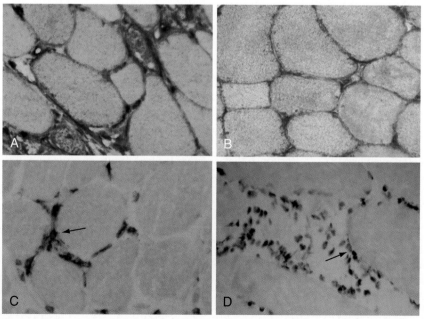

Figure 85-3 HLA-ABC, CD8+ T cell, and granzyme B staining of polymyositis biopsy. HLA expression is evident on muscle fibers, infiltrating cells, and endothelial cells **(A)**. HLA cell surface and sarcoplasmic staining is shown on muscle fibers **(B)**, CD8+ T cells **(C,** *arrow*), and granzyme B–positive cells **(D)** surrounding muscle fibers *(arrow)*.

vessels, predominating in DM. However, several studies have shown that the degree of inflammation does not consistently correlate with the severity of the structural changes in the muscle fibers or with the severity of the clinical disease,[106] suggesting that nonimmune processes also play a role in disease pathogenesis. A role for nonimmune processes is supported by the following observations: First, marked structural changes in the muscle fibers occur in the absence of any inflammatory cells.[107,108] Second, there is a lack of correlation between the degree of inflammation and the degree of muscle weakness.[109] Third, some myositis patients do not respond, even to powerful anti-inflammatory therapy.[110,111] Fourth, steroid treatment may eliminate inflammatory cells in myositis muscle tissue, but this removal alone may not substantially improve the clinical disease, suggesting that immunosuppressive therapies modulate disease activity but do not change other mediators of the disease process.[112] Finally, the clinical disease may progress when identifiable inflammation has subsided,[113] suggesting a role for nonimmune mechanisms in the pathogenesis of myositis. Thus the exact contribution of immune-mediated pathways to muscle damage is currently unknown.

Class I Major Histocompatibility Complex

Normal skeletal muscle cells do not constitutively express or display MHC class I molecules, although they can be induced to do so by proinflammatory cytokines such as IFN-γ or TNF[107,114-116] or by the alarmin HMGB1.[139] In contrast, in human IIMs, the early and widespread appearance of MHC class I in non-necrotic muscle cells is a striking feature, even in muscle cells distant from the lymphocytic infiltration.[107,108,117] MHC class I staining is usually observed on the sarcolemma of muscle fibers, but some fibers also show staining in both the sarcolemma and the sarcoplasm (see Figure 85-3A and B). In some patients, the expression is restricted to a few clusters (often in early disease), whereas in others, almost every fiber is positively stained, particularly in late-phase and treatment-resistant cases. The biologic significance of these observations has been explored by generating a conditional transgenic mouse model overexpressing syngenic mouse MHC class I. The overexpression of MHC class I molecules in the skeletal muscle of mice results in the development of clinical, biochemical, histologic, and immunologic features that resemble human myositis and provides a close model of the human disease. The disease in these mice is inflammatory, limited to skeletal muscles, self-sustaining, more severe in females, and often accompanied by MSAs.[118] Recent studies in this model further suggest that MHC class I overexpression leads to endoplasmic reticulum stress, muscle atrophy, and decrease in force generation capacity of skeletal muscle, implicating the role for MHC class I muscle weakness in myositis.[119,120]

A number of observations in human myositis patients and in the mouse model of myositis suggest that MHC class I molecules themselves may mediate muscle fiber damage and dysfunction in the absence of lymphocytes. For instance, in human myositis, the induction of MHC class I antigen in muscle fibers occurs early, preceding inflammatory cell infiltration.[121,122] MHC class I staining of human myositis biopsies shows both a cell surface and a sarcoplasmic

reticulum pattern of internal reactivity, demonstrating that some of the MHC class I molecules may be retained in the endoplasmic reticulum (ER) of these fibers.[78,108,123] Persistent MHC class I overexpression in muscle fibers may exist in the absence of an inflammatory infiltrate.[113] The controlled induction of MHC class I in the mouse model is followed by muscle weakness before mononuclear cell infiltration.[118] It has recently been shown that in vivo gene transfer of MHC class I plasmids attenuates muscle regeneration and differentiation.[124] Together, these observations, and particularly the obvious retention of MHC class I within the cell in both human and murine disease, indicate that the muscle fiber damage seen in myositis may not be solely mediated by immune attack (e.g., CTLs, autoantibodies); it may also be mediated through nonimmunologic mechanisms such as the ER stress response and hypoxia.

Because MHC class I assembly occurs in the ER and because upregulation in myositis muscle fibers is widespread, even in the absence of visible inflammatory infiltrate, it is likely that ER stress plays a role in the muscle fiber damage and dysfunction associated with human myositis. The ER is intimately involved in the folding, exporting, and processing of newly synthesized proteins. When there is an imbalance between the protein load in the ER and the cell's ability to process that load, a series of signaling pathways that adapt cells to ER stress is activated. This ER stress response can be provoked by a variety of pathophysiologic conditions including ischemia, hyperhomocysteinemia, viral infections, and mutations that impair protein folding, as well as by excess accumulation of protein in the ER.[125,126] Cells self-protect against ER stress by initiating at least four functionally distinct responses: (1) upregulation of the nuclear factor κB (NFκB) pathway (ER overload response); (2) upregulation of genes encoding ER chaperone proteins such as Bip/GRP78 and GRP94, as a means of increasing protein folding activity and preventing protein aggregation; (3) translational attenuation to reduce the load of protein synthesis and to prevent the further accumulation of unfolded proteins (unfolded protein response); and (4) cell death, which occurs when the ER's functions are severely impaired. This cell death event is mediated by transcriptional activation of the gene for CHOP/GADD153, a member of the C/EBP family of transcription factors,[127] and by the activation of ER-associated caspase 12.[128]

In myositis, it appears that overexpression of MHC class I in myofibers initiates a series of cell autonomous changes that contribute to myofiber pathology. Recent investigations have indicated that overexpression of MHC class I on muscle fibers results in activation of the NFκB and ER stress response pathway in human inflammatory myopathies and in the mouse model of myositis.[78,129] NFκB can be activated within minutes by a variety of stimuli including inflammatory cytokines such as TNF and IL-1, T cell activation signals, and stress inducers. It is likely that in human myositis, NFκB activates both classic (proinflammatory cytokines) and nonclassic (ER stress response) pathways.[78,129-132] Further, there is evidence that downstream target genes (e.g., MHC class I, intercellular adhesion molecule [ICAM], monocyte chemoattractant protein [MCP]-1) regulated by the NFκB pathway are highly upregulated in myositis patients.[123,133,134] Recent studies have indicated that NFκB p65 is activated both in human myositis biopsies and in the

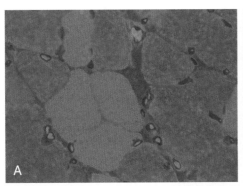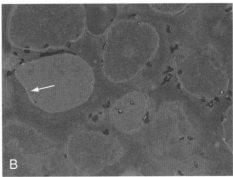

Figure 85-4 Nuclear factor κB (NFκB) expression in normal and myositis biopsy. Immunofluorescence staining with rabbit anti-NFκB and anti–rabbit Texas red and counterstaining with 4, 6-diamino-2-phenylindole (blue nuclei). Note the cytoplasmic expression of NFκB in normal muscle (**A**) and a subsarcolemmal pattern in the myositis biopsy (**B**; *arrow*). *(From Nagaraju K, Casciola-Rosen L, Lundberg I, et al: Activation of the endoplasmic reticulum stress response in autoimmune myositis: potential role in muscle fiber damage and destruction, Arthritis Rheum 52:1824–1835, 2005.)*

mouse model,[78,129,135,136] suggesting that this pathway may be directly involved in muscle fiber damage (Figure 85-4). NFκB is a potential therapeutic target in myositis, and the use of NFκB pathway inhibitors significantly reduces the pathology associated with several autoimmune diseases including diabetes, multiple sclerosis, inflammatory bowel disease, and rheumatoid arthritis, suggesting that this pathway is a critical player in the effector phase of autoimmune pathology. Thus it appears that MHC class I expression on muscle fibers links the immune and nonimmune mechanisms of muscle fiber damage.

Cytokines and Hypoxia

A number of other effector molecules produced in muscle tissue by inflammatory cells, endothelial cells, and muscle fibers are thought to play a role in the pathogenesis of myositis.[75] Most of the data assembled relate to cytokines, but some data related to chemokines are also available. The most consistently demonstrated cytokines in muscle tissue from patients with IIMs are cytokines with proinflammatory properties: IL-1α, IL-1β, TNF, and IFN-α. Recently, IL-10, IL-13, epidermal growth factor (EGF), vascular endothelial growth factor (VEGF), fibroblast growth factor (FGF), CCL3 (macrophage inflammatory protein [MIP-1α]), CCL4 (MIP-1β) and CCL11 (eotaxin), IL-15, and IL-15Rα were also demonstrated to be significantly upregulated and granulocyte colony-stimulating factor (G-CSF) downregulated in patients with IIMs relative to normal subjects.[137,138] Further, the DNA-binding high mobility group box 1 (HMGB1) was found to exhibit both extranuclear and extracellular patterns in the muscle tissue of patients with PM and DM. Stimulation with IFN-γ showed an increased HMGB1 expression in muscle nuclei and the myoplasm. Exposure to HMGB1 induced a reversible upregulation of MHC class I in the muscle fibers and irreversible decrease in Ca^{2+} release from the sarcoplasmic reticulum during fatigue, implicating a role of HMGB1 and MHC class I early in the pathogenesis of IIMs.[139] In addition to inducing the upregulation of MHC class I and II molecules on muscle fibers, cytokines may have a direct effect on muscle fiber function, as has been demonstrated for TNF.[140] The relative importance of the various cytokines and chemokines in patients with myositis is still uncertain, but these molecules

are potential biomarker candidates in this disease as exemplified by a recent study showing serum IL-6 production and the type I IFN gene signature in the peripheral blood correlating with disease activity in DM patients.[141]

Microvessel involvement was first observed in DM but has also become evident in PM. The endothelial cells in both subsets show increased expression of adhesion molecules and proinflammatory cytokines such as IL-1α. This phenotype can be induced by tissue hypoxia, which may result from capillary loss and local tissue inflammation. Muscle tissue hypoxia can contribute to the clinical symptoms and muscle fatigue and might be associated with disease mechanisms in inflammatory myopathies.[75] A recent study reported the expression of VEGF receptor in muscle fibers and HIF-2α reactivity in endothelial cells of PM and IBM patients DM patients showed hypoxia-inducible factor (HIF)-1α and HIF-1β expression in endothelial cells, whereas expression of HIF-2α, erythropoietin receptor, VEGF, and VEGF-R were also observed on muscle fiber. These observations suggest that deprivation of blood supply by immune-mediated mechanisms might trigger the upregulation of hypoxia-related proteins as an adaptive response.[142] The hypoxia hypothesis is further supported by the clinical improvement observed after exercise, but a causal connection still needs to be established. In addition, magnetic resonance spectroscopic analysis, before and after a work load, has demonstrated reduced levels of energy substrates that are important for muscle contraction such as adenosine triphosphate and phosphocreatine, when compared with levels in healthy individuals. This finding supports the hypothesis that an acquired metabolic disturbance occurs in chronic inflammatory myopathies and that this disturbance can contribute to impaired muscle performance.

Proposed Mechanisms of Muscle Damage

Currently available data suggest that both immune (cell-mediated and humoral) and nonimmune (ER stress, hypoxia) mechanisms play a role in muscle fiber damage and dysfunction in myositis. ER stress, hypoxia, and the NFκB pathway are highly active within the skeletal muscle of myositis patients, and the proinflammatory NFκB pathway connects the immune and nonimmune components contributing to muscle damage. The relative contribution of

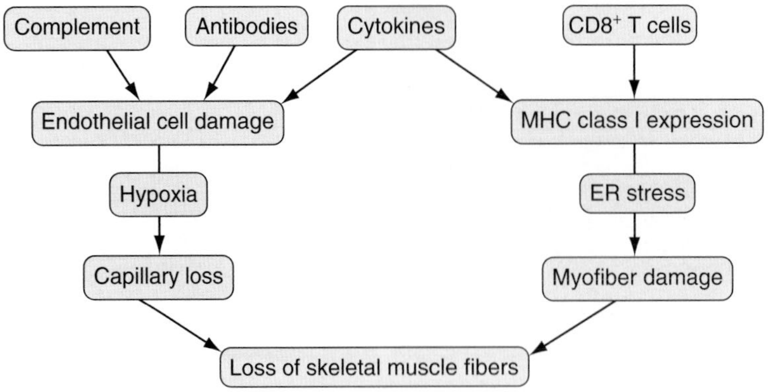

Figure 85-5 Mechanisms of muscle fiber damage in myositis. ER, endoplasmic reticulum; MHC, major histocompatibility complex.

each of these pathways to muscle fiber damage is presently unclear (Figure 85-5). Therefore use of specific drugs to inhibit these pathways, either alone or in combination, would help define their roles in myositis and potentially serve as effective therapeutic agents.

CLINICAL FEATURES

The inflammatory myopathies may occur as distinct disease entities, or they may coexist with some other rheumatic disease. This observation is true for all three subsets of myositis, but it is most often seen in PM and DM. The rheumatic diseases most often associated with inflammatory myopathies are systemic sclerosis, mixed connective tissue disease, Sjögren's syndrome, and SLE; however, rheumatoid arthritis may also be associated with inflammatory myopathies. IBM may be associated with Sjögren's syndrome, SLE, and other autoimmune diseases.[143,144] Because the clinical features of IBM differ somewhat from those of PM and DM, they are presented separately.

Polymyositis and Dermatomyositis

The predominant symptoms in patients with PM or DM are muscle weakness and low muscle endurance. The weakness is most pronounced in proximal muscle groups—typically in the neck, pelvic, thigh, and shoulder muscles—with a symmetric distribution. Patients generally experience more problems performing repetitive movements than with single-strength exercises, and they report difficulty walking uphill or upstairs, working with their arms above their shoulders, or rising from chairs. The onset is often subacute, occurring over a few weeks, or it may be insidious, developing over several months. If untreated, the muscle weakness progresses slowly, and in the most severe cases, patients may become wheelchair dependent. Problems with swallowing and nutrition may occur as a result of impaired contractility of the throat muscles, possibly leading to aspiration pneumonia. In rare cases patients develop difficulty breathing because of weakness of the diaphragm or thoracic muscles, and they may require assisted ventilation. Other striated muscles may be involved, such as in the lower part of the esophagus (causing reflux problems) or the sphincter ani (causing incontinence).

Skin

Dermatomyositis is characterized by the presence of certain types of rashes[145]; the same types are often seen in both children and adults. The most specific skin manifestations are Gottron's papules and the heliotrope rash (Figure 85-6). Gottron's papules are slightly elevated violaceous, pink, or dusky red papules located over the dorsal side of the metacarpal or interphalangeal joints. These papules may also occur over the extensor side of the wrist, elbow, or knee joints. Gottron's papules are considered to be pathognomonic of DM. A macular rash (without papules) with the same distribution as Gottron's papules is called *Gottron's sign* (see Figure 85-6C and D). The heliotrope rash is a periorbital red or violaceous erythema of one or both eyelids, often with edema (see Figure 85-6B). Linear erythema overlying the extensor surfaces of joints is also relatively specific to DM (Figure 85-7A). Many patients with DM have photosensitive rashes, typically located on the face or scalp or over the neck (the so-called **V** sign), although this rash is not specific to DM (Figure 85-7B and C). Another common rash in DM is located over the shoulders (shawl sign; Figure 85-7D) or over the hips (holster sign). Pruritus is common. Patients with DM often have skin lesions on their fingers such as periungual erythema, nail-fold telangiectasias, and cuticular overgrowth (Figure 85-8C). Other less common skin manifestations are panniculitis, livedo reticularis, and nonscarring alopecia. Vasculitis may be seen in children with DM but rarely in adults.

In general, the skin rash is moderate, with local erythema. In rare cases, a severe, diffuse erythema (erythroderma) may occur, occasionally with vesiculobullous lesions or ulcers. The skin rash may precede the muscle symptoms by months or even years, and in some patients, the skin manifestations may be the only clinical sign of DM; this condition is often called amyopathic DM or DM sine myositis (see later). The pattern of the rash over the knuckles and dorsum of the hand is distinct, in that the rash generally affects the phalanges but spares knuckles in SLE, and vice versa in DM (Figure 85-8A and B). However, no histopathologic skin features are specific for DM; most of the features are also seen in patients with SLE. Thus skin biopsy is rarely helpful in distinguishing between these two disorders. The cutaneous manifestations may fail to respond to

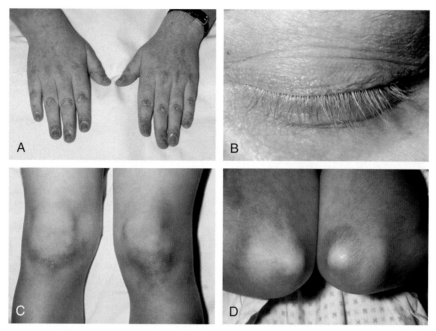

Figure 85-6 Characteristic features of dermatomyositis skin changes. **A,** Gottron's papules. **B,** Heliotrope rash. **C,** Gottron's sign on knee and **D,** elbow. *(Courtesy Dr. Paul Plotz.)*

immunosuppressive treatment, despite improvement in muscle symptoms. Thus it is possible that different molecular pathways or disease mechanisms cause the skin rash and the muscle inflammation.

Calcinosis, which can be severe, is found mainly in juvenile DM but is occasionally seen in adults. The calcinosis occurs predominantly in sites that have been subject to friction or trauma such as the elbows or knees. Sometimes the calcinosis can be extensive and erupt, leading to ulcers. It is most often localized to the subcutaneous tissue but can also develop in the skin, fascia, or muscle and can be visualized by radiography, computed tomography (CT), or

magnetic resonance imaging (MRI). The calcinosis seems to progress as long as there is active inflammatory disease. Also, once it has developed, it is often treatment resistant. Some data, however, suggest that the progress of calcinosis can be inhibited by effectively treating the inflammatory process in the skin and muscle.[146]

Another type of skin pathology seen in inflammatory myopathies is called mechanic's hands. This rash is often associated with the presence of antisynthetase autoantibodies and can be seen in both PM and DM. The rash is a hyperkeratotic, scaling, fissuring of the fingers, particularly on the radial side of the index fingers (Figure 85-9).

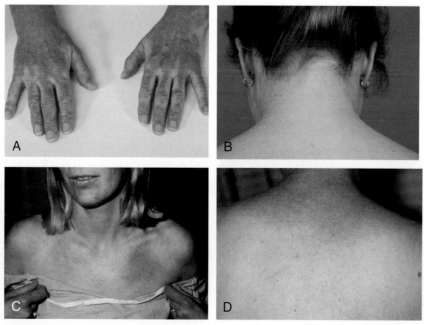

Figure 85-7 Characteristic features of dermatomyositis skin changes. **A,** Linear erythema. **B,** Scalp rash. **C,** V-like sign. **D,** Shawl sign. *(Courtesy Dr. Paul Plotz.)*

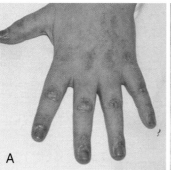
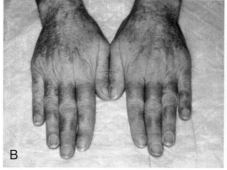
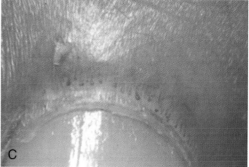

Figure 85-8 Erythematous rashes on the hand in dermatomyositis and systemic lupus erythematosus. **A,** Note the changes on the knuckles and dorsum of the hand in dermatomyositis (Gottron's sign). **B,** Rash is absent on the knuckles but present on the phalanges in lupus. **C,** Capillary nail-fold changes in dermatomyositis. *(Courtesy Dr. Paul Plotz.)*

Lungs

Lung involvement is frequent in PM and DM and is a major risk factor for morbidity and mortality. Clinical symptoms such as dyspnea and cough are common. Lung involvement can be caused by weakness of the respiratory muscles or inflammation of the lung tissue (interstitial lung disease). Weakness of the respiratory muscles may lead to restrictive lung disease, and involvement of the pharyngeal muscles is a risk factor for aspiration pneumonia. Interstitial lung disease, caused by inflammation in the small airways, is common in PM and DM and is often associated with antisynthetase autoantibodies; it may be present in up to 70% of patients when investigated with sensitive techniques such as high-resolution CT and measurement of pulmonary function and diffusion capacity.[147] In most cases, the changes are present at the time of diagnosis of myositis; they rarely develop after immunosuppressive treatment has started. The severity of interstitial lung disease may vary from mild or even asymptomatic to rapidly progressive (Hamman-Rich–like) with a fatal outcome. In most cases, the interstitial lung disease is mild and has a slowly progressive course. In some cases, improvement in lung function is seen with immunosuppressive treatment. The course and outcome vary, depending on the histopathology, suggesting that different disease mechanisms cause interstitial lung disease.

In general, the clinical course and histopathology of interstitial lung disease in myositis are no different from those in idiopathic interstitial lung disease. The most common histopathologic finding is nonspecific interstitial pneumonia, but other entities such as cryptogenic organizing pneumonia, bronchiolitis obliterans organizing pneumonia, diffuse alveolar damage, and usual interstitial pneumonia are also found. Some studies suggest that bronchiolitis obliterans organizing pneumonia responds favorably to corticosteroids, whereas histopathologic changes compatible with diffuse alveolar damage, usual interstitial pneumonia, or acute interstitial pneumonia respond poorly to corticosteroids or other immunosuppressive therapies and have a poor prognosis.

Arthritis

Joint pain and arthritis are common in patients with PM or DM. The most common form of arthritis is a symmetric arthritis of the small joints of the hands and feet. This arthritis is typically nonerosive but can sometimes be erosive and destructive. Most frequently, arthritis is seen in patients with anti–Jo-1 antibodies and other antisynthetase autoantibodies, but it is also seen in patients with overlapping syndromes of other rheumatic diseases.

Heart

Cardiovascular disease is a risk factor for death among patients with PM and DM. However, clinically evident heart involvement is rare, perhaps indicating that cardiac

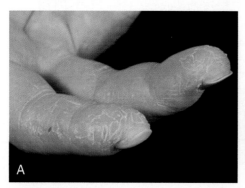
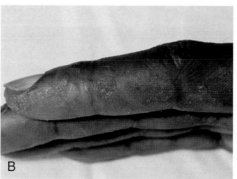

Figure 85-9 Mechanic's hands in a white **(A)** and a black **(B)** patient. Note the characteristic skin changes on the lateral side of the fingers. *(Courtesy Dr. Paul Plotz.)*

involvement may be overlooked in these conditions. Subclinical manifestations are frequently discovered when patients with PM or DM are evaluated. The most frequently reported subclinical manifestations are conduction abnormalities and arrhythmias detected by electrocardiogram (ECG). The underlying pathophysiologic mechanisms that may lead to cardiac manifestations in patients with PM or DM are myocarditis and coronary artery disease, as well as involvement of the small vessels of the myocardium.

Examination with ECG is recommended in newly diagnosed patients with PM or DM. Serum tests such as CK-MB to detect cardiac involvement are unreliable in patients with inflammatory myopathies because CK-MB can be released from regenerating skeletal muscle fibers, a common feature in biopsies from patients with PM or DM. The CK-MB/total CK ratio may be greater than 3%, a threshold value that is used to define myocardial damage. A more specific marker for myocardial damage in myositis patients is increased serum levels of cardiac isoform troponin I. The other cardiac troponin isoforms, troponin C and troponin T, are less specific and are also expressed in adult skeletal muscle; increased serum levels have been reported in various muscle disorders.

Gastrointestinal Tract

Difficulty swallowing is frequent in patients with inflammatory myopathies, particularly those with IBM. Muscle weakness occasionally becomes severe and causes problems with nutrition and aspiration pneumonia. The pathophysiology is related to weakness in the tongue, pharyngeal muscles, and sometimes the lower esophagus. Reflux that requires special care is common, occurring in 15% to 50% of patients. Constipation, diarrhea, and stomach pain are common symptoms and may result from disturbed motility of the gut or GI tract inflammation. Vasculitis in the blood vessels of the GI tract is rare but may be complicated by intestinal bleeding.

Antisynthetase Syndrome

A new classification system is based on the presence of MSAs, rather than clinical and histopathologic changes. The most common of these antibodies are the antisynthetase autoantibodies directed against aminoacyl-tRNA synthetases. A clinically distinct subset of myositis, often called *antisynthetase syndrome*, has been identified in patients with antisynthetase autoantibodies.[42,63] The most common of the antisynthetase autoantibodies is anti–Jo-1, which is directed against histidyl-tRNA synthetase. This autoantibody is present in approximately 20% of patients with PM or DM but is only rarely found in patients with IBM.[79] Antisynthetase syndrome is characterized by the presence of antisynthetase autoantibodies and a set of clinical features that includes myositis, interstitial lung disease, Raynaud's phenomenon, nonerosive symmetric polyarthritis of the small joints, and mechanic's hands (see Figure 85-9). These patients often have fever at disease onset and during flares of disease. Antisynthetase syndrome can be seen in patients with PM or DM but is more often seen in patients without skin rashes other than mechanic's hands.

Amyopathic Dermatomyositis

A subset of DM is called clinically amyopathic DM. These patients have a skin rash, which is typical of DM, but no clinical signs of muscle involvement.[148] The proposed definition is based on a skin biopsy consistent with DM and a duration of 6 months or longer in the absence of clinical or laboratory evidence of myositis. Some of these patients do have subclinical myositis based on MRI or biopsy findings at presentation; others develop clinically overt myositis sometime later. Patients without clinically overt myositis, however, may develop extramuscular manifestations such as interstitial lung disease, which may be severe. Amyopathic DM may be associated with malignancies, as is the case for classic DM. The frequency of this subset is uncertain, but some recent studies suggest that this form of DM may be more common than previously thought.

Juvenile Dermatomyositis

The incidence of juvenile dermatomyositis (JDM) is between 1.7 and 3 per million children. The disease onset has two peaks—at age 6 and 11 years. JDM is more common in girls than in boys in Europe and North America; in Japan and Saudi Arabia, this difference is less prominent. The most common clinical manifestations at disease onset are muscle weakness, easy fatigability, skin rash, malaise, and in some cases fever.[146] The skin rash is often pathognomonic and similar to adult DM, with the most typical skin manifestation being heliotrope discoloration of the upper eyelids, Gottron's papules, periungual erythema, and capillary loop abnormalities. Calcinosis, cutaneous ulceration, and lipodystrophy are more common in juvenile cases than in adults. Calcinosis is seen in 30% to 70% of children with JDM. The calcinosis is most often located at sites exposed to trauma and can be seen in the skin, fascia, or muscles. In some children, the calcinosis becomes prominent and causes contractures and ulcerations. Lipodystrophy occasionally develops, and other metabolic abnormalities such as insulin resistance and hepatomegaly are sometimes seen. Vasculopathy that affects the GI tract with ulceration, perforation, or hemorrhage is rare but seems to be more common in children than in adults with DM. Because this can be a serious sign, screening for GI involvement should be included in the evaluation of patients with JDM. Interstitial lung disease is rarely seen in JDM cases.

The overall prognosis is variable, but some patients have a good prognosis. Patients with JDM may go into remission, allowing the discontinuation of immunosuppressive treatment. Side effects of immunosuppressive treatment such as growth failure are common. In many patients, however, the disease remains chronic, with persisting disease activity into adulthood.

Inclusion Body Myositis

IBM is distinguished from PM and DM on the basis of both clinical and histopathologic features.[149,150] Sporadic IBM is a distinct entity from familial hereditary inclusion body myopathy, which shares some clinical and histopathologic features but lacks signs of inflammation in muscle tissue.

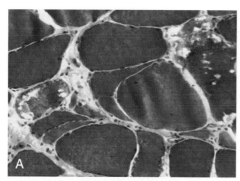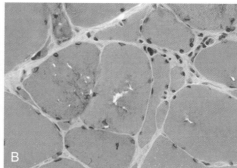

Figure 85-10 Trichrome and hematoxylin and eosin staining of inclusion body myositis biopsy. Note the red-rimmed inclusions (**A**) and marked variation in muscle fiber size (**A** and **B**). *(Courtesy Dr. Paul Plotz.)*

IBM was identified in the 1960s as a subset of inflammatory myopathies, distinct from PM, primarily on the basis of typical histopathologic features that include sarcoplasmic and nuclear inclusions and rimmed vacuoles.[16,17] A characteristic clinical phenotype was later identified, characterized by an insidious onset of muscle weakness over months to years, muscle weakness localized predominantly to the thigh muscles and finger flexors, and resistance to glucocorticoid treatment. IBM patients often have a history of frequent falling. Sporadic IBM cases are sometimes misdiagnosed as PM because the classic histopathologic changes (rimmed vacuoles and inclusions) may not be evident in early biopsies (Figure 85-10). A slowly progressive clinical course, development of severe muscle atrophy in the thighs and forearms, and resistance to treatment with immunosuppressive drugs should raise the suspicion of IBM, and a second muscle biopsy should be considered.

In contrast to PM and DM, IBM is more frequent in men than in women, and it is seen mainly in individuals older than 50 years. The onset is more insidious than that of PM or DM. Patients with IBM rarely have pain. The most frequent initial symptoms are difficulty climbing stairs and walking uphill and frequent falls as a result of weakness in the knee extensor muscles. Muscle weakness may become prominent, and even walking across a threshold may become a problem. Difficulty swallowing may also be an early clinical feature, reflecting the involvement of the pharyngeal muscles. The course is slowly progressive, leading to muscle atrophy that can be striking, particularly in the thigh and forearm muscles. Severe weakness may develop, and many patients become wheelchair dependent. Extramuscular organ involvement is rare, although a subgroup of patients with IBM has sicca symptoms and may develop a secondary Sjögren's syndrome.[151] There are also occasional case reports of IBM in patients with other chronic inflammatory diseases such as SLE, systemic sclerosis, and interstitial pneumonitis. Autoantibodies are rarely present in IBM patients.

IBM is usually resistant to treatment with glucocorticoids and other immunosuppressive agents. Because of this resistance to treatment, some have questioned whether IBM is an autoimmune disease or a degenerative muscle disease supported by the abnormal accumulation of proteins such as amyloid-β in muscle fibers. This issue is still under debate and subject to ongoing research in several institutions around the world.

Myositis Associated with Malignancies

An association between DM and malignancies was observed in several early case reports. The clinical implications of this association, irrespective of the pathophysiologic mechanisms involved, are that it is imperative to screen for tumors in patients with DM at the time of diagnosis and at relapse, particularly if the symptoms do not respond to conventional immunosuppressive treatment. A myositis-specific autoantibody that is associated with DM and malignancies in adults, p155/140, has been identified, but its sensitivity and specificity in the context of myositis is not known.[151a,151b] However, so far this autoantibody can only be detected by immunoprecipitation, which limits its use in clinical practice. The types of malignancies vary and include not only hematologic malignancies such as lymphoma but also solid tumors such as lung, ovarian, breast, and colon cancer. The screening for malignancies should include, at minimum, a careful clinical examination, routine blood tests, and chest radiograph. For women, mammography and a gynecologic examination should be conducted as well. If any abnormalities are found, these should guide a more thorough investigation for malignancies.

CLASSIFICATION AND DIAGNOSTIC CRITERIA

At present, there are no prospectively validated diagnostic or classification criteria for myositis. Dividing diseases into homogeneous subsets serves several important functions including allowing us to estimate disease incidence and prevalence, understand disease pathogenesis and natural history, and evaluate the patient's response to therapy and prognosis. More than 3 decades ago, Bohan and Peter[14,15] proposed a set of five criteria to facilitate the diagnosis of IIM patients (Table 85-4). They classified IIMs into five groups: primary idiopathic PM, primary idiopathic DM, IIMs associated with malignancy, childhood IIMs associated with vasculitis, and IIMs associated with collagen vascular diseases. Exclusion criteria include signs of central or peripheral neurologic disease; family history of muscle disease (although familial myositis has been reported in dozens of cases); and symptoms and signs suggestive of muscular dystrophy, granulomatous myositis, infections (including trichinosis, schistosomiasis, trypanosomiasis,

Table 85-4 Bohan and Peter Criteria for Polymyositis and Dermatomyositis

Exclude all other myopathies
Symmetric proximal muscle weakness
Increase in serum muscle enzymes, such as CK, AST, ALT, aldolase, and LDH
Abnormal electromyographic findings, such as short, small, polyphasic motor units; fibrillations; positive sharp waves; insertional irritability; and bizarre high-frequency repetitive discharges
Abnormal muscle biopsy findingssuch as mononuclear infiltration, regeneration, degeneration, and necrosis
Skin rashes, such as heliotrope rash, Gottron's sign, and Gottron's papules

ALT, alanine transaminase; AST, aspartate transaminase; CK, creatine kinase; LDH, lactate dehydrogenase.

staphylococcal infection, and toxoplasmosis), drug-induced myopathy, toxic myopathy, rhabdomyolysis, metabolic disorders, endocrinopathies, myasthenia gravis, or myositis after viral infection (influenza or rubella). A weakness of the Bohan and Peter classification is that it overdiagnoses PM patients and loosely defines overlap syndromes.

Despite several drawbacks, these criteria have served well in diagnosing and defining patients for research purposes for the past 3 decades. IBM was later recognized as a separate disease entity characterized by a slow onset and progression involving finger flexors or the quadriceps muscles.[149,150] It can occur as a stand-alone entity or with other connective tissue diseases, and patients are often resistant to steroid therapy. Other focal and diffuse forms of myositis such as orbital myositis, focal nodular myositis, macrophagic myositis, and eosinophilic myositis are relatively rare.

Since Bohan and Peter proposed their classification criteria, advances in clinical research have led to the identification of certain autoantibodies that are strikingly associated with some clinical phenotypes of myositis (see Table 85-3). The identification of clinical features associated with MSAs and MAAs has led to the proposal of a serologic approach to complement the Bohan and Peter classification system. Others have suggested that the Bohan and Peter criteria be modified to add MSA as a criterion.[152] However, the inclusion of MSA has some limitations: these antibodies are not present in all patients, the immunoprecipitation techniques that are the "gold standard" for identifying these antibodies are available in only a few commercial laboratories, and the enzyme-linked immunosorbent assays often used can give false-positive or false-negative results.

Ongoing debate and dialogue within the scientific community about the nature of the diagnostic and classification criteria that could better define these disorders is extensive.[73,153,154] Some emphasize a focus on histopathologic features and others on autoantibody profiles. Certainly, the addition of autoantibody profiles, characteristic histopathologic and immunohistochemical features, and imaging techniques such as MRI would significantly strengthen the current criteria and better define these disorders. The most frequently used subclassification is based on differences in clinical, immunologic, and histopathologic features and identifies three subtypes of inflammatory myopathies: PM, DM, and IBM[155] (Table 85-5).

Table 85-5 Clinical and Laboratory Features of Idiopathic Inflammatory Myopathy Subgroups

Diagnostic Features	Dermatomyositis	Polymyositis	Inclusion Body Myositis
Clinical features			
Age	Children and adults	Adults[a]	Adults > 50 yr
Disease onset	Subacute	Subacute	Chronic
Muscle weakness	Proximal	Proximal	Selective pattern[b]
Symmetry	Symmetric	Symmetric	Asymmetric
Systemic features	Yes[c]	Yes[c]	Yes[d]
Skin changes	Yes[e]	No	No
Calcinosis	Yes[f]	Rarely	No
Associated connective tissue disease	Yes[g]	Yes[g]	Yes[h]
Associated malignancy[i]	Yes	Yes	Yes
Laboratory features			
Serum enzymes[j]	Normal to high	Normal to high	Normal to high
Abnormal EMG[k]	Yes	Yes	Yes
Abnormal muscle biopsy	Perifascicular atrophy, capillary depletion, patchy MHC class I expression and microinfarcts	CD8+ T cell invasion of non-necrotic fibers and MHC class I expression on fibers	CD8+ T cell invasion, MHC expression, vacuolated fibers, and tubulofilamentous inclusions in fibers

[a]Rarely in children.
[b]Early involvement of finger flexor, wrist flexor or wrist extensor weakness, and involvement of quadriceps femoris.
[c]Some patients have dysphagia, synovitis, and interstitial lung disease.
[d]Some patients have dysphagia.
[e]Gottron's sign and heliotrope rash.
[f]Especially in children.
[g]Overlap with scleroderma, systemic lupus erythematosus, rheumatoid arthritis, Sjögren's syndrome, and mixed connective tissue disease.
[h]Associated with Sjögren's syndrome but less frequently associated with other connective tissue diseases.
[i]Dermatomyositis is more frequently associated with cancer than are polymyositis and inclusion body myositis and not overrepresented in polymyositis or inclusion body myositis.
[j]Serum creatine kinase, aspartate transaminase, lactate dehydrogenase, and aldolase vary from normal to very high levels.
[k]Myopathic motor unit potentials with spontaneous discharges in dermatomyositis, with and without spontaneous discharges in polymyositis, and mixed pattern of short- and long-duration motor unit potentials in inclusion body myositis.
EMG, electromyogram; MHC, major histocompatibility complex.

PHYSICAL EXAMINATION

Although most patients present with muscle weakness or fatigue, the IIMs are systemic connective tissue diseases and other organs are frequently involved; therefore a full clinical examination should be conducted when patients present with muscle symptoms. This could also be helpful in distinguishing IIMs from noninflammatory myopathies.

The muscle problems reported by many patients consist of not only muscle weakness but also muscle fatigue or reduced muscle function. Thus the evaluation must differentiate between strength and fatigue by evaluating muscle strength and testing repetitive movements for muscle fatigue. In the early phases, atrophy is usually not a pronounced phenomenon in PM or DM. In later phases, a moderate symmetric atrophy of proximal muscles may be present. Asymmetric atrophies indicate conditions other than inflammatory myopathies. Patients with IBM often develop more severe atrophy of the quadriceps muscles and the flexor muscles of the forearms; they may also develop deformities in the finger joints and experience difficulty making fists.

Muscle strength can be tested in various ways. A quick screening test for weakness in proximal lower leg muscles is to ask the patient to stand up from a sitting or squatting position without support. A more standardized test that is easy to perform in the clinic is the manual muscle test, with grading according to the Medical Research Council (MRC) scale. There are many variants of this test, but a short form, addressing eight muscles on the dominant side, is recommended as part of the disease activity score by the International Myositis Assessment and Clinical Studies (IMACS).[156] In most patients with PM or DM, muscle strength as assessed by the manual muscle test is good in most of the tested muscle groups. Typically, moderate muscle weakness is seen in the neck flexors and hip girdle muscles. Testing that involves a number of repetitions is often a more sensitive method of detecting muscle impairment. The Functional Index in Myositis-2 is a myositis-specific outcome measure that assesses a number of repetitions. With this test, proximal muscle groups are more involved than are distal muscles. This index is often used by physical therapists.[157] In patients with IBM, knee extensors and finger flexors are often weak.

The skin should also be examined to detect changes including those in nail folds and the scalp. Joints can be affected by arthritis, and heart and lung changes should be carefully looked for.

LABORATORY EVALUATION

Laboratory evaluations are critical components of both diagnosis and patient management. Combinations of laboratory tests are generally used during patient evaluations. Because no laboratory test is highly specific for IIMs, the results of these tests are usually interpreted in the clinical context.

Biochemical

Measuring serum levels of muscle enzymes is an important part of the evaluation of myositis patients. Increased levels of muscle-derived serum enzymes reflect ongoing damage to the muscle parenchyma. These measurements help differentiate IIMs from conditions such as steroid myopathy and denervation, in which atrophy is a prominent feature.[158] Measurement of the serum CK level is traditionally the first step in the assessment of patients with IIM. CK exists as MM (skeletal muscle), MB (cardiac muscle), and BB (brain) isoforms in serum. In comparison with other serum muscle enzymes, CK appears to be a relatively specific and sensitive indicator of the degree of muscle fiber injury. However, the range varies significantly among patients, with levels being near normal in some patients and elevated by several hundred-fold in others.

Generally, 80% to 90% of adult myositis patients show an increase in CK during the initial evaluation. However, a certain proportion of patients, especially those in advanced stages of the disease, show normal or relatively modest elevations in CK, in part because of a lack of muscle mass or the presence of inhibitors of CK activity.[159,160] Normal CK is relatively more common in DM than in PM. In the absence of CK elevation, it is usually easier to diagnose DM than PM because of the presence of skin rashes in the former. It is also known that CK levels are generally lower in IBM patients than in those with PM or DM. Therefore a normal CK level does not exclude a diagnosis of IIM, particularly IBM or JDM.

Constantly elevated levels of CK are often a sign of inflammatory activity. A rise in CK level is generally correlated with overall disease activity over time, but not with strength or functional measures of disease activity.[161,162] CK measurements are usually not useful for monitoring disease exacerbations, and they should always be evaluated in the clinical context. CK levels may normalize without clinical improvement, or they may increase without clinical worsening; however, increasing levels point to a potential flare and warrant closer clinical evaluation. CK elevations are not specific for myositis because this enzyme is also elevated in other muscle diseases including muscular dystrophies, rhabdomyolysis, hypothyroidism, and many drug-induced myopathies. It is important to note that serum levels of CK-MB can be elevated in patients with myositis as a result of the regeneration of skeletal muscle fibers; they are not specific for heart involvement in these patients. The cardiac isoform troponin I has the highest specificity as an indicator of myocardial involvement and is the most reliable serum marker for detecting myocardial damage in patients with inflammatory muscle disease.[163]

Measurement of other serum muscle enzymes including aldolase, aspartate transaminase (AST), alanine transaminase (ALT), and lactate dehydrogenase (LDH) significantly improves the chance of diagnosing myositis, especially in patients with active disease and normal CK levels. Aldolase, LDH, and AST are better correlated with disease activity in JDM patients. The main disadvantage of these enzymes is that they are also elevated in liver diseases; therefore the muscle source needs to be identified before interpreting the data.[164]

The serum myoglobin level is a sensitive index of muscle fiber membrane integrity and can therefore be used to assess the degree of disease activity. The advantage of the myoglobin assay is that it involves a nonenzymatic immunologic reaction. Disadvantages are that a significant range of serum myoglobin levels occurs in myositis patients because of circadian variation,[165] and the test is less readily available than CK for routine use. Elevation of other serum components such as troponin, creatine, neopterin, manganese superoxide dismutase, hyaluronate, and soluble CD30 has been shown to correlate with disease activity, but assays of these components have not been validated for use in clinical practice and they are not available for routine analyses.

Immunologic

The immune response to self-antigens is a common feature of several systemic autoimmune rheumatic diseases including IIMs. ANAs are found in approximately 60% to 70% of myositis patients. The autoantibody response in IIMs is directed to ubiquitous nuclear and cytoplasmic antigens. The presence of these antibodies is usually assessed by an indirect immunofluorescence assay. ANAs are more frequently found in patients with PM and DM, especially those with overlap syndrome. These are less frequently seen in IBM patients or those with malignancy-associated myositis. High-titer ANA is a particularly valuable finding for differentiating IIMs from dystrophies. Many IIM patients show speckled nuclear ANA patterns, and about 10% of IIM patients also show exclusive cytoplasmic patterns in indirect immunofluorescence staining.[166] Many of the MSAs are associated with distinctive clinical features such as skin rash or interstitial lung disease (Table 85-6). Certain MSAs such as anti–Jo-1 are more frequently associated with PM; others such as Mi-2 are more frequent in DM.

Histologic

Muscle biopsy is the "gold standard" for the diagnosis of inflammatory myopathies and a critical component of the definitive diagnosis of IIMs.[167,168] For optimal biopsy results, it is important to select a muscle that is moderately weak. The histologic features can be grouped into general features that are common to all IIMs and specific features unique to a particular subgroup. The general features include necrosis,

regeneration, degeneration, variation in fiber diameter, increase in connective tissue, and inflammation. The features specific to DM include loss of capillaries, alterations in the morphology of capillaries, capillary necrosis with the deposition of complement products (e.g., membrane attack complex) on the vessel walls, and, rarely, muscle infarcts. Another specific histopathologic finding, albeit a late sign, is perifascicular atrophy. The infiltrates typically have a perivascular distribution. The inflammatory infiltrates are dominated by a high percentage of CD4 T cells and macrophages at the sites of inflammation, with B cells occasionally in evidence. Although perifascicular atrophy is the hallmark of the histologic changes seen in DM, it may not be visible if a biopsy is acquired early in the course of the disease. In early DM, the MHC class I expression is patchy and the perifascicular areas are usually stained.

The features of PM include the presence of macrophages and activated CD8+ T cells in muscle fibers and the expression of MHC class I molecules on muscle fibers. Mononuclear cell invasion around non-necrotic muscle fibers in endomysial areas is a characteristic feature of IIMs. The histologic features of IBM resemble those of PM but also include unique features such as red-rimmed vacuoles and inclusions (cytoplasmic or nuclear) and amyloid deposits.[150] An increased number of cytochrome-c oxidase–negative fibers can also be seen, but this change is not specific for IBM. In IBM, electron microscopy usually demonstrates 15- to 21-nm cytoplasmic and intranuclear tubulofilaments, which are not found in DM or PM. It is not uncommon to find biopsies that are negative for both rimmed vacuoles and tubulofilamentous inclusions. In this situation, if the suspicion for IBM is high, it is best to obtain another sample or to treat the patient with steroids. Nonresponsiveness to treatment further supports the diagnosis of IBM in an otherwise typical patient. Inflammation surrounding necrotic fibers is a feature of some muscular dystrophies (e.g., facioscapulohumeral muscular dystrophy, limb-girdle muscular dystrophy type IIB, Duchenne's muscular dystrophy), where it is secondary to muscle cell degeneration. Thus the presence of a mononuclear infiltration surrounding

Table 85-6 Immunologic Features of Idiopathic Inflammatory Myopathies

Feature	Dermatomyositis	Polymyositis	Inclusion Body Myositis
B cell infiltration	+	–/+	–/+
T cell infiltration	+	+	+
CD8+ T cell infiltration in non-necrotic fibers	–/+	+	+
Vascular membrane attack complex	+	–	–
Immunoglobulin deposition on blood vessels	+	–	–
Major histocompatibility complex class I expression on muscle fibers	–/+[a]	+	+
Cytokines and chemokines	+	+	+
Cell adhesion molecules	+	+	+
Antinuclear antibodies	+	+	+[b]
Anti–Jo 1 antibodies[c,d]	+	+	–/+
Anti–signal recognition particle antibodies[d]	–/+	+	–/+
Anti–Mi-2 antibodies[e]	+	–/+	–/+
Anti–PM-Scl antibodies[f]	+	+	–

[a]Mostly in perifascicular areas and necrotic fibers.
[b]Less frequently, but 20% higher than in normal population.
[c]Frequency varies among ethnicities; more frequent in polymyositis (22%) than dermatomyositis (16%) or inclusion body myositis (5%).
[d]Present only in a proportion of polymyositis (14%), dermatomyositis (5%), and inclusion body myositis (3%) patients.
[e]Present only in a proportion of polymyositis (9%), dermatomyositis (21%), and inclusion body myositis (8%) patients.
[f]Present only in a proportion of polymyositis (7%) and dermatomyositis (6%) patients.

Table 85-7 Histologic Features of Idiopathic Inflammatory Myopathies

Feature	Dermatomyositis	Polymyositis	Inclusion Body Myositis
Necrosis of muscle fibers	+	+	+
Variation in fiber diameter	+	+	+
Regeneration of muscle fibers	+	+	+
Proliferation of connective tissue	+	+	+
Infiltration of mononuclear cells*	+	+	+
Perivascular and perimysial inflammation	+	–/+	–/+
Endomysial inflammation	–/+	+	+
Perifascicular atrophy	+	–	–
Abnormally dilated capillaries	+	–/+	–
Reduced capillary density	+	–/+	–
Deposition of complement on vessel walls	+	–/+	–
Microinfarcts	+	–	–
Invasion of non-necrotic fibers by cytotoxic T lymphocytes and macrophages	–	+	+
Expression of major histocompatibility complex class I on muscle fibers	–/+	+	+
Rimmed vacuoles with amyloid deposits and tubulofilaments†	–	–	+
Angulated or atrophic and hypertrophic fibers	–	–	+
Ragged red or cytochrome oxidase–negative fibers	–	–	+

*Inflammation is absent in a small proportion of polymyositis and dermatomyositis biopsies.
†Also seen in chronic neurogenic conditions and distal myopathies.

non-necrotic muscle fibers confirms the diagnosis of IBM or PM. The common and unique immunologic and histologic features of the various subgroups are listed in Tables 85-6 and 85-7, respectively.

Molecular

One of the more tangible deliverables of the human genome product has been the development and use of microarrays for messenger RNA (mRNA) profiling. In the commonly used form of microarray, about 1 million DNA probes are placed on 1 cm² glass slides, allowing the query of each gene of the genome. Although all genes are shared among all cells, only certain genes are expressed (turned on) in any specific cell at any specific time. Messenger RNA expression profiling using microarrays allows genome-wide assessment of the response of each gene, with a comparison of normal and pathologic states.

Muscle is routinely biopsied as part of the clinical workup of muscle disease, and muscle histopathology is an important part of the diagnosis of inflammatory myopathies. Diagnostic muscle biopsies have been used for mRNA expression profiling in a series of studies, with comparisons between inflammatory myopathies (JDM, PM, IBM) and dystrophic myopathies (Duchenne's muscular dystrophy).[169,170] These comparisons are important because they differentiate between inflammation associated with downstream myofiber degeneration or regeneration (dystrophies) and inflammatory processes that may initiate the inflammatory myopathies.

Microarrays have provided considerable new insights into DM. Early on, mRNA profiling in DM showed a predominance of type I IFN-responsive pathways, suggesting the possible persistence of an antiviral response.[169] Particularly prevalent was the dramatic expression of the IFN-inducible MxA gene. This signature was confirmed and extended,[171] supporting an important role of the innate immune response, with prominent plasmacytoid dendritic cell infiltration in DM compared with the other inflammatory myopathies. The beneficial effect of intravenous immunoglobulin (IVIG) in DM has been queried by microarrays to define the drug-responsive genes, then compared with the lack of response in IBM.[172] This study suggested that IVIG suppressed a relatively small subset of inflammatory responses in DM muscle including complement (C1q) and inflammatory cell migration proteins (ICAM-1). Microarrays have helped elucidate an unexpectedly important role for innate immunity in DM. They have also provided new insights into the humoral immunity in PM and IBM. Specifically, mRNA expression profiling showed a high proportion of immunoglobulin transcripts as differentially expressed (59% of all detected genes in IBM and 33% in PM).[173] Plasma cells, defined as those terminally differentiated B cells expressing CD138 but not CD19 or CD20, were then shown to be a key differentiating cell type within IBM and PM muscle.

IMAGING

Muscles

Ultrasonograophy, CT, and MRI are the three general imaging techniques used to evaluate skeletal muscle. MRI has emerged as the method of choice for the examination of soft tissue muscle abnormalities because it efficiently visualizes and quantifies inflammation, fat infiltration, calcification, and alterations in muscle size and localizes pathologic changes in specific muscle groups (Figure 85-11). MRI examinations can be done on large volumes and can be helpful guides for muscle biopsy sampling. MRI is a potential outcome tool to be used in the longitudinal analysis of responses to therapy and in clinical trials, although its sensitivity to changes has not been validated.[174-177]

Ultrasonography is useful for detecting abnormal vascularization, and rates of blood flow can be monitored effectively with color Doppler imaging. The main disadvantage of ultrasonography is its inability to visualize deep-seated muscles in cross-section. Moreover, image analyses are more subjective than with MRI and depend to a greater degree

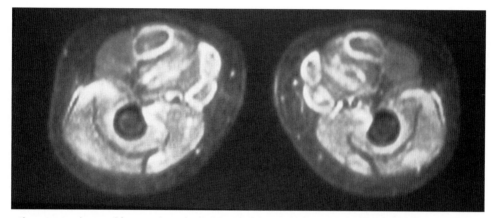

Figure 85-11 Magnetic resonance images (short tau inversion recovery) of the thigh. Note the symmetric inflammation in the affected muscle, seen as bright areas relative to unaffected muscle.

on the experience of the examiner.[178] Ultrasound muscle examinations are much more frequent in countries where physicians are responsible for performing such examinations and maintaining uniform standards for their evaluation. Ultrasonography provides a safe, noninvasive, easily portable, and relatively inexpensive approach to the evaluation of muscle abnormalities.[179]

CT is the modality of choice for identifying calcifications in soft tissues (e.g., JDM), but it is not useful for detecting inflammatory changes in muscle tissue. Cross-sectional CT images allow quantification of muscle atrophy and fat replacement in deep muscles that may not be generally accessible to ultrasonography. A combination of MRI and P-31 magnetic resonance spectroscopy examinations produces the most comprehensive and accurate evaluation of patients.[174]

Lungs

Radiography and high-resolution CT of the lungs are important for detecting lung involvement and should be considered at the time of myositis diagnosis because the prevalence of interstitial lung disease is high. In contrast, conventional radiography may not always be sensitive enough to detect interstitial lung disease. These are also important tests for assessing the effects of immunosuppressive treatment.

ELECTROMYOGRAPHY

Electromyogram (EMG) changes are usually nonspecific but are a useful indicator of myopathic changes. The major abnormalities include abnormal electrical irritability, decrease in the mean duration of motor unit potentials or increase in the percentage of polyphasic motor unit potentials (short duration), and rapid firing of the motor unit potentials in relation to the level of activity. Later in the course of the disease, fibers are lost from some motor units and recruitment is reduced. Abnormal electrical irritability in DM and PM involves increased insertional activity, trains of positive sharp waves, and fibrillation potentials. Spontaneous electrical activity is a reasonable measure of disease activity in DM and PM. EMG abnormalities correlate with alterations in muscle strength and serum muscle enzymes[180]

and are a useful measure when serum levels and muscle strength are uninterpretable. The inflammation in IIMs is often patchy, and EMG is useful in determining which muscle should be sampled for biopsy. Because EMG can cause histopathologic changes that complicate the interpretation of the biopsy, it is best to perform EMG on one side and obtain the muscle biopsy from the same muscle on the contralateral side. Even for IBM, in which the disease is often asymmetric, this technique is useful as long as the contralateral muscle is also weak.

LUNG FUNCTION TESTS

Pulmonary function tests are an important means of obtaining an objective assessment of respiratory involvement. Typically, patients demonstrate a restrictive ventilatory impairment, with decreased total lung capacity, functional residual capacity, residual volume, forced expiratory volume in 1 second (FEV_1), and forced vital capacity (FVC), but with a normal or elevated FEV_1/FVC ratio and reduced diffusing capacity for carbon monoxide. Pulmonary function tests are also important in estimating disease severity and response to therapy, in concert with radiographic examination.

DIFFERENTIAL DIAGNOSIS

The differential diagnosis of IIMs and other myopathies is important because the clinical associations and response to therapeutic interventions differ significantly. A variety of myopathies closely mimic IIMs (Table 85-8).

Dystrophic Myopathies

Dysferlinopathy

Genetic defects in the dysferlin gene result in limb-girdle muscular dystrophy type 2B and distal muscular dystrophy of the Miyoshi type. These diseases can appear in the late teens or early 20s, and the weakness in the limb-girdle type 2B phenotype first assumes a pelvifemoral distribution: the quadriceps muscle is affected first, followed by weakness in the arms in the later stages of the disease. A relatively acute

Table 85-8 Differential Diagnosis of Inflammatory Myopathies

Disease	Key Diagnostic Features	Disease	Key Diagnostic Features
Dystrophic Myopathies		**Infectious Myopathies**	
Dysferlinopathy (Miyoshi myopathy and LGMD2B)	Mutations in dysferlin gene Progressive proximal (LGMD2B) and distal (Miyoshi myopathy) muscle weakness Onset in late teens to early 20s Increased CK levels Inflammation in muscle biopsy Nonresponsiveness to steroids	HIV myopathy	Progressive myopathy Proximal symmetric muscle weakness Endomysial inflammation Increased serum CK levels
		Parasitic Myopathies	
Facioscapulohumeral muscular dystrophy	Partial deletion in D4Z4 repeats near chromosome 4q telomere at 4q35 Initial facial and shoulder girdle weakness progresses to pelvic girdle and extremities Normal serum CK levels or modest elevation	Protozoal myopathy	Clinical features of idiopathic inflammatory myopathies Focal or diffuse inflammation Myocarditis Increased serum CK levels
		Drug-Induced Myopathies	
Becker's dystrophy	Mutations in dystrophin gene X-linked recessive disorders Limb-girdle weakness and cardiomyopathy High serum CK levels	Zidovudine myopathy	Proximal muscle weakness Increased serum lactate levels Ragged red fibers and abnormal mitochondria in muscle Improves with drug discontinuation
Proximal myotonic myopathy	CCTG expansion in intron 1 of ZNF9 gene Autosomal dominant Proximal muscle weakness	Statin myopathy	Necrotizing myopathy Acute or subacute painful proximal myopathy Increased serum CK levels
Sarcoglycanopathy	Mutations in sarcoglycans (α, β, γ, and δ) Limb-girdle weakness and cardiomyopathy High serum CK levels	Corticosteroid myopathy	Proximal and distal weakness Type 2 atrophy and vacuolar changes in muscle Increased serum CK levels
Metabolic Myopathies		D-Penicillamine, interferon-α, and procainamide-induced myopathy	Proximal muscle weakness and pain Inflammation and necrosis in muscle Skin changes Increased serum CK levels
Acid maltase deficiency	Mutations in acid α-glucosidase Proximal muscle weakness Respiratory muscle involvement Abnormal irritability on EMG Increased serum CK levels	**Neuromuscular Diseases**	
McArdle's disease	Mutations in myophosphorylase gene Exercise intolerance Fixed proximal muscle weakness Increased serum CK levels	Motoneuron disease	Upper and lower motoneuron signs Asymmetric weakness with denervation atrophy Fasciculations and fatigability Fibrillations and enlarged motor unit potentials on EMG Modest elevation in serum CK levels
Mitochondrial Myopathies	Mutations in complex I-IV, complex V, and coenzyme Q10 genes Myopathy with limb-girdle weakness Exercise intolerance and fatigue Increased serum CK levels	Spinal muscular atrophy	Symmetric muscle weakness and atrophy Neurogenic changes on EMG and biopsy Normal serum CK levels
Endocrine Myopathies		Myasthenia gravis	Abnormal weakness and fatigability Decremental EMG response Antiacetylcholine receptor antibodies Positive anticholinesterase drug test
Cushing's syndrome	Insidious onset Proximal muscle weakness Normal serum CK, AST, and LDH levels		
Thyrotoxic myopathy	Subacute onset of proximal muscle weakness Normal serum CK levels or modest elevation Respiratory muscle weakness		

AST, aspartate transaminase; CK, creatine kinase; EMG, electromyogram; HIV, human immunodeficiency virus; LDH, lactate dehydrogenase; LGMD, limb-girdle muscular dystrophy.

onset with elevated levels of serum muscle enzymes points to PM as a differential diagnosis. The weakness in the Miyoshi phenotype occurs predominantly in the gastrocnemius and soleus muscles, thereby affecting the ability to walk on the toes. The weakness is slowly progressive, with loss of ambulation generally occurring in the fourth decade, but earlier in some cases. Serum CK levels are high during the active phase of the disease. In general, the muscle biopsy is dystrophic, with significant mononuclear cell infiltration and small sarcolemmal defects with thickened basal lamina structures over the defects.[181]

Facioscapulohumeral Muscular Dystrophy

A partial deletion of the D4Z4 repeats near the chromosome 4q telomere at 4q35 leads to the facioscapulohumeral phenotype. The initial weakness usually affects the facial muscles, and the onset is insidious. Shoulder weakness is commonly seen because of the weakness of the scapular fixator muscles. The weakness is generally slowly progressive, with typical myopathic changes on the EMG such as brief, small-amplitude, polyphonic voluntary motor unit potentials. The presence of perivascular, endomysial, and perimysial inflammation is a common feature.[182] Serum CK levels are elevated and vary with age and sex.

Dystrophinopathies

These X-linked recessive disorders are caused by mutations in the dystrophin gene. Milder forms of Becker's muscular dystrophy manifest as myalgias, muscle cramps, exercise intolerance, mild limb-girdle weakness, and quadriceps myopathy. The severe Becker's phenotype that presents before age 8 years is indistinguishable from the Duchenne's phenotype. An elevation in serum CK levels is seen in asymptomatic patients. The mean age at loss of ambulation is usually in the fourth decade. Histologic features include variation in fiber size, central nuclei, regeneration, necrosis, hypercontracted fibers, and endomysial fibrosis. In Becker's dystrophy the number of necrotic and regenerating fibers is decreased compared with the Duchenne phenotype, and the incidence of hypercontracted and central nuclei increases with age.[183] A plasma membrane defect in non-necrotic fibers and endomysial inflammation with macrophage, T cell, mast cell, and eosinophil infiltration are also characteristic features of this disease.

Proximal Myotonic Myopathy

CCTG expansion in intron 1 of the zinc finger transcription factor (ZNF9) gene results in type II myotonic dystrophy. The myotonia is usually absent or minimal but is detectable by EMG. The weakness is mainly proximal, with minimal or no facial involvement. Smooth muscle, cardiac, and diaphragmatic involvement is common in this disease. First-degree heart block is the most common abnormality, and sudden death is well documented.[184] Muscle biopsies show nonspecific features such as central nuclei, sarcoplasmic masses, and atrophy of type I fibers.

Sarcoglycanopathy

Mutations in sarcoglycans (α, β, γ, and δ) result in limb-girdle muscular dystrophy types IIC to IIF. Sarcoglycanopathies often start in childhood, with a median age of onset of 6 to 8 years. These diseases present initially as pelvic muscle weakness including a waddling gait and difficulty performing common tasks such as getting up from the floor, climbing the stairs, and running. The trunk muscles are prominently affected, and upper extremity involvement usually follows lower extremity involvement. Distal muscles are generally spared until later in the disease process.[185] These progressive disorders result in high levels of serum CK early in the disease; the levels decrease when patients become wheelchair bound by 12 to 16 years of age. Dilated cardiomyopathy is often seen in these disorders, and muscle biopsies show marked regeneration and necrosis.

Neuromuscular Disorders

Motoneuron Diseases

These diseases including amyotrophic lateral sclerosis (ALS) are progressive, degenerative disorders of motoneurons in the spinal cord, brain stem, and cerebral motor cortex that manifest clinically as amyotrophy and exaggerated reflexes. These diseases are characterized by a selective loss of function of upper or lower motoneurons, finally leading to a progressive loss of both types of motoneurons over time. EMG shows fibrillation and fasciculation potentials in the muscles of the lower and upper limbs or in the bulbar muscles. Muscle biopsies show the presence of denervation atrophy and secondary myopathic changes in chronically denervated muscles. IBM is the primary muscle disorder most likely to be confused with ALS, and muscle biopsy helps differentiate the two. Serum CK levels are slightly elevated, particularly in the early stages of the disease and in men who are physically active.

Spinal Muscular Atrophy

Late-onset forms of spinal muscular atrophy (SMA) are characterized by progressive muscle weakness and atrophy and reduced tendon reflexes. EMG and muscle testing reveal neurogenic changes in the muscle. Typical muscle biopsy findings include small and large groups of atrophic fibers in the chronic and severe forms of SMA, respectively. Histochemical changes show fiber type grouping, indicating reinnervation. Serum CK levels are slightly increased in juvenile-onset cases and normal in other forms of SMA. EMG shows abnormal spontaneous electrical activity (fibrillations, positive sharp waves, fasciculations), suggesting ongoing denervation.

Myasthenia Gravis

The clinical manifestations of myasthenia gravis include abnormal weakness that is worsened by repeated or sustained exertion and fatigability. Proximal muscles are usually more severely affected than distal muscles. This is a generalized disease that exhibits external ocular muscle involvement, positive anticholinesterase drug tests, and a decremental EMG response. Patients are often positive for antiacetylcholine receptor antibodies.

Metabolic Myopathies

Acid Maltase Deficiency

This autosomal recessive glycogen storage disease is caused by acid maltase gene mutations. The disease has infantile, childhood, and adult variants. The infantile form manifests in the first few months after birth as rapidly progressive weakness and hypotonia, with death occurring as a result of cardiorespiratory failure. The childhood form manifests as a myopathy in which the weakness is usually greater in the proximal than in the distal muscles; the disease progresses relatively slowly, and patients die of respiratory failure. The adult form presents in the 20s as a progressive myopathy that resembles PM or limb-girdle muscular dystrophy, with additional respiratory symptoms. Serum muscle enzymes (CK, AST, and LDH) are increased in all three forms of the disease, and EMG indicates myopathy in all three cases. Histologic examination reveals a vacuolar myopathy, with the vacuoles displaying a high glycogen content and strongly positive staining for acid phosphatase; necrotic and regenerating fibers are uncommon.

McArdle's Disease

McArdle's disease is the most common of the nonlysosomal muscle glycogenoses. Exercise intolerance is the characteristic feature of this disease, and it often manifests as early fatigue, myalgia, and stiffness of exercising muscle that is relieved by resting. The EMG is normal in some patients; it shows nonspecific myopathic changes in others. Forearm ischemic exercise testing shows virtually no increase in venous lactate in most patients. Serum CK levels, however, are variably elevated in these patients. Muscle biopsies show subsarcolemmal deposits of glycogen at the periphery of the fibers.

Mitochondrial Myopathies

Mitochondrial diseases are heterogeneous and often present a diagnostic challenge. It has been suggested that myopathy is due to mutations in mitochondrial DNA in the skeletal muscle.[186] The clinical course of the pure myopathy varies from rapidly progressive to almost reversible disease, with disease onset occurring from infancy through adulthood. The weakness is facioscapulohumeral and more proximal than distal, with involvement of the orbicularis and extraocular muscles. Patients often complain of exercise intolerance and fatigue and have recurrent episodes of myoglobinuria. Muscle biopsy plays a critical role in the diagnosis of these conditions, especially the use of special histochemical stains that detect succinate dehydrogenase, Cox staining, and Gomori trichrome staining.

Endocrine Myopathies

Cushing's Syndrome

Cushing's syndrome is an endogenous glucocorticoid excess disease that manifests as muscle weakness and wasting. Chronic corticosteroid treatment results in similar manifestations and significant loss of strength within a few weeks of treatment. Muscle biopsy shows increased vacuolations and glycogen accumulation in type II muscle. The onset of weakness is usually insidious. The weakness is primarily proximal, with more severe involvement in the legs than in the arms. These patients generally show normal serum muscle enzyme levels (CK, AST, and LDH). Muscle wasting can often be reversed if the glucocorticoid levels are returned to the normal range.

Hyperthyroid and Hypothyroid Myopathy

Myopathic thyroid disease is characterized primarily by proximal muscle weakness and muscle wasting. When distal weakness occurs, it often follows proximal myopathy. Exercise intolerance, fatigue, and breathlessness are common complaints, and weakness of the respiratory muscles results in respiratory insufficiency and the need for ventilatory support. Patients often have difficulty rising from a sitting position or lifting their arms above their heads. Serum muscle enzymes (CK, AST, and ALT) are often normal or low in hyperthyroidism and elevated in hypothyroidism. EMG findings are variable, with short-duration motor unit potentials and increased polyphasic potentials in proximal muscles; fibrillations and fasciculations are uncommon. Muscle biopsy shows atrophy in fiber types, nerve terminal damage, fatty infiltration, and isolated fiber necrosis, with macrophage and lymphocyte infiltration.

Infectious Myopathies

Human Immunodeficiency Virus Myopathy

Neuromuscular manifestations are common in human immunodeficiency virus (HIV)–induced myopathy. The clinical features typically include a myopathy of subacute onset that progresses slowly. The myopathy often starts as proximal symmetric muscle weakness with or without muscle wasting, similar to that in IIMs. Histologic features include muscle fiber necrosis, inflammation, and vacuolated muscle fibers, with a significant increase in serum CK levels. EMG shows spontaneous activity, with fibrillation potentials, positive sharp waves, and brief, low-amplitude polyphasic motor unit potentials.

HTLV-1 Myopathy

Myositis associated with human T-lymphotropic virus I (HTLV-I) has been noted in certain areas of the world (e.g., Japan, Jamaica). In these patients, symptoms of PM and IBM occur either alone or in combination with tropical spastic paraparesis.[187] Typical features include weakness and increases in serum CK levels. Histologic findings include interstitial inflammation, muscle fiber necrosis in PM and endomysial inflammation, vacuoles, amyloid deposits, and tubulofilaments in IBM.

Parasitic Myopathies

Diseases caused by various parasites—protozoa (e.g., toxoplasmosis, trypanosomiasis, sarcocystosis, malaria), cestodes (e.g., cysticercosis, echinococcosis, coenurosis, sparganosis), and nematodes (trichinellosis, taxocariasis, racunculiasis)—can cause myositis. The clinical features include nonspecific complaints such as myalgia and focal swelling, as well as typical features of PM and DM. Each parasitic infection shows typical changes on muscle biopsy (e.g., the presence of tachyzoites and toxoplasma cysts along with perimysial and endomysial inflammation). A combination of muscle biopsy and serologic findings is useful in making a diagnosis.

Drug-Induced Myopathies

Drugs can induce myopathic changes either by acting directly on the muscle or by indirectly influencing various factors required for muscle cell survival and growth.

Zidovudine Myopathy

Nucleoside analogues such as zidovudine are used to treat HIV because they act as false substrates for the viral reverse transcriptase. These drugs also cause myalgias, proximal muscle weakness, and fatigue and are sometimes associated with increased levels of serum CK. EMG shows typical myopathic changes. Histologically, muscle fibers show ragged red fibers; atrophic fibers show marked sarcoplasmic changes, with rod-body formation. Pronounced abnormalities in mitochondria, myofilaments, and tubules are also noted by electron microscopy. It has been suggested that these drugs also inhibit mitochondrial DNA polymerase, thus producing the mitochondrial abnormalities. Discontinuation of therapy improves muscle strength and function. In these patients, zidovudine-induced mitochondrial myopathy may coexist along with HIV-induced T cell–mediated inflammatory myopathy.[188]

Statin Myopathy

Statins are lipid-lowering drugs (e.g., lovastatin, simvastatin) that are known to cause necrotizing myopathy. These HMG-CoA reductase inhibitors generally suppress specific cholesterol synthesis and lower plasma concentrations of low-density lipoprotein. The clinical features of this condition include myalgia, cramps, and acute and subacute painful proximal myopathy, with histologic features varying from mild, discrete, and unspecific to muscle fiber necrosis, mononuclear cell infiltration, and myophagocytosis and regeneration. A mild increase in serum CK levels is also noted. Other agents that are known to cause necrotizing myopathy include fibric acid derivatives (clofibrate, gemfibrozil); nicotinic acid; organophosphate poisoning; and ε-aminocaproic acid.

Other Drugs

D-penicillamine is known to induce clinical features reminiscent of DM; recovery usually occurs after withdrawal of the drug. Agents such as IFN-α that are used to treat viral hepatitis and certain malignant tumors are also known to induce clinical features that resemble PM. Amphiphilic drugs such as chloroquine, hydroxychloroquine, and amiodarone are also known to induce cytoplasmic vacuoles, necrosis, and longitudinal branching of muscle fibers.[189] Drugs that affect microtubules such as colchicines and vincristine also induce myopathic changes, with the appearance of characteristic autophagic vacuoles in muscle fibers.

MANAGEMENT AND OUTCOME

The recommended treatment for patients with PM or DM is based on a combination of pharmacologic therapy and physical exercise. The optimal pharmacologic treatment in PM and DM is unclear. Few controlled trials have been undertaken, so recommendations are based on clinical observations from case series. With these limitations in mind, a suggested outline of treatment for patients with PM or DM is depicted in Figure 85-12. In addition to providing treatment, it is important to give patients adequate information about their disease and its treatment. This educational component is best provided by a rheumatology team and patient support groups.

Pharmacologic Treatment

The initial pharmacologic treatment in PM and DM is high-dose glucocorticoids: 0.75 to 1 (up to 2) mg/kg body weight per day for 4 to 12 weeks. Most experts recommend that glucocorticoid treatment be combined with another immunosuppressive drug to reduce the side effects of the glucocorticoids and to boost the immunosuppressive effect. The most frequently used immunosuppressive agents are azathioprine and methotrexate. In the extension phase of one of the few double-blind, placebo-controlled trials that have been reported, the combination of azathioprine and glucocorticoids, as compared with prednisone alone, was associated with better functional ability and a lower requirement for prednisone after 1 and 3 years.[190,191] The recommended azathioprine dosage is 2 mg/kg per day. The dosing regimen for methotrexate is similar to that for rheumatoid arthritis—up to 25 mg weekly, although there have been reports of higher doses. Pulmonary involvement related to myositis does not seem to be a contraindication for methotrexate.

The combination of methotrexate and azathioprine proved to be successful in a few patients with refractory myositis in a prospective, randomized, open-label crossover study comparing two aggressive approaches. There are also newer reports that mycophenolate mofetil might be effective. In patients with interstitial lung disease, cyclophosphamide could be of value. There are also a few reports that cyclosporine A or tacrolimus can be beneficial in these cases.[192,193] In treatment-resistant DM, a high dose of IVIG was found to have a beneficial effect on muscle strength when compared with placebo; however, the therapeutic effect was temporary, and repeated infusions were required.[194] In patients with severe, rapidly progressive disease that might be life threatening, high-dose pulses of intravenous methylprednisolone have been reported to be beneficial. Pharmacologic treatment including tapering of the corticosteroid dose should be guided by clinical outcome measures. As discussed earlier, the most appropriate outcome measures are muscle endurance and muscle strength. Side effects of glucocorticoids in these high doses are frequent. Prophylaxis against osteoporosis is recommended with vitamin D and calcium and, when clinically indicated, bisphosphonates. Steroid myopathy is another possible consequence of glucocorticoid treatment that is particularly problematic in patients with inflammatory myopathies. There is no specific test to verify steroid myopathy, but in the absence of active clinical disease, steroid myopathy could contribute to muscle weakness. If steroid myopathy is suspected, tapering of the glucocorticoid dose with careful evaluation of the clinical response is recommended. Glucocorticoids may also cause hypokalemia, and if this is not corrected, it may be associated with muscle weakness and incorrectly interpreted as myositis activity.

The depletion of B cells has recently emerged as a new strategy in autoimmune diseases. One approach is to use rituximab (monoclonal antibody against CD20). There are

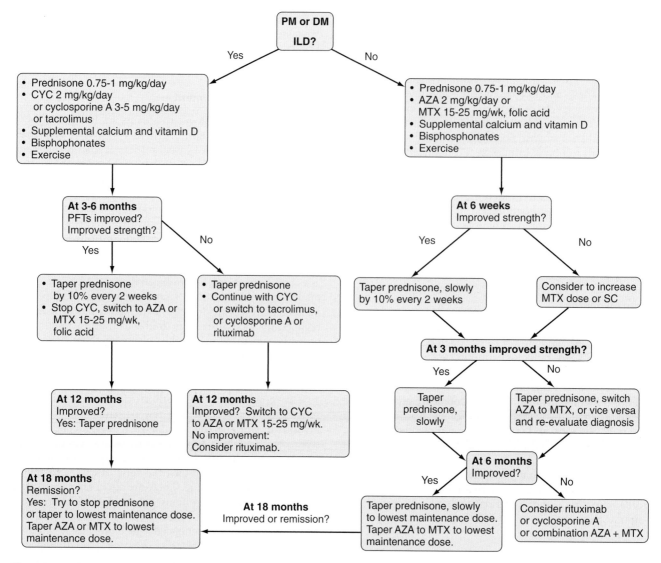

Figure 85-12 Treatment algorithm for adult patients with polymyositis (PM) or dermatomyositis (DM). AZA, azathioprine; CYC, cyclophosphamide; ILD, interstitial lung disease; MTX, methotrexate; PFT, pulmonary function test; SC, subcutaneous.

a few case series suggesting a beneficial effect of depleting B cells in patients with DM or PM.[195-197] A large international multicenter trial of B cell depletion is currently under way. Use of anti-TNF treatments produced mixed results. For example, treatment with infliximab at 3 mg/kg resulted in improved muscle function in patients with juvenile DM. However, interpretation of the data from this trial was complicated by the fact that all patients were concomitantly being treated with a tapering dose of prednisone during the trial.[198] A second, larger trial examining the use of infliximab in patients with PM, DM, or IBM found that only 30% of patients experienced an improvement in disease symptoms, while the remaining participants suffered from adverse side effects or worsening of the disease.[199]

IBM is usually nonresponsive to glucocorticoids. There are occasional case reports of "stabilization" for a period of months, but this condition probably reflects the natural history of the disease. Prolonged administration of glucocorticoids to IBM patients may actually lead to worsening of clinical aspects of the disease, despite the improvement in

CK levels and reduced T cell numbers in biopsies. Prednisone treatment also increases the number of amyloid-containing fibers.

A few small studies have shown some beneficial effect of methotrexate, anti–T lymphocyte globulin, or mycophenolate. Anabolic steroids and oxandrolone may have some beneficial effects on muscle strength, although this benefit needs to be confirmed in larger studies. Most experts consider their use justified in combination with glucocorticoids for a limited period in patients who have inflammatory infiltrates on muscle biopsy, or in combination with a more aggressive immunosuppressive treatment (e.g., methotrexate, azathioprine) in patients with another connective tissue disease.

Nonpharmacologic Treatment

With immunosuppressive treatment, approximately 75% of patients improve, but few recover normal muscle function, even in the absence of muscle inflammation. In previous decades, patients with myositis were cautioned against exercise due to concerns over possible muscle damage and inflammation, but recent publications have demonstrated that combining exercise and immunosuppressive therapy is a safe approach and has clear beneficial effects on muscle function.[200] In a pair of small studies of immunosuppressed myositis patients, it was demonstrated that personalized submaximal exercise programs improved muscle function without causing any increase in inflammation. This was true for patients who had individually tailored exercise regimens[201] and self-administered home exercise routines.[202] Examinations of patient biopsies both before and after exercise indicated that the patients showed improved muscle strength due to an increase in the proportion of slow twitch (type I) muscle fibers and reduction of inflammation and fibrosis.[202,203] Combining exercise and immunosuppressive therapy is a safe approach and has clear beneficial effects on muscle function.[198] The exercise regimen should be individualized and supervised by a physiotherapist to avoid the overuse of muscles. Physical exercise is now recommended as combination therapy with immunosuppressive treatment.

Assessing Disease Activity and Outcome

The most important variable to measure in myositis patients is muscle performance or physical function. However, it is equally important to evaluate whether impaired muscle function reflects disease activity or irreversible muscle damage.

Muscle Examination

Manual Muscle Test. There are several tools to measure muscle performance, but the most often used method in clinical practice and clinical trials is the manual muscle test with the MRC scale (see earlier). The drawback is that these tools measure muscle strength but not muscle endurance, which is often a major problem in PM or DM. Further, they have not been validated in adults with inflammatory myopathies. Previously, the number of muscle groups tested using the manual muscle test varied and different scales were used (5 or 10 grade). Recently, a consensus was reached to assess eight muscle groups on the dominant side using a 0- to 10-point scale, where 0 is no muscle contraction, 5 is ability to hold the test position without any added pressure, and 10 is ability to hold the test position against strong pressure. The points between these scores are based on gradual increased resistance against the examiner's pressure. The eight muscle groups tested are neck flexors, shoulder abduction (deltoid middle), biceps brachii, wrist extensors, knee extensors (quadriceps), dorsiflexion of ankle, gluteus maximus, and gluteus medius. The score achieved varies between 0 and 80.

Functional Index in Myositis. The Functional Index in Myositis and its revised form, the Functional Index in Myositis-2, were developed as outcome measures for patients with PM or DM. This test measures the number of repetitions that can be performed in defined muscle groups.[157,162] It is a more sensitive method of measuring impaired muscle function in patients with PM or DM.[157] The drawback is

that it takes a longer time to perform than the manual muscle test, and it may be difficult to use in everyday clinical practice. Preferably, the Functional Index in Myositis-2 is administered by a physiotherapist and can be combined with the manual muscle test.

Extramuscular Involvement

In some patients, extramuscular symptoms predominate among the clinical features. These symptoms may require other assessment tools such as those used to evaluate interstitial lung disease. For monitoring the effects of treatment of interstitial lung disease, high-resolution CT and pulmonary function tests are recommended.

Disease Activity and Damage

It is also important to distinguish whether symptoms are caused by active inflammatory disease or are a consequence of organ damage. IMACS, an international collaboration, made a consensus recommendation that outcome measures for patients with myositis include tools that measure disease activity, damage, and quality of life. The IMACS network developed one outcome measure to assess myositis disease activity and one to measure organ damage: the myositis disease activity assessment tool and the myositis damage index, respectively.[156] The disease activity outcome measure is a core set that consists of the six variables listed in Table 85-9. The damage index is recorded by the physician on the basis of the patient's history and covers several organ systems that can be affected in patients with inflammatory myopathies. To assess the impact on general health, the generic Short Form 36, a self-administered health-related quality of life questionnaire, is recommended. These outcome measures have been developed for clinical trials and research but can also be useful in clinical practice. More detailed information about these outcome measures can be found on the IMACS website: https://dir-apps.niehs.nih.gov/imacs.

IMACS has also reached a consensus on what constitutes improvement. Improvement is based on the disease activity core set and is defined as greater than 20% improvement in three of the six variables of the core set, with two or fewer of the variables (except the manual muscle test) worsening by less than 25%. However, this definition of improvement must be validated in longitudinal studies.

Table 85-9 Disease Activity Measure: Core Set

Physician's overall assessment of disease activity on a visual analogue scale (VAS)
Patient's or parent's overall assessment of disease activity (VAS)
Functional assessment (health assessment questionnaire)
Muscle strength testing (manual muscle test)
Serum levels of at least 2 of 4 muscle enzymes (CK, LDH, AST, ALT)
Extramuscular score (myositis disease activity assessment VAS [MYOACT] or myositis intention to treat activity index [MITAX]), in which disease activity in 7 organ systems (general symptoms, skin, joints, gastrointestinal tract, pulmonary, heart, and muscles) is scored

ALT, alanine transaminase; AST, aspartate transaminase; CK, creatine kinase; LDH, lactate dehydrogenase.

Selected References

14. Bohan A, Peter JB: Polymyositis and dermatomyositis (first of two parts), *N Engl J Med* 292:344–347, 1975.

15. Bohan A, Peter JB: Polymyositis and dermatomyositis (second of two parts), *N Engl J Med* 292:403–407, 1975.

16. Yunis E, Samaha F: Inclusion body myositis, *Lab Invest* 25:240–248, 1971.

17. Carpenter S, Karpati G, Heller I, Eisen A: Inclusion body myositis: a distinct variety of idiopathic inflammatory myopathy, *Neurology* 28:8–17, 1978.

18. Oddis C, Conte C, Steen V: Incidence of polymyositis-dermatomyositis: a 20 year study of hospital diagnosed cases in Allegheny County, PA 1963-1982, *J Rheumatol* 17:1329–1334, 1990.

19. Mastaglia FL, Phillips BA: Idiopathic inflammatory myopathies: Epidemiology, classification, and diagnostic criteria, *Rheum Dis Clin North Am* 28:723–741, 2002.

21. Patrick M, Buchbinder R, Jolley D, et al: Incidence of inflammatory myopathies in Victoria, Australia, and evidence of spatial clustering, *J Rheumatol* 26:1094–1100, 1999.

25. Badrising UA, Maat-Schieman M, van Duinen SG, et al: Epidemiology of inclusion body myositis in the Netherlands: a nationwide study, *Neurology* 55:1385–1387, 2000.

26. Amato A, Barohn R: Idiopathic inflammatory myopathies, *Neurol Clin* 15:615–648, 1997.

28. Andras C, Ponyi A, Constantin T, et al: Dermatomyositis and polymyositis associated with malignancy: a 21-year retrospective study, *J Rheumatol* 35(3):438–444, 2008.

30. Hill CL, Zhang Y, Sigurgeirsson B, et al: Frequency of specific cancer types in dermatomyositis and polymyositis: a population-based study, *Lancet* 357:96–100, 2001.

31. Buchbinder R, Forbes A, Hall S, et al: Incidence of malignant disease in biopsy-proven inflammatory myopathy: a population-based cohort study, *Ann Intern Med* 134:1087–1095, 2001.

34. Rider LG, Gurley RC, Pandey JP, et al: Clinical, serologic, and immunogenetic features of familial idiopathic inflammatory myopathy, *Arthritis Rheum* 41:710–719, 1998.

36. O'Hanlon TP, Carrick DM, Arnett FC, et al: Immunogenetic risk and protective factors for the idiopathic inflammatory myopathies: distinct HLA-A, -B, -Cw, -DRB1 and -DQA1 allelic profiles and motifs define clinicopathologic groups in caucasians, *Medicine (Baltimore)* 84:338–349, 2005.

38. O'Hanlon TP, Rider LG, Mamyrova G, et al: HLA polymorphisms in African Americans with idiopathic inflammatory myopathy: allelic profiles distinguish patients with different clinical phenotypes and myositis autoantibodies, *Arthritis Rheum* 54(11):3670–3681, 2006.

40. Badrising UA, Schreuder GM, Giphart MJ, et al: Associations with autoimmune disorders and HLA class I and II antigens in inclusion body myositis, *Neurology* 63:2396–2398, 2004.

41. Furuya T: Association of HLA class 1 and class 2 alleles with myositis in Japanese patients, *J Rheumatol* 25:1109–1114, 1998.

42. Love LA, Leff RL, Fraser DD, et al: A new approach to the classification of idiopathic inflammatory myopathy: myositis-specific autoantibodies define useful homogeneous patient groups, *Medicine (Baltimore)* 70:360–374, 1991.

43. Artlett CM, Cox LA, Jimenez SA: Detection of cellular microchimerism of male or female origin in systemic sclerosis patients by polymerase chain reaction analysis of HLA-Cw antigens, *Arthritis Rheum* 43:1062–1067, 2000.

44. Reed AM, Picornell YJ, Harwood A, Kredich DW: Chimerism in children with juvenile dermatomyositis, *Lancet* 356:2156–2157, 2000.

46. Travers RL, Hughes GR, Cambridge G, Sewell JR: Coxsackie B neutralisation titres in polymyositis/dermatomyositis, *Lancet* 1:1268, 1977.

48. Leff RL, Love LA, Miller FW, et al: Viruses in idiopathic inflammatory myopathies: absence of candidate viral genomes in muscle, *Lancet* 339:1192–1195, 1992.

49. Behan WM, Behan PO, Draper IT, Williams H: Does *Toxoplasma* cause polymyositis? Report of a case of polymyositis associated with toxoplasmosis and a critical review of the literature, *Acta Neuropathol (Berl)* 61:246–252, 1983.

52. Cossermelli W, Friedman H, Pastor EH, et al: Polymyositis in Chagas's disease, *Ann Rheum Dis* 37:277–280, 1978.

55. Andersson J, Nyberg P, Dahlstedt A, et al: CBA/J mice infected with *Trypanosoma cruzi* as an experimental model for human polymyositis, *Muscle Nerve* 27:442–448, 2003.

56. Okada S: Global surface ultraviolet radiation intensity may modulate the clinical and immunologic expression of autoimmune muscle disease, *Arthritis Rheum* 48:2285–2293, 2003.

57. Sigurgeirsson B, Lindelof B, Edhag O, Allander E: Risk of cancer in patients with dermatomyositis or polymyositis: a population-based study, *N Engl J Med* 326:363–367, 1992.

58. Casciola-Rosen L: Autoimmune myositis: new concepts for disease initiation and propagation, *Curr Opin Rheumatol* 17:699–700, 2005.

59. Casciola-Rosen L, Nagaraju K, Plotz P, et al: Enhanced autoantigen expression in regenerating muscle cells in idiopathic inflammatory myopathy, *J Exp Med* 201:591–601, 2005.

60. Rosen A, Casciola-Rosen L: Stem cells in inflammatory disease, *Curr Opin Rheumatol* 18:618–619, 2006.

61. Limaye VS, Lester S, Blumbergs P, Roberts-Thomson PJ: Idiopathic inflammatory myositis is associated with a high incidence of hypertension and diabetes mellitus, *Int J Rheum Dis* 13(2):132–137, 2010.

63. Love LA, Miller FW: Noninfectious environmental agents associated with myopathies, *Curr Opin Rheumatol* 5:712–718, 1993.

65. Sinzinger H, Schmid P, O'Grady J: Two different types of exercise-induced muscle pain without myopathy and CK-elevation during HMG-Co-enzyme-A-reductase inhibitor treatment, *Atherosclerosis* 143:459–460, 1999.

66. Argov Z: Drug-induced myopathies, *Curr Opin Neurol* 13:541–545, 2000.

67. Mammen AL, Chung T, Christopher-Stine L, et al: Autoantibodies against 3-hydroxy-3-methylglutaryl-coenzyme A reductase in patients with statin-associated autoimmune myopathy, *Arthritis Rheum* 63(3):713–721, 2011.

69. Klein R, Rosenbach M, Kim EJ, et al: Tumor necrosis factor inhibitor-associated dermatomyositis, *Arch Dermatol* 146(7):780–784, 2010.

70. Ishikawa Y, Yukawa N, Ohmura K, et al: Etanercept-induced anti-Jo-1-antibody-positive polymyositis in a patient with rheumatoid arthritis: a case report and review of the literature, *Clin Rheumatol* 29(5):563–566, 2010.

71. Gherardi RK, Coquet M, Cherin P, et al: Macrophagic myofasciitis lesions assess long-term persistence of vaccine-derived aluminium hydroxide in muscle, *Brain* 124:1821–1831, 2001.

72. Lyon MG, Bloch DA, Hollak B, Fries JF: Predisposing factors in polymyositis-dermatomyositis: results of a nationwide survey, *J Rheumatol* 16:1218–1224, 1989.

73. Dalakas MC, Hohlfeld R: Polymyositis and dermatomyositis, *Lancet* 362:971–982, 2003.

74. Lundberg IE: The physiology of inflammatory myopathies: an overview, *Acta Physiol Scand* 171:207–213, 2001.

75. Lundberg IE: New possibilities to achieve increased understanding of disease mechanisms in idiopathic inflammatory myopathies, *Curr Opin Rheumatol* 14:639–642, 2002.

76. Nagaraju K: Immunological capabilities of skeletal muscle cells, *Acta Physiol Scand* 171:215–223, 2001.

77. Nagaraju K: Update on immunopathogenesis in inflammatory myopathies, *Curr Opin Rheumatol* 13:461–468, 2001.

78. Nagaraju K, Casciola-Rosen L, Lundberg I, et al: Activation of the endoplasmic reticulum stress response in autoimmune myositis: potential role in muscle fiber damage and dysfunction, *Arthritis Rheum* 52:1824–1835, 2005.

80. Vazquez-Abad D, Rothfield NF: Sensitivity and specificity of anti-Jo-1 antibodies in autoimmune diseases with myositis, *Arthritis Rheum* 39:292–296, 1996.

81. Arnett FC, Targoff IN, Mimori T, et al: Interrelationship of major histocompatibility complex class II alleles and autoantibodies in four ethnic groups with various forms of myositis, *Arthritis Rheum* 39:1507–1518, 1996.

82. Mierau R, Dick T, Bartz-Bazzanella P, et al: Strong association of dermatomyositis-specific Mi-2 autoantibodies with a tryptophan at position 9 of the HLA-DR beta chain, *Arthritis Rheum* 39:868–876, 1996.

83. Targoff IN, Reichlin M: The association between Mi-2 antibodies and dermatomyositis, *Arthritis Rheum* 28:796–803, 1985.

84. Miller FW, Twitty SA, Biswas T, Plotz PH: Origin and regulation of a disease-specific autoantibody response: antigenic epitopes, spectrotype stability, and isotype restriction of anti-Jo-1 autoantibodies, *J Clin Invest* 85:468–475, 1990.

85. Oddis CV, Okano Y, Rudert WA, et al: Serum autoantibody to the nucleolar antigen PM-Scl: clinical and immunogenetic associations, *Arthritis Rheum* 35:1211–1217, 1992.

86. Blaszczyk M, Jablonska S, Szymanska-Jagiello W, et al: Childhood scleromyositis: an overlap syndrome associated with PM-Scl antibody, *Pediatr Dermatol* 8:1–8, 1991.

88. Cambridge G, Ovadia E, Isenberg DA, et al: Juvenile dermatomyositis: serial studies of circulating autoantibodies to a 56kD nuclear protein, *Clin Exp Rheumatol* 12:451–457, 1994.

89. Emslie-Smith AM, Engel AG: Microvascular changes in early and advanced dermatomyositis: a quantitative study, *Ann Neurol* 27:343–356, 1990.

90. Kissel JT, Mendell JR, Rammohan KW: Microvascular deposition of complement membrane attack complex in dermatomyositis, *N Engl J Med* 314:329–334, 1986.

91. Nagaraju K, Rider LG, Fan C, et al: Endothelial cell activation and neovascularization are prominent in dermatomyositis, *J Autoimmune Dis* 3:2, 2006.

92. Greenberg SA, Pinkus JL, Pinkus GS, et al: Interferon-alpha/beta-mediated innate immune mechanisms in dermatomyositis, *Ann Neurol* 57(5):664–678, 2005.

93. Salajegheh M, Kong SW, Pinkus JL, et al: Interferon-stimulated gene 15 (ISG15) conjugates proteins in dermatomyositis muscle with perifascicular atrophy, *Ann Neurol* 67(1):53–63, 2010.

94. Kissel JT, Halterman RK, Rammohan KW, Mendell JR: The relationship of complement-mediated microvasculopathy to the histologic features and clinical duration of disease in dermatomyositis, *Arch Neurol* 48:26–30, 1991.

95. Arahata K, Engel AG: Monoclonal antibody analysis of mononuclear cells in myopathies. III. Immunoelectron microscopy aspects of cell-mediated muscle fiber injury, *Ann Neurol* 19:112–125, 1986.

96. Goebels N, Michaelis D, Engelhardt M, et al: Differential expression of perforin in muscle-infiltrating T cells in polymyositis and dermatomyositis, *J Clin Invest* 97:2905–2910, 1996.

97. Mantegazza R, Andreetta F, Bernasconi P, et al: Analysis of T cell receptor repertoire of muscle-infiltrating T lymphocytes in polymyositis: Restricted V alpha/beta rearrangements may indicate antigen-driven selection, *J Clin Invest* 91:2880–2886, 1993.

98. Bender A, Ernst N, Iglesias A, et al: T cell receptor repertoire in polymyositis: clonal expansion of autoaggressive CD8+ T cells, *J Exp Med* 181:1863–1868, 1995.

99. Hohlfeld R, Engel AG: Coculture with autologous myotubes of cytotoxic T cells isolated from muscle in inflammatory myopathies, *Ann Neurol* 29:498–507, 1991.

100. Behrens L, Bender A, Johnson MA, Hohlfeld R: Cytotoxic mechanisms in inflammatory myopathies: co-expression of Fas and protective Bcl-2 in muscle fibres and inflammatory cells, *Brain* 120:929–938, 1997.

101. Nagaraju K, Casciola-Rosen L, Rosen A, et al: The inhibition of apoptosis in myositis and in normal muscle cells, *J Immunol* 164:5459–5465, 2000.

102. Li M, Dalakas MC: Expression of human IAP-like protein in skeletal muscle: a possible explanation for the rare incidence of muscle fiber apoptosis in T-cell mediated inflammatory myopathies, *J Neuroimmunol* 106:1–5, 2000.

103. Pandya JM, Fasth AE, Zong M, et al: Expanded T cell receptor Vbeta-restricted T cells from patients with sporadic inclusion body myositis are proinflammatory and cytotoxic CD28null T cells, *Arthritis Rheum* 62(11):3457–3466, 2010.

105. Waschbisch A, Schwab N, Ruck T, et al: FOXP3+ T regulatory cells in idiopathic inflammatory myopathies, *J Neuroimmunol* 225(1-2):137–142, 2010.

106. DeVere R, Bradley WG: Polymyositis: its presentation, morbidity and mortality, *Brain* 98:637–666, 1975.

107. Emslie-Smith AM, Arahata K, Engel AG: Major histocompatibility complex class I antigen expression, immunolocalization of interferon subtypes, and T cell-mediated cytotoxicity in myopathies, *Hum Pathol* 20:224–231, 1989.

108. Englund P, Nennesmo I, Klareskog L, Lundberg IE: Interleukin-1alpha expression in capillaries and major histocompatibility complex class I expression in type II muscle fibers from polymyositis and dermatomyositis patients: important pathogenic features independent of inflammatory cell clusters in muscle tissue, *Arthritis Rheum* 46:1044–1055, 2002.

109. Plotz PH, Dalakas M, Leff RL, et al: Current concepts in the idiopathic inflammatory myopathies: polymyositis, dermatomyositis, and related disorders, *Ann Intern Med* 111:143–157, 1989.

110. Adams E: A pilot study: use of fludarabine for refractory dermatomyositis and polymyositis, and examination of endpoint measures, *J Rheumatol* 26:352–360, 1999.

111. Nawata Y, Kurasawa K, Takabayashi K, et al: Corticosteroid resistant interstitial pneumonitis in dermatomyositis/polymyositis: prediction and treatment with cyclosporine, *J Rheumatol* 26:1527–1533, 1999.

112. Lundberg I, Kratz AK, Alexanderson H, Patarroyo M: Decreased expression of interleukin-1alpha, interleukin-1beta, and cell adhesion molecules in muscle tissue following corticosteroid treatment in patients with polymyositis and dermatomyositis, *Arthritis Rheum* 43:336–348, 2000.

113. Nyberg P, Wikman AL, Nennesmo I, Lundberg I: Increased expression of interleukin 1alpha and MHC class I in muscle tissue of patients with chronic, inactive polymyositis and dermatomyositis, *J Rheumatol* 27:940–948, 2000.

115. Nagaraju K, Raben N, Merritt G, et al: A variety of cytokines and immunologically relevant surface molecules are expressed by normal human skeletal muscle cells under proinflammatory stimuli, *Clin Exp Immunol* 113:407–414, 1998.

116. Hohlfeld R, Engel AG: HLA expression in myoblasts, *Neurology* 41:2015, 1991.

117. Karpati G, Pouliot Y, Carpenter S: Expression of immunoreactive major histocompatibility complex products in human skeletal muscles, *Ann Neurol* 23:64–72, 1988.

118. Nagaraju K, Raben N, Loeffler L, et al: Conditional up-regulation of MHC class I in skeletal muscle leads to self-sustaining autoimmune myositis and myositis-specific autoantibodies, *Proc Natl Acad Sci USA* 97:9209–9214, 2000.

119. Nagaraju K, Casciola-Rosen L, Lundberg I, et al: Activation of the endoplasmic reticulum stress response in autoimmune myositis: potential role in muscle fiber damage and dysfunction, *Arthritis Rheum* 52(6):1824–1835, 2005.

120. Li CK, Knopp P, Moncrieffe H, et al: Overexpression of MHC class I heavy chain protein in young skeletal muscle leads to severe myositis. Implications for juvenile myositis, *Am J Pathol* 175:1030–1040, 2009.

123. Bartoccioni E, Gallucci S, Scuderi F, et al: MHC class I, MHC class II and intercellular adhesion molecule-1 (ICAM-1) expression in inflammatory myopathies, *Clin Exp Immunol* 95:166–172, 1994.

124. Pavlath GK: Regulation of class I MHC expression in skeletal muscle: deleterious effect of aberrant expression on myogenesis, *J Neuroimmunol* 125:42–50, 2002.

125. Kaufman RJ: Stress signaling from the lumen of the endoplasmic reticulum: coordination of gene transcriptional and translational controls, *Genes Dev* 13:1211–1233, 1999.

126. Mori K: Tripartite management of unfolded proteins in the endoplasmic reticulum, *Cell* 101:451–454, 2000.

128. Nakagawa T, Zhu H, Morishima N, et al: Caspase-12 mediates endoplasmic-reticulum-specific apoptosis and cytotoxicity by amyloid-beta, *Nature* 403:98–103, 2000.

129. Vattemi G, Engel WK, McFerrin J, Askanas V: Endoplasmic reticulum stress and unfolded protein response in inclusion body myositis muscle, *Am J Pathol* 164:1–7, 2004.

130. Lundberg I, Brengman JM, Engel AG: Analysis of cytokine expression in muscle in inflammatory myopathies, Duchenne dystrophy, and non-weak controls, *J Neuroimmunol* 63:9–16, 1995.

131. Lundberg I, Ulfgren AK, Nyberg P, et al: Cytokine production in muscle tissue of patients with idiopathic inflammatory myopathies, *Arthritis Rheum* 40:865–874, 1997.

133. De Bleecker JL, Engel AG: Expression of cell adhesion molecules in inflammatory myopathies and Duchenne dystrophy, *J Neuropathol Exp Neurol* 53:369–376, 1994.

134. Nagaraju K, Raben N, Villalba ML, et al: Costimulatory markers in muscle of patients with idiopathic inflammatory myopathies and in cultured muscle cells, *Clin Immunol* 92:161–169, 1999.

135. Chevrel G, Granet C, Miossec P: Contribution of tumour necrosis factor alpha and interleukin (IL) 1beta to IL6 production, NF-kappaB nuclear translocation, and class I MHC expression in muscle cells: in vitro regulation with specific cytokine inhibitors, *Ann Rheum Dis* 64:1257–1262, 2005.

136. Monici MC, Aguennouz M, Mazzeo A, et al: Activation of nuclear factor-kappaB in inflammatory myopathies and Duchenne muscular dystrophy, *Neurology* 60:993–997, 2003.

137. Loell I, Lundberg IE: Can muscle regeneration fail in chronic inflammation: a weakness in inflammatory myopathies? *J Intern Med* 269(3):243–257, 2011.

139. Grundtman C, Bruton J, Yamada T, et al: Effects of HMGB1 on in vitro responses of isolated muscle fibers and functional aspects in skeletal muscles of idiopathic inflammatory myopathies, *FASEB J* 24(2):570–578, 2010.

140. Reid MB, Lannergren J, Westerblad H: Respiratory and limb muscle weakness induced by tumor necrosis factor-alpha: involvement of muscle myofilaments, *Am J Respir Crit Care Med* 166:479–484, 2002.

146. Ramanan AV, Feldman BM: Clinical features and outcomes of juvenile dermatomyositis and other childhood onset myositis syndromes, *Rheum Dis Clin North Am* 28:833–857, 2002.

147. Fathi M, Dastmalchi M, Rasmussen E, et al: Interstitial lung disease, a common manifestation of newly diagnosed polymyositis and dermatomyositis, *Ann Rheum Dis* 63:297–301, 2004.

153. Tanimoto K, Nakano K, Kano S, et al: Classification criteria for polymyositis and dermatomyositis, *J Rheumatol* 22:668–674, 1995.

154. Miller F, Rider L, Plotz P, et al: Diagnostic criteria for polymyositis and dermatomyositis, *Lancet* 362:1762–1763, 2003.

155. Dalakas M: Polymyositis, dermatomyositis and inclusion body myositis, *N Engl J Med* 325:1487–1498, 1991.

156. Miller FW, Rider LG, Chung YL, et al: Proposed preliminary core set measures for disease outcome assessment in adult and juvenile idiopathic inflammatory myopathies, *Rheumatology (Oxford)* 40:1262–1273, 2001.

157. Alexanderson H, Broman L, Tollback A, et al: Functional index-2: Validity and reliability of a disease-specific measure of impairment in patients with polymyositis and dermatomyositis, *Arthritis Rheum* 55:114–122, 2006.

158. Askari A, Vignos PJ Jr, Moskowitz RW: Steroid myopathy in connective tissue disease, *Am J Med* 61:485–492, 1976.

162. Josefson A, Romanus E, Carlsson J: A functional index in myositis, *J Rheumatol* 23:1380–1384, 1996.

166. Targoff IN: Update on myositis-specific and myositis-associated autoantibodies, *Curr Opin Rheumatol* 12:475–481, 2000.

167. Dalakas MC: Muscle biopsy findings in inflammatory myopathies, *Rheum Dis Clin North Am* 28:779–798, 2002.

170. Greenberg SA, Sanoudou D, Haslett JN, et al: Molecular profiles of inflammatory myopathies, *Neurology* 59:1170–1182, 2002.

171. Greenberg SA, Pinkus JL, Pinkus GS, et al: Interferon-alpha/beta-mediated innate immune mechanisms in dermatomyositis, *Ann Neurol* 57:664–678, 2005.

172. Raju R, Dalakas MC: Gene expression profile in the muscles of patients with inflammatory myopathies: effect of therapy with IVIG and biological validation of clinically relevant genes, *Brain* 128:1887–1896, 2005.

174. Park JH, Vital TL, Ryder NM, et al: Magnetic resonance imaging and P-31 magnetic resonance spectroscopy provide unique quantitative data useful in the longitudinal management of patients with dermatomyositis, *Arthritis Rheum* 37:736–746, 1994.

180. Sandstedt PE, Henriksson KG, Larrsson LE: Quantitative electromyography in polymyositis and dermatomyositis, *Acta Neurol Scand* 65:110–121, 1982.

198. Riley P, McCann LJ, Maillard SM, et al: Effectiveness of infliximab in the treatment of refractory juvenile dermatomyositis with calcinosis, *Rheumatology (Oxford)* 47(6):877–880, 2008.

199. Dastmalchi M, Grundtman C, Alexanderson H, et al: A high incidence of disease flares in an open pilot study of infliximab in patients with refractory inflammatory myopathies, *Ann Rheum Dis* 67(12):1670–1677, 2008.

201. Alexanderson H, Dastmalchi M, Esbjornsson-Liljedahl M, et al: Benefits of intensive resistance training in patients with chronic polymyositis or dermatomyositis, *Arthritis Rheum* 57(5):768–777, 2007.

202. Dastmalchi M, Alexanderson H, Loell I, et al: Effect of physical training on the proportion of slow-twitch type I muscle fibers, a novel nonimmune-mediated mechanism for muscle impairment in polymyositis or dermatomyositis, *Arthritis Rheum* 57(7):1303–1310, 2007.

203. Nader GA, Dastmalchi M, Alexanderson H, et al: A longitudinal, integrated, clinical, histological and mRNA profiling study of resistance exercise in myositis, *Mol Med* 16(11-12):455–464, 2010.

Full references for this chapter can be found on www.expertconsult.com.

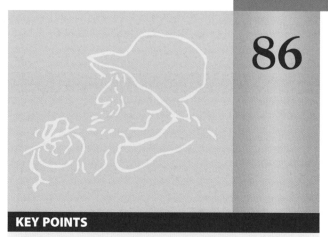

86 Overlap Syndromes

ROBERT BENNETT

The clustering of symptoms and signs into readily recognizable groupings has an important historic precedence in the classification of disease. With the progress of knowledge, such groupings may become more precisely defined in terms of distinctive pathology, specific laboratory findings, and genetic associations. According to current nosology, there are six autoimmune connective tissue diseases (AICTDs):

1. Systemic lupus erythematosus (SLE)
2. Scleroderma (Scl)
3. Polymyositis (PM)
4. Dermatomyositis (DM)
5. Rheumatoid arthritis (RA)
6. Sjögren's syndrome

All six classic AICTDs are descriptive syndromes without a "gold standard" for diagnosis. The diagnosis of a well-differentiated AICTD is usually readily apparent without recourse to extensive investigations. However, in the early stages, there are often common features such as Raynaud's phenomenon, arthralgias, myalgias, esophageal dysfunction, and positive tests for antinuclear antibodies (ANA). In such cases the diagnosis is not always so obvious; this is often referred to as undifferentiated connective tissue disease (UCTD).[1] About 35% of such patients have clinical overlap syndromes, whereas most differentiate into a clinical picture consistent with the traditional description of an AICTD. In some instances one AICTD evolves into another AICTD over time.

The propensity for differentiation into a classic AICTD or the maintenance of an overlap state is often associated with distinctive serologic profiles and major histocompatibility (MHC) linkages. Although most rheumatologists generally feel more comfortable thinking in terms of the classic AICTD paradigms, a case can be advanced for using serologic profiles and human leukocyte antigen (HLA) typing to better understand the clinical features and prognoses. In this respect a careful analysis of the overlap syndromes and their serologic associations has provided insights for understanding the clinical heterogeneity of the AICTDs.[2] Researchers have reported numerous clinical correlations of autoantibodies (Table 86-1).

EPIDEMIOLOGY

The reported prevalence of AICTDs is variable, depending on methodology, nature of referral bias, and ethnicity.[3] It is generally accepted that Sjögren's syndrome has the highest prevalence (0.5 to 3.6%), with SLE being much lower at about 15 to 50 per 100,000. Scleroderma, polymyositis, and dermatomyositis are relatively rare AICTDs, occurring in fewer than 10 per 100,000. Experts are increasingly realizing that overlap syndromes of scleroderma and myositis are more common than the "pure" forms of the disease.[4] There are no epidemiology studies of overlap syndromes, apart from Japan, where the reported prevalence of mixed connective tissue disease (MCTD) was 2.7 per 100,000. The syndrome of MCTD usually occurs as an isolated finding, but there are reports of a familial occurrence. Unlike SLE, precipitation by sun exposure has not been described in patients with MCTD. Likewise, drug exposure has not been related to the onset of MCTD, although a transient appearance of anti-RNP antibodies has been seen at the initiation

Table 86-1 Correlations of Autoantibodies with Clinical Features

Autoantigen	Clinical Associations
Rheumatoid factor	RA, erosive arthritis, cryoglobulinemia
Anticyclic citrullinated protein	RA
Nucleosome	SLE, Scl, MCTD
Proteasome	SLE, PM/DM, Sjögren's syndrome, multiple sclerosis
Sm snRNP	SLE
Histones H1, H2A, H2B, H3, H4	SLE, UCTD, RA, PBC, generalized morphea
Ribosomal P	SLE psychosis
dsDNA	SLE, glomerulonephritis, vasculitis
ACL/β_2-glycoprotein	SLE, thrombosis, thrombocytopenia, miscarriages
β_2-glycoprotein–independent ACL	MCTD (not associated with APL syndrome)
68-kD peptide of U1-RNP	MCTD, Raynaud's, pulmonary hypertension
U1 snRNP	MCTD, SLE, PM
hnRNP-A2 (also called RA-33)	MCTD, RA, erosive arthritis in SLE and Scl
Ro/La	Sjögren's, SLE, congenital heart block, photosensitivity, PBC
Fodrin	Sjögren's, glaucoma, moyamoya disease
Platelet-derived growth factor	Diffuse and limited Scl
Topoisomerase I (Scl-70)	Diffuse Scl with prominent organ involvement
Centromere	Limited Scl, CREST, Raynaud's, pulmonary hypertension, PBC
Th/To	Limited Scl
U3-snRNP	Limited Scl
hnRNP-I	Scl (early diffuse and limited)
RNA polymerases I and III	Scl (diffuse with renovascular hypertension)
Fibrillarin	Severe generalized Scl
Ku	Myositis overlap, primary pulmonary hypertension, Graves' disease
U5-snRNP	Myositis overlap
PM/Scl	Myositis overlap with arthritis, skin lesions, mechanic's hands
Signal recognition particle	Myositis overlap (severe course with cardiac disease)
Antisynthetases (Jo-1, PL-7, PL-12)	Myositis overlap with arthritis and interstitial lung disease
Mi-2	Dermatomyositis
Proteinase-3	Granulomatosis with polyangiitis (formerly Wegener's granulomatosis), pulmonary capillaritis
Myeloperoxidase	Churg-Straus, pauci-immune glomerulonephritis
Endothelial cell	Pulmonary hypertension, severe digital gangrene
α-Enolase	Behçet's, RA, MCTD, Scl, Takayasu's
Angiotensin-converting enzyme 2	AICTDs with vasculopathy

ACL, anticardiolipin; AICTDs, autoimmune connective tissue diseases; APL, antiphospholipid syndrome; CREST, syndrome of calcinosis, Raynaud's phenomenon, esophageal dysmotility, sclerodactyly, and telangiectasia; DM, dermatomyositis; hn, heterogeneous nuclear; MCTD, mixed connective tissue disease; PBC, primary biliary cirrhosis; PM, polymyositis; RA, rheumatoid arthritis; RNP, ribonucleoprotein particle; Scl, scleroderma; SLE, systemic lupus erythematosus; sn, small nuclear; UCTD, undifferentiated connective tissue disease.

of procainamide therapy.[5] Vinyl chloride and silica are the only environmental agents that have been associated with MCTD so far.

AUTOIMMUNITY IN OVERLAP SYNDROMES

Compelling evidence indicates that autoimmunity is often antigen driven by components of subcellular particles, in particular spliceosomes, nucleosomes, and proteasomes.[6]

Autoimmunity to Spliceosomal Components

Certain components of the spliceosome are common targets of autoimmunity in the AICTDs.[7] Furthermore, it appears that post-translational modifications of these molecules, as occurs during apoptosis, are often associated with increased immunogenicity.[8] Spliceosomes are complex nuclear particles made up of some 300 distinct proteins and 5 RNAs, which are involved in the processing of premessenger RNA (pre-mRNA) into mature "spliced RNA."[9] Two major spliceosomal subunits are antigenic targets in autoimmunity: (1) small nuclear ribonucleoprotein protein particles (snRNPs) and (2) heterogeneous nuclear RNP particles (hnRNPs).

The snRNPs contain small RNA species ranging in size from 80 to 350 nucleotides that are complexed with proteins.[6] These RNAs contain a high content of uridine and are therefore called U-RNAs; 5 different U-RNAs were defined on the basis of immunoprecipitation (U1, U2, U4, U5, and U6). Autoantibodies to these complexes are mainly directed to the protein components. Anti-Sm antibodies precipitate five proteins with molecular weights of 28,000 (B'B), 16,000 (D), 13,000 (E), 12,000 (F), and 11,000 (G); five of these polypeptides are common to the U1, U2, U4, U5, and U6 RNAs. Anti-RNP antibodies precipitate three proteins with molecular weights of 68,000 (70K), 33,000 (A'), and 22,000 (C); these polypeptides are uniquely associated with U1 RNA (Figure 86-1). The clinical correlates considered to be distinctive of MCTD are associated with the 70-kD specificity with an immunodominant epitope embracing amino acid residue 125 flanked by important conformational residues at positions 119-126 (see Figure 86-1). On the other hand, SLE is associated with anti-Sm antibodies.

The hnRNPs are among the most abundant proteins in the eukaryotic cell nucleus. They contain pre-mRNA associated with 30 small proteins that are all structurally related and have molecular weights of 33 to 43 kD. Nine hnRNP core proteins have been designated A1, A2, B1a, B1b, B1c, B2, C1, C2, and C3. An antibody termed anti-RA33, which

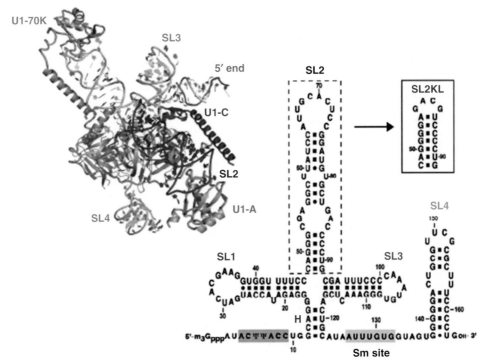

Figure 86-1 The spliceosome is made up of five small nuclear RNAs (snRNAs) complexed with proteins to form a small nuclear ribonucleoprotein particle (snRNP). This subcellular structure is responsible for splicing introns from pre-mRNA to form mRNA via a 59-splice recognition site. Antibodies to various spliceosomal constituents are a common feature of autoimmune rheumatic disorders with a tendency to associate with different clinical profiles (see Table 86-1). The U1 small nuclear RNP (U1-snRNP) particle of the spliceosome is composed of U1-RNA, RNP proteins (70 kD, A, and C), and common Sm proteins (B′B, D, E, F, and G). The structure of U1-RNA consists of single-stranded RNA and double-stranded RNA called stem loops (SL) 1, 2, 3, and 4. An electron density map of the functional core of U1-snRNP at 5.5 Å resolution has enabled the spatial visualization of the RNA and placement of the seven Sm proteins, U1-C, and U1-70K into the map. A striking feature is the amino (N)-terminal polypeptide of U1-70K, which extends over a distance of 180 Å from its RNA binding domain, wraps around the core domain consisting of the seven Sm proteins, and finally contacts U1-C, which is crucial for 59-splice-site recognition. *(Modified from Newman J: Structural studies of the spliceosome,* Curr Opin Struct Biol *20:82–89, 2010; and Pomeranz AD: Crystal structure of human spliceosomal U1 snRNP at 5.5 A resolution,* Nature *458:457–480, 2009.)*

targets the 33-kD hnRNP-A2, is particularly interesting because it is found in about one-third of sera from patient with RA, SLE, and MCTD.[10] It also has associations with patient subsets of erosive arthritis in SLE, scleroderma, and MCTD and predicts the eventual development of RA in patients with early polyarthritis.[11] Importantly, this association with anti-RA33 is not seen in scleroderma (sine erosions), PM, or overlaps of PM/Scl or PM/DM. The antigenic epitopes of hnRNP-A2 contain two RNA binding regions at the N-terminal end and a glycine-rich C-terminal region. Certain disease subsets target these two RNA binding regions differently. For instance, RA and SLE sera preferentially react with the complete second RNA binding domain, whereas MCTD sera target an epitope that spans both RNA binding domains.

Autoimmunity to Nucleosomal Components

Nucleosomes are the compact building blocks of chromatin and consist of an octamer of two copies of histones H2A, H2B, H3, and H4, wrapped around approximately 146 base pairs of DNA (Figure 86-2). During apoptosis endonucleases cleave chromatin with the liberation of nucleosomal particles. Following the release into the cytoplasm, nucleosomes migrate to the surface of the dying cell[12] and thus become accessible to B cell receptors. The development of autoimmunity has been linked to defective phagocytosis of

apoptotically released constituents.[12] Nucleosomal antibodies are directed to antigenic determinants on the intact nucleosome rather than its individual components, DNA and histones. In a study of 496 patients with 13 different AICTDs and 100 patients with hepatitis C, antinucleosome antibodies were found in the sera of patients with SLE (71.7%), Scl (45.9%), and MCTD (45.0%).[13]

Autoimmunity to Proteasomal Components

The 26S proteasome is a large subcellular particle involved in the degradation of proteins that have been tagged with ubiquitin, resulting in the generation of peptides for presentation by the MHC class I molecules (Figure 86-3). There is good evidence that it is the target of an autoimmune response in AICTD. Antibodies to proteasomal subunits have been reported in patients with autoimmune myositis, systemic lupus erythematosus, and primary Sjögren's syndrome. Circulating 20S proteasomes (c20S) subunits appear to have an association with disease activity in MCTD and SLE.[14]

Generation of Autoimmunity

The antibody response to just one component of an intracellular structure such as a spliceosome will result in the uptake of the entire particle by antigen-presenting cells

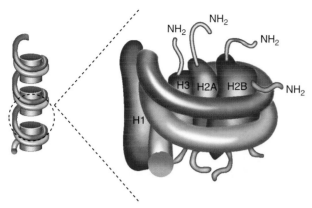

Figure 86-2 The nucleosome is the fundamental repeating unit of chromatin. The central part of the nucleosome is composed of a tetramer composed of two molecules of histones H3 and H4, flanked by two dimers of histones H2A and H2B. This central core is surrounded by two super-helical turns, consisting of 146 base pairs of histone-free DNA. Histone H1 is located at the point where DNA enters and exits the nucleosome. Antibodies to the nucleosome arise early in the evolution of systemic lupus erythematosus—before anti-DNA and antihistone antibodies. Thus the nucleosome is thought to be an important early autoantigen in the development of epitope spreading. Nucleosome antibodies are also found in scleroderma and mixed connective tissue disease. *(From Amoura Z, Koutouzov S, Piette C, et al: The role of nucleosomes in lupus,* Curr Opin Rheumatol *12:369–373, 2000.)*

(APCs). Thus all the proteins making up the particle will be subject to antigen processing with potential peptide presentation linked to their affinity to class II HLA antigens. Depending on the polymorphisms of the individual HLA molecules, there will be a diversification of the antibody response to include some of these other antigens. This process is called *epitope spreading* and is considered pivotal in the development of the linked antibody responses that are observed in different connective tissue diseases (CTDs).[15] For instance, it has been shown that the induction of an immune response to one component of a U-RNP complex can induce a diversified autoantibody response to other components of the complex.[16] In this way an immune response becomes modified over time, and this change has been associated with changes in the clinical picture.

The interaction between T cell receptors and peptides presented by HLA molecules is a critical event in the generation of autoimmunity. The 70-kD and anti-U1-RNP antibody responses are associated with the HLA DR4 and DR2 phenotype.[17] In a transgenic murine model of MCTD, the majority of T cells targeted a limited number of epitopes residing within the RNA binding domain of the 70-kD antigen.[18] DNA sequencing of HLA-DB genes has revealed that DR2- and DR4-positive patients share a common set of amino acids in the beta chain at positions 26, 28, 30, 31, 32, 70, and 73 that form a pocket for antigen binding. It is hypothesized that these two HLA subtypes represent a critical genetic specificity for the presentation of antigenic peptides to their cognate T cell receptors. The shared epitope on HLA-DR4/DR2 that is associated with an anti-U1-RNP response is different from the shared epitope associated with HLA-DR4/DR1 in RA patients.[19] The 70-kD polypeptide has several different epitopes, the most consistent sequence being KDK DRD RKR RSS RSR.[20] This region is preferentially targeted by MCTD sera but not by SLE sera.[21] The autoimmune response to the spliceosome in these three

disorders is characterized by differential degrees of epitope spreading. The widest range of antibodies, to both snRNP and hnRNP, is seen in SLE; a more restricted antispliceosomal antibody repertoire to snRNP and hnRNP is seen in MCTD; and in RA the antispliceosomal antibody repertoire is restricted to hnRNP.[22] In general the autoimmune rheumatic diseases are characterized by the production of autoantibodies that recognize evolutionarily conserved molecules. The mechanism whereby these "hidden" intracellular molecules become autoantigens is an area of ongoing research. The two main theories are apoptotic modification[23] and molecular mimicry.[24]

Proteins modified during apoptosis can be presented to the immune system in ways that bypass tolerance to self-proteins.[6] Although rheumatic disease autoantigens are not unified by common structure or function, they have the common feature of becoming clustered and concentrated in the surface blebs of apoptotic cells. A population of smaller blebs contains fragmented endoplasmic reticulum and ribosomes, as well as the ribonucleoprotein Ro. Larger blebs (apoptotic bodies) contain nucleosomal DNA, Ro, La, and the small nuclear ribonucleoproteins.[25] During the process of apoptosis several enzyme systems are upregulated with resulting post-translational modifications of the cleaved proteins. These modifications, which include citrullination, phosphorylation, dephosphorylation, transglutamination, and conjugation to ubiquitin, render the molecules more antigenic. For instance, the U1-70K protein is cleaved by the enzyme caspase-3, converting it into a C-terminally truncated fragment, which contains a major B cell epitope that is preferentially recognized by autoimmune sera.[26]

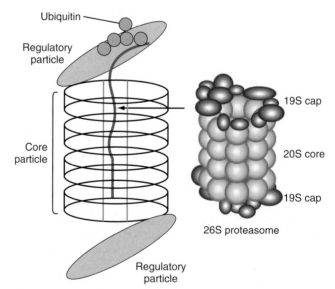

Figure 86-3 Most proteins in the cytosol and nucleus are degraded via the proteasome-ubiquitin pathway. The 26S proteasome is a huge complex of 2.5 mega-daltons, made up of approximately 35 different subunits. It contains a proteolytic core complex, the 20S proteasome, and one or two 19S regulatory complexes that associate with the termini of the barrel-shaped 20S core. The function of proteasomes is twofold: (1) to degrade intracellular proteins that have been tagged with ubiquitin and (2) to generate antigenic peptides for presentation by the major histocompatibility complex class I molecules. Antibodies to proteasomal subunits have been reported in several autoimmune diseases (especially systemic lupus erythematosus and polymyositis/dermatomyositis), and elevated levels of proteasomes have been correlated with disease activity.

The initial stimulus for a first antibody response may be a *non–self-protein* possessing a peptide region that mimics a self-epitope—so-called molecular mimicry. Environmental stressors such as infection, toxins, drugs, and ultraviolet light may, under some circumstances, induce accelerated apoptosis. A critical limitation to molecular mimicry is the necessity for the antigenic sequence to undergo TCR recognition. Helper T lymphocytes (CD4+) usually recognize peptides of 12 to 16 amino acids in the context of HLA class II molecules. However, in some instances smaller peptides may be recognized. They can be *more* immunostimulatory than the parent ligand. Thus antigen recognition by T cells is highly degenerate and expands the potential for molecular mimicry. The universe of molecules containing a pentapeptide, for example, is much greater than for 12 amino residue peptide. Once an immune response to one component of an immunogenic molecular complex has been elicited, other proteins/epitopes of the complex may become antigenic by the same process of epitope spreading.[15]

UNDIFFERENTIATED CONNECTIVE TISSUE DISEASE

KEY POINTS

Nearly all patients with a UCTD have Raynaud's phenomenon in combination with an unexplained synovitis.

Nail-fold capillary microscopy is useful in evaluating the potential pathology.

Antibody profiles are useful in predicting the eventual clinical features:
   U1-RNP antibodies predict the differentiation into MCTD.
   DNA antibodies predict the differentiation into SLE.
   Nucleolar antibodies predict the differentiation into systemic sclerosis (SSc).

Synthetase and PM/Scl antibodies predict the differentiation into a myositis overlap syndrome.

Rheumatologists frequently see patients who present with a weakly positive ANA and nonspecific symptoms such as arthralgias, fatigue, and cold sensitivity. The critical question in such patients is "will they develop a connective tissue disease?" or "do they have fibromyalgia?"

The answer to this question is not always straightforward because fibromyalgia is not a diagnosis of exclusion[27]; it is a common comorbidity with the well-defined CTDs and is often associated with cold-induced vasospasm.[28] An algorithm for diagnosing UCTDs is given in Figure 86-4. In the early stages of a CTD, there may be just one or two suspicious clinical and laboratory features, but a definitive diagnosis cannot always be made. In such cases a working diagnosis of undifferentiated connective tissue disease (UCTD) may be appropriate.[29] Most patients with this UCTD have Raynaud's phenomenon with or without an unexplained polyarthralgia and a positive ANA with usually just a single autoantibody specificity, often anti-Ro and anti-RNP.[30] A 5-year follow-up study of 665 patients with UCTD reported that only 34% developed a well-defined CTD (RA—13.1%, Sjögren's—6.8%, SLE—4.2%, MCTD—4%, Scl—2.8%, systemic vasculitis—3.3%, and

Table 86-2 Disorders Associated with Increased Fibrosis

Localized
Morphea
Scleredema
Scleromyxedema
Eosinophilic fasciitis
Peyronie's disease
Dupuytren's contracture
Pachydermoperiostitis
Idiopathic pulmonary fibrosis
Sclerosing cholangitis
Primary biliary cirrhosis
Cryptogenic fibrosis

Systemic
Scleroderma
Metastatic carcinoid
Retroperitoneal fibrosis
Graft-versus-host disease
Nephrogenic systemic fibrosis
Amyloidosis

PM/DM—0.5%).[31] Certain combinations of features are predictive for the development of an established CTD: Polyarthritis plus U1-RNP antibodies predict MCTD, sicca symptoms plus anti-SSA/SSB antibodies predict Sjögren's syndrome, Raynaud's phenomenon plus a nucleolar ANA pattern predict Scl, polyarthritis plus high levels of rheumatoid factor (RF) predict RA, and fever/serositis plus a homogeneous ANA pattern or anti-dsDNA antibodies predict progression into SLE (Table 86-2). The identification of a pathologic nail-fold capillary pattern can provide some early indication that the UCTD may progress to systemic sclerosis (SSc) or MCTD (Figure 86-5).[32] Low levels of vitamin D are also reported to be a risk factor for the development of UCTDs and should be evaluated and corrected in all such patients.[33]

SCLERODERMA OVERLAPS

KEY POINTS

Scleroderma overlap syndromes include scleroderma variants such as calcinosis, Raynaud's phenomemon, esophageal involvement, sclerodactyly, and telangiectasia (CREST), myositis associated with sclerodactyly, and MCTD.

Raynaud's phenomenon is often the first clinical feature of SSc overlaps and must be distinguished from primary cold Raynaud's (i.e., cold-induced vasospasm).

The finding of thickened and dilated capillaries on nail-fold microscopy and pathologic autoantibodies (e.g., Scl-70, anticentromere, PM/Scl, U1-RNP) are important clues about the development of an overlap syndrome.

CREST has a common overlap with primary biliary cirrhosis.

Pulmonary fibrosis and pulmonary hypertension are the main causes of morbidity/mortality.

Scleroderma-like disorders (e.g., eosinophilic fasciitis, scleromyxedema, nephrogenic fibrosis, scleredema) need to be considered in the differential diagnosis of scleroderma overlaps.

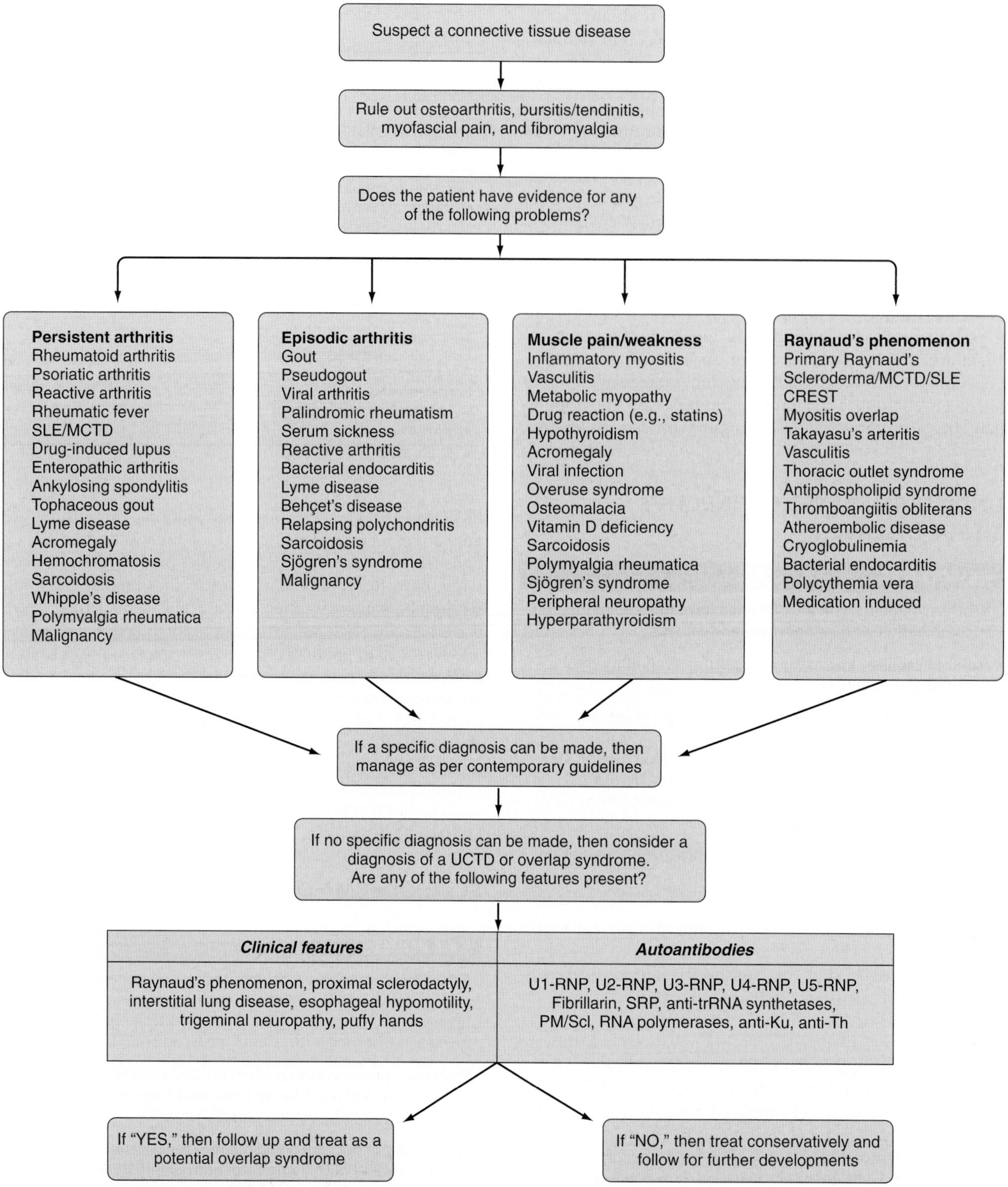

Figure 86-4 Algorithm for evaluating patients with undifferentiated connective tissue disease (UCTD). CREST, calcinosis, Raynaud's phenomenon, esophageal dysmotility, sclerodactyly, and telangiectasia; MCTD, mixed connective tissue disease; SLE, systemic lupus erythematosus.

Several fibrotic conditions may mimic scleroderma (see Table 86-2). Scleroderma itself has a widespread heterogeneity of disease expression ranging from a diffuse cutaneous disease, with a poor prognosis, to a limited cutaneous involvement, with generally a good prognosis. Furthermore, some patients with Scl have a prominent overlap with other connective tissue diseases.[34] In many cases, these overlaps occur in patients who do not have prominent skin involvement (sine scleroderma) or with the limited form of the disease—CREST. Approximately 90% of patients with Scl have a positive ANA. Scleroderma-related antibodies include topoisomerase I (Scl-70), anticentromere (ACA),

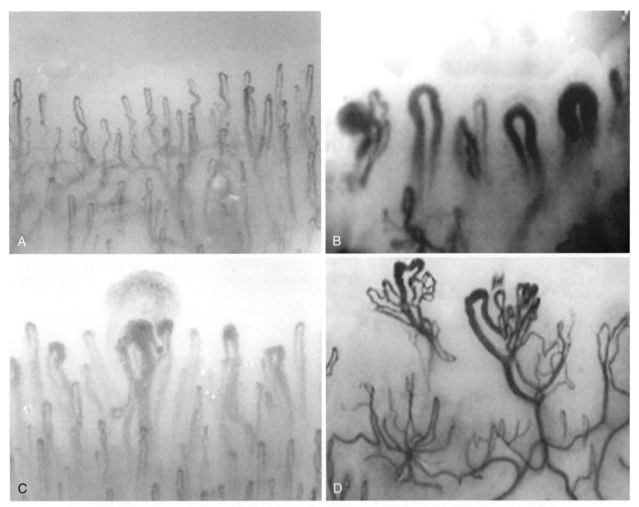

Figure 86-5 Nail-fold capillaroscopy in patients with systemic sclerosis and mixed connective tissue disease (MCTD). **A,** Normal capillaries. **B,** MCTD patient showing dilated and thickened capillary loops. **C,** Early scleroderma with irregular capillaries and mild dropout. **D,** Advanced scleroderma with capillary dropout and neoangiogenesis. *(Modified from Cutolo M, Sulli A, Pizzorni C, Smith V: Capillaroscopy as an outcome measure for clinical trials on the peripheral vasculopathy in SSc—is it useful?* Int J Rheumatol *pii:784947, 2010.)*

hnPNP-I, RA33, p23, p25, RNA polymerase I (RNAP-1), RNA polymerase III, U1-RNP, PM/Scl, fibrillarin, histone, Ku, endothelial cell, and Th/To[35] (see Table 86-1).

A German registry for scleroderma has reported on patterns of organ involvement in two subsets of 1483 SSc patients.[36] Limited distal skin involvement (distal to the knee and elbows) was seen in 46% (the lcSSc group), and 33% had progressive widespread scleroderma (rapid involvement of trunk, face, and extremities—the dcSSc group). An overlap syndrome was seen in 11%, and 8% were undifferentiated. The extent of organ involvement varied between subgroups. For instance, musculoskeletal involvement was seen in 68% of the overlap group compared with 57% of the dcSSc group. Pulmonary fibrosis (56%) and pulmonary hypertension (19%) were most common in the dcSSc group, but pulmonary hypertension was seen in 15% of the dcSSc group.

Specific antibody profiles tend to be associated with distinctive patterns of morbidity and mortality.[37] Patients possessing anticentromere, anti-U3 snRNP, and anti-Th/To antibodies tend to have the limited form of Scl, whereas anti-Scl-70, ACA, and anti-RNAP are associated with diffuse skin involvement and systemic disease. Anti-PM/Scl antibodies are associated with a myositis/Scl overlap and a tendency to develop pulmonary interstitial disease.[38] About 60% of patients with scleroderma have obvious synovitis, and 35% are positive for RF. Erosive arthritis in Scl has an association with anti-RA33; the Scl component in such overlap patients is often an incomplete form of CREST.[39] The limited form of scleroderma has a well-documented overlap with primary biliary cirrhosis (PBC). The distinctive antibody association of scleroderma with PBC is antimitochondrial antibodies.[40] Conversely, anticentromere antibodies have been found in 10% to 29% of patients with PBC; approximately half developed some features of the CREST syndrome. Hence a serologic overlap between the two syndromes is more prevalent in the clinical overlap. Low-grade muscle involvement is not uncommon in scleroderma, being described in between 50% and 80% of patients. A European review of 114 scleroderma overlap patients reported a 95% PM/Scl antibody positivity[41] with 80% having an inflammatory myositis. This "scleromyositis" differed from MCTD by coexistent features of dermatomyositis (myalgia, myositis, Gottron sign, heliotrope rash, calcinosis), but no overlap SLE features, as is characteristic of classic MCTD. Many of these patients had a deforming arthritis of the hands. In general they had a chronic benign course, and most were steroid responsive. Scleroderma lupus overlaps are less common. However, Scl patients often have antinuclear antibodies other than ACA and Scl-70.

Nonscleroderma fibrotic disorder may be mistaken for a scleroderma overlap at initial presentation (see Table 86-2); although these disorders may have some systemic involvement, they seldom exhibit overlap features with other AICTDs.

Nephrogenic systemic fibrosis (NSF) is a fibrotic disorder that develops in some patients following exposure to gadolinium-containing contrast agents; most patients have pre-existing renal disease.[42] Histologically there is fibroblast proliferation, thickened collagen bundles, and deposits of mucin, similar to those observed in scleromyxedema. The clinical presentation is a rapid progression with confluence of initially focal areas of indurated skin (Figure 86-6). The face is usually spared, but joint contractures may occur at the elbows and knees, and systemic involvement with pulmonary and neurologic symptoms can develop in refractory

cases. NSF is usually nonresponsive to corticosteroids and immunosuppressive therapy.

Eosinophilic fasciitis presents with limited scleroderma-like skin changes involving the extremities (see Figure 86-6). The correct diagnosis is suggested by finding a peripheral eosinophilia and a hypergammaglobulinemia.[43] The definitive diagnosis is established by a full-thickness skin biopsy that shows a diffuse inflammation of the fascia. Initial treatment is with corticosteroids (prednisone 0.5 to 1 mg/kg) tapering according to the clinical response; some patients need to continue moderate-dose corticosteroids for up to 2 years. Methotrexate and mycophenalate may be used in refractory cases.

Scleromyxedema is characterized by cutaneous mucinosis and is often associated with a gammopathy, usually IgM and light chains.[44] The mucinous skin lesions appear as waxy papules on the face, neck, and limbs. If the papules coalesce, it may be mistaken for scleroderma (see Figure 86-6). Systemic involvement may occur with dysphagia, proximal muscle weakness, pulmonary, cardiac, and renal complications. It is difficult to manage; corticosteroids are usually tried initially, in refractory cases some benefit has

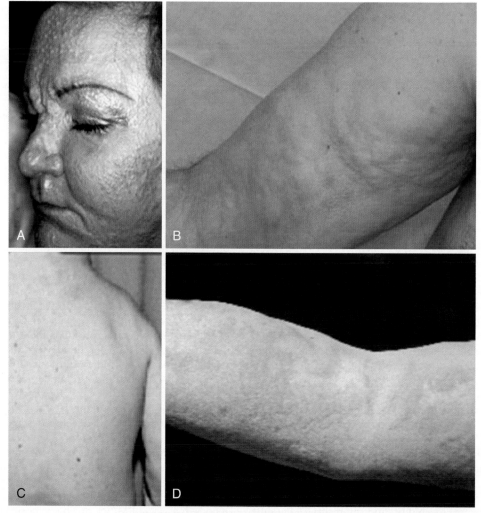

Figure 86-6 Four examples of fibrosing disorders. **A,** Scleromyxedema (mucinous skin lesions appear as waxy papules on the face). **B,** Eosinophilic fasciitis (induration of skin and subcutaneous tissues). **C,** Scleredema (diffuse subcutaneous edema with swelling over right trapezius). **D,** Nephrogenic systemic fibrosis (coalescence of indurated nodules with joint contracture). *(Modified from Boin F, Hummers LK: Scleroderma-like fibrosing disorders, Rheum Dis Clin North Am 34:199–220, 2008.)*

been reported for intravenous immunoglobulin and thalidomide.

Scleredema is a cutaneous mucinosis that often starts with a febrile episode and resolves spontaneously.[45] More chronic scleredema has been associated with paraprotein-emias including multiple myeloma and diabetes mellitus. The dermis is thickened with increased collagen glycosyl-ation, as in diabetic stiff skin syndrome. The face and neck are commonly involved, and there is relative sparing of the hands and feet (see Figure 86-6). Systemic organ involve-ment is rare, but a monoclonal gammopathy is sometimes seen. Such cases need to be worked up for lymphoma. Refractory cases have been helped by local radiotherapy.

MYOSITIS OVERLAPS

KEY POINTS

Myositis overlap syndromes are more common than the classic descriptions of PM or DM.

Amino-acyl trRNA synthetase antibodies (ARS) are associated with myositis, arthritis, and interstitial lung disease.

Arthritis and interstitial lung disease may antedate the appearance of myositis in patients with ARS.

Antibodies to synthetases, signal recognition particle (SRP), and nucleoporin tend to be associated with corticosteroid unresponsiveness.

Antibodies to U1-RNP, PM/Scl, or Ku are associated with corticosteroid responsiveness.

Antibodies to 155-kD and 140-kD proteins have been associated with an increased risk of myositis-associated malignancy.

Polymyositis (PM), dermatomyositis (DM), and inclusion body myositis (IBM) are the classic idiopathic inflammatory myopathies (IIM), yet the same clinical picture and inves-tigational findings may be found in patients with SLE, Scl, MCTD, and Sjögren's syndrome. Such overlaps, especially with scleroderma, have been reported as being more common in the classic description of polymyositis.[4] When clinical overlaps emerge, they are most commonly associ-ated with specific autoantibodies, namely anti-PM-Scl, anti-Ku, U1-RNP, Jo-1, SRP, and ARS.[46] The arthropathy associated with polymyositis is characterized by deforming subluxations (particularly of the distal interphalangeals and thumbs) with only minor erosive changes. Another myositis overlap syndrome is seen in patients with amino-acyl trRNA synthetase antibodies (ARS).[47] This is a family of enzymes that catalyze the transfer of a specific amino acid to its cognate transfer RNA—the commonest association is with anti-Jo-1 (histidine-trRNA synthetase). The clinical syndromes associated with the various antisynthetase anti-bodies are similar, with remissions and exacerbations characterized by inflammatory myositis, fever, Raynaud's syndrome, and skin problems (mechanic's hands).[48] The arthritis of ARS may initially mimic RA with an inflamma-tory arthritis and nodules; erosions, however, do not occur.[49] Interstitial lung disease may be a presenting clinical feature of patients with ARS antibodies, with myopathy occurring

much later. The association of myositis in patients with anti-U1-RNP antibodies is usually seen in the context of MCTD.[50] Antibodies to the signal recognition particle (SRP) have been reported in 4% of patients with Scl/PM overlap; these patients usually have a severe, rapidly pro-gressive myositis with prominent muscle fiber necrosis without much inflammatory cell infiltration.[51]

A 2006 clinical and longitudinal study of 100 consecu-tive French Canadian patients with idiopathic IIM con-cluded that the original Bohan and Peter classification of inflammatory myopathies should be abandoned because 60% of patients with IIM were found to have an overlap syndrome.[4] In this study an overlap syndrome was based on the presence of an inflammatory myopathy as per the Bohan and Peter classification,[52] plus at least one clinical overlap feature (Table 86-3), or one of the following autoantibodies: synthetases, centromere, topo I, RNA-polymerases I or III, Th, U1-RNP, U2-RNP, U3-RNP, U5-RNP, PM/Scl, Ku, SRP and nucleoporins (see Table 86-3). The distinction between classic PM/DM and an overlap syndrome was reported to be of prognostic/therapeutic significance because classic PM nearly always pursued a chronic course with 50% of patients being initially unresponsive to corticosteroid therapy. Pure dermatomyositis was almost always chronic, but most had an initial response to corticosteroids. On the other hand, myositis overlap syndromes (usually with scleroderma features) were almost always responsive to cor-ticosteroids (≈90% response rate). When overlap patients were divided according to antibody subsets, antisynthetase, SRP, and nucleoporin autoantibodies were markers for treatment-resistant myositis, whereas autoantibodies to U1-RNP, PM/Scl, or Ku were markers for corticosteroid responsiveness. Patients with autoimmune myositis, espe-cially dermatomyositis, are at risk of developing cancer,[53] and it has been problematic as to how far and how often one should pursue a malignancy workup. It is now apparent that the finding of an antibody against 155-kD and 140-kD protein specificities (anti-155/140 antibody) signifies a sig-nificant risk for the co-occurrence of a malignancy and points to the need for a thorough cancer workup.[54]

MIXED CONNECTIVE TISSUE DISEASE

KEY POINTS

The clinical overlap features of MCTD (i.e., Scl, SLE, and IIM) seldom occur concurrently but develop sequentially over the course of months or years.

Raynaud's phenomenon is seen in nearly all patients with MCTD; if Raynaud's syndrome is absent, the diagnosis should be reconsidered.

About 25% of MCTD patients develop renal involvement—usually membranous glomerulonephritis. Proliferative glomerulonephritis is uncommon in MCTD.

Serious CNS involvement is rare in MCTD; the commonest findings are trigeminal neuropathy and sensorineural hearing loss.

Pulmonary hypertension is the commonest cause of death in MCTD patients and should be screened for on an ongoing basis.

Table 86-3 Suggested Classification for Inflammatory Myopathies

Abbreviation	Description
PM	Pure polymyositis
DM	Pure dermatomyositis
OM	Overlap myositis: myositis with at least 1 clinical overlap feature and/or an overlap autoantibody
CAM	Cancer-associated myositis: with clinical paraneoplastic features and without an overlap autoantibody or anti-Mi-2

Bohan and Peter's[52] Definition of Myositis

1. Symmetric proximal muscle weakness.
2. Elevation of serum skeletal muscle enzymes.
3. Electromyographic triad of short, small, polyphasic motor unit potentials; fibrillations, positive sharp waves, and insertional irritability; and bizarre, high-frequency repetitive discharges.
4. Muscle biopsy abnormalities of degeneration, regeneration, necrosis, phagocytosis, and an interstitial mononuclear infiltrate.
5. Typical skin rash of DM including the heliotrope rash, Gottron sign, and Gottron papules.

Definite myositis: 4 criteria (without the rash) for PM, 3 or 4 criteria (plus the rash) for DM.
Probable myositis: 3 criteria (without the rash) for PM, 2 criteria (plus the rash) for DM.
Possible myositis: 2 criteria (without the rash) for PM, 1 criterion (plus the rash) for DM.

Definition of Clinical Overlap Features

Inflammatory myopathy plus at least 1 or more of the following clinical findings: polyarthritis, Raynaud's phenomenon, sclerodactyly, scleroderma proximal to metacarpophalangeal joints, typical SSc-type calcinosis in the fingers, lower esophageal or small-bowel hypomotility, DLCO lower than 70% of the normal predicted value, interstitial lung disease on chest radiogram or computed tomography scan, discoid lupus, anti-native DNA antibodies plus hypocomplementemia, 4 or more of 11 American College of Rheumatology criteria for systemic lupus erythematosus, antiphospholipid syndrome.

Definition of Overlap Autoantibodies

Antisynthetases (Jo-1, PL-7, PL-12, OJ, EJ, KS); scleroderma-associated autoantibodies (scleroderma-specific antibodies: centromeres, topoisomerase I, RNA polymerases I or III, Th; and antibodies associated with scleroderma overlap: U1-RNP, U2-RNP, U3-RNP, U5-RNP, Pm-Scl, Ku, and other autoantibodies (signal recognition particle, nucleoporins).

Definition of Clinical Paraneoplastic Features

Cancer within 3 yr of myositis diagnosis, plus absence of multiple clinical overlap features; plus, if cancer was cured, myositis was cured as well.

Modified from Troyanov Y, Targoff IN, Tremblay JL, et al: Novel classification of idiopathic inflammatory myopathies based on overlap syndrome features and autoantibodies: analysis of 100 French Canadian patients, *Medicine (Baltimore)* 84:231–249, 2005.

MCTD was described by Sharp and colleagues[55] in a 1971 paper reporting an overlap of SLE, Scl, and PM. This was the first overlap syndrome defined in terms of a specific antibody—namely antibodies to a ribonuclease-sensitive extractable nuclear antigen (ENA). Over the past 38 years, many studies have explored the clinical correlates of this antibody system (now called U1-RNP).

Serologic Features

The basic premise of the MCTD concept is that the presence of high-titer anti-U1-RNP antibodies modifies the expression of an AICTD in ways that are relevant to prognosis and treatment.[56] The first clue to diagnosing MCTD is usually a positive ANA with a high-titer speckled pattern. The titer is often greater than 1 : 1000 and sometimes greater than 1 : 10,000. This finding should prompt the measurement of antibodies to U1-RNP, Sm, Ro, and La. It is also pertinent to note whether the serum contains antibodies to dsDNA and histones because patients destined to follow a course most consistent with MCTD have sera with predominant U1-RNP reactivity. Antibodies to dsDNA, Sm, and Ro are occasionally seen as a transient phenomenon in patients with MCTD. But when they are found consistently, as the *predominant* antibody system, the clinical picture is usually more consistent with classic SLE. Antibodies to the 70-kD antigen, especially in its apoptotic form, are most closely associated with the clinical correlates of MCTD.[8]

Clinical Features

Diagnosis

MCTD is an overlap syndrome that embraces features of SLE, Scl, and PM/DM.[57] These overlap features seldom occur concurrently; it usually takes several years before enough overlapping features have appeared to be confident that MCTD is the most appropriate diagnosis.[58] The commonest clinical associations with U1-RNP antibodies in the early phase of the disease are hand edema, arthritis, Raynaud's phenomenon, inflammatory muscle disease, and sclerodactyly. No American College of Rheumatology (ACR) criteria are available for the diagnosis of MCTD, but a comparative study reported that two criteria sets, those of Alarcon-Segovia and Kahn, had the best sensitivity and specificity (62.5% and 86.2%, respectively)[59] (Table 86-4). The sensitivity could be improved to 81.3% if the term "myalgia" was substituted for "myositis."[60] Some patients initially diagnosed as MCTD will evolve into a clinical picture most consistent with SLE or RA; in one long-term follow-up, more than half of the subjects continued to satisfy criteria for MCTD.[61] A comparison of the clinical and serologic features of MCTD with SLE, RA, Scl, and PM/DM is given in Table 86-5.

Early Symptoms

In the early stages most patients destined to develop MCTD cannot be differentiated from the other classic AICTDs.

Table 86-4 Diagnostic Criteria for Mixed Connective Tissue Disease

	Alarcón-Segovia Criteria	Kahn Criteria
Serologic criteria	Anti-RNP at hemagglutination titer of ≥1:1600	High-titer anti-RNP corresponding to a speckled ANA of ≥1:1200 titer
Clinical criteria	1. Swollen hands 2. Synovitis 3. Myositis (biologically proven) 4. Raynaud's phenomenon 5. Acrosclerosis	1. Swollen fingers 2. Synovitis 3. Myositis 4. Raynaud's phenomenon
MCTD present if:	Serologic criterion accompanied by 3 or more clinical criteria, one of which must include synovitis or myositis	Serologic criterion accompanied by Raynaud's phenomenon and 2 or more of the 3 remaining clinical criteria

ANA, antinuclear antibody; MCTD, mixed connective tissue disease; RNP, ribonucleoprotein particle.
From Alarcon-Segovia D, Cardiel MH: Comparison between 3 diagnostic criteria for mixed connective tissue disease. Study of 593 patients, *J Rheumatol* 16(3):328–334, 1989.

The assumption that a diagnosis of MCTD implies a *simultaneous* presence of features usually seen in SLE, Scl, and PM is erroneous. It is unusual to see such an overlap during the early course of MCTD, but with the progress of time the overlapping features usually occur sequentially. Early in the course of the disease most patients complain of easy fatigability, poorly defined myalgias, arthralgias, and Raynaud's phenomenon; at this point in time a diagnosis of RA, SLE, or undifferentiated connective tissue disease (UCTD) seems most appropriate.[1] If such a patient is found to have swollen hands or puffy fingers (Figure 86-7) in association with a high-titer speckled ANA, he or she should be carefully followed for the evolution of overlap features (see Table 86-3). A high titer of anti-RNP antibodies in a patient with UCTD is a powerful predictor for a later evolution into MCTD. Less commonly there is an acute onset of MCTD, which gives little clue to the subsequent course; such presentations have included polymyositis, acute arthritis, aseptic meningitis, digital gangrene, high fever, acute abdomen, and trigeminal neuropathy.[62]

Fever

Fever may be a prominent feature of MCTD in the absence of an obvious cause. Fever of unknown origin has been the initial presentation of MCTD; after careful evaluation, fever in MCTD can usually be traced to a coexistent myositis, aseptic meningitis, serositis, lymphadenopathy, or intercurrent infection.

Joints

Joint pain and stiffness is an early symptom in nearly all patients who develop the MCTD syndrome. Over the past 2 decades it has become increasingly apparent that joint involvement in MCTD is more common and more severe than in classic SLE.[63] About 60% of patients eventually develop an obvious arthritis, often with deformities commonly seen in RA such as ulnar deviation, swan neck, and boutonnière changes.[64] Radiographs usually show a characteristic absence of severe erosive changes; they often

Table 86-5 Differential Features of the Classic Autoimmune Connective Tissue Diseases

Clinical Feature	SLE	RA	Scl	PM	MCTD
Pleurisy/pericarditis	++++	+	+	−	+++
Erosive joint disease	±	++++	+	±	+
Raynaud's phenomenon	++	−	++++	+	++++
Inflammatory myositis	+	+	+	++++	+++
Sclerodactyly	±	−	++++	−	++
Nonacral skin thickening	−	−	+++	−	−
Interstitial pulmonary fibrosis	+	+	+++	++	+
Pulmonary hypertension	++	±	+	+	+++
Butterfly rash	++++	−	−	−	++
Oral ulcers	+++	−	−	−	++
Seizures/psychosis	+++	−	−	−	−
Trigeminal neuropathy	+	−	++	−	+++
Peripheral neuropathy	++	+	±	−	++
Transverse myelopathy	+++	+	−	−	++
Aseptic meningitis	+++	+	−	−	+++
Diffuse proliferative glomerulonephritis	++++	−	−	−	+
Membranous glomerulonephritis	+++	−	−	−	++
Renovascular hypertension	+	−	++++	−	+++
Inflammatory vasculitis	++	+	+	+	+
Noninflammatory vasculopathy	−	−	++++	−	+++
Esophageal dysmotility	+	±	++++	+	+++

MCTD, mixed connective tissue disease; PM, polymyositis; RA, rheumatoid arthritis; Scl, scleroderma; SLE, systemic lupus erythematosus.

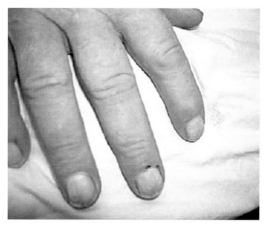

Figure 86-7 The hand of a man with mixed connective tissue disease. The fingers have a generally puffy appearance with a fusiform proximal interphalangeal swelling of the third finger from an inflammatory arthritis. There is a periungual infarct at the nail fold of the third finger. *(Modified from Pope JE: Other manifestations of mixed connective tissue disease,* Rheum Dis Clin North Am *31:519–533, 2005.)*

develop a flexor tenosynovitis, bone edema, and pericapsular inflammation reminiscent of a seronegative spondyloarthropathy (Figure 86-8). A positive RF is found in 50% to 70% of patients; indeed, patients may be diagnosed as having RA and fulfill ACR criteria for RA.

Skin and Mucous Membranes

Most patients with MCTD develop mucocutaneous changes sometime during the course of the syndrome. Raynaud's phenomenon is the commonest problem and one of the earliest manifestations of MCTD.[66] It may be accompanied by puffy, swollen digits and sometimes total hand edema.[62] In some patients, skin changes commonly associated with classic SLE are prominent findings, particularly malar rash and discoid plaques. Other problems have included buccal ulceration, sicca complex, orogenital ulceration, livedo vasculitis, subcutaneous nodules, and nasal septal perforation.

Muscle

Myalgia is a common symptom in patients with the MCTD syndrome. In most patients there is no demonstrable weakness, EMG abnormalities, or muscle enzyme changes. It is often unclear whether the symptom represents a low-grade myositis, physical deconditioning, or an associated

resemble Jaccoud's arthropathy. However, a destructive arthritis including an arthritis mutilans is a well-established association.[64] Small marginal erosions, often with a well-demarcated edge, are the most characteristic radiologic features in patients with severe joint disease.[65] Some patients

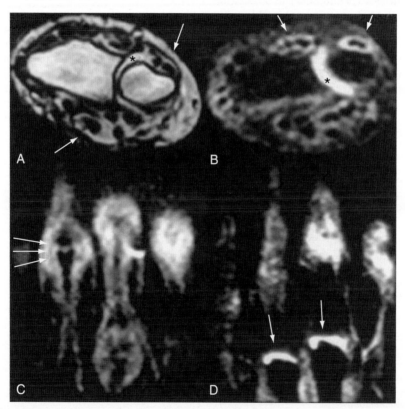

Figure 86-8 Hand magnetic resonance images of two females aged 25 and 32 with mixed connective tissue disease and hand arthritis. **A,** Patient 1 has synovitis/effusion around the ulnar styloid *(asterisk)* and tenosynovitis of the flexor and extensor tendons *(arrows)* (T1-weighted gadolinium-enhanced sequence on axial plane). **B,** Patient 2 has intense synovitis of the radioulnar joint *(asterisk)* and extensor tenosynovitis *(arrows)* causing thickening of the dorsum of the hand (T1-weighted short tau inversion recovery [STIR] sequence on axial plane). **C,** Patient 1 has synovitis/effusion, and pericapsular edema is seen in the second proximal interphalangeal joint. The distended capsule is indicated by arrows. **D,** Patient 2 has intracapsular synovial effusion or synovitis of the third and fourth metacarpophalangeal joints *(arrows)*. (Both **C** and **D** are T1-weighted STIR sequences in the coronal plane.) *(From Cimmino MA, Lozzelli A, Garlaschi G, et al: Magnetic resonance imaging of the hand in mixed connective tissue disease,* Ann Rheum Dis *62:380–381, 2003.)*

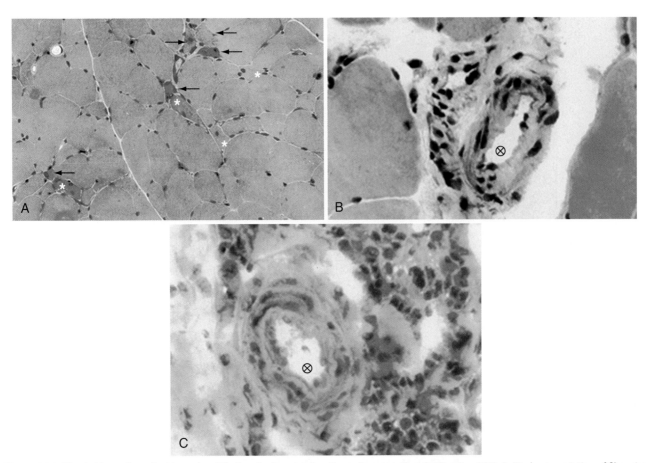

Figure 86-9 Muscle biopsy from the biceps brachii of a mixed connective tissue disease patient (H&E stain, ×300). **A,** Moderate variation of fiber size and degenerated fibers (→) with mononuclear cell infiltration. **B** and **C** show perivascular inflammatory infiltration and thickening of vessel walls. *(Modified from Vianna M, Borges MT, Borba EF, et al: Myositis in mixed connective tissue disease: a unique syndrome characterized by immuno-histopathologic elements of both polymyositis and dermatomyositis,* Arq Neuro-Psiquiatr *62:923–934, 2004.)*

fibromyalgia syndrome. The inflammatory myopathy associated with MCTD is similar histologically to IIM, with features of both the vascular involvement of DM and the cell-mediated changes of PM[67] (Figure 86-9). In most patients myositis occurs as an acute flare against a background of general disease activity. Such patients usually respond well to a short course of high-dose corticosteroid therapy. Another scenario is that of a low-grade inflammatory myopathy, which is often insidious in its onset; these patients often have a poor therapeutic response to corticosteroids. Some patients with PM associated with MCTD develop an impressive fever[62]; other patients may give a history of febrile myalgias that were diagnosed as "flu."

Heart

All three layers of the heart may be involved in MCTD.[68] An abnormal electrocardiogram (ECG) is noted in about 20% of patients. The most common ECG changes are right ventricular hypertrophy, right atrial enlargement, and interventricular conduction defects. Pericarditis is the commonest clinical manifestation of cardiac involvement, reported in 10% to 30% of patients. Pericardial tamponade is rare. Involvement of the myocardium is increasingly recognized. In some patients myocardial involvement is secondary to

pulmonary hypertension (PAH); this occurs in some 20% of patients and is often asymptomatic in its early stages.[69] The early detection of pulmonary hypertension is increasingly important because there are now more effective therapeutic options. PAH is probably underdiagnosed in its early stages; in a community rheumatology practice setting an elevation of the estimated right ventricular systolic pressure (ERVSP), consistent with the diagnosis of PAH, was found in 13% of previously undiagnosed subjects.[70] This diagnosis should be suspected in patients with increasing exertional dyspnea. Two-dimensional echocardiography with Doppler flow studies is the most useful screening test, with a definitive diagnosis requiring cardiac catheterization showing a mean resting pulmonary artery pressure greater than 25 mm Hg at rest. The development of pulmonary hypertension has been correlated with a nail-fold capillary pattern similar to that seen in Scl, antiendothelial cell antibodies, anticardiolipin antibodies, and anti-U1-RNP antibodies.[71] Both left and right ventricular dysfunction appears to be a common finding that is not always associated with PAH; regular echocardiographic evaluations are recommended for all MCTD patients, especially those with PAH. Elevated levels of anti-U1-RNP antibodies, antiendothelial cell antibodies, serum thrombomodulin, and Willebrand factor are prognostic clues to the development of PAH.[72]

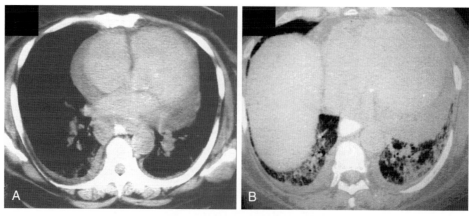

Figure 86-10 Computed tomography scans of a patient with mixed connective tissue disease and pulmonary hypertension (**A,** upper zones; **B,** lower zones). There are bilateral pleural effusions and enlarged bilateral mediastinal lymph nodes in the right paratracheal region and left perivascular areas. The pulmonary artery has a diameter greater than that of the ascending aorta—consistent with the diagnosis of pulmonary hypertension. Both hilar pulmonary arteries are also enlarged. A fairly large pericardial effusion is present. The lung windows show evidence of a diffuse abnormality with linear opacities and some areas of ground-glass attenuation in the upper zones. At the lung bases there are more confluent opacities, both reticular and ground glass, and some air-space consolidation. No honeycombing is identified, and there is no distortion of the lung architecture. *(From Saito Y, Terada M, Ishida T, et al: Pulmonary involvement in mixed connective tissue disease: comparison with other collagen vascular diseases using high resolution CT, J Comput Assist Tomogr 26:349–357, 2002.)*

Lung

Lung involvement occurs in up to 75% of patients.[73] Early symptoms that should prompt further investigations are dry cough, dyspnea, and pleuritic chest pain.[74] Interstitial lung disease (ILD) occurs in up to 50% of subjects. High-resolution computed tomography (HRCT) is the most sensitive test to determine the presence of ILD (Figure 86-10).[75] The commonest HRCT findings are septal thickening and ground-glass opacities. Untreated ILD is usually progressive with the development of severe pulmonary fibrosis in 25% of subjects after 4 years of follow-up.[76] Pulmonary hypertension (PAH) is prognostically the most severe form of pulmonary involvement in MCTD. Unlike Scl, where pulmonary hypertension is often secondary to an interstitial pulmonary fibrosis, PAH in MCTD is usually caused by a bland intimal proliferation and medial hypertrophy of pulmonary arterioles[77] (Figure 86-11).

Kidney

In the initial description of MCTD, renal involvement was considered to be rare.[57] After some 4 decades of observations, it is now evident that renal involvement occurs in about 25% of patients.[78] However, high titers of anti-U1 RNP antibodies are relatively protective against the development of diffuse proliferative glomerulonephritis, irrespective of whether they occur in a setting of classic SLE or MCTD. When patients with MCTD do develop renal changes, it usually takes the form of a membranous glomerulonephritis.[79] This is often asymptomatic but may sometimes cause an overt nephrotic syndrome.[86] The development of diffuse proliferative glomerulonephritis or parenchymal interstitial disease has been rarely recorded in MCTD. There is increasing recognition that MCTD patients are at risk of developing a renovascular hypertensive crisis similar to the scleroderma kidney.

Gastrointestinal

Gastrointestinal involvement is a major feature of the overlap with scleroderma, occurring in about 60% to 80% of patients.[63] The commonest abdominal problem in MCTD is disordered motility in the upper gastrointestinal tract. There have been case reports of hemoperitoneum, hematobilia, duodenal bleeding, megacolon, pancreatitis, ascites, protein-losing enteropathy, primary biliary cirrhosis, portal hypertension, pneumatosis intestinalis, and autoimmune hepatitis.[80] Abdominal pain in MCTD may result from

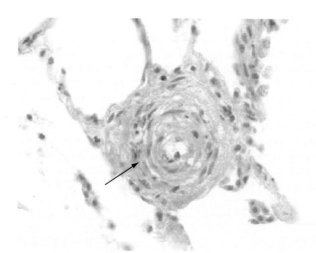

Figure 86-11 Intimal hyperplasia and smooth muscle hypertrophy without accompanying inflammation are the characteristic features of the vasculopathy of mixed connective tissue disease. When it occurs in the lung, as shown here, it may give rise to severe pulmonary hypertension. (Note absence of pulmonary fibrosis.) The plexiform lesion *(arrow)* is a characteristic pathologic finding in this disease process. *(From Bull TM, Fagan KA, Badesch DB: Pulmonary vascular manifestations of mixed connective tissue disease, Rheum Dis Clin North Am 31:451–464, 2005.)*

bowel hypomotility, serositis, mesenteric vasculitis, colonic perforation, and pancreatitis. Malabsorption syndrome can occur secondarily to small bowel dilation with bacterial overgrowth. Liver involvement in the form of chronic active hepatitis and Budd-Chiari syndrome has been described. Pseudodiverticula, identical to those seen in SCC, may be seen along the antimesenteric border of the colon.

Nervous System

In keeping with Sharp's original description, CNS involvement has not been a conspicuous feature of MCTD. The commonest problem is a trigeminal neuropathy.[81] In a review of 81 cases of trigeminal neuropathy seen in a neurologic clinic, the most frequently associated CTDs were undifferentiated connective tissue disease (47%), mixed connective tissue disease (26%), and scleroderma (19%). A sensorineural hearing loss has been reported in nearly 50% of MCTD patients.[82] In contrast to CNS involvement in classic SLE, frank psychosis and convulsions have rarely been reported in MCTD.[81] Headaches are a relatively common symptom; in the majority of patients they are vascular in origin with many of the components of classic migraine. In a subset of these patients, signs of meningeal irritation develop and examination of the cerebrospinal fluid (CSF) reveals the changes of aseptic meningitis.[83] Aseptic meningitis in MCTD has also been described as a hypersensitivity reaction to nonsteroidal anti-inflammatory drugs, in particular sulindac and ibuprofen. There are isolated reports of transverse myelitis, cauda equina syndrome, cerebral hemorrhage, retinal vasculitis, optic neuropathy, progressive multifocal leukoencephalopathy, cold-induced brain ischemia, myasthenia gravis, polyradiculopathy, demyelinating disorder, and peripheral neuropathy. Elevated CSF levels of anti-U1-RNP antibodies, with a predominance of anti-70-kD antibodies, have been reported in both SLE and MCTD patients with diffuse central neuropsychiatric involvement.[84] Many patients with AICTDs have changes on brain magnetic resonance imaging that are referred to as unspecific bright objects (UBOs). In many instances UBOs occur in the absence of neurologic symptoms. However, there is a modest correlation between the density and positioning of UBOs; in MCTD these lesions tend to cluster at the corticomedullary junction and periventricular region.[85]

Blood Vessels

Raynaud's phenomenon is an early feature of nearly all patients who are eventually diagnosed as having MCTD.[66] A bland intimal proliferation and medial hypertrophy affecting medium- and small-sized vessels is the characteristic vascular lesion of MCTD[86] (see Figure 86-11) and is the characteristic pathology in pulmonary hypertension and renovascular crises. Both nail-fold capillary microscopy[87] and color Doppler[88] are useful in distinguishing benign primary Raynaud's from secondary involvement in MCTD and other AICTDs (see Figure 86-5). Fingernail capillaroscopy is abnormal in most MCTD patients with the same pattern of capillary dilation and dropout that has been reported in Scl.[89] An angiographic study reported a high prevalence of medium-size vessel occlusions[90] (Figure 86-12). Endothelial cell and anticardiolipin antibodies have been reported to be associated with endothelial dysfunction and the development of atherosclerosis in MCTD.[91]

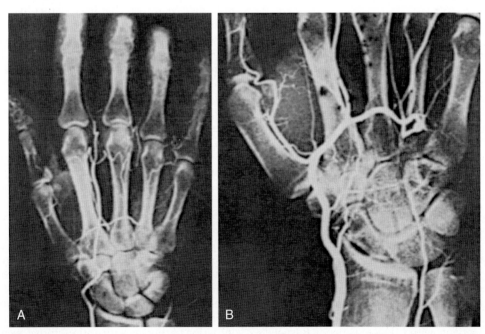

Figure 86-12 A, Digital angiogram showing multiple arterial occlusions with collateral formation. **B,** Digital angiogram showing ulnar artery occlusions. *(From Peller JS, Gabor GT, Porter JM, Bennett RM: Angiographic findings in mixed connective tissue disease: correlation with fingernail capillary photomicroscopy and digital photoplethysmography findings,* Arthritis Rheum *28:768, 1985. Reprinted with permission of the American College of Rheumatology.)*

Blood

Hematologic abnormalities are a common finding in MCTD. Anemia is found in 75% of patients, and the usual profile is most consistent with the anemia of chronic inflammation.[63] A positive Coombs test is seen in about 60% of patients, but an overt hemolytic anemia is uncommon.[92] As in SLE, a leukopenia affecting mainly the lymphocyte series is seen in about 75% of patients and tends to correlate with disease activity. Less common associations have been thrombocytopenia, thrombotic thrombocytopenia purpura, and red cell aplasia. Hypocomplementemia has been described in several studies[63]; it is not as prevalent as in classic SLE and has not been correlated with any particular clinical situation. Positive tests for RF have been found in about 50% of patients.[93] The presence of RF is associated with more severe degrees of arthritis, especially if anti-A2/RA33 are also present.[11] Anticardiolipin antibodies or lupus anticoagulants, or both, have also been reported. Unlike the anticardiolipin antibodies found in SLE, they are β2-glycoprotein independent and tend to be associated with thrombocytopenia rather than thrombotic events.[94]

Pregnancy

Reports of maternal and fetal morbidity in MCTD are quite diverse.[95] In a comparison study of patients with MCTD and SLE, the fertility rates in both diseases were unaltered, whereas the parity and fetal wastage was increased in both.[96] Some studies have reported an exacerbation of MCTD during pregnancy and postpartum flares,[96] whereas others have not. Antiendothelial antibodies have been linked to spontaneous abortion in MCTD.[97] A single case of neonatal "lupus" has been reported, suggesting a pathogenic role for the transplacental passage of anti-U1-RNP antibodies.[98]

Juvenile Mixed Connective Tissue Disease

MCTD may first become apparent in childhood. The average age of onset in one report was 10.7 years.[99] Polyarthritis and Raynaud's phenomena are the most common presenting features. There tends to be a progression of organ involvement with 20% involvement at 5 years and 48% at 10 years. Significant myocarditis, glomerulonephritis, thrombocytopenia, seizures, hemolytic uremic syndrome, an acute coronary syndrome, and aseptic meningitis have been described in isolated cases.

MANAGEMENT OF CONNECTIVE TISSUE DISEASE OVERLAPS

The rational management of overlap CTDs is confounded by the absence of controlled trials. Recommendations for management are based on conventional treatments for SLE, PM/DM, RA, and Scl.[100] General guidelines for treating specific features of the overlap CTDs are given in Table 86-6. Nearly all patients with CTDs experience Raynaud's phenomenon. Apart from advice on minimizing cold exposure, most patients should be tried on calcium channel blockers (e.g., nifedipine). The use of topical nitrates, endothelin antagonists (e.g., bosentan), phosphodiesterase-5

inhibitors (e.g., tadalafil), and prostaglandin analogues (e.g., iloprost) should be considered in severe refractory cases.[101] Pulmonary hypertension is the main cause of death in MCTD, and patients should be evaluated at regular intervals for the development of this complication because early intervention is the key to effective management. Recent advances in the treatment of pulmonary hypertension have led to reduced morbidity and mortality.[77] Overall effective management requires anticoagulation and vasodilator therapy such as calcium channel blockers or prostacyclin analogues. Long-term treatment with intravenous epoprostenol or prostacyclin improves exercise capacity, hemodynamics, and survival in many patients,[102] as does therapy with inhaled iloprost.[103] Evidence indicates that some patients respond to a regimen of intravenous cyclophosphamide and corticosteroids.[104] Bosentan, an oral endothelin-1 antagonist, has been reported to improve dyspnea and slow PAH progression in MCTD.[105]

The management of overlap syndromes has not been the subject of controlled trials. Therefore management is based on an analysis of the clinical features and the application of management strategies used in the usual treatment of presenting features in terms of inflammatory arthritis, Raynaud's, inflammatory muscle disease, serositis, interstitial lung disease, pulmonary hypertension, and the gastrointestinal features of scleroderma. By definition, the clinical features of an overlap syndrome will be quite diverse and often change over time. Thus a constant reappraisal of management strategies is necessary at each patient visit.

Many of the problems causing morbidity in overlap syndromes tend to be intermittent and responsive to corticosteroids (e.g., aseptic meningitis, myositis, pleurisy, pericarditis, and myocarditis). On the other hand, nephrotic syndrome, Raynaud's phenomenon, deforming arthropathy, acrosclerosis, and peripheral neuropathies are usually steroid resistant. Many of the scleroderma-like gastrointestinal problems can be managed according to the usual practice in scleroderma such as management of renal crisis with angiotensin-converting enzyme inhibitors, Raynaud's phenomenon with calcium channel blockers, and gastrointestinal reflux disease with proton pump inhibitors.[101] Fibrotic lung disease is notoriously resistant to corticosteroids and immunosuppressives; there is some evidence that a new class of drugs, the tyrosine kinase inhibitors (e.g., imatinib), may be effective in some patients.[106]

In patients with steroid-resistant thrombocytopenia, refractory myositis, or hemolytic anemia, it is worth considering the use of intravenous gammaglobulin[107] or danazol.[108]

Successful autologous peripheral blood stem cell transplantation has been reported in a patient with refractory myositis and MCTD.[109] Over the long term, concern usually mounts over the total corticosteroid burden and the possibility of inducing an iatrogenic steroid myopathy, nosocomial infection, aseptic necrosis of bone, or accelerated osteoporosis. Routine evaluation of bone mineral density is warranted to detect early presymptomatic osteoporosis and initiation of therapy with antiresorptive agents. Unless contraindicated, all patients should take supplementary calcium and vitamin D. In patients requiring long-term corticosteroids it would seem reasonable to use antimalarials[110] or methotrexate[111] in an attempt to minimize the cumulative

Table 86-6 Guidelines for Managing Overlap Syndromes

Problems	Treatments
Fatigue, arthralgias, myalgias	NSAIDs, antimalarials, low-dose prednisone (<10 mg/day); trial use of modafinil
Arthritis	NSAIDs, antimalarials, methotrexate. Consider TNF inhibition[a]
Raynaud's phenomenon	Keep warm, avoid finger trauma, avoid β-blockers, stop smoking; dihydropyridine calcium channel blocker (e.g., nifedipine); α-sympatholytic (e.g., prazosin); consider endothelin receptor antagonist (e.g., bosentan) in recalcitrant cases
Acute-onset digital gangrene	Local chemical sympathectomy (infiltration of lidocaine at base of involved digit), anticoagulation, topical nitrates; consider hospitalization for intra-arterial prostacyclin; start endothelin receptor antagonist therapy
Pleurisy	NSAID or short course of prednisone (≈20 mg/day)
Pericarditis	NSAID or short course of prednisone (≈20 mg/day); tamponade will require percutaneous or surgical drainage
Aseptic meningitis	Discontinue NSAIDs[b] and give short course of high-dose prednisone, about 60 mg/day
Myositis	Acute onset, severe: prednisone 60-100 mg/day Chronic, low grade: prednisone, 10-30 mg/day[c] Consider methotrexate and/or IVIG in recalcitrant cases
Membranous glomerulonephropathy	Mild: no treatment required Progressive proteinuria: trial of ACE inhibitor; trial of low-dose aspirin combined with dipyridamole Severe: trial of prednisone 15-60 mg/day plus monthly pulse cyclophosphamide or daily chlorambucil
Nephrotic syndrome	Steroids alone are seldom effective. Low-dose aspirin combined with dipyridamole to prevent thrombotic complications; ACE inhibitor to reduce protein loss; trial of prednisone 15-60 mg/day plus monthly pulse cyclophosphamide or daily chlorambucil; dialysis or transplantation may be required
Scleroderma-like renal crisis	ACE inhibitor
Myocarditis	Trial of steroids and cyclophosphamide[d]; avoid digoxin[e]
Incomplete heart block	Avoid chloroquine[f]
Asymptomatic pulmonary hypertension	Trial of steroids and cyclophosphamide, low-dose aspirin and ACE inhibitors; consider endothelin receptor antagonist (oral bosentan)
Symptomatic pulmonary hypertension	Intravenous prostacyclin, ACE inhibitors, anticoagulation, endothelin receptor antagonist (oral bosentan); trial of sildenafil; heart-lung transplantation
Vascular headache	Trial of propranolol and/or alternate-day aspirin, 350 mg Symptomatic use of a triptan (e.g., sumatriptin, eletriptan)
Autoimmune anemia/thrombocytopenia	High-dose steroids (≈prednisone 80 mg/day) with taper dependent on clinical course. Consider danazol, IVIG, and immunosuppression in recalcitrant cases
Thrombotic thrombocytopenic purpura	Immediate infusion of fresh-frozen plasma; may require plasma exchange and transfusion of platelet-depleted RBCs; consider splenectomy in recalcitrant cases
Dysphagia	Mild: no treatment With reflux: proton pump inhibitor; consider Nissen fundoplication Severe: calcium channel antagonist, alone or in combination with an anticholinergic agent
Intestinal dysmotility	Prokinetic agents such as metoclopramide and erythromycin Small bowel bacterial overgrowth: tetracycline, erythromycin
Osteoporosis	Ca/Vit D supplements, estrogen replacement or raloxifene; bisphosphonates[g]; nasal calcitonin; carboxyl-truncated PTH analogues such as hPTH-(1-34).
Heartburn/Dyspepsia	Raise head of bed, discontinue smoking, lose weight and avoid caffeine; H_2 antagonists, H^+ proton pump blockers; trial of metoclopramide; consider *Helicobacter pylori* infection in recalcitrant cases
Trigeminal neuropathy	No effective therapy for numbness; trial of an antiepileptic (e.g., gabapentin) or tricyclic antidepressant (e.g., nortryptiline) for pain

[a]Has been associated with flares in MCTD and SLE.
[b]Sulindac and ibuprofen have been associated with a hypersensitivity aseptic meningitis.
[c]Remain alert for steroid myopathy, aseptic necrosis of bone, and accelerated osteoporosis.
[d]Cardiotoxic at high doses.
[e]Predisposes to ventricular arrhythmias.
[f]Predisposes to complete heart block.
[g]Cannot be used if esophagus is more than mildly involved.
ACE, angiotensin-converting enzyme; IVIG, intravenous immunoglobulin; NSAID, nonsteroidal anti-inflammatory drug; PTH, parathyroid hormone; RBC, red blood cell; TNF, tumor necrosis factor.

steroid burden. Antimalarials should be used with caution in overlap patients with a fascicular or bundle branch block due to the risk of causing a complete heart block[112] or an idiosyncratic hepatitis.[113] Digitalis is relatively contraindicated in patients with myocarditis due to the risk of inducing ventricular arrhythmias. As in SLE, the tumor necrosis factor inhibitor etanercept has been reported to exacerbate MCTD.[114] Rituximab has been beneficial in some patients with severe refractory antisynthetase syndrome.[115] Patients with severe hand deformities may be helped by soft tissue release operations and selected joint fusions.

The management of pregnancy presents several special problems in patients with overlap CTDs. Doria and colleagues[116] have provided the following general advice:

1. Patients should be correctly informed about the risk of becoming pregnant.

2. Pregnancies should be planned when the disease is in remission because it increases the probability of successful maternal and fetal outcome.

3. Patients should be regularly monitored during gestation and postpartum by a multidisciplinary team including a rheumatologist, an obstetrician, and a neonatologist.

4. In the case of disease relapse an adequate treatment, even aggressive if necessary, should be recommended because active disease can be more detrimental for a fetus than drugs.

There is often a tendency to assume that all patients with overlap CTDs should be on long-term corticosteroids; this mistake is compounded by the assumption that all medical problems in these patients are related to their underlying overlap CTDs. For instance, apparent flares of discomfort and pain in overlap CTDs may be due to myofascial pain syndrome or fibromyalgia and are thus unresponsive to corticosteroids. Likewise, the feeling of malaise and easy fatigability may be related to a reactive depression or the fact that the patient has become deconditioned. Premature atherosclerosis is now well recognized as a cause of increased morbidity and mortality in AICTDs,[117] and all patients with overlap syndromes need ongoing evaluation for risk factors and appropriate advice and therapy for hypertension and hyperlipidemia. The management of patients with overlap CTDs requires continuing reassessment of an ever-changing pattern of clinical problems and a constant alertness to the iatrogenic disease. As with any disease of unknown etiology, effective management of patients with the overlap CTDs presents a constant and ever-evolving challenge.

OUTCOME

The prognosis for overlap syndromes is often better than the classic AICTDs. For instance, Troyanov reported on the follow-up of 100 patients with idiopathic inflammatory myopathy. It was found that the long-term course after treatment with prednisone, with a dose/duration that initially resulted in good symptomatic improvement, was strikingly different; all PM patients (100%) and most DM patients (92%) progressed to chronic myositis, whereas only 58% of overlap patients developed persistent muscle disease.[4] The tendency for overlap patients to develop chronic disease was more common in those with antisynthetase and nucleoporin antibodies and less with antibodies to U1-RNP, PM/Scl, or Ku. Patients with three or four U1 snRNP antibodies (i.e., anti-70 kD, anti-A, anti-C, and anti-U1 snRNA) tended to have minimal renal disease compared with patients with just one or two reactivities.[118] Antibodies to 155-kD and 140-kD proteins in myositis are a risk factor for the development of cancer.[119] There is unequivocal evidence that patients with high-titer U1-RNP antibodies have a low prevalence of serious renal disease and life-threatening neurologic problems; in this sense MCTD can be favorably compared with classic SLE. However, not all patients with MCTD have a favorable prognosis and death may occur from progressive pulmonary hypertension and its cardiac sequelae. A 38-year follow-up of 47 MCTD patients at the University of Missouri reported a favorable course in 62% and continuing active disease in 38%. Eleven (23%) patients had a fatal outcome related to pulmonary hypertension in nine patients and two deaths unrelated to MCTD.[120] It is evident that the course of overlap syndromes is unpredictable; many patients do follow a relatively benign course, but it is major organ involvement that ultimately dictates the morbidity and mortality of the disease.

References

1. LeRoy EC, Maricq H, Kahaleh M: Undifferentiated connective tissue syndrome, *Arthritis Rheum* 23:341–343, 1980.
2. Rahman A, Stollar BD: Origin and structure of autoantibodies and antigens in autoimmune rheumatic diseases, *Lupus* 17(3):232–235, 2008.
3. Gaubitz M: Epidemiology of connective tissue disorders, *Rheumatology (Oxford)* 45(Suppl 3):iii3–iii4, 2006.
4. Troyanov Y, Targoff IN, Tremblay JL, et al: Novel classification of idiopathic inflammatory myopathies based on overlap syndrome features and autoantibodies: analysis of 100 French Canadian patients, *Medicine (Baltimore)* 84(4):231–249, 2005.
5. Winfield JB, Koffler D, Kunkel HG: Development of antibodies to ribonucleoprotein following short term therapy with procainamide, *Arthritis Rheum* 18:531, 1975.
6. Kattah NH, Kattah MG, Utz PJ: The U1-snRNP complex: structural properties relating to autoimmune pathogenesis in rheumatic diseases, *Immunol Rev* 233(1):126–145, 2010.
7. McClain MT, Ramsland PA, Kaufman KM, James JA: Anti-sm autoantibodies in systemic lupus target highly basic surface structures of complexed spliceosomal autoantigens, *J Immunol* 168(4):2054–2062, 2002.
8. Hoffman RW, Maldonado ME: Immune pathogenesis of mixed connective tissue disease: a short analytical review, *Clin Immunol* 128(1):8–17, 2008.
9. Pomeranz Krummel DA, Oubridge C, Leung AK, et al: Crystal structure of human spliceosomal U1 snRNP at 5.5 A resolution, *Nature* 458(7237):475–480, 2009.
10. Steiner G, Skriner K, Hassfeld W, Smolen JS: Clinical and immunological aspects of autoantibodies to RA33/hnRNP-A/B proteins—a link between RA, SLE and MCTD, *Mol Biol Rep* 23(3-4):167–171, 1996.
11. Hassfeld W, Steiner G, Graninger W, et al: Autoantibody to the nuclear antigen RA33: a marker for early rheumatoid arthritis, *Br J Rheumatol* 32(3):199–203, 1993.
12. Radic M, Marion T, Monestier M: Nucleosomes are exposed at the cell surface in apoptosis, *J Immunol* 172(11):6692–6700, 2004.
13. Amoura Z, Koutouzov S, Chabre H, et al: Presence of antinucleosome autoantibodies in a restricted set of connective tissue diseases: antinucleosome antibodies of the IgG3 subclass are markers of renal pathogenicity in systemic lupus erythematosus, *Arthritis Rheum* 43(1):76–84, 2000.
14. Majetschak M, Perez M, Sorell LT, et al: Circulating 20S proteasome levels in patients with mixed connective tissue disease and systemic lupus erythematosus, *Clin Vaccine Immunol* 15(9):1489–1493, 2008.
15. Deshmukh US, Bagavant H, Lewis J, et al: Epitope spreading within lupus-associated ribonucleoprotein antigens, *Clin Immunol* 117(2): 112–120, 2005.
16. Monneaux F, Muller S: Key sequences involved in the spreading of the systemic autoimmune response to spliceosomal proteins, *Scand J Immunol* 54(1-2):45–54, 2001.
17. Genth E, Zarnowski H, Mierau R, et al: HLA-DR4 and Gm(1,3;5,21) are associated with U1-nRNP antibody positive connective tissue disease, *Ann Rheum Dis* 46:189–196, 1987.
18. Greidinger EL, Zang YJ, Jaimes K, et al: CD4+ T cells target epitopes residing within the RNA-binding domain of the U1-70-kDa small nuclear ribonucleoprotein autoantigen and have restricted TCR diversity in an HLA-DR4-transgenic murine model of mixed connective tissue disease, *J Immunol* 180(12):8444–8454, 2008.
19. Merryman PF, Crapper RM, Lee S, et al: Class II major histocompatibility complex gene sequences in rheumatoid arthritis: the third diversity region of both DR beta 1 and DR beta 2 genes in two DR1, DRw10-positive individuals specify the same inferred amino acid sequence as the DR beta 1 and DR beta 2 genes of a DR4(Dw14) haplotype, *Arthritis Rheum* 32:251–258, 1989.

20. James JA, Scofield RH, Harley JB: Basic amino acids predominate in the sequential autoantigenic determinants of the small nuclear 70K ribonucleoprotein, *Scand J Immunol* 39:557–566, 1994.

21. Barakat S, Briand JP, Abuaf N, et al: Mapping of epitopes on U1 snRNP polypeptide A with synthetic peptides and autoimmune sera, *Clin Exp Immunol* 86:71–78, 1991.

22. Hassfeld W, Steiner G, Studnicka-Benke A, et al: Autoimmune response to the spliceosome. An immunologic link between rheumatoid arthritis, mixed connective tissue disease, and systemic lupus erythematosus, *Arthritis Rheum* 38(6):777–785, 1995.

23. Mahoney JA, Rosen A: Apoptosis and autoimmunity, *Curr Opin Immunol* 17(6):583–588, 2005.

24. Mihara S, Suzuki N, Takeba Y, et al: Combination of molecular mimicry and aberrant autoantigen expression is important for development of anti-Fas ligand autoantibodies in patients with systemic lupus erythematosus, *Clin Exp Immunol* 129(2):359–369, 2002.

25. Casciola-Rosen LA, Anhalt G, Rosen A: Autoantigens targeted in systemic lupus erythematosus are clustered in two populations of surface structures on apoptotic keratinocytes, *J Exp Med* 179(4):1317–1330, 1994.

26. Hof D, Cheung K, de Rooij DJ, et al: Autoantibodies specific for apoptotic U1-70K are superior serological markers for mixed connective tissue disease, *Arthritis Res Ther* 7(2):R302–R309, 2005.

27. Wolfe F, Smythe HA, Yunus MB, et al: The American College of Rheumatology 1990 Criteria for the Classification of Fibromyalgia. Report of the Multicenter Criteria Committee, *Arthritis Rheum* 33(2):160–172, 1990.

28. Okano Y, Steen VD, Medsger TA Jr: Autoantibody reactive with RNA polymerase III in systemic sclerosis, *Ann Intern Med* 119:1005–1013, 1993.

29. Mosca M, Tani C, Neri C, et al: Undifferentiated connective tissue diseases (UCTD), *Autoimmun Rev* 6(1):1–4, 2006.

30. Vaz CC, Couto M, Medeiros D, et al: Undifferentiated connective tissue disease: a seven-center cross-sectional study of 184 patients, *Clin Rheumatol* 28(8):915–921, 2009.

31. Bodolay E, Csiki Z, Szekanecz Z, et al: Five-year follow-up of 665 Hungarian patients with undifferentiated connective tissue disease (UCTD), *Clin Exp Rheumatol* 21(3):313–320, 2003.

32. Smith V, De Keyser F, Pizzorni C, et al: Nailfold capillaroscopy for day-to-day clinical use: construction of a simple scoring modality as a clinical prognostic index for digital trophic lesions, *Ann Rheum Dis* 70(1):180–183, 2011.

33. Zold E, Szodoray P, Gaal J, et al: Vitamin D deficiency in undifferentiated connective tissue disease, *Arthritis Res Ther* 10(5):R123, 2008.

34. Pope JE: Scleroderma overlap syndromes, *Curr Opin Rheumatol* 14(6):704–710, 2002.

35. Steen VD: Autoantibodies in systemic sclerosis, *Semin Arthritis Rheum* 35(1):35–42, 2005.

36. Hunzelmann N, Genth E, Krieg T, et al: The registry of the German Network for Systemic Scleroderma: frequency of disease subsets and patterns of organ involvement, *Rheumatology (Oxford)* 47(8):1185–1192, 2008.

37. Ho KT, Reveille JD: The clinical relevance of autoantibodies in scleroderma, *Arthritis Res Ther* 5(2):80–93, 2003.

38. Hanke K, Bruckner CS, Dahnrich C, et al: Antibodies against PM/Scl-75 and PM/Scl-100 are independent markers for different subsets of systemic sclerosis patients, *Arthritis Res Ther* 11(1):R22, 2009.

39. Zimmermann C, Steiner G, Skriner K, et al: The concurrence of rheumatoid arthritis and limited systemic sclerosis: clinical and serologic characteristics of an overlap syndrome, *Arthritis Rheum* 41(11):1938–1945, 1998.

40. Akimoto S, Ishikawa O, Muro Y, et al: Clinical and immunological characterization of patients with systemic sclerosis overlapping primary biliary cirrhosis: a comparison with patients with systemic sclerosis alone, *J Dermatol* 26(1):18–22, 1999.

41. Jablonska S, Blaszczyk M: Scleroderma overlap syndromes, *Adv Exp Med Biol* 455:85–92, 1999.

42. Chen AY, Zirwas MJ, Heffernan MP: Nephrogenic systemic fibrosis: a review, *J Drugs Dermatol* 9(7):829–834, 2010.

43. Bischoff L, Derk CT: Eosinophilic fasciitis: demographics, disease pattern and response to treatment: report of 12 cases and review of the literature, *Int J Dermatol* 47(1):29–35, 2008.

44. Boin F, Hummers LK: Scleroderma-like fibrosing disorders, *Rheum Dis Clin North Am* 34(1):199–220, 2008.

45. Beers WH, Ince A, Moore TL: Scleredema adultorum of Buschke: a case report and review of the literature, *Semin Arthritis Rheum* 35(6):355–359, 2006.

46. Ghirardello A, Zampieri S, Tarricone E, et al: Clinical implications of autoantibody screening in patients with autoimmune myositis, *Autoimmunity* 39(3):217–221, 2006.

47. Dugar M, Cox S, Limaye V, et al: Clinical heterogeneity and prognostic features of South Australian patients with anti-synthetase autoantibodies, *Intern Med J* 41:674–679, 2010.

48. Marguerie C, Bunn CC, Beynon HL, et al: Polymyositis, pulmonary fibrosis and autoantibodies to aminoacyl-tRNA synthetase enzymes, *Q J Med* 77(282):1019–1038, 1990.

49. Mumm GE, McKown KM, Bell CL: Antisynthetase syndrome presenting as rheumatoid-like polyarthritis, *J Clin Rheumatol* 16(7):307–312, 2010.

50. Bennett RM: Overlap syndromes. In: Firestein GS, Budd RC, Harris ED Jr, et al, editors: *Textbook of rheumatology*, ed 8, Philadelphia, 2009, WB Saunders, pp 1381–1399.

51. Takada T, Hirakata M, Suwa A, et al: Clinical and histopathological features of myopathies in Japanese patients with anti-SRP autoantibodies, *Mod Rheumatol* 19(2):156–164, 2009.

52. Bohan A, Peter JB, Bowman RL, Pearson CM: Computer-assisted analysis of 153 patients with polymyositis and dermatomyositis, *Medicine (Baltimore)* 56(4):255–286, 1977.

53. Chen YJ, Wu CY, Huang YL, et al: Cancer risks of dermatomyositis and polymyositis: a nationwide cohort study in Taiwan, *Arthritis Res Ther* 12(2):R70, 2010.

54. Chinoy H, Payne D, Poulton KV, et al: HLA-DPB1 associations differ between DRB1*03 positive anti-Jo-1 and anti-PM-Scl antibody positive idiopathic inflammatory myopathy, *Rheumatology (Oxford)* 48(10):1213–1217, 2009.

55. Sharp GC, Irvin WS, LaRoque RL, et al: Association of autoantibodies to different nuclear antigens with clinical patterns of rheumatic disease and responsiveness to therapy, *J Clin Invest* 50:350–359, 1971.

56. Aringer M, Smolen JS: Mixed connective tissue disease: what is behind the curtain? *Best Pract Res Clin Rheumatol* 21(6):1037–1049, 2007.

57. Sharp GC, Irvin WS, Tan EM, et al: Mixed connective tissue disease: an apparently distinct rheumatic disease syndrome associated with a specific antibody to an extractable nuclear antigen, *Am J Med* 52:148–159, 1972.

58. Bennett RM: Mixed connective tissue disease and overlap syndromes. In: Harris ED, et al, editors: *Textbook of rheumatology*, ed 7, Philadelphia, 2004, WB Saunders, pp 1241–1529.

59. Alarcon-Segovia D, Cardiel MH: Comparison between 3 diagnostic criteria for mixed connective tissue disease. Study of 593 patients, *J Rheumatol* 16(3):328–334, 1989.

60. Amigues JM, Cantagrel A, Abbal M, Mazieres B: Comparative study of 4 diagnosis criteria sets for mixed connective tissue disease in patients with anti-RNP antibodies. Autoimmunity Group of the Hospitals of Toulouse, *J Rheumatol* 23(12):2055–2062, 1996.

61. van den Hoogen FH, Spronk PE, Boerbooms AM, et al: Long-term follow-up of 46 patients with anti-(U1)snRNP antibodies, *Br J Rheumatol* 33:1117–1120, 1994.

62. Bennett RM, O'Connell DJ: Mixed connective tisssue disease: a clinicopathologic study of 20 cases, *Semin Arthritis Rheum* 10(1):25–51, 1980.

63. Pope JE: Other manifestations of mixed connective tissue disease, *Rheum Dis Clin North Am* 31(3):519–533, vii, 2005.

64. Bennett RM, O'Connell DJ: The arthritis of mixed connective tissue disease, *Ann Rheum Dis* 37(5):397–403, 1986.

65. Udoff EJ, Genant HK, Kozin F, Ginsberg M: Mixed connective tissue disease: the spectrum of radiographic manifestations, *Radiology* 124(3):613–618, 1977.

66. Grader-Beck T, Wigley FM: Raynaud's phenomenon in mixed connective tissue disease, *Rheum Dis Clin North Am* 31(3):465–481, 2005.

67. Vianna MA, Borges CT, Borba EF, et al: Myositis in mixed connective tissue disease: a unique syndrome characterized by immunohistopathologic elements of both polymyositis and dermatomyositis, *Arq Neuropsiquiatr* 62(4):923–934, 2004.

68. Lundberg IE: Cardiac involvement in autoimmune myositis and mixed connective tissue disease, *Lupus* 14(9):708–712, 2005.

69. Sullivan WD, Hurst DJ, Harmon CE, et al: A prospective evaluation emphasizing pulmonary involvement in patients with mixed connective tissue disease, *Medicine (Baltimore)* 63(2):92–107, 1984.

70. Wigley FM, Lima JA, Mayes M, et al: The prevalence of undiagnosed pulmonary arterial hypertension in subjects with connective tissue disease at the secondary health care level of community-based rheumatologists (the UNCOVER study), *Arthritis Rheum* 52(7):2125–2132, 2005.

71. Vegh J, Szodoray P, Kappelmayer J, et al: Clinical and immunoserological characteristics of mixed connective tissue disease associated with pulmonary arterial hypertension, *Scand J Immunol* 64(1):69–76, 2006.

72. Vegh J, Szodoray P, Kappelmayer J, et al: Clinical and immunoserological characteristics of mixed connective tissue disease associated with pulmonary arterial hypertension, *Scand J Immunol* 64(1):69–76, 2006.

73. Hant FN, Herpel LB, Silver RM: Pulmonary manifestations of scleroderma and mixed connective tissue disease, *Clin Chest Med* 31(3):433–449, 2010.

74. Bull TM, Fagan KA, Badesch DB: Pulmonary vascular manifestations of mixed connective tissue disease, *Rheum Dis Clin North Am* 31(3):451–464, vi, 2005.

75. Colin G, Nunes H, Hatron PY, et al: [Clinical study of interstitial lung disease in mixed connective tissue disease], *Rev Mal Respir* 27(3):238–246, 2010.

76. Vegh J, Szilasi M, Soos G, et al: [Interstitial lung disease in mixed connective tissue disease], *Orv Hetil* 146(48):2435–2443, 2005.

77. Coghlan JG, Pope J, Denton CP: Assessment of endpoints in pulmonary arterial hypertension associated with connective tissue disease, *Curr Opin Pulm Med* 16(Suppl 1):S27–S34, 2010.

78. Kitridou RC, Akmal M, Turkel SB, et al: Renal involvement in mixed connective tissue disease: a longitudinal clinicopathologic study, *Semin Arthritis Rheum* 16(2):135–145, 1986.

79. Bennett RM, Spargo BH: Immune complex nephropathy in mixed connective tissue disease, *Am J Med* 63(4):534–541, 1977.

80. Takahashi A, Abe K, Yokokawa J, et al: Clinical features of liver dysfunction in collagen diseases, *Hepatol Res* 40:1092–1097, 2010.

81. Bennett RM, Bong DM, Spargo BH: Neuropsychiatric problems in mixed connective tissue disease, *Am J Med* 65(6):955–962, 1986.

82. Hajas A, Szodoray P, Barath S, et al: Sensorineural hearing loss in patients with mixed connective tissue disease: immunological markers and cytokine levels, *J Rheumatol* 36(9):1930–1936, 2009.

83. Okada J, Hamana T, Kondo H: Anti-U1RNP antibody and aseptic meningitis in connective tissue diseases, *Scand J Rheumatol* 32(4):247–252, 2003.

84. Sato T, Fujii T, Yokoyama T, et al: Anti-U1 RNP antibodies in cerebrospinal fluid are associated with central neuropsychiatric manifestations in systemic lupus erythematosus and mixed connective tissue disease, *Arthritis Rheum* 62:3730–3740, 2010.

85. Schedel J, Kuchenbuch S, Schoelmerich J, et al: Cerebral lesions in patients with connective tissue diseases and systemic vasculitides: are there specific patterns? *Ann N Y Acad Sci* 1193(1):167–175, 2010.

86. Alpert MA, Goldberg SH, Singsen BH, et al: Cardiovascular manifestations of mixed connective tissue disease in adults, *Circulation* 68(6):1182–1193, 1983.

87. Maricq HR, LeRoy EC, D'Angelo WA, et al: Diagnostic potential of in vivo capillary microscopy in scleroderma and related disorders, *Arthritis Rheum* 23:183, 1980.

88. Schmidt WA, Krause A, Schicke B, Wernicke D: Color Doppler ultrasonography of hand and finger arteries to differentiate primary from secondary forms of Raynaud's phenomenon, *J Rheumatol* 35(8):1591–1598, 2008.

89. Lambova SN, Muller-Ladner U: The role of capillaroscopy in differentiation of primary and secondary Raynaud's phenomenon in rheumatic diseases: a review of the literature and two case reports, *Rheumatol Int* 29(11):1263–1271, 2009.

90. Peller JS, Gabor GT, Porter JM, Bennett RM: Angiographic findings in mixed connective tissue disease. Correlation with fingernail capillary photomicroscopy and digital photoplethysmography findings, *Arthritis Rheum* 28(7):768–774, 1985.

91. Soltesz P, Bereczki D, Szodoray P, et al: Endothelial cell markers reflecting endothelial cell dysfunction in patients with mixed connective tissue disease, *Arthritis Res Ther* 12(3):R86, 2010.

92. Segond P, Yeni P, Jacquot JM, Massias P: Severe autoimmune anemia and thrombopenia in mixed connective tissue disease, *Arthritis Rheum* 21:995, 1986.

93. Mimura Y, Ihn H, Jinnin M, et al: Rheumatoid factor isotypes in mixed connective tissue disease, *Clin Rheumatol* 25(4):572–574, 2006.

94. Komatireddy GR, Wang GS, Sharp GC, Hoffman RW: Antiphospholipid antibodies among anti-U1-70 kDa autoantibody positive patients with mixed connective tissue disease, *J Rheumatol* 24(2):319–322, 1997.

95. Kitridou RC: Pregnancy in mixed connective tissue disease, *Rheum Dis Clin North Am* 31(3):497–508, vii, 2005.

96. Kaufman RL, Kitridou RC: Pregnancy in mixed connective tissue disease: comparison with systemic lupus erythematosus, *J Rheumatol* 9(4):549–555, 1982.

97. Bodolay E, Bojan F, Szegedi G, et al: Cytotoxic endothelial cell antibodies in mixed connective tissue disease, *Immunol Lett* 20(2):163–167, 1989.

98. Fujiwaki T, Urashima R, Urushidani Y, et al: Neonatal lupus erythematosus associated with maternal mixed connective tissue disease, *Pediatr Int* 45(2):210–213, 2003.

99. Tsai YY, Yang YH, Yu HH, et al: Fifteen-year experience of pediatric-onset mixed connective tissue disease, *Clin Rheumatol* 29(1):53–58, 2010.

100. Kim P, Grossman JM: Treatment of mixed connective tissue disease, *Rheum Dis Clin North Am* 31(3):549–565, viii, 2005.

101. Levien TL: Advances in the treatment of Raynaud's phenomenon, *Vasc Health Risk Manag* 6:167–177, 2010.

102. Galie N, Manes A, Branzi A: Medical therapy of pulmonary hypertension. The prostacyclins, *Clin Chest Med* 22(3):529–537, x, 2001.

103. Vegh J, Soos G, Csipo I, et al: Pulmonary arterial hypertension in mixed connective tissue disease: successful treatment with Iloprost, *Rheumatol Int* 26(3):264–269, 2006.

104. Sanchez O, Sitbon O, Jais X, et al: Immunosuppressive therapy in connective tissue diseases-associated pulmonary arterial hypertension, *Chest* 130(1):182–189, 2006.

105. Naclerio C, D'Angelo S, Baldi S, et al: Efficacy of bosentan in the treatment of a patient with mixed connective tissue disease complicated by pulmonary arterial hypertension, *Clin Rheumatol* 29:687–690, 2009.

106. Distler JH, Distler O: Tyrosine kinase inhibitors for the treatment of fibrotic diseases such as systemic sclerosis: towards molecular targeted therapies, *Ann Rheum Dis* 69(Suppl 1):i48–i51, 2010.

107. Godeau B, Chevret S, Varet B, et al: Intravenous immunoglobulin or high-dose methylprednisolone, with or without oral prednisone, for adults with untreated severe autoimmune thrombocytopenic purpura: a randomised, multicentre trial, *Lancet* 359(9300):23–29, 2002.

108. Blanco R, Martinez-Taboada VM, Rodriguez-Valverde V, et al: Successful therapy with danazol in refractory autoimmune thrombocytopenia associated with rheumatic diseases, *Br J Rheumatol* 36(10):1095–1099, 1997.

109. Myllykangas-Luosujarvi R, Jantunen E, Kaipiainen-Seppanen O, et al: Autologous peripheral blood stem cell transplantation in a patient with severe mixed connective tissue disease, *Scand J Rheumatol* 29(5):326–327, 2000.

110. Wallace DJ: Antimalarials—the 'real' advance in lupus, *Lupus* 10(6):385–387, 2001.

111. Sato EI: Methotrexate therapy in systemic lupus erythematosus, *Lupus* 10(3):162–164, 2001.

112. Nolan RJ, Shulman ST, Victorica BE: Congenital complete heart block associated with maternal mixed connective tissue disease, *J Pediatr* 95(3):420–422, 1979.

113. Giner Galvan V, Oltra MR, Rueda D, et al: Severe acute hepatitis related to hydroxychloroquine in a woman with mixed connective tissue disease, *Clin Rheumatol* 26(6):971–972, 2007.

114. Richez C, Blanco P, Dumoulin C, Schaeverbeke T: Lupus erythematosus manifestations exacerbated by etanercept therapy in a patient with mixed connective tissue disease, *Clin Exp Rheumatol* 23(2):273, 2005.

115. Sem M, Molberg O, Lund MB, Gran JT: Rituximab treatment of the anti-synthetase syndrome: a retrospective case series, *Rheumatology (Oxford)* 48(8):968–971, 2009.

116. Doria A, Iaccarino L, Ghirardello A, et al: Pregnancy in rare autoimmune rheumatic diseases: UCTD, MCTD, myositis, systemic vasculitis and Behçet disease, *Lupus* 13(9):690–695, 2004.

117. Hahn BH, Grossman J, Chen W, McMahon M: The pathogenesis of atherosclerosis in autoimmune rheumatic diseases: roles of inflammation and dyslipidemia, *J Autoimmun* 28(2-3):69–75, 2007.

118. Kaneko Y, Suwa A, Hirakata M, et al: Clinical associations with autoantibody reactivities to individual components of U1 small nuclear ribonucleoprotein, *Lupus* 19(3):307–312, 2010.

119. Chinoy H, Fertig N, Oddis CV, et al: The diagnostic utility of myositis autoantibody testing for predicting the risk of cancer-associated myositis, *Ann Rheum Dis* 66(10):1345–1349, 2007.

120. Burdt MA, Hoffman RW, Deutscher SL, et al: Long-term outcome in mixed connective tissue disease: longitudinal clinical and serologic findings, *Arthritis Rheum* 42(5):899–909, 1999.

The references for this chapter can also be found on www.expertconsult.com.

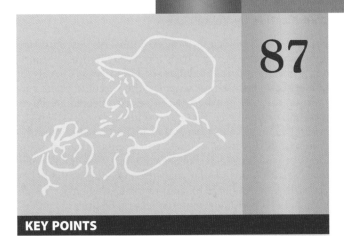

87

Classification and Epidemiology of Systemic Vasculitis

JOHN H. STONE

CLASSIFICATION

Few disorders in medicine are more challenging in diagnosis and treatment than the systemic vasculitides. These heterogeneous disorders are linked by the common finding of destructive inflammation within the walls of blood vessels. Current classification schemes recognize approximately 20 primary forms of vasculitis and several major categories of secondary vasculitis (e.g., other rheumatologic diseases, malignancy, infection) (Table 87-1). Over the past half century, numerous comprehensive classification schemes have been attempted.[1] No attempt has been entirely satisfactory because understanding of these conditions continues to evolve. All vasculitis classification schemes are works in progress, susceptible to change as new information emerges.

Current classification schemes are understood best in light of their nosologic predecessors. The first "modern" case of systemic vasculitis was recognized in the 1860s by Kussmaul and Maier.[2] That case, which involved medium-sized, muscular arteries, has served as the reference point for classifying many subsequently recognized forms of vasculitis. Because of the importance of that first report in the understanding and classification of vasculitis, the case is described in detail here.

First Modern Case: "Periarteritis Nodosa"

In 1866 Kussmaul and Maier reported the case of a 27-year-old tailor who died during a month-long hospital stay.[2,3] On presentation, the patient was strong enough to climb two flights of stairs to the clinic but "afterward felt so weak that he immediately had to go to bed." He complained of numbness on the volar aspect of his thumb and the two neighboring fingers on the right hand. Over the ensuing days, "the general weakness increased so rapidly that he was unable to leave the bed, [and] the feeling of numbness also appeared in the left hand." Muscle paralysis progressed quickly: "Before our eyes, a young man developed a general paralysis of the voluntary muscles ... [He] had to be fed by attendants, and within a few weeks was robbed of the use of most of his muscles."[2,3]

The patient's weakness, caused by vasculitic neuropathy (mononeuritis multiplex), was accompanied by tachycardia, abdominal pains, and the appearance of cutaneous nodules over his trunk. His death was described as follows: "He was scarcely able to speak, lay with persistent severe abdominal and muscle pains, opisthotonically stretched, whimpering, and begged the doctors not to leave him ... Death occurred ... at 2 o'clock in the morning." At autopsy, grossly visible nodules were present along the patient's medium-sized arteries. Kussmaul and Maier[2] suggested the name "periarteritis nodosa" for this disease because of the apparent localization of inflammation to the perivascular sheaths and outer layers of the arterial walls, leading to nodular thickening of the vessels. The name was later revised to polyarteritis nodosa (PAN), to reflect the widespread arterial involvement of this disease and the fact that inflammation in PAN extends through the entire thickness of the vessel wall.[4,5]

Polyarteritis Nodosa as a Reference Point

In addition to its status as the first form of vasculitis recognized, several features of PAN make it a logical reference

Table 87-1 Classification Scheme of Vasculitides According to Size of Predominant Blood Vessels Involved

Primary Vasculitides
Predominantly Large Vessel Vasculitides
Takayasu's arteritis
Giant cell arteritis (temporal arteritis)
Cogan's syndrome
Behçet's disease*
Predominantly Medium Vessel Vasculitides
Polyarteritis nodosa
Cutaneous polyarteritis nodosa
Buerger's disease
Kawasaki disease
Primary angiitis of the central nervous system
Predominantly Small Vessel Vasculitides
Immune complex mediated
Goodpasture's disease (anti–glomerular basement membrane disease)†
Cutaneous leukocytoclastic angiitis ("hypersensitivity vasculitis")
Henoch-Schönlein purpura
Hypocomplementemic urticarial vasculitis
Essential cryoglobulinemia‡
Erythema elevatum diutinum
ANCA-associated disorders§
Granulomatosis with polyangiitis (formerly Wegener's granulomatosis‡)
Microscopic polyangiitis‡
Churg-Strauss syndrome‡
Renal-limited vasculitis
Secondary Forms of Vasculitis
Miscellaneous Small Vessel Vasculitides
Connective tissue disorders‡ (rheumatoid vasculitis, lupus erythematosus, Sjögren's syndrome, inflammatory myopathies)
Inflammatory bowel disease
Paraneoplastic
Infection
Drug-induced vasculitis: ANCA-associated, other

*May involve small, medium, and large blood vessels.

  †Immune complexes formed in situ, in contrast to other forms of immune complex–mediated vasculitis.

  ‡Frequent overlap of small and medium blood vessel involvement.

  §Not all forms of these disorders are always associated with ANCA.
ANCA, antineutrophil cytoplasmic antibody.

point for the classification of inflammatory vascular disease. Other forms of vasculitis can usually be differentiated from PAN through their contrasts to one or more of the following PAN characteristics:

- The general confinement of the disease to medium-sized vessels* as opposed to capillaries and postcapillary venules (small vessels) and the aorta and its major branches (large vessels)
- The exclusive involvement of arteries, with sparing of veins
- The tendency to form microaneurysms
- The absence of lung involvement
- The lack of granulomatous inflammation
- The absence of associated autoantibodies (e.g., antineutrophil cytoplasmic antibodies [ANCAs],

---

*The fact of vessel size overlap in vasculitis syndromes is acknowledged and discussed subsequently.

anti–glomerular basement membrane [anti-GBM] antibodies, or rheumatoid factor)
- The association of some cases with hepatitis B virus (HBV) infection

Classification by Vessel Size

Because the etiologies of most forms of vasculitis are unknown, the most valid basis for classifying the vasculitides is the size of the predominant blood vessels involved. Under such classification schemes, the vasculitides are categorized initially by whether the vessels affected are large, medium, or small (see Table 87-1 and Figure 87-1). "Large" generally denotes the aorta and its major branches (and the corresponding vessels in the venous circulation in some forms of vasculitis, e.g., Behçet's disease). "Medium" refers to vessels that are smaller than the major aortic branches yet still large enough to contain four elements: (1) an intima, (2) a continuous internal elastic lamina, (3) a muscular media, and (4) an adventitia. In clinical terms, medium vessel vasculitis (see Table 87-1) is generally macrovascular (i.e., involves vessels large enough to be observed in gross pathologic specimens or visualized by angiography). "Small vessel" vasculitis, which incorporates all vessels below macroscopic disease, includes capillaries, postcapillary venules, and arterioles. Such vessels all are typically less than 500 μm in outer diameter. Because glomeruli may be viewed simply as differentiated capillaries, forms of vasculitis that cause glomerulonephritis are considered to be small vessel vasculitides. Table 87-2 presents the typical clinical manifestations associated with small, medium, and large vessel vasculitides.

All discussions of vasculitis classification schemes involving vessel size must acknowledge the frequent occurrence of overlap. Although PAN primarily involves medium-sized arteries, palpable purpura—a manifestation of small vessel disease—is observed in some cases. Despite the possibility of vessel size overlap within individual cases, the categorization of a patient's vasculitis as primarily large, medium, or small vessel in nature remains enormously useful in focusing the differential diagnosis and initiating plans for treatment.

Additional Considerations in Classification

Many other considerations are important in the classification of vasculitis (Table 87-3): (1) the patient's demographic profile (see Epidemiology section), (2) the disease's tropism for particular organs, (3) the presence or absence of granulomatous inflammation, (4) the participation of immune complexes in disease pathophysiology, (5) the finding of characteristic autoantibodies in the patients' serum (e.g., ANCAs, anti-GBM antibodies, or rheumatoid factor), and (6) the detection of certain infections known to cause specific forms of vasculitis.

The organ tropisms of these disorders are illustrated by the following examples. Granulomatosis with polyangiitis (formerly Wegener's granulomatosis) and herein abbreviated GPA, classically involves the kidneys, upper airways, and lungs. In contrast, Henoch-Schönlein purpura often affects the kidneys, but never the nose or sinuses and almost never the lungs. In contrast to both of these forms of

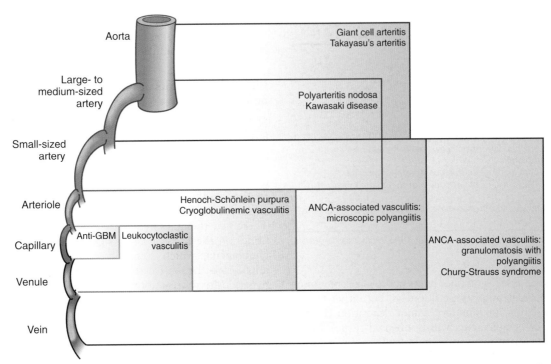

Figure 87-1 Classification by blood vessel size. ANCA, antineutrophil cytoplasmic antibody; GBM, glomerular basement membrane.

vasculitis, Cogan's syndrome is defined by the simultaneous occurrence of ocular inflammation (most often interstitial keratitis) and sensorineural hearing loss (and, in 10% of cases, a large vessel vasculitis). The histopathologic findings in these three disorders are equally distinctive, ranging from granulomatous inflammation of small to medium vessels (GPA), to IgA deposition in small vessels (Henoch-Schönlein purpura), to large vessel vasculitis centered on the adventitia (Cogan's syndrome).

The granulomatous features of some forms of vasculitis resemble chronic infections (e.g., infections caused by fungi or mycobacteria) or the inflammation induced by the presence of a foreign body. Granulomatous inflammation is more likely to be found in some organs (e.g., the lung) than in others (e.g., the kidney or skin). Some patients without evidence of granulomatous inflammation at early points in their courses later exhibit such features as their diseases unfold. Patients initially diagnosed with cutaneous leukocytoclastic angiitis or microscopic polyangiitis may be reclassified as having GPA if disease manifestations appear in new organs and granulomatous inflammation is found on biopsy specimens. Table 87-4 presents forms of vasculitis commonly associated with granulomatous inflammation.

Immune complexes are essential to the pathophysiology of some small and medium vessel vasculitides. Immune complex–mediated tissue injury does not produce a single clinical syndrome, but rather applies to many forms of vasculitis and overlaps with injuries caused by other immune mechanisms. Anti-GBM disease (Goodpasture's disease) is a unique form of immune complex disease in which the immune complexes form in situ rather than in the circulation.[6] Complexes of IgA1 are found in Henoch-Schönlein purpura. Immune complexes comprising IgG, IgM, complement components, and the hepatitis C virion characterize most cases of mixed cryoglobulinemia. HBV surface antigen/antibody complexes are present in the circulation and involved tissues of patients with HBV-associated PAN. Rheumatoid factor and complement proteins are found within organs involved by rheumatoid vasculitis.

In contrast, other small and medium vessel vasculitides such as GPA, microscopic polyangiitis, and Churg-Strauss syndrome are disorders associated with "pauci-immune"

Table 87-2 Typical Clinical Manifestations of Large, Medium, and Small Vessel Involvement by Vasculitis

Large	Medium	Small
Limb claudication	Cutaneous nodules	Purpura
Asymmetric blood pressures	Ulcers	Vesiculobullous lesions
Absence of pulses	Livedo reticularis	Urticaria
Bruits	Digital gangrene	Glomerulonephritis
Aortic dilation	Mononeuritis multiplex	Alveolar hemorrhage
Renovascular hypertension	Microaneurysms	Cutaneous extravascular necrotizing granulomas
	Renovascular hypertension	Splinter hemorrhages
		Uveitis/episcleritis/scleritis

Constitutional symptoms: fever, weight loss, malaise, arthralgias/arthritis (common to vasculitides of all vessel sizes)

Table 87-3 Considerations in the Classifications of Systemic Vasculitis

Size of predominant blood vessels affected
Epidemiologic features
Age
Gender
Ethnic background
Pattern of organ involvement
Pathologic features
Granulomatous inflammation
Immune complex deposition versus pauci-immune histopathology
Linear staining along glomerular basement membrane
Presence of ANCA, anti-GBM antibodies, or rheumatoid factor in serum
Demonstration of a specific associated infection (hepatitis B or hepatitis C)

ANCA, antineutrophil cytoplasmic antibody; GBM, glomerular basement membrane.

inflammation. "Pauci-immune" refers not to a lack of immunologic involvement in these disorders, but rather to the absence of significant immunoreactant deposition (immunoglobulin or complement) within diseased tissues. Many (but not all) patients with pauci-immune forms of vasculitis have ANCAs in their serum. Three decades before the description of ANCAs, Godman and Churg[7] observed pathologic links between these three entities, noting that the disorders "group themselves into a compass, [ranging from] necrotizing and granulomatous processes with angiitis, through mixed forms, to vasculitis without granulomata."

ANCAs (see Chapter 89) are directed against antigens that reside within the primary granules of neutrophils and monocytes.[8] Two types of ANCAs seem to be relevant to vasculitis: (1) ANCAs directed against proteinase-3 (PR3), a serine protease found within the primary granules of neutrophils and monocytes; and (2) ANCAs directed against myeloperoxidase and another serine protease found within the same granules. Although rigorous serologic assays for these antibodies are helpful in diagnosis, evidence for a primary etiologic role of these antibodies in human forms of pauci-immune vasculitis is still lacking. In contrast, anti-GBM antibodies have been proven to play a major role in the pathogenesis of Goodpastures's disease.[9] In RA, systemic rheumatoid vasculitis occurs only in patients who are rheumatoid factor positive. Rheumatoid factor is believed to play an essential role in the immune complex nature of that disease complication. Finally, although the causes of most forms of vasculitis are unknown, several infections have

Table 87-4 Forms of Vasculitis Associated with Granulomatous Inflammation

Giant cell arteritis
Takayasu's arteritis
Cogan's syndrome
Granulomatosis with polyangiitis
Churg-Strauss syndrome
Primary angiitis of the central nervous system*
Buerger's disease†
Rheumatoid vasculitis

*Sometimes granulomatous.
†Giant cells occur within inflammatory thrombi (and are diagnostic of Buerger's disease) but do not occur within the blood vessel wall.

been linked definitively with specific forms of these diseases (e.g., HBV with some cases of PAN, hepatitis C with type II mixed cryoglobulinemia).

Historical Attempts at Classification and Nomenclature

For decades after this initial description of vasculitis, most forms of systemic inflammatory vascular disease were termed *periarteritis nodosa*. In the 1900s, two major factors led to the recognition of new forms of vasculitis: (1) the use of microscopy in the evaluation of pathologic specimens became routine, and (2) horse serum and sulfonamides came to be employed in the treatment of many medical conditions. These new therapies frequently induced small vessel vasculitides on the basis of serum sickness or "hypersensitivity" phenomena, which were observed readily through the microscope. In some cases, the histopathologic findings of hypersensitivity reactions (e.g., serum sickness) were confused with periarteritis nodosa. The gradual recognition that these syndromes represented departures from PAN spurred interest in the first classification scheme for necrotizing angiitis.

In 1952 Zeek[10] identified five major categories of necrotizing angiitis. The Zeek classification included (1) hypersensitivity angiitis, (2) allergic granulomatous angiitis (Churg-Strauss syndrome), (3) rheumatic arteritis (vasculitis associated with fulminant rheumatic fever), (4) periarteritis nodosa, and (5) temporal arteritis. This classification scheme omitted several forms of systemic vasculitis that were known but not yet described in the English medical literature (e.g., GPA, Takayasu's arteritis).

Sources of Confusion in Classification

Two forms of vasculitis, now termed *microscopic polyangiitis* and *cutaneous leukocytoclastic angiitis*, have been consistent sources of confusion in vasculitis nosology. In the current understanding of systemic vasculitides, these two conditions are separate entities. Microscopic polyangiitis affects capillaries, veins, and arteries (in contrast to PAN) and is recognized to be a disorder associated with ANCAs in approximately 70% of cases.[11] In 1923 Wohlwill[12] observed unequivocal evidence of small vessel involvement in cases of vasculitis that he still considered part of the spectrum of "periarteritis nodosa." Davson and colleagues[13] remarked on two forms of "periarteritis nodosa" with differential effects on the kidney—one with a predilection for medium-sized, muscular arteries and the other with a predilection for small vessels including glomerulonephritis. Davson and colleagues[13] termed this latter form *microscopic periarteritis nodosa*. Swayed by human and animal models of hypersensitivity that showed small vessel disease involving the kidneys, lungs, and other organs,[14,15] Zeek chose to group microscopic periarteritis nodosa under the heading of *hypersensitivity vasculitis*.[10]

Over the next several decades, hypersensitivity vasculitis came to refer to an immune complex–mediated small vasculitis of the skin that spared internal organs and often followed drug exposures.[16] The Chapel Hill Consensus Conference (CHCC)[17] (see later) recommended eliminating the term *hypersensitivity* altogether because evidence for hypersensitivity is lacking in many cases. Participants in the CHCC preferred the term *cutaneous leukocytoclastic angiitis* because of the disorder's typical confinement to the skin and the usual predominant cell type—the neutrophil. Although cutaneous leukocytoclastic angiitis can mimic the skin features of microscopic polyangiitis, cutaneous leukocytoclastic angiitis does not involve the kidneys, lungs, peripheral nerves, and other internal organs and is not associated with ANCAs.

In 1990 the American College of Rheumatology (ACR) performed a study designed to establish criteria for the classification of vasculitis, through the identification of features that distinguished one form of vasculitis from others.[18,19] An important caveat: This study was *not* designed to establish criteria for diagnosis, but rather to facilitate research by permitting the inclusion of similar types of patients in studies. Patients with giant cell arteritis, Takayasu's arteritis, PAN, GPA, Churg-Strauss syndrome, Henoch-Schönlein purpura, and hypersensitivity vasculitis were included in this study.[16,20-25] The findings of the ACR study remain useful for the purposes of the study's original intention—the insurance of uniform inclusion criteria for patients in research studies. The passage of time and the development of new insights have shown the need for updates, however. First, because the study was performed before the days of reliable and widely available assays for ANCAs, ANCA positivity was not considered as a possible classification criterion. Second, the ACR classification criteria study did not include microscopic polyangiitis as a separate disease, but rather lumped such patients under the heading of PAN.[22] Third, the study did not define classification criteria for such rarer forms of vasculitis as Cogan's syndrome and Behçet's syndrome. As noted subsequently, Behçet's syndrome is rare in North America but not in countries bordering the Old Silk Route. Classification criteria for this disease have been defined.[26]

In 1994 the CHCC reviewed the nomenclature of systemic vasculitides. Formal diagnostic criteria were not attempted, but definitions were created for 10 forms of vasculitis (in addition to the 7 forms of vasculitis included in the ACR study, microscopic polyangiitis, Kawasaki disease, and "essential" cryoglobulinemic vasculitis were defined). The CHCC emphasized the important role that ANCAs play in the diagnosis of several forms of vasculitis and carefully distinguished microscopic polyangiitis from classic PAN. The conference defined classic PAN as necrotizing inflammation of medium-sized or small arteries without glomerulonephritis.[17] Microscopic polyangiitis was defined as a necrotizing vasculitis with few or no immune deposits that (1) affects small blood vessels (capillaries, venules, or arterioles), (2) often includes glomerulonephritis and pulmonary capillaritis, and (3) is often associated with either myeloperoxidase ANCAs or PR-3 ANCAs.

The classification of vasculitis continues to evolve. In the years since the CHCC, it has become clear that hepatitis C plays a major role in 90% of cases that formerly were termed *essential mixed cryoglobulinemia*. Some cases of this syndrome are not associated with hepatitis C infections, however, and probably have some other infectious etiology. Similarly, with the availability of the HBV vaccine, increasingly fewer cases of PAN are associated with this infection. Most PAN cases have no known cause. As emphasized by Churg,[27] cases of PAN currently termed *idiopathic* do not represent a single entity but almost certainly include several different disorders. Some of these, as indicated by low serum complement levels and measurable immune complexes in the blood, are mediated by immune complex deposition. Others seem to be independent of this mechanism. Finally, although *cutaneous leukocytoclastic angiitis* may be preferable to *hypersensitivity vasculitis* in describing small vessel vasculitis confined to the skin, the term fails to acknowledge the few cases in which lymphocytic infiltrates predominate and the nonspecific term "lymphocytic vasculitis" is used.

EPIDEMIOLOGY

Accurate definition of the epidemiology of vasculitis confronts several challenges, as follows: (1) the uncommon nature of many forms of vasculitis; (2) the frequent difficulties in making the correct diagnosis of vasculitis (and in distinguishing one form of vasculitis from another); (3) the fact that the etiologies of most types of vasculitis remain unknown; and (4) historical uncertainty with regard to the classification of these conditions. Nevertheless, in recent years, the epidemiology of some forms of vasculitis has been defined with reasonable precision. Table 87-5 presents the major epidemiologic features of several forms of systemic vasculitis.

Geography

The epidemiologic features of systemic vasculitis vary tremendously by geography. This variation may reflect

Table 87-5 Epidemiology of Selected Forms of Vasculitis

| Disease | Incidence | | Age/Gender/Ethnic Predispositions |
	United States	Elsewhere	
Giant cell arteritis	240/1 million	240/1 million (Scandinavia)	Age > 50, mean age 72; females 3:1/Northern European ancestry
Takayasu's arteritis	3/1 million	200-300/1 million (India)	Age <40; females 9:1/Asian
Behçet's disease	3/1 million	3000/1 million (Turkey)	Silk Route countries
Polyarteritis nodosa	7/1 million	7/1 million (Spain)	Slight male predominance
Kawasaki disease	100/1 million*	900/1 million (Japan)	Children of Asian ancestry
Granulomatosis with polyangiitis	4/1 million	8.5/1 million (United Kingdom)	Whites >> blacks
Henoch-Schönlein purpura	In children: 135-180/1 million; in adults: 13/1 million		Only 10% of cases occur in adults

*Among children younger than 5 years of age.
From Gonzalez-Gay MA, Garcia-Porrua C: Epidemiology of the vasculitides, *Rheum Dis Clin North Am* 27:729–750, 2001.

genetics, differences in environmental exposures dictated by continent and latitude, and the prevalence of other disease risk factors. Although Behçet's syndrome is rare in North Americans (affecting only approximately 1 in 300,000), the condition is perhaps several hundred times more common among inhabitants of countries that border the ancient Silk Route.[26,28] Similarly, although Takayasu's arteritis is rare in the United States—on the order of 3 new cases per 1 million people per year—the disease is reportedly the most common cause of renal artery stenosis in India, where the incidence may be 200 to 300 per million per year. Several studies indicate that the prevalence of giant cell arteritis in Olmsted County, Minnesota; is similar to that of Scandinavian countries, with an annual incidence rate of approximately 240 cases for every 1 million individuals older than age 50 years.[29] The similar prevalence calculations across these countries probably reflect shared genetic risk factors for this condition because many of the current inhabitants of Olmsted County are descended from Scandinavia and northern Europe. On the basis of 2010 U.S. Census data, the prevalence of giant cell arteritis in the United States is on the order of 200,000 cases.

Age, Gender, and Ethnicity

Age is an important consideration in the epidemiology of vasculitis. Of patients with Kawasaki disease, 80% are younger than age 5 years.[30] In contrast, giant cell arteritis virtually never occurs in patients younger than age 50, and the mean age of patients with that disease is 72. Age also may affect disease severity and outcome. In Henoch-Schönlein purpura, most cases in children (who comprise 90% of all cases) have self-limited courses, resolving within several weeks. In adults, Henoch-Schönlein purpura may have a higher likelihood of chronicity and a greater likelihood of a poor renal outcome.[31]

The distribution of gender varies across many forms of vasculitis. Buerger's disease is the only form of vasculitis with a striking male predominance. The predilection of this disease for men may be explained by the greater prevalence of smoking among men in most societies. In contrast, Takayasu's arteritis has an overwhelming tendency to occur in women (a 9:1 female-to-male ratio), a fact that presently has no explanation. Pauci-immune forms of vasculitis such as GPA occur in men and women with approximately equal frequencies, but there is some evidence for a female predominance in patients with the limited form of the disease and a male predominance among patients with severe GPA.[32]

For some forms of vasculitis, there are striking variations in tendencies to affect specific ethnic groups. Giant cell arteritis and GPA occur with an overwhelming predominance in whites.[33-35] Takayasu's arteritis and Kawasaki disease have higher incidences in patients of Asian ancestry.

Genes

Although genetic risk factors are undoubtedly important in the susceptibility to some forms of vasculitis, familial cases are rare (with the exception of giant cell arteritis; see later). The rarity of familial cases in vasculitis indicates that the genetics of these disorders are polygenic and complex. The

strongest link between any single gene and vasculitis is the association of HLA-B51 with Behçet's disease. In Behçet's disease, 80% of Asian patients have the *HLA-B51* gene.[28] The prevalence of *HLA-B51* is significantly higher among patients with Behçet's disease in Japan than among nondisease controls (55% vs. < 15%). Among the sporadic cases of Behçet's disease involving white patients in the United States, however, *HLA-B51* occurs in less than 15% of cases. In addition to increasing the risk of disease susceptibility in some patients, *HLA-B51* increases disease severity. Patients with this gene are more likely to have posterior uveitis, central nervous system involvement, or other severe manifestations.

Reports of familial aggregation in giant cell arteritis are common. Genetic studies have indicated roles for HLA class II alleles such as HLA-DRB1*0401 and HLA-DRB1*0101, albeit the specific associations have varied from study to study.[36,37] Other work indicates that certain tumor necrosis factor microsatellite polymorphisms may contribute to disease susceptibility.[38]

The greatest progress in understanding the relationship of genetics to systemic vasculitis has come in the area of rheumatoid vasculitis. The contribution of the "shared epitope" found on class II human leukocyte antigen (HLA) molecules (DR4) to the development of rheumatoid arthritis (RA) has been appreciated for 2 decades.[39] Possession of the shared epitope is now known to substantially increase the risk of extraarticular manifestations in RA including vasculitis, at least in Northern European populations. A gene dosage effect for extra-articular RA with severe organ manifestations has been noted; patients with two copies of shared epitope alleles have a substantially higher risk of extra-articular disease manifestations, many of which are mediated by vasculitis.[40] One study reported an association between rheumatoid vasculitis and 0401/0404.[41]

In a case-control study of patients with severe extra-articular RA compared with RA patients without extra-articular disease manifestations, the presence of two HLA-DRB1*04 alleles encoding the shared epitope was associated with extra-articular RA (odds ratio [OR], 1.79; 95% confidence interval [CI], 1.04 to 3.08) and rheumatoid vasculitis (OR, 2.44; 95% CI, 1.22 to 4.89).[42] In a meta-analysis of HLA-DRB1 genotyping studies of patients with rheumatoid vasculitis,[43] rheumatoid vasculitis was found to be associated with the genotypes 0401/0401, 0401/0404, and 0401/0101.

An association between rheumatoid vasculitis and class I HLA molecules has also been reported. An analysis of 159 patients with severe extra-articular RA (46 of whom had vasculitis) and 178 RA patients without extra-articular disease reported a strong association between the HLA-C3 allele and vasculitis.[44] Among vasculitis patients, the allele frequency of HLA-C3 was 0.411 compared with 0.199 in RA patients without extra-articular disease (P < .001). The odds ratio for vasculitis in patients with HLA-C3 was 4.15 (95% CI, 2.14 to 8.08).

The association between HLA-C3 and vasculitis was not due to linkage disequilibrium with HLA-DRB1, suggesting that these two genetic risk factors operate through different pathways. HLA-C3 was a strong predictor of vasculitis in patients lacking HLA-DRB1*04 shared epitope alleles, suggesting that HLA-C and HLA-DR genes influence the RA disease process through different pathways. Linkage disequilibrium with other genes in the major histocompatibility complex (MHC) could not be excluded in this study, however.

In GPA, the allele frequency of a functional polymorphism, 620W, in the intracellular tyrosine phosphatase gene *PTPN22* was found to be increased significantly among ANCA-positive patients compared with healthy controls.[45] Analyses of families with multiple autoimmune disorders have identified this allele as a risk factor for type 1 diabetes, seropositive RA, systemic lupus erythematosus, and autoimmune thyroid disease. In GPA, the allelic association was particularly strong among patients with generalized disease (i.e., vasculitis involving the kidney, lung, eye, and peripheral nervous system).

Study of the relationships between genes and systemic vasculitis is in its infancy. Substantial progress can be anticipated in this area in the future.

Environment

Several environmental and occupational exposures have been linked to the development of vasculitis. Medications and certain infections have well-known associations with vasculitides. As examples, antibiotics such as the penicillins and cephalosporins are common causes of hypersensitivity vasculitis (see Chapter 91), and virtually any medication can trigger this syndrome. Hepatitis B and C have well-recognized links to polyarteritis nodosa and mixed cryoglobulinemia, respectively. Moreover, both medications and infections can serve as triggers for Henoch-Schönlein purpura.

The strongest environmental exposure, now linked convincingly to Buerger's disease and to rheumatoid vasculitis, is cigarette smoking. Buerger's disease does not occur in the absence of cigarette smoking. The relationship between smoking and Buerger's disease is usually one of primary exposure (usually heavy), but cases related to second-hand smoke have been alleged.

In a case-control study of patients with recent-onset RA, the interactions among smoking, shared epitope genes, and antibodies to citrullinated proteins were studied.[46] A dose-dependent relationship between smoking and the occurrence of anti–cyclic citrullinated peptide antibodies was found. The presence of shared epitope genes was a risk factor for RA only among patients who were positive for anticyclic citrullinated protein. A major gene-environment interaction between smoking and HLA-DR SE genes was evident in the large subgroup of patients who possessed anticyclic citrullinated protein antibodies: The combination of smoking history and double copies of shared epitope alleles increased the risk of RA 21-fold. Smoking may trigger RA-specific immune reactions to citrullinated proteins in the context of shared epitope genes.

Associations have been reported, but not confirmed, between exposure to inhaled silica dust and some types of pauci-immune vasculitis.[47] Precise definitions of the relationships between exposures and vasculitis are complicated by difficulties in obtaining reliable measurements of the levels of such exposures, the likelihood of recall bias among patients who are diagnosed with vasculitis, and the choice of appropriate control groups.

Finally, estimates of disease prevalence in vasculitis may be subject to revision because of changing disease definitions. In the ACR classification criteria study, manifestations of small and medium vessel involvement were included in the criteria for PAN.[22] Four years later, the CHCC defined PAN as a form of arterial inflammation limited to medium-sized vessels, sparing capillaries, arterioles, and venules.[17] Under this definition, classic PAN is believed to be a rare condition. Applying the CHCC definition retrospectively, not a single case of classic PAN was reported over a 6-year period in the region of the Norwich Health Authority (United Kingdom), an area that included a population of more than 400,000.[48,49]

The epidemiologic differences among individual types of vasculitis raise compelling questions about the etiologies of these diseases. Ultimately, better insights into the pathogenesis of these conditions should explain these epidemiologic differences and facilitate the development of more refined classification schemes.

Relevant Websites

The Johns Hopkins Vasculitis Center: http://vasculitis.med.jhu.edu
The Cleveland Clinic Foundation Center for Vasculitis: www.clevelandclinic.org/arthritis/vasculitis/default.htm
The Vasculitis Foundation: www.vasculitisfoundation.org/
The Vasculitis Clinical Research Consortium: http://rarediseasesnetwork.epi.usf.edu/vcrc/
The National Institute of Allergy and Infectious Disease: http://www.niaid.nih.gov

References

1. Lie JT: Nomenclature and classification of vasculitis: plus ça change, plus c'est la même chose, *Arthritis Rheum* 37:181–186, 1994.
2. Kussmaul A, Maier R: Ueber eine bisher nicht beschriebene eigenthümliche Arterienerkrankung (Periarteritis nodosa), die mit morbus brightii und rapid fortschreitender allgemeiner muskellähmung einhergeht, *Dtsch Arch Klin Med* 1:484–518, 1866.
3. Matteson E: *Polyarteritis nodosa: commemorative translation on the 130-year anniversary of the original article by Adolf Kussmaul and Rudolf Maier*, Rochester Minn, 1996, Mayo Foundation.
4. Ferrari E: Ueber polyarteritis acuta nodosa (sogenannte periarteritis nodosa) und ihre beziehungen zur polymyositis und polyneuritis acuta, *Beitr Pathol Anat* 34:350–386, 1903.
5. Dickson W: Polyarteritis acuta nodosa and periarteritis nodosa, *J Pathol Bacterial* 12:31–57, 1908.
6. Salama AD, Pusey CD: Immunology of anti-glomerular basement membrane disease, *Curr Opin Nephrol Hypertension* 11:279–286, 2002.
7. Godman GC, Churg J: Wegener's granulomatosis: pathology and review of the literature, *Arch Pathol* 58:533–553, 1954.
8. Hoffman GS, Specks U: Antineutrophil cytoplasmic antibodies, *Arthritis Rheum* 41:1521–1537, 1998.
9. Salama AD, Levy JB, Lightstone L, et al: Goodpasture's disease, *Lancet* 358:917–920, 2001.
10. Zeek PM: Periarteritis nodosa: a critical review, *Am J Clin Pathol* 22:777–790, 1952.
11. Guillevin L, Durand-Gasselin B, Cevallos R, et al: Microscopic polyangiitis: clinical and laboratory findings in 85 patients, *Arthritis Rheum* 42:421–430, 1999.
12. Wohlwill F: On the only microscopically recognizable form of periarteritis nodosa, *Virchow's Archiv für pathologische Anatomie und Physiologie* 246:377–411, 1923.
13. Davson J, Ball J, Platt R: The kidney in periarteritis nodosa, *QJM* 17:175–192, 1948.
14. Rich AR: The role of hypersensitivity in periarteritis nodosa, *Bull Johns Hopkins Hosp* 71:123–140, 1942.
15. Zeek P, Smith C, Weeter J: Studies on periarteritis nodosa, III: the differentiation between the vascular lesions of periarteritis nodosa and hypersensitivity, *Am J Pathol* 24:889–917, 1948.

16. Calabrese LH, Michel BA, Bloch DA, et al: The American College of Rheumatology 1990 criteria for the classification of hypersensitivity vasculitis, *Arthritis Rheum* 33:1094–1100, 1990.

17. Jennette JC, Falk RJ, Andrassy K, et al: Nomenclature of systemic vasculitides: proposal of an international consensus conference, *Arthritis Rheum* 37:187–192, 1994.

18. Hunder GG, Arend WP, Bloch DA, et al: The American College of Rheumatology 1990 criteria for the classification of vasculitis: introduction, *Arthritis Rheum* 33:1065–1067, 1990.

19. Bloch DA, Michel BA, Hunder GG, et al: The American College of Rheumatology 1990 criteria for the classification of vasculitis: patients and methods, *Arthritis Rheum* 33:1068–1073, 1990.

20. Hunder GG, Bloch DA, Michel BA, et al: The American College of Rheumatology 1990 criteria for the classification of giant cell arteritis, *Arthritis Rheum* 33:1122–1128, 1990.

21. Arend WP, Michel BA, Bloch DA, et al: The American College of Rheumatology 1990 criteria for the classification of Takayasu's arteritis, *Arthritis Rheum* 33:1129–1134, 1990.

22. Lightfoot RW Jr, Michel BA, Bloch DA, et al: The American College of Rheumatology 1990 criteria for the classification of polyarteritis nodosa, *Arthritis Rheum* 33:1088–1093, 1990.

23. Leavitt RY, Fauci AS, Bloch DA, et al: The American College of Rheumatology 1990 criteria for the classification of Wegener's granulomatosis, *Arthritis Rheum* 33:1101–1107, 1990.

24. Masi AT, Hunder GG, Lie JT, et al: The American College of Rheumatology 1990 criteria for the classification of Churg-Strauss syndrome (allergic granulomatosis and angiitis), *Arthritis Rheum* 33:1094–1100, 1990.

25. Mills JA, Michel BA, Bloch DA, et al: The American College of Rheumatology 1990 criteria for the classification of Henoch-Schönlein purpura, *Arthritis Rheum* 33:1114–1121, 1990.

26. International Study Group for Behçet's disease: criteria for diagnosis of Behçet's disease, *Lancet* 335:1078–1080, 1990.

27. Churg J: Nomenclature of vasculitic syndromes: a historical perspective, *Am J Kidney Dis* 18:148–153, 1991.

28. Sakane T, Tekeno M, Suzuki N, et al: Behçet's disease, *N Engl J Med* 341:1284–1291, 1999.

29. Salvarani C, Gabriel SE, O'Fallon WM, et al: The incidence of giant cell arteritis in Olmsted County, Minnesota: apparent fluctuations in a cyclic pattern, *Ann Intern Med* 123:192–194, 1995.

30. Barron KS, Shulman ST, Rowley A, et al: Report of the National Institutes of Health Workshop on Kawasaki's Disease, *J Rheumatol* 26:170–190, 1999.

31. Blanco R, Martinez-Taboada VM, Rodriguez-Valverde V, et al: Henoch-Schönlein purpura in adulthood and childhood: two different expressions of the same syndrome, *Arthritis Rheum* 40:859–864, 1997.

32. The Wegener's Granulomatosis Etanercept Trial Research Group: Limited versus severe Wegener's granulomatosis: baseline data on patients in the Wegener's Granulomatosis Etanercept Trial, *Arthritis Rheum* 48:2299–2309, 2003.

33. Regan MJ, Green WR, Stone JH: Ethnic disparity in the incidence of temporal arteritis: a 32-year experience at an urban medical center, *Arthritis Rheum* 47:S108, 2002.

34. Falk RJ, Hogan S, Carey TS, et al: Clinical course of anti-neutrophil cytoplasmic autoantibody-associated glomerulonephritis and systemic vasculitis. The Glomerular Disease Collaborative Network, *Ann Intern Med* 113:656–663, 1990.

35. Hoffman GS, Kerr GS, Leavitt RY, et al: Wegener's granulomatosis: an analysis of 158 patients, *Ann Intern Med* 116:488–498, 1992.

36. Weyand CM, Hunder GG, Hickok KC, et al: HLA-DRB1 alleles in polymyalgia rheumatica, giant cell arteritis, and rheumatoid arthritis, *Arthritis Rheum* 37:514–520, 1994.

37. Rauzy O, Fort M, Nourhashemi F: Relation between HLA DRB1 alleles and corticosteroid resistance in giant cell arteritis, *Ann Rheum Dis* 57:380–382, 1998.

38. Mattey DL, Hajeer AH, Dababneh A, et al: Association of giant cell arteritis and polymyalgia rheumatica with different tumor necrosis factor microsatellite polymorphisms, *Arthritis Rheum* 43:1749–1755, 2000.

39. Gregersen PK, Silver J, Winchester RJ: The shared epitope hypothesis: an approach to understanding the molecular genetics of susceptibility to rheumatoid arthritis, *Arthritis Rheum* 30:1205–1213, 1987.

40. Weyand CM, Xie C, Goronzy JJ: Homozygosity for the HLA-DRB1 allele selects for extra-articular manifestations in rheumatoid arthritis, *J Clin Invest* 89:2033–2039, 1992.

41. Voskuhl AE, Hazes JMW, Schreuder GMT, et al: HLA-DRB1, DQA1, and DQB1 genotypes and risk of vasculitis in patients with rheumatoid arthritis, *J Rheumatol* 24:852–855, 1997.

42. Turesson C, Schaid DJ, Weyand CM, et al: The impact of HLA-DRB1 genes on extra-articular disease manifestations in rheumatoid arthritis, *Arthritis Res Ther* 7:R1386–R1393, 2005.

43. Gorman JD, David-Vaudey E, Pai M, et al: Particular HLA-DRB1 shared epitope genotypes are strongly associated with rheumatoid vasculitis, *Arthritis Rheum* 50:3476–3484, 2004.

44. Turesson C, Schaid DJ, Weyand CM, et al: Association of HLA-C3 and smoking with vasculitis in patients with rheumatoid arthritis, *Arthritis Rheum* 54:2776–2783, 2006.

45. Jagiello P, Aries P, Arning L, et al: The PTPN22 620W allele is a risk factor for Wegener's granulomatosis, *Arthritis Rheum* 52:4039–4043, 2005.

46. Klareskog L, Stolt P, Lundberg K, et al: A new model for an etiology of rheumatoid arthritis: smoking may trigger HLA-DR (shared epitope)-restricted immune reactions to autoantigens modified by citrullination, *Arthritis Rheum* 54:38–46, 2006.

47. Hogan SL, Satterly KK, Dooley MA, et al: Silica exposure in anti-neutrophil cytoplasmic autoantibody-associated glomerulonephritis and lupus nephritis, *J Am Soc Nephrol* 12:134–142, 2001.

48. Watts R, Carruthers D, Scott D: Epidemiology of systemic vasculitis: changing incidence or definition? *Semin Arthritis Rheum* 25:28–34, 1995.

49. Gonzalez-Gay MA: Garcia-Porrua J: Epidemiology of the vasculitides, *Rheum Dis Clin North Am* 27:729–750, 2001.

The references for this chapter can also be found on www.expertconsult.com.

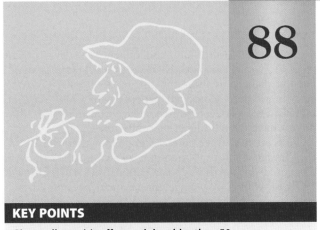

88

Giant Cell Arteritis, Polymyalgia Rheumatica, and Takayasu's Arteritis

DAVID B. HELLMANN

KEY POINTS

Giant cell arteritis affects adults older than 50 years.

The most common manifestations of giant cell arteritis are constitutional symptoms, headache, jaw claudication, and visual symptoms; almost all untreated patients have an elevated erythrocyte sedimentation rate.

The diagnosis of giant cell arteritis is usually confirmed by temporal artery biopsy.

Early treatment of giant cell arteritis can prevent blindness.

Polymyalgia rheumatica can occur by itself or with giant cell arteritis.

Polymyalgia rheumatica responds to prednisone 10 to 20 mg/day, whereas giant cell arteritis requires an initial dose of prednisone of approximately 60 mg/day.

Takayasu's arteritis most frequently affects the aorta and its major branches in young women.

Giant cell arteritis (GCA) and polymyalgia rheumatica (PMR) are discussed together because they affect similar epidemiologic subsets of patients and often occur together in the same individual. Although GCA is a disease of older people and Takayasu's arteritis is a disease of younger people, their shared predilection for causing vasculitis of large arteries and their nearly identical histopathologic changes prompt their inclusion in the same chapter.

GIANT CELL ARTERITIS AND POLYMYALGIA RHEUMATICA

American College of Rheumatology Criteria

Classification criteria for the diagnosis of GCA have been proposed by the American College of Rheumatology (ACR) (Table 88-1).[1] Three classification schemes have been proposed for PMR (Table 88-2).[2,3,3a] The provisional criteria for 2012 were developed in part to incorporate information from ultrasound evaluation.

Definitions

Giant Cell Arteritis

GCA is the most common form of systemic vasculitis in adults.[4] The disease affects primarily the extracranial branches of the carotid artery in patients older than 50 years. The most feared complication of GCA is irreversible loss of vision. Because the cause of GCA is unknown, various names—including temporal arteritis, cranial arteritis, and granulomatous arteritis—have been used to highlight different salient features.[5] All the names for this disease have both merits and shortcomings. The designation *temporal arteritis* or *cranial arteritis*, for example, conveys how frequently the temporal arteries or other cranial arteries are involved but fails to capture GCA's more widespread nature. Although *granulomatous arteritis* and GCA pay homage to an important pathologic finding, this focus is undeserved because giant cells are absent in about half the cases and may be present in other forms of vasculitis. With no perfect name available, this chapter bows to convention and refers to this disease as GCA.

Polymyalgia Rheumatica

Polymyalgia rheumatica, a term suggested by Barber, is a syndrome characterized by aching in the proximal portions of the extremities and torso. Because there are no specific diagnostic tests or pathologic findings, PMR is defined by its clinical features. The features included in most definitions of PMR are as follows (1) aching and morning stiffness lasting half an hour or longer in the shoulder, hip girdle, neck, or some combination; (2) duration of these symptoms for 1 month or longer; (3) age older than 50 years; and (4) laboratory evidence of systemic inflammation such as an elevated erythrocyte sedimentation rate (ESR).[2] Some definitions also include a rapid response to small doses of glucocorticoids such as prednisone 10 mg/day.[6] The presence of another specific disease other than GCA such as rheumatoid arthritis (RA), chronic infection, polymyositis, or malignancy excludes the diagnosis of PMR.

Epidemiology

The incidence of GCA varies widely in different populations, from less than 0.1 per 100,000 to 77 per 100,000 persons aged 50 years and older.[4,7-11] The greatest risk factor for developing GCA is aging; the disease almost never occurs before age 50, and its incidence rises steadily thereafter. The average age at diagnosis has risen over the past half century, from 74.7 years in the 1950s to 79.2 years now.[12] Nationality, geography, and race are also important, with the highest incidence figures found in Scandinavians and in Americans of Scandinavian descent. The lowest incidence of GCA is reported in Japanese, northern Indians, and African-Americans. In western Europe, GCA is more common in the northern latitudes than the southern ones. The incidence of GCA has been increasing over the past

Table 88-1 American College of Rheumatology Classification Criteria for Giant Cell Arteritis

Criterion*	Definition
Age at disease onset ≥ 50 yr	Development of symptoms or findings beginning at age 50 or older
New headache	New onset or new type of localized pain in the head
Temporal artery abnormality	Temporal artery tenderness to palpation or decreased pulsation, unrelated to arteriosclerosis of cervical arteries
Elevated ESR	ESR ≥50 mm/hr by the Westergren method
Abnormal artery biopsy	Biopsy specimen with artery showing vasculitis characterized by a predominance of mononuclear cell infiltration or granulomatous inflammation, usually with multinucleated giant cells

*For purposes of classification, a patient with vasculitis is said to have giant cell (temporal) arteritis if at least three of these five criteria are present. The presence of any three or more criteria yields a sensitivity of 93.5% and a specificity of 91.2%.

ESR, erythrocyte sedimentation rate.

From Hunder GG, Bloch DA, Michel BA, et al: The American College of Rheumatology 1990 criteria for the classification of giant cell arteritis, *Arthritis Rheum* 33:1125, 1990.

20 to 40 years, possibly because of greater physician awareness.[4,7] Some studies have reported seasonal variations and clustering of cases, with peaks about 7 years apart.[7,10] The prevalence of GCA in Olmsted County, Minnesota, home to many Scandinavian immigrants, is 200 per 100,000 population aged 50 years or older. Autopsy studies suggest that GCA may be more common than is clinically apparent. Östberg[13] found arteritis in 1.6% of 889 postmortem cases in which sections of the temporal artery and two transverse sections of the aorta were examined.

Genetic susceptibility to the development of GCA was initially suggested by reports of GCA in families[14] and, more recently, by studies demonstrating an association with genes in the human leukocyte antigen (HLA) class II region.[15] Sixty percent of GCA patients have HLA-DRB1*04 haplotype variants, which have a common sequence motif in the second hypervariable region of the B1 molecule.[15] This motif differs from that found in patients with RA.[15] The low prevalence of these alleles in African-Americans may explain why blacks develop GCA relatively infrequently. To date, GCA is the form of systemic vasculitis most closely associated with HLA class II genes. Susceptibility to GCA and PMR has also been associated with polymorphisms of genes for tumor necrosis factor, intercellular adhesion molecules, and interleukin 18 (IL-18).[4]

The existence of environmental risk factors has been suggested by the geographic clustering of GCA cases. Smoking appears to increase the risk of developing GCA sixfold in women.[16] Circumstantial evidence links the development of GCA to a variety of infectious agents including *Mycoplasma pneumoniae*, varicella-zoster virus, parvovirus B19, and parainfluenza virus type I.[10,11] The results of examining temporal artery biopsy specimens with polymerase chain reaction methods to detect parvovirus B19 or herpesvirus DNA have been negative or inconsistent.[17] The reported association between GCA and *Chlamydia pneumoniae* infection has not withstood close scrutiny.[18]

Gender and health status also influence the development of GCA. Women are affected about twice as often as men.[10] Having diabetes reduces the risk of developing GCA by 50% in women.[2] Although patients with GCA have an increased risk of developing thoracic aortic aneurysms, they do not have overall higher mortality rates.[10]

PMR is two to three times more common than GCA.[4,8,9,19] In Olmsted County, Minnesota, 245 cases of PMR were diagnosed during the 22-year period from 1970 through 1991, providing an average annual incidence rate of 52.5 cases per 100,000 persons aged 50 years or older.[19] The prevalence of PMR (active plus remitted cases) was

Table 88-2 Diagnostic* and Classification Criteria for Polymyalgia Rheumatica

Diagnostic Criteria of Chuang and Colleagues[2] (1982)

Age 50 yr or older
Bilateral aching and stiffness for 1 mo or more and involving two of the following areas: neck or torso, shoulders or proximal regions of the arms, and hips or proximal aspects of the thighs
ESR > 40 mm/hr
Exclusion of all other diagnoses except giant cell arteritis

Diagnostic Criteria of Healey[3] (1984)

Pain persisting for at least 1 mo and involving two of the following areas: neck, shoulders, and pelvic girdle
Morning stiffness lasting > 1 hr
Rapid response to prednisone (≤20 mg/day)
Absence of other diseases capable of causing the musculoskeletal symptoms
Age older than 50 yr
ESR > 40 mm/hr

Classification Criteria of Dasgupta and Colleagues[3a] (2012)

Age 50 years or older, bilateral shoulder aching and abnormal C-reactive protein and/or ESR[†]

	Points without US (0-6)	Points with US‡ (0-8)
Morning stiffness duration >45 min	2	2
Hip pain or limited range of motion	1	1
Absence of rheumatoid factor or anticitrullinated protein antibody	2	2
Absence of other joint involvement	1	1
At least one shoulder with subdeltoid bursitis and/or biceps tenosynovitis and/or glenohumeral synovitis (either posterior or axillary) and at least one hip with synovitis and/or trochanteric bursitis	Not applicable	1
Both shoulders with subdeltoid bursitis, biceps tenosynovitis or glenohumeral synovitis	Not applicable	1

*For each set of criteria, all the findings must be present for polymyalgia rheumatica to be diagnosed.

†A score of 4 or more is categorized as polymyalgia rheumatica in the algorithm without US, and a score of 5 or more is categorized as polymyalgia rheumatica in the algorithm with US.

‡Optional ultrasound criteria.

ESR, erythrocyte sedimentation rate; US, ultrasound.

From Salvarani C, Cantini F, Boiardi L, Hunder GG: Polymyalgia rheumatic and giant-cell arteritis, *N Engl J Med* 347:261, 2002; and Dasgupta B, Cimmino MA, Kremers HM, et al: 2012 provisional classification criteria for polymyalgia rheumatica: a European League Against Rheumatism/American College of Rheumatology collaborative initiative, *Arthritis Rheum* 64:943–954, 2012.

approximately 600 per 100,000 persons aged 50 years and older.[19] PMR is associated with the same *HLA-DR4* genes as GCA.[15,20]

Cause, Pathology, and Pathogenesis

The causes of GCA and PMR are unknown. Because pathologic studies have provided important clues to the pathogenesis, they are discussed first.

In GCA, inflammation is found most often in medium-size muscular arteries that originate from the arch of the aorta.[10,13,21,22] The inflammation tends to affect the arteries in a segmental fashion (possibly leading to "skip lesions" within arteries), but long portions of arteries may be involved.[23] In patients who died during the active phase of GCA, the greatest frequency of severe involvement was noted in the superficial temporal arteries, vertebral arteries, and ophthalmic and posterior ciliary arteries.[24] The internal carotid, external carotid, and central retinal arteries were affected somewhat less frequently.[24] In other postmortem studies, lesions were commonly found in the proximal and distal aorta and internal and external carotid, subclavian, brachial, and abdominal arteries.[13] Because GCA affects vessels with an internal elastic lamina and vasa vasorum, and because intracranial arteries lose these structures after penetrating the dura, it is not surprising that GCA rarely involves intracranial arteries.[24-26] In some patients with GCA, follow-up biopsy or autopsy surveys showed the persistence of mild chronic inflammation, even though symptoms had resolved.[2]

Early in the disease, collections of lymphocytes are confined to the region of the internal or external elastic lamina or adventitia. The inflammation may be limited to the vasa vasorum in some cases.[3] Intimal thickening with prominent cellular infiltration is a hallmark of more advanced cases. In heavily involved areas, all layers are affected (Figure 88-1). Transmural inflammation of portions of the arterial wall (including the elastic laminae) and granulomas containing multinucleated histiocytic and foreign body giant cells, histiocytes, lymphocytes (which are predominantly CD4+ T cells), and some plasma cells and fibroblasts are found.[22,27,28] Eosinophils may be seen, but polymorphonuclear leukocytes are rare. Thrombosis may develop at sites of active inflammation; later, these areas may recanalize. The inflammatory process is usually most marked in the inner portion of the media adjacent to the internal elastic lamina. Fragmentation and disintegration of elastic fibers occur, closely associated with an accumulation of giant cells (Figure 88-2). However, giant cells are seen in only about half of routinely examined specimens; therefore they are not required to make the diagnosis if other features are compatible. In contrast to some other forms of systemic vasculitis (e.g., polyarteritis nodosa, microscopic polyangiitis, granulomatosis with polyangiitis [GPA] [formerly Wegener's granulomatosis]), fibrinoid necrosis is rarely if ever observed in GCA.[3]

Immunohistochemical studies demonstrate inflammatory changes that are specific for each layer of the affected artery.[11,22,28-31] Dendritic cells, which can present antigen and activate T cells, are found in the adventitia, along with two separate lineages of CD4+ T cells: (1) Th1 cells that secrete interferon-γ (IFN-γ) and interleukin-2 (IL-2) and (2) Th17 cells that secrete interleukin-17 (IL-17) family

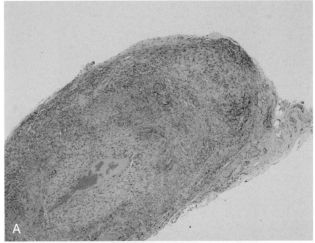

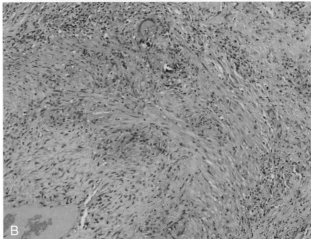

Figure 88-1 Giant cell arteritis. **A,** Cross-section of a temporal artery showing transmural inflammation with mononuclear cells and giant cells (hematoxylin and eosin, ×10). **B,** Higher-power (×100) view demonstrating giant cells infiltrating the media. *(Courtesy Dr. Frederic Askin.)*

members including IL-17A.[32-34] The adventitial T cells show evidence of clonal expansion. The adventitia is also infiltrated with macrophages that secrete IL-1, IL-6, and transforming growth factor-β (TGF-β). The media is populated mostly by macrophages that, in contrast to those in other layers, produce matrix metalloproteinases and oxygen free radicals. Closer to the intima, the macrophages secrete nitric oxide and unite to form syncytia—the giant cells—which produce platelet-derived growth factor (PDGF) and substances that stimulate intimal proliferation.[22,35]

Although microscopic examination of arteries in PMR is usually normal, immunohistochemical studies of apparently uninvolved temporal arteries reveal upregulation of the same macrophage-related inflammatory cytokines found in GCA.[22] The T cell cytokine IFN-γ is abundantly expressed in GCA and is absent in arteries from patients having only PMR. Pathologically, relatively little else has been found in the arteries of patients with PMR. Granulomatous myocarditis and hepatitis have been noted.[36] Muscle biopsy specimens may be normal or show nonspecific type II muscle atrophy. However, a number of reports have shown the presence of lymphocytic synovitis in the knees, sternoclavicular joints, and shoulders and evidence of a similar

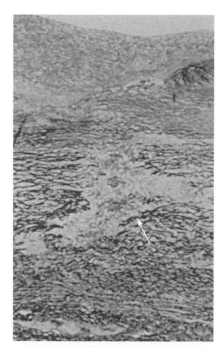

Figure 88-2 Giant cell arteritis involving the proximal aorta in a patient who died of a ruptured ascending aorta. This section of the ascending aorta is distal to the ruptured portion and shows destruction of elastic fibers *(arrow)* (elastic van Gieson stain, ×64). Neighboring sections stained with hematoxylin and eosin showed infiltrations of mononuclear leukocytes in the areas of disrupted fibers.

reaction in sacroiliac joints.[37,38] Synovitis (mostly subclinical) was shown in bone scans demonstrating an increased uptake of technetium pertechnetate in the joints of 2 of 25 patients with PMR.[37] More sensitive studies using magnetic resonance imaging (MRI) and ultrasonography have convincingly demonstrated that in PMR, the principal foci of inflammation are the bursae surrounding the shoulder more than the glenohumeral joint itself.[5] Sera from patients with GCA, PMR, or both demonstrate evidence of systemic inflammation, with increased levels of circulating immune complexes during active disease[39] and elevated levels of IL-6 and IL-1.[7]

These observations, together with the results from experiments in which temporal arteries from patients with GCA have been implanted into mice with severe combined immunodeficiency (SCID), suggest that GCA results from an adaptive immune response in the wall of an artery.[22,33] In this model (Figure 88-3) the key initiating event is activation of dendritic cells located in the adventitia, the only arterial layer normally penetrated by the vasa vasorum. In large and medium-size arteries, immunohistochemical studies reveal that the dendritic cells in temporal arteries have a specific phenotype and express fascin and CD11c.[22,32] Dendritic cells express Toll-like receptors (TLRs) that normally serve as sentinels, monitoring for any immunologic breach of the adventitia.[40] In GCA, activation of TLRs on dendritic cells appears to be the initial triggering event.[32,40,41] Of the many different types of TLRs, TLR-2 and TLR-4 might be the most important in GCA. Although the exact trigger of the adaptive immune response in GCA is not known, experiments in the GCA-SCID mouse model have shown that blood-borne lipopolysaccharide serves as an effective TLR ligand in temporal arteries. Other

constituents of microorganisms or some self-antigens (e.g., oxidized lipids) might also be TLR ligands that activate the arterial dendritic cells.

Once its TLRs have been engaged, dendritic cells differentiate from the resting to the active state and release cytokines such as IL-6 and IL-18, which recruit, activate, and retain CD4+ T cells in the blood vessel. The crucial role of dendritic cells in activating T cells and maintaining vasculitis has been demonstrated in the GCA-SCID mouse model: Depleting the dendritic cells markedly reduces the T cell infiltrate and suppresses the vasculitis. As noted, two separate populations of CD4+ T cells become activated and expand: IFN-γ producing Th1 cells and IL-17 producing Th17 cells. IFN-γ causes macrophages to migrate, differentiate, and form granulomas.[34,40] Production of matrix metalloproteinases and lipid peroxidation agents by macrophages in the media results in the destruction of elastic laminae. The vessel attempts to counter the tissue destruction by elaborating a variety of growth factors including PDGF, vascular endothelial growth factor (VEGF), and TGF-β, which prompt smooth muscle cells in the media to revert from a contractile phenotype to a secretory one and migrate to the intima. Proliferation of the intimal smooth muscle cells results in occlusion of the lumen.[22,32]

PMR appears to result from a similar but less intense adaptive immune response in blood vessels (as evidenced by the in situ production of many inflammatory cytokines). According to this model, both PMR and GCA begin with the activation of dendritic cells at the adventitia-media border.[32,41] However, the distinguishing feature of PMR is the absence of T cells producing IFN-γ. Without IFN-γ to

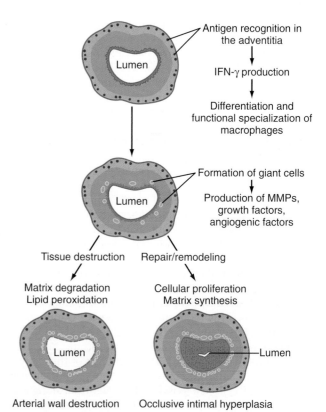

Figure 88-3 Proposed model for the pathogenesis of giant cell arteritis. IFN-γ, interferon-gamma; MMPs, matrix metalloproteinases.

stimulate the recruitment and differentiation of macrophages, the level of arterial inflammation in PMR remains subclinical. Thus the development of GCA appears to require both vascular dendritic cell activation and a disease-inducing repertoire of T cells.[22,32,41] The constitutional symptoms of PMR and GCA are attributed to the high levels of inflammatory cytokines (e.g., IL-1, IL-6) found in the sera. Whether these serum cytokine elevations result from blood vessel inflammation alone or from some other source of inflammation is not yet clear. The attractiveness of this model is increased by its ability to explain why subsets of clinical features occur together.

Clinical Features

The mean age at onset of GCA and PMR is approximately 79 years, with a range of about 50 to 90 years of age.[10,12] Younger patients with PMR have been described occasionally. Women are affected about twice as often as men.[19] Although the onset of the disease is usually insidious, typically evolving over weeks or months, in one-third of cases, the disease begins so abruptly that some patients recall the very day they became ill.[10,36]

Giant Cell Arteritis

Classic Manifestations. The most common manifestations of GCA are constitutional symptoms, headache, visual symptoms, jaw claudication, and PMR[10] (Table 88-3). Almost all patients experience one or more constitutional symptoms including fatigue, weight loss, malaise, and fever.

Besides constitutional symptoms, headache is the most common symptom in GCA, being present in nearly three-quarters of patients.[42] The pain is typically described as boring in quality, of moderate severity, and most commonly appreciated in the temporal area. However, the description of the headache varies enormously. It can be mild to so severe that the patient seeks immediate relief by presenting to the emergency department. The pain may localize to any part of the skull including the occiput (owing to involvement of the occipital artery).[10,13] The most consistent characteristic is that the patient experiences the headache as something new and unusual. In untreated patients, the headache may subside over weeks, even though the disease

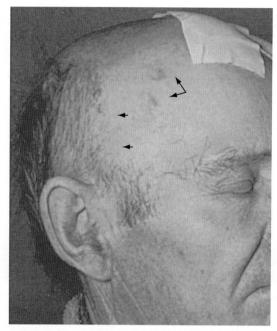

Figure 88-4 Giant cell arteritis (GCA) involving the temporal artery. Short segments of curved artery were erythematous and tender *(long arrows)*. The bandage on the scalp covers a similar artery that was biopsied and showed GCA. A previous biopsy specimen of a proximal segment of the right temporal artery, which was normal on physical examination, was normal histologically. The faint scar from that biopsy can be seen above and anterior to the right ear *(short arrows)*.

activity continues. Often, the headache of GCA is not associated with any particular findings on physical examination. Abnormalities of the temporal artery—including enlargement, nodular swelling, tenderness, or loss of pulse—develop in only about half of patients (Figure 88-4). Some patients note tenderness of the scalp, which can be aggravated by brushing or combing the hair.

Visual symptoms are common in GCA, especially loss of vision and diplopia. Vision loss can be unilateral or (less commonly) bilateral, transient or permanent, and partial or complete.[43] Vision loss lasting more than a few hours usually does not reverse. Loss of vision often reflects an anterior ischemic optic neuropathy caused by occlusive arteritis of the posterior ciliary artery, the chief blood supply to the head of the optic nerve. The posterior ciliary artery is a branch of the ophthalmic artery (which derives, in turn, from the internal carotid artery). Less frequently, vision loss in GCA stems from a retinal artery occlusion. Regardless of the site of the culprit lesion, vision loss in GCA is usually profound, with more than 80% of patients unable to see hand waving.[43] GCA patients who present with fever or other systemic symptoms are less likely to develop vision loss.[44,45] One possible explanation of this protective effect of fever and other systemic manifestations is that patients with prominent systemic inflammation demonstrate more extensive angiogenesis in temporal artery biopsies.[6] The angiogenesis associated with increased inflammation may result in the development of collateral circulation that reduces the chance of ischemic events.[6]

The early funduscopic appearance in the setting of blindness caused by anterior ischemic optic neuropathy is that of ischemic optic neuritis: slight pallor and edema of the optic

Table 88-3 Symptoms of Giant Cell Arteritis

Symptom	Frequency (%)
Headache	76
Weight loss	43
Fever	42
Fatigue	39
Any visual symptom	37
Anorexia	35
Jaw claudication	34
Polymyalgia rheumatica	34
Arthralgia	30
Unilateral visual loss	24
Bilateral visual loss	15
Vertigo	11
Diplopia	9

Modified from Smetana GW, Shmerling RH: Does this patient have temporal arteritis? *JAMA* 287:92, 2002. Data from a review of 2475 patients reported in the literature.

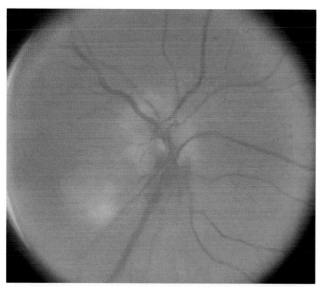

Figure 88-5 Ophthalmoscopic appearance of the acute phase of anterior ischemic optic neuropathy seen in patients with giant cell arteritis and loss of vision. The optic disc is pale and swollen, the retinal veins are dilated, and several flame-shaped hemorrhages and a cotton-wool spot (retinal infarct) are visible. (*Courtesy Dr. Neil R. Miller.*)

disc, with scattered cotton-wool patches and small hemorrhages[43] (Figure 88-5). Later, optic atrophy occurs. Rarely, blindness may be the initial symptom; however, it tends to follow other symptoms by several weeks or even months. Ophthalmoscopic examination in patients without eye involvement is generally normal. In most reports, the incidence of blindness is 20% or less.[6,43,46] In a series of 245 patients from the modern era, 34 (14%) had some permanent loss of vision.[46] In 32 of these patients, the deficit developed before glucocorticoid therapy was begun; in the other 2, vision loss occurred after therapy was started. Vision loss progressed in 3 of the 32 after therapy was initiated, and it improved in 5. At 5 years' follow-up, among the patients who had visual deficits caused by GCA at the time glucocorticoids were started, the risk of additional loss of vision was 13% over the follow-up period. If no loss had occurred at the beginning of glucocorticoid therapy, there was only a 1% risk of new loss of vision over the subsequent 5 years.

Another potential ocular complication of GCA is ophthalmoplegia. Diplopia usually results from ocular motor nerve palsies caused by ischemia and usually resolves after therapy is started. Oculomotor nerve involvement in GCA usually spares the pupil.[43] Rarely, arterial lesions cause infarction of the occipital cortex and vision loss.

Intermittent claudication may occur in the muscles of mastication (jaw claudication), the extremities, and occasionally the muscles of the tongue or those involved in swallowing.[10] In the jaw muscles, the discomfort is noted, especially when chewing meat, and may involve the muscles on one side of the mandible more than those on the other. In some instances, facial artery involvement results in spasm of the jaw muscles. More marked vascular narrowing may lead to gangrene of the scalp or tongue.

Atypical Manifestations. Approximately 40% of patients present with disease manifestations that are considered atypical[33,47-49] (Table 88-4). In these patients, headache, jaw claudication, visual symptoms, and PMR do not occur or are less prominent.

Fever occurs in up to 40% of patients with GCA, but it is usually low grade and overshadowed by other classic symptoms. However, 15% of GCA patients may present with fever of unknown origin (FUO) in which the temperature spikes are high, dominating the clinical picture.[6,36] Although GCA causes only 2% of all cases of FUO, it is responsible for 16% of all such fevers in individuals older than 65 years.[36] Approximately two-thirds of patients experience shaking chills and drenching sweats, features often attributed to infection or malignancy. The median temperature is 39.1° C, and the maximum 39.8° C. The white blood cell count in GCA-induced FUO is usually normal or nearly so (at least before the initiation of prednisone).

Neurologic problems occur in approximately 30% of patients.[1,50] These are diverse, but most common are neuropathies and transient ischemic attacks or strokes. Hemiparesis or brain stem events are due to narrowing or occlusion of the carotid or vertebrobasilar artery. GCA preferentially involves the posterior circulation; the 3 : 2 ratio of anterior to posterior strokes and transient ischemic attacks seen in the normal population reaches nearly 1 : 1 in patients with GCA.[51] Delirium, reversible dementia, and myelopathy have also been reported. However, the assignment of an exact cause to ischemic central nervous system events is often challenging, given the older population in which GCA occurs. The neuropathies of GCA include mononeuropathies and peripheral polyneuropathies and may affect the upper or lower extremities. Presumably, they are secondary to the involvement of nutrient arteries, but little pathologic documentation is available. Among the vasculitides, GCA has a nearly unique propensity for involving the C5 nerve root, resulting in loss of shoulder abduction.[25] Mononeuropathies affecting the hands and feet, so typical of polyarteritis and other forms of vasculitis, develop less often in GCA.

Table 88-4   Atypical Manifestations of Giant Cell Arteritis

Fever of unknown origin
Respiratory symptoms (especially cough)
Otolaryngeal manifestations
Glossitis
Lingual infarction
Throat pain
Hearing loss
Large artery disease
Aortic aneurysm
Aortic dissection
Limb claudication
Raynaud's phenomenon
Neurologic manifestations
Peripheral neuropathy
Transient ischemic attack, stroke
Dementia
Delirium
Myocardial infarction
Tumor-like lesions
Breast mass
Ovarian and uterine mass
Syndrome of inappropriate antidiuretic hormone secretion
Microangiopathic hemolytic anemia

Prominent respiratory tract symptoms occur in about 10% of patients.[52] These include cough with or without sputum, sore throat, and hoarseness. When these symptoms are severe or an initial manifestation of GCA, they may direct the attention of the examining physician away from the underlying arteritis. Vasculitis may induce these symptoms by causing ischemia or hyperirritability of the affected tissues. Otolaryngeal manifestations of GCA include throat pain, dental pain, tongue pain, glossitis, and ulceration or infarction of the tongue.[52,53]

Clinical evidence of large artery involvement occurs in 10% to 15% of cases at presentation and in up to 27% eventually.[3,38,54] Positron emission tomography (PET) studies using fluorodeoxyglucose (FDG) revealed that subclinical involvement of large arteries occurs in the vast majority of GCA patients. One PET study, for example, showed that 88% of 35 patients had increased FDG uptake in large arteries, with subclavian involvement in 7% and aortic involvement in 54%.[55]

Generally, clinically evident disease can be divided into early (within a year of diagnosis) and late (years after diagnosis) stages. Usually, early disease consists chiefly of large artery stenosis resulting in upper extremity claudication; bruits over the carotid, subclavian, axillary, and brachial arteries; absent or decreased pulses in the neck or arms; and Raynaud's phenomenon (Figure 88-6).[54] Angiographic features that suggest GCA are smooth-walled arterial stenoses or occlusions alternating with areas of normal or increased caliber in the absence of irregular plaques and ulcerations, located especially in the carotid, subclavian, axillary, and brachial arteries. Late disease most frequently involves thoracic aortic aneurysm.[54] The tendency for aneurysm to develop late was confirmed in one series of 41 patients in which the average time between diagnosis of GCA and recognition of this complication was 7 years.[39] Thoracic aortic aneurysm is 17 times more likely to develop in patients with GCA than in persons without this disease. To place this risk in context, thoracic aortic aneurysms are twice as likely to complicate GCA as lung cancer is to result from smoking. Abdominal aortic aneurysm is also 2.4 times more common in patients with GCA.[3,39] In aggregate,

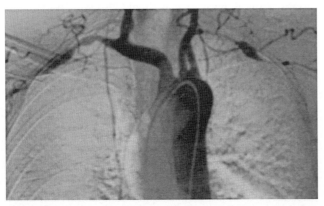

Figure 88-6 Arch aortogram showing giant cell arteritis of large arteries. Both subclavian and axillary arteries are affected. Smooth-walled segmental constrictions alternate with areas of normal caliber or aneurysmal dilation. *(From Klein RG, Hunder GG, Stanson AW, Sheps SG: Large artery involvement in giant cell [temporal] arteritis, Ann Intern Med 83:806, 1975.)*

nearly one out of five patients (18%) with GCA develops an aortic aneurysm or dissection.[54] Patients with large artery disease often do not have headache or other classic manifestations of GCA, and less than 50% have an abnormal temporal artery biopsy. Computed tomography (CT) angiography and magnetic resonance angiography (MRA) are the imaging modalities most commonly used to detect large artery disease in GCA.

In women, GCA can uncommonly present as a breast or ovarian mass.[49,56] The mass lesions in these tissues result from granulomatous inflammation in and around the arteries. Angina pectoris, congestive heart failure, and myocardial infarction secondary to coronary arteritis occur rarely.

Clinical Subsets. Studies suggest that GCA is not just one disease but rather a number of clinical subsets that are explained by the differential expression of inflammatory cytokines.[57] Ischemic events including blindness, stroke, and large artery disease occur more commonly in patients who express high levels of IFN-γ and low levels of IL-6.[57] In contrast, patients who produce high amounts of IL-6 are more likely to have strong inflammatory features (such as fever and constitutional symptoms) and are less likely to develop vision loss or other ischemic events.[57-59]

Polymyalgia Rheumatica

As in GCA, PMR patients are characteristically in good health before their disease begins.[10] Systemic manifestations such as malaise, low-grade fever, and weight loss are present in more than half the patients and may be the initial symptoms. High, spiking fevers are uncommon in PMR in the absence of GCA.[36] Arthralgias and myalgias may develop abruptly or evolve insidiously over weeks or months.[2] Malaise, fatigue, and depression, along with aching and stiffness, may be present for months before the diagnosis is made. In most patients, the shoulder girdle is the first to become symptomatic; in the remainder, the hip or neck is involved at the onset. The discomfort may begin in one shoulder or hip but usually becomes bilateral within weeks. Symptoms center on the proximal limb, axial musculature, and tendinous attachments. Morning stiffness resembling that of RA and "gelling" after inactivity are usually prominent. If the symptoms are severe, aching is more persistent. Although movement of the joints accentuates the pain, it is often felt in the proximal extremities rather than in the joints.[2] Distal joint pain and swelling occur in some cases including diffuse distal extremity swelling with pitting edema.[60] Pain at night is common, and movement during sleep may awaken the patient. Muscle strength is generally unimpaired, although pain with movement makes the interpretation of strength-testing maneuvers difficult. Pain with movement also makes it difficult for patients to get out of bed or the bathtub. In the later stages of the syndrome, muscle atrophy may develop, and contracture of the shoulder capsule may result in limitation of passive and active motion.

As noted, the presence of bursal inflammation and synovitis in PMR has been described by many authors and is undoubtedly the cause of many of the findings in this condition.[5] A careful examination may reveal transient synovitis of the knees, wrists, and sternoclavicular joints.

The shoulders and hips are covered by heavy muscles, and minimal effusions of slight synovitis are not palpable on physical examination. Synovitis has been documented by biopsies, synovial analysis, joint scintiscans, ultrasonography, and MRI.[36-38]

Relationship between Polymyalgia Rheumatica and Giant Cell Arteritis

Evidence that PMR and GCA are related and should be considered different manifestations of a common disease process is abundant.[10,22] The associations with age, ethnicity, geographic region, and HLA class II alleles are the same in both disorders. Moreover, both disorders involve overproduction of many of the same inflammatory cytokines. Between 30% and 50% of patients with GCA develop PMR. Approximately 10% to 15% of patients who appear to have only PMR have positive temporal artery biopsies. In the absence of symptoms of GCA (e.g., headache, jaw claudication, visual symptoms, high fever), PMR by itself does not appear to cause vision loss and responds to low doses of glucocorticoids (see later).[10]

Laboratory Studies

Except for the findings on arterial biopsy, laboratory results in PMR and GCA are similar (Table 88-5). A mild to moderate normochromic anemia is usually present in both diseases during their active phases. Leukocyte and differential counts are generally normal. A markedly elevated ESR and C-reactive protein (CRP) level are characteristic of both. An ESR higher than 100 mm/hr (Westergren method) is common, but untreated biopsy-proven cases of GCA may be associated with normal or nearly normal levels. In a study of 167 GCA patients, 10.8% presented with an ESR of less than 50 mm/hr and 3.6% had a rate of less than 30 mm/hr. Rare individuals appear to be unable to develop an elevated ESR during any inflammatory process including active GCA. The ESR is also liable to be relatively low or normal in patients who have been receiving corticosteroids for another condition.[61] Thus a normal ESR does not exclude GCA, especially in a patient with otherwise classic symptoms and findings. Platelet counts are often increased.

Nonspecific changes in plasma proteins are often present and include a decrease in the concentration of albumin and an increase in α_2-globulins, fibrinogen, and other acute-phase reactant proteins. Slight increases in γ-globulins and complement may be present. Results of tests for antinuclear antibodies and rheumatoid factor are generally negative.

Liver function test results are mildly abnormal in approximately one-third of patients with GCA and in a slightly smaller fraction of those with PMR. An increased alkaline phosphatase level is the most common abnormality, but increases in aspartate transaminase and prolonged prothrombin time may also be found. Liver biopsy specimens are generally normal; granulomatous hepatitis has been observed.[36] Renal function and urinalysis are usually normal. Red blood cell casts are found in some instances, but their presence does not correlate with clinical large artery involvement.[23]

Levels of serum creatine kinase and other enzymes reflecting muscle damage are normal. Electromyograms are usually normal, and muscle biopsy shows normal histologic features or only the mild atrophy characteristic of disuse.

Synovial fluid analyses reported in GCA or PMR show evidence of mild inflammation including increased synovial fluid leukocyte counts, with a mean of 2900 cells/mm³ but a range from 300 to 20,000 cells/mm³, with 40% to 50% being polymorphonuclear leukocytes. Synovial fluid complement levels are usually normal. In some instances, synovial biopsy has shown lymphocytic synovitis.[37,38]

Serum IL-6 levels are elevated in patients with PMR and GCA and appear to closely parallel the inflammatory activity.[62] Levels of factor VIII or von Willebrand factor are elevated in patients with GCA and PMR.

Differential Diagnosis

The diagnosis of GCA should be considered in any patient older than 50 years who experiences loss of vision, diplopia, new form of headache, jaw claudication, PMR, FUO, unexplained constitutional symptoms, anemia, and a high ESR. GCA can cause so many forms of cranial discomfort (e.g., headache, scalp tenderness, jaw claudication, pain of the throat, gums, and tongue) that the disease should also be considered in any patient older than 50 who develops new, unexplained "above-the-neck" pain. The protean manifestations of GCA mean that it should also be considered in the differential diagnosis of an older patient presenting with dry cough, stroke, arm claudication, or acute C5 radiculopathy accompanied by other classic symptoms or findings of GCA.

Only a few individual symptoms or findings substantially increase or decrease the likelihood of a patient having this disease[42] (Table 88-6). For example, jaw claudication, diplopia, abnormal temporal artery signs, scalp tenderness, and ESR greater than 50 mm/hr increase the likelihood that a patient has GCA.[42] In one series of 373 patients, the presence of either jaw claudication or diplopia increased the likelihood of a positive biopsy by more than threefold; the presence of both jaw claudication and double vision had a 100% positive predictive value for a diagnostic temporal artery biopsy.[63] Conversely, the absence of headache or temporal artery abnormalities on physical examination, the presence of synovitis, and a normal ESR reduce the likelihood of GCA.

Table 88-5 Physical Findings and Laboratory Abnormalities in Giant Cell Arteritis

Feature	Frequency (%)
Any temporal artery abnormality	65
Prominent or enlarged temporal artery	47
Absent temporal artery pulse	45
Scalp tenderness	31
Any funduscopic abnormality	31
Abnormal ESR	96
ESR >50 mm/hr	83
ESR >100 mm/hr	39
Anemia	44

ESR, erythrocyte sedimentation rate.
Modified from Smetana GW, Shmerling RH: Does this patient have temporal arteritis? *JAMA* 287:92, 2002.

Table 88-6 Likelihood Ratios* for Symptoms, Signs, and Laboratory Findings in Giant Cell Arteritis

Finding	Positive Likelihood Ratio (95% CI)	Negative Likelihood Ratio (95% CI)
Symptoms		
Jaw claudication	4.2 (2.8-6.2)	0.72 (0.65-0.81)
Diplopia	3.4 (1.3-8.6)	0.95 (0.91-0.99)
Weight loss	1.3 (1.1-1.5)	0.89 (0.79-1.0)
Any headache	1.2 (1.1-1.4)	0.7 (0.57-0.85)
Fatigue	NS	NS
Anorexia	NS	NS
Arthralgia	NS	NS
Polymyalgia rheumatica	NS	NS
Fever	NS	NS
Visual loss	NS	NS
Signs		
Beaded temporal artery	4.6 (1.1-18.4)	0.93 (0.88-0.99)
Tender temporal artery	2.6 (1.9-3.7)	0.82 (0.74-0.92)
Any temporal artery abnormality	2.0 (1.4-3.0)	0.53 (0.38-0.75)
Scalp tenderness	1.6 (1.2-2.1)	0.93 (0.86-1.0)
Synovitis	0.41 (0.23-0.72)	1.1 (1.0-1.2)
Optic atrophy	NS	NS
Laboratory Results		
ESR abnormal	1.1 (1.0-1.2)	0.2 (0.08-0.51)
ESR >50 mm/hr	1.2 (1.0-1.4)	0.35 (0.18-0.67)
ESR >100 mm/hr	1.9 (1.1-3.3)	0.8 (0.68-0.95)
Anemia	NS	NS

*Based on literature review, with the number of patients for each variable ranging from 68 to 2475.

CI, confidence interval; ESR, erythrocyte sedimentation rate; NS, not significant.

Modified from Smetana GW, Shmerling RH: Does this patient have temporal arteritis? *JAMA* 287:92, 2002.

A large number of disorders can mimic GCA (Table 88-7). There are many causes of monocular vision loss besides vasculitis including arteriosclerosis-induced thromboembolic disease.[43] Patients with nonarteritic vision loss do not have other GCA-related symptoms, signs, or findings. The funduscopic examination may help by revealing Hollenhorst plaques in cases caused by cholesterol emboli. Anterior ischemic optic neuropathy, the most common cause of vision loss in GCA, can also be caused by arteriosclerosis. Nonarteritic optic neuropathy invariably produces a small optic disc and cup-to-disc ratio, whereas GCA-related optic neuropathy results in an optic disc of variable size.[43] Thus a normal size or large cup in a patient with anterior ischemic optic neuropathy suggests GCA until proved otherwise.[43]

Constitutional symptoms with anemia and an elevated ESR in an older person may also be produced by occult infections (e.g., tuberculosis, bacterial endocarditis, human immunodeficiency virus [HIV]) or malignancy (especially lymphoma and multiple myeloma). These diagnoses highlight the value of selective serologic tests, imaging studies, and immunoelectrophoresis in appropriate patients. Systemic amyloidosis can closely mimic GCA, being one of the few disorders other than GCA that causes jaw claudication. The amyloid deposits in the temporal artery may not be detected unless the specimen is stained with Congo red. Polyarthritis in an older patient is much more likely caused by RA than by GCA. In one study of 520 GCA patients, less than 2% developed polyarthritis before GCA was diagnosed.

Criteria for the classification of GCA have been formulated and can help differentiate this arteritis from other forms of vasculitis[64] (see Table 88-1). Takayasu's arteritis, like GCA, can affect the aorta and the major arterial branches to the head and arms. Takayasu's arteritis, however, is a disease of young women. Antineutrophil cytoplasmic antibody (ANCA)-associated granulomatous vasculitis can affect the temporal artery and, along with systemic amyloidosis, is an exception to the rule that jaw claudication is pathognomonic for GCA. AGV, however, almost always produces telltale involvement of the respiratory tract or kidneys and is associated with ANCAs. Polyarteritis nodosa can also affect the temporal artery and should be considered if the biopsy does not contain giant cells and the patient has other features atypical for GCA such as mesenteric arteritis. Fibrinoid necrosis of the vasa vasorum occurs in polyarteritis but rarely, if ever, in GCA. Primary angiitis of the central nervous system differs from GCA in that it affects the intracranial arteries.

The diagnosis of PMR is clinical and depends on eliciting the symptoms and findings noted earlier. Two sets of criteria for the diagnosis have been proposed[2,3] (see Table 88-2). Several disorders can mimic PMR (see Table 88-7). Distinguishing early RA from PMR can be difficult, especially in the 15% of patients who are rheumatoid factor negative and in those few RA patients who have not yet developed prominent synovitis of the small joints of the hands and feet. Patients with polymyositis complain much more of weakness than of pain—the opposite symptom pattern reported by patients with PMR. In addition, in polymyositis, levels

Table 88-7 Differential Diagnosis of Giant Cell Arteritis and Polymyalgia Rheumatica

Disease Type	Specific Entities
Giant Cell Arteritis	
Occult infections	Tuberculosis, bacterial endocarditis, human immunodeficiency virus
Malignancy	Lymphoma and multiple myeloma
Systemic amyloidosis	—
Other forms of vasculitis	Takayasu's arteritis, antineutrophil cytoplasmic antibody–associated granulomatous vasculitis, polyarteritis nodosa, primary angiitis of the central nervous system
	Other vascular disorders causing anterior ischemic optic neuropathy
Polymyalgia Rheumatica	
Early rheumatoid arthritis	—
Polymyositis	—
Chronic infections	Bacterial endocarditis
Fibromyalgia	
Complication of medication	Statins
Endocrine disorders	Hypothyroidism
Remitting, seronegative synovitis with pitting edema	

of muscle enzymes are elevated and electromyograms are abnormal. Although patients with neoplasms may have generalized musculoskeletal aching, there is no association between PMR and malignant neoplasia. Therefore a search for an underlying tumor is not necessary unless some clinical evidence for a tumor is present or the patient has an atypically poor response to low-dose prednisone.

Some patients with chronic infections such as bacterial endocarditis may have findings simulating PMR, and blood cultures should be obtained in patients with fever. Patients with fibromyalgia usually do not have typical morning stiffness and have laboratory test results that are normal or nearly so. Rarely, the stiffness of early Parkinson's disease can be confused with PMR if the bradykinesia and tremor of Parkinson's disease are subtle or absent. Lumbar spinal stenosis sometimes causes patients to complain of pain and stiffness in the hip girdle area. The absence of symptoms above the waist helps differentiate it from PMR. Cholesterol-lowering statin drugs can produce myalgia with or without muscle enzyme elevations but rarely mimic PMR. Hypothyroidism in the elderly can mimic many conditions including PMR. A peculiar syndrome of remitting, seronegative synovitis with pitting edema (designated RS$_3$PE syndrome) may be difficult to differentiate from PMR, and they may be related disorders. Patients with the RS$_3$PE syndrome develop acute symmetric polysynovitis of distal joints with pitting edema of the hands and feet. The RS$_3$PE syndrome and PMR both respond to nonsteroidal anti-inflammatory drugs (NSAIDs) and low-dose prednisone.[10,64]

Diagnostic Evaluation in Giant Cell Arteritis

Temporal artery biopsy is the "gold standard" for diagnosing GCA.[10,65] Because GCA does not involve the artery in a continuous fashion, temporal artery biopsy should be directed to the symptomatic side, if evident. Removing a small (1- to 2-cm) section of temporal artery is usually adequate in patients who have palpable abnormalities of the vessel.[66] Otherwise, the surgeon should try to excise a 4- to 6-cm sample, and the pathologist should examine multiple sections.[10] In skilled hands, temporal artery biopsy is virtually free of morbidity or mortality. Scalp necrosis can rarely complicate active GCA but has not developed as a consequence of temporal artery biopsy.[65]

Temporal artery biopsies performed at institutions experienced in treating GCA are sensitive and have a high negative predictive value. At the Mayo Clinic, the sensitivity of temporal artery biopsy is approximately 90% to 95%, meaning that only 5% to 10% of patients with negative biopsies will subsequently be proved (by additional biopsy, angiography, or autopsy) to have GCA and require corticosteroid therapy.[65] The sensitivity figures noted previously include some patients who underwent bilateral temporal artery biopsy. Estimates of the value of bilateral biopsies vary.[64,67,68] Of 234 cases of biopsy-proven GCA, unilateral biopsy was positive in 86% and the second biopsy was positive in 14%.[64] Other studies indicate that a second temporal artery biopsy improves the diagnostic yield by only 3% to 5%.[68]

Management of a patient with a negative unilateral biopsy depends on how strongly the patient's clinical picture suggests GCA (Figure 88-7). When GCA is still strongly

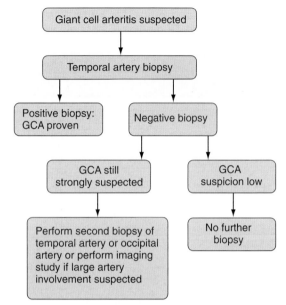

Figure 88-7 Algorithm for diagnosing giant cell arteritis (GCA).

suspected, a second biopsy or an imaging test (see later) should be considered. Opting for a second temporal artery biopsy probably makes most sense in patients who have jaw claudication or diplopia. Patients with chiefly occipital headache may be best diagnosed by biopsy of the occipital artery.[69] Patients who have signs of subclavian and axillary disease manifested by arm claudication, unequal arm blood pressures, and supraclavicular or axillary bruits may be diagnosed by angiogram, MRA, or CT scan.[57] Typically, patients with extracranial GCA have smooth, tapered stenosis or occlusion of the subclavian, axillary, and proximal brachial arteries. In one series, temporal artery biopsy was positive in only 58% of patients with larger artery involvement.[57] MRI and CT are the best-established methods for detecting aortic involvement by GCA.[10]

Other imaging techniques have been proposed to assist in the diagnosis of GCA. Color duplex ultrasonography showed abnormalities of the temporal artery in 28 of 30 patients with GCA (sensitivity of 93%).[70] The most characteristic finding was a dark halo around the lumen of the temporal artery (Figure 88-8). However, the diagnostic value of ultrasonography is undermined by the absence of expertise with this technique at most medical centers and conflicting estimates of its sensitivity and specificity.[71-73] One meta-analysis of 2036 patients in 23 studies estimated that the sensitivity and specificity of the halo sign were 69% and 82%, respectively. Another study found that ultrasonography did not improve the diagnostic accuracy of a carefully performed physical examination.[74] High-resolution MRI can demonstrate contrast enhancement and mural thickening of superficial cranial arteries in GCA. Small studies have found a sensitivity of 91% and a specificity of 73% compared with temporal artery biopsy.[71-73] Best results are achieved with 3-Tesla MRI scanners.[73] PET has shown promise in detecting occult involvement of the aorta and great vessels by GCA; however, estimates of sensitivity have varied from 65% to 100% and specificity from 77% to 99%.[71,73] PET scanning cannot image small arteries that are near highly metabolic tissues such as the brain and thus

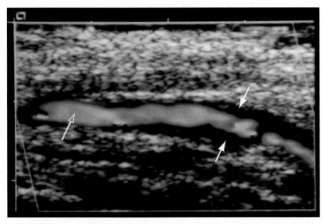

Figure 88-8 Color duplex ultrasound examination of a swollen, tender temporal artery in a patient with giant cell arteritis. The variably thickened artery wall is visible as a clear "halo" *(solid arrows)* around the lumen in the center *(open arrow). (Courtesy Dr. Gene Hunder.)*

cannot be used to study superficial extracranial arteries. Repeated PET scans do not predict the risk of relapse.[73] For the rare patient who has a compelling story for GCA but negative, bilateral temporal artery biopsies, one should reconsider conditions that mimic GCA described earlier (e.g., ask the pathologist to stain the biopsied arteries with Congo red to rule out systemic amyloidosis). If no other diagnosis becomes evident, then it is reasonable to search for occult large vessel disease with an imaging test such as a PET scan or MRA to look for occult aortic disease. Rarely, a patient's clinical picture strongly indicates GCA despite negative biopsies and imaging. In this case the patient can be treated for GCA while watching vigilantly for the emergence of another disease.

Treatment and Course

Most authorities recommend starting glucocorticoid therapy as soon as the diagnosis of GCA is strongly suspected. The main goal of treatment is to prevent loss of vision. Because vision loss is almost always permanent, it seems prudent to initiate corticosteroid therapy as early as possible, even before the biopsy is performed. Fortunately, the diagnostic yield of temporal artery biopsy is not altered by corticosteroid therapy for at least 2 weeks and perhaps longer.[75]

Initial Treatment for Giant Cell Arteritis

An initial dose of prednisone 40 to 60 mg/day or equivalent is adequate in nearly all cases.[10] Dividing the dose for the first 1 to 2 weeks may accelerate the rate of improvement. If the patient does not respond promptly, the dose should be increased. One double-blind, placebo-controlled, randomized trial involving 27 GCA patients suggested that initiating treatment with intravenous methylprednisolone (15 mg/kg of ideal weight per day) for 3 days allowed more rapid tapering of oral corticosteroids and increased the likelihood of achieving a sustained remission.[76] The small size of that study and the possible overreliance on laboratory tests to define relapse raise questions about the generalizability of these results. High-dose, intravenous-pulse methylprednisolone (1000 mg/day) for 3 days has also been tried

in patients with recent loss of vision. Unfortunately, the loss remains permanent in the vast majority of patients. The occlusive nature of the vasculitis argues against any role of acute thrombolytic therapy in the treatment of blindness.

Because all patients with GCA require months of glucocorticoid therapy, measures to prevent osteoporosis should be started early, as outlined in Table 88-8. In addition, because traditional risk factors for atherosclerosis (e.g., smoking, hypertension, diabetes, hypercholesterolemia) might increase the risk of vision loss or stroke in GCA,[45] reducing or eliminating these risk factors is an important part of overall management.

Subsequent Treatment for Giant Cell Arteritis

The initial effective dose of prednisone should be continued until all reversible symptoms, signs, and laboratory abnormalities have reverted to normal.[10] This usually takes 2 to 4 weeks. After that, the dose can be gradually reduced by a maximum of 10% of the total dose each week or every 2 weeks.[10] The decision to reduce prednisone should be based on a composite assessment of the patient's symptoms, signs, and laboratory markers of inflammation. The ESR and serum concentration of CRP are generally the most convenient and helpful laboratory markers of inflammation. The ESR is reliable only if performed promptly after the blood sample is obtained. Serum levels of IL-6 appear to be the most sensitive marker of activity of GCA, but this test is not widely available.[77] CRP may be slightly more sensitive than ESR in detecting flares.[77] At some point during drug tapering, the ESR or CRP may rise above normal again, and further reductions of prednisone should be temporarily interrupted. If, over the next week or so, the patient does not develop signs or symptoms of active GCA, reductions in prednisone (at smaller decrements and at longer intervals) can usually be resumed. Doses of 10 to 20 mg/day or more are often required for several months before further reductions are possible. However, making the prednisone dose a slave to the levels of inflammatory markers without regard to the patient's overall clinical context risks corticosteroid-related side effects. Gradual reductions allow the identification of the minimal suppressive dose and help avoid exacerbations resulting from too-rapid tapering. Even with a gradual reduction of prednisone, more than 50% of

Table 88-8 Measures to Prevent Corticosteroid-Induced Osteoporosis in Giant Cell Arteritis or Polymyalgia Rheumatica

Avoid or stop smoking
Reduce alcohol consumption if excessive
Participate in weight-bearing exercise
Supplement diet with calcium (1000 to 1500 mg/day)
Supplement diet with vitamin D (800 IU/day)
Measure BMD at lumbar spine and hip
If BMD is normal, repeat BMD annually
If BMD is not normal (i.e., T score below −1), prescribe bisphosphonate

BMD, bone mineral density.
Modified from American College of Rheumatology Ad Hoc Committee on Glucocorticoid-Induced Osteoporosis: Recommendations for the prevention and treatment of glucocorticoid-induced osteoporosis, *Arthritis Rheum* 44:1496, 2001.

patients experience flares of disease activity during the first year.[78] These exacerbations can usually be handled by increasing the prednisone 10 mg above the last dose at which the disease was controlled.

Most patients with GCA have a chronic disease that requires prednisone treatment for at least 1 year and often for several years; a minority of patients run a self-limited course of only several months.[10] Glucocorticoids can eventually be reduced and discontinued in some patients. Many patients require low doses of prednisone for several years or more to control musculoskeletal symptoms.

The nearly universal experience of serious side effects associated with daily corticosteroids has prompted the search for alternative steroid-sparing treatments. Unfortunately, to date, none has been convincingly effective. Alternate-day prednisone, for example, is not effective initial therapy for GCA. The combination of weekly low-dose oral methotrexate and prednisone was steroid sparing in one placebo-controlled, double-blind treatment trial but not in another.[78] These conflicting results argue against using methotrexate in combination with prednisone as initial therapy for GCA. Methotrexate may be worth adding to the treatment regimen of a patient who has experienced several exacerbations despite slow tapering of prednisone. Although open-label studies suggested that anti–tumor necrosis factor (TNF) agents might be effective in a granulomatous vasculitic process, neither infliximab nor etanercept is effective in GCA.[79,80] In fact, in a treatment trial of patients with GPA, etanercept in combination with cyclophosphamide increased the number of solid tumors compared with cyclophosphamide alone. Similarly, cytotoxic drugs, dapsone, antimalarials, and cyclosporine have not been clearly shown to be effective, but they may be considered in patients who cannot achieve an acceptably low dose of prednisone.[10]

No prospective, double-blind trials have tested the potential adjunctive role of aspirin or anticoagulants in the treatment of GCA. However, aspirin is theoretically appealing because, in experimental models of GCA, it inhibits IFN-γ production more effectively than prednisone.[81] In addition, two retrospective studies found that GCA patients taking low-dose aspirin or anticoagulant therapy had a threefold to fivefold lower risk of developing an ischemic event such as vision loss.[82,83] Together, these studies suggest that it is reasonable to add low-dose aspirin in GCA patients who do not have an excessive risk of gastrointestinal bleeding.

Arm claudication from GCA affecting the subclavian and axillary arteries usually improves or resolves with corticosteroid therapy. Rare GCA patients with severe upper extremity claudication unresponsive to corticosteroid therapy may benefit from balloon angioplasty. In one series of 10 patients, all improved initially after angioplasty but 50% developed symptomatic restenosis over 2 months.[84] In all cases, recurrent stenosis developed in vascular lesions that were greater than 3 cm long.[84]

Thoracic aortic aneurysm is greatly increased in patients with GCA. Although it can be present at the outset, aneurysms are usually noted late in the disease course, an average of 7 years after onset. Some authorities have recommended annual chest radiographs to detect thoracic aortic aneurysms.

Treatment for Polymyalgia Rheumatica

Patients with PMR without symptoms or signs or biopsy evidence of GCA are usually treated initially with prednisone 10 to 20 mg/day or equivalent.[85] A systematic review of 30 studies recommended starting treatment with prednisone at 15 mg/day: Lower initial doses were less effective and higher doses were more toxic.[86] Salicylates and NSAIDs have been used but are less appealing; salicylates and NSAIDs adequately control symptoms in only a minority of patients with milder symptoms and add to overall adverse drug reactions when they are used with glucocorticoids.[2,7] Prednisone therapy usually results in rapid (often overnight) and dramatic improvement of the musculoskeletal aching and stiffness and a more gradual return of the ESR and CRP level to normal. A minority of patients with isolated PMR fails to respond to prednisone 20 mg/day after 1 week and may require up to 30 mg/day as initial treatment. Studies suggest that these resistant cases are more likely to have ESRs greater than 50 mm/hr and high levels of IL-6. Failure to respond to prednisone 30 mg/day for 1 week should prompt a search for an alternative diagnosis (Figure 88-9). Lower doses of prednisone might not suppress an underlying arteritis if it is present. Thus the patient must be observed carefully even though the aching improves. In patients with PMR, the dose should be reduced gradually as soon as symptoms permit. Pretreatment ESR, CRP, and IL-6 concentrations and initial responses to therapy appear to be helpful in dividing patients into subsets with different treatment requirements.[85] If the laboratory test results become normal while the patient is receiving a smaller dose, the likelihood of an underlying active vasculitis seems to be much less, and the risk of vascular complications is smaller. However, this is not true in all instances because active arteritis has been observed even though the ESR improved.

Once the symptoms, signs, and laboratory abnormalities of PMR have resolved (usually after 2 to 3 weeks of therapy), the daily dose of prednisone can be slowly tapered. Some experts recommend tapering prednisone by 2.5 mg every week until 10 mg/day is reached, at which point the decrements should be reduced by 1 mg each month.[86] Flares are common, necessitating a dose increase to achieve remission before attempting a slower taper. The minority of patients with PMR succeed in tapering off prednisone in less than 1 year. Many require at least 2 years of low-dose prednisone.[87]

Some, but not all, studies suggest that oral methotrexate (10 mg once a week for 48 weeks) can reduce the long-term need for corticosteroids in patients with PMR.[86,88] It is not yet known whether the small but statistically significant reduction in prednisone use achieved with methotrexate results in a clinically important reduction in prednisone-related side effects.

TAKAYASU'S ARTERITIS

Takayasu's arteritis (TA), also known as *pulseless disease* or *occlusive thromboaortopathy*, is a form of vasculitis of unknown cause that chiefly affects the aorta and its major branches, most frequently in young women.[89,90] The disease is named for the Japanese ophthalmologist who in 1908 described a young woman with peculiar retinal arteriovenous

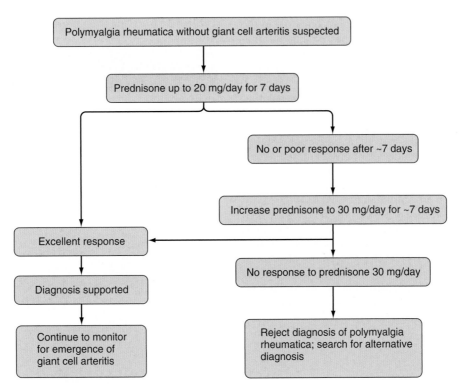

Figure 88-9 Algorithm for diagnosing polymyalgia rheumatica without giant cell arteritis.

anastomoses caused by retinal ischemia from large vessel vasculitis.[1]

American College of Rheumatology Criteria

The ACR classification criteria for the diagnosis of TA are listed in Table 88-9.

Epidemiology

Although TA has been described worldwide, it occurs most commonly in Japan, China, India, and Southeast Asia; the disease is also prevalent in Mexico. Whereas the incidence of TA in Japan is nearly 150 per million per year, it is only 0.2 to 2.6 per million in western Europe and North America. TA affects women eight times more frequently than men. The median age of onset is 25 years; however, approximately 25% of cases begin before age 20, and 10%

Table 88-9 American College of Rheumatology Classification Criteria for Takayasu's Arteritis*

Onset before age 40 yr
Limb claudication
Decreased brachial artery pulse
Unequal arm blood pressure (>10 mm Hg)
Subclavian or aortic bruit
Angiographic evidence of narrowing or occlusion of aorta or its primary branches, or large limb arteritis

*The presence of three or more of the six criteria is sensitive (91%) and specific (98%) for the diagnosis of Takayasu's arteritis.

American College of Rheumatology 1990 criteria for the classification of Takayasu arteritis, *Arthritis Rheum* 33:1129, 1990. From Hellmann DB: Takayasu arteritis. In Imboden JB, Hellmann DB, Stone JH, editors: *Current rheumatology diagnosis and treatment,* New York, 2004, Lange Medical Books/McGraw-Hill, p 245.

to 20% present after age 40.[89] Immunogenetic studies in Japanese patients suggest an association with several HLAs, especially HLA-Bw52, Dw12, DR2, and DQw1. Different HLA associations have been found in Koreans and Indians. No HLA association has been found in North American patients. In Mexican patients, TA has been associated with previous exposure to *Mycobacterium tuberculosis.*

Cause and Pathogenesis

The cause of TA is unknown. The nearly identical pathology in TA and GCA has invited speculation that the model of immunopathogenesis of GCA described earlier (see Figure 88-3) applies to TA as well.[22,40] Indeed, some have argued that TA and GCA represent a spectrum within the same disease. Like GCA, TA is thought to result from an autoimmune process that targets large elastic-containing arteries. Both feature panarteritis involving infiltration of dendritic cells; T cells (including $\alpha\beta$, $\gamma\delta$, and cytotoxic); natural killer cells; and macrophages. In TA, the majority of lymphocytes are perforin-secreting killer lymphocytes such as T cells and natural killer cells. The T cell receptors in TA, as in GCA, are oligoclonal, suggesting that the vasculitis is driven in both diseases by a T cell response to a specific but unknown antigen.[91] Chronic inflammation of the vessel wall leads to aneurysm formation, stenosis, or thrombosis more frequently in TA than in GCA. Dissection occurs in TA but is rare and less frequent than in syphilitic aortitis.[92] The late phase of TA, like that of GCA, is characterized by intima proliferation with superimposed atherosclerosis, medial necrosis with scarring, and adventitial fibrosis. As in GCA, the inflammatory involvement in TA can be continuous or segmental, with skip areas of normal vessel interposed between involved areas.[92] It is possible that the humoral immune system may play some role in the pathogenesis of TA; most TA patients possess antiendothelial cell antibodies that can damage vessels by inducing endothelial inflammatory cytokine production, adhesion molecules, and apoptosis.

The geographic clustering of cases has suggested that genetics and environmental factors participate in the pathogenesis of TA. However, immunogenetic studies (described earlier) have not identified any other universally shared genetic risk factors. The young age of onset and the female predominance in TA and in systemic lupus erythematosus have invited speculation about the influence of female hormones in promoting an autoimmune disease process. In some countries, the apparent association of TA with high rates of exposure to tuberculosis has suggested an infectious cause. An animal model of TA has been produced in mice using a herpesvirus that infects the smooth muscle cells of the media. In that model, the media of large elastic arteries serves as an immunoprivileged site that allows the herpesvirus to propagate a chronic inflammatory response in the aorta and its major branches.[93]

Clinical Features

Symptoms and Signs

Although the presenting manifestations of TA are protean, the vast majority of patients present with symptoms and signs of vascular insufficiency (from stenosis, occlusion, or aneurysm); systemic inflammation; or both[74,89] (Table 88-10). In a North American series of 60 patients followed at the National Institutes of Health, the most common presenting vascular symptoms were claudication (35%), reduced or absent pulse (25%), carotid bruit (20%), hypertension (20%), carotidynia (20%), lightheadedness (20%), and asymmetric arm blood pressures (15%).[89] Stroke, aortic regurgitation, and visual abnormalities were present at onset in less than 10% of patients. The extreme manifestations of retinal ischemia noted in Takayasu's original patient are rarely seen now.[89] Permanent loss of vision, the major concern in GCA, rarely develops in TA.

Claudication affects the arms at least twice as frequently as the legs. For many young women, arm claudication first reveals itself as arm pain or fatigue experienced while trying to hold a hair dryer. Overall, bruit is the most common sign, eventually found in 80% of patients. Although bruit over the carotid artery is most frequent, it can also be found in the supraclavicular, infraclavicular, axillary, flank, chest, abdominal, and femoral areas. One-third of patients have multiple bruits.[89] Unequal arm blood pressures eventually develop in half of all patients. Headache, which is common in TA, does not correlate with carotid or vertebral disease, which develops in nearly 40% of patients.[89,94]

Constitutional, musculoskeletal, and other symptoms of systemic inflammation are also common presenting complaints.[74,89] About one in five TA patients presents with fever and malaise, which can be accompanied by night sweats and weight loss. A few patients who have minimal or no signs of vascular insufficiency may appear to have FUO for weeks or months before the diagnosis of TA becomes evident. A minority of patients present with

Table 88-10 Clinical Features of Takayasu's Arteritis

Feature	At Presentation (%)	Ever Present (%)
Vascular	50	100
Bruit		80
Claudication (upper extremity)	30	62
Claudication (lower extremity)	15	32
Hypertension	20	33
Unequal arm blood pressures	15	50
Carotidynia	15	32
Aortic regurgitation		20
Central nervous system	30	57
Lightheadedness	20	35
Visual abnormality	10	30
Stroke	5	10
Musculoskeletal	20	53
Chest wall pain	10	30
Joint pain	10	30
Myalgia	5	15
Constitutional	33	43
Malaise	20	30
Fever	20	25
Weight loss	15	20
Cardiac	15	38
Aortic regurgitation	8	20
Angina	2	12
Congestive heart failure	2	10

Data based on a study of 60 North American patients reported by Kerr GS, Hallahan CW, Giordano A, et al: Takayasu arteritis, *Ann Intern Med* 120:919, 1994. From Hellmann DB: Takayasu arteritis. In Imboden JB, Hellmann DB, Stone JH, editors: *Current rheumatology diagnosis and treatment*, New York, 2004, Lange Medical Books/McGraw-Hill, p 243.

myalgia or arthralgia (see Table 88-10). Some patients have striking midthoracic back pain, perhaps as a result of aortic inflammation irritating nociceptive nerve fibers.

Cardiac involvement occurs eventually in nearly one-third of patients (see Table 88-10).[89] Aortic regurgitation develops in 20% of patients as a result of aortic root dilation. Aortic regurgitation is important because it frequently progresses and may lead to left ventricular dilation with secondary mitral regurgitation and congestive heart failure. Aortic valve replacement is often required eventually. Angina can develop as a result of coronary artery disease. TA of the coronary arteries most often produces ostial lesions but can also produce either diffuse vasculitis of the coronary arteries or aneurysms.[95-97] Myocarditis also occurs in TA and causes potentially reversible congestive heart failure. Pericarditis is rare. TA is, along with Behçet's disease, one of the few forms of vasculitis that can affect the large pulmonary arteries. Although TA of the pulmonary arteries is rare (<3%), affected patients can present with cough, chest wall pain, dyspnea, or hemoptysis.

Unlike polyarteritis or GPA, TA rarely causes peripheral neuropathies. Cutaneous manifestations develop in less than 10% of patients with TA.[89] Erythema nodosum is most common, but purpura, livedo reticularis, and ulceration may rarely occur. As in GCA, a minority of TA patients with active disease have a persistent, dry cough.

Laboratory Findings

At presentation, the ESR is more frequently elevated (80%) than the CRP (≈50%).[74] Mild anemia and hypergammaglobulinemia are common. The white blood cell count is usually normal or slightly elevated. The platelet count is elevated in one-third of patients and may exceed 500,000/μL in those with active disease. The serum creatinine and urinalysis are usually normal. Any renal abnormalities are usually secondary to hypertension; unlike ANCA-associated vasculitis, TA rarely causes glomerulonephritis.

Imaging Studies

Vascular abnormalities in TA can be imaged by conventional angiography, MRI, MRA, CT angiography, or ultrasonography[24,71,73,89,98] (Figures 88-10 to 88-12). Each imaging technique has advantages and disadvantages (Table 88-11). The earliest detectable abnormality in TA is thickening of the vessel wall from inflammation. MRI, ultrasonography, and, to a lesser degree, CT can detect this early vessel wall thickening. Conventional angiography is invasive and provides the least sensitive method for visualizing wall thickness; however, conventional angiography is the "gold standard" for precisely delineating the stenoses, occlusions,

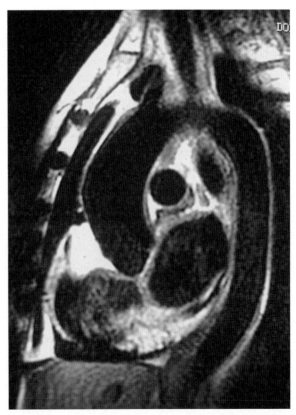

Figure 88-11   Magnetic resonance image (sagittal section) through the chest showing thickening of the ascending and descending thoracic aorta in a 26-year-old woman with Takayasu's arteritis. *(From Hellmann DB: Takayasu arteritis. In Imboden J, Hellmann DB, Stone JH, editors:* Current rheumatology: diagnosis & treatment, *New York, 2004, McGraw-Hill, p 244.)*

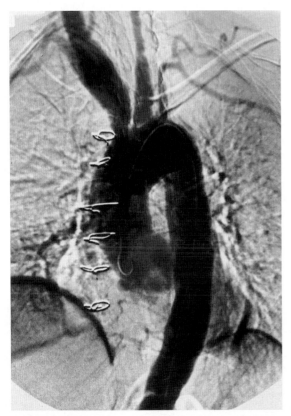

Figure 88-10   Angiogram showing multiple changes of Takayasu's arteritis including dilation of the aortic root (with surgical wires from previous aortic valve replacement), aneurysmal dilation of the innominate and right carotid arteries, and occlusion of the distal left common carotid artery. *(From Hellmann DB, Flynn JA: Clinical presentation and natural history of Takayasu's arteritis and other inflammatory arteritides. In Perler BA, Becker GJ, editors:* Vascular intervention: a clinical approach, *New York, 1998, Thieme Medical and Scientific Publisher, pp 249–256.)*

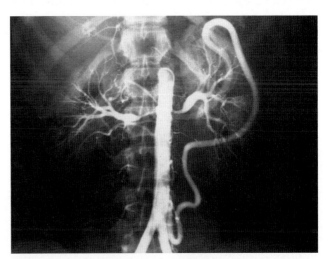

Figure 88-12   Angiogram showing bilateral renal artery stenosis. A large left colic branch of the inferior mesenteric artery provides collateral circulation to the gut. *(From Hellmann DB, Flynn JA: Clinical presentation and natural history of Takayasu's arteritis and other inflammatory arteritides. In Perler BA, Becker GJ, editors:* Vascular intervention: a clinical approach, *New York, 1998, Thieme Medical and Scientific Publisher, pp 249–256.)*

Table 88-11 Comparison of Imaging Techniques in Takayasu's Arteritis

Technique	Advantages	Disadvantages
Conventional angiography	"Gold standard" image quality Allows CAP measurement Allows angioplasty at same time	Invasive Radiation exposure Does not visualize vessel wall thickness
Magnetic resonance angiography	Excellent image quality Noninvasive No ionizing radiation exposure Visualizes vascular wall thickness	Image quality not "gold standard" Cannot use in patients with pacemaker CAP measurement not possible
Ultrasonography	Noninvasive No ionizing radiation exposure Can visualize vessel wall edema	Image quality not "gold standard" Image quality affected by obesity Operator dependent CAP measurement not possible
Computed tomography angiography	Excellent image quality	Ionizing radiation exposure CAP measurement not possible Intravenous contrast agent required
Positron emission tomography	Can measure intensity of vascular inflammation	Ionizing radiation exposure Vascular anatomy not well seen CAP measurement not possible Intravenous contrast agent required

CAP, central arterial blood pressure.

and aneurysms that characterize the latter stages of TA. Also, only conventional angiography allows the direct measurement of central arterial blood pressure, which may be otherwise unobtainable in patients with stenotic lesions affecting all four extremities. Although MRA does not provide the same level of detail as conventional angiography, it comes close. Because MRA is not invasive and does not involve ionizing radiation, it has become the preferred imaging method for assessing the extent of vascular involvement and damage, both initially and during follow-up. The role of MRI in assessing disease activity is not clear because vessel wall edema and contrast enhancement have not correlated well with clinical measures of disease activity.[73] Although PET scanning would be expected to be more sensitive than angiography in the early detection of vascular inflammation that precedes the development of stenoses, its sensitivity may be no greater than MRI. PET scanning has no established role in following disease activity in TA. Indeed, one study of 28 TA patients showed that PET scans did not correlate with clinical, biologic, or MRI assessment of disease activity.[99]

The most common sites of lesions in TA are the aorta (65%) and the left subclavian arteries (93%)[89] (Table 88-12). The left subclavian artery is affected slightly more frequently than the right. Carotid, renal, and vertebral arteries are also commonly affected.[89] Lesions may be stenotic (93%), occluded (57%), dilated (16%), or aneurysmal (7%). Stenotic lesions are about four times more common than aneurysmal lesions.[89] Stenotic segments often extend a few centimeters and may be followed by areas of dilation (see Figure 88-10). The majority of patients (53%) have vascular lesions above and below the diaphragm. However, the frequency distribution of aortic lesions varies considerably from country to country.[89]

Diagnosis and Diagnostic Tests

The ACR has established classification criteria for the diagnosis of TA (see Table 88-9). In clinical practice, the diagnosis of TA is almost always secured by an imaging procedure (see Table 88-11) that demonstrates the characteristic

abnormalities of the aorta and its major branches (Figure 88-13). Rarely, the diagnosis is first suggested when a pathologist finds granulomatous inflammation in a section of aorta or other larger artery that was removed or biopsied during a vascular surgery procedure. Unfortunately, the diagnosis of TA is often delayed; the delay averaged 44 months in one large series. The most frequent impediment to a speedy diagnosis is a physician's failure to consider TA in the differential diagnosis. Although the rarity of TA helps explain its omission from diagnostic consideration, another reason is that some patients have striking features of inflammation that camouflage or overshadow the somewhat more familiar vascular abnormalities. Indeed, a few patients with TA present chiefly with FUO. Most of these patients have other, albeit subtle, manifestations of TA such as bruits, diminished pulses, unequal arm blood pressures, or aortic regurgitation. In other patients with more striking vascular abnormalities, the physician might be lured into focusing on familiar and dramatic abnormalities such as anemia or thrombocytopenia. Thus instead of ordering an imaging test that would explain the patient's unequal and low blood pressure in the left arm, the physician mistakenly

Table 88-12 Frequency of Blood Vessel Involvement in Takayasu's Arteritis

Blood Vessel	% Abnormal
Aorta	65
Aortic arch or root	35
Abdominal aorta	47
Thoracic aorta	17
Subclavian artery	93
Common carotid artery	58
Renal artery	38
Vertebral artery	35
Celiac axes	18
Common iliac artery	17
Pulmonary artery	5

Data based on a study of 60 North America patients reported by Kerr GS, Hallahan CW, Giordano A, et al: Takayasu arteritis, *Ann Intern Med* 120:919, 1994. From Hellmann DB: Takayasu arteritis. In Imboden JB, Hellmann DB, Stone JH, editors: *Current rheumatology diagnosis and treatment*, New York, 2004, Lange Medical Books/McGraw-Hill, p 245.

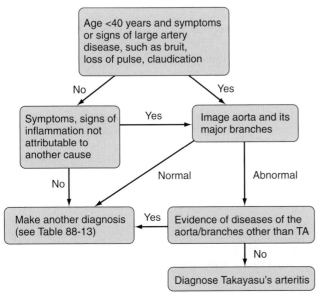

Figure 88-13 Algorithm for the diagnosis of Takayasu's arteritis (TA).

Table 88-14 Comparison of Giant Cell Arteritis and Takayasu's Arteritis

Feature	Giant Cell Arteritis	Takayasu's Arteritis
Female-male ratio	2:1	8:1
Age range (yr)	≥50	<40
Average age of onset (yr)	72	25
Visual loss	10%-30%	Rare
Involvement of aorta or its major branches	25%	100%
Histopathology	Granulomatous arteritis	Granulomatous arteritis
Pulmonary artery involvement	No	Occasionally
Renal hypertension	Rare	Common
Claudication	Uncommon	Common
Ethnic groups with highest incidence	Scandinavians	Asians
Corticosteroid responsive	Yes	Yes
Bruits present	Minority	Majority
Surgical intervention needed	Rare	Common

diverts the patient to a hematologist, gastroenterologist, or oncologist for additional blood tests and procedures that further delay the diagnosis.

Many of these delays can be prevented by remembering that TA should be included in the differential diagnosis of any person younger than 40 years who presents with FUO, aortic regurgitation, hypertension, or unequal or absent pulses. Delays in diagnosis can also be reduced by carefully searching for unequal or absent upper extremity pulses and by listening for bruits not only over the carotid arteries but also above and below the clavicle (for subclavian artery bruits) and over the abdomen and flanks (for renal and other mesenteric artery bruits). Recognizing that anemia and thrombocytosis can be manifestations of active inflammatory disorders such as vasculitis can also help speed the diagnosis of TA.

Once an imaging test demonstrates disease of the aorta or its major branches, the differential diagnosis narrows to a set of disorders that are usually easily differentiated (Table 88-13). Most rheumatic diseases that can affect the aorta are distinguished by their associated features. For example,

Table 88-13 Differential Diagnosis of Takayasu's Arteritis: Other Diseases That Can Affect the Aorta

Disease Type	Specific Entities
Rheumatic	Giant cell arteritis, Cogan's syndrome, relapsing polychrondritis, ankylosing spondylitis, rheumatoid arthritis, systemic lupus erythematosus, Buerger's disease, Behçet's disease
Infectious	Syphilis, tuberculosis
Other	Atherosclerosis, ergotism, radiation-induced damage, retroperitoneal fibrosis, inflammatory bowel disease, sarcoidosis, neurofibromatosis, congenital coarctation, Marfan's syndrome, Ehlers-Danlos syndrome, IgG4-related systemic disease

From Hellmann DB: Takayasu arteritis. In Imboden JB, Hellmann DB, Stone JH, editors: *Current rheumatology diagnosis and treatment,* New York, 2004, Lange Medical Books/McGraw-Hill, p 243.

Cogan's syndrome typically produces ocular inflammation (especially keratitis) and vestibuloauditory dysfunction. The one rheumatic disease that can be difficult to distinguish from TA is GCA (Table 88-14). Usually, the patient's age and the distribution of lesions allow their rapid differentiation, but distinguishing TA beginning after age 40 from GCA affecting chiefly the major branches of the aorta can be difficult or even impossible. The similarity of treatment (see later) diminishes the practical importance of solving this diagnostic dilemma.

Infections of the aorta are rare in most countries. Tertiary syphilis can be excluded by a negative fluorescent treponemal antibody test (the rapid plasma reagin test is falsely negative in about one-quarter of patients with late syphilis). Other diseases of the aorta (see Table 88-14) are usually readily separated from TA by the history and physical examination. There has been growing appreciation for a small subset of patients who have noninfectious aortitis that is difficult to categorize. At one center, noninfectious aortitis was found in 8% of patients undergoing resection of the ascending aorta.[100] Although nearly 70% had giant cells, only a minority neatly fit a diagnosis of TA or GCA. A fraction of the cases of thoracic or abdominal aortitis are caused by a recently recognized inflammatory condition known as IgG4-related disease (IgG4-RD) associated with high levels of IgG4.[101]

Treatment

Medical Therapy

Corticosteroids are the cornerstone of treatment of active TA.[89] Prednisone, at a dose of 0.5 to 1 mg/kg per day, is indicated for the treatment of active disease. Criteria for active disease include new onset or worsening of two or more of the following: (1) fever or other systemic features (in the absence of other cause); (2) elevated ESR; (3) symptoms or signs of vascular ischemia or inflammation (e.g., claudication, absent pulse, carotidynia); and (4) typical angiographic lesions.[89] Although about 85% of TA patients present with active disease, about 15% do not.[74] The initial dose of prednisone is continued for 4 to 12 weeks before commencing a gradual taper, as is done when treating GCA (see earlier). Although nearly two-thirds of patients achieve remission, more than half later relapse. Relapses are especially common as the prednisone dose falls below 20 mg per day.

Relapses can be treated by increasing the prednisone dose or adding an immunosuppressive agent. No agent used for TA has been evaluated in a double-blind, placebo-controlled trial. However, open trials have suggested that weekly oral methotrexate (started at 0.3 mg/kg per week, with the initial dose not to exceed 15 mg/wk) is a moderately effective corticosteroid-sparing drug.[102] Methotrexate can be gradually increased to 25 mg/wk. The emphasis is on lowering the corticosteroid dose because methotrexate seldom allows the elimination of prednisone completely; most patients continue to require at least 5 to 10 mg/day of prednisone. Small open trials have provided even more encouraging results about the effectiveness of anti-TNF inhibitors (etanercept and infliximab) in treating patients with refractory TA.[103] These trials emphasize that although these agents can treat TA, they rarely cure it: relapses are likely when the treatment is stopped.[103] Tocilizumab, which blocks the IL-6 receptor, has also been reported effective in individual patients.[104] Caution should be used when interpreting these results because similar open-label studies in GCA and PMR were also positive.

Small studies and series suggest that other corticosteroid-sparing drugs include azathioprine (2 mg/kg per day), mycophenolate mofetil (2000 mg/day), and cyclophosphamide (2 mg/kg per day).[89,105] The toxicity of cyclophosphamide in young women is so high that it is rarely used in TA.[89]

To prevent osteoporosis, patients on chronic corticosteroids should take calcium and vitamin D and perform weight-bearing exercises (see Table 88-8). In postmenopausal women, a bisphosphonate should be added if the bone mineral density is low (see Table 88-8). In premenopausal women, caution in use of bisphosphonates is advised: Their usefulness is less clear and recent use can harm a fetus. Modifiable risk factors for atherosclerosis—especially hypertension, smoking, inactivity, diabetes, and hyperlipidemia—should be treated maximally.

Surgical Therapy

TA is the form of vasculitis most frequently requiring revascularization procedures.[89,106,107] Unfortunately, medical therapy rarely reduces or reverses stenotic lesions. Treating stenotic or aneurysmal lesions may require bypass surgery (especially of stenotic cervicobrachial arteries, coronary arteries, or renal arteries); aortic valve replacement (for aortic regurgitation); or percutaneous transluminal angioplasty (especially for stenotic renal arteries causing hypertension).

A review of the experience with vascular interventions in TA supports several general recommendations. First, the mere presence of stenosis does not necessitate intervention. The gut, for example, has such rich collaterals that even critical stenoses of the celiac, superior, or inferior mesenteric arteries usually produce no symptoms and require no surgical intervention. Moreover, many patients with arm claudication will develop collateral circulation and improve substantially over time with medical therapy alone. For upper extremity vascular insufficiency, patiently waiting for a response to medical therapy usually pays higher dividends than undertaking rapid surgical intervention. Second, whenever possible, surgical intervention should be deferred until TA is in remission; procedures done during active disease often produce disappointing results. Third, bypass surgery yields better results than angioplasty. With bypass graft procedures, autologous vessels give better results than synthetic grafts (restenosis rates of 9% vs. 36%). Patients who undergo aortic surgery are liable to develop anastomotic aneurysms; such aneurysms developed in nearly 14% of patients followed for 20 years.[106,108] Although angioplasty gives good short-term results, long-term results are often disappointing except for very short stenotic segments.[108] The experience with conventional stents has been mostly disappointing.

Outcome and Prognosis

Twenty percent of TA patients have a self-limited disease. The rest have a relapsing-remitting or progressive course requiring chronic corticosteroid and/or immunosuppressive therapy. Nearly two-thirds of patients experience new angiographic lesions. In one study from the National Institutes of Health, 74% of patients experienced some form of morbidity and 47% were permanently disabled.[89] In a Japanese study of 120 patients, survival at 15 years was 83%.[108] Age of onset older than 35 years; development of major complications (i.e., retinopathy, hypertension, aortic regurgitation, and aneurysm); or a progressive course was associated with decreased survival. Congestive heart failure and renal failure are the most common causes of death.[106] Pregnancy appears to be relatively well tolerated in the presence of good medical care and in the absence of abdominal aortic involvement.[89,109]

References

1. Hunder GG, Bloch DA, Michel BA, et al: The American College of Rheumatology 1990 criteria for the classification of giant cell arteritis, *Arthritis Rheum* 33:1122, 1990.
2. Chuang T-Y, Hunder GG, Ilstrup DM, Kurland LT: Polymyalgia rheumatica: a 10-year epidemiologic and clinical study, *Ann Intern Med* 97:672, 1982.
3. Healey LA: Long-term follow-up of polymyalgia rheumatica: evidence for synovitis, *Semin Arthritis Rheum* 13:322, 1984.
3a. Dasgupta B, Cimmino MA, Kremers HM, et al: 2012 provisional classification criteria for polymyalgia rheumatica: a European League Against Rheumatism/American College of Rheumatology collaborative initiative, *Arthritis Rheum* 64:943–954, 2012.
4. Gonzalez-Gay MA, Vazquez-Rodriguez TR, Lopez-Diaz MJ, et al: Epidemiology of giant cell arteritis and polymyalgia rheumatica, *Arthritis Rheum* 61:15, 2009.
5. Hunder GG: The early history of giant cell arteritis and polymyalgia rheumatica, *Mayo Clin Proc* 81:1071, 2006.
6. Healey LA, Wilske KR: *The systemic manifestations of temporal arteritis*, New York, 1978, Grune & Stratton.
7. Salvarani C, Gabriel SE, O'Fallon WM, Hunder GG: The incidence of giant cell arteritis in Olmsted County, Minnesota: apparent fluctuations in cyclic pattern, *Ann Intern Med* 123:192, 1995.
8. Nordborg E, Bengtsson B-A: Epidemiology of biopsy-proven giant cell arteritis (GCA), *J Intern Med* 227:233, 1990.
9. Barrier J, Pion P, Massari R, et al: Epidemiologic approach to Horton's disease in Department of Loire-Atlantique: 110 cases in 10 years (1970-1979), *Rev Med Interne* 3:13, 1983.

10. Salvarani C, Cantini F, Boiardi L, Hunder GG: Polymyalgia rheumatica and giant cell arteritis, *N Engl J Med* 347:261, 2002.
11. Levine SM, Hellmann DB: Giant cell arteritis, *Curr Opin Rheumatol* 14:3, 2002.
12. Kermani TA, Schäfer VS, Crowson CS, et al: Increase in age at onset of giant cell arteritis: a population-based study, *Ann Rheum Dis* 69:780, 2010.
13. Östberg G: On arteritis with special reference to polymyalgia arteritica, *Acta Pathol Microbiol Scand (A)* 237(Suppl):1, 1973.
14. Liang GC, Simkin PA, Hunder GG, et al: Familial aggregation of polymyalgia rheumatica and giant cell arteritis, *Arthritis Rheum* 17:19, 1974.
15. Weyand CM, Hunder NN, Hicok KC, et al: HLA-DRB1 alleles in polymyalgia rheumatica, giant cell arteritis, and rheumatoid arthritis, *Arthritis Rheum* 37:514, 1994.
16. Duhaut P, Pinede L, Demolombe-Rague S, et al: Giant cell arteritis and cardiovascular risk factors, *Arthritis Rheum* 41:1960, 1998.
17. Álvarez-Lafuente R, Fernández-Gutiérrez B, Jover JA, et al: Human parvovirus B19, varicella zoster virus, and human herpes virus 6 in temporal artery biopsy specimens of patients with giant cell arteritis: analysis with quantitative real time polymerase chain reaction, *Ann Rheum Dis* 6:780, 2005.
18. Regan MJ, Wood BJ, Hsieh YH, et al: *Chlamydia pneumoniae* and temporal arteritis: failure to detect the organism by PCR in 180 cases and controls, *Arthritis Rheum* 46:1056, 2002.
19. Salvarani C, Gabriel SE, O'Fallon WM, Hunder GG: Epidemiology of polymyalgia rheumatica in Olmsted County, Minnesota, 1970-1991, *Arthritis Rheum* 38:369, 1995.
20. Sakkas LI, Loqueman N, Panayi GS, et al: Immunogenetics of polymyalgia rheumatica, *Br J Rheumatol* 29:331, 1990.
21. Bongartz T, Matteson EL: Large-vessel involvement in giant cell arteritis, *Curr Opin Rheumatol* 18:10, 2006.
22. Weyand CM, Goronzy JJ: Medium- and large-vessel vasculitis, *N Engl J Med* 39:160, 2003.
23. Klein RG, Campbell RJ, Hunder GG, Carney JA: Skip lesions in temporal arteritis, *Mayo Clin Proc* 51:50, 1976.
24. Wilkinson IMS, Russell RWR: Arteries of the head and neck in giant cell arteritis: a pathological study to show the pattern of arterial involvement, *Arch Neurol* 27:378, 1972.
25. Caselli RJ, Hunder GG: Neurologic aspects of giant cell (temporal) arteritis, *Rheum Dis Clin North Am* 19:941, 1993.
26. Reich KA, Giansiracusa DF, Strongwater SL: Neurologic manifestations of giant cell arteritis, *Am J Med* 89:67, 1990.
27. Cid MC, Campo E, Ercilla G, et al: Immunohistochemical analysis of lymphoid and macrophage cell subsets and the immunological activation markers in temporal arteritis, *Arthritis Rheum* 32:884, 1989.
28. Weyand CM, Garonzy JJ: Arterial wall injury in giant cell arteritis, *Arthritis Rheum* 42:844, 1999.
29. Wagner AD, Garonzy JJ, Weyand CM: Functional profile of tissue-infiltrating and circulating CD68⁺ cells in giant cell arteritis: evidence for two components of the disease, *J Clin Invest* 113, 1994.
30. Weyand CM, Hicok KC, Hunder GG, et al: Tissue cytokine patterns in patients with polymyalgia rheumatica and giant cell arteritis, *Ann Intern Med* 121:484, 1994.
31. Grunewald J, Andersson R, Rydberg L, et al: CD4⁺ and CD8⁺ T cell expansions using selected TCR V and J gene segments at the onset of giant cell arteritis, *Arthritis Rheum* 37:1221, 1994.
32. Weyand CM, Ma-Krupa W, Pryshchep O, et al: Vascular dendritic cells in giant cell arteritis, *Ann N Y Acad Sci* 1062:195, 2005.
33. Shmerling RH: An 81-year-old woman with temporal arteritis, *JAMA* 295:2525, 2006.
34. Weyand CM, Younge BR, Goronzy JJ: IFN-γ and IL-17: the two faces of T-cell pathology in giant cell arteritis, *Curr Opin Rheumatol* 23:43–49, 2010.
35. Kaiser M, Weyand CM, Bjornsson J, et al: Platelet-derived growth factor, intimal hyperplasia, and ischemic complications in giant cell arteritis, *Arthritis Rheum* 1:623, 1998.
36. Calamia KT, Hunder GG: Giant cell arteritis (temporal arteritis) presenting as fever of undetermined origin, *Arthritis Rheum* 2:11, 1981.
37. O'Duffy JD, Hunder GG, Wahner HW: A follow-up study of polymyalgia rheumatica: evidence of chronic axial synovitis, *J Rheumatol* 7:685, 1980.
38. Chou CT, Schumacher HR Jr: Clinical and pathologic studies of synovitis in polymyalgia rheumatica, *Arthritis Rheum* 27:1107, 1984.
39. Papaioannou CC, Gupta RC, Hunder GG, McDuffie FC: Circulating immune complexes in giant cell arteritis polymyalgia rheumatica, *Arthritis Rheum* 23:1021, 1980.
40. Piggott K, Biousse V, Newman NJ, et al: Vascular damage in giant cell arteritis, *Autoimmunity* 2:596, 2009.
41. Ma-Krupa W, Kwan M, Goronzy JJ, Weyand CM: Toll-like receptors in giant cell arteritis, *Clin Immunol* 115:38, 2005.
42. Smetana GW, Shmerling RH: Does this patient have temporal arteritis? *JAMA* 287:92, 2002.
43. Miller NR: Visual manifestations of temporal arteritis. In Stone JH, Hellmann DB, editors: *Rheumatic disease clinics of North America*, Philadelphia, 2001, WB Saunders, pp 781.
44. Nesher G, Berkun Y, Mates M, et al: Risk factors for cranial ischemic complications in giant cell arteritis, *Medicine* 83:114, 2004.
45. Gonzalez-Gay MA, Piñeiro A, Gomez-Gigirey A, et al: Influence of traditional risk factors of atherosclerosis in the development of severe ischemic complications in giant cell arteritis, *Medicine* 83:342, 2004.
46. Aiello PD, Trautmann JC, McPhee TJ, et al: Visual prognosis in giant cell arteritis, *Ophthalmology* 100:550, 1993.
47. Healy LA, Wilske KR: Presentation of occult giant cell arteritis, *Arthritis Rheum* 23:641, 1980.
48. Hellmann DB: Occult manifestations of giant cell arteritis, *Med Rounds* 2:296, 1989.
49. Hernández-Rodriguez J, Tan CD, Rodriguez ER, et al: Gynecologic vasculitis: an analysis of 163 patients, *Medicine* 88:169, 2009.
50. Hollenhorst RW, Brown JR, Wagener HP, Shick RM: Neurologic aspects of temporal arteritis, *Neurology* 10:490, 1960.
51. Gonzalez-Gay MA, Varquez-Rodriguez TR, Gomez-Acebo I, et al: Strokes at time of disease diagnosis in a series of 287 patients with biopsy-proven giant cell arteritis, *Medicine* 88:227, 2009.
52. Larson TS, Hall S, Hepper NGG, Hunder GG: Respiratory tract symptoms as a clue to giant cell arteritis, *Ann Intern Med* 101:594, 1984.
53. Hamilton CR, Shelley WM, Tumulty PA: Giant cell arteritis: including temporal arteritis and polymyalgia rheumatica, *Medicine* 50:1, 1971.
54. Nuenninghoff DM, Hunder GG, Christianson TJ, et al: Incidence and predictors of large-vessel complication (aortic aneurysm, aortic dissection, and/or large-artery stenosis) in patients with giant cell arteritis: a population-based study over 50 years, *Arthritis Rheum* 48:3522, 2003.
55. Blockmans D, de Ceuninck L, Vanderschueren S, et al: Repetitive 18F-fluorodeoxyglucose positron emission tomography in giant cell arteritis: a prospective study of 35 patients, *Arthritis Rheum* 55:131, 2006.
56. Kariv R, Sidi Y, Gur H: Systemic vasculitis presenting as a tumorlike lesion: four case reports and an analysis of 79 reported cases, *Medicine* 79:349, 2000.
57. Brack A, Martinez-Taboada V, Stanson A, et al: Disease pattern in cranial and large-vessel giant cell arteritis, *Arthritis Rheum* 42:311, 1999.
58. Liozon E, Herrmann F, Ly K, et al: Risk factors for visual loss in giant cell (temporal) arteritis: a prospective study of 174 patients, *Am J Med* 111:211–217, 2001.
59. Cid MC, Font C, Oristrell J, et al: Association between strong inflammatory response and low risk of developing visual loss and other cranial ischemic complications in giant cell (temporal) arteritis, *Arthritis Rheum* 41:26, 1998.
60. Salvarani C, Gabriel S, Hunder GG: Distal extremity swelling with pitting edema in polymyalgia rheumatica: report of nineteen cases, *Arthritis Rheum* 39:73, 1996.
61. Wise CM, Agudelo CA, Chmelewski WL, et al: Temporal arteritis with low erythrocyte sedimentation rate: a review of five cases, *Arthritis Rheum* 34:1571, 1991.
62. Roche NE, Fulbright JW, Wagner AD, et al: Correlation of interleukin-6 production and disease activity in polymyalgia rheumatica and giant cell arteritis, *Arthritis Rheum* 36:1286, 1993.
63. Younge BR, Cook BE Jr, Bartley GB, et al: Initiation of glucocorticoid therapy: before or after temporal artery biopsy? *Mayo Clin Proc* 79:483, 2004.
64. McCarty DJ, O'Duffy D, Pearson L, Hunter JB: Remitting seronegative symmetrical synovitis with pitting edema: RS₃PE syndrome, *JAMA* 25:2763, 1985.

65. Hall S, Hunder GG: Is temporal artery biopsy prudent? *Mayo Clin Proc* 59:793, 1984.
66. Gonzalez-Gay MA: The diagnosis and management of patients with giant cell arteritis, *J Rheumatol* 32:1186, 2005.
67. Breuer GS, Nesher G, Nesher R: Rate of discordant findings in bilateral temporal artery biopsy to diagnose giant cell arteritis, *J Rheumatol* 36:79, 2009.
68. Boyev LR, Miller NR, Green WR: Efficacy of unilateral versus bilateral temporal artery biopsies for the diagnosis of giant cell arteritis, *Am J Ophthalmol* 128:211, 1999.
69. Jundt JW, Mock D: Temporal arteritis with normal erythrocyte sedimentation rates presenting as occipital neuralgia, *Arthritis Rheum* 3:217, 1991.
70. Schmidt WA, Kraft HE, Vorpahl L, et al: Color duplex ultrasonography in the diagnosis of temporal arteritis, *N Engl J Med* 337:1336, 1997.
71. Hall JK: Giant-cell arteritis, *Curr Opin Ophthalmol* 19:5, 2008.
72. Karassa FB, Matsagas MI, Schmidt WA, et al: Meta-analysis: test performance in ultrasonography for giant-cell arteritis, *Ann Intern Med* 12:359, 2005.
73. Blockmans D, Bley T, Schmidt W: Imaging for large-vessel vasculitis, *Curr Opin Rheumatol* 21:19, 2009.
74. Park M-C, Lee S-W, Park Y-B, et al: Clinical characteristics and outcomes of Takayasu's arteritis: analysis of 108 patients using standardized criteria for diagnosis, activity assessment, and angiographic classification, *Scand J Rheumatol* 3:28, 2005.
75. Achkar AA, Lie JT, Hunder GG, et al: How does previous corticosteroid treatment affect the biopsy findings in giant cell (temporal) arteritis? *Ann Intern Med* 120:987, 1994.
76. Mazlumzadeh M, Hunder GG, Easley KA, et al: Treatment of giant cell arteritis using induction therapy with high-dose glucocorticoids: a double-blind, placebo-controlled, randomized prospective clinical trial, *Arthritis Rheum* 54:3310, 2006.
77. Weyand CM, Fulbright JW, Hunder GG, et al: Treatment of giant cell arteritis: interleukin-6 as a biologic marker of disease activity, *Arthritis Rheum* 3:101, 2000.
78. Hoffman GS, Cid MC, Hellmann DB, et al: A multicenter, randomized, double-blind, placebo-controlled trial of adjuvant methotrexate treatment for giant cell arteritis, *Arthritis Rheum* 46:1309, 2002.
79. Hoffman GS, Cid MC, Rendt-Zagar KE, et al: Infliximab for maintenance of glucocorticosteroid-induced remission of giant cell arteritis: a randomized trial, *Ann Intern Med* 16:621, 2007.
80. Martínez-Taboada VM, Rodríguez-Valverde V, Carreño L, et al: A double-blind placebo controlled trial of etanercept in patients with giant cell arteritis and corticosteroid side effects, *Ann Rheum Dis* 67:625, 2008.
81. Weyand CM, Kaiser M, Yang H, et al: Therapeutic effects of acetylsalicylic acid in giant cell arteritis, *Arthritis Rheum* 46:457, 2002.
82. Nesher G: Low-dose aspirin and prevention of cranial ischemic complications in giant cell arteritis, *Arthritis Rheum* 50:1332, 2004.
83. Lee MS, Smith SD, Galor A, Hoffman GS: Antiplatelet and anticoagulant therapy in patients with giant cell arteritis, *Arthritis Rheum* 54:3306, 2006.
84. Both M, Aries PM, Müller-Hülsbeck S, et al: Balloon angioplasty of arteries of the upper extremities in patients with extracranial giant-cell arteritis, *Ann Rheum Dis* 65:1124, 2006.
85. Weyand CM, Fulbright JW, Evans JM, et al: Corticosteroid requirements in polymyalgia rheumatica, *Arch Intern Med* 159:577, 1999.
86. Hernández-Rodriguez J, Cid MC, López-Soto A, et al: Treatment of polymyalgia rheumatica. A systemic review, *Arch Intern Med* 169:1839, 2009.
87. Narvaez J, Nolla-Sole JM, Clavaguera MT, et al: Longterm therapy in polymyalgia rheumatica: effect of coexistent temporal arteritis, *J Rheumatol* 26:195, 1999.
88. Caporali R, Cimmino MA, Ferraccioli G, et al: Prednisone plus methotrexate for polymyalgia rheumatica: a randomized, double-blind, placebo-controlled trial, *Ann Intern Med* 141:493, 2004.
89. Kerr GS, Hallahan CW, Giordano J, et al: Takyasu arteritis, *Ann Intern Med* 120:919, 1994.
90. Takayasu M: A case of a peculiar change in the central retinal vessels, *Acta Soc Ophthalmol Jpn* 12:55, 1908.
91. Seko Y, Minota S, Kawasaki A, et al: Perforin-secreting killer cell infiltration and expression of a 65-kD heat-shock protein in aortic tissue of patients with Takayasu's arteritis, *J Clin Invest* 93:750, 1994.
92. Tavora F, Burke A: Review of isolated ascending aortitis: differential diagnosis, including syphilitic, Takayasu's and giant cell aortitis, *Pathology* 38:302, 2006.
93. Dal Canto AJ, Swanson PE, O'Guin AK, et al: IFN-gamma action in the media of the great elastic arteries, a novel immunoprivileged site, *J Clin Invest* 107:R15, 2001.
94. Maksimowicz-McKinnon K, Clark TM, Hoffman GS: Takayasu arteritis and giant cell arteritis. A spectrum within the same disease? *Medicine* 88:221, 2009.
95. Talwar KK, Kuman K, Chopra P, et al: Cardiac involvement in nonspecific aortoarteritis (Takayasu's arteritis), *Am Heart J* 122:1666, 1991.
96. Malik IS, Harare O, Al-Nahhas A, et al: Takayasu's arteritis: management of left main stem stenosis, *Heart* 89:e9, 2003.
97. Endo M, Tomizawa Y, Nishida H, et al: Angiographic findings and surgical treatment of coronary artery involvement in Takayasu arteritis, *J Thorac Cardiovasc Surg* 125:570, 2003.
98. Andrews J, Al-Nahhas A, Pennell DJ, et al: Non-invasive imaging in the diagnosis and management of Takayasu's arteritis, *Ann Rheum Dis* 63:995, 2004.
99. Arnaud L, Haroche J, Malek Z, et al: Is ^{18}F-fluorodeoxyglucose positron emission tomography scanning a reliable way to assess disease activity in Takayasu arteritis? *Arthritis Rheum* 60:1193, 2009.
100. Liang KP, Chowdhary VR, Michet CJ, et al: Noninfectious ascending aortitis: a case series in 64 patients, *J Rheumatol* 36:2290, 2009.
101. Stone JR: Aortitis, periaortitis, and retroperitoneal fibrosis, as manifestations of IgG-related systemic disease, *Curr Opin Rheumatol* 23:88, 2011.
102. Hoffman GS, Leavitt RY, Kerr GS, et al: Treatment of glucocorticoid-resistant or relapsing Takayasu arteritis with methotrexate, *Arthritis Rheum* 37:578, 1994.
103. Molloy ES, Langford CA, Clark TM, et al. Anti-tumour necrosis factor therapy in patients with refractory Takayasu arteritis: long-term follow-up, *Ann Rheum Dis* 67:1567, 2008.
104. Salvarani C, Magnani L, Catanoso M, et al: Tocilizumab: a novel therapy for patients with large-vessel vasculitis, *Rheumatology (Oxford)* 51:151–156, 2012.
105. Koening CL, Langford CA: Novel therapeutic strategies for large vessel vasculitis, *Rheum Dis Clin North Am* 32:173, 2006.
106. Miyata T, Sato O, Koyama H, et al: Long-term survival after surgical treatment of patients with Takayasu's arteritis, *Circulation* 108:1474, 2003.
107. Matsuura K, Ogino H, Kobayashi J, et al: Surgical treatment of aortic regurgitation due to Takayasu arteritis: long-term morbidity and mortality, *Circulation* 112:3707, 2005.
108. Ogino H, Matsuda H, Minatoya K, et al: Overview of late outcome of medical and surgical treatment for Takayasu arteritis, *Circulation* 118:2738, 2008.
109. Sharma BK, Jain S, Visishta K: Outcome of pregnancy in Takayasu arteritis, *Int J Cardiol* 75(Suppl):S159, 2000.

The references for this chapter can also be found on www.expertconsult.com.

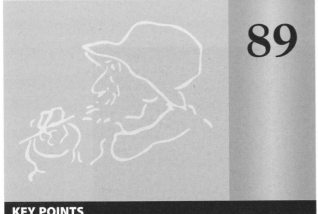

89 Antineutrophil Cytoplasm Antibody–Associated Vasculitis

CAROLINE O.S. SAVAGE • LORRAINE HARPER

KEY POINTS

Granulomatosis with polyangiitis (GPA), microscopic polyangiitis (MPA), and allergic granulomatosis with polyangiitis (AGPA) are forms of vasculitis that affect small to medium-sized vessels and share a number of clinical, pathologic, and laboratory features.

Animal models, in vitro studies, and clinical studies support a pathogenic role for antineutrophil cytoplasm antibodies (ANCAs) in most patients.

Testing for ANCAs and more specific autoantibodies by immunoassay is a useful tool in the diagnosis of small vessel vasculitis, but its role in disease monitoring is more controversial.

GPA can affect any organ or tissue but has a predilection for the upper and lower respiratory tracts and the kidneys. GPA is most commonly associated with ANCA positivity by immunofluorescence and positive testing for the proteinase-3 antigen.

MPA can be distinguished from other forms of small vessel vasculitis by the absence of granuloma formation and the predominance of perinuclear ANCA staining by immunofluorescence and positive testing for the myeloperoxidase antigen.

AGPA can be distinguished from other forms of small vessel vasculitis on the basis of a prior history of adult-onset asthma or allergic rhinitis and tissue eosinophilia with necrotizing vasculitis and extravascular granuloma formation.

Combination therapy with glucocorticoids and cyclophosphamide is required for the treatment of systemic small vessel vasculitis; methotrexate may be substituted for cyclophosphamide in non–organ-threatening disease. In those with severe disease, plasma exchange should be used as an adjuvant. Rituximab may be an alternative induction agent for those unable to receive cyclophosphamide. Patients with AGPA without any adverse prognostic signs may be treated with steroids alone.

Upon induction of disease remission, cyclophosphamide should be switched to less toxic immunosuppressive agents, such as azathioprine, for maintenance of remission.

With current therapeutic regimens, long-term outlook has improved, with 78% of patients surviving 5 years.

CLASSIFICATION OF THIS GROUP OF VASCULITIDES

(American College of Rheumatology [ACR] and European League Against Rheumatism [EULAR] Criteria for Disease)

The primary systemic vasculitides involve small and medium-sized vessels and are associated with autoantibodies that target neutrophil cytoplasm antigens (antineutrophil cytoplasm antibodies [ANCAs]). Thus they are frequently referred to as ANCA-associated vasculitides (AAVs), although the terminology ANCA disease has also been proposed.[1] The presence of ANCA suggests that AAVs are autoimmune diseases. Individual disease descriptions include granulomatosis with polyangiitis (GPA), formerly known as Wegener's granulomatosis; microscopic polyangiitis (MPA); allergic granulomatosis with polyangiitis (AGPA), formerly known as Churg-Strauss syndrome; and renal-limited pauci-immune necrotizing and crescentic glomerulonephritis (RLV). The name changes have been recommended by the Boards of the ACR, the American Society of Nephrology, and EULAR, which wished a shift from eponyms to disease-descriptive or cause-based nomenclature.

The major autoantigens to which ANCAs are directed within neutrophils and monocytes include two enzyme proteins identified in the 1980s as autoantigens, namely, proteinase-3 (PR3), myeloperoxidase (MPO) (Figure 89-1), and, more recently, lysosome-associated membrane protein 2 (LAMP2).[2-4] Confirmation of the presence of antibodies directed against LAMP2 in AAV is awaited, so this antibody subclass is not routinely tested for in current clinical practice.

The initial descriptions of GPA, MPA, and AGPA occurred in the 1930s, 1940s, and 1950s, respectively. However, the term polyarteritis nodosa (PAN) was often used during this period in a generic manner to cover these conditions, particularly MPA, despite the fact that Kussmaul and Meyer had clearly described PAN in 1866 as a systemic condition in which inflammation of medium-sized muscular arteries occurs, leading to aneurysm formation and ischemic tissue or organ infarction.[5] The AAVs, in contrast, are generally considered disorders affecting both small and medium-sized arteries. In 1990, the ACR published classification criteria for seven types of vasculitis that included GPA and AGPA, but not MPA, thereby helping to begin to unravel the complexities of vasculitis classification. Four criteria were selected for GPA:

- Abnormal urinary sediment (red cell casts or greater than five red blood cells per high-power field)
- Abnormal findings on chest radiograph (nodules, cavities, or fixed infiltrates)
- Oral ulcers or nasal discharge
- Granulomatous inflammation on biopsy[6]

The presence of two or more of these four criteria was associated with a sensitivity of 88.2% and a specificity of 92%. It is worth bearing in mind that these criteria were

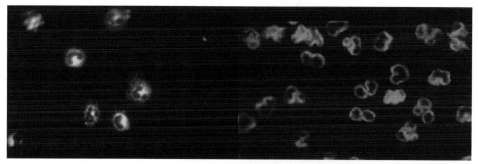

Figure 89-1 Immunofluorescence of diffuse or cytoplasmic antineutrophil cytoplasm antibody (c-ANCA; *left*), which is highly correlated with antibodies to proteinase-3 (PR3), and the less specific perinuclear pattern (p-ANCA; *right*), which is indicative of antibodies to myeloperoxidase (MPO). Although immunofluorescence was once the standard for ANCA testing, current standards require confirmatory antigen-specific testing for PR3 and MPO. *(Courtesy Dr. C.G.M. Kallenberg.)*

based on clinical features of 85 patients with GPA who were compared with 722 control patients with other forms of vasculitis.

Six criteria were selected for AGPA:
1. Asthma
2. Eosinophilia greater than 10% on differential blood cell count
3. Mononeuropathy (including multiplex) or polyneuropathy
4. Nonfixed pulmonary infiltrates on chest radiograph
5. Paranasal sinus abnormality
6. Biopsy containing a blood vessel with extravascular eosinophils[7]

The presence of four or more of these six criteria gave a sensitivity of 85% and a specificity of 99.7%. The criteria for AGPA were based on clinical findings in 20 patients compared with 787 controls with other forms of vasculitis.

The next major step forward was development of definitions for forms of vasculitis by the Chapel Hill Consensus Conference (CHCC) in 1994, which included GPA, MPA, and AGPA in the 10 types of vasculitis considered.[8] These are shown in totality in Table 89-1. Neither the ACR classification criteria nor the CHCC definitions included ANCA as a criterion. Lack of classification criteria for MPA prompted development of an algorithm by international consensus that has been validated in two separate populations, covering GPA, MPA, and AGPA, as well as PAN.[9,10]

The ACR classification criteria and the CHCC definitions were not designed as diagnostic criteria. Indeed, the positive predictive value of the ACR classification criteria can be as low as 29% in clinical practice.[11] Although attempts have been made to develop diagnostic criteria based on the CHCC, these Sorensen criteria have not been validated.[12] Indeed, believing the ACR criteria for AGPA, PAN, and some other vasculitides, and the CHCC definitions for GPA, MPA, and PAN to no longer be fit for purpose, EULAR convened an expert consensus group to consider re-evaluating definitions, classifications, and diagnostic criteria in systemic vasculitis. Seventeen points to consider were formulated before the development of classification criteria and definitions in the systemic vasculitides that related to biopsy, laboratory testing, diagnostic radiology, nosology, definitions, and the research agenda.[13] Not all of the points were relevant to AAV. Those that were relevant included the following:

- Histology point 1: Although histology is fundamental to the diagnosis of vasculitis and exclusion of its mimics, biopsy of affected organs is not always possible, and yields vary significantly according to conditions and target organs.
- Laboratory testing point 4: ANCA testing plays an important diagnostic role in suspected small vessel vasculitis.
- Diagnostic radiology point 10: Computed tomography (CT) and magnetic resonance imaging (MRI) may be useful in diagnosing ear, nose, and throat (ENT) involvement associated with GPA/AGPA.
- Nosology points 12 to 14: The nomenclature in use for distinguishing between "disease definitions," "classification," and "diagnostic" criteria is confusing and should be clarified wherever possible. Nosology of different forms of vasculitis should be a reflection of their etiopathogenesis, wherever this has been determined. In the absence of this, definition must rely on a clear, accurate description of the salient features of the condition. The use of eponyms should be reviewed if a more rational approach to nomenclature can be developed, based on etiopathogenesis, but their retention is necessary at present to avoid confusion.
- Definitions point 15: Age is worthy of inclusion in the definitions of some forms of vasculitis, but its role should not be overstated.
- Research agenda points 16 and 17: Future criteria initiatives should include all forms of vasculitis, providing definitions of less common syndromes not covered by CHCC. The development of a classification tree will provide the foundation for future criteria.

EPIDEMIOLOGY

Determining the incidence and prevalence of AAV is challenging given the uncommon occurrence of the disorders, difficulties in case ascertainment, the slow evolution of classification criteria and definitions fit for epidemiologic purposes, and the clinicopathologic overlaps that occur between the component diseases designated ANCA-associated diseases (GPA, MPA, AGPA) and their limited variants, including RLV. Most studies have been carried out in populations of European ancestry using data that were collected

Table 89-1 Classification of Vasculitis as Adopted by the Chapel Hill Consensus Conference on the Nomenclature of Systemic Vasculitis*

	Histopathology	Comments
Large Vessel Vasculitis		
Giant cell (temporal) arteritis	Granulomatous arteritis of the aorta and its major branches, with a predilection for the extracranial branches of the carotid artery	Often involves the temporal artery Usually occurs at >50 yr of age Often associated with polymyalgia rheumatica
Takayasu's arteritis	Granulomatous inflammation of the aorta and its major branches	Usually occurs at <50 yr of age
Medium-Sized Vessel Vasculitis		
Polyarteritis nodosa† (classic polyarteritis nodosa)	Necrotizing inflammation of medium-sized or small arteries without glomerulonephritis or vasculitis in arterioles, capillaries, or venules	
Kawasaki disease	Arteritis involving large, medium-sized, and small arteries, associated with mucocutaneous lymph node syndrome	Coronary arteries often involved Aorta and veins may be involved Usually occurs in children
Small Vessel Vasculitis		
Granulomatosis with polyangiitis‡	Granulomatous inflammation involving the respiratory tract and necrotizing vasculitis affecting small to medium-sized vessels (capillaries, venules, arterioles, arteries)	Necrotizing glomerulonephritis common
Allergic granulomatosis with polyangiitis‡	Eosinophil-rich and granulomatous inflammation involving the respiratory tract and necrotizing vasculitis affecting small to medium-sized vessels, associated with asthma and blood eosinophilia	
Microscopic polyangiitis‡	Necrotizing vasculitis with few or no immune deposits affecting small vessels (capillaries, venules, arterioles)	Necrotizing arteritis involving small and medium-sized arteries may be present Necrotizing glomerulonephritis very common Pulmonary capillaritis often occurs
Henoch-Schönlein purpura	Vasculitis with IgA-dominant immune deposits affecting small vessels (capillaries, venules, arterioles)	Typically involves skin, gut, and glomeruli Associated with arthralgia or arthritis
Essential cryoglobulinemic vasculitis	Vasculitis with cryoglobulin immune deposits affecting small vessels (capillaries, venules, arterioles) and associated with cryoglobulins in serum	Skin and glomeruli often involved
Cutaneous leukocytoclastic angiitis	Isolated cutaneous leukocytoclastic angiitis without systemic vasculitis	

*Large arteries include the aorta and the largest branches directed toward major body regions (e.g., the extremities, head and neck). Medium-sized arteries are the main visceral arteries (e.g., renal, hepatic, coronary, mesenteric). Small arteries are distal arterial radicles that connect with arterioles. Note that some small and large vessel vasculitides may involve medium-sized arteries, but large and medium-sized vessel vasculitides do not involve vessels smaller than arteries.

†Preferred term.

‡Strongly associated with antineutrophil cytoplasm antibodies.

retrospectively. Despite these difficulties, collective studies suggest that the AAVs have an incidence of around 10 to 20 per million and prevalence rates that have been increasing over the past two decades (summarized in Reference 14). The peak age of onset is 65 to 74 years; the disease is very rare in childhood, and most studies suggest a slightly higher occurrence in men than in women (1.5:1.0).

Within the spectrum of ANCA-associated disease are interesting geographic and population differences in the relative incidence of GPA versus MPA or AGPA, or between MPO-ANCA and PR3-ANCA positivity. In populations of European ancestry, GPA appears to have an incidence of around 2 to 10 per million, depending on the geographic location, with the higher 8 to 10 per million incidence being reported in more northerly countries and lower incidences of 3 to 6.6 per million in Greece and Spain.[15-17] A similar inverse relationship between GPA and MPA has been observed in the southern hemisphere,[18] and a possible link to ultraviolet exposure has been proposed.[19]

However, in a Japanese population studied for occurrence of primary renal vasculitis, more than 90% had MPO-ANCA, but PR3-ANCA was not observed, and neither GPA nor AGPA was diagnosed clinically.[20] In China, MPA also seems to be more common than GPA[10]; high rates of MPA have also been reported in a Peruvian population and in Kuwait, where the incidence of MPA was reported as 24 per million.[21,22]

Considering epidemiologic studies for GPA in greater detail, studies from Finland, Norway, and Sweden have suggested an increased incidence over the past two to three decades,[23-25] but others from Germany and the United Kingdom and a later Swedish study have not.[26-28] Overall, it is most likely that methodological factors account for reported differences, with no significant increase in incidence occurring during the past two decades. Prevalence figures for GPA have been increasing, which probably reflects improved treatment regimens. In a primary care–based population in the United Kingdom, the prevalence increased from 28.8 per million in 1990 to 64.8 per million in 2005.[15] Prevalence figures are now available for several populations in Europe, the United States, and the southern hemisphere over various time periods (summarized in Reference 14).

Epidemiologic studies in MPA have variously shown an increased incidence or not over the past two decades. It is possible that earlier suggestions of an increased incidence reflected increasing awareness of MPA and its differentiation from PAN and GPA. An interesting increase in cases of MPA in Japan followed the Kobe earthquake in 1995.[29]

AGPA is the least common of the AAVs, with an incidence around 1.0 to 3.0 per million, although this increases in patients with asthma to 34.6 per million person-years.[30] AGPA affects a similar age of population as GPA and MPA, but its occurrence is more common in women than in men. An association has been noted between the development of AGPA and the administration of leukotriene inhibitors or the anti-immunoglobulin (Ig)E monoclonal antibody omalizumab, possibly due to unmasking of previously unrecognized disease with reduction of corticosteroid dose.[31,32]

Environmental factors are relevant to AAV.[33] There appears to be a higher incidence of GPA in rural as compared with urban areas.[34] No clear seasonal variation trends have been identified. Infection as a trigger for autoimmune disease in general, and for AAV in particular, is often hypothesized. The closest association is between *Staphylococcus aureus* and GPA, with nasal carriage of *S. aureus* being linked to a higher incidence of disease relapse.[35] Silica exposure has been linked to AAV in several studies, including a case-control study in the United States.[36] Exposure to several drugs, including propylthiouracil, has also been associated with AAV.[37] Cocaine abuse has been linked to a midline destructive granulomatous disease that mimics GPA.[38]

GENETICS

Evidence of a heritable risk for AAV comes from recent studies suggesting a modestly increased risk of disease in first-degree relatives,[39] similar to that found in rheumatoid arthritis (RA). Children of patients with GPA have an increased risk of RA,[40] suggesting familial clustering of genes associated with inflammatory autoimmune disease. Occasional familial cases of GPA are also reported in the literature.[41,42] Given the relatively modest risk of disease in family members, it is likely that several genes contribute a small effect on disease development. Undertaking genetic studies in AAV is challenging owing to the rarity of the disease as the statistical power of genetic association studies is determined by the number of cases and controls included in the analysis. A number of candidate genes, often involving the immune response, have been identified. However, many association studies have produced inconsistent results because of the small number of cases studied. More recent studies have used larger numbers of patients with evidence of validation of results by duplication in separate cohorts of patients. Large cohorts of patients are being assembled to allow performance of genome-wide association studies, in which thousands of genes across the genome are compared.

Consistent genetic associations with multiple autoimmune conditions have been restricted to three gene regions: human leukocyte antigen (HLA) class II region, CTLA, and the *PTPN22* gene. HLA genes are exceedingly polymorphic, and small studies suggest associations between GPA and HLA compared with healthy controls. However, most of these studies are of poor reliability because of their small size and lack of replication in independent cohorts. Recently, a larger study of 150 German patients with GPA identified an association with the HLA-DPB1*0401 allele. In contrast, the *0301 allele frequency was significantly decreased.[43] The extended haplotype DPB1*0401/RXB03 showed stronger association, suggesting that this genomic region confers significant risk for development of GPA. Among other functions, the retinoid X receptor β protein forms heterodimers with vitamin D receptors. Vitamin D receptor is important for the effects of the active vitamin D metabolite 1,25-dihydroxycholecalciferol. Active vitamin D has potent immunomodulatory properties, which include inhibition of cytokine transcription and differentiation of T cells toward a T regulatory (Treg) cell phenotype.[44] This association has been replicated in a larger cohort of 282 GPA patients.[45] The association with *0401 was present only in ANCA-positive GPA patients. Other studies have shown associations with HLA-DR. A relatively large study (304 AAV patients and 9872 controls) has shown associations with HLA-DR4,[46] and another showed that HLA-DRB1*04 was increased in frequency in GPA patients with end-stage renal failure.[47]

Different HLA associations have been found in AGPA with disease associating with HLA-DRB4 alleles, while HLA-DRB3 afforded disease protection.[48] No association of AGPA with HLA-DPB has been described.[49] Different HLA associations suggest that AGPA and GPA may be different disease entities despite many similarities. This is supported by observations that showed association of the extended IL-10.2 haplotype with ANCA-negative AGPA but not GPA.[49]

Cytotoxic T lymphocyte–associated antigen 4 (CTLA4) is expressed mainly on activated CD4+ T cells and inhibits T cell function. Polymorphisms in the *CTLA4* gene have been associated with several autoimmune diseases.[50] Several studies have shown associations with polymorphisms in the *CTLA4* gene. The most widely implicated CTLA4 polymorphism for risk of autoimmunity is the +49 single nucleotide polymorphism (SNP) (alanine-to-threonine substitution in the leader peptide), which appears to affect cell surface expression of CTLA4 in response to T cell activation.[51,52] The CT60 SNP appears to affect the expression of soluble CTLA4 and to alter the signaling threshold of CD4+ T cells.[53] Both of these SNPs have been associated with disease in patients with AAV.[54-57]

PTPN22 encodes the lymphoid tyrosine phosphatase LYP, which forms a complex with the kinase Csk and is a critical negative regulator of signaling through the T cell receptor. The R620W variation, which has been associated with autoimmunity, disrupts the interaction between Lck and LYP, leading to reduced phosphorylation of LYP, which ultimately contributes to gain-of-function inhibition of T cell signaling.[58] Two studies have shown an association of the PTPN22 620W allele with AAV,[57,59] suggesting that this is likely to contribute to the risk of AAV, as in other autoantibody-associated autoimmune diseases.

Numerous other candidate genes have been investigated in patients with AAV. Alpha1 antitrypsin (A1AT) is the major inhibitor of PR3. The *A1AT* gene is highly polymorphic. The deficiency alleles S and Z are increased in patients with AAV.[60-63] However, most individuals with A1AT homozygous for the Z allele do not develop AAV.[64]

PR3 is expressed on the membrane of neutrophils and appears to be genetically determined.[65] Patients with GPA tend to have higher percentages of neutrophils expressing PR3 than healthy controls,[66] particularly those with relapsing disease.[67] However, increased expression does not appear related to 564 promoter polymorphism of the *PR3* gene.[68,69] The percentage of neutrophils expressing PR3 may be influenced by HLA antigens, although the mechanism of this is unclear. In one study, a group of 34 HLA antigens was found to predict 64% of the variability in PR3 membrane expression.[70] This study requires replication in an independent cohort of patients. Less support has been found for a genetic association affecting the expression of MPO. A recent meta-analysis showed no association with the functional promoter polymorphism (G-463A) in the MPO gene.[71]

Many other genes have been investigated, but results are conflicting owing to the small size of the studies and require further investigation. However, it is clear that existing studies suggest a complex model of genetic variability. Future studies need collaboration between groups to increase the number of available cases of these rare diseases.

CLINICAL FEATURES

The three types of AAV may all be associated with marked constitutional upset comprising fevers, night sweats, myalgia, and arthralgia. Systemic vasculitis may also lead to certain commonality of features that may occur in some, but not all, patients. Thus nail-fold hemorrhages, purpuric rashes, and cutaneous ulcers may be observed.

Microscopic Polyangiitis

The first descriptions of MPA were provided in 1948 by Davson, Ball, and Platt, who described an illness that they termed *microscopic polyarteritis*, distinguishing it from polyarteritis nodosa by its marked segmental necrotizing glomerulonephritis and greater propensity to involve small vessels.[72]

The pathology of MPA is of a fibrinoid necrotizing vasculitis with few or no immune deposits that primarily affects small vessels such as capillaries, arterioles, or venules, although spread to include small and medium-sized arteries may occur. A focal segmental necrotizing glomerulonephritis is very common and may progress into a full blown crescentic glomerulonephritis.[73] However, in view of the sometimes indolent nature of the disease, evidence of chronic damage with obsolete glomeruli and tubulointerstitial fibrosis may be present at the time of the first diagnostic kidney biopsy.[74] Examination of the kidney by immunohistology or electron microscopy reveals few or no immune deposits, although careful inspection may indicate that some complement fragments are present.[75] Within the

lungs, a pulmonary capillaritis may develop, and, following rupture of capillaries, blood can spill into alveolar spaces and thrombosis may occur within capillaries themselves. Marked neutrophilic infiltration of the alveolar wall is usually seen; this ultimately undergoes fibrinoid necrosis. Type II epithelial cell hyperplasia and lymphoplasmacytic infiltration can develop.

The pathophysiologic understanding of MPA advanced considerably after the strong association between MPA and ANCA was recognized, particularly ANCA directed toward myeloperoxidase (MPO).[2,76] A small percentage of patients have ANCA directed toward proteinase-3 (PR3). ANCAs are believed to bind to their target antigen on the surface of primed neutrophils, leading to further neutrophil activation with release of proinflammatory granule contents and reactive oxygen species, as well as increasing adherence and damage to endothelial cells (Figure 89-2) (reviewed in Reference 77). Studies in mouse and rat species have provided direct evidence that anti-MPO antibodies induce systemic vasculitis, including necrotizing glomerulonephritis,[78,79] and can promote neutrophil-endothelial cell interactions in vivo.[80,81]

The clinical features of MPA have been recognized for many years[82-85] and are summarized in Table 89-2. The most commonly affected organs are the kidneys and the lungs. Symptoms can involve the ears, nose, or throat, but distinction from GPA then needs to be considered. The presentation can be insidious with symptoms of deteriorating renal function on the background of mild features that can be attributed to a low-grade vasculitis; alternatively, it may be severe and acute with rapidly progressive glomerulonephritis and pulmonary hemorrhage, presenting as a pulmonary renal syndrome; or it may appear to be limited to the kidney, sometimes being described as renal-limited vasculitis.

Renal manifestations include microscopic hematuria, an abnormal renal sediment with red cell casts, proteinuria that is not usually of nephrotoxic proportions (i.e., is less than 3.5 g per 24 hours), and variable loss of kidney function. The presence of red cell casts is always indicative of an active glomerulonephritis, and the presence of red cells in a patient with long-standing disease may be due to active disease or to damage in the absence of disease activity, or indeed to other conditions affecting the lower urinary tract, including cystitis or bladder malignancy, as a result of cyclophosphamide therapy.[86] Loss of renal function can be very rapid, occurring over days or weeks. Dialysis may be required,

Table 89-2 Principal Clinical Features of Microscopic Polyangiitis

Clinical Feature	Percentage*
Constitutional symptoms	76-79
Fever	50-72
Renal disease	100
Arthralgias	28-65
Purpura	40-44
Pulmonary disease (hemorrhage, infiltrates, effusion)	50
Neurologic disease (central, peripheral)	28
Ear, nose, throat involvement	30

*Percentage of a population totaling 150 patients from four studies.[82-85]

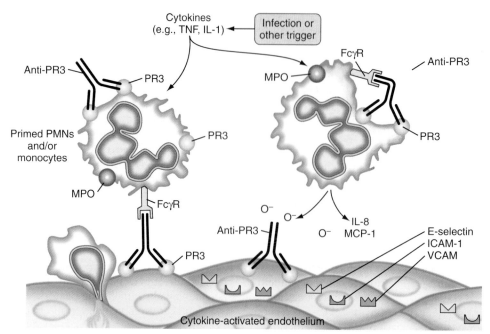

Figure 89-2 Schematic representation of the immune mechanisms hypothetically involved with antineutrophil cytoplasm antibody (ANCA) enhancement of vascular injury. An infectious trigger or another environmental stimulus leads to a burst of cytokines, which prime the neutrophils or monocytes, possibly leading to local upregulation of adhesion molecules on endothelium. The priming process within the inflammatory cells leads to enhanced expression of ANCA antigens on the cell surface. Activated neutrophils or monocytes may degranulate and release reactive oxygen species (O) and lysosomal enzymes, leading to endothelial injury and further activation of the endothelial cell surface. The magnitude of this effect is influenced by the specificity of ANCA for proteinase-3 (PR3) or myeloperoxidase (MPO), as well as different epitopes of these respective antigens. The reaction may be further influenced by the immunoglobulin G (IgG) and Fcγ receptor phenotype engaged. Products released from degranulated inflammatory cells become bound to endothelial cells and further serve as targets of ANCA. Release of chemotactic chemokines such as interleukin-8 (IL-8) and macrophage chemoattractant protein-1 (MCP-1), in conjunction with other adhesion molecules, serves to augment chemotaxis and inflammatory cell transmigration. Thus, the scheme provides the prerequisites for endothelial and vascular injury induced by ANCA, that is, the presence of ANCA, expression of target antigens for ANCA on primed neutrophils and monocytes, interaction between primed neutrophils and endothelium via adhesion molecules, and finally, activation of endothelial cells and ultimate efflux of inflammatory cells to extravascular and perivascular tissues. FcγR, Fcγ receptor; ICAM-1, intercellular adhesion molecule-1; PMN, polymorphonuclear leukocyte; TNF, tumor necrosis factor.

but some recovery of renal function may occur following treatment. In patients who remain on dialysis, the likelihood of relapse is less than before dialysis, so the need for immunosuppression may be less.[87] Although kidney involvement is present in most patients, it is not invariable.

Lung involvement occurs in up to a third of patients.[82-85] Clinical features include cough, dyspnea, pleurisy, and hemoptysis. Onset may be insidious or acute and severe. Widespread pulmonary hemorrhage can occur without overt hemoptysis. Chest radiograph findings may be patchy or diffuse, reflecting alveolar infiltrates. Repeated episodes of lung hemorrhage can lead to pulmonary fibrosis.

Granulomatosis with Polyangiitis

GPA is a granulomatous disorder, often associated with fibrinoid necrotizing vasculitis, which was first described in 1931 by Klinger,[88] with pathologic refinement added to the description by Wegener in 1936.[89]

The pathology of GPA comprises granulomas and necrosis, as well as the vasculitis, which is similar to that occurring in MPA.[73] Pathologic biopsy material is taken more frequently from the nasal mucosa, lung, skin, or kidney. All features are not usually present in any one biopsy specimen, given the small sample of material that may be available, so findings may be compatible with the diagnosis but not diagnostic. In the lung, open biopsies generally are more likely

to be diagnostic than transbronchial biopsies.[90,91] Renal pathology is similar between MPA and GPA, and granulomas are rarely seen in the kidney (Figure 89-3); sometimes intense periglomerular leukocytic infiltration has the appearance of pseudogranulomas.[92]

The pathophysiology of GPA, as with MPA, is believed to be inherently autoimmune[93] and driven by PR3-ANCA in a manner very similar to that proposed for MPO-ANCA,[77] with PR3-ANCA being highly specific for GPA.[76,94] However, a good animal model is not available for anti-PR3 antibodies, so direct evidence for a role in development of vasculitis, or indeed in granuloma formation, is not available as with anti-MPO antibodies; this may reflect differences in expression of PR3 on murine neutrophils. However, the ex vivo effects of MPO-ANCA and PR3-ANCA on human neutrophils are very similar (reviewed in Reference 77). B cells and T cells are also acknowledged to play important roles in the AAV diseases, with recent demonstration of responsiveness to anti–B cell therapies placing increased interest in the role that B cells play.[95,96] T cell subset abnormalities have repeatedly been described in MPA and GPA, but the nature of the factors responsible for these changes has not been defined.

The clinical features of GPA are driven by a predilection for the upper and lower respiratory tracts, as well as for the kidneys. GPA may occur as a disease limited to the respiratory tract without evidence of systemic involvement, when

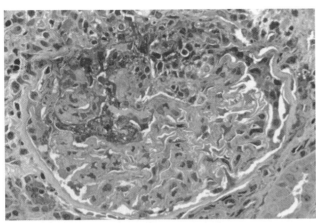

Figure 89-3 Antineutrophil cytoplasm antibody–associated crescentic glomerulonephritis. This toluidine blue–stained plastic section demonstrates a glomerulus with a cellular crescent. Bowman's space is partially obliterated by a proliferation of epithelial cells and macrophages. All types of crescentic glomerulonephritis appear similar by light microscopy, and immunofluorescence is needed to distinguish among pauci-immune, immune complex, and anti–glomerular basement membrane subtypes. *(Courtesy Dr. J. Myles.)*

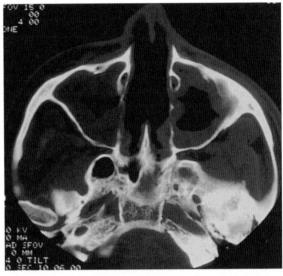

Figure 89-5 Computed tomography scan of the sinuses, revealing the presence of chronic sinusitis.

it is referred to as limited GPA; such presentation is usually as a granulomatous disorder without vasculitic features. In a recent study, 10% of patients evolved to develop generalized disease within a median time of 6 years.[97] Upper airway disease is the most common presenting feature of GPA, occurring in more than 70% and eventually being present in more than 90% of patients.[90,98] Serous otitis media and conductive and sensorineural hearing loss may occur; vertigo is rare. Nasal involvement causes mucosal swelling with obstruction, crusting, septal perforations, serosanguineous discharge, and epistaxis; a saddle nose deformity due to collapse of the cartilaginous portion of the nasal septum may develop (Figure 89-4). Sinusitis is common and will occur in more than 80% at some point during the illness (Figure 89-5)[99]; bony erosion may develop and can be

detected better using CT scanning of the sinuses than by plain radiography. *S. aureus* may infect sinuses and is commonly carried on the diseased nasal mucosa, where it may be one factor contributing to disease relapse.[35] Laryngotracheal disease may cause hoarseness but may also progress to severe stridor and upper airway obstruction, usually following subglottic stenosis (Figure 89-6). Direct laryngoscopy may reveal an ulcerated friable mucosa, and tracheal tomograms, CT, or MRI can help to further delineate the extent of the stenosis. In occasional patients, subglottic stenosis can precede the development of other features of the disease by years; in others, subglottic stenosis may develop despite apparently effective control of the disease.

Pulmonary involvement will affect around 90% of patients at some point during the course of disease.[90] Symptoms are similar to those associated with MPA, although some patients may have asymptomatic disease that is detected only after imaging. In addition to the capillaritis (Figure 89-7) and vasculitis that occur in MPA, patients with GPA are burdened with granulomatous disease that causes development of nodules of chronic granulation tissue

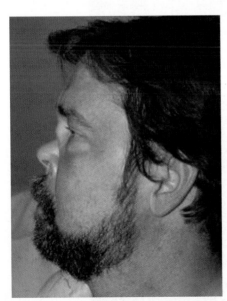

Figure 89-4 Saddle-nose deformity in a patient with granulomatosis with polyangiitis. *(Courtesy Dr. G. Hoffman.)*

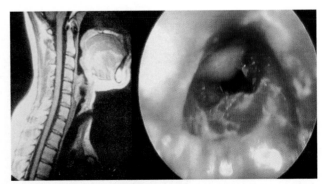

Figure 89-6 Subglottic stenosis in a patient with granulomatosis with polyangiitis. Magnetic resonance imaging *(left)* and endoscopic view *(right)*. *(Right, Courtesy Dr. G.S. Hoffman; from Hoffman GS, Kerr GS, Leavitt RY, et al: Wegener granulomatosis: an analysis of 158 patients,* Ann Intern Med *116:488–498, 1992.)*

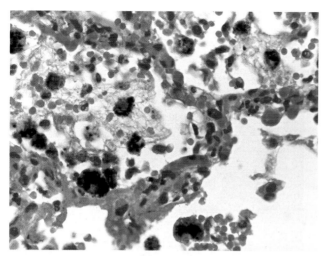

Figure 89-7 Capillaritis. Alveolar septa with congestion, neutrophilic infiltrate, and fibrinoid necrosis of capillary walls. Adjacent alveolar spaces contain hemosiderin-laden macrophages, consistent with a history of pulmonary hemorrhage (hematoxylin and eosin, ×40). *(Courtesy Dr. C. Farver.)*

allow the test to be undertaken. Depending on the progress of the disease, pulmonary function tests may show an obstructive or a restrictive component, particularly if fibrosis has developed following repeated episodes of hemorrhage or cyclophosphamide-induced pneumonitis.[102]

The features of renal involvement in systemic GPA are similar clinically and pathologically to those in MPA. Renal involvement probably occurs in around 80% of patients at some time during the course of the illness,[90,99] although determining the precise frequency overall is difficult. However, it should never be assumed that limited disease excludes the future development of renal and systemic disease because, as already noted, a proportion of patients will develop systemic disease at some point.[97] The lower urinary tract may also be affected with necrotizing vasculitis of the bladder, necrotizing urethritis, orchitis, epididymitis, prostatitis, and penile necrosis (reviewed in Reference 103). Urinary obstruction may develop, particularly with involvement of the ureters. Cystoscopy should be undertaken if unexplained persistent hematuria is present, to exclude bladder malignancy or other complications.

The eye may be affected in several ways during the course of GPA in 28% to 58% of patients.[104,105] Keratitis, conjunctivitis, episcleritis, scleritis, uveitis, retrobulbar granulomatous disease with proptosis, ocular palsies, lacrimal duct obstruction, optic neuritis, and retinal vascular occlusion may all occur.[104-106] Proptosis and optic neuritis are feared because they are particularly likely to lead to visual loss. Both CT and MRI may be helpful in defining retrobulbar disease (Figure 89-9). In patients treated with high doses of corticosteroids, cataracts may occur as a complication.

Both the peripheral and the central neurologic system can be affected in GPA.[107] Peripheral neuropathy may manifest as a mononeuritis multiplex or, less commonly, as a distal and symmetric polyneuropathy. Nerve conduction

that can cavitate centrally.[100] The most common radiographic findings are pulmonary infiltrates and nodules (Figure 89-8). Infiltrates may be fleeting in nature but may be extensive, particularly when associated with severe pulmonary hemorrhage. Small nodules that are not apparent radiologically may be detected by CT scanning. Imaging may also demonstrate pleural effusion and mediastinal or hilar lymph node enlargement. Infection may be superimposed on the disease background; it is important to exclude this by culture and by bronchoscopy if necessary.[101] If pulmonary hemorrhage is recent, the carbon monoxide diffusion capacity may be reduced if a patient is well enough to

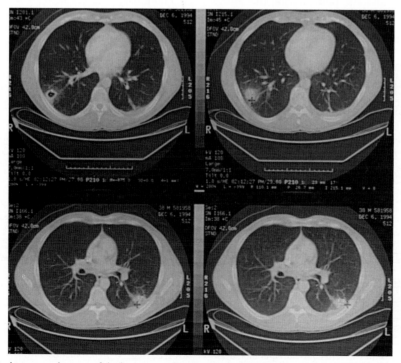

Figure 89-8   Computed tomography scan of the lungs, revealing the presence of nodules. The right-sided pulmonary nodule is cavitary.

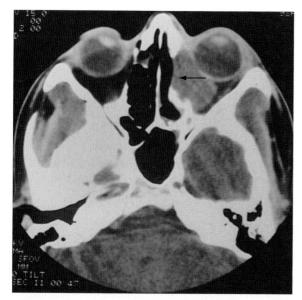

Figure 89-9 Computed tomography scan of the orbits, revealing the presence of a retro-orbital mass (orbital pseudotumor).

studies may be helpful in verifying the presence and extent of neuropathy, and biopsy of a nerve, usually the sural nerve, may establish the presence of vasculitis. Central nervous system disease occurs in a minority of patients—around 10%—but can be severe, particularly when a cerebral vasculitis is present.[108] Chronic pachymeningitis, cerebral hemorrhage and thrombosis, pituitary involvement, cerebral nerve involvement, brain stem lesions, spinal cord involvement, and subarachnoid or subdural hemorrhage may occur. Substantiating the presence of cerebral vasculitis may be difficult because small vessels are affected and angiography is of little utility. However, CT and MRI may help to define infarctions, hemorrhages, mass lesions, meningeal involvement, and white matter changes (Figure 89-10). Lumbar puncture may be necessary if subarachnoid hemorrhage is suspected or to exclude the presence of meningeal infection.

Cardiac involvement through coronary artery vasculitis and involvement of the myocardium by granulomatous disease may occur, and magnetic resonance angiography and contrast-enhanced MRI may be useful in its detection.[109] Increased risk of cardiovascular disease is noted in patients with AAV, including GPA.[110,111]

Symptomatic involvement of the gastrointestinal tract is not usually a major feature of GPA, or indeed of MPA. However, abdominal pain, bleeding, and diarrhea can occur as a result of the disease itself or through the effects of treatment, for example, corticosteroids can cause peptic ulceration and mycophenolate mofetil may cause diarrhea. The vasculitic process itself may lead to ulcerations, or even perforations, in the small or large intestine. A number of unusual presentations include involvement of the tongue and salivary glands (parotic, sublingual, or submandibular),[112] pancreatic involvement that may mimic pancreatic cancer,[113] and cholecystitis and hepatic granulomatous disease that can cause liver failure.[114] Splenic involvement with vasculitis, granulomas, and necrosis is present in many patients in older autopsy series.[115]

Allergic Granulomatosis with Polyangiitis

This syndrome was described by Churg and Strauss in 1951.[116] It has three salient histopathologic features, namely, necrotizing vasculitis, tissue infiltration by eosinophils, and extravascular granulomas (Figure 89-11). To improve recognition of this disorder, Lanham suggested that diagnosis be based on clinical features comprising asthma, peak eosinophil count greater than 1500 cells/mL, and systemic vasculitis involving two or more organs.[117,118] None of these clinical or pathologic features is entirely specific for AGPA, and they may not all be present or detectable concurrently.

The pathogenesis of AGPA is unknown, but a strong association has been noted with allergy and atopic disorders, including allergic rhinitis, nasal polyposis, and asthma. Around 70% of patients have elevated IgE levels,[117] as well as eosinophilia of peripheral blood and tissue. The association with leukotriene inhibitors was described in the epidemiology section. Although ANCAs may be present and, if so, usually are directed to MPO, up to 60% of patients may be negative for ANCA.[119,120] ANCA positivity is suggested to be associated with a higher incidence of renal disease, alveolar hemorrhage, mononeuritis multiplex, and purpura.[119,120]

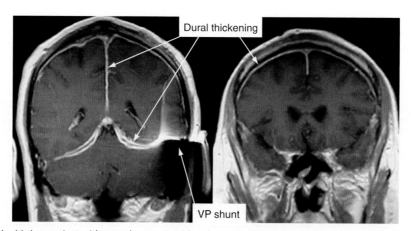

Figure 89-10 Pachymeningitis in a patient with granulomatosis with polyangiitis. Magnetic resonance imaging findings. VP, ventriculoperitoneal.

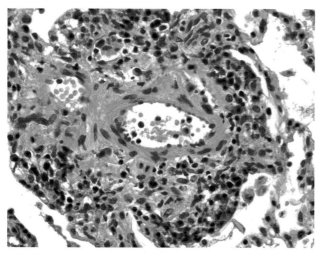

Figure 89-11 Churg-Strauss syndrome. Transmural eosinophilic infiltrate with scattered plasma cells and lymphocytes involving a small artery in the lung of a patient with Churg-Strauss syndrome (hematoxylin and eosin, ×40). *(Courtesy Dr. C. Farver.)*

In some patients, AGPA appears to unfold in distinct phases: a prodrome with allergic features, followed by the vasculitic phase, and then dominance of the clinical picture by allergic disease.[117] Asthma with pulmonary infiltrates on radiologic examination is typical, and infiltrates may have a lobar, interstitial, or nodular appearance. Pulmonary effusions can develop with eosinophils in the pleural fluid. Alveolar hemorrhage is a serious complication, as it is in other AAVs. Peripheral neuropathy occurs in around two-thirds of patients, taking the form of a mononeuritis multiplex with symmetric or asymmetric polyneuropathy. Cranial nerves can be affected, and occasionally central nervous system (CNS) disease develops. AGPA can affect the kidney, but less commonly than with MPA and GPA; the pathophysiology is similar, albeit with the presence of eosinophils. Lower urinary tract involvement may occur. As with other forms of AAV, multiple other organs can be affected occasionally, including the heart, gastrointestinal tract, and eye. Arthralgia and skin disease also occur as in other AAVs, although in AGPA, inflammatory skin nodules with the characteristic histopathology can develop. Features associated with a less favorable prognosis include creatininemia (>140 mmoles/L [1.58 mg/dL]), proteinuria (>1 g/day), or central nervous system, gastrointestinal, or myocardial involvement according to the Five Factor Score developed by Guillevin and colleagues.[121]

DIAGNOSIS AND DIAGNOSTIC TESTS

Diagnosis depends on clinical recognition of potentially vasculitic or granulomatous disease patterns, backed up by histology, serology, and appropriate imaging tests.

A broad summary of factors that aid differential diagnosis between AAVs is given in Table 89-3.

Whenever possible, diagnosis should be confirmed by pathologic examination of affected tissues; for MPA, this is usually done via biopsy of kidney, lung, or skin; for GPA, nasal or paranasal mucosal biopsy may be helpful also, although such biopsies are usually "consistent with" rather than "diagnostic of" GPA, because vasculitis, necrosis, and granulomas are encountered together in only a minority of cases; for AGPA, biopsy of nerve or muscle may be helpful if those tissues are involved clinically. Confirmation of diagnosis by histology gives confidence to embarking on a course of therapy that may have serious adverse effects. In the case of the kidney, the biopsy may also yield some prognostic information, depending on the percentage of normal glomeruli present.[122] Histologic classification of renal lesions into focal, crescentic, mixed, and sclerotic has been proposed to aid prognostic evaluation.[123]

Laboratory results may confirm the presence of an acute phase response, define the nature and extent of individual organ involvement, or contribute to diagnostic evaluation through detection or not of a range of immune antibody products. Leukocytosis, normocytic normochromic anemia, thrombocytosis, and elevated erythrocyte sedimentation rate and C-reactive protein may be indicative of an acute inflammatory state. In AGPA, peripheral eosinophilia in excess of 1500 cells/mL is often present, although occasional patients may have marked tissue eosinophilia without blood eosinophilia.

Detection of PR3- and MPO-ANCA now occurs by antigen-specific enzyme-linked immunosorbent assay (ELISA), widely available as routine laboratory testing. As a screening assay, indirect immunofluorescence (IIF) using ethanol-fixed human neutrophils reveals two major staining patterns of antibody binding to neutrophils comprising a cytoplasmic pattern (cANCA) and a perinuclear pattern (pANCA) (see Figure 89-1). The cANCA pattern usually equates to specificity for PR3-ANCA, and pANCA usually equates to MPO-ANCA. Guidelines for testing for ANCA have been agreed by international consensus,[124] and if these guidelines are adhered to, the chance of missing a case of AAV are low while indiscriminant testing is avoided.[125] The combination of IIF and ELISA testing increases specificity.[76] Thus, when the IIF test was combined with ELISA testing

Table 89-3 Differential Diagnostic Features of the Antineutrophil Cytoplasm Antibody–Associated Vasculitides

Feature	Microscopic Polyangiitis	GPA	AGPA	Comments
Glomerulonephritis	+++	+++	+	Progressive renal failure uncommon in AGPA
Pulmonary infiltrates or nodules	++	+++	+++	Asthma and eosinophilia in AGPA
Alveolar hemorrhage	++	++	+	
Upper airway disease	+	+++	++	Ear, nose, and throat disease usually favors GPA
Skin, purpura	+++	+	++	
Peripheral nerve involvement	+	++	+++	Often a prominent feature of AGPA
Central nervous system involvement	+	+	+	

+++, very commonly seen; ++, seen often; +, uncommon finding; AGPA, allergic granulomatosis with polyangiitis; GPA, granulomatosis with polyangiitis.

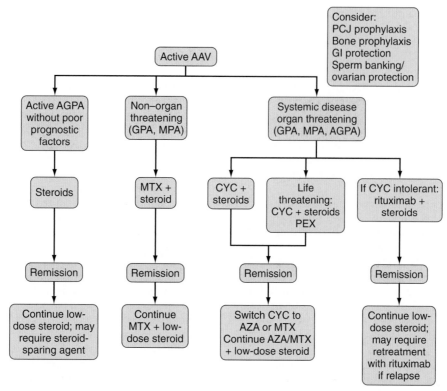

Figure 89-12 Treatment algorithm for antineutrophil cytoplasm antibody (ANCA)-associated vasculitides. AAV, ANCA-associated vasculitis; AGPA, allergic granulomatosis with polyangiitis; AZA, azathioprine; CYC, cyclophosphamide; GI, gastrointestinal; GPA, granulomatosis with polyangiitis; MPA, microscopic polyangiitis; MTX, methotrexate; PCJ, *Pneumocystis jiroveci*; PEX, plasma exchange; WG, Wegener's granulomatosis.

(cANCA/anti-PR3 positive, pANCA/anti-MPO positive), diagnostic specificity increased to 99%. The sensitivity of the combination of cANCA plus anti-PR3 or pANCA plus anti-MPO for GPA or MPA was 73% and 67%, respectively. The question of the status of ANCA-negative patients arises also because around 10% of patients may be negative; the reasons for this may include low titer antibody levels, a poorly performing IIF or ELISA test, or genuinely ANCA-negative disease. However, if clinical and pathologic features are consistent with AAV, patients generally should be treated along similar lines.

Both at the initiation of therapy and during monitoring, a number of tools are available to measure the extent of disease activity and the damage caused through effects of disease or treatment. Chief among these following their validation and use in multicenter randomized prospective clinical trials are the Birmingham Vasculitis Activity Score (now in its third iteration) and the Vasculitis Damage Index.[126-128] Other outcome measures include the Five Factor Score (FFS) and the Disease Extent Index (reviewed in Reference 129).

TREATMENT

The natural history of untreated AAV is rapidly progressive and usually fatal, with a 2-year mortality of 85%. The introduction of cyclophosphamide-based regimens to treat AAV in the 1970s has dramatically improved patient survival to around 80% at 5 years.[130] The aim of treatment is to induce and then maintain disease remission and prevent relapse, using agents with the lowest adverse event profile.

Treatment is tailored according to the disease severity at presentation, and more aggressive immunosuppression is required in the presence of life- or organ-threatening disease.[131] An algorithm for therapy is shown in Figure 89-12.

Induction of Remission

Cyclophosphamide, an alkylating immunosuppressant agent, with glucocorticoids is considered the "standard of care" as induction therapy for those with generalized disease.[132] Treatment should be continued for 3 to 6 months with remission rates following induction treatment varying from 35% to 93% in GPA and from 75% to 89% in MPA.[133] Cyclophosphamide treatment is not without its complications. As with all immunosuppression, risk of infection is present. Other adverse events associated with cyclophosphamide in patients with GPA have included hemorrhagic cystitis, bladder cancer, bone marrow suppression, lymphoma, myelodysplasia, and infertility.[86,90] A dose-response relationship between cyclophosphamide and the risk of bladder cancer has been demonstrated,[134] suggesting the need to treat with the lowest possible cumulative dose. There is therefore a need to balance the toxicity of treatment with the morbidity and mortality associated with disease.

One approach to limiting the cumulative cyclophosphamide dose has involved the use of pulsed cyclophosphamide versus the more traditional continuous daily regimens. A meta-analysis of three small, randomized studies suggested that pulsed intravenous cyclophosphamide was preferable to daily oral cyclophosphamide in terms of remission and reduced adverse events.[135] A more recent randomized controlled trial in 149 patients with generalized disease performed by the European Vasculitis Study Group (EUVAS) showed no statistically significant difference in the time to remission or in the proportion of patients attaining remission at 9 months between those randomized to pulse cyclophosphamide compared with daily oral cyclophosphamide, despite an absolute lower cumulative dose of cyclophosphamide that was associated with a lower rate of leukopenia in the pulsed limb. This study did not have sufficient duration of follow-up and was not powered to detect a difference in relapse rates.[136]

Other immunosuppressants may be used as alternatives to cyclophosphamide. Rituximab, an anti-CD20 chimeric monoclonal antibody that depletes B cells, has been shown to be effective in inducing remission in AAV in two randomized controlled trials. RITUXVAS compared cyclophosphamide- and rituximab-based regimens in newly diagnosed patients with severe AAV; the median glomerular filtration rate (GFR) at entry was 18 mL/min.[137] Forty-four patients were randomly assigned to receive two pulses of cyclophosphamide and four of rituximab or six to ten pulses of cyclophosphamide. Both groups received the same prednisolone dose and were followed for a minimum of 12 months. At 12 months, no differences were noted between the two groups in terms of remission rates, times to remission, or severe adverse events. The RAVE trial also supports the use of rituximab as an induction agent in AAV. This multicenter, randomized, double-blind, placebo-controlled trial, involving 197 ANCA-positive patients, of whom 52% had renal disease and 28% had alveolar hemorrhage, compared rituximab with cyclophosphamide during induction. Both limbs received the same reducing glucocorticoid regimen. Rituximab was shown to be noninferior to cyclophosphamide in the rate of disease remission at 6 months in the absence of corticosteroid therapy. In this study, rituximab may have been superior to cyclophosphamide in inducing remission in patients with relapsing disease. The rate of adverse events was the same between the two treatment limbs.[138] Of course, both trials were limited by the follow-up time, and long-term outcome trials are required.

ANCA levels fall with rituximab treatment, but this fall often occurs more slowly than the improvement in renal disease activity.[95,139] Induction of remission in patients is generally associated with complete peripheral B cell depletion following rituximab. B cell depletion, although to a lesser extent, also occurs with cyclophosphamide.[138] However, in studies of patients with relapsing disease, it has been shown that measurement of B cells peripherally is not a good surrogate marker for the risk of relapse because relapses may occur before the peripheral B cell population has recovered.[139]

Methotrexate has been identified as another alternative agent to cyclophosphamide in the induction phase of limited disease in the absence of vital organ involvement and with serum creatinine less than 150 µmol/L. The NORAM trial, involving 100 patients with newly diagnosed AAV, compared methotrexate with cyclophosphamide. Treatment was tapered and withdrawn in both limbs at 12 months. This study demonstrated noninferiority in the remission rate at 6 months between patients treated with

oral methotrexate versus those treated with oral cyclophosphamide. If treated with methotrexate, time to remission was longer in those with more extensive disease or lung involvement, suggesting that methotrexate is more appropriate in patients with limited early disease. The rate of leukopenia was significantly lower among those in the methotrexate limb. Relapse rates at 18 months were unacceptably high in both limbs, suggesting that immunosuppression should be continued for longer than 12 months.[140]

A small study of 35 patients recently suggested that mycophenolate mofetil may be useful as an alternative agent to cyclophosphamide for induction therapy in those with generalized disease and moderate renal impairment.[141] A larger, multicenter, randomized trial is being conducted by EUVAS to address this question (www.vasculitis.org).

Maintenance of Remission

It has been suggested that cyclophosphamide is used for the induction of remission, and another immunosuppressant agent, with fewer associated adverse events, is used to maintain remission. Four major agents have been used in this way: methotrexate, azathioprine, mycophenolate mofetil, and leflunomide. CYCAZAREM, a multicenter, randomized, controlled trial, compared azathioprine with cyclophosphamide to maintain remission, and compared relapse rates within 18 months of diagnosis. Investigators showed that following the induction of remission with cyclophosphamide for a minimum of 3 months, no difference in relapse rates was observed between the two limbs.[142] Although in this trial no difference in adverse events between the two treatment limbs was reported, azathioprine is considered to be less toxic than cyclophosphamide. A retrospective study using historical controls also suggested that relapse rates were no different in those treated with azathioprine compared with cyclophosphamide during the maintenance phase of treatment. This study suggested that switching to azathioprine in patients with PR3-AAV, who remained ANCA-positive at the time of remission, was associated with a high risk of relapse.[143]

Following induction of remission with cyclophosphamide, methotrexate is as effective as azathioprine in maintaining remission and may be used in those with normal renal function.[144]

Small case series have suggested that mycophenolate mofetil is well tolerated when used as maintenance therapy.[145,146] However, results from a large study of 154 adult patients randomized to receive azathioprine or mycophenolate for the maintenance of remission (IMPROVE study) suggested that azathioprine may be associated with fewer total relapses than mycophenolate.[147] However, no difference was observed in the number of major relapses or in damage sustained during the study as measured by the vasculitis damage index. No difference in adverse events was described in this study.

In a multicenter trial, following induction of remission with cyclophosphamide and prednisolone, 54 patients with GPA were randomized to receive leflunomide or methotrexate as maintenance therapy. This study was terminated prematurely owing to the high incidence of major relapse in those treated with methotrexate, but findings suggested that leflunomide was effective in preventing major relapses.

Conversely, leflunomide was associated with more adverse events than occurred with methotrexate. A dose of 30 mg/day of leflunomide was used; therefore, this may not be an appropriate dose.[148]

Guidelines suggest that patients with AAV should continue on maintenance therapy for at least 24 months, maybe longer, following successful remission.[149] The IMPROVE study continued therapy for 40 months and reported relapse rates of almost 50%.[147]

Adjuvant Therapy

Adjunct plasmapheresis in adult patients presenting with severe progressive renal failure (creatinine >500 μmol/L) has been shown, in the MEPEX study, to be superior to methylprednisolone in reducing the number of patients who remain dialysis dependent.[150] The underpinning principle of plasma exchange is the removal of circulating autoantibodies, with the by-product being the removal of other plasma proteins, including coagulation factors. No randomized trials have examined the use of plasma exchange in diffuse alveolar hemorrhage (DAH). A single retrospective review of 20 patients who presented with DAH associated with AAV treated with plasma exchange showed improved outcome with no complications of therapy compared with historical controls.[151] A randomized trial conducted by EUVAS aims to investigate the efficacy of plasma exchange in addition to standard immunosuppressive therapy in AAV with pulmonary hemorrhage or renal involvement (GFR <50 mL/min) (www.vasculitis.org).

Alternative Agents

Alternative agents may be used for those who fail to respond to first-line treatment, or when there is cyclophosphamide intolerance. Rituximab has been shown to be effective in patients with refractory disease in whom maximal treatment with conventional therapy had not previously resulted in remission. Antilymphocyte therapies may also be effective in refractory disease. Treatment with antithymocyte globulin, which consists of polyclonal antibodies directed against T cell surface antigens and results in rapid T cell depletion, has been shown to be of benefit in a small pilot study of 15 patients.[152] Deoxyspergualin is an antiproliferative agent with lymphocyte and macrophage inhibitory functions. In a study of patients with relapsing or refractory AAV treated for 6 months with deoxyspergualin, 42 of 44 patients achieved at least partial remission and 45% achieved full remission. However, relapse occurred in 44% with a median time of 170 days, and 53% developed severe or life-threatening treatment-related adverse events.[153] Campath, a humanized anti-CD52 antibody that depletes lymphocytes and monocytes, has shown benefit in refractory disease. However, it should be used with caution in those older than 50 years and dialysis dependent at the time of treatment.[154]

Intravenous immunoglobulin (IVIG) has been used to induce remission in AAV. In a double-blind controlled trial, 34 patients were randomized to receive a single course of IVIG or a placebo, alongside conventional treatment. Those who received IVIG had significantly reduced Birmingham Vasculitis Activity Score (BVAS) at 3 months compared with the placebo limb, but this effect was not maintained beyond 3 months.[155] Six months of IVIG treatment has been shown to be effective in inducing remission in the context of disease relapse,[156] with a study of six patients also suggesting effectiveness of IVIG as sole therapy.[157] IVIG may be useful where significant immunosuppression should be avoided.

EULAR has recently produced guidelines to help guide the management of patients with AAV[131] (Table 89-4). However, it must be noted that most studies have excluded patients with AGPA.

Treatment of Allergic Granulomatosis with Polyangiitis

Patients without poor prognostic disease according to the FFS can be managed by corticosteroids alone.[158] However, relapse is common, with 35% of patients relapsing with a mean follow-up of 56 months. Long-term steroids were necessary in 79% mainly owing to asthma. In patients with one or more poor prognostic factors, induction therapy with corticosteroids and cyclophosphamide is necessary.[121] No maintenance therapy was prescribed in this study, and relapses were common, occurring in 74%. As with those patients without poor prognostic factors, long-term use of steroids occurred in the majority (81%), even after a median follow-up of 8 years.

Table 89-4 EULAR Recommendations on the Management of AAV (12 of 15 Applicable to AAV)

1. Manage in collaboration with, or at, centers of expertise
2. ANCA testing should be performed only in an appropriate clinical context
3. A positive biopsy is strongly supportive of vasculitis—recommend the procedure to assist diagnosis and further evaluation for patients suspected of having vasculitis
4. Structured clinical assessment, urinalysis, and other basic laboratory tests at each clinical visit
5. Categorize according to different levels of severity to assist treatment decisions
6. Cyclophosphamide (oral or IV) and glucocorticoids for remission induction
7. Combination of methotrexate and glucocorticoid as a less toxic alternative to cyclophosphamide for the induction of remission in non–organ-threatening or non–life-threatening ANCA-associated vasculitis
8. Use of high-dose glucocorticoids as an important part of remission induction therapy; high dose continued for the first month (usual practice to start at 1 mg/kg/day). Dosage should not be reduced to <15 mg/day in first month
9. Plasma exchange for selected patients with rapidly progressive severe renal disease to improve renal survival
10. Remission maintenance therapy with a combination of low-dose glucocorticoid therapy and azathioprine/leflunomide/methotrexate
11. Alternative immunomodulatory therapy choices should be considered for patients who do not achieve remission or relapse on maximal doses of standard therapy
12. Investigation of persistent unexplained hematuria in patients with prior exposure to cyclophosphamide

AAV, antineutrophil cytoplasm antibody–associated vasculitides; ANCA, antineutrophil cytoplasm antibody; EULAR, European League Against Rheumatism.

From Mukhtyar C, Guillevin L, Cid MC, et al: EULAR recommendations for the management of primary small and medium vessel vasculitis, *Ann Rheum Dis* 68:310–317, 2009.

Patient survival with these regimens is good; those without adverse prognostic signs have 5-year survival of 97%,[158] and those with more severe disease have 92% survival at 8 years.[121] However, the optimal duration of maintenance therapy is unknown, and many require long-term therapy for asthma symptoms.

Up to 10% of patients are refractory to conventional therapy. New therapies are under investigation. Rituximab has been effective in a few cases[159,160]; however it has been reported to provoke severe bronchospasm.[161] Small open-label studies are in progress to assess the efficacy and safety of rituximab and mepolizumab, an anti-IL-5 monoclonal antibody, in AGPA.

Adverse Events

Despite improvement in survival resulting from improved treatment strategies, a recent EUVAS short-term outcome study, which included 524 patients prospectively recruited into four clinical trials, reported a 1-year mortality probability of 11.1%.[162] The cause of death was related to an adverse event of treatment in 59%, and infection was the overwhelming factor. Active vasculitis accounted for only 14% of deaths. This study highlights the burden of using nonselective immunosuppressant agents, which suppress the whole immune system, not just the production of ANCA. Patients receiving such treatments, including glucocorticoids, are at increased risk for opportunistic infection, with respiratory tract infection and generalized septicemia being the most common infections in the EUVAS study previously discussed. Factors predictive of infection include age, severity of renal dysfunction, leukopenia, and intensity and duration of immunosuppression. Guidelines advocate the use of prophylaxis against *Pneumocystis jiroveci* in patients receiving cyclophosphamide.[131] Influenza vaccinations have been shown to be safe and effective in AAV without association with relapse in a retrospective study of 230 patients.[163] Rituximab is associated with an impaired secondary humoral response, making immunization ineffective during treatment.[164]

Other adverse events are specific to treatments. Glucocorticoids are known to have a broad adverse event profile, including steroid-associated diabetes, avascular necrosis, and ocular cataract formation; monitoring for all of these should be provided during treatment. Prophylaxis against osteoporosis[131] and peptic ulceration has become routine, especially in those receiving high-dose corticosteroids. The adverse events associated with cyclophosphamide have already been highlighted. Concomitant treatment with mesna, which binds to the toxic metabolite of cyclophosphamide, is advised on the first day of a cyclophosphamide pulse and in oral regimens[131] to reduce the risk of bladder toxicity.[86] Male and female infertility is a recognized complication of cyclophosphamide therapy in autoimmune disease.[149,165] In females, infertility is related to high cumulative doses and older age at treatment.[165] Minimizing the dose of cyclophosphamide is important, as is the continuing development of methods of fertility preservation.[166,167] Patients should be counseled as to the risk of infertility, and cryopreservation of sperm and oocytes should be offered if appropriate.[149]

Adverse events can also be attributable to the disease itself. In a study of 198 patients, followed for a median of 6.1 years, it was shown that AAV is associated with increased risk of venous thromboembolism, especially when the disease is active.[168] Avoidance of classic risk factors for venous thromboembolism is therefore important, as is the use of prophylaxis during prolonged immobility. Because patients are now surviving their acute illness, the long-term consequences of disease activity need to be considered, along with the already discussed burden of therapy.

OUTCOME

Over the past 30 years, treatment has improved outcomes for patients with AAV. Most patients respond to treatment, and 85% achieve remission. Older age may predict treatment resistance.[169] Patient survival is reported as 45% to 91% at 5 years and as 75% to 88% at 10 years compared with 80% mortality at 2 years if left untreated.[133]

Despite advances in therapy, patients continue to have substantially higher mortality than a matched background population, as was shown by a recent study of long-term outcomes of patients recruited to EUVAS studies.[130] The mortality rate ratio was 2.6 compared with the normal population, with advanced renal failure, increasing age, and a high BVAS being the main predictors of an adverse outcome. Several other studies have identified increasing age and worsening renal function as poor prognostic markers.[170,171] In this study, no difference in survival was reported between patients with GPA and those with MPA in contrast to other studies.[170,172] Mortality is highest in the first year, with 1-, 2-, and 5-year survival of 88%, 85%, and 78%. Disease and therapy-related deaths, particularly infection, account for most deaths in the first year. Infection remains an important cause of death even beyond 1 year, but malignancy and cardiovascular disease are also common.[130]

End-stage kidney disease (ESKD) is not uncommon in patients with AAV; approximately 20% of those presenting who have evidence of renal involvement will develop ESKD by 5 years. In a multivariate analysis, renal survival was best predicted by presenting serum creatinine and percentage of normal glomeruli in the diagnostic biopsy.[122] Patients who develop ESKD should be considered for transplantation. Using United Network for Organ Sharing (UNOS) data from 1996-2007, 919 patients with ESKD secondary to GPA were identified. Adjusted outcomes for graft loss, death, and functional graft loss were better in those patients with GPA compared with other causes of ESKD.[173] Outcome in those patients who remain on dialysis is similar to that with other causes of ESKD.[87]

Cardiovascular disease is more common in patients with AAV than in the healthy population or in patients with matched levels of chronic kidney disease.[110,111] It is currently unclear whether this is related to persistent inflammation or to therapy with prolonged steroid use. Malignancy rates in treated AAV patients are also higher than in the healthy population, particularly nonmelanoma skin and bladder cancer and acute myeloid leukemia.[86,174-176] The cumulative dose of cyclophosphamide is important in determining risk of cancer; patients receiving more than 36 g are at greatest risk.[174] Preliminary results from the EUVAS group suggest that the philosophy of minimizing cyclophosphamide usage may be proving correct; a follow-up study of patients recruited to clinical trials revealed only nonmelanoma skin cancer to be substantially increased compared with the healthy population.[176a]

The clinical course in patients with AAV is difficult to predict; approximately 50% of patients will relapse over 5 years. Predictors of relapse have included anti-PR3 antibodies, lung and upper respiratory involvement,[177] age,[178] nasal carriage of *S. aureus*,[35] and absence of severe renal involvement.[178,179] Patients with ESKD have lower rates of relapse.[87,162] Daily oral cyclophosphamide may be more effective than intermittent cyclophosphamide but at the expense of higher risk of death and adverse events.[179-181]

Using microarray analysis of purified T cells, a CD8+ T cell transcription signature has been identified that can identify patients at risk of relapse. The subset of genes defining the poor prognostic group was enriched for genes involved in the interleukin (IL)-7 receptor pathway and T cell receptor signaling, and for genes expressed by memory T cells. A model using only three genes—*ITAG2*, *PTPN22*, and *NOTCH1*—was predictive of the poor prognostic group. However, this signature was not discernible following treatment.[182] Confirmation of this signature by others raises the possibility of individualized therapy.

SUMMARY

Understanding of the causes and pathogenic mechanisms underlying AAV has progressed apace over the past 20 years. The central place of ANCA and immune processes is appreciated. The mortality incurred by patients suffering from AAV has fallen steadily, but the chronic relapsing nature of the disease, without definitive treatments that offer cure, continues to extract a heavy toll on the health of afflicted individuals of all ages. Understanding of the most efficacious ways with which to control disease using corticosteroids, cyclophosphamide, other immune suppressants, and plasma exchange has increased through use of randomized prospective clinical trials. However, although rituximab holds promise, no therapy has yet been licensed for AAV. Despite the rarity of the condition, the large unmet need for safe, effective therapies remains a challenge to pharmaceutical companies, particularly because mechanisms underpinning the disease are understood sufficiently to provide realistic targets for new therapies.

Selected References

1. Falk RJ, Jennette JC: ANCA disease: where is this field heading? *J Am Soc Nephrol* 21:745–752, 2010.
2. Falk RJ, Jennette JC: Anti-neutrophil cytoplasmic autoantibodies with specificity for myeloperoxidase in patients with systemic vasculitis and idiopathic necrotising and crescentic glomerulonephritis, *N Engl J Med* 318:1651–1657, 1988.
3. Goldschmeding R, van der Schoot CE, ten Bokkel Huinink D, et al: Wegener's granulomatosis autoantibodies identify a novel diisopropylfluorphosphate-binding protein in the lysosomes of normal human neutrophils, *J Clin Invest* 84:1577–1587, 1989.
4. Kain R, Exner M, Brandes R, et al: Molecular mimicry in pauci-immune focal necrotizing glomerulonephritis, *Nat Med* 14:1088–1096, 2008.
6. Leavitt RY, Fauci AS, Bloch DA, et al: The American College of Rheumatology 1990 criteria for the classification of Wegener's granulomatosis, *Arthritis Rheum* 33:1101–1107, 1990.

7. Masi A, Hunder GG, Lie JT, et al: The American College of Rheumatology 1990 criteria for the classification of Churg-Strauss syndrome (allergic granulomatosis and angiitis), *Arthritis Rheum* 33:1094–1100, 1990.
8. Jennette JC, Falk RJ, Andrassy K, et al: Nomenclature of systemic vasculitides: the proposal of an International Consensus Conference, *Arthritis Rheum* 37:187–192, 1994.
9. Watts R, Lane S, Hanslik T, et al: Development and validation of a consensus methodology for the classification of the ANCA-associated vasculitides and polyarteritis nodosa for epidemiological studies, *Ann Rheum Dis* 66:222–227, 2007.
10. Liu LJ, Chen M, Yu F, et al: Evaluation of a new algorithm in classification of systemic vasculitis, *Rheumatology (Oxford)* 47:708–712, 2008.
13. Basu N, Watts R, Bajema I, et al: EULAR points to consider in the development of classification and diagnostic criteria in systemic vasculitis, *Ann Rheum Dis* 2010, published online as 10.136/ard.2009.119032.
14. Ntatsaki E, Watts RA, Scott DG: Epidemiology of ANCA-associated vasculitis, *Rheum Dis Clin N Am* 36:447–461, 2010.
15. Watts RA, Al-Taiar A, Scott DG, et al: Prevalence and incidence of Wegener's granulomatosis in the UK general practice research database, *Arthritis Rheum* 61:1412–1416, 2009.
20. Fujimoto S, Uezono S, Hisanaga S, et al: Incidence of ANCA-associated primary renal vasculitis in the Miyazaki Prefecture: the first population-based, retrospective, epidemiologic survey in Japan, *Clin J Am Soc Nephrol* 1:1016–1022, 2006.
29. Yashiro M, Muso E, Itoh-Ihara T, et al: Significantly high regional morbidity of MPO-ANCA-related angiitis and/or nephritis with respiratory tract involvement after the 1995 great earthquake in Kobe (Japan), *Am J Kidney Dis* 35:889–895, 2000.
30. Harrold LR, Andrade SE, Go AS, et al: Incidence of Churg-Strauss syndrome in asthma drug users: a population based perspective, *J Rheumatol* 32:1076–1080, 2005.
32. Bibby S, Healy B, Steele R, et al: Association between leukotriene receptor antagonist therapy and Churg-Strauss syndrome: an analysis of the FDA AERS data-base, *Thorax* 65:132–138, 2010.
33. Chen M, Kallenberg CG: The environment, geoepidemiology and ANCA-associated vasculitides, *Autoimmun Rev* 9:A293–A298, 2010.
36. Hogan SL, Cooper GS, Savitz DA, et al: Association of silica exposure with anti-neutrophil cytoplasmic autoantibody small-vessel vasculitis: a population-based, case-control study, *Clin J Am Soc Nephrol* 2:290–299, 2007.
39. Knight A, Sandin S, Askling J: Risks and relative risks of Wegener's granulomatosis among close relatives of patients with the disease, *Arthritis Rheum* 58:302–307, 2008.
40. Hemminki K, Li X, Sundquist J, et al: Familial associations of rheumatoid arthritis with autoimmune diseases and related conditions, *Arthritis Rheum* 60:661–668, 2009.
43. Jagiello P, Gencik M, Arning L, et al: New genomic region for Wegener's granulomatosis as revealed by an extended association screen with 202 apoptosis-related genes, *Hum Genet* 114:468–477, 2004.
44. Jeffery LE, Burke F, Mura M, et al: 1,25-Dihydroxyvitamin D3 and IL-2 combine to inhibit T cell production of inflammatory cytokines and promote development of regulatory T cells expressing CTLA-4 and FoxP3, *J Immunol* 183:5458–5467, 2009.
45. Heckmann M, Holle JU, Arning L, et al: The Wegener's granulomatosis quantitative trait locus on chromosome 6p21.3 as characterised by tagSNP genotyping, *Ann Rheum Dis* 67:972–979, 2008.
46. Stassen PM, Cohen-Tervaert JW, Lems SP, et al: HLA-DR4, DR13(6) and the ancestral haplotype A1B8DR3 are associated with ANCA-associated vasculitis and Wegener's granulomatosis, *Rheumatology (Oxford)* 48:622–625, 2009.
47. Gencik M, Borgmann S, Zahn R, et al: Immunogenetic risk factors for anti-neutrophil cytoplasmic antibody (ANCA)-associated systemic vasculitis, *Clin Exp Immunol* 117:412–417, 1999.
48. Vaglio A, Martorana D, Maggiore U, et al: HLA-DRB4 as a genetic risk factor for Churg-Strauss syndrome, *Arthritis Rheum* 56:3159–3166, 2007.
49. Wieczorek S, Hellmich B, Gross WL, et al: Associations of Churg-Strauss syndrome with the HLA-DRB1 locus, and relationship to the genetics of antineutrophil cytoplasmic antibody-associated vasculitides: comment on the article by Vaglio et al, *Arthritis Rheum* 58:329–330, 2008.

50. Brand O, Gough S, Heward J: HLA, CTLA-4 and PTPN22: the shared genetic master-key to autoimmunity? *Expert Rev Mol Med* 7:1–15, 2005.

54. Kamesh L, Heward JM, Williams JM, et al: CT60 and +49 polymorphisms of CTLA 4 are associated with ANCA-positive small vessel vasculitis, *Rheumatology (Oxford)* 48:1502–1505, 2009.

55. Zhou Y, Huang D, Paris PL, et al: An analysis of CTLA-4 and proinflammatory cytokine genes in Wegener's granulomatosis, *Arthritis Rheum* 50:2645–2650, 2004.

56. Slot MC, Sokolowska MG, Savelkouls KG, et al: Immunoregulatory gene polymorphisms are associated with ANCA-related vasculitis, *Clin Immunol* 128:39–45, 2008.

57. Carr EJ, Niederer HA, Williams J, et al: Confirmation of the genetic association of CTLA4 and PTPN22 with ANCA-associated vasculitis, *BMC Med Genet* 10:121, 2009.

59. Jagiello P, Aries P, Arning L, et al: The PTPN22 620W allele is a risk factor for Wegener's granulomatosis, *Arthritis Rheum* 52:4039–4043, 2005.

60. Mahr AD, Edberg JC, Stone JH, et al: Alpha 1-antitrypsin deficiency-related alleles Z and S and the risk for Wegener's granulomatosis, *Arthritis Rheum* 62:3760–3767, 2010.

64. Audrain MAP, Sesboue R, Baranger TAR, et al: Analysis of antineutrophil cytoplasmic antibodies (ANCA): frequency and specificity in a sample of 191 homozygous (PiZZ) alpha1-antitrypsin-deficient subjects, *Nephrol Dial Transplant* 16:39–44, 2001.

65. Schreiber A, Busjahn A, Luft FC, et al: Membrane expression of proteinase 3 is genetically determined, *J Am Soc Nephrol* 14:68–75, 2003.

66. Witko-Sarsat V, Lesavre P, Lopez S, et al: A large subset of neutrophils expressing membrane proteinase 3 is a risk factor for vasculitis and rheumatoid arthritis, *J Am Soc Nephrol* 10:1224–1233, 1999.

67. Rarok AA, Stegeman CA, Limburg PC, et al: Neutrophil membrane expression of proteinase 3 (PR3) is related to relapse in PR3-ANCA-associated vasculitis, *J Am Soc Nephrol* 13:2232–2238, 2002.

68. Abdgawad M, Hellmark T, Gunnarsson L, et al: Increased neutrophil membrane expression and plasma level of proteinase 3 in systemic vasculitis are not a consequence of the −564 A/G promoter polymorphism, *Clin Exp Immunol* 145:63–70, 2006.

69. Pieters K, Pettersson A, Gullberg U, et al: The −564 A/G polymorphism in the promoter region of the proteinase 3 gene associated with Wegener's granulomatosis does not increase the promoter activity, *Clin Exp Immunol* 138:266–270, 2004.

70. von Vietinghoff S, Busjahn A, Schönemann C, et al: Major histocompatibility complex HLA region largely explains the genetic variance exercised on neutrophil membrane proteinase 3 expression, *J Am Soc Nephrol* 17:3185–3191, 2006.

71. Rajp C, Adu D, Savage CO: Meta-analysis of myeloperoxidase G-463/A polymorphism in anti-neutrophil cytoplasmic autoantibody-positive vasculitis, *Clin Exp Immunol* 149:251–256, 2007.

73. Jennette JC, Falk RJ: Renal and systemic vasculitis. In Johnson RJ, Feehally J, editors: *Comprehensive clinical nephrology*, London, 2000, Harcourt Publishers Ltd., pp 5.28–5.41.

74. Franssen CFM, Gans ROB, Arends B, et al: Differences between anti-myeloperoxidase and anti-proteinase 3-associated renal disease, *Kidney Int* 47:193–199, 1995.

75. Xing GQ, Chen M, Liu G, et al: Complement activation is involved in renal damage in human antineutrophil cytoplasmic autoantibody associated pauci-immune vasculitis, *J Clin Immunol* 29:282–291, 2009.

76. Hagen EC, Daha MR, Hermans J, et al: Diagnostic value of standardized assays for anti-neutrophil cytoplasmic antibodies in idiopathic systemic vasculitis, *Kidney Int* 53:743–753, 1998.

77. Ferraro A, Hassan B, Savage COS: Pathogenic mechanisms of antineutrophil antibody-associated vasculitis, *Exp Rev Clin Immunol* 3:543–555, 2007.

78. Xiao H, Heeringa P, Hu P, et al: Antineutrophil cytoplasmic autoantibodies specific for myeloperoxidase (MPO-ANCA) cause glomerulonephritis and vasculitis in mice, *J Clin Invest* 110:955–963, 2002.

79. Little MA, Smyth L, Salama AD, et al: Experimental autoimmune vasculitis: an animal model of anti-neutrophil cytoplasmic autoantibody-associated systemic vasculitis, *Am J Pathol* 174:1212–1220, 2009.

80. Little MA, Smyth CL, Yadav R, et al: Antineutrophil cytoplasm antibodies directed against myeloperoxidase augment leukocyte-microvascular interactions in vivo, *Blood* 106:2050–2058, 2008.

81. Nolan SL, Kalia N, Nash GB, et al: Murine antineutrophil cytoplasmic antibodies increase leukocyte-endothelial cell interactions in vivo with a critical role for Fcγ receptors, *J Am Soc Nephrol* 19:973–984, 2008.

82. Serra A, Cameron JS, Turner DR, et al: Vasculitis affecting the kidney: presentation, histopathology and long-term outcome, *Q J Med* 210:181–207, 1984.

83. Savage COS, Winearls CG, Evans DJ, et al: Microscopic polyarteritis: presentation, pathology and prognosis, *Q J Med* 56:467–483, 1985.

84. D'Agati V, Chandler P, Nash ME, et al: Idiopathic microscopic polyarteritis nodosa: ultrastructural observations on the renal vasculature and glomerular lesions, *Am J Kidney Dis* 7:95–110, 1986.

85. Adu D, Howie AJ, Scott DGI, et al: Polyarteritis and the kidney, *Q J Med* 62:221–237, 1987.

86. Talar-Williams C, Hijazi YM, Walther MM, et al: Cyclophosphamide-induced cystitis and bladder cancer in patients with Wegener granulomatosis, *Ann Intern Med* 124:477–484, 1996.

87. Weidanz F, Day CJ, Hewins P, et al: Recurrences and infections during continuous immunosuppressive therapy after beginning dialysis in ANCA-associated vasculitis, *Am J Kidney Dis* 50:36–46, 2007.

90. Hoffman GS, Kerr GS, Leavitt RY, et al: Wegener's granulomatosis: an analysis of 158 patients, *Ann Intern Med* 116:488–498, 1992.

91. Travis WD, Hoffman GS, Leavitt RY, et al: Surgical pathology of the lung in Wegener's granulomatosis: review of 87 open lung biopsies from 67 patients, *Am J Surg Pathol* 15:315–333, 1991.

92. Rastaldi MP, Ferrario F, Tunesi S, et al: Intraglomerular and interstitial leukocyte infiltration, adhesion molecules, and interleukin-1 alpha expression in 15 cases of antineutrophil cytoplasmic autoantibody-associated renal vasculitis, *Am J Pathol* 27:48–57, 1996.

93. Hewins P, Cohen Tervaert JW, Savage COS, et al: Is Wegener's granulomatosis an autoimmune disease? *Curr Opin Rheumatol* 12:3–10, 2000.

94. van der Woude FJ, Rasmussen N, Lobatto S, et al: Autoantibodies against neutrophils and monocytes: tool for diagnosis and marker of disease activity in Wegener's granulomatosis, *Lancet* i:425–429, 1985.

95. Ferraro A, Drayson M, Savage COS, et al: Levels of autoantibodies, unlike antibodies to all extrinsic antigen groups, fall following B cell depletion with rituximab, *Eur J Immunol* 38:292–298, 2008.

96. Berden AE, Kallenberg CGM, Savage COS, et al: Cellular immunity in Wegener's granulomatosis: characterizing T lymphocytes, *Arthritis Rheum* 60:1578–1587, 2009.

97. Holle JU, Gross WL, Holl-Ulrich K, et al: Prospective long-term follow-up of patients with localised Wegener's granulomatosis: does it occur as persistent disease stage? *Ann Rheum Dis* 69:1934–1939, 2010.

98. Murty GE: Wegener's granulomatosis: otorhinolaryngological manifestations, *Clin Otolaryngol* 15:385–393, 1990.

99. Fauci AS, Haynes BF, Katz P, et al: Wegener's granulomatosis: prospective clinical and therapeutic experience with 85 patients for 21 years, *Ann Intern Med* 98:76–85, 1983.

102. Thickett DR, Richter AG, Nathani N, et al: Pulmonary manifestations of anti-neutrophil cytoplasmic antibody (ANCA)-positive vasculitis, *Rheumatology (Oxford)* 45:261–268, 2006.

103. Duna GF, Galperin C, Hoffman GS: Wegener's granulomatosis, *Rheum Dis Clin N Am* 21:949–986, 1995.

104. Pakrou N, Selva D, Leibovitch I: Wegener's granulomatosis: ophthalmic manifestations and management, *Semin Arthritis Rheum* 35:284–292, 2006.

105. Harper SL, Letko E, Samson CM, et al: Wegener's granulomatosis: the relationship between ocular and systemic disease, *J Rheumatol* 28:1025–1032, 2001.

107. Nishino H, Rubino FA, DeRemee RA, et al: Neurological involvement in Wegener's granulomatosis: an analysis of 324 consecutive patients at the Mayo Clinic, *Ann Neurol* 33:4–9, 1993.

108. Seror R, Mahr A, Ramanoelina J, et al: Central nervous system involvement in Wegener granulomatosis, *Medicine (Baltimore)* 85:54–65, 2006.

109. Mavrogeni S, Manoussakis MN, Karagiorga TC, et al: Detection of coronary artery lesions and myocardial necrosis by magnetic resonance in systemic necrotizing vasculitides, *Arthritis Rheum* 61:1121–1129, 2009.

110. Morgan MD, Turnbull J, Selamet U, et al: Increased incidence of cardiovascular events in patients with antineutrophil cytoplasmic

antibody-associated vasculitides: a matched-pair cohort study, *Arthritis Rheum* 60:3493–3500, 2009.

111. Faurschou M, Mellemkjaer L, Sorensen IJ, et al: Increased morbidity from ischemic heart disease in patients with Wegener's granulomatosis, *Arthritis Rheum* 60:1187–1192, 2009.

117. Lanham JG, Elkon KB, Pusey CD, et al: Systemic vasculitis with asthma and eosinophilia: a clinical approach to the Churg-Strauss syndrome, *Medicine (Baltimore)* 63:65–81, 1984.

119. Sinico RA, Di Toma L, Maggiore U, et al: Prevalence and clinical significance of antineutrophil cytoplasmic antibodies in Churg-Strauss syndrome, *Arthritis Rheum* 52:2926–2935, 2005.

120. Sablé-Fourtassou R, Cohen P, Mahr A, et al: Antineutrophil cytoplasmic antibodies and the Churg-Strauss syndrome, *Ann Intern Med* 43:632–638, 2005.

121. Cohen P, Pagnoux C, Mahr A, et al: Churg-Strauss syndrome with poor-prognosis factors: a prospective multicenter trial comparing glucocorticoids and six or twelve cyclophosphamide pulses in forty-eight patients, *Arthritis Rheum* 57:686–693, 2007.

122. Day CJ, Howie AJ, Nightingale P, et al: Prediction of ESRD in pauci-immune necrotizing glomerulonephritis: quantitative histomorphometric assessment and serum creatinine, *Am J Kidney Dis* 55:250–258, 2010.

123. Berden AE, Ferrario F, Hagen EC, et al: Histopathologic classification of ANCA-associated glomerulonephritis, *J Am Soc Nephrol* 21:1628–1636, 2010.

124. Savige J, Gillis D, Benson E, et al: International consensus statement on testing and reporting of antineutrophil cytoplasmic antibodies (ANCA), *Am J Clin Pathol* 111:507–513, 1999.

125. Robinson PC, Steele RE: Appropriateness of antineutrophil cytoplasmic antibody testing in a tertiary hospital, *J Clin Pathol* 62:743–745, 2009.

126. Mukhtyar C, Lee R, Brown D, et al: Modification and validation of the Birmingham Vasculitis Activity Score (version 3), *Ann Rheum Dis* 68:1827–1832, 2009.

129. Suppiah R, Robson J, Luqmani R: Outcome measures in ANCA-associated vasculitis, *Rheum Dis Clin N Am* 36:587–607, 2010.

130. Flossmann O, Berden AE, de Groot K, et al: Long-term patient survival in ANCA-associated vasculitis, *Ann Rheum Dis* 70:488–494, 2011.

131. Mukhtyar C, Guillevin L, Cid MC, et al: EULAR recommendations for the management of primary small and medium vessel vasculitis, *Ann Rheum Dis* 68:310–317, 2009.

133. Mukhtyar C, Hellmich B, Bacon P, et al: Outcomes from studies of antineutrophil cytoplasm antibody associated vasculitis: a systematic review by the European League Against Rheumatism systemic vasculitis task force, *Ann Rheum Dis* 67:1004–1010, 2008.

135. de Groot K, Adu D, Savage COS: The value of pulse cyclophosphamide in ANCA-associated vasculitis: meta-analysis and critical review, *Nephrol Dial Transplant* 16:2018–2027, 2001.

136. de Groot K, Harper L, Jayne DR, et al: Pulse versus daily oral cyclophosphamide for induction of remission in antineutrophil cytoplasmic antibody-associated vasculitis: a randomized trial, *Ann Intern Med* 150:670–680, 2009.

137. Jones RB, Tervaert JW, Hauser T, et al: Rituximab versus cyclophosphamide in ANCA-associated renal vasculitis, *N Engl J Med* 363:211–220, 2010.

138. Stone JH, Merkel PA, Spiera R, et al: Rituximab versus cyclophosphamide for ANCA-associated vasculitis, *N Engl J Med* 363:221–232, 2010.

139. Jones RB, Ferraro AJ, Chaudhry AN, et al: A multicenter survey of rituximab therapy for refractory antineutrophil cytoplasmic antibody-associated vasculitis, *Arthritis Rheum* 60:2156–2168, 2009.

140. De Groot K, Rasmussen N, Bacon PA, et al: Randomized trial of cyclophosphamide versus methotrexate for induction of remission in early systemic antineutrophil cytoplasmic antibody-associated vasculitis, *Arthritis Rheum* 52:2461–2469, 2005.

141. Hu W, Liu C, Xie H, et al: Mycophenolate mofetil versus cyclophosphamide for inducing remission of ANCA vasculitis with moderate renal involvement, *Nephrol Dial Transplant* 23:1307–1312, 2008.

142. Jayne DRW, Rasmussen N, Andrassy K, et al: A randomized trial of maintenance therapy for vasculitis associated with antineutrophil cytoplasmic autoantibodies, *N Engl J Med* 349:36–44, 2003.

144. Pagnoux C, Mahr A, Hamidou MA, et al: Azathioprine or methotrexate maintenance for ANCA-associated vasculitis, *N Engl J Med* 359:2790–2803, 2008.

147. Hiemstra TF, Walsh M, Mahr A, et al: Mycophenolate mofetil vs azathioprine for remission maintenance in antineutrophil cytoplasmic antibody-associated vasculitis: a randomized controlled trial, *JAMA* 304:2381–2388, 2010.

149. Lapraik C, Watts R, Bacon P, et al: BSR and BHPR guidelines for the management of adults with ANCA associated vasculitis, *Rheumatology (Oxford)* 46:1615–1616, 2007.

150. Jayne DRW, Gaskin G, Rasmussen N, et al: Randomised trial of plasma exchange or high dose methyl prednisolone as adjunctive therapy for severe renal vasculitis, *J Am Soc Nephrol* 18:2180–2188, 2007.

151. Klemmer PJ, Chalermskulrat W, Reif MS, et al: Plasmapheresis therapy for diffuse alveolar hemorrhage in patients with small-vessel vasculitis, *Am J Kidney Dis* 42:1149–1153, 2003.

152. Schmitt WH, Hagen EC, Neumann I, et al: Treatment of refractory Wegener's granulomatosis with antithymocyte globulin (ATG): an open study in 15 patients, *Kidney Int* 65:1440–1448, 2004.

153. Flossmann O, Baslund B, Bruchfeld A, et al: Deoxyspergualin in relapsing and refractory Wegener's granulomatosis, *Ann Rheum Dis* 68:1125–1130, 2009.

154. Walsh M, Chaudhry A: Long-term follow-up of relapsing/refractory anti-neutrophil cytoplasm antibody associated vasculitis treated with the lymphocyte depleting antibody alemtuzumab (CAMPATH-1H), *Ann Rheum Dis* 67:1322–1327, 2008.

155. Jayne DRW, Chapel H, Adu D, et al: Intravenous immunoglobulin for ANCA-associated systemic vasculitis with persistent disease activity, *Q J Med* 93:433–439, 2000.

156. Martinez V, Cohen P, Pagnoux C, et al: Intravenous immunoglobulins for relapses of systemic vasculitides associated with antineutrophil cytoplasmic autoantibodies: results of a multicenter, prospective, open-label study of twenty-two patients, *Arthritis Rheum* 58:308–317, 2008.

158. Ribi C, Cohen P, Pagnoux C, et al: Treatment of Churg-Strauss syndrome without poor-prognosis factors: a multicenter, prospective, randomized, open-label study of seventy-two patients, *Arthritis Rheum* 58:586–594, 2008.

162. Little MA, Nightingale P, Verburgh CA, et al: Early mortality in systemic vasculitis: relative contribution of adverse events and active vasculitis, *Ann Rheum Dis* 69:1036–1043, 2010.

166. Dooley MA, Nair R: Therapy insight: preserving fertility in cyclophosphamide-treated patients with rheumatic disease, *Nat Clin Pract Rheumatol* 4:250–257, 2008.

172. Weidner S, Geuss S, Hafezi-Rachti S, et al: ANCA-associated vasculitis with renal involvement: an outcome analysis, *Nephrol Dial Transplant* 19:1403–1411, 2004.

174. Faurschou M, Sorensen IJ, Mellemkjaer L, et al: Malignancies in Wegener's granulomatosis: incidence and relation to cyclophosphamide therapy in a cohort of 293 patients, *J Rheumatol* 35:100–105, 2008.

176. Westman KW, Bygren PG, Olsson H, et al: Relapse rate, renal survival, and cancer morbidity in patients with Wegener's granulomatosis or microscopic polyangiitis with renal involvement, *J Am Soc Nephrol* 9:842–852, 1998.

177. Hogan SL, Falk RJ, Chin H, et al: Predictors of relapse and treatment resistance in antineutrophil cytoplasmic antibody-associated small-vessel vasculitis, *Ann Intern Med* 143:621–631, 2005.

178. Koldingsnes W, Nossent JC: Baseline features and initial treatment as predictors of remission and relapse in Wegener's granulomatosis, *J Rheumatol* 30:80–88, 2003.

179. Pierrot-Deseilligny Despujol C, Pouchot J, Pagnoux C, et al: Predictors at diagnosis of a first Wegener's granulomatosis relapse after obtaining complete remission, *Rheumatology (Oxford)* 49:2181–2190, 2011.

182. McKinney EF, Lyons PA, Carr EJ, et al: A CD8+ T cell transcription signature predicts prognosis in autoimmune disease, *Nat Med* 16:586–591, 2010.

Full references for this chapter can be found on www.expertconsult.com.

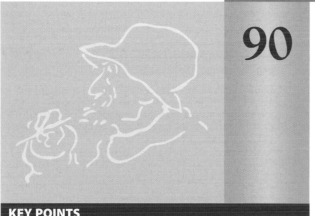

90

Polyarteritis Nodosa and Related Disorders

RAASHID LUQMANI

KEY POINTS

Polyarteritis nodosa (PAN), characterized by vasculitis of medium-sized arteries with few or no immune deposits, is relatively rare, especially in comparison with patients with microscopic polyangiitis or granulomatosis with polyangiitis.

One form of PAN is caused by hepatitis B virus and usually responds well to antiviral therapy, plasma exchange, and/or glucocorticoids.

Non–hepatitis B–associated PAN should be treated aggressively with cyclophosphamide and glucocorticoids, using the same approach as for systemic small vessel vasculitis.

The true incidence and prevalence of nonhepatitis PAN is around 1 per million per annum.

A significant reduction in the incidence of PAN has occurred due to a decreasing incidence of hepatitis B infection.

Presenting features of PAN include insidious onset of weight loss, purpuric skin lesions together with mononeuritis multiplex, and symptoms of mesenteric ischemia.

Glomerular renal disease is absent in PAN and should prompt consideration of other diagnoses.

Hematuria with renal impairment is rare but can occur in the presence of renal infarction.

There is much confusion regarding the term "cutaneous PAN," which in some cases may represent a subset of patients with early PAN; in others it is a distinct condition.

Buerger's disease, thromboangiitis obliterans, affects both sexes and involves the upper and lower extremities.

The role of tobacco use in Buerger's disease is clearly established but not understood.

Rare forms of vasculitis are described, but the evidence base for treatment is limited.

POLYARTERITIS NODOSA

Definition and Classification

The term *periarteritis nodosa* was originally introduced in 1866 and subsequently used to describe any form of systemic vasculitis.[1] The term has been modified to polyarteritis nodosa (PAN), and the definition has been improved to consist of "necrotizing inflammation of medium-sized or small arteries without glomerulonephritis or vasculitis in arterioles, capillaries, or venules."[2]

The American College of Rheumatology (ACR) criteria, which can be used to classify patients as having PAN, in order to distinguish them from patients with other forms of primary systemic vasculitis, do not differentiate between PAN and microscopic polyangiitis (MPA); both conditions are included under the umbrella of PAN. Three of 10 criteria (listed in Table 90-1) are required.[3]

The sensitivity of the ACR criteria for PAN (or MPA) is 82.2%, with a specificity of 86.6% when used to classify the disease.[3] Definitions of vasculitis (including PAN) were published in 1994 by the Chapel Hill Consensus Conference (CHCC).[2] Microscopic polyangiitis, granulomatosis with polyangiitis (GPA) (formerly Wegener's granulomatosis), and Churg-Strauss syndrome were distinguished from PAN on the basis of the pathologic findings of small vessel involvement in the former three diseases; by contrast, small vessel involvement is absent in PAN.

There has been, and still is, much confusion in the terms used to describe patients with different forms of vasculitis. It is worth considering this for a moment because, on reviewing patients who have previously been given the label of "PAN," the clinical features at presentation might actually suggest another form of vasculitis, typically MPA or GPA. In an attempt to rationalize the naming of different forms of vasculitis, the European Medicines Agency (EMEA) produced an algorithm to assist in the classification of patients with systemic small and medium vessel primary systemic vasculitis.[4] A decision tree approach was used, effectively putting PAN at the bottom of the tree.[4] In other words, patients were assigned to any other form of vasculitis, and only as a last resort, if no other diagnosis was made, the term *PAN* was applied. Perhaps this might seem a rather negative view of the condition, but because of the overuse of the term PAN in preference to others in the past, the true incidence and prevalence of PAN are actually low.

The EMEA algorithm is particularly useful because MPA is a more common condition than PAN but is absent from the ACR classification criteria (it is considered part of PAN), whereas in the CHCC definition PAN and MPA are treated as separate entities. There are important differences between PAN and MPA in terms of pathogenesis, organ involvement, tendency to relapse, and prognosis.[5] In the CHCC definition PAN is a medium vessel disease; by comparison, MPA is predominantly a small vessel disease that includes glomerulonephritis and pulmonary capillaritis.[2]

Patients are assessed using the EMEA algorithm if they have a clinical diagnosis of an antineutrophil cytoplasm antibody (ANCA)-associated vasculitis or PAN. In the algorithm, PAN is regarded as a diagnosis of exclusion. The first part of the algorithm is to determine whether the patient fulfills the Lanham[6] or ACR criteria[7] for Churg-Strauss syndrome (CSS). If they do, they are classified as having CSS. If not, the next step is to determine whether

Table 90-1 American College of Rheumatology Criteria for Classification of Polyarteritis Nodosa (and Microscopic Polyangiitis)

Weight loss ≥4 kg
Livedo reticularis
Testicular pain or tenderness
Myalgias, weakness, or leg tenderness
Mononeuropathy or polyneuropathy
Diastolic blood pressure >90 mm Hg
Elevated blood urea nitrogen or creatinine
Hepatitis B virus
Arteriographic abnormality
Biopsy of small or medium-sized artery containing polymorphonuclear neutrophils

From Lightfoot RW, Michel BA, Bloch DA, et al: The American College of Rheumatology 1990 criteria for the classification of polyarteritis nodosa, *Arthritis Rheum* 33:1088–1093, 1990.

they fulfill the ACR criteria or CHCC definition for GPA[2,8] either by direct evidence with histology or with appropriate surrogate markers and a positive ANCA. If they fulfill these requirements, they are classified as having GPA. If not, they proceed down the algorithm to see whether they fulfill a definition of MPA.[2] This is either by histology showing small vessel vasculitis or glomerulonephritis and no surrogate markers for GPA or with surrogate markers of glomerulonephritis and a positive ANCA. Only when CSS, GPA, and MPA are excluded is a diagnosis of PAN possible in this schema. To fulfill the definition of PAN in this algorithm, there must be histology or angiographic features consistent with the diagnosis. Any remaining patients are determined to be unclassifiable. The initial validation of the algorithm made use of paper cases assessed by a number of experts in vasculitis. In fact, every case was assigned to one of the conditions, without the need to describe any case as unclassifiable. This may not reflect clinical practice, where some patients appear to have an overlap between different forms of vasculitis or incomplete forms of a vasculitis. This is an important issue and has started to be addressed by a recent task force on classification and diagnostic tests in vasculitis.[9]

The French Vasculitis Study Group proposed a set of predictive items (Table 90-2) to be used as diagnostic criteria.[10] The items were derived from 949 patients with known

Table 90-2 Predictive Variables for Classification of Polyarteritis Nodosa (PAN)

Variable	Positive Prediction for PAN	Negative Prediction for PAN
Positive hepatitis B serology	+	
Arteriographic abnormalities	+	
Mononeuropathy or polyneuropathy	+	
Positive antineutrophil cytoplasm antibody		+
Asthma		+
Ear, nose, or throat signs		+
Glomerulopathy		+
Cryoglobulinemia		+

Modified from Henegar C, Pagnoux C, Puéchal X, et al: A paradigm of diagnostic criteria for polyarteritis nodosa: analysis of a series of 949 patients with vasculitides, *Arthritis Rheum* 58(5):1528–1538, 2008.

vasculitis (including 262 described as having PAN) and not from undifferentiated patients, and therefore they are actually another form of classification criteria.

The combination of nonspecific constitutional symptoms and ischemic symptoms in one or more organ systems should alert the physician to the possibility of a systemic vasculitis. PAN typically presents with nonspecific symptoms such as fever, weight loss, and myalgia in combination with single or multiorgan manifestations resulting from ischemia or infarction. The commonest organ manifestation is neurologic with mononeuritis multiplex, followed by skin lesions, abdominal pain from mesenteric ischemia, and renal infarction. Testicular pain due to ischemic orchitis is a classic feature of PAN but is rare at presentation. Some patients may present with an acute surgical abdomen due to bowel, liver, spleen, or pancreatic infarction. Myocardial infarction, ischemic cardiomyopathy, optic ischemia, and ischemic complications of the female genital tract are possible but unusual.

Epidemiology

The epidemiology of PAN has changed over time. Effective hepatitis B virus (HBV) immunization programs, improved blood screening for HBV, and major changes in definition and classification of vasculitis have resulted in a substantial reduction in incidence of PAN. Before the CHCC definition in 1994, MPA was included in the incidence and prevalence estimates. The impact of this is highlighted in a study comparing the incidence of PAN in three European regions: 4.4 to 9.7 per million by the ACR criteria versus 0 to 0.9 per million with the CHCC definition.[11]

The incidence of PAN is 2 to 9 per million in Europe and the United States by ACR criteria.[12] A higher incidence of 16 per million (by CHCC definition) is reported in Kuwait[13] and 77 per million described in an Alaskan population endemic for HBV, although it was based on only 13 actual cases of HBV PAN (in a study performed before ACR criteria or CHCC definitions).[14] The prevalence of PAN by ACR criteria is 31 to 33 per million in Western Europe[15-17]; 2 to 9 per million in Germany by CHCC definition.[18] A small study from Australia assessed the incidence and prevalence of different sorts of vasculitis between 1995 and 2005 in one area, suggesting a fall in the incidence of PAN from 2.3 per million per annum to 1.1 per million per annum.[19] A study from 2009 assessed the incidence and survival of patients with different forms of vasculitis and estimated the incidence of PAN to be 0.9 (between 0 and 1.7) per million per annum. This compares with an almost 10-fold difference in incidence of GPA and MPA (between 9.8 and 10.1 per million per annum).[20]

PAN can occur at any age, but the commonest age range at diagnosis is 40 to 60 years. There is no clear gender difference.[17] In a multiethnic population from France, patients with European ancestry had a higher prevalence of PAN compared with those without.[16]

Etiology and Pathogenesis

PAN is often related to infection with hepatitis B.[21] The incidence of HBV-related PAN follows HBV infection rates, previously accounting for 7% to 38.5% of patients diagnosed with PAN.[16,22] The prevalence of HBV-related PAN has reduced in recent years as a result of vaccination for HBV and improved screening of blood products.[16,23] PAN develops in 1% to 5% of patients with HBV infection,[14] which confers an approximately 1000-fold increase in risk compared with the background population.[12] By contrast, in Alaska, an area endemic for HBV, there is a substantial increased annual incidence of HBV PAN (77 per million), primarily due to vertical transmission.[14] Documented exposure to HBV occurs from blood products, intravenous drug use, and sexual contact. Screening of blood products for HBV and mass vaccination against the virus has successfully reduced the incidence of HBV PAN, as shown in French patients with the proportion of PAN due to HBV falling from 38.5% in the 1970s to 17.4% by the period 1997-2002.[24]

In HBV-related PAN the postulated mechanism of vasculitis includes direct vessel injury by replicating virus or deposition of immune complexes. Deposition of immune complexes leads to activation of the complement cascade, resulting in an inflammatory response and subsequent endothelial damage. The vasculitis typically occurs within the first few months following HBV infection and may be the first presenting feature of this infection. Evidence for the pathogenic nature of HBV and immune complexes is supported by the effectiveness of a treatment strategy to eradicate HBV with antiviral therapy and removal of immune complexes by plasmapheresis without the need for long-term immunosuppression.[24,25]

Saadoun and colleagues[26] described 31 patients who had hepatitis C virus (HCV)-associated vasculitis, which they classified as PAN according to ACR criteria and CHCC definitions. This cohort, representing approximately one-fifth of their HCV vasculitis patients, had more frequent fever, weight loss, severe hypertension, gastrointestinal tract involvement, severe acute sensory-motor multifocal mononeuropathy, kidney and liver microaneurysms, and increased C-reactive protein compared with other HCV vasculitis patients. By contrast, their response to therapy was more successful.

In the remainder of patients with PAN, the etiology is unknown. Genetic, infectious, and environmental agents are thought to be important, but there is no conclusive evidence.[11] The fact that idiopathic PAN responds to immunosuppressive therapy suggests an immunologic mechanism. In idiopathic PAN the role of immune complexes is unclear. There is evidence of endothelial dysfunction, an increase in inflammatory cytokines, and an increase in expression of adhesion molecules. There is a propensity for the inflammatory lesions to occur at the sites of bifurcation in vessels, where there is most likely to be turbulent flow. Following the inciting event, there is focal and segmental necrotizing inflammation of medium- and small-sized arteries. This leads to intimal proliferation with subsequent thrombosis, resulting in ischemia or infarction of the organ or tissue supplied by these arteries.

There are case reports describing the development of PAN in patients with pre-existing hairy cell leukemia.[27,28] Most cases had undergone splenectomy before the development of PAN. Potential mechanisms for the association between hairy cell leukemia and PAN include cross-reactivity of antibodies between the tumor cells and the endothelium, direct damage of the endothelium by tumor cells, and local production of proinflammatory cytokines triggering vessel wall damage.[28]

Pathologic Features

Due to the protean manifestations of the disease, a number of different sites can be biopsied. Sampling should be directed by the pattern of clinical involvement suggested by the history or physical examination. Muscle, peripheral nerves, kidney, testis and rectum, when involved, provide the best yield. Skin involvement and a positive skin biopsy do not always indicate evidence of systemic involvement[29-31] (see section on cutaneous PAN).

A biopsy of a medium-sized artery will show "focal and segmental" transmural necrotizing inflammation[30,31] (Figure 90-1). If there are any clinical or laboratory features indicating involvement of small vessels, further assessment should be undertaken because it suggests an alternative form of vasculitis such as MPA.[32]

Inflammatory change at the bifurcation of vessels is reported to be common. The coexistence of different stages of inflammation and scarring, as well as normal vessel wall, is typical in PAN. Areas of acute inflammation will usually have a pleomorphic cellular infiltrate of lymphocytes, neutrophils, macrophages, and eosinophils. Aneurysms can occur at the site of active lesions, and this morphologic appearance is what led to the term "nodosa" (Figure 90-2). Proliferative scarring in other areas may lead to vessel narrowing.[30-33]

Clinical Features

PAN can present at any age, but it typically occurs in the age range of 40 to 60. There is no significant gender difference. The diagnosis can be difficult to make because individual features can occur in a variety of other diseases. Table

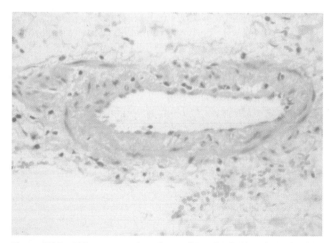

Figure 90-1 This cross-section of a medium-sized artery demonstrates transmural inflammation with infiltrating lymphocytes typical of polyarteritis nodosa. The lesion is at an early stage, before occlusion of the whole vessel or weakness of the vessel wall leading to aneurysm formation.

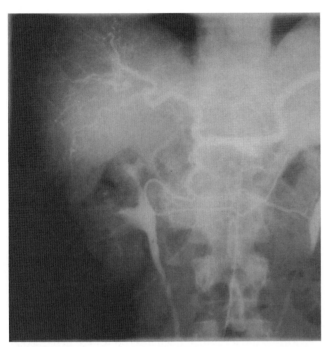

Figure 90-2 This celiac axis angiogram from a patient with polyarteritis nodosa demonstrates an irregular vascular pattern with small aneurysms in the hepatic vessels.

90-3 summarizes the clinical findings in PAN. The presence of nonspecific constitutional symptoms such as fever, weight loss, joint and muscle pains (found in 65% to 80% of cases of PAN), and ischemic symptoms in one or more organ system should raise the possibility of a systemic vasculitis.[17,24] Organ-specific manifestations may be present at the onset of disease, or there may be a more low-grade course, resulting in the development of specific organ involvement months to years later. Involvement of organs may be in isolation or as multisystem disease. In a Swedish series, the most common manifestations occurred at disease onset: nervous system (55%), skin (44%), abdominal (33%), and renal (11%).[17] A review of 348 patients diagnosed as having PAN since the 1960s[34] suggested that their mean age of diagnosis was 51 and the most frequent symptoms were generalized features in more than 90% of cases, neurologic features in 79%, skin involvement in 50%, abdominal involvement in 36%, hypertension in 35%, renal artery microaneurysms in 66%, and histologically proven PAN in 70%. The subset of 123 patients with hepatitis B–associated PAN was more likely to suffer peripheral neuropathy, abdominal pain, cardiomyopathy, orchitis, and hypertension compared with 225 non-HBV PAN patients. The relapse rate was 22% over a follow-up of 6 years (28% for non–HBV-related PAN compared with 11% for HBV PAN). The mortality rate was 25% overall (20% for

Table 90-3 Organ Involvement in Polyarteritis Nodosa (PAN)

System	Comment	Frequency	Reference
Constitutional	Fever and weight loss (current and previous)	>90%	34
Musculoskeletal	Arthritis, arthralgia, myalgia, or weakness; when muscle is involved, it provides a useful site for biopsy	24%-80%	17,24
Skin	Purpura, nodules, livedo reticularis, ulcers, bullous or vesicular eruptions, and segmental skin edema	44%-50%	17,34-36
Cardiovascular	Cardiac ischemia, cardiomyopathy, hypertension	35%	24,30,34
Ear, nose, and throat	No involvement. Nasal crusting, sinusitis, and hearing loss suggest an alternative diagnosis such as granulomatosis with polyangiitis	None	
Respiratory	Lung involvement not seen in PAN; abnormal respiratory findings suggest alternative diagnosis	None	
Abdominal	Pain is an early feature of mesenteric artery involvement. Progressive involvement may cause bowel, liver, or splenic infarction; bowel perforation; or bleeding from a ruptured arterial aneurysm. Less common presentations include appendicitis, pancreatitis, or cholecystitis as a result of ischemia or infarction The presence of abdominal tenderness or peritonitis and blood loss on rectal examination should be assessed	33%-36%	17,34
Renal	Vasculitis involving the renal arteries is present in many cases but does not commonly give rise to clinical features. It can present with renal impairment, renal infarcts, or rupture of renal arterial aneurysms. Glomerular ischemia may result in mild proteinuria or hematuria, but red cell casts are absent because glomerular inflammation is not a feature. If there is evidence of glomerular inflammation, then an alternative diagnosis such as microscopic polyangiitis or granulomatosis with polyangiitis must be considered. Hypertension is a manifestation of renal ischemia causing activation of the renin-angiotensin system	11%-66%	17,34
Nervous system	Mononeuritis multiplex, with sensory symptoms preceding motor deficits. Central nervous system involvement is a less frequent finding and can present with encephalopathy, seizures, and stroke	55%-79%	17,34
Ocular	Visual impairment, retinal hemorrhage, and optic ischemia	Rare	24,30
Other	Breast or uterine involvement is rare; testicular pain from ischemic orchitis is a characteristic feature, albeit an uncommon presentation	Rare	37,38

non-HBV PAN compared with 34% in HBV-PAN). Five-year relapse-free survival was higher in patients with HBV-related PAN (67% compared with 59%). The conclusion was that non-HBV PAN in particular had a high mortality, especially involving the elderly, and was worse in those patients with skin manifestations.

Clinical Assessment of Patients

In patients where vasculitis is suspected, a thorough history and physical examination is necessary to identify the potential organ systems involved. Use of the Birmingham Vasculitis Activity Score as a checklist of important features of the disease is recommended[39] to guide further targeted investigation and to be used subsequently in devising a management plan for treatment. Table 90-3 lists the typical features to be assessed in suspected PAN.

Laboratory Testing

No specific laboratory tests are available to diagnose PAN, but some may be useful to support the diagnosis, identify organs that may be affected, and rule out alternative diagnoses (Table 90-4).

Radiology

The angiogram is the imaging modality of choice, but increasingly it is being replaced by less invasive, safer techniques. The classic findings are multiple small aneurysms, vessel ectasia, and focal occlusive lesions in medium-sized vessels, typically in the renal and mesenteric arteries. The reported sensitivity of angiography is as high as 89% and specificity 90% when performed in individuals suspected of having vasculitis.[40] Magnetic resonance (MR) or computed tomography (CT) angiography are less invasive alternatives to conventional angiography but are much less sensitive in demonstrating microaneurysms.[41] They do have the advantage of being able to demonstrate areas of renal infarction and other potential pathology. In the setting of high suspicion of PAN and normal CT or MR angiography, it is still necessary to proceed to conventional angiography. Doppler ultrasound can identify renal and hepatic aneurysms related to PAN.[42] A plain chest radiograph may be useful for excluding other diseases such as other vasculitides that may affect the lungs and also to exclude infection.

Polyarteritis Nodosa in Children

Pediatric cases of polyarteritis are also well described. In a review of 110 patients, with a mean age of 9 (male-to-female ratio equal), one-third were classified as having cutaneous PAN. Only 5% had classic PAN associated with hepatitis B surface antigen, whereas 80% were described as having MPA associated with ANCA and 57% had systemic PAN.[43]

Microscopic Polyangiitis versus Polyarteritis Nodosa

A comparison of patients with PAN and MPA showed a difference in the skin manifestations of the 162 patients

---

Table 90-4 Investigations for Patients with Suspected Polyarteritis Nodosa (PAN)

Test	Supports Diagnosis of PAN	Supports an Alternative Diagnosis	Comment
Elevated C-reactive protein	+		Supports the presence of systemic inflammation
Elevated sedimentation rate	+		Supports the presence of systemic inflammation
Elevated serum creatinine	+/–	+/–	Raised serum creatinine, typically without hematuria or proteinuria on urinalysis, may indicate renal ischemia or infarction. Significant proteinuria or hematuria (especially red cell casts) would suggest glomerular disease, which is *not* a feature of PAN
Abnormal liver function tests	+		May suggest hepatitis, either from HBV or as a result of ischemic hepatitis from PAN affecting the hepatic arteries
Positive HBV serology	+		Seen in HBV PAN
Anemia	+		Due to chronic inflammation or from gastrointestinal blood loss
Positive ANCA		+	A positive ANCA would suggest an alternative type of vasculitis such as granulomatosis with polyangiitis or MPA
Elevated creatine kinase	+/–	+/–	Normal or mildly elevated, despite any muscle involvement
Blood cultures		+	To exclude endocarditis or other infective mimic of vasculitis
Positive HCV serology and cryoglobulins		+	HCV associated with a skin limited manifestation of PAN, but typically it is associated with a small vessel vasculitis related to cryoglobulinemia
Positive rheumatoid factor and ACPA		+	To rule out rheumatoid arthritis, especially in the context of a patient presenting predominantly with arthritis
Positive ANA and anti-dsDNA		+	In patients with clinical features consistent with SLE or other connective tissue disease
HIV positive		+	

ACPA, anticitrullinated protein antibody; ANA, antinuclear antibody; ANCA, antineutrophil cytoplasm antibody; dsDNA, double-stranded deoxyribonucleic acid; ESR, erythrocyte sedimentation rate; HBV, hepatitis B virus; HCV, hepatitis C virus; HIV, human immunodeficiency virus; MPA, microscopic polyangiitis; SLE, systemic lupus erythematosus.

with MPA and 248 with PAN.[44] There was a greater frequency of purpura (26%) in MPA compared with only 19% in PAN. By contrast, urticaria was more common in PAN (6% vs. 1.2%). The presence or absence of HBV infection–influenced skin manifestations were less common (only 30%) in HBV-positive patients compared with HBV-negative patients (54%). Histologic examination of the skin, however, was identical in patients with either MPA or PAN. (See Chapter 89 for more details on MPA.)

Cutaneous Polyarteritis Nodosa

The term *cutaneous* PAN usually implies a separate entity from PAN that is limited to the skin, but there is some uncertainty as to whether these are actually just early cases of PAN and whether progression to PAN will occur. Cutaneous PAN is defined as a skin-limited form of PAN that is usually considered a separate clinical entity to systemic PAN. Pathologically the findings on skin biopsy are indistinguishable between the two.[31] In a retrospective review of cutaneous PAN patients from a Japanese group, 22 patients with histologically proven cutaneous vasculitis were followed: 32% had a peripheral neuropathy, and 27% had myalgia, suggesting a need to revise the current criteria to differentiate between the two entities of cutaneous PAN and PAN. It was suggested that the two conditions were indeed separate, but cutaneous PAN is not confined to the skin.[45] HCV infection has been associated with cutaneous PAN in one retrospective study of 16 patients, in which 5 individuals were found to have HCV infection.[46]

Hepatitis B Virus Polyarteritis Nodosa

Hepatitis B vasculitis occurs in individuals with chronic hepatitis B antigenemia, most of whom have active liver disease.[21] The manifestations vary considerably, from diffuse small vessel vasculitis predominantly in the skin to larger vessel lesions typical of PAN. Clinical symptoms may include the entire spectrum of vasculitic manifestations, from purpura and other rashes to abdominal pain, hypertension, renal disease, and stroke. HBV-associated PAN is an increasingly rare condition as a result of better immunization programs against hepatitis B. A cohort of 115 patients with PAN was reviewed on the basis of inclusion into studies between 1972 and 2002.[24] Treatment of hepatitis B–related PAN with steroids plus an antiviral agent plus plasmapheresis resulted in 81% of patients achieving remission and a subsequent 10% relapse rate. However, 36% did subsequently die. Seroconversion of hepatitis B antibody status was associated with complete remission and

no relapse. In patients who were ANCA negative, the major cause of death was gut involvement. Plasmapheresis achieved not only a control of disease in combination with steroids and antiviral therapy but facilitated seroconversion to prevent secondary long-term complications from HBV infections such as liver involvement.

Non–Hepatitis B Virus Polyarteritis Nodosa

The French Vasculitis Study Group has combined data on PAN and microscopic polyangiitis focusing more on the severity of disease manifestations rather than the type of disease in their studies of treatment or outcome. For example, Ribi and colleagues[50] described the outcome of 124 patients with a new diagnosis of either PAN or MPA in whom the outcome was likely to be good (based on a lack of poor prognostic factors as measured by the Five Factor Score). All patients were treated with corticosteroids only followed by either azathioprine or cyclophosphamide if they relapsed. Ninety-eight of these patients achieved remission with steroids alone, but 46 of these patients relapsed. Primary treatment with steroids failed to control the disease in 26 patients, and 49 of the original 124 patients required additional immunosuppression. Similar rates of improvement were documented by using either azathioprine or cyclophosphamide. Therefore despite the absence of poor prognostic factors, only around 50% of patients could be managed with corticosteroids alone. A study of plasma exchange in 62 patients with a mixture of Churg-Strauss syndrome and what was described as PAN suggested that there was no clinical benefit from adding plasma exchange to standard treatment with pulse intermittent high-dose cyclophosphamide and steroid. This study from the mid-1990s describes patients with "PAN," but most of these patients probably had MPA.[51] Table 90-5 lists treatment regimens for non-HBV PAN that are based on the European League Against Rheumatism guidelines on management of small and medium vessel vasculitis.[52]

Treatment of Polyarteritis Nodosa

Uncontrolled vasculitis accounts for 58% to 73% of deaths occurring within the first year of diagnosis.[47-49] Management of non-HBV PAN should be appropriate to the severity of the disease as defined by the five-factor prognostic score and includes aggressive immunosuppression with corticosteroids and cyclophosphamide in patients with Five Factor Score values of at least one.[49] Patients with HBV-related PAN should be treated with high-dose corticosteroids followed by combination plasma exchange and antiviral agents to

Table 90-5 Pulsed Cyclophosphamide and Methylprednisolone for Non–Hepatitis B Virus Polyarteritis Nodosa

Phase	Drug	Dose	Route	Frequency	Duration
Induction	Cyclophosphamide	15 mg/kg per pulse	IV	Every 2 wk × 3, then every 3 wk ×3-6	3-6 mo
Induction	Methylprednisolone	10 mg/kg	IV	Every 2 wk x 3, then every 3 wk x3-6	
Maintenance	Azathioprine	2 mg/kg/day	Oral	Daily	18-24 mo
Maintenance	Prednisone	7.5 mg/day	Oral	Daily	18-24 mo

Modified from Mukhtyar C, Guillevin L, Cid MC, et al: EULAR recommendations for management of primary small and medium vessel vasculitis, *Ann Rheum Dis* 68:310–317, 2009.

reduce early mortality from vasculitis and late mortality from the consequences of chronic hepatitis.[24]

Outcome

Earlier diagnosis and initiation of treatment has improved outcomes. In non-HBV PAN the 7-year survival rate is 79%, compared with a 5-year survival rate of 72.5% in HBV-related PAN. This is similar to the rates in vasculitis associated with ANCAs.[53] The relapse rate in HBV-related PAN is low (<10%) compared with non–HBV-related PAN (19.4% to 57% relapse rates).[24,49] Delayed diagnosis (>3 months) increases the risk of relapse but does not affect mortality risk.[54] Seroconversion rates from hepatitis B e-antigen positive to hepatitis B e-antibody positive (i.e., eradication of active viral infection) is achieved in just under 50% of patients treated with glucocorticoids, antiviral agents, plus limited plasmapheresis.[24]

A prognostic tool designed for use in PAN is effectively used to distinguish patients with higher or lower risk of poor outcome. This simple clinical score (the Five Factor Score), assessed at diagnosis, consists of assessment of the following abnormalities: proteinuria (<1 g/day), elevated creatinine (>1.58 mg/dL), gastrointestinal involvement, central nervous system involvement, and cardiomyopathy.[55] Allocating 1 point per item, there is a reduced survival for patients with higher scores (86% survival for 0 points, 69% survival for 1 point, 47% survival for 2 or more points) at onset when followed up for 6 years.[55] Mortality can also be predicted using the Birmingham Vasculitis Activity Score, a clinical index of disease activity.[39,49] Older age at diagnosis has been shown to be an important adverse predictor of survival in the first year and after 5 years of follow-up.[47,56]

COGAN'S SYNDROME

Cogan's syndrome[57] is a rare form of vasculitis. The median age at onset is 25 years.[58,59] Patients typically present with red painful eyes and/or hearing loss concurrently or within 4 months in 75% of patients. Most patients do not develop features of more widespread systemic vasculitis, with the exception of aortitis and aneurysm or aortic insufficiency, occurring in about 12% of patients.[60] In atypical Cogan's syndrome, where the ocular manifestation is episcleritis, scleritis, iritis, uveitis, or chorioretinitis rather than interstitial keratitis, there is a worse prognosis and a higher frequency of aortic and other systemic manifestations.[61] Eye symptoms usually consist of photophobia with red and irritable eyes. The audiovestibular symptoms are rapid in onset with partial or complete hearing loss (often bilateral), vertigo, and ataxia. Although the vertigo and ataxia may improve, the hearing loss is usually permanent. About 50% of cases will have constitutional features such as weight loss, fever, lymphadenopathy, hepatosplenomegaly, and purpura. Aortic involvement is the most serious manifestation of Cogan's syndrome and accounts for most deaths. Ophthalmic and audiovestibular features may precede aortic involvement by months to several years. Rarely, patients develop widespread vasculitis, with purpura and gangrene.[62]

Pathology

A mixture of acute and chronic inflammation is present in large blood vessels, especially around the internal elastic lamina. The main findings are an infiltration of neutrophils, eosinophils, mononuclear cells, and fibrosis. Occasionally granulomas containing giant cells can be found in the lesions.

Clinical Features

The diagnosis of Cogan's syndrome is largely based on clinical features, supported by the histologic abnormalities and exclusion of other conditions. Definitive serologic markers do not exist. Most patients have leukocytosis, anemia, thrombocytosis, and an elevated sedimentation rate during active phases of their disease. Patients with aortitis show aortic root dilation and aortic insufficiency on echocardiography or magnetic resonance imaging. Rare case reports demonstrate the presence of autoantibodies such as antiendothelial cell antibodies[63] and anti-myeloperoxidase (MPO) antibodies,[64] but their role in the disease is unknown.

Treatment

There is no clear evidence base because there are no prospective studies of treatment in this rare disease. Interstitial keratitis usually responds to topical corticosteroids. Most experts manage the acute audiovestibular symptoms with high doses of glucocorticoids, with a prompt response within a month (or none at all in resistant cases). Cytotoxic drugs,[65] methotrexate,[66] and cyclosporine[67] have been used to treat the condition. The course is variable: For some patients there is only a single episode, and they are free of active disease thereafter. The more typical course is one of waxing and waning symptoms for months or years. Most patients sustain permanent hearing loss, and almost half lose hearing entirely; by contrast, few have permanent effects on vision.[60] Cochlear implantation can successfully restore some hearing in these patients. Aortic valve replacement and surgical repair of aortic aneurysms may be required, but as in Takayasu's arteritis,[68] it would probably be best to ensure that there is no active disease at the time of surgery.

BUERGER'S DISEASE

Buerger's disease, also known as *thromboangiitis obliterans*, is an inflammatory vaso-occlusive disease that predominantly affects the vascular supply to the lower limbs in young adult male tobacco smokers, although women and older adults[69] can also be affected. The average age at onset is 35 years. Tobacco, especially cigarette smoking, is clearly important, but the mechanism of action remains unknown. There is no clear human leukocyte antigen association.[70] Antibodies directed against collagen, elastin, and laminin have been reported in some patients.[71,72] The presence of high levels of antiendothelial cell antibodies has been described in patients with active disease, but not in patients in remission.[73] ANCAs directed against MPO, lactoferrin, and elastase have also been associated with severe cases.[74] More recently a link to periodontal disease and anticardiolipin antibody has been reported.[75]

Pathology

In most cases Buerger's disease affects small arteries and veins in the distal extremities, but there are case reports of visceral arterial involvement including coronary, pulmonary, and mesenteric arteries. There is a transmural infiltration of polymorphonuclear leukocytes and lymphocytes with preservation of the internal elastic lamina.[76] Thrombosis is prominent, and microabscesses can be found in the vessel wall and surrounding tissue. The infiltrating cells are enriched in CD3+ T cells; CD68+ macrophages and dendritic cells have been reported to be increased during disease activity.[77]

Clinical Features

Buerger's disease typically begins with bilateral pain and ischemia in both lower extremities, although the upper extremities may be the site of initial symptoms. At first, the symptoms can be mild, with paresthesia or pain on exposure to cold. Most cases evolve rapidly, however, with increasing ischemic (claudicant) limb pain, digital cyanosis, splinter hemorrhages, and skin vesicles. Digital ulcers often occur, especially after minor trauma.[78] The disease typically begins distally, with symptoms worse in the tips of the toes (and fingers), but it progresses to larger, more proximal vessels over several years. Usually Buerger's disease does not cause proximal leg claudication. Superficial phlebitis occurs in about one-third of patients and may be the first symptom. Typical angiographic changes include multiple bilateral areas of narrowing or occlusion in the digital, palmar, plantar, ulnar, radial, tibial, and peroneal arteries. Small collateral vessels around the occlusion can appear to be corkscrew shaped. More proximal lesions resemble atherosclerotic occlusion. Although these findings are typical, none are pathognomonic; in the absence of pathologic confirmation, the differential diagnosis includes premature atherosclerosis; hyperviscosity syndrome; scleroderma and other rheumatic diseases; Takayasu's arteritis; embolic disease including cholesterol emboli and atrial myxomas; ergot toxicity; and thoracic outlet syndrome.

Treatment

The most important treatment is to stop smoking. In patients who are unable to comply with this, nicotine substitutes may be used at least in the short term.[79]

Affected limbs must be protected from trauma and cold. Ulcers and cellulitis often require antibiotics and local wound management. Anecdotal use of calcium channel blockers and pentoxifylline reportedly has been beneficial in some, but not all, patients. Sympathectomy seems to provide little or no long-term benefit and is not usually recommended.[80] Intravenous prostacyclin is effective and superior to aspirin[81] and also superior to lumbar sympathectomy for rest pain or ischemic ulcers[80] on the basis of two large randomized controlled trials. Recent approaches using bone marrow–derived mesenchymal stem cells, basic fibroblast growth factor, and granulocyte colony-stimulating factor have been effective in treatment of leg ulcers and ischemia in small open-label studies.[82-85] A radical surgical approach using omental grafting is reported in large open-label surgical studies to offer more than 90% success in improving the severe ischemic complications.[86]

In patients who continue to smoke, about half require amputation, often multiple times as more proximal vessels are involved.[87] If they stop smoking, most patients will stop getting worse, but a few still require amputation. However, the ischemic limb may be a source of pain and ulceration for many years.

SUSAC'S SYNDROME

This is another rare condition affecting a wide age range from children to older adults.[88,89] The etiology is unknown. The presentation is usually with sudden onset of sensorineural hearing loss in the context of encephalopathy and branch retinal artery occlusion.[88] The differential diagnosis would include Cogan's syndrome and GPA. The pathogenetic mechanisms suggest an endotheliopathy rather than a true vasculitis. Nevertheless, treatment with immunosuppressive agents including glucocorticoids and cytotoxic agents is reported to improve some patients, but there are no controlled trials.[89] The diagnosis rests on the combination of clinical features and exclusion of other causes. The outcome is variable, but most patients recover some hearing.[90]

VIRUS-INDUCED VASCULITIS

The most common virus-associated vasculitis today is HCV-associated cryoglobulinemia (see Chapter 91). The majority of patients with cryoglobulinemia have concomitant hepatitis C infection (see Chapter 91). Treatment with immunosuppressive drugs has been only moderately successful; many patients die as a result of vasculitis or liver disease. Saadoun and colleagues[26] describe their cohort of 72 patients treated with combination antiviral therapy. Patients responded well to a combination of interferon-α and ribavirin; however, 40% required glucocorticoids, around 12% had plasmapheresis, and 6% received immunosuppressive drugs for severe complications. The mortality was just over 10%. The vasculitis resulting from human immunodeficiency virus infection is discussed in Chapter 113. Although the most common rheumatic manifestation of parvovirus B19 infection is arthritis (see Chapter 114), some children with chronic parvovirus B19 infection have been reported to develop a vasculitis similar to PAN. It is not clear, given the high incidence of the infection in children, whether the presence of the virus is coincidental or causative in the few cases of vasculitis described.[91]

References

1. Kussmaul A, Maier R: Uber eine bisher nicht beschriebene eigenthumliche arterier krankung (periarteritis nodosa), die mit morbus brightii und rapid fortschreitender allgemeiner muskellahmung einhergeht, *Deutsches Arch Klin Med* 1:484–517, 1866.
2. Jennette JC, Falk RJ, Andrassy K, et al: Nomenclature of systemic vasculitides. Proposal of an international consensus conference, *Arthritis Rheum* 37(2):187–192, 1994.

3. Lightfoot RW, Michel BA, Bloch DA, et al: The American College of Rheumatology 1990 criteria for the classification of polyarteritis nodosa, *Arthritis Rheum* 33:1088, 1990.

4. Watts R, Lane S, Hanslik T, et al: Development and validation of a consensus methodology for the classification of the ANCA-associated vasculitides and polyarteritis nodosa for epidemiological studies, *Ann Rheum Dis* 66(2):222–227, 2007.

5. Lhote F, Cohen P, Guillevin L: Polyarteritis nodosa, microscopic polyangiitis and Churg-Strauss syndrome, *Lupus* 7:238–258, 1998.

6. Lanham JG, Elkon KB, Pusey CD, et al: Systemic vasculitis with asthma and eosinophilia: a clinical approach to the Churg-Strauss syndrome, *Medicine (Baltimore)* 63:65–81, 1984.

7. Masi AT, Hunder GG, Lie JT, et al: The American College of Rheumatology 1990 criteria for the classification of Churg-Strauss syndrome (allergic granulomatosis and angiitis), *Arthritis Rheum* 33:1094–1100, 1990.

8. Leavitt RY, Fauci AS, Bloch DA, et al: The American College of Rheumatology 1990 criteria for the classification of Wegener's granulomatosis, *Arthritis Rheum* 33(8):1101–1107, 1990.

9. Basu N, Watts R, Bajema I, et al: EULAR points to consider in the development of classification and diagnostic criteria in systemic vasculitis, *Ann Rheum Dis* 69:1744–1750, 2010.

10. Henegar C, Pagnoux C, Puéchal X, et al: A paradigm of diagnostic criteria for polyarteritis nodosa: analysis of a series of 949 patients with vasculitides, *Arthritis Rheum* 58(5):1528–1538, 2008.

11. Watts RA, Lane SE, Scott DG, et al: Epidemiology of vasculitis in Europe, *Ann Rheum Dis* 60:1156–1157, 2001.

12. Watts RA, Scott DG: Epidemiology of vasculitis. In Bridges L, Ball G, editors: *Vasculitis,* Oxford, UK, 2008, Oxford University Press, pp 7–22.

13. el-Reshaid K, Kapoor MM, el-Reshaid W, et al: The spectrum of renal disease associated with microscopic polyangiitis and classic polyarteritis nodosa in Kuwait, *Nephrol Dial Transplant* 12:1874–1882, 1997.

14. McMahon BJ, Heyward WL, Templin DW, et al: Hepatitis B–associated polyarteritis nodosa in Alaskan Eskimos: clinical and epidemiologic features and long-term follow-up, *Hepatology* 9:97–101, 1989.

15. Koldingsnes W, Nossent H: Epidemiology of Wegener's granulomatosis in northern Norway, *Arthritis Rheum* 3:2481–2487, 2000.

16. Mahr A, Guillevin L, Poissonnet M, et al: Prevalences of polyarteritis nodosa, microscopic polyangiitis, Wegener's granulomatosis, and Churg-Strauss syndrome in a French urban multiethnic population in 2000: a capture-recapture estimate, *Arthritis Rheum* 51:92–99, 2004.

17. Mohammad AJ, Jacobsson LT, Mahr AD, et al: Prevalence of Wegener's granulomatosis, microscopic polyangiitis, polyarteritis nodosa and Churg-Strauss syndrome within a defined population in southern Sweden, *Rheumatology (Oxford)* 46:1329–1337, 2007.

18. Reinhold-Keller E, Zeidler A, Gutfleisch J, et al: Giant cell arteritis is more prevalent in urban than in rural populations: results of an epidemiological study of primary systemic vasculitides in Germany, *Rheumatology (Oxford)* 39:1396–1402, 2000.

19. Ormerod AS, Cook MC: Epidemiology of primary systemic vasculitis in the Australian Capital Territory and south-eastern New South Wales, *Intern Med J* 38(11):816–823, 2008.

20. Mohammad AJ, Jacobsson LT, Westman KW, et al: Incidence and survival rates in Wegener's granulomatosis, microscopic polyangiitis, Churg-Strauss syndrome and polyarteritis nodosa, *Rheumatology (Oxford)* 48(12):1560–1565, 2009.

21. Gocke DJ, Hsu K, Morgan C, et al: Association between polyarteritis nodosa and Australia antigen, *Lancet* 2:1149–1153, 1970.

22. Guillevin L, Lhote F, Cohen P, et al: Polyarteritis nodosa related to hepatitis B virus: a prospective study with long-term observation of 41 patients, *Medicine (Baltimore)* 74:238–253, 1995.

23. Pagnoux C, Cohen P, Guillevin L: Vasculitides secondary to infections, *Clin Exp Rheumatol* 24(2 Suppl 41):S71–S81, 2006.

24. Guillevin L, Mahr A, Callard P, et al: Hepatitis B virus-associated polyarteritis nodosa: clinical characteristics, outcome, and impact of treatment in 115 patients, *Medicine (Baltimore)* 84:313–322, 2005.

25. Guillevin L, Lhote F, Leon A, et al: Treatment of polyarteritis nodosa related to hepatitis B virus with short term steroid therapy associated with antiviral agents and plasma exchanges. A prospective trial in 33 patients, *J Rheumatol* 20(2):289–298, 1993.

26. Saadoun D, Resche-Rigon M, Thibault V, et al: Antiviral therapy for hepatitis C virus–associated mixed cryoglobulinemia vasculitis: a long-term followup study, *Arthritis Rheum* 54(11):3696–3706, 2006.

27. Wooten MD, Jasin HE: Vasculitis and lymphoproliferative diseases, *Semin Arthritis Rheum* 26:564–574, 1996.

28. Hasler P, Kistler H, Gerber H: Vasculitides in hairy cell leukemia, *Semin Arthritis Rheum* 25:134–142, 1995.

29. Morgan AJ, Schwartz RA: Cutaneous polyarteritis nodosa: a comprehensive review, *Int J Dermatol* 49(7):750–756, 2010.

30. Colmegna I, Maldonado-Cocco JA: Polyarteritis nodosa revisited, *Curr Rheumatol Rep* 7:288–296, 2005.

31. Lie JT: Illustrated histopathologic classification criteria for selected vasculitis syndromes. American College of Rheumatology Subcommittee on Classification of Vasculitis, *Arthritis Rheum* 33:1074–1087, 1990.

32. Jennette JC, Falk RJ: The role of pathology in the diagnosis of systemic vasculitis, *Clin Exp Rheumatol* 25(1 Suppl 44):S52–S56, 2007.

33. Stone JH: Polyarteritis nodosa, *JAMA* 288:1632–1639, 2002.

34. Pagnoux C, Seror R, Henegar C, et al: Clinical features and outcomes in 348 patients with polyarteritis nodosa: a systematic retrospective study of patients diagnosed between 1963 and 2005 and entered into the French Vasculitis Study Group Database, *Arthritis Rheum* 62(2):616–626, 2010.

35. Gibson LE: Cutaneous vasculitis update, *Dermatol Clin* 19:603–615, 2001.

36. Gibson LE, Su WP: Cutaneous vasculitis, *Rheum Dis Clin North Am* 21:1097–1113, 1995.

37. Ng WF, Chow LT, Lam PW: Localized polyarteritis nodosa of breast—report of two cases and a review of the literature, *Histopathology* 23:535–539, 1993.

38. Teichman JM, Mattrey RF, Demby AM, et al: Polyarteritis nodosa presenting as acute orchitis: a case report and review of the literature, *J Urol* 149:1139–1140, 1993.

39. Luqmani RA, Bacon PA, Moots RJ, et al: Birmingham vasculitis activity score (BVAS) in systemic necrotizing vasculitis, *Q J Med* 87:671–678, 1994.

40. Hekali P, Kajander H, Pajari R, et al: Diagnostic significance of angiographically observed visceral aneurysms with regard to polyarteritis nodosa, *Acta Radiol* 32:143–148, 1991.

41. Ozaki K, Miyayama S, Ushiogi Y, et al: Renal involvement of polyarteritis nodosa: CT and MR findings, *Abdom Imaging* 34:265–270, 2009.

42. Ozcakar ZB, Yalcinkaya F, Fitoz S, et al: Polyarteritis nodosa: successful diagnostic imaging utilizing pulsed and color Doppler ultrasonography and computed tomography angiography, *Eur J Pediatr* 165:120–123, 2006.

43. Ozen S, Anton J, Arisoy N, et al: Juvenile polyarteritis: results of a multicenter survey of 110 children, *J Pediatr* 145(4):517–522, 2004.

44. Kluger N, Pagnoux C, Guillevin L, et al: Comparison of cutaneous manifestations in systemic polyarteritis nodosa and microscopic polyangiitis, *Br J Dermatol* 159(3):615–620, 2008.

45. Nakamura T, Kanazawa N, Ikeda T, et al: Cutaneous polyarteritis nodosa: revisiting its definition and diagnostic criteria, *Arch Dermatol Res* 301(1):117–121, 2009.

46. Soufir N, Descamps V, Crickx B, et al: Hepatitis C virus infection in cutaneous polyarteritis nodosa: a retrospective study of 16 cases, *Arch Dermatol* 135:1001–1002, 1999.

47. Bourgarit A, Le Toumelin P, Pagnoux C, et al: Deaths occurring during the first year after treatment onset for polyarteritis nodosa, microscopic polyangiitis, and Churg-Strauss syndrome: a retrospective analysis of causes and factors predictive of mortality based on 595 patients, *Medicine (Baltimore)* 84:323–330, 2005.

48. Cohen RD, Conn DL, Ilstrup DM: Clinical features, prognosis, and response to treatment in polyarteritis, *Mayo Clin Proc* 55:146–155, 1980.

49. Gayraud M, Guillevin L, le Toumelin P, et al: Long-term followup of polyarteritis nodosa, microscopic polyangiitis, and Churg-Strauss syndrome: analysis of four prospective trials including 278 patients, *Arthritis Rheum* 44:666–675, 2001.

50. Ribi C, Cohen P, Pagnoux C, et al: Treatment of polyarteritis nodosa and microscopic polyangiitis without poor-prognosis factors: a prospective randomized study of one hundred twenty-four patients, *Arthritis Rheum* 62(4):1186–1197, 2010.

51. Guillevin L, Lhote F, Cohen P, et al: Corticosteroids plus pulse cyclophosphamide and plasma exchanges versus corticosteroids plus pulse cyclophosphamide alone in the treatment of polyarteritis nodosa and Churg-Strauss syndrome patients with factors predicting poor prognosis. A prospective, randomized trial in sixty-two patients, *Arthritis Rheum* 38(11):1638–1645, 1995.

52. Mukhtyar C, Guillevin L, Cid MC, et al: EULAR Recommendations for management of primary small & medium vessel vasculitis, *Ann Rheum Dis* 68:310–317, 2009.

53. Phillip R, Luqmani R: Mortality in systemic vasculitis: a systematic review, *Clin Exp Rheum* 26:S51, S94–104, 2008.
54. Agard C, Mouthon L, Mahr A, et al: Microscopic polyangiitis and polyarteritis nodosa: how and when do they start? *Arthritis Rheum* 49:709–715, 2003.
55. Guillevin L, Lhote F, Gayraud M, et al: Prognostic factors in polyarteritis nodosa and Churg-Strauss syndrome: a prospective study in 342 patients, *Medicine (Baltimore)* 75:17–28, 1996.
56. Guillevin L, Le Thi Huong D, Godeau P, et al: Clinical findings and prognosis of polyarteritis nodosa and Churg-Strauss angiitis: a study in 165 patients, *Br J Rheumatol* 27:258–264, 1988.
57. Cogan DG: Syndrome of nonsyphilitic interstitial keratitis and vestibuloauditory symptoms, *Arch Ophthalmol* 33:144–149, 1945.
58. Vollertsen RS, McDonald TJ, Younge BR, et al: Cogan's syndrome: 18 cases and a review of the literature, *Mayo Clin Proc* 61:344–361, 1986.
59. Haynes BF, Kaiser-Kupfer MI, Mason P, et al: Cogan syndrome: studies in thirteen patients, long-term follow-up, and a review of the literature, *Medicine (Baltimore)* 59:426–441, 1980.
60. Gluth MB, Baratz KH, Matteson EL, Driscoll CL: Cogan syndrome: a retrospective review of 60 patients throughout a half century, *Mayo Clin Proc* 81(4):483–488, 2006.
61. Grasland A, Pouchot J, Hachulla E, et al: Typical and atypical Cogan's syndrome: 32 cases and review of the literature, *Rheumatology (Oxford)* 43(8):1007–1015, 2004.
62. Vollertsen RS: Vasculitis and Cogan's syndrome, *Rheum Dis Clin North Am* 16:433–439, 1990.
63. Ottaviani F, Cadoni G, Marinelli L, et al: Anti-endothelial cell autoantibodies in patients with sudden hearing loss, *Laryngoscope* 109:1084–1087, 1999.
64. Yamanishi Y, Ishioka S, Takeda M, et al: Atypical Cogan's syndrome associated with antineutrophil cytoplasmic antibodies, *Br J Rheumatol* 35:601–603, 1996.
65. Van Doornum S, McColl G, Walter M, et al: Prolonged prodrome, systemic vasculitis, and deafness in Cogan's syndrome, *Ann Rheum Dis* 60:69–71, 2001.
66. Richardson B: Methotrexate therapy for hearing loss in Cogan's syndrome, *Arthritis Rheum* 37:1559–1561, 1994.
67. Hammer M, Witte T, Mugge A, et al: Complicated Cogan's syndrome with aortic insufficiency and coronary stenosis, *J Rheumatol* 21:552–555, 1994.
68. Mukhtyar C, Guillevin L, Cid MC, et al: EULAR Recommendations for the management of large vessel vasculitis, *Ann Rheum Dis* 68:318–323, 2009.
69. Olin JW, Young JR, Graor RA, et al: The changing clinical spectrum of thromboangiitis obliterans (Buerger's disease), *Circulation* 82(5 Suppl):IV3–8, 1990.
70. Olin JW: Thromboangiitis obliterans, *Curr Opin Rheumatol* 6:44–49, 1994.
71. Adar R, Papa MZ, Halpern Z, et al: Cellular sensitivity to collagen in thromboangiitis obliterans, *N Engl J Med* 308:1113–1116, 1983.
72. Hada M, Sakihama T, Kamiya K, et al: Cellular and humoral immune responses to vascular components in thromboangiitis obliterans, *Angiology* 44:533–540, 1993.
73. Eichhorn J, Sima D, Lindschau C, et al: Antiendothelial cell antibodies in thromboangiitis obliterans, *Am J Med Sci* 315:17–23, 1998.
74. Halacheva KS, Manolova IM, Petkov DP, et al: Study of antineutrophil cytoplasmic antibodies in patients with thromboangiitis obliterans (Buerger's disease), *Scand J Immunol* 48:544–550, 1998.

75. Chen YW, Nagasawa T, Wara-Aswapati N, et al: Association between periodontitis and anti-cardiolipin antibodies in Buerger disease, *J Clin Periodontol* 36(10):830–835, 2009.
76. Lie JT: Diagnostic histopathology of major systemic and pulmonary vasculitic syndromes, *Rheum Dis Clin North Am* 16:269–292, 1990.
77. Kobayashi M, Ito M, Nakagawa A, et al: Immunohistochemical analysis of arterial cell wall infiltration in Buerger's disease (endarteritis obliterans), *J Vasc Surg* 29:451–458, 1999.
78. Joyce JW: Buerger's disease (thromboangiitis obliterans), *Rheum Dis Clin North Am* 16:463–470, 1990.
79. Kawallata H, Kanekura T, Gushi A, et al: Successful treatment of digital ulceration in Buerger's disease with nicotine chewing gum, *Br J Dermatol* 140:187–188, 1999.
80. Bozkurt AK, Köksal C, Demirbas MY, et al: A randomized trial of intravenous iloprost (a stable prostacyclin analogue) versus lumbar sympathectomy in the management of Buerger's disease, *Int Angiol* 25(2):162–168, 2006.
81. Fiessinger JN, Schäfer M: Trial of iloprost versus aspirin treatment for critical limb ischaemia of thromboangiitis obliterans. The TAO Study, *Lancet* 335(8689):555–557, 1990.
82. Matoba S, Tatsumi T, Murohara T, et al: Long-term clinical outcome after intramuscular implantation of bone marrow mononuclear cells (Therapeutic Angiogenesis by Cell Transplantation [TACT] trial) in patients with chronic limb ischemia, *Am Heart J* 156(5):1010–1018, 2008.
83. Dash NR, Dash SN, Routray P, et al: Targeting nonhealing ulcers of lower extremity in human through autologous bone marrow-derived mesenchymal stem cells, *Rejuvenation Res* 12(5):359–366, 2009.
84. Hashimoto T, Koyama H, Miyata T, et al: Selective and sustained delivery of basic fibroblast growth factor (bFGF) for treatment of peripheral arterial disease: results of a phase I trial, *Eur J Vasc Endovasc Surg* 38(1):71–75, 2009.
85. Kawamoto A, Katayama M, Handa N, et al: Intramuscular transplantation of G-CSF-mobilized CD34(+) cells in patients with critical limb ischemia: a phase I/IIa, multicenter, single-blinded, dose-escalation clinical trial, *Stem Cells* 27(11):2857–2864, 2009.
86. Agarwal VK: Long-term results of omental transplantation in chronic occlusive arterial disease (Buerger's disease), *Int Surg* 90(3):167–174, 2005.
87. Jiménez-Ruiz CA, Dale LC, Astray Mochales J, et al: Smoking characteristics and cessation in patients with thromboangiitis obliterans, *Monaldi Arch Chest Dis* 65(4):217–221, 2006.
88. Susac JO: Susac's syndrome: the triad of microangiopathy of the brain and retina with hearing loss in young women, *Neurology* 44(4):591–593, 1994.
89. Rennebohm R, Susac JO, Egan RA, Daroff RB: Susac's syndrome—update, *J Neurol Sci* 299:86–91, 2010.
90. Aubart-Cohen F, Klein I, Alexandra JF, et al: Long-term outcome in Susac syndrome, *Medicine (Baltimore)* 86(2):93–102, 2007.
91. Finkel TH, Torok TJ, Ferguson PJ, et al: Chronic parvovirus B19 infection and systemic necrotizing vasculitis: opportunistic infection or aetiological agent? *Lancet* 343:1255–1258, 1994.

The references for this chapter can also be found on www.expertconsult.com.

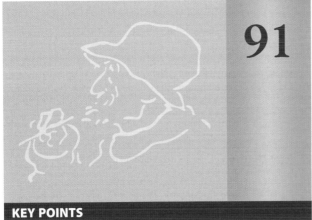

91

Immune Complex–Mediated Small Vessel Vasculitis

JOHN H. STONE

KEY POINTS

Vasculitis mediated by immune complexes (ICs) includes a heterogeneous group of disorders linked by inefficient or dysregulated clearance of ICs.

The most common types of IC-mediated vasculitis are hypersensitivity vasculitis, Henoch-Schönlein purpura (HSP), and mixed cryoglobulinemia. Rarer forms of this condition include hypocomplementemic urticarial vasculitis and erythema elevatum diutinum.

Connective tissue disorders such as systemic lupus erythematosus, Sjögren's syndrome, and rheumatoid arthritis can be associated with IC-mediated vasculitis.

Cutaneous involvement of small blood vessels is the most prominent feature in the majority of cases, but extracutaneous involvement occurs in some forms.

The classic cutaneous finding in small vessel vasculitis is palpable purpura, but a variety of other skin lesions may be found including pustules, vesicles, urticaria, and small ulcerations.

Direct immunofluorescence studies of involved blood vessels demonstrate characteristic types and patterns of immunoglobulin (Ig) and complement deposition.

Hypersensitivity vasculitis usually results from a reaction to a medication or an infection.

HSP is associated with purpura, arthritis, glomerulonephritis, and colicky abdominal pain. IgA deposition is found within blood vessel walls.

Cryoglobulinemic vasculitis is most often associated with long-standing hepatitis C virus infection. The term *mixed cryoglobulinemia* is sometimes used for this disorder because the immunoreactants involved in the disease include both IgG and IgM.

The inflammation within blood vessel walls that characterizes vasculitis frequently leads to cellular destruction, damage to the vascular structures, compromise of blood flow to organs, and organ dysfunction. It has been known for decades that immune complex (IC)–mediated mechanisms play critical roles in many forms of systemic vasculitis, particularly those that involve primarily small blood vessels. As described in Chapter 87, the use of horse serum and sulfonamides as therapeutic agents for infectious diseases in the early 1900s frequently led to small vessel vasculitis on the basis of serum sickness or hypersensitivity phenomena. *Hypersensitivity angiitis,* often confused with the pauci-immune form of vasculitis now termed *microscopic polyangiitis* (see Chapter 89),[1] was one of five disorders included in the original classification of the vasculitides in 1952.[2]

This chapter focuses on forms of small vessel vasculitis that are mediated by IC deposition. These disorders include hypersensitivity vasculitis, Henoch-Schönlein purpura (HSP), mixed cryoglobulinemia, hypocomplementemic urticarial vasculitis, and erythema elevatum diutinum. In addition, forms of vasculitis associated with connective tissue diseases, particularly systemic lupus erythematosus (SLE), Sjögren's syndrome, and rheumatoid vasculitis, are discussed briefly. Anti–glomerular basement membrane disease and the pauci-immune forms of vasculitis such as those associated with antineutrophil cytoplasmic antibodies, are discussed elsewhere (see Chapter 89). Throughout this chapter, the terms *vasculitis* and *angiitis* are used interchangeably when referring to inflammation involving small blood vessels (capillaries, venules, arterioles).

Because all forms of IC-mediated vasculitis share certain elements of pathogenesis, have many cutaneous findings in common, and have overlapping differential diagnoses, these aspects of the disorders are considered together. The epidemiology, cause, distinctive pathophysiologic mechanisms, unique clinical features, and approaches to treatment are discussed separately for each condition. Treatments are also summarized in Table 91-1.

PATHOGENESIS

Arthus Reaction

The Arthus reaction, described after the injection of horse serum into rabbits, forms the basis of our understanding of IC-mediated diseases.[3] The formation of ICs in the Arthus reaction initiates complement activation and an influx of inflammatory cells, followed by thrombus formation and hemorrhagic infarction in the areas of most intense inflammation. ICs, formed by the combination of antibody and antigen, are continuously created (and usually cleared swiftly and efficiently) by the reticuloendothelial system as a means of neutralizing foreign antigens. Under some circumstances, however, ICs escape clearance and become deposited within joints, blood vessels, and other tissues, inciting inflammation and causing disease. ICs deposited in the blood vessel walls lead to vasculitis. Similarly, those deposited within small blood vessels of the kidney—the glomeruli—cause glomerulonephritis.[4]

Immunogenicity

The fate of formed ICs is governed by several major factors including antigen load, antibody response, efficiency of the reticuloendothelial system, physical properties of the blood vessels (including flow dynamics and previous endothelial

Table 91-1 Potential Treatment Approaches for Different Forms of Immune Complex–Mediated Vasculitis

Disease	Preferred Treatment Approach
Hypersensitivity vasculitis	Removal of the offending agent
	Brief (2- to 4-wk) course of glucocorticoids for severe cases
Henoch-Schönlein purpura	No treatment required in the majority of cases, particularly children (symptomatic therapy only)
	Moderate glucocorticoid doses (prednisone 20-40 mg/day) are of variable utility but may be used empirically in patients with disabling symptoms
	Pulse glucocorticoids (e.g., 1 g methylprednisolone/day) employed with anecdotal success for refractory purpura when moderate glucocorticoid doses have failed
	Refractory glomerulonephritis may require high-dose glucocorticoids, azathioprine, mycophenolate mofetil, or cyclophosphamide
Cryoglobulinemia	Combined antiviral therapies and B cell depletion strategies synergistic in treating mixed cryoglobulinemia associated with hepatitis C
	Rituximab possibly effective in treating idiopathic mixed cryoglobulinemia
Hypocomplementemic urticarial vasculitis	Low-dose prednisone (5-20 mg/day), hydroxychloroquine, dapsone
	Higher doses of glucocorticoids in patients with serious internal organ involvement or ulcerative skin lesions
	Anecdotal reports of success with tumor necrosis factor inhibition
Erythema elevatum diutinum	Dapsone or sulfapyridine
Connective tissue disease	Hydroxychloroquine, low-dose prednisone (5-20 mg/day), azathioprine
Rheumatoid vasculitis	High-dose glucocorticoids plus cyclophosphamide for widespread necrotizing vasculitis
	Anecdotal experience suggests that tumor necrosis factor inhibition or rituximab might be effective in combination with glucocorticoids

damage), and solubility of the ICs themselves. The ratio of antibody to antigen determines the solubility of ICs. Large ICs, formed when antibody and antigen are present in approximately equal proportions, are identified and removed easily by the reticuloendothelial system. In contrast, small ICs are formed in conditions of antibody excess. Small ICs remain in the serum and do not elicit an immune response within tissues. However, when there is a slight antigen excess, ICs precipitate from the serum and become trapped within certain vascular beds. Following the deposition of ICs in tissue, a cascade of pathologic events ensues: complement fixation, neutrophil recruitment, local inflammation, lysosomal release, oxygen free radical generation, and tissue injury.

CUTANEOUS MANIFESTATIONS

Small blood vessels generally include capillaries, postcapillary venules, and nonmuscular arterioles—vessels that are typically less than 50 μm in diameter. These are found principally within the superficial papillary dermis (Figure 91-1). Medium-sized blood vessels, those between 50 and 150 μm in diameter, contain muscular walls and are located principally in the deep reticular dermis, near the junction of the dermis and subcutaneous tissues. Vessels larger than 150 μm in diameter are not commonly found in the skin.

Figure 91-1, which demonstrates the location and size of blood vessels involved in various types of cutaneous vasculitis, illustrates the types of blood vessels affected by several forms of IC-mediated disease. A blood vessel's size correlates closely with its depth in the skin layers: The larger the vessel, the deeper its location. Although telltale signs of vasculitis may be evident on inspection of the skin's surface, the epidermis is avascular. Therefore the pathologic findings in cutaneous vasculitides lie within the dermis and subcutaneous tissues.

Palpable purpura, synonymous with small vessel vasculitis, is the most common cutaneous finding in IC-mediated vasculitis (Figure 91-2). Purpuric lesions result from the extravasation of erythrocytes through damaged blood vessel walls into tissue. Many other skin manifestations are possible in these conditions including vesicles, pustules, urticaria, superficial ulcerations, nonpalpable lesions (macules and patches), and splinter hemorrhages (Figure 91-3). These lesions frequently occur in combination, and careful examination usually reveals a purpuric component. Purpuric lesions *do not blanch* when pressure is applied to the skin. Following resolution, purpuric lesions may leave postinflammatory hyperpigmentation, particularly if repeated bouts occur (see Figure 91-3F).

In IC-mediated vasculitis, purpuric lesions are usually distributed in a symmetric fashion over dependent regions of the body, particularly the lower legs, because of the increased hydrostatic pressure in these areas. Purpuric lesions are not always palpable to the touch, and the

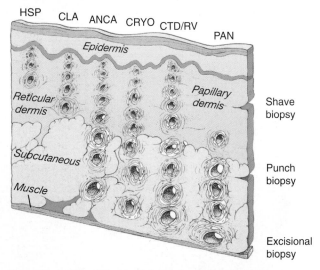

Figure 91-1 Size of the blood vessels involved in forms of cutaneous vasculitis. The types of vasculitis with an immune complex–mediated pathogenesis include Henoch-Schönlein purpura (HSP), cutaneous leukocytoclastic angiitis (CLA), mixed cryoglobulinemia (CRYO), and connective tissue disease/rheumatoid vasculitis (CTD/RV). ANCA, antineutrophil cytoplasmic antibody; PAN, polyarteritis nodosa.

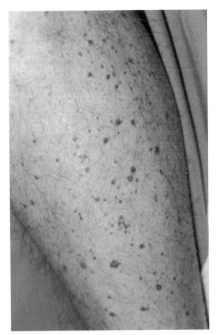

Figure 91-2 Hypersensitivity vasculitis. Palpable purpura in a patient with hypersensitivity vasculitis.

existence of palpable purpura does not necessarily imply an IC-mediated pathophysiology; pauci-immune forms of vasculitis such as granulomatosis with polyangiitis (GPA) (formerly Wegener's granulomatosis), microscopic polyangiitis, and Churg-Strauss syndrome, for example, may present with

identical skin findings (albeit distinctive histopathology; see Chapter 89).

PATHOLOGIC FEATURES

Full pathologic assessment of cutaneous vasculitis involves examination of a skin biopsy specimen by both light microscopy and direct immunofluorescence (DIF). DIF is a particularly critical procedure in the evaluation of small vessel vasculitides. DIF studies must be planned at the time the biopsy is performed because they require a fresh skin biopsy sample.

Light Microscopy

Figure 91-4A displays the light microscopy findings of cutaneous vasculitis. The optimal time for skin biopsy is 24 to 48 hours after the appearance of a lesion. Biopsies should be obtained from a nonulcerated site. For ulcerated lesions—usually more of an issue with medium vessel vasculitides—biopsies should be taken from the ulcer's edge. The cellular infiltrates in cutaneous vasculitis are usually made up of a combination of neutrophils and lymphocytes, but most cases demonstrate a predominance of one cell type or the other. Lymphocyte-rich infiltrates may be seen in specimens taken from either new (<12 hours) or old (>48 hours) lesions, regardless of the underlying type of vasculitis. Even in connective tissue disorders such as Sjögren's syndrome, the typical finding is a leukocytoclastic vasculitis rather than a lymphocytic vasculitis.[5]

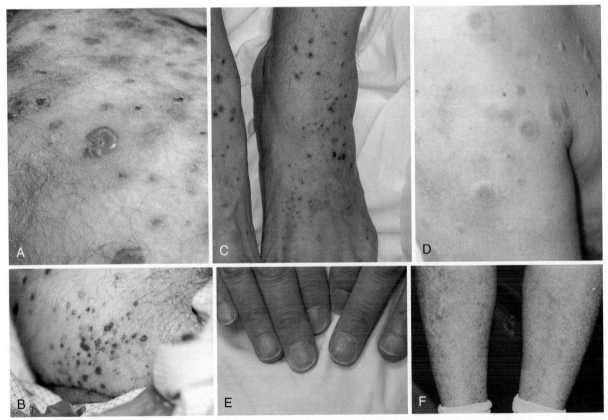

Figure 91-3 Cutaneous findings of immune complex–mediated small vessel vasculitis. **A,** Vesicles. **B,** Pustules. **C,** Superficial ulcerations. **D,** Urticaria. **E,** Splinter hemorrhages. **F,** Hyperpigmentation.

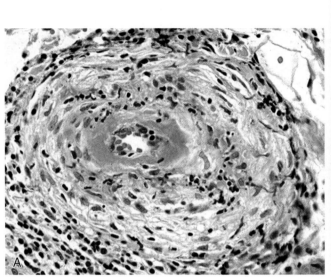

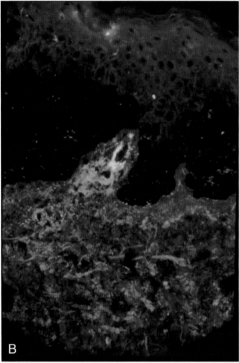

Figure 91-4 Skin biopsy findings in immune complex–mediated small vessel vasculitis. **A,** Light microscopy. **B,** Direct immunofluorescence demonstrating IgA deposits.

The essential histologic feature in any form of cutaneous vasculitis is the disruption of blood vessel architecture by an inflammatory infiltrate within and around the vessel walls. Endothelial swelling and proliferation, leukocytoclasis (degranulation of neutrophils, leading to the production of nuclear "dust"; see Figure 91-4), and extravasation of erythrocytes may be evident in the biopsy but are not essential to the diagnosis.

Direct Immunofluorescence

Although the diagnosis of cutaneous vasculitis rests on routine histology, the features revealed by hematoxylin and eosin stains do not distinguish between pauci-immune and IC-mediated disorders. DIF studies complement the histologic information, provide the only way of diagnosing HSP with certainty, and yield important clues regarding the nature of the underlying disease. The performance of *separate* biopsies for histologic and DIF analyses is recommended if sufficient lesions exist. With DIF studies, frozen sections are incubated with fluorescein-labeled anti–human immunoglobulin (Ig) G, IgM, IgA, and C3. The staining patterns of these immunoreactants may provide insight into not only the diagnosis but also the pathophysiology of certain conditions. Figure 91-4B displays the typical DIF findings in a skin lesion from a patient with IC-mediated vasculitis.

DIFFERENTIAL DIAGNOSIS

The differential diagnosis of IC-mediated small vessel vasculitis is shown in Table 91-2. There are three main groups of disorders in the differential diagnosis of IC-mediated small vessel vasculitis: other forms of IC-mediated disorders, forms of small vessel vasculitis that are not mediated through

ICs, and vasculitis mimickers that involve small blood vessels. A diagnostic algorithm that includes the critical laboratory and radiographic tests is shown in Figure 91-5.

CLINICAL SYNDROMES

Hypersensitivity Vasculitis (Cutaneous Leukocytoclastic Angiitis)

The term *hypersensitivity vasculitis* (see Chapter 87) generally refers to an IC-mediated small vessel vasculitis of the skin that spares internal organs and usually follows drug exposures or infections. The Chapel Hill consensus conference recommended eliminating the term *hypersensitivity vasculitis* in favor of *cutaneous leukocytoclastic angiitis* because of the disorder's usual confinement to the skin and its predominant cell type, the neutrophil.[1] However, *hypersensitivity vasculitis* remains firmly embedded in the medical literature. The disease is characterized pathologically by IC deposition in capillaries, postcapillary venules, and arterioles. A similar illness—serum sickness—is a systemic illness that includes rash and prominent arthralgias or arthritis; it occurs 1 to 2 weeks after exposure to a drug or foreign antigen.

In 1990 the American College of Rheumatology (ACR) performed a study designed to identify features that distinguished one form of vasculitis from others.[6] The resulting ACR classification criteria for hypersensitivity vasculitis are shown in Table 91-3.[7] The key historical element in evaluating a patient with possible hypersensitivity vasculitis is identifying exposures that may have triggered the reaction. However, in approximately half of all patients with presumed hypersensitivity vasculitis, no inciting agent can be identified.

Table 91-2 Differential Diagnosis of Immune Complex–Mediated Vasculitis

Immune Complex–Mediated Vasculitides

Hypersensitivity vasculitis
Henoch-Schönlein purpura
Mixed cryoglobulinemia
Urticarial vasculitis
Erythema elevatum diutinum
Connective tissue disease, rheumatoid vasculitis

Pauci-Immune Vasculitides

Granulomatosis with polyangiitis
Churg-Strauss syndrome
Microscopic polyangiitis

Miscellaneous Small Vessel Vasculitides

Behçet's disease
Malignancy associated
Infection
Inflammatory bowel disease

Vasculitis Mimickers

Hemorrhage
   Pigmented purpuric dermatoses
   Scurvy
   Immune thrombocytopenic purpura
Thrombosis
   Antiphospholipid syndrome
   Thrombotic thrombocytopenic purpura
   Livedoid vasculopathy (atrophie blanche)
   Warfarin-induced skin necrosis
   Purpura fulminans
   Disseminated intravascular coagulation
Embolism
   Cholesterol emboli
   Atrial myxomas
Vascular wall pathology
   Calciphylaxis
   Amyloidosis
Infection
   Infective endocarditis
   Leprosy (Lucio's phenomenon)

A long list of medications, infections, and other exposures may lead to the syndrome of hypersensitivity vasculitis. The typical history for a drug-induced hypersensitivity vasculitis is the occurrence of clinical symptoms approximately 7 to 14 days after starting a new medication. Although virtually any medication can be associated with the induction of a hypersensitivity vasculitis, antibiotics (particularly penicillins and cephalosporins) are the most common offenders. Other common culprits are diuretics and antihypertensive agents, but when confronted with a patient with a potential drug-induced vasculitis it is critical to examine and potentially discontinue any medication added within a recent timeframe. Drug-induced hypersensitivity vasculitides begin to resolve within days of removal of the offending agent.

Thorough efforts are also required to exclude disease in organs other than the skin, the finding of which would implicate another form of vasculitis (see Figure 91-5). For example, although hypersensitivity vasculitis can mimic the skin features of microscopic polyangiitis, it does not involve the kidneys, lungs, peripheral nerves, or other internal organs and is not associated with antineutrophil cytoplasmic antibodies.

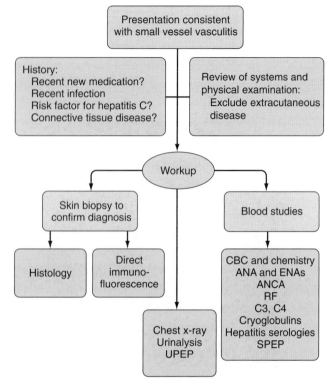

Figure 91-5 Diagnostic algorithm for immune complex–mediated small vessel vasculitis. The critical diagnostic test is usually a skin biopsy with hematoxylin and eosin staining and direct immunofluorescence. ANA, antinuclear antibody; ANCA, antineutrophil cytoplasmic antibody; CBC, complete blood count; ENA, extractable nuclear antigen; RF, rheumatoid factor; SPEP, serum protein electrophoresis; UPEP, urine protein electrophoresis.

Removal of the inciting agent is the most critical therapy for hypersensitivity vasculitis when the likely agent can be identified. In patients who have been exposed to multiple medications, determining the inciting agent may be difficult and may require the withdrawal of multiple agents simultaneously until the syndrome clears, typically in 1 to 2 weeks.

The prognosis for patients with hypersensitivity vasculitis depends on the inciting cause. Treatment with glucocorticoids is reserved for patients with extensive disease and can usually be discontinued within several weeks. Patients who experience repeated disease flares may need low-dose glucocorticoids to prevent recurrences.

Table 91-3 American College of Rheumatology 1990 Criteria* for the Classification of Hypersensitivity Vasculitis

Age >16 yr
Use of a possible offending medication in temporal relation to symptoms
Palpable purpura
Maculopapular rash
Biopsy of a skin lesion showing neutrophils around an arteriole or venule

*The presence of three or more criteria has a sensitivity of 71% and specificity of 84% for the diagnosis of hypersensitivity vasculitis.

From Calabrese LH, Michel BA, Bloch DA, et al: American College of Rheumatology 1990 criteria for the classification of hypersensitivity vasculitis, *Arthritis Rheum* 33:1108–1113, 1990.

Henoch-Schönlein Purpura

HSP is an IC-mediated form of small vessel vasculitis that is strongly associated with IgA deposition within blood vessel walls. Many cases of HSP occur after upper respiratory tract infections. Multiple bacterial, viral, and other infectious agents have been suggested as the cause of HSP, but the true cause remains unknown. The 1990 ACR criteria for the classification of HSP are shown in Table 91-4.[8]

A major risk factor for HSP (as well as IgA nephropathy, which has renal findings identical to those of HSP) is aberrant glycosylation of O-linked glycans in the hinge region of a fraction of IgA1 molecules.[9] Rather than terminating with galactose, the aberrant galactose-deficient O-glycans end with N-acetylgalactosamine (GalNAc) or sialylated GalNAc. The terminal GalNAc moiety on the aberrantly glycosylated IgA1 may in turn be recognized by antiglycan antibodies, leading to the formation of circulating immune complexes that deposit in the skin, joints, kidneys, and other organs. However, a high serum Gd-IgA1 level is not sufficient for the development of clinical symptoms. A "second hit" in the form of another environmental or inherited risk factor is required to produce HSP. This probably explains why multiple types of infections and many different drugs (e.g., antibiotics) have been linked etiologically with HSP.

The hallmarks of HSP include an upper respiratory tract infection followed by a syndrome characterized by a purpuric rash, arthralgias, abdominal pain, and renal disease. HSP is usually viewed as a disease of childhood, and the majority of cases affect children younger than 5 years. However, adults can also be affected by HSP and have a greater tendency toward a prolonged disease course (with recurrent bouts of purpura) than do children.[10] Colicky abdominal pain, presumably secondary to gastrointestinal vasculitis, is a common characteristic of HSP and frequently occurs within a week after the onset of rash. Sometimes the gastrointestinal symptoms of HSP precede the onset of purpura, leading to a diagnostic quandary and occasionally to exploratory surgery. Endoscopy may demonstrate purpura in the upper or lower intestinal tract. Mild glomerulonephritis is common and generally self-limited, although some patients develop end-stage renal disease.

In children with mild manifestations, the clinical history alone may be sufficient to confirm the diagnosis. In more serious cases (e.g., in the presence of renal involvement) or when there is sufficient doubt about the diagnosis, biopsy of an involved organ is essential. Unlike in other forms of

Table 91-4 American College of Rheumatology 1990 Criteria* for the Classification of Henoch-Schönlein Purpura

Palpable purpura
Age at onset <20 yr
Bowel angina
Vessel wall granulocytes on biopsy

*The presence of two criteria identified Henoch-Schönlein purpura with a sensitivity of 87% and a specificity of 88% in a group of individuals with forms of systemic vasculitis.

From Mills JA, Michel BA, Bloch DA, et al: The American College of Rheumatology 1990 criteria for the classification of Henoch-Schönlein purpura, *Arthritis Rheum* 33:1114–1121, 1990.

IC-mediated disease, however, DIF reveals florid IgA deposition. In the proper clinical setting, this finding is diagnostic of HSP. Other forms of small vessel vasculitis may have small quantities of IgA within blood vessels, but IgA is not the predominant immunoreactant in such cases.

In mild cases of HSP, no specific therapy is necessary. Even for patients with glomerulonephritis, it has been difficult to demonstrate that treatment with glucocorticoids or immunosuppressive agents significantly alters the outcome. Despite this, it is prudent to treat aggressive renal involvement with an immunosuppressive regimen including high-dose glucocorticoids and another immunosuppressive agent such as cyclophosphamide, azathioprine, or mycophenolate mofetil, depending on disease severity.

Recurrences of skin disease, often consisting of multiple episodes occurring over many months, are not unusual. However, even in patients with recurrent disease, the rule is for the disorder to subside and to resolve completely over a few months to a year. In a minority of patients, some evidence of permanent renal damage persists in the form of proteinuria and hematuria. Less than 5% of patients develop renal failure as a result of HSP.

Cryoglobulinemic Vasculitis

Cryoglobulins are immunoglobulins characterized by a tendency to precipitate from serum under conditions of cold.[11] Such proteins, detectable to a varying degree in a wide array of inflammatory conditions, do not always cause disease. In some patients, however, cryoglobulins bind to circulating antigen (e.g., portions of the hepatitis C virion), deposit in the walls of small and medium-sized blood vessels, and activate complement, leading to cryoglobulinemic vasculitis.

In contrast to most other forms of IC-mediated vasculitis, cryoglobulinemia tends to involve small- and medium-sized blood vessels. Thus the syndrome of cryoglobulinemic vasculitis can be associated with the development of large cutaneous ulcers, digital ischemia, and livedo racemosa—findings characteristic of disturbances in medium-sized vessels. The Chapel Hill Consensus Conference provided a consensus definition for mixed cryoglobulinemia (Table 91-5).[1]

Three major types of cryoglobulinemia are recognized, defined by the specific kinds of immunoglobulins with which they are associated (Table 91-6). Type I, characterized by a monoclonal gammopathy (generally IgG or IgM), differs substantially from types II and III in its clinical presentation and disease associations. Type I cryoglobulinemia, associated with Waldenström's macroglobulinemia or, less frequently, multiple myeloma, is more likely to cause syndromes related to hyperviscosity (dizziness, confusion, headache, and stroke) than necrotizing vasculitis. In contrast to the monoclonal nature of type I cryoglobulinemia, types II and III are known as *mixed cryoglobulinemias* because they are composed of both IgG and IgM. In type II cryoglobulinemia, more than 90% of cases are caused by hepatitis C infection and the cryoproteins consist of monoclonal IgM and polyclonal IgG. Cases of type II cryoglobulinemia not associated with hepatitis C are sometimes termed *mixed essential cryoglobulinemia* because their cause is not known. Type III cryoglobulinemia, typically associated with polyclonal IgG and polyclonal IgM, is associated with many

Table 91-5 Chapel Hill Consensus Conference Definitions of Immune Complex–Mediated Forms of Vasculitis

Disease	Definition
Cutaneous leukocytoclastic angiitis	Isolated cutaneous leukocytoclastic angiitis without systemic vasculitis or glomerulonephritis
Henoch-Schönlein purpura	Vasculitis with immunoglobulin A–dominant immune deposits, affecting small blood vessels (capillaries, venules, arterioles); typically involves skin, gut, and glomeruli and is associated with arthralgias or arthritis
Essential cryoglobulinemia	Vasculitis with cryoglobulin immune deposits, affecting small blood vessels (capillaries, venules, arterioles) and associated with cryoglobulins in serum; skin and glomeruli often involved

From Jennette JC, Falk RJ, Andrassy K, et al: Nomenclature of systemic vasculitides: proposal of an international consensus conference, *Arthritis Rheum* 37:187–192, 1994.

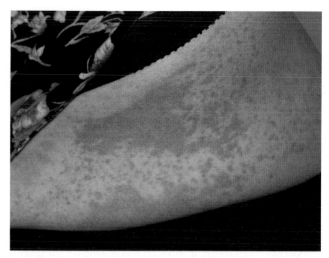

Figure 91-6 Confluent purpura in mixed cryoglobulinemia. Extensive purpuric lesions are often so numerous that they form confluent areas of cutaneous involvement.

forms of chronic inflammation including infection and autoimmune disease.

Type II and III cryoglobulinemias often present with a triad of signs and symptoms: purpura, arthralgias, and myalgias. The purpura may be extensive and confluent (Figure 91-6), sometimes involving the trunk, upper extremities, and even the face; in most cases, however, the rash is confined to the lower extremities. Other organ systems commonly involved in mixed cryoglobulinemia are the kidneys and peripheral nerves. Mixed cryoglobulinemia may cause membranoproliferative glomerulonephritis that resembles lupus nephritis histopathologically. It may also cause a vasculitic neuropathy, usually with sensory symptoms predominating over motor symptoms. Finally, in rare cases, cryoglobulinemia is associated with alveolar hemorrhage.

Skin biopsy is the most straightforward method of confirming the diagnosis. Light microscopy of purpuric lesions demonstrates leukocytoclastic vasculitis. In addition, DIF studies reveal various types of immunoglobulin and complement deposition, depending on the type. In type II cryoglobulinemia, for example, DIF reveals IgG and IgM deposition, as well as complement components. Serologic testing may also yield clues to the presence of mixed cryoglobulinemia. To assay for serum cryoglobulins, the blood is collected in a prewarmed apparatus, allowed to clot at 37° C before processing, and then refrigerated at 4° C for several days. The percentage of the serum occupied by the cryoprecipitate is referred to as the "cryocrit." The difficulties involved in performing cryoglobulin assays often lead to false-negative results. Nonspecific serologic testing may also implicate mixed cryoglobulinemia. As noted, cryoglobulins detected are not always associated with disease.

A strong clue is the presence of an extremely low level of C4, reduced out of proportion to C3. In addition, the monoclonal component of type II cryoglobulins almost invariably has rheumatoid factor activity (i.e., binds to the Fc portion of IgG). Thus essentially all patients with type II cryoglobulinemia have high titers of rheumatoid factor. As markers of clinical disease activity, C4 levels, rheumatoid factor titers, and cryocrits all fare poorly, often remaining abnormal in the face of clinically improved disease.

Treatment of cryoglobulinemia has seen substantial progress in recent years. Until recently, antiviral therapies with the combination of interferon-α and ribavirin were believed to be the optimal treatment for mixed cryoglobulinemia. Dual strategies that combine antiviral therapies and B cell depletion approaches with rituximab appear to be synergistic in treating this condition and leading to long-term treatment responses.[12] The rationale behind rituximab use in cryoglobulinemia is that peripheral B lymphocyte depletion will lead to a reduction in plasma cells that produce cryoglobulins. Studies of these treatment modalities have suggested that disease relapses are associated with the absence of virologic control and peripheral B cell recovery, implying

Table 91-6 Types of Cryoglobulins

Cryoglobulin	RF Positivity	Monoclonality	Associated Diseases
Type I	No	Yes (IgG or IgM)	Hematopoietic malignancy (multiple myeloma, Waldenström's macroglobulinemia)
Type II	Yes	Yes (polyclonal IgG, monoclonal IgM)	Hepatitis C Other infection Sjögren's syndrome SLE
Type III	Yes	No (polyclonal IgG and IgM)	Hepatitis C Other infection Sjögren's syndrome SLE

Ig, immunoglobulin; RF, rheumatoid factor; SLE, systemic lupus erythematosus.

the need to combine the two treatment strategies. The optimal timing of antiviral and B cell depletion strategies is not clear. However, one reasonable approach is to initiate antiviral strategies first and then to employ rituximab within several weeks. Patients who present with overwhelming illness such as the unusual patient with alveolar hemorrhage or with symptoms of hyperviscosity are candidates for plasma exchange, with the goal of removing the pathogenic immune complexes as quickly as possible. One approach is to perform plasma exchange every other day with concomitant immunosuppressive therapy or B cell depletion for a total of seven exchanges or until there is sufficient clinical improvement. The prognosis of patients with cryoglobulinemia generally depends on the underlying cause. The outcome of type I cryoglobulinemia relates closely to the success in treating the cause. Type II or III cryoglobulinemia secondary to hepatitis C can be treated effectively if the viral infection is responsive to therapy. If patients do not tolerate antiviral therapy well or if the treatment is ineffective, they may require low to moderate doses of prednisone to control the disease.

Hypocomplementemic Urticarial Vasculitis

In contrast to common urticaria, the lesions of urticarial vasculitis (UV) last more than 48 hours, do not blanch when pressure is applied to the skin, and may leave postinflammatory hyperpigmentation. Unlike common urticaria, the lesions of UV are frequently associated with moderate pain, burning, and tenderness in addition to pruritus. Whereas common urticaria typically resolves completely within 24 to 48 hours, the lesions of UV may take days to resolve completely, often leaving residual hyperpigmentation; they may worsen without therapy.

Three different syndromes of UV are recognized: normocomplementemic UV, hypocomplementemic UV, and the hypocomplementemic urticarial vasculitis syndrome (HUVS). Normocomplementemic UV is typically a self-limited subset of hypersensitivity vasculitis. In chronic cases, normocomplementemic UV must be distinguished carefully from neutrophilic urticaria, a persistent form of urticaria not associated with vasculitis. In contrast, hypocomplementemic UV is more likely to be a chronic disorder that has certain overlapping features with SLE: low serum complements, autoantibodies, and an interface dermatitis characterized by immunoreactant deposition (complement and immunoglobulins) at the dermal-epidermal junction in a pattern essentially identical to the lupus band test. Finally, HUVS is a severe form of the disease associated with extracutaneous disease and an array of organ system findings atypical of SLE.[13] For example, HUVS may be associated with uveitis, chronic obstructive pulmonary disease (COPD), and angioedema.

The skin lesions in UV tend to be centripetal, favoring the trunk and proximal extremities more than dependent regions. The lesions are painful and associated with a burning sensation rather than the pruritus of common urticaria. Biopsy of an urticarial wheal in UV demonstrates evidence of leukocytoclastic vasculitis including injury to the endothelial cells of the postcapillary venules, erythrocyte extravasation, leukocytoclasis, fibrin deposition, and a perivascular neutrophilic (or, less commonly, lymphocytic)

infiltrate. DIF demonstrates IC deposition around blood vessels in the superficial dermis and a striking deposition of immunoglobulins and complement along the dermal-epidermal junction. In the proper setting, these findings (interface dermatitis and immunoreactant deposition within blood vessels) are diagnostic of hypocomplementemic UV. HUVS, in contrast, is a clinical diagnosis based on the presence of UV and the occurrence of typical features in extracutaneous organ systems.

Some cases of hypocomplementemic UV respond to therapies commonly used for the treatment of SLE including low-dose prednisone, hydroxychloroquine, dapsone, or other immunomodulatory agents. Serious cases of HUVS, particularly those presenting with glomerulonephritis or other forms of serious organ involvement, may require high doses of glucocorticoids or biologic agents such as inhibitors of tumor necrosis factor. Both COPD and cardiac valve abnormalities are associated with HUVS and may require specific treatment as well.

The prognosis of UV is linked to the disorder with which it is associated. SLE, COPD, angioedema, and valvular abnormalities are all known to occur in association with this disorder and may strongly influence both quality and quantity of life.

Erythema Elevatum Diutinum

Erythema elevatum diutinum (EED) is a rare, distinctive form of leukocytoclastic vasculitis limited to the skin.[14] The disorder is distinctive because of the unusual distribution of skin lesions (found symmetrically over the extensor surfaces of joints) and the prompt response to sulfone medications. The cutaneous findings are typical of any small vessel vasculitis, with a predominance of papules, plaques, and nodules. Early lesions are often pink or yellowish and then become red or purple (Figure 91-7). The natural history of untreated lesions is to persist for years, becoming doughy or hard with time. The lesions have a predilection for the skin overlying the small joints of the hands and the knees; they can also affect the buttocks. The trunk is generally spared.

The principal histopathologic findings of EED are leukocytoclastic vasculitis with fibrinoid necrosis. Although an IC basis is suspected in this disorder, DIF studies are not distinctive. EED has been associated with various connective tissue diseases (CTDs), rheumatoid arthritis, other forms of vasculitis such as GPA, human immunodeficiency virus infections, and paraproteinemias (particularly IgA). EED typically responds promptly to dapsone or sulfapyridine, but chronic therapy may be required because skin lesions recur after cessation of treatment.

Connective Tissue Disease–Associated Vasculitis

Vasculitis rarely occurs in CTDs without overt manifestations of the underlying disorder. The forms of CTD typically complicated by vasculitis include those related to SLE: lupus itself, mixed CTD, Sjögren's syndrome, and overlap CTD. Although vasculitis clearly occurs in some CTD settings, it is commonly overdiagnosed to explain perplexing disease features in patients with known rheumatic illnesses. For example, neuropsychiatric SLE is generally not caused

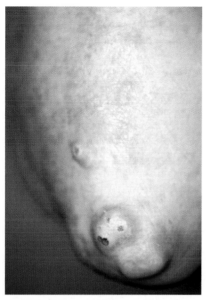

Figure 91-7 Erythema elevatum diutinum. Nodules typically form over the extensor surfaces of the knuckles and other joints.

by a true vasculitis but rather by other mechanisms that remain poorly defined. Whenever possible, the clinical hypothesis of vasculitis should be confirmed by biopsy.

Cutaneous vasculitis in CTDs is associated almost invariably with hypocomplementemia and high titers of antinuclear antibodies (ANAs). DIF examination of skin lesions shows granular IgG and C3 deposition in and around dermal vessels, with or without IgM, reflecting the contribution of ICs to disease pathogenesis. The phenomenon of the "in vivo ANA" is also observed in keratinocytes and dermal cells in DIF studies (Figure 91-8).

Vasculitis in patients with SLE-related disorders is more likely than other forms of vasculitis to be associated with a lymphocytic predominance. One variant of CTD-associated cutaneous vasculitis, the so-called benign

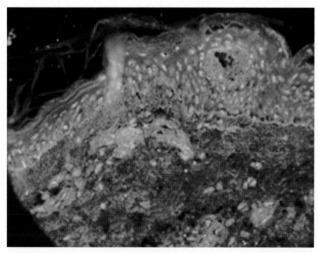

Figure 91-8 Direct immunofluorescence study in connective tissue disease–associated vasculitis, revealing tissue deposits of IgG and an "in vivo antinuclear antibody" phenomenon. This phenomenon is caused by the binding of immunoreactants to targets within the nuclei of epidermal cells.

hypergammaglobulinemia of Waldenström, is usually a true lymphocytic vasculitis. Patients with this disorder invariably have anti-Ro antibodies, and many have subclinical Sjögren's syndrome. Lymphocytic vasculitis typically demonstrates less disruption of blood vessel architecture than does leukocytoclastic vasculitis, perhaps because lymphocytes contain fewer of the destructive enzymes found within neutrophil granules. Fibrinoid necrosis, for example, is rare in lymphocytic vasculitis. True lymphocytic vasculitis is nearly always confined to the small blood vessels of the superficial papillary dermis. Even in Sjögren's syndrome, however, the histopathology encountered in most cases is that of leukocytoclastic vasculitis.

Rheumatoid Vasculitis

Rheumatoid vasculitis (RV) must be distinguished from the isolated digital (periungual) vasculitis that, in the absence of severe involvement, does not require intensive, vasculitis-specific therapy. Isolated digital vasculitis in patients with rheumatoid arthritis, characterized by splinter-like lesions in the periungual region (Bywaters' lesions), is not necessarily associated with a poorer prognosis than rheumatoid arthritis without digital vasculitic lesions and does not require specific therapy for vasculitis. In contrast, RV is a potentially devastating complication that may involve both medium and small blood vessels and requires the most aggressive therapeutic interventions. Many clinical manifestations of RV are indistinguishable from polyarteritis nodosa, although microaneurysms are less common in RV. RV classically occurs in patients with nodular, rheumatoid factor–positive, joint-destructive disease who have few clinical indications of active synovitis at the time vasculitis begins. However, RV occasionally complicates early disease.

The most common presentation of RV includes purpuric lesions with or without evidence of concomitant medium vessel vasculitis. DIF examination of the skin lesions shows granular IgM and C3 deposition in vessels, consistent with an IC-mediated pathophysiology in which rheumatoid factor, complement, and cryoglobulins may all participate. Deep cutaneous ulcers near the malleoli are a hallmark of RV and require scrupulous local care, as well as judicious immunosuppression. Mononeuritis multiplex often complicates RV. High-dose glucocorticoids, tumor necrosis factor inhibitors, rituximab, and cyclophosphamide have been employed in the treatment of rheumatoid vasculitis.

References

1. Jennette JC, Falk RJ, Andrassy K, et al: Nomenclature of systemic vasculitides. Proposal of an international consensus conference, *Arthritis Rheum* 37:187–192, 1994.
2. Zeek PM: Periarteritis nodosa: a critical review, *Am J Clin Pathol* 22:777–790, 1952.
3. Arthus M: Injections repetees de serum de cheval cuez le lapin, *Seances et Memoire de la Societe de Biologie* 55:817–825, 1903.
4. Nangaku M, Couser WG: Mechanisms of immune-deposit formation and the mediation of immune renal injury, *Clin Exp Nephrol* 9:183–191, 2005.
5. Ramos-Casals M, Anaya JM, Garcia-Carrasco M, et al: Cutaneous vasculitis in primary Sjögren syndrome: classification and clinical significance of 52 patients, *Medicine (Baltimore)* 83:96, 2004.
6. Hunder GG, Arend WP, Bloch DA, et al: The American College of Rheumatology 1990 criteria for the classification of vasculitis: introduction, *Arthritis Rheum* 33:1065–1067, 1990.

7. Calabrese LH, Michel BA, Bloch DA, et al: American College of Rheumatology 1990 criteria for the classification of hypersensitivity vasculitis, *Arthritis Rheum* 33:1108–1113, 1990.

8. Mills JA, Michel BA, Bloch DA, et al: The American College of Rheumatology 1990 criteria for the classification of Henoch-Schönlein purpura, *Arthritis Rheum* 33:1114–1121, 1990.

9. Mestecky J, Tomana M, Moldoveanu Z, et al: Role of aberrant glycosylation of IgA1 molecules in the pathogenesis of IgA nephropathy, *Kidney Blood Press Res* 31:29–37, 2008.

10. Blanco R, Martinez-Taboada VM, Rodriguez-Valverde V, et al: Henoch-Schönlein purpura in adulthood and childhood: two different expressions of the same syndrome, *Arthritis Rheum* 40:859–864, 1997.

11. Wintrobe MM, Buell MV: Hyperproteinemia associated with multiple myeloma: with report of a case in which an extraordinary hyperproteinemia was associated with thrombosis of the retinal veins and symptoms suggesting Raynaud's disease, *Bull Johns Hopkins Hosp* 52:156, 1933.

12. Ramos-Casals M, Stone JH, Cinta-Cid M, Bosch X: The cryoglobulinaemias, *Lancet* 379:348–360, 2012.

13. Davis MD, Brewer JD: Urticarial vasculitis and hypocomplementemic urticarial vasculitis syndrome. *Immunol Allergy Clin North Am* 24:183–213, 2004.

14. Wahl CE, Bouldin MB, Gibson LE: Erythema elevatum diutinum: clinical, histopathologic, and immunohistochemical characteristics of six patients, *Am J Dermatopathol* 27:397–400, 2005.

The references for this chapter can also be found on www.expertconsult.com.

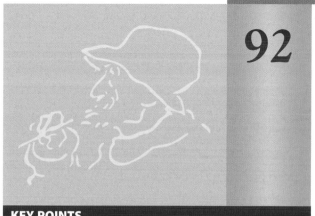

92

Primary Angiitis of the Central Nervous System

RULA A. HAJJ-ALI • CAROL A. LANGFORD

EPIDEMIOLOGY

Vasculitis affecting the central nervous system (CNS) most commonly occurs as a manifestation of a primary systemic vasculitis or as a secondary vasculitis in settings such as connective tissue diseases or infections. When the disease is confined only to the CNS (brain, meninges, and the spinal cord), it is referred to as *primary angiitis of the central nervous system* (PACNS).

PACNS is a rare disease, first reported as a distinct clinical pathologic entity in 1959 by Cravioto and Feigin.[1] The disease was initially described as "noninfectious granulomatous angiitis with a predilection for the nervous system" that is fatal. Other reports of similar clinicopathologic phenotypes emerged in the literature, and "granulomatous angiitis of the central nervous system" was proposed to describe this

entity.[2,3] Subsequently, different terms surfaced in the literature such as *isolated angiitis of the CNS* to encompass cases that were characterized by nongranulomatous pathologic findings.[4] Currently, PACNS is a well-accepted terminology of this disease that emphasizes the sole involvement of the CNS.[5,6] Following the description of diagnostic criteria for PACNS proposed by Calabrese and Mallek in 1988[5] and the potential for effective treatment,[7] there was a tremendous increase of published cases in the literature such that more than 500 cases have now been described worldwide.[8,9]

Because of its rarity and our evolving understanding of PACNS, the true incidence of PACNS is difficult to calculate.[9] In the recent era, the estimated annual incidence rate of PACNS is 2.4 cases per 1 million person-years.[9] Middle-aged men are often affected by PACNS with a median age at onset of approximately 50 years with a male-to-female ratio of around 2:1.[5,6,9]

GENETICS

The pathogenesis of PACNS is not well understood. To date, there has been no evidence to suggest a genetic predisposition, although this remains under active investigation.

CLINICAL FEATURES

Great progress has been made toward understanding the clinical features of PACNS despite the many challenges that include the lack of highly specific diagnostic modalities, the sparse material for research, and the lack of controlled clinical trials. In the recent era, specific clinical and pathologic subsets of PACNS that have prognostic implications have been identified.[10-13]

Proposed Criteria for Primary Angiitis of the Central Nervous System

In 1988 Calabrese and Mallek[5] proposed diagnostic criteria for PACNS that emphasized the importance of ruling out mimics when diagnosing PACNS. These criteria include (1) the presence of an unexplained neurologic deficit after thorough clinical and laboratory evaluation; (2) documentation by cerebral angiography and/or tissue examination of an arteritic process within the central nervous system; and (3) no evidence of a systemic vasculitides or any other condition to which the angiographic or pathologic features could be secondary.

In 2009 Birnbaum and Hellmann[12] proposed changes to the criteria described by Calabrese and colleagues, incorporating the levels of diagnostic certainty in their assessment. They proposed the term *definite diagnosis of PACNS* if there is confirmation of vasculitis on tissue biopsy and a *probable diagnosis of PACNS* when the diagnosis is based on high probability findings on an angiogram in the absence of tissue confirmation but with consideration of cerebrospinal fluid (CSF) profiles and neurologic symptoms to discriminate between PACNS and its mimics.

Although the original criteria by Calabrese served as a platform of literature-based research, their interpretation has changed fundamentally as advancement of our diagnostic modalities has revealed many unexplained neurologic diseases. The importance of ruling out mimics of PACNS remains essential in the diagnostic approach of patients with suspected PACNS.

Clinical Subsets

The original pathologic reports of PACNS as a granulomatous angiitis imposed a histologic-based nomenclature on the disease that led to the original name of *granulomatous angiitis of the* CNS (GACNS). Until the 1980s, PACNS was considered largely a homogeneous entity with a uniform clinical picture and grave prognosis. This paradigm was challenged with the introduction of direct vascular imaging as a diagnostic tool and recognition that nongranulomatous pathologic findings occur in PACNS.

Initial attempts at subclassification of PACNS described three broad subsets: GACNS, benign angiopathy of the CNS (BACNS), and "atypical" PACNS.[14] BACNS has since become recognized to be a part of the reversible cerebral vasoconstriction syndrome (RCVS)[11] with the other PACNS subsets now being defined by pathologic or radiographic features.

Granulomatous Angiitis of the Central Nervous System

GACNS is a subset of PACNS described as a clinicopathologic entity characterized by granulomatous angiitis confined to the brain. This is a rare subset of PACNS, in which patients clinically present with chronic insidious headaches along with diffuse and focal neurologic deficits. Because the disease is confined to the brain, meninges, or the spinal cord, signs and symptoms of systemic inflammatory diseases are usually lacking. The diagnosis of this subset is confirmed by the findings of granulomatous angiitis on pathology (Figure 92-1). Typically the CSF findings include those of an aseptic meningitis picture with negative staining for microorganisms. GACNS predominantly affects middle-aged men. The most common findings on neuroimaging include infarcts, most often bilateral, as well as high-

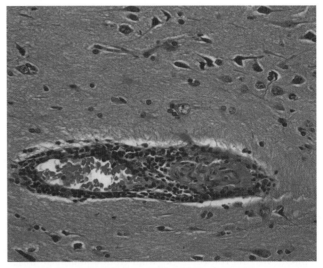

Figure 92-1 Histopathologic findings of patients with granulomatous angiitis of the central nervous system vasculitis.

intensity T2-weighted fluid attenuation inversion recovery (FLAIR) lesions on magnetic resonance imaging (MRI) in the subcortical white matter and deep gray matter. Cerebral angiogram is not the diagnostic modality of choice given its poor spatial resolution of detecting small vessel vasculitis, which mainly occurs in GACNS.

Atypical Central Nervous System Vasculitis

This subset of PACNS comprises multiple manifestations of PACNS that are clinically, radiologically, or pathologically distinct from GACNS. Atypical PACNS represents the most frequent and heterogeneous subset of PACNS. Included in this subset are patients with specific presentations such as lesions or those with pathologic findings of lymphocytic infiltration rather than granulomatous angiitis.

Masslike Presentation. Masslike (ML) presentation is a rare manifestation of PACNS occurring in less than 5% of the cases. This presentation has gained attention after the recent report of a series of 38 patients with histologically confirmed PACNS that presented with a solitary cerebral mass.[15] Typically the diagnosis is unanticipated and is confirmed after the pathologic examination from either biopsy samples or surgical excision of the mass. Unfortunately, there are no specific features on clinical assessment, neuroimaging, cerebral angiography, or CSF examination that could reliably distinguish ML-PACNS from other, more common causes of a solitary cerebral mass. Appropriate stains and cultures to rule out mycobacterial, fungal, or other infections and immunohistochemistry/gene rearrangement studies to exclude lymphoproliferative disease are essential to secure the diagnosis and exclude concomitant infectious or malignant processes.

Cerebral Amyloid Angiitis. Amyloid protein, in particular amyloid-β peptide, a fragment of the amyloid precursor peptide, can deposit in the brain, causing disease ranging from Alzheimer's disease to cerebral amyloid angiopathy (CAA). CAA-related inflammation and angiocentric inflammatory reaction in CAA is referred to as amyloid-β–related angiitis (ABRA).[16] Patients with ABRA tend to be older and more prone to hallucinations and mental status changes than other PACNS patients. MRI cannot distinguish between ABRA and other forms of PACNS, although there is a higher occurrence of cerebral hemorrhage in ABRA. ABRA carries a poor outcome, which could be related to older age and comorbidities.

Angiographically Defined Central Nervous System Vasculitis. The poor specificity of the cerebral angiogram poses a major challenge in the diagnosis of PACNS. When the diagnosis of PACNS is based on angiographic findings, a thorough evaluation should be performed to rule out mimics, especially RCVS.[17,18]

Spinal Cord Presentation. Spinal cord presentation of PACNS is a rare subset in which disease is present only in the spinal cord. The diagnosis is usually made by biopsy.[19]

Nongranulomatous PACNS. Pathologic findings of lymphocytic infiltration rather than granulomatous findings can occur in PACNS. In this category, the emphasis should be in ruling out secondary causes of CNS vasculitis such as infectious or lymphoproliferative diseases; adequate staining and immunophenotyping should always be carefully carried out in this category.

DIAGNOSIS AND DIAGNOSTIC TESTS

> **KEY POINTS**
>
> Spinal fluid, brain and vascular imaging, and brain biopsy are central to the diagnosis of PACNS and in ruling out other diseases.
>
> In PACNS 80% to 90% of patients have abnormal spinal fluid.
>
> Abnormalities on cerebral angiogram are not specific for PACNS and can be seen in a wide range of other settings.
>
> Reversible cerebral vasoconstriction syndrome is an important mimic of PACNS characterized by thunderclap headaches, normal CSF, and abnormal cerebral angiogram in which the changes resolve within 12 weeks.
>
> Other important entities in the differential of PACNS include infection, lymphoproliferative disease, primary systemic vasculitis, connective tissue disease, and thromboembolic disease.

The diagnosis of PACNS is challenging due to the nonspecific clinical presentation, the lack of highly specific laboratory and radiologic tests, and the difficulty in obtaining pathologic material.

Diagnostic Tests

Laboratory Findings

Elevation of acute phase reactants, anemia, and thrombocytosis are not typical of PACNS and, if present, should raise the possibility of a primary systemic vasculitis or other underlying disease. Laboratory testing to rule out connective tissue diseases and thromboembolic abnormalities should be performed. Infectious workup with appropriate cultures, serologies, and polymerase chain reaction testing

should be directed by clinical and diagnostic findings and host risk factors.

Cerebrospinal Fluid Analysis

CSF is an important tool in the evaluation of PACNS. Although CSF findings are nonspecific in PACNS, its value also lies in ruling out other entities. Obtaining appropriate CSF cultures, microbiologic stains, cytology, and flow cytometry are crucial in ruling infectious and neoplastic disease. Elevated protein, modest lymphocytic pleocytosis, and occasionally oligoclonal bands and elevated IgG synthesis characterize the CSF in 80% to 90% of patients with pathologically documented PACNS.[5,20,21] The median CSF white blood cell count is around 20 cells/μL, and the median CSF protein is approximately 120 mg/dL.[5,9]

Radiologic Evaluation

MRI is a sensitive modality for the diagnosis of PACNS reaching 90% to 100%.[9,22] Abnormalities include infarcts in 50% of patients, commonly affecting the cortex and the subcortex bilaterally.[9,23] Affected areas include subcortical white matter, followed by deep gray matter, deep white matter, and the cerebral cortex.[24] Hyperintense lesions on T2-weighted sequences are common but not specific for PACNS.[25] Other abnormalities include mass lesions in 5% of patients[15]; leptomeningeal enhancement in 8% of the cases[9]; and gadolinium-enhanced intracranial lesions in about one-third of patients.[9]

Cerebral vasculature imaging by catheter-directed dye angiogram or through magnetic resonance angiography (MRA) is an important modality in the diagnosis of PACNS. Alternating areas of dilatation and stenosis characterize the angiographic findings in PACNS and typically involve the vasculature on both sides but sometimes can involve single vessels.[26] Other angiographic features include smooth tapering of one or multiple vessels. Although cerebral angiograms may visualize abnormalities in medium-sized vessels, they have limited sensitivity to detect abnormalities in small vessels that are less than 500 μm in diameter. Although cerebral angiography is valuable, its specificity for the diagnosis of PACNS can be as low as 25%.[27] The reported "typical" angiographic findings for vasculitis are not specific to PACNS and can be encountered in atherosclerosis, radiation vasculopathy, or vascular spasm.[26,27] Moreover, cerebral angiogram carries a poor positive predictive value in the diagnosis of PACNS in that the angiographic findings seen in RCVS can be consistent with those found in PACNS.[28] Vascular studies should therefore be interpreted with caution and should not be considered the diagnostic "gold standard" in PACNS.

Brain Biopsy

Brain biopsy is thought to carry a low morbidity and mortality in patients with PACNS[14] and is an important part of the evaluation to confirm the diagnosis and rule out mimics. When a brain biopsy is performed, an alternative diagnosis is identified in 30% to 40% of the cases.[29] The interpretation of the brain biopsy results should take into consideration the potential for false-negative results because of the patchy degree of involvement and the small amount of tissue that can often be obtained. The finding of vasculitis on pathologic examination does not exclude the diagnosis of infection or malignancy, and appropriate stains and markers should be pursued for accurate diagnosis.

Differential Diagnosis

The differential diagnosis algorithm of PACNS is large due to the lack of highly specific clinical features, laboratory, or imaging findings (Table 92-1). Excluding other entities that can have similar findings is critical in confirming a diagnosis of PACNS. Certain disease categories in particular should be considered and warrant further detailed discussion.

Reversible Cerebral Vasoconstriction Syndromes

RCVS is the leading mimic of PACNS, which is important to distinguish because it carries different implications for treatment and outcome (Table 92-2). RCVS comprises a group of disorders characterized by acute-onset headaches and reversible cerebrovasoconstriction.[11] These disorders include Call-Fleming syndrome, drug-induced angiopathy, migraine angiitis, BACNS, postpartum angiopathy, and drug-induced vasospasm. The clinical features of RCVS include acute onset of severe headaches, with or without neurologic deficit, with evidence of cerebral vasoconstriction that is reversible. The headaches are usually recurrent thunderclap headaches and can be precipitated by straining and coughing. RCVS can be associated with strokes (39%), generalized tonic-clonic seizures (17%), convexity subarachnoid hemorrhage (34%), lobar hemorrhage (20%), and brain edema (38%).[18] RCVS occurs more frequently in women than men. In contrast to PACNS, CSF analysis is generally normal in RCVS except where there is a concomitant disorder or subarachnoid bleeding. The diagnosis of RCVS is usually brought into consideration when cerebral vascular imaging reveals multiple areas of smooth or tapered arterial narrowing followed by segments of normal-caliber or distended arteries. Typically, arterial narrowing involves multiple intracerebral arteries and their branches in both hemispheres resulting in severe arterial narrowing. The diagnosis of RCVS is secured when repeat vascular imaging reveals reversibility of the cerebral vascular abnormalities, often occurring in about 6 to 12 weeks, which is in contrast to the fixed angiographic abnormalities encountered in PACNS. There is a lack of controlled trials to direct treatment of RCVS. Calcium channel blockers are used for symptomatic treatment of the headaches, with no evidence that they alter the clinical outcome. Some experts use glucocorticoid therapy but with no evidence that this improves the outcome.

Primary Systemic Vasculitides

Primary systemic vasculitides such as granulomatosis with polyangiitis (GPA) (formerly Wegener's granulomtosis), microscopic polyangiitis, Churg-Strauss syndrome (CSS), polyarteritis nodosa, or Behçet syndrome (BS) can affect the CNS leading to inflammation and vasculitis. In GPA, CNS disease occurs in 7% to 11% of patients and presents

Table 92-1 Differential Diagnosis of Primary Angiitis of the Central Nervous System

Secondary Cerebral Vasculitis
Primary Systemic Vasculitides
Granulomatosis with polyangiitis Microscopic polyangiitis Churg-Strauss syndrome Polyarteritis nodosa Behçet syndrome
Connective Tissue Diseases
Systemic lupus erythematosus Sjögren's syndrome Inflammatory myositis Rheumatoid arthritis Mixed connective tissue disease
Other Multisystem Inflammatory Disorders
Sarcoidosis Susac's syndrome
Infection
Bacterial, mycobacterial, fungal, viral, protozoal
Malignancy
Central nervous system lymphoma Glioma Angiocentric lymphoma Lymphomatoid granulomatosis Metastatic malignancy
Vasospastic Disorders
Reversible cerebral vasoconstrictive syndrome Drug exposures
Other Arterial Disease
Atherosclerosis Fibromuscular dysplasia Moyamoya Dissection
Hypercoagulable States
Antiphospholipid antibody syndrome Thrombotic thrombocytopenic purpura
Strokelike Syndromes
CADASIL Mitochondrial diseases Sickle cell disease Fabry's disease Sneddon's syndrome
Leukoencephalopathies
Progressive multifocal leukoencephalopathy Reversible posterior leukoencephalopathy syndrome
Cerebral Hemorrhage
Hypertensive Aneurysmal Amyloid angiopathy Arteriovenous malformation
Embolic Disease
Thrombus Cholesterol emboli Myxoma Endocarditis Air emboli

CADASIL, cerebral autosomal dominant arteriopathy with subcortical infarcts and leukoencephalopathy.

Table 92-2 Differentiating Clinical and Radiological Features between Reversible Cerebral Vasoconstrictive Syndrome (RCVS) and Primary Angiitis of the Central Nervous System (PACNS)

Feature	RCVS	PACNS
Gender	Female predominant	Male predominant
Cerebrospinal fluid	Normal	Abnormal
Normal magnetic resonance image	10%-15%	Very rare
Abnormal angiogram	100%	40%-50%
Headache pattern	Recurrent thunderclap	Insidious, chronic
Infarct pattern	Watershed	Small, scattered
Lobar hemorrhage	Common	Extremely rare
Convexity subarachnoid hemorrhage	Common	Very rare

in three different ways: direct invasion of granuloma from extracranial sites, remote intracranial granuloma, and rarely because of CNS vasculitis.[30] The diagnosis of CNS vasculitis is often made on the basis of radiologic findings and by exclusion of other etiologies of the neurologic deficits, especially infection.[31] As in GPA, the diagnosis of CNS vasculitis in CSS is often presumed without a histologic confirmation when other mimics are excluded. Neuroophthalmologic manifestations including amaurosis fugax, superior oblique palsy, ischemic optic neuropathy, fourth cranial palsy, and scattered areas of retinal infarction are common presentations of CNS vasculitis in CSS.[32,33] In BS, CNS involvement occurs in 14% of cases manifesting as meningoencephalitis involving the brain stem and rarely as a consequence of thrombosis and inflammation of the dural venous sinuses.[34-36] Pathologic evaluation in neuro-BS typically shows a mononuclear infiltration around the small vessels of the brain including the venous system, which is not a typical finding in PACNS.[37] True CNS vasculitis rarely occurs in BS.[38]

Connective Tissue Diseases

The brain is a common target in connective tissue diseases. In systemic lupus erythematosus (SLE), CNS involvement occurs in 14% to 80% of adults and 22% to 95% of children.[39] Multifocal microinfarcts, cortical atrophy, gross infarcts, hemorrhage, ischemic demyelination, and patchy multiple-sclerosis-like demyelination are typical findings in neuropsychiatric lupus. The most common microscopic brain finding in SLE is microvasculopathy, described as "healed vasculitis" consistent with hyalinization, thickening, and thrombus formation.[40,41] Rheumatoid arthritis, Sjögren's syndrome, and mixed connective tissue disease rarely affect the CNS in a vasculitic pattern.[42] CNS vasculitis is typically a late occurrence in these diseases.

Infections

Infections are one of the most important entities that should be ruled out when considering PACNS. Vasculitis can occur in the setting of human immunodeficiency syndrome (HIV), often presenting as multifocal cerebral ischemia with pathologic findings of angiocentric lymphoproliferative lesions.[43] In addition, HIV can result in granulomatous arteritis[44] or can affect the brain secondary to co-infections such as syphilis. *Treponema pallidum* infection can affect vessels in the subarachnoid space and result in thrombosis, ischemia, and infarction that can mimic PACNS.[45] Other infectious agents that have predilection to brain include varicellazoster virus (VZV). VZV affects the brain either by involvement of large cerebral vessels, often affecting the proximal segments of the anterior and middle cerebral arteries in immunocompetent individuals, or small vessel disease in immunocompromised patients.[46] History of VZV rash is usually elicited before the CNS involvement but not always. The diagnosis of VZV angiitis is confirmed by finding VZV DNA in CSF or the presence of reduced serum/CSF ratios of VZV immunoglobulin G (IgG).[47] Tuberculosis affecting the CNS is an important cause of CNS vasculitis in endemic areas and should be carefully excluded. Hepatitis C,[48] West Nile virus,[49] parvovirus B19,[50] and rarely herpes simplex virus[51] can cause CNS vasculitis. Cytomegalovirus can cause CNS vasculitis as an opportunistic infection in immunocompromised individuals.[52] Rarely cysticercosis can involve middle-sized cerebral arteries.[53] A travel history and history of exposures are important features of the workup of patients with suspected PACNS.

Lymphoproliferative Diseases

Lymphoproliferative disease with predilection to the vascular wall such as lymphomatoid granulomatosis (LG) can cause CNS vasculitis leading to multiple small cortical infarcts and pathologic findings of multifocal angiocentric, angiodestructive lymphoma.[54] Concomitant HIV infection is common with LG and should be ruled out.[55] Rarely, LG is associated with other systemic autoimmune diseases such as Sjögren's syndrome.[56] Other lymphoproliferative diseases such as CNS lymphoma and intravascular lymphoma can mimic PACNS.

Miscellaneous

Atherosclerotic involvement of the intracerebral arteries is common and is often a consideration in the workup of PACNS. The poor specificity of the cerebral angiogram poses a major limitation in differentiating inflammatory causes from other vasculopathies. However, the lack of inflammatory changes of the CSF and the presence of multiple atherosclerotic risk factors should raise the suspicion for atherosclerotic disease. Other entities such as antiphospholipid antibody syndrome, hypercoagulable states, and thromboembolic etiologies should be carefully ruled out. The workup of PACNS should include transesophageal echocardiogram and hypercoagulable profile to rule out thromboembolic etiologies, especially in patients presenting with recurrent strokes. Other rare diseases that mimic the angiographic findings of PACNS include Moyamoya disease, small vessel arterial dissection, cerebral autosomal dominant arteriopathy with subcortical infarcts and leukoencephalopathy (CADASIL), radiation vasculopathy, and thromboangiitis obliterans.[57]

TREATMENT

KEY POINTS

No standardized trials have been conducted on the treatment of PACNS.

GACNS is typically treated initially with glucocorticoids and cyclophosphamide.

The treatment of PACNS subsets besides GACNS is based on the diagnostic subset and severity of neurologic impairment.

The treatment of PACNS is guided by expert opinion and reports of case series, as well as from extrapolation from controlled trials in primary systemic vasculitis. To date, there have been no controlled trials in the treatment of PACNS. Because of this, it is not possible to have a specific treatment algorithm and therapy is based on the subtype and neurologic severity.

The report of successful treatment of GACNS with a combination of cyclophosphamide and glucocorticoids led to the regular use of this regimen.[7] Generally, patients are treated with a combination of cyclophosphamide and high-dose glucocorticoids for 3 to 6 months until remission is achieved. Then cyclophosphamide is stopped and switched to a maintenance agent following the same principles that are used in small vessel vasculitis.[58] Maintenance therapy usually consists of either azathioprine or mycophenolate mofetil and rarely methotrexate given its low CNS penetration. The duration of maintenance therapy in PACNS is not well defined.

The treatment of atypical PACNS varies highly. Multiple factors affect the treatment regimen in atypical PACNS, and the treatment is usually individualized taking into consideration the degree of the neurologic deficit and the features of the diagnosis. All atypical PACNS cases are treated with high dose of glucocorticoids initially, and the decision to add other immunosuppressive agents is individually based. ABRA and ML-PACNS are two PACNS subsets in which cyclophosphamide is considered at the outset of the treatment.

Assessing disease status and defining remission are crucial steps in the course of treatment of PACNS. Permanent deficits occurring after the initial event in PACNS should not be erroneously considered as lack of remission. Disease is considered in remission when there is stability or improvement of the clinical and radiologic features. Serial MRI should be obtained to help in the assessment of disease activity. Adjunctive therapy for osteoporosis prevention and prophylaxis for opportunistic infections should be incorporated into the treatment plan.

OUTCOME

KEY POINTS

PACNS has an estimated mortality rate of 10% to 17%.

Moderate to severe disability occurs in up to 20% of patients with PACNS.

Originally, PACNS was described as a fatal disease by Cravioto,[7] but an improved outlook became possible following the description of treatment with glucocorticoids and cyclophosphamide. From recent reports, the estimated mortality rate of PACNS varies between 10% and 17%[9,59] with one study finding that survival correlated with the initial findings of infarcts and gadolinium-enhanced lesions on MRI.[9] Salvarani and colleagues[9] and Hajj-Ali and colleagues[59] reported that 20% of patients with PACNS had moderate to severe disability as assessed by the modified Rankin disability scores and the Barthel index, respectively. Salvarani and colleagues[9] reported an improvement in disability scores over time.

SUMMARY

Considerable progress has been made in our understanding of PACNS. Our ability to recognize disease mimics have substantially increased our accuracy in the diagnosis of PACNS. The identification of RCVS in particular has clarified many of the cases that were erroneously diagnosed as PACNS. Effective diagnosis and management of PACNS requires a multidisciplinary team to evaluate the clinical features, obtain and interpret diagnostic tests, and determine the most effective regimen that will treat the underlying disease and minimize therapeutic toxicity.

There remains a great need for controlled trials to further guide treatment for patients with PACNS in their initial and maintenance phases. Prospective evaluation of long-term cohorts is necessary to better determine the rates of disability and long-term outcome of PACNS.

References

1. Cravioto H, Feigin I: Noninfectious granulomatous angiitis with predilection for the nervous system, *Neurology* 9:599–609, 1959.
2. McCormick HM, Neubuerger KT: Giant-cell arteritis involving small meningeal and intracerebral vessels, *J Neuropathol Exp Neurol* 17:471–478, 1958.
3. Budzilovich GN, Feigin I, Siegel H: Granulomatous angiitis of the nervous system, *Arch Pathol* 76:250–256, 1963.
4. Moore PM: Diagnosis and management of isolated angiitis of the central nervous system, *Neurology* 39:167–173, 1989.
5. Calabrese LH, Mallek JA: Primary angiitis of the central nervous system. Report of 8 new cases, review of the literature, and proposal for diagnostic criteria, *Medicine (Baltimore)* 67:20–39, 1988.
6. Lie JT: Primary (granulomatous) angiitis of the central nervous system: a clinicopathologic analysis of 15 new cases and a review of the literature, *Hum Pathol* 23:164–171, 1992.
7. Cupps TR, Moore PM, Fauci AS: Isolated angiitis of the central nervous system. Prospective diagnostic and therapeutic experience, *Am J Med* 74:97–105, 1983.
8. Molloy ES, Hajj-Ali RA: Primary angiitis of the central nervous system, *Curr Treat Options Neurol* 9:169–175, 2007.
9. Salvarani C, Brown RD Jr, Calamia KT, et al: Primary central nervous system vasculitis: analysis of 101 patients, *Ann Neurol* 62:442–451, 2007.
10. Neel A, Paganoux C: Primary angiitis of the central nervous system, *Clin Exp Rheumatol* 27:S95–S107, 2009.
11. Calabrese LH, Dodick DW, Schwedt TJ, Singhal AB: Narrative review: reversible cerebral vasoconstriction syndromes, *Ann Intern Med* 146:34–44, 2007.
12. Birnbaum J, Hellmann DB: Primary angiitis of the central nervous system, *Arch Neurol* 66:704–709, 2009.
13. Calabrese LH: Vasculitis of the central nervous system, *Rheum Dis Clin North Am* 21:1059–1076, 1995.
14. Calabrese LH, Duna GF, Lie JT: Vasculitis in the central nervous system, *Arthritis Rheum* 40:1189–1201, 1997.

15. Molloy ES, Singhal AB, Calabrese LH: Tumour-like mass lesion: an under-recognised presentation of primary angiitis of the central nervous system, *Ann Rheum Dis* 67:1732–1735, 2008.

16. Eng JA, Frosch MP, Choi K, et al: Clinical manifestations of cerebral amyloid angiopathy-related inflammation, *Ann Neurol* 55:250–256, 2004.

17. Ducros A, Boukobza M, Porcher R, et al: The clinical and radiological spectrum of reversible cerebral vasoconstriction syndrome. A prospective series of 67 patients, *Brain* 130:3091–3101, 2007.

18. Singhal AB, Hajj-Ali RA, Topcuoglu MA, et al: Reversible cerebral vasoconstriction syndromes: analysis of 139 cases, *Arch Neurol* 68:1005–1012, 2011.

19. Salvarani C, Brown RD Jr, Calamia KT, et al: Primary CNS vasculitis with spinal cord involvement, *Neurology* 70:2394–2400, 2008.

20. Pou Serradell A, Maso E, Roquer J, et al: [Isolated angiitis of the central nervous system. Clinical and neuropathological study of 2 cases], *Rev Neurol (Paris)* 151:258–266, 1995.

21. Stone JH, Pomper MG, Roubenoff R, et al: Sensitivities of noninvasive tests for central nervous system vasculitis: a comparison of lumbar puncture, computed tomography, and magnetic resonance imaging, *J Rheumatol* 21:1277–1282, 1994.

22. Calabrese LH: Therapy of systemic vasculitis, *Neurol Clin* 15:973–991, 1997.

23. Hurst RW, Grossman RI: Neuroradiology of central nervous system vasculitis, *Semin Neurol* 14:320–340, 1994.

24. Pomper MG, Miller TJ, Stone JH, et al: CNS vasculitis in autoimmune disease: MR imaging findings and correlation with angiography, *AJNR Am J Neuroradiol* 20:75–85, 1999.

25. Bekiesinska-Figatowska M: T2-hyperintense foci on brain MR imaging, *Med Sci Monit* 10(Suppl 3):80–87, 2004.

26. Alhalabi M, Moore PM: Serial angiography in isolated angiitis of the central nervous system, *Neurology* 44:1221–1226, 1994.

27. Duna GF, Calabrese LH: Limitations of invasive modalities in the diagnosis of primary angiitis of the central nervous system, *J Rheumatol* 22:662–667, 1995.

28. Kadkhodayan Y, Alreshaid A, Moran CJ, et al: Primary angiitis of the central nervous system at conventional angiography, *Radiology* 233:878–882, 2004.

29. Alrawi A, Trobe JD, Blaivas M, Musch DC: Brain biopsy in primary angiitis of the central nervous system, *Neurology* 53:858–860, 1999.

30. Nishino H, Rubino FA, Parisi JE: The spectrum of neurologic involvement in Wegener's granulomatosis, *Neurology* 43:1334–1337, 1993.

31. Seror R, Mahr A, Ramanoelina J, et al: Central nervous system involvement in Wegener granulomatosis, *Medicine (Baltimore)* 85:54–65, 2006.

32. Weinstein JM, Chui H, Lane S, et al: Churg-Strauss syndrome (allergic granulomatous angiitis). Neuro-ophthalmologic manifestations, *Arch Ophthalmol* 101:1217–1220, 1983.

33. Vitali C, Genovesi-Ebert F, Romani A, et al: Ophthalmological and neuro-ophthalmological involvement in Churg-Strauss syndrome: a case report, *Graefes Arch Clin Exp Ophthalmol* 234:404–408, 1996.

34. Al-Araji A, Sharquie K, Al-Rawi Z: Prevalence and patterns of neurological involvement in Behcet's disease: a prospective study from Iraq, *J Neurol Neurosurg Psychiatry* 74:608–613, 2003.

35. Al-Araji A, Kidd DP: Neuro-Behcet's disease: epidemiology, clinical characteristics, and management, *Lancet Neurol* 8:192–204, 2009.

36. Akman-Demir G, Serdaroglu P, Tasci B: Clinical patterns of neurological involvement in Behcet's disease: evaluation of 200 patients. The Neuro-Behcet Study Group, *Brain* 122(Pt 11):2171–2182, 1999.

37. Hirohata S: Histopathology of central nervous system lesions in Behcet's disease, *J Neurol Sci* 267:41–47, 2008.

38. Zouboulis CC, Kurz K, Bratzke B, Orfanos CE: [Adamantiades-Behcet disease: necrotizing systemic vasculitis with a fatal outcome], *Hautarzt* 42:451–454, 1991.

39. Brey RL: Neuropsychiatric lupus: clinical and imaging aspects, *Bull NYU Hosp Jt Dis* 65:194–199, 2007.

40. Ellis SG, Verity MA: Central nervous system involvement in systemic lupus erythematosus: a review of neuropathologic findings in 57 cases, 1955–1977, *Semin Arthritis Rheum* 8:212–221, 1979.

41. Hanly JG, Walsh NM, Sangalang V: Brain pathology in systemic lupus erythematosus, *J Rheumatol* 19:732–741, 1992.

42. Neamtu L, Belmont M, Miller DC, et al: Rheumatoid disease of the CNS with meningeal vasculitis presenting with a seizure, *Neurology* 56:814–815, 2001.

43. Montilla P, Dronda F, Moreno S, et al: Lymphomatoid granulomatosis and the acquired immunodeficiency syndrome, *Ann Intern Med* 106:166–167, 1987.

44. Yankner BA, Skolnik PR, Shoukimas GM, et al: Cerebral granulomatous angiitis associated with isolation of human T-lymphotropic virus type III from the central nervous system, *Ann Neurol* 20:362–364, 1986.

45. Kakumani PL, Hajj-Ali RA: A forgotten cause of central nervous system vasculitis, *J Rheumatol* 36:655, 2009.

46. Pierot L, Chiras J, Debussche-Depriester C, et al: Intracerebral stenosing arteriopathies. Contribution of three radiological techniques to the diagnosis, *J Neuroradiol* 18:32–48, 1991.

47. Gilden DH: Varicella zoster virus vasculopathy and disseminated encephalomyelitis, *J Neurol Sci* 195:99–101, 2002.

48. Dawson TM, Starkebaum G: Isolated central nervous system vasculitis associated with hepatitis C infection, *J Rheumatol* 26:2273–2276, 1999.

49. Alexander JJ, Lasky AS, Graf WD: Stroke associated with central nervous system vasculitis after West Nile virus infection, *J Child Neurol* 21:623–625, 2006.

50. Bilge I, Sadikoglu B, Emre S, et al: Central nervous system vasculitis secondary to parvovirus B19 infection in a pediatric renal transplant patient, *Pediatr Nephrol* 20:529–533, 2005.

51. Schmitt JA, Dietzmann K, Muller U, Krause P: [Granulomatous vasculitis—an uncommon manifestation of herpes simplex infection of the central nervous system], *Zentralbl Pathol* 138:298–302, 1992.

52. Koeppen AH, Lansing LS, Peng SK, Smith RS: Central nervous system vasculitis in cytomegalovirus infection, *J Neurol Sci* 51:395–410, 1981.

53. Barinagarrementeria F, Cantu C: Frequency of cerebral arteritis in subarachnoid cysticercosis: an angiographic study, *Stroke* 29:123–125, 1998.

54. Kleinschmidt-DeMasters BK, Filley CM, Bitter MA: Central nervous system angiocentric, angiodestructive T-cell lymphoma (lymphomatoid granulomatosis), *Surg Neurol* 37:130–137, 1992.

55. Katsetos CD, Fincke JE, Legido A, et al: Angiocentric CD3(+) T-cell infiltrates in human immunodeficiency virus type 1-associated central nervous system disease in children, *Clin Diagn Lab Immunol* 6:105–114, 1999.

56. Khanna D, Vinters HV, Brahn E: Angiocentric T cell lymphoma of the central nervous system in a patient with Sjögren's syndrome, *J Rheumatol* 29:1548–1550, 2002.

57. No YJ, Lee EM, Lee DH, Kim JS: Cerebral angiographic findings in thromboangiitis obliterans, *Neuroradiology* 47:912–915, 2005.

58. Molloy ES, Langford CA: Advances in the treatment of small vessel vasculitis, *Rheum Dis Clin North Am* 32:157–172, 2006.

59. Hajj-Ali R, Villa-Forte AL, Abou-Chebel A, et al: Long term outcome of patients with primary angiitis of the central nervous system (PACNS), *Arthritis Rheum* 43:S162, 2000.

The references for this chapter can also be found on www.expertconsult.com.

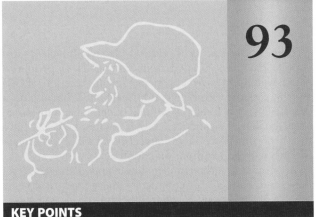

93 Behçet's Disease

WILLIAM S. KAUFMAN •
ELIZABETH KAUFMAN McNAMARA •
JOSEPH L. JORIZZO

KEY POINTS

Behçet's disease is a complex multisystem disease characterized by oral and genital ulcers and other systemic features.

Diagnosis is based on the International Criteria for Behçet's Disease including oral aphthae, genital aphthae, ocular lesions, cutaneous lesions, and a positive pathergy test.

Cutaneous lesions should display a neutrophilic vascular reaction on histopathologic examination.

Treatment is based on the degree of systemic involvement and ranges from topical corticosteroids to thalidomide to systemic immunosuppressive agents and tumor necrosis factor inhibitors.

Prognosis is variable, and patients typically have periods of exacerbations and remissions.

Behçet's disease is a chronic, complex multisystem disease characterized clinically by oral aphthae, genital aphthae, cutaneous lesions, and ophthalmic, neurologic, or rheumatologic manifestations. The first description of Behçet's disease was probably by Hippocrates in the fifth century BC,[1] and the first modern account was presented in 1937 by the Turkish dermatologist Hulusi Behçet, who reported on a patient with recurrent oral and genital aphthae and uveitis.[2]

EPIDEMIOLOGY

Behçet's disease is seen worldwide, with the highest prevalence reported in Turkey (80 to 370 patients per 100,000 inhabitants)[3] and Japan (13.6 per 100,000).[4] The prevalence and often the severity is increased in the Middle East and the Mediterranean (i.e., the "Silk Route").[5,6] The remainder of the Asian continent has a prevalence of 7 to 30 patients per 100,000 inhabitants.[7] It is relatively uncommon in northern Europe (0.27 to 1.18 per 100,000 inhabitants) and the United States (0.12 to 0.33 patients per 100,000 inhabitants).[3,5,7] Patients commonly fulfill the diagnostic criteria in their mid-20s to 30s.[8] In the past, Behçet's disease was thought to predominantly affect males, but current epidemiologic data show a more equal male-to-female ratio.[9] Overall, the male-to-female ratio has decreased over the past 20 years with males being more affected in the Middle East and a female predominance existing in Korea, China, the United States, and northern Europe.[7]

CAUSE AND PATHOGENESIS

Although the pathogenesis of Behçet's disease remains unclear, many factors have been implicated. Heredity, immunologic factors, infectious agents, inflammatory mediators, and clotting factors likely contribute.

Genetics

The onset of Behçet's disease is believed to be sporadic, though familial clustering, families with multiple affected members, has been reported. Individuals with a first-degree relative with the disease are at an increased risk of developing the disease.[10] Additionally, children of individuals with Behçet's disease may have an earlier age of onset, suggesting genetic anticipation, which is due to a progressive increase in nucleotide repeats through consecutive generations.[11] Familial occurrence differs regionally throughout the world and is more common in Korea, Israel, Turkey, and Arab countries, compared with Japan, China, and Europe.[7]

Studies have shown a significant association between the human leukocyte antigen (HLA)-B51 and Behçet's disease.[12,13] HLA-B51–positive patients are at an increased risk of developing Behçet's disease (odds ratio of 5.9).[14] This association is more common in the Middle East, Mediterranean, and Japan, though not seen as often in Western nations. Disease prognosis also appears to be more severe in HLA-B51–positive patients.[7] The role of HLA-B51 in Behçet's remains unclear. It may be that HLA-B51 is not directly involved in causing the disease but is closely linked to disease-related genes.[15] Candidate genes have been localized to chromosome 6 and include the major histocompatibility complex class I chain-related gene A (MICA) and, more specifically, the MICA6 allele; perth block (PERB); new organization associated with HLA-B (NOB); and transporter associated with antigen processing genes (TAP).[15,16] Other hypotheses suggest that HLA-B51 may contribute to the onset of Behçet's disease by serving as a heterologous antigen either through original antigen presentation or through viral or bacterial molecular mimicry.[15,17] A recent genome-wide association study confirmed the HLA-B51 relationship and also identified a second, independent association within the MHC class I region.[18]

Although Behçet's disease has many features in common with the spondyloarthropathies, especially those associated with inflammatory bowel disease (IBD), the disorder in IBD patients generally evolves in a pattern resembling reactive arthritis, with an erosive axial arthritis; erosive arthritis and HLA-B27 are not associated with Behçet's disease.[19]

Immune Mechanisms

Immune mechanisms play a major role in Behçet's disease. Heat shock proteins, cytokines, alterations in neutrophil and macrophage activity, and autoimmune mechanisms have all been implicated.[15] Heat shock proteins are released in response to stress and may be involved in stimulating a T helper type 1 immune response through interaction with Toll-like receptors.[20] Specifically, immunoglobulin M–type, 47-kD cell surface heat shock protein against α-enolase has been identified in patients with Behçet's disease.[21] Although most of the T lymphocytes thought to be involved in this reaction are of the $\gamma\delta$ type, the diversity of T lymphocytes seen in the disease suggests a response to multiple antigens, which may account for the various symptoms seen in Behçet's.[22] Cytokines such as interleukin (IL)-1, IL-8, IL-12, IL-17, and tumor necrosis factor (TNF) seem to be involved in the pathogenesis. Although elevated cytokine levels may serve as an indicator of disease severity, it should be appreciated that plasma TNF levels may rise and fall as an acute-phase reactant along with C-reactive protein and the erythrocyte sedimentation rate.[23] The production of these proinflammatory cytokines, which are responsible for the chronic inflammation observed, may be the result of activated macrophages.[15,24] In addition to macrophage activation, neutrophil chemotaxis and phagocytosis are increased in the lesions of Behçet's disease.[15,25] This increased activity of neutrophils leads to tissue injury in the form of the neutrophilic vascular reaction seen in lesions such as aphthae, pustular cutaneous lesions, and erythema nodosum–like lesions. Circulating immune complexes also play a role in precipitating the characteristic neutrophilic vascular reaction.[26] Finally, the role of endothelial cell dysfunction in the pathogenesis of Behçet's disease has been suggested by decreased levels of prostacyclin in the serum of Behçet's disease patients. Increased nitric oxide concentrations in the serum, synovial fluid, and aqueous humor of individuals with Behçet's may play a role in endothelial activation, resulting in vascular inflammation and thrombosis.[27,28] Elevated homocysteine levels have been cited as the cause of the increased nitric oxide concentrations, suggesting that hyperhomocysteinemia may represent an acquired risk factor for Behçet's, which is potentially reversible.[29-31]

Infectious Agents

Several studies have suggested a role for various infectious agents in the pathogenesis of Behçet's disease; however, no organisms have been consistently isolated. Antistreptococcal antibodies have been isolated in the serum of patients with Behçet's disease.[32] Higher concentrations of *Streptococcus sanguis* have also been found in the oral flora of patients with Behçet's disease and may play a role in the development of aphthae, which is often the initial manifestation.[33] In addition to streptococcal antigens, other bacteria such as *Escherichia coli* and *Staphylococcus aureus* may have a role in Behçet's disease through the activation of lymphocytes.[34] Additionally, a lipoprotein of *Mycoplasma fermentans* has been found in patients with Behçet's. This lipoprotein (MALP-404) contains the specific peptide motif, which is capable of being presented by *HLA-B51*.[35] Studies have also indicated that there is a higher rate of *Helicobacter pylori* cytotoxin-associated gene-A antibodies in Behçet's patients. These antibodies may cause endothelial damage via cross-reaction with endothelial antigens. *H. pylori* eradication in these patients has been shown to decrease disease severity.[36]

Herpes simplex virus (HSV) deoxyribonucleic acid (DNA) has been isolated from the nuclei of peripheral blood lymphocytes by polymerase chain reaction (PCR) assay in patients with Behçet's disease.[19] HSV has also been detected by PCR in biopsy samples of genital and intestinal ulcers of Behçet's patients.[34] Other studies, however, have shown no difference in the detection of HSV in Behçet's patients with and without oral aphthae.[37]

In summary, although the cause and pathogenesis of Behçet's disease are not completely understood, they likely involve an infectious or environmental trigger and subsequent inflammatory response in a genetically predisposed individual. The article by Zouboulis and May[15] provides an excellent overview of the current understanding of the pathogenesis of Behçet's disease.

CLINICAL FEATURES

Aphthae

Oral aphthae, or canker sores (Figure 93-1), are often the initial feature of Behçet's disease and constitute a requisite diagnostic feature (although many believe that Behçet's occurs in the absence of oral aphthae). Oral ulcerations usually occur in crops of more than 3 to 10s of lesions, but individual lesions may occur on the buccal mucosa, gingiva, lips, and tongue. Aphthae tend to be painful and shallow, and they heal without scarring over 1 to 3 weeks.[38] Genital ulcers typically occur on the scrotum and penis in males and on the vulva or vaginal mucosa in females. These aphthae are similar in appearance to oral lesions, but they have a greater tendency to scar and may recur less frequently.[38] Lesions in the oral mucosa are generally easy to distinguish from oral HSV, but with genital lesions, HSV should be excluded by viral culture or PCR before lesions are accepted as a diagnostic criterion.

Cutaneous Lesions

Several cutaneous manifestations of Behçet's disease have been described: erythema nodosum–like lesions, pyoderma gangrenosum–like lesions, Sweet's syndrome–like lesions, cutaneous small vessel vasculitis, and pustular vasculitic

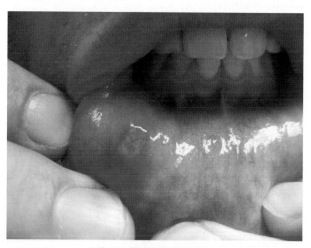

Figure 93-1 Oral aphtha.

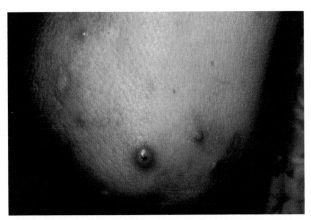

Figure 93-2 Pustular vasculitis lesions representing a neutrophilic vascular reaction.

lesions (Figure 93-2) including lesions induced by trauma—the so-called pathergy lesion.[38] Pathergy signifies the development of erythematous pustules or papules 24 to 48 hours following puncture of the skin with a 20- to 21-gauge sterile needle.[39] Specimens from all these lesions demonstrate a neutrophilic vascular reaction on histopathologic analysis.[40] Acneiform or pseudofolliculitis lesions should be considered nonspecific, nondiagnostic findings because of their common occurrence in acne vulgaris and folliculitis.

Ophthalmic Features

A variety of ocular manifestations have been reported in Behçet's patients including anterior and posterior uveitis, retinal vasculitis, and hypopyon, with secondary glaucoma, cataract formation, decreased visual acuity, and synechiae formation.[41] Ocular involvement occurs in 83% to 95% of men and 67% to 73% of women with Behçet's disease.[41] Although ocular involvement is not commonly the presenting feature of Behçet's disease, it is a major source of serious morbidity, and close ophthalmologic evaluation and follow-up are critical to prevent blindness in these patients.[42] BenEzra and Cohen[43] suggested that if ocular disease does not present within a few years of diagnosis, it is unlikely to be a major problem.

Arthritis

The arthritis of Behçet's disease is typically a nonerosive, inflammatory, symmetric, or asymmetric oligoarthritis, although polyarticular and monoarticular forms are also seen. The most commonly involved joints are the knees, wrists, ankles, and elbows.[44] The prevalence of arthritis among different populations ranges from 40% to 60%, and joint erosions are not observed.[42] Dilsen and colleagues[45] reported that 10% of patients with Behçet's disease had a sacroiliitis. However, HLA-B27–positive patients were not excluded from their series, and occult IBD was not excluded, as required by O'Duffy and Goldstein.[46] Other studies have shown no significant difference in the occurrence of sacroiliitis between patients with Behçet's disease and the normal population. HLA-B27–positive patients with erosive sacroiliitis should be included in the reactive arthritis or enteropathic arthritis disease spectrum, given the erosive, axial

nature of the arthritis in the HLA-B27 pattern. This contrasts with the classically nonerosive, nonaxial nature of the arthritis in Behçet's disease. Oral aphthae, ocular lesions, erythema nodosum–like lesions, pustular vasculitis, and pyoderma gangrenosum all occur in patients with IBD.

Other Systemic Manifestations

Central nervous system (CNS) involvement is most commonly characterized by brain stem or corticospinal tract syndromes (neuro-Behçet's syndrome), venous sinus thrombosis, increased intracranial pressure secondary to venous sinus thrombosis or aseptic meningitis, isolated behavioral symptoms, or isolated headache.[47] Rarely, ruptured aneurysms, peripheral neuropathy, optic neuritis, and vestibular involvement can occur.[47] Poor prognosis is associated with a progressive course, parenchymal or brain stem involvement, cerebellar symptoms, and cerebrospinal fluid abnormalities.[48] Cranial and peripheral nerve involvement may also occur.

Patients with Behçet's disease may have gastrointestinal lesions resembling orogenital aphthae. These occur most commonly in the ileocecal region and in the ascending colon, transverse colon, or esophagus.[30] Large aphthae may lead to perforation. Presenting symptoms include abdominal pain, diarrhea, and melena. It is important to distinguish IBD from Behçet's disease.[49] Aphthae may also affect the bladder.

Pulmonary abnormalities are uncommon in Behçet's disease. Pulmonary artery aneurysms occur most frequently, followed by other complications secondary to vasculitis affecting the small pulmonary vessels. Aneurysm, thrombosis, hemorrhage, and infarction can result and cause death in patients with Behçet's disease.[31]

Renal manifestations are not common. They vary from minimal changes to proliferative glomerulonephritis and rapidly progressive crescentic glomerulonephritis. The pathogenesis likely involves immune complex deposition.[50]

Cardiac complications include myocardial infarction, pericarditis, arterial and venous thromboses, and aneurysm formation. Thromboses more commonly involve the venous system, sometimes leading to superior and inferior vena cava obstruction.[40] Cardiac manifestations, either occlusive or aneurysmal, are postulated to occur due to a vasculitis of the vasa vasorum, which induces a thickening of the media and splitting of elastic fibers.[51] Atherosclerosis does not appear to occur at an increased rate, as is seen in many autoimmune diseases such as systemic lupus erythematosus.[52] Mortality in Behçet's disease is low and is usually related to pulmonary or CNS involvement or to bowel perforation.[9]

Limited data are available evaluating Behçet's in pregnancy. One case-control study reported more remissions than exacerbations during and after pregnancy with higher rates of pregnancy complications but no changes in neonatal outcomes.[53]

HISTOPATHOLOGY

Histopathologic analysis of specimens from the cutaneous lesions seen in Behçet's disease reveals a neutrophilic vascular reaction or even fully developed leukocytoclastic vasculitis. Microscopic examination of dermal capillary or venule walls shows neutrophilic infiltrates, nuclear dust, and extravasation of erythrocytes, with or without fibrinoid necrosis.[54] Immune complex–mediated vasculitis is the likely mechanism in the development of Behçet's disease.[55] A previously reported finding of lymphocytic vasculitis in patients with Behçet's disease is thought to represent an older lesion.[40]

Biopsy specimens of synovial membranes reveal a neutrophilic reaction, with occasional plasma cells and lymphocytes. Immunofluorescence microscopy may show immunoglobulin G (IgG) deposition along the synovial membrane.[42] Reports of synovial fluid analysis in patients with Behçet's disease show leukocyte counts ranging from 300 to 36,200 cells/mm³, with a predominance of neutrophils and normal glucose levels.[56] Synovitis is included as one of the O'Duffy-Goldstein criteria for the diagnosis of Behçet's disease.[57]

DIAGNOSIS

The diagnosis of Behçet's disease can be difficult, particularly in patients with only a limited number of common features of the disease. Clinicians and investigators must rely on clinical criteria because there are no pathognomonic laboratory findings. Several sets of diagnostic criteria have been proposed including those by O'Duffy and Goldstein,[57] Mason and Barnes,[58] and a Japanese study group.[59] In 2008 the International Team for the Revision of International Criteria for Behçet's Disease revised the established criteria on the basis of the presence of various disease manifestations including oral aphthae, cutaneous lesions, positive

Table 93-1 Revised International Criteria for Behçet's Disease*

Oral aphthosis	1 point
Skin manifestations (pseudofolliculitis, skin aphthosis)	1 point
Vascular lesions (phlebitis, large vein thrombosis, aneurysm, arterial thrombosis)	1 point
Positive pathergy test	1 point
Genital aphthosis	2 points
Ocular lesions	2 points

*Diagnosis of Adamantiades-Behçet's disease is made with a score of 3 points.

Modified from International Team for the Revision of International Criteria for Behçet's Disease: Clinical manifestations of Behçet's disease. The ITR-ICBD report, *Clin Exp Rheumatol* 26(Suppl 50): S1–18, 2008.

pathergy, genital aphthae, and ocular involvement.[60] Each manifestation contributes 1 or 2 points with a diagnosis confirmed in an individual with a score of 3 or more points (Table 93-1). A diagnostic algorithm based on the Revised International Criteria for Behçet's disease is presented in Figure 93-3.

Although not required by diagnostic criteria, IBD, systemic lupus erythematosus, reactive arthritis, and herpetic infections should first be excluded because the presenting manifestations of these conditions are often similar to those of Behçet's disease. Recurrent aphthous stomatitis and complex aphthosis, defined as recurrent oral and genital aphthae or almost constant, multiple (three or more) oral aphthae, should also be considered in the differential diagnosis of patients presenting with oral or genital aphthae.[61]

The O'Duffy-Goldstein criteria mandate the presence of recurrent oral aphthae plus at least two of the following: genital aphthae, synovitis, posterior uveitis, cutaneous

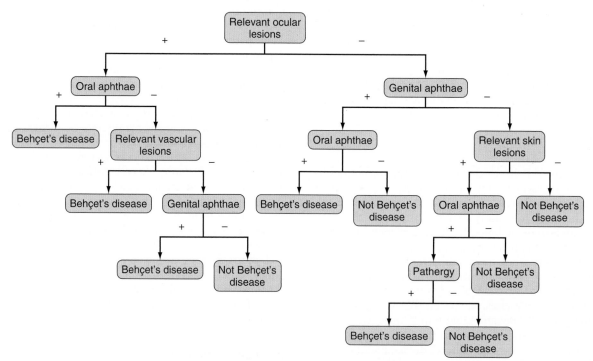

Figure 93-3 Revised international criteria for Behçet's disease: diagnosis of Adamantiades-Behçet's disease–classification tree format. *(Modified from International Team for the Revision of International Criteria for Behçet's Disease: Clinical manifestations of Behçet's disease. The ITR-ICBD report,* Clin Exp Rheumatol *26(Suppl 50):S1–18, 2008.)*

pustular vasculitis, and meningoencephalitis. Patients who have only two of these findings, one being recurrent oral aphthae, are considered to have an incomplete form of Behçet's disease. Another concern with regard to the International Criteria for Behçet's is the inclusion of acneiform lesions, which are a common nonspecific finding in both adolescents and adults. Therefore our group advocates histologic confirmation of vessel-based histology to exclude acne lesions and the use of both the O'Duffy and the International Study Group criteria to exclude patients with IBD and enteropathic arthritis.[62]

The initial evaluation should include referral for ophthalmologic consultation to identify insidious ocular involvement. Patients who have arthralgias, gastrointestinal symptoms, or neurologic abnormalities may require radiographic studies and evaluation by appropriate subspecialists. Cutaneous pustular lesions, erythema nodosum–like lesions, and pyoderma gangrenosum–like lesions should be biopsied (for both histologic evaluation and culture) to confirm the clinical diagnosis.

TREATMENT

Therapeutic options should be based on the degree of disease involvement (Tables 93-2 and 93-3).[38]

Mucocutaneous Disease

Patients with oral and genital aphthae can be treated with intralesional, superpotent topical, or aerosolized (not inhaled) corticosteroids. Topical tacrolimus can also be used, often in combination with superpotent topical corticosteroids. Other palliative therapies include oral tetracycline solutions, topical anesthetics, and rinses containing chlorhexidine gluconate. Oral colchicine, 1 to 2 mg daily, can decrease the size and frequency of mucocutaneous lesions.[63,64] Doses can be adjusted according to the degree of gastrointestinal upset experienced by the patient. Dapsone in a dose of 50 to 150 mg/day is often helpful alone[65] or in combination with colchicine.[61] Patients must be monitored for the development of hemolytic anemia and

Table 93-2 Treatment of Behçet's Disease

Mucocutaneous Disease Only
Topical, intralesional, or aerosolized corticosteroids
Topical sucralfate
Local anesthetics
Topical tacrolimus
Colchicine (1-2 mg/day)
Dapsone (50-150 mg/day)
Combinations of these agents

Severe Mucocutaneous Disease
Thalidomide (50-150 mg/day)
Methotrexate (2.5-25 mg/wk)
Prednisone
Interferon-α (3 million–9 million U/wk)

Systemic Disease
Prednisone
Azathioprine (50-200 mg twice daily)
Chlorambucil (4-6 mg/day)
Cyclophosphamide
Cyclosporine
Mycophenolate mofetil (1-1.5 g twice daily)
Intravenous immunoglobulin
Rituximab (severe ocular disease)[75]
Anti–tumor necrosis factor agents

Table 93-3 Modified EULAR 2008 Recommendations for the Management of Behçet's Disease (BD)

No.	Recommendation
1	Any patient with BD and inflammatory eye disease affecting the posterior segment should be on a treatment regimen that includes azathioprine, *or equivalent mycophenolate,** and systemic corticosteroids.
2	If the patient has severe eye disease defined as >2 lines of drop in visual acuity on a 10/10 scale and/or retinal disease (retinal vasculitis or macular involvement), it is recommended that either cyclosporine A or infliximab be used in combination with azathioprine and corticosteroids; alternatively, IFN-α with or without corticosteroids could be used instead. *Rituximab is also an effective treatment for severe eye disease.*[75]
3	There is no firm evidence to guide the management of major vessel disease in BD. For the management of acute deep vein thrombosis in BD immunosuppressive agents such as corticosteroids, azathioprine, cyclophosphamide, or cyclosporine A are recommended. For the management of pulmonary and peripheral arterial aneurysms, cyclophosphamide and corticosteroids are recommended.
4	Similarly, there are no controlled data on, or evidence of benefit from, uncontrolled experience with anticoagulants, antiplatelet, or antifibrinolytic agents in the management of deep vein thrombosis or for the use of anticoagulation for the arterial lesions of BD.
5	There is no evidence-based treatment that can be recommended for the management of gastrointestinal involvement of BD. Agents such as sulfasalazine, corticosteroids, azathioprine, TNF antagonists, and thalidomide should be tried first before surgery, except in emergencies.
6	In most patients with BD, arthritis can be managed with colchicine.
7	There are no controlled data to guide the management of CNS involvement in BD. For parenchymal involvement, agents to be tried may include corticosteroids, IFN-α, azathioprine, cyclophosphamide, methotrexate, and TNF antagonists. For dural sinus thrombosis corticosteroids are recommended.
8	Cyclosporine A should not be used in BD patients with CNS involvement unless necessary for intraocular inflammation.
9	The decision to treat skin and mucosa involvement will depend on the perceived severity by the doctor and the patient. Mucocutaneous involvement should be treated according to the dominant or codominant lesions present. Topical measures (i.e., local corticosteroids) should be the first line of treatment for isolated oral and genital ulcers. Colchicine should be preferred when the dominant lesion is erythema nodosum. *Dapsone may also be used.* Leg ulcers in BD might have different causes. Treatment should be planned accordingly. *Thalidomide*, azathioprine, IFN-α, and TNF antagonists may be considered in resistant cases.

*Our modifications to the recommendations are noted in italics.

CNS, central nervous system; EULAR, European League Against Rheumatism; IFN-α, interferon-alpha; TNF, tumor necrosis factor.
From Hatemi, G, Silman, A, Bang, D, et al: EULAR recommendations for the management of Behçet disease, *Ann Rheum Dis* 67:1656, 2008.

methemoglobinemia; the glucose-6-phosphate dehydrogenase level should be checked in all patients before beginning therapy with dapsone. Etanercept has also been shown to improve mucosal and skin manifestations of Behçet's disease.[66]

Severe Mucocutaneous Disease

Patients who fail to respond to conservative therapy as outlined for mucocutaneous disease may require thalidomide. Its mechanism of action is thought to be mediated by modulation of TNF and other cytokines. Previous studies have shown that thalidomide is an effective agent for the treatment of severe mucocutaneous lesions of Behçet's disease.[67,68] Thalidomide is known to cause severe birth defects, and all patients and prescribing physicians must adhere to the System for Thalidomide Education and Prescribing Safety (STEPS) protocol including monthly follow-up visits.[69] Patients receiving thalidomide can be monitored with nerve conduction studies for the development of peripheral neuropathy, if doing so is warranted on the basis of the clinical neurologic evaluation. Of note, the cost of treatment increased drastically when thalidomide was approved for the treatment of multiple myeloma.

Low-dose oral methotrexate (2.5 to 25 mg/wk) and low-dose prednisone are alternatives for patients with severe mucocutaneous involvement.[64,70] Patients receiving methotrexate should be monitored for the development of hepatotoxicity and leukopenia. The risk of rebound after the tapering or discontinuation of systemic prednisone greatly limits its use for mucocutaneous disease alone. In addition, interferon-α is effective for severe mucocutaneous lesions and some systemic manifestations.[71,72] A review of the safety and efficacy of interferon-α by Zouboulis and Orfanos[71] recommended a 3-month high-dose regimen of 9 million units three times per week, followed by a low, maintenance dose of 3 million units three times per week. Patients do experience the usual flulike symptoms associated with this therapy.

Systemic Disease

Patients with systemic disease such as ocular and cardiovascular abnormalities require immunosuppressive therapy, particularly in view of the risk of morbidity and mortality resulting from untreated disease. Systemic corticosteroids may be used alone or in combination with other immunosuppressive agents such as azathioprine, interferon-α, cyclosporine, cyclophosphamide, and chlorambucil.[64,73] The standard of care for eye disease is prednisone plus azathioprine.[74] If this combination is not successful, one of the aforementioned immunosuppressive agents or mycophenolate mofetil can be substituted for azathioprine.[73] Rituximab has also been effective in the treatment of severe ocular manifestations of Behçet's disease.[75] Several of these immunosuppressive agents have associated hematologic toxicity, as well as the potential for the development of associated malignancies; therefore close monitoring is essential. There have also been reports of Behçet's disease treated with anti-TNF agents. A double-blind, placebo-controlled trial showed that etanercept was successful in suppressing most of the mucocutaneous manifestations of Behçet's disease.[76]

Other reports support the efficacy of adalimumab and infliximab.[77,78] In 2008 the European League Against Rheumatism (EULAR) developed a standard of recommendations for the management of the various systemic manifestations of Behçet's disease (see Table 93-3).

OUTCOME

Behçet's disease has a variable clinical course in most patients with a pattern of exacerbations and remissions. A delay in diagnosis after the initial manifestation of Behçet's disease is common. Most patients present initially with mucocutaneous manifestations, and evidence of ocular and neurologic involvement may appear several years after diagnosis. Patients with the finding of complex aphthosis may represent a forme fruste of Behçet's disease, and they should be monitored for the development of additional abnormalities fulfilling the diagnostic criteria through regular follow-up and referral to appropriate specialists.[61] The greatest morbidity is associated with ocular manifestations (two-thirds of patients), vascular disease (one-third of patients), and CNS disease (10% to 20% of patients).[79] The most common cause of morbidity is ocular involvement; manifestations such as posterior uveitis and retinal vasculitis can cause blindness. Mortality in Behçet's disease is low and is usually related to pulmonary or CNS involvement or to bowel perforation.[9]

References

1. Feigenbaum A: Description of Behçet's syndrome in the Hippocratic third book of endemic diseases, *Br J Ophthalmol* 40:355, 1956.
2. Behçet H: Uber rezidivierende Aphthose durch ein Virus verursachte Geschwure am Mund, am Auge, und an den Genitalien, *Dermatol Wochenschr* 105:1152–1157, 1937.
3. Zoubloulis CC: Epidemiology of Adamantiades-Behçet's disease [abstract], *Ann Med Interne (Paris)* 150:488–498, 1999.
4. Kontogiannis V, Powell RJ: Behçet's disease, *Postgrad Med J* 76:629–637, 2000.
5. Dilsen N: History and development of Behçet's disease [abstract], *Rev Rhum Engl Ed* 63:512–519, 1996.
6. Sakane T, Takeno M: Novel approaches to Behçet's disease, *Expert Opin Investig Drugs* 9:1993–2005, 2000.
7. Zouboulis CC, Turnbull JR, Martus P: Univariate and multivariate analyses comparing demographic, genetic, clinical, and serological risk factors for severe Adamantiades-Behçet's disease, *Adv Exp Med Biol* 528:123, 2003.
8. Hegab S, Al-Mutawa S: Immunopathogenesis of Behçet's disease, *Clin Immunol* 96:174–186, 2000.
9. Zouboulis CC: Epidemiology of Adamantiades-Behçet's disease. In Bang D, Lang E-S, Lee S, editors: *Behçet's disease: Proceedings of the 8th and 9th International Conference on Behçet's Disease*, Seoul, 2000, Design Mecca, pp 43–47.
10. Akpolat T, Koc Y, Yeniay I, et al: Familial Behçet's disease, *Eur J Med* 1:391, 1992.
11. Fresko I, Soy M, Hamuryudan V, et al: Genetic anticipation in Behçet's syndrome, *Ann Rheum Dis* 57:45, 1998.
12. Yazici H, Chamberlain MA, Schreuder I, et al: HLA antigens in Behçet's disease: a reappraisal by a comparative study of Turkish and British patients, *Ann Rheum Dis* 39:344–348, 1980.
13. Ohno S, Ohguchi M, Hirose S, et al: Close association of HLA-BW51 with Behçet's disease, *Arch Ophthalmol* 100:1455–1458, 1982.
14. de Menthon M, Lavalley MP, Maldini C, et al: HLA-B51/B5 and the risk of Behçet's disease: a systematic review and meta-analysis of case-control genetic association studies, *Arthritis Rheum* 61:1287, 2009.
15. Zouboulis CC, May T: Pathogenesis of Adamantiades-Behçet's disease, *Adv Exp Med Biol* 528:161–171, 2003.
16. Zierhut M, Mizuki N, Ohno S, et al: Immunology and functional genomics of Behçet's disease, *Cell Mol Life Sci* 60:1903–1922, 2003.

17. Fietta P: Behçet's disease: Familial clustering and immunogenetics, *Clin Exp Rheumatol* 23:S96, 2005.

18. Remmers EF, Cosan F, Kirino Y, et al: Genome-wide association study identifies variants in the MHC class I, IL10, and IL23R-IL12RB2 regions associated with Behçet's disease, *Nature Genet* 42: 698–702, 2010.

19. O'Duffy JD, Taswell HF, Elveback LR: HL-A antigens in Behçet's disease, *J Rheumatol* 3:1–3, 1976.

20. Direskeneli H., Saruhan-Direskeneli G: The role of heat shock proteins in Behçet's disease, *Clin Exp Rheumatol* 21(4 Suppl 30):S44-S48, 2003.

21. Lee EB, Kim JY, Lee YJ, et al: TNF and TNF receptor polymorphisms in Korean Behçet's disease patients, *Hum Immunol* 64:614, 2003.

22. Hasan A, Fortune F, Wilson A, et al: Role of gamma delta T cells in the pathogenesis and diagnosis of Behçet's disease, *Lancet* 347:789–794, 1996.

23. Katsantonis J, Adler Y, Orfanos CE, Zouboulis CC: Adamantiades-Behçet's disease: serum IL-8 is a more reliable marker for disease activity than C-reactive protein and erythrocyte sedimentation rate, *Dermatology* 201:37–39, 2000.

24. Sahin S, Lawrence R, Direskeneli H, et al: Monocyte activity in Behçet's disease, *Br J Rheumatol* 35:424–429, 1996.

25. Takeno M, Kariyone A, Yamashita N, et al: Excessive function of peripheral blood neutrophils from patients with Behçet's disease and from HLA-B51 transgenic mice, *Arthritis Rheum* 38:426–433, 1955.

26. Gupta RC, O'Duffy JD, McDuffie FC, et al: Circulating immune complexes in active Behçet's disease, *Clin Exp Immunol* 34:213–218, 1978.

27. Direskeneli H, Keser G, D'Cruz D, et al: Anti-endothelial cell antibodies, endothelial proliferation and von Willebrand factor antigen in Behçet's disease, *Clin Rheumatol* 14:55, 1995.

28. Duygulu F, Evereklioglu C, Calis M, et al: Synovial nitric oxide concentrations are increased and correlated with serum levels in patients with active Behçet's disease: a pilot study, *Clin Rheumatol* 24:324, 2005.

29. Ates A, Aydintug O, Olmez U, et al: Serum homocysteine level is higher in Behçet's disease with vascular involvement, *Rheumatol Int* 25:42, 2005.

30. Ozkan Y, Yardim-Akaydin S, Sepici A, et al: Assessment of homocysteine, neopterin and nitric oxide levels in Behçet's disease, *Clin Chem Lab Med* 45:73, 2007.

31. Sarican T, Ayabakan H, Turkmen S, et al: Homocysteine: an activity marker in Behçet's disease? *J Dermatol Sci* 45:121, 2007.

32. Mizushima Y: Behçet's disease, *Curr Opin Rheumatol* 3:32–35, 1991.

33. Isogai E, Ohno S, Kotake S, et al: Chemiluminescence of neutrophils from patients with Behçet's disease and its correlation with an increased proportion of uncommon serotypes of *Streptococcus sanguis* in the oral flora, *Arch Oral Biol* 35:43–48, 1990.

34. Direskeneli H: Behçet's disease: Infectious aetiology, new autoantigens, and HLA-B51, *Ann Rheum Dis* 60:996–1002, 2001.

35. Zouboulis CC, Turnbull JR, Mühlradt PF: High seroprevalence of anti-Mycoplasma fermentans antibodies in patients with malignant aphthosis, *J Invest Dermatol* 121:211, 2003.

36. Inanc N, Mumcu G, Birtas E, et al: Serum mannose-binding lectin levels are decreased in Behçet's disease and associated with disease severity, *J Rheumatol* 32:287, 2005.

37. Lee S, Bang D, Cho YH: Polymerase chain reaction reveals herpes simplex virus DNA in saliva of patients with Behçet's disease, *Arch Dermatol Res* 288:179–183, 1996.

38. Ghate JV, Jorizzo JL: Behçet's disease and complex aphthosis, *J Am Acad Dermatol* 40:1–8, 1999.

39. Dinc A, Karaayvaz M, Caliskaner AZ, et al: Dermographism and atopy in patients with Behçet's disease, *J Investig Allerg Clin Immunol* 10:368, 2000.

40. Jorizzo JL, Abernethy JL, White WL, et al: Mucocutaneous criteria for the diagnosis of Behçet's disease: an analysis of clinicopathologic data from multiple international centers, *J Am Acad Dermatol* 32:968–976, 1995.

41. Bhisitkul RB, Foster CS: Diagnosis and ophthalmological features of Behçet's disease, *Int Ophthalmol Clin* 36:127–134, 1996.

42. Kaklamani VG, Vaiopoulos G, Kaklamanis PG: Behçet's disease. *Semin Arthritis Rheum* 27:197–215, 1998.

43. BenEzra D, Cohen E: Treatment and visual prognosis in Behçet's disease, *Br J Ophthalmol* 70:589–592, 1986.

44. Moral F, Hamuryudan V, Yurdakul S, et al: Inefficacy of azapropazone in the acute arthritis of Behçet's syndrome: a randomized, double blind, placebo controlled study, *Clin Exp Rheumatol* 13:493–495, 1995.

45. Dilsen N, Konice M, Aral O: Why Behçet's disease should be accepted as a seronegative arthritis. In Lehner T, Barnes CG, editors: *Recent advances in Behçet's disease.* International Congress and Symposium Series no. 103. London, 1986, Royal Society of Medicine Services, pp 281–284.

46. O'Duffy JD, Goldstein NP: Neurologic involvement in seven patients with Behçet's disease, *Am J Med* 61:17–18, 1976.

47. Siva A, Kantarci OH, Saip S, et al: Behçet's disease: diagnostic and prognostic aspects of neurological involvement, *J Neurol* 248:95–103, 2001.

48. Akman-Demir G, Serdaroglu P, Tasçi B (Neuro-Behçet Study Group): Clinical patterns of neurological involvement in Behçet's disease: evaluation of 200 patients, *Brain* 122:2171–2181, 1999.

49. Sakane T, Takeno M, Suzuki N, et al: Behçet's disease, *N Engl J Med* 341:1284–1291, 1999.

50. El Ramahi KM, Al Dalaan A, Al Shaikh A, et al: Renal involvement in Behçet's disease: review of 9 cases, *J Rheumatol* 25:2254–2260, 1998.

51. Du LTH., Wechsler B, Piette J, et al: Long-term prognosis of arterial lesions in Behçet's disease. In Wechsler B, Godeau P, editors: *Behçet's disease: Proceedings of the 6th International Conference on Behçet's Disease.* Paris, France, 30 June-1 July, 1993. Amsterdam, 1993, Elsevier Science, pp 557–562.

52. Kural-Seyahi E, Fresko I, Seyahi N, et al: The long-term mortality and morbidity of Behçet syndrome: a 2-decade outcome survey of 387 patients followed at a dedicated center, *Medicine (Baltimore)* 82:60, 2003.

53. Jadaon J, Shushan A, Ezra Y, et al: Behçet's disease and pregnancy, *Acta Obstet Gynecol Scand* 84:939, 2005.

54. Ackerman AB: Behçet's disease. In Ackerman AB, Chongchitnant N, Sanchez J, et al, editors: *Histologic diagnosis of inflammatory skin diseases: an algorithmic method based on pattern analysis,* ed 2, Baltimore, 1997, Williams & Wilkins, pp 229–232.

55. Lakhanpal S, Tani K, Lie JT, et al: Pathologic features of Behçet's syndrome: a review of Japanese autopsy registry data, *Hum Pathol* 16:790, 1985.

56. Yurdakul S, Yazici H, Tuzun Y, et al: The arthritis of Behçet's disease: a prospective study, *Ann Rheum Dis* 42:505–515, 1983.

57. O'Duffy JD, Goldstein NP: Neurologic involvement in seven patients with Behçet's disease, *Am J Med* 61:17–18, 1976.

58. Mason RM, Barnes CG: Behçet's syndrome with arthritis, *Ann Rheum Dis* 28:95–103, 1969.

59. Behçet's Disease Research Committee of Japan: Behçet's disease: a guide to diagnosis of Behçet's disease, *Jpn J Ophthalmol* 18:291–294, 1974.

60. International Team for the Revision of International Criteria for Behçet's Disease: Clinical manifestations of Behçet's disease. The ITR-ICBD report, *Clin Exp Rheumatol* 26(Suppl 50):S1–18, 2008.

61. Letsinger JA, McCarty MA, Jorizzo JL: Complex aphthosis: a large case series with evaluation algorithm and therapeutic ladder from topicals to thalidomide, *J Am Acad Dermatol* 52:500–508, 2005.

62. Zouboulis CC: Adamantiades-Behçet's disease. In Wolff K, et al, editors: *Fitzpatrick's dermatology in general medicine,* 7th ed, New York, 2008, McGraw-Hill, pp 1620–1623.

63. Yurdakul S, Mat C, Tuzun Y, et al: A double-blind trial of colchicine in Behçet's syndrome, *Arthritis Rheum* 44:2686–2692, 2001.

64. Kaklamani VG, Kaklamanis PG: Treatment of Behçet's disease: an update, *Semin Arthritis Rheum* 30:299–312, 2001.

65. Sharquie KE, Najim RA, Abu-Raghif AR: Dapsone in Behçet's disease: a double-blind, placebo-controlled, cross-over study, *J Dermatol* 29:267–279, 2002.

66. Melikoglu M, Fresko I, Mat C, et al: Short-term trial of etanercept in Behçet's disease: a double blind, placebo controlled study, *J Rheumatol* 32:98, 2005.

67. Hamuryudan V, Mat C, Saip S, et al: Thalidomide in the treatment of the mucocutaneous lesions of Behçet's syndrome: a randomized double-blinded, placebo controlled trial, *Ann Intern Med* 128:443–450, 1998.

68. De Wazieres B, Gil H, Vuitton DA, et al: Treatment of recurrent orogenital ulceration with low doses of thalidomide, *Clin Exp Rheumatol* 17:393, 1999.

69. Housman TS, Jorizzo JL, McCarty AM, et al: Low-dose thalidomide therapy for refractory cutaneous lesions of lupus erythematosus, *Arch Dermatol* 139:50–54, 2003.

70. Jorizzo JL, White WL, Wise CM, et al: Low-dose weekly methotrexate for unusual neutrophilic vascular reactions: cutaneous polyarteritis nodosa and Behçet's disease, *J Am Acad Dermatol* 24:973–978, 1991.

71. Zouboulis CC, Orfanos CE: Treatment of Adamantiades-Behçet disease with systemic interferon alpha, *Arch Dermatol* 134:1010–1016, 1998.

72. O'Duffy JD, Calamia K, Cohen S, et al: Alpha interferon treatment of Behçet's disease, *J Rheumatol* 25:1938–1944, 1998.

73. Lee AD, Ravitskiy L, Green JJ, Jorizzo JL: Behçet's disease. In Lebwohl MG, Heymann WR, Berth-Jones J, Coulson I, editors: *Treatment of skin disease: comprehensive therapeutic strategies*, ed 3, Oxford, 2010, Elsevier Ltd, pp 86–88.

74. Yazici H, Pazarli H, Barnes CG, et al: A controlled trial of azathioprine in Behçet syndrome, *N Engl J Med* 322:281–285, 1990.

75. Davatchi F, Shams H, Rezaipoor M, et al: Rituximab in intractable ocular lesions of Behçet's disease; randomized single-blind control study (pilot study), *Int J Rheum Dis* 13:246–252, 2010.

76. Melikoglu M, Fresko I, Mat C, et al: Short-term trial of etanercept in Behçet's disease: a double blind, placebo controlled study, *J Rheumatol* 32:98–105, 2005.

77. Alexis AF, Strober BE: Off-label dermatologic uses of anti-TNF-α therapies, *J Cutan Med Surg* 9:296–302, 2005.

78. Van Laar JA, Missotten T, van Daele PL, et al: Adalimumab: a new modality for Behçet's disease? *Ann Rheum Dis* 66:565–566, 2007.

79. Zouboulis CC, Vaiopoulos G, Marcomichelakis N, et al: Onset signs, clinical course, prognosis, treatment and outcome of adult patients with Adamantiades-Behçet's disease in Greece, *Clin Exp Rheumatol* 21:S19, 2003.

The references for this chapter can also be found on www.expertconsult.com.

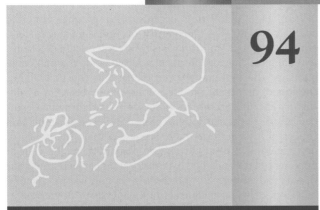

94

Etiology and Pathogenesis of Hyperuricemia and Gout ◧

ROBERT T. KEENAN • JOHANNES NOWATZKY • MICHAEL H. PILLINGER

KEY POINTS

Uric acid is the biologically active end product of human purine metabolism.

Serum urate concentrations are determined by the balance between urate production and elimination; hyperuricemia results from urate overproduction, urate underexcretion, or a combination of both.

Specific organic anion transporters (OATs) have recently been identified as playing a central role in the excretion of urate by the kidney.

Hyperuricemia is defined as serum urate levels greater than 6.8 mg/dL, the limit of its solubility in serum.

Gout pathogenesis requires the accumulation of monosodium urate at levels sufficient to drive the precipitation of crystals, resulting in the initiation of an inflammatory response.

Monosodium urate crystals activate the NLRP3 (NALP3) inflammasome, a multimolecular cytosolic complex that processes and generates interleukin-1β (IL-1β), IL-18, and IL-33.

The initiation of gouty inflammation by local white blood cells induces an influx of neutrophils into the joint; when these neutrophils encounter urate crystals, they become activated and propagate further inflammation.

Low-level inflammation is present in chronic gout and tophaceous gout; macrophages continue to produce cytokines and proteases, thereby facilitating cartilage and bone destruction.

The ancient disease gout has a complex pathogenesis, and its modern relevance is underscored by a rise in prevalence by as much as fourfold in the past half century. Indeed, gout is now the most common inflammatory arthritis in the United States.[1] Gout is a disease of both metabolism and inflammation/immunity. Gout pathogenesis requires the intersection of two distinct processes: (1) the intrinsic formation of uric acid, in the form of urate, at levels sufficient to drive the precipitation of urate into crystallized forms and (2) an inflammatory response to the crystals so formed. How these processes occur and under what circumstances they cross from adaptive to pathologic responses are the subjects of this chapter.

EVOLUTIONARY CONSIDERATIONS

KEY POINT

High baseline levels of serum urate in humans may be the result of evolutionary pressures in an era when hyperuricemia provided survival benefits.

The metabolic production of uric acid is ubiquitous among mammals and many other forms of animal life, and it is important to recognize that urate generation is not a priori pathologic. Indeed, the production of uric acid may serve one, or possibly a multitude of beneficial roles, an area of interest to molecular immunologists and molecular anthropologists alike.

Uric Acid as a Danger Signal

Uric acid is a breakdown product of purine metabolism. As such, it represents a metabolic waste molecule that might, in theory, be nothing more than a nuisance requiring excretion. However, studies by Shi and colleagues[2] and others suggest that evolution has co-opted this waste-generating process to play an important and perhaps critical role in organismal immunity. It had long been appreciated that the lysates of damaged mammalian cells can serve effectively as adjuvants—that is, can promote immune responses to injected antigens. Recently Shi and colleagues[2] used classical biochemical techniques to demonstrate that the major endogenous adjuvant found in damaged cells was uric acid. These investigators further demonstrated that uric acid had the capacity to promote T cell activation in response to antigen and that aggressive urate-lowering treatment could abrogate murine immune responses. Thus uric acid may serve as a *danger signal* to promote immune responses. As first proposed by Matzinger, *a danger signal* is an intrinsically produced molecule, typically issued by an altered or damaged cell in order to alert the immune system to the need for an immunologic response.[3] Viewed from this perspective, the production of uric acid in a virally infected cell, for example, might serve as an upstream "second signal" to promote antigen presentation by a professional antigen-presenting cells such as dendritic cells, macrophages, or B cells. Indeed, although damaged or dying cells tend to have limited ability to manufacture proteins, their output of uric acid characteristically increases during cellular breakdown. The uric acid danger signal might also play an important role in tumor immunity, and at least one mouse model suggests that modulation of uric acid levels may directly affect immune tumor rejection.[4] Although these observations require more study, they are consistent with a paradigm in which urate production at the local cellular level may play an important role in immunity and homeostasis.

Uric Acid and Human Evolution

Most mammals have serum urate levels in a range roughly between 0.5 and 2 mg/dL. In contrast, humans and other primates, including some New World monkeys, typically demonstrate serum urate levels between 4 and 6 mg/dL. The genetic and biochemical basis for these increases is well appreciated. During the Miocene era (10 to 25 million years ago), mutations in various primate and some monkey species resulted in inactivation of the uricase gene, which codes for the enzyme that degrades uric acid to allantoic acid. Genetic studies indicate that the uricase gene experienced nonsense mutations during that period, not once but multiple times across multiple hominoid lineages (Figure 94-1).[5,6] The occurrence of multiple independent loss-of-function mutations has led some biologists to hypothesize that increases

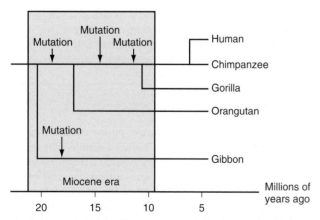

Figure 94-1 Mutations affecting the uricase gene. During the Miocene era, hominoid species experienced not one but multiple different mutations, resulting in the loss of uricase activity. The survival of multiple species harboring different mutations suggests that loss of uricase may have conveyed a survival advantage, even as it established the necessary precondition for hyperuricemia and gout. (*Modified with permission from Wu XW, Muzny DM, Lee CC, Caskey CT: Two independent mutational events in the loss of urate oxidase during hominoid evolution, J Mol Evol 34:78–84, 1992. © Springer-Verlag GmbH.*)

in urate generation may have conferred a survival benefit for these particular species. Several compelling, and not necessarily mutually exclusive, hypotheses have been proposed.

Ames and colleagues[7] noted the fact that these same primate species had also been subject to a unique deletion of the gene permitting organisms to produce ascorbic acid, an event that apparently occurred in the Eocene era, some 10 to 20 million years before the uricase deletions. In mammals that do produce ascorbic acid, this molecule serves as the pre-eminent antioxidant in the body. Thus the loss of ascorbate production may have been an evolutionary liability, for which increases in urate provided compensation, particularly as a protectant against aging and cancer.[7] Other authors have suggested that the effects of urate may have been particularly important in the central nervous system and that hyperuricemia provided an evolutionary advantage by promoting hominoid intellectual function, either through its antioxidant effects or via activation of neurostimulatory adenosine receptors (in a manner similar to that of caffeine).[8] Although the antioxidant theory would appear compelling, critics have pointed out that (1) the production of urate itself generates oxidant molecules, diminishing any possible urate benefit; (2) intracellular urate may have pro-oxidant effects[9]; and (3) the human/primate capacity for antioxidation may be large even in the absence of soluble antioxidants; for example, human red cell membranes have extensive antioxidant capacities.[10]

Other investigators have examined the specific evolutionary pressures exerted on primate species during the Miocene era, in an attempt to understand the potential advantages of urate elevations. Johnson and colleagues[12] pointed out that the Miocene era was an important era in hominoid evolution and that the hominoid diet during that time appears to have been mainly vegetarian and extremely low in salt. They suggest that hominoids during that period may have experienced a "hypotensive crisis," particularly in the face of the transition to upright walking. They further postulate that an elevation in serum uric acid levels provided a mechanism for restoring normotension, primarily through urate-induced renovascular injury.[11,12] To model this hypothesis, these investigators exposed rats to a low-salt diet, resulting in hypotension. When treated with the uricase inhibitor oxonic acid (to mimic the primate uricase loss), the rats' urate levels rose and their blood pressures normalized. The effects of uricase inhibition on blood pressure could be reversed through the use of the urate-lowering agent allopurinol. These observations imply that what may once have been a homeostatic adaptation could now contribute to essential hypertension in today's salt-rich era. In support of the latter hypothesis, Feig and colleagues[13] identified adolescents with premature essential hypertension and hyperuricemia and treated them with the urate-lowering agent allopurinol. The result was normalization in blood pressure that reversed after allopurinol discontinuation.

Although the loss of uricase promoted serum urate increases in humans and other hominoids, the levels of serum urate so achieved were not sufficient to promote urate crystallization and gout. Rather, uricase inactivation created the circumstances under which additional increases in urate production, or impairments in urate excretion, can result in serum urate concentrations exceeding the solubility threshold. Accordingly, we next review the mechanisms of urate production and excretion, as well as the events that may tip the scales toward pathologic hyperuricemia.

URIC ACID PRODUCTION AND EXCRETION: NORMAL LEVELS AND HYPERURICEMIA

Uric acid is a breakdown product of purines, and uric acid generation therefore depends directly on both intrinsic purine production and purine intake. In humans, uric acid is an end-product metabolite; consequently the depletion of uric acid depends directly on its excretion. The balance between uric acid production and excretion determines the serum urate level. Most individuals maintain a relatively stable uric acid level between 4 and 6.8 mg/dL and a total body uric acid pool of approximately 1000 mg.[14] However, it is increasingly appreciated that individuals with high serum uric acid levels may deposit uric acid either occultly or in the form of appreciable masses (tophi), with the consequence that the total body urate pool may be significantly higher than in nonhyperuricemics.[15] Such occult deposition of uric acid (total body urate burden) may have implications for treatment because they may form a "buffering reservoir" of urate that resists initial treatment with urate-lowering agents.

Urate Production: Purine Metabolism and Intake

KEY POINT

Uric acid is the end product of human purine metabolism.

In addition to the intrinsic synthesis and extrinsic intake of purines, uric acid production also depends on the metabolic processes that convert purines into uric acid. Next, we review purine and uric acid synthesis; purine intake is discussed later following Diet and Uric Acid.

Purine Biosynthesis

Purines are heterocyclic aromatic compounds, consisting of conjoined pyrimidine and imidazole rings (Figure 94-2). In mammals, the most common expression of purines is found in the form of deoxyribonucleic acid (DNA) and ribonucleic acid (RNA) (containing the purines adenine and guanine), as well as single-molecule nucleotides (adenosine triphosphate [ATP], adenosine diphosphate [ADP], adenosine monophosphate [AMP], cyclic AMP, and to a lesser extent, guanosine triphosphate [GTP] and cyclic glucose monophosphate [GMP]). Purines are also critical elements of the energy metabolism molecules NADH, NADPH, and coenzyme Q. Purines may also serve as direct neurotransmitters; for example, adenosine may interact with receptors

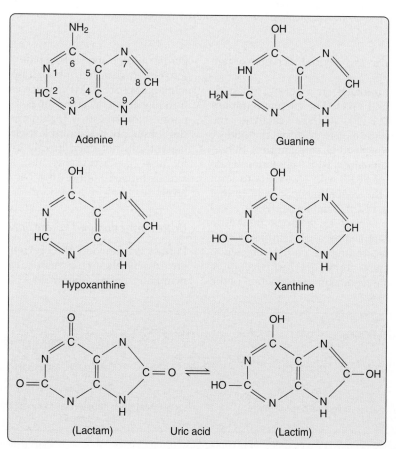

Figure 94-2 Structure of uric acid and common purines. All purine bases may exist in the lactam form in a reversible manner as shown for uric acid.

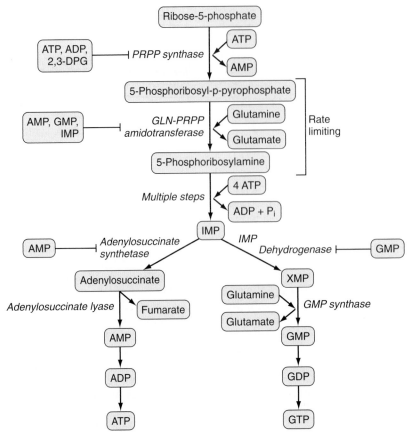

Figure 94-3 Purine biosynthesis. See text for details. ADP, adenosine diphosphate; AMP, adenosine monophosphate; ATP, adenosine triphosphate; 2,3-DPG, 2,3-diphosphoglycerate; GDP, guanosine diphosphate; GLN, glutamine; GMP, guanosine monophosphate; GTP, guanosine triphosphate; IMP, inosine monophosphate; PRPP, phosphoribosyl pyrophosphate; XMP, xanthine monophosphate.

to modulate cardiovascular and central nervous system function.[16]

Purine biosynthesis is initiated on a core of ribose-5-phosphate (Figures 94-3 and 94-4). The enzyme phosphoribosyl pyrophosphate (PRPP) synthase catalyzes the addition of a pyrophosphate moiety to form the adduct PRPP. This reaction is thought to be rate limiting. Subsequently, the enzyme glutamine-PRPP amidotransferase catalyzes the interaction of PRPP with glutamine to form 5-phosphoribosyl amine, the commitment step in purine biosynthesis. Glutamine-PRPP amidotransferase and PRPP synthase are both subject to feedback inhibition by IMP, AMP, and GMP, providing a mechanism to slow purine biosynthesis in the setting of purine sufficiency. 5-phosphoribosyl amine next forms the backbone for a series of molecular additions, ending in the formation of the

purine inosine monophosphate (IMP). IMP is converted into either adenosine monophosphate (AMP) or guanosine monophosphate (GMP), which can then be phosphorylated into higher-energy compounds. Collectively, the process of purine biosynthesis is highly energy dependent, requiring the consumption of multiple molecules of ATP. Thus purine biosynthesis not only directly increases the substrate load for urate generation but also increases the turnover of already-formed purines that contribute to increased urate levels.[17]

Urate Formation and Purine Salvage

Purines generated by the previously described mechanisms are susceptible to enzymatic catabolism, presumably to maintain purine homeostasis (Figure 94-5). Purines

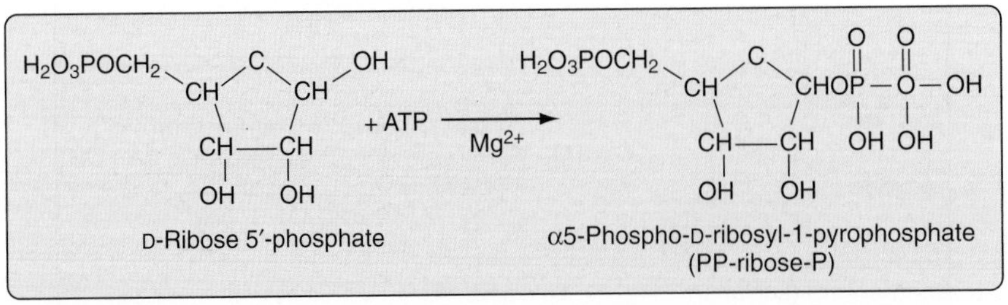

Figure 94-4 Formation of phosphoribosyl pyrophosphate by phosphoribosyl pyrophosphate synthase. In some patients, this reaction proceeds too rapidly, promoting hyperuricemia on the basis of primary overproduction of uric acid.

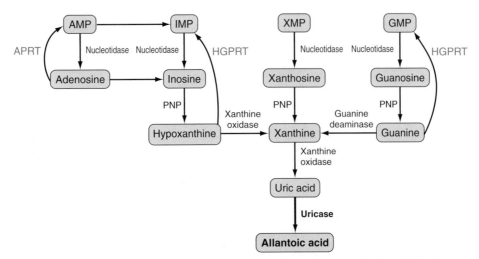

Figure 94-5 Uric acid synthesis and purine salvage. Catabolism of purines, especially inosine monophosphate (IMP) and guanosine monophosphate (GMP), results in urate synthesis via the common substrate xanthine. Xanthine oxidase is necessary for urate synthesis from any purine and so serves as a target for agents that inhibit uric acid synthesis (e.g., allopurinol, febuxostat). Purine salvage via hypoxanthine guanine phosphoribosyl transferase (HGPRT) returns hypoxanthine and guanine to IMP and GMP, respectively. HGPRT deficiencies result in not only increases in hypoxanthine and guanine and subsequent uric acid synthesis but also in the depletion of nucleotides that provide feedback inhibition on purine biosynthesis. *Denoted in bold,* mammals other than primates and some monkeys possess uricase, which converts uric acid to allantoic acid for further degradation. APRT, adenine phosphoribosyl transferase; AMP, adenosine monophosphate; PNP, purine nucleotide phosphorylase; XMP, xanthine monophosphate.

susceptible to degradation include the monophosphate nucleotides GMP and IMP. These molecules are converted by nucleotidases to their purine base forms, guanosine and inosine. In contrast to GMP and IMP, AMP is not susceptible to nucleotidase activity. However, AMP can undergo conversion, through the activity of adenylate deaminase, into IMP for further degradation. Additionally, adenosine deaminase can convert adenosine to inosine for inclusion in the degradative pathway. Further catabolism of both guanosine and inosine is mediated by the common enzyme purine nucleoside phosphorylase (PNP). Guanosine is converted to guanine, whereas inosine is converted to hypoxanthine. Both guanine and hypoxanthine are subsequently converted to xanthine, by the enzymes guanine deaminase and xanthine oxidase (also known as *xanthine dehydrogenase*), respectively. Xanthine from either source is then converted directly to uric acid, again by the action of xanthine oxidase. As noted earlier, organisms other than humans and primates including New World monkeys possess an additional enzyme—uricase (urate oxidase), which converts uric acid to allantoic acid, a relatively soluble compound that can be further degraded to urea. Lacking this enzyme, human and primate purine metabolism ceases with the production of uric acid.[18]

Presumably because purine synthesis is energy expensive for the cell, evolution has dictated that mechanisms exist to recover purines before they completely traverse the degradative pathway. These pathways, collectively known as *purine salvage,* are intimately connected to the feedback regulation of purine synthesis. The major enzyme responsible for purine salvage, hypoxanthine/guanine phosphoribosyl transferase (HGPRT), catalyzes the transfer of a phosphoribose from PRPP to either hypoxanthine or guanine, to form inosinate or guanylate, respectively (Figure 94-6). These products are then available for reinclusion in the available purine pool. A second salvage enzyme is adenine phosphoribosyl transferase (APRT), which restores

adenine to adenylate. However, as described earlier, most adenosine/adenine breakdown occurs via conversion to inosinic acid. The failure of APRT deficiencies to alter uric acid production suggests that APRT plays only a minor or redundant role in purine salvage.[19]

Urate Overproduction: Primary and Secondary Causes

> **KEY POINT**
>
> Hyperuricemia may result from urate overproduction owing to primary or secondary causes.

Primary Urate Overproduction

In some patients, inborn errors of metabolism lead to urate overproduction and subsequent hyperuricemia. Several of these deserve mention. First, a small number of individuals possess PRPP synthase enzymes that are hyperactive. The result is increased generation of PRPP. Because under normal circumstances PRPP concentrations are below the Km of glutamine-PRPP amidotransferase for this substrate, increased PRPP levels drive amidotransferase activity and accelerate purine biosynthesis.

The second well-described class of abnormality occurs within the purine salvage pathway. Deficiencies of HGPRT result in impaired purine salvage and increased substrate for uric acid generation. Additionally, because purine salvage normally results in nucleotide monophosphate generation, patients with purine salvage failure experience lower levels of nucleotide monophosphates, as well as loss of feedback inhibition of both PRPP synthase and glutamine-PRPP amidotransferase. As a result, purine salvage failure resulting from HGPRT deficiency is accompanied by purine overproduction.

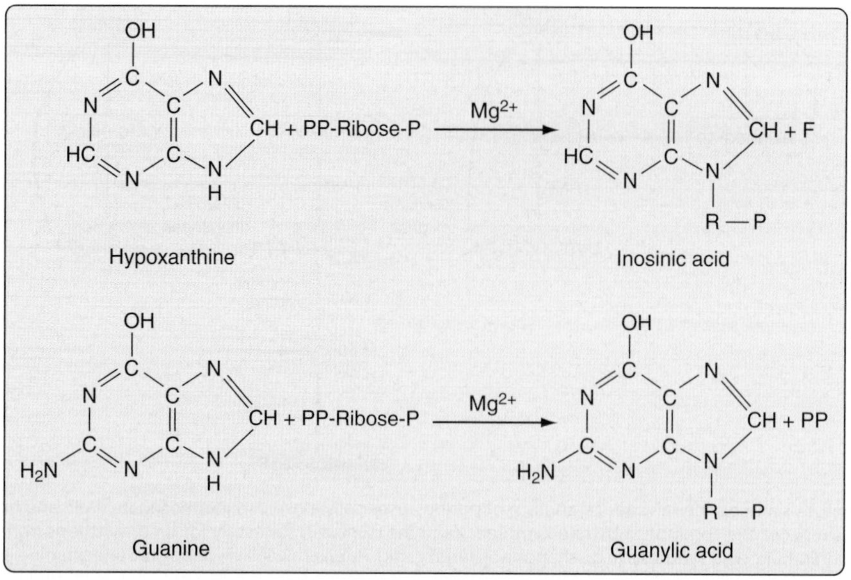

Figure 94-6 Action of hypoxanthine guanine phosphoribosyl transferase (HGPRT). Loss of HGPRT activity results in hyperuricemia and, in severe cases, the neurologic deficits of Lesch-Nyhan syndrome.

Two major variants of HGPRT deficiency have been described. Complete HGPRT deficiency, better known as *Lesch-Nyhan syndrome,* is an X-linked recessive disorder characterized by extremely high levels of serum urate, gouty attacks, nephrolithiasis, mental retardation, movement, and behavioral disorders including self-mutilating behavior. The disorder can occasionally arise by de novo mutation; female carriers are generally asymptomatic but may have elevated serum urate levels. In contrast to the gouty attacks and nephrolithiasis, which are direct consequences of hyperuricemia, the neurologic findings in Lesch-Nyhan syndrome are independent of hyperuricemia and unresponsive to urate-lowering drugs. Life expectancy can be greatly reduced, and these patients rarely come to the attention of adult rheumatologists.[20]

In contrast to Lesch-Nyhan patients, individuals with Kelley-Seegmiller syndrome have a partial deficiency of HGPRT.[21] Kelley-Seegmiller patients typically present with hyperuricemia and gout and have limited or no neurologic symptoms.[22] Several variants of Kelley-Seegmiller syndrome have been described, based on the extent of HGPRT inactivity and the presence/absence of neurologic findings. The mutations seen in the Kelley-Seegmiller variants tend to occur in regions of the *HGPRT* gene other than those identified in Lesch-Nyhan patients (whose mutations typically localize to the PRPP-binding region); whether such differences influence the presence/absence of neurologic symptoms has not been determined.[23]

Several hereditary defects of energy metabolism also promote hyperuricemia, mainly as a consequence of ATP consumption. Patients with glucose-6-phosphatase deficiency (type I glycogen storage, or von Gierke's disease) demonstrate a high rate of both purine and ATP turnover. The lactic acidemia that secondarily occurs in patients with glucose-6-phosphatase deficiency may also contribute to hyperuricemia, by promoting decreased renal urate excretion (see later).[24] In fructose-1-phosphate aldolase deficiency, patients lack the capacity to metabolize

fructose-1-phosphate. Fructose-1-phosphate accumulation causes feedback inhibition of fructokinase and fructose accumulation in the blood. As an apparent consequence of these changes, AMP accumulates and promotes hyperuricemia by the mechanisms described earlier.[25] The role of fructose intake in patients without inborn errors of fructose metabolism is discussed further later.

Secondary Urate Overproduction and Hyperuricemia

A number of secondary causes can lead to urate overproduction and hyperuricemia. In most cases, these conditions induce increased cell turnover, with resultant purine generation and breakdown. Chief among these must be counted diseases of erythropoietic, lymphopoietic, and myelopoietic cell turnover, of both malignant and nonmalignant varieties. Among the erythropoietic diseases causing hyperuricemia, autoimmune, and other hemolytic anemias (red cell destruction with increased red cell generation), sickle cell disease,[26,27] polycythemia vera,[28] and ineffective erythropoiesis (e.g., in pernicious and other forms of megaloblastic anemia, thalassemia, and other hemoglobinopathies) must be included.[29] Patients with myeloproliferative and lymphoproliferative disorders including myelodysplastic syndrome, myeloid metaplasia, leukemias, lymphomas, and paraproteinemic diseases such as multiple myeloma and Waldenström's macroglobulinemia are also at increased risk for hyperuricemia.[30,31] In some cases, particularly in the pediatric setting, hyperuricemia and concomitant renal failure may be the first presentation of these malignancies.[32] Indeed, the level of hyperuricemia may correlate with the degree of disease and cell turnover. Patients with essential thrombocytosis may also be at increased risk for hyperuricemia.[33] An association between solid tumors and hyperuricemia has been reported[34]; given the slower turnover of solid tumor cells, solid tumor hyperuricemia tends to be less common and less severe than that seen in malignancies of bone marrow–derived cells.

Tumor lysis syndrome represents a unique form of tumor-related hyperuricemia, in which cell death induced by chemotherapy results in not only hyperuricemia but also hyperphosphatemia, hyperkalemia, and hypocalcemia, often resulting in acute renal failure and arrhythmias. Although tumor lysis syndrome occurs most commonly during treatment for hematologic malignancies, it may also occur during treatment of solid tumors.[35] Although not well documented in the literature, the authors have noted hyperuricemia subsequent to the use of granulocyte colony-stimulating factor for myelofibrosis-associated anemia. Such use of colony-stimulating factors may secondarily contribute to the new onset of gout.[36]

Although somewhat more controversial, the increased cell turnover in patients with psoriasis has also been associated with elevated levels of serum urate.[37,38] An association between sarcoidosis and hyperuricemia has also been proposed,[31] again presumably relating to increased cell turnover and/or metabolic activity. However, the epidemiologic evidence supporting sarcoidosis as a cause of hyperuricemia is less than convincing.[39]

Conditions leading directly to the physiologic consumption/degradation of ATP also contribute to the potential for secondary purine turnover leading to hyperuricemia. Thus strenuous and prolonged exercise, particularly to levels driving anaerobic respiration, may induce transient serum urate elevations.[40,41] *Status epilepticus* is likely to mimic these events. A number of acute illnesses including myocardial infarction and sepsis are also accompanied by ATP catabolism and may result in transient hyperuricemia.[34] Patients with hereditary myopathies including metabolic myopathies such as glycogen storage disease types III, V, and VII (debranching enzyme deficiency, myophosphorylase deficiency, and muscle phosphofructokinase deficiency, respectively), as well as mitochondrial myopathies (including carnitine palmitoyltransferase deficiency and myoadenylate deaminase deficiency), are susceptible to increases in serum urate levels after even moderate exercise.[34,42,43] In these individuals, a limited ability to synthesize ATP on demand apparently results in a rapid turnover of established ATP pools during exercise, with resultant purine and uric acid formation. Patients with medium-chain acyl-coenzyme A dehydrogenase deficiency, a defect of fatty acid metabolism, have also been shown to have elevated levels of serum urate, although the mechanism for this effect is not entirely clear.[44]

Urate Excretion: Gastrointestinal and Renal Mechanisms

KEY POINT

Urate excretion occurs via the gut and the kidneys. In the kidneys, a complex series of urate transport proteins mediates a net elimination of sodium urate.

In most patients, serum urate level is maintained within a narrow range. Accordingly, mechanisms must exist to ensure disposal of urate, either by metabolism or excretion. As noted earlier, humans possess little or no capacity to metabolize urate; therefore urate excretory mechanisms play a critical role in homeostasis. The gastrointestinal tract and the kidneys each participate in urate excretion.

Gastrointestinal Excretion of Urate

Uric acid elimination via the gastrointestinal tract has been recognized for more than 50 years but has been relatively little studied. On the basis of radiolabeled urate tracer studies, Sorensen estimated that in healthy individuals, the gastrointestinal tract is responsible for the excretion of 20% to 30% of the daily uric acid burden.[45-47] Thus gastrointestinal excretion of uric acid may represent a minor pathway for urate excretion under most circumstances. Gastrointestinal uric acid excretion may become more important in settings of renal insufficiency, however, particularly in view of animal studies suggesting that uric acid excretion via the gut may increase in a compensatory manner in the setting of renal failure and decreased renal uric acid excretion.[48] Mechanisms of uric acid transport into the gut appear to include exocrine secretion (saliva, gastric, and pancreatic juices), as well as direct bowel secretory mechanisms.[34] Uric acid is apparently excreted into the gut in its native form and then undergoes degradation by intestinal flora.[47]

Renal Excretion of Uric Acid: Normal Mechanisms

In all but the most extreme circumstances of renal failure, the kidney comprises the primary organ for uric acid excretion. The mechanisms of renal urate excretion are complex and involve multiple steps. In the bloodstream, uric acid (in the form of urate anion) is considered to be completely or nearly completely unbound to plasma proteins. As a result, nearly 100% of the urate load entering the renal afferent arteriole undergoes ultrafiltration by the glomerulus. As discussed further later, decreases in glomerular function therefore reduce urate filtration and promote rises in serum urate levels.

Subsequent to ultrafiltration, urate (initially in a monovalent ion form) undergoes several distinct handling steps: (1) a *resorption step*, in which as much as 90% to 98% of the filtered urate undergoes reclamation; (2) a *secretion step*, in which most of the urate resorbed in step 1 is retransferred back into the tubule lumen; and (3) a possible additional *resorption step* in which a smaller amount of uric acid is then resorbed. The net result is excretion of approximately 10% of the filtered load. In fully functioning nephrons, these steps are responsive to serum urate levels, such that rises in serum urate induce increased renal excretion and maintenance of total body urate homeostasis. Early studies, particularly in mouse models, suggested that these three steps might occur in anatomic sequence, in the proximal tubule, descending loop of Henle, and distal convoluted tubule, respectively. However, studies in humans over the past decade including both genetic and physiologic approaches suggest that these functions are likely to overlap and to occur mainly in the proximal tubule. Moreover, these same studies have emphasized the importance of organic anion transporters (OATs) and other active and passive transport molecules in the movements of urate in both directions across the proximal tubule (Figure 94-7).[49,50]

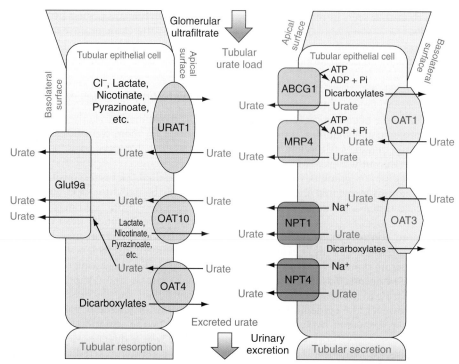

Figure 94-7 Renal tubular handling of urate. Both urate resorption and urate secretion are handled by the epithelial cells of the proximal tubule. For simplicity, resorption is shown on the *left* and secretion on the *right* of the figure. *Resorption:* multiple apical transporters (URAT1, OAT4, OAT10) move urate from the proximal tubule ultrafiltrate into the epithelial cytosol. Of these, URAT1 appears to be most important. Both inorganic (Cl⁻) and organic (e.g., lactate, nicotinate, pyrazinoate) counter-ions promote urate transport at this step; therefore rises in organic acid levels can promote urate retention and hyperuricemia. Urate is subsequently transported from the cell to the interstitium by the basolateral transporter Glut9a. *Secretion:* The organic anion transporters OAT1 and OAT3 move urate from the interstitium to the epithelial cell interior, using dicarboxylates as counter-ions. Urate within the epithelial cell is moved out to the tubular fluid by multiple transporters. Urate secretion by some transporters (ABCG1, MRP4) is adenosine triphosphate (ATP) dependent, whereas other transporters (NPT1, 4) move urate via cotransport of Na⁺. Accordingly, sodium depletion can promote hyperuricemia. ADP, adenosine diphosphate.

Urate Resorption. Urate resorption in the proximal tubule depends on the action of several apical surface transporters and at least one resorption transporter at the basolateral surface (see Figure 94-7). In humans, the most important of the apical-surface transporters appears to be URAT1 (gene, *SLC22A12*). URAT1 acts as a urate/anion exchanger to transfer urate from the tubule lumen to the epithelial cytosol. The major inorganic counter-ion for URAT1 activity is Cl⁻. However, organic anions such as lactate, pyrazinoate, and nicotinate can substitute for chloride, with potential clinical consequences as discussed later. The importance of URAT1 to renal urate resorption is indicated by the fact that patients with inactivating mutations of URAT1 excrete nearly 100% of their filtered urate and demonstrate low serum urate levels (along with increased urinary uric acid levels and risk for uric acid kidney stones).[51-53] Moreover, several well-established urate-lowering drugs including probenecid, benzbromarone, and losartan act by inhibiting URAT1. Conversely, other mutations in the URAT1 gene appear to convey a risk for increased urate resorption and hyperuricemia, presumably through a gain-of-function mutation.

OAT4 (gene, *SLC22A11*) and OAT10 (gene, *SLC22A8*) are two other apical anion transporters involved in renal uric acid resorption. Like URAT1, OAT10 is an anion exchange transporter; counter-ions that can promote urate transport by OAT10 include lactate, pyrazinoate, and nicotinate, a fact of clinical importance (see later). In contrast,

although OAT4 also transports urate from the tubular lumen to the cytosol of renal epithelial cells, the counter-ions it employs tend to be dicarboxylates.[49,54]

Urate transport by URAT1, OAT4, and OAT10 would lead to accumulation of urate intracellularly and presumably to gradients that would eventually impair further urate uptake if a mechanism did not exist to transport intracellular urate out of the cell at the basolateral surface. This function appears to be served by Glut9a (gene, *SLC2A9*; also confusingly known as *URATv1*), which was first identified as a glucose transport family protein but has little or no glucose transport capacity. Instead, Glut9a is an effective transporter of urate from the renal epithelial cell out into the renal interstitium.[55,56] A number of different inactivating mutations of Glut9a have been identified in both humans and mice; in each case the result is impaired urate resorption, increased urate excretion, and hypouricemia.[55,57-61] Glut9a and its splice variant, Glut9b, are also expressed on other cells including chondrocytes, leukocytes, intestinal cells, and hepatocytes; the role of Glut9 proteins on these cells is actively being explored.[62,63]

Urate Secretion. Other transport proteins in the renal tubule epithelium regulate the excretion of urate from the peritubular fluid into the tubular lumen (see Figure 94-7). At the basolateral surface, OAT1 and OAT3 (genes, *SLC22A6* and *SLC22A8*, respectively) transport urate from the interstitium into the epithelial cell cytosol. These transporters act via exchange with dicarboxylate anions and transport not only urate, but other organic anions and some drugs.[64] At the apical surface of proximal tubule cells, two proteins have been identified that serve as urate-extruding transporters. The multidrug resistance protein MRP4 (gene, *ABCC4*) mediates ATP-dependent urate transport.[65] Whether energy failure promotes hyperuricemia by impairing MRP4 has not been established but would seem plausible. ABCG2 (gene, *ABCG2*) also directly mediates urate excretion.[66,67] Genetic association studies have implicated two other anion transport proteins as playing a role in apical urate transport outside of the cell, namely, NPT1 (gene, *SCL17A1*) and NPT4 (gene, *SLC17A3*).[66,68-70] Additionally, genetic studies have implicated nontransporter proteins as playing roles in urate excretion including PDZK1, CARMIL, NHERF1, SMCT1, SLC5A8, SMCT2, and SLC2A12. It is thought that some of these proteins may contribute to a macromolecular complex regulating urate transport.[71]

Renal Causes of Hyperuricemia

> **KEY POINT**
>
> Decreased renal excretion of urate, owing to intrinsic or secondary causes, results in elevated levels of serum urate.

Many patients with hyperuricemia underexcrete urate; that is, for any given serum urate level, their degree of renal urate excretion is inadequate and less than is seen in normal controls (Figure 94-8). The mechanisms of urate underexcretion are various and stem from either primary or secondary renal effects.

Primary Urate Underexcretion

In a subset of patients, hereditary defects of renal tubule urate excretion result in hyperuricemia. With the identification of the aforementioned renal urate transporters, the underlying basis for some of these defects has become apparent. For example, up to 10% of gout cases in white Europeans may be attributable to hyperuricemia induced by defects in the urate exporter ABCG2.[66,67] Gain-of-function mutations of other transport-related proteins (e.g., PDZK1, CARMIL, NHERF1) may actually promote tubular urate resorption mediated by URAT1 activity. Patients with such intrinsic tubular defects leading to net urate underexcretion frequently display normal renal filtration and normal serum creatinine levels.

Familial juvenile hyperuricemic nephropathy (FJHN), also known as *medullary cystic kidney disease* (MDCK), constitutes a group of autosomal dominant disorders characterized by early hyperuricemia and progressive chronic kidney disease.[72] The hyperuricemia typically precedes the renal insufficiency and is considered to be primary. Three variants are recognized, designated MDCK 1, 2, and 3. In MDCK2, mutations in the uromodulin gene result in underproduction and/or misproduction of uromodulin (Tamm-Horsfall protein), the most prevalent protein secreted by the kidney.[73-75] The probable importance of uromodulin deficiencies to FJHN has recently been underlined by the observation that although patients with the MDCK1 and 3 subtypes of FJHN have mutations that are not in the uro-

modulin gene, they nevertheless display a phenotype of decreased uromodulin expression.[76] The mechanisms through which uromodulin deficiencies predispose to hyperuricemia are not yet understood, but mice transgenic for human uromodulin mutations develop renal tubular abnormalities and concentrating defects.[77]

Secondary Causes of Renal Urate Underexcretion

A large number of underlying causes can result in nephrogenic retention of urate and subsequent hyperuricemia. These include acute or chronic renal failure, the effects of toxins and drugs, and systemic illnesses that alter renal urate handling directly or indirectly.[78]

Age and Gender. Classic studies by French and colleagues[79] documented that serum urate levels tend to be low in children. In males, urate levels increase precipitously at puberty, a time when females experience only a slight increase in serum urate. For women, a gradual increase over the subsequent years, followed by another rise at menopause, finally brings the serum urate near to that of men, consistent with Hippocrates' astute aphorisms that "a young man does not take the gout until [around the time] he indulges in coition" and that "a woman does not take the gout, unless her menses be stopped."[79,80] This discrepancy between men and women, in the period between puberty and menses, suggests strongly that sex hormones play a role in urate regulation. Indeed, studies suggest that in women, estrogenic hormones may promote renal urate excretion.[81]

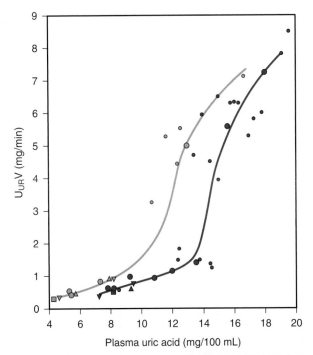

Figure 94-8 Plasma uric acid versus renal urate excretion in underexcreters versus normal controls. The *red line* and symbols represent urate underexcreters; the *blue line* and symbols represent normal controls. For any given plasma urate level, the urate underexcreting patients demonstrate a lower degree of urinary urate; they thus require higher serum urates to produce urate-comparable urate excretion. (Large and small circles represent mean and representative individual data for the experiment, respectively.) $U_{UR}V$, urine urate excretion rate. *(From Wyngaarden JB: Gout, Adv Metabol Dis 2:2, 1965.)*

Conversely, an active role for androgens in promoting hyperuricemia may be inferred from Hippocrates' assertion that "Eunichs do not take the gout" and from studies indicating that androgens and estrogens have opposing effects on renal organic anion transporters.[82] In pregnant women, increases in serum urate levels are characteristic of pre-eclampsia, a reproductive emergency consisting of hypertension and proteinuria. The hyperuricemia of pre-eclampsia is thought to result from that condition's renal dysfunction; hyperuricemia in pre-eclampsia does not lead to gout but is considered by some investigators to secondarily contribute to pre-eclamptic renal dysfunction.[83]

Systemic Illnesses (Table 94-1). Renal insufficiency (i.e., reduction in glomerular filtration rate), whether acute or chronic and for whatever reason, promotes urate underexcretion and hyperuricemia. The mechanisms of hyperuricemia in patients with renal insufficiency are complex but depend first and foremost on decreased delivery of a filtered urate load to the renal tubule. At high levels of azotemia such as are rarely seen in this era of dialysis (blood urea nitrogen >100 mg/dL), hyperuricemia is practically universal. Lesser degrees of renal failure are more variably accompanied by hyperuricemia because decreases in glomerular filtration rate (GFR) promote some compensatory increase in renal tubule urate secretion. The effects of renal insufficiency on hyperuricemia may be more apparent in patients who also possess other risk factors for elevated urate

Table 94-1 Systemic Conditions Promoting Hyperuricemia

Overproduction
Hemolytic anemia
Sickle cell disease
Polycythemia vera
Megaloblastic anemia
Thalassemia
Myelodysplastic syndrome
Leukemia
Lymphoma
Multiple myeloma
Waldenström's macroglobulinemia
Essential thrombocytosis
Solid tumors
Tumor lysis syndrome
Psoriasis
Sarcoidosis
Metabolic myopathies
Mitochondrial myopathies
Underexcretion
Renal insufficiency
Dehydration/volume depletion
Lactic acidosis
Ketoacidosis
Both Overproduction and Underexcretion
Myocardial infarction
Congestive heart failure
Sepsis
Metabolic States
Hyperthyroidism
Hypothyroidism
Hyperparathyroidism
Hypoparathyroidism
Obesity

levels. An association between congestive heart failure and hyperuricemia has also been reported. Although the effect direction of this relationship has not been well established, it is likely that the reduced renal perfusion seen in congestive heart failure can promote urate retention.

Various forms of organic (metabolic) acidoses may promote renal underexcretion of urate. Thus patients suffering lactic acidosis (e.g., in hypoxia, sepsis, liver or kidney disease, postsurgery or myocardial infarction, during excessive anaerobic exercise, or in response to certain drugs such as metformin) may become hyperuricemic. Similarly, patients experiencing ketoacidosis (e.g., alcoholic or diabetic ketoacidosis, starvation ketosis) may also develop hyperuricemia. Lactic acidosis may also occur secondarily to ketoacidosis. Although the mechanisms of these effects were previously considered to result from direct competition between the organic acids and urate for tubular excretion, they are probably better considered from the perspective of recent discoveries in renal urate transport (described earlier). In particular, organic acids serve as exchange anions for the apical surface renal urate transporters URAT1 and OAT10. Such acids therefore provide a motive force for increased urate resorption in the proximal tubule.

Dehydration (volume depletion) on any basis promotes hyperuricemia.[84] Once again, the mechanisms are complex but include decreased renal perfusion and subsequently decreased urate filtration and delivery to the proximal tubule. Subsequent sodium retention will reduce tubular urate secretion, probably at the Na$^+$/urate co-transporters NPT1 and NPT4. Patients exposed to low-sodium diets may also retain urate in an effort to retain sodium.

Several metabolic and/or endocrinologic conditions have been associated with hyperuricemia, although whether these represent independent associations has not been determined. These include hypothyroidism and hyperthyroidism, and hypoparathyroidism and hyperparathyroidism. Obesity is associated with hyperuricemia,[85] and weight loss has been shown to reduce both serum urate levels[86] and risk of gout.[87] Although it is conceivable that adiposity itself may promote hyperuricemia, this relationship is complex because adiposity may also reflect diet and thyroid status. Patients who have undergone renal transplant experience increases in prevalence of hyperuricemia and gout (2% to 13%). It is likely that the hyperuricemia in renal transplant patients is not related to the transplant per se, but to other factors such as intrinsic renal insufficiency, diuretic use, and especially the use of cyclosporine to suppress rejection (discussed further later).[88] Reciprocally, some studies suggest that hyperuricemia in transplant patients may contribute to worsening renal function.

Drugs (Table 94-2). Diuretics are among the most commonly used agents to treat hypertension and congestive heart failure, and it has long been appreciated that many diuretics promote hyperuricemia and subsequent gout.[89,90] Despite early assessments suggesting otherwise,[91] the increase in gout risk owing to diuretic use is substantial and may range as high as 3- to 20-fold.[92] The mechanisms through which diuretics raise serum urate are incompletely elucidated but include the induction of sodium wasting and volume depletion, with a resultant decrease in the fractional excretion of urate.[93] However, individual diuretics may also have more specific and direct effects on renal urate

Table 94-2 Drugs Promoting Hyperuricemia

Diuretics
Thiazide diuretics
Loop diuretics
Organic Acids
Salicylates (low-dose)
Nicotinic acid
Pyrazinamide
Other
Cyclosporine
Ethambutol
Ethanol
Colony-stimulating factors (?)

handling. For example, loop diuretics such as furosemide and bumetanide interact directly with the tubular urate transporter NPT4,[70] and both thiazide and loop diuretics inhibit the renal urate exporter MRP4.[94] Indeed, despite the volume-depleting effects of diuresis, not all diuretics promote hyperuricemia. For example, the potassium-sparing diuretics triamterene, amiloride, and spironolactone do not raise urate. Interestingly, some diuretics actually lower serum urate levels, apparently by directly promoting renal urate excretion even as they induce volume depletion. One such drug was tienilic acid, an effective diuretic and antihyperuricemic that was withdrawn from use owing to hepatotoxicity.

Several drugs that are weak organic acids may raise serum urate by serving as counter-ions to promote urate retention by URAT1 and OAT10. These drugs have also been assumed to inhibit tubular secretion, possibly by acting as urate competitors. Among these agents is the lipid-lowering drug nicotinic acid, which may not only block urate secretion but also promote urate formation.[90] Low-dose salicylates including the low doses of aspirin used for cardioprotection may also raise urate by impairing renal urate efflux.[94] At high doses salicylates become uricosuric, apparently through the inhibition of URAT1.[95] The antituberculous agent pyrazinamide is the most potent urate-retaining agent known.[90] Pyrazinamide is metabolized to pyrazinoate and subsequently to 5-hydroxypyrazinoate[96]; it is likely that these organic anions act in a manner similar to nicotinate and salicylate. Another antituberculous agent, ethambutol, can also reduce renal tubular urate excretion and promote hyperuricemia. However, the mechanism of ethambutol's action is not well established.[97]

The immunosuppressant cyclosporine is well known to promote decreased renal urate excretion and hyperuricemia. The mechanism of cyclosporine-induced hyperuricemia is presumed to depend, at least in part, on the common cyclosporine effect of decreasing renal glomerular filtration; reciprocally, hyperuricemia may exacerbate the nephrotoxic cyclosporine effects.[98] However, tacrolimus, whose mechanism of immune action is not dissimilar to that of cyclosporine, and which also can impair renal function, does not promote similar hyperuricemia. Moreover, cyclosporine's effect on urate retention appears to exceed its effects on renal filtration, suggesting a probable direct effect on tubular urate transport.[90,99] Most studies of cyclosporine's effects on urate have been performed in patients who have undergone

renal transplant; cyclosporine's effects on urate in other settings are less well established.

Toxins. Several toxins can affect the kidney to promote hyperuricemia. Chief among these is lead. Lead exposure is endemic to Western society, but there have been a number of periods during which lead exposure may have been excessive (e.g., during the Roman Empire). A connection between lead exposure, hyperuricemia, and gout has been suspected at least since the 18th century.[100] In the 20th century, a large cohort of patients with lead-induced hyperuricemia (saturnine gout) was recognized during and after the era of Prohibition, predominantly in the Southeastern United States and relating to the home brewing of whiskey (moonshine, or white lightning) using lead-lined vessels (typically, automobile radiators). Lead consumption results in distribution to a reservoir in bone and may have adverse effects on the central nervous system as well. In the kidney, lead poisoning leads to interstitial and perivascular fibrosis, as well as glomerular and tubular degeneration.[101,102] Although patients with lead nephropathy do experience mild to moderate renal insufficiency, their clearance of urate is excessively limited, indicating a tubular defect in urate excretion.[103] Suggestions that lead exposure may also promote purine turnover are provocative but have been less well supported.[104] Although saturnine gout is currently a relatively rare condition, epidemiologic data suggest that it may be more prevalent than commonly assumed.[105] In patients with moonshine nephropathy, associated lifestyle factors (e.g., alcohol consumption, obesity) may play a significant role in the genesis of the hyperuricemia.[106]

Patients with chronic beryllium poisoning, usually as a result of an occupational exposure, may also suffer diminished renal urate excretion and hyperuricemia.[107]

Diet and Uric Acid

> **KEY POINT**
>
> Diet can have significant effects on serum urate levels, both by serving as a source of dietary purines and by altering the metabolic production and/or renal excretion of uric acid.

A number of dietary components can affect serum urate levels, mainly by leading to urate overproduction. Several other dietary components may have the capacity to lower serum urate levels.

Purine-Rich Foods

Purine-rich foods comprise a major source of daily purine load and hence a major source of generated urate. However, not all purine-rich foods convey equivalent risk: seafood and red meat, particularly organ meats, convey an increased risk for hyperuricemia, whereas consumption of purine-rich, leafy-green vegetables apparently does not.[108] Earlier authors emphasized the limited effect of purine intake, with studies suggesting that alterations in purine intake may result in, at most, changes in serum urate of about 1 mg/dL.[78,109] However, such studies have rarely accounted for the role of renal urate excretion in the context of diet. Thus it is worth considering whether, for a patient who is intrinsically unable to excrete serum urate, an increased dietary purine load may produce more profound increases in serum urate levels than would be seen in a patient with normal excretory capacities.

In contrast to purine ingestion, protein consumption does not increase the risk of hyperuricemia and/or gout, a point of occasional confusion for practitioners, because many high-purine foods are also high in protein.[108]

Fructose

Osler recognized the ability of fructose to provoke gouty attacks as early as 1901.[110] Little was made of this observation, however, until the 1960s and 1970s, when it was demonstrated that fructose loads, administered orally or intravenously, cause transient rises in serum urate levels, particularly in gout patients.[111,112] These effects are reproduced with consumption of sucrose (which contains fructose), but not glucose or galactose. Biochemical analysis of fructose metabolism has provided insight into the mechanisms of fructose-induced hyperuricemia (Figure 94-9). The first step in fructose metabolism (not shared with glucose or galactose) is the donation of a phosphate from ATP to form fructose-1-phosphate (enzyme phosphofructokinase), generating ADP. ADP is then converted to AMP (enzyme adenylate kinase), which in turn can be degraded via several steps to uric acid. In addition, fructose in effect serves as a phosphate "sink" because the donated phosphate is no longer available for the regeneration of ATP from AMP and ADP. Because both Pi and ATP inhibit the purine degradation pathway (inhibition of AMP deaminase and 5′ nucleotidase, respectively), depletion of these compounds promotes the formation of uric acid as well.[113] Depletion of ADP/AMP may also impair feedback inhibition and promote purine biosynthesis. Epidemiologic studies confirm a role for fructose consumption in hyperuricemia; patients who consume excessive fructose in the form of fructose-sweetened soft drinks or fruit juices demonstrate both higher serum urate levels and increased incidence of gout.[114-117] The probable importance of fructose may be underscored by the fact that the rise in gout prevalence over the past several decades has occurred in parallel with an increased industrial use of fructose, rather than dextrose (glucose), as a major additive in soft drinks and prepared foods.

Alcoholic Beverages

Ethanol ingestion is associated with incidence of gout, and ample physiologic and epidemiologic data confirm that ethanol consumption promotes the development of hyperuricemia.[118-122] Ethanol is a particularly effective agent for raising serum urate levels because it works through multiple mechanisms. Chief among these is the requirement for ATP degradation during ethanol metabolism, resulting in increased purine turnover and urate generation.[123,124] The ability of binge alcohol consumption to induce increases in lactate levels also contributes to hyperuricemia by decreasing renal urate excretion, likely through effects on URAT1 as discussed earlier.[125,126] Ethanol consumption also promotes a diuresis, probably via antidiuretic hormone suppression[127]; as noted earlier, dehydration and volume depletion can promote renal urate retention. At high levels of acute-on-chronic alcohol consumption ketoacidosis may ensue, particularly in the setting of transient starvation and/or vomiting[128]; in such settings uric acid secretion may be inhibited, or uric acid resorption promoted by 3-hydroxybutyrate and acetoacetate, in much the same manner as lactic acid.[129] As a dietary matter, some alcoholic beverages, particularly beers and ales, are high in purines, mainly in the form of guanosine. Indeed, consumption of ethanol-free beer derivatives transiently raises serum urate levels, although not to the extent of beer itself.[130] The importance of purine load in alcoholic beverages may be underlined by the fact that, in contrast to beer, moderate wine consumption (<2 glasses/day) does not appear to increase serum urate levels.[122,131] As noted earlier, saturnine gout contracted from lead-adulterated moonshine may also contribute to ethanol-induced hyperuricemia.

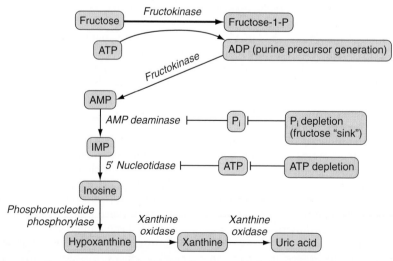

Figure 94-9 Fructose and the generation of uric acid. Ingested fructose is converted to fructose-1-phosphate, a process that uses adenosine triphosphate (ATP), generates adenosine diphosphate (ADP), and sequesters inorganic phosphate (fructose/phosphate "sink"). The ADP generated then serves as a substrate for urate generation, while the depletion of ATP and Pi results in decreased feedback inhibition of the enzymes that mediate uric acid synthesis. AMP, adenosine monophosphate; IMP, inosine monophosphate.

Other Dietary Components

Recent data, both epidemiologic and physiologic, indicate that consumption of low-fat dairy products is independently associated with reduced serum urate levels and risk of gout.[108] In physiologic studies, consumption of milk or milk proteins has a direct uricosuric effect that results in serum urate lowering.[132] Interestingly, dairy products may also have anti-inflammatory effects.[133] Regular heavy coffee consumption (4 to 6 cups daily) may have urate-lowering properties that are independent of caffeine[134-136]; these effects appear to be concordant with a reduced risk of incident gout.[137] In contrast, intermittent coffee consumption may be transiently prohyperuricemic, possibly as a result of caffeine-induced diuresis and volume depletion. Increased intake of vitamin C has been associated with decreased serum urate levels, possibly via a uricosuric effect.[138]

CRYSTAL FORMATION: THE TRANSITION FROM HYPERURICEMIA TO GOUT

> **KEY POINT**
>
> **Monosodium crystal formation involves physicochemical processes but may be regulated by synovial fluid proteins and immunoglobulins.**

Soluble urate does not induce gouty attacks; only crystallized urate promotes acute inflammation. Urate crystallization is therefore a critical step in the progression from hyperuricemia to frank gout.[139]

Uric acid is a weak organic acid (pKa1 of 5.75 [position 9] and pKa2 of 10.3 [position 3]). At physiologic pH (7.4), approximately 98% of uric acid exists in the form of monosodium urate (MSU) monohydrate. At concentrations greater than 6.8 mg/dL, MSU exceeds its apparent solubility limit in serum, the definition of hyperuricemia. Exceeding the urate solubility threshold potentiates the precipitation of needle-shaped crystals and results in inflammatory responses. However, Sir William Roberts recognized that not all patients with hyperuricemia developed gout and drew a distinction between hyperuricemia and the crystallization of MSU.[140] Epidemiologic studies also suggest that urate crystal formation and consequent development of acute gout may occur in a minority of subjects with hyperuricemia.[141] Therefore factors other than hyperuricemia must influence the formation of urate crystals.

In vitro models have shed light on the relationship between urate crystallization and environmental factors such as pH, temperature, salt content, vibration, and large molecules.[142-144] The fact that urate may more readily precipitate at both lower pH and lower temperature, for example, provides a possible rationale for the fact that gout attacks are most commonly seen in the first metatarsophalangeal joint, a joint that is both circumferentially exposed (i.e., relatively low in temperature) and at the farthest point of the systemic circulation.

Given that crystal formation and gouty attacks most commonly occur within the confines of the joint, other investigators have emphasized a possible role for joint biology per se in the formation of MSU crystals. For example,

some investigators have suggested that soluble urate is excreted more slowly from the joint than other serum elements, providing a possible mechanism for urate concentration within the joint space.[145] Once urate crystals are formed, the fenestrated endothelium of the synovium might permit the joint space to serve as a crystal "trap," preventing crystals from being dispersed and/or dissolved in the wider circulation. Other investigators have emphasized the possible role of cartilage itself in the precipitation of urate, particularly in the setting of aging and/or osteoarthritis.[146] Potential mechanisms through which aging cartilage might facilitate MSU nucleation/crystallization include changes in the proportions and/or chemical properties of cartilage glycoaminoglycans and proteoglycans, as well as increases in intracellular and extracellular lipid content of articular cartilage.[146-148] One recent report suggests that osteoarthritis chondrocytes may actually secrete urate into the joint space, promoting local urate excesses in the synovial fluid.[149]

Several investigators have suggested that urate crystallization may be an immune-assisted process. Kam and colleagues[150] proposed that IgG antibody-binding to MSU monomers, previously assumed to be nonspecific, may permit the stacking of MSU crystals to occur despite dispersion forces that exist in fluid and tissue. More recently, Kanevets and colleagues[151] postulated a role for urate crystal–specific IgM antibodies in the nucleation and formation of urate crystals.

Although urate precipitation is the sine qua non of acute gout, not all urate precipitation may lead directly to acute gouty arthritis. Imaging studies confirm that, in patients with asymptomatic hyperuricemia, urate crystals may nonetheless deposit in both cartilage and synovium.[152] These deposits are of consequence not only for their potential to directly damage tissue (see Chronic Tophaceous Gout later) but also for their role as a reservoir of uncoated and potentially inflammatory urate crystals. Thus local trauma, long recognized as a possible antecedent to acute gouty attacks, may physically release cartilage-deposited crystals into the joint space, where they can initiate inflammation. In addition, the acute lowering of serum and synovial fluid urate levels (e.g., during initiation of urate-lowering drugs) is well documented to precipitate gouty attacks[153] by a mechanism that is most likely akin to that in which glacial melting causes the sloughing off of icebergs and the exposure of previously hidden surfaces.

ACUTE GOUT ATTACKS: THE INFLAMMATORY RESPONSE TO MONOSODIUM URATE CRYSTALS

> **KEY POINT**
>
> **Uric acid crystals activate both complement and resident synovial leukocytes, inciting neutrophil influx that itself promotes further inflammation.**

Uric acid in its crystalline form is a potent trigger of inflammation. The phlogistic potential of crystalline urate in human gout was established dramatically in the 1960s by Faires and McCarty, who self-injected urate crystals into their knee joints and subsequently experienced attacks of acute inflammation.[154,155] In the clinic, the diagnosis of gout is made on joint aspiration, when examination of synovial fluid under polarized light microscopy demonstrates the presence of urate crystals, neutrophils, and particularly intracellular urate crystals, confirming directed neutrophil phagocytic activity.[156] However, the inflammatory mechanisms of gout are complex and involve not only neutrophils but other cell types, numerous inflammatory mediators, and well-organized sequences of events.[157]

Uric Acid Crystals and Complement Activation

Complement activation by the alternative pathway is a continuous process in body fluids, in which C3 component activation in the fluid phase is followed by rapid C3b deposition onto nearby surfaces.[158] On most cell surfaces C3 is routinely inactivated by regulatory proteins. In contrast, the polyanionic surfaces of uric acid crystals provide opportunities for unconstrained C3 deposition and subsequent activation of downstream complement components. Weissmann and others[159,160] have demonstrated the ability of urate crystals to activate complement from C2-depleted serum, confirming activation of the alternative pathway. Interestingly, other groups have confirmed that uric acid crystals also activate complement by the classical pathway (i.e., via C1 activation). Crystal activation of the classical pathway may occur in two ways. First, uric acid crystals may activate the classical pathway by an immunoglobulin-independent, C-reactive protein (CRP)-dependent pathway.[159,161,162] In addition, it has been shown repeatedly that urate crystals possess the ability to bind antibodies. The specificity of IgG binding, as well as the question of whether antibodies bound to urate crystals can lead to additional activation of the classical pathway, is not fully resolved.[159,162,163] One result of crystal-induced complement cascades is to produce C5a, a potent vasodilator and chemoattractant for inflammatory cells such as neutrophils.[164,165] A study by Tramontini and colleagues suggests that urate crystal complement activation may also lead to generation of soluble complement membrane attack complexes, which may activate local cells to promote inflammation.[165] Other proteins of potential import to inflammation including fibronectin and kininogen may also adhere to urate crystals.[166]

Cellular Response to Crystals

Cell Recognition of Crystalline Urate

MSU crystals interact with, and potently stimulate, a range of inflammatory cells. How crystals activate cells remains an open question, but three major mechanisms have been proposed: (1) crystal recognition via Toll-like receptors (TLRs), (2) interactions between urate crystals and cholesterol rafts in the cell membrane, and (3) direct phagocytic mechanisms.

TLRs are critical for innate immunity and permit organisms to rapidly recognize bacteria and viruses on the basis of stereotypical features (pathogen-associated molecular patterns [PAMPs]), rather than characteristics unique to the specific invader. Because crystalline urate might theoretically be treated as a foreign molecule, several investigators have examined whether urate crystals can activate TLRs.

In TLR2- and TLR4-knockout mice, decreased IL1-β and tumor necrosis factor (TNF) production, as well as decreased neutrophil influx in the air pouch inflammation model, argue strongly for a role for TLRs in urate crystal responses.[167] Impairment of urate-driven inflammation in CD14 knockout mice also appears to support a role for TLRs (CD14 is essential for TLR2- and TLR4-dependent signaling).[168] Interestingly, Joosten and colleagues suggest that TLR2 activation by MSU crystals requires simultaneous exposure of the receptors to C18:0 free fatty acids, suggesting a synergistic effect.[169] However, other researchers have observed no effect of multiple TLR knockouts on murine models of urate-induced inflammation.[170] The role of TLRs in urate signaling therefore remains something of an open question.

Other authors have emphasized the ability of MSU crystals to electrostatically interact with cholesterol.[171] Cholesterol-rich regions of plasma membranes (lipid rafts) are characteristically rich in signaling molecules and represent hot spots for cellular activation. Receptor-independent interactions between crystalline MSU and lipid rafts have been demonstrated in dendritic cells, resulting directly in cell activation. The mechanism behind this effect appears to relate to hydrogen bond–dependent aggregation of lipid rafts; aggregation of transmembrane receptors within the rafts then results in activation of immunoreceptor tyrosine-based activation motifs (ITAMs), followed by activation of the signaling molecule Syk.[172,173] Syk activation in turn can induce cell activation including phosphoinositol-3 (PI-3) kinase signaling, cytoskeletal rearrangement, and crystal phagocytosis.

As noted earlier, MSU crystals may become coated by immunoglobulins and other serum proteins and may serve as a substrate for complement activation. Thus protein-coated urate crystals may also activate cells via their ability to engage immunoglobulin, complement, and possibly other cell surface receptors. Consistent with this model, IgG- but not IgM-coated urate crystals have been observed to incite greater inflammatory responses than those that are uncoated.[174]

Intracellular Responses to Urate Crystal Encounters

Activation of cells by urate crystals results in the activation of a number of intracellular signaling molecules associated with inflammatory responses. In addition to Syk, these include PI-3 kinase; the ERK, JNK, and p38 mitogen-activated protein (MAP) kinases; phospholipases C and D; rho-family proteins; and nuclear factor κB (NFκB). Depending on the cell type in question, activation of these molecules will result in specific phenotype alterations including cytoskeletal alterations, production of cytokines and lipid mediators, and induction of phagocytosis and superoxide generation.[175-180] Additional responses, secondary to these initial ones, include vasodilation and vascular leakiness, the upregulation of adhesion molecules on endothelial and inflammatory cell surfaces, and cellular chemotaxis, discussed later.

It has long been appreciated that urate crystals can induce macrophages to produce IL-1β and that IL-1β so produced is central to the development of gouty inflammation.[176] However, the mechanism of urate-induced IL-1β upregulation remained, until recently, unknown. The NLRP3 (formerly NALP3, CIAS1, or cryopyrin) inflammasome is a multimolecular, cytosolic complex whose primary purpose is to generate IL-1β, as well as IL-18 and IL-33 (see also Chapter 18).[181] The pro form of IL-1β is cleaved into activated IL-1β by the inflammasome-associated enzyme caspase-1, which may also play a role in IL-1β secretion. In a seminal study, Martinon and colleagues[182] documented the ability of MSU crystals to activate the NLRP3 inflammasome and stimulate IL-1β generation (Figure 94-10). Subsequent inflammatory responses (e.g., TNF production) appear to occur secondary to autoengagement of cell surface IL-1β receptors. The importance of the inflammasome in crystal inflammation has been well documented in mouse models: Macrophages from mice lacking inflammasome components generate diminished levels of IL-1β on MSU crystal exposure, and intraperitoneal injection of urate crystals into inflammasome-deficient mice, as well as mice deficient in IL-1β receptors, leads to significantly decreased neutrophil recruitment.[182] Moreover, the ability of IL-1β-directed therapies to abrogate both human gout and murine crystal-induced inflammation speaks to the centrality of IL-1β in the inflammatory response to urate crystals.[183]

To date, there is no definitive explanation as to how urate crystals activate the NLRP3 inflammasome. Leading theories center on the inflammasome as an internal sensor for cell stress resulting from either (1) oxidative stress or shifts in ion concentration, and/or (2) lysosomal disruption.[184,185] In one proposed model, crystal-induced damage

to the plasma membrane promotes cellular potassium efflux and the resultant hypokalic state activates the inflammasome directly.[186] Additionally, crystal activation of the phagocyte NADPH oxidase leads to the generation of reactive oxygen species (ROS), which may then be directly or indirectly sensed by the inflammasome. The ability of large urate crystals to provoke incomplete or frustrated phagocytosis—in which a phagocyte surrounds but cannot fully engulf a target—may lead to an activated state (including oxidase activation) that also contributes to inflammasome activation.[184] The second proposed mechanism of inflammasome activation by MSU crystals is based on the ability of phagocytosed urate crystals to rupture the membranes of phagolysosomes, either by mechanical or physicochemical effects.[187] Phagolysosome rupture would lead to cytosolic acidification and intracellular release of cathepsin B, each of which has been proposed as a NLRP3 inflammasome activator.[185] These various mechanisms may not be mutually exclusive and may act synergistically (e.g., lysosomal disintegration and cathepsin-B release may themselves promote the production of ROS).

Initiation and Propagation of the Acute Gouty Attack

The clinical picture of acute gout is one of rapid, almost explosive development of an inflammatory response. Accordingly, cellular changes during the acute attack must reflect the accelerating nature of the inflammation.

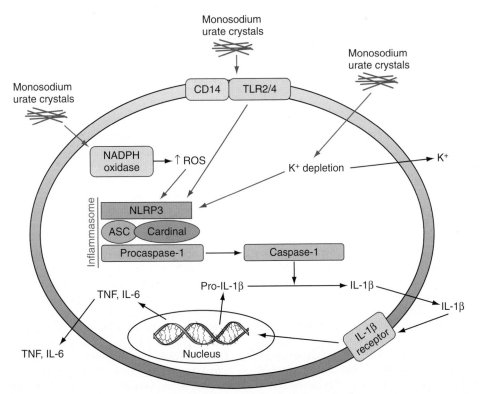

Figure 94-10 Activation of the NOD-like receptor family, pyrin domain containing 3 (NLRP3) inflammasome by monosodium urate crystals. Activation of the inflammasome by urate crystals results in activation of caspase-1, which cleaves and activates interleukin-1β (IL-1β) and promotes IL-1β secretion. In turn, IL-1β can engage its receptors to secondarily promote the synthesis and secretion of other cytokines such as tumor necrosis factor (TNF) and IL-6. Three possible mechanisms of inflammasome activation by urate crystals are illustrated: (1) production of reactive oxygen species (ROS), (2) activation of Toll-like receptors 2 and 4 (TLR2/4), and (3) potassium depletion, which may be sensed by the inflammasome. The precise roles of these and other mechanisms of inflammasome activation by urate crystals remain a matter of investigation. ASC, apoptosis-associated speck-like protein containing a caspase-recruitment domain.

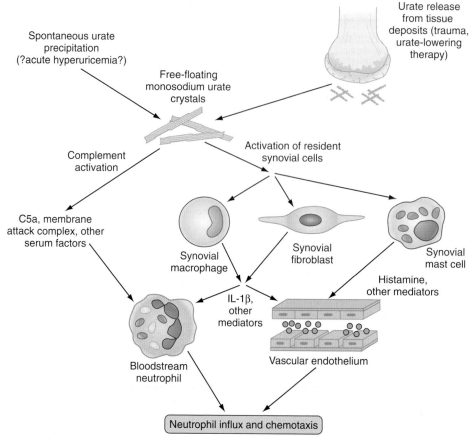

Figure 94-11   Initial phases of urate crystal–induced activation. The presence of "fresh" urate crystals, resulting either from spontaneous precipitation or the liberation of crystals from established pools, results in direct complement activation and activation of resident cells in the synovium including macrophages, fibroblasts, and mast cells. Activated cells produce interleukin-1β (IL-1β) and other cytokines, as well as multiple other mediators (not all illustrated) that in turn activate both bloodstream neutrophils and endothelial cells. Not illustrated, these responses permit neutrophils to adhere to and traverse the endothelium, resulting in neutrophil influx and the further propagation of inflammation as neutrophils undergo direct activation by urate crystals. See text for additional details.

Beginning with the appearance/release of urate crystals, the initial phase of gouty inflammation must depend on already-available local mediators, as well as cells that are both (1) capable of urate responses and (2) already in place within the joint. Clearly, immunoglobulin binding and the activation of complement on the crystal surface must be one such early response. Interaction of the crystal with local tissue cells, facilitated in part by IgG and complement opsonization, is also likely to play an early role. Best studied among the early cell type responses is that of the synovial macrophage, a resident cell in the synovial membrane. Macrophage activation in response to crystals results in synthesis and secretion of important cytokines such as IL-1β, TNF, IL-6, and the chemokine IL-8 (CXCL8), as well as release of potentially tissue-destroying matrix metalloproteinases and toxic oxygen radicals.[175,176,188,189] Activation of synovial macrophages is contemporaneous with their phagocytosis of urate crystals. Human synovial fibroblasts are also capable of responding to urate crystals, leading to the generation of both inflammatory mediators and metalloproteinases.[190] Finally, mast cells are also resident within the synovium and appear to be important in the early phases of acute gouty responses, as their depletion diminishes inflammation in murine models of crystal-induced inflammation.[191] Mast cells increase in number and activity in the lining

of experimental air pouches after MSU crystal injection, suggesting that additional mast cells may be secondarily attracted to the inflammatory site (Figure 94-11).[192]

These early events promote the influx of both additional bloodstream monocyte/macrophages and polymorphonuclear neutrophils, the predominant cell in the inflamed gouty joint. Cytokines and other inflammatory mediators produced in the early phase of the crystal response act on the vascular endothelium to promote vasodilation and leakiness and to upregulate the expression of adhesion molecules such as selectins and ICAMs (intercellular adhesion molecules) on the vascular surface of endothelial cell.[193] These same cytokines also promote neutrophil activation within the bloodstream, particularly the upregulation of the integrin adhesion molecule CD11b/CD18. A role for the crystal-generated complement component C5a in the activation of bloodstream neutrophils is also likely because C5a can potently stimulate CD11b/CD18 activation and neutrophil adhesiveness.[194] The result is that neutrophils and (in far fewer numbers) monocytes first adhere tightly to the endothelium and then exit the vasculature, followed by chemotaxis up the C5a complement gradient, leading to encounter with, and phagocytosis of, the provoking urate crystals. The mechanisms of neutrophil activation by crystals include those discussed earlier and appear to importantly include interactions with CD11b/CD18 (which is also a complement receptor) and the IgG receptor FcγRIIIB. Subsequent neutrophil intracellular signaling events include phosphorylation and/or activation of a number of tyrosine kinases including Lyn, Syk, Tec, and Src; activation of PI-3 kinase; and activation of phospholipase C.[195] Activation of MAP kinases is probably also involved because these kinases regulate neutrophil adhesion and superoxide generation.[194]

Neutrophils encountering urate crystals can rapidly promote additional inflammation and additional neutrophil influx via several mechanisms (Figure 94-12). First, neutrophils stimulated by urate crystals generate a number of inflammatory mediators and potent neutrophil chemoattractants including IL-1β, IL-8, leukotriene B$_4$ (LTB$_4$), S100A8/A9, prostaglandin E$_2$, and crystal-induced chemotactic factor.[195] Of these, IL-8 and LTB$_4$ are potent chemoattractants. They play a particularly important role in amplifying the chemoattractant gradient and promoting additional neutrophil influx. Second, neutrophils stimulated by crystals release a wide range of products capable of directly damaging local tissues including oxygen radicals and metalloproteinases such as MMP-8. Although these mediators are intended for digestion of foreign particles within phagolysosomes, the large size of many urate crystals results in incomplete ("frustrated") phagocytosis of the crystals, with the result that lysosomal contents are released into an unsealed phagolysosome and can escape to promote extracellular tissue damage ("regurgitation during feeding"). This process appears to be facilitated by crystals coated with immunoglobulins.[174] Alternatively, when uncoated crystals are phagocytosed, their ability to interact with the cholesterol-rich bilayers of the phagolysosome results in phagolysosome rupture, cellular necrosis, and direct release

of toxic neutrophil contents.[187] In either case, the result is the potential for tissue damage and rapidly accelerating inflammation.

Resolution of the Acute Gouty Attack

One of the more interesting features of the acute gouty attack is that, particularly in the early years of the disease, most such attacks are self-limited.[196] Multiple effects have been invoked to explain this phenomenon. Urate crystals may become coated with synovial fluid proteins (e.g., apolipoproteins B and E), inhibiting their ability to provoke inflammation.[197] In this context, it is worth noting that between acute attacks, some crystals may be present in the joint despite the absence of inflammation, suggesting the potential for such crystals to become inactive. Additional research has been focused on the clearance of crystals from the joint during the resolution phase of acute attacks, when the joint fluid crystal burden typically falls. Some authors have emphasized the ability of macrophages to clear urate crystals and of macrophages to clear apoptotic neutrophils that have ingested crystals, resulting in decreased crystal burden.[198,199] The enzymatic products of inflammatory cells may degrade proinflammatory cytokines, and persistent receptor stimulation may result in receptor downregulation. The stress of the gouty attack may promote adrenocorticotropic hormome (ACTH) secretion; in addition to its ability to induce glucocorticoid release, ACTH can bind directly to melanocyte-stimulating hormone receptors to provoke anti-inflammatory effects.[200-202]

More recent investigations have emphasized the local, active events through which inflammation may be resolved. For example, in vivo studies using the urate crystal–induced mouse air pouch model of inflammation suggest that local

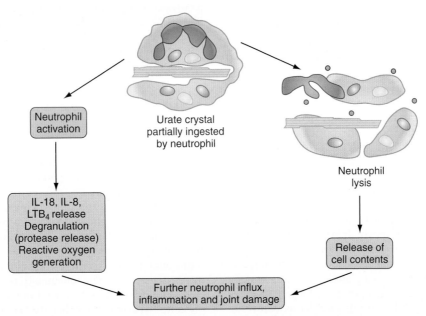

Figure 94-12 Propagation of the acute gouty response by activated neutrophils. Neutrophils that enter the joint migrate toward and phagocytose crystals. In the case of crystals coated with immunoglobulins and complement, the resultant activation results in synthesis and/or release of inflammatory mediators such as interleukin (IL)-1β, IL-8, and tumor necrosis factor, as well as proteases and reactive oxygen species. In the case of uncoated crystals, the crystal frequently interacts with, and lyses the membrane of the phagolysosome, spilling toxic contents and leading to cell lysis. In both cases, the result is local tissue damage and recruitment of additional neutrophils from the bloodstream in an explosive inflammatory cycle. LTB$_4$, leukotriene B$_4$.

upregulation of expression of PGD$_2$ and 15d-PGJ$_2$ (a spontaneous dehydration product of PGD$_2$) contributes to the resolution of crystal-mediated inflammation, probably through the ability of these molecules to activate the peroxisome proliferator activating receptor-γ (PPAR-γ).[203,204] Urate crystals also stimulate the expression of PPAR-γ itself, setting the stage for enhanced suppression of inflammation. 15d-PGJ$_2$ inhibits secretion of IL-1β, IL-6, and IL-12, as well as TNF from macrophages, and downregulates the expression of inducible nitric oxide synthase. Other targets of 15d-PJG^2 include PGD receptors and the NFκB pathway. 15d-PGJ$_2$ also inhibits CXC chemokine production, alters cellular adhesion molecules, and stimulates apoptosis of endothelial cells. Other anti-inflammatory molecules (e.g., IL-10) are also upregulated, and the more recently identified and potent anti-inflammatory resolvins and lipoxins are almost certainly involved.[205]

In considering the resolution of acute gouty inflammation, it is important to recognize the biologic programs that delay the production of anti-inflammatory molecules until the appropriate phase in the sequence. For example, PGD$_2$ and 15d-PGJ$_2$ production initially declines on exposure to urate crystals, apparently facilitating the inflammatory response, but then rebounds during the resolution phase.[206] Similarly, the generation of anti-inflammatory lipoxins requires the accumulation of at least two active cell types (either neutrophils and activated endothelium, or neutrophils and activated platelets), an evolutionary adaptation that creates an intrinsic delay before the anti-inflammatory effects are initiated.[207] Finally, a late-phase, anti-inflammatory release of TGF-β by macrophages that have phagocytosed urate crystals appears to require cellular maturation because monocytes that are newly arrived to the gouty joint generate proinflammatory rather than anti-inflammatory mediators.

Chronic Gouty Arthritis and Tophaceous Gout

The natural history of gout may include eventual progression to a state characterized by chronic inflammation and/ or the establishment of macroscopic urate deposits known as *tophi*. Even during the asymptomatic, intercritical periods of gout, low-grade chronic inflammation can persist, with continuous phagocytosis of crystals by leukocytes.[208] In patients with longstanding gout, intercritical inflammation can become frankly apparent and the cytokines, chemokines, proteases, and oxidants that participate in acute inflammation can contribute to chronic synovitis, cartilage loss, and bone erosion, signaling the progression to chronic gouty arthritis.[209]

Although tophi are composed primarily of MSU crystals, they are complex structures in which urate (1) is embedded in a matrix of lipids, proteins, and mucopolysaccharides and (2) drives a persistent inflammatory state.[147] A tophus can alternatively be conceived of as a granuloma of mononucleated and multinucleated macrophages arranged in three distinguishable zones. MSU crystals and debris constitute the central zone. Surrounding the central zone is the corona zone, consisting of macrophages, mast cells, and plasma cells. This biologically active corona is thought to account for the ultrasonographic finding of an anechoic rim that circumscribes a tophus.[210] Eventually, the corona and

central zones may become encased by a connective tissue layer, the fibrovascular zone. Within this zone, macrophages express surface markers of recent migration, maturation, apoptosis, continuous recruitment, and proinflammatory activation.[211,212]

Tophi are important not only for their role as reservoirs of crystalline urate but also for their ability to damage the tissues in which they reside (see Figure 95-6). Mechanical factors, induction of lytic enzymes, and synthesis of proinflammatory cytokines all contribute to the tophus's ability to promote erosion and joint destruction.[146] Tophus macrophages produce IL-1β, TNF, IL-6, IL-17, matrix metalloproteinases (MMP)-2, and MMP-9, and macrophage colony-stimulating factor (M-CSF).[211] These molecules promote further inflammation and tissue damage, as well as promote the maturation and activation of osteoclasts that actively resorb bone. For example, M-CSF interacts with M-CSF receptors on osteoblast progenitor cells to promote osteoclastogenesis. Tophus expression of IL-1β and other cytokines has been shown to decrease the anabolic effects of osteoblasts by decreasing the 1,25-dihdroxyvitamin D$_3$-dependent activity of alkaline phosphatase and osteocalcin.[209] Both IL-1β and TNF may directly promote bone erosions through the elucidation of matrix metalloproteinases and may also upregulate the RANK/RANK ligand system, the major promoter of osteoclastogenesis and osteoclast activation. Additionally, MSU crystals on the cartilage surface activate chondrocytes to release IL-1β, nitric oxide, and MMPs, causing further joint damage and cartilage destruction. Even in asymptomatic patients, the inflammatory and erosive processes persist; damage may not be apparent until late in the process.

NONGOUT EFFECTS OF HYPERURICEMIA

> **KEY POINT**
>
> Even in the absence of gout, hyperuricemia and soluble serum urate are biologically active and may have previously unappreciated clinical effects.

In addition to its roles in acute and chronic gouty arthritis, hyperuricemia may have other adverse as well as beneficial effects. Several investigators have demonstrated that soluble urate is biologically active, with effects on renal and vascular function. Among its mechanisms of action, soluble urate inhibits synthesis of the potent vasodilator nitric oxide; induces smooth muscle cell proliferation by activating mitogen-activated protein kinases; and stimulates cyclooxygenase-2 and platelet-derived growth factor synthesis, all contributing to arterial vasoconstriction.[213,214] Soluble urate has also been shown to directly stimulate the renin-angiotensin system in the kidney and to induce renal interstitial and tubular inflammation.[215,216] As noted earlier (see Evolutionary Considerations), these effects may promote hypertension; other studies suggest that hyperuricemia may also contribute to the risk for both renal insufficiency and myocardial infarction, though additional research is necessary to better assess the direction of causality.[217] Several recent clinical trials suggest that lowering serum urate levels may reduce the risk of myocardial infarction and slow the progression of renal failure.[218,219] Hyperuricemia may also promote insulin resistance in adipose cells, potentially serving as a risk factor for diabetes and metabolic syndrome.[220,221] Urate may also play a role and/or serve as a biomarker in osteoarthritis (OA).[149,222] In contrast to the adverse effects of serum urate, accumulating evidence suggests that hyperuricemia may protect against neurologic diseases such as dementia, multiple sclerosis, and Parkinson's and Huntington's diseases.[223-226] Recognition of uric acid's biologic complexity will likely lead to a better understanding of its impact on the immune, cardiovascular, endocrine, neurologic, and musculoskeletal systems.

Selected References

2. Shi Y, Evans JE, Rock KL: Molecular identification of a danger signal that alerts the immune system to dying cells, *Nature* 425(6957):516–521, 2003.
3. Matzinger P: The danger model: a renewed sense of self, *Science* 296(5566):301–305, 2002.
4. Hu DE, Moore AM, Thomsen LL, Brindle KM: Uric acid promotes tumor immune rejection, *Cancer Res* 64(15):5059–5062, 2004.
7. Ames BN, Cathcart R, Schwiers E, Hochstein P: Uric acid provides an antioxidant defense in humans against oxidant- and radical-caused aging and cancer: a hypothesis, *Proc Natl Acad Sci U S A* 78(11):6858–6862, 1981.
8. Orowan E: The origin of man, *Nature* 175(4459):683–684, 1955.
10. Hershfield MS, Roberts LJ 2nd, Ganson NJ, et al: Treating gout with pegloticase, a PEGylated urate oxidase, provides insight into the importance of uric acid as an antioxidant in vivo, *Proc Natl Acad Sci U S A* 107(32):14351–14356, 2010.
11. Watanabe S, Kang DH, Feng L, et al: Uric acid, hominoid evolution, and the pathogenesis of salt-sensitivity, *Hypertension* 40(3):355–360, 2002.
12. Johnson RJ, Titte S, Cade JR, Rideout BA, Oliver WJ: Uric acid, evolution and primitive cultures, *Semin Nephrol* 25(1):3–8, 2005.
13. Feig DI, Soletsky B, Johnson RJ: Effect of allopurinol on blood pressure of adolescents with newly diagnosed essential hypertension: a randomized trial, *JAMA* 300(8):924–932, 2008.
15. Choi HK, Al-Arfaj AM, Eftekhari A, et al: Dual energy computed tomography in tophaceous gout, *Ann Rheum Dis* 68(10):1609–1612, 2009.
20. Lesch M, Nyhan WL: A familial disorder of uric acid metabolism and central nervous system function, *Am J Med* 36:561–570, 1964.
21. Kelley WN, Greene ML, Rosenbloom FM, et al: Hypoxanthine-guanine phosphoribosyltransferase deficiency in gout, *Ann Intern Med* 70(1):155–206, 1969.
31. Smyth CJ: Disorders associated with hyperuricemia, *Arthritis Rheum* 18(6 Suppl):713–719, 1975.
38. Eisen AZ, Seegmiller JE: Uric acid metabolism in psoriasis, *J Clin Invest* 40:1486–1494, 1961.
46. Sorensen LB: Role of the intestinal tract in the elimination of uric acid, *Arthritis Rheum* 8(5):694–706, 1965.
49. So A, Thorens B: Uric acid transport and disease, *J Clin Invest* 120(6):1791–1799, 2010.
51. Enomoto A, Kimura H, Chairoungdua A, et al: Molecular identification of a renal urate anion exchanger that regulates blood urate levels, *Nature* 417(6887):447–452, 2002.
55. Anzai N, Ichida K, Jutabha P, et al: Plasma urate level is directly regulated by a voltage-driven urate efflux transporter URATv1 (SLC2A9) in humans, *J Biol Chem* 283(40):26834–26838, 2008.
61. Preitner F, Bonny O, Laverriere A, et al: Glut9 is a major regulator of urate homeostasis and its genetic inactivation induces hyperuricosuria and urate nephropathy, *Proc Natl Acad Sci U S A* 106(36):15501–15506, 2009.
67. Woodward OM, Kottgen A, Coresh J, et al: Identification of a urate transporter, ABCG2, with a common functional polymorphism causing gout, *Proc Natl Acad Sci U S A* 106(25):10338–10342, 2009.
79. French JG, Dodge HJ, Kjelsberg MO, et al: A study of familial aggregation of serum uric acid levels in the population of Tecumseh, Michigan, 1959-1960, *Am J Epidemiol* 86(1):214–224, 1967.

80. Hippocrates: *Aphorisms* (website). http://classics.mit.edu/Hippocrates/aphorisms.6.vi.html. Accessed April 27, 2012.
84. Feinstein EI, Quion-Verde H, Kaptein EM, Massry SG: Severe hyperuricemia in patients with volume depletion, *Am J Nephrol* 4(2):77–80, 1984.
85. Cea-Soriano L, Rothenbacher D, Choi HK, Garcia Rodriguez LA: Contemporary epidemiology of gout in the UK general population, *Arthritis Res Ther* 13(2):R39, 2011.
87. Choi HK, Atkinson K, Karlson EW, Curhan G: Obesity, weight change, hypertension, diuretic use, and risk of gout in men: the health professionals follow-up study, *Arch Intern Med* 165(7):742–748, 2005.
88. Clive DM: Renal transplant-associated hyperuricemia and gout, *J Am Soc Nephrol* 11(5):974–979, 2000.
90. Scott JT: Drug-induced gout, *Baillieres Clin Rheumatol* 5(1):39–60, 1991.
92. Singh JA, Reddy SG, Kundukulam J: Risk factors for gout and prevention: a systematic review of the literature, *Curr Opin Rheumatol* 23(2):192–202, 2011.
94. El-Sheikh AA, van den Heuvel JJ, Koenderink JB, Russel FG: Effect of hypouricaemic and hyperuricaemic drugs on the renal urate efflux transporter, multidrug resistance protein 4, *Br J Pharmacol* 155(7):1066–1075, 2008.
95. Shin HJ, Takeda M, Enomoto A, et al: Interactions of urate transporter URAT1 in human kidney with uricosuric drugs, *Nephrology (Carlton)* 16(2):156–162, 2011.
96. Weiner IM, Tinker JP: Pharmacology of pyrazinamide: metabolic and renal function studies related to the mechanism of drug-induced urate retention, *J Pharmacol Exp Ther* 180(2):411–434, 1972.
97. Postlethwaite AE, Bartel AG, Kelley WN: Hyperuricemia due to ethambutol, *N Engl J Med* 286(14):761–762, 1972.
100. Poor G, Mituszova M: Saturnine gout, *Baillieres Clin Rheumatol* 3(1):51–61, 1989.
101. Morgan JM, Hartley MW, Miller RE: Nephropathy in chronic lead poisoning, *Arch Intern Med* 118(1):17–29, 1966.
103. Ball GV, Sorensen LB: Pathogenesis of hyperuricemia in saturinine gout, *N Engl J Med* 280(22):1199–1202, 1969.
108. Choi HK, Liu S, Curhan G: Intake of purine-rich foods, protein, and dairy products and relationship to serum levels of uric acid: the Third National Health and Nutrition Examination Survey, *Arthritis Rheum* 52(1):283–289, 2005.
109. Gutman AB, Yu TF: Current principles of management in gout, *Am J Med* 13(6):744–759, 1952.
110. Osler W: *The principles and practice of medicine*, ed 4, New York, 1901, D. Appleton and Company.
111. Perheentupa J, Raivio K: Fructose-induced hyperuricaemia, *Lancet* 2(7515):528–531, 1967.
113. Mayes PA: Intermediary metabolism of fructose, *Am J Clin Nutr* 58(5 Suppl):754S–765S, 1993.
114. Gao X, Qi L, Qiao N, et al: Intake of added sugar and sugar-sweetened drink and serum uric acid concentration in US men and women, *Hypertension* 50(2):306–312, 2007.
115. Choi JW, Ford ES, Gao X, Choi HK: Sugar-sweetened soft drinks, diet soft drinks, and serum uric acid level: the Third National Health and Nutrition Examination Survey, *Arthritis Rheum* 59(1):109–116, 2008.
116. Choi HK, Willett W, Curhan G: Fructose-rich beverages and risk of gout in women, *JAMA* 304(20):2270–2278, 2010.
117. Choi HK, Curhan G: Soft drinks, fructose consumption, and the risk of gout in men: prospective cohort study, *BMJ* 336(7639):309–312, 2008.
120. Grunst J, Dietze G, Wicklmayr M: Effect of ethanol on uric acid production of human liver, *Nutr Metab* 21(Suppl 1):138–141, 1977.
121. Gibson T, Rodgers AV, Simmonds HA, Toseland P: Beer drinking and its effect on uric acid, *Br J Rheumatol* 23(3):203–209, 1984.
122. Choi HK, Curhan G: Beer, liquor, and wine consumption and serum uric acid level: the Third National Health and Nutrition Examination Survey, *Arthritis Rheum* 51(6):1023–1029, 2004.
124. Puig JG, Fox IH: Ethanol-induced activation of adenine nucleotide turnover. Evidence for a role of acetate, *J Clin Invest* 74(3):936–941, 1984.
125. Lieber CS: Hyperuricemia induced by alcohol, *Arthritis Rheum* 8(5):786–798, 1965.
127. Roberts KE: Mechanism of dehydration following alcohol ingestion, *Arch Intern Med* 112:154–157, 1963.

128. Fulop M: Alcoholic ketoacidosis, *Endocrinol Metab Clin North Am* 22(2):209–219, 1993.

130. Yamamoto T, Moriwaki Y, Takahashi S, et al: Effect of beer on the plasma concentrations of uridine and purine bases, *Metabolism* 51(10):1317–1323, 2002.

132. Dalbeth N, Wong S, Gamble GD, et al: Acute effect of milk on serum urate concentrations: a randomised controlled crossover trial, *Ann Rheum Dis* 69(9):1677–1682, 2010.

133. Dalbeth N, Gracey E, Pool B, et al: Identification of dairy fractions with anti-inflammatory properties in models of acute gout, *Ann Rheum Dis* 69(4):766–769, 2010.

134. Kiyohara C, Kono S, Honjo S, et al: Inverse association between coffee drinking and serum uric acid concentrations in middle-aged Japanese males, *Br J Nutr* 82(2):125–130, 1999.

136. Choi HK, Curhan G: Coffee, tea, and caffeine consumption and serum uric acid level: the Third National Health and Nutrition Examination Survey, *Arthritis Rheum* 57(5):816–821, 2007.

138. Gao X, Curhan G, Forman JP, et al: Vitamin C intake and serum uric acid concentration in men, *J Rheumatol* 35(9):1853–1858, 2008.

142. Kippen I, Klinenberg JR, Weinberger A, Wilcox WR: Factors affecting urate solubility in vitro, *Ann Rheum Dis* 33(4):313–317, 1974.

143. Fiddis RW, Vlachos N, Calvert PD: Studies of urate crystallisation in relation to gout, *Ann Rheum Dis* 42(Suppl 1):12–15, 1983.

144. Loeb JN: The influence of temperature on the solubility of monosodium urate, *Arthritis Rheum* 15(2):189–192, 1972.

145. McGill NW, Dieppe PA: The role of serum and synovial fluid components in the promotion of urate crystal formation, *J Rheumatol* 18(7):1042–1045, 1991.

146. Schlesinger N, Thiele RG: The pathogenesis of bone erosions in gouty arthritis, *Ann Rheum Dis* 69(11):1907–1912, 2010.

147. Katz WA, Schubert M: The interaction of monosodium urate with connective tissue components, *J Clin Invest* 49(10):1783–1789, 1970.

149. Denoble AE, Huffman KM, Stabler TV, et al: Uric acid is a danger signal of increasing risk for osteoarthritis through inflammasome activation, *Proc Natl Acad Sci U S A* 108(5):2088–2093, 2011.

151. Kanevets U, Sharma K, Dresser K, Shi Y: A role of IgM antibodies in monosodium urate crystal formation and associated adjuvanticity, *J Immunol* 182(4):1912–1918, 2009.

153. Becker MA, Schumacher HR Jr, Wortmann RL, et al: Febuxostat compared with allopurinol in patients with hyperuricemia and gout, *N Engl J Med* 353(23):2450–2461, 2005.

154. Seegmiller JE, Howell RR, Malawista SE: The inflammatory reaction to sodium urate: its possible relationship to the genesis of acute gouty arthritis, *JAMA* 180(6):469–475, 1962.

155. Faires JS, McCarty DJ: Acute arthritis in man and dog after intrasynovial injection of sodium urate crystals, *Lancet* 2:682–685, 1962.

157. Pessler F, Mayer CT, Jung SM, et al: Identification of novel monosodium urate crystal regulated mRNAs by transcript profiling of dissected murine air pouch membranes, *Arthritis Res Ther* 10(3):R64, 2008.

159. Fields TR, Abramson SB, Weissmann G, et al: Activation of the alternative pathway of complement by monosodium urate crystals, *Clin Immunol Immunopathol* 26(2):249–257, 1983.

160. Doherty M, Whicher JT, Dieppe PA: Activation of the alternative pathway of complement by monosodium urate monohydrate crystals and other inflammatory particles, *Ann Rheum Dis* 42(3):285–291, 1983.

161. Giclas PC, Ginsberg MH, Cooper NR: Immunoglobulin G independent activation of the classical complement pathway by monosodium urate crystals, *J Clin Invest* 63(4):759–764, 1979.

162. Russell IJ, Papaioannou C, McDuffie FC, et al: Effect of IgG and C-reactive protein on complement depletion by monosodium urate crystals, *J Rheumatol* 10(3):425–433, 1983.

163. Hasselbacher P: Binding of IgG and complement protein by monosodium urate monohydrate and other crystals, *J Lab Clin Med* 94(4):532–541, 1979.

164. Hasselbacher P: C3 activation by monosodium urate monohydrate and other crystalline material, *Arthritis Rheum* 22(6):571–578, 1979.

165. Russell IJ, Mansen C, Kolb LM, Kolb WP: Activation of the fifth component of human complement (C5) induced by monosodium urate crystals: C5 convertase assembly on the crystal surface, *Clin Immunol Immunopathol* 24(2):239–250, 1982.

166. Terkeltaub R, Tenner AJ, Kozin F, Ginsberg MH: Plasma protein binding by monosodium urate crystals. Analysis by two-dimensional gel electrophoresis, *Arthritis Rheum* 26(6):775–783, 1983.

167. Liu-Bryan R, Scott P, Sydlaske A, et al: Innate immunity conferred by Toll-like receptors 2 and 4 and myeloid differentiation factor 88 expression is pivotal to monosodium urate monohydrate crystal-induced inflammation, *Arthritis Rheum* 52(9):2936–2946, 2005.

168. Scott P, Ma H, Viriyakosol S, et al: Engagement of CD14 mediates the inflammatory potential of monosodium urate crystals, *J Immunol* 177(9):6370–6378, 2006.

170. Chen CJ, Shi Y, Hearn A, et al: MyD88-dependent IL-1 receptor signaling is essential for gouty inflammation stimulated by monosodium urate crystals, *J Clin Invest* 116(8):2262–2271, 2006.

171. Weissmann G, Rita GA: Molecular basis of gouty inflammation: interaction of monosodium urate crystals with lysosomes and liposomes, *Nat New Biol* 240(101):167–172, 1972.

174. Kozin F, Ginsberg MH, Skosey JL: Polymorphonuclear leukocyte responses to monosodium urate crystals: modification by adsorbed serum proteins, *J Rheumatol* 6(5):519–526, 1979.

175. di Giovine FS, Malawista SE, Thornton E, Duff GW: Urate crystals stimulate production of tumor necrosis factor alpha from human blood monocytes and synovial cells. Cytokine mRNA and protein kinetics, and cellular distribution, *J Clin Invest* 87(4):1375–1381, 1991.

176. Di Giovine FS, Malawista SE, Nuki G, Duff GW: Interleukin 1 (IL 1) as a mediator of crystal arthritis. Stimulation of T cell and synovial fibroblast mitogenesis by urate crystal-induced IL 1, *J Immunol* 138(10):3213–3218, 1987.

177. Abramson S, Hoffstein ST, Weissmann G: Superoxide anion generation by human neutrophils exposed to monosodium urate, *Arthritis Rheum* 25(2):174–180, 1982.

178. Serhan CN, Lundberg U, Weissmann G, Samuelsson B: Formation of leukotrienes and hydroxy acids by human neutrophils and platelets exposed to monosodium urate, *Prostaglandins* 27(4):563–581, 1984.

179. Pouliot M, James MJ, McColl SR, et al: Monosodium urate microcrystals induce cyclooxygenase-2 in human monocytes, *Blood* 91(5):1769–1776, 1998.

181. Martinon F: Update on biology: uric acid and the activation of immune and inflammatory cells, *Curr Rheumatol Rep* 12(2):135–141, 2010.

182. Martinon F, Petrilli V, Mayor A, et al: Gout-associated uric acid crystals activate the NALP3 inflammasome, *Nature* 440(7081):237–241, 2006.

184. Martinon F, Mayor A, Tschopp J: The inflammasomes: guardians of the body, *Annu Rev Immunol* 27:229–265, 2009.

186. Petrilli V, Papin S, Dostert C, et al: Activation of the NALP3 inflammasome is triggered by low intracellular potassium concentration, *Cell Death Differ* 14(9):1583–1589, 2007.

187. Hoffstein S, Weissmann G: Mechanisms of lysosomal enzyme release from leukocytes. IV. Interaction of monosodium urate crystals with dogfish and human leukocytes, *Arthritis Rheum* 18(2):153–165, 1975.

188. Guerne PA, Terkeltaub R, Zuraw B, Lotz M: Inflammatory microcrystals stimulate interleukin-6 production and secretion by human monocytes and synoviocytes, *Arthritis Rheum* 32(11):1443–1452, 1989.

189. Terkeltaub R, Zachariae C, Santoro D, et al: Monocyte-derived neutrophil chemotactic factor/interleukin-8 is a potential mediator of crystal-induced inflammation, *Arthritis Rheum* 34(7):894–903, 1991.

190. Wigley FM, Fine IT, Newcombe DS: The role of the human synovial fibroblast in monosodium urate crystal-induced synovitis, *J Rheumatol* 10(4):602–611, 1983.

191. Getting SJ, Flower RJ, Parente L, et al: Molecular determinants of monosodium urate crystal-induced murine peritonitis: a role for endogenous mast cells and a distinct requirement for endothelial-derived selectins, *J Pharmacol Exp Ther* 283(1):123–130, 1997.

193. Chapman PT, Yarwood H, Harrison AA, et al: Endothelial activation in monosodium urate monohydrate crystal-induced inflammation: in vitro and in vivo studies on the roles of tumor necrosis factor alpha and interleukin-1, *Arthritis Rheum* 40(5):955–965, 1997.

195. Popa-Nita O, Naccache PH: Crystal-induced neutrophil activation, *Immunol Cell Biol* 88(1):32–40, 2010.

196. Cronstein BN, Terkeltaub R: The inflammatory process of gout and its treatment, *Arthritis Res Ther* 8(Suppl 1):S3, 2006.

197. Terkeltaub RA, Dyer CA, Martin J, Curtiss LK: Apolipoprotein (apo) E inhibits the capacity of monosodium urate crystals to stimulate

neutrophils. Characterization of intraarticular apo E and demonstration of apo E binding to urate crystals in vivo, *J Clin Invest* 87(1):20–26, 1991.

198. Yagnik DR, Hillyer P, Marshall D, et al: Noninflammatory phagocytosis of monosodium urate monohydrate crystals by mouse macrophages. Implications for the control of joint inflammation in gout, *Arthritis Rheum* 43(8):1779–1789, 2000.

199. Landis RC, Yagnik DR, Florey O, et al: Safe disposal of inflammatory monosodium urate monohydrate crystals by differentiated macrophages, *Arthritis Rheum* 46(11):3026–3033, 2002.

200. Getting SJ, Christian HC, Flower RJ, Perretti M: Activation of melanocortin type 3 receptor as a molecular mechanism for adrenocorticotropic hormone efficacy in gouty arthritis, *Arthritis Rheum* 46(10):2765–2775, 2002.

203. Akahoshi T, Namai R, Murakami Y, et al: Rapid induction of peroxisome proliferator-activated receptor gamma expression in human monocytes by monosodium urate monohydrate crystals, *Arthritis Rheum* 48(1):231–239, 2003.

204. Scher JU, Pillinger MH: 15d-PGJ(2): The anti-inflammatory prostaglandin? *Clin Immunol* 114(2):100–109, 2005.

205. Serhan CN, Krishnamoorthy S, Recchiuti A, Chiang N: Novel anti-inflammatory–pro-resolving mediators and their receptors, *Curr Top Med Chem* 11:629–647, 2011.

206. Murakami Y, Akahoshi T, Hayashi I, et al: Inhibition of monosodium urate monohydrate crystal-induced acute inflammation by retrovirally transfected prostaglandin D synthase, *Arthritis Rheum* 48(10):2931–2941, 2003.

207. Serhan CN, Savill J: Resolution of inflammation: the beginning programs the end, *Nat Immunol* 6(12):1191–1197, 2005.

208. Pascual E, Batlle-Gualda E, Martinez A, et al: Synovial fluid analysis for diagnosis of intercritical gout, *Ann Intern Med* 131(10):756–759, 1999.

209. Choi HK, Mount DB, Reginato AM: Pathogenesis of gout, *Ann Intern Med* 143(7):499–516, 2005.

210. Carter JD, Kedar RP, Anderson SR, et al: An analysis of MRI and ultrasound imaging in patients with gout who have normal plain radiographs, *Rheumatology (Oxford)* 48(11):1442–1446, 2009.

212. Palmer DG, Highton J, Hessian PA: Development of the gout tophus. An hypothesis, *Am J Clin Pathol* 91(2):190–195, 1989.

213. Corry DB, Eslami P, Yamamoto K, et al: Uric acid stimulates vascular smooth muscle cell proliferation and oxidative stress via the vascular renin-angiotensin system, *J Hypertens* 26(2):269–275, 2008.

215. Mazzali M, Hughes J, Kim YG, et al: Elevated uric acid increases blood pressure in the rat by a novel crystal-independent mechanism, *Hypertension* 38(5):1101–1106, 2001.

217. Pillinger MH, Goldfarb DS, Keenan RT: Gout and its comorbidities, *Bull NYU Hosp Jt Dis* 68(3):199–203, 2010.

219. Whelton A, MacDonald PA, Zhao L, et al: Renal function in gout: long-term treatment effects of febuxostat, *J Clin Rheumatol* 17(1):7–13, 2011.

222. Nowatzky J, Howard R, Pillinger MH, Krasnokutsky S: The role of uric acid and other crystals in osteoarthritis, *Curr Rheumatol Rep* 12(2):142–148, 2010.

223. Alonso A, Rodriguez LA, Logroscino G, Hernan MA: Gout and risk of Parkinson disease: a prospective study, *Neurology* 69(17):1696–1700, 2007.

224. Euser SM, Hofman A, Westendorp RG, Breteler MM: Serum uric acid and cognitive function and dementia, *Brain* 132(Pt 2):377–382, 2009.

225. Guerrero AL, Gutierrez F, Iglesias F, et al: Serum uric acid levels in multiple sclerosis patients inversely correlate with disability, *Neurol Sci* 32(2):347–350, 2011.

226. Auinger P, Kieburtz K, McDermott MP: The relationship between uric acid levels and Huntington's disease progression, *Mov Disord* 25(2):224–228, 2010.

Full references for this chapter can be found on www.expertconsult.com.

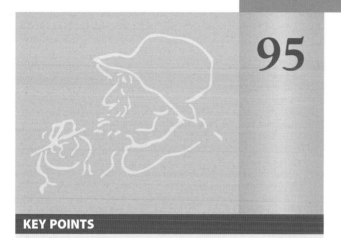

95

Clinical Features and Treatment of Gout

CHRISTOPHER M. BURNS •
ROBERT L. WORTMANN

Gout has been called the "king of diseases" and the "disease of kings." Today, the term *gout* is used to represent a heterogeneous group of diseases found exclusively in humans that include the following characteristics:

- Elevated serum urate concentration (hyperuricemia)
- Recurrent attacks of acute arthritis in which monosodium urate monohydrate crystals are demonstrable in synovial fluid leukocytes
- Aggregates of sodium urate monohydrate crystals (tophi) deposited chiefly in and around joints, which sometimes lead to deformity and crippling
- Renal disease involving glomerular, tubular, and interstitial tissues and blood vessels
- Uric acid nephrolithiasis

These manifestations can occur in various combinations.[1,2]

Hyperuricemia denotes an elevated level of urate in the blood. This occurs in an absolute (or physiochemical) sense when the serum urate concentration exceeds the limit of solubility of monosodium urate in the serum, which is 6.8 mg/dL at 37° C. Thus a value greater than 6.8 mg/dL indicates supersaturation of body fluids. The serum urate concentration is elevated in a relative sense when it exceeds the upper limit of an arbitrary normal range, which is usually defined as the mean serum urate value plus two standard deviations in a sex- and age-matched healthy population. In most epidemiologic studies, the upper limit has been rounded off at 7 mg/dL in men and 6 mg/dL in women. A serum urate value in excess of 7 mg/dL begins to carry an increased risk of gouty arthritis or renal stones.

EPIDEMIOLOGY

Hyperuricemia is fairly common, with prevalence ranging between 2.6% and 47.2% in various populations.[3,4] A variety of factors appears to be associated with high serum urate concentrations. In adults, serum urate levels correlate strongly with the serum creatinine and urea nitrogen levels, body weight, height, age, blood pressure, and alcohol intake.[5] In epidemiologic studies, body bulk (as estimated by body weight, surface area, or body mass index) has proved to be one of the most important predictors of hyperuricemia in people of many different races and cultures, with rare exceptions.[6-8]

Serum urate concentrations vary with age and sex. Children normally have a concentration in the range of 3 to 4 mg/dL because of high renal uric acid clearance.[9] At puberty, serum urate concentrations increase by 1 to 2 mg/dL in males, and this higher level is generally sustained throughout life. In contrast, females exhibit little change in the serum urate concentration until menopause, when concentrations increase and approach those seen in adult men. The mechanism of lower serum urate levels in women is a consequence of sex hormones and is related to a higher fractional excretion of urate secondary to lower tubular urate postsecretory reabsorption.[10]

The incidence of gout varies among populations, with an overall prevalence ranging from less than 1% to 15.3%.[5]

This upper limit appears to be increasing.[11,12] The prevalence increases substantially with age and with increasing serum urate concentration. The annual incidence rate of gout is 4.9% for urate levels greater than 9 mg/dL, 0.5% for values between 7 and 8.9 mg/dL, and 0.1% for values less than 7 mg/dL.[13] For serum urate values greater than 9 mg/dL, the cumulative incidence of gout reaches 22% after 5 years.

ENVIRONMENTAL FACTORS

KEY POINTS

Many environmental factors are associated with gout including alcohol consumption, particularly beer, and diet.

Certain foods clearly promote hyperuricemia and gout including alcohol, seafood, and red meat.

The consumption of some foods may be protective, especially milk and yogurt.

An association between alcohol consumption and gout has been recognized for centuries. The risk of developing gout varies by the type of alcohol ingested.[14] Beer, which is purine rich, carries the highest risk; this risk is substantially greater than that for liquor. Moderate wine drinking does not increase the risk of gout. The quantity of alcohol also strongly correlates with gout. Compared with men who did not consume alcohol, the relative risk of gout was 1.32 for an alcohol intake of 10 to 14.9 g/day, 1.49 for 15 to 29.9 g/day, 1.96 for 30 to 49.9 g/day, and 2.53 for 50 g/day and higher, with calculations based on 12.8 g of alcohol per 12 oz serving of regular beer, 11.3 g per 12 oz. serving of light beer, 11 g per 4 oz. serving of wine, and 14 g per shot of liquor.

Diet also influences hyperuricemia and gout. Serum urate levels increase with meat or seafood intake and decrease with dairy intake.[15] Men in the highest quintile of seafood consumption have a 51% higher risk of developing gout, and those in the highest quintile of meat intake have a 41% higher risk. However, consumption of oatmeal and purine-rich vegetables (e.g., peas, mushrooms, lentils, spinach, cauliflower) is not associated with an increased risk for gout. The consumption of milk one or more times a day or yogurt consumption at least once every other day is associated with lower serum urate levels.

GENETICS

KEY POINTS

Rare forms of early hyperuricemia and gout have a clear genetic and metabolic basis.

Gout often runs in families, probably because of inherited factors affecting serum urate levels through renal urate clearance.

Recent genome-wide association studies have identified polymorphisms in several candidate genes encoding urate transporters in the renal proximal tubules as determinants of serum urate levels and the risk of gout.

Since antiquity, gout has been recognized as a familial disorder. The familial incidences reported range from 11% to 80%.[16] In two large series, one English and one American, about 40% of gouty subjects gave a positive family history of gout. These wide discrepancies may be attributed in part to variations in diligence and pursuit of genealogic data. When all available data are considered, they suggest that serum urate concentrations are controlled by polygenic traits. Several rare forms of hyperuricemia and gout such as hypoxanthine phosphoribosyltransferase deficiency, phosphoribosyl-1-pyrophosphate synthetase overactivity, and familial hyperuricemia nephropathy have a clear genetic basis, most presenting in childhood or early adulthood[17] (see later).

But the vast majority of gout patients do not have one of these discrete inborn errors of metabolism as explanations for their disease. In most gout patients, the mechanism of hyperuricemia is simply inefficient renal excretion of uric acid.[18,19] It stands to reason then that some of the familial predisposition to gout is related to inherited variations in renal urate handling. With the recent advances in our understanding of the transport of uric acid in the renal proximal tubule, some of this variability is being clarified. Genome-wide association studies (GWASs) have identified genetic variations of the *SLC2A9/GLUT9* and *ABCG2* genes as important determinants of serum urate levels (see Chapter 94).[20] Curiously, the data for the role of polymorphisms in URAT1 (*SLC22A12*), a key urate transporter involved in renal proximal tubule urate reabsorption, are thus far inconsistent.[21-25] Glucose transporter 9 (GLUT9, *SLC2A9*) is an electrogenic hexose transporter whose splicing variants mediate reabsorption of uric acid, along with glucose and fructose, at the renal proximal tubule epithelial cell, first at the apical membrane, then through the basolateral membrane, and on into the circulation.[26-29] Polymorphisms in *SLC2A9* are associated with a lower serum uric acid, with stronger effects seen in women, possibly accounting for 0.5% to 2% of the variance in serum urate concentration in men and 3.4% to 8.8% in women.[22,27,30-32] In five of six populations studied by GWAS, *SLC2A9* polymorphisms were associated with a decreased incidence of self-reported gout, particularly in women.[27,30,31] Indeed, three patients with renal hypouricemia have been identified with loss-of-function mutations in *SLC2A9*.[28,33] The implication is that certain polymorphisms in *SLC2A9* enhance renal uric acid excretion, lower serum urate levels, and are therefore protective against gout, particularly in women.

A gene product of *ABCG2*, human adenosine triphosphate (ATP)-binding cassette, subfamily G, 2, appears to be a secretory urate transporter located in the renal proximal tubule apical border.[34] Polymorphisms in *ABCG2* are associated with a higher serum urate concentration in humans, with a more potent influence in men, potentially accounting for 1.6% to 2.1% of the variance in serum urate concentration in men and 0.5% to 0.8% in women.[23,31] One *ABCG2* polymorphism, rs2231142, has been associated with a higher incidence of gout only in males (odds ratio [OR], 2.03 for self-reported gout).[31] In a transfection model in *Xenopus* oocytes, the common mutation in human *ABCG2* encoded by rs2231142, Q141K, resulted in a 53% decrease in urate transport compared with the wild-type gene product.[34] The implication is that certain polymorphisms in *ABCG2* result in reduced proximal tubule urate secretion, increased serum urate concentrations, and a higher incidence of gout, at least in men.

Because the impact of comorbidities and environmental influences such as diet and lifestyle is so significant in gout, it remains to be seen whether risk contribution from genetic variation is clinically relevant, either directly or due to an unexpected interaction with these other factors. An example of the latter is the potential influence the urate-fructose/glucose exchange transporter *SCL2A9* polymorphisms may have on the well-described association of heavy consumption of soft drinks with elevated serum urate levels and gout.[35-38]

CLINICAL FEATURES

KEY POINTS

The three stages of gout are asymptomatic hyperuricemia, acute and intercritical gout, and chronic gouty arthritis.

A period of asymptomatic hyperuricemia lasts up to 20 years before the initial attack of gout or nephrolithiasis.

The first gout attack generally occurs at age 40 to 60 in men and after age 60 in women.

Many drugs raise serum urate levels and predispose to gout attacks, especially diuretics.

Most attacks of gout, especially early in the course, are monoarticular, with a predilection for the first metatarsophalangeal joint (podagra) and have a characteristic abrupt and painful onset.

The differential diagnosis for acute gout is usually infectious arthritis or other crystal-induced synovitis, particularly pseudogout.

Ultrasonography appears to be a useful adjunct in the diagnosis of acute and chronic gout.

In untreated or undertreated individuals, chronic gout is characterized by the development of tophi and progressive joint damage.

Throughout its natural history, gout passes through three stages: (1) asymptomatic hyperuricemia, (2) episodes of acute gouty arthritis separated by asymptomatic intervals (termed *intercritical* or *interval gout*), and (3) chronic gouty arthritis, the period when tophi often become apparent.

The basic pattern of clinical gout begins with acute attacks of intensely painful arthritis. The first attack is usually monoarticular and associated with few constitutional symptoms. Later, attacks may become polyarticular and are associated with fever. Attacks vary in duration but are time limited. Over time, attacks recur at shorter intervals, last longer, and eventually resolve incompletely. This leads to the development of chronic arthritis that slowly progresses to a crippling disease on which acute exacerbations are superimposed.

Asymptomatic Hyperuricemia

Asymptomatic hyperuricemia is a condition in which the serum urate level is high, but gout—manifested by arthritis or uric acid nephrolithiasis—has not yet occurred. Most people with hyperuricemia remain asymptomatic throughout their lifetimes. The tendency toward acute gout increases with the serum urate concentration. The risk of nephrolithiasis increases with the serum urate level and with the magnitude of urinary uric acid excretion. The phase of asymptomatic hyperuricemia ends with the first attack of gouty arthritis or urolithiasis. In most instances, this occurs after at least 20 years of sustained hyperuricemia. Between 10% and 40% of gouty subjects have one or more attacks of renal colic before the first articular event.

Acute Gouty Arthritis

The first attack of acute gouty arthritis usually occurs between age 40 and 60 years in men and after age 60 in women. Onset before age 25 should raise the possibility of an unusual form of gout, perhaps one related to a specific enzymatic defect that causes marked purine overproduction, an inherited renal disorder, or the use of cyclosporine.

A single joint is involved in about 85% to 90% of first attacks, with the first metatarsophalangeal joint being the most commonly affected site. The initial attack is polyarticular in 3% to 14%. Acute gout is predominantly a disease of the lower extremities, but eventually, any joint of any extremity may be involved. Ninety percent of patients experience acute attacks in the great toe at some time during the course of their disease. Next in order of frequency are the insteps, ankles, heels, knees, wrists, fingers, and elbows. Acute attacks rarely affect the shoulders, hips, spine, sacroiliac joints, sternoclavicular joints, acromioclavicular joints, or temporomandibular joints.[39,40] Acute gouty bursitis, tendinitis, or tenosynovitis can also occur.[41,42] Urate deposition and subsequent gout appear to have a predilection for previously damaged joints such as in Heberden's nodes of older women.[43] The differential diagnosis is usually septic arthritis or other crystal-induced arthritis, but a broader differential should be considered in confusing cases (Table 95-1).

Some patients report a history of short, trivial episodes of "ankle sprains," sore heels, or twinges of pain in the great toe before the first dramatic gouty attack. In most patients, however, the initial attack occurs with explosive suddenness and commonly begins at night after the individual has gone to sleep feeling well. Within a few hours of onset, the affected part becomes hot, dusky red, swollen, and extremely tender. Occasionally, lymphangitis may develop. Systemic signs of inflammation may include leukocytosis, fever, and elevation of the erythrocyte sedimentation rate. Radiographs usually show only soft tissue swelling during early episodes.

The course of untreated acute gout is highly variable. Mild attacks may subside in several hours or persist for only a day or two and never reach the intensity described for the classic attack. Severe attacks may last days to weeks. The skin over the joint often desquamates as the erythema subsides. With resolution, the patient becomes asymptomatic and enters the intercritical period.

Table 95-1 Differential Diagnosis of Gout

Acute Gouty Arthritis
Other crystal arthritis, especially CPPD, or pseudogout, but also basic calcium phosphate (hydroxyapatite) and others
Septic arthritis including gonorrhea
Trauma
Cellulitis
Lyme arthritis
Reactive arthritis
Psoriatic arthritis
Sarcoidosis
Unusual presentations of other inflammatory arthritides including rheumatoid arthritis

Chronic Gouty Arthritis
Rheumatoid or other chronic inflammatory arthritis
CPPD
(Inflammatory) osteoarthritis
Lyme disease
Indolent infections including mycobacterial

CPPD, calcium pyrophosphate disease.

Drugs may precipitate acute gout by either increasing or decreasing serum urate levels acutely. The occurrence of gout after the initiation of antihyperuricemic therapy is well established. In fact, the more potent the urate-lowering effect, the more likely there is to be an acute attack.[44] Drug-induced gout secondary to increased serum urate levels occurs on occasion with diuretic therapy, intravenous heparin, and cyclosporine.[45-47] Diuretic therapy in the elderly appears to be a particularly important precipitating factor for gouty arthritis. Other provocative factors include trauma, alcohol ingestion, surgery, dietary excess, hemorrhage, foreign protein therapy, infections, and radiographic contrast exposure.[48,49] The risk of a patient with gout developing an attack during hospitalization is 20%.[50]

The definitive diagnosis of gout is best established by aspiration of the joint and identification of intracellular needle-shaped crystals that have negative birefringence with compensated polarized light microscopy. However, various alternatives have been proposed for a presumptive diagnosis. These include the triad of acute monoarticular arthritis, hyperuricemia, and a dramatic response to colchicine therapy,[51] a set of criteria proposed by the American College of Rheumatology (Table 95-2) in 1977,[52] and 10 "propositions" for diagnosis by a European League Against Rheumatism (EULAR) panel of experts in 2006 (Table 95-3).[53] There are limitations to using any of these schemes. First, although the diagnosis of acute gouty arthritis can be strongly suggested by the typical presentation, not all inflammation of the great toe (podagra) in hyperuricemic patients is caused by gout.[54] Second, some patients with gout are normouricemic at the time of an acute attack, a phenomenon related to alcohol use or a consequence of interleukin (IL)-6 generation by the acute inflammatory process.[55-57] Third, diseases other than gout can occasionally improve with colchicine therapy; these include pseudogout, hydroxyapatite calcific tendinitis, sarcoid arthritis, erythema nodosum, serum sickness, rheumatoid arthritis, and familial Mediterranean fever.[16] Finally, the simultaneous presence of both gout and septic arthritis can be confusing clinically, with the former masking the latter.[58]

The use of ultrasonagraphy as a means of diagnosing acute and chronic gout is gaining favor. The characteristic finding is a superficial, hyperechoic, irregular band on the surface of articular cartilage, the so-called "double contour sign" or "urate icing," in one study seen in 92% of gouty joints and in no joints of patients with other types of arthritis.[59,60] Also characteristic is nonhomogeneous tophaceous material surrounded by an anechoic rim. Further support for ultrasound comes from the demonstration of resolution of these findings in a small number of gout patients on urate-lowering therapy who maintained a serum urate less than or equal to 6 mg/dL for at least 7 months.[61] Recent studies presented in abstract form have indicated excellent concordance between ultrasound readers in identifying changes, the presence of these findings even in those with asymptomatic hyperuricemia, and the superiority of ultrasound over conventional radiography in detecting gouty erosions.[62-64] Ultrasound now appears to be a technology that will be an important ancillary approach to the diagnosis and treatment of gout. Magnetic resonance imaging is much more sensitive than even ultrasound at detecting gouty erosions in patients with gout and normal plain radiographs.[65-67] Computed tomography (CT) scan is also sensitive for the detection of erosions and tophi, and three-dimensional CT may have utility in the quantitation of the size of tophi during clinical trials in gout.[67]

Intercritical Gout

The terms *intercritical gout* and *interval gout* have been applied to the periods between gouty attacks. Some patients never have a second attack. However, most patients suffer a second attack within 6 months to 2 years. In Gutman's series,[68] 62% had recurrences within the first year, 16% in 1 to 2 years, 11% in 2 to 5 years, and 4% in 5 to 10 years; 7% had experienced no recurrence in 10 or more years. The frequency of gout attacks usually increases over time in untreated patients. Later attacks have a less explosive onset, are polyarticular, become more severe, last longer, and abate more slowly. Nevertheless, recovery is complete.

Table 95-2 Criteria for the Classification of Acute Gouty Arthritis

The presence of characteristic urate crystals in the joint fluid, or a tophus proved to contain urate crystals by chemical means or polarized light microscopy, or the presence of 6 of the following 12 clinical, laboratory, and radiographic phenomena:
More than 1 attack of acute arthritis
Maximal inflammation developed within 1 day
Attack of monoarticular arthritis
Joint redness observed
First metatarsophalangeal joint painful or swollen
Unilateral attack involving first metatarsophalangeal joint
Unilateral attack involving tarsal joint
Suspected tophus
Hyperuricemia
Asymmetric swelling within a joint (radiograph)
Subcortical cysts without erosions (radiograph)
Negative culture of joint fluid for microorganisms during attack of joint inflammation

Adapted from Wallace SL, Robinson H, Masi AT, et al: Preliminary criteria for the classification of acute arthritis of primary gout, *Arthritis Rheum* 20:895–900, 1977.

Table 95-3 Propositions and Strength of Recommendation (SOR): Order According to Topic (Clinical, Urate Crystals, Biochemical, Radiographic, and Risk Factors/Comorbidities)

	Proposition	SOR (95% CI) VAS 100	A-B%*
1	In acute attacks the rapid development of severe pain, swelling, and tenderness that reaches its maximum within just 6-12 hr, especially with overlying erythema, is highly suggestive of crystal inflammation though not specific for gout	88 (80-96)	93
2	For typical presentations of gout (such as recurrent podagra with hyperuricemia), a clinical diagnosis alone is reasonably accurate but not definitive without crystal confirmation	95 (91-98)	100
3	Demonstration of MSU crystals in synovial fluid or tophus aspirates permits a definitive diagnosis of gout	96 (93-100)	100
4	A routine search for MSU crystals is recommended in all synovial fluid samples obtained from undiagnosed inflamed joints	90 (83-97)	87
5	Identification of MSU crystals from asymptomatic joints may allow definite diagnosis in intercritical periods	84 (78-91)	93
6	Gout and sepsis may coexist, so when septic arthritis is suspected, Gram stain and culture of synovial fluid should still be performed even if MSU crystals are identified	93 (87-99)	93
7	Although being the most important risk factor for gout, serum uric acid levels do not confirm or exclude gout because many people with hyperuricemia do not develop gout, and during acute attacks serum levels may be normal	95 (92-99)	93
8	Renal uric acid excretion should be determined in selected gout patients, especially those with a family history of young-onset gout, onset of gout under age 25, or with renal calculi	72 (62-81)	60
9	Although radiographs may be useful for differential diagnosis and may show typical features in chronic gout, they are not useful in confirming the diagnosis of early or acute gout	86 (79-94)	93
10	Risk factors for gout and associated comorbidity should be assessed including features of the metabolic syndrome (obesity, hyperglycemia, hyperlipidemia, hypertension)	93 (88-98)	100

*A-B%: percentage of strongly to fully recommended, based on the EULAR ordinal scale (A = fully recommended, B = strongly recommended, C = moderately recommended, D = weakly recommended, E = not recommended).

CI, confidence interval; MSU, monosodium urate; VAS, visual analogue scale (0-100 mm, 0 = not recommended at all, 100 = fully recommended).

From Zhang W, Doherty M, Pascual E, et al: EULAR evidence based recommendations for gout. Part I: diagnosis. Report of a task force of the standing committee for international clinical studies including therapeutics (ESCISIT), *Ann Rheum Dis* 65:1301, 2006.

Radiographic changes may develop during the intercritical period despite no sign of tophi on physical examination. These changes are more likely in patients with more severe hyperuricemia and more frequent acute attacks.[50,69]

The diagnosis of gout in a hyperuricemic patient with a history of acute attacks of monoarthritis may be difficult or inconclusive during the intercritical phase. Aspiration of an asymptomatic joint, however, can be a useful adjunct in the diagnosis of gout if urate crystals are demonstrated. Joint fluids obtained from gouty patients during the intercritical phase revealed monosodium urate crystals in 12.5% to 90% of joints.[70] Such crystals in asymptomatic joints are often associated with mild synovial fluid leukocytosis, which suggests the potential to contribute to joint damage even in the intervals between attacks.

Chronic Gouty Arthritis

Eventually, the patient may enter a phase of chronic polyarticular gout with no pain-free intercritical periods. At this stage, gout may be easily confused with other types of arthritis or other conditions.[71-73] The time from the initial attack to the beginning of chronic symptoms or visible tophaceous involvement is highly variable in studies of untreated patients. Hensch reported intervals ranging from 3 to 42 years, with an average of 11.6 years between the first attack and the development of chronic arthritis.[74] Ten years after the first attack, about half the individuals were still free of obvious tophi and most of the remainder had only minimal deposits. Thereafter, the proportion of those with nontophaceous involvement slowly declined, to 28% after 20 years. Two percent of the patients had severe crippling disease some 20 years after the initial attack.

The rate of formation of tophaceous deposits correlates with both the degree and the duration of hyperuricemia. The principal determinant is the serum urate level.[50] Gutman[75] found the mean serum urate concentration to be 9.1 mg/dL in 722 patients without tophi, 10 to 12 mg/dL in 456 patients with minimal to moderate tophi, and greater than 11 mg/dL in 11 patients with extensive tophaceous involvement. The rate of tophus formation also increases with the severity of renal disease and the use of diuretics.[45]

Tophaceous gout is the consequence of the chronic inability to eliminate urate as rapidly as it is produced. As the urate pool expands, deposits of urate crystals appear in cartilage, synovial membranes, tendons, soft tissues, and elsewhere. Tophi are rarely present at the time of an initial attack of primary gout[76,77]; they are more likely to be present in gout secondary to myeloproliferative diseases, in juvenile gout-complicating glycogen storage diseases (GSDs), in Lesch-Nyhan syndrome, or after allograft transplantation in patients treated with cyclosporine.[16,78]

Tophi can occur in a variety of locations. Tophaceous deposits may produce irregular, asymmetric, moderately discrete tumescence of the fingers (Figure 95-1), hands, knees, or feet. Tophi also form along the ulnar surfaces of the forearm, as saccular distentions of the olecranon bursa (Figure 95-2), in the antihelix of the ear (Figure 95-3), or as fusiform enlargements of the Achilles tendon (Figure 95-4). The process of tophaceous deposition advances insidiously. Although the tophi themselves are relatively painless, acute inflammation can occur around them. Eventually, extensive destruction of the joints and large subcutaneous tophi may lead to grotesque deformities, particularly of the hands and feet, and to progressive crippling (Figure 95-5).

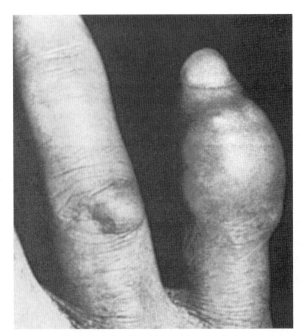

Figure 95-1 Tophus of the fifth digit, with a smaller tophus over the fourth proximal interphalangeal joint.

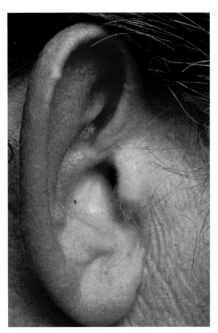

Figure 95-3 Tophus of the helix of the ear adjacent to the auricular tubercle.

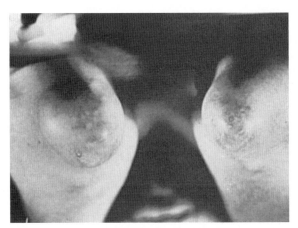

Figure 95-2 Saccular tophaceous enlargements of the oclecranon bursae, with small cutaneous deposits of urate.

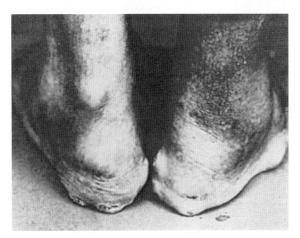

Figure 95-4 Tophi of Achilles tendons and their insertions in a patient with gout.

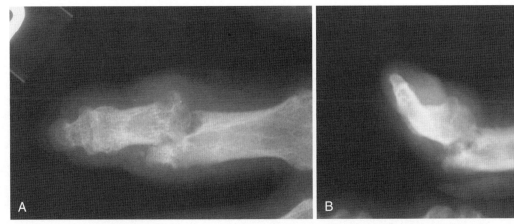

Figure 95-5 **A** and **B,** Radiographs demonstrating severe destructive changes in tophaceous gout.

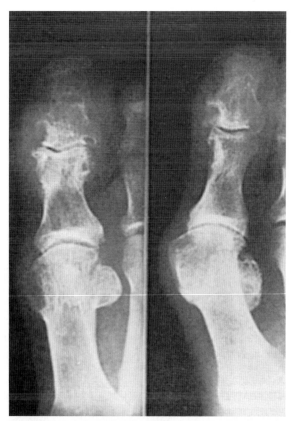

Figure 95-6 Radiographs show changes typical of bony tophi including soft tissue distortion, erosions with sclerotic margins, and overwhelming edges. Joint space narrowing is minimal, despite the large erosions. (*From Nakayama DA, Barthelemy C, Carrera G, et al: Tophaceous gout: a clinical and radiographic assessment,* Arthritis Rheum *27:468, 1984.*)

The tense, shiny, thin skin overlying the tophus may ulcerate and extrude white, chalky, or pasty material composed of urate crystals. Secondary infection of tophi is rare.

Typical radiographic changes, particularly erosions with sclerotic margins and overhanging edges of bone, occur with the development of tophi (Figure 95-6).[79] These may be difficult to distinguish from erosions of other causes, but the presence of a thin, overhanging calcified edge is strong evidence of gout. Calcifications can be seen in some tophi, and bony ankylosis may rarely occur. Ultrasonography, magnetic resonance imaging, and computed tomography can demonstrate tophi, with the last providing the most specific images.[59-68,80]

Tophi can produce a marked limitation of joint movement by involvement of the joint structure directly or of a tendon serving the joint. Any joint can be involved, although those of the lower extremity are affected primarily. Spinal joints do not escape urate deposition,[73,81] but acute gouty spondylitis is unusual. Symptoms related to nerve or spinal cord compression by tophi have rarely been observed. Tophi rarely occur in myocardium, valves, cardiac conduction system, various parts of the eye, and larynx.[82,83]

ASSOCIATED CONDITIONS

KEY POINTS

Gout is associated with obesity, hypertriglyceridemia, glucose intolerance and the metabolic syndrome, hypertension, atherosclerosis, and hypothyroidism.

Renal insufficiency is frequently associated with hyperuricemia and gout.

Hyperuricemia is a common cause of nephrolithiasis, and rarely, chronic hyperuricemia may cause urate nephropathy and acute hyperuricemia may lead to uric acid nephropathy in the tumor lysis syndrome.

Alcohol use, lead intoxication, and cyclosporine treatment are associated with hyperuricemia and gout.

A diagnosis of gout should prompt a search for the coexistence of these associated conditions.

The association of gout with obesity and overeating is well recognized.[84] In 6000 subjects, hyperuricemia was found in only 3.4% of those with a relative weight at or below the 20th percentile, in 5.7% of those between the 21st and 79th percentiles, and in 11.4% of those at or above the 80th percentile.[85]

Hypertriglyceridemia has been reported in 75% to 80% of patients with gout,[86] and hyperuricemia is found in more than 80% of patients with hypertriglyceridemia.[16] However, studies have been unable to show a correlation between serum urate and cholesterol values or a unique lipid phenotype.[87] Gouty patients who drink alcohol excessively have mean serum triglyceride levels that are higher than those of their obesity-matched controls and of non–alcohol-drinking gouty patients.[88]

Hyperuricemia has been reported in 2% to 50% of patients with diabetes mellitus, and gouty arthritis has been reported in less than 0.1% to 9%.[89] Abnormal glucose tolerance tests have been noted in 7% to 74% of patients with gout, depending, in part, on the criteria used.[90]

Hyperuricemia has been reported in 22% to 38% of patients with untreated hypertension. This figure increases to 67% when diuretic therapy and renal disease are present.[16] Hyperuricemia may be an indication of a potential risk for hypertension in adolescent males.[91] Hypertension is present in one-fourth to one-half of patients with classic gout, but the presence of hypertension is unrelated to the duration of gout.[84,85] Elevated serum urate concentrations are associated with increased tubular reabsorption of sodium.[90] The serum urate concentration also correlates inversely with renal blood flow and urate clearance and correlates directly with both renovascular and total resistance. Therefore the association between hypertension and hyperuricemia may be related to the reduction of renal blood flow in hypertension. In addition, uric acid causes smooth muscle proliferation in vitro and vascular disease in animal models through a mechanism that involves complex intracellular signaling, mitogen-activated protein kinase activation, and platelet-derived growth factor expression.[92,93]

The association between hyperuricemia and the manifestations of atherosclerosis has led to speculation that hyperuricemia is a risk factor for coronary artery disease. Some studies show no clear associations among blood pressure, blood glucose, or serum cholesterol and serum urate concentration when adjustments are made for the effects of age, sex, and relative weight[85,94-97]; the serum urate concentrations of persons with coronary heart disease are not significantly different from the mean levels of the population.[97,98] Other studies, however, maintain that hyperuricemia is an independent risk factor for coronary artery disease.[99,100]

The term *metabolic syndrome* has been applied to a cluster of abnormalities including resistance to insulin-stimulated glucose uptake, hyperinsulinemia, hypertension, and dyslipoproteinemia that are characterized by high levels of plasma triglycerides and high-density lipoprotein cholesterol. Hyperuricemia closely correlates with the degree of insulin resistance[97-103] and therefore is a likely feature of metabolic syndrome. Metabolic syndrome has been associated with coronary artery disease, and hyperuricemia as a component of metabolic syndrome may explain the previously recognized association between coronary artery disease and hyperuricemia. A recent study concluded that the relationship between hyperuricemia and acute myocardial infarction is independent, but patients who experience gouty arthritis are at an increased risk for myocardial infarction. This association could not be explained by renal function, metabolic syndrome, diuretic use, or traditional cardiovascular risk factors.[104]

Alcohol consumption has long been associated with hyperuricemia and gout. In susceptible persons, alcohol use can precipitate acute gouty arthritis. An epidemiologic study in Saudi Arabia, where alcohol consumption is rare, revealed an 8.42% prevalence of hyperuricemia but no cases of gout among the study group.[105] Both a decrease in the renal excretion of uric acid and an increase in uric acid production seem to be important factors in this association.[106] Ethanol increases uric acid production by accelerating the turnover of ATP. Among alcoholic beverages, beer may have more potent effects on uric acid production because of its high guanosine content.[14]

There appears to be a significant increased prevalence of hypothyroidism among both female and male patients with gouty arthritis.[107] Hyperuricemia may also be more prevalent in patients with hypothyroidism. Thyroid replacement therapy is associated with a decrease in serum urate concentration caused by an increased uric acid diuresis—a change not explained solely by a change in creatinine clearance.[108] Although the cause of hyperuricemia and gout in patients with hypothyroidism is unknown, it is speculated that urate metabolism is mediated by thyroid-stimulating hormone receptors in extrathyroidal tissues including the kidney and that these modulate urate homeostasis.

Studies of acutely ill patients in intensive care units indicate that markedly increased serum urate concentrations, in the vicinity of 20 mg/dL, are associated with hypotensive events and a poor prognosis.[109] This finding may be related to two factors. First, ischemic tissue may foster the degradation of ATP to purine end products, thereby enhancing the production of urate. The finding of increased plasma ATP degradation products associated with hyperuricemia and adult respiratory distress syndrome supports this possibility.[110] Second, the conversion of hypoxanthine to uric acid by xanthine oxidase during ischemia produces oxidant radicals, which are themselves associated with tissue injury.[111] It is possible that inhibition of xanthine oxidase with allopurinol may be a useful therapy in this setting.

Maternal serum urate concentrations normally decrease during pregnancy until the 24th week and then increase until 12 weeks after delivery.[112] An increase in the serum urate level occurs in preeclampsia and toxemia of pregnancy, owing to a decrease in the renal clearance of urate.[113] Perinatal mortality is markedly increased when maternal plasma urate levels are raised, usually in association with early-onset preeclampsia. The highest mortality rate is seen with serum urate concentrations higher than 6 mg/dL and diastolic blood pressures greater than 110 mm Hg. Labor itself is associated with an increased serum urate level, and it remains elevated for 1 to 2 days after delivery.

Gout is rarely seen in patients with rheumatoid arthritis, systemic lupus erythematosus, or ankylosing spondylitis.[41,114-116] The basis for the decreased concurrence of these disorders is unclear, although the long-term use of nonsteroidal anti-inflammatory drugs (NSAIDs) or corticosteroids may mask the clinical features of gout in some of these patients.

Renal Disease

After gouty arthritis, renal problems appear to be the most frequent complication of hyperuricemia. Twenty percent to 40% of patients with gout have albuminuria, which is usually mild and often intermittent. Hyperuricemia alone may be implicated as the cause of chronic kidney disease only when the concentration of urate chronically exceeds 13 mg/dL in men or 10 mg/dL in women.[117] Before the routine treatment of asymptomatic hypertension, renal failure accounted for 10% of the deaths in patients with gout. Whether moderate hyperuricemia has a direct harmful effect on renal function is unclear. Some evidence suggests that urate damages the kidneys and leads to hypertension.[92,93]

The term *urate nephropathy* is used to describe the deposition of urate crystals in the interstitium of the medulla and pyramids, with a surrounding giant cell reaction—a distinctive histologic finding characteristic of the gouty kidney (Figure 95-7). Factors such as coexistent hypertension, chronic lead exposure, ischemic heart disease, and primary pre-existing renal insufficiency probably play important roles in the pathogenesis of this pathology. Although urate nephropathy appears to exist as a distinct entity, it is not believed to be an important contributor to renal function in most gouty patients.[16,118]

In contrast, *uric acid nephropathy* is the term used to describe acute renal failure resulting from the precipitation of large quantities of uric acid crystals in the collecting ducts and ureters. This complication most commonly occurs in patients with leukemia and lymphoma as a result of rapid malignant cell turnover, often during chemotherapy.[119,120] This syndrome (also termed *acute tumor lysis syndrome*) has

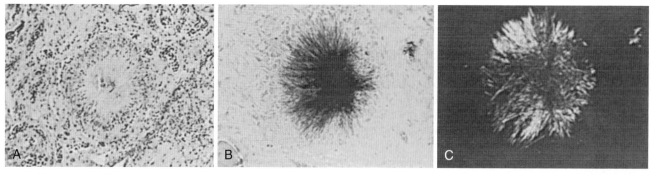

Figure 95-7 **A,** Urate deposit in the medulla of the kidneys as seen in an alcohol-fixed section stained with hematoxylin and eosin (×250). **B,** Adjacent section of the deposit shown in **A,** stained with methenamine silver (×250). **C,** Adjacent section of the deposit shown in **A** seen with polarized light (×250).

been more clearly defined as hyperuricemia, lactic acidosis, hyperkalemia, hyperphosphatemia, and hypocalcemia and is most commonly observed in patients with aggressive, rapidly proliferating tumors including lymphoproliferative disorders and metastatic medulloblastoma. Uric acid nephropathy is less commonly found with other neoplasms, after epileptic seizures, after vigorous exercise with heat stress, and after angiography and coronary artery bypass surgery.[16]

In the tumor lysis syndrome, the large amount of nucleic acid in nucleotides liberated with massive cytolysis is converted rapidly to uric acid. Typically, there is marked hyperuricemia, with a mean serum urate level of 20 mg/dL (range, 12 to 80 mg/dL). The pathogenesis of acute renal failure in uric acid nephropathy is related to the precipitation of uric acid in the distal tubules and collecting ducts, the sites of maximal acidification and concentration of urine. Oliguria, or even anuria, and azotemia may occur. There may be "gravel" or "sand" noted in the urine. The ratio of urinary uric acid to creatinine in these patients typically exceeds 1; in patients with most other causes of acute renal failure, the ratio is 0.4 ± 0.3.[120]

Nephrolithiasis occurs in 10% to 25% of patients with primary gout, a prevalence greater than that in the general population. The likelihood of stones in a given patient with gout increases with the serum urate concentration and with amounts of urinary uric acid excretion.[121,122] It exceeds 50% with a serum urate value above 13 mg/dL or with urinary uric acid excretion rates in excess of 1100 mg every 24 hours.

Uric acid calculi account for approximately 10% of all stones in patients in the United States; elsewhere, rates range from as low as 5% up to 40% in Israel and Australia, respectively.[16] Uric acid stones can occur in patients with no history of gouty arthritis, and only 20% in this group are hyperuricemic. Other renal stone disease is associated with

hyperuricemia and gout. Gouty subjects also have an increased incidence of stones that contain calcium. In addition, about 30% of patients with recurrent calcium stone disease have either an increased urinary uric acid excretion rate or hyperuricemia. A causative link between uric acid and recurrent calcium oxalate stones is provided by reports of reduced stone frequency in patients treated with allopurinol.

Finally, the report of uric acid as the major constituent of a stone obtained from a patient with no apparent abnormalities of uric acid metabolism should suggest the possibility that the constituent is actually 2,8-dihydroxyadenine and that the patient has adenine phosphoribosyltransferase deficiency.[123] This is because x-ray diffraction is required to distinguish uric acid from 2,8-dihydroxyadenine.

Familial juvenile hyperuricemic nephropathy (FJHN), sometimes called *familial juvenile gouty nephropathy,* was first described in 1960.[124] This disorder is inherited as an autosomal dominant trait with a high degree of penetrance and is usually associated with gout. Renal disease typically develops in the second decade of life and progresses to end-stage renal failure by midlife.[125-127] Histologic examination of kidney tissue reveals tubulointerstitial inflammation and splitting of thickened tubular basement membranes. The primary diagnostic criterion is a reduced fractional excretion of urate (defined as uric acid clearance factored by creatinine clearance × 100 equal to 5% or less; normal is 8% to 18%).[128] The dramatically low fractional excretion of urate and the early onset of disease are conspicuous characteristics of FJHN and distinguish it from other autosomal dominant hyperuricemic disorders that usually appear later in life (Table 95-4). Genotype mapping has linked the gene for FJHN to chromosome 16p12-p11.[126]

Autosomal dominant medullary cystic kidney disease (ADMCKD) is another hereditary nephropathy that usually includes gout among its constellation of symptoms. The

Table 95-4 Genetics of Renal Diseases Associated with Gout

Condition	Inheritance	Chromosomal Location	Gene
FJHN	AD	16p12.3	Uromodulin
		17cenq21.3	Hepatic nuclear factor 1β
MCKD type 1	AD	1q21	?
MCKD type 2	AD, AR	16p12.3	Uromodulin

AD, autosomal dominant; AR, autosomal recessive; FJHN, familial juvenile hyperuricemic nephropathy; MCKD, medullary cystic kidney disease.

onset of renal dysfunction occurs later than in those with FJHN. Renal histology reveals numerous corticomedullary and intramedullary cysts in the kidneys and increased medullary connective tissue. At least two loci appear to be responsible for ADMCKD. One, termed ADMCKD1, is located on chromosome 1; the other, ADMCKD2, is a 16p locus. ADMCKD2 and FJHN loci map to approximately the same region of chromosome 16p.[129]

The chromosome 16p12 locus that harbors the candidate interval for FJHN and ADMCKD2 contains six candidate genes, including the uromodulin gene (UMOD).[130-132] UMOD encodes the Tamm-Horsfall protein, a glycosylphosphatidylinositol-anchored glycoprotein localized to the thick ascending limb of the loop of Henle. Amorphous deposits of uromodulin are present in the renal interstitium of patients with medullary cystic kidney disease.[133] Four different mutations in exon 4 have been identified in the UMOD gene. Because mutations in the same gene are responsible for both FJHN and ADMCKD, the two entities appear to be allelic variants in UMOD that cause decreased urinary concentrations of Tamm-Horsfall protein, with resulting hyperuricemia and progressive renal failure.[134]

Lead Intoxication

Hyperuricemia and gout are well-recognized complications of chronic lead intoxication, with the prevalence of gout in patients with plumbism ranging between 6% and 50%.[135] Although a renal defect is recognized, it has not been well defined.[136,137] Some patients with primary gout have increased blood lead levels compared with age- and sex-matched controls, despite the absence of a history of overt lead exposure.[138] This suggests that occult chronic lead intoxication may play a causative role in some cases of primary gout (up to 36% of some gout populations).[135] In addition, patients with gout who have renal impairment seem to have an increased quantity of mobilized lead compared with gouty patients with normal renal function.[139] These observations suggest an important role for lead in the pathogenesis of gouty nephropathy.

Cyclosporine-Induced Hyperuricemia and Gout

Cyclosporine interferes with the renal excretion of uric acid. Hyperuricemia and gout occur with increased frequency among transplant recipients treated with cyclosporine and are even more common when diuretics are used concomitantly.[78,140] However, serum urate levels do not correlate directly with cyclosporine levels or with the degree of hypertension or renal insufficiency. The onset of gout may occur soon after transplantation, with a mean of about 17 months. Gouty attacks may be typical and monoarticular, or they may affect unusual sites such as the shoulder, hip, or sacroiliac joints. Polyarticular attacks and an accelerated course, with early development of tophi, may also be observed. Nephrolithiasis develops in about 3% of renal transplant patients. All calculi from azathioprine-treated patients are composed of calcium compounds, whereas 60% of the calculi from those treated with cyclosporine contain uric acid.[141]

CLASSIFICATION OF HYPERURICEMIA AND GOUT

> ### KEY POINTS
>
> Primary hyperuricemia and gout are caused by decreased renal uric acid excretion in more than 90% and overproduction of urate in less than 10% of affected patients.
>
> Secondary hyperuricemia and gout are usually related to decreased renal urate clearance as a direct or indirect consequence of the primary disease process.
>
> Four known specific inborn errors of purine metabolism with overproduction of urate account for less than 1% of cases of secondary hyperuricemia and gout.

The concentration of urate in body fluids is determined by the balance between production and elimination. Accordingly, hyperuricemia may be caused by an excessive rate of urate production, a decrease in the renal excretion of uric acid, or a combination of both events.

Hyperuricemia and gout may be classified as follows (Table 95-5):

Primary: These cases appear to be innate, neither secondary to an acquired disorder nor the result of a subordinate manifestation of an inborn error that leads initially to a major disease unlike gout. Some cases of primary gout have a genetic basis; others do not.

Secondary: These cases develop in the course of another disease or as a consequence of drug use.

Idiopathic: In these cases, a more precise classification cannot be assigned.

Further subdivisions within each major category are based on the identification of overproduction, underexcretion, or both, as responsible for the hyperuricemia. Evidence of overproduction of urate is provided by determination of the 24-hour urinary uric acid excretion. For adults ingesting a purine-free diet, a total excretion of up to 600 mg/day is considered within the normal range.[142] For patients on regular diets, a value in excess of 1000 mg/day is clearly abnormal and an indication of overproduction, and values between 800 and 1000 mg/day are considered borderline. It has been suggested that overproduction of uric acid can be assessed simply by determining the ratio of uric acid to creatinine in the urine or the $C_{urate}/C_{creatinine}$ ratio. However, comparison of these two ratios with the 24-hour urinary uric acid excretion reveals a poor correlation in most patients.[143,144] Exceptions include patients with specific enzymatic deficiencies or with rapid cell lysis during chemotherapy for leukemia or lymphoma.

Primary Gout

Renal mechanisms are responsible for the hyperuricemia in most cases of gout. Genetic factors exert an important control in the renal clearance of urate.[145] A careful comparison of uric acid clearances and excretion rates over a wide but comparable range of filtered loads of urate indicates that most gouty subjects have a lower ratio of urate-to-inulin clearance (C_{urate}/C_{inulin} ratio) than do

Table 95-5 Classification of Hyperuricemia and Gout

Type	Metabolic Disturbance	Inheritance
Primary		
Molecular defects undefined		
Underexcretion (90% of primary gout)	Not established	Polygenic
Overproduction (10% of primary gout)	Not established	Polygenic
Associated with specific enzyme defects		
PRPP synthetase variants; increased activity	Overproduction of PRPP and uric acid	X-linked
HPRT deficiency, partial	Overproduction of uric acid; increased purine biosynthesis de novo driven by surplus PRPP; Kelley-Seegmiller syndrome	X-linked
Secondary		
Associated with Increased Purine Biosynthesis De Novo		
HPRT deficiency, "virtually complete"	Overproduction of uric acid; increased purine biosynthesis de novo driven by surplus PRPP; Lesch-Nyhan syndrome	X-linked
Glucose-6-phosphatase deficiency or absence	Overproduction plus underexcretion of uric acid; glycogen storage disease type I (von Gierke's disease)	Autosomal recessive
Fructose-1-phosphate aldolase deficiency	Overproduction plus underexcretion of uric acid	Autosomal recessive
Associated with Increased ATP Degradation		
Associated with increased nucleic acid turnover	Overproduction of uric acid	Most not familial
Associated with decreased renal excretion of uric acid	Decreased filtration of uric acid, inhibited tubular secretion of uric acid, or enhanced tubular reabsorption of uric acid	Some autosomal dominant; some not familial; most unknown
Idiopathic		Unknown

ATP, adenosine triphosphate; HPRT, hypoxanthine phosphoribosyltransferase; PRPP, phosphoribosylpyrophosphate.

nongouty subjects.[142,145,146] The excretion rates and the capacity of the excretory mechanism for uric acid are the same for gouty subjects and nongouty individuals (see Figure 94-8). The excretion curve, however, is shifted. Gouty subjects require serum urate values 2 or 3 mg/dL higher than those of controls to achieve equivalent uric acid excretion rates. Theoretically, the shift in the excretion curve in gouty subjects may result from reduced filtration of urate, enhanced reabsorption, or decreased secretion. Patients classified as exhibiting an overproduction of uric acid represent less than 10% of the gouty population.

Secondary Gout

Numerous secondary causes of hyperuricemia and gout can be attributed to a decrease in the renal excretion of uric acid. A reduction in the glomerular filtration rate leads to a decrease in the filtered load of urate and, consequently, to hyperuricemia. Patients with renal disease are hyperuricemic on this basis. Other factors such as decreased secretion of urate have been postulated in patients with some types of renal disease (e.g., polycystic kidney disease, lead nephropathy). Gout is a rare complication of the secondary hyperuricemia that results from renal insufficiency. When it occurs in this setting, there is likely to be a positive family history.

Diuretic therapy currently represents one of the most important causes of secondary hyperuricemia in humans. Diuretic-induced volume depletion leads to a decreased filtered load and enhanced tubular reabsorption of urate. A number of other drugs lead to hyperuricemia by a renal mechanism. These agents include low-dose aspirin, pyrazinamide, nicotinic acid, ethambutol, ethanol, and cyclosporine.

Decreased renal excretion of uric acid is thought to be an important mechanism for the hyperuricemia associated with several disease states. Volume depletion may be an important factor in patients with hyperuricemia associated with adrenal insufficiency or nephrogenic diabetes insipidus. An accumulation of organic acids leads to hyperuricemia. This is the case in starvation, alcoholic ketosis, diabetic ketoacidosis, maple syrup urine disease, and lactic acidosis of any cause (e.g., hypoxemia, respiratory insufficiency, chronic beryllium disease, acute alcohol intoxication). The renal basis of the hyperuricemia in conditions such as chronic lead intoxication, hypoparathyroidism, pseudohypoparathyroidism, and hypothyroidism remains unclear.

Secondary gout can also result from urate overproduction. Four specific defects cause urate overproduction as a consequence of accelerated de novo purine biosynthesis: hypoxanthine phosphoribosyltransferase (HPRT) deficiency, phosphoribosylpyrophosphate synthetase overactivity, glucose-6-phosphatase deficiency, and fructose-1-phosphate aldolase deficiency.

TREATMENT

KEY POINTS

Asymptomatic hyperuricemia is generally not treated, but its identification should lead to a search for the cause and/or associated conditions.

Episodes of acute gouty arthritis can be treated with colchicine, NSAIDs, adrenocorticotropic hormone, and systemic or intra-articular steroids.

Prophylaxis against acute attacks with colchicine or NSAIDs can be effective but does not change the underlying process in the absence of concomitant urate-lowering therapy.

Starting urate-lowering therapy after a single attack of gout remains debatable, but recurrent attacks of gout, urate nephrolithiasis, tophaceous gout, and/or evidence of gout-induced joint damage are all accepted indications.

Xanthine oxidase inhibitors and uricosurics are effective at lowering serum urate levels in most patients.

Uricases such as pegloticase should be reserved for refractory tophaceous gout.

A serum urate of less than 6 mg/dL should be targeted.

Prophylaxis with colchicine, NSAIDs, or less preferably, systemic steroids should be continued for at least 6 months after initiation of urate-lowering therapy.

Long-term compliance with the treatment regimen remains a major issue in gout; forming a therapeutic alliance with the patient is critical.

Lifestyle modifications may help somewhat in the control of gout, especially reduced alcohol consumption, but are more important for the management of associated conditions such as obesity and hyperlipidemia.

The therapeutic aims in gout are as follows (Figure 95-8):

1. To terminate the acute attack as promptly and gently as possible
2. To prevent recurrences of acute gouty arthritis
3. To prevent or reverse complications of the disease resulting from the deposition of sodium urate or uric acid crystals in joints, kidneys, or other sites
4. To prevent or reverse associated features of the illness that are deleterious such as obesity, hypertriglyceridemia, and hypertension

Asymptomatic Hyperuricemia

The presence of hyperuricemia is rarely an indication for specific antihyperuricemic drug therapy. Rather, the finding of hyperuricemia should cause the following questions to be addressed:

1. What is the cause of the hyperuricemia?
2. Are associated findings present?
3. Has damage to tissues or organs occurred as a result?
4. What, if anything, should be done?

Hyperuricemia may be the initial clue to the presence of a previously unsuspected disorder. In 70% of hyperuricemic patients, an underlying cause can be readily defined by history and physical examination. The nature of the underlying cause may be useful in predicting the potential consequences, if any, of the elevated serum urate concentration. Therefore an underlying cause should be sought in every patient with hyperuricemia.

Whether to treat hyperuricemia uncomplicated by articular gout, urolithiasis, or nephropathy is an exercise in clinical judgment, and universal agreement is lacking. When considering whether to treat asymptomatic hyperuricemia with urate-lowering agents, the following data are pertinent:

- Although there are intriguing data from animal models to the contrary,[147] there is no good evidence that renal function is adversely affected by elevated serum urate concentrations.
- The renal disease that accompanies hyperuricemia is most often related to inadequately controlled hypertension.

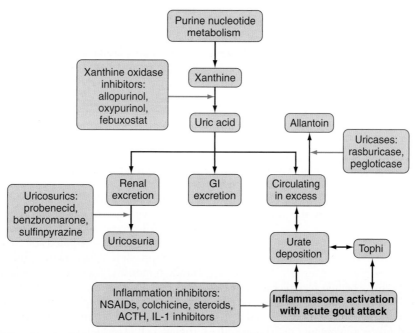

Figure 95-8 Treatment options for gout, including inhibitors of inflammation used for acute attacks and the available approaches for lowering serum urate when appropriate. Some inflammation inhibitors may also be used for prophylaxis when initiating urate lowering therapy. See text for details. *Red arrows* indicate inhibitory effects; *green arrows* indicate promoting effects. ACTH, adrenocorticotropic hormone; GI, gastrointestinal; IL-1, interleukin-1; NSAID, nonsteroidal anti-inflammatory drug.

- Although debate exists regarding whether hyperuricemia is an independent risk factor for coronary artery disease,[97-100] there is no evidence that correction of hyperuricemia has an effect on the development of heart disease.

Thus it seems prudent not to treat hyperuricemia with specific antihyperuricemic agents until symptoms develop. Rare exceptions include individuals with a known hereditary cause of uric acid overproduction or patients at risk for acute uric acid nephropathy.

It is, however, strongly recommended that the cause of hyperuricemia be determined and any associated factors related to the process such as obesity, hyperlipidemia, alcoholism, and, especially, hypertension, be addressed. Fenofibrate and losartan might be appropriate agents for the treatment of hypertriglyceridemia and hypertension, respectively, in hyperuricemic individuals because each has modest uricosuric effects.[148,149]

Acute Gouty Arthritis

The acute gouty attack may be successfully terminated by any of several drugs. For practical purposes, the choice in most situations is among colchicine, an NSAID, a corticosteroid preparation, or adrenocorticotropic hormone (ACTH). In response to the recognition of the critical role IL-1β plays in the initiation of gout attacks, trials of biologic inhibitors of IL-1β for both the treatment and prophylaxis of acute gout have been undertaken with promising results.[150-154] Although approved for the treatment of tumor necrosis factor (TNF) receptor–associated periodic fever syndromes, these expensive agents remain unapproved for gout at this writing. The timing of therapy initiation is more important than the choice of drug for acute gout.[155] With any of these agents, the sooner the drug is started, the more rapidly a complete response will be attained. Generally, colchicine is preferred for patients in whom the diagnosis of gout is not confirmed, whereas NSAIDs are preferred when the diagnosis is secure. If a patient cannot take medications by mouth or has active peptic ulcer disease, the choice is among intra-articular glucocorticoid, parenteral glucocorticoid, or ACTH. Local application of ice packs may help control the pain of an acute attack.[156] In some cases, analgesics including narcotics may be added as well. Drugs that affect serum urate concentrations including antihyperuricemic agents should not be changed (either started or stopped) during an acute attack. Just as sudden fluctuations in serum urate levels tend to precipitate an acute attack, an inflammatory reaction that is already in progress may be substantially worsened by a major change in the serum urate concentration.

Colchicine

Traditionally, the oral dosing schedule for colchicine was 0.5 or 0.6 mg taken hourly until one of three things occurred: joint symptoms eased; nausea, vomiting, or diarrhea developed; or the patient had taken a maximum of 10 doses. If 10 doses were taken without benefit, the clinician questioned the accuracy of the diagnosis. Many clinicians have

recommended that doses be taken every 2 to 6 hours to reduce side effects.[157] In 2009 the U.S. Food and Drug Administration (FDA) approved Colcrys (URL Pharma, Inc.) as the first single-ingredient oral colchicine product for the treatment of acute gout flares and the prophylaxis of gout flares, as well as for familial Mediterranean fever in adults and children 4 years of age or older. The FDA ordered a halt to the marketing of unapproved single-ingredient colchicine preparations other than Colcrys. The new recommendation for colchicine is the use of a low-dose regimen of 1.2 mg followed by 0.6 mg in 1 hour, for a total of 1.8 mg per attack. That protocol was based on the results of a randomized controlled trial of 184 patients with acute gout flares of less than 12 hours' duration that compared low-dose (74 patients) with high-dose colchicine (4.8 mg total over 6 hours; 52 patients) and with placebo (58 patients) with a primary endpoint of at least a 50% reduction in pain within 24 hours.[158] The low-dose approach resulted in comparable peak plasma concentrations and early gout flare control with much fewer side effects, particularly diarrhea and vomiting, compared with the high-dose approach. It should be noted that these were patients who started treatment within 12 hours of attack onset, and there was still a greater than 30% failure to achieve the primary endpoint in both treatment arms. The appropriate dosing of colchicine for attacks of greater duration remains unclear. The low-dose recommendations are in line with those of a EULAR panel of experts.[159] On the basis of two randomized trials, the recommended dosing for prophylaxis is 0.6 mg once or twice a day.[160,161] Patients with severe renal insufficency should be started at 0.3 mg a day. The marketing of unapproved, injectable colchicine was prohibited by the FDA in 2008 due to an unacceptable safety profile, with the potential for serious adverse events including death with intravenous administration.

Peak plasma concentrations of colchicine occur within 2 hours of oral administration. Although its plasma half-life is 4 hours, levels can be detected in neutrophils 10 days after ingestion. Colchicine has a low therapeutic index, with steady-state plasma concentrations after acute treatment ranging from 0.5 to 3 ng/mL and with toxic effects occurring at approximately 3 ng/mL.[162] Therefore in most patients, the side effects precede or coincide with the improvement in joint symptoms. These side effects develop in 50% to 80% of patients using the old, high-dose regimen and include increased peristalsis, cramping abdominal pain, diarrhea, nausea, and vomiting. The drug must be stopped promptly at the first sign of gastrointestinal side effects.[163]

Colchicine derives its effectiveness from its ability to interfere with acute inflammatory reactions in a variety of ways. Colchicine blocks the processing of IL-1β[164] and inhibits E-selectin–mediated adhesiveness to neutrophils.[165] Its action diminishes neutrophil L-selectin expression, random motility, chemotaxis, phospholipase A₂ activation, and IL-1 expression, as well as the stimulated elaboration of platelet-activating factor, crystal-induced chemotactic factor, and leukotriene B₄. Colchicine also inhibits endothelial cell ICAM-1 expression and mast cell histamine release and downregulates TNF receptors on macrophages and endothelial cells.

Nonsteroidal Anti-inflammatory Drugs

In a patient with an established diagnosis of uncomplicated gout, the preferred agent is an NSAID and indomethacin has been the traditional choice. Although this drug may be effective in doses as low as 25 mg four times a day, an initial dose of 50 to 75 mg, followed by 50 mg every 6 to 8 hours, with a maximum dose of 200 mg in the first 24 hours, has generally been recommended. To prevent relapse, it is reasonable to continue this dose for an additional 24 hours and then taper to 50 mg every 6 to 8 hours for the next 2 days. Clinical trials have shown that oral naproxen, fenoprofen, ibuprofen, sulindac, piroxicam, and ketoprofen, as well as intramuscular ketorolac, are also effective. In fact, all members of this family of drugs can be highly effective in the treatment of acute gouty arthritis including the cyclooxygenase-2 (COX-2) selective agents.[166]

Corticosteroids

Intra-articular glucocorticoids are useful in the treatment of acute gout limited to a single joint or bursa.[155,167] Oral, intramuscular, or intravenous glucocorticoids can also provide relief, but these agents are usually reserved for patients who are intolerant of colchicine or NSAIDs or who have medical conditions such as peptic ulcer disease or renal disease that contraindicate their use. Doses of glucocorticoids have been systematically studied, and generally, high doses (prednisone 20 to 60 mg/day) are necessary. Lower doses may not be effective, as evidenced by gout flares occurring in organ transplant patients who are taking maintenance prednisone at doses of 7.5 to 15 mg a day.[168] Anecdotally, rebound attacks were reported as steroids were withdrawn.

Adrenocorticotropic Hormone

Single injections of intramuscular ACTH gel (25 to 80 IU) can terminate an acute gout attack.[169] More often, however, repeated administration is required every 24 to 72 hours. This treatment is effective postoperatively and may be more effective than glucocorticoids, possibly related to the mechanism of action. In addition to stimulating the adrenal cortex to produce corticosteroids, ACTH interferes with the acute inflammatory response through activation of melanocortin receptor-3.[170] Unfortunately, ACTH preparations, when available at all, have become prohibitively expensive.

Prophylaxis

The practice of giving small daily doses of colchicine as prophylaxis to prevent acute attacks is up to 85% effective.[171] Colchicine 0.6 mg one to three times a day is generally well tolerated, although the drug may produce a reversible axonal neuromyopathy.[172] This complication causes proximal muscle weakness with or without painful paresthesia and elevated serum levels of creatine phosphokinase. This is most often seen in patients with hypertension, renal dysfunction, or liver disease who are also using diuretics. Rhabdomyolysis may also occur in these settings and is more common in individuals who are also taking a statin (HMG-CoA reductase inhibitor) or cyclosporine.[173]

In patients who are unable to tolerate even one colchicine tablet per day, indomethacin or another NSAID has been used prophylactically at low doses (e.g., 25 mg indomethacin twice a day or naproxen 250 mg/day), with some success.[174] Maintenance doses of colchicine or an NSAID may make the difference between frequent incapacitation and uninterrupted daily activities. Prophylaxis is usually continued until the serum urate value has been maintained well within the normal range and there have been no acute attacks for 3 to 6 months. It is important to warn patients that colchicine discontinuation may be followed by an exacerbation of acute gouty arthritis and advise them what to do should an attack occur. Finally, prophylactic treatment is not recommended unless the clinician also uses urate-lowering agents. Prophylactic colchicine may block the acute inflammatory response but does not alter the deposition of crystals in tissues. When deposition continues without the warning signs of recurrent bouts of acute arthritis, tophi and destruction to cartilage and bone can occur without notice.

Control of Hyperuricemia

Elimination of hyperuricemia with antihyperuricemic agents can prevent and reverse urate deposition. Today, opinion differs as to when in the course of gout the clinician should start antihyperuricemic therapy. Some physicians regard the first gouty attack as a late event in a disorder marked by years of antecedent silent deposition of urate crystals in cartilage and other connective tissue. Others believe that because tophi and symptomatic chronic gouty arthritis develop in only a minority of cases and ordinarily develop slowly after many years of recurrent acute attacks, unnecessary or premature medication can be avoided without demonstrable penalty. In practice, it is rare to have a patient who never experiences a second attack.[59] The probability of such a benign course is greatest in patients who have only minimally elevated serum urate concentrations and normal 24-hour urinary uric acid values. Arguably, a case can be made for initiating antihyperuricemia therapy after the second attack in most patients.[175]

Antihyperuricemic drugs provide a definitive method for controlling hyperuricemia. Although it is important to treat and prevent acute attacks of gouty arthritis with anti-inflammatory agents, it is the long-term control of hyperuricemia that ultimately modifies the manifestations of the gouty diathesis. Once started, treatment with specific urate-lowering agents is lifelong and the dose must be sufficient to maintain the serum urate level below 6.8 mg/dL, preferably between 5 and 6 mg/dL. Lowering the serum urate level from 11 mg/dL to 7.5 mg/dL may seem encouraging, but this change does not reverse the process. It merely slows the rate at which crystals continue to deposit. Generally, the lower the serum urate level achieved during antihyperuricemic therapy, the faster the reduction in tophaceous deposits.[176] The 5 to 6 mg/dL target is recommended because it is far enough below the saturation level of 6.8 mg/dL that it provides some margin for fluctuations in serum levels and avoids excessive exposure to the medication, which might increase the chance of toxicity.

Reduction to target levels may be achieved pharmacologically by the use of xanthine oxidase inhibitors, uricosuric agents, or uricases. Xanthine oxidase, the enzyme that catalyzes the oxidation of hypoxanthine to xanthine and xanthine to uric acid, is inhibited by allopurinol, oxypurinol, and febuxostat. Probenecid, sulfinpyrazone, and benzbromarone are uricosuric agents that reduce serum urate concentrations by enhancing the renal excretion of uric acid. Rasburicase and pegloticase nezymatically convert urate to allantoin, which is much more soluble and readily excreted in the urine. These antihyperuricemic drugs do not have anti-inflammatory properties.

For those patients with gout who excrete less than 800 mg of uric acid per day and have normal renal function, reduction of the serum urate concentration can be achieved equally well with a xanthine oxidase inhibitor or a uricosuric drug. These agents are equally effective in preventing the deterioration of renal function in patients with primary gout.[177] In most cases, allopurinol is the drug of choice because it can be used with fewer restrictions compared with uricosuric agents.

In general, the ideal candidate for uricosuric agents is a gouty patient who is younger than 60 years and has normal renal function (creatinine clearance >80 mL/min), uric acid excretion of less than 800 mg per 24 hours on a general diet, and no history of renal calculi. Patients prescribed uricosuric agents should be counseled to avoid salicylate use at doses greater than 81 mg/day.[178]

In certain situations, an inhibitor of xanthine oxidase is clearly the drug of choice in a gouty patient. Gouty individuals who excrete larger quantities of uric acid in their urine or who have a history of renal calculi of any type should be treated with a xanthine oxidase inhibitor (Table 95-6). The incidence of renal calculi is about 35% in patients with primary gout who excrete more than 700 mg/day of uric acid.[122] There is also a greater risk for uric acid stones on initiation of uricosuric therapy. In addition, patients with tophi generally should receive a xanthine oxidase inhibitor to decrease the load of urate that must be handled by the kidney. Patients with gout and mild renal insufficiency can be given either type of agent, but probenecid and sulfinpyrazone would not be expected to work when the glomerular filtration rate is less than 50 mL/min. Allopurinol is effective in the presence of renal

Table 95-6 Indications for Xanthine Oxidase Inhibitor

Hyperuricemia Associated with Increased Uric Acid Production
Urinary uric acid excretion of 1000 mg or more in 24 hr
Hyperuricemia associated with HPRT deficiency or PRPP synthetase overactivity
Uric acid nephropathy
Nephrolithiasis
Prophylaxis before cytolytic therapy
Intolerance or Reduced Efficacy of Uricosuric Agents
Gout with renal insufficiency (GFR < 60 mL/min)
Allergy to uricosurics

GFR, glomerular filtration rate; HPRT, hypoxanthine phosphoribosyltransferase; PRPP, phosphoribosylpyrophosphate.

Table 95-7 Maintenance Doses of Allopurinol Based on Creatinine Clearance Measurement*

Creatinine Clearance (mL/min)	Allopurinol Dose (mg)
0	100 every 3 days
10	100 every 2 days
20	100 daily
40	150 daily
60	200 daily
80	250 daily
100	300 daily
120	350 daily
140	400 daily

*These doses represent those that might be selected when initiating therapy with allopurinol. However, urate levels should be checked and the dosage adjusted so that the patient is taking the lowest dose that maintains the serum urate level below 5 to 6 mg/dL.

From Hande KR, Noone RM, Stone WJ: Severe allopurinol toxicity: description and guidelines for presentation in patients with renal insufficiency, *Am J Med* 76:47, 1984.

insufficiency, but doses may have to be decreased in that situation. Febuxostat needs no adjustment in mild to moderate renal insufficiency. A final indication for a xanthine oxidase inhibitor is the failure of uricosuric agents to produce a serum urate concentration lower than 6 mg/dL or patient intolerance of the uricosuric agent. A xanthine oxidase inhibitor and a uricosuric drug may be used in combination for a patient with tophaceous gout in whom it is not possible to reduce the serum urate below 6 mg/dL with a single agent. In most settings, if allopurinol does not cause the serum urate to drop below 6 mg/dL, it is the result of insufficient dosing or poor patient compliance.

Xanthine Oxidase Inhibitors

Allopurinol is a substrate for xanthine oxidase and is converted to oxypurinol by that enzyme activity. Oxypurinol is also an inhibitor of xanthine oxidase. Allopurinol is metabolized in the liver and has a half-life of 1 to 3 hours, but oxypurinol, which is excreted in the urine, has a half-life of 12 to 17 hours. Because of these pharmacokinetic properties, allopurinol is dosed on a daily basis and the dosage required to reduce serum urate levels is lower in patients with decreased glomerular filtration rates.

In 1984 guidelines for allopurinol dosing based on creatinine clearance were published (Table 95-7).[179] It is now apparent that these guidelines are useful for selecting the initial dosage of allopurinol, but they do not provide the effective maintenance dose for many individuals and following them does not protect against cutaneous hypersensitivity reactions.[179-182]

Allopurinol should be used at the lowest dose that lowers the serum urate level below 5 to 6 mg/dL. The most commonly prescribed dose is 300 mg/day, but this is insufficient to adequately reduce serum urate to the target level in 21% to 55% of individuals.[44,183,184] Thus higher doses, with a maximum of 800 mg/day, may be required. The sudden lowering of serum urate concentrations that accompanies the initiation of allopurinol therapy may trigger acute gout attacks. This risk can be minimized by beginning prophylactic colchicine or an NSAID (see the previous discussion) 2 weeks before the first dose of allopurinol. Alternatively, the clinician can start allopurinol at a dose of 50 to 100 mg/

day and increase it by similar increments weekly until the desired target is reached.

About 20% of patients who take allopurinol report side effects, with 5% discontinuing the medication. Common side effects include gastrointestinal intolerance and skin rashes. The occurrence of a rash does not necessarily mean the drug should be discontinued. If the rash is not severe, the allopurinol can be withheld temporarily and resumed after the rash has cleared. Oxypurinol has been tried in patients who are sensitive to allopurinol, but its use is limited by poor gastrointestinal absorption and a high prevalence of cross-reactivity with allopurinol. Oral and intravenous protocols for desensitization to allopurinol have been successful in some patients following cutaneous reactions.[174,185]

Other adverse reactions include fever, toxic epidermal necrolysis, alopecia, bone marrow suppression with leukopenia or thrombocytopenia, agranulocytosis, aplastic anemia, granulomatous hepatitis, jaundice, sarcoid-like reaction, and vasculitis. The most severe reaction is the allopurinol hypersensitivity syndrome, which may include fever, skin rash, eosinophilia, hepatitis, progressive renal insufficiency, and death.[180,186] Autopsies reveal diffuse vasculitis involving multiple organs. This is most likely to develop in individuals with pre-existing renal dysfunction and in those taking diuretics.

Allopurinol is involved in relatively few drug-drug interactions. Its use potentiates the actions of other agents that are inactivated by xanthine oxidase. The most important of these are azathioprine and 6-mercaptopurine. In addition, allopurinol can reduce the activity of hepatic microsomal drug-metabolizing enzymes and prolong the half-lives of warfarin and theophylline. Rash may be more common in patients using allopurinol and ampicillin, and bone marrow suppression may be increased in those also taking cyclophosphamide.

Febuxostat (Uloric, Takeda Pharmaceuticals America, Inc.) was recently approved for use in the treatment of gout on the basis of one phase II, three phase III, and two open-label extension trials.[44,150,187-191] Febuxostat is a potent xanthine oxidase inhibitor that differs from allopurinol in that it is of another chemical class and is a selective inhibitor of enzyme activity. These properties indicate that it would be an excellent alternative for individuals who are intolerant of or hypersensitive to allopurinol. In fact, febuxostat appeared to outperform allopurinol in achieving target serum urates in the clinical trials. Importantly, though, allopurinol doses were fixed and clearly too low in these trials, and therefore it is impossible to make firm conclusions about the comparative efficacy of these two agents. In the United States, febuxostat doses of 40 or 80 mg a day have been approved, whereas in Europe, doses of 80 and 120 mg a day are recommended. The dosage of febuxostat does not need to be adjusted in individuals with mild to moderate renal insufficiency. The same precautions apply as with allopurinol in terms of use with other agents metabolized by xanthine oxidase including azathioprine and 6-mercaptopurine. Diarrhea, dizziness, headache, liver function test abnormalities, and altered thyroid function tests were the most common side effects noted in the clinical trials. Cardiovascular events were numerically higher with febuxostat than with other treatments, but when total drug exposures were taken into account, the incidence was the same.[192] In Europe, the use of febuxostat in patients with ischemic heart disease or congestive heart failure is not recommended. After the FDA-required CONFIRMS trial[189] did not detect increased cardiovascular risk with febuxostat, the FDA approved dosing of 40 mg and 80 mg daily in the United States. Takeda, under guidance from the FDA, has committed to cardiovascular postmarketing. Gout flares were higher early on with febuxostat compared with allopurinol, emphasizing again the need for prophylaxis of up to 6 months when initiating urate-lowering therapy.

Febuxostat and allopurinol have similar safety profiles. Patients with hypersensitivity reactions to allopurinol who were given febuxostat were able to tolerate the new drug.[193] Febuxostat should be considered mainly for patients intolerant to allopurinol, for those whose gout is not controlled with other urate-lowering treatments, and for those with renal insufficiency (creatinine clearance >30 mL/min). Febuxostat should be tried before an attempt at allopurinol desensitization. Finally, febuxostat should be used before uricosuric drugs in patients with nephrolithiasis.

Uricosuric Agents

Administration of a uricosuric agent increases the rate of renal uric acid excretion.[194] In the kidney, there are separate transport systems for the secretion and reabsorption of organic ions including uric acid. Because urate is reabsorbed by a renal tubular brush border anion transporter, the reabsorption of urate can be inhibited when uricosuric agents are present in the lumen and compete with urate for the transporter. This inhibition of reabsorptive anion transporter requires high doses of uricosuric agents. Because the secretory transport system is quantitatively much smaller than that for reabsorption and is located in the basolateral membrane of the tubule, when uricosuric agents are taken in low doses, they actually decrease the renal excretion of uric acid and raise serum urate levels by inhibiting the secretory transport system.

Probenecid and sulfinpyrazone are the most widely used uricosuric agents available in the United States. Benzbromarone is used for this purpose in other countries as well. However, many other agents can reduce serum urate levels by enhancing the renal excretion of uric acid (see Table 95-8).

Probenecid is readily absorbed from the gastrointestinal tract. Its half-life in plasma is dose dependent, varying from

Table 95-8 Drugs That Are Uricosuric in Humans

Acetohexamide	Glycerol guaiacolate
Amflutizole	Glycine
Ascorbic acid	Glycopyrrolate
Azapropazone	Iodopyracet
Azauridine	Iopanoic acid
Benzbromarone	Losartan
Calcitonin	Meclofenamic acid
Calcium ipodate	Orotic acid
Citrate	Outdated tetracyclines
Dicumarol	Phenolsulfonphthalein
Diflunisal	Probenecid
Estrogens	Salicylates
Fenofibrate	Sulfinpyrazone

6 to 12 hours. This can be prolonged by the concomitant use of allopurinol. Probenecid is metabolized in vivo, with less than 5% of the administered dose recovered in the urine. The maintenance dosage of probenecid ranges from 500 mg to 3 g per day and is administered two or three times a day. Acute gouty attacks may accompany the initiation of this medication, and, as with all uricosuric agents, patients using probenecid are at increased risk for developing renal calculi. With long-term use, up to 18% of individuals develop gastrointestinal complaints and 5% develop hypersensitivity and rash. Although serious toxicity is rare, approximately one-third of individuals eventually become intolerant of probenecid and discontinue its use. Probenecid alters the metabolism of several other agents by several mechanisms (Table 95-9). Concomitant use of probenecid can increase the potency of some agents by decreasing their renal excretion, delaying their metabolism, or impairing their hepatic uptake. It may decrease the effectiveness of other medications by reducing their volume of distribution.

Sulfinpyrazone is completely absorbed from the gastrointestinal tract and has a half-life of 1 to 3 hours. Most of the drug is excreted in the urine as the parahydroxyl metabolite, which is also uricosuric. Sulfinpyrazone is usually given at a dosage of 300 to 400 mg/day divided into three or four doses. The rates of tolerability and types of adverse reactions are similar to those with probenecid. Unfortunately, sulfinpyrazone is no longer readily available.

Benzbromarone is more potent than probenecid and sulfinpyrazone.[177] It is well tolerated and effective in cyclosporine-treated renal transplant patients. It can be used in those with moderate renal dysfunction (creatinine clearance approximately 25 mL/min).

Table 95-9 Effects of Probenecid on Metabolism of Other Drugs

Decreased Renal Excretion
p-Aminohippuric acid
Phenolsulfonphthalein
Salicylic acid and its acyl and phenolic glucuronides
Phlorizin and its glucuronide
Acetazolamide
Dapsone and its metabolites
Sulfinpyrazone and its parahydroxyl metabolite
Indomethacin
Ampicillin
Penicillin
Cephradine
Reduced Volume of Distribution
Ampicillin
Ancillin
Nafcillin
Cephaloridine
Impairment of Hepatic Uptake
Bromsulfophthalein
Indocyanine green
Rifampicin
Delayed Metabolism
Heparin

Uricases

Uricase was lost to man and some nonhuman primates via a missense mutation in the gene encoding the enzyme (see Chapter 94).[195] Pegloticase is a pegylated mammalian (porcine-like) recombinant uricase, recently approved by the FDA at a dosage of 8 mg intravenously every 2 weeks for the treatment of severe tophaceous gout.[150,196] With intravenous administration of 0.5 mg to 12 mg, the plasma uricase activity increases linearly with doses up to 8 mg, with an enzymatic activity half-life of 6.4 to 13.8 days. With intravenous doses of 4 mg or more, the serum urate falls dramatically in 24 to 72 hours, from a mean of 11.1 mg/dL to 1 mg/dL and stays low for 21 days after infusion.[197] Pegloticase was studied in a phase I, a phase II open-label trial (41 patients), and two replicate phase III randomized control trials (212 patients total).[198-202] In the phase III trials, subjects with treatment-failure gout were randomly assigned to either pegloticase 8 mg intravenously every 2 weeks or 4 weeks or placebo.[201] Pegloticase was significantly more effective than placebo at achieving the primary endpoint of a plasma urate concentration lower than 6 mg/dL for 80% of the time in months 3 and 6 of the trial. It also seemed clear that, when tolerated, pegloticase was efficacious at reducing tophi (Figure 95-9).[200,202] Colchicine or NSAIDs were used for gout prophylaxis, and oral fexofenadine and acetaminophen, as well as hydrocortisone 200 mg intravenously before infusion, were used for infusion reaction prophylaxis. Despite that, gout flares, infusion reactions, and serious adverse events were significantly more frequent in patients given pegloticase than in other patients. The most common reason for withdrawal was infusion reaction.

Important relations were noted among immunogenicity, infusion reactions, and efficacy.[203] High-titer antibodies to pegloticase and/or polyethylene glycol were associated with loss of response and infusion reactions. In fact, 96% of patients with antibodies to poly(ethylene glycol) from the groups assigned every-2-week or every-4-week pegloticase were nonresponders, and 50% and 76%, respectively, had infusion reactions. These antibodies did not neutralize uricase activity in vitro. The development of these anti-pegloticase antibodies was associated with a loss of response in patients coinciding with a rise in plasma urate concentrations above 6 mg/dL.[204] Tellingly, 71% of infusion reactions occurred after this loss of response. In the group assigned pegloticase every 2 weeks, cessation of treatment when concentrations of plasma urate were higher than 6 mg/dL would have avoided 91% of infusion reactions.[204] Because of this observation, the FDA has recommended that clinicians follow serum urates carefully and stop pegloticase when the serum urate rises above 6 mg/dL. An open-label extension study with 151 patients supported the conclusions from the phase III trials.[205] Gout attacks continued to decline in patients, most patients maintained target serum urates, and an additional 20 patients, beyond the 32 patients in the randomized trials, had complete resolution of at least one tophus. Unfortunately, infusion reactions remained common and sometimes serious, frequently leading to discontinuation, particularly in those who had only received placebo in the randomized trials.

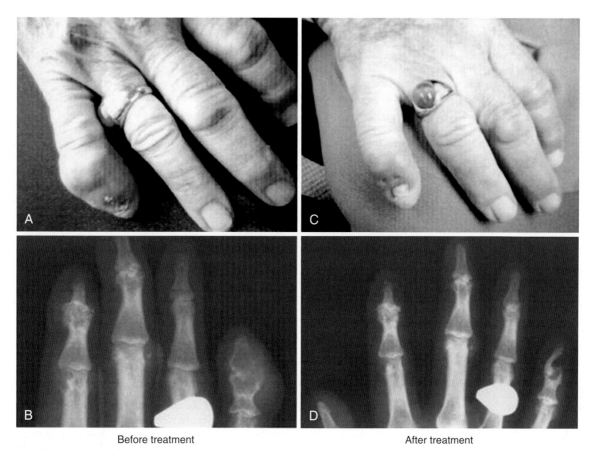

Before treatment   After treatment

Figure 95-9 Photographic and radiographic evidence of tophus resolution after pegloticase treatment. **A,** Large draining tophus on fifth distal interphalangeal (DIP) joint, before treatment. **B,** Corresponding radiograph showing soft tissue swelling and bony erosions in fifth DIP joint, before treatment. **C,** Resolution of tophus on fifth DIP joint after 12 weeks of treatment. **D,** Corresponding radiograph showing resolution of soft tissue swelling in fifth DIP joint, a decrease in bony erosions, and thickening of bone cortex at this joint, 15 months after termination of therapy. *(From Baraf HS, Matsumoto AK, Maroli AN, Waltrip RW: Resolution of gouty tophi after twelve weeks of pegloticase treatment,* Arthritis Rheum 58:3632, 2008.)

All patients in the pegloticase randomized trials had some cardiovascular risk factor.[201] There was a concern for an independent cardiovascular side effect signal in patients treated with pegloticase, but the FDA's independent analysis concluded that the number of events was too small to lend support to a definite cardiovascular signal.[206] The FDA approved pegloticase for use in treatment-failure gout in October 2010. Pegloticase will have a more limited target population than febuxostat. Terkeltaub has proposed guidelines for the use of uricases in gout.[207] They are appropriate for patients with tophaceous gout with a large excess of total body urate and persisting gout attacks, or with damaging arthropathy, who have failed or are intolerant of conventional therapy. Presumably, many patients who fit this description can now be given and will respond to febuxostat, but others will not. The notion of debulking the urate load is a good way to conceptualize the pegloticase strategy and emphasizes it as adjunctive therapy, best followed by other urate-lowering therapy when possible. A clear advantage is that pegloticase can reduce tophi dramatically and more quickly than conventional treatment[200,202,205] (see Figure 95-9). Problems with immunogenicity continue, and the continuous use of pegloticase may be restricted by antibody development. At least 25% of patients develop antibodies, with subsequent infusion reactions, restricted

efficacy, or drug withdrawal. Anaphylaxis occurs in about 5% of treated patients. Gout flares are sometimes severe and are frequent, occurring despite prophylaxis in more than 80% of treated patients. The required concomitant infusion of corticosteroids with peglotocase may further restrict its use in patients with conditions such as diabetes or glaucoma, and pegloticase should not be given to patients with glucose-6-phosphate dehydrogenase deficiency because it may induce hemolysis.

Despite the potential downsides of pegloticase, previously these often terribly symptomatic patients had no options. Hopefully, monitoring for a rising serum urate concentration as a sign of antibody development and impending infusion reaction will allow for safer administration.[204] Encouraging data recently presented in abstract form suggest that a subset of patients who normalize their serum urate within the first 6 months of pegloticase treatment can be safely maintained on therapy long term, with a median follow-up of 2.5 years.[208] In addition to ongoing clinical improvement, the frequency of infusion reactions was low in this group, even in subjects with breaks in treatment of up to 6 months. Nevertheless, this is a drug that should be administered at centers familiar with its use and with an established capability of dealing with serious infusion reactions including anaphylaxis.

COMPLIANCE WITH TREATMENT

Because the disease processes involved in gout are so well understood, the diagnosis can be definitively established. Once gout is diagnosed, the available therapies are so effective that it should be a readily treated and easily managed disease. However, too many patients including those who are accurately diagnosed do not do well. Failure of antihyperuricemic therapy to attain the target urate level is usually due to improper prescribing or poor compliance.[180] Compliance is often a problem when treating chronic asymptomatic conditions, and associated alcoholism can be a factor. Perhaps more important is the fact that patients may need to take up to three different medications on three different schedules to control their symptoms and treat the disease.

It is believed that if patients understand why they are taking medications, they are more likely to be compliant. Toward this end, an analogy has been developed that helps some patients become more compliant.[209] In this analogy, urate crystals are compared with matches. The patient is told that "when the match strikes," it causes a gout attack. To "put out the fire," the patient takes an NSAID or colchicine. Although this resolves the attack, "the matches are still there." To eliminate future attacks, the patient is given prophylactic colchicine, "which makes the matches damp and harder to strike," and allopurinol (or a uricosuric agent), "which actually removes the matches from the body."

MANAGEMENT OF GOUT AFTER ORGAN TRANSPLANTATION

The management of patients with gout after organ transplantation requires careful consideration. The use of glucocorticoids, azathioprine, or cyclosporine and the precarious status of renal function in many patients pose complex problems. Colchicine and NSAIDs may be inappropriate for the management of acute gouty arthritis in this setting because of their potential toxicities. Intra-articular glucocorticoid injections may be most helpful, and one may be forced to rely more heavily on pain medications in this setting. Prophylactic colchicine can be used in patients with normal renal function, but treatment must be monitored closely. The combination of colchicine and cyclosporine has induced rhabdomyolysis.[173]

When considering chronic therapy, it is helpful to lower the doses of cyclosporine and eliminate the use of diuretics, if possible. Uricosuric agents can be used safely, but their usefulness declines if renal function is poor. Allopurinol can be used in patients with abnormal renal function, but the dose may need to be reduced. Febuxostat may be safer in this setting but has not been studied. But both allopurinol and febuxostat may have severe interactions with azathioprine. Azathioprine is metabolized by xanthine oxidase, and because these drugs inhibit that enzyme, the breakdown of azathioprine is slowed, increasing the effective dose. If care is not taken, significant bone marrow toxicity can result. Thiopurine S-methyltransferase (TPMT) studies should be obtained before starting azathioprine. When azathioprine and allopurinol are used together, they can be started at 25

and 50 mg/day, respectively.[210] Revised dosing for febuxostat in such a situation has not been determined. Complete blood counts and serum urate level concentrations are then monitored weekly when using allopurinol, and the dose is adjusted to bring the serum urate concentration to less than 6 mg/dL. As an alternative to azathioprine, mycophenolate mofetil has been used effectively with allopurinol in some transplant patients.[211]

Uricase has been used to drastically lower serum urate levels and shrink tophi in a small number of patients with gout after cardiac transplantation.[212] This treatment has been associated with significant allergic reactions including anaphylaxis, bronchospasm, and hemolytic anemia. The newer preparations of uricase such as pegloticase may avoid those complications and prove more effective.[213]

ANCILLARY FACTORS

In addition to anti-inflammatory agents, colchicine prophylaxis, and antihyperuricemic therapy, other factors may be decisive in determining whether the following develop: recurrent attacks, chronic gouty arthritis, kidney stones, or nephropathy. Today, dietary purine restriction solely to control serum urate levels is rarely advised. A totally purine-free diet reduces the urinary excretion of uric acid by only 200 to 400 mg/day and lowers the mean serum urate value by about 1 mg/dL. In addition, the antihyperuricemic agents available today are so effective that this type of dietary manipulation is rarely necessary. Nevertheless, beneficial results have been reported with a diet of moderate calorie and carbohydrate restriction and a proportionally increased intake of protein and unsaturated fat.[214] Some subjects with gout are susceptible to acute attacks after the consumption of alcoholic beverages or rich foods. Others describe idiosyncratic responses such as acute gout after eating a particular food, but such relationships are rare and questionable. A diet designed to avoid indiscretions known to precipitate acute gouty attacks in a particular individual is recommended.

In addition, diet is important with regard to other medical problems.[215] Many gouty patients are overweight, and restoration of ideal body weight through regulated calorie restriction is recommended. In addition, at least 75% of patients with primary gout have hypertriglyceridemia. The initial step in managing hypertriglyceridemia is reduction to ideal body weight and elimination of alcohol ingestion.

Many patients with gout consume liberal amounts of alcohol. Acute excesses may lead to exacerbations of hyperuricemia secondary to temporary hyperlactacidemia, and chronic ingestion of alcohol may stimulate increased purine production.[106] The added purine load resulting from regular ingestion of beer may also be a contributing factor. Patients should be warned about the deleterious effects of excessive alcohol intake. Compliance with medication is also much worse among patients who consume alcohol.

About one-third of gouty subjects are hypertensive. The complications of hypertension are potentially more serious than those of hyperuricemia, and the clinician should not hesitate to use whatever drugs are necessary to control the hypertension. Many hypertensive gouty patients require a thiazide diuretic. If this medication is necessary to control hypertension, it should be used, with the recognition that the dosage of concomitant antihyperuricemic therapy may need to be adjusted to maintain appropriate control of serum urate levels.

Selected References

1. Wyngaarden JD, Kelley WN: *Gout and hyperuricemia*, New York, 1976, Grune & Stratton.
2. Wortmann RL, Schumacher HR Jr, Becker MA, Ryan LM: *Crystal-induced arthropathies: gout, pseudogout, and apatite-associated syndromes*, New York, 2006, Informa Healthcare.
5. Mikuls TR, Saag KG: New insights into gout epidemiology, *Curr Opin Rheumatol* 18:199, 2006.
11. Arromlee E, Michet CJ, Crowson CS, et al: Epidemiology of gout: is the incidence rising? *J Rheumatol* 29:2403, 2002.
12. Wallace KL, Riedel AA, Joseph-Ridge N, Wortmann RL: Increased prevalence of gout and hyperuricemia over 10 years among older adults in a managed care population, *J Rheumatol* 31:1582, 2004.
14. Choi H, Atkinson KK, Karlson E, et al: Alcohol intake and risk incidence of gout in men: a prospective study, *Lancet* 363:1277, 2004.
15. Choi HK, Liu S: Intake of purine-rich foods, protein, and dairy products and relationship to serum levels of uric acid: the Third National Health and Nutrition Examination Survey, *Arthritis Rheum* 52:283, 2005.
16. Wortmann RL, Kelley WN: Gout and hyperuricemia. In Ruddy S, Harris ED Jr, Sledge CB, editors: *Kelley's textbook of rheumatology*, ed 6, Philadelphia, 2001, WB Saunders.
17. Zaka R, Williams CJ: New developments in the epidemiology and genetics of gout, *Curr Rheumatol Rep* 8:215, 2006.
18. Wyngaarden JB, Kelley WN: Disposition of uric acid in primary gout. In Wyngaarden JB, Kelley WN, editors: *Gout and hyperuricemia*, New York, 1976, Grune & Stratton, pp 149–157.
19. Simkin PA: New standards for uric acid excretion: evidence for an inducible transporter, *Arthritis Care Res* 49:735, 2003.
20. Choi HK, Zhu Y, Mount DB: Genetics of gout, *Curr Opin Rheumatol* 22:144, 2010.
21. Enomoto A, Kimura H, Chairoungdu A, et al: Molecular identification of a renal urate anion exchanger that regulates blood urate levels, *Nature* 417:447, 2002.
22. Wallace C, Newhouse SJ, Braund P, et al: Genome-wide association study identifies genes for biomarkers of cardiovascular disease: serum urate and dyslipidemia, *Am J Hum Genet* 82:139, 2008.
23. Kolz M, Johnson T, Sanna S, et al: Meta-analysis of 28,141 individuals identifies common variants within five new loci that influence uric acid concentrations, *PLoS Genet* 5:e1000504, 2009.
24. Iwai N, Mino Y, Hosoyamada M, et al: A high prevalence of renal hypouricemia caused by inactive *SLC22A12* in Japanese, *Kidney Int* 66:935, 2004.
25. Shima Y, Teruya K, Ohta H: Association between intronic SNP in urate-anion exchanger gene, *SLC22A12*, and serum uric acid levels in Japanese, *Life Sci* 79:2234, 2006.
26. Augustin R, Carayannopoulos MO, Dowd LO, et al: Identification and characterization of human glucose transporter-like protein-9 (GLUT9): alternative splicing alters trafficking, *J Biol Chem* 279:16229, 2004.
27. Vitart V, Rudan I, Hayward C, et al: *SLC2A9* is a newly identified urate transporter influencing serum urate concentration, urate excretion and gout, *Nat Genet* 40:437, 2008.
28. Anzai N, Ichida K, Jutabha P, et al: Plasma urate level is directly regulated by a voltage-driven urate efflux transporter URATv1 (SLC2A9) in humans, *J Biol Chem* 283:26834, 2008.
29. Caulfield MJ, Munroe PB, O'Neill D, et al: SLC2A9 is a high-capacity urate transporter in humans, *PLoS Med* 5:e197, 2008.
30. Doring A, Gieger C, Mehta D, et al: SLC2A9 influences uric acid concentrations with pronounced sex-specific effects, *Nat Genet* 40:430, 2008.
31. Dehghan A, Kottgen A, Yang Q, et al: Association of three genetic loci with uric acid concentration and risk of gout: a genome-wide association study, *Lancet* 372:1953, 2008.
33. Matsuo H, Chiba T, Nagamori S, et al: Mutations in glucose transporter 9 gene SLC2A9 cause renal hypouricemia, *Am J Hum Genet* 83:744, 2008.
34. Woodward OM, Kottgen A, Coresh J, et al: Identification of a urate transporter, ABCG2, with a common functional polymorphism causing gout, *Proc Natl Acad Sci USA* 106:10338, 2009.
35. Brandstatter A, Kiechl S, Kollerits B, et al: Sex-specific association of the putative fructose transporter SLC2A9 variants with uric acid levels is modified by BMI, *Diabetes Care* 31:1662, 2008.
36. Choi HK, Curhan G: Soft drinks, fructose consumption, and the risk of gout in men: prospective cohort study, *Br Med J* 336:309, 2008.
37. Choi JW, Ford ES, Gao X, Choi HK: Sugar-sweetened soft drinks, diet soft drinks, and serum uric acid level: the Third National Health and Nutrition Examination Survey, *Arthritis Rheum* 59:109, 2008.
38. Gao X, Qi L, Qiao N, et al: Intake of added sugar and sugar-sweetened drink and serum uric acid concentration in US men and women, *Hypertension* 50:306, 2007.
44. Becker MA, Schumacher HR, Wortmann RL, et al: A study comparing safety and efficiency of oral febuxostat and allopurinol in subjects with hyperuricemia and gout, *N Engl J Med* 353:2450, 2005.
45. Hunter DJ, York M, Chaisson CE, et al: Recent diuretic use and the risk of recurrent gout attacks: the online case-crossover gout study, *J Rheumatol* 33:1341, 2006.
52. Wallace SL, Robinson H, Masi AT, et al: Preliminary criteria for the classification of acute arthritis of primary gout, *Arthritis Rheum* 20:897, 1977.
53. Zhang W, Doherty M, Pascual E, et al: EULAR evidence based recommendations for gout. Part I: diagnosis. Report of a task force of the standing committee for international clinical studies including therapeutics (ESCISIT), *Ann Rheum Dis* 65:1301, 2006.
56. Tsutani H, Yoshio N, Takanori U: Interleukin 6 reduces serum urate concentrations, *J Rheumatol* 27:554, 2000.
57. Urano W, Yamanaka H, Tsutani H, et al: The inflammatory process in the mechanism of decreased serum uric acid concentration during acute gouty arthritis, *J Rheumatol* 29:1950, 2002.
59. Thiele RG, Schlesinger N: Diagnosis of gout by ultrasound, *Rheumatology (Oxford)* 46:1116, 2007.
60. Wright SA, Filippucci E, McVeigh C, et al: High-resolution ultrasonography of the first metatarsal phalangeal joint in gout: a controlled study, *Ann Rheum Dis* 66:859, 2007.
61. Thiele RG, Schlesinger N: Ultrasonography shows disappearance of monosodium urate crystal deposition on hyaline cartilage after sustained normouricemia is achieved, *Rheumatol Int* 30:495, 2010.
62. Howard RNG, Pillinger MH, Gyftopoulos S, et al: Concordance between ultrasound readers determining presence of monosodium urate crystal deposition in knee and toe joints, *Arthritis Rheum* 62:S672, 2010.
63. Solano C, Rodríguez-Henríquez PJ, Hofmann F, et al: Asymptomatic hyperuricemia: ultrasonographic findings, *Arthritis Rheum* 62:S671, 2010.
64. Thiele RG, Schlesinger N: Ultrasound detects more erosions in gout than conventional radiography, *Arthritis Rheum* 62:S638, 2010.
65. Carter JD, Kedar RP, Anderson SR, et al: An analysis of MRI and ultrasound imaging in patients with gout who have normal plain radiographs, *Rheumatology (Oxford)* 48:1442, 2009.
66. Thiele RG: Role of ultrasound and other advanced imaging in the diagnosis and management of gout, *Curr Rheumatol Rep* 13:146, 2011.
67. Dalbeth N, McQueen FM.: Use of imaging to evaluate gout and other crystal deposition disorders, *Curr Opin Rheumatol* 21:124, 2009.
68. Gutman AB: Gout. In Beeson PB, McDermott W, editors: *Textbook of medicine*, ed 12, Philadelphia, 1958, WB Saunders; p 595.
69. McCarthy GM, Barthelemy CR, Verum JA, et al: Influence of antihyperuricemia therapy and radiographic progression of gout, *Arthritis Rheum* 34:1489, 1991.
70. Pascual E, Battle-Gualda E, Martinez A, et al: Synovial fluid analysis for diagnosis of intercritical gout, *Ann Intern Med* 131:756, 1999.
78. Beathge BA, Work J, Landreneau MD, et al: Tophaceous gout in patients with renal transplants treated with cyclosporine A, *J Rheumatol* 20:718, 1993.
80. Gentili A: The advanced imaging of gouty tophi, *Curr Rheum Rep* 8:231, 2006.
84. Choi HK, Atkinson K, Karlson EW, et al: Obesity weight change, hypertension, diuretic use, and risk of gout in white men: The Health Professionals Follow-up Study, *Arch Intern Med* 165:742, 2005.
88. Tsutsumi S, Yamamoto T, Moriwaki Y, et al: Decreased activities of lipoprotein lipase and hepatic triglyceride lipase in patients with gout, *Metabolism* 50:952, 2001.

91. Feig DI, Johnson RJ: Hyperuricemia in childhood primary hypertension, *Hypertension* 42:247, 2003.

93. Kang DH, Nakagawa T, Feng L, et al: A role for uric acid in the progression of renal disease, *J Am Soc Nephrol* 13:1288, 2002.

94. Mazzali M, Kanellis J, Han L, et al: Hyperuricemia induces primary renal arteriolopathy in rats by a blood pressure-independent mechanism, *Am J Physiol Renal Physiol* 282:F991, 2002.

97. Culleton BF, Larson MG, Kannel WB, Levy D: Serum uric acid and the risk for cardiovascular disease and death: The Framingham Heart Study, *Ann Intern Med* 131:7, 1999.

99. Fang J, Alderman MH: Serum uric acid and cardiovascular mortality: The NHANES I Epidemiologic Follow-up Study, 1971-1992, *JAMA* 283:2404, 2000.

100. Verdecchia P, Schillaci G, Reboldi GP, et al: Relation between serum uric acid and risk of cardiovascular disease in hypertension: The PIUMA Study, *Hypertension* 36:1072, 2000.

101. Chou P, Lin K-C, Lin Y-H, et al: Gender differences in the relationship of serum uric acid with fasting serum insulin and plasma glucose in patients without diabetes, *J Rheumatol* 28:571, 2001.

102. Takahashi S, Moriwaki Y, Tsutsumi Z, et al: Increased visceral fat accumulation further aggravates the risks of insulin resistance in gout, *Metabolism* 50:393, 2001.

103. Ford ES, Giles WH, Dietz WH: Prevalence of metabolic syndrome among US adults: findings of the Third National Health and Nutrition Examination Survey, *JAMA* 287:356, 2002.

104. Krishnan E, Baker JF, Furst DE, Schumacher HR: Gout and the risk of acute myocardial infarction, *Arthritis Rheum* 54:2688, 2006.

107. Giordano N, Santacroce C, Mattii G, et al: Hyperuricemia and gout in thyroid endocrine disorders, *Clin Exp Rheumatol* 19:661, 2001.

117. Fessel WJ: Renal outcomes of gout and hyperuricemia, *Am J Med* 67:74, 1979.

126. Kamatani N, Moritani M, Yamanaka H, et al: Localization of a gene for familial juvenile hyperuricemic nephropathy causing underexcretion type gout to 16p12 by genome-wide linkage analysis of a large family, *Arthritis Rheum* 43:925, 2000.

127. Stacey JM, Turner JJO, Harding B, et al: Genetic mapping studies of familial juvenile hyperuricemic nephropathy on chromosome 16p13-p11, *J Clin Endocrinol Metab* 88:464, 2003.

129. Hart TC, Gorry MC, Hart PS, et al: Mutations of the UMOD gene are responsible for medullary cystic kidney disease 2 and familial juvenile hyperuricemic nephropathy, *J Med Genet* 39:882, 2002.

131. Bleyer AJ, Trachtman H, Sandhu J, et al: Renal manifestations of a mutation in the uromodulin (Tamm-Horsfall protein) gene, *Am J Kidney Dis* 42:E20, 2003.

132. Kudo E, Kamatani N, Tezuka O, et al: Familial juvenile hyperuricemic nephropathy: detection of mutations in the uromodulin gene in five Japanese families, *Kidney Int* 65:1589, 2004.

133. Turner JJ, Stacey JM, Harding B, et al: Uromodulin mutations cause familial juvenile hyperuricemic nephropathy, *J Clin Endocrinol Metab* 88:1398, 2003.

134. Rezende-Lima W, Parreira KS, Garcia-Gonzalez M, et al: Homozygosity for uromodulin disorders: FJHN and MCKD-type 2, *Kidney Int* 66:558, 2004.

136. Lin J-L, Tan D-T, Ho H-H, et al: Environmental lead exposure and urate excretion in the general population, *Am J Med* 113:563, 2002.

137. Marsden PA: Increased body lead burden—cause or consequence of chronic renal insufficiency? *N Engl J Med* 348:345, 2002.

138. Batuman V: Lead nephropathy, lead, and hypertension, *Am J Med Sci* 305:241, 1993.

140. Burack DA, Griffith BP, Thompson ME, Kahl LE: Hyperuricemia and gout among heart transplant recipients receiving cyclosporine, *Am J Med* 92:141, 1992.

144. Moriwaki Y, Yamamoto T, Takahashi S, et al: Spot urine uric acid to creatinine ratio used in the estimation of uric acid excretion in primary gout, *J Rheumatol* 28:1306, 2001.

147. Nakagawa T, Mazzali M, Kang DH, et al: Hyperuricemia causes glomerular hypertrophy in the rat, *Am J Nephrol* 23:2, 2002.

148. Yamamoto T, Moriwaki Y, Tukahashi S, et al: Effect of finafibrate on plasma concentration and urinary excretion of purine bases and oxypurinal, *J Rheumatol* 28:2294, 2001.

149. Wurzner G, Gester JC, Chiolero A, et al: Comparative effects of losartan and irbesartan on serum uric acid in hypertensive patients with hyperuricemia and gout, *J Hypertens* 19:1855, 2001.

150. Burns CM, Wortmann RL: Gout therapeutics: new drugs for an old disease, *Lancet* 2010; doi:10.1016/S0140-6736(10)60665-60664.

151. So A, De Smedt T, Revaz S, Tschopp J: A pilot study of IL-1 inhibition by anakinra in acute gout, *Arthritis Res Ther* 9:R28, 2007.

152. Terkeltaub R, Sundy JS, Schumacher HR, et al: The IL-1 inhibitor rilonacept in treatment of chronic gouty arthritis: results of a placebo-controlled, monosequence crossover, nonrandomized, single-blind pilot study, *Ann Rheum Dis* 68:1613, 2009.

154. So A, De Meulemeester M, Andrey Pikhlak A, et al: Canakinumab for the treatment of acute flares in difficult-to-treat gouty arthritis: results of a multicenter, phase II, dose-ranging study, *Arthritis Rheum* 62:3064, 2010.

155. Schlesinger N, Baker DG, Schumacher HR Jr: How well have diagnostic tests and therapies for gout been evaluated? *Curr Opin Rheumatol* 11:441, 1999.

157. Kim KY, Schumacher H, Hunsche E, et al: A literature review of the epidemiology and treatment of acute gout, *Clin Ther* 25:1593, 2003.

158. Terkeltaub RA, Furst DE, Bennett K, et al: High versus low dosing of oral colchicine for early acute gout flare: twenty-four-hour outcome of the first multicenter, randomized, double-blind, placebo-controlled, parallel-group, dose-comparison colchicine study, *Arthritis Rheum* 62:1060, 2010.

159. Zhang W, Doherty M, Bardin T, et al: EULAR Standing Committee for International Clinical Studies Including Therapeutics. EULAR evidence based recommendations for gout. Part II: Management. Report of a task force of the EULAR Standing Committee for International Clinical Studies Including Therapeutics (ESCISIT), *Ann Rheum Dis* 65:1312, 2006.

160. Paulus HE, Schlosstein LH, Godfrey RG, et al: Prophylactic colchicine therapy of intercritical gout. A placebo-controlled study of probenecid-treated patients, *Arthritis Rheum* 17:609, 1974.

161. Borstad GC, Bryant LR, Abel MP, et al: Colchicine for prophylaxis of acute flares when initiating allopurinol for chronic gouty arthritis, *J Rheumatol* 31:2429, 2004.

164. Martinon F, Petrilli V, Mayor A, et al: Gout-associated uric acid crystals activate the NALP3 inflammasome, *Nature* 440:237, 2006.

165. Ryckman C, Gilbert C, De Medicis R, et al: Monosodium urate monohydrate crystals induce the release of the proinflammatory protein S100A8/A9 from neutrophils, *J Leukoc Biol* 76:433, 2004.

168. Clive DM: Renal transplant-associated hyperuricemia and gout, *J Am Soc Nephrol* 11:974, 2000.

170. Getting SJ, Christian HC, Flower RJ, Perritti M: Activation of melanocortin type 3 receptor as a molecular mechanism for adrenocorticotropic hormone efficacy in gouty arthritis, *Arthritis Rheum* 46:2765, 2002.

171. Yu TF, Gutman AB: Efficacy of colchicine prophylaxis: prevention of recurrent gouty arthritis over a mean period of five years in 208 gouty subjects, *Ann Intern Med* 55:179, 1961.

173. Chattopadhyay I, Shetty HMG, Routledge PA, et al: Colchicine induced rhabdomyolysis, *Postgrad Med J* 77:191, 2001.

176. Perez-Ruiz F, Calabozo M, Pijoan JI, et al: Effect of urate-lowering therapy on the velocity of size reduction of tophi in chronic gout, *Arthritis Care Res* 47:356, 2002.

177. Perez-Ruiz F, Calabozo C, Herrero-Betes A, et al: Improvement in renal function in patients with chronic gout after proper control of hyperuricemia and gouty bouts, *Nephron* 86:287, 2000.

179. Hande KR, Noone RM, Stone WJ: Severe allopurinol toxicity: description and guidelines for presentation in patients with renal insufficiency, *Am J Med* 76:47, 1984.

180. Stamp L, Sharples K, Gow P, et al: The optional use of allopurinol: an audit of allopurinol use in South Auckland, *Aust N Z J Med* 30:567, 2000.

181. Perez-Ruiz F, Hernando I, et al: Correction of allopurinol dosing should be based on clearance of creatinine, but not plasma creatinine levels: another insight to allopurinol-related toxicity, *J Clin Rheumatol* 11:129, 2005.

182. Dalbeth N, Kumar S, Stamp L, Gow P: Dose adjustment of allopurinol according to creatinine clearance does not provide adequate control of hyperuricemia in patients with gout, *J Rheumatol* 33:1646, 2006.

184. Li-Yu J, Clayburne G, et al: Treatment of chronic gout: can we determine when urate stores are depleted enough to prevent attacks of gout? *J Rheumatol* 28:577, 2001.

187. Becker MA, Schumacher HR Jr, Wortmann RL, et al: Febuxostat, a novel nonpurine selective inhibitor of xanthine oxidase: a twenty-eight-day, multicenter, phase II, randomized, double-blind,

placebo-controlled, dose-response clinical trial examining safety and efficacy in patients with gout, *Arthritis Rheum* 52:916, 2005.

188. Schumacher HR, Becker MA, Wortmann RL, et al: Effects of febuxostat versus allopurinol and placebo in reducing serum urate in subjects with hyperuricemia and gout: a 28-week, phase III, randomized, double-blind, parallel group trial, *Arthritis Care Res* 59:1540, 2008.

189. Becker M, Schumacher HR Jr, Espinoza L, et al: A phase 3 randomized, controlled, multicenter, double-blind trial (RCT) comparing efficacy and safety of daily febuxostat (FEB) and allopurinol (ALLO) in subjects with gout, *Arthritis Rheum* 58:S4029, 2008.

190. Schumacher Jr HR, Becker MA, Lloyd E, et al: Febuxostat in the treatment of gout: 5-yr findings of the FOCUS efficacy and safety study, *Rheumatology* 48:188, 2009.

191. Becker MA, Schumacher HR, MacDonald PA, et al: Clinical efficacy and safety of successful longterm urate lowering with febuxostat or allopurinol in subjects with gout, *J Rheumatol* 36:1273, 2009.

193. Becker MA, Schumacher HR, Wortmann RL, et al: Allopurinol intolerant patients treated with febuxostat for 4 years, *Arthritis Rheum* 54:S646, 2006.

196. Sherman MR, Saifer MGP, Perez-Ruiz F: PEG-uricase in the management of treatment-resistant gout and hyperuricemia, *Adv Drug Deliv Rev* 60:59, 2008.

199. Sundy JS, Becker MA, Baraf HSB, et al: Reduction of plasma urate levels following treatment with multiple doses of pegloticase (polyethylene glycol-conjugated uricase) in patients with treatment failure gout, *Arthritis Rheum* 58:2882, 2008.

200. Baraf HS, Matsumoto AK, Maroli AN, Waltrip RW: Resolution of gouty tophi after twelve weeks of pegloticase treatment, *Arthritis Rheum* 58:3632, 2008.

201. Sundy JS, Baraf HS, Becker MA, et al: Efficacy and safety of intravenous pegloticase (PGL) in treatment failure gout (TFG): results from GOUT1 and GOUT2, *Ann Rheum Dis* 68:318, 2009.

203. Becker MA, Treadwell EL, Baraf HS, et al: Immunoreactivity and clinical response to pegloticase (PGL): pooled data from GOUT1 and GOUT2, PGL phase 3 randomized, double blind, placebo-controlled trials, *Arthritis Rheum* 58:S880, 2008.

204. Wright D, Sundy JS, Rosario-Jansen T: Routine serum uric acid (SUA) monitoring predicts antibody-mediated loss of response and infusion reaction risk during pegloticase therapy, *Arthritis Rheum* 60:S413, 2009.

205. Sundy JS, Baraf HS, Gutierrez-Urena SR, et al: Chronic use of pegloticase: study and efficacy update, *Arthritis Rheum* 60:S417, 2009.

207. Terkeltaub R: Learning how and when to employ uricase as bridge therapy in refractory gout, *J Rheumatol* 34:1955, 2007.

208. Hamburger SA, Lipsky PE, Simon LS: Safety and efficacy of long-term pegloticase (KRYSTEXXA) treatment in adult patients with chronic gout refractory to conventional therapy, *Arthritis Rheum* 62:L12, 2010.

209. Wortmann RL: The treatment of gout: the use of an analogy, *Am J Med* 105:513, 1998.

210. Perez-Ruiz F, Alonso-Ruiz A, Calabozo M, Duruelo J: Treatment of gout after transplantation, *Br J Rheumatol* 37:580, 1998.

214. Dessein PH, Shipton EA, Stanwix AE, et al: Beneficial effects of weight loss associated with moderate calorie/carbohydrate restriction, and increased proportional intake of protein and unsaturated fat on serum urate and lipoprotein levels in gout: a pilot study, *Ann Rheum Dis* 59:539, 2000.

215. Fam AG: Gout, diet and the insulin resistance syndrome, *J Rheumatol* 29:1350, 2002.

Full references for this chapter can be found on www.expertconsult.com.

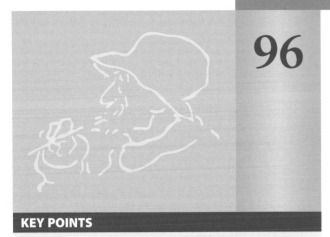

96

Calcium Crystal Disease: Calcium Pyrophosphate Dihydrate and Basic Calcium Phosphate

ROBERT TERKELTAUB

KEY POINTS

Dysregulated chondrocyte differentiation to hypertrophy and inorganic pyrophosphate (PP$_i$) metabolism are central in pathogenesis of calcium pyrophosphate dihydrate (CPPD) crystal deposition disease.

Autosomal dominant familial CPPD crystal deposition disease has been linked in multiple kindreds to certain mutations in *ANKH*, a gene encoding a PP$_i$ transporter.

NLRP3 (cryopyrin) inflammasome activation and consequent caspase-1 activation and interleukin (IL)-1β processing and secretion drive cell responses to CPPD crystals and CPPD crystal-induced inflammation.

Degenerative arthropathy caused by CPPD crystal deposition disease often involves joints uncommonly affected by primary osteoarthritis such as the metacarpophalangeal, wrist, and elbow joints.

Diagnosis of CPPD deposition disease before age 55, particularly if CPPD deposition is polyarticular, should prompt differential diagnostic consideration of a primary metabolic or familial disorder, and hyperparathyroidism should always be considered in CPPD deposition disease presenting in patients older than the age of 55.

High-resolution ultrasound appears particularly helpful in diagnosis of CPPD crystal deposition disease, partly because radiographic chondrocalcinosis is not detectable in all joints affected by the disease.

Basic calcium phosphate (BCP) crystal deposition in articular cartilage is intimately linked with osteoarthritis, particularly with osteoarthritis of increased severity.

BCP crystals (unlike urate and CPPD crystals) do not demonstrate birefringence, and specialized methods are required to conclusively identify BCP crystals in specimens from the joint.

ACR AND EULAR CRITERIA FOR DISEASE

Table 96-1 features proposed diagnostic criteria for calcium pyrophosphate dihydrate (CPPD) deposition disease, adapted by the author from the proposed European League Against Rheumatism (EULAR) criteria[1] and the original criteria proposed in the past by Daniel J McCarty and colleagues. The diagnosis is based on detection of CPPD crystals by one or more methods. These include not only standard clinically applied radiography but also high-resolution ultrasound to detect hyaline articular cartilage or fibrocartilage calcifications characteristic of CPPD crystal deposition (termed *chondrocalcinosis*). However, identification of CPPD crystals via compensated polarized light

microscopic analysis of synovial fluid in the absence of joint infection or other cause of arthritis is the gold standard for diagnosis of CPPD crystal deposition disease, particularly for acute CPPD crystal-associated arthritis (termed *pseudogout*). Detection of typical CPPD crystals in tissue sections also can be accomplished whether specimens are fixed in formaldehyde or ethanol, unlike the case for monosodium urate crystals (which dissolve in formaldehyde). On occasion, specialized crystal analytic approaches including x-ray energy spectroscopy and powder diffraction analysis or atomic force microscopy may be helpful in establishing or confirming CPPD crystal deposition. In assessing the form of deposited crystals in calcifications, determination of the calcium/phosphate ratios and the spacing of x-ray powder diffraction lines provide the most specific information.

Consensus clinical diagnostic criteria for articular basic calcium phosphate (BCP) crystal deposition disorders are not in place. Importantly, BCP crystals (unlike urate and CPPD) do not demonstrate global birefringence, though the aggregated particles of basic calcium phosphate crystals demonstrate edge birefringence. Hence diagnosis is predicated on detection of (1) radiographic detection of calcifications characteristic of BCP crystals, (2) synovial fluid crystals that stain strongly for the calcium-binding dye Alizarin red S (which only weakly stains CPPD crystals), (3) BCP crystals confirmed by transmission electron microscopy or specialized crystal analytic approaches (including those mentioned earlier for CPPD and discussed later).

EPIDEMIOLOGY

KEY POINTS

The true prevalence of both CPPD crystal deposition disease and pathologic articular BCP crystal deposition is not known due to limits of radiographic detection.

Chondrocalcinosis including asymptomatic disease increases progressively in prevalence with aging.

Idiopathic/sporadic chondrocalcinosis is rare before age 55, particularly in the absence of a history of joint trauma or knee meniscectomy.

In the past, studies of the prevalence of both CPPD crystal deposition disease[2-5] and various forms of articular BCP crystal deposition disease have been predominantly based on characteristic plain radiographic features of the disease

📷 Supplemental images available on the Expert Consult Premium Edition website.

Table 96-1 Proposed Diagnostic Criteria for Calcium Pyrophosphate Dihydrate (CPPD) Crystal Deposition Disease

Criteria
I. Demonstration of CPPD crystals, obtained by biopsy or aspirated synovial fluid, by definitive means (such as characteristic x-ray diffraction powder pattern)
II. A. Identification of monoclinic or triclinic crystals showing a weak positive birefringence (or no birefringence) by compensated polarized light microscopy
B. Presence of typical calcifications on radiographs (as discussed in text): heavy punctate and linear calcifications in fibrocartilages, articular (hyaline) cartilages, and joint capsules, especially if bilaterally symmetric
C. Presence of typical findings for CPPD crystal deposition in articular hyaline cartilage or fibrocartilage by high-resolution ultrasound
III. A. Acute arthritis, especially of knees, wrists, or other large joints
B. Chronic arthritis, especially of knee, hip, wrist, carpus, elbow shoulder, and metacarpophalangeal joints, particularly if accompanied by acute exacerbations

Diagnostic Categories
A. Definite: criteria I or IIA must be fulfilled
B. Probable: criteria IIA or IIB or IIC must be fulfilled
C. Possible: criteria IIIA or IIIB suggests possible underlying CPPD deposition disease

Modified from McCarty DJ: Crystals and arthritis, *Dis Month* 6:255, 1994.

in limited numbers of joints. This is an incompletely sensitive and specific approach.[2] Other studies have been based on results of synovial fluid analyses, but definitive studies based on pathologic findings on examination of articular cartilages, or imaging approaches superior to plain radiography, have not been done. As such, the true prevalence of both CPPD crystal deposition disease and pathologic articular BCP crystal deposition is not known.

It is clear that chondrocalcinosis including asymptomatic disease increases progressively in prevalence with aging.[2-5] Idiopathic/sporadic chondrocalcinosis is rare before age 55, particularly in the absence of a history of joint trauma or knee meniscectomy. Studies of prevalence based on radiographs have estimated higher prevalence of chondrocalcinosis when the hands, wrists, pelvis, and knees have been surveyed. Indeed, most elderly patients with chondrocalcinosis of the knee also have detectable chondrocalcinosis in other joints. Knee meniscal fibrocartilage calcification alone has been detected in 16% of women aged 80 to 89 and in 30% of women older than 89,[6] figures comparable with those obtained in other studies.[7] In a radiographic survey study of hands, wrists, pelvis, and knees of patients admitted to a geriatrics ward, there was a 44% prevalence of chondrocalcinosis in patients older than 84, a 36% prevalence in the 75- to 84-year-olds, and a prevalence of 15% in 65- to 74-year-olds[8]; studies of U.K. and Italian community cohorts have been limited to analyses of fewer regions (the knee, or knee and pelvis, respectively) and have yielded lower numbers for prevalence.[2-5]

In a large U.K. community study the age-, sex-, and knee pain–adjusted prevalence of knee chondrocalcinosis was 4.5% for those older than age 40.[3] In some studies, women have appeared somewhat more commonly affected by CPPD crystal deposition disease than men,[1] but in the recent U.K.

study, there was no sex predisposition, although strong association between osteoarthritis (OA) and chondrocalcinosis was confirmed.[3] This appeared to be linked more to the presence of osteophytes rather than joint space narrowing with OA. Interestingly, an association between chondrocalcinosis and diuretic use was uncovered, proposed to be due to the capacity of diuretics to induce hypomagnesemia.[3]

CPPD crystal deposition disease is not uniform in epidemiology between populations. In a random sample of Beijing residents older than 60 years of age, radiographic chondrocalcinosis was compared with whites in the American Framingham OA Study.[9] Chinese had a much lower prevalence of knee chondrocalcinosis, and wrist chondrocalcinosis was particularly rare in Chinese elderly.[9] These findings were unexpected because there is an excess of knee OA in Beijing, and chondrocalcinosis and OA are quite commonly associated in the knee joint.

GENETICS

> **KEY POINTS**
>
> The vast majority of CPPD crystal deposition disease is idiopathic/sporadic, but early-onset familial disease also occurs.
>
> Linkage of familial CPPD crystal deposition disease to the gene *ANKH* on chromosome 5p (which encodes a transmembrane protein with functions including PP_i transport) is well established.

The vast majority of CPPD crystal deposition disease is idiopathic/sporadic, but early-onset (defined as onset before age 55) familial disease also occurs.[10] Two major chromosomal linkages, 8q and 5p, have been identified in studies of familial CPPD deposition disease. Linkage with chromosome 8q of both early-onset OA and chondrocalcinosis was given the designation CCAL1, but chromosome 5p-linked chondrocalcinosis (CCAL2) is broadly distributed and has been studied in greater detail than 8q chondrocalcinosis.[10-12] Linkage of familial CPPD crystal deposition disease to the gene *ANKH* on chromosome 5p (which encodes a transmembrane protein with inorganic pyrophosphate [PP_i] transport and other apparent functions discussed later) has been established in these studies.[10-12] A search for *ANKH* mutation in 95 subjects with sporadic chondrocalcinosis uncovered a unique mutation (ΔE590) in one subject.[11] Homozygosity for a single nucleotide substitution (−4 G to A) in the *ANKH* 5′-untranslated region that promotes increased *ANKH* messenger RNA expression was present in approximately 4% of British subjects previously thought to have idiopathic/sporadic chondrocalcinosis of aging.[13]

Familial chondrocalcinosis is heterogeneous, and, as one example, prominent CPPD and hydroxyapatite (HA) crystal deposits and cartilage and periarticular calcifications in association with OA were described in a kindred not yet linked to a specific chromosomal locus.[14] A syndrome of spondyloepiphyseal dysplasia tarda, brachydactyly, precocious OA, and intra-articular calcifications with CPPD and/ or HA crystals, as well as periarticular calcifications, was linked to mutation of the procollagen type II gene in indigenous natives of the Chiloe Island region of Chile.[15] This population has a high prevalence of familial CPPD deposition disease. Families affected with diffuse idiopathic skeletal hyperostosis (DISH) and/or chondrocalcinosis have been identified in the Azores Islands, possibly reflecting an unidentified, shared pathogenic mechanism.[16]

PATHOGENESIS

KEY POINTS

The loose avascular connective tissue matrices of articular hyaline cartilage, fibrocartilaginous menisci, and of certain ligaments and tendons are particularly susceptible to pathologic calcification.

Joint cartilage pathologic calcification reflects complex interplay between organic and inorganic biochemistry of P_i and PP_i metabolism, aging, dysregulated chondrocyte growth factor responsiveness and differentiation, and other factors.

The loose avascular connective tissue matrices of articular hyaline cartilage, fibrocartilaginous menisci, and of certain ligaments and tendons are particularly susceptible to calcification. Calcium-containing crystals deposited in the pericellular matrix of cartilage are often in the form of CPPD (chemical formula, $Ca_2P_2O_7 \cdot H_2O$; calcium-to-phosphate ratio, 1). Crystals of BCP including partially carbonate-substituted HA ($Ca_5[PO_4]_3OH \cdot 2H_2O$; calcium-to-phosphate ratio, 1.67) also may be deposited pathologically in articular cartilage, particularly in OA. Importantly, physiologic (and noninflammatory) deposition of HA is essential because HA is the principal mineral phase laid down in growth cartilage and in bone.

Inflammatory conditions also may result from deposition of HA, as well as the closely related BCP crystals, octacalcium phosphate (OCP) ($Ca_8H_2[PO_4]_6 \cdot 5H_2O$; calcium-to-phosphate ratio, 1.33) and tricalcium phosphate or "whitlockite" ($Ca_3[PO_4]_2$; calcium-to-phosphate ratio, 1.5) in periarticular structures such as the rotator cuff (calcific tendinitis) and subacromial bursa of the shoulder (see Chapter 46). CPPD and BCP crystal deposition, reviewed here, are by far the most prevalent arthropathies associated with calcium-containing crystals. Articular calcium oxalate crystal deposition is less common.

Articular cartilage, unlike growth plate cartilage, is specialized to avoid the process of matrix calcification. However, the matrix of articular hyaline cartilage, like that of fibrocartilaginous menisci, lends itself well to pathologic calcification,[17] particularly in association with certain changes in extracellular matrix composition and hydration in aging and OA.[18] Joint cartilage calcification reflects complex interplay between organic and inorganic biochemistry, ion transport, aging, genetics, inflammation, oxidative stress, and dysregulated chondrocyte growth factor responsiveness and differentiation. Pathologic cartilage calcification can reflect deficiencies of certain physiologic calcification inhibitors or upregulation of mediators that actively drive certain patterns of tissue injury culminating in calcification within degenerating cartilage.[19,20]

Alteration of the concentrations of calcium, inorganic phosphate (P_i,), PP_i, and the solubility products of these ions are clearly at work in promoting CPPD and BCP crystal formation.[19] The levels of ambient magnesium and the composition of the chondrocyte extracellular matrix influence the dynamics of CPPD crystal formation and help to determine whether predominantly monoclinic or triclinic CPPD crystals are predominantly formed.[21,22] Significantly, monoclinic CPPD crystals are more inflammatory than triclinic CPPD crystals.[23] Matrix effects for CPPD and BCP crystals, studied in experimental gel systems, include promotion of CPPD formation by adenosine triphosphate (ATP) and corticosteroids in conjunction with matrix type I collagen and osteopontin, whereas type II collagen and intact proteoglycans appear to suppress ATP-driven CPPD crystal formation in vitro.[21,22] Experimental systems to analyze CPPD and BCP crystal deposition have commonly employed isolated matrix vesicle cell fragments from chondrocytes that are enriched in promineralizing constituents and provide a nidus for intiation of calcification, specifically with BCP crystals.[21] Matrix vesicles are important in cartilage growth plate calcification, but it is not yet clear whether CPPD and BCP crystal formation in articular cartilages is driven more by matrix vesicle–mediated effects or nucleation of crystals in association with changes in extracellular matrix constituents, or both pathways. However, CPPD crystals are too large (micron size) to form within matrix vesicles. It should be noted that loci of pericellular concentration of PP_i may be necessary to drive CPPD crystal formation at low micromolar PP_i concentrations developing in cartilages with chondrocalcinosis.

Besides physical effects of calcium, P_i, and PP_i on crystal nucleation and propagation, these same solutes exert a variety of mineralization-regulating effects on gene expression, differentiation, and viability in chondrocytes, mediated partly by calcium-sensing receptors and sodium-dependent inorganic phosphate co-transport in chondrocytes.[24-27] Noxious effects of excess PP_i on chondrocytes including induction of matrix metalloproteinase-13 (MMP-13) expression[28] and promotion of apoptosis[29] support the clinical terminology *pyrophosphate arthropathy* to describe chronic cartilage degenerative manifestations of CPPD crystal deposition disease.

Dysregulated Inorganic Pyrophosphate Metabolism in Pathologic Articular Cartilage Calcification

PP_i is a potent inhibitor of the nucleation and propagation of BCP crystals.[19] Concordantly, maintenance of physiologic extracellular PP_i levels by chondrocytes and certain other cells serves to suppress calcification with HA, as illustrated in mouse models of deficient PP_i generation and transport,[25] and a variant of human infantile arterial calcification associated with periarticular calcification.[30] The relatively unique capacity of chondrocytes to produce copious amounts of extracellular PP_i is double-edged (Figure 96-1), as supersaturation of cartilage extracellular matrix with PP_i is a major factor in promoting CPPD crystal deposition.[19,31,32] Furthermore, excess PP_i generation can promote BCP crystal deposition by providing a source for increased extracellular P_i generation via PP_i hydrolysis by the ecto-enzyme tissue-nonspecific alkaline phosphatase (TNAP)[19,25] (see Figure 96-1). Depending on cartilage ATP and PP_i

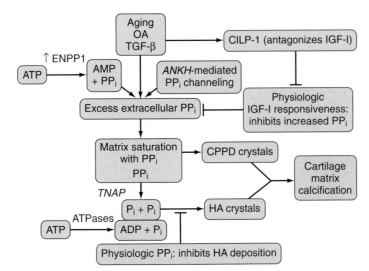

Figure 96-1 Proposed inorganic pyrophosphate (PP_i)-dependent mechanisms stimulating calcium pyrophosphate dihydrate (CPPD) and hydroxyapatite (HA) crystal deposition in aging and osteoarthritis (OA). Roles of adenosine triphosphate (ATP) and PP_i metabolism and inorganic phosphate (P_i) generation in pathologic cartilage calcification. This model accounts for the association of extracellular PP_i excess with both CPPD and basic calcium phosphate (HA) crystal deposition in OA and chondrocalcinosis, as well as the paradoxical association of extracellular PP_i deficiency (from defective *ANKH* or ectonucleotide pyrophosphatase/phosphodiesterase 1 [ENPP1] expression) with pathologic calcification of articular cartilage with HA crystals in vivo. Factors driving pathologic calcification are indicated in green and physiologic factors suppressing calcification in red. Excess PP_i generation in aging cartilages in idiopathic CPPD deposition disease of aging and in OA cartilages is mediated in part by increased ENPP1. In idiopathic chondrocalcinosis of aging, mean cartilage PP_i and nucleotide pyrophosphatase phosphodiesterase (NPP) catalytic activity levels are double normal. ENPP1 is markedly increased at sites of meniscal cartilage calcification in vivo, and NPP1 directly induces PP_i elevation and matrix calcification by chondrocytes in vitro. Depending on extracellular availability of substrate PP_i and the activity of the pyrophosphatase tissue-nonspecific alkaline phosphatase (TNAP), the availability of substrate ATP and the activity of ATPases, as well as other factors such as substantial local Mg^{2+} concentrations and HA crystal deposition, as opposed to CPPD deposition, may be stimulated. In this model, excess extracellular PP_i also may result from heightened "leakiness" of intracellular PP_i via increased *ANKH* expression in OA and abnormal *ANKH* function in familial chondrocalcinosis. Also illustrated is the role in cartilage calcification in OA and aging of increased expression of cartilage intermediate layer protein-1 (CILP-1), which inhibits the capacity of insulin-like growth factor-I (IGF-I) to suppress elevation of extracellular PP_i. AMP, adenosine monophosphate; TGF-β, transforming growth factor-beta.

concentrations, as well as the level of activity of P_i-generating ATPases and TNAP, CPPD and HA crystal formation may be jointly promoted in cartilage, an event that commonly occurs clinically in OA.

Role of ENPP1 and *ANKH* in Inorganic Pyrophosphate Metabolism in Chondrocalcinosis

Sporadic aging-associated CPPD crystal deposition disease is consistently linked with excess chondrocyte PP_i-generating nucleotide pyrophosphatase phosphodiesterase (NPP) activity and augmented PP_i generation by chondrocytes.[19,31,32] In this context, the NPP family isoenzymes ectonucleotide pyrophosphatase/phosphodiesterase 1 (ENPP1) (formerly known as *NPP1* and *plasma cell membrane glycoprotein-1 [PC-1]*) and ENPP3 (formerly known as *B10*) actively generate PP_i by hydrolysis of nucleoside triphosphates including ATP.[19,31,32] ENPP1 plays a central role in sustaining and augmenting extracellular PP_i in chondrocytes and certain other cells (see Figure 96-1). A substantial portion of ATP used by chondrocytes to generate extracellular PP_i is provided by the mitochondria.[19]

ENPP1 is one of a family of enzymes that share NPP catalytic activity and modular type II transmembrane ectoenzyme structures.[19,33] ENPP1 plays by far the greatest role in augmenting extracellular PP_i in chondrocytes.[31,32] Significantly, marked and total ENPP1 deficiency states in vivo and in vitro are associated with up to 50% less plasma and extracellular PP_i.[24,30] In contrast, in idiopathic

chondrocalcinosis, cartilage NPP activity and PP_i levels may average approximately double those of normal subjects.[34]

Increased ENPP1 expression is associated with both calcification and apoptosis in degenerative human cartilages.[31] In more advanced osteoarthritis, decreased cartilage ENPP1 has been described and promotes BCP crystal deposition.[34a] Direct upregulation of ENPP1 in chondrocytic cells stimulates calcification, as well as apoptosis.[35] These effects are not shared by ENPP3, which likely has other intracellular "housekeeping" functions in chondrocytes.[31] ENPP2, which is also expressed in normal cartilages, functions more actively in physiology as a lysophospholipase D, and ENPP2 only modestly stimulates chondrocytes to calcify in vitro.[31]

ANKH encodes a multiple-pass transmembrane protein that functions in PP_i channeling[36-39] (Figure 96-2) and possibly ATP release[40] and regulation of P_i metabolism and uptake by the type III sodium-dependent P_i co-transporter Pit-1.[41] *ANKH* promotes bidirectional movement of PP_i at the plasma membrane in vitro,[38] but the gradient for *ANKH*-stimulated PP_i movement in chondrocytes (which generate abundant PP_i both by their robust ENPP1 expression and intense matrix biosynthetic activity) is from the intracellular to the extracellular space.[19] Indeed, *ANKH* transport of PP_i generated intracellularly by ENPP1[28] may be the primary means to regulate extracellular PP_i levels.[19] Modeling of the PP_i channeling function of *ANKH* has proposed 10 or 12 membrane-spanning domains in *ANKH* with an alternating inside/out orientation and with a central channel to accommodate the passage of PP_i.[36,38] (see Figure 96-2).

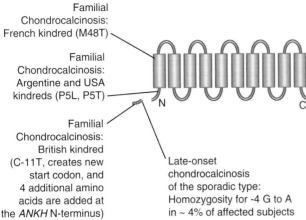

Familial Chondrocalcinosis: French kindred (M48T)

Familial Chondrocalcinosis: Argentine and USA kindreds (P5L, P5T)

Familial Chondrocalcinosis: British kindred (C-11T, creates new start codon, and 4 additional amino acids are added at the *ANKH* N-terminus)

Late-onset chondrocalcinosis of the sporadic type: Homozygosity for -4 G to A in ~ 4% of affected subjects

Figure 96-2 Model for multiple-pass membrane protein structure of *ANKH* and for *ANKH* mutations associated with chromosome 5p-linked autosomal dominant familial chondrocalcinosis and heritable late-onset chondrocalcinosis. The figure schematizes the putative multiple-pass transmembrane protein structure of *ANKH*, which appears to promote bidirectional inorganic pyrophosphate (PP$_i$) movement between the cytosol to the extracellular space. The gradient for *ANKH*-stimulated PP$_i$ movement in chondrocytes (which generate abundant PP$_i$ both by high specific activity of ectonucleotide pyrophosphatase/phosphodiesterase 1 and robust matrix biosynthesis) is from the intracellular to the extracellular space. Distinct mutations in *ANKH* promote differences in age of onset and phenotypes in familial chondrocalcinosis. The figure summarizes sites of known *ANKH* mutations clustered near the N-terminus that are associated with chromosome 5p-linked autosomal dominant familial chondrocalcinosis (calcium pyrophosphate dihydrate [CPPD] crystal deposition disease), and all, except the French kindred M48T (which increases intracellular PP$_i$ and disrupts the association of *ANKH* with the inorganic phosphate transporter Pit-1), may act in part by increasing extracellular PP$_i$. A C-terminal domain *ANKH* mutation ΔE590 linked with one case of sporadic chondrocalcinosis is not depicted; *ANKH*ΔE590 appears to indirectly suppress PP$_i$ catabolism by association with impairing tissue-nonspecific alkaline phosphatase expression. The figure also depicts the −4 G to A transition in the 5'-untranslated region of *ANKH* for which homozygosity is seen in approximately 4% of late-onset chondrocalcinosis of the sporadic type, suggesting a heritable subset of otherwise typical late-onset chondrocalcinosis. As a group, the N-terminally clustered *ANKH* mutations linked to human chondrocalcinosis promote chronic low-grade extracellular PP$_i$ excess resulting in CPPD crystal formation.

ANKH is clearly implicated in the pathogenesis of familial and idiopathic/sporadic chondrocalcinosis,[10,13] and increased *ANKH* expression in cartilage is a factor in secondary chondrocalcinosis in OA[28] (see Figure 96-1). In this context, expression of wild-type *ANKH* is highly regulated and *ANKH* is increased in OA and chondrocalcinotic cartilages.[28] Interestingly, hypoxia, via effects of the transcription factor hypoxia inducible factor-1α, suppresses *ANKH* expression.[42] It is conceivable that increased permeability to oxygen of fibrillated and fissured cartilage in OA favors increased *ANKH* expression. *ANKH*, in conjunction with signaling via extracellular P$_i$ likely derived from PP$_i$, promotes chondrocyte maturation to the procalcifying hypertrophic differentiation state.[43] Figure 96-1 presents a model in which secondary alterations in chondrocyte expression of both wild-type *ANKH* and ENPP1 drive PP$_i$ supersaturation in cartilage in idiopathic/sporadic and OA-associated CPPD crystal deposition disease.

Mutations at different locations in *ANKH* can affect function and the skeleton in a manner including autosomal dominant chondrocalcinosis[10,37-39] and certain other phenotypes. These include murine progressive ankylosis in the *ank/ank* mouse and human craniometaphyseal dysplasia associated with apparent decrease of the capacity to transport PP$_i$ within bone and effects on bone resorption and remodeling, putatively mediated in part by direct and indirect effects on osteoclasts.[36,39,44] In a consanguineous family with mental retardation, deafness, and ankylosis, with painful small joint soft tissue calcifications, progressive spondyloarthropathy, osteopenia, and mild hypophosphatemia, the homozygous ANK missense mutation L244S was detected in all patients.[45] The mutant ANK protein was expressed and localized to the plasma membrane, but fibrosis and mineralization of articular soft tissues developed in homozygotes, with heterozygous carriers of the L244S mutation showing mild osteoarthritis without metabolic alterations.[45]

Clinical heterogeneity even for chondrocalcinosis associated with *ANKH* mutations[10] suggests differing functional effects of *ANKH* mediated by specific regions of the molecule. All the N-terminally clustered *ANKH* mutations identified to cause familial chondrocalcinosis (see Figure 96-2) appear to increase PP$_i$ transport.[38] However, some *ANKH* mutations have distinct effects on chondrocyte differentiation.[13] The M48T *ANKH* mutant in the French kindred appears functionally unique by association with increased intracellular PP$_i$[46] and also interrupts the interaction of *ANKH* with the sodium/phosphate co-transporter Pit-1.[47] This may be functionally significant because elevated P$_i$ increases both *ANKH* and Pit-1 expression and because *ANKH* and Pit-1 co-localize in chondrocytes.[47] In addition are the P$_i$ effects on chondrocyte differentiation discussed later. In 5p familial chondrocalcinosis, subtle gain of function of intrinsic *ANKH* PP$_i$ channeling activity may lead to chronic, low-grade chondrocyte "PP$_i$ leakiness," thereby causing matrix supersaturation with PP$_i$, CPPD crystal deposition, and cartilage degeneration.[10,37,48] An alternative mechanism of disrupting PP$_i$ metabolism may be promoted by the *ANKH* mutation ΔE590 linked with a case of sporadic chondrocalcinosis[11] because *ANKH*ΔE590 appears to indirectly suppress PP$_i$ catabolism by association with impairing TNAP expression.[49]

Effects of Imbalance of Chondrocyte Growth Factor Responses on Inorganic Pyrophosphate Metabolism in Chondrocalcinosis

The chondrocyte growth factor transforming growth factor (TGF)-β stimulates ATP release by chondrocytes,[40] as well as ENPP1 expression and ENPP1 subcellular movement to the plasma membrane, which drive elevation of extracellular PP$_i$.[32,50] Interleukin (IL)-1β suppresses both ENPP1 expression and extracellular PP$_i$ in chondrocytes and blocks the effects of TGF-β on PP$_i$.[32,50] The capacity of TGF-β to raise chondrocyte PP$_i$ rises with aging, as does TGF-β–stimulated NPP activity,[51] whereas growth-promoting effects of TGF-β decrease with aging in articular chondrocytes.[52] The anabolic chondrocyte growth factor insulin-like growth factor-I (IGF-I) normally suppresses extracellular PP$_i$ (as well as ATP release)[40] in chondrocytes[53] (see Figure 96-1). Moreover, chondrocyte IGF-I resistance is characteristic of OA and aging cartilages[54] (see Figure 96-1). IGF-I induces expression of cartilage intermediate layer protein (CILP) (see Figure 96-1), a secreted cartilage matrix molecule. CILP's expression rises in aging and OA and is most abundant in the middle zone of articular cartilage where CPPD crystal deposition is most prevalent. Significantly, the CILP-1, but not the CILP-2 isoform, promotes increased extracellular PP_i in chondrocytes indirectly by antagonizing IGF-I at the receptor level.[54]

CPPD Deposition Disease Secondary to Primary Metabolic Disorders: Relationship to Inorganic Pyrophosphate Metabolism and Chondrocyte Differentiation

Hypophosphatasia, hypomagnesemic conditions (including the Gitelman's variant of Bartter's syndrome), hemochromatosis, and hyperparathyroidism are the best-characterized primary metabolic disorders linked to secondary CPPD crystal deposition disease.[55] Increased joint fluid PP_i levels in each of these conditions suggests at least one common thread in the pathogenesis of chondrocalcinosis via cartilage PP_i excess.[56] Magnesium is a cofactor for pyrophosphatase activity, and iron excess can suppress pyrophosphatase activity. Hypercalcemia may promote CPPD crystal deposition in hyperparathyroidism (and in familial hypocalciuric hypercalcemia)[57] by effects beyond cartilage matrix supersaturation with ionized calcium such as calcium function as a cofactor in ENPP1 catalytic activity, as well as chondrocyte-activating effects mediated by the calcium-sensing receptor.[27] In addition, normal articular chondrocytes express parathyroid hormone/parathyroid-hormone-related protein (PTH/PTHrP) receptors, and functional responses of chondrocytes to PTH can promote proliferation, altered matrix synthesis, and mineralization.[58,59]

Hypophosphatasia is due to deficient activity of TNAP, consequently with effects including limitation of hydrolysis PP_i to generate P_i.[25] TNAP is a major physiologic antagonist of ENPP1-mediated elevation of extracellular PP_i.[25] Conversely, physiologic ENPP1-induced PP_i generation antagonizes the essential promineralizing effects of TNAP mediated by P_i generation,[25] and cartilage PP_i excess presumably drives chondrocalcinosis in hypophosphatasia. *Enpp1* knockout mice and mice homozygous for the ENPP1 truncation mutant *ttw* demonstrate marked articular cartilage calcification with HA and OA, as well as ankylosing spinal ligament hyperostosis and synovial joint ossific fusion; extracellular PP_i levels and mineralization disturbances in soft tissues (but not long bones) of *Enpp1* knockout and TNAP-deficient mice are mutually corrected by cross-breeding.[25]

Inflammation, Hypertrophic Chondrocyte Differentiation, and Transglutaminase 2 in Joint Cartilage Calcification

Regulated changes in chondrocyte differentiation and viability appear to be a mechanistically unified process that promotes joint cartilage HA and CPPD crystal deposition, as well as OA.[60] Such changes include development of foci of chondrocyte maturation to hypertrophy,[60] with the presence of hypertrophy, as seen in histopathology of the knee cartilage in Figure 96-3, and apoptosis of chondrocytes typically found adjacent to cartilage calcifications.[61,62] Articular

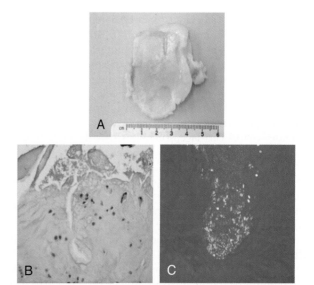

Figure 96-3 Calcium pyrophosphate dihydrate (CPPD) crystal deposition arthropathy of the knee joint. **A,** Femoral condyle. There are extensive foci of chalky white particulate deposits within the articular cartilage. This is characteristic of CPPD crystal deposition. **B,** Histology of CPPD crystal deposition within the hyaline articular cartilage. The hypertrophic chondrocytes adjacent to the crystal aggregates are within enlarged chondrons (hematoxylin and eosin, original magnification ×250). **C,** Polarized light microscopy of CPPD crystal aggregates within the hyaline articular cartilage. The individual crystals have rod and rhomboid shapes and are positively birefringent (original magnification ×250). *(Courtesy Dr. Ken Pritzker, Mount Sinai Hospital Pathology Department, University of Toronto, Ontario, Canada.)*

chondrocyte hypertrophy[60] is associated with heightened PP_i generation; increased production of calcifying, membrane-limited cell fragments known as matrix vesicles[63]; and certain other calcification-promoting changes in differentiation including alteration of extracellular matrix composition, such that osteopontin (which promotes CPPD crystal formation) is increased and normal collagen subtype composition in the matrix is lost.[64] Altered TGF-β signal transduction in aging and OA may be involved in promoting chondrocyte hypertrophy.[65]

P_i taken up by Pit-1 sodium-dependent co-transport and calcium sensing can modulate chondrocyte hypertrophic differentiation and apoptosis, as well as PP_i-modulating responses to TGF-β.[19,31,66-69] Local upregulation of PTHrP expression also may be one of the shared features driving sequential chondrocyte proliferation and altered differentiation in growth plate chondrocytes and articular chondrocytes.[27] Chondrocyte apoptosis also promotes calcification partly through the calcifying potential of apoptotic bodies functioning as "inside-out" matrix vesicles on release from dying chondrocytes.[70-72] Mitochondrial dysfunction, a central factor in tissue aging and an apparent mediator of OA progression in aging,[73,74] also can stimulate cartilage matrix degeneration and calcification. Mitochondria are remarkably specialized to regulate calcification, and apoptosis is critically regulated by mitochondrial function. Moreover, chondrocyte ATP depletion is driven via suppression of mitochondrial oxidative phosphorylation by nitric oxide (NO) as OA evolves in aging, thereby promoting increased ATP scavenging by NPP activity and consequent augmentation of extracellular PP_i.[74]

Inflammation-associated chondrocyte hypertrophy is driven by hypoxia-inducible factor-2α and Indian hedgehog,[60] as well as by multiple cytokines and calgranulins, oxidative stress, P_i transport, and receptor for advanced glycation end products (RAGE) signaling, and it is modulated by transglutaminase 2 (TG2) release. Chondrocyte hypertrophy and inflammation jointly drive chondrocalcinosis and progression of OA. For example, IL-1β, which is increased in OA cartilage, stimulates articular chondrocytes to calcify the matrix.[51,64] NO stimulates both apoptosis and calcification in chondrocytes.[71] IL-1β stimulates inducible nitric oxide synthase (iNOS) expression and increased NO generation, as well matrix alterations. IL-1β (as well as TNF, donors of NO, and the potent oxidant peroxynitrite) also induces increased chondrocyte transglutaminase (TG) activity mediated through the TG family enzymes, factor XIIIA and TG2.[51,64]

TG2 and factor XIIIA, which function in part to crosslink proteins by transamidation, are markers of growth plate chondrocyte hypertrophy.[51,64] Significantly, there is upregulation of TG2 and factor XIIIA expression in hypertrophic cells in the superficial and deep zones of knee OA articular cartilage and the central (chondrocytic) zone of OA menisci.[51] Moreover, increased factor XIIIA and TG2 activities both directly stimulate calcification by chondrocytes.[51] OA severity–related, donor age–dependent, and marked age–dependent IL-1-induced increases in TG activity occur in chondrocytes from human knee menisci.[51] TG2 is essential for IL-1β to stimulate articular chondrocytes to calcify in vitro.[64] In addition, the closely related inflammatory chemokines CXCL1 and CXCL8, which are both increased in OA cartilage, induce TG2[75] and chondrocyte hypertrophic differentiation and calcification that requires TG2.[75] Distinct TG2-independent and TG2-dependent mechanisms promote articular chondrocyte hypertrophy and calcification in vitro, and increased TG2 release is sufficient to promote chondrocyte hypertrophy.[64,76] TG2 also promotes activation of TGF-β.[77]

The multiligand RAGE mediates several chronic degenerative diseases accompanied by low-grade inflammation.[78] RAGE ligands include S100/calgranulins, a class of small, calcium-binding polypeptides, several of which are expressed by chondrocytes. Normal human knee cartilages demonstrate constitutive RAGE and S100A11 expression, and both RAGE and S100A11 expression are increased in OA cartilages. CXCL8 and TNF induce S100A11 release in cultured chondrocytes.[78] Furthermore, S100A11 induces chondrocyte hypertrophy in vitro,[78] and it does so in a manner dependent on S100A11 homodimerization catalyzed by TG2-mediated transamidation and antagonized by the alternative S100A11 receptor CD36.[79,80] CXCL1-induced and TNF-induced chondrocyte hypertrophy require RAGE signaling.[78]

Special Pathogenic Aspects of Articular and Periarticular Basic Calcium Phosphate Crystal Deposition

CPPD and BCP crystal deposition can develop in different zones of articular cartilage and probably in distinct phases of cartilage degenerative disease such as ongoing loss of viability in hypertrophic chondrocytes. In addition, abundant cartilage NO production may promote mitochondrial dysfunction, chondrocyte extracellular ATP depletion,[74] and lowering of extracellular PP_i, consequently favoring HA over CPPD crystal deposition.[81] The observation that OA and HA crystal deposition in articular cartilage (and arteries)[30] are both promoted by extracellular PP_i deficiency states strikingly illustrates the deleterious effects of deprivation of physiologic extracellular PP_i levels.[19] Yet it is noted that joint fluid PP_i and NPP activity are elevated in HA-associated shoulder arthropathy (Milwaukee shoulder syndrome [MSS]),[82] consistent with the model in Figure 96-1.

Pathologic BCP crystal deposition may occur in periarticular sites, as well as numerous organs and soft tissues. Significantly, the shoulder is the most common articular region affected by symptomatic BCP crystal deposition, in part reflecting unique shoulder structure-function (see Chapter 46). Degenerative changes promoted by biomechanical stress promote calcific tendinitis in the body of the rotator cuff.[82] Such tendon calcifications can remain asymptomatic and also can eventually resorb, but the degenerative changes can predispose to tendon rupture. Osteopontin, a factor that normally restrains BCP crystal deposition (and is regulated by PP_i and P_i),[24] can be detected in fibroblast-like cells and multinucleated macrophages surrounding areas of calcification in calcific tendinitis.[83] In this regard, osteopontin promotes oxidative stress, MMP activation, and macrophage recruitment and osteoclast activation.[24] The presence of multinucleated cells with cathepsin K expression and osteoclast-like functions at sites of tendon calcification[84] suggests a mechanism for both resorption of BCP crystal deposits and tendon degeneration.

Crystal-Induced Inflammation

Some of the crystals deposited in cartilage (Supplemental Figure 96-1 on www.expertconsult.com) can subclinically traffic to joint fluid and synovium, and the crystals can directly stimulate chondrocytes, synovial lining cells, and intra-articular leukocytes.[85-91] Inflammation triggered by CPPD and BCP crystals thereby contributes to cartilage degradation and can potentiate worsening of OA.[85-91] Many proinflammatory mechanisms active in gout also likely mediate synovitis and cartilage degeneration associated with CPPD and BCP crystal deposition.[85-91] In this regard, CPPD and BCP crystals activate cells partly via nonspecific activation of signal transduction pathways (e.g., mitogen activated protein kinase activation) and induce cellular release of cyclooxygenase- and lipoxygenase-derived metabolites of arachidonic acid and cytokines including tumor necrosis factor (TNF), IL-1, and CXCL8.[85-91] Innate immune recognition of extracellular CPPD crystals by Toll-like receptor 2 (TLR2)[92] and CPPD crystal-induced activation of the intracellular NLRP3 (cryopyrin) inflammasome, resulting in caspase-1 activation and IL-1β processing and release, drive cell responses to CPPD crystals in vitro and CPPD crystal-induced inflammation in vivo.[93]

The ingress of neutrophils into the joint is central in triggering acute crystal-induced synovitis, and effects on neutrophil-endothelial interaction likely represent a major locus for prophylactic effects of nanomolar concentrations of colchicine for the acute arthritis of pseudogout.[95] CXCL8 and related chemokines that bind the CXCL8 receptor CXCR2 (including CXCL1) appear to be critical in initiating and perpetuating neutrophil ingress in acute crystal-induced inflammation.[96] Despite the fact that BCP and CPPD crystals share the capacity to activate certain cell signaling pathways and to induce several MMPs, BCP crystals generally trigger much less neutrophil influx into the joint than do CPPD crystals. Concordantly, free intra-articular BCP crystals likely induce less proinflammatory cytokine expression than do CPPD and monosodium urate crystals,[97-99] though OCP crystals could be more inflammatory than hydroxyapatite crystals.[100]

CLINICAL FEATURES

KEY POINTS

In the elderly, CPPD deposition can mimic conditions including gout, infectious arthritis, primary osteoarthritis, RA, or polymyalgia rheumatica. It can also present as fever of unknown origin.

Pseudogout is a major cause of acute monoarticular or oligoarticular arthritis in the elderly; attacks typically involve a large joint, most often the knee, and less often the wrist or ankle, and, unlike gout, rarely the first metatarsophalangeal joint.

Chronic degenerative arthropathy in CPPD deposition disease commonly affects certain joints that are typically spared in primary OA (e.g., metacarpophalangeal joints, wrists, elbows, glenohumeral joints).

Calcium Pyrophosphate Dihydrate Deposition Disease

Most elderly individuals with CPPD deposition disease in the United States have a primary (idiopathic/sporadic) disorder (Table 96-2). Idiopathic chondrocalcinosis generally appears only after the fifth decade of life. But patients with a history of repetitive joint trauma of knee meniscectomy

Table 96-2 Causes of Calcium Pyrophosphate Dihydrate Crystal Deposition Disease

High Prevalence
Idiopathic in association with aging (most frequent)
Complication of primary osteoarthritis
Long-term consequence of mechanical joint trauma or knee meniscectomy

Moderate Prevalence
Familial
Associated with systemic metabolic disease (hyperparathyroidism, dialysis-dependent renal failure, hemochromatosis, hypomagnesemia)

Low Prevalence (Largely Based on Case Reports)
X-linked hypophosphatemic rickets
Familial hypocalciuric hypercalcemia
Ochronosis
Gout
Articular amyloidosis
Myxedematous hypothyroidism
Osteochondrodysplasias and spondyloepiphyseal dysplasias
Neuropathic joints
Wilson's disease

Table 96-3 Common Clinical Presentations of Calcium Pyrophosphate Dihydrate (CPPD) Crystal Deposition Disease

Asymptomatic or incidental finding (e.g., asymptomatic knee fibrocartilage chondrocalcinosis in the elderly)
Recurrent acute inflammatory monoarticular arthritis (pseudogout) (e.g., wrist, knee, including provocation by trauma, concurrent medical or surgical illness, or intra-articular hyaluronan)
Pseudoseptic arthritis
Recurrent acute hemarthrosis
Chronic degenerative arthritis (pseudo-osteoarthritis or pseudo-neuropathic arthritis)
Chronic symmetric inflammatory polyarthritis (pseudorheumatoid arthritis)
Systemic illness (pseudo-polymyalgia rheumatica, fever of unknown origin)
Destructive arthritis in dialysis-dependent renal failure
Carpal tunnel syndrome
Tumoral and pseudotophaceous CPPD crystal deposits
Central nervous system disease complicating ligamentum flavum or transverse ligament of atlas involvement (cervical canal stenosis, cervical myelopathy, meningismus, foramen magnum syndrome, odontoid fracture)

may present with nonsystemic (monoarticular) chondrocalcinosis before age 55. Familial forms of CPPD crystal deposition disease also have been widely documented, as discussed later. The clinical presentation of familial chondrocalcinosis is often manifested in the third and fourth decades of life, but familial disease can sometimes be detected before age 20 or first present clinically at advanced age. CPPD crystal deposition disease is also a common manifestation of a variety of hereditary and metabolic conditions (including hyperparathyroidism, dialysis-dependent renal failure, and hemochromatosis)[55] in which the CPPD-related arthropathy can present earlier than age 55. For unclear reasons, hemochromatosis can present predominantly with CPPD crystal deposition disease or as OA. The weight of evidence from controlled studies suggests that hypothyroidism (with the probable exception of myxedematous hypothyroidism) is not associated with a significantly increased prevalence of CPPD crystal deposition disease, though both disorders are clearly prevalent in aging.[55,101,102] It has been suggested that initiation of thyroxine supplementation therapy may trigger pseudogout.[103]

The clinical manifestations of CPPD deposition disease vary widely[104] (Table 96-3). Quite commonly, the disease can be asymptomatic. Alternatively, it can mimic OA (pseudo-osteoarthritis), gout (pseudogout) (Supplemental Figure 96-2 on www.expertconsult.com), acute-onset or insidious rheumatoid arthritis (RA) (pseudorheumatoid arthritis) (Figure 96-4), or present as "pseudo-neuropathic" arthropathy. Patients with CPPD crystal deposition disease also commonly present with episodes of hemarthrosis, often post-traumatic and in the knee. The contributions of the forms of CPPD deposited (e.g., monoclinic vs. triclinic crystals) and of host factors to these wide differences in clinical manifestations are not clear. Overall, only a small fraction of patients with CPPD deposition disease have prolonged, recurring polyarticular inflammation. Progressive degenerative arthropathy is more common. Though CPPD deposition disease appears to be a common and significant public health problem in the elderly, the disease and health-related quality of life impact and the long-term course of CPPD-

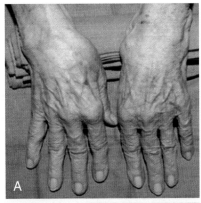
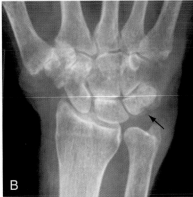

Figure 96-4 Idiopathic symmetric pseudorheumatoid calcium pyrophosphate dihydrate (CPPD) deposition arthropathy in an elderly female. This 84-year-old female presented with a history of past right carpal tunnel syndrome and with chronic symmetric proliferative synovitis of both wrists and second and third metacarpophalangeal (MCP) joints, with physical findings of synovial and dorsal extensor tenosynovial swelling of the wrists and synovial swelling at the second to third MCP joints **(A).** Changes on hand and wrist plain radiographs consistent with the diagnosis of CPPD deposition disease, presented for the right wrist **(B),** included cystic changes in multiple carpal bones including the scaphoid and lunate, linear calcification on the ulnar side of the carpus (arrow) typical for the chondrocalcinosis of CPPD deposition, and mild narrowing of the radiocarpal joint indicative of cartilage loss.

associated degenerative arthropathy in an unselected population have not been adequately evaluated.

Acute Synovitis

Pseudogout is a major cause of acute monoarticular or oligoarticular arthritis in the elderly. The attacks typically involve a large joint, most often the knee and less often the wrist or ankle, and, unlike gout, rarely the first metatarsophalangeal joint. Acute attacks of inflammatory pseudogout in patients with CPPD deposition disease typically have a sudden onset and can be excruciatingly painful, with pronounced periarticular erythema, warmth, and swelling, comparable to gout. In addition, arthritis in some attacks of pseudogout can be migratory or can be additive, polyarticular, and bilateral. Polyarticular pseudogout is particularly common in association with familial chondrocalcinosis and hyperparathyroidism.

Pseudogout can be provoked by minor trauma or intercurrent medical or surgical conditions including pneumonia, myocardial infarction, cerebrovascular accident, and pregnancy. Parathyroid surgery for hyperparathyroidism

frequently triggers pseudogout attacks. In addition, pseudogout of the knee can be precipitated by arthroscopy or by intra-articular administration of hyaluronan[105] that could reflect proinflammatory mechanisms triggered through the hyaluronan receptor CD44. Parenteral administration of granulocyte colony-stimulating factor (G-CSF)[106] and of bisphosphonates[107] also can trigger pseudogout, the former likely by ignition of smoldering subclinical intra-articular inflammation, the latter theoretically via pyrophosphatase inhibition because bisphosphonates are nonhydrolyzable analogues of PP_i.

Acute and subacute pseudogout can be associated with fever, chills, elevated erythrocyte sedimentation rate, and systemic leukocytosis, particularly with polyarticular involvement and in the elderly.[108] Leukocyte counts in the synovial fluid are substantially elevated, and intraleukocytic CPPD crystals are most often (but not universally) detectable by compensated polarized light microscopy in pseudogout. The attacks typically last for 7 to 10 days but also can be clustered and last for weeks to months. Occasionally the leukocyte count in pseudogout can exceed 50,000 per mm³ (pseudoseptic arthritis).

Chronic Degenerative and Inflammatory Arthropathies

Acute pseudogout attacks may be interspersed with chronic arthropathy in CPPD crystal deposition disease, though it has been suggested that acute flares of pseudogout may become less common in those with established chronic degenerative CPPD deposition arthropathy.[109] Chronic degenerative arthropathy in CPPD deposition disease commonly affects certain joints that are typically spared in primary OA (e.g., metacarpophalangeal joints, wrists, elbows, glenohumeral joints). The development of cartilage degenerative changes in CPPD deposition disease in both typical and atypical joints for primary OA suggests one or more systemic abnormalities.

Degenerative cartilage disease associated with sporadic CPPD crystal deposition disease may present as destructive arthropathy of the knees, hips, and/or shoulders, particularly in elderly females (Figures 96-5 and 96-6). The CPPD crystal arthropathy–associated degenerative disease can be less or more destructive than that observed in primary OA. For example, patients with primary OA and CPPD crystals have been reported to require knee replacement surgery more often than with primary OA without crystals.[110] In another study, 60% of patients undergoing joint replacement had CPPD or BCP crystals (and commonly both) in their knee synovial fluids, and higher mean radiographic scores correlated with the presence of calcium-containing crystals.[111] However, prospective analysis of CPPD deposition disease that principally involved the knee has suggested that radiographic worsening of degenerative changes may be slow.[112] The disease also may not appear to be clinically progressive in the involved knee after substantial periods of follow-up in a subset of patients, though clinical involvement may spread to other joints in the same time frame.[112] Most patients develop changes in radiographic extent of chondrocalcinosis over time. But there is no clear correlation between the extent of calcification and progression of CPPD deposition arthropathy. There may be a relatively

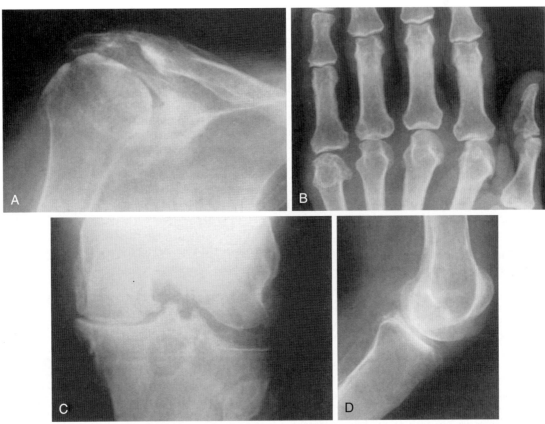

Figure 96-5 Radiographic features of calcium pyrophosphate dihydrate arthropathy. **A,** Destructive shoulder arthropathy. **B,** Metacarpophalangeal joint arthropathy. **C,** Knee degenerative joint disease with large subchondral bone cyst. **D,** Wraparound patella (same patient shown in **A**).

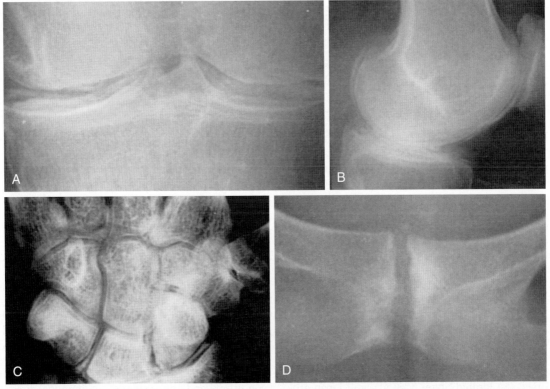

Figure 96-6 Chondrocalcinosis of the most commonly affected joints in calcium pyrophosphate dihydrate deposition disease. **A,** Linear calcifications observed in knee menisci and fibrocartilage. **B,** Lateral view showing calcification of the articular cartilage as a line parallel to the femoral condyles. **C,** Calcification of intercarpal joints and triangular ligament. **D,** Calcification of the symphysis pubis fibrocartilage associated with subchondral bone erosions and subchondral increased bone density.

good prognosis for initial presentation of CPPD deposition disease in the knee as acute pseudogout attacks alone.[112]

Pseudorheumatoid involvement in a small subset of patients with CPPD deposition disease presents as a chronic, bilateral, symmetric deforming inflammatory polyarthropathy (see Figure 96-4). Many of these patients have bilateral wrist and metacarpophalangeal joint involvement. Wrist tenosynovitis and carpal tunnel syndrome, cubital tunnel syndrome, and tendon rupture may develop. Ingestion of CPPD crystals by synovial lining cells and lysosomal catabolism of such ingested crystals stimulates synovial proliferation, in part via solubilization of the crystalline calcium. Such effects may contribute to regional synovial and periarticular tenosynovial proliferation promoted by CPPD crystal deposition.[84]

Other Clinical Forms of Calcium Pyrophosphate Dihydrate Crystal Deposition

Concentrated (tumoral or pseudotophaceous) CPPD crystal deposition can occur in periarticular structures including tendons, ligaments, bursae, and occasionally in bone.[104,113] CPPD deposits in tendons (e.g., Achilles, triceps, and obturator tendons) are usually fine and linear on radiographs. Pseudotophaceous deposits of CPPD crystals have been detected in the temporal bone, around the knee and hip, and in the acromioclavicular, temporomandibular, elbow, and small hand joints.[113] Peripheral tumoral CPPD crystal deposits may sometimes present with acute arthritic attacks. Rarely, tumoral CPPD deposits around the knee can mimic osteonecrosis.[114] Tumoral CPPD crystal deposition is typically associated with tissue chondroid metaplasia and behaves like a benign but locally aggressive chondroid tumor, with some of the connective tissue invasion and destruction likely mediated by CPPD crystal-induced cell activation.

Axial skeletal CPPD crystal deposition occasionally involves the intervertebral disks, sacroiliac joints, and lumbar facet joints, and radiographic findings such as linear calcification and spinal ankylosis may appear.[115] Meningismus and clinical manifestations resembling herniated intervertebral disk, ankylosing spondylitis, and acute pseudogout of lumbar facet joints have been observed.[115,116] In addition, CPPD deposits within the ligamentum flavum or the transverse ligament of atlas can be sizeable and can progress to cause cervical canal stenosis, cervical myelopathy, and foramen magnum syndrome.[117-119] Odontoid fracture due to the calcification of the atlantoaxial joint may occur in CPPD deposition disease.[117-120] Thus CPPD deposition disease can factor in the differential diagnosis of patients with neurologic disturbances and painful cervical mass, especially in the elderly.

Familial Chondrocalcinosis

Familial CPPD deposition disease has been described in numerous countries and ethnic groups including kindreds from Czechoslovakia, Holland, France, England, Germany, Sweden, Israel, the United States, Canada, and Japan and may be most prevalent in Chile and Spain. In one English kindred with CPPD disease linked to *ANKH* mutation on chromosome 5p, recurrent childhood seizures were strongly

associated with later development of CPPD deposition disease.[121] For linkages to *ANKH* on chromosome 5p, some families manifest early-onset polyarthritis, which can include ankylosing intervertebral and sacroiliac joint disease. In others a late-onset chondrocalcinosis occurs, and the disease can be oligoarticular, mild in intensity and destructiveness, and nearly indistinguishable from idiopathic CPPD deposition disease.[12,38,48] Kindreds from Argentina and the Alsace region of France linked to 5p did share similar phenotypic features of chondrocalcinosis including early age at onset (third decade of life), common but not universal premature OA, some cases of pseudorheumatoid arthritic peripheral joint disease, and radiographic evidence of fibrocartilage and hyaline cartilage calcifications typical of CPPD deposition.[122] The most commonly affected joints in these kindreds were the knees and wrists, with involvement of the pubic symphysis and intervertebral disks also described.[122]

CLINICAL FEATURES OF ARTICULAR BASIC CALCIUM PHOSPHATE CRYSTAL DISEASE

KEY POINTS

Unlike urate and CPPD crystal deposition, acute synovitis due to HA crystal deposition is unusual. Acute inflammatory syndromes including subacromial bursitis and a form of pseudopodagra described in young women may occur in association with periarticular HA crystal deposition in bursae, tendons, ligaments, and soft tissues.

Patients with advanced chronic renal failure, particularly on dialysis, may develop symptomatic articular and periarticular BCP crystal deposition, which may be destructive and involve the axial skeleton. They may resemble or be associated with CPPD deposition disease.

Clinical Features of Pathologic Basic Calcium Phosphate Crystal Deposition in Joint Tissues

Unlike the case for urate and CPPD crystal deposition, acute synovitis due to HA crystal deposition is unusual. But acute inflammatory syndromes including subacromial bursitis and a form of pseudopodagra described in young women[123] may occur in association with periarticular HA crystal deposition in bursae, tendons, ligaments, and soft tissues. Patients with advanced chronic renal failure, particularly on dialysis, may develop symptomatic articular and periarticular BCP crystal deposition (Figure 96-7), which may be destructive and involve the axial skeleton.[124] In some cases of dialysis-dependent renal failure, destructive arthropathy associated with BCP crystal deposition may resemble or be associated with CPPD deposition disease, and monosodium urate crystal deposits in the joint also may occur in the setting. Hyperparathyroidism can promote BCP-associated arthropathy[125] and periarticular disease including calcific bursitis (see Figure 96-7). Clinically significant periarticular HA crystal deposition also may occur in certain post-traumatic conditions and the systemic autoimmune diseases scleroderma and dermatomyositis.

BCP crystal deposition has a particular predilection for the shoulder (see Chapter 46), where it may manifest as

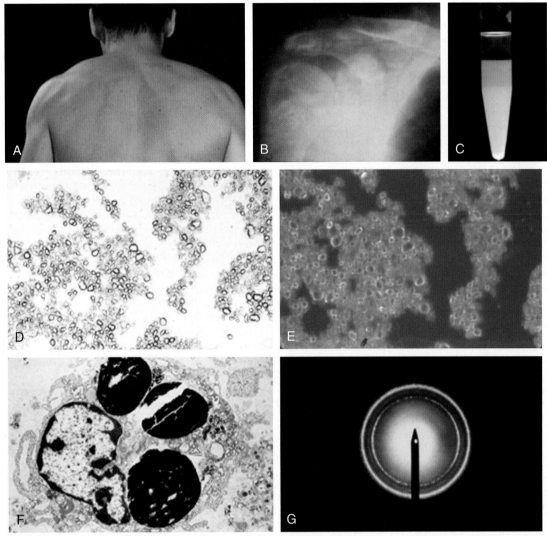

Figure 96-7 Hydroxyapatite crystal-associated calcific bursitis of the shoulder in a patient with chronic renal failure and secondary hyperparathyroidism. **A,** Chronic soft tissue swelling involving the right shoulder due to calcific right shoulder subacromial bursitis in a middle-aged male with a history of chronic renal failure on hemodialysis. Note the convex contour of the right shoulder compared with the left. **B,** Radiograph showing extensive calcification both within the rotator cuff and the expanded subacromial bursa surrounding the right shoulder joint. Incidental note is made of the resorption of the distal end of the clavicle consistent with the secondary hyperparathyroidism in this patient. **C,** Subacromial bursa fluid from the right shoulder. Note the milk-white appearance with a chalky sediment of the particulate material in the fluid after centrifugation consistent with crystal deposition disease. **D,** Microscopic appearance of bursa fluid aggregates of basic calcium phosphate crystals in the absence of special stains. The particles are irregular but have approximately spherical profiles. (Unstained. Magnification ×250.) **E,** Appearance of the bursa fluid under polarized light microscopy. Importantly, the aggregated particles of basic calcium phosphate crystals demonstrate edge birefringence but do not display intrusive birefringence, as seen in the figure. (Unstained. Magnification ×250.) **F,** Electron photomicrograph of a mononuclear phagocyte from this bursa fluid that contained phagocytosed electron dense (dark black) spherical aggregates of crystals of the basic calcium phosphate hydroxyapatite in three phagolysosomes oriented vertically to the right of the nucleus. Hundreds of tiny needle-shaped hydroxyapatite crystals are clumped in each of these dense aggregates. For perspective, the size of the mononuclear phagocyte is approximately 20 microns, and an individual (nonaggregated) hydroxyapatite crystal is approximately 0.04 × 0.01 × 0.01 microns in size. (Transmission electron microscopy. Magnification ×1000.) **G,** Electron diffraction pattern of hydroxyapatite crystal aggregates. The diffraction rings are indicative of a powder pattern (i.e., small crystals). The position of the bright rings with d-spacings = 3.44 and 2.81 Å are characteristic of hydroxyapatite (calcium apatite). *(Courtesy Dr. Ken Pritzker, Mount Sinai Hospital Pathology Department, University of Toronto, Ontario, Canada.)*

calcific tendinitis of the rotator cuff or as a destructive process associated with rotator cuff tear, which is most prevalent in the elderly and more common in females.[126] Abundant intra-articular BCP crystalline material is typically present in the distinctive noninflammatory syndrome of rotator cuff tear and marked cartilage degeneration, an entity termed MSS, *cuff tear arthropathy,* or *apatite-associated destructive arthritis.*[126] Mechanical instability of the shoulder due to rotator cuff tear may be the driving force in many of these patients, with consequent release of BCP crystals from

bone fragments into the joint space promoting secondary synovitis and connective tissue destruction. The process may be bilateral but is generally worse on the side of the dominant hand. Substantial glenohumeral joint effusions are typically seen, and synovial fluid is often blood stained but contains, at most, relatively low numbers of mononuclear leukocytes. Joints other than the shoulder such as the knee and hip can be affected by a condition similar to MSS, sometimes in the same individual with shoulder involvement. In contrast to primary OA, lateral tibiofemoral compartment involvement is common in BCP-associated destructive knee arthropathy. Concurrent CPPD deposition, biomechanical abnormalities, chronic renal failure, and neuropathic factors appear to be predisposing factors. A kindred with familial OA and apparent Milwaukee shoulder-knee syndrome (MSKS) had an unusual type of degenerative joint disease with both intra-articular and periarticular calcifications.[127]

Aging itself is a factor in articular cartilage BCP crystal deposition.[128] Multiple studies of synovial fluids and cartilage specimens from OA including recent work that has taken advantage of high-resolution means for BCP crystal detection[129] have suggested that deposition of intra-articular BCP crystalline material including HA in the pericellular matrix of chondrocytes and the capacity of joint cartilages to form such deposits are intimately linked with OA, as well as increased chondrocyte hypertrophy and severity of OA.[111,130-132] One limitation of some of these studies is that cartilages were fixed before analysis, and calcifications can develop as a fixation artifact. However, unequivocally, cartilage and synovial fluid BCP crystals, frequently in conjunction with CPPD crystals, are commonly detectable in advanced disease of the knee at the time of total joint replacement for OA.[111,132] Traffic of crystals from articular cartilage to synovium can promote calcific synovial crystal deposits at or just beneath the synovial surface, and synovium-derived rice bodies can give rise to BCP crystal deposits released into the joint space.[133,134]

Collectively, the abundance of HA and CPPD crystals in OA joints is likely significant under many clinical circumstances because HA and CPPD crystal-induced synovial proliferation, cytotoxic effects on chondrocytes, and synovial and chondrocyte MMP expression have the potential to promote OA progression.[132,133] Better surveys of joint tissues with advanced methods for detection of BCP crystals,[132,135,136] in particular, will be necessary to improve understanding of the clinical impact of these calcific crystals on OA.

DIAGNOSIS AND DIAGNOSTIC TESTS

KEY POINTS

Presence of radiographic evidence for chondrocalcinosis is a common finding in the aged and does not necessarily indicate that the patient's symptomatic articular problem is due to CPPD deposition disease, which is often asymptomatic.

The use of compensated polarized light microscopy is essential to confirm the presence of positively birefringent CPPD crystals, though it should be noted that some CPPD crystals are nonbirefringent.

Patients with arthritis in whom CPPD deposition disease is part of the differential diagnosis can be screened by plain radiographs, but high-resolution ultrasound of the affected joint is a useful and sensitive alternative approach.

Differential Diagnosis

CPPD deposition disease can imitate a number of other conditions and vice versa (see Table 96-3), which mandates

attention to fulfillment of diagnostic criteria for CPPD deposition disease (see Table 96-1) and necessitates careful adherence to a diagnostic algorithm (Figure 96-8). Conversely, it is important to note that presence of radiographic evidence for chondrocalcinosis is a common finding in the aged and does not necessarily indicate that the patient's symptomatic articular problem is due to CPPD deposition disease, which is often asymptomatic. The demonstrable presence of CPPD crystals in synovial fluid or in tissues using compensated polarized light microscopy (as discussed earlier for gout vs. pseudogout) is definite evidence for CPPD deposition disease. Though weakly birefringent relative to urate crystals and often rhomboid in shape, CPPD crystals can be rod shaped and intracellular, thereby resembling urate crystals. Thus the use of compensated polarized light microscopy is essential to confirm the presence of positively birefringent CPPD crystals, though it should be noted that some CPPD crystals are nonbirefringent.[137] The appearance and number of CPPD crystals can change with storage. Therefore clinicians should examine relatively fresh specimens collected in vials free of calcium-chelating anticoagulants such as EDTA. Cytocentrifugation increases sensitivity of detection of rare CPPD crystals, as observed in one study that highlighted approximately 75% to 78% of synovial fluid samples (of subjects with gout and OA) having both urate and CPPD crystals.[138]

The ability of pseudogout to mimic septic arthritis (pseudoseptic arthritis) and vice versa underscores the diagnostic importance of arthrocentesis with appropriate synovial fluid crystal analysis and, in many instances, concomitant exclusion of joint infection. Significantly, crystal deposits can be "enzymatically strip-mined" by inflammation associated with joint sepsis. Hence CPPD (as well as other crystals) may be observed free in the joint fluid and within synovial fluid leukocytes in an infected joint.

Diagnosis of CPPD deposition disease before age 55, particularly if CPPD deposition is widespread, should prompt differential diagnostic consideration of a primary metabolic or familial disorder (see Table 96-2). In the elderly, presentation of CPPD deposition as diffuse pain and fever of unknown origin[66] can mimic infection, polymyalgia rheumatica, and RA. A false-positive rheumatoid factor (RF) test is common in the elderly (≥30% positivity). Thus patients with pseudorheumatoid CPPD deposition disease are often RF seropositive.

Differential Diagnostic Considerations for Basic Calcium Phosphate Crystal Deposition

BCP crystals may be detected as nonbirefringent globular clumps within leukocytes in some synovial and bursal fluids (see Figure 96-7), and BCP crystal clumps stain with the calcium-binding dye Alizarin red S under light microscopy.[139,140] CPPD crystals can also be detected using Alizarin red S but stain more weakly than BCP crystals. Relative paucity of osteophytes (so-called *atrophic degenerative arthritis*) on plain radiographs and the sizeable glenohumeral joint effusions with abundant synovial fluid BCP crystalline material associated with MSS help distinguish MSS from primary OA of the glenohumeral joint. However, destructive, neuropathic shoulder arthropathy due to syringomyelia or alcoholism sometimes merits consideration in the

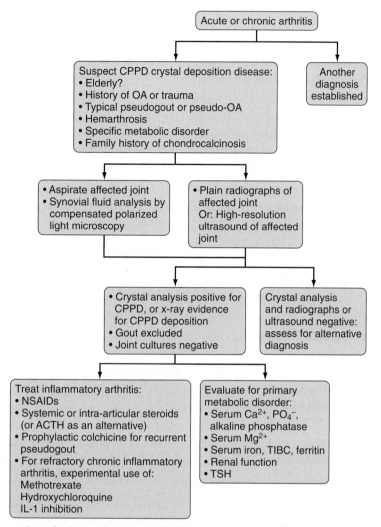

Figure 96-8 Algorithm for diagnosis, evaluation, and treatment of calcium pyrophosphate dihydrate (CPPD) deposition disease. The algorithm is discussed in detail in the text. Treatment options are in line with those recently advanced by the European League Against Rheumatism. ACTH, adrenocorticotropic hormone; IL-1, interleukin-1; NSAIDs, nonsteroidal anti-inflammatory drugs; OA, osteoarthritis; TIBC, total iron binding capacity; TSH, thyroid-stimulating hormone. *(From Guerne P-A, Terkeltaub R: Calcium pyrophosphate dihydrate crystal deposition: epidemiology, clinical features, diagnosis, and treatment. In Terkeltaub R, editor: Gout and other crystal arthropathies, Philadelphia, 2011, Elsevier.)*

differential diagnosis of MSS (see Chapter 47). Oxalate crystal deposition arthropathy can be a major differential diagnostic consideration with BCP-associated arthritis and periarticular calcifications in dialysis-dependent renal failure.

Chronic CPPD Deposition Arthropathy, BCP Crystal-Associated Arthritis, and Use of Plain Radiographs in Diagnosis

Chronic arthritis in CPPD deposition disease has several clinical and plain radiographic features helpful in differentiating it from OA. These include involvement at sites uncommon for primary OA such as the wrist, metacarpophalangeal joints, elbow, or shoulder, as well as radiographic heavy punctate and linear calcifications in fibrocartilages, articular (hyaline) cartilages, and joint capsules, especially if bilaterally symmetric (see Figures 96-5 and 96-6). It should be noted that faint or atypical calcifications may be due to BCP-related vascular calcifications. Deposition of nonpathologic dicalcium phosphate dihydrate (DCPD)

$(CaHPO_4 \cdot 2H_2O$, calcium-to-phosphate ratio, 1) ("brushite") crystals has been thought to cause some atypical calcifications, but brushite crystals can arise as an artifact of acid preparation of calcified tissue for pathologic analyses.[141]

CPPD crystal deposits often appear as broad linear streaks or linear "chunks" in articular hyaline and fibrocartilages on plain radiographs, whereas BCP crystal deposits in articular cartilage require high-resolution radiography for detection. Only a pattern of "atrophic" degenerative arthritis without osteophytes and variable subchondral bone thickening may be seen on plain radiographs of BCP arthritis in the shoulder and other large joints.

Patients with arthritis in whom CPPD deposition disease is part of the differential diagnosis can be screened radiologically by obtaining an anteroposterior (AP) view of each knee, an AP view of the pelvis (to detect symphysis pubis involvement, which is quite common), and posteroanterior (PA) views of both hands that include visualization of both wrists (see Figures 96-5 and 96-6). Calcific deposits may or may not be detectable by x-ray screening of these areas in

CPPD deposition disease. In this circumstance, radiographic evidence other than chondrocalcinosis may point to the correct diagnosis.[142] For example, radiographic findings suggestive of CPPD deposition disease, as opposed to primary OA, include radiocarpal or marked patellofemoral joint space narrowing, especially if isolated (such as the patella "wrapped around" the femur), as well as scaphoid-lunate widening and femoral cortical erosion superior to the patella. Severe progressive degeneration in the knee with subchondral bony collapse (microfractures) and fragmentation with formation of intra-articular radiodense bodies is a feature of CPPD presenting as a "pseudoneuropathic" joint. CPPD deposition disease involving the metacarpophalangeal joints can be distinguished radiographically from RA by metacarpal squaring associated with "beaklike" osteophytes and subchondral cyst formation. Tendon calcifications (e.g., Achilles, triceps, and obturator tendons) are a valuable differential diagnostic feature of CPPD deposition. Osteophyte formation is more variable with CPPD deposition disease than with OA. Clearly, x-ray findings may not correlate with pathologic and clinical manifestations in CPPD disease. For example, the correlation between radiographic and pathologic findings was only 39.2% in a study of patients via knee arthroscopy.[143]

High-Resolution Ultrasound and Advanced Imaging for Diagnosis of CPPD and BCP Crystal Deposition Diseases

Ultrasound can clearly detect aggregated BCP-related calcifications outside of joint cartilages including in the rotator cuff of the shoulder. In addition, in small, preliminary studies, high-resolution ultrasound (e.g., in the 6 to 13 MHz range using the current generation of equipment) detection of CPPD crystal deposits in joints has correlated well with positive results for synovial fluid analysis and has detected CPPD in some patients in whom plain radiographs were negative in the affected joint.[144-149] Preliminary criteria proposed for CPPD calcifications by ultrasound are summarized in Table 96-4, and Figure 96-9 (and Supplemental Figure

Table 96-4 Preliminary Criteria for Calcium Pyrophosphate Dihydrate (CPPD) Crystal Deposition Diagnosis by High-Resolution Ultrasound

1. All CPPD deposits are hyperechoic and present as one of the following patterns:
   Thin hyperechoic bands, parallel to the surface of the hyaline cartilage (frequently observed in the knee)
   A "punctate" pattern, composed of several thin hyperechoic spots, more common in fibrous cartilage and in tendons
   Homogeneous hyperechoic nodular or oval deposits localized in bursae and articular recesses (frequently mobile)
2. CPPD crystal deposit calcifications always have a sparkling appearance and create posterior shadowing only when they reach dimensions of greater than 10 mm. In contrast, calcifications that present a hypoechoic appearance with posterior shadowing even at an early stage (2-3 mm in diameter) are considered as crystalline deposits of another nature, most commonly due to basic calcium phosphate crystal deposition disease.

Modified from Frediani B, Filippou G, Falsetti P, et al: Diagnosis of calcium pyrophosphate dihydrate crystal deposition disease: ultrasonographic criteria proposed, *Ann Rheum Dis* 64:638–640, 2005.

96-3 on www.expertconsult.com) illustrates characteristic ultrasound features of CPPD deposits. Further validation is necessary for reliance on ultrasound without radiography in CPPD diagnosis.

The ultrasound approach is likely most specific for detection of CPPD crystal deposition in fibrocartilages (e.g., triangular fibrocartilage of the wrist and the midzones of articular hyaline cartilages (see Figure 96-9). Ultrasound, without use of synovial fluid analysis in diagnosis of acute pseudogout, runs the risk of missing other conditions such as infectious arthritis. Gout can generally be differentiated, particularly because redundant hyperechoic contouring of the cartilage surface is seen more in gout, whereas CPPD crystal deposition disease is typically visualized within the cartilage.[145] Because enthesopathies other than CPPD disease can also give rise to calcification of tendons and plantar fascia, the diagnostic value for CPPD disease of ultrasound detection of calcification in plantar fascia and Achilles tendon[150] is not yet clear.

Limitations of ultrasound include difficulty in visualizing crystal deposits in deep recesses of the joint space, the need for a high-resolution machine of the current generation, dependence on the skill of the ultrasonographer, and aforementioned issues with specificity of findings.

Dual-energy computed tomography has not been specifically studied for CPPD detection but is useful for specific discrimination of urate from BCP deposits.[151] Magnetic resonance imaging (MRI) is not yet a reliable approach for detecting CPPD crystal deposition disease due to a lack of mobile protons in CPPD crystals, and nonenhanced MRI is less sensitive in detecting knee meniscal fibrocartilage calcification than hyaline cartilage calcification.[152]

Laboratory Diagnostic Tests for CPPD and BCP Crystal Deposition Disease

Conventional radiography or ultrasound is usually the first method to evaluate patients with suspected chondrocalcinosis, but thorough laboratory evaluation of the newly diagnosed CPPD disease patient routinely includes serum levels of calcium, phosphorus, magnesium, alkaline phosphatase, ferritin, iron and total iron-binding capacity, and thyroid-stimulating hormone (TSH) (see Figure 96-8).

Specialized techniques beyond Alizarin red S staining such as x-ray diffraction, Raman spectroscopy, Fourier transform intrared spectroscopy, atomic force microscopy, or transmission electron microscopy showing electron-dense clumps of needle-like crystals may be necessary to confirm BCP crystal deposition (see Figure 96-7).[129]

Cytocentrifugation can increase sensitivity of CPPD detection in synovial fluid.[138] Under conditions where synovial fluid specimens are not fresh (or stored at 4° C for analysis after significant delay[153]), Gram stain and Diff Quik staining methods for crystal analysis in synovial fluids have been suggested to provide information beyond that from compensated polarized light microscopy.[154,155] Demonstration of CPPD crystals in articular tissues (see Figure 96-3) can be difficult in specimens stained with hematoxylin and eosin because the acidity of hematoxylin solutions promotes decalcification. However, the decalcifying effect of hematoxylin can be diminished by limiting the staining period with Mayer's hematoxylin to 3 minutes.[156]

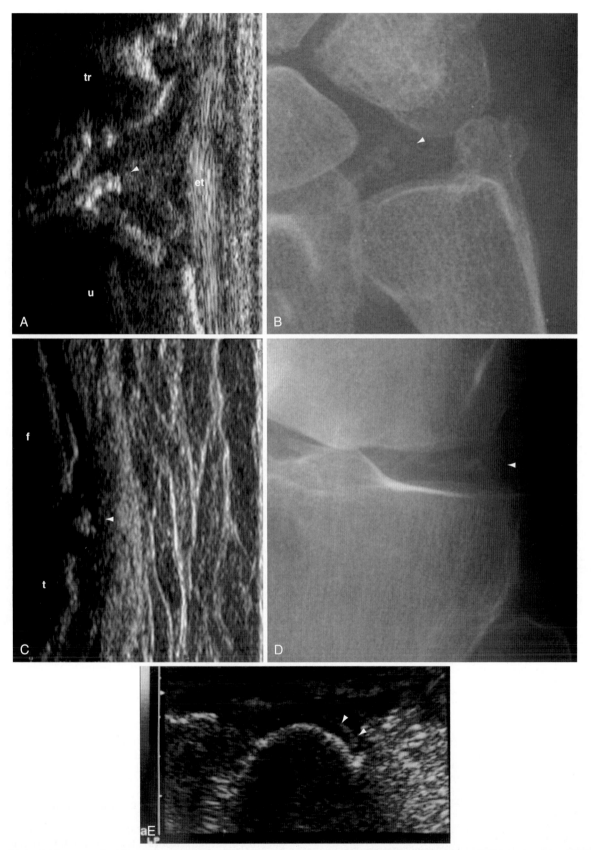

Figure 96-9 Calcium pyrophosphate dihydrate (CPPD) deposition disease detected by high-resolution ultrasound (US) versus plain radiography. **A** and **B,** Triangular fibrocartilage of the wrist. Longitudinal **(A)** lateral scan and **(B)** corresponding wrist radiograph showing hyperechoic rounded deposits within the substance of the fibrocartilage. **C** and **D,** Meniscal calcification of the knee as it appears on US **(C)** and corresponding radiograph **(D).** *Arrowhead,* fibrocartilage calcification; et, extensor carpi ulnaris tendon; f, femur; t, tibia; tr, triquetrum bone; u, ulna. **A** was obtained with a Diasus (Dynamic Imaging, Livingstone, United Kindom) using an 8- to 16-MHz linear probe. **C** was obtained using a Logiq 9 (General Electric Medical Systems, Milwaukee, Wisc) using a 4D16L probe. **E,** Ultrasonographic manifestations of hyaline cartilage CPPD crystal deposition disease as hyperechoic linear band parallel to the femoral condyle in a posterior location *(arrowheads). (**D,** From Grassi W, Meenagh G, Pascual E, Filippucci E: "Crystal clear"—sono-graphic assessment of gout and calcium pyrophosphate deposition disease,* Semin Arthritis Rheum *36(3):197–202, 2006; **E,** From Foldes K: Knee chondrocal-cinosis: an ultrasonographic study of the hyalin cartilage,* Clin Imaging *26(3):194–196, 2002.)*

TREATMENT

KEY POINTS

CPPD deposition disease treatment involves alleviation and prophylaxis of acute arthritic attacks, but therapy to lessen chronic and anatomically progressive sequelae of crystal deposition is not well developed for CPPD disease.

The approach to pseudogout treatment is similar to that for acute gout.

Calcium Pyrophosphate Dihydrate Deposition Disease

A treatment algorithm is presented at the bottom of Figure 96-8 that is consonant with the preliminary EULAR guidelines.[156a] As in gout (see Chapter 95), therapeutic approaches to patients with CPPD deposition disease involve treatment and prophylaxis of acute arthritic attacks, but therapy to lessen chronic and anatomically progressive sequelae of crystal deposition is not well developed for CPPD (Table 96-5). Reduced meniscal calcification was reported over a 10-year period in association with administration of oral magnesium to a patient with secondary CPPD deposition disease caused by hypomagnesemia.[157] However, there is no specific treatment validated to prevent or lessen crystal deposition of idiopathic CPPD deposition disease. Metabolic disorders that secondarily cause CPPD crystal deposition obviously require treatment. However, the potential benefits for prevention of chondrocalcinotic cartilage degeneration in the appropriate treatment of

Table 96-5 Therapeutics for Calcium Pyrophosphate Dihydrate (CPPD) Crystal Deposition Disease

Proven Benefits
NSAIDs or COX-2 inhibitors
Intra-articular corticosteroids
Systemic corticosteroids
ACTH
Prophylactic low-dose colchicine
Possible Benefits Already Observed Clinically
Methotrexate for refractory chronic inflammation and recurrent pseudogout
Oral magnesium (for patients with hypomagnesemia)
Theoretic Benefits
Phosphocitrate
Caspase-1 or IL-1 antagonism for CPPD crystal-induced inflammation
Hydroxychloroquine for refractory chronic inflammation
TLR2 antagonism for CPPD-associated degenerative arthropathy
Oral calcium supplementation to suppress PTH levels
ANKH anion channel blockade (probenecid)
NPP1 inhibition
TG2 inhibition
Polyphosphates
Promotion of crystal dissolution by alkaline phosphatase or polyamines

ACTH, adrenocorticotropic hormone; COX-2, cyclooxygenase-2; IL-1, interleukin-1; NPP1, nucleotide pyrophosphate phosphodiesterase 1; NSAIDs, nonsteroidal anti-inflammatory drugs; PTH, parathyroid hormone; TG2, transglutaminase 2; TLR2, Toll-like receptor 2.

hemochromatosis and hyperparathyroidism are unclear because the ability to detect chondrocalcinosis radiologically is usually indicative of advanced crystal deposition disease.

Episodes of pseudogout generally respond to nonsteroidal anti-inflammatory drugs (NSAIDs) (including cyclooxygenase-2 inhibitors) and/or intra-articular steroids, though sometimes more slowly than in gout. Systemic glucocorticosteroids or adrenocorticotropic hormone (ACTH),[158,159] generally given as described for acute gout (see Chapter 95), appear effective in most cases of acute pseudogout. The response to colchicine bolus is less consistent than that usually seen in acute gout. Intravenous colchicine is not recommended as treatment for pseudogout and was withdrawn from active marketing in 2008 by the U.S. Food and Drug Administration. However, pseudogout episodes can be diminished in frequency by low-dose daily colchicine prophylaxis, as for gouty arthritis. The self-limited nature of most acute pseudogout attacks in the knee can sometimes be accelerated by simple arthrocentesis and thorough drainage of the joint effusion, but there are currently no data for measures such as tidal irrigation in CPPD deposition disease, unlike the case for MSS.[160,161]

Hydroxychloroquine[162] has been suggested to be of some benefit to patients with refractory chronic polyarticular CPPD deposition disease and to reduce flares of pseudogout, and it has theoretic benefits by potentially stabilizing phagolysosomes to suppress NLRP3 inflammasome activation in response to CPPD crystal uptake. Methotrexate was promising to patients with refractory chronic polyarticular CPPD deposition disease and to reduce flares of pseudogout, though in an exploratory study limited to five consecutive patients, and with patients prior to methotrexate as their own controls.[163] IL-1 antagonism (e.g., with off-label use of anakinra) has had anecdotal success,[164,165] whereas breakthrough pseudogout has been reported during TNF antagonist therapy.[166] Collectively, at this time, there is insufficient evidence basis for hydroxychlorquine, methotrexate, and IL-1 antagonism as standard therapies for refractory inflammation in CPPD crystal deposition disease.

Effective cartilage-preserving therapy is still lacking in idiopathic chronic progressive CPPD deposition disease. Only limited evidence suggests that OA patients with cartilage calcification respond distinctly to arthroscopic irrigation and daily low-dose colchicines,[167-169] but further substantiation is necessary. There is currently no evidence to support arthroscopic débridement as a treatment modality for CPPD deposition disease. There is insufficient evidence for beneficial effects of intra-articular hyaluronan therapy in CPPD deposition disease of the knee, and risks of precipitating pseudogout appear significant with this treatment modality, as cited earlier.

Basic Calcium Phosphate Crystal Arthropathies

NSAIDs and local glucocorticoid injection (Table 96-6) are effective treatment options for BCP crystal-associated calcific tendinitis and subacromial bursitis (see Chapter 46). BCP crystal–associated inflammation of the rotator cuff and subacromial bursa of the shoulder can be successfully treated using needle aspiration, irrigation, and steroid injections. Ultrasound-guided techniques, which promote resorption of

Table 96-6 Therapeutics for Articular and Periarticular Basic Calcium Phosphate (BCP) Crystal Deposition

Proven Benefits
NSAIDs or selective COX-2 inhibitors
Local corticosteroid injection
Local irrigation
High-frequency therapeutic ultrasound to degrade BCP crystal deposits

Theoretic Benefits
Phosphocitrate
Modulators of ANKH (e.g., probenecid), ENPP1, or transglutaminase 2

COX-2, cyclooxygenase-2; ENPP1, ectonucleotide pyrophosphatase/phosphodiesterase 1; NSAIDs, nonsteroidal anti-inflammatory drugs.

rotator cuff and bursal calcifications, can enhance the success of such approaches.[170,171] Tidal irrigation may be of benefit for symptoms and function in MSS.[152,160]

Future Directions in Treatment

A potential factor that helps suppress the prevalence of chondrocalcinosis in China is high oral calcium intake, which can limit PTH production by the parathyroid. Specifically, calcium levels in tap water in Beijing were 12- to 20-fold higher than that in Framingham, whereas no difference was found in levels of magnesium in the aforementioned study of China versus USA chondrocalcinosis prevalence by Zhang and colleagues.[9] Deficient calcium intake in aging is a major public health problem in Western countries. It is possible that chondrocalcinosis is more of an environmentally mediated finding than previously recognized, via subclinical variability in calcium intake and parathyroid function. Given the current lack of effective, rational therapies to prevent or lessen idiopathic CPPD crystal deposition, further study of the potential prophylactic and therapeutic benefits of dietary calcium supplementation on chondrocalcinosis is warranted.

The potential to develop therapies for both CPPD and BCP crystal–associated arthropathies based on new molecular targets has been elevated by identification of ANKH, ENPP1, and TG2 as specific molecular mediators of cartilage calcification. Intriguingly, the anion transport inhibitor probenecid suppresses ANKH-induced and TGF-β–induced increases in extracellular PP$_i$ in vitro.[36,38,172] Prevention of CPPD deposition by polyphosphates or promotion of CPPD dissolution by depot alkaline phosphatase and by pyrophosphatase activation-promoting polyamines could provide alternative therapeutic approaches.[173-175] However, incomplete CPPD crystal dissolution by intra-articular lavage of patients with chondrocalcinosis of the knees with disodium EDTA and magnesium ions in the past was a therapeutic failure in that insignificant amounts of CPPD were removed and all subjects developed postlavage attacks of pseudogout mediated by crystal shedding.[176]

The PP$_i$ analogue phosphocitrate, a natural compound in mammalian mitochondria and in the urinary tract, is a potent inhibitor of HA crystal formation.[177] Phosphocitrate inhibits nitric oxide–induced calcification of cartilage and also inhibits both HA and CPPD crystal-associated cell

stimulation including induction of MMP-3 in fibroblasts.[178] Systemic phosphocitrate treatment suppresses ankylosing ossification in murine progressive ankylosis of ank/ank mice.[179] Moreover, an analogue of phosphocitrate (CaNaPC) decreased both the abundant meniscal cartilage HA deposition and the continuous progression of OA in the Hartley guinea pig model of spontaneous knee OA.[180] The CaNaPC treatment did not exert therapeutic effects in a rabbit knee hemimeniscectomy model of OA in which there was an absence of intra-articular calcification.[180] Such results suggest that phosphocitrate acts on calcification-mediated mechanisms of dysregulation of joint biomechanics and cartilage degeneration without exerting nonspecific chondroprotective effects. Further clinical development of phosphocitrate would be of interest but has been slowed in part by low bioavailability unless given parenterally.[177]

The use of bisphosphonates as PP$_i$ analogues can be beneficial in some cases of soft tissue calcification with HA. Lastly, the identified roles of TLR2 in chondrocyte responsiveness to CPPD crystals,[92] of TLR4 in hydroxyapatite crystal–induced inflammatory responses,[181] and of NLRP3 inflammasome-mediated caspase-1 activation and IL-1β processing in CPPD crystal–induced inflammation[93] suggest certain mediators of innate immunity including TLR2, TLR4, caspase-1, and IL-1β to be potential therapeutic targets for human forms of CPPD and hydroxyapatite crystal-driven inflammation and connective tissue destruction.

OUTCOME

> **KEY POINTS**
>
> It is not clear whether the presence of CPPD crystals in primary knee OA is a predictive factor for more frequent knee replacement surgery, despite the fact that CPPD crystals are frequently found in OA knee tissues at the time of total joint arthroplasty.
>
> There is no clear correlation between the extent of calcification and progression of primary CPPD deposition arthropathy.

The presence of CPPD crystals in primary knee OA had been proposed to be a predictive factor for more frequent knee replacement surgery.[110] Moreover, mean radiographic scores directly correlated with the presence of calcium-containing crystals in OA in patients at the time of total joint arthroplasty.[111] However, degenerative cartilage disease associated with sporadic CPPD crystal deposition disease may be less destructive than that observed in primary OA. For example, prospective analysis of CPPD deposition disease of the knee suggested that radiographic worsening of degenerative arthritis was slow to progress.[67] Typically, changes in radiographic extent of chondrocalcinosis are observed over time,[67] but there is no clear correlation between the extent of calcification and progression of CPPD deposition arthropathy.

In the Boston OA Knee Study (BOKS) and in the Health, Aging and Body Composition (Health ABC) Study[182] the relationship between chondrocalcinosis and the progression of knee OA was prospectively evaluated longitudinally using MRI. In BOKS, knees with chondrocalcinosis had a decreased risk of cartilage loss compared with knees without chondrocalcinosis and there was no difference in risk in Health ABC. Stratification by the presence of intact or damaged knee menisci produced comparable results within each cohort. In a Thai study, CPPD crystal deposition disease was identified radiographically and/or by synovial fluid analysis in 52.9% of 102 patients undergoing total knee arthroplasty.[183] Patients with and without chondrocalcinosis did not differ in difficulties in performing daily activities or treatment, and those with chondrocalcinosis did not undergo knee arthroplasty at an earlier age than those without chondrocalcinosis.

In the setting of OA, the processes leading to matrix calcification had been regarded to reflect passive secondary consequences of advanced cartilage pathology. Moreover, joint inflammation induced by deposited crystals was thought to be the primary determinant of the clinical impact of chondrocalcinosis on the progression of OA. The aforementioned studies and advances in understanding the pathogeneses of OA and chondrocalcinosis paint a different picture of the impact of chondrocalcinosis in OA. In essence, the dysregulated cartilage matrix repair that generates cartilage calcification may be as effective (or in some cases more effective) at slowing cartilage tissue failure than other phenotypes of cartilage repair in OA.

Websites

Wellcome Trust Centre for Human Genetics: www.well.ox.ac.uk

Teaching resource page for radiographic images of BCP and CPPD arthropathies:
www.orthopaedicweblinks.com/Teaching_Resources/Radiology/more3.html

Selected References

1. Zhang W, Doherty M, Bardin T, et al: European League Against Rheumatism recommendations for calcium pyrophosphate deposition. Part I: terminology and diagnosis, *Ann Rheum Dis* 70:563–570, 2011.
2. Richette P, Bardin T, Doherty M: An update on the epidemiology of calcium pyrophosphate dihydrate crystal deposition disease, *Rheumatology (Oxford)*. 48:711–715, 2009.
3. Neame RL, Carr AJ, Muir K, et al: UK community prevalence of knee chondrocalcinosis: evidence that correlation with osteoarthritis is through a shared association with osteophyte, *Ann Rheum Dis* 62:513–518, 2003.
4. Ramonda R, Musacchio E, Perissinotto E, et al: Prevalence of chondrocalcinosis in Italian subjects from northeastern Italy. The Pro.V.A. (PROgetto Veneto Anziani) study, *Clin Exp Rheumatol* 27:981–984, 2009.
5. Salaffi F, De Angelis R, Grassi W, et al: Investigation Group (MAPPING) study. Prevalence of musculoskeletal conditions in an Italian population sample: results of a regional community-based study. I. The MAPPING study, *Clin Exp Rheumatol* 23(6):819–828, 2005.
9. Zhang Y, Terkeltaub R, Nevitt M, et al: Lower prevalence of chondrocalcinosis in Chinese subjects in Beijing than in white subjects in the United States: The Beijing Osteoarthritis Study, *Arthritis Rheum* 54:3508–3512, 2006.
10. Zaka R, Williams CJ: Genetics of chondrocalcinosis, *Osteoarthritis Cartilage* 13:745–750, 2005.
11. Pendleton A, Johnson MD, Hughes A, et al: Mutations in ANKH cause chondrocalcinosis, *Am J Hum Genet* 71:933–940, 2002.
12. Williams JC, Zhang Y, Timms A, et al: Autosomal dominant familial calcium pyrophosphate dihydrate deposition disease is caused by mutation in the transmembrane protein ANKH, *Am J Hum Genet* 71:985–991, 2002.
13. Zhang Y, Johnson K, Russell RG, et al: Association of sporadic chondrocalcinosis with a -4-basepair G-to-A transition in the 5'-untranslated region of ANKH that promotes enhanced expression of ANKH protein and excess generation of extracellular inorganic pyrophosphate, *Arthritis Rheum* 52:1110–1117, 2005.
14. Pons-Estel BA, Gimenez C, Sacnun M, et al: Familial osteoarthritis and Milwaukee shoulder associated with calcium pyrophosphate and apatite crystal deposition, *J Rheumatol* 27:471–480, 2000.
16. Bruges-Armas J, Couto AR, Timms A, et al: Ectopic calcification among families in the Azores: clinical and radiologic manifestations in families with diffuse idiopathic skeletal hyperostosis and chondrocalcinosis, *Arthritis Rheum* 54:1340–1349, 2006.
19. Terkeltaub R: Inorganic pyrophosphate (PPi) generation and disposition in pathophysiology, *Am J Physiol: Cell Physiol* 281:C1–C11, 2001.
24. Johnson K, Goding J, van Etten D, et al: Linked deficiencies in extracellular inorganic pyrophosphate and osteopontin expression mediate pathologic calcification in PC-1 null mice, *Am J Bone Min Res* 18:994–1004, 2003.
25. Hessle L, Johnson KA, Anderson HC, et al: Tissue-nonspecific alkaline phosphatase and plasma cell membrane glycoprotein-1 are central antagonistic regulators of bone mineralization, *Proc Natl Acad Sci U S A* 99:9445–9449, 2002.
26. Wang D, Canaff L, Davidson D, et al: Alterations in the sensing and transport of phosphate and calcium by differentiating chondrocytes, *J Biol Chem* 276:33995–34005, 2001.
27. Burton DW, Foster M, Johnson KA, et al: Chondrocyte calcium-sensing receptor expression is up-regulated in early guinea pig knee osteoarthritis and modulates PTHrP, MMP-13, and TIMP-3 expression, *Osteoarthritis Cartil* 13:395–404, 2005.
28. Johnson K, Terkeltaub R: Upregulated ank expression in osteoarthritis can promote both chondrocyte MMP-13 expression and calcification via chondrocyte extracellular PPi excess, *Osteoarthritis Cartil* 12:321–335, 2004.
29. Johnson K, Pritzker K, Goding J, et al: The nucleoside triphosphate pyrophosphohydrolase (NTPPPH) isozyme PC-1 directly promotes cartilage calcification through chondrocyte apoptosis and increased calcium precipitation by mineralizing vesicles, *J Rheumatol* 28:2681–2691, 2001.
30. Rutsch F, Ruf N, Vaingankar S, et al: Mutations in ENPP1 are associated with 'idiopathic' infantile arterial calcification, *Nat Genet* 34:379–381, 2003.
31. Johnson K, Hashimoto S, Lotz M, et al: Up-regulated expression of the phosphodiesterase nucleotide pyrophosphatase family member PC-1 is a marker and pathogenic factor for knee meniscal cartilage matrix calcification, *Arthritis Rheum* 44:1071–1081, 2001.
33. Terkeltaub R: Physiologic and pathologic functions of the NPP nucleotide pyrophosphatase/phosphodiesterase family focusing on NPP1 in calcification, *Purinergic Signaling* 2:371–377, 2006.
35. Johnson K, Pritzker K, Goding J, et al: The nucleoside triphosphate pyrophosphohydrolase (NTPPPH) isozyme PC-1 directly promotes cartilage calcification through chondrocyte apoptosis and increased calcium precipitation by mineralizing vesicles, *J Rheumatol* 28:2681–2691, 2001.
36. Ho A, Johnson M, Kingsley DM: Role of the mouse ank gene in tissue calcification and arthritis, *Science* 289:265–270, 2000.
37. Zaka R, Stokes D, Dion AS, et al: P5L mutation in Ank results in an increase in extracellular PPi during proliferation and non-mineralizing hypertrophy in stably transduced ATDC5 cells, *Arthritis Res Ther* 8:R164, 2006.
38. Williams CJ, Pendleton A, Bonavita G, et al: Mutations in the amino terminus of ANKH in two US families with calcium pyrophosphate dihydrate crystal deposition disease, *Arthritis Rheum* 48:2627–2631, 2003.
39. Gurley KA, Reimer RJ, Kingsley DM: Biochemical and genetic analysis of ANK in arthritis and bone disease, *Am J Hum Genet* 79:1017–1029, 2006.
40. Costello JC, Rosenthal AK, Kurup IV, et al: Parallel regulation of extracellular ATP and inorganic pyrophosphate: roles of growth factors, transduction modulators, and ANK, *Connect Tissue Res* 52:139–146, 2011.
41. Wang J, Tsui HW, Beier F, et al: The CPPDD-associated ANKH M48T mutation interrupts the interaction of ANKH with the sodium/phosphate cotransporter PiT-1, *J Rheumatol* 36:1265–1272, 2009.

42. Zaka R, Dion AS, Kusnierz A, et al: Oxygen tension regulates the expression of ANK (progressive ankylosis) in an HIF-1-dependent manner in growth plate chondrocytes, *J Bone Miner Res* 24:1869–1878, 2009.

43. Wang W, Xu J, Du B, et al: Role of the progressive ankylosis gene (ank) in cartilage mineralization, *Mol Cell Biol* 25:312–323, 2005.

44. Nürnberg P, Thiele H, Chandler D, et al: Heterozygous mutations in ANKH, the human ortholog of the mouse progressive ankylosis gene, result in craniometaphyseal dysplasia, *Nat Genet* 28:37–41, 2001.

45. Morava E, Kohnisch J, Drijvers JM, et al: Autosomal recessive mental retardation, deafness, ankylosis, and mild hypophosphatemia associated with a novel ANKH mutation in a consanguineous family, *J Clin Endocrinol Metab* 96:E189–E198, 2011.

47. Wang J, Tsui HW, Beier F, et al: The CPPDD-associated ANKH M48T mutation interrupts the interaction of ANKH with the sodium/phosphate cotransporter PiT-1, *J Rheumatol* 36:1265–1272, 2009.

48. Williams CJ, Pendleton A, Bonavita G, et al: Mutations in the amino terminus of ANKH in two US families with calcium pyrophosphate dihydrate crystal deposition disease, *Arthritis Rheum* 48:2627–2631, 2003.

49. Wang J, Tsui HW, Beier F, et al: The ANKH deltaE490 mutation in calcium pyrophosphate dihydrate crystal deposition disease (CPPDD) affects tissue non-specific alkaline phosphatase (TNAP) activities, *Open Rheumatol J* 2:23–30, 2008.

51. Johnson K, Hashimoto S, Lotz M, et al: IL-1 induces pro-mineralizing activity of cartilage tissue transglutaminase and factor XIIIa, *Am J Pathol* 159:149–163, 2001.

54. Johnson K, Farley D, Hu S-I, et al: One of two chondrocyte-expressed isoforms of cartilage intermediate layer protein functions as an IGF-I antagonist, *Arthritis Rheum* 48:1302–1314, 2003.

57. Volpe A, Guerriero A, Marchetta A, et al: Familial hypocalciuric hypercalcemia revealed by chondrocalcinosis, *Joint Bone Spine* 76:708–710, 2009.

60. Husa M, Liu-Bryan R, Terkeltaub R: Shifting HIFs in osteoarthritis, *Nat Med* 16:641–644, 2010. Erratum in: Nat Med 2010;16:828.

64. Johnson K, Van Etten D, Nanda N, et al: Distinct transglutaminase II/TG2-independent and TG2-dependent pathways mediate articular chondrocyte hypertrophy, *J Biol Chem* 278:18824–18832, 2003.

66. Cecil DL, Rose DM, Terkeltaub R, et al: Role of interleukin-8 in PiT-1 expression and CXCR1-mediated inorganic phosphate uptake in chondrocytes, *Arthritis Rheum* 52:144–154, 2005. Erratum in: Arthritis Rheum 2006;54:2320.

67. Adams CS, Shapiro IM: The fate of the terminally differentiated chondrocyte: evidence for microenvironmental regulation of chondrocyte apoptosis, *Crit Rev Oral Biol Med* 13:465–473, 2002.

68. Hamade T, Bianchi A, Sebillaud S, et al: Inorganic phosphate (Pi) modulates the expression of key regulatory proteins of the inorganic pyrophosphate (PPi) metabolism in TGFβ1-stimulated chondrocytes, *Biomed Mater Eng* 20:209–215, 2010.

73. Terkeltaub R, Johnson K, Murphy A, et al: The mitochondrion in osteoarthritis, *Mitochondrion* 1:301–319, 2002.

74. Johnson K, Svensson CI, Etten DV, et al: Mediation of spontaneous knee osteoarthritis by progressive chondrocyte ATP depletion in Hartley guinea pigs, *Arthritis Rheum* 50:1216–1225, 2004.

75. Merz D, Liu R, Johnson K, et al: IL-8/CXCL8 and growth-related oncogene alpha/CXCL1 induce chondrocyte hypertrophic differentiation, *J Immunol* 171:4406–4415, 2003.

76. Johnson KA, Terkeltaub RA: External GTP-bound transglutaminase 2 is a molecular switch for chondrocyte hypertrophic differentiation and calcification, *J Biol Chem* 280:15004–15012, 2005.

78. Cecil DL, Johnson K, Rediske J, et al: Inflammation-induced chondrocyte hypertrophy is driven by receptor for advanced glycation end products, *J Immunol* 175:8296–8302, 2005.

79. Cecil DL, Appleton CT, Polewski MD, et al: The pattern recognition receptor CD36 is a chondrocyte hypertrophy marker associated with suppression of catabolic responses and promotion of repair responses to inflammatory stimuli, *J Immunol* 182:5024–5031, 2009.

80. Cecil DL, Terkeltaub R: Transamidation by transglutaminase 2 transforms S100A11 calgranulin into a procatabolic cytokine for chondrocytes, *J Immunol* 180:8378–8385, 2008.

83. Takeuchi E, Sugamoto K, Nakase T, et al: Localization and expression of osteopontin in the rotator cuff tendons in patients with calcifying tendinitis, *Virchows Arch* 438:612–617, 2001.

84. Nakase T, Takeuchi E, Sugamoto K, et al: Involvement of multinucleated giant cells synthesizing cathepsin K in calcified tendinitis of the rotator cuff tendons, *Rheumatology (Oxford)* 39:1074–1077, 2000.

85. Liu R, O'Connell M, Johnson K, et al: Extracellular signal-regulated kinase 1/extracellular signal-regulated kinase 2 mitogen-activated protein kinase signaling and activation of activator protein 1 and nuclear factor kappaB transcription factors play central roles in interleukin-8 expression stimulated by monosodium urate monohydrate and calcium pyrophosphate crystals in monocytic cells, *Arthritis Rheum* 43:1145–1155, 2000.

86. Morgan MP, McCarthy GM: Signaling mechanisms involved in crystal-induced tissue damage, *Curr Opin Rheumatol* 14:292–297, 2002.

87. Sun Y, Wenger L, Brinckerhoff CE, et al: Basic calcium phosphate crystals induce matrix metalloproteinase-1 through the Ras/mitogen-activated protein kinase/c-Fos/AP-1/metalloproteinase 1 pathway. Involvement of transcription factor binding sites AP-1 and PEA-3, *J Biol Chem* 277:1544–1552, 2002.

88. Molloy ES, Morgan MP, Doherty GA, et al: Microsomal prostaglandin E2 synthase 1 expression in basic calcium phosphate crystal-stimulated fibroblasts: role of prostaglandin E2 and the EP4 receptor, *Osteoarthritis Cartil* 17:686–692, 2009.

89. Molloy ES, Morgan MP, Doherty GA, et al: Mechanism of basic calcium phosphate crystal-stimulated cyclo-oxygenase-1 upregulation in osteoarthritic synovial fibroblasts, *Rheumatology (Oxford)* 47:965–971, 2008.

90. Molloy ES, Morgan MP, Doherty GA, et al: Mechanism of basic calcium phosphate crystal-stimulated matrix metalloproteinase-13 expression by osteoarthritic synovial fibroblasts: inhibition by prostaglandin E2, *Ann Rheum Dis* 67:1773–1779, 2008.

91. Molloy ES, Morgan MP, McDonnell B, et al: BCP crystals increase prostacyclin production and upregulate the prostacyclin receptor in OA synovial fibroblasts: potential effects on mPGES1 and MMP-13, *Osteoarthritis Cartil* 15:414–420, 2007.

92. Liu-Bryan R, Pritzker K, Firestein GS, et al: TLR2 signaling in chondrocytes drives calcium pyrophosphate dihydrate and monosodium urate crystal-induced nitric oxide generation, *J Immunol* 174:5016–5023, 2005.

93. Martinon F, Petrilli V, Mayor A, et al: Gout-associated uric acid crystals activate the NALP3 inflammasome, *Nature* 440:237–241, 2006.

100. Narayan S, Pazar B, Ea HK, et al: Octacalcium phosphate crystals induce inflammation in vivo through interleukin-1 but independent of the NLRP3 inflammasome in mice, *Arthritis Rheum* 63:422–433, 2011.

104. Canhao H, Fonseca JE, Leandro MJ, et al: Cross-sectional study of 50 patients with calcium pyrophosphate dihydrate crystal arthropathy, *Clin Rheumatol* 20:119–122, 2001.

105. Bernardeau C, Bucki B, Lioté F: Acute arthritis after intra-articular hyaluronate injection: onset of effusions without crystals, *Ann Rheum Dis* 60:518–520, 2000.

107. Wendling D, Tisserand G, Griffond V, et al: Acute pseudogout after pamidronate infusion, *Clin Rheumatol* 27:1205–1206, 2008.

109. Schlesinger N, Hassett AL, Neustadter L, et al: Does acute synovitis (pseudogout) occur in patients with chronic pyrophosphate arthropathy (pseudo-osteoarthritis)? *Clin Exp Rheumatol* 27:940–944, 2009.

110. Reuge L, Lindhoudt DV, Geerster J: Local deposition of calcium pyrophosphate crystals in evolution of knee osteoarthritis, *Clin Rheumatol* 20:428–431, 2001.

111. Derfus BA, Kurian JB, Butler JJ, et al: The high prevalence of pathologic calcium crystals in pre-operative knees, *J Rheumatol* 29:570–574, 2002.

113. Yamakawa K, Iwasaki H, Ohjimi Y, et al: Tumoral calcium pyrophosphate dihydrate crystal deposition disease, *Pathology* 197:499–506, 2001.

116. Fujishiro T, Nabeshima Y, Yasui S, et al: Pseudogout attack of the lumbar facet joint: a case report, *Spine* 27:396–398, 2002.

117. Pascal-Moussellard H, Cabre P, Smadja D, et al: Myelopathy due to calcification of the cervical ligamenta flava: a report of two cases in the West Indian patients, *Eur Spine J* 8:238–240, 1999.

118. Cabre P, Pascal-Moussellard H, Kaidomar S, et al: Six cases of ligamentum cervical flavum calcification in blacks in the French West Indies, *Joint Bone Spine* 68:158–165, 2001.

119. Assaker R, Louis E, Boutry N, et al: Foramen magnum syndrome secondary to calcium pyrophosphate crystal deposition in the transverse ligament of atlas, *Spine* 26:1396–1400, 2001.

120. Kakitsubata Y, Boutin RD, Theodorou DJ, et al: Calcium pyrophosphate dihydrate crystal deposition in and around the atlantoaxial joints: association with type 2 odontoid fractures in nine patients, *Radiology* 216:213–219, 2000.

126. Halverson PB: Crystal deposition disease of the shoulder (including calcific tendonitis and Milwaukee shoulder syndrome), *Curr Rheumatol Rep* 5:244–247, 2003.

127. Pons-Estel BA, Gimenez C, Sacnun M, et al: Familial osteoarthritis and Milwaukee shoulder associated with calcium pyrophosphate and apatite crystal deposition, *J Rheumatol* 27:471–480, 2000.

128. Mitsuyama H, Healey RM, Terkeltaub RA, et al: Calcification of human articular knee cartilage is primarily an effect of aging rather than osteoarthritis, *Osteoarthritis Cartil* 15:559–565, 2007.

129. Yavorskyy A, Hernandez-Santana A, McCarthy G, et al: Detection of calcium phosphate crystals in the joint fluid of patients with osteoarthritis—analytical approaches and challenges, *Analyst* 133:302–318, 2008.

130. Fuerst M, Bertrand J, Lammers L, et al: Calcification of articular cartilage in human osteoarthritis, *Arthritis Rheum* 60:2694–2703, 2009.

131. Fuerst M, Lammers L, Schäfer F, et al: Investigation of calcium crystals in OA knees, *Rheumatol Int* 30:623–631, 2010.

132. McCarthy GM, Cheung HS: Point: hydroxyapatite crystal deposition is intimately involved in the pathogenesis and progression of human osteoarthritis, *Curr Rheumatol Rep* 11:141–147, 2009.

133. van Linthoudt D, Beutler A, Clayburne G, et al: Morphometric studies on synovium in advanced osteoarthritis: is there an association between apatite-like material and collagen deposits? *Clin Exp Rheumatol* 15:493–497, 1997.

134. Li-Yu J, Clayburne GM, Sieck MS, et al: Calcium apatite crystals in synovial fluid rice bodies, *Ann Rheum Dis* 61:387–390, 2002.

135. Rosenthal AK, Fahey M, Gohr C, et al: Feasibility of a tetracycline-binding method for detecting synovial fluid basic calcium phosphate crystals, *Arthritis Rheum* 58:3270–3274, 2008.

136. Rosenthal AK, Mattson E, Gohr CM, et al: Characterization of articular calcium-containing crystals by synchrotron FTIR, *Osteoarthritis Cartil* 16:1395–1402, 2008.

137. Ivorra J, Rosas J, Pascual E: Most calcium pyrophosphate crystals appear as non-birefringent, *Ann Rheum Dis* 58:582–584, 1999.

138. Robier C, Neubauer M, Quehenberger F, et al: Coincidence of calcium pyrophosphate and monosodium urate crystals in the synovial fluid of patients with gout determined by the cytocentrifugation technique, *Ann Rheum Dis* 70:1163–1164, 2011.

142. Steinbach LS, Resnick D: Calcium pyrophosphate dihydrate crystal deposition disease: imaging perspective, *Curr Probl Diagn Radiol* 29:209–229, 2000.

144. Filippucci E, Scire CA, Delle Sedie A, et al: Ultrasound imaging for the rheumatologist. XXV. Sonographic assessment of the knee in patients with gout and calcium pyrophosphate deposition disease, *Clin Exp Rheumatol* 28:2–5, 2010.

145. Grassi W, Meenagh G, Pascual E, et al: "Crystal clear"—sonographic assessment of gout and calcium pyrophosphate deposition disease, *Semin Arthritis Rheum* 36:197–202, 2006.

146. Frediani B, Filippou G, Falsetti P, et al: Diagnosis of calcium pyrophosphate dihydrate crystal deposition disease: ultrasonographic criteria proposed, *Ann Rheum Dis* 64:638–640, 2005.

147. Foldes K: Knee chondrocalcinosis: an ultrasonographic study of the hyalin cartilage, *Clin Imaging* 26:194–196, 2002.

148. Sofka CM, Adler RS, Cordasco FA: Ultrasound diagnosis of chondrocalcinosis in the knee, *Skeletal Radiol* 31:43–45, 2002.

149. Monteforte P, Brignone A, Rovetta G: Tissue changes detectable by sonography before radiological evidence of elbow chondrocalcinosis, *Int J Tissue React* 22:23–25, 2000.

150. Falsetti P, Frediani B, Acciai C, et al: Ultrasonographic study of Achilles tendon and plantar fascia in chondrocalcinosis, *J Rheumatol* 31:2242–2250, 2004.

151. Choi HK, Al-Arfaj AM, Eftekhari A, et al: Dual energy computed tomography in tophaceous gout, *Ann Rheum Dis* 68:1609–1612, 2009.

152. Abreu M, Johnson K, Chung CB, et al: Calcification in calcium pyrophosphate dihydrate (CPPD) crystalline deposits in the knee: anatomic, radiographic, MR imaging, and histologic study in cadavers, *Skeletal Radiol* 33:392–398, 2004.

160. Halverson PB, Ryan LM: Tidal lavage in Milwaukee shoulder syndrome: do crystals make the difference? *J Rheumatol* 34:1446–1447, 2007.

161. Epis O, Caporali R, Scire CA, et al: Efficacy of tidal irrigation in Milwaukee shoulder syndrome, *J Rheumatol* 34:1545–1550, 2007.

163. Chollet-Janin A, Finckh A, Dudler J, et al: Methotrexate as an alternative therapy for chronic calcium pyrophosphate deposition disease: an exploratory analysis, *Arthritis Rheum* 56:688–692, 2007.

164. Announ N, Palmer G, Guerne PA, et al: Anakinra is a possible alternative in the treatment and prevention of acute attacks of pseudogout in end-stage renal failure, *Joint Bone Spine* 76:424–426, 2009.

165. McGonagle D, Tan AL, Madden J, et al: Successful treatment of resistant pseudogout with anakinra, *Arthritis Rheum* 58:631–633, 2008.

166. Josefina M, Ana CJ, Ariel V, et al: Development of pseudogout during etanercept treatment, *J Clin Rheumatol* 13:177, 2007.

175. Kannampuzha JV, Tupy JH, Pritzker KP: Mercaptopyruvate inhibits tissue-nonspecific alkaline phosphatase and calcium pyrophosphate dihydrate crystal dissolution, *J Rheumatol* 36:2758–2765, 2009.

177. Cheung HS: Phosphocitrate as a potential therapeutic strategy for crystal deposition disease, *Curr Rheumatol Rep* 3:24–28, 2001.

180. Cheung HS, Sallis JD, Demadis KD, et al: Phosphocitrate blocks calcification-induced articular joint degeneration in a guinea pig model, *Arthritis Rheum* 54:2452–2461, 2006.

181. Grandjean-Laquerriere A, Tabary O, Jacquot J, et al: Involvement of toll-like receptor 4 in the inflammatory reaction induced by hydroxyapatite particles, *Biomaterials* 28:400–404, 2007.

182. Neogi T, Nevitt M, Niu J, et al: Lack of association between chondrocalcinosis and increased risk of cartilage loss in knees with osteoarthritis: results of two prospective longitudinal magnetic resonance imaging studies, *Arthritis Rheum* 54:1822–1828, 2006.

183. Viriyavejkul P, Wilairatana V, Tanavalee A, et al: Comparison of characteristics of patients with and without calcium pyrophosphate dihydrate crystal deposition disease who underwent total knee replacement surgery for osteoarthritis, *Osteoarthritis Cartil* 13:232–235, 2006.

Full references for this chapter can be found on www.expertconsult.com.

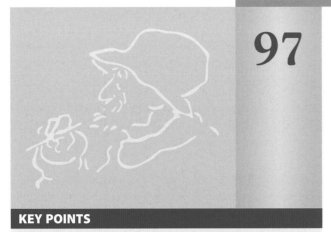

97

Familial Autoinflammatory Syndromes

ANNA SIMON • JOS W.M. van der MEER • JOOST P.H. DRENTH

KEY POINTS

Autoinflammatory disorders are characterized by recurrent or chronic inflammation without signs of infection or autoimmunity.

Dysregulation of the interleukin-1β (IL-β) pathway is central to many autoinflammatory syndromes, especially the cryopyrin-associated periodic syndromes, deficiency of the IL-1 receptor antagonist, and familial Mediterranean fever.

The need for a definite diagnosis in the familial autoinflammatory syndromes has increased because of advances in treatment options.

A severe complication is type amyloid A amyloidosis, which often leads to renal failure; the risk of this complication is greatly reduced when patients receive adequate treatment.

In a substantial portion of patients presenting with a clear autoinflammatory phenotype, the diagnosis can remain elusive, which indicates that other disorders remain to be discovered.

Because of the central role of IL-1β in many autoinflammatory diseases, a trial of IL-1β inhibiting therapy can be warranted for diagnostic and therapeutic purposes.

The familial autoinflammatory syndromes, often referred to as *hereditary periodic fever syndromes,* comprise rare hereditary disorders with a common phenotype of lifelong, recurrent inflammatory episodes, characterized by inflammatory symptoms such as fever, abdominal pain, diarrhea, rash, or arthralgia.[1] Between the fever episodes, patients with most of these syndromes generally feel healthy and function normally. Routine laboratory investigations during a fever attack invariably reveal a severe acute-phase response with a high erythrocyte sedimentation rate, leukocytosis, and high concentrations of acute-phase proteins such as C-reactive protein (CRP) and serum amyloid A (SAA). The inflammatory episodes occur without an obvious trigger, although some patients note a relationship to physical stimuli (e.g., exposure to cold), emotional stress, or the menstrual cycle. The episodes resolve spontaneously in days or weeks. Patients go undiagnosed for years, generating a high level of discouragement and frustration for patients and physicians when no diagnosis is made.[2,3] The term *autoinflammatory,* coined by McDermott and colleagues in 1999,[4] describes the phenotype of recurrent, acute inflammatory responses. It is preferable to the term *autoimmune* in these cases because typical autoimmune phenomena are not found; the defect is located more in the innate immune system than the acquired immune system.[5]

Several genetically distinct types of hereditary autoinflammatory syndromes are recognized. Despite the common phenotype described previously, these can often be differentiated clinically by specific characteristics, in particular mode of inheritance, age of onset, average duration of the fever episodes and the fever-free interval, geographic region of origin of the patient, and occurrence of long-term complications such as amyloidosis or deafness (Table 97-1 and Figure 97-1). A significant number of patients with a periodic fever phenotype still do not fit into this genetically based classification, probably representing additional (genetic) defects that can lead to autoinflammatory disease. This chapter describes the seven best characterized familial autoinflammatory syndromes at this time in detail.

DIFFERENTIAL DIAGNOSIS

When a patient has had recurrent fever episodes for more than 2 years, it is increasingly unlikely that these are caused by an infection or a malignant disorder. The differential diagnosis at that time may include numerous inflammatory disorders such as juvenile rheumatoid arthritis, adult-onset Still's disease, inflammatory bowel disease, Schnitzler syndrome, and Behçet's disease, in addition to the hereditary periodic fever syndromes (Table 97-2). Because the hereditary syndromes are rare (except for familial Mediterranean fever [FMF] in individuals with a distinct ethnic background), the more common diagnoses should usually be excluded first.

The mainstay of the diagnosis of hereditary autoinflammatory syndromes is clinical assessment, with a detailed medical and family history, and preferably at least one observation of the patient during a fever episode because physical examination of the patient in a period of remission is seldom abnormal. Another helpful clue, although not pathognomonic, is often gained from knowing the patient's ethnic origin. This clinical assessment often yields enough information to build a differential diagnosis of the specific familial autoinflammatory syndromes (see Table 97-1) to determine the direction of genetic testing (Figure 97-2).

When the specific diagnosis remains elusive, a trial treatment with an interleukin-1 (IL-1) inhibitor (e.g., anakinra) can give a diagnostic clue. A significant proportion of patients that suffer from an autoinflammatory disease "not otherwise specified" respond well to treatment with anakinra; we even use the (temporary) label of "anakinra-responsive disease" for this category in daily practice.

Table 97-1 Differential Diagnosis of Familial Autoinflammatory Syndromes

	Familial Mediterranean Fever (FMF)	Mevalonate Kinase (MKD) Deficiency — Hyper-immunoglobulin D Syndrome (HIDS)	Mevalonate Kinase (MKD) Deficiency — Mevalonic Aciduria	Tumor Necrosis Factor Receptor-Associated Periodic Syndrome (TRAPS)	Cryopyrin-Associated Periodic Syndrome (CAPS) — Familial Cold Autoinflammatory Syndrome (FCAS)	Cryopyrin-Associated Periodic Syndrome (CAPS) — Muckle-Wells Syndrome (MWS)	Cryopyrin-Associated Periodic Syndrome (CAPS) — Chronic Infantile Neurologic Cutaneous and Articular Syndrome (CINCA)	Deficiency of IL-1 Receptor Antagonist (DIRA)
Mode of Inheritance	Autosomal recessive	Autosomal recessive	Autosomal recessive	Autosomal dominant	Autosomal dominant	Autosomal dominant	Autosomal dominant	Autosomal recessive
Age at Onset (yr)	<20	<1	<1	<20	<1	<20	<1	Birth, <4 wk
Duration of attack (days)*	<2	4-6	4-5	>14	<2	1-2	?	Continuous
Cutaneous Involvement	Erysipelas-like erythema	Maculopapular rash	Morbilliform rash	Migratory rash, overlying area of myalgia	Cold-induced urticaria-like lesions	Urticaria-like rash	Urticaria-like lesions	Generalized pustulosis
Musculoskeletal Involvement	Monoarthritis common	Arthralgia, occasional oligoarthritis	Arthralgia common	Severe myalgia common; occasional frank monoarthritis	Arthralgia common; occasional mild myalgia	Lancing limb pain, arthralgia common; arthritis can occur	Epiphyseal bone formation	Sterile pustulous osteomyelitis
Abdominal Involvement	Sterile peritonitis common	Splenomegaly, severe pain common	Splenomegaly, pain may occur	Severe pain common	None	May occur	Hepatosplenomegaly	
Eye Involvement	Uncommon	Uncommon	Uncommon	Conjunctivitis and periorbital edema common	Conjunctivitis	Conjunctivitis; sometimes optic nerve elevation	Papilledema with possible loss of vision, uveitis	
Distinguishing Clinical Symptoms	Erysipelas-like erythema	Prominent cervical lymphadenopathy	Dysmorphic features, neurologic symptoms	Migratory nature of myalgia and rash, periorbital edema	Cold-induced urticaria-like lesions	Sensorineural hearing loss	Chronic aseptic meningitis, sensorineural hearing loss, arthropathy	
Gene Involved	MEFV	MVK	MVK	TNFRSF1A	CIAS1 = NLRP3	CIAS1 = NLRP3	CIAS1 = NLRP3	IL-1RN
Protein Involved	Pyrin (marenostrin)	Mevalonate kinase	Mevalonate kinase	Type 1 tumor necrosis factor receptor	Cryopyrin	Cryopyrin	Cryopyrin	IL-1RA

*Duration may vary; this is a typical duration.

Note: For details on Blau syndrome, DIRA, and pyogenic sterile arthritis, pyoderma gangrenosum, and acne (PAPA) syndrome, see text.

Modified from Hull KM, Shoham N, Chae JJ, et al: The expanding spectrum of systemic autoinflammatory disorders and their rheumatic manifestations, *Curr Opin Rheumatol* 15:61-69, 2003.

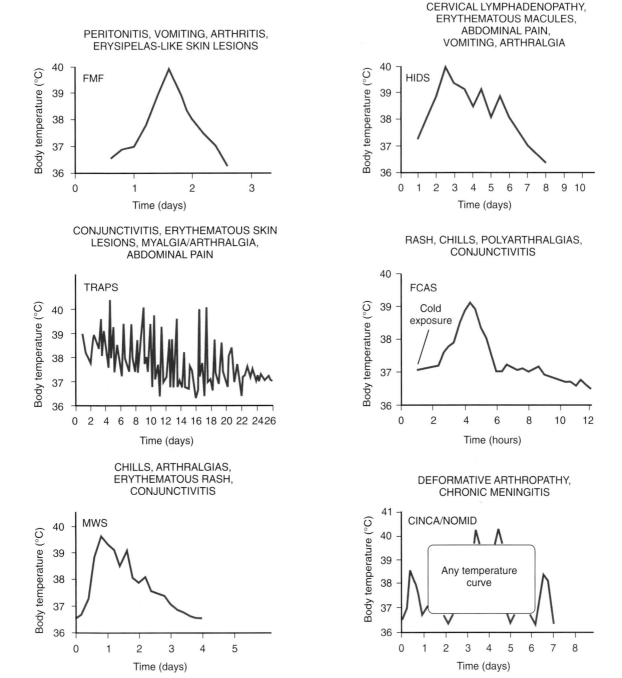

Figure 97-1 Characteristic patterns of body temperature during inflammatory attacks in the familial autoinflammatory syndromes. Interindividual variability for each syndrome is considerable, and even for the individual patient, the fever pattern may vary greatly from episode to episode. Note the different time scales on the x-axes. CINCA/NOMID, chronic infantile neurologic cutaneous and articular syndrome/neonatal-onset multisystemic inflammatory disease; FCAS, familial cold autoinflammatory syndrome; HIDS, hyper-IgD syndrome; MWS, Muckle-Wells syndrome; TRAPS, tumor necrosis factor receptor–associated periodic syndrome.

FAMILIAL MEDITERRANEAN FEVER

Epidemiology

FMF (Mendelian inheritance in men [MIM] 249100) is the most prevalent disorder among the hereditary autoinflammatory syndromes, with more than 10,000 patients affected worldwide. It occurs primarily in people originating from the Mediterranean basin including Armenians, Sephardic Jews, Arabs, and Turks. FMF is an autosomal recessively inherited disorder. Most families reported with an apparent autosomal dominant inheritance pattern of FMF[6] represent examples of pseudodominant inheritance owing to consanguinity combined with the high carrier frequency of FMF mutations in certain populations[6-8]; however, at least three families studied do seem to show a true dominant inheritance, even after extensive genetic analysis.[8]

Table 97-2 Differential Diagnosis of Periodic Fever

1. Hereditary (see Table 97-1)
2. Nonhereditary
   a. Infectious
      i. Hidden infectious focus (e.g., aortoenteric fistula, Caroli's disease)
      ii. Recurrent reinfection (e.g., chronic meningococcemia, host defense defect)
      iii. Specific infection (e.g., Whipple's disease, malaria)
   b. Noninfectious inflammatory disorder, e.g.:
      i. Adult-onset Still's disease
      ii. Juvenile chronic rheumatoid arthritis
      iii. Periodic fever, aphthous stomatitis, pharyngitis, and adenitis
      iv. Schnitzler syndrome
      v. Behçet's syndrome
      vi. Crohn's disease
      vii. Sarcoidosis
      viii. Extrinsic alveolitis
      ix. Humidifier lung, polymer fume fever
   c. Neoplastic
      i. Lymphoma (e.g., Hodgkin's disease, angioimmunoblastic lymphoma)
      ii. Solid tumor (e.g., pheochromocytoma, myxoma, colon carcinoma)
   d. Vascular (e.g., recurrent pulmonary embolism)
   e. Hypothalamic
   f. Psychogenic periodic fever
   g. Factitious or fraudulent

Etiology

In 1997 two groups independently traced the genetic background of FMF to a hitherto unknown gene on the short arm of chromosome 16, dubbed the MEditterranean FeVer (MEFV) gene.[9,10] At least 80 disease-linked mutations in the MEFV gene have been described so far, most of which are clustered in the tenth exon of this gene (for details see the online mutation database at http://fmf.igh.cnrs.fr/infevers/). Most are missense mutations that produce a single amino acid change in the protein (Figure 97-3). There are six common mutations, accounting for almost 99% of all FMF chromosomes: M694V (occurring in 20% to 65% of cases, depending on the population examined[11]), V726A (in 7% to 35%), M680I, M694I, V694I, and E148Q. For the first three mutations mentioned here, a founder effect has been established,[10] pointing to common ancestors at least 2500 years ago. The high frequency of the mutated MEFV gene in more than one Middle Eastern population has led to the hypothesis that heterozygous carriers have an as-yet-unknown advantage, possibly a heightened (inflammatory) resistance to an as-yet-unidentified endemic pathogen of the Mediterranean basin.[10] In about 30% of patients, only one or no mutations in the MEFV gene can be detected; the etiology in these patients still needs to be determined.

Pathogenesis

The MEFV gene encodes for a protein of 781 amino acids, known as *pyrin* or *marenostrin*. Pyrin is expressed as a cytoplasmic protein in mature monocytes in association with microtubules[12] but is predominantly found in the nucleus in granulocytes, dendritic cells, and synovial fibroblasts.[13] The expression of pyrin is induced by inflammatory mediators such as interferon-α and tumor necrosis factor (TNF).[14] The pyrin domain is shared by many proteins involved in apoptosis and inflammation and is a member of the death-domain superfamily that includes death domains, death-effector domains, and caspase-recruitment domains. Pyrin binds specifically to other proteins that contain a pyrin domain, which include the adapter protein "apoptosis-associated specklike-like protein with a CARD" (ASC).

The proinflammatory cytokine interleukin (IL)-1β is central in the pathogenesis of FMF. This cytokine is expressed as an inactive precursor, which is cleaved by caspase-1 to yield the active IL-1β. Caspase-1 itself first needs to be activated through the interaction with a protein complex termed an *inflammasome*. Several inflammasomes have been described so far. The major inflammasome complex involved in the activation of caspase-1 and IL-1β is the cryopyrin or NLRP3 inflammasome.[15,16] Two hypotheses have been proposed regarding the effect of pyrin on IL-1β processing. The "sequestration hypothesis" holds that pyrin has an inhibitory effect on caspase-1–mediated activation of IL-1β, through its prevention of the formation of the cryopyrin inflammasome by competitive binding of the adapter protein ASC and procaspase-1 and binding caspase-1.[17,18] Under this hypothesis, FMF mutations are thought to interfere with the inhibiting interactions of pyrin, resulting in decreased regulation of IL-1β activation.[18] The second hypothesis, proposed by Yu and colleagues,[19] suggests that pyrin can form its own specific inflammasome for activation of IL-1β, although not all the components of this proposed inflammasome have been specified so far. The FMF mutations would increase the sensitivity of this putative pyrin inflammasome. Apart from its role in regulation of IL-1β, there is also conflicting evidence for the effect of pyrin on regulation of nuclear factor κB (NFκB) or apoptosis, varying from inhibition to stimulation.[1]

Clinical Features

In approximately 90% of FMF patients, symptoms start before age 20 years.[20] The inflammatory attacks of FMF usually last 1 to 3 days The frequency can vary widely; 2 to 4 weeks is the most common interval (see Figure 97-1). Symptoms of serositis (i.e., peritonitis, pleuritis, synovitis) are the main feature of FMF attacks, usually accompanied by fever. Abdominal pain of 1 or 2 days' duration occurs in 95% of patients, varying in severity from severe peritonitis resembling an acute abdomen to only mild abdominal pain without overt peritonitis.[21] Arthritis (rarely destructive) is often confined to one large joint such as the knee, ankle, or wrist and may be the only symptom. Chest pain resulting from pleuritis is usually unilateral and associated with a friction rub or transient pleural effusion. Skin involvement occurs in approximately 30% of patients, most often as erysipelas-like skin lesions on the shins or feet (Figure 97-4).[22] Other, more uncommon, symptoms are pericarditis, occurring in less than 1%[23]; acute scrotal swelling and tenderness[24]; aseptic meningitis; and severe protracted myalgia, especially of the legs.

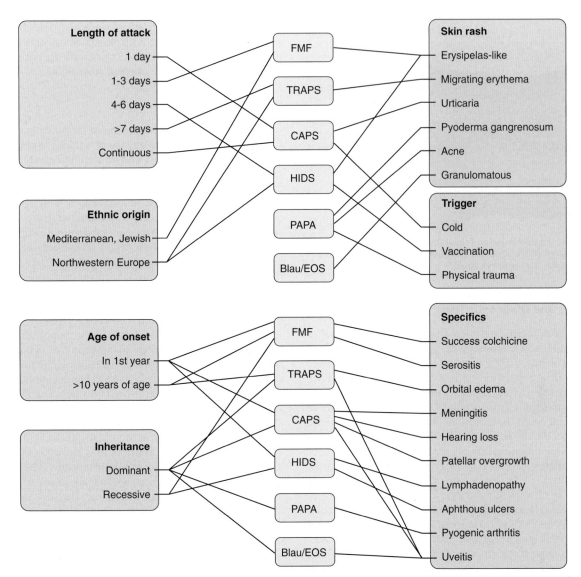

Figure 97-2 Differential diagnosis of the familial autoinflammatory syndromes. First exclude other, more common causes of fever and inflammation in the patient. When a familial autoinflammatory syndrome seems likely, check the clinical characteristics found in the patient on the right and left of the diagram, and assign one point to each syndrome that is linked to these characteristics by a line (one characteristic could lead to or point to more than one syndrome). The final combined score assigns a rank for the likelihood of the disorders in this patient and offers help in deciding on the correct subsequent diagnostic tests. This algorithm is not evidence based but is solely derived from expert opinion. CAPS, cryopyrin-associated periodic syndrome; EOS, early-onset sarcoidosis; FMF, familial Mediterranean fever; HIDS, hyper-IgD syndrome; PAPA, pyogenic sterile arthritis, pyoderma gangrenosum, and acne; TRAPS, tumor necrosis factor receptor–associated periodic syndrome.

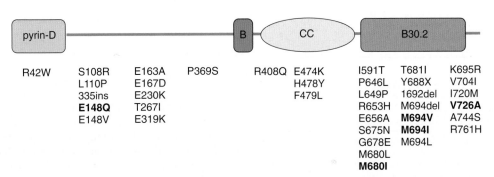

Figure 97-3 Schematic representation of pyrin (marenostrin) protein, with four conserved domains including a pyrin domain, a B-box (B), coiled-coil domain (CC), and a B30.2 domain. Indicated are mutations as found in familial Mediterranean fever, with the five most common missense mutations in bold type. For complete listing of all currently known mutations, see INFEVERS website: http://fmf.igh.cnrs.fr/infevers/.

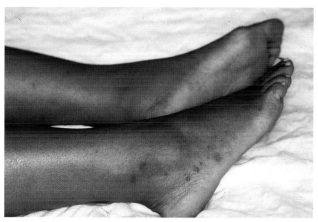

Figure 97-4 Erysipelas-like eruption in a patient with a familial Mediterranean fever attack. *(Courtesy Professor A. Livneh, Heller Institute of Medical Research, Tel Hashomer, Israel.)*

Diagnosis and Diagnostic Tests

FMF is still primarily a clinical diagnosis. There is a set of validated diagnostic criteria with a reported sensitivity and specificity of 96% to 99% (Table 97-3).[25] These criteria were validated in a population with a high prevalence of FMF and low prevalence of the other autoinflammatory disorders, however, and the ethnic origin of the patient needs to be taken into account. In molecular diagnostic testing, genetic laboratories usually screen for the five most common mutations and rare mutations are missed. *MEFV* mutations occur on both alleles in only 70% of typical cases,[26] whereas in the remaining 30%, only one or no mutation can be detected, even after sequencing. There is also evidence of reduced penetrance. Despite these limitations, molecular testing can be used as a confirmatory test. Whether or not the results are positive, treatment with colchicine is warranted in symptomatic cases of fitting ethnic origin fulfilling the diagnostic criteria.[27,28] No specific biologic marker is available to distinguish an inflammatory FMF attack from an infectious fever or appendicitis. During an inflammatory

Table 97-3 Diagnostic Criteria for Familial Mediterranean Fever*

Major Criteria
Typical attacks[†] with peritonitis (generalized)
Typical attacks with pleuritis (unilateral) or pericarditis
Typical attacks with monoarthritis (hip, knee, ankle)
Typical attacks with fever alone
Incomplete abdominal attack

Minor Criteria
Incomplete attacks[‡] involving chest pain
Incomplete attacks involving monoarthritis
Exertional leg pain
Favorable response to colchicine

*Requirements for diagnosis of familial Mediterranean fever are ≥1 major criteria or ≥2 minor criteria.
  [†]Typical attacks are defined as recurrent (≥3 of the same type), febrile (≥38° C), and short (lasting between 12 hours and 3 days).
  [‡]Incomplete attacks are defined as painful and recurrent attacks not fulfilling the criteria for a typical attack.
  From Livneh A, Langevitz P, Zemer D, et al: Criteria for the diagnosis of familial Mediterranean fever, *Arthritis Rheum* 40:1879–1885, 1997.

attack, there is an acute-phase response, which includes elevation of SAA, CRP, and plasma fibrinogen and polymorphonuclear leukocytosis. Proteinuria in patients with FMF is highly suggestive of renal amyloidosis.

Treatment

Colchicine is the first-line treatment for patients with FMF. Colchicine prevents inflammatory attacks completely in 60% to 75% of patients, and it significantly reduces the number of attacks in an additional 20% to 30%.[29] The average dose in adults is 1 mg daily, but this may be increased to 3 mg in cases in which no response is seen at the lower dose. This regimen is usually well tolerated; gastrointestinal side effects including diarrhea and abdominal pain generally resolve with dose reduction. More serious side effects such as myopathy, neuropathy, and leukopenia are rare and occur primarily in patients with renal or liver impairment. During a fever attack, oral or intramuscular nonsteroidal anti-inflammatory drugs (NSAIDs) can be used for pain relief. Glucocorticoids have limited efficacy.

Compliance with colchicine use is important because colchicine has been shown to prevent the occurrence of amyloidosis. Since the introduction of colchicine therapy, the incidence of amyloidosis in FMF has decreased dramatically, whereas in areas with a high prevalence of FMF where colchicine is not routinely available, such as Armenia, amyloidosis is still common. Colchicine's principal effect at the cellular level is to depolymerize microtubules by interacting with tubulin, inhibiting motility and exostosis of intracellular granules. It has a powerful antimitotic effect, causing metaphase arrest. It has been speculated, in cases of infertility in patients treated with colchicine, that this medication causes azoospermia. Colchicine does not have a significant adverse effect on sperm production or function, however.[30] Unfounded fear of teratogenic effects of colchicine often wrongly leads to cessation of this drug in young women who want to get pregnant, with a subsequent increased frequency and severity of attacks, which enhances problems with fertility and pregnancy. Colchicine has proved to be safe, even in early pregnancy, and treatment should not be interrupted for this reason.[31,32] It can also be used while breastfeeding.[29]

In about 5% to 10% of patients, FMF is refractory to colchicine use. Lidar and colleagues[33] used parenteral colchicine in such refractory cases, but this can be toxic. More recently, the IL-1β inhibitor anakinra has been shown to be effective in several case reports and series.[34-38]

Outcome

Recurrent attacks of peritonitis may lead to intra-abdominal or pelvic adhesions, resulting in complications such as small bowel obstruction. Another serious long-term complication of FMF is amyloid A (AA) amyloidosis. This amyloidosis is primarily found in the kidneys, resulting in renal failure, but can also occur in the gastrointestinal tract, liver, and spleen, and eventually in the heart, testes, and thyroid. The prevalence of amyloidosis varies, especially depending on the ethnic origin, but it is high in untreated patients. It is common among Sephardic Jews but rare in Ashkenazi Jews.[39]

For a variety of reasons including peritoneal adhesions and ovulatory dysfunction, subfertility in women is common.[31] In men, subfertility secondary to azoospermia (sometimes secondary to testicular amyloidosis) or impairment of sperm penetration has been found.[20]

HYPER–IMMUNOGLOBULIN D SYNDROME (MEVALONATE KINASE DEFICIENCY)

Epidemiology

Hyper-IgD syndrome (HIDS) (MIM 260920), also known as *mevalonate kinase deficiency*, is an autosomal recessively inherited disorder, but it is far less prevalent than FMF. The International Hyper-IgD Syndrome Registry, based in Nijmegen, the Netherlands, in which clinical information is collected from physicians worldwide, currently holds data on approximately 220 patients. Approximately 75% of these patients are from Western Europe, and 50% are from the Netherlands and France.[40] Most HIDS patients are of Caucasian origin. These observations can be explained partly by a founder effect.[41] In the Netherlands, the carrier frequency of the most common mevalonate kinase mutation is 1:153.[42] Men and women are affected in equal numbers.[40]

Etiology

HIDS is caused by mutations in the gene encoding for the enzyme mevalonate kinase, located on the long arm of chromosome 12 (for details, see the online mutation database available at http://fmf.igh.cnrs.fr/infevers/).[43-45] Patients with classic HIDS are most often compound heterozygotes for two missense mutations (Figure 97-5). Two mutations (V377I and I268T) account for more than 85% of the patients described to date.[40]

The term *variant type HIDS*, which we proposed for patients with an autoinflammatory disease and high immunoglobulin (Ig)D without mevalonate kinase deficiency,[45] has been largely abandoned. Many patients with fever syndromes have a raised IgD and this subclass is heterogeneous. It seems more useful to designate these patients as "autoinflammatory disease not otherwise specified" to indicate that a more specific diagnosis may still be found in the future.

Pathogenesis

Mevalonate kinase is part of the isoprenoid pathway; it is the step after 3-hydroxy-3-methyl-glutaryl–coenzyme A (HMG-CoA) reductase, phosphorylating mevalonic acid. The isoprenoid pathway has many diverse end products that include cholesterol, dolichol, and ubiquinone, and it leads to isoprenylation of proteins, with a post-translational modification directing these proteins such as Rho and Ras to the cell membrane.[46]

HIDS mutations lead to a constantly diminished activity of mevalonate kinase to about 5% to 15% of normal levels, and these levels decrease further during a fever attack.[47] Because of this reduced enzyme activity, the substrate mevalonic acid accumulates in serum and urine. Higher levels are found during the episodes of fever. There does not seem to be a dramatic shortage of any specific end product; concentrations of cholesterol, ubiquinone, and dolichol in patients are normal to slightly decreased.[1]

Another syndrome was already linked to mutations in the mevalonate kinase gene before the discovery of HIDS[48]—classic mevalonic aciduria. Patients with mevalonic aciduria carry specific mutations that cause a more severe reduction of mevalonate kinase enzyme activity, reducing it to undetectable levels. These patients constantly produce large amounts of mevalonic acid and often have more than 1000 times as much mevalonic acid in their urine than do HIDS patients.[49] Patients with mevalonic aciduria also have a more severe phenotype. Classic mevalonic aciduria and HIDS seem to be two extremes of a continuous spectrum of disease related to mevalonate kinase deficiency.[50]

The pathogenetic link between mevalonate kinase deficiency and inflammation is still unclear, but there is increasing evidence for a connection between the isoprenoid pathway and inflammation. Inhibition of the isoprenoid pathway by statins, the inhibitors of HMG-CoA reductase (the enzymatic step before that of mevalonate kinase), can have anti-inflammatory effects, ranging from increased apoptosis of inflammatory cells to reduction of expression of cytokines.[51,52] In other settings, statins seem to be proinflammatory, most notably in a study in which stimulation with *Mycobacterium tuberculosis* or mitogens in combination with statins increased caspase-1 activation and IL-1β secretion by monocytes, through a decrease of geraniolgeraniol.[15] The ex vivo production of IL-1β is increased in HIDS,[53,54]

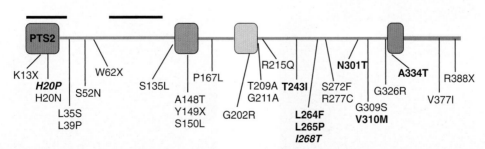

Figure 97-5 Mevalonate kinase, with four conserved domains represented by colored boxes. Indicated are missense mutations, nonsense mutations, and two deletions, which have been identified in mevalonate kinase deficiency. In bold are mutations found in mevalonic aciduria patients; in bold and italic are mutations found in classic hyper-IgD syndrome and mevalonic aciduria. For complete listing of all currently known mutations, see INFEVERS website: http://fmf.igh.cnrs.fr/infevers/.

whereas treatment with the IL-1 blocker anakinra is beneficial.[55,56] Current evidence points to a link between the mevalonate pathway and IL-1 through alterations of isoprenylation of the small GTPase Rac1, phosphoinositide 3-kinase (PI3K), and protein kinase B (PKB).[57] A defect in apoptosis may also contribute to the pathogenesis of HIDS. Lymphocytes from HIDS patients (who had no fever at the time of blood sampling) showed a decrease in apoptosis when stimulated with anisomycin, which was not found in patients with TNF receptor–associated periodic syndrome (TRAPS) or FMF patients.[58] Such a decrease in apoptosis would result in increased survival of lymphocytes and may delay the resolution of the inflammatory response. An ordinarily innocuous stimulus in HIDS patients would more easily lead to a full-blown fever episode.

The cause of the characteristic high serum concentrations of IgD in this syndrome, which have led to its name, is still unexplained.

Clinical Features

Ninety percent of patients with HIDS experience their first fever episode in the first year of life,[40] and these episodes become most frequent in childhood and adolescence. The high fevers may lead to seizures, especially in young children. Vaccination, minor trauma, surgery, and physical or emotional stress are factors that provoke a fever episode, although often a triggering factor is not obvious.[40] The fevers often begin with cold chills and a sharp increase in body temperature. They are almost always accompanied by cervical lymphadenopathy and abdominal pain with vomiting and diarrhea. Other frequent symptoms are headache, myalgia, and arthralgia. Apart from the lymphadenopathy, physical signs frequently consist of splenomegaly and a skin rash with erythematous macules and papules (Figure 97-6) or petechiae (Figure 97-7).[40] Sometimes there are also signs of frank arthritis (principally large joints) and hepatomegaly. About 40% of patients report painful aphthous ulcers

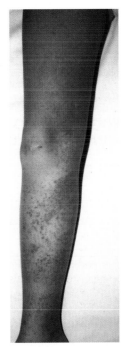

Figure 97-7 Petechiae on the leg of a hyper-IgD syndrome patient during a febrile attack.

in the mouth, vagina, or scrotum (Figure 97-8). The fever disappears spontaneously after 3 to 5 days, although it may take longer before the symptoms in joints or skin disappear completely. These inflammatory attacks occur, on average, once every 4 to 6 weeks, although this may vary from patient to patient or in an individual patient.

Patients with mevalonic aciduria, the metabolic disorder that is also caused by mevalonate kinase gene mutations, experience similar but more severe inflammatory episodes as HIDS patients. In addition, these patients suffer from psychomotor retardation, ataxia, failure to thrive, cataracts, and dysmorphic facies. Patients with classic mevalonic aciduria usually die in early childhood.[49] An intermediary clinical phenotype between classic mevalonic aciduria and HIDS has been described.[50]

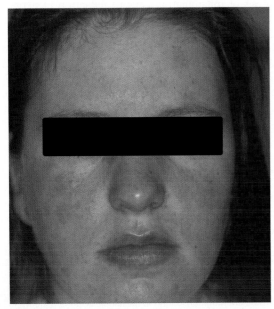

Figure 97-6 Facial erythematous macules and papules in a hyper-IgD syndrome patient during an attack.

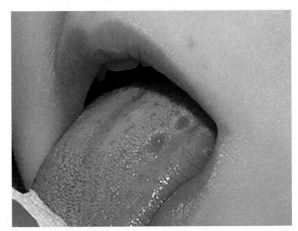

Figure 97-8 Aphthous ulceration detected on the tongue of a patient with hyper-IgD syndrome. *(Courtesy Dr. K. Antila, North Carelian Central Hospital, Joensuu, Finland.)*

Table 97-4 Diagnostic Indicators of Hyper–Immunoglobulin D Syndrome

At Time of Attacks
Elevated erythrocyte sedimentation rate and leukocytosis
Abrupt onset of fever (≥38.5° C)
Recurrent attacks
Lymphadenopathy (especially cervical)
Abdominal distress (e.g., vomiting, diarrhea, pain)
Skin manifestations (e.g., erythematous macules and papules)
Arthralgias and arthritis
Splenomegaly
Constantly Present
Elevated IgD (≥100 U/mL) measured on 2 occasions at least 1 mo apart*
Elevated IgA (≥2.6 g/L)
Specific Features
Mutations in mevalonate kinase gene
Decreased mevalonate kinase enzyme activity

*Extremely high serum concentrations of IgD are characteristic but not obligatory.

Diagnosis and Diagnostic Tests

HIDS is diagnosed on the basis of a combination of characteristic clinical findings and continuously elevated IgD concentrations (>100 IU/mL) (Table 97-4). There are numerous caveats concerning IgD serum concentration, however: Values may be normal in young patients (especially patients younger than 3 years old),[59] persistently normal levels have been reported in a few patients with HIDS,[43] and patients with other familial autoinflammatory syndromes may also have elevated IgD concentrations, although these are usually only slightly elevated. More than 80% of HIDS patients combine a high concentration of IgD with high IgA levels.[59,60] During fever attacks, a brisk acute-phase response is observed including leukocytosis, high levels of SAA and CRP, and activation of the cytokine network.[53,61]

The diagnosis of HIDS can be confirmed by DNA analysis of the mevalonate kinase gene. The best approach is to start with screening for the two most prevalent mutations, V377I and I268T. If this screening is negative, but the clinical suspicion remains high, sequencing of the entire gene can be considered. A good alternative is the measurement of urinary mevalonic acid concentrations during an attack, which are slightly elevated. Gas chromatography–mass spectroscopy is necessary to detect this slight increase, however.[62] The measurement of mevalonate kinase enzyme activity is complicated and time-consuming and should be reserved for research purposes.

Treatment

There is no established treatment regimen for HIDS. Anakinra is effective in reducing disease severity in a number of case reports[55,56,63-65] and is currently the most promising therapy. A double-blind, placebo-controlled, crossover trial of the HMG-CoA reductase inhibitor simvastatin showed a beneficial effect of this drug, with a reduction in number of days of illness in five out of six patients[66]; however, in clinical practice the beneficial effect is not impressive. Favorable preliminary experience with the TNF antagonist etanercept has been reported.[55,67,68]

Some individual patients have been reported to have benefited from treatment with corticosteroids, colchicine, intravenous immunoglobulin, or cyclosporine, but these results have not been repeated in most patients.[40] Thalidomide did not have an effect on disease activity in a placebo-controlled trial.[69]

Outcome

The long-term outcome in HIDS is relatively benign in most patients. In some patients, the fever episodes occur less frequently and become less severe later in life, starting from late adolescence.[40] Joint destruction is rare, but abdominal adhesions are seen, resulting from repeated abdominal inflammation or (unnecessary) diagnostic laparotomy because of suspected acute abdomen.

Until more recently, no cases of amyloidosis had been seen in HIDS patients since its first description in 1984. Since 2004, four HIDS patients 19 to 27 years old have been reported who developed renal failure because of AA amyloidosis.[40,70-72] Regular screening for proteinuria also may be advisable in HIDS patients, especially patients with frequent and severe fever episodes.

TUMOR NECROSIS FACTOR RECEPTOR–ASSOCIATED PERIODIC SYNDROME

Epidemiology

TRAPS (MIM 142680) has an autosomal dominant inheritance pattern. It was originally described in a large family from Irish and Scottish descent as "familial Hibernian fever."[73] It is found primarily in patients from northwestern Europe but also has been described in families from Australia, Mexico, Puerto Rico, Portugal, and the Czech Republic.[74] Any ethnic group may be affected. Other abandoned nomenclature for this syndrome includes "autosomal dominant familial periodic fever"[75] and "familial perireticular amyloidosis."[76]

Etiology

Mutations are found in the gene for the type I TNF receptor (TNFRSF1A), which is located on the short arm of chromosome 12.[4] These are mainly single-nucleotide missense substitutions, located in exons 2, 3, and 4, which encode for the extracellular domain of TNFRSF1A. Many of these mutations disrupt one of the highly conserved cysteine residues involved in extracellular disulfide bonds of the 55-kD type I TNF receptor protein (Figure 97-9) (for details, see the online mutation database available at http://fmf.igh.cnrs.fr/infevers/).[77]

There are some general genotype-phenotype correlations, especially when mutations are grouped in cysteine and noncysteine mutations. Noncysteine mutations have, overall, a lower penetrance than cysteine mutations, and amyloidosis is seen far more often in association with cysteine mutations.[78] Two missense mutations in TNFRSF1A, P46L and R92Q, have a particularly low penetrance and

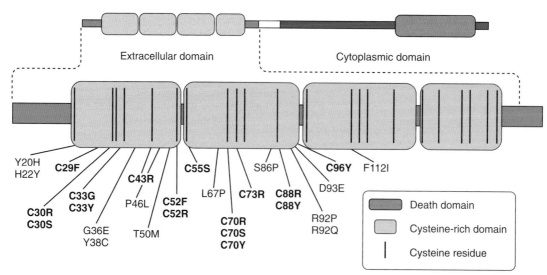

Extracellular domain   Cytoplasmic domain

Y20H
H22Y   **C29F**   **C55S**   S86P   **C96Y**   F112I

C43R   **C33G**   L67P   **C73R**   **C88R**   D93E
            C33Y   P46L   **C52F**   **C88Y**
C30R   **C52R**
C30S   G36E   T50M   **C70R**   R92P
        Y38C   **C70S**   R92Q
                C70Y

	Death domain
	Cysteine-rich domain
|	Cysteine residue

Figure 97-9   Schematic representation of the tumor necrosis factor (TNF) receptor type 1 protein (TNFRSF1A), depicting mutations found in TNF receptor–associated periodic syndrome up to this time (except for one intron mutation affecting a splice site). Mutations disrupting cysteine residues are in boldface type. For complete listing of all currently known mutations, see INFEVERS website: http://fmf.igh.cnrs.fr/infevers/.

are found in approximately 1% to 10% of control chromosomes.[78-80] R92Q has been observed in higher prevalence in a group of patients with arthritis. It is thought that the clinical manifestations of patients with an R92Q mutation depend on other so-far-unidentified modifying genes, environmental factors, or both.[77,78]

Pathogenesis

TNF is a pleiotropic molecule, which induces cytokine secretion, activation of leukocytes, fever, and cachexia. Activation of the TNF receptor by TNF causes cleavage and shedding of its extracellular part into the circulation, where it acts as an inhibitor of TNF. However, TRAPS-associated mutations in the TNF receptor lead not to an increase but rather to a loss of TNF-signaling function including less binding of TNF,[81,82] less cell surface expression,[82-85] and decreased TNF-induced NFκB-activation.[84,86,87] The mutated *TNFRSF1A* is retained intracellularly, pooled in the endoplasmic reticulum.[82,83,87,88] Mutant *TNFR1* cannot associate with the wild-type version but can form aggregates by self-interaction.[82,83] This cytoplasmic receptor aggregation results in ligand-independent signaling.[87,89] Mitochrondrial-derived reactive oxygen species appear to mediate this effect.[90] This new hypothesis also might offer an explanation for the observation that blocking IL-1β works better in some TRAPS patients than blocking TNF.[87,91]

An alternative hypothesis, the "shedding hypothesis," was postulated on the finding of reduced shedding, which leads to prolonged TNF signaling and uncontrolled inflammation. Not all TRAPS mutations cause decreased shedding, however, and although serum concentrations of the shedded soluble *TNFRSF1A* in TRAPS patients during periods without symptoms are often found to be significantly reduced compared with normal subjects, this is not always the case.[1] The hypothesis of reduced shedding, although attractive by its simplicity, is not supported as the sole cause of the fever attacks in TRAPS, and additional mechanisms seem to be at work.

Clinical Features

The clinical features can vary much more between individual TRAPS patients than is generally seen in FMF or HIDS.[74,77] The age of onset can vary, even within the same family, with a documented range of 2 weeks to 53 years old.[74,92] There is also a large variation in duration and frequency of the fever episodes in TRAPS. On average, attacks last 3 to 4 weeks and recur two to six times each year, but episodes also may be limited to a few days (see Figure 97-1). Although the index patient, through whom the diagnosis is made, often displays well-defined inflammatory attacks, affected family members may have less typical symptoms such as episodic mild arthritis.

During inflammatory attacks, a high, spiking fever can be accompanied by skin lesions, myalgia and arthralgia, abdominal distress, and ocular symptoms. The most common cutaneous manifestation is a centrifugal, migratory, erythematous patch, which may overlie a local area of myalgia (Figure 97-10),[93] but urticarial plaques also may be seen.

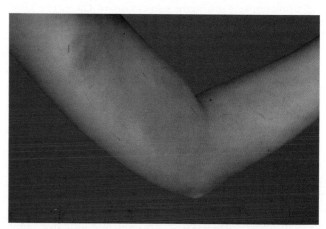

Figure 97-10   Migrating erythematous rash during a tumor necrosis factor receptor–associated periodic syndrome attack. *(Courtesy Dr. T. Fiselier, University Medical Center St. Radboud, Nijmegen, The Netherlands.)*

Myalgia is often located primarily in the muscles of the thighs, but it may migrate during the fever episode, affecting all of the limbs and the torso, face, and neck. Arthralgia primarily affects large joints including hips, knees, and ankles. Frank synovitis is rarer, and when it does occur it is nonerosive, asymmetric, and monoarticular.[74] Abdominal pain occurs in 92% of TRAPS patients during inflammatory attacks; other gastrointestinal symptoms often seen include vomiting and constipation. Ocular involvement is characteristic in TRAPS, and it may involve conjunctivitis, periorbital edema, or periorbital pain in one or both eyes. Severe uveitis and iritis have been described, and any TRAPS patient with ocular pain should be examined for these complications.[74,93] Other, less frequently observed symptoms during fever attacks in TRAPS are chest pain, breathlessness, pericarditis, and testicular and scrotal pain, which may be caused by inflammation of the tunica vaginalis. One case report described a patient who presented with psychosis without fever.[94] It has been suggested from observation in one of the first families with TRAPS that this disorder is associated with an increased incidence of indirect inguinal hernias,[95] but this has not been shown in other patients. Lymphadenopathy is rare in TRAPS.

Diagnosis and Diagnostic Tests

As in the other familial autoinflammatory syndromes, laboratory investigations during inflammatory attacks show a clear acute-phase response, and even in between fever attacks, such an inflammatory response may be measured. The IgD level may be elevated, but the value is almost always less than 100 IU/mL.[92,95]

Hull and colleagues[74] proposed a set of clinical diagnostic criteria for TRAPS (Table 97-5). These criteria are not validated by epidemiologic measures, but they may be used as a first step in evaluation of patients. TRAPS is ultimately a genetic diagnosis, defined by a missense mutation in the gene for *TNFRSF1A*. Clinical penetrance of TRAPS mutations is not 100%, however, even for cysteine mutations, and asymptomatic carriers are common. Also, the finding of an R92Q or P46L variant in this gene would pose a difficulty. Because they have many characteristics of a

Table 97-5 Diagnostic Indicators of Tumor Necrosis Factor Receptor–Associated Periodic Syndrome

1. Recurrent episodes of inflammatory symptoms spanning >6 mo duration (several symptoms generally occur simultaneously)
   a. Fever
   b. Abdominal pain
   c. Myalgia (migratory)
   d. Rash (erythematous macular rash occurs with myalgia)
   e. Conjunctivitis or periorbital edema
   f. Chest pain
   g. Arthralgia or monoarticular synovitis
2. Episodes last >5 days on average (although variable)
3. Responsive to glucocorticosteroids but not colchicine
4. Affects family members in autosomal dominant pattern (although may not always be present)
5. Any ethnicity may be affected

From Hull KM, Drewe E, Aksentijevich I, et al: The TNF receptor-associated periodic syndrome (TRAPS): emerging concepts of an autoinflammatory disorder, *Medicine (Baltimore)* 81:349–368, 2002.

polymorphism rather than a direct disease-causing mutation (see etiology), it is debatable whether such a finding should lead to a diagnosis of TRAPS.

Treatment

In mild cases of TRAPS, NSAIDs are often sufficient. NSAIDs and glucocorticoids in high doses (>20 mg/day of oral prednisone) alleviate the symptoms of fever and inflammation in most TRAPS patients, although they do not alter the frequency of attacks. They can be used beneficially at times of attack, and glucocorticoids usually can be tapered in the course of 1 or 2 weeks, as tolerated. There is no response to colchicine or immunosuppressive drugs such as azathioprine, cyclosporine, thalidomide, or cyclophosphamide.[74]

Anti-TNF and anti-IL-1 biologic therapy is much more effective in reducing symptoms. Use of etanercept, a fusion product of TNFRSF1B (the receptor that is not defective) has been partially successful.[74,78,96,97] A study with twice-weekly administration of etanercept (25 mg for adults or 0.4 mg/kg for children) in nine TRAPS patients with various mutations revealed an overall 66% response rate as determined by decreased number of attacks over a 6-month period.[74] Another study with the same dosage of etanercept for 24 weeks in seven TRAPS patients also showed a clear beneficial effect without serious adverse events.[96] A similar regimen of etanercept reversed the nephrotic syndrome in a patient with amyloidosis.[98]

Drewe and colleagues[99] described one patient whose symptoms were resistant to administration of etanercept, who responded favorably to use of oral sirolimus (4 to 6 mg daily). Infliximab, a monoclonal antibody against TNF, has been shown to be less effective than etanercept in TRAPS and seems to cause increased symptoms.[96,99,100] Intravenous infusion of a synthetic TNFRSF1A fusion protein was tried in one patient by Drewe and colleagues,[96] but this seemed to provoke a severe attack.

Blocking IL-1β with anakinra is even more effective than blocking TNF in several case reports and case series.[91,101-103]

Outcome

Reactive AA amyloidosis is the principal systemic complication of TRAPS. It occurs in about 15% to 25% of patients[78,104] and generally leads to renal impairment. Amyloidosis in a patient with TRAPS places other affected family members at high risk for this complication. It is principally associated with *TNFRSF1A* mutations affecting cysteine residues.[78] Because proteinuria is the initial manifestation of renal amyloidosis, it is advisable to screen urine samples from TRAPS patients regularly by dipstick examination, especially affected family members of a TRAPS patient with amyloidosis.

CRYOPYRIN-ASSOCIATED PERIODIC SYNDROME

Cryopyrin-associated periodic syndrome (CAPS) encompasses three clinical syndromes that all have been traced to mutations in one common gene: Muckle-Wells syndrome (MWS), familial cold autoinflammatory syndrome (FCAS), and chronic infantile neurologic cutaneous and articular syndrome (CINCA), also known as *neonatal-onset multisystemic inflammatory disease* (NOMID). After the recognition of the genetic defect, it became clear that there is considerable overlap among these three disorders.[105] FCAS, MWS, and CINCA/NOMID might represent a spectrum of disease, with FCAS the mildest and CINCA the most severe form. Given their common genotype, they are discussed under one heading here, but clinical features and outcomes are dealt with separately.

Epidemiology

All three syndromes are rare, autosomal dominantly inherited syndromes. Most articles on FCAS, first described in 1940, describe large families from Europe and North America with extensive pedigrees, but sporadic cases have been described. There seems to be a founder effect in American families of Northern European extraction.[106] MWS was first described in 1962 and has since been described in large families, although it does occur in isolated cases and small nuclear families. CINCA is rare, and, to date, some 70 cases and only a few families have been described.

Etiology

The first indications that MWS and FCAS are allelic stem from early linkage studies showing that FCAS and MWS were linked to the same region on the long arm of chromosome 1 (1q44).[107,108] In 2001, the gene for FCAS and MWS was identified. In a large-scale, positional cloning effort using three families with FCAS and one family with MWS, missense mutations in a new gene were found.[109] This gene, *CIAS1*, encodes for a protein denoted cryopyrin at discovery, but now by consensus known as NLRP3 (other names that have been used are NALP3 and PYPAF). Later studies showed that *CIAS1* mutations were also associated with CINCA.[110,111] Practically all mutations are missense mutations found in exon 3 of the *CIAS1* gene, which encodes for the NOD domain of NLRP3.[112] (Figure 97-11) (for

details, see the online mutation database available at http://fmf.igh.cnrs.fr/infevers/).

Pathogenesis

NLRP3 or cryopyrin was a previously unknown protein at the time of the discovery of the mutations involved in these syndromes. Since that time, it has become the focus of numerous studies, which have led to a new concept—the inflammasome.[113] NLRP3 is a member of the nucleotide-binding oligomerization domain–leucine-rich repeat (NOD-LRR) protein family.[114] It consists of a pyrin domain (PYD), a NOD (also known as NACHT domain), and a LRR domain. NLRP3 is mainly expressed in monocytes and neutrophils but is also found in human chondrocytes.[109,111,115]

NLRP3 is thought to be an intracellular sensor of pathogens or danger signals, regulating innate immunity. On stimulation with various ligands, which include bacterial RNA, imidazoquinolone compounds, gram-positive bacterial toxins nigericin and maitotoxin, adenosine triphosphate, and uric acid crystals, NLRP3 forms interactions with adapter proteins ASC and cardinal, which results in a multiprotein complex termed the *NLRP3 inflammasome*. The NLRP3 inflammasome activates caspase-1, which subsequently cleaves pro-IL-1β to the active IL-1β.[116,117]

There is conflicting evidence for a role of NLRP3 in regulation of transcription factor NFκB.[1] Possibly, the ultimate effect on NFκB is determined by interaction of multiple proteins. Four more recent publications by independent groups that each developed an NLRP3-deficient mouse showed no effect, however, on NFκB activation in these mice, whereas they did show a clear deficiency in caspase-1–mediated IL-1β activation.[1]

Monocytes from patients with mutations in the NOD of NLRP3 show increased activation of caspase-1 and subsequently increased release of IL-1β.[117,118] The key role of IL-1β in CAPS is confirmed by the success of treatment with the IL-1 blocker anakinra in all three clinical syndromes (see treatment section).

The exact effect of the NLRP3 mutations is still unclear. An attractive hypothesis involves a possible autoinhibitory loop of NLRP3.[118] Mutations in the NOD could interfere

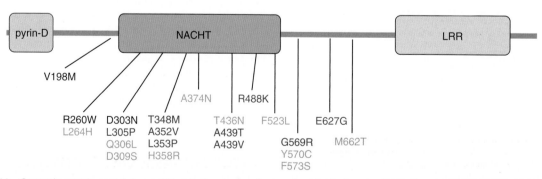

Figure 97-11 Cryopyrin protein, containing an N-terminal pyrin domain, a nucleotide binding site (NACHT), and a leucine-rich repeat (LRR) domain. Indicated are missense mutations identified in patients with familial cold autoinflammatory syndrome *(red)*, Muckle-Wells syndrome *(green)*, or chronic infantile neurologic cutaneous and articular syndrome *(blue)*, and mutations found in common in two or all of these clinical syndromes *(black)*. For complete listing of all currently known mutations, see INFEVERS website: http://fmf.igh.cnrs.fr/infevers/.

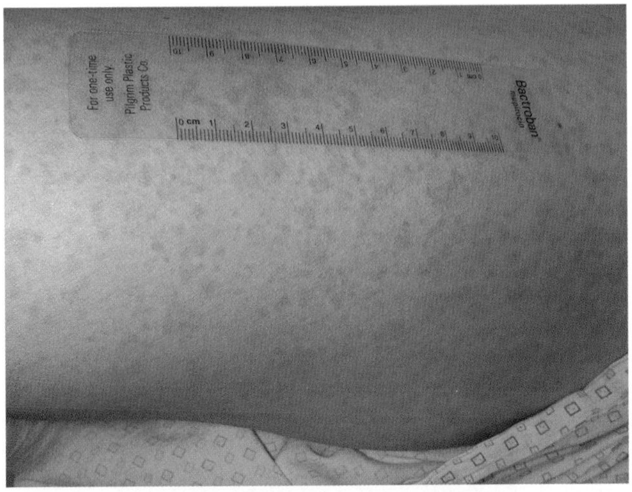

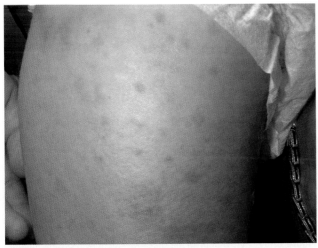

Figure 97-12 Fine, confluent, erythematous macules on the upper leg of a patient with familial cold autoinflammatory syndrome. *(Courtesy Dr. Johnstone, Medical College of Georgia, Augusta, Ga.)*

with this autoinhibitory mechanism of NLRP3, leading to undue and excessive activation of caspase-1 and IL-1β.[1]

Clinical Features and Outcome

Familial Cold Autoinflammatory Syndrome

FCAS (MIM 120100) is characterized by episodes of rash, fever, and arthralgia after generalized exposure to cold (see Figure 97-1). The disease occurs in large families as an autosomal dominant inherited disorder with an almost complete penetrance.[106] The rash usually starts on the exposed extremities and, in most episodes, extends to the remainder of the body. It consists of erythematous macules and plaques (Figures 97-12 and 97-13), urticarial lesions, and sometimes petechiae[119] and can cause a burning or itchy sensation. In one case report, FCAS was associated with Raynaud's disease.[120] In some cases, localized edematous swelling of extremities is reported. Arthralgia, present in 93% of cases, most often affects the hands, knees, and ankles but can also involve feet, wrists, and elbows.[121] Frank arthritis is not

seen. Most patients (84%) also report conjunctivitis during a fever episode. Other symptoms include myalgia, profuse sweating, drowsiness, headache, extreme thirst, and nausea.

A typical feature of FCAS is the requirement of cold exposure to trigger the symptoms. The delay between cold and onset of symptoms varies from 10 minutes to 8 hours.[121] When Hoffman and colleagues[122] provoked an inflammatory attack in FCAS patients by generalized cold exposure in a cold room, they saw that patients developed rash, fever, and arthralgia within 1 to 4 hours. The occurrence of these symptoms could be blocked by pretreatment with the IL-1β inhibitor anakinra.[122]

The subsequent fever attack varies in length, depending on the degree of cold exposure; generally it lasts a few hours to a maximum of 3 days. These episodes start at an early age, with 95% of patients having had their first fever episode in the first year of life—60% even within the first days of life. The symptoms tend to become less severe with advancing age.[119] Type AA amyloidosis complicated by renal insufficiency has been described in at least three FCAS families.[121]

Muckle-Wells Syndrome

MWS (MIM 191900) is a rare autosomal dominant inflammatory disorder with incomplete penetrance. Patients have recurrent episodes of fever, abdominal pain, myalgia, urticarial rash (Figures 97-14 and 97-15), and conjunctivitis, frequently accompanied by arthralgia, arthritis with limb pain, or both. Attacks start in adolescence and can be provoked by hunger, fatigue, and sometimes exposure to cold.[123] The inflammatory episodes generally last 24 to 48 hours (see Figure 97-1) and start with ill-defined malaise and transient chills and rigor, followed by aching or lancinating pains in the distal limbs and larger joints. Arthralgia is a common feature of the attacks, but synovitis of the large joints is less common.[124] The rash consists of usually aching and sometimes pruritic erythematous papules 1 to 7 cm in diameter. In a few cases, genital and buccal aphthous ulcers have been seen.[125] Ocular symptoms include uveitis and conjunctivitis. Symptoms typically start in adolescence, although they have been reported at an earlier age. Late-onset development of perceptive deafness is common in MWS. Bone

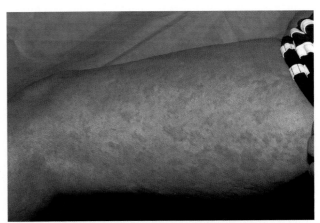

Figure 97-13 Detail of upper leg with fine, confluent, erythematous macules in familial cold autoinflammatory syndrome. *(Courtesy Dr. Johnstone, Medical College of Georgia, Augusta, Ga.)*

Figure 97-14 Urticarial skin rash in a patient with Muckle-Wells syndrome. *(Courtesy Dr. D. L. Kastner, National Institutes of Health, Bethesda, Md.)*

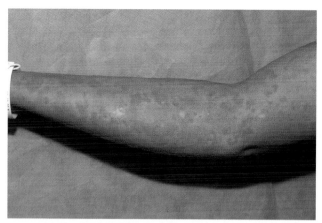

Figure 97-15 Urticarial skin rash on the arm of a patient with Muckle-Wells syndrome. *(Courtesy Dr. D. L. Kastner, National Institutes of Health, Bethesda, Md.)*

involvement such as clubbing of nails and pes cavus can be seen as well. Most often, patients have a positive family history for the disease, which is indicative of autosomal dominant inheritance, but isolated cases have been reported. The most feared complication of the inflammatory attacks is type AA amyloidosis, which affects the kidneys first, leading to proteinuria and subsequent rapid progression to renal failure.

Chronic Infantile Neurologic Cutaneous and Articular Syndrome

CINCA or NOMID (MIM 607115) is a rare congenital disorder defined by the presence of the triad of (1) neonatal-onset skin lesions, (2) chronic aseptic meningitis, and (3) recurrent fever along with joint symptoms.[126] The key clinical feature of CINCA is a skin rash accompanied by peculiar joint manifestations and central nervous system involvement. The symptoms in CINCA begin right after birth or in the first months of life with a generalized skin rash. The disease follows an unpredictable course with persistent non-pruritic and migratory rash with fever, hepatosplenomegaly, and lymphadenopathy. Central nervous system involvement is not obvious from the outset, although some patients present with seizures, spasticity, or transient episodes of hemiplegia. In most patients, there are signs of chronic persistent aseptic meningitis.[127] Cerebrospinal fluid analysis may show mild pleocytosis, and there may be increased intracranial pressure. Brain imaging shows mild ventricular dilation, prominent sulci, central atrophy, and, in long-standing cases, calcifications of fauces and dura.

In older children, headache is often a prominent feature as a sign of chronic meningitis. Mental retardation is present in almost all cases. Progressive sensorineural impairment leading to high-frequency hearing loss can be seen in a few cases. Ocular manifestations are prominent, with optic disc changes such as optic disc edema, pseudopapilledema, and optic atrophy, as well as anterior segment manifestations such as chronic anterior uveitis.[128] These symptoms may lead to visual impairment. Hoarseness, especially in older children, is typical. Joint and bone symptoms are a prominent feature of CINCA, and these manifest as bone inflammation, which gives rise to major arthropathies secondary

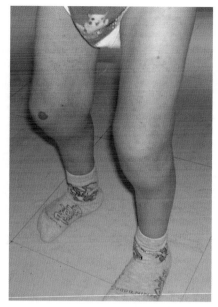

Figure 97-16 Severe deformational arthropathy of the knees in a patient with chronic infantile neurologic cutaneous and articular syndrome. *(Courtesy Dr. A. M. Prieur, Hôpital Necker-Enfants Malades, Paris.)*

to epiphyseal and metaphyseal disorganization. Growth cartilage alterations such as enlarged epiphyses and patellar overgrowth can be an impressive feature of the disease (Figures 97-16 and 97-17). Erosive changes occur, especially in the phalanges of hands and feet. There are typical dysmorphic features such as frontal bossing and a saddle nose. These common physical features are the reason CINCA patients give the impression that totally unrelated patients are siblings. The prognosis of these patients is grave; 20% die in childhood because of infections, vasculitis, and amyloidosis.[126]

Diagnosis and Diagnostic Tests

Diagnosis starts with a thorough patient and family history (see Table 97-1). Hoffman and colleagues[121] suggested a set

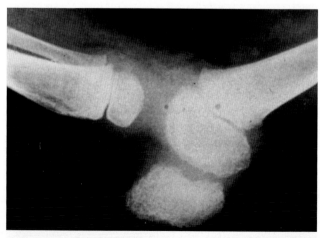

Figure 97-17 Radiograph of the knee in a patient with chronic infantile neurologic cutaneous and articular syndrome showing greatly enlarged epiphyses and patella with punctate increased density. *(Courtesy Dr. A. M. Prieur, Hôpital Necker-Enfants Malades, Paris.)*

Table 97-6 *Diagnostic Criteria for Familial Cold Autoinflammatory Syndrome*

1. Recurrent intermittent episodes of fever and rash that primarily follow generalized cold exposures
2. Autosomal dominant pattern of disease inheritance
3. Age of onset < 6 mo
4. Duration of most attacks <24 hr
5. Presence of conjunctivitis associated with attacks
6. Absence of deafness, periorbital edema, lymphadenopathy, and serositis

From Hoffman HM, Wanderer AA, Broide DH: Familial cold autoinflammatory syndrome: phenotype and genotype of an autosomal dominant periodic fever, *J Allergy Clin Immunol* 108:615–620, 2001.

of diagnostic criteria for FCAS after studying six large families with this syndrome (Table 97-6), but these have not been validated in an independent cohort. Laboratory examination during a fever episode in CAPS shows an acute-phase response with polymorphonuclear leukocytosis and increased erythrocyte sedimentation rate, but this does not differentiate among the periodic fever disorders. Symptoms such as an urticarial rash after cold exposure highly favor a diagnosis of FCAS. The ice cube test (i.e., holding an ice cube to a patch of skin to provoke urticaria), which is diagnostic in acquired cold urticaria, is negative in FCAS. Typical facial features such as frontal bossing and a long pediatric history including chronic aseptic meningitis point to CINCA/NOMID.

Genetic testing of the *CIAS1* gene can subsequently help to establish the genetic diagnosis. Usually, exon 3 of this gene is screened for mutations. There seems to be genetic heterogeneity in CINCA because not all patients have *CIAS1* mutations.

Treatment

Since the advent of IL-1 inhibition, it is the treatment of choice for patients with severe forms of cryopyrin-associated periodic syndrome.[129] Previously, high-dose oral corticosteroids were often used and found to be beneficial in some patients. NSAIDs, disease-modifying antirheumatic drugs, and cytotoxic drugs generally do not help.

IL-1 inhibition by anakinra was shown to be beneficial for patients with any of the cryopyrin-associated periodic syndromes in a number of case reports and case series.[129,130] The largest study was by Goldbach-Mansky and colleagues,[130] who studied 18 patients with CINCA/NOMID, 12 of whom had mutations in the cryopyrin gene. All of them had a rapid and sustained response to daily subcutaneous injection of anakinra (1 to 2 mg/kg body weight), with decrease of symptoms, acute-phase response, and leptomeningeal lesions as seen on MRI. Mirault and colleagues[131] described improvement of sensorineural deafness in a patient with MWS on treatment with anakinra.

Lachmann and colleagues published the results of a trial of the new IL-1β antibody canakinumab in patients with CAPS,[132] demonstrating the efficacy of an injection of 150 mg canakinumab once every 2 months. The first reports of the new IL-1 inhibitor IL-1-trap are also promising.[129]

BLAU SYNDROME/EARLY-ONSET SARCOIDOSIS

Epidemiology

Blau syndrome,[133] also known as *familial granulomatous arthritis* (OMIM 186580), and early-onset sarcoidosis (OMIM 609464) (BS/EOS) are now recognized as the same disorder.[134,135] "Pediatric granulomatous arthritis" has been suggested as a new name to describe this syndrome,[136] although this might, erroneously, give the impression that the disease occurs only in children. Little is known about its epidemiology, although it is thought to occur worldwide.[134]

Etiology

The inheritance pattern of BS/EOS is autosomal dominant. In many cases, a de novo mutation is found, which explains the relatively high incidence of sporadic cases. These sporadic cases were often classified as early-onset sarcoidosis precisely because of the absence of affected relatives, but Blau syndrome and early-onset sarcoidosis have now been shown to be caused by mutations in the nucleotide-binding oligomerization domain 2/caspase recruitment domain 15 gene (*NOD2/CARD15*).[135,137,138] Mutations are mostly located in exon 4 of *NOD2/CARD15*. The predominant mutations are two missense mutations at position 334 (R334Q and R334W)[136] (for details, see the online mutation database available at http://fmf.igh.cnrs.fr/infevers/).

Pathogenesis

The NOD2/CARD15 protein is considered to be an intracellular sensor for pathogenic components, analogous to the Toll-like receptors. Activation of NOD2/CARD15 results in a wide array of downstream effects that are still not well understood, including activation of NFκB and mitogen-activated protein kinase pathways, turning on an innate immune response of diverse cytokines (e.g., IL-1β) and defensins.[139]

Seven of the nine different mutations of *NOD2/CARD15* linked to BS/EOS are located in the NOD domain of the protein, similar to the mutations in cryopyrin (NLRP3) in the cryopyrin-associated syndromes. The two most common mutations affect a codon at a homologous position in the NOD domain to the location of the cryopyrin R260W mutation.[140] This suggests a similar pathophysiologic effect on the function of the protein.

Polymorphisms in another part of this same *NOD2/CARD15* gene on chromosome 16 are associated with increased susceptibility to Crohn's disease[141]; the risk of developing Crohn's disease is increased 40-fold in individuals homozygous for these polymorphisms. Whether these polymorphisms result in a gain or loss of function of this protein is debated. There are some shared features between the two diseases: Both are characterized by granulomatous inflammation, and although bowel inflammation is not seen in Blau syndrome, Crohn's disease can manifest with uveitis, arthritis, and skin rash.

Clinical Features and Outcome

The clinical phenotype of BS/EOS consists of recurrent granulomatous inflammations. The three typical sites affected are joints, eyes, and skin. The granulomatous arthritis is most often polyarticular, with a synovitis or tenosynovitis.[134] The uveitis associated with this disorder tends to follow a chronic, persistent course. It can be an acute anterior uveitis, but it often extends to a panuveitis.[136] Cataracts, secondary glaucoma, and significant visual impairment can result. Involvement of the skin results in a papular, erythematous skin rash with associated dermal granulomas, usually generalized and intermittent, on trunk and extremities.[142] Other symptoms include campylodactyly (contracture of multiple interphalangeal joints), cranial neuropathies, fever, and arteritis.[137] In some severely affected patients, granulomatous inflammation can disseminate at an advanced stage into a systemic disease, with granulomas in liver, lung, and kidney.[136] Onset is generally before age 5. In familial cases, genetic anticipation is often observed (i.e., the course of disease tends to be more severe in later generations). The major long-term complications are joint deformity and visual impairment.[134]

Diagnosis

The most important aspect of diagnosis is the histologic evidence of granulomas at the site of inflammation. This evidence can be obtained by biopsy of any involved site, of which skin is least invasive. One study showed that skin biopsy was diagnostic in all cases with the typical skin rash, whereas synovial biopsy was not positive in all patients, perhaps owing to sampling error.[136] Genetic testing is available for NOD2/CARD15 mutations, but in some series, not all patients with a typical clinical phenotype carried a mutation in this gene.[137]

Treatment

There are no controlled studies of management of BS/EOS patients. There tends to be a poor response to NSAIDs. A good response to the TNF inhibitor infliximab was reported in case reports,[143,144] one of which also noted that etanercept did not have the same effect. IL-1 blockade by anakinra was also reported as beneficial in a case description,[145] although in two other cases anakinra was not effective.[146] Thalidomide was effective in two children in Japan.[147] The panuveitis is usually managed by topical, subconjunctival, or systemic corticosteroids.[134]

PYOGENIC STERILE ARTHRITIS, PYODERMA GANGRENOSUM, AND ACNE SYNDROME

Epidemiology

Pyogenic sterile arthritis, pyoderma gangrenosum, and acne (PAPA) syndrome (MIM 604416) is an autosomal dominant disorder first described by Lindor and colleagues.[148] Fewer than 20 families have been reported.

Etiology/Pathogenesis

Wise and colleagues[149] identified mutations in the CD2-binding protein 1 (CD2BP1) gene as the cause of PAPA syndrome. CD2BP1, also known as *proline-serine-threonine phosphatase interacting protein 1* (PSTPIP1), is highly expressed in neutrophils[112] (see the online mutation database available at http://fmf.igh.cnrs.fr/infevers/).

PSTPIP1 can form interactions with pyrin, the protein mutated in FMF.[150] The mutations in PAPA syndrome result in hyperphosphorylation of PSTPIP1,[150-152] which increases the strength of the interaction between PSTPIP1 and pyrin. This increased interaction of PSTPIP1 and pyrin leads to increased IL-1β production. This activity correlated with a higher IL-1β production in response to lipopolysaccharide stimulation of peripheral blood leukocytes from a PAPA patient ex vivo compared with a healthy control.[150] It places PAPA syndrome in the same pathogenic pathway as FMF. Other studies report an increased production of TNF.[153,154] Dysregulated apoptosis may also be involved.[155]

Clinical Features and Outcome

The episodic inflammation in this syndrome includes, as the name aptly indicates, symptoms of pyogenic sterile arthritis, pyoderma gangrenosum, and severe cystic acne. Lesions generally occur at the site of mild physical trauma, but sometimes no obvious trigger can be discerned.[148] The inflammation can be severe and eventually may lead to destruction of joints, muscle, and skin. Fever is not prominent in this syndrome. Onset is usually from age 1 to 16 years.[148,156] The acne generally starts early in puberty and persists in adulthood.

Diagnosis

No specific diagnostic test exists. Diagnosis is based on a finding of the typical constellation of symptoms and a positive family history. A specialized DNA diagnostics department would be able to perform the genetic test for PAPA syndrome. At this time, it is unknown whether this genetic test would detect all patients or whether other genes could be involved.

Treatment

Diverse anecdotal evidence is only available on treatment options in PAPA syndrome. High-dose steroids generally have a positive effect on the pyoderma gangrenosum but may be associated with increased acne.[148] Pyogenic arthritis is often responsive to glucocorticoids intra-articularly and orally.[156] Varying results have been reported with anticytokine treatment. The TNF inhibitor etanercept was reported to be beneficial,[153,157] as was the IL-1 inhibitor anakinra.[150,158,159] Stichweh and colleagues[160] reported on a patient with severe pyoderma gangrenosum, however, who did not respond to either etanercept or anakinra, but in whom the other TNF inhibitor infliximab did prove successful.

DEFICIENCY OF THE IL-1 RECEPTOR ANTAGONIST

Deficiency of the IL-1 receptor antagonist (DIRA) is the latest discovery of a monogenetic disorder in the group of autoinflammatory diseases.[161,162] It was found in nine patients from six families, one from Newfoundland, Canada, three from the Netherlands, one from Puerto Rico, and one consanguineous family from Lebanon.

All patients were homozygous for mutations affecting the gene encoding the IL-1 receptor antagonist (IL-1ra), designated *IL1RN*.[161] These mutations resulted in an absence of secretion of IL-1ra. IL-1ra is an endogenous inhibitor of the inflammatory cytokines IL-1α and IL-1β. The patients showed signs of unopposed IL-1 signaling leading to overproduction of other inflammatory cytokines and chemokines.

The clinical phenotype is present at birth or in the first month of life. Features include primarily cutaneous pustulosis and sterile pustulous osteomyelitis. Patients do not present with fever. Two children died of multiorgan failure secondary to severe inflammatory response syndrome (SIRS) at the ages of 2 months and 21 months, and a third child died at 9.5 years of complications of pulmonary hemosiderosis with progressive intestinal fibrosis.

The diagnosis is made by a combination of the clinical features and an impressive response to anakinra. Anakinra is a synthetic version of IL-1ra and thus supplements the missing protein in DIRA. Treatment with anakinra suppresses all disease symptoms, although in one patient inflammatory markers remained elevated.

CONCLUSION

The familial autoinflammatory syndromes are characterized by recurrent episodes of fever and inflammation. This group of disorders should be considered in a patient with a history of years of such inflammatory attacks with symptom-free intervals in between (except for CINCA/NOMID, in which some symptoms and morphologic features persist). Dysregulation of the IL-1β pathway is central to many familial autoinflammatory syndromes, especially CAPS, FMF, and DIRA. Increasing availability of IL-1 inhibitors has revolutionized treatment options in many of these diseases.

The discovery of the causative genes has had an enormous impact in the field of periodic fevers. This discovery has been made possible because of the accurate phenotypic characterization of patients with periodic fever. Careful analysis and proper clustering of these patients is indispensable to allow the elucidation of the genetic background and the evaluation of possible treatment options (Table 97-7). Central periodic fever registries have afforded the opportunity to appreciate previously unrecognized symptoms, to give insight into the long-term prognosis, and to allow better evaluation of drug regimens. Despite these efforts at classification, however, many patients with periodic fever do not fall in one of the previously mentioned disease categories. It is to be expected that in the future other periodic fever syndromes and corresponding genes will be discovered.

Table 97-7 Summary of Treatment Options

Disorder	Treatment Options
FMF	Colchicine In refractory cases or intolerance of colchicine: intravenous colchicine; IL-1 inhibition (anakinra)
HIDS	Simvastatin; etanercept; IL-1 inhibition (anakinra)
TRAPS	NSAIDs; etanercept; IL-1 inhibition (anakinra)
CAPS	IL-1 inhibition (anakinra, canakinumab, IL-1 trap)
BS/EOS	Corticosteroids; infliximab?
PAPA	High-dose steroids; IL-1 inhibition (anakinra); etanercept; infliximab

BS/EOS, Blau syndrome/early-onset sarcoidosis; CAPS, cryopyrin-associated periodic syndrome; FMF, familial Mediterranean fever; HIDS, hyper-IgD syndrome; IL-1, interleukin-1; NSAIDs, nonsteroidal anti-inflammatory drugs; PAPA, pyogenic sterile arthritis, pyoderma gangrenosum, and acne; TRAPS, tumor necrosis factor receptor–associated periodic syndrome.

Selected References

1. Masters SL, Simon A, Aksentijevich I, Kastner DL: Horror autoinflammaticus: the molecular pathophysiology of autoinflammatory disease (*), *Annu Rev Immunol* 27:621–668, 2009.
4. McDermott MF, Aksentijevich I, Galon J, et al: Germline mutations in the extracellular domains of the 55 kDa TNF receptor, TNFR1, define a family of dominantly inherited autoinflammatory syndromes, *Cell* 97:133–144, 1999.
5. Kastner DL, Aksentijevich I, Goldbach-Mansky R: Autoinflammatory disease reloaded: a clinical perspective, *Cell* 140:784–790, 2010.
9. A candidate gene for familial Mediterranean fever. The French FMF Consortium, *Nat Genet* 17:25–31, 1997.
10. Consortium TIF: Ancient missense mutations in a new member of the RoRet gene family are likely to cause familial Mediterranean fever, *Cell* 90:797–807, 1997.
13. Diaz A, Hu C, Kastner DL, et al: Lipopolysaccharide-induced expression of multiple alternatively spliced MEFV transcripts in human synovial fibroblasts: a prominent splice isoform lacks the C-terminal domain that is highly mutated in familial Mediterranean fever, *Arthritis Rheum* 50:3679–3689, 2004.
14. Centola M, Wood G, Frucht DM, et al: The gene for familial Mediterranean fever, MEFV, is expressed in early leukocyte development and is regulated in response to inflammatory mediators, *Blood* 95:3223–3231, 2000.
15. Simon A, van der Meer JW: Pathogenesis of familial periodic fever syndromes or hereditary autoinflammatory syndromes, *Am J Physiol Regul Integr Comp Physiol* 292:R86–R98, 2007.
16. Drenth JP, van der Meer JW: The inflammasome—a linebacker of innate defense, *N Engl J Med* 355:730–732, 2006.
17. Chae JJ, Komarow HD, Cheng J, et al: Targeted disruption of pyrin, the FMF protein, causes heightened sensitivity to endotoxin and a defect in macrophage apoptosis, *Mol Cell* 11:591–604, 2003.
18. Chae JJ, Wood G, Masters SL, et al: The B30.2 domain of pyrin, the familial Mediterranean fever protein, interacts directly with caspase-1 to modulate IL-1beta production, *Proc Natl Acad Sci U S A* 103:9982–9987, 2006.
19. Yu JW, Wu J, Zhang Z, et al: Cryopyrin and pyrin activate caspase-1, but not NF-kappaB, via ASC oligomerization, *Cell Death Differ* 13:236–249, 2006.
20. Ben Chetrit E, Levy M: Familial Mediterranean fever, *Lancet* 351:659–664, 1998.
21. Simon A, van der Meer JW, Drenth JP: Familial Mediterranean fever—a not so unusual cause of abdominal pain, *Best Pract Res Clin Gastroenterol* 19:199–213, 2005.
25. Livneh A, Langevitz P, Zemer D, et al: Criteria for the diagnosis of familial Mediterranean fever, *Arthritis Rheum* 40:1879–1885, 1997.
29. Ben Chetrit E, Levy M: Colchicine: 1998 update, *Semin Arthritis Rheum* 28:48–59, 1998.
30. Haimov-Kochman R, Ben Chetrit E: The effect of colchicine treatment on sperm production and function: a review, *Hum Reprod* 13:360–362, 1998.

31. Ehrenfeld M, Brzezinski A, Levy M, Eliakim M: Fertility and obstetric history in patients with familial Mediterranean fever on long-term colchicine therapy, *Br J Obstet Gynaecol* 94:1186–1191, 1987.

32. Rabinovitch O, Zemer D, Kukia E, et al: Colchicine treatment in conception and pregnancy: two hundred thirty-one pregnancies in patients with familial Mediterranean fever, *Am J Reprod Immunol* 28:245–246, 1992.

34. Ozen S, Bilginer Y, Ayaz NA, Calguneri M: Anti-interleukin 1 treatment for patients with familial Mediterranean fever resistant to colchicine, *J Rheumatol* 38:516–518, 2011.

35. Alpay N, Sumnu A, Caliskan Y, et al: Efficacy of anakinra treatment in a patient with colchicine-resistant familial Mediterranean fever, *Rheumatol Int* 2010 Apr 13 [Epub ahead of print].

36. Moser C, Pohl G, Haslinger I, et al: Successful treatment of familial Mediterranean fever with Anakinra and outcome after renal transplantation, *Nephrol Dial Transplant* 24:676–678, 2009.

37. Roldan R, Ruiz AM, Miranda MD, Collantes E: Anakinra: new therapeutic approach in children with familial Mediterranean fever resistant to colchicine, *Joint Bone Spine* 75:504–505, 2008.

38. Calligaris L, Marchetti F, Tommasini A, Ventura A: The efficacy of anakinra in an adolescent with colchicine-resistant familial Mediterranean fever, *Eur J Pediatr* 167:695–696, 2008.

40. van der Hilst JC, Bodar EJ, Barron KS, et al: Long-term follow-up, clinical features, and quality of life in a series of 103 patients with hyperimmunoglobulinemia D syndrome, *Medicine (Baltimore)* 87:301–310, 2008.

43. Houten SM, Kuis W, Duran M, et al: Mutations in MVK, encoding mevalonate kinase, cause hyperimmunoglobulinaemia D and periodic fever syndrome, *Nat Genet* 22:175–177, 1999.

44. Drenth JPH, Cuisset L, Grateau G, et al: Mutations in the gene encoding mevalonate kinase cause hyper-IgD and periodic fever syndrome. International Hyper-IgD Study Group, *Nat Genet* 22:178–181, 1999.

49. Hoffmann GF, Charpentier C, Mayatepek E, et al: Clinical and biochemical phenotype in 11 patients with mevalonic aciduria, *Pediatrics* 91:915–921, 1993.

50. Simon A, Kremer HP, Wevers RA, et al: Mevalonate kinase deficiency: evidence for a phenotypic continuum, *Neurology* 62:994–997, 2004.

53. Drenth JP, van Deuren M, van der Ven-Jongekrijg J, et al: Cytokine activation during attacks of the hyperimmunoglobulinemia D and periodic fever syndrome, *Blood* 85:3586–3593, 1995.

54. Drenth JP, Goertz J, Daha MR, van der Meer JW: Immunoglobulin D enhances the release of tumor necrosis factor-alpha, and interleukin-1 beta as well as interleukin-1 receptor antagonist from human mononuclear cells, *Immunology* 88:355–362, 1996.

55. Bodar EJ, van der Hilst JC, Drenth JP, et al: Effect of etanercept and anakinra on inflammatory attacks in the hyper-IgD syndrome: introducing a vaccination provocation model, *Neth J Med* 63:260–264, 2005.

56. Korppi M, Van Gijn ME, Antila K: Hyperimmunoglobulinemia D and periodic fever syndrome in children. Review on therapy with biological drugs and case report, *Acta Paediatr* 100:21–25, 2011.

57. Kuijk LM, Beekman JM, Koster J, et al: HMG-CoA reductase inhibition induces IL-1beta release through Rac1/PI3K/PKB-dependent caspase-1 activation, *Blood* 112:3563–3573, 2008.

58. Bodar EJ, van der Hilst JC, van Heerde W, et al: Defective apoptosis of peripheral-blood lymphocytes in hyper-IgD and periodic fever syndrome, *Blood* 109:2416–2418, 2007.

61. Simon A, Bijzet J, Voorbij HA, et al: Effect of inflammatory attacks in the classical type hyper-IgD syndrome on immunoglobulin D, cholesterol and parameters of the acute phase response, *J Intern Med* 256:247–253, 2004.

63. Cailliez M, Garaix F, Rousset-Rouviere C, et al: Anakinra is safe and effective in controlling hyperimmunoglobulinaemia D syndrome-associated febrile crisis, *J Inherit Metab Dis* 29:763, 2006.

64. Rigante D, Ansuini V, Bertoni B, et al: Treatment with anakinra in the hyperimmunoglobulinemia D/periodic fever syndrome, *Rheumatol Int* 27:97–100, 2006.

65. Nevyjel M, Pontillo A, Calligaris L, et al: Diagnostics and therapeutic insights in a severe case of mevalonate kinase deficiency, *Pediatrics* 119:e523–527, 2007.

66. Simon A, Drewe E, van der Meer JW, et al: Simvastatin treatment for inflammatory attacks of the hyperimmunoglobulinemia D and periodic fever syndrome, *Clin Pharmacol Ther* 75:476–483, 2004.

67. Takada K, Aksentijevich I, Mahadevan V, et al: Favorable preliminary experience with etanercept in two patients with the hyperimmunoglobulinemia D and periodic fever syndrome, *Arthritis Rheum* 48:2645–2651, 2003.

68. Topaloglu R, Ayaz NA, Waterham HR, et al: Hyperimmunoglobulinemia D and periodic fever syndrome; treatment with etanercept and follow-up, *Clin Rheumatol* 27:1317–1320, 2008.

69. Drenth JP, Vonk AG, Simon A, et al: Limited efficacy of thalidomide in the treatment of febrile attacks of the hyper-IgD and periodic fever syndrome: a randomized, double-blind, placebo-controlled trial, *J Pharmacol Exp Ther* 298:1221–1226, 2001.

70. Obici L, Manno C, Muda AO, et al: First report of systemic reactive (AA) amyloidosis in a patient with the hyperimmunoglobulinemia D with periodic fever syndrome, *Arthritis Rheum* 50:2966–2969, 2004.

71. Lachmann HJ, Goodman HJ, Andrews PA, et al: AA amyloidosis complicating hyperimmunoglobulinemia D with periodic fever syndrome: a report of two cases, *Arthritis Rheum* 54:2010–2014, 2006.

72. Siewert R, Ferber J, Horstmann RD, et al: Hereditary periodic fever with systemic amyloidosis: is hyper-IgD syndrome really a benign disease? *Am J Kidney Dis* 48:e41–45, 2006.

74. Hull KM, Drewe E, Aksentijevich I, et al: The TNF receptor-associated periodic syndrome (TRAPS): emerging concepts of an autoinflammatory disorder, *Medicine (Baltimore)* 81:349–368, 2002.

77. Kimberley FC, Lobito AA, Siegel RM, Screaton GR: Falling into TRAPS–receptor misfolding in the TNF receptor 1-associated periodic fever syndrome, *Arthritis Res Ther* 9:217, 2007.

82. Todd I, Radford PM, Draper-Morgan KA, et al: Mutant forms of tumour necrosis factor receptor I that occur in TNF-receptor-associated periodic syndrome retain signalling functions but show abnormal behaviour, *Immunology* 113:65–79, 2004.

83. Lobito AA, Kimberley FC, Muppidi JR, et al: Abnormal disulfide-linked oligomerization results in ER retention and altered signaling by TNFR1 mutants in TNFR1-associated periodic fever syndrome (TRAPS), *Blood* 108:1320–1327, 2006.

84. Siebert S, Amos N, Fielding CA, et al: Reduced tumor necrosis factor signaling in primary human fibroblasts containing a tumor necrosis factor receptor superfamily 1A mutant, *Arthritis Rheum* 52:1287–1292, 2005.

85. Huggins ML, Radford PM, McIntosh RS, et al: Shedding of mutant tumor necrosis factor receptor superfamily 1A associated with tumor necrosis factor receptor-associated periodic syndrome: differences between cell types, *Arthritis Rheum* 50:2651–2659, 2004.

86. Siebert S, Fielding CA, Williams BD, Brennan P: Mutation of the extracellular domain of tumour necrosis factor receptor 1 causes reduced NF-kappaB activation due to decreased surface expression, *FEBS Lett* 579:5193–5198, 2005.

87. Simon A, Park H, Maddipati R, et al: Concerted action of wild-type and mutant TNF receptors enhances inflammation in TNF receptor 1-associated periodic fever syndrome, *Proc Natl Acad Sci U S A* 107:9801–9806, 2010.

90. Bulua AC, Simon A, Maddipati R, et al: Mitochondrial reactive oxygen species promote production of proinflammatory cytokines and are elevated in TNFR1-associated periodic syndrome (TRAPS), *J Exp Med* 208:519–533, 2011.

91. Simon A, Bodar EJ, van der Hilst JC, et al: Beneficial response to interleukin 1 receptor antagonist in traps, *Am J Med* 117:208–210, 2004.

101. Gattorno M, Pelagatti MA, Meini A, et al: Persistent efficacy of anakinra in patients with tumor necrosis factor receptor-associated periodic syndrome, *Arthritis Rheum* 58:1516–1520, 2008.

102. Sacre K, Brihaye B, Lidove O, et al: Dramatic improvement following interleukin 1beta blockade in tumor necrosis factor receptor-1-associated syndrome (TRAPS) resistant to anti-TNF-alpha therapy, *J Rheumatol* 35:357–358, 2008.

103. Obici L, Meini A, Cattalini M, et al: Favourable and sustained response to anakinra in tumour necrosis factor receptor-associated periodic syndrome (TRAPS) with or without AA amyloidosis, *Ann Rheum Dis* 70:1511–1512, 2010.

109. Hoffman HM, Mueller JL, Broide DH, et al: Mutation of a new gene encoding a putative pyrin-like protein causes familial cold autoinflammatory syndrome and Muckle-Wells syndrome, *Nat Genet* 29:301–305, 2001.

110. Aksentijevich I, Nowak M, Mallah M, et al: De novo CIAS1 mutations, cytokine activation, and evidence for genetic heterogeneity in patients with neonatal-onset multisystem inflammatory disease

(NOMID): a new member of the expanding family of pyrin-associated autoinflammatory diseases, *Arthritis Rheum* 46:3340–3348, 2002.

112. Hull KM, Shoham N, Chae JJ, et al: The expanding spectrum of systemic autoinflammatory disorders and their rheumatic manifestations, *Curr Opin Rheumatol* 15:61–69, 2003.

113. Martinon F, Tschopp J: Inflammatory caspases: linking an intracellular innate immune system to autoinflammatory diseases, *Cell* 117:561–574, 2004.

114. Ting JP, Kastner DL, Hoffman HM: CATERPILLERs, pyrin and hereditary immunological disorders, *Nat Rev Immunol* 6:183–195, 2006.

116. Martinon F, Burns K, Tschopp J: The inflammasome: a molecular platform triggering activation of inflammatory caspases and processing of proIL-1beta, *Mol Cell* 10:417–426, 2002.

117. Agostini L, Martinon F, Burns K, et al: NALP3 forms an IL-1beta-processing inflammasome with increased activity in Muckle-Wells autoinflammatory disorder, *Immunity* 20:319–325, 2004.

118. Dowds TA, Masumoto J, Zhu L, et al: Cryopyrin-induced interleukin 1beta secretion in monocytic cells: enhanced activity of disease-associated mutants and requirement for ASC, *J Biol Chem* 279:21924–22198, 2004.

126. Prieur AM: A recently recognised chronic inflammatory disease of early onset characterised by the triad of rash, central nervous system involvement and arthropathy, *Clin Exp Rheumatol* 19:103–106, 2001.

127. Prieur AM, Griscelli C, Lampert F, et al: A chronic, infantile, neurological, cutaneous and articular (CINCA) syndrome. A specific entity analysed in 30 patients, *Scand J Rheumatol Suppl* 66:57–68, 1987.

129. Hoffman HM: Therapy of autoinflammatory syndromes, *J Allergy Clin Immunol* 124:1129–1138; quiz 39-40, 2009.

130. Goldbach-Mansky R, Dailey NJ, Canna SW, et al: Neonatal-onset multisystem inflammatory disease responsive to interleukin-1beta inhibition, *N Engl J Med* 355:581–592, 2006.

132. Lachmann HJ, Kone-Paut I, Kuemmerle-Deschner JB, et al: Use of canakinumab in the cryopyrin-associated periodic syndrome, *N Engl J Med* 360:2416–2425, 2009.

133. Blau EB: Familial granulomatous arthritis, iritis, and rash, *J Pediatr* 107:689–693, 1985.

134. Becker ML, Rose CD: Blau syndrome and related genetic disorders causing childhood arthritis, *Curr Rheumatol Rep* 7:427–433, 2005.

136. Rose CD, Wouters CH, Meiorin S, et al: Pediatric granulomatous arthritis: an international registry, *Arthritis Rheum* 54:3337–3344, 2006.

138. Miceli-Richard C, Lesage S, Rybojad M, et al: CARD15 mutations in Blau syndrome, *Nat Genet* 29:19–20, 2001.

141. Eckmann L, Karin M: NOD2 and Crohn's disease: loss or gain of function? *Immunity* 22:661–667, 2005.

143. Milman N, Andersen CB, Hansen A, et al: Favourable effect of TNF-alpha inhibitor (infliximab) on Blau syndrome in monozygotic twins with a de novo CARD15 mutation, *APMIS* 114:912–919, 2006.

144. Borzutzky A, Fried A, Chou J, et al: NOD2-associated diseases: Bridging innate immunity and autoinflammation, *Clin Immunol* 134:251–261, 2010.

145. Arostegui JI, Arnal C, Merino R, et al: NOD2 gene-associated pediatric granulomatous arthritis: clinical diversity, novel and recurrent mutations, and evidence of clinical improvement with interleukin-1 blockade in a Spanish cohort, *Arthritis Rheum* 56:3805–3813, 2007.

148. Lindor NM, Arsenault TM, Solomon H, et al: A new autosomal dominant disorder of pyogenic sterile arthritis, pyoderma gangrenosum, and acne: PAPA syndrome, *Mayo Clin Proc* 72:611–615, 1997.

149. Wise CA, Gillum JD, Seidman CE, et al: Mutations in CD2BP1 disrupt binding to PTP PEST and are responsible for PAPA syndrome, an autoinflammatory disorder, *Hum Mol Genet* 11:961–969, 2002.

150. Shoham NG, Centola M, Mansfield E, et al: Pyrin binds the PSTPIP1/CD2BP1 protein, defining familial Mediterranean fever and PAPA syndrome as disorders in the same pathway, *Proc Natl Acad Sci U S A* 100:13501–13506, 2003.

153. Cortis E, De Benedetti F, Insalaco A, et al: Abnormal production of tumor necrosis factor (TNF)-alpha and clinical efficacy of the TNF inhibitor etanercept in a patient with PAPA syndrome [corrected], *J Pediatr* 145:851–855, 2004.

155. Baum W, Kirkin V, Fernandez SB, et al: Binding of the intracellular Fas ligand (FasL) domain to the adaptor protein PSTPIP results in a cytoplasmic localization of FasL, *J Biol Chem* 280:40012–40024, 2005.

156. Tallon B, Corkill M: Peculiarities of PAPA syndrome, *Rheumatology (Oxford)* 45:1140–1143, 2006.

157. Tofteland ND, Shaver TS: Clinical efficacy of etanercept for treatment of PAPA syndrome, *J Clin Rheumatol* 16:244–245, 2010.

158. Dierselhuis MP, Frenkel J, Wulffraat NM, Boelens JJ: Anakinra for flares of pyogenic arthritis in PAPA syndrome, *Rheumatology (Oxford)* 44:46–48, 2005.

159. Brenner M, Ruzicka T, Plewig G, et al: Targeted treatment of pyoderma gangrenosum in PAPA (pyogenic arthritis, pyoderma gangrenosum and acne) syndrome with the recombinant human interleukin-1 receptor antagonist anakinra, *Br J Dermatol* 161:1199–1201, 2009.

160. Stichweh DS, Punaro M, Pascual V: Dramatic improvement of pyoderma gangrenosum with infliximab in a patient with PAPA syndrome, *Pediatr Dermatol* 22:262–265, 2005.

161. Aksentijevich I, Masters SL, Ferguson PJ, et al: An autoinflammatory disease with deficiency of the interleukin-1-receptor antagonist, *N Engl J Med* 360:2426–2437, 2009.

162. Reddy S, Jia S, Geoffrey R, et al: An autoinflammatory disease due to homozygous deletion of the IL1RN locus, *N Engl J Med* 360:2438–2444, 2009.

Full references for this chapter can be found on www.expertconsult.com.

PART 15 | CARTILAGE, BONE, AND HERITABLE CONNECTIVE TISSUE DISORDERS

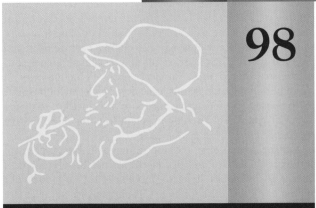

98 | Pathogenesis of Osteoarthritis

PAUL E. Dı CESARE •
DOMINIK R. HAUDENSCHILD •
JONATHAN SAMUELS •
STEVEN B. ABRAMSON

KEY POINTS

Osteoarthritis is a degenerative joint disease, occurring primarily in older individuals, characterized by erosion of the articular cartilage, hypertrophy of bone at the margins (i.e., osteophytes), subchondral sclerosis, and a range of biochemical and morphologic alterations of the synovial membrane and joint capsule.

Risk factors for developing osteoarthritis include age, joint location, obesity, genetic predisposition, joint malalignment, trauma, and gender.

Morphologic changes in early osteoarthritis include articular cartilage surface irregularity, superficial clefts within the tissue, and altered proteoglycan distribution.

Morphologic changes in late osteoarthritis include deepened clefts, increase in surface irregularities, and eventual articular cartilage ulceration, exposing the underlying bone. Chondrocytes form clusters or clones in an attempt at self-repair. In addition, marginal osteophytes can form.

The matrix metalloproteinase family of proteinases degrades proteoglycans (aggrecanases) and collagen (collagenases).

A suboptimal repair response of normal articular cartilage to injury typically results in secondary osteoarthritis.

Chondrocytes sense and respond to mechanical and physicochemical stimuli via several regulatory pathways.

Mediators classically associated with inflammation during the course of osteoarthritis include interleukin-1β and tumor necrosis factor.

Nitric oxide, produced by the inducible isoform of nitric oxide synthase, is a major catabolic factor produced by chondrocytes in response to proinflammatory cytokines.

Expression of inducible cyclooxygenase-2 is increased in osteoarthritis chondrocytes.

Low-grade inflammation occurs in osteoarthritic synovial tissues and contribute to disease pathogenesis.

Most current treatments aim to improve the signs and symptoms of osteoarthritis.

Osteoarthritis (OA) is a degenerative joint disease, occurring primarily in older persons, characterized by erosion of the articular cartilage, hypertrophy of bone at the margins (i.e., osteophytes), subchondral sclerosis, and a range of biochemical and morphologic alterations of the synovial membrane and joint capsule. Pathologic changes in the late stages of OA include softening, ulceration, and focal disintegration of the articular cartilage; synovial inflammation may also occur. Typical clinical symptoms are pain and stiffness, particularly after prolonged activity.

In industrialized societies OA is the leading cause of physical disability, increases in health care usage, and impaired quality of life. The impact of arthritic conditions is expected to grow as the population both increases and ages in the coming decades.[1] Despite its prevalence, the precise etiology, pathogenesis, and progression of OA remain beyond our understanding, primarily due to multiple confounding factors. Without a clear-cut picture of how OA arises at the cellular or molecular level, many still consider it a result of "wear and tear," an inevitable consequence of aging. In fact, the accompanying biochemical, structural, and metabolic changes in joint cartilage have been well documented. It is now known, for example, that cytokines, mechanical trauma, and altered genetics are involved in its pathogenesis and that these factors can initiate a degradative cascade that results in many of the characteristic alterations of articular cartilage in OA. More recently it has become apparent that OA is a disease process that affects the entire joint structure including cartilage, synovial membrane, subchondral bone, ligaments, and periarticular muscles. OA is thus better considered a group of overlapping disorders of various etiologies arising from a combination of systemic factors (e.g., genetics) and local factors (e.g., biomechanically or biochemically mediated events) that gradually converge to produce a condition with definable morphologic and clinical outcomes.[2]

OA may be classified as primary or secondary according to its cause or major predisposing factor; what they all have in common is altered cartilage physiology. Primary OA is the most common type and has no identifiable etiology or predisposing cause. Secondary OA, although it has an identifiable underlying cause, is pathologically indistinguishable from primary OA. The most common causes of secondary OA are metabolic conditions (e.g., calcium crystal deposition, hemochromatosis, acromegaly); anatomic factors (e.g., leg length inequality, congenital hip dislocation); traumatic events (e.g., major joint trauma, chronic joint injury, joint surgery); or the sequelae of inflammatory disorders (e.g., ankylosing spondylitis, septic arthritis). In the case of secondary OA arising from inflammatory joint disease, cartilage degeneration most likely results initially from degradative enzymes released from the synovium or leukocytes within the joint space and later from the mechanical attrition of a biomechanically altered extracellular matrix. Distinguishing between primary and secondary OA may be difficult because the clinical presentation and symptoms are often so similar.

ETIOLOGIC FACTORS IN OSTEOARTHRITIS

Major factors affecting degree of risk for developing OA include age, joint location, obesity, genetic predisposition, joint malalignment, trauma, and gender.

Age

Age is the risk factor most strongly correlated with OA.[3,4] OA is the most common chronic disease in later life; more than 80% of persons older than age 75 years are affected, and OA increases progressively with age at all joint sites. Radiologic changes in OA increase as individuals age,[5] although these changes do not always correlate with clinical symptoms or disability.[6,7] Although clearly an age-related disease, OA is not, however, an inevitable consequence of aging. Age-related morphologic and structural changes in articular cartilage include fraying, softening, and thinning of the articular surface; decreased size and aggregation of matrix proteoglycans; and loss of matrix tensile strength and stiffness. These age-related tissue changes are most likely due to a decrease in the chondrocytes' ability to maintain and repair the tissue, as chondrocytes themselves undergo age-related decreases in mitotic and synthetic activity, exhibit decreased responsiveness to anabolic growth factors, and synthesize smaller and less uniform large aggregating proteoglycans and fewer functional link proteins.[4]

There also appears to be a direct correlation between chondrocyte apoptosis and cartilage degradation leading to OA. Age does appear to be an independent factor that predisposes articular chondrocytes to apoptosis because the expression levels of specific proapoptotic genes (Fas, FasL, caspase-8, and p53) is higher in aged cartilage.[8,9]

Joint Location

Although osteoarthritis occurs most commonly in weight-bearing joints,[10] age affects joints differentially.[11] A study comparing tensile fracture stress of cartilage in the femoral head and in the talus showed that it decreased progressively with age in the former but not in the latter.[12] Joint-specific age-related viability in articular cartilage may explain why OA is more common in hip and knee joints with increasing age but occurs rarely in the ankle.

Obesity

Obesity is another important risk factor for OA.[13-15] Greater body mass index in both women and men has been shown to be associated with an increased risk of knee (but not hip) OA.[7,16,17] An increase in mechanical forces across weight-bearing joints is probably the primary factor leading to joint degeneration. Obesity not only increases the forces at weight-bearing joints but may also change posture, gait, and physical activity level, any or all of which may further contribute to altered joint biomechanics.[18] The majority of obese patients exhibit varus knee deformities, which results in increased joint reactive forces in the medial compartment of the knee, thereby accelerating the degenerative process.[19]

Particularly in elderly obese individuals, heavy physical activity is an additional risk factor for the development of knee OA, whereas light to moderate activity does not appear to increase risk for knee OA and may in fact alleviate symptomatic knee OA by reducing body mass index.[7,16,17] Similarly, weight loss can reduce both radiographic knee OA progression and clinical symptoms. Recent evidence indicates that in obese patients with OA, significant weight loss dramatically improves functional status, with short-term results equivalent to those of patients who have undergone joint replacement.[20]

Yet recent work suggests that the association between obesity and osteoarthritis lies beyond the mechanical loading from a higher body mass index. Adipose tissue is now recognized as a metabolically active contributor to inflammatory cascades. Activated adipose tissue increases the synthesis of proinflammatoy cytokines including leptin, adiponectin, resistin, interleukin-1 (IL-1), IL-6, and tumor necrosis factor (TNF), while some regulatory cytokine levels such as IL-10 are decreased.[21,22] Specifically, the discovery of the obesity gene and its product leptin may have important implications for the onset and progression of OA and increase our understanding of the link between obesity and OA. The fact that women have a greater proportion of total body fat and relatively higher levels of adipose-derived systemic leptin concentrations than men may partially account for the gender disparity in OA patients. Leptin, however, is produced not only by adipose cells but also by osteoblasts and chondrocytes, suggesting that local leptin production may play a role in OA. Significant levels of leptin were observed in the cartilage and osteophytes of subjects with OA, yet few chondrocytes produced leptin in the cartilage of healthy subjects. Leptin has also been demonstrated to induce anabolic activity in the chondrocytes of rats and thus may ultimately confer structural joint changes.[23,24]

Genetic Predisposition

Because of the prevalence of OA in the general population and its extensive clinical heterogeneity, the genetic contribution to its pathogenesis has been difficult to analyze.[25,26] Two major cohorts (the Framingham Study and the Baltimore Longitudinal Study on Aging) support a genetic contribution to OA, with evidence for a major recessive gene and a multifactorial component, representing either polygenic or environmental factors.[27,28] Twin pair and family risk studies have indicated that the heritable component of OA may be on the order of 50% to 65%.[26,29,30] Moreover, family, twin, and population studies have indicated differences among genetic influences that determine the site of OA (hip, spinal, knee, hand).[28,31,32] Further evidence supporting a genetic predisposition to OA is the demonstration of a significantly higher concordance for OA between monozygotic twins than between dizygotic twins. Genetic studies have identified multiple gene variations associated with an increased risk of OA.[33]

Inherited forms of OA may be caused by mutations in several genes that are expressed in cartilage including those encoding types II, IV, V, and VI collagens, as well as cartilage oligomeric matrix protein (COMP).[34,35] Recently it was reported that mice deficient in the type IX collagen gene and the matrilin 3 gene (human equivalent condition not yet reported) developed age-dependent OA-like changes in the knee and temporal mandibular joints.[36,37] Moreover, candidate genes in OA have been identified that are not structural proteins. The haplotype of a vitamin D receptor (VDR) that plays a vital role in controlling bone mineral density appears to be associated with a twofold risk of knee OA[38-40]—although the VDR locus is close to the COL2A1 locus on chromosome 12q, so the association may be due to linkage disequilibrium with the latter.[25] In addition, the locus of the insulin-like growth factor 1 (IGF-1) gene has been associated with radiographic OA, as has an aggrecan polymorphic allele with hand OA.[25]

In population studies, genome-wide linkage scans have highlighted up to seven chromosomal regions that may harbor OA susceptibility genes.[41] Chromosome 2q was positive in several scans, suggesting that this chromosome is likely to harbor one or more susceptibility genes. In a study of affected sibling pairs, a region of linkage stretching from 2q12 to 2q21 was reported for OA of the distal interphalangeal joint and a previous study of affected sibling pairs in the United Kingdom demonstrated a broader region of linkage, stretching from 2q12 to 2q31.[41,42] Two IL-1 genes (*IL1A* and *IL1B*) and the gene encoding IL-1Ra (*IL1RN*) are located on chromosome 2q13 within a 430-kb genomic fragment. Given the importance of IL-1 in the perpetuation of cartilage damage in OA, it is possible that a proportion of the genetic susceptibility to OA may be encoded for by variation in the activity of interleukins, and that for chromosome 2q this susceptibility could reside within the IL-1 gene clusters. Loughlin and colleagues,[41] however, have provided evidence that the IL-1 gene cluster harbors susceptibility for knee OA, but not for hip OA. These and other epidemiologic studies have highlighted potential differences in the degree of OA heritability among different joint groups and between the two sexes.[43,44]

Genomic and postgenomic technology, in addition to defining susceptibility genotypes, will also lead to the discovery of genes and gene products that are overexpressed in OA tissues and that contribute to disease pathogenesis and progression.[45-47] Studies of differential gene expression in diseased tissue, in addition to elucidating pathogenic processes that lead to novel therapies, could also have two additional benefits: (1) identification of unique biomarkers that can be used for OA diagnosis or management and (2) identification of candidate susceptibility genotypes such as polymorphic variations of cytokines or growth factors that may predispose to disease progression.[48]

Joint Malalignment and Trauma

Joint malalignment or trauma may lead to rapid development of OA, or it may initiate a slow process that results in symptomatic OA years later. Probably as a result of progressive reduction in periarticular blood flow and the resultant decrease in rate of remodeling at the osteochondral junction, joints become increasingly congruent with age.[49,50] Altered joint geometry may interfere with nutrition of the cartilage, or it may alter load distribution, either or which may result in altered biochemical composition of the cartilage, irrespective of age.[51,52] Local factors such as stresses related to joint use and joint deformity also influence the development of OA.

Joint incongruence (e.g., malreduced intra-articular fractures, developmental dysplasia of the hip, recurrent dislocation of the patella) can lead to early-onset OA.[53] Repetitive, high-impact sports are strongly associated with joint injury and increase the risk for lower limb OA.[54] Repetitive trauma at a subfracture level has been shown to accelerate remodeling in the zone of calcified cartilage, with reduplication of the tidemark and thinning of the noncalcified zone, resulting in stiffening of the subchondral bone, increased wear of the overlying cartilage, and ultimately development of OA.[55-57] Regular exercise is important in maintaining articular cartilage structure and metabolic function. Recreational running and low-impact activities have not been shown to increase the risk of OA.

Articular cartilage is remarkably resistant to damage by shear forces; it is, however, highly vulnerable to repetitive impact loading.[58] When joints are subjected to in vitro cyclic loads that are easily borne by subchondral bone, cartilage degeneration still results.[59] This vulnerability accounts for the high frequency of OA in shoulders and elbows of pneumatic drill operators and baseball pitchers, ankles of ballet dancers, metacarpophalangeal joints of boxers, and knees of basketball players. The risk for knee osteoarthritis among participants in sports, however, may be more closely related to previous knee injury than to participation in sport alone.[60]

The major forces on articular cartilage, in addition to weight bearing, are due to the contraction of the muscles that stabilize or move the joint.[61] For example, in normal walking, 4 to 5 times the body weight may be transmitted through the knee, and in squatting it is up to 10 times the body weight.[39] Articular cartilage is believed to be too thin to be an effective shock absorber under these high loads. What protects the joint under physiologic conditions of impact loading is joint motion, with the associated lengthening of muscles under tension and deformation of the subchondral bone.[40,62] Cancellous subchondral bone functions as a major shock absorber due to its material properties.[56] Two-thirds of subchondral bone stiffness derives from bony trabeculae, about one-third from intraosseous fluid.[63] In the normal unloaded joint, the opposing surfaces are not congruous; under loading, both the cartilage and the bone deform so that a larger proportion of the opposing surfaces comes into contact, increasing joint congruity and resulting in a force distribution over the largest possible area.[64]

Excessive loads may cause microfractures of subchondral trabeculae that heal via callus formation and remodeling, resulting in stiffer-than-normal bone that is less effective as a shock absorber and predisposing articular cartilage to degeneration.

Whether subchondral sclerosis precedes the onset of OA or is a change secondary to cartilage degeneration is not known. Indirect evidence supports the theory that biomechanical changes in subchondral bone may be important in OA.[63,65,66] Foss, for example, reported cases of femoral osteoporosis (which is associated with softening and greater compliance of the subchondral bone) that may have protected the hip from OA.[67] Conversely, in vitro studies have shown that stiffening of the cancellous bone with methacrylate, reducing its deformability, leads to cartilage degeneration with repetitive impact loading.[68]

Gender

Women are about twice as likely as men to develop OA. Although women have a lower prevalence of OA than men before age 50 years, there is a marked increase in prevalence among women after 50, particularly in the knee.[69] Radiographic and interview data from the National Health and Nutrition Examination Survey (NHANES III), a representative cross-sectional health examination survey of the U.S. population, reported that the lifetime prevalence of radiographic knee osteoarthritis was 37.4% and that the prevalence of symptomatic knee osteoarthritis was 12.1% in adults age 60 years and older; prevalence was greater among women than men (42.1% vs. 31.2%), and women had significantly more Kellgren-Lawrence grade 3 and 4 changes (12.9% vs. 6.5% in men).[70] Women have a greater number of joints involved and are more likely to exhibit clinical symptoms of morning stiffness, joint swelling, and nocturnal pain. The gender differences in OA incidence after age 50 may be the result of postmenopausal estrogen deficiency. Articular chondrocytes possess functional estrogen receptors, suggesting that these cells can be regulated by estrogen. Nuclear estrogen receptors (ERs) have been detected in articular chondrocytes of humans,[71,72] rats,[72,73] monkeys,[72,74] pigs,[75] and human growth plate chondrocytes.[76]

Recent epidemiologic studies have linked estrogen replacement therapy (ERT) with a lower-than-expected risk of knee and hip OA in postmenopausal women. Clinical investigations of the association between OA and hormonal level in women have involved measurement of circulating estrogen levels in postmenopausal women, general radiographic evaluation of postmenopausal women, and examination of the effect of ERT on such variables as knee OA and cartilage volume.[77-80] In a study of more than 4000 women age 65 years or older that assessed pelvis radiographs for hip OA, Nevitt and colleagues[77] showed that women using oral estrogen faced a significantly reduced risk of hip OA. Estrogen users for 10 years or longer had a greater reduction in risk of developing hip OA than users for less than 10 years. Zhang and colleagues,[79] using weight-bearing radiographs in female participants in the Framingham Osteoarthritis Study (n = 831; mean age, 73 years; age range, 63 to 93) to study the rate of knee OA, reported a modest but nonsignificant greater protective effect for

radiographically detected OA in women who were on ERT. A prospective cohort study using anteroposterior weight-bearing knee radiographs of women (mean age, 71 years; age range, 63 to 91) from the Framingham Study categorized patients into three groups according to estrogen use at biennial examination: never users (n = 349), past users (n = 162), and current users (n = 40). When both incident and progressive radiographic knee OA cases were combined, current ERT users were found to have 60% less risk for knee OA than never users. Wluka and colleagues[80] reported on the longer-term use of ERT and its association with knee cartilage volume (measured by magnetic resonance imaging [MRI]) in postmenopausal women; results showed that after adjusting for confounders, women using long-term ERT had more knee cartilage than controls. Beneficial effects of ERT on the severity of knee OA in ovariectomized monkeys have also been demonstrated.[81]

CHANGES IN OSTEOARTHRITIS

Morphologic Changes

In early OA, the articular cartilage surface becomes roughened and irregular, and superficial clefts within the tissue become apparent. Histologically, the surface is fibrillated and small cracks are apparent but limited to the upper layers of the surface zone. These changes show evidence of mechanical wear and are often accompanied by matrix swelling and chondrocyte proliferation or, to a limited extent, apoptosis near the articular surface. Proteoglycan distribution is altered, as revealed by histochemical staining. As OA progresses, the articular cartilage surface becomes more irregular and the superficial clefts within the tissue become enlarged and extend beyond the superficial zone and into the middle zone of cartilage. The previously isolated and focal portions of damaged cartilage become increasingly contiguous. Portions of the superficial zone are completely missing in focal lesions. As the condition worsens, the clefts deepen, surface irregularities increase, and the articular cartilage eventually ulcerates, exposing the underlying bone. As the disease continues to progress, the joint articulates on exposed bone, causing eburnation and thickening of the bone. The eburnated bone becomes denser and more metabolically active in response.

Early Reparative, Proliferative, and Hypertrophic Changes

Attempts at local self-repair can be seen as an initial increase in the number of chondrocytes in the form of clusters or clones, with as many as 50 or more cells in a cluster[39] (Figure 98-1). In healthy cartilage, chondrocytes are quiescent and neither commit to proliferation nor to further hypertrophic differentiation. In contrast, in the early stages of OA, proliferating chondrocytes in clusters express higher levels of matrix proteins including aggrecan and type II collagen,[83] as well as stem cell markers[84] and markers of hypertrophic differentiation.[83] The chondrocyte clusters with proliferative and hypertrophic markers are a hallmark of OA and are also prominent in animal models of OA and three-dimensional cell cultures.[85] In addition to being a repair response, chondrocyte clusters are thought to contribute to

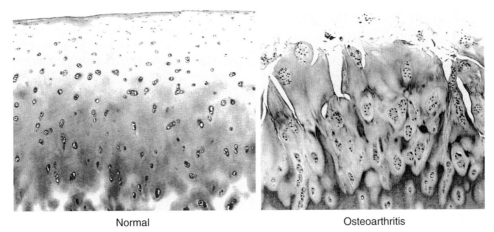

Normal   Osteoarthritis

Figure 98-1   Histologic sections of normal *(left)* and osteoarthritic *(right)* articular cartilage obtained from the femoral head. The osteoarthritic cartilage has surface irregularities, with clefts to the radial zone and cloning of chondrocytes.

OA pathogenesis and progression through the release of matrix-degrading enzymes, growth factors, and inflammatory cytokines that affect surrounding chondrocytes and joint tissues.[85]

Osteophyte Formation

Osteophytes consist of newly formed fibrocartilage and bone and are most commonly formed at the peripheral margins of joints at the interface between cartilage and the periosteum. Osteophytes are thought to arise through chondrogenic differentiation of progenitor cells, most commonly from within the periosteum.[86] As such, osteophytes may be a cellular repair response to the altered growth factor environment after joint injury, and in certain cases osteophytes can contribute to the stability of the joints.[87,88] The connection between osteophyte formation and the repair response is further strengthened by animal models of OA in which the early stages of osteophyte formation can be histologically apparent as early as 3 days after joint injury. Many growth factors that enhance in vitro chondrogenic differentiation of stem cells are also present in osteophytes, including members of the transforming growth factor (TGF)-β superfamily,[89] bone morphogenetic proteins (BMPs),[90] IGF, and fibroblast growth factor,[86] and TGF-β can induce osteophyte formation in animal models.[91] As OA progresses, the osteophytes can limit movement and become painful.

Hypocellularity

A reduction in cell number is observed in aging cartilage, and the reduced synthetic capability of hypocellular cartilage is a contributing factor to the initiation and progression of OA. In healthy adult femoral cartilage, the cell density varies between 24,000/mm^3 in the surface zone and 8000/mm^3 in the deep zone, with an average of 1.65% of the cartilage volume consisting of cells.[92] This number is greatly reduced in OA, through cell death via necrosis or apoptosis.[93] Necrosis can result from direct mechanical damage to cells and is not generally an active process, whereas apoptosis is an active energy-consuming process. Apoptotic chondrocyte death can be initiated by many factors that are involved in the initiation and progression of arthritis

including mechanical damage or injury, changes in cell-matrix interactions, oxidative stress resulting from nitric oxide or other reactive oxygen species, impaired mitochondrial function, and signal transduction pathways such as CD95/CD95 ligand. These pathways ultimately converge, and the execution of apoptotic cell death is mediated by the activation of caspases. Inhibition of apoptosis by interfering with caspase activation following injury is being explored as a chondroprotective intervention to prevent secondary OA following injury. Compromised regulation of cellular senescence and autophagy can also cause cell death. The role of autophagy in inflammation and pathogenesis has been gaining the attention of researchers.[94] In some circumstances cell death can be mediated by the autophagic degradation of the damaged organelles. In cartilage, autophagy can be protective, and its reduction in OA corresponds with increased apoptotic markers.[95]

ALTERATIONS IN CARTILAGE MATRIX METABOLISM

Biochemical Changes

These morphologic changes are accompanied by changes in the biochemical composition of the cartilage, which vary from early to later stages in the disease process. In early OA, the water content of the articular cartilage significantly increases, causing the tissue to swell and altering its biomechanical properties. This phenomenon suggests that there has been weakening of the collagen network; the type II collagen fibers have a smaller diameter than normal cartilage, and the normally tight weave in the midzone is slackened and distorted.[96-101]

In later stages of OA, type I collagen concentration within the extracellular matrix increases and the proteoglycan concentration falls to 50% or less than normal, with less aggregation and shorter glycosaminoglycan side chains.[98,102] Keratan sulfate concentration decreases, and the ratio of chondroitin-4-sulfate to chondroitin-6-sulfate increases, reflecting synthesis by chondrocytes of a proteoglycan profile more typical of immature cartilage.[103] Proteoglycan concentration in the cartilage diminishes progressively until the end stages, when histologic staining detects little or none.[104]

Our understanding of how the biochemical changes progress from the early to the later stages of OA is evolving. One of the first steps in cartilage degradation is a decrease in the density of proteoglycans. This step is thought to be at least partly reversible.[105] However, decreased proteoglycan density opens up the cartilage porosity to make it more permeable to collagenases and other proteases, and it exposes collagen fibrils. This initiates a vicious circle of positive-feedback loops that further promote cartilage degradation. For example, epitopes on collagen become accessible to the DDR2 receptor on the cell surface, which then increases MMP-13 production through activation of the Ras/Raf/MEK/ERK and p38 signal cascades.[106] The partially digested matrix components themselves have cytokine-like activity that enhances the inflammatory response and promotes matrix degradation. The destruction of the collagenous cartilage component is thought to be irreversible.

Calcium crystals (e.g., calcium pyrophosphate dihydrate, basic calcium phosphate crystals) are commonly found in the cartilage of the elderly, and often crystal arthropathy coexists with OA.[107] That calcium crystals play a role in causing or worsening OA is supported by clinical and laboratory studies, but the relationship is complex and it is unclear whether these crystals are directly involved in OA pathogenesis.[108-110] Pyrophosphate (PP) is produced from adenosine triphosphate (ATP) by the exoenzyme nucleoside pyrophosphohydrolase.[111] High levels of PP in synovial fluid from OA patients correlate directly with the severity of joint damage.[112,113] Young or proliferating chondrocytes are a major source of PP, whereas resting chondrocytes from normal adult cartilage secrete little.[111] Thus the increased PP secretion in OA cartilage might indicate increased chondrocyte metabolic activity toward matrix repair.[114] The presence of CPPD may alter the biomechanical properties of the cartilage extracellular matrix and lead to cartilage breakdown. Hemochromatosis (hemosiderin), Wilson's disease (copper), ochronotic arthropathy (homogentisic acid polymers), gouty arthritis (crystals of monosodium urate), and calcium pyrophosphate dihydrate (CPPD) crystal deposition disease are further examples of conditions in which the abnormal entity may alter the cartilage extracellular matrix, leading to either direct or indirect chondrocyte injury by increasing the stiffness of the tissue and thereby precipitating the development of OA.

Metabolic Changes

Early OA is characterized by increased synthesis of proteoglycans, collagen, noncollagenous proteins, hyaluronate, and cell replication.[104,115] This "activation" of chondrocytes is thought to be an attempt to repair the cartilage matrix, although it is not always effective and yields a matrix of inferior quality that is more susceptible to degradation.[116] However, both anabolic and catabolic processes increase as cells attempt to repair or maintain tissue integrity[98] and it is the imbalance between synthesis and degradation that is important in the pathogenesis of OA.[117] In later stages of OA, there is a decrease in the synthesis of matrix

per cell and a decrease in cell number. Furthermore, the quality of the synthesized matrix is reduced with respect to the composition and distribution of their glycosaminoglycans, the size of the proteoglycan subunit, and their ability to aggregate with hyaluronic acid.[98,100,103,118,119] In addition to the reduced matrix production and hypocellularity, there is increased synthesis and activation of matrix degrading enzymes, as well as an overall decrease in the concentrations of enzyme inhibitors such as tissue inhibitors of metalloproteinases (TIMPs). Eventually OA progresses when the chondrocytic anabolic repair processes cannot keep pace with catabolic processes.[98,104] The complex interaction between matrix synthesis and degradation explains why OA typically is slowly progressive and at times remains static by morphologic criteria, but ultimately it results in the overall degradation of cartilage matrix. The following sections summarize the major anabolic and catabolic factors relevant to cartilage degradation and the pathogenesis of OA.

Anabolic Factors (Transforming Growth Factor-β, Bone Morphogenetic Proteins) and Cartilage Repair

TGF-β is essential for the formation and maintenance of cartilage (reviewed in Reference 120). Interference with TGF-β function in cartilage leads to OA in multiple animal models[121] and in human genetic susceptibility to OA.[122] TGF-β affects cartilage homeostasis at multiple levels: It enhances stem cell chondrogenesis to increase the pool of cells available for cartilage synthesis, and it increases matrix production in existing chondrocytes. TGF-β also increases synthesis of anticatabolic factors such as TIMPs and PAI-1, proteins that inhibit the activation of latent proteinases in cartilage. TGF-β attenuates the cellular response to inflammatory cytokines including IL-1β and TNF,[120] and TGF-β signaling through the Smad2/3 pathway can inhibit terminal differentiation and hypertrophy in chondrocytes. However, TGF-β activity can also contribute to the pathogenesis and progression of OA. For example, TGF-β signaling induces osteophyte formation in animal models. In aging cells and cells in which the ratio of the TGF-β receptors ALK1 and ALK5 is altered, TGF-β can also have opposing effects such as activating MMP-13 and inducing terminal hypertrophic differentiation in chondrocytes.[123]

BMPs are structurally related to TGF-β but generally activate a different set of receptors and intracellular signaling molecules. BMPs influence all stages of embryonic chondrogenesis and can promote chondrogenic differentiation of adult MSCs.[124] Recent genetic evidence suggests that impaired BMP signaling affects OA susceptibility, with the most progress reported for BMP-14 (GDF-5).[125,126] There is good evidence that a reduction of BMP-7 (OP-1) is evident in osteoarthritic cartilage,[127] with possible regulation occurring through both inhibitory microRNA[128] and promoter methylation.[129] Supplementation of BMP-7 in joints reduces experimental arthritis in animals and was proven safe in a phase I clinical trial, with no findings of ectopic bone formation in the enrolled patients during the study.[130] However, as described for TGF-β earlier, BMP signaling through certain receptors can also enhance terminal differentiation and hypertrophy in chondrocytes, processes that are hallmarks of OA progression.

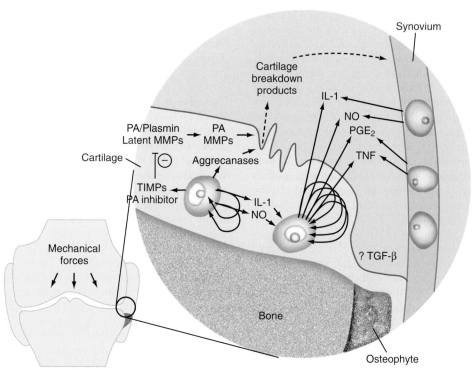

Figure 98-2 Schematic of pathogenic mechanisms of osteoarthritis. Mechanical stress initiates altered metabolism characterized by the release of matrix metalloproteinases (MMPs), proinflammatory cytokines, and mediators such as nitric oxide (NO) and prostaglandin E_2 (PGE$_2$). Cartilage break-down products play a role by stimulating the release of cytokines from synovial lining cells and by inducing MMP production by chondrocytes. Per-petuation of cartilage damage is amplified by the autocrine and paracrine actions of interleukin (IL)-1β and tumor necrosis factor (TNF) produced by chondrocytes. PA, plasminogen activator; TGF-β, transforming growth factor-β; TIMPs, tissue inhibitors of metalloproteinases.

Catabolic Factors and Cartilage Degradation

In addition to new matrix synthesis, cartilage remodeling also involves a degree of proteolysis. This occurs via the induction of an array of proteases, particularly matrix metal-loproteinases (MMPs). In OA, the cytokines IL-1 and TNF stimulate the synthesis and secretion of many proteases and MMPs (Figure 98-2).[105] IL-1 is synthesized by mononuclear cells (including synovial lining cells) in the inflamed joint and by chondrocytes as an autocrine activity.[131-133] The enzymes stimulated by IL-1 and TNF include latent colla-genase, latent stromelysin, latent gelatinase, aggrecanase, and tissue plasminogen activator (TPA).[134-137] Plasminogen is either synthesized by the chondrocyte or enters the matrix by diffusion from the synovial fluid. TPA converts plasmino-gen to plasmin, a serine proteinase that can activate latent cartilage-degrading enzymes. A downstream mediator of IL-1- and TNF-induced cartilage degradation that is gaining increasing attention is hypoxia-inducible factor 2α (Hif2α).[138,139] Hif2α is a transcription factor strongly upreg-ulated in OA cartilage and mouse models of OA. It directly induces the expression of many cartilage-degrading enzymes including MMPs 1, 3, 9, and 12, as well as a disintegrin and metalloproteinase with thrombospondin motif (ADAMTS-4) and (indirectly) ADAMTS-5. In addition, a high level of Hif2α decreases the protective role of autophagy, increases the extent of cell death, and activates the RUNX2 and IHH pathways that further contribute to cartilage matrix degra-dation. The different classes of proteinases that are acti-vated by these cytokines in OA are discussed in more detail later.

Classes of Proteinases (Metalloproteinases, Aggrecanases, Serine and Cysteine Proteases)

In OA, the synthesis and secretion of matrix-degrading enzymes by chondrocytes markedly increases.[104,115,140-142] There are four classes of proteases, which are grouped by the catalytic mechanisms of peptide bond cleavage: metallopro-teinases, cysteine proteinases, serine proteinases, and aspar-tyl proteinases. Of these, the first three have clearly defined roles in the degradation of cartilage during the progression of OA.

Metalloproteinases

Metalloproteinases have an enzymatic site that requires a metal ion (often zinc) for activity. Cartilage contains two families of metalloproteinases, namely ADAMTSs and MMPs. Early cartilage degeneration in OA is most likely the result of metalloproteinase enzymatic activity. Both families of metalloproteinases are upregulated in osteo-arthritic cartilage, and both are highly expressed in OA car-tilage at lesional sites. As the MMPs and ADAMTSs play major roles in the degradation of cartilage extracellular matrix, several MMPs and ADAMTSs are candidate targets for disease modification.[143]

The control of metalloproteinase activity in OA is complex, with regulation occurring at three different levels: synthesis and secretion, activation of latent enzyme, and inactivation by proteinase inhibitors.[144] Most metallopro-teinases are not constitutively expressed, but their transcrip-tion is induced after stimulation with cytokine and growth factor signaling. Once transcribed, the transcript stability and translation of several metalloproteinases are regulated by microRNA (miR). For example, microRNA-27b (miR-27b) regulates MMP-13 expression.[145] Also, miR-140 levels are decreased in OA, which reduces its repression of ADAMTS-5.[146] Several of these miRNAs are controlled by the same cytokines and growth factors that maintain cartilage homeostasis including IL-1 and TGF-β. Although the miR field is still in its infancy, it is already evident that several miRs are involved in the pathogenesis of OA by affecting transcript stability and protein translation. Once translated into proteins, almost all MMPs are expressed as inactive proenzymes (zymogens) that require further processing for full proteolytic activity. Most MMPs contain an N-terminal prodomain that blocks or otherwise inhibits the catalytic site. The primary MMP activators are serine- and cysteine-dependent proteases (e.g., the plasminogen/plasmin cascade or furin-like proprotein convertases and cathepsin B, respectively), as well as membrane-type MMPs.[118,147,148] Activated MMPs can then be inactivated nonspecifically by α2 macroglobulin and with more specificity by the tissue inhibitor of metalloproteinase (TIMP) family of proteins.

MMPs have historically been further divided into three groups on the basis of their substrate specificities; collagenases cleave across all three chains of the native triple-helical collagens, whereas gelatinases preferably cleave denatured collagen and stromelysins have much broader substrate specificities.[149] However, there is considerable overlap in substrates between these classifications; for example, MMP-1 (interstitial collagenase), MMP-3 (stromelysin 1), and MMP-13 (collagenase-3) are all capable of cleaving aggrecan core protein.[150] MMPs can degrade other cartilage extracellular matrix molecules in addition to collagen. If combined with plasmin, which has the capability of activating many MMPs, MMPs can rapidly destroy cartilage altogether.

Collagenases

Collagenases typically make the first cleavage in triple-helical collagen, allowing its further degradation by other proteases. Degradation of collagens is thought to be the first irreversible step in the pathogenesis of OA because it significantly reduces the mechanical properties of cartilage. The best-studied MMPs capable of cleaving native collagens are MMP-13 and MMP-1, although MMP-8 and MMP-28 are also involved in breaking down type II collagen. Of the MMPs that degrade native collagen, MMP-13 may be the most important in OA because it preferentially degrades type II collagen.[151] Mice deficient in MMP-13 resist developing OA and have reduced cartilage erosion even after proteoglycan loss.[152] Expression of MMP-13 greatly increases in OA[153]; overall collagenase activity also markedly increases in human osteoarthritic cartilage cultures, suggesting that it is a major factor in OA progression and cartilage matrix degradation.[154,155] The resultant collagen fragments may then be susceptible to further cleavage by such other enzymes as MMP-2 (gelatinase A), MMP-9 (gelatinase B), MMP-3, and cathepsin B (a cysteine proteinase).

Aggrecanases

The aggrecanases are metalloproteases that belong to a family of extracellular proteases known as ADAMTS.[156] Two aggrecanases, ADAMTS-4 and ADAMTS-5, appear to be major enzymes in cartilage degradation in arthritis.[157] The roles of these enzymes appear reversed in human and mouse OA—whereas ADAMTS-4 is predominantly associated with aggrecan degradation in human OA, in mouse models of OA ADAMTS-5 is more important.[158-160] Recombinant ADAMTS-4 and ADAMTS-5 cleave aggrecan at five distinct sites along the core protein, and all resultant fragments have been identified in cartilage explants undergoing matrix degradation. The G1 region of aggrecan is highly resistant to proteases; however, a glutamate-alanine bond within the extended region between G1 and G2 is remarkably susceptible to proteolytic degradation.[161] Aggrecanase proteolytic activity can be modulated by altered expression, by activation by proteolytic cleavage at a furin-sensitive site, by binding to the aggrecan substrate through the C-terminal thrombospondin motif, by activation through post-translational processing of a portion of the C-terminus, and by inhibition of activity by the endogenous inhibitor, tissue inhibitor of metalloproteinase 3 (TIMP-3). ADAMTS-4 and ADAMTS-5 activity is also detected in joint capsule and synovium and may be upregulated in arthritic synovium at either the message level or through posttranslational processing. In addition to ADAMTS-4 and ADAMTS-5, several MMPs are also capable of cleaving aggrecan in vitro (MMP-1, MMP-2, MMP-3, MMP-7, MMP-8, MMP-9, MMP-13, and MMP-28), as are ADAMTS-1, ADAMTS-8, ADAMTS-9, and ADAMTS-15.[162] It has been shown that ADAMTS-7 and ADAMTS-12 both bind to and degrade COMP (a prominent noncollagenous protein in cartilage) and that the latter is highly upregulated in osteoarthritic cartilage.[163,164] ADAMTS-4, ADAMTS-19, and ADAMTS-20 also have been shown to degrade COMP in vitro; however, their in vivo activity in osteoarthritis has yet to be determined.[165,166]

A specific hyaluronidase has not been found in articular cartilage matrix, but one or several lysosomal enzymes that can cleave both hyaluronic acid and chondroitin-6-sulfate have been implicated.[147] There are six or seven potential hyaluronidases in the human genome, and of these, hyaluronidase-1, hyaluronidase-2, hyaluronidase-3, and PH-20 are likely to be active in cartilage.[167] However, experimental evidence to date suggests that these enzymes are either exclusively lysosomal or can exist both in the lysozome and at the plasma membrane. Thus although there is convincing evidence of extracellular degradation of hyaluronan, the precise role of the hyaluronidases in this process has not yet been clearly identified. The decrease in chondroitin sulfate chain length in osteoarthritic cartilage may be due to digestion by synovial fluid hyaluronidase, which may diffuse into the matrix as its permeability increases.[103] Evidence to support this theory is the finding that the hyaluronic acid concentration in OA cartilage is low, even though its rate of synthesis is considerably greater than normal.[104,115] These degradative enzymes serve to disrupt the proteoglycan aggregate. The early result of the MMP-induced tissue degradation is thinning of the collagen fibers, loosening of the tight collagen network, and the consequent cartilage matrix swelling seen in OA.

Enzyme Inhibitors (Tissue Inhibitor of Metalloproteinases, Plasminogen Activator Inhibitor-1)

The balance of active and latent enzymes is controlled to some extent by at least two enzyme inhibitors: tissue inhibitor of metalloproteinases (TIMP) and plasminogen activator inhibitor-1 (PAI-1).[141,168,169] TIMP and PAI-1 are synthesized in increased amounts under the regulation of transforming growth factor-β.[170-172] If insufficient concentrations of or degraded TIMP or PAI-1 are present in the matrix along with active enzymes, then increased matrix degradation occurs. Expression profiling of all known members of the MMP, ADAMTS, and tissue inhibitor of metalloproteinases (TIMP) gene families in normal cartilage and cartilage from patients with OA has revealed that several members are regulated in OA. Genes that showed increased expression in OA were MMP-2, MMP-9, MMP-13, MMP-16, MMP-28, ADAMTS-2, ADAMTS-12, ADAMTS-14, ADAMTS-16, and TIMP-3 (all at $P < .05$). Genes with decreased expression in OA were MMP-1, MMP-3, MMP-10; ADAMTS-1, ADAMTS-5, ADAMTS-9, and ADAMTS-15; and TIMP-1 and TIMP-4.[173] These results illustrate the complexity of the events that occur within the extracellular matrix regarding regulation of tissue-degrading enzymes.

Alterations in Matrix Synthesis

Much of what is known about changes in the extracellular matrix in early OA comes from animal models (e.g., the rabbit partial meniscectomy model, the canine anterior cruciate ligament–deficient model).[174,175] These animal models represent secondary OA, produced by internal derangement of the joint, and therefore may not precisely simulate the state of affairs in primary OA. In a recent review, models for spontaneous osteoarthritis were reviewed and their preclinical utility was compared.[176] Of particular interest is an iodoacetate model, validated as the first pain model of osteoarthritis, in which intra-articular injection of iodoacetate in rats has been shown to lead to cartilage degeneration associated with pain and manifesting as time- and concentration-dependent alterations in hindlimb weight bearing.[177,178] That not all animal models of osteoarthritis are equivalent becomes clear when one considers the differences in therapeutic response between young and old animals and between spontaneous and surgical models.[179]

In the dog model, the first alteration seen within days after joint destabilization is an increase in cartilage water content.[180] Initially, water content increases locally, in the tibial plateau and femoral condyle cartilage, but it soon spreads to the entire joint cartilage. Proteoglycans are more readily extractable from the matrix of experimental animals than from that of controls, and this is reflected in the serum biomarker profile after acute injury in patients.[181] These matrix changes are also seen in spontaneously occurring dog and steer OA and in experimentally induced rabbit OA.[180,182,183] The increase in water content in osteoarthritic cartilage is due to loss of the collagen network's elastic

restraint, enabling the hydrophilic proteoglycans to swell more than normally.[184] In early-stage OA, proteoglycan concentration may increase and the cartilage may consequently become thicker than normal and exhibit increased staining for proteoglycans.[185-187] Shortly after the increase in cartilage water, newly synthesized proteoglycans are characterized by a higher proportion of chondroitin sulfate and a lower proportion of keratan sulfate and proteoglycan aggregation is impaired.[175,180] These abnormal changes in extracellular matrix occur before fibrillation or any other gross morphologic changes are evident and result in a generalized decrease in stiffness that occurs in grossly normal cartilage adjacent to fibrillated areas.[188] As OA progresses, focal cartilage ulcerations develop. Proteoglycan loss is accompanied by a decrease in its ability to aggregate, persistence in abnormal glycosaminoglycan composition, and a decrease in chondroitin sulfate chain length. Once proteoglycan loss reaches a critical threshold, water content, which initially increased, falls below normal.[189]

Chondrocyte Senescence

The term *senescence* was originally coined to describe the replicative limit of primary cells cultured in vitro, and the concept has evolved to include premature senescence or senescence-like changes in differentiated postmitotic cells. Senescent cells have a unique phenotype that affects both the proteins expressed by senescent cells and their responses to extracellular stimuli. Furthermore, the impact of senescence is not limited to the cells undergoing senescence; rather, the senescent cells have an impact on surrounding cells through the paracrine effects of the altered protein secretions.[190]

Premature chondrocyte senescence in OA is thought to be enhanced by oxidative injury.[191] The inflammatory cytokines IL-1β and TNF that are active in OA induce oxidative stress in chondrocytes, thereby contributing to the potential for oxidative injury that leads to senescence. Oxidative injury is also induced with excessive mechanical shear and injurious loading of explants, and this may contribute to the accumulation of senescent chondrocytes in aged cartilage.[192] TGF-β can influence both growth arrest and senescence in cultured cells, and senescent cells can overexpress TGF-β, but this effect has mostly been demonstrated in endothelial cells and not cells of mesenchymal origin. In summary, although it is clearly evident that many of the cellular mechanisms controlling senescence are also active in disease progression including OA, a causal link between senescence and OA has yet to be identified.

BIOMECHANICS AND DISEASE MECHANISMS OF OSTEOARTHRITIS

Biomechanical Changes

Two long-standing biomechanical theories of the pathogenesis of OA hold that mechanical stresses injure chondrocytes, causing them to release degradative enzymes, and that mechanical stresses initially damage the collagen network (as opposed to the cells per se)[193,194]—in either case, the result is that matrix breaks down. Extracellular matrix breakdown in osteoarthritic cartilage leads to (1) loss of compressive stiffness and elasticity, resulting in greater mechanical stress on chondrocytes; and (2) an increase in hydraulic permeability, resulting in loss of interstitial fluid during compression and increased diffusion of solutes through the matrix (including the movement of degradative enzymes and their inhibitors). One important consequence is disruption of normal fluid film joint lubrication and loading dynamics due to alterations in inflammatory synovial fluid.[195-197] Joint friction, wear, lubrication, and contact mechanics are further negatively affected by the loss of cartilage proteoglycans and superficial zone protein (also called *lubricin*).[198-202]

Response of Cartilage to Mechanical Injury

The response of normal articular cartilage to injury typically results in suboptimal repair; these injuries can often result in secondary OA.[203,204] Articular cartilage produces a repair tissue with neither the original structure nor properties of normal cartilage.[205-208] Chondrocytes in areas surrounding an injured zone are unable to migrate, proliferate, repopulate, or regenerate repair tissue with similar structure, function, and biomechanical properties of normal hyaline cartilage.[189,205,209]

That articular cartilage lacks regenerative power has a long history of documentation.[210] In 1851 Redfern reported that articular cartilage wounds healed with fibrous tissue, which he believed arose from chondrocyte intercellular substance.[211] Fisher and Ito in the 1920s proposed that cartilage repair is effected by fibrous tissue resulting from proliferation of cells from bone marrow, synovial membrane, and occasionally surrounding articular cartilage.[212,213] It was later observed that the fibrous tissue regenerate subsequently transforms into fibrocartilage, with occasional foci of imperfect hyaline cartilage.[214-217] The common findings of these investigators were that articular cartilage lacks regenerative potential and that the regenerative fibrous tissue and fibrocartilage tissue must have originated from undifferentiated mesenchymal tissue arising from bone marrow, synovium, or the superficial layer of articular cartilage.[210]

One reason the reparative process of cartilage significantly differs from those of other tissues is that it is avascular. The healing response in vascularized tissues consists of three main phases: necrosis, inflammation, and repair.[203,208] Cartilage undergoes the initial phase of necrosis in response to injury, although typically less cell death occurs than in vascularized tissues because of chondrocytes' relative insensitivity to hypoxia.[203,208] The inflammatory phase, primarily mediated (in other tissues) by the vascular system, is largely absent in partial-thickness injuries (i.e., lesions that do not cross the tidemark), and the repair phase is severely limited given the lack of vascularity and a preceding inflammatory response. Thus no local hyperemia results, no fibrin network is produced, no subsequent clot develops to act as a scaffold for the ingrowth of repair tissue, no mediators nor cytokines are released that can stimulate cellular migration and proliferation, and no inflammatory cells, which have mitotic and reparative potential, are recruited.[189,208] In lesions that do not cross the tidemark, the burden of repair falls on the chondrocytes[208] in a process that has been termed *intrinsic repair*.[218] Although fetal cartilage is capable of mitotic activity and replication, adult chondrocytes have little potential

for replication and intrinsic repair.[216,217] Articular cartilage lesions that cross the tidemark may undergo extrinsic repair via differentiation and proliferation of mesenchymal stem cells from para-articular connective tissues; typically, however, a fibrocartilaginous regenerate results.[218]

There are three categories of articular cartilage injury: (1) microdamage or repetitive trauma to the matrix and cells; (2) partial-thickness or superficial injuries or chondral fractures, articular surface injuries that do not penetrate the subchondral plate; and (3) osteochondral (full-thickness or deep penetrating) injuries, which extend through the tidemark and into the underlying subchondral bone.[203,205,208] The host response to each type of injury differs in both timing and quality of repair.

Microdamage to the chondrocytes and/or extracellular matrix without gross disruption of the articular surface can be caused by a single severe impact or repetitive blunt trauma.[203,205,208] Repetitive loading of rabbit cartilage produces a surface loss of proteoglycans and an increase in chondrocyte metabolic activity.[219] Proteoglycans become more easily extractable from the articular cartilage, with a greater percentage of nonaggregated forms.[189] The cellular, metabolic, and biochemical changes after repetitive blunt trauma resemble those in the early stages of OA: increased hydration; cellular degeneration and/or death; disruption of the collagen ultrastructure resulting in marked variation in the size and arrangements of fibers, fissuring and ulceration of the articular surface, thickening of the subchondral bone, and softening of the cartilage with loss of its compressive and tensile stiffness.[189,205,220-223] Trauma induces the release of degradative enzymes and proinflammatory factors (e.g., nitric oxide, TNF, IL-1) that frequently cause degradation of the surrounding matrix.[219,224,225] Eventually the material properties of the cartilage are altered—cartilage matrix thins and subchondral bone stiffens—which in turn often accelerate the degenerative process.[189] The point at which accumulated microdamage becomes irreversible is unknown, although it has been demonstrated that lost proteoglycans and matrix components may be restored if damage to chondrocytes and the collagen network is limited and the repetitive trauma halted.[205]

Necrosis of neighboring chondrocytes follows chondral fractures and superficial lacerations, injuries that do not cross the tidemark.[203,208,226] Within 48 to 72 hours, surviving chondrocytes bordering the defect exhibit increased synthesis rates of extracellular matrix molecules and type II collagen, sometimes accompanied by cell proliferation and formation of clusters or clones in the periphery of the injured zone.[189,208,226,227] The increased metabolism and mitotic activity is transient, however, and is followed by a fall in metabolic rate back to normal levels, typically resulting in a suboptimal repair.[189,208] Chondrocytes proliferating on the border of the injured zone do not migrate into the defect, which remains unfilled by the newly synthesized matrix.[189,205,209] In some cases, superficial lacerations in otherwise normal joints may not progress to full-thickness loss of cartilage or OA.[189]

Lesions that cross the articular cartilage tidemark and disrupt the underlying subchondral plate elicit the three-phase repair response normally encountered in vascularized tissues. A hematoma forms in the defect that becomes organized into a fibrin clot, activating an inflammatory response.

Transformation of the fibrin clot into vascular fibroblastic repair tissue[208,227] is accompanied by release of cytokines important in stimulating a repair response (e.g., TGF-β, platelet-derived growth factor, insulin-like growth factor, BMPs).[206] These cytokines help set in motion the recruitment, proliferation, and differentiation of undifferentiated cells into a fibrin network that serves as a scaffold for fibrocartilaginous repair tissue.[206,228,229] The origin of these mesenchymal stem cells has been determined to be the underlying bone marrow rather than the adjacent residual articular surface.[227,229,230] These cells progressively differentiate into chondroblasts, chondrocytes, and osteoblasts and synthesize cartilage and bone matrices. At 6 to 8 weeks postinjury, the repair tissue contains a high proportion of chondrocyte-like cells surrounded by a matrix consisting of proteoglycans and type II collagen, with a lesser amount of type I collagen.[230-232] Cells in the deeper layers of the defect differentiate into osteoblasts and subsequently undergo endochondral ossification to heal the subchondral bone defect.[189]

This regenerative tissue eventually undergoes a transformation to a more fibrocartilaginous repair accompanied by a shift in the synthesis of collagen from type II to type I.[209,226,228,229,232] Typically, within 1 year from injury, the repair tissue resembles a mixture of fibrocartilage and hyaline cartilage, with a substantial component (20% to 40%) of type I collagen.[231] The size of the osteochondral defect is an important factor in the quality of repair; as a general rule, the smaller the defect, the better the repair.[233] Depending on the joint, there exists a critical size defect that will not repair. Fibrocartilaginous repair is susceptible to early degenerative changes because it lacks the biomechanical properties to withstand normal physiologic joint loads.[229,231]

Mechanotransduction and Gene Expression

Chondrocytes can sense and respond to mechanical stimuli via several regulatory pathways (e.g., upstream signaling, transcription, translation, post-translational modification, vesicular transport).[234] Chondrocytes can remodel extracellular matrix in response to alterations in functional demand, as physical forces influence the synthesis, assembly, and degradation of the extracellular cartilage matrix. High magnitude or duration loads can also cause chondrocyte death and collagen damage, and chondrocytes in the superficial zone appear to be more vulnerable to load-induced injury than those in the middle and deep zones.[235,236] Normal stimuli help chondrocytes maintain the extracellular matrix; abnormal stimuli can disrupt this balance.

Mechanotransduction influences the cell-mediated feedback between physical stimuli, the molecular structure of newly synthesized matrix molecules, and the resulting biomechanical tissue properties.[237] Cell-matrix interactions via integrins are believed to be one of the important mediators in mechanotransduction in chondrocytes. In a study on the expression of COMP to long-term cyclic compression, it was found that uniaxial unconfined dynamic compression significantly upregulated COMP expression, which could be blocked by incubation with anti-α1-integrin antibodies.[238] Studies of bovine articular cartilage explants showed that cyclic loading increased protein synthesis by as much as 50% above free-swelling controls and had an inhibitory influence on proteoglycan synthesis, whereas static compression reduced biosynthetic activity.[239] Fibronectin and COMP were the most affected noncollagenous extracellular proteins; static compression caused a significant increase in fibronectin synthesis versus free-swelling control levels, and cyclic compression caused a significant increase in synthesis of COMP and fibronectin.

Human articular chondrocytes use the α5β1 integrin as a mechanoreceptor. Mechanical stimulation initiates a signal cascade involving stretch-activated ion channels, the actin cytoskeleton, and focal adhesion complex molecules.[240] The result is an anabolic response, manifested by increased aggrecan and decreased MMP-3 expression. Mechanical stimulation also activates Rho and Rho kinase pathways, which are linked to changes in the actin cytoskeleton.[241,242] Stimulation of the Rho/ROCK pathway in this context is an anabolic stimulus that leads to nuclear translocation and activation of Sox9, which is a "master regulator" of cartilage gene expression.[243] Indian hedgehog (Ihh) protein is a key signaling molecule that controls chondrocyte proliferation and differentiation and may also be an essential mediator of mechanotransduction in cartilage: Cyclic mechanical stress was shown to induce Ihh expression by chondrocytes.[244]

Dysregulation of these anabolic pathways is thought to contribute to the progression of OA. For example, although the α5β1 integrin is also mechanosensitive in OA chondrocytes, the downstream signaling pathways differ, leading instead to increased cartilage breakdown.[245] Integrins and integrin-associated signaling pathways are at least partly regulated by mechanical stimulation by activation of plasma membrane apamin-sensitive Ca2+-activated K+ channels; the result is membrane hyperpolarization after cyclic mechanical stimulation.[246] Chondrocytes from normal articular cartilage exhibit membrane hyperpolarization response to cyclic pressure-induced strain, whereas chondrocytes from osteoarthritic cartilage respond by membrane depolarization and exhibit no changes in aggrecan or MMP-3 messenger RNA following mechanical stimulation.[247,248] The different signaling pathways responding to mechanical stimulation in healthy versus OA chondrocytes may affect the disease outcome.

In addition to cell and matrix deformation, fluid flow is also sensed by chondrocytes. A study using a tissue shear-loading model to uncouple fluid flow from cell and matrix deformation demonstrated that deformation of cells and pericellular matrix alone stimulated protein and proteoglycan synthesis.[249]

ABNORMALITIES OF BONE

Osteophyte Formation

Osteophytes—bony proliferations at the joint margins and in the floor of cartilage lesions—are in part responsible for the pain and restriction of joint movement in OA. Human osteoarthritic joint osteophytes synthesize cartilage with significant amounts of type I collagen and nonaggregating proteoglycans.[250] In experimentally induced OA, osteophytes may develop even though the articular cartilage appears grossly normal.[251] Osteophytes may result from penetration of blood vessels into the basal layers of degenerating cartilage or as a result of abnormal healing of stress fractures in the subchondral trabeculae near the joint margins.[252,253] In the OA dog model, periarticular osteophyte formation begins in the marginal zone, where synovium merges with periosteum and articular cartilage, as early as 3 days after induction of knee instability.[254] Bony proliferation may result from venous congestion; in human hip OA, phlebography has demonstrated the formation of medullary varices, presumably due to changes in the medullary sinusoids, which may be compressed by subchondral cysts and thickened subchondral trabeculae.[255,256] Subchondral cysts in OA may be created by entry of synovial fluid under pressure through defects in the cartilage or may develop in necrotic areas of subchondral bone.[257] The increased venous pressure caused by the cysts and remodeled trabeculae may account for some of the pain in OA. Immobilization and glucocorticoids (but not bisphosphonates) have been shown to decrease the size and prevalence of osteophytes in experimental models of OA.[258-261]

Subchondral Bone Sclerosis

Increased remodeling and hardening of subchondral bone is evident early in osteoarthritis and can sometimes be detected before loss of cartilage thickness is evident radiologically.[262] An advancing tidemark of calcified cartilage is observed in OA, which changes the mechanical interface between subchondral bone and cartilage and is associated with increased subchondral vascularity. The increased calcification results in a thinning cartilage layer, which increases the mechanical stress in the adjacent cartilage. In combination with subchondral bone sclerosis, the altered mechanical environment and rapid bone remodeling may be contributing factors in cartilage degradation and OA pathogenesis.

Bone Marrow Lesions

Bone marrow lesions (detectable by MRI) are associated with OA, and studies suggest that they contribute to the pain felt by OA patients.[263] The presence of bone marrow lesions is predictive of OA progression, the development of cartilage defects and degradation, and the need for joint replacement.[264] The relationship between bone marrow lesions and cartilage degeneration in OA is still under investigation. For example, a longitudinal study also found that the presence of cartilage defects predicts progression of bone marrow lesions. The study authors suggest that it "remains unclear whether bone marrow lesions precede, accompany, or follow cartilage damage and volume loss in OA."[264]

Fibrosis and necrosis of the underlying bone marrow are common histologic features of the lesions visible by MRI, as are high bone turnover, altered trabecular structure, and edema. Unlike cartilage loss, bone marrow lesions are not a permanent structural change in OA. Several reports demonstrate that these lesions can resolve or at least regress, although it is more commonly observed that bone marrow lesion scores increase over time.[265] It has been postulated that edema-like lesions are less severe and reversible, whereas more advanced fibrotic and necrotic lesions are not.[266] There is a possibility that synovial fluid entering the subchondral bone marrow through intra-articular defects leads to an altered growth factor and cytokine environment that affects bone turnover. These findings suggest that there may be an altered biomechanical property of the subchondral tissues, which in turn would affect the biomechanical stresses experienced by the adjacent cartilage.

ROLE OF INFLAMMATORY MEDIATORS IN DISEASE PROGRESSION

Although levels of inflammatory cytokines such as IL-1, IL-6, and TNF are elevated in the serum of patients with knee osteoarthritis,[267] these and other classic inflammatory mediators are activated within the joint tissues themselves during the course of OA. These cytokines autocatalytically stimulate their own production and induce chondrocytes to produce proteases, chemokines, nitric oxide, and eicosanoids such as prostaglandins and leukotrienes. The action of these inflammatory mediators within cartilage is predominantly to drive catabolic pathways, inhibit matrix synthesis, and promote cellular apoptosis. Thus although osteoarthritis is not conventionally considered an inflammatory disease, "inflammatory" mediators from the affected tissues perpetuate disease progression and therefore represent potential targets for disease modification.

Inflammatory Molecules Produced by Articular Cartilage

Cytokines and Chemokines

A characteristic feature of established osteoarthritis is the increased production of proinflammatory cytokines such as IL-1β and TNF by articular chondrocytes. Both IL-1β and TNF exert comparable catabolic effects on chondrocyte metabolism, decreasing proteoglycan collagen synthesis and increasing aggrecan release via the induction of degradative proteases.[142,268-273] IL-1β and TNF also induce chondrocytes and synovial cells to produce other inflammatory mediators such as IL-8, IL-6, nitric oxide, and prostaglandin E_2. The actions of both cytokines are in part mediated by the activation of the transcription factor nuclear factor κB (NFκB), which further increases their own expression and that of other catabolic proteins such as inducible nitric oxide synthase and COX-2, thus creating an autocatalytic cascade that promotes self-destruction of articular cartilage[274-276] (Figure 98-3). Mounting evidence suggests that NFκB mediates chondrocytes' proinflammatory stress responses in OA and also controls these cells' differentiation, making NFκB activating factors attractive OA therapeutic targets for many reasons.[277]

IL-1β and TNF are both synthesized intracellularly as precursors, converted through proteolytic cleavage to their mature forms by caspases—membrane-bound IL-1β–converting enzyme (ICE) and TNF-converting enzyme (TACE)—and released extracellularly in their active forms.[278] The expression of both ICE and TACE has been shown to be upregulated in OA cartilage.[251-253] Inhibitors of both ICE and TACE are of interest as future therapeutic small-molecule antagonists of downstream IL-1β and TNF expression, respectively.

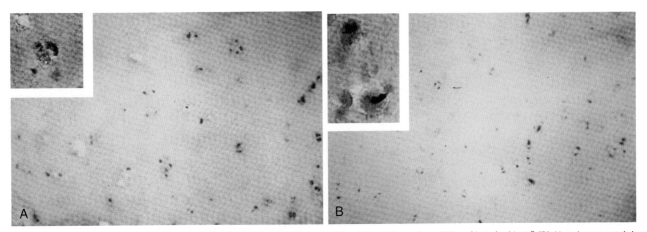

Figure 98-3 Immunostaining of osteoarthritic cartilage specimen for inducible nitric oxide synthase (**A**) and interleukin-1β (**B**). Note intense staining of chondrocytes in the superficial zones for both inflammatory proteins. *(From Melchiorri C, Meliconi R, Frizziero L, et al: Enhanced and coordinated in vivo expression of inflammatory cytokines and nitric oxide synthase by chondrocytes from patients with osteoarthritis, Arthritis Rheum 41:2165–2174, 1998.)*

The actions of IL-1 are dependent on the engagement of two specific cell surface receptors (IL-1Rs), designated type I and type II. The type I receptor, which spans the plasma membrane, is responsible for signal transduction, whereas the type II receptor is a "decoy" receptor, expressed at the cell membrane but unable to signal. A relative deficit of the ratio of IL-1Ra (the competitive inhibitor to the IL-1/IL-1R complex) to IL-1 has been described in OA synovial tissue, which may permit increased IL-1 activity.[279,280] Addition of IL-1Ra, or soluble type I and II IL-1 receptors, to OA explant cultures blocks prostaglandin E₂ (PGE₂) synthesis, collagenase production, and nitric oxide (NO) production[273,281]; addition of these antagonists in culture also results in an increase in aggrecan content, likely by inhibiting degradation of newly synthesized molecules.[282] One recent study showed that chondrocytes with abnormal morphology, from macroscopically intact cartilage representative of early OA, demonstrated increased levels of cell-associated IL-1 and loss of type VI collagen.[283]

Encouraging results with IL-1Ra have also been reported in vivo, where gene therapy or the intra-articular administration of IL-1Ra has been shown to retard the progression of OA in experimental animal models.[284,285] Other lines of evidence also point to IL-1β as an essential link in the pathogenesis of cartilage damage including proteoglycan loss by intra-articular injection of IL-1.[284] Clinical trials using IL-1β antagonists in OA are few and have been inconclusive. One multicenter trial with double-blinded doses of intra-articular IL-1Ra to 14 OA patients resulted in decreased pain without significant adverse events or acute injection reactions.[286] No long-term studies of structure-modifying effects of such therapies have been reported, however.

Osteoarthritic cartilage is also the site of increased production of both CXC and CC chemokines. These include IL-8, monocyte chemoattractant protein-1 (MCP-1), and RANTES (regulated on activation, normal T-cell expressed and secreted; aka CCL5) chemokine, as well as the receptors CCR-2 and CCR-5.[287-289] The expression of chemokines is low or undetectable in normal chondrocytes unless stimulated with cytokines such as IL-1 or IL-17.[290] Chemokines are detected by immunohistochemistry in the superficial and midzones of the tissue, as has been demonstrated for such other inflammatory mediators as inducible nitric oxide synthase (iNOS), IL-1β, and TNF.[288] RANTES induces expression of its own receptor, CCR-5, suggesting an autocrine/paracrine pathway of the chemokine within the cartilage. MCP-1 and RANTES promote chondrocyte catabolic activities including induction of nitric oxide synthase, increased MMP-3 expression, inhibition of proteoglycan synthesis, and enhancement of proteoglycan release.[288,291] Consistent with these effects, treatment of normal articular cartilage with RANTES increases the release of glycosaminoglycans and profoundly reduces the intensity of safranin O staining.[288]

Proteinases

A presumed key action of cytokines and chemokines produced in osteoarthritis is to promote cartilage proteolysis via the induction of a wide array of proteases, in particular MMPs. The two main families of MMP enzymes are (1) the collagenases that break down type II collagen (especially MMP-1, MMP-8, MMP-13, and MMP-28) and proteoglycans (MMP-3, which also cleaves pro-MMPs into their active forms) and (2) the aggrecanase (ADAMTS) family, which mediate aggregan degradation in cartilage.[173,184] Both families of MMPs are expressed in OA cartilage at lesional sites, where it is presumed that they play a major role in degradation of the extracellular matrix. A recent comprehensive analysis of specific metalloproteinases that are overexpressed by OA cartilage and synovium has revealed several MMPs and ADAMTSs that may be candidates as targets for disease modification.[143] Among the most interesting is MMP-13, which is overexpressed in murine and human OA cartilage and is the most efficient protease capable of cleaving type II collagen.[228,292] Similarly, the aggrecanase ADAMTS-5 has surfaced as the aggrecanase required for aggrecan loss in experimental OA[159] and inflammatory joint disease.[160] It has been demonstrated that mice lacking ADAMTS-5 are protected from developing OA.[159]

The expression and degradation of noncollagenous proteins and nonaggregating proteoglycans are also altered in OA cartilage and may have a direct or indirect effect on modulating the catabolic state of the chondrocyte.[293] These groups of molecules are likely to have important structural and/or biologic functions.[294,295] From their interactions with other extracellular matrix constituents, they can influence the supramolecular assembly of the cartilage matrix and as a result affect the physical properties of the tissue; by interacting directly with chondrocytes and/or neighboring cells, they can provide biologic signals on matrix properties and thereby influence cellular function.[296]

Nitric Oxide

Nitric oxide, produced by the inducible isoform of nitric oxide synthase (iNOS), is a major catabolic factor produced by chondrocytes in response to proinflammatory cytokines such as IL-1β and TNF.[287] Considerable evidence indicates that the overproduction of nitric oxide by chondrocytes plays a role in the perpetuation of cartilage destruction in OA[297-299] (Figure 98-4). Increased concentrations of nitrites have been demonstrated in the synovial fluid of patients with OA, and iNOS has been demonstrated in OA synoviocytes and chondrocytes by in situ hybridization and immunohistochemistry.[300,301] Although normal cartilage does not express iNOS or produce nitric oxide without stimulation by cytokines such as IL-1, OA cartilage explants spontaneously produce large amounts of nitric oxide[297]; iNOS is also upregulated from chondrocytes by cartilage compression.[302,303]

Nitric oxide exerts multiple effects on chondrocytes that promote articular cartilage degradation.[304] These include (1) inhibition of collagen and proteoglycan synthesis[304]; (2) activation of metalloproteinases[305]; (3) increased susceptibility to injury by other oxidants (e.g., H_2O_2)[306]; and (4) apoptosis.[304] Several studies have implicated nitric oxide as an important mediator in chondrocyte apoptosis, a feature common in progressive OA.[306,307] Immunohistochemistry of joint tissue obtained from patients with OA reveals

colocalization of iNOS protein and apoptosis in articular cartilage cells.[308] There is evidence that apoptosis results from the formation of peroxynitrite, a toxic free radical produced by the reaction of nitric oxide and superoxide anion. Peroxynitrite reacts with tyrosine residues on proteins, which can be detected by antibodies to nitrotyrosine. Immunostaining of OA cartilage reveals that chondrocytes that are highly positive for IL-1β also stain for nitrotyrosine, consistent with overproduction of peroxynitrate and oxidative damage.[301] The importance of nitric oxide has been corroborated in animal models of OA. In the Pond-Nuki canine model, the inhibition of nitric oxide reduced the progression of cartilage lesions.[309]

Transforming Growth Factor-β

In most respects, TGF-α acts as a counterregulatory molecule that opposes the effects of inflammatory mediators in cartilage. TGF-β₁ has been shown to downregulate proteolytic MMP-1 and MMP-13, as well as IL-1 and TNF receptors on OA chondrocytes.[310] TGF-β₂ selectively suppresses the cleavage of type II collagen by collagenases in OA cartilage in culture and limits MMP and proinflammatory cytokine expression.[268] Recent studies using the murine knee osteoarthritis model indicate that TGF-β₃ protects articular cartilage, as histologic staining for this molecule revealed a lack of TGF-β₃ in damaged cartilage in comparison with normals. Although premature osteophyte chondrocyte clusters express high levels of TGF-β₃, other data suggest that bone morphogenic protein 2 (BMP-2) is more responsible for the development of late osteophyte development.[311] Of note, TGF-β₁ may also exert selected catabolic effects via the stimulation of ADAMTS-4 expression.[310]

Hyaluronic Acid

Hyaluronic acid (HA) has been investigated as a marker of cartilage degradation that can be detected in synovial fluid and serum (see Biomarkers of Osteoarthritis later),[312] but it also appears to play a role in limiting the progression of arthritis. A recent study by Karna and colleagues found that HA in vitro counteracts the ability of IL-1β to inhibit collagen biosynthesis. At the transcriptional and posttranscriptional levels, chondrocyte cultures with IL-1β upregulated collagen synthesis markers, whereas HA negated this effect.[313] The same group found that HA similarly protects against IL-1–induced inhibition of collagen synthesis in human skin fibroblasts at the level of the insulin-like growth factor I receptor.[314]

Prostaglandins

The expression of inducible cyclooxygenase-2 (COX-2) is increased in OA chondrocytes, which spontaneously produce PGE₂ ex vivo.[289] The effects of prostaglandins on chondrocyte metabolism are complex, and include enhanced type II collagen synthesis, activation of metalloproteinases, and promotion of apoptosis.[315] In cartilage explants, IL-1β induces COX-2 expression and PGE₂ production coordinates with proteoglycan degradation. COX-2 inhibition prevents IL-1β–induced proteoglycan degradation, which can be reversed by the addition of PGE₂ to cultures.[316] In

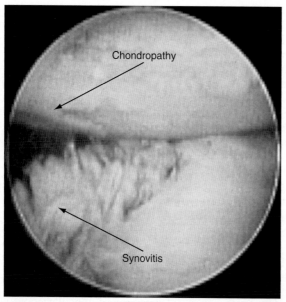

Figure 98-4 Arthroscopic view of osteoarthritic lesion of the femoral condyle (designated chondropathy). Note that proliferative synovitis is localized to the area of the osteoarthritic lesion. *(Courtesy Maxime Dougados.)*

contrast, in vitro evidence has accumulated that selected nonsteroidal anti-inflammatory drugs (NSAIDs) may interfere with proteoglycan synthesis.[317] Of note, another study concluded that up to 30% of PGE$_2$ expression in OA synovial tissue stems from the COX-1 pathway.[318] Whether any differences exist between the effects of COX-1– and COX-2–derived prostaglandins on cartilage metabolism is unknown.

F-spondin

A novel mediator in OA cartilage, F-spondin is a neuronal extracellular matrix glycoprotein that appears to regulate cartilage degradation through the TGF-β and PGE$_2$ pathways. One recent article reported a sevenfold increase in expression in human OA cartilage and a significant upregulation in knee cartilage surgical specimens from rats with OA. Addition of F-spondin in vitro to OA cartilage tissue led to increased levels of activated TGF-β and production of PGE$_2$, as well as accelerated collagen degradation and reduced proteoglycan synthesis, which are both dependent on these two molecules.[319]

Alterations in Bone

The inflammatory mediators produced by bone in OA are less well understood than those produced by cartilage and synovium. Biomechanical and biochemical factors seem to influence the remodeling, but the underlying pathogenesis has yet to be identified. Nitric oxide plays a role in bone cell function, which could have implications for OA insofar as it contributes to alterations in subchondral bone. The endothelial isoform, endothelial cell nitric oxide synthase (ecNOS), is constitutively expressed in bone, where it seems to play a key role in regulating osteoblast activity and bone formation. ecNOS also mediates the effects of mechanical loading on the skeleton, where it acts along with prostaglandins to promote bone formation and suppress bone resorption.[320] In contrast, such proinflammatory cytokines as IL-1 and TNF induce iNOS in bone cells, and NO derived from this pathway potentiates bone loss.[287] Osteophyte formation and subchondral bone remodeling likely result from local production of anabolic growth factors such as insulin-like growth factor 1 (IGF-1) and mostly TGF-β, which is highly expressed in osteophytes of the femoral head in OA patients.[321,322] Areas of increased radionuclide uptake ("hot spots") on bone scintigraphy have also been reported to identify OA joints more likely to progress by radiographic criteria—and/or to require surgical intervention—over a 5-year period.[216]

Alterations in Synovial Tissue

Synovial lining inflammation and synovial effusions have emerged as another key feature of OA pathophysiology. OA has traditionally been classified as a noninflammatory arthritis, largely because the synovial fluid leukocyte count in OA is typically fewer than 2000 cells/mm^3. Such parameters can be misleading because low-grade inflammatory processes nevertheless occur in osteoarthritic synovial tissues and contribute to disease pathogenesis, and some degree of synovitis has been observed even in early OA.

This localized synovitis may be subclinical because arthroscopic studies suggest that localized proliferative and inflammatory changes of the synovium occur in up to 50% of OA patients, and the activated synovium may produce proteases and cytokines that accelerate damage to the adjacent cartilage.[323] More recently, musculoskeletal ultrasound has provided a reliable noninvasive method to detect both synovial hypertrophy and even small effusions in OA patients, using both grayscale and power Doppler methods.[324]

Many of the clinical symptoms and signs seen in OA joints (e.g., joint swelling and effusion, stiffness, occasionally redness) reflect synovial inflammation. Synovial histologic changes include synovial hypertrophy and hyperplasia with an increased number of lining cells, often accompanied by infiltration of the sublining tissue with scattered foci of lymphocytes. In contrast to rheumatoid arthritis (RA), synovial inflammation in OA is mostly confined to areas adjacent to pathologically damaged cartilage and bone. This activated synovium can release proteinases and cytokines that may accelerate destruction of nearby cartilage.[322] Although synovial macrophages and macrophage-produced mediators result in key inflammatory cascades and cartilage destruction in both OA and RA, it appears there may be differences between the diseases in levels of the cytokines and how they mediate destruction of the cartilage.[325]

As described earlier, the metalloproteinases that degrade cartilage are produced not only by the cartilage itself but also by the synovium. Although cartilage destruction might be directed by the chondrocytes, some degree of synovitis exists in patients even with mild OA. A comprehensive analysis by Davidson and colleagues reported several proinflammatory genes significantly elevated in the synovium that had not previously been reported.[143] Cartilage breakdown products, derived from the articular surface as a result of mechanical or enzymatic destruction of the cartilage, can provoke the release of collagenase and other hydrolytic enzymes from synovial cells and macrophages (Figure 98-5).[326,327] Cartilage breakdown products are also believed to result in mononuclear cell infiltration and vascular hyperplasia in the synovial membrane in OA.[328-330]

A consequence of the low-grade inflammatory processes is the induction of synovial IL-1β and TNF, which are likely contributors to the degradative cascade.[287] There are also reports of increased numbers of immune cells in synovial tissue including activated B cells and T lymphocytes, as well as evidence that OA patients express cellular immunity to the cartilage proteoglycan link protein and C1 domain.[331,332] Histologic changes in OA synovium usually demonstrate mild or moderate synovitis characterized by an increase in the number of inflammatory mononuclear cells in the sublining tissue including activated B cells and T lymphocytes.[333-338]

A recent study of 10 patients with early OA (arthroscopic specimens) and 15 patients undergoing total knee arthroplasty revealed that synovial tissues from early OA had higher levels of IL-1β and TNF and increased mononuclear cell infiltration compared with late OA.[339]

Along the lines of acute episodes of OA, the inflammation may result from crystal-induced synovitis (either calcium apatite or calcium pyrophosphate dihydrate). "Milwaukee shoulder syndrome" represents a rapidly destructive form of OA with evidence of inflammation in the synovial

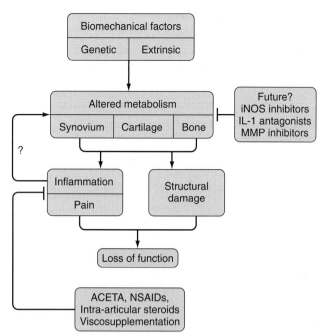

Figure 98-5 Multiple factors that predispose to, initiate, and perpetuate osteoarthritis. In the future, structure-modifying treatments will be targeted to the biochemical processes that promote disease progression. ACETA, acetaminophen; IL-1, interleukin-1; iNOS, inducible nitric oxide synthase; MMP, matrix metalloproteinase; NSAIDs, nonsteroidal anti-inflammatory drugs.

membrane but minimal synovial fluid leukocytosis. It is typically associated with rotator cuff degeneration, severe shoulder OA, and hydroxyapatite crystal deposition in the synovial membrane.[340] The synovial fluid typically contains few cells and high levels of active collagenase. It is theorized that crystals released from the degenerating tendons trigger the release of collagenase from synovial mononuclear cells that leads to cartilage breakdown; cartilage breakdown products then further activate release of enzymes from the synovium. This inflammation is typically associated with increases in synovial IL-1 and TNF that further proteinate the degradative cascade.[341]

Biomarkers of Osteoarthritis

The aims of biomarker research in OA are early detection before irreversible damage occurs, predicting OA progression, and monitoring response to therapeutic intervention.[342] The OA Biomarkers Network, funded by the National Institutes of Health, has established the "BIPED" biomarker classification with five separate categories of surrogate markers: **b**urden of disease, **i**nvestigative, **p**rognostic, **e**fficacy of intervention, and **d**iagnostic.[322] Examples of burden of disease and prognosis for hip and knee OA include serum COMP, serum hyaluronic acid, and urinary CTXII.[343] A recent survey revealed that this classification scheme was not adopted as often as anticipated, and therefore the authors undertook a systematic review of the primary OA biomarker literature to standardize the findings according to the BIPED classification.[344]

The major structural components in cartilage are type II collagen and aggrecan, which are relatively unique to cartilage. Additional constituents of articular cartilage include the proteins COMP, cartilage intermediate layer protein (CILP), cartilage link protein, matrilin, minor collagens (types I, V, VI, IX, and XI), and hyaluronic acid. In healthy cartilage these molecules have a relatively slow turnover rate, whereas OA is characterized by enhanced synthesis and enzymatic degradation of most of these molecules. Therefore much focus in OA biomarkers has been on detecting markers of cartilage matrix synthesis and degradation.[345] The biomarkers have been made more specific through the detection of "neo-epitopes," or degraded cartilage matrix fragments generated by specific proteases enhanced in OA. The turnover of subchondral bone is also enhanced in OA, although biomarkers of bone turnover have proven less specific in identifying OA, perhaps because of the continuous bone remodeling in the skeleton as a whole. In addition to markers of matrix degradation and turnover, recent advances in the proteomics and microRNA fields have enabled detection of new OA biomarkers using unbiased screening of serum constituents in arthritic patients.[128] The slow progression of primary OA is causing researchers to refocus the search for OA biomarkers on more rapidly progressing secondary OA after acute injury.[181]

One study of 62 patients with knee OA compared MRI findings at baseline and 1 year, as well as levels of serum hyaluronic acid, osteocalcin, cartilage glycoprotein 39, COMP, and urine C-telopeptide of type II collagen. The researchers suggested that a single measurement of serum HA or short-term increases in urine CTXII would identify patients at greatest risk for progression of OA.[346]

Although OA is not considered an inflammatory disease in the traditional sense, it definitely involves inflammatory processes, and these hold promise as biomarkers for OA. For example, elevated levels of the inflammatory marker C-reactive protein (CRP) appear to be predictive of radiographic progression of long-term knee OA.[287] In a study of 1025 women, higher levels of serum CRP were associated with a statistically significant increase in both prevalent and incident knee OA and greater knee OA severity; women with bilateral knee OA had higher CRP levels than those with unilateral knee OA. Compared with women who did not develop knee OA, those who did had a higher baseline CRP than at their index test 2.5 years earlier.[347] In another study of women (age 44 to 67 years), CRP levels were statistically greater in 105 women with knee OA than in 740 women without OA. These results must be interpreted with caution because a recent study concluded that after adjustment of CRP levels to the patient's body mass index, serum CRP levels were no longer correlated to OA.[348] In summary, these and other studies report that inflammation markers such as CRP are modestly but significantly increased in early knee OA and can be predictive of OA that will progress over time.[89]

Several studies have identified COMP levels as helpful assessors of the potential for, presence of, and progression of OA.[349,350] This noncollagenous extracellular matrix protein, synthesized by both cartilage and synovium with TGF-β₁ stimulation,[351] is abundant in articular cartilage.[352-355] Both the degradation and tissue distribution of COMP exhibit marked differences in normal and OA human knee articular cartilage. Synovial fluid COMP levels are higher in individuals with knee pain or injury,[356] anterior cruciate ligament or meniscal injuury,[356,357] and OA[356,358] than in demographically matched healthy individuals. Similarly, serum levels of COMP are often higher in patients with more rapidly progressive joint damage,[275,289,291] with some studies showing this specifically in hip OA[293,359] and knee OA.[290] Although COMP is one of the most useful serum markers for OA, the lack of specificity to OA and relatively high natural variations in serum COMP levels currently necessitate use of additional markers. The development of specific reagents to detect degradative products of COMP may increase its utility as an OA biomarker.[350] As with other biomarkers based on anabolic and catabolic processes in cartilage, serum COMP levels indicate a specific stage of OA.

Hyaluronic acid (HA) is a marker of cartilage degradation that can be detected in synovial fluid and serum,[312] even though the majority of circulating HA originates from extracartilaginous sources. HA levels reflect synovial activity, whereas proteoglycan levels reflect cartilage turnover.[312,360] In addition, higher serum HA levels have been correlated with the number of joints involved and degree of clinical disability. These findings support the theory that serum HA levels reflect synovial hyperactivity. An animal model in which the anterior cruciate ligament was transected to induce OA also demonstrated a rise in serum HA level within 7 days after joint injury, a rise sustained at 13 weeks; the rise in synovial fluid HA levels correlated with serum levels.[361] Serum HA levels, which may also serve as a predictor of OA disease progression,[293,362] correlated with radiographic evidence of disease progression over a 5-year time interval because patients whose disease progressed had higher levels than at the outset.[343]

SUMMARY

Osteoarthritis, although classically conceived of as a degenerative consequence of aging, is a disease with an increasingly well-characterized molecular pathophysiology. Biomechanical factors, particularly in the context of genetic predisposition, obesity, and malalignment, result in chemical alterations within the joint that promote cartilage degradation. Early, anabolic changes, characterized by proliferation of chondrocytes and increased matrix production, are followed by a predominantly catabolic state, characterized by decreased matrix synthesis, increased proteolytic degradation of matrix, and chondrocyte apoptosis. Many of the features of the chondrocyte in the catabolic state are related to the production of inflammatory mediators by synovium and chondrocytes that act locally to perpetuate cartilage degradation. Although current treatments improve the signs and symptoms of disease, further characterization of the altered metabolism in synovium, cartilage, and bone that promote disease progression should lead to future treatments that prevent structural damage in osteoarthritis.

Selected References

2. Sarzi-Puttini P, Cimmino MA, Scarpa R, et al: Osteoarthritis: an overview of the disease and its treatment strategies, *Semin Arthritis Rheum* 35(1 Suppl 1):1–10, 2005.
9. Robertson CM, Pennock AT, Harwood FL, et al: Characterization of pro-apoptotic and matrix-degradative gene expression following induction of osteoarthritis in mature and aged rabbits, *Osteoarthritis Cartil* 14(5):471–476, 2006.

21. Iannone F, Lapadula G: Obesity and inflammation—targets for OA therapy, *Curr Drug Targets* 11(5):586–598, 2010.
22. Sowers MR, Karvonen-Gutierrez CA: The evolving role of obesity in knee osteoarthritis, *Curr Opin Rheumatol* 22(5):533–537, 2010.
36. Hu K, Xu L, Cao L, et al: Pathogenesis of osteoarthritis-like changes in the joints of mice deficient in type IX collagen, *Arthritis Rheum* 54(9):2891–2900, 2006.
39. Sokoloff L: *The biology of degenerative joint disease*. Chicago, 1969, University of Chicago Press.
44. Abramson SB, Attur M: Developments in the scientific understanding of osteoarthritis, *Arthritis Res Ther* 11(3):227, 2009.
60. Thelin N, Holmberg S, Thelin A: Knee injuries account for the sports-related increased risk of knee osteoarthritis, *Scand J Med Sci Sports* 16(5):329–333, 2006.
70. Dillon CF, Rasch EK, Gu Q, Hirsch R: Prevalence of knee osteoarthritis in the United States: arthritis data from the Third National Health and Nutrition Examination Survey 1991-94, *J Rheumatol* 33(11):2271–2279, 2006.
71. Ushiyama T, Ueyama H, Inoue K, et al: Expression of genes for estrogen receptors alpha and beta in human articular chondrocytes, *Osteoarthritis Cartil* 7(6):560–566, 1999.
83. Buckwalter JA, Mankin HJ, Grodzinsky AJ: Articular cartilage and osteoarthritis, *Instr Course Lect* 54:465–480, 2005.
84. Grogan SP, Miyaki S, Asahara H, et al: Mesenchymal progenitor cell markers in human articular cartilage: normal distribution and changes in osteoarthritis, *Arthritis Res Ther* 11(3):R85, 2009.
85. Lotz MK, Otsuki S, Grogan SP, Sah R, Terkeltaub R, D'Lima D: Cartilage cell clusters, *Arthritis Rheum* 62(8):2206–2218, 2010.
86. van der Kraan PM, Blaney Davidson EN, van den Berg WB: Bone morphogenetic proteins and articular cartilage: to serve and protect or a wolf in sheep's clothing? *Osteoarthritis Cartil* 18(6):735–741, 2010.
87. Pottenger LA, Phillips FM, Draganich LF: The effect of marginal osteophytes on reduction of varus-valgus instability in osteoarthritic knees, *Arthritis Rheum* 33(6):853–858, 1990.
88. Danielsson LG: Incidence and prognosis of coxarthrosis, *Clin Orthop* 1993(287):13–18, 1964.
90. Davidson ENB, Vitters EL, van Beuningen HM, et al: Resemblance of osteophytes in experimental osteoarthritis to transforming growth factor β-induced osteophytes: limited role of bone morphogenetic protein in early osteoarthritic osteophyte formation, *Arthritis Rheum* 56(12):4065–4073, 2007.
92. Hunziker E: Quantitative structural organization of normal adult human articular cartilage, *Osteoarthritis Cartil* 10(7):564–572, 2002.
94. Levine B, Mizushima N, Virgin HW: Autophagy in immunity and inflammation, *Nature* 469(7330):323–335, 2011.
95. Caramés B, Taniguchi N, Otsuki S, et al: Autophagy is a protective mechanism in normal cartilage, and its aging-related loss is linked with cell death and osteoarthritis, *Arthritis Rheum* 62(3):791–801, 2010.
96. Maroudas AI: Balance between swelling pressure and collagen tension in normal and degenerate cartilage, *Nature* 260(5554):808–809, 1976.
98. Mankin HJ, Brandt KD: Biochemistry and metabolism of articular cartilage in osteoarthritis. In Moskowitz RW, Howell DS, Goldberg VM, et al, editors: *Osteoarthritis: diagnosis and medical/surgical management*, ed 2, Philadelphia, 1992, WB Saunders, pp 109–154.
102. Inerot S, Heinegard D, Audell L, Olsson SE: Articular-cartilage proteoglycans in aging and osteoarthritis, *Biochem J* 169(1):143–156, 1978.
104. Mankin HJ, Dorfman H, Lippiello L, Zarins A: Biochemical and metabolic abnormalities in articular cartilage from osteo-arthritic human hips. II. Correlation of morphology with biochemical and metabolic data, *J Bone Joint Surg Am* 53(3):523–537, 1971.
105. Goldring MB, Otero M, Tsuchimochi K, et al: Defining the roles of inflammatory and anabolic cytokines in cartilage metabolism, *Ann Rheum Dis* 67(Suppl 3):iii75–iii82, 2008.
106. Xu L, Servais J, Polur I, et al: Attenuation of osteoarthritis progression by reduction of discoidin domain receptor 2 in mice, *Arthritis Rheum* 62(9):2736–2744, 2010.
108. Rosenthal AK: Calcium crystal deposition and osteoarthritis, *Rheum Dis Clin North Am* 32(2):401–412, vii, 2006.
109. Wu CW, Terkeltaub R, Kalunian KC: Calcium-containing crystals and osteoarthritis: implications for the clinician, *Curr Rheumatol Rep* 7(3):213–219, 2005.

111. Howell DS, Muniz OE, Morales S. 5' Nucleotidase and pyrophosphate (Ppi)-generating activities in articular cartilage extracts in calcium pyrophosphate deposition disease (CPPD) and in primary osteoarthritis (OA). In Peyron JG, editor: *Epidemiology of osteoarthritis*. Paris, 1980, Ciba-Geigy, p 99.

116. Umlauf D, Frank S, Pap T, Bertrand J: Cartilage biology, pathology, and repair, *Cell Mol Life Sci* 67(24):4197–4211, 2010.

119. Teshima R, Treadwell BV, Trahan CA, Mankin HJ: Comparative rates of proteoglycan synthesis and size of proteoglycans in normal and osteoarthritic chondrocytes, *Arthritis Rheum* 26(10):1225–1230, 1983.

120. Derynck R, Miyazono Ko: *The TGF-[beta] family*. Cold Spring Harbor, NY, 2007, Cold Spring Harbor Laboratory Press.

121. Blaney Davidson EN, van der Kraan PM, van den Berg WB: TGF-β and osteoarthritis, *Osteoarthritis Cartil* 15(6):597–604, 2007.

122. Nakajima M, Kizawa H, Saitoh M, et al: Mechanisms for asporin function and regulation in articular cartilage, *J Biol Chem* 282(44):32185–32192, 2007.

123. van der Kraan PM, Blaney Davidson EN, van den Berg WB: A role for age-related changes in TGFbeta signaling in aberrant chondrocyte differentiation and osteoarthritis, *Arthritis Res Ther* 12(1):201, 2010.

124. Reddi AH: Bone morphogenetic proteins: from basic science to clinical applications, *J Bone Joint Surg Am* 83A(Suppl 1, Part 1):S1–S6, 2001.

125. Egli RJ, Southam L, Wilkins JM, et al: Functional analysis of the osteoarthritis susceptibility-associated GDF5 regulatory polymorphism, *Arthritis Rheum* 60(7):2055–2064, 2009.

126. Lories RJU, Luyten FP: Bone morphogenetic protein signaling and arthritis, *Cytokine Growth Factor Rev* 20(5-6):467–473, 2009.

128. Koutsopoulos S, Iliopoulos D, Malizos KN, et al: Integrative microRNA and proteomic approaches identify novel osteoarthritis genes and their collaborative metabolic and inflammatory networks, *PLoS One* 3(11):e3740, 2008.

129. Loeser RF, Im HJ, Richardson B, et al: Methylation of the OP-1 promoter: potential role in the age-related decline in OP-1 expression in cartilage, *Osteoarthritis Cartil* 17(4):513–517, 2009.

130. Hunter DJ, Pike MC, Jonas BL, et al: Phase 1 safety and tolerability study of BMP-7 in symptomatic knee osteoarthritis, *BMC Musculoskelet Disord* 11(1):232, 2010.

132. Ollivierre F, Gubler U, Towle CA, et al: Expression of IL-1 genes in human and bovine chondrocytes: a mechanism for autocrine control of cartilage matrix degradation, *Biochem Biophys Res Commun* 141(3):904–911, 1986.

136. Ratcliffe A, Tyler JA, Hardingham TE: Articular cartilage cultured with interleukin 1. Increased release of link protein, hyaluronate-binding region and other proteoglycan fragments, *Biochem J* 238(2):571–580, 1986.

138. Yang S, Kim J, Ryu J-H, et al: Hypoxia-inducible factor-2α is a catabolic regulator of osteoarthritic cartilage destruction, *Nature Med* 16(6):687–693, 2010.

139. Husa M, Liu-Bryan R, Terkeltaub R: Shifting HIFs in osteoarthritis, *Nature Med* 16(6):641–644, 2010.

140. Mort JS, Billington CJ: Articular cartilage and changes in arthritis: matrix degradation, *Arthritis Res* 3(6):337–341, 2001.

144. Hedbom E, Hauselmann HJ: Molecular aspects of pathogenesis in osteoarthritis: the role of inflammation, *Cell Mol Life Sci* 59(1):45–53, 2002.

145. Akhtar N, Rasheed Z, Ramamurthy S, et al: MicroRNA-27b regulates the expression of matrix metalloproteinase 13 in human osteoarthritis chondrocytes, *Arthritis Rheum* 62(5):1361–1371, 2010.

146. Miyaki S, Nakasa T, Otsuki S, et al: MicroRNA-140 is expressed in differentiated human articular chondrocytes and modulates interleukin-1 responses, *Arthritis Rheum* 60(9):2723–2730, 2009.

148. Sapolsky AI, Howell DS: Further characterization of a neutral metalloprotease isolated from human articular cartilage, *Arthritis Rheum* 25(8):981–988, 1982.

149. Tallant C, Marrero A, Gomis-Ruth FX: Matrix metalloproteinases: fold and function of their catalytic domains, *Biochim Biophys Acta* 1803(1):20–28, 2010.

150. Little CB, Hughes CE, Curtis CL, et al: Matrix metalloproteinases are involved in C-terminal and interglobular domain processing of cartilage aggrecan in late stage cartilage degradation, *Matrix Biol* 21(3):271–288, 2002.

151. Knauper V, Lopez-Otin C, Smith B, et al: Biochemical characterization of human collagenase-3, *J Biol Chem* 271(3):1544–1550, 1996.

152. Little CB, Barai A, Burkhardt D, et al: Matrix metalloproteinase 13-deficient mice are resistant to osteoarthritic cartilage erosion but not chondrocyte hypertrophy or osteophyte development, *Arthritis Rheum* 60(12):3723–3733, 2009.

155. Ehrlich MG, Houle PA, Vigliani G, Mankin HJ: Correlation between articular cartilage collagenase activity and osteoarthritis, *Arthritis Rheum* 21(7):761–766, 1978.

156. Tang BL: ADAMTS: a novel family of extracellular matrix proteases, *Int J Biochem Cell Biol* 33(1):33–44, 2001.

158. Yatabe T, Mochizuki S, Takizawa M, et al: Hyaluronan inhibits expression of ADAMTS4 (aggrecanase-1) in human osteoarthritic chondrocytes, *Ann Rheum Dis* 68(6):1051–1058, 2009.

159. Glasson SS, Askew R, Sheppard B, et al: Deletion of active ADAMTS5 prevents cartilage degradation in a murine model of osteoarthritis, *Nature* 434(7033):644–648, 2005.

160. East CJ, Stanton H, Golub SB, et al: ADAMTS-5 deficiency does not block aggrecanolysis at preferred cleavage sites in the chondroitin sulfate-rich region of aggrecan, *J Biol Chem* 282(12):8632–8640, 2007.

162. Tortorella MD, Malfait F, Barve RA, et al: A review of the ADAMTS family, pharmaceutical targets of the future, *Curr Pharm Des* 15(20):2359–2374, 2009.

163. Liu CJ, Kong W, Ilalov K, et al: ADAMTS-7: a metalloproteinase that directly binds to and degrades cartilage oligomeric matrix protein, *FASEB J* 20(7):988–990, 2006.

164. Liu CJ, Kong W, Xu K, et al: ADAMTS-12 associates with and degrades cartilage oligomeric matrix protein, *J Biol Chem* 281(23):15800–15808, 2006.

167. Bastow ER, Byers S, Golub SB, et al: Hyaluronan synthesis and degradation in cartilage and bone, *Cell Mol Life Sci* 65(3):395–413, 2007.

173. Kevorkian L, Young DA, Darrah C, et al: Expression profiling of metalloproteinases and their inhibitors in cartilage, *Arthritis Rheum* 50(1):131–141, 2004.

176. Poole R, Blake S, Buschmann M, et al: Recommendations for the use of preclinical models in the study and treatment of osteoarthritis, *Osteoarthritis Cartil* 18(Suppl 3):S10–S16, 2010.

178. Pomonis JD, Boulet JM, Gottshall SL, et al: Development and pharmacological characterization of a rat model of osteoarthritis pain, *Pain* 114(3):339–346, 2005.

179. Ameye LG, Young MF: Animal models of osteoarthritis: lessons learned while seeking the "Holy Grail", *Curr Opin Rheumatol* 18(5):537–547, 2006.

181. Catterall JB, Stabler TV, Flannery CR, Kraus VB: Changes in serum and synovial fluid biomarkers after acute injury (NCT00332254), *Arthritis Res Ther* 12(6):R229, 2010.

189. Mankin HJ, Mow VC, Buckwalter JA, et al: Form and function of articular cartilage. In Simon S, editor: *Orthopaedic basic science*. Chicago, 1994, American Academy of Orthopaedic Surgeons, pp 1–44.

190. Muller M: Cellular senescence: molecular mechanisms, in vivo significance, and redox considerations, *Antioxidants Redox Signaling*. 11(1):59–98, 2009.

191. Krasnokutsky S, Attur M, Palmer G, et al: Current concepts in the pathogenesis of osteoarthritis, *Osteoarthritis Cartil* 16:S1–S3, 2008.

195. Hlavacek M: The role of synovial fluid filtration by cartilage in lubrication of synovial joints—I. Mixture model of synovial fluid, *J Biomech* 26(10):1145–1150, 1993.

196. Mow VC, Ateshian GA, Spilker RL: Biomechanics of diarthrodial joints: a review of twenty years of progress, *J Biomech Eng* 115(4B):460–467, 1993.

198. Neu CP, Reddi AH, Komvopoulos K, et al: Increased friction coefficient and superficial zone protein expression in patients with advanced osteoarthritis, *Arthritis Rheum* 62(9):2680–2687, 2010.

202. Hlavacek M: The influence of the acetabular labrum seal, intact articular superficial zone and synovial fluid thixotropy on squeeze-film lubrication of a spherical synovial joint, *J Biomech* 35(10):1325–1335, 2002.

203. Chen FS, Frenkel SR, Di Cesare PE: Repair of articular cartilage defects: part I. Basic science of cartilage healing, *Am J Orthop* 28(1):31–33, 1999.

204. Frenkel SR, Di Cesare PE: Degradation and repair of articular cartilage, *Front Biosci* 4:D671–D685, 1999.

208. Mankin HJ: The response of articular cartilage to mechanical injury, *J Bone Joint Surg Am* 64(3):460–466, 1982.

212. Fisher T: Some researches into the physiological principles underlying the treatment of injuries and diseases of the articulations, *Lancet* 2:541–548, 1923.

218. Grande DA, Singh IJ, Pugh J: Healing of experimentally produced lesions in articular cartilage following chondrocyte transplantation, *Anat Rec* 218(2):142–148, 1987.

220. Poulet B, Hamilton RW, Shefelbine S, Pitsillides AA: Characterizing a novel and adjustable noninvasive murine joint loading model, *Arthritis Rheum* 63(1):137–147, 2011.

223. Lee SH, Abramson SA: Stepped-care guide to osteoarthritis therapy, *Orthop Spec Ed* 2(2):7–10, 1996.

231. Furukawa T, Eyre DR, Koide S, Glimcher MJ: Biochemical studies on repair cartilage resurfacing experimental defects in the rabbit knee, *J Bone Joint Surg Am* 62(1):79–89, 1980.

236. Lin PM, Chen CT, Torzilli PA: Increased stromelysin-1 (MMP-3), proteoglycan degradation (3B3- and 7D4) and collagen damage in cyclically load-injured articular cartilage, *Osteoarthritis Cartil* 12(6):485–496, 2004.

237. Grodzinsky AJ, Levenston ME, Jin M, Frank EH: Cartilage tissue remodeling in response to mechanical forces, *Annu Rev Biomed Eng* 2:691–713, 2000.

241. Haudenschild DR, Nguyen B, Chen J, et al: Rho kinase-dependent CCL20 induced by dynamic compression of human chondrocytes, *Arthritis Rheum* 58(9):2735–2742, 2008.

242. Haudenschild DR, D'Lima DD, Lotz MK: Dynamic compression of chondrocytes induces a Rho kinase-dependent reorganization of the actin cytoskeleton, *Biorheology* 45(3-4):219–228, 2008.

243. Haudenschild DR, Chen J, Pang N, et al: Rho kinase-dependent activation of SOX9 in chondrocytes, *Arthritis Rheum* 62(1):191–200, 2010.

248. Millward-Sadler SJ, Wright MO, Lee H, et al: Altered electrophysiological responses to mechanical stimulation and abnormal signalling through alpha5beta1 integrin in chondrocytes from osteoarthritic cartilage, *Osteoarthritis Cartil* 8(4):272–278, 2000.

262. Goldring MB, Goldring SR: Articular cartilage and subchondral bone in the pathogenesis of osteoarthritis, *Ann N Y Acad Sci* 1192(1):230–237, 2010.

264. Dore D, Martens A, Quinn S, et al: Bone marrow lesions predict site-specific cartilage defect development and volume loss: a prospective study in older adults, *Arthritis Res Ther* 12(6):R222, 2010.

265. Daheshia M, Yao JQ: The bone marrow lesion in osteoarthritis, *Rheumatol Int* 31(2):143–148, 2010.

266. Leydet-Quilici H, Le Corroller T, Bouvier C, et al: Advanced hip osteoarthritis: magnetic resonance imaging aspects and histopathology correlations, *Osteoarthritis Cartil* 18(11):1429–1435, 2010.

267. Stannus O, Jones G, Cicuttini F, et al: Circulating levels of IL-6 and TNFalpha are associated with knee radiographic osteoarthritis and knee cartilage loss in older adults, *Osteoarthritis Cartil* 18(11):1441–1447, 2010.

268. Tchetina EV, Kobayashi M, Yasuda T, et al: Chondrocyte hypertrophy can be induced by a cryptic sequence of type II collagen and is accompanied by the induction of MMP-13 and collagenase activity: implications for development and arthritis, *Matrix Biol* 26(4):247–258, 2007.

274. Vaillancourt F, Morquette B, Shi Q, et al: Differential regulation of cyclooxygenase-2 and inducible nitric oxide synthase by 4-hydroxynonenal in human osteoarthritic chondrocytes through ATF-2/CREB-1 transactivation and concomitant inhibition of NF-kappaB signaling cascade, *J Cell Biochem* 100(5):1217–1231, 2007.

276. Lianxu C, Hongti J, Changlong Y: NF-kappaBp65-specific siRNA inhibits expression of genes of COX-2, NOS-2 and MMP-9 in rat IL-1beta-induced and TNF-alpha-induced chondrocytes, *Osteoarthritis Cartilage* 14(4):367–376, 2006.

277. Marcu KB, Otero M, Olivotto E, et al: NF-kappaB signaling: multiple angles to target OA, *Curr Drug Targets* 11(5):599–613, 2010.

283. Murray DH, Bush PG, Brenkel IJ, Hall AC: Abnormal human chondrocyte morphology is related to increased levels of cell-associated IL-1β and disruption to pericellular collagen type VI, *J Orthop Res* 28(11):1507–1514, 2010.

286. Chevalier X, Giraudeau B, Conrozier T, et al: Safety study of intraarticular injection of interleukin 1 receptor antagonist in patients with painful knee osteoarthritis: a multicenter study, *J Rheumatol* 32(7):1317–1323, 2005.

302. Fermor B, Weinberg JB, Pisetsky DS, Guilak F: The influence of oxygen tension on the induction of nitric oxide and prostaglandin E2 by mechanical stress in articular cartilage, *Osteoarthritis Cartil* 13(10):935–941, 2005.

303. Piscoya JL, Fermor B, Kraus VB, et al: The influence of mechanical compression on the induction of osteoarthritis-related biomarkers in articular cartilage explants, *Osteoarthritis Cartil* 13(12):1092–1099, 2005.

311. Blaney Davidson EN, Vitters EL, van der Kraan PM, van den Berg WB: Expression of transforming growth factor-beta (TGFbeta) and the TGFbeta signalling molecule SMAD-2P in spontaneous and instability-induced osteoarthritis: role in cartilage degradation, chondrogenesis and osteophyte formation, *Ann Rheum Dis* 65(11):1414–1421, 2006.

313. Karna E, Miltyk W, Palka JA, et al: Hyaluronic acid counteracts interleukin-1-induced inhibition of collagen biosynthesis in cultured human chondrocytes, *Pharmacol Res* 54(4):275–281, 2006.

314. Nawrat P, Surazynski A, Karna E, Palka JA: The effect of hyaluronic acid on interleukin-1-induced deregulation of collagen metabolism in cultured human skin fibroblasts, *Pharmacol Res* 51(5):473–477, 2005.

319. Atttur MG, Palmer GD, Al-Mussawir HE, et al: F-spondin, a neuroregulatory protein, is up-regulated in osteoarthritis and regulates cartilage metabolism via TGF-beta activation, *FASEB J* 23(1):79–89, 2009.

324. D'Agostino MA, Conaghan P, Le Bars M, et al: EULAR report on the use of ultrasonography in painful knee osteoarthritis. Part 1: prevalence of inflammation in osteoarthritis, *Ann Rheum Dis* 2005 64(12): 1703–1709.

339. Benito MJ, Veale DJ, FitzGerald O, et al: Synovial tissue inflammation in early and late osteoarthritis, *Ann Rheum Dis* 64(9):1263–1267, 2005.

344. van Spil WE, DeGroot J, Lems WF, et al: Serum and urinary biochemical markers for knee and hip-osteoarthritis: a systematic review applying the consensus BIPED criteria, *Osteoarthritis Cartil* 18(5):605–612, 2010.

346. Bruyere O, Genant H, Kothari M, et al: Longitudinal study of magnetic resonance imaging and standard X-rays to assess disease progression in osteoarthritis, *Osteoarthritis Cartil* 15(1):98–103, 2007.

348. Kerkhof HJM, Bierma-Zeinstra SMA, Castano-Betancourt MC, et al: Serum C reactive protein levels and genetic variation in the CRP gene are not associated with the prevalence, incidence or progression of osteoarthritis independent of body mass index, *Ann Rheum Dis* 69(11):1976–1982, 2010.

349. Jordan JM: Update on cartilage oligomeric matrix protein as a marker of osteoarthritis, *J Rheumatol* 32(6):1145–1147, 2005.

350. Tseng S, Reddi AH, Di Cesare PE: Cartilage oligomeric matrix protein (COMP): a biomarker of arthritis, *Biomark Insights* 4:33–44, 2009.

Full references for this chapter can be found on www.expertconsult.com.

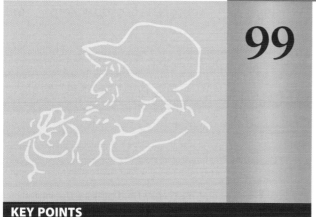

99 Clinical Features of Osteoarthritis

AMANDA E. NELSON • JOANNE M. JORDAN

KEY POINTS

Osteoarthritis is the most common form of arthritis, typically affecting the hands, hips, knees, spine, and feet.

Osteoarthritis can be defined radiographically, clinically, or symptomatically.

As more sensitive measures of damage from osteoarthritis become available, such as improved imaging and molecular biomarkers, definitions may change.

Pain and functional limitations contribute substantially to disability in osteoarthritis.

Mortality is increased among individuals with osteoarthritis compared with the general population.

Osteoarthritis (OA), the most common form of arthritis, is found worldwide and is strongly associated with aging. It affected 27 million adults in the United States in 2005.[1] OA of the knee and hip has significant functional impact due to effects on ambulation and mobility and is associated with considerable medical costs, accounting for 97% of the 455,000 total knee replacements and 83% of the 233,000 total hip replacements for arthritis in 2004.[2] Given the aging of our society and the obesity epidemic, the burden of OA can only be expected to increase over the next 20 years.[3]

OA affects all of the structures in and around a joint and should be considered a failure of the total joint. Historically, the emphasis in OA research has been on cartilage degeneration, but more recent work has expanded this view to an improved understanding of the role of subchondral bone, synovium, ligaments/tendons, meniscus, muscle, and nerve tissues in the disease process.[4,5] The late- or end-stage joint, clinically recognizable as OA, likely represents a final common pathway of many different factors including genetics, environment, and biomechanical contributors.

EPIDEMIOLOGY OF OSTEOARTHRITIS

OA can be defined pathologically, radiographically, or clinically. The American College of Rheumatology (ACR) criteria for the classification of OA of the hand, hip, and knee are shown in Table 99-1.[6-8] For the hand, only clinical criteria are used, with a sensitivity of 92% and specificity of 98%. For the hip, the sensitivity and specificity of the ACR criteria are estimated to be 91% and 89%, whereas for the knee they are 91% and 86%, respectively. Due to their high specificity, these criteria are most useful for differentiating OA from inflammatory arthropathy, but less so for differentiating early OA from healthy controls. Compared with radiographic definitions, the ACR criteria tend to underestimate prevalence of OA.[9,10]

The presence of radiographic OA usually requires the presence of a definite osteophyte or joint space narrowing on plain radiographs, although magnetic resonance imaging (MRI)-based definitions are under development.[11] Clinical OA is usually defined by abnormalities on physical examination consistent with OA such as nodal changes in the hands, limited and painful internal rotation of the hip, or crepitus with knee movement. Symptomatic OA is usually defined as pain, aching, or stiffness in a joint with radiographic OA. Definitions can vary according to joint site, frequency or intensity of symptoms, and time span over which symptoms are assessed.

Prevalence of Radiographic Osteoarthritis

Because of the multiple different definitions of OA, prevalence estimates vary. The first National Health and Nutrition Examination Survey (NHANES I) found that 12% of the U.S. population had clinically defined OA in at least one joint. A few population-based studies have estimated the prevalence of radiographic OA at the knee, recently reviewed by Lawrence and colleagues.[1] Despite variations based on radiographic technique and participant age, these studies estimate that radiographic knee OA is present in 14% to 37% of U.S. adults and is more frequent in women.[12-14] For radiographic hip OA, available estimates vary more widely, from less than 1% to 27%, depending on the population being studied.[15] Radiographic hand OA is common, especially in older individuals, but it may not be symptomatic or functionally limiting. One large study found radiographic OA of at least one joint in 67% of women and 55% of men aged 55 years and older, with 28% having radiographic OA in at least two of three hand joint sites (distal or proximal interphalangeal or carpometacarpal).[16] A recent review of radiographic findings in foot OA reported a prevalence of 12% to 35% for first metatarsophalangeal OA.[17]

Prevalence of Symptomatic Osteoarthritis

A summary of prevalence estimates for symptomatic OA (symptoms in the presence of radiographic OA) at the hands, knees, and hips is presented in Table 99-2.[1] On the basis of these findings, Lawrence and colleagues[1] estimated that more than 9 million U.S. adults are affected by symptomatic knee OA and more than 13 million have symptomatic hand OA.

Table 99-1 American College of Rheumatology Radiologic and Clinical Criteria for Osteoarthritis

Hand[8]

1. Hand pain, aching, or stiffness on most days of prior mo
2. Hard tissue enlargement of ≥2 of 10 selected joints*
3. Fewer than 3 swollen MCP joints
4. Hard tissue enlargement of ≥2 DIP joints
5. Deformity of ≥2 of 10 selected joints*
Diagnosis requires items 1-3 and either 4 or 5
*10 selected joints: DIP 2-3, PIP 2-3, and CMC 1 bilaterally

Knee: Clinical[6]

1. Knee pain for most days of prior mo
2. Crepitus with active joint motion
3. Morning stiffness lasting ≤30 min
4. Bony enlargement of the knee on examination
5. Age ≥38 yr
Diagnosis requires 1 + 2 + 4, or 1 + 2 + 3 + 5, or 1 + 4 + 5

Knee: Clinical and Radiographic

1. Knee pain for most days of prior mo
2. Osteophytes at joint margins
3. Synovial fluid typical of osteoarthritis
4. Age ≥40 yr
5. Morning stiffness lasting ≤30 min
6. Crepitus with active joint motion
Diagnosis requires: 1 + 2, or 1 + 3 + 5 + 6, or 1 + 4 + 5 + 6

Hip: Clinical and Radiographic[7]

1. Hip pain for most days of the prior mo
2. ESR ≤20 mm/hr
3. Radiographic femoral and/or acetabular osteophytes
4. Radiographic hip joint space narrowing
Diagnosis requires: 1 + 2 + 3, or 1 + 2 + 4, or 1 + 3 + 4

CMC, carpometacarpal; DIP, distal interphalangeal; ESR, erythrocyte sedimentation rate; MCP, metacarpophalangeal; PIP, proximal interphalangeal.
From Altman R, Asch E, Bloch D, et al: Development of criteria for the classification and reporting of osteoarthritis. Classification of osteoarthritis of the knee. Diagnostic and Therapeutic Criteria Committee of the American Rheumatism Association, *Arthritis Rheum* 29(8):1039–1049, 1986; Altman R, Alarcon G, Appelrouth D, et al: The American College of Rheumatology criteria for the classification and reporting of osteoarthritis of the hip, *Arthritis Rheum* 34(5):505–514, 1991; and Altman R, Alarcon G, Appelrouth D, et al: The American College of Rheumatology criteria for the classification and reporting of osteoarthritis of the hand, *Arthritis Rheum* 33(11):1601–1610, 1990.

Primary and Secondary Osteoarthritis

Historically, osteoarthritis was considered to be "primary" in the absence of an injury history or other joint disease and "secondary" if a predisposing disorder was present (Table 99-3). However, as more and more local risk factors for OA

Table 99-2 Prevalence of Symptomatic Osteoarthritis (OA)

Site (Age in Yrs)	Source	% with Symptomatic OA		
		Male	Female	Total
Hands (≥26)	Framingham[89]	3.8	9.2	6.8
Knees				
≥26	Framingham[13]	4.6	4.9	4.9
≥45	Framingham[13]	5.9	7.2	6.7
≥45	Johnston County[14]	13.5	18.7	16.7
≥60	NHANES III[12]	10.0	13.6	12.1
Hips (≥45)	Johnston County[90]	8.7	9.3	9.2

NHANES, National Health and Nutrition Examination Survey.
From Lawrence RC, Felson DT, Helmick CG, et al:. Estimates of the prevalence of arthritis and other rheumatic conditions in the United States. Part II, *Arthritis Rheum* 58(1):26–35, 2008.

Table 99-3 Etiologies of Secondary Osteoarthritis

Metabolic

Crystal-associated arthritis
   Calcium pyrophosphate or apatite deposition
Acromegaly
Ochronosis
Hemochromatosis
Wilson's disease
Hyperparathyroidism
Ehlers-Danlos
Gaucher's disease
Diabetes

Mechanical/Local Factors

Slipped capital femoral epiphysis
Epiphyseal dysplasias
Legg-Calvé-Perthes disease
Congenital dislocation
Femoroacetabular impingement
Congenital hip dysplasia
Limb-length inequality
Hypermobility syndromes
Avascular necrosis/osteonecrosis

Traumatic

Joint trauma (e.g., ACL tear)
Fracture through joint
Prior joint surgery (i.e., meniscectomy, ACL)
Charcot joint (neuropathic arthropathy)

Inflammatory

Rheumatoid arthritis or other inflammatory arthropathies
Crystalline arthropathy (gout)
History of septic arthritis

ACL, anterior cruciate ligament.
Modified from Altman R, Asch E, Bloch D, et al: Development of criteria for the classification and reporting of osteoarthritis. Classification of osteoarthritis of the knee. Diagnostic and Therapeutic Criteria Committee of the American Rheumatism Association, *Arthritis Rheum* 29(8):1039–1049, 1986.

have been identified (such as femoroacetabular impingement at the hip and malalignment at the knee) and a broader range of associated factors have been discovered (genetic, biomechanical, and environmental factors), the division between primary and secondary is less clear. Many individuals who develop secondary OA are likely predisposed to the condition with or without the identified inciting event; other individuals who have a disorder that is linked to secondary OA may not develop clinical OA. It may be most useful to think of OA as a common pathway through which an individual's genetics, history of injury or other joint damage, mechanical factors, and psychosocial milieu act on the joint, in some cases leading to an "end-stage" or "failed" joint.

CLINICAL FEATURES

General Symptoms and Signs

OA most commonly affects the knees, hands, feet, hips, and spine. These joints may be symptomatic or may be affected only on radiographs. Individuals with OA generally describe pain in the joint(s) that is worse with activity, with limited morning stiffness (<30 minutes), and pain and stiffness with rest. This stiffness after inactivity, or "gelling" phenomenon, is often a main complaint, although morning stiffness is generally less severe and of shorter duration than that seen in systemic inflammatory arthropathies. Affected joints in OA often demonstrate bony enlargement and crepitus on examination, with concomitant reductions in range of motion. There may be soft tissue swelling or effusion, although these tend to be much less dramatic than in inflammatory arthritis. Pain complaints may be more or less than expected on the basis of structural damage.[18,19] The effects of depression, disturbed sleep, and other psychosocial factors on the pain experience in OA are being increasingly recognized.[20-23]

Joint-Specific Symptoms and Signs: Knee

Knee OA is characterized by the insidious onset of pain with gelling and limited range of motion. Individuals with knee OA often describe pain and limitation with walking, transferring (as from seated to standing), and especially stair climbing. These complaints are often associated with a sensation of instability or "giving out" at the knee. A "locking" sensation at the knee can be a consequence of stiffness, loose bodies in the joint space, or meniscal lesions. Knees with OA often have demonstrable crepitus and bony enlargement. Pain may be elicited by palpation of the medial or lateral joint line, or both. Effusions, when present, are often cool and generally without redness. They can be associated with popliteal bursa enlargement (Baker's cyst) when large. Associated pain over the anserine bursa, or even the greater trochanter, is often seen in knee OA and may be related to altered biomechanics.[24] Appreciation of such soft tissue symptoms is important because these may be amenable to corticosteroid injections with subsequent pain relief.

Malalignment, most often varus, is often seen in severe disease but can be present even in fairly mild/early disease. Clinically evident varus thrust may be a risk factor for progression.[25] Other signs of severe disease include flexion deformities or joint instability. Quadriceps weakness represents an early modifiable risk factor for knee OA progression, particularly in women,[26,27] and in late stages of disease may be apparent as muscle atrophy.[28,29] Alterations in proprioception and vibratory sense have been demonstrated in association with knee OA, although the relation of these factors to progression and pain is still unclear.[30-32]

Patellofemoral OA can strongly contribute to pain and disability at the knee but is often overlooked.[33] OA of the patellofemoral joint is characterized by pain with ascending or descending stairs and is often located anteriorly. It can be seen in isolation or in association with tibiofemoral OA. The relation between patellofemoral OA and commonly seen patellofemoral pain disorders in younger individuals remains to be elucidated.[34]

Joint-Specific Symptoms and Signs: Hip

OA of the hip can present with groin pain, which is fairly specific[35] but may be described more vaguely as pain in the thigh, buttock, low back, or even in the ipsilateral knee. Therefore it is important to assess for other causes of pain in the "hip" including spinal pain (lumbar disk degeneration, spinal stenosis, facet joint OA, sacroiliac pain); trochanteric bursitis; altered gait due to knee pathology; meralgia paresthetica (lateral femoral cutaneous nerve entrapment); thigh claudication from vascular causes; or even intrapelvic causes. It is also important to consider other causes of hip and groin pain such as occult femoral neck fracture or avascular necrosis. Persons affected by hip OA have limitations in walking, bending, and transferring, as well as stair climbing. Internal rotation of the affected hip is often limited and can be quite painful, even in early disease, often evident to the patient as difficulty putting on socks, tying shoes, or trimming toenails. Visible deformity, hip flexion contracture, or severe limitations of range of motion are indicators of more advanced disease, which may also be associated with shortening of the affected limb due to superior migration of the femoral head. In young individuals presenting with groin pain that is worsened by sitting, with pain and limitation when internally rotating and adducting the hip in the flexed position, femoroacetabular impingement is a consideration.[36]

Joint-Specific Symptoms and Signs: Hand

The hands often provide the first clue to a diagnosis of OA. Evident bony enlargement of the distal interphalangeal (DIP) joints, called Heberden's nodes, and proximal interphalangeal (PIP) joints, called Bouchard's nodes, can be appreciated (Figure 99-1). These nodes may be acutely inflamed with warmth and tenderness or may be bland, hard enlargements and are often more marked in the dominant hand. Some patients, most commonly elderly women, have erosive osteoarthritis characterized by episodic inflammation, pain, and swelling. It remains a matter of debate whether this type of OA is part of the continuum or is in itself a separate disease entity.[37,38] OA involvement of the first carpometacarpal (CMC) joint is particularly problematic and can lead to significant pain, limitations in functionality of the hand, and reduced grip strength.[39,40] CMC squaring, representing deformity of the joint due to osteophyte formation and joint space narrowing, can be seen on examination. Bilateral involvement of multiple joints, both within (multiple PIPs) and across (both DIPs and PIPs) joint groups, is frequent. Metacarpophalangeal joints are affected more commonly than previously recognized,[41-43] although prominent involvement of these joints should prompt consideration of inflammatory arthropathies or secondary causes of OA such as hemochromatosis.[44] Again, soft tissue findings such as deQuervain's tenosynovitis should be considered because they are associated with hand OA, can mimic or aggravate symptoms, and are amenable to conservative management.

Joint-Specific Symptoms and Signs: Spine

Facet joint arthritis is a common finding, is associated with back pain, and has many features in common with OA of other diarthrodial joints,[45] although few studies of this finding in association with OA at other sites have been reported.[46] Osteophytosis of the spine is nearly ubiquitous in older individuals, although it is often asymptomatic.[47] Lumbar disk degeneration (LDD), characterized by disk space narrowing, end-plate sclerosis, and herniation, is often seen in association with radiographic osteophytosis,[48] although the relationship between LDD and osteoarthritis of other joint sites remains controversial.[49] Clinical

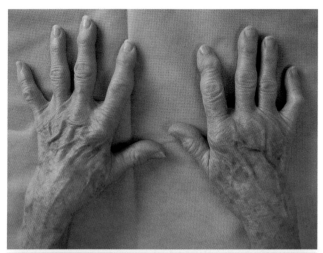

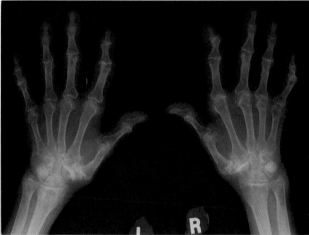

Figure 99-1 Hands of a 79-year-old woman showing clinical *(top)* and radiographic *(bottom)* features of osteoarthritis (OA). This patient has Heberden's and Bouchard's nodes of multiple digits; radiographs show osteophytes, joint space narrowing, and cysts typical of OA, as well as "gull-wing" deformities at the third proximal interphalangeal joints suggestive of erosive OA.

symptoms in the cervical spine can include pain in the neck, often accompanied by radiation down the arms, sometimes with weakness or paresthesias due to compression of the cervical nerves secondary to osteophytic encroachment on intervertebral foramina or the spinal column. Large anterior cervical spine osteophytes can cause dysphagia due to compression of the esophagus.[50] Similarly, in the lumbosacral spine, osteophytes and disk space narrowing can lead to sciatic nerve impingement with pain, burning, numbness, and/or weakness down one or both legs. Diffuse idiopathic skeletal hyperostosis, or DISH, is characterized by exuberant osteophytosis and calcification of spinal ligaments and entheses, leading to an appearance likened to flowing candle wax.[51] Individuals with DISH can be asymptomatic and identified only by radiographic appearance or can present in a fashion similar to OA or LDD.

Joint-Specific Symptoms and Signs: Shoulder

The shoulder is a common source of pain in patients with OA, although the symptoms are more often due to osteophytosis and narrowing of the acromioclavicular and/or sternoclavicular joints than the glenohumeral joint itself. Other maladies common in older adults such as subacromial bursitis, rotator cuff pathology, and adhesive capsulitis should be assessed. Rotator cuff damage, in particular, can predispose to glenohumeral OA. Pathology at the cervical spine can present as pain in the shoulder region, so the shoulder evaluation should include an assessment of the cervical spine. Milwaukee shoulder syndrome is a destructive arthropathy of the glenohumeral joint associated with large effusions, which on aspiration often reveal high red blood cell content and basic calcium crystals.[52]

Joint-Specific Symptoms and Signs: Other Joints

Osteoarthritis of the foot has been largely neglected in the literature to date. OA of the first metatarsophalangeal (MTP) joint is characterized by pain and hallux valgus (bunion) deformity and has radiographic features (joint space narrowing, osteophytosis) similar to OA at other joints. Loss of function at the first MTP joint due to ankylosis (hallux rigidus) can lead to altered gait. Other joints that can be affected by OA but are often not part of epidemiologic studies include the ankles (talonavicular and subtalar) and temporomandibular joint (TMJ). Elbow OA is rare and may be the result of trauma, vibration damage, or other entities such as pseudogout.

Polyarticular Osteoarthritis

It has been recognized for more than 100 years that OA can co-occur in multiple joint sites.[53] Although the term *generalized* OA (GOA) has been used to describe this disease entity, there is no universally understood or accepted definition of what constitutes GOA (Figure 99-2). Kellgren and Moore in 1952 provided the first clinical description of GOA, involving primarily Heberden's nodes and the CMC joints, with the spine, knees, hips, and feet involved in descending frequency.[54] Later studies have defined GOA as more than three or more than five joint sites affected,[55] affected joint counts,[56,57] multiple hand joint involvement,[58] nodal hand OA with other joint involvement,[43] or summed scores of OA across multiple joints.[59,60] It remains unclear which joints should be included in such definitions, particularly whether lumbar disk degeneration and hip OA are part of the same disease entity as other joints. Clinically, it is important to recognize and consider that a patient with OA in one joint is likely to have involvement at other sites and to assess the impact of that individual's overall OA burden on their functional status, rather than focusing on a single joint.

DIAGNOSTIC TESTING

Diagnostic Approach

The diagnosis of OA is a clinical one, and laboratory testing is rarely required. Similarly, if the diagnosis is clear on the basis of history and clinical findings, radiographs are often not required. The purpose of additional diagnostic testing in OA is primarily to exclude potentially treatable underlying conditions such as metabolic or inflammatory arthropathies.

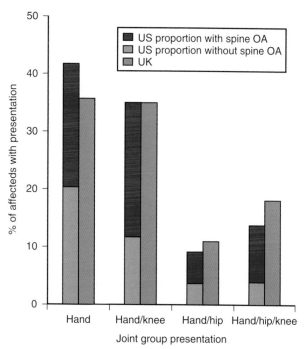

Figure 99-2 Frequency of multiple joint involvement with radiographic osteoarthritis (OA) in the Genetics of Generalized Osteoarthritis Study. The frequencies of radiographic OA at various sites and sites in combination are shown for the United States in *blue*. For the United Kingdom they are shown in *green* for the 1963 participants meeting specified hand radiographic OA criteria. The groups represented are mutually exclusive. The frequency of spine OA (only assessed by U.S. sites) in combination with these phenotypes is indicated by the *red bars*. *(Modified from Kraus VB, Jordan JM, Doherty M, et al: The Genetics of Generalized Osteoarthritis (GOGO) study: study design and evaluation of osteoarthritis phenotypes, Osteoarthritis Cartil 15:120–127, 2007.)*

Laboratory Testing

There is rarely an indication for testing rheumatoid factor, antinuclear antibodies, or other serologic studies in the setting of clinically suspected OA, and such tests should be reserved for a patient in whom there are findings suggestive of an inflammatory arthropathy. Complete blood count, chemistry panel including glucose and creatinine, and liver function tests should be obtained before initiation of pharmacologic therapy for OA, especially in older individuals with comorbid medical conditions, due to an increased risk of adverse events in this population. In cases where there is prominent involvement of the metacarpophalangeal (MCP) joints, evaluation for hypothyroidism and hemochromatosis may be warranted.

Synovial Fluid

The synovial fluid in OA is typically normal or mildly inflammatory, appearing clear and colorless to slightly yellowish. The leukocyte cell count is typically less than or equal to 2000 cells/mm^3 (<2 cells seen across 10 high-power fields).[61] Fluid is often obtained in the course of a symptomatic joint injection, although diagnostic aspiration may be done in the setting of an effusion. Concomitant calcium pyrophosphate crystal disease can be identified, although other calcium crystals, or hydroxyapatite, are not seen on routine preparations.

Molecular Biomarkers

Quantitative determination of the products of cartilage and bone metabolism has provided several putative biomarkers of OA pathophysiology. As an example, one such biomarker, urinary C-telopeptide fragments of type II collagen (u-CTXII), is associated with the occurrence and progression of radiographic OA, independent of other risk factors.[46,62] Such biomarkers, obtained from serum, urine, or synovial fluid, may eventually provide a method for early diagnosis and monitoring of treatment effect, although they are currently used primarily in research. Interested readers are referred to a comprehensive review of biomarkers by van Spil and colleagues.[63]

Imaging: Conventional Radiography, General Considerations

Conventional radiography is widely available and relatively inexpensive, making this modality useful to confirm the diagnosis and exclude others, primarily when there is clinical uncertainty regarding the diagnosis, when the joint involved is atypical, or when evidence exists to suggest other diagnoses such as inflammatory arthritis, fractures, Paget's disease, osteonecrosis, infection, or malignancy. Radiographs of joints affected by osteoarthritis typically show osteophytes, joint space narrowing, sclerosis, and cysts of subchondral bone.[64] The Kellgren-Lawrence (KL) grading system remains the most commonly used for research purposes.[65] KL grades range from 0 (no osteophytes or joint space narrowing) to 4 (severe joint space narrowing with subchondral sclerosis); a grade of 2 is generally considered diagnostic of osteoarthritis. The KL system relies on osteophytes and may underestimate OA in individuals with a more atrophic subtype (where joint space narrowing is more severe than osteophytosis, particularly at the hip). Other grading systems, such as the Osteoarthritis Research Society International (OARSI) grading system, view osteophytes and joint space narrowing separately and assign separate scores (Figure 99-3).[66] The choice of grading system depends on the goal of the study and the joint site of interest.

Imaging: Conventional Radiography, Specific Joint Issues

Imaging of the knees should be bilateral and in weight bearing, and for clinical purposes it should generally be anteroposterior (AP). Lateral, posteroanterior, or sunrise views may be necessary in some circumstances. Alignment, although best determined from full-limb views, can be estimated from routine knee films.[67] An AP pelvis view should be obtained to assess hip OA and can be supine or weight bearing. Additional views such as frog-leg or lateral images may be indicated for specific hip pathology or to assess for femoroacetabular impingement or congenital abnormalities. An atrophic subtype of hip OA, characterized by joint space narrowing with either mild or absent osteophytosis, has been described,[68] and alternative radiographic definitions for hip OA (other than KL grading) have been proposed and used in research to address this issue.[10,69] For hand OA, a posteroanterior view of both hands including the

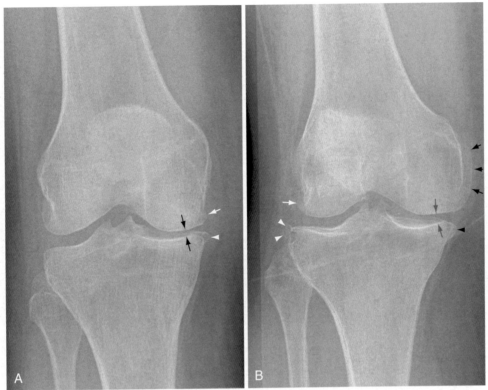

Figure 99-3 Examples of semiquantitative radiographic assessment with use of the Kellgren-Lawrence and Osteoarthritis Research Society International (OARSI) grading schemes. **A,** Kellgren-Lawrence grade 3. No lateral femoral and tibial osteophytes are seen (OARSI grade 0). A medial femoral osteophyte: OARSI grade 1 *(white arrow)*; a medial tibial osteophyte: OARSI grade 2 *(white arrowhead)*; lateral tibiofemoral joint-space width: OARSI grade 0; and medial tibiofemoral joint-space narrowing: OARSI grade 2 *(black arrows)* are depicted. **B,** Kellgren-Lawrence grade 2. A lateral femoral osteophyte: OARSI grade 2 *(white arrow)*; a lateral tibial osteophyte: OARSI grade 2 *(white arrowheads)*; a medial femoral osteophyte: OARSI grade 3 *(short black arrows)*; a medial tibial osteophyte: OARSI grade 2 *(black arrowhead)*; a normal lateral tibiofemoral joint-space width: OARSI grade 0; and medial tibiofemoral joint-space width: OARSI grade 1 *(long black arrows)* are shown. *(From Guermazi A, Hunter DJ, Roemer FW: Plain radiography and magnetic resonance imaging diagnostics in osteoarthritis: validated staging and scoring,* J Bone Joint Surg Am *91(Suppl 1):54–62, 2009.)*

wrists will reveal the characteristic features of OA. If there is an erosive component to hand OA, radiographs may demonstrate central erosions and "gull-wing" deformities of the interphalangeal joints. Marked destructive changes at the DIP joints may indicate another inflammatory disorder such as psoriatic arthritis or, rarely, multicentric reticulohistiocytosis. Prominent involvement of the MCP joints may indicate a metabolic process such as hemochromatosis or calcium pyrophosphate deposition disease. Conventional radiography of the lateral lumbar spine can show facet OA, disk space narrowing, and osteophytosis.

Imaging: Advanced Modalities

Other imaging modalities, such as MRI, can be useful to exclude avascular necrosis, stress fractures, other occult fractures, infectious processes, or inflammatory arthropathy. MRI is increasingly used in OA research as a means to obtain information about structural changes earlier in the disease process, before findings are apparent on conventional radiographs. Bone marrow lesions identified on knee MRI, for example, have been shown to correlate with pain, meniscal lesions, bone attrition, and progressive cartilage damage (Figure 99-4).[5,70-72] However, due to a lack of effective treatment options in OA; growing evidence that surgical interventions such as knee arthroscopy, which are often

a response to findings on MRI, are overused and generally ineffective[73]; and the cost associated with these studies, they are generally not indicated in routine clinical practice at present. Ultrasound is gaining in popularity and may have a role at the bedside in detecting small effusions, identifying early cartilage changes, differentiating inflammatory from noninflammatory arthropathies, and as a therapeutic adjunct to allow more accurate aspirations and placement of intraarticular injections.[74-77]

OUTCOME

Performance Measures and Functional Assessment

Although not routinely used in clinical practice, there are several validated tools for assessing functional status in OA that are widely used in research settings. Results on standardized performance-based tests such as determination of walking speed and time to stand from a chair five times unassisted have been shown to correlate with the severity and number of affected joints in OA.[78,79] Questionnaire-based measures such as the Stanford Health Assessment Questionnaire (HAQ) disability index (for overall function), Western Ontario and McMaster Universities Arthritis Index (WOMAC, focused on lower extremity joints,

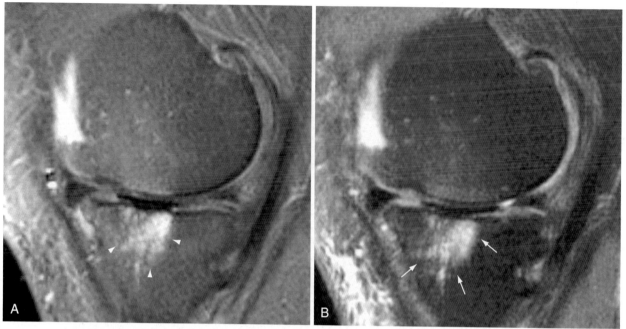

Figure 99-4 Subchondral bone marrow lesion (BML) in osteoarthritis. **A,** Sagittal proton density fat suppressed (FS) image. Tibial BML is depicted as diffuse hyperintensity *(arrowheads)*. **B,** T1-weighted FS image after intravenous gadolinium diethylene triamine penta-acetic acid administration shows BML with similar extent *(arrows)*. *(From Roemer FW, Frobell R, Hunter DJ, et al: MRI-detected subchondral bone marrow signal alterations of the knee joint: terminology, imaging appearance, relevance and radiological differential diagnosis, Osteoarthritis Cartil 17:1115–1131, 2009.)*

Table 99-4), and Australian/Canadian Hand Osteoarthritis Index (AUSCAN, for hand-specific function), are often used to assess the functional impact of OA on affected individuals for research purposes.[80-82]

Time to Total Joint Replacement

Total joint replacement is a "hard" endpoint in OA, but its use as an outcome measure is hampered by a variety of factors affecting an individual patient's decision to undergo this procedure including insurance coverage, procedure availability, comorbid conditions, ability to rehabilitate the joint, and patient preference.[83,84] Therefore efforts are ongoing to identify a composite index that would define the "need for total joint replacement," which could be used as an outcome measure.[85,86]

Mortality in Osteoarthritis

Moderate evidence indicates increased mortality in individuals with OA compared with the general population.[87] The apparent modestly increased mortality risk, determined through a review of nine studies, appears to be primarily due to cardiovascular and gastrointestinal causes. One study showed an increased mortality risk with increasing numbers of joint groups affected by OA, as well as reduced survival in individuals with hand, bilateral knee, or cervical spine involvement, but not in those with OA of the hip, foot, or lumbar spine.[88] Contributors to increased mortality risk include a combination of reduced physical activity among individuals with OA, comorbid conditions, and/or adverse medication effects such as are seen with acetaminophen and nonsteroidal anti-inflammatory drugs.[87]

Table 99-4 Western Ontario and McMaster Universities Arthritis Index (WOMAC)

Pain Subscale
How much pain do you have …
Walking on a flat surface?
Going up or down stairs?
At night while in bed?
Sitting or lying?
Standing upright?

Stiffness Subscale
How severe is your stiffness …
After first waking in the morning?
After sitting, lying down, or resting later in the day?

Function Subscale
What degree of difficulty do you have with …
Descending stairs?
Ascending stairs?
Rising from sitting?
Standing?
Bending to floor?
Walking on a flat surface?
Getting in or out of a car?
Going shopping?
Putting on socks or stockings?
Rising from bed?
Taking off socks or stockings?
Lying in bed?
Getting in and out of the bath?
Sitting?
Getting on or off the toilet?
Heavy domestic duties?
Light domestic duties?

Modified from Bellamy N, Buchanan WW, Goldsmith CH, et al: Validation study of WOMAC: a health status instrument for measuring clinically important patient relevant outcomes to antirheumatic drug therapy in patients with osteoarthritis of the hip or knee, *J Rheumatol* 15(12):1833–1840, 1988.

SUMMARY

OA is a highly prevalent and debilitating condition, with increasing prevalence along with the aging of our society and the ongoing obesity epidemic. OA is readily recognized on clinical grounds, although further diagnostic testing and imaging are indicated in some cases to assess for potentially treatable underlying conditions. Pain is the most common reason for a patient with OA to seek medical advice, and examination often reveals loss of function. Assessment of the patient's pain symptoms and functional limitations, in the framework of that individual's goals, is necessary to formulate an appropriate plan of care in the absence of disease-modifying medications. Current research in OA, in addition to ongoing efforts in both pharmacologic and non-pharmacologic therapeutic development, is focused on optimizing incident case and progressor definitions and understanding the whole-body burden of OA.

References

1. Lawrence RC, Felson DT, Helmick CG, et al: Estimates of the prevalence of arthritis and other rheumatic conditions in the United States. Part II, *Arthritis Rheum* 58(1):26–35, 2008.
2. American Academy of Orthopaedic Surgeons (AAOS): *The burden of musculoskeletal disease in the United States*, Rosemont, Ill, 2008, AAOS, pp 71–96.
3. Hootman JM, Helmick CG: Projections of US prevalence of arthritis and associated activity limitations, *Arthritis Rheum* 54(1):226–229, 2006.
4. Burr DB: The importance of subchondral bone in the progression of osteoarthritis, *J Rheumatol Suppl* 70:77–80, 2004.
5. Lo GH, Hunter DJ, Nevitt M, et al, for the OAI Investigators Group: Strong association of MRI meniscal derangement and bone marrow lesions in knee osteoarthritis: data from the osteoarthritis initiative, *Osteoarthritis Cartil* 17(6):743–747, 2008.
6. Altman R, Asch E, Bloch D, et al: Development of criteria for the classification and reporting of osteoarthritis. Classification of osteoarthritis of the knee. Diagnostic and Therapeutic Criteria Committee of the American Rheumatism Association, *Arthritis Rheum* 29(8):1039–1049, 1986.
7. Altman R, Alarcon G, Appelrouth D, et al: The American College of Rheumatology criteria for the classification and reporting of osteoarthritis of the hip, *Arthritis Rheum* 34(5):505–514, 1991.
8. Altman R, Alarcon G, Appelrouth D, et al: The American College of Rheumatology criteria for the classification and reporting of osteoarthritis of the hand, *Arthritis Rheum* 33(11):1601–1610, 1990.
9. McAlindon TE, Dieppe P: Osteoarthritis: definitions and criteria, *Ann Rheum Dis* 48:531–532, 1989.
10. Croft P, Cooper C, Coggon D: Case definition of hip osteoarthritis in epidemiologic studies, *J Rheumatol* 21(4):591–592, 1994.
11. Hunter DJ, Arden N, Conaghan PG, et al: Definition of osteoarthritis on MRI: results of a Delphi exercise, *Osteoarthritis Cartil* 18(Suppl 2), S174–S175, Abstract, 2010.
12. Dillon CF, Rasch EK, Gu Q, Hirsch R: Prevalence of knee osteoarthritis in the United States: arthritis data from the Third National Health and Nutrition Examination Survey 1991-94, *J Rheumatol* 33(11):2271–2279, 2006.
13. Felson DT, Naimark A, Anderson J, et al: The prevalence of knee osteoarthritis in the elderly. The Framingham Osteoarthritis Study, *Arthritis Rheum* 30(8):914–918, 1987.
14. Jordan JM, Helmick CG, Renner JB, et al: Prevalence of knee symptoms and radiographic and symptomatic knee osteoarthritis in African Americans and Caucasians: The Johnston County Osteoarthritis Project, *J Rheumatol* 34(1):172–180, 2007.
15. Dagenais S, Garbedian S, Wai EK: Systematic review of the prevalence of radiographic primary hip osteoarthritis, *Clin Orthop Relat Res* 467(3):623–637, 2009.
16. Dahaghin S, Bierma-Zeinstra SM, Ginai AZ, et al: Prevalence and pattern of radiographic hand osteoarthritis and association with pain and disability (the Rotterdam study), *Ann Rheum Dis* 64(5):682–687, 2005.
17. Trivedi B, Marshall M, Belcher J, Roddy E: A systematic review of radiographic definitions of foot osteoarthritis in population-based studies, *Osteoarthritis Cartil* 18(8):1027–1035, 2010.
18. Neogi T, Felson DT, Niu J, et al: Radiographic features of osteoarthritis are strongly associated with knee pain in two cohorts: MOST and Framingham, *Arthritis Rheum* 58(9 Suppl):S436, 2008. (Abstract).
19. Hannan MT, Felson DT, Pincus T: Analysis of the discordance between radiographic changes and knee pain in osteoarthritis of the knee, *J Rheumatol* 27(6):1513–1517, 2000.
20. Hawker GA, Gignac MA, Badley E, et al: A longitudinal study to explain the pain-depression link in older adults with osteoarthritis, *Arthritis Care Res (Hoboken)* 63:1382–1390, 2011.
21. Silva A, Andersen ML, Tufik S: Sleep pattern in an experimental model of osteoarthritis, *Pain* 140(3):446–455, 2008.
22. Smith MT, Quartana PJ, Okonkwo RM, Nasir A: Mechanisms by which sleep disturbance contributes to osteoarthritis pain: a conceptual model, *Curr Pain Headache Rep* 13(6):447–454, 2009.
23. Keefe FJ, Somers TJ: Psychological approaches to understanding and treating arthritis pain, *Nat Rev Rheumatol* 6(4):210–216, 2010.
24. Segal NA, Felson DT, Torner JC, et al: Greater trochanteric pain syndrome: epidemiology and associated factors, *Arch Phys Med Rehabil* 88(8):988–992, 2007.
25. Chang A, Hochberg M, Song J, et al: Frequency of varus and valgus thrust and factors associated with thrust presence in persons with or at higher risk for knee osteoarthritis, *Arthritis Rheum* 62(5):1403–1411, 2010.
26. Segal NA, Glass NA, Torner J, et al: Quadriceps weakness predicts risk for knee joint space narrowing in women in the MOST cohort, *Osteoarthritis Cartil* 18(6):769–775, 2010.
27. Baker KR, Xu L, Zhang Y, et al: Quadriceps weakness and its relationship to tibiofemoral and patellofemoral knee osteoarthritis in Chinese: the Beijing osteoarthritis study, *Arthritis Rheum* 50(6):1815–1821, 2004.
28. Slemenda C, Brandt KD, Heilman DK, et al: Quadriceps weakness and osteoarthritis of the knee, *Ann Intern Med* 127(2):97–104, 1997.
29. Ikeda S, Tsumura H, Torisu T: Age-related quadriceps-dominant muscle atrophy and incident radiographic knee osteoarthritis, *J Orthop Sci* 10(2):121–126, 2005.
30. Felson DT, Gross KD, Nevitt MC, et al: The effects of impaired joint position sense on the development and progression of pain and structural damage in knee osteoarthritis, *Arthritis Rheum* 61(8):1070–1076, 2009.
31. Shakoor N, Agrawal A, Block JA: Reduced lower extremity vibratory perception in osteoarthritis of the knee, *Arthritis Rheum* 59(1):117–121, 2008.
32. van der EM, Steultjens M, Harlaar J, et al: Joint proprioception, muscle strength, and functional ability in patients with osteoarthritis of the knee, *Arthritis Rheum* 57(5):787–793, 2007.
33. Duncan R, Peat G, Thomas E, et al: Does isolated patellofemoral osteoarthritis matter? *Osteoarthritis Cartil* 17(9):1151–1155, 2009.
34. Thomas MJ, Wood L, Selfe J, Peat G: Anterior knee pain in younger adults as a precursor to subsequent patellofemoral osteoarthritis: a systematic review, *BMC Musculoskelet Disord* 11:201, 2010.
35. Khan AM, McLoughlin E, Giannakas K, et al: Hip osteoarthritis: where is the pain? *Ann R Coll Surg Engl* 86(2):119–121, 2004.
36. Reid GD, Reid CG, Widmer N, Munk PL: Femoroacetabular impingement syndrome: an underrecognized cause of hip pain and premature osteoarthritis? (Review) *J Rheumatol* 37:1395–1404, 2010.
37. Bijsterbosch J, Watt I, Meulenbelt I, et al: Clinical and radiographic disease course of hand osteoarthritis and determinants of outcome after 6 years, *Ann Rheum Dis* 70:68–73, 2010.
38. Bijsterbosch J, Watt I, Meulenbelt I, et al: Clinical burden of erosive hand osteoarthritis and its relationship to nodes, *Ann Rheum Dis* 69(10):1784–1788, 2010.
39. Dominick KL, Jordan JM, Renner JB, Kraus VB: Relationship of radiographic and clinical variables to pinch and grip strength among individuals with osteoarthritis, *Arthritis Rheum* 52(5):1424–1430, 2005.

40. Bijsterbosch J, Visser W, Kroon HM, et al: Thumb base involvement in symptomatic hand osteoarthritis is associated with more pain and functional disability, *Ann Rheum Dis* 69(3):585–587, 2010.

41. Chaisson CE, Zhang Y, McAlindon TE, et al: Radiographic hand osteoarthritis: incidence, patterns, and influence of pre-existing disease in a population based sample, *J Rheumatol* 24(7):1337–1343, 1997.

42. Kalichman L, Cohen Z, Kobyliansky E, Livshits G: Patterns of joint distribution in hand osteoarthritis: contribution of age, sex, and handedness, *Am J Hum Biol* 16(2):125–134, 2004.

43. Kraus VB, Jordan JM, Doherty M, et al: The genetics of generalized osteoarthritis (GOGO) study: study design and evaluation of osteoarthritis phenotypes, *Osteoarthritis Cartil* 15(2):120–127, 2007.

44. Hirsch JH, Killien FC, Troupin RH: The arthropathy of hemochromatosis, *Radiology* 118:591–596, 1976.

45. Kalichman L, Hunter DJ: Lumbar facet joint osteoarthritis: a review, *Semin Arthritis Rheum* 37(2):69–80, 2007.

46. Meulenbelt I, Kloppenburg M, Kroon HM, et al: Urinary CTX-II levels are associated with radiographic subtypes of osteoarthritis in hip, knee, hand, and facet joints in subject with familial osteoarthritis at multiple sites: the GARP study, *Ann Rheum Dis* 65(3):360–365, 2006.

47. Sarzi-Puttini P, Atzeni F, Fumagalli M, et al: Osteoarthritis of the Spine, *Semin Arthritis Rheum* 34(6, Suppl 2):38–43, 2004.

48. Battie MC, Videman T: Lumbar disc degeneration: epidemiology and genetics, *J Bone Joint Surg Am* 88(Suppl 2):3–9, 2006.

49. Pye SR, Reid DM, Lunt M, et al: Lumbar disc degeneration: association between osteophytes, end-plate sclerosis and disc space narrowing, *Ann Rheum Dis* 66(3):330–333, 2007.

50. Kos MP, van Royen BJ, David EF, Mahieu HF: Anterior cervical osteophytes resulting in severe dysphagia and aspiration: two case reports and literature review, *J Laryngol Otol* 123(10):1169–1173, 2009.

51. Cammisa M, De SA, Guglielmi G: Diffuse idiopathic skeletal hyperostosis, *Eur J Radiol* 27(Suppl 1):S7–11, 1998.

52. McCarty DJ, Halverson PB, Carrera GF, et al: "Milwaukee shoulder"—association of microspheroids containing hydroxyapatite crystals, active collagenase, and neutral protease with rotator cuff defects. I. Clinical aspects, *Arthritis Rheum* 24(3):464–473, 1981.

53. Adams R: *A treatise on rheumatic gout, or chronic rheumatic arthritis of all the joints*, ed 2. London, 1873, John Churchill.

54. Kellgren JH, Moore R: Generalized osteoarthritis and Heberden's nodes, *Br Med J* 1(4751):181–187, 1952.

55. Lawrence JS: Generalized osteoarthrosis in a population sample, *Am J Epidemiol* 90(5):381–389, 1969.

56. Felson DT, Couropmitree NN, Chaisson CE, et al: Evidence for a Mendelian gene in a segregation analysis of generalized radiographic osteoarthritis: the Framingham Study, *Arthritis Rheum* 41(6):1064–1071, 1998.

57. Hirsch R, Lethbridge-Cejku M, Scott WW, et al: Association of hand and knee osteoarthritis: evidence for a polyarticular disease subset, *Ann Rheum Dis* 55:25–29, 1996.

58. Doherty M, Watt I, Dieppe P: Influence of primary generalised osteoarthritis on development of secondary osteoarthritis, *Lancet* 2(8340):8–11, 1983.

59. Meulenbelt I, Kloppenburg M, Kroon HM, et al: Urinary CTX-II levels are associated with radiographic subtypes of osteoarthritis in hip, knee, hand, and facet joints in subject with familial osteoarthritis at multiple sites: the GARP study, *Ann Rheum Dis* 65(3):360–365, 2006.

60. Kraus VB, Kepler TB, Stabler T, et al: First qualification study of serum biomarkers as indicators of total body burden of osteoarthritis, *PLoS One* 5(3):e9739, 2010.

61. Clayburne G, Baker DG, Schumacher HR Jr: Estimated synovial fluid leukocyte numbers on wet drop preparations as a potential substitute for actual leukocyte counts, *J Rheumatol* 19(1):60–62, 1992.

62. Reijman M, Hazes JMW, Bierma-Zeinstra SMA, et al: A new marker for osteoarthritis—Cross-sectional and longitudinal approach, *Arthritis Rheum* 50(8):2471–2478, 2004.

63. van Spil WE, DeGroot J, Lems WF, et al: Serum and urinary biochemical markers for knee and hip-osteoarthritis: a systematic review applying the consensus BIPED criteria, *Osteoarthritis Cartil* 18(5):605–612, 2010.

64. Guermazi A, Hunter DJ, Roemer FW: Plain radiography and magnetic resonance imaging diagnostics in osteoarthritis: validated staging and scoring, *J Bone Joint Surg Am* 91 (Suppl 1):54–62, 2009.

65. Kellgren JH, Lawrence JS: Radiological assessment of osteo-arthrosis, *Ann Rheum Dis* 16:494–502, 1957.

66. Burnett SJ, Hart DJ, Cooper C, Spector TD: *A radiographic atlas of osteoarthritis*. London, 1994, Springer-Verlag.

67. Kraus VB, Vail TP, Worrell T, McDaniel G: A comparative assessment of alignment angle of the knee by radiographic and physical examination methods, *Arthritis Rheum* 52(6):1730–1735, 2005.

68. Conrozier T, Merle-Vincent F, Mathieu P, et al: Epidemiological, clinical, biological and radiological differences between atrophic and hypertrophic patterns of hip osteoarthritis: a case-control study, *Clin Exp Rheumatol* 22(4):403–408, 2004.

69. Arden NK, Lane NE, Parimi N, et al: Defining incident radiographic hip osteoarthritis for epidemiologic studies in women, *Arthritis Rheum* 60(4):1052–1059, 2009.

70. Roemer FW, Neogi T, Nevitt MC, et al: Subchondral bone marrow lesions are highly associated with, and predict subchondral bone attrition longitudinally: the MOST study, *Osteoarthritis Cartil* 18(1):47–53, 2010.

71. Kothari A, Guermazi A, Chmiel JS, et al: Within-subregion relationship between bone marrow lesions and subsequent cartilage loss in knee osteoarthritis, *Arthritis Care Res (Hoboken)* 62(2):198–203, 2010.

72. Felson DT, Niu J, Guermazi A, et al: Correlation of the development of knee pain with enlarging bone marrow lesions on magnetic resonance imaging, *Arthritis Rheum* 56(9):2986–2992, 2007.

73. Kirkley A, Birmingham TB, Litchfield RB, et al: A randomized trial of arthroscopic surgery for osteoarthritis of the knee, *N Engl J Med* 359(11):1097–1107, 2008.

74. Iagnocco A: Imaging the joint in osteoarthritis: a place for ultrasound? *Best Pract Res Clin Rheumatol* 24(1):27–38, 2010.

75. Epis O, Iagnocco A, Meenagh G, et al: Ultrasound imaging for the rheumatologist. XVI. Ultrasound-guided procedures, *Clin Exp Rheumatol* 26(4):515–518, 2008.

76. Moller I, Bong D, Naredo E, et al: Ultrasound in the study and monitoring of osteoarthritis, *Osteoarthritis Cartil* 16(Suppl 3):S4–S7, 2008.

77. Meenagh G, Filippucci E, Iagnocco A, et al: Ultrasound imaging for the rheumatologist VIII. Ultrasound imaging in osteoarthritis, *Clin Exp Rheumatol* 25(2):172–175, 2007.

78. Purser JL, Renner JB, Woodard J, Jordan JM: Osteoarthritis and walking speed in the Johnston County Osteoarthritis Project, *Arthritis Rheum* 54(9):S153, 2006.

79. Elliott AL, Kraus VB, Fang F, et al: Joint-specific hand symptoms and self-reported and performance-based functional status in African-Americans and Caucasians: The Johnston County Osteoarthritis Project, *Ann Rheum Dis* 66:1622–1626, 2007.

80. Fries JF, Spitz PW, Young DY: The dimensions of health outcomes: the Health Assessment Questionnaire, disability and pain scales, *J Rheumatol* 9(5):789–793, 1982.

81. Bellamy N, Campbell J, Haraoui B, et al: Dimensionality and clinical importance of pain and disability in hand osteoarthritis: development of the Australian/Canadian (AUSCAN) Osteoarthritis (OA) Hand Index, *Osteoarthritis Cartil* 10(11):855–862, 2002.

82. Bellamy N, Buchanan WW, Goldsmith CH, et al: Validation study of WOMAC: a health status instrument for measuring clinically important patient relevant outcomes to antirheumatic drug therapy in patients with osteoarthritis of the hip or knee, *J Rheumatol* 15(12):1833–1840, 1988.

83. March L, Cross M, Tribe K, et al: Cost of joint replacement surgery for osteoarthritis: the patients' perspective, *J Rheumatol* 29(5):1006–1014, 2002.

84. Hawker GA, Wright JG, Glazier RH, et al: The effect of education and income on need and willingness to undergo total joint arthroplasty, *Arthritis Rheum* 46(12):3331–3339, 2002.

85. Gossec L, Hawker G, Davis AM, et al: OMERACT/OARSI Initiative to define states of severity and indication for joint replacement in hip and knee osteoarthritis, *J Rheumatol* 34(6):1432–1435, 2007.

86. Dougados M, Hawker G, Lohmander S, et al: OARSI/OMERACT criteria of being considered a candidate for total joint replacement in knee/hip osteoarthritis as an endpoint in clinical trials evaluating

potential disease modifying osteoarthritic drugs, *J Rheumatol* 36(9): 2097–2099, 2009.

87. Hochberg MC: Mortality in osteoarthritis, *Clin Exp Rheumatol* 26 (5 Suppl 51):S120–S124, 2008.

88. Cerhan JR, Wallace RB, El-Khoury GY, et al: Decreased survival with increasing prevalence of full-body, radiographically defined osteoarthritis in women, *Am J Epidemiol* 141(3):225–234, 1995.

89. Zhang Y, Niu J, Kelly-Hayes M, et al: Prevalence of symptomatic hand osteoarthritis and its impact on functional status among the elderly, *Am J Epidemiol* 156(11):1021–1027, 2002.

90. Jordan JM, Helmick CG, Renner JB, et al: Prevalence of hip symptoms and radiographic and symptomatic hip osteoarthritis in African Americans and Caucasians: the Johnston County Osteoarthritis project, *J Rheumatol* 36(4):809–815, 2009.

The references for this chapter can also be found on www.expertconsult.com.

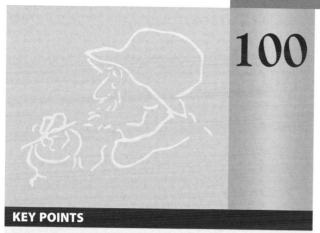

100

Treatment of Osteoarthritis

CARLOS J. LOZADA

KEY POINTS

Osteoarthritis (OA) is the most common form of arthritis.

Pain is the most common symptom in patients with OA.

The management plan should be individualized, accounting for factors such as sources of pain and extent of accompanying inflammatory features.

Nonpharmacologic interventions such as weight loss and exercise should be an integral part of the management plan for OA.

Currently available pharmacologic interventions are directed at symptomatic relief.

Investigation continues into potential disease-modifying interventions in OA.

Osteoarthritis (OA) is the most common form of arthritis. It is often referred to by other names such as *arthrosis, osteoarthrosis,* or simply *arthritis.* Because its incidence increases with age, OA is becoming an increasingly important health issue with the "graying" of the world's population.

OA can be defined radiographically or clinically. The most useful definition, however, includes symptoms and radiographic changes. If a purely radiographic definition is used, it can be demonstrated that almost all individuals older than 75 years have OA.[1] Although the epidemiology of OA is well covered in Chapter 99, it has been estimated that between 10% and 30% of those affected with OA are significantly disabled, making OA the leading cause of chronic disability in the United States.[2] This leads to substantial direct and indirect costs.

Traditional treatment paradigms for OA have conceded the inexorable progression of the disease and concentrated on pain management.[3] A simplistic but potentially useful algorithm is provided in Figure 100-1. As the population ages, there will be increasing societal pressure on physicians, particularly rheumatologists, to improve the available treatments for OA.[4-6] Researchers have turned to the investigation of agents that might delay the progression of OA. Particular investigational agents have included collagenase inhibitors, nutritional supplements, and polysaccharides, although many novel molecular entities are now under exploration.[7]

PATIENT ASSESSMENT

Appropriate management of OA begins with an accurate diagnosis. As with most rheumatic illnesses, obtaining a good history is of paramount importance. Symptoms should be carefully described, particularly pain. Duration, location, and any alleviating or exacerbating factors should be ascertained. Distinct features such as stiffness or gelling and the description of events such as "locking" or "giving way" of a joint can help direct the physical examination.

The physical examination seeks to confirm the diagnostic suspicion and establish the causes of symptoms. Laboratory evaluations are not helpful in establishing the diagnosis of OA but can help in excluding alternative diagnoses. They are also useful in determining which therapeutic approaches are appropriate for a particular patient because conditions such as renal insufficiency or anemia can be identified.

Radiographs are not necessary for diagnosis in the majority of patients but can identify coexistent conditions such as chondrocalcinosis that may require further workup or modification of the therapeutic plan.

SOURCE OF PAIN

The main symptom in OA is pain. It has many potential sources in and around the joint. These include focal synovitis, synovial effusions, subchondral bone pain receptors, and periarticular tendons and bursae. Factors complicating the determination of the source of pain may include varus or valgus deformity, weight issues, and the emotional impact of chronic pain. Once the source or sources of pain are accurately identified, a treatment plan can be formulated.

MANAGEMENT

The management of OA can be divided into nonpharmacologic interventions (Table 100-1), pharmacologic interventions, and surgical options. Pharmacologic interventions can be further subdivided into symptomatic therapy and potential structure- or disease-modifying therapy.

Nonpharmacologic Interventions

Psychosocial Interventions

As in other types of arthritis, patient education is an important first step in OA therapy. The patient should be an integral part of the decision-making team. To do this effectively, the patient should understand the nature of OA including its natural history and treatment options. It is often reassuring for the patient to realize that OA is a common, slowly progressive ailment and is not typically as disabling or deforming as the inflammatory arthritides. A significant number of patients have already tried nonprescription medications or nutraceutical remedies before

Video available on the Expert Consult Premium Edition website.

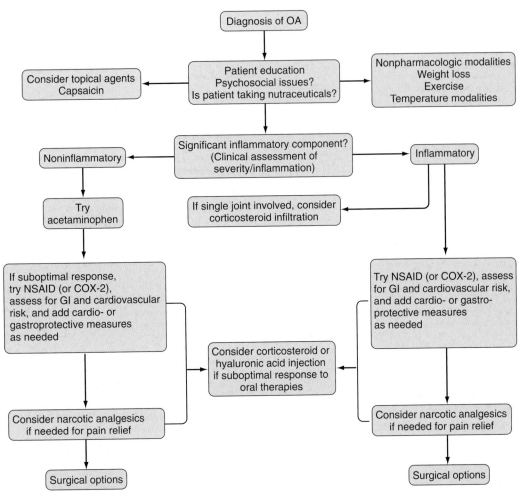

Figure 100-1 Algorithm for the management of osteoarthritis (OA). COX, cyclooxygenase; GI, gastrointestinal; NSAID, nonsteroidal anti-inflammatory drug.

seeing a physician and will want to discuss these options. Physicians should emphasize that treatment includes non-pharmacologic and pharmacologic interventions. Organizations such as the Arthritis Foundation can be valuable sources of information geared toward patients and can provide helpful reading materials.

Some patients may develop significant emotional disturbances related to the pain and changes in normal daily activities that can stem from OA. These may include mood disorders such as depression or sleep disorders. Worsened measures of mental health have been associated with increased OA pain and risk of flares.[8] Suspicion of either condition should lead to an evaluation by a psychiatrist or a primary physician who regularly manages these types of disorders.

Weight Loss

Obesity is an important risk factor in the development of OA of the knee.[9,10] Further, higher body mass index (BMI) has been associated with an increased risk of progression of OA of the knee.[11] This can be compounded by malalignment—namely, varus and valgus deformities that modulate the effect of weight on knee OA.[12] In one study, BMI was associated with OA severity in those with varus deformity but not in those with valgus.

Regimens of weight loss and exercise have been associated with improvement in pain and disability in OA of the knee.[13] Weight loss alone has been associated with a decrease in the odds of developing symptomatic knee OA.[14] One study suggested that a reduction in the percentage of body fat, rather than weight, may be significant in reducing pain from OA of the knee.[15] The symptom-relieving effects of weight loss have been shown to last as long as 1 year.[16] The

Table 100-1 Nonpharmacologic Management of Osteoarthritis

Conventional Options
Patient education
Arthritis self-help courses
Weight loss
Temperature modalities
Exercise
Orthotics
Modified activities of daily living

Unconventional Options
Transcutaneous electrical nerve stimulation
Pulsed electromagnetic fields
Static magnets
Acupuncture
Spa therapy
Yoga

combination of weight loss and exercise can be superior to either intervention alone.[17]

Temperature Modalities

Topical applications of heat or cold can be a helpful adjunct to the therapeutic plan. These are more effectively used in superficial joints such as the knees than in deep ones such as the hip. An acute injury such as a sprained ankle calls for cold applications for the first 2 to 3 days.[18] In a setting of chronic pain, most patients prefer warm applications, although if superior pain relief is obtained from cold applications, these can be continued.

Warm applications can be in the form of warm soaks or heating pads. Individual sessions should not exceed a temperature of 45° C or last more than approximately 30 minutes.[19] The application of warmth should be avoided over certain areas such as close to the testicles and in patients with poor vascular supply, neuropathy, or cancer. Benefits of warm applications include decreased pain and stiffness, along with relief of muscle spasm and prevention of contractures.

Exercise

Periarticular structures, particularly muscles, influence the expression of OA. This is likely due to their role in providing stability to the joints and in dampening some of the forces acting across joints. Quadriceps muscle weakness has been postulated as a risk factor for OA of the knee.[20] Quadriceps strengthening exercises have been advanced as fundamental to the management of conditions such as chondromalacia patellae.[21]

Both the dynamic and isometric exercise arms of a 16-week study of patients with knee OA showed equivalent improvement in symptoms and physical functioning.[22] Walking can be beneficial, and supervised fitness-walking regimens can improve function in those with OA of the knee.[21] Home-based exercise interventions also significantly improve symptoms in those with knee OA.[23,24] Finally, community-based aquatic exercise programs such as aquatic aerobics have merit.[25]

Orthotics and Bracing

Orthotics—ranging from insoles to braces—can be effective in providing symptomatic relief and are probably underused by most physicians. Studies have demonstrated that lateral wedged insoles provide substantial relief to those with medial compartment knee OA, particularly those with varus deformity.[26] In some studies, those with milder symptoms obtained greater benefit.[27] Knee braces have been evaluated as well. Valgus bracing of patients with medial compartment OA can reduce pain and increase levels of activity.[28] In one study, medial taping of the patella reduced the pain of those with patellofemoral compartment OA by 25%.[29]

Heel lifts have been tried in those with hip OA. In an uncontrolled study, most patients reported diminished symptoms. Time to improvement lengthened with the radiographic stage of OA.[30] For those with calcaneal spurs or foot joint OA in general, appropriate athletic-type

footwear is recommended. A good athletic shoe should provide medial arch support and calcaneal cushioning, as well as good mediolateral stability.

Those with carpometacarpal joint arthritis should initially be offered conservative management including the use of splints. In one trial, 70% of patients treated with a 7-month intervention that included the use of splints were able to improve their symptoms considerably and avoid surgical intervention.[31]

Cane/Walking Aid

The appropriate use of a cane (walking stick) can be an important adjunct, particularly in OA of the hip. It has been estimated that a cane can provide up to a 40% reduction in hip contact forces during ambulation.[32] The cane should be used in the hand contralateral to the affected hip or knee[33] and should be advanced with the affected limb while walking. The appropriate cane size is that which results in about a 20-degree flexion of the elbow during use.[34] A useful approximation is a cane that is equal to the distance from the floor to the patient's greater trochanter.

Modification in Activities of Daily Living

Physician advice and occupational therapy can provide useful insights into modifications of daily activities to reduce OA symptoms. These interventions can range from using an elevated toilet seat or shower bench in someone with lower extremity OA to using appliances designed to open jars in patients with hand OA. Assistance from occupational therapists can be valuable.

Other Interventions

Other modalities have been tried in OA. These are unconventional and include magnetic field application, acupuncture, and yoga-based regimens. These are not accepted as standard therapy for OA, but some deserve further study. A significant number of these interventions are being used by patients on their own and should be formally studied not only for evidence of any benefit but also to ensure that there are no harmful effects.

Studies of transcutaneous electrical nerve stimulation (TENS) have generally been small. A review of TENS studies in OA of the knee concluded that a trend toward symptom improvement existed, warranting larger, well-controlled studies.[35] In one randomized, controlled study, patients had initial symptom reduction, but at 1-year follow-up, only two patients continued to use the device.[36] TENS use for 3 weeks was compared with three weekly hyaluronic acid injections in 60 patients with OA of the knee. Pain relief was observed in both groups through the 6 months of follow-up. There was superior improvement in the Western Ontario McMaster Universities Osteoarthritis Index (WOMAC) physical function subscale score for the hyaluronic acid group.[37]

Pulsed electromagnetic fields have been tested in double-blind, placebo-controlled trials. These fields are applied through the daily use of a brace-type device. In one study, a primary endpoint of pain reduction was not achieved.[38] Another study did not meet its primary endpoint but reported an improvement in knee stiffness in subjects younger than 65 years, without an accompanying reduction in pain.[39]

The use of static magnets in chronic knee pain has become popular with some patients. In one double-blind, randomized, placebo-controlled trial of 43 patients, the WOMAC pain and physical function subscales, along with a 50-foot walk, demonstrated a statistically significant benefit of static magnets at 2 weeks.[40] Another 29-patient double-blind, placebo-controlled trial in knee OA reported a benefit over placebo after 4 hours of use, but there were no significant differences between groups at 6 weeks of continued treatment.[41] The potential mechanism for any effect remains unclear, and larger, longer-term studies are necessary before any clinical benefit can be postulated.

Acupuncture is being formally tested in a National Institutes of Health (NIH)–sponsored multicenter clinical trial. It has been difficult to develop appropriate controls to test acupuncture's clinical efficacy. Most recent studies have tried to employ "sham" methods in the control arm such as the use of blunted, telescopic needles.[42] Early clinical trials[43,44] and one literature review[45] concluded that acupuncture shows promise in the treatment of knee pain from OA. A double-blind, randomized, placebo-controlled trial of acupuncture as adjunctive therapy in OA of the knee enrolled 570 patients in two outpatient clinics. Reduction in knee pain in the true acupuncture group was superior to that in the sham acupuncture group at 26 weeks by WOMAC function score, WOMAC pain score, and patient global assessment. Twenty-five percent of the patients in each of the acupuncture groups were unavailable for analysis at 26 weeks, however.[46]

The most recent and largest randomized, double-blind, placebo-controlled trial of acupuncture in knee OA showed a benefit of both sham and "traditional" methods of acupuncture over physiotherapy and as-needed nonsteroidal anti-inflammatory drugs (NSAIDs); however, there were no significant differences between the sham and "traditional" arms of the studies in terms of OA symptom relief. The beneficial pain-relieving effect seen in slightly more than half the patients in each of these arms appeared to be secondary to the use of the needles themselves rather than the specific locations where they were placed.

Spa therapy also has advocates. It has been touted for low back pain and for lower extremity OA.[47] However, randomized, controlled studies are lacking.[48] Yoga has also shown some symptomatic benefit in OA of the hands on the basis of limited testing.[49]

Pharmacologic Interventions

Topical Agents

Topical agents for the management of OA are available without a prescription in the United States (Table 100-2). The two most widely used types are preparations containing capsaicin and those containing topical NSAIDs.

Capsaicin is a pungent ingredient found in red peppers (such as hot chili peppers). The mechanism of action is thought to be through selective stimulation of unmyelinated type C afferent neurons, causing the release of substance P. This release reversibly depletes the stores of

Table 100-2 Symptom-Relieving Pharmacologic Therapies for Osteoarthritis

Topical
Capsaicin
Topical NSAID preparations
Topical lidocaine preparations

Systemic
Acetaminophen
Nonselective NSAIDs
Cyclooxygenase-2–specific inhibitors
Tramadol
Narcotic analgesics

Intra-articular
Corticosteroids
Hyaluronic acid derivatives

NSAID, nonsteroidal anti-inflammatory drug.

substance P, a neurotransmitter of peripheral pain sensations.[50] Capsaicin preparations are available in concentrations of 0.025% or 0.075% in either ointment or, more recently, "roll-on" form, and they can be applied up to four times daily. They have been tested in controlled, double-blind studies in OA of the hands and knees.[51,52] Patient response is quite variable, with some obtaining significant pain relief and others not being able to tolerate the burning or stinging sensation produced by its application. Usually, the counterirritant sensation decreases gradually with repeated use, but pain relief remains. Although safe overall, capsaicin products can be irritating if they come in contact with mucosal surfaces, particularly the eyes. Patients should wear disposable gloves, if possible, when applying the agents. There may be some reddening of the skin where the compound is applied.

Topical NSAID preparations are popular worldwide for the treatments of OA.[53,54] Safety concerns about traditional oral NSAIDs were the driving force in the use of these topical agents,[55] although questions remain as to their absorption and the degree of relief obtained. Results of placebo-controlled trials in OA of the knee have been conflicting. Some demonstrated symptomatic relief with topical application of gels containing NSAIDs such as diclofenac,[56,57] whereas others showed only trends favoring the NSAID or no difference at all. In one trial, diclofenac gel was compared with placebo in 238 patients with OA of the knee over 3 weeks. The primary outcome was average pain with movement on days 1 to 14. The group on diclofenac gel had statistically superior improvement in this variable compared with those on placebo. WOMAC scores for function, pain, and disability were also significantly superior to placebo at weeks 2 and 3.[58] Transdermal diclofenac patches are also available and can be applied twice daily to painful articular locations. Patients were also randomized to receive eltenac or placebo gel over 4 weeks. Eltenac is a nonselective NSAID that is structurally similar to diclofenac. The primary endpoint was global pain on a visual analogue scale (VAS). At 4 weeks, there was a trend, but no statistical difference, favoring the eltenac gel. Two patients in the active treatment group and two in the placebo group had local itching, reddening, or both in the application area. There are also menthol- and salicylate-based over-the-counter topical preparations, but there are no published trials supporting their use in OA. Finally, lidocaine has gained popularity as a topical agent for musculoskeletal pain. Transdermal lidocaine 5% patches are available for management of pain and can be applied to up to three articular and periarticular locations at a time as an analgesic agent for 12-hour periods.

Systemic Agents

Non-narcotic Analgesics. Acetaminophen (paracetamol) has often been touted as the initial systemic intervention for the management of OA. This is mainly due to its favorable side effect profile but also to a perception of its equivalent efficacy to NSAIDs. This perception derives from studies of OA in which patients were not stratified in terms of degree of symptoms. In one study, acetaminophen 4 g/day was equivalent to ibuprofen 1200 or 2400 mg/day, with the notable exception of pain at rest.[59] A meta-analysis of 10 randomized, controlled trials concluded that acetaminophen is effective in the relief of pain associated with OA. However, the effect was small, and there was no improvement in overall WOMAC score. This suggests that acetaminophen may be effective for the relief of pain and should not be expected to have a strong effect on stiffness or function.[60] More recently, it has been noted that NSAIDs may have superior efficacy in patients with more symptomatic or inflammatory presentations because acetaminophen has no anti-inflammatory effects at approved doses.[61] A recent database review concluded that the available evidence suggests that NSAIDs have superior efficacy in symptomatic relief in those with hip or knee OA and also in those with moderate to severe levels of pain from OA.[62] Particular concerns in patients taking acetaminophen include the concomitant use of alcohol or over-the-counter products containing acetaminophen. Either of these situations can lead to the possibility of hepatic toxicity through toxic metabolites.

Nonsteroidal Anti-inflammatory Drugs. NSAIDs are the most commonly prescribed medications for the treatment of OA. Nonselective NSAIDs work through nonspecific inhibition of cyclooxygenase isoforms 1 and 2 (COX-1 and COX-2). COX-1 is constitutively expressed in renal and gastrointestinal (GI) tissues, among others. COX-2 is inducible in inflammatory responses. The major side effects of NSAIDs are GI toxicities (gastritis, peptic ulcer disease) and renal toxicities (interstitial nephritis, prostaglandin inhibition–related renal insufficiency). Because GI tissues have a higher expression of COX-1, a selective COX-2 inhibitor might spare patients the GI side effects. Unfortunately, COX-2 is expressed in renal tissue, and COX-2–specific drugs such as traditional NSAIDs have potential adverse renal effects. This is especially true in those with baseline renal insufficiency. Concerns about cardiovascular risks led to the voluntary withdrawal of rofecoxib from the market in the United States. There have also been concerns about celecoxib at a dose of 200 mg twice daily, owing to an increased relative risk for myocardial infarction in an adenomatous polyp trial[63]; this, however, has not been confirmed in six observational studies.[64] All NSAIDs and COX-2–specific agents have received "black box" warnings in their package inserts addressing cardiovascular risk. Alternative mechanisms of action of NSAIDs such as interference with receptors in the cell membrane phospholipid bilayers have been proposed.[65]

Nonselective NSAIDs are widely used for the management of OA. They include ibuprofen, naproxen, and diclofenac. NSAIDs are usually analgesic at lower doses but have both analgesic and anti-inflammatory effects at their higher recommended doses. They are prescribed either in fixed doses or "as needed" and are quite effective as symptom modifiers; however, they have no structure- or disease-modifying effects. NSAIDs should be used in the smallest dose that provides satisfactory symptom relief because GI toxicity has been linked to dosage. Adverse GI events have also been linked to patient age, previous history of peptic ulcers or bleeding, and the presence of comorbid conditions such as heart disease.

To reduce the potential for adverse GI events, misoprostol can be added to the therapeutic regimen. It is a prostaglandin E_2 analogue that has been shown to reduce the GI side effects of NSAIDs when used at 200 μg three times a day.[66] Diarrhea is a potential side effect. The use of a concomitant proton pump inhibitor may reduce upper GI endoscopic ulceration rates from NSAIDs, although no study has attempted to show a decrease in events such as symptomatic ulcers or bleeds.[67] Over-the-counter doses of H_2 blockers and antacids have not been shown to reduce either endoscopic or serious clinical GI events. COX-2–specific inhibitors are the latest drugs used in an attempt to reduce the GI adverse event profile of OA therapy.

COX-2–specific inhibitors are highly selective for COX-2 in vitro. Currently, only one such agent is available in the United States, celecoxib. Others such as etoricoxib are available elsewhere. These agents have been shown to reduce the rate of endoscopic ulceration by more than 50% when compared with nonselective NSAIDs. Celecoxib significantly reduces the rates of symptomatic ulcers, bleeds, perforations, and obstructions in patients not concurrently on aspirin.[68,69] It remains unclear how substantial the gastrointestinal benefits of these compounds are to patients taking aspirin. Because COX-2–specific agents can inhibit endothelial prostacyclin but do not affect platelet thromboxane, cardiovascular safety remains an area of investigation.[70,71]

Combination COX-lipoxygenase inhibitors are still investigational. It remains to be seen how these will compare with traditional NSAIDs and with COX-2 inhibitors in terms of both safety and efficacy.[72] Animal studies have hinted at the possibility of a structure- and disease-modifying effect.[73]

Narcotic Analgesics. Although several options exist for the management of pain in OA, some patients obtain suboptimal pain relief. If a patient has failed to respond to other nonpharmacologic and pharmacologic modalities and has no additional identifiable causes of pain (such as fibromyalgia), a narcotic analgesic should be considered.

The pain of OA is generally responsive to narcotic analgesics. Because of concerns about potential addiction, appropriate patient selection is important. Narcotic analgesics such as codeine and propoxyphene have been used effectively in patients with OA, especially in combination with non-narcotic analgesics (e.g., acetaminophen). Potential side effects include nausea, constipation, and somnolence.

Tramadol is an oral medication with mild suppressive effects on the mu opioid receptor. It also inhibits the uptake of norepinephrine and serotonin[74] and is not thought to have significant addictive tendencies.[75] It is available alone or in combination with acetaminophen and is not a controlled-schedule medication in the United States.[76] Tramadol has been used for the symptomatic relief of OA.[77] Seizures and allergic reactions are potential side effects.[78] A warning of increased risk of suicide in certain patients, similar to that on antidepressants, has been added to the label. The incidence of nausea can be reduced by slowly escalating the dose until the desired pain relief is achieved.

One study compared tramadol and acetaminophen with the combination of codeine and acetaminophen.[79] Patients with OA or chronic low back pain were randomized to receive tramadol and acetaminophen (37.5 mg and 325 mg, respectively) or codeine and acetaminophen (30 mg and 300 mg, respectively) for 4 weeks. Pain relief and changes in pain intensity were equivalent in both groups. Those on codeine and acetaminophen had a significantly higher incidence of somnolence (24% vs. 17%) and constipation (21% vs. 11%). The tramadol-acetaminophen combination also provides symptomatic relief as add-on therapy in OA patients receiving NSAIDs or COX-2 agents as baseline therapy.[80]

Extended-release narcotic analgesics have been tested in clinical trials in OA. This approach is intended to achieve a lower level of peak-to-trough variability in the plasma concentration of the narcotic. An extended-release, once-a-day preparation of tramadol relieves pain in OA of the knee and hip.[81] Extended-release oxymorphone dosed twice a day also provides relief in those with moderate to severe pain from OA of the hip or knee, as demonstrated by a VAS and the WOMAC composite index, as well as the subscales for pain, stiffness, and physical function.[82]

Transdermal fentanyl, a narcotic analgesic, has been used in the treatment of moderately to severely symptomatic knee and hip OA. It relieved pain and improved function in clinical trials as judged by a VAS and the WOMAC physical function subscale.[83]

Intra-articular Agents

Corticosteroids. Although there is no role for systemic corticosteroids in OA, local intra-articular corticoid preparations have a long history in the management of OA. Corticosteroids have been shown to downregulate the expression of adhesion molecules. This, in turn, can reduce cellular infiltration into the joint and subsequent inflammation. Corticosteroid injections slow macrophage-like cell infiltration of the synovium in OA.[84] The dose of steroid injected is determined by the volume of the joint being injected, with larger joints such as the knee receiving higher doses. The risk of joint infection is low if proper technique is employed. Postinjection flares due to corticosteroid crystal synovitis can occur.

There is a relative dearth of information from clinical trials of intra-articular corticosteroid injections. However, in one study, symptomatic benefit from corticosteroid injection for OA of the knee was demonstrated in a double-blind trial at 1 and 4 weeks postinjection.[85] Another trial attempted to assess the possible disease-modifying effects of corticosteroids by randomizing 68 patients to corticosteroid or saline injections of the knee every 3 months for 2 years. At the study's end, there was no significant difference in rate of joint space narrowing; thus no case could be made for a disease-modifying effect of corticosteroid injections. There was a trend favoring pain relief in the corticosteroid group as measured by the pain subscale of the WOMAC.[86] A review of published studies of intra-articular corticosteroid injections in OA concluded that the short-term symptomatic benefits have been well established, with few adverse events, but long-term benefits have not been confirmed.[87]

The specific corticosteroid compound used, the frequency of injections, and other factors related to the use of corticosteroid injections in OA vary widely and are heavily influenced by the training program the rheumatologist attended and where he or she practices.[88] In general, corticosteroid injections are believed to be most effective in patients with evidence of inflammation, effusions, or both. Because of concerns over possible deleterious effects, usually no more than four corticosteroid injections per year are given in a particular joint. Further discussion of arthrocentesis can be found in Chapter 54.

Hyaluronic Acid Derivatives. Synthetic and naturally occurring hyaluronic acid derivatives are administered intra-articularly. Although often mentioned as potential structure-modifying agents, these products are presently considered symptom-modifying drugs. Their molecular weights vary (from <100,000 to >1 million Svedberg units), depending on the preparation. They reportedly reduce pain for prolonged periods and may improve mobility.[89] Improvement in overall physical functioning has also been reported.[90] The mechanisms of action are not known. However, there is evidence of an anti-inflammatory effect (particularly at high molecular weight), a short-term lubricant effect, an analgesic effect by direct buffering of synovial nerve endings, and a stimulating effect on synovial lining cells, leading to the production of normal hyaluronic acid.[91]

Several preparations have been approved in the United States for OA of the knee. The injection regimens vary from five weekly injections to one injection depending on the product selected by the clinician for use.[92] Pain relief has been the primary outcome in these studies with relief at 26 weeks postinjection for some. In one study, three weekly hyaluronic acid intra-articular injections provided comparable pain relief to a single corticosteroid intra-articular injection at 1-week follow-up; at 45 days' follow-up, hyaluronic acid was superior to the corticosteroid.[93] In a Canadian study, 102 patients with OA of the knee were randomized to three weekly intra-articular injections of hylan G-F (Synvisc), hylan G-F plus an NSAID, or NSAID alone. At 26 weeks, both groups receiving hylan G-F were significantly better than the group receiving NSAIDs alone.[94]

Substantial clinical responses to the saline injections used as placebo in hyaluronic acid trials have sometimes made data interpretation challenging. In a double-blind, placebo-controlled trial, 495 patients with knee OA were randomized to receive five intra-articular injections of hyaluronic acid (Hyalgan) given 1 week apart, placebo, or naproxen (500 mg orally twice a day) and followed for 26 weeks.[95] Patients in the group receiving hyaluronic acid had significantly greater improvement in pain on the 50-foot walk compared with placebo, and more of them had a 20-mm or greater reduction in pain as judged by a VAS. At the conclusion of the trial, more hyaluronic acid–treated patients (47.6%) had slight pain or were pain free compared with placebo-treated (33.1%) or naproxen-treated (36.9%) patients. As expected, GI adverse events were significantly more common in the naproxen group than the hyaluronic acid and placebo groups.

Hyaluronic acid preparations have been tested in other randomized trials, with symptomatic relief of OA of the ankles, shoulders, and hips being reported.[96-98] One multicenter, randomized, double-blind study, reported as an abstract, revisited the issue of disease modification with hyaluronic acid. Patients received three courses of three intra-articular knee injections of either hyaluronan or saline over the course of 1 year. Joint space width was assessed using standing, weight-bearing radiographs; 273 patients completed the trial and had complete data collection. This study failed to demonstrate a disease-modifying effect for hyaluronan therapy because the primary endpoint was not met. Both the active treatment group and the placebo group had similar joint space narrowing during the study period. In those with a joint space width of 4.6 mm or greater at entry, hyaluronan use led to slightly less joint space narrowing than saline (placebo, 0.55 mm ± 1.04; hyaluronan, 0.13 mm ± 1.05; $P = .02$).[99] These results have not been confirmed in other trials. Hyaluronic acid products continue to be actively investigated in shoulder joint OA, periarthritis,[100] and adhesive capsulitis.[101]

Nutraceuticals

Two nutritional supplements—glucosamine and chondroitin sulfate—have received significant attention (Table 100-3). Health food stores and the lay press rather dubiously proposed them as "cures for arthritis." The mechanism of action of glucosamine sulfate is uncertain. Some in vitro experiments have shown stimulation of the synthesis of cartilage glycosaminoglycans and proteoglycans.[102,103] Others have shown that glucosamine and N-acetylglucosamine inhibit interleukin (IL)-1β– and tumor necrosis factor (TNF)–induced nitric oxide production in normal human articular chondrocytes.[104] N-acetylglucosamine also suppresses the production of IL-1β and stimulates IL-6 and COX-2.

Glucosamine

Urinary excretion of glucosamine (and other glycosaminoglycans) has been investigated and found to be elevated in

Table 100-3 Nutraceuticals for Osteoarthritis

Glucosamine
Chondroitin sulfate
Ginger extracts
Avocado and soy unsaponifiables
Cat's claw
Shark cartilage
S-adenosyl methionine

both OA and rheumatoid arthritis.[105] Supplementation with glucosamine sulfate, an intermediate in mucopolysaccharide synthesis, has been tried both orally and intramuscularly as therapy for OA. Glucosamine sulfate (400 mg injected intramuscularly twice weekly for 6 weeks) reduced the severity of disease as judged by the Lequesne index when compared with placebo.[106] A randomized, double-blind, parallel-group study in knee OA compared 500 mg oral glucosamine sulfate three times a day with 400 mg ibuprofen three times a day for 4 weeks. The response to ibuprofen was more rapid, but at 4 weeks, there was no statistically significant difference in the response rate (reduction of at least 2 points in the Lequesne index).[107] No group in the study received higher, anti-inflammatory doses of ibuprofen. An NIH-sponsored trial is currently under way in the United States to more thoroughly study the symptom-relieving and possible structure-modifying properties of glucosamine. Meanwhile, some already advocate the use of glucosamine as part of the first line of therapy for symptomatic OA.[108]

Glucosamine has also been compared with acetaminophen in an industry-sponsored trial. In the GUIDE trial, 318 patients with knee OA were randomized to glucosamine sulfate soluble powder 1500 mg once a day, acetaminophen 1000 mg three times a day, or placebo for 6 months. The main efficacy parameter was the 6-month change in the Lequesne index. At 6 months, the glucosamine group achieved significantly greater efficacy versus placebo. Those on acetaminophen failed to achieve a statistically significant benefit versus placebo by either the Lequesne index or WOMAC. There was no statistically significant difference between those on glucosamine and those on placebo on the basis of WOMAC outcomes.[109] Another clinical trial randomized 80 patients with knee OA to either glucosamine sulfate 1500 mg/day or placebo for 6 months. There was no difference between glucosamine and placebo in the primary variable of patients' global assessment of pain in the affected knee.[110] Another trial used a unique Internet-based recruiting system and followed 205 patients with knee OA randomized to glucosamine sulfate 1500 mg/day or placebo for 12 weeks.[111] The primary endpoint was the pain subscale of the WOMAC. At study conclusion, there was no difference in the groups with regard to pain, physical function, or overall WOMAC scores. Stratification by severity of OA, glucosamine product used, or use of NSAIDs did not alter the results. The Cochrane review of glucosamine therapy in OA analyzed a pool of 20 studies and 2570 patients. Pain and function improved by 28% and 21%, respectively, by the Lequesne index, compared with placebo. There was no improvement in the overall WOMAC pain and function scales. There has been speculation that these inconsistencies in study results may be due to a lack of standardization in glucosamine preparations.[112]

A recent discontinuation trial has added to the uncertainty about glucosamine's efficacy. It found that 137 patients who had been clinically classified as moderate responders to glucosamine sulfate were equally likely to experience an OA flare whether they continued or discontinued the glucosamine. No statistically significant differences between the groups were noted in pain and WOMAC function scores after 6 months.[113]

Combination products containing both glucosamine and chondroitin have become popular in the United States, despite a dearth of clinical trial data. One small, placebo-controlled trial randomized patients with knee OA to receive a regimen of glucosamine hydrochloride (1000 mg), chondroitin sulfate (800 mg), and manganese ascorbate (152 mg) twice a day or placebo.[114] Patients were evaluated at baseline and then every 2 months for 6 months using the Lequesne index of OA severity. At 4 and 6 months, those with mild to moderate radiographic OA of the knee showed significant improvement by the Lequesne index compared with those on placebo. In those with severe radiographic OA of the knee, no significant symptomatic benefit could be demonstrated. The study did not evaluate patients for structure or disease modification.

In the Glucosamine/Chondroitin Arthritis Intervention Trial (GAIT),[115] 1583 patients with OA of the knee were randomized to placebo, glucosamine hydrochloride 1500 mg/day, chondroitin sulfate 1200 mg/day, celecoxib 200 mg/day, or glucosamine hydrochloride and chondroitin sulfate. The primary endpoint was the percentage of patients achieving at least 20% improvement on the WOMAC pain subscale at 6 months. The only statistically significant response was seen in those on celecoxib versus placebo (70.1% vs. 60.1%; $P =.008$). Patients were then stratified for baseline severity by WOMAC pain scores, most of them falling into the mild OA pain category. In a subgroup analysis, in those with moderate to severe OA pain (WOMAC pain, 301 to 400 mm), the combination of glucosamine hydrochloride and chondroitin sulfate was more efficacious than placebo as measured by a dichotomous response rate (positive = 50% improvement in pain): 79.2% versus 54.3% ($P =.002$). Analysis of the radiographic data from this trial failed to support the notion of a disease-modifying/slowing role for glucosamine, chondroitin sulfate, or the combination of these compounds.

From these results, it appears that patient selection may be important in maximizing any potential benefit from glucosamine or chondroitin therapy. The GAIT study also had a particularly high placebo response rate, which may reflect the enrollment of patients with less symptomatic OA and may have affected the results. It also used a glucosamine hydrochloride preparation instead of the glucosamine sulfate used in most other studies, particularly those that have demonstrated efficacy. This raises the question of whether the choice of glucosamine hydrochloride negatively affected efficacy in the trial. However, one small (142 patients) Chinese trial randomized patients with OA of the knee to glucosamine sulfate 1500 mg/day or glucosamine hydrochloride 1440 mg/day for 1 month.[116] No efficacy differences were noted, with a clear majority of patients in each treatment arm achieving symptomatic improvement by Lequesne scores. The study had no placebo arm. Safety assessments continued for 2 additional weeks, with no significant adverse events reported. At present, it is still unclear whether glucosamine hydrochloride preparations have the same potential clinical benefits as glucosamine sulfate preparations. Additional investigations are necessary.

Two European trials tried to address the subject of disease modification with glucosamine. In one study, 212 patients with OA of the knee were randomized to receive placebo or glucosamine sulfate (1500 mg/day) and were followed prospectively for 3 years.[117] Fluoroscopically positioned, standing anteroposterior radiographs of the knees were taken at enrollment, 1 year, and 3 years. At 3 years, the treatment group had a joint space reduction of 0.06 mm, whereas the placebo group had a reduction of 0.31 mm. Whether this is a clinically meaningful difference in joint space is unclear. Those taking glucosamine also showed symptomatic benefit on the order of 20% to 25%, whereas those taking placebo had a slight worsening of symptoms, as judged by the WOMAC. There were no significant adverse events attributed to the use of the glucosamine sulfate. A second group of researchers randomized 202 patients to receive placebo or glucosamine sulfate (1500 mg/day) for 3 years.[118] The width of the narrowest medial joint space of the tibiofemoral joint was measured serially, using visual assessments with a 0.1-mm graduated magnifying glass on standardized full-extension, weight-bearing antero-posterior radiographs of each knee. At 3 years, there was a significant difference in joint space width, with a decrease of 0.19 mm in the placebo group and an increase of 0.04 mm in the glucosamine sulfate group. Also, significantly greater improvements in the WOMAC score and the Lequesne index were seen in the glucosamine group. The favorable results of these studies have been questioned because of the radiographic technique used to assess joint space. At issue is whether the joint space seen on standing films of the knee might be significantly affected by the symptoms of OA (i.e., pain) and whether a semiflexed film would be preferable. In one study, investigators obtained baseline radiographs (after analgesic or NSAID washout) using both standing-extended and semiflexed, fluoroscopically positioned techniques in 19 patients with knee OA.[119] Radiographs were then repeated 2 to 8 weeks later after reinstitution of analgesic or NSAID therapy. Joint space width increased with effective pain relief in highly symptomatic patients if measured by standing-extended radiographs. Using the semiflexed technique, there were no significant changes in joint space width related to severity of pain or responsiveness to pain therapy. This suggests that data obtained using the standing-extended radiographic technique may need to be revisited because the results may represent a therapeutic intervention's effect on symptoms (pain) rather than a disease-modifying effect. More recent, ongoing trials have changed to the semiflexed, fluoroscopically positioned knee radiograph to assess potential disease modification.[120]

Chondroitin Sulfate

Oral chondroitin sulfate, a glycosaminoglycan composed of units of glucosamine with attached sugar molecules (molecular mass of around 14,000), has also been used as therapy for hip and knee OA. Its mechanism of action is unknown. A double-blind, placebo-controlled study included a 3-month treatment phase followed by a 2-month treatment-free phase. The major outcome parameter was NSAID consumption. Those receiving chondroitin sulfate used fewer NSAIDs than the controls both at the completion of treatment and in the treatment-free phase.[121] Another study compared chondroitin sulfate to diclofenac sodium. One group received chondroitin sulfate (400 mg three times a day) and the other diclofenac sodium (50 mg three times a day). Each group was also changed over to placebo at some point. The chondroitin group received the active drug for 3 months, whereas the diclofenac group received it for only 1 month before being switched to placebo. For months 4 through 6, both groups took only placebo. The diclofenac group had a quicker response to therapy, whereas the chondroitin group had a more prolonged improvement as measured by the Lequesne index, VAS for pain, four-point scale for pain, and paracetamol use (rescue medication).[114,122] This study raises questions because of the different lengths of treatment with active drug in each group. Further studies are necessary.

One study evaluated chondroitin sulfate as a disease-modifying intervention. Three hundred patients were enrolled and randomized to chondroitin sulfate 800 mg daily or placebo for 2 years.[123] Joint space width was assessed using anteroposterior semiflexed radiographs. Pain and function were assessed as secondary endpoints. In the placebo group, the mean change in joint space width was 0.07 mm/year, while in the treatment group, the mean change was 0.00. A similar difference was noted when the minimum joint space width was evaluated. The differences were statistically significant (mean joint space width, $P = .04$; minimum joint space width, $P = .05$), but the clinical relevance remains unclear. The changes in radiographic progression were not matched by similar differences when pain and function were analyzed. The treatment group achieved improvement in all WOMAC subscales of pain, function, and stiffness, but a statistically significant difference could not be shown. It has been suggested that the overall low baseline WOMAC scores created difficulties in assessing for clinical improvement.

Other Nutraceuticals

Ginger extracts have been popular "natural" remedies for OA for some time.[124] Most of the world's ginger comes from China, and its "medicinal" use dates back more than 2000 years. Ginger actually contains small amounts of salicylate.[125] In some animal models, ginger has been shown to have inhibitory effects on COX and lipoxygenase.[126] One study with 247 evaluable patients revealed a small but statistically significant reduction in knee pain on standing (63% vs. 50%; $P = .048$) after taking ginger.[127] Reduction in knee pain after a 50-foot walk was also significant. Use of acetaminophen was reduced in the ginger-extract group, but the difference was not statistically significant. The extract was well tolerated, except for GI events such as dyspepsia, nausea, and eructation, which were increased over placebo. The question remains whether benefits observed represent a clinically relevant effect.

Some of the more unusual agents proposed as structure or disease modifiers in OA are oral preparations of avocado and soy unsaponifiables (ASUs). These compounds are derived from unsaponifiable residues of avocado and soya oils mixed in a 1:2 ratio. In vitro studies on cultured chondrocytes showed partial reversal of IL-1β effects. The roles of IL-1β in OA are thought to include inhibition of prostaglandin synthesis by chondrocytes and stimulation of matrix metalloproteinases (MMPs) and nitric oxide production. MMPs and nitric oxide can degrade cartilage matrix and cause chondrocyte apoptosis. Use of ASUs also reportedly results in inhibited production of IL-6, IL-8, and MMPs and stimulation of collagen synthesis. Increased aggrecan synthesis has been reported as well.[128] The mechanism of action is unknown, as is the active ingredient in ASUs.[129] Symptomatic benefit in double-blind human trials in OA of the hip and knee has been reported.[130] However, a double-blind, placebo-controlled trial in OA of the hip failed to show disease modification in the overall population, although a post hoc analysis reported benefit in those with more advanced OA at baseline. Some abstract presentations have suggested structure or disease modification in human hip OA.[131]

Other nutritional supplements such as cat's claw and shark cartilage have become entrenched in regional and international popular cultures. Many people take them, despite limited or no data to support their use. A small, placebo-controlled trial showed improvement of OA pain with activity in those taking cat's claw extracts.[132] Shark cartilage contains a small amount of chondroitin sulfate.[133] S-adenosyl methionine (SAMe), a methyl group donor and oxygen radical scavenger, is often touted as a remedy for OA, although little evidence of its effectiveness has been published.[134,135] In one double-blind, placebo-controlled study, two centers reported differing results. One center reported reductions in overall pain and rest pain, whereas the other showed no significant difference between the test group and placebo group.[136] Another small, double-blind, placebo-controlled crossover study of 61 patients compared oral SAMe 1200 mg/day with oral celecoxib 200 mg/day for 16 weeks. After the first month of phase I, celecoxib provided superior pain relief that was statistically significant. By the end of the second month, however, there was no statistically significant difference between the groups.[137] There is insufficient evidence to recommend the use of these products in the treatment of OA.

Other Potential Structure- or Disease-Modifying Therapies

The term *chondroprotective* has been used to describe structure- or disease-modifying agents. This is a misnomer, however, because the goal is to protect the entire joint (not only the cartilage) from the arthritic process. A workshop of the Osteoarthritis Research Society recommended that the term *structure-modifying drugs* be used for medications that previously would have been classified as chondroprotective.[138] These drugs are intended to prevent, retard, stabilize, or even reverse the development of OA. Recently, the term *disease-modifying osteoarthritis drug* (DMOAD) has been used for any such agent (Table 100-4). Such a disease-modifying effect in OA would require prolonged observation, given the typically slow progression of OA. Therefore clinical trials in this area have been challenging, with most being designed for at least 2½ to 3 years of follow-up. Progress in the methodology used to assess structure and disease modification may shorten the length of these trials. Radiographic assessments of joint space such as fluoroscopically positioned anteroposterior radiographs of the knee or magnetic resonance imaging may be useful in this regard.[139]

Unfortunately, to date, no drug has been conclusively proved to be structure or disease modifying. Although this chapter focuses on medication-based therapies, other

Table 100-4 Potential Structure- and Disease-Modifying Drugs in Osteoarthritis

Tetracyclines
Metalloproteinase or collagenase inhibitors
Glucosamine
Diacerein
Growth factor and cytokine manipulation (IL-1Ra, TGF-β)
Gene therapy (IL-1Ra, IL-1RII)
Chondrocyte and stem cell transplantation

IL-1Ra, interleukin-1 receptor antagonist; IL-1RII, interleukin-1 receptor type II; TGF-β, transforming growth factor-beta.

approaches such as osteochondral grafts of chondrocytes, donation of stem cells, or both, with eventual differentiation into bone and cartilage, are in various stages of development.[140] Potential structure- or disease-modifying interventions under investigation include collagenase inhibitors, polysaccharides, and growth factor and cytokine manipulation.

Tetracyclines, apart from any antimicrobial effect, are inhibitors of tissue metalloproteinases, perhaps owing to their ability to chelate calcium and zinc ions. There has also been research into the potential role of nitric oxide in the mechanism of action of the tetracyclines.[141] Minocycline, a tetracycline-family antibiotic, has been used in the management of rheumatoid arthritis.[142] Doxycycline, another tetracycline derivative, has been shown to inhibit articular cartilage collagenase activity.[143,144] Doxycycline has also reduced the severity of OA in canine models. In one study, there was preservation of medial femoral condyle cartilage in treated dogs compared with the untreated group. Other lesions such as medial trochlear ridge cartilage damage, superficial fibrillation of the medial tibial plateau, and osteophytosis were unaffected by treatment. Collagenolytic activity and gelatinolytic activity, however, were reduced to 20% and 25% of their previous levels, respectively, compared with untreated dogs. In an in vitro model, doxycycline not only reduced collagenase and gelatinase activity in cartilage but also prevented proteoglycan loss, cell death, and deposition of type X collagen matrix.[145]

A multicenter, double-blind, placebo-controlled trial using doxycycline for structure or disease modification in obese female subjects with OA of the knee has been completed. In this study, 431 obese women with unilateral OA of the knee were treated with doxycycline 100 mg twice daily or placebo. The primary endpoint was radiographic progression. The minimum joint space width was assessed by fluoroscopically positioned anteroposterior, semiflexed, standing radiographs. Pain and function were evaluated as secondary endpoints. Progression of minimum joint space width at 30 months was 0.3 ± 0.60 mm in the treatment group and 0.45 ± 0.70 mm in the placebo group ($P = .017$). Imaging of the contralateral knee was also performed at baseline and at 30 months. Progression in the contralateral knees was no different between the groups.[146] Secondary outcomes of pain and function were also recorded by WOMAC, VAS, 50-foot walk pain, and global assessment. Mean overall scores for pain were not significantly different between the groups. However, the frequency with which patients reported 20% or greater increase in knee pain was less in the treatment group ($P < .05$). Although a small disease-modifying effect was demonstrated in the target

knee, no such effect could be demonstrated in the contralateral knee. Thus the implications of these findings for clinical practice are uncertain. Other compounds with collagenase-inhibiting properties are being developed and investigated as structure- or disease-modifying agents not only in OA but also in rheumatoid arthritis.[147]

Glycosaminoglycan polysulfuric acid (GAGPS; Arteparon or Adequan) has been purported to work by reducing the activity of collagenase. It is a highly sulfated glycosaminoglycan, with a molecular weight ranging from 2000 to 16,000,[148] derived from bovine tracheal cartilage. In a canine model of OA, GAGPS was administered intra-articularly twice weekly for 4 weeks.[149] Four weeks after completion of the GAGPS treatment, medial femoral condylar lesions had developed to a lesser degree in the treated group than in saline-treated dogs. Swelling, an indicator of collagen network integrity, remained near control levels in the treatment group. In humans, OA of the knee was studied in a 5-year trial. There was improvement in multiple measured parameters including less time lost from work.[150] Another double-blind, placebo-controlled trial evaluated GAGPS in 80 patients with OA of the knee; patients received two series of five intra-articular injections of 25 mg (0.5 mL) GAGPS at 1-week intervals. At 14 weeks, 31% of the GAGPS group had improvement as judged by the Lequesne index, compared with 15% in the placebo group.[151] Potential allergy and heparin-like effects were observed. GAGPS is available in the United States for equine, but not human, use.

Another extract, a glycosaminoglycan-peptide complex (GP-C) known as *Rumalon*, has been investigated. It is a highly sulfated polysaccharide derived from bovine tracheal cartilage and bone marrow and is administered intramuscularly.[152] It has been shown to increase the levels of tissue inhibitor of metalloproteinases (TIMPs).[153] A randomized, placebo-controlled trial selected patients with hip or knee OA to receive 10 courses of injections of placebo or GP-C (2 mL) over 5 years (two courses per year). Each course consisted of 15 injections given twice weekly. GP-C failed to demonstrate a structure- or disease-modifying effect.[154] In addition, there were no statistical differences favoring the active treatment group when measured by the Lequesne index, pain on passive motion, or consumption of NSAIDs. GP-C is available in parts of Europe and South America.

Pentosan polysulfate (Cartrofen) is a purified extract of beech hemicellulose administered intramuscularly or orally as a calcium salt. It can inhibit granulocyte elastase and has inhibited the catabolism of aggrecan in cartilage explants.[155] Experimental studies in animal models suggest that it helps preserve cartilage proteoglycan content and retards cartilage degradation.[156,157] However, a recent blinded, placebo-controlled study using an oral preparation in a dog model failed to demonstrate either a symptomatic benefit or a structure- or disease-modifying effect.[158]

Diacerein and its active metabolite rhein are anthraquinones related to senna compounds.[159] They inhibit the synthesis of IL-1β in human OA synovium in vitro, as well as the expression of IL-1 receptors on chondrocytes.[160] No effects have been reported on TNF or its receptors. Collagenase production and articular damage have been reduced in animal models.[161-163] Early human clinical trials have shown improved pain scores compared with placebo and comparable efficacy to NSAIDs but a slower onset of action. Diarrhea is the main potential side effect. On the strength of these prior trials, diacerein has been proposed as a slow-acting symptom-modifying and perhaps structure- or disease-modifying drug for OA.

A double-blind, randomized, placebo-controlled trial looking at the efficacy and safety of diacerein enrolled 484 patients with symptomatic knee OA.[164] They were randomized to receive placebo, diacerein 25 mg twice a day, diacerein 50 mg twice a day, or diacerein 75 mg twice a day. Using intent-to-treat analysis, diacerein 100 mg/day was significantly superior to placebo ($P < .05$) by the primary endpoint—patients' assessment of pain on movement at week 24 (-18.3 ± 19.3 mm vs. -10.9 ± 19.3 mm). It was also superior on the basis of WOMAC and disability scores. However, no statistical difference was detected in the primary endpoint between placebo and 50 mg/day diacerein (-15 ± 21.0 mm) or 150 mg/day diacerein (-14.3 ± 23.7 mm).

There have also been investigations into the potential structure- or disease-modifying attributes of diacerein in OA.[165] In one study, 507 patients with OA of the hip (according to American College of Rheumatology criteria) were randomized to receive either diacerein (50 mg orally twice a day) or placebo for 3 years. Patients were followed with yearly pelvic radiographs to assess hip joint space. Using completer analysis, the diacerein patients showed a significantly lower rate of radiographic progression (0.18 vs. 0.23 mm/year). Using intent-to-treat analysis, a smaller proportion of those taking diacerein had significant joint space loss (defined as loss of ≥ 0.5 mm) during the study (50.7% vs. 60.4%). Unfortunately, almost 50% of the patients failed to complete the 3-year study. In the placebo group, the principal reason for discontinuation was lack of efficacy, whereas in the diacerein group, it was adverse effects such as diarrhea. Curiously, the symptom-relieving effect of diacerein observed in prior studies could not be confirmed in this one. A recent meta-analysis of clinical trials of diacerein in OA concluded that available clinical evidence supports pain relief in hip and knee OA. There was no analysis of a disease-modifying effect.[166]

Potential methods of intervention in OA include growth factor and cytokine manipulation.[167] Cytokines such as IL-1 and TNF are produced by the synovium and contribute to inflammation within osteoarthritic joints.[168] Moreover, there may be deficient expression of naturally occurring anti-inflammatory compounds such as IL-1 receptor antagonist (IL-1Ra) by the chondrocytes of patients with OA.[169] In some cases, increased nitric oxide production by OA articular chondrocytes may inhibit IL-1Ra synthesis.[170] In a dog model of OA, IL-1Ra therapy reduced the expression of collagenase-1 in cartilage.[171] The severity of cartilage lesions is also diminished.[172] In a rabbit model of OA, transfer of the IL-1Ra gene to joints prevented OA progression.[173] The effect of IL-1 blockade in humans with OA through the use of IL-1Ra is currently being investigated. Induction of repair in partial-thickness articular cartilage lesions by the timed release of transforming growth factor-β using liposomes has been attempted in an animal model. There was an increase in the cellularity of the defects, which were populated by cells of mesenchymal origin from the synovial membrane. The repaired cartilage resembled hyaline cartilage, and its integrity persisted up to 1 year after surgery.[174] Combination therapy is another alternative. In a study of canine-induced OA, sodium pentosan polysulfate, when combined with insulin-like growth factor-I, reduced stromelysin activity and increased TIMP.[175]

Initial attempts at gene therapy are intriguing. The control of genes such as TIMP and MMPs would, in theory, provide the opportunity to modulate the patient's disease. As previously noted, gene expression of IL-1Ra has already been tried in rabbits and dogs, as well as in an equine model of OA using an adenovirus vector.[176] Use of gene transfer–mediated overexpression of IL-1β decoy receptor has also been contemplated.[177] Chondrocyte and stem cell transplants into articular cartilage defects have been tried as well. Chondrocytes transplanted (expressing a previously transfected β-galactosidase gene) into human cartilage explants survived up to 45 days in vitro in one trial.[178,179] Transfection of chondrocytes with the galactosidase gene has been successful both before and after transplantation.

Surgical Intervention

Surgical interventions in OA usually consist of osteotomies or joint replacements. Osteotomies can be effective pain-relieving interventions and can delay the need for joint replacement surgery in selected patients. These tend to be younger subjects with OA.

Joint replacement surgery (joint arthroplasty) is effective in providing pain relief and restoring function in many patients with OA. Hip and knee joint replacements are most common. Indications for surgery include pain that is refractory to the previously discussed interventions and significant impairment of the patient's daily life. Therefore patients should be the key decision makers because they are the ones who must weigh the severity of symptoms and impairment. Patients undergoing replacement surgery should be deemed able to undertake the rehabilitation necessary to regain reasonable use of the joint involved. Infections are rare but do occur. Joint replacements have a typical life span of between 10 and 15 years. Revision surgery may be necessary, particularly in a relatively young patient who outlives the useful life of the prosthesis.

Other potential rationales for surgical intervention in OA include removal of loose bodies, stabilization of joints, redistribution of joint forces (e.g., osteotomy), and relief of neural impingement (e.g., spinal stenosis, herniated disk). The value of arthroscopic débridement or lavage in OA has been questioned. A recent randomized, blinded trial failed to demonstrate significant symptomatic benefit in OA of the knee.

SUMMARY

The treatment of OA includes a variety of possible nonpharmacologic and pharmacologic interventions. Treatment should be tailored to the individual and consists of a combination of modalities. These provide symptom relief but have no proven effect on the progression of disease. Structure and disease modification has yet to be achieved in OA. Trials that are under way could determine whether this is a realistic goal. Claims of structure or disease modification in OA should not be made for any drugs until well-designed, double-blind, placebo-controlled trials demonstrate that this is so. It is hoped that with the eventual advent of disease-modifying OA drugs, treatment will eventually consist of a combination of symptom-relieving and disease-modifying interventions.

Selected References

1. Lawrence JS, Bremmer JM, Bier F: Osteo-arthrosis: prevalence in the population and relationship between symptoms and x-ray changes, *Ann Rheum Dis* 25:1–24, 1966.
2. Peyron JG, Altman RD: The epidemiology of osteoarthritis. In Moskowitz RW, Howell DS, Goldberg M, Mankin HI, editors: *Osteoarthritis: diagnosis and medical/surgical management*, ed 2, Philadelphia, 1992, WB Saunders, pp 15–37.
3. Lozada CJ, Altman RD: Osteoarthritis: a comprehensive approach to management, *J Musculoskeletal Med* 14:26–38, 1997.
4. Hochberg MC, Altman RD, Brandt RD, et al: Guidelines for the medical management of osteoarthritis. I. Osteoarthritis of the hip, *Arthritis Rheum* 38:1535–1540, 1995.
5. Hochberg MC, Altman RD, Brandt KD, et al: Guidelines for the medical management of osteoarthritis. II. Osteoarthritis of the knee, *Arthritis Rheum* 38:1541–1546, 1995.
6. American College of Rheumatology Subcommittee on Osteoarthritis Guidelines: Recommendations for the medical management of osteoarthritis of the hip and knee: 2000 update, *Arthritis Rheum* 43:1905–1915, 2000.
8. Wise BL, Niu J, Zhang Y, et al: Psychological factors and their relation to osteoarthritis pain, *Osteoarthritis Cartil* 18:883–887, 2010.
10. Sturmer T, Gunther KP, Brenner H: Obesity, overweight and patterns of osteoarthritis: The Ulm Osteoarthritis Study, *J Clin Epidemiol* 53:307–313, 2000.
11. Cooper C, Snow S, McAlindon TE, et al: Risk factors for the incidence and progression of radiographic knee osteoarthritis, *Arthritis Rheum* 43:995–1000, 2000.
12. Sharma L, Lou C, Cahue S, Dunlop DD: The mechanism of the effect of obesity in knee osteoarthritis: the mediating role of malalignment, *Arthritis Rheum* 43:568–575, 2000.
13. Messier SP, Loeser RF, Mitchell MN, et al: Exercise and weight loss in obese older adults with knee osteoarthritis: a preliminary study, *J Am Geriatr Soc* 48:1062–1072, 2000.
14. Felson DT, Zhang Y, Anthony JM, et al: Weight loss reduces the risk for symptomatic knee osteoarthritis in women, *Ann Intern Med* 116:535–539, 1992.
15. Toda Y, Toda T, Takemura S, et al: Change in body fat, but not body weight or metabolic correlates of obesity, is related to symptomatic relief of obese patients with knee osteoarthritis after a weight control program, *J Rheumatol* 25:2181–2186, 1998.
16. Christensen R, Astrup A, Bliddal H, et al: Sustained weight loss as a treatment of osteoarthritis in obese patients: long-term results from a randomized trial, *Ann Rheum Dis* 64(Suppl III):66, 2005.
17. Messier SP, Loeser RF, Miller GD, et al: Exercise and dietary weight loss in overweight and obese older adults with knee osteoarthritis: the arthritis, diet and activity promotion trial, *Arthritis Rheum* 50:1501–1510, 2005.
18. Swezey RL: Essentials of physical management and rehabilitation in arthritis, *Semin Arthritis Rheum* 3:349–368, 1974.
19. Lehman JF, DeLateur BJ: Diathermy and superficial heat, laser, and cold therapy. In Kottke FJ, Lehman JF, editors: *Krusen's handbook of physical medicine and rehabilitation*, ed 4, Philadelphia, WB Saunders, 1990, pp 283–367.
20. Slemenda C, Heilman DK, Brandt KD, et al: Reduced quadriceps strength relative to body weight: a risk factor for knee osteoarthritis in women? *Arthritis Rheum* 41:1951–1959, 1998.
21. Bentley G, Dowd G: Current concepts of etiology and treatment of chondromalacia patellae, *Clin Orthop* 189:209–228, 1984.
22. Topp R, Woolley S, Hornyak J III, et al: The effect of dynamic versus isometric resistance training on pain and functioning among adults with osteoarthritis of the knee, *Arch Phys Med Rehabil* 83:1187–1195, 2002.
23. Kovar PA, Allegrante JP, MacKenzie R, et al: Supervised fitness walking in patients with osteoarthritis of the knee, *Ann Intern Med* 116:529–534, 1992.
24. Thomas KS, Muir KR, Doherty M, et al: Home based exercise programme for knee pain and knee osteoarthritis: randomised controlled trial, *BMJ* 325:752, 2002.
25. Belza B, Topolski T, Kinne S, et al: Does adherence make a difference? Results from a community-based aquatic exercise program, *Nurs Res* 51:285–291, 2002.
26. Kerrigan DC, Lelas JL, Goggins J, et al: Effectiveness of a lateral-wedge insole on knee varus torque in patients with knee osteoarthritis, *Arch Phys Med Rehabil* 83:889–893, 2002.
27. Keating EM, Faris PM, Ritter MA, Kane J: Use of lateral heel and sole wedges in the treatment of medial osteoarthritis of the knee, *Orthop Rev* 22:921–924, 1993.
28. Pollo FE, Otis JC, Backus SI, et al: Reduction of medial compartment loads with valgus bracing of the osteoarthritic knee, *Am J Sports Med* 30:414–421, 2002.
29. Cushnaghan J, McCarthy C, Dieppe P: Taping the patella medially: a new treatment for osteoarthritis of the knee joint? *BMJ* 308:753–755, 1994.
30. Ohsawa S, Ueno R: Heel lifting as a conservative therapy for osteoarthritis of the hip: based on the rationale of Pauwels' intertrochanteric osteotomy, *Prosthet Orthot Int* 21:153–158, 1997.
31. Berggren M, Joost-Davidsson A, Lindstrand J, et al: Reduction in the need for operation after conservative treatment of osteoarthritis of the first carpometacarpal joint: a seven year prospective study, *Scand J Plast Reconstr Surg Hand Surg* 35:415–417, 2001.
32. Brand RA, Crowninshield RD: The effect of cane use on hip contact force, *Clin Orthop* 147:181–184, 1980.
33. Chan GN, Smith AW, Kirtley C, Tsang WW: Changes in knee moments with contrateral versus ipsilateral cane usage in females with knee osteoarthritis, *Clin Biomech* 20:396–404, 2005.
34. Blount WP: Don't throw away the cane, *J Bone Joint Surg Am* 38:695–708, 1956.
35. Osiri M, Welch V, Brosseau L, et al: Transcutaneous electrical nerve stimulation for knee osteoarthritis, *Cochrane Database Syst Rev* 4:CD002823, 2000.
36. Taylor P, Hallett M, Flaherty L: Treatment of osteoarthritis of the knee with transcutaneous electrical nerve stimulation, *Pain* 11:233–240, 1981.
37. Paker N, Tekdos D, Kesiktas N, Soy D: Comparison of the therapeutic efficacy of TENS versus intra-articular hyaluronic acid injection in patients with knee osteoarthritis: a prospective, randomized study, *Adv Ther* 23:342–353, 2006.
38. Pipitone N, Scott DL: Magnetic pulse treatment for knee osteoarthritis: a randomised, double-blind, placebo-controlled study, *Curr Med Res Opin* 17:190–196, 2001.
39. Thamsborg G, Florescu A, Oturai P, et al: Treatment of knee osteoarthritis with pulsed electromagnetic fields: a randomized, double-blind, placebo-controlled study, *Osteoarthritis Cartil* 13:575–581, 2005.
40. Hinman MR, Ford J, Heyl H: Effects of static magnets on chronic knee pain and physical function: a double-blind study, *Altern Ther Health Med* 8:50–55, 2002.
42. White AR, Filshie J, Cummings TM: International Acupuncture Research Forum: clinical trials of acupuncture: consensus recommendations for optimal treatment, sham controls and blinding, *Complement Ther Med* 9:237–245, 2001.
43. Tillu A, Tillu S, Vowler S: Effect of acupuncture on knee function in advanced osteoarthritis of the knee: a prospective, non-randomised controlled study, *Acupunct Med* 20:19–21, 2002.
44. Berman BM, Singh BB, Lao L, et al: A randomized trial of acupuncture as an adjunctive therapy in osteoarthritis of the knee, *Rheumatology (Oxford)* 38:346–354, 1999.
45. Ezzo J, Hadhazy V, Birch S, et al: Acupuncture for osteoarthritis of the knee: a systematic review, *Arthritis Rheum* 44:819–825, 2001.
46. Berman BM, Lao L, Langenberg P, et al: Effectiveness of acupuncture as adjunctive therapy in osteoarthritis of the knee: a randomized, controlled trial, *Ann Intern Med* 141:901–910, 2004.
47. Guillemin F, Virion JM, Escudier P, et al: Effect on osteoarthritis of spa therapy at Bourbonne-les-Bains, *Joint Bone Spine* 68:499–503, 2001.
48. Ernst E, Pittler MH: [How effective is spa treatment? A systematic review of randomized studies], *Dtsch Med Wochenschr* 123:273–277, 1998.
49. Garfinkel M, Schumacher HR Jr: Yoga, *Rheum Dis Clin North Am* 26:125–132, 2000.

50. Rains C, Bryson HM: Topical capsaicin: a review of its pharmacological properties and therapeutic potential in post-herpetic neuralgia, diabetic neuropathy and osteoarthritis, *Drugs Aging* 7:317–328, 1995.

51. McCarthy GM, McCarty DJ: Effect of topical capsaicin in the therapy of painful osteoarthritis of the hands, *J Rheumatol* 19:604–607, 1992.

52. Deal CL, Schnitzer TJ, Lipstein E, et al: Treatment of arthritis with topical capsaicin: a double-blind trial, *Clin Ther* 13:383–395, 1991.

53. Dreiser RL, Tisne-Camus M: DHEP plasters as a topical treatment of knee osteoarthritis: a double-blind placebo-controlled study, *Drugs Exp Clin Res* 19:117–123, 1993.

56. Grace D, Rogers J, Skeith K, Anderson K: Topical diclofenac versus placebo: a double blind, randomized clinical trial in patients with osteoarthritis of the knee, *J Rheumatol* 26:2659–2663, 1999.

57. Niethard FU, Gold MS, Solomon GS, et al: Efficacy of topical diclofenac diethylamine gel in osteoarthritis of the knee, *J Rheumatol* 32:2384–2392, 2005.

58. Sandelin J, Harilainen A, Crone H, et al: Local NSAID gel (eltenac) in the treatment of osteoarthritis of the knee: a double blind study comparing eltenac with oral diclofenac and placebo gel, *Scand J Rheumatol* 26:287–292, 1997.

59. Bradley JD, Brandt KD, Katz BP, et al: Comparison of an antiinflammatory dose of ibuprofen, an analgesic dose of ibuprofen, and acetaminophen in the treatment of patients with osteoarthritis of the knee, *N Engl J Med* 325:87–91, 1991.

60. Zhang W, Jones A, Doherty M: Does paracetamol (acetaminophen) reduce the pain of osteoarthritis? A meta-analysis of randomized controlled trials, *Ann Rheum Dis* 63:901–907, 2005.

61. Pincus T, Koch GG, Sokka T, et al: A randomized, double-blind crossover clinical trial of diclofenac plus misoprostol versus acetaminophen in patients with osteoarthritis of the hip or knee, *Arthritis Rheum* 44:1587–1598, 2001.

62. Towheed TE, Maxwell L, Judd MG, et al: Acetaminophen for osteoarthritis, *Cochrane Database Syst Rev* 1:CD004257, 2006.

63. Solomon SD, McMurrray JV, Pfeffer MA, et al: Cardiovascular risk associated with celecoxib in a clinical trial for colorectal adenoma prevention, *N Engl J Med* 352:1071–1080, 2005.

64. Solomon DH: Selective cyclooxygenase 2 inhibitors and cardiovascular events, *Arthritis Rheum* 52:1968–1978, 2005.

65. Abramson SB, Weissmann G: The mechanism of action of nonsteroidal antiinflammatory drugs, *Arthritis Rheum* 32:1, 1989.

66. Graham DY, Agrawal NM, Roth SH: Prevention of NSAID-induced gastric ulcer with misoprostol: multicenter, double-blind, placebo-controlled trial, *Lancet* 2:1277–1280, 1988.

67. Hawkey CJ, Karrasch JA, Szczepanski L, et al: Omeprazole compared with misoprostol for ulcers associated with nonsteroidal antiinflammatory drugs: Omeprazole versus Misoprostol for NSAID-Induced Ulcer Management (OMINUM) Study Group, *N Engl J Med* 338:727–734, 1998.

68. Bombardier C, Laine L, Reicin A, et al: Comparison of upper gastrointestinal toxicity of rofecoxib and naproxen in patients with rheumatoid arthritis: VIGOR Study Group, *N Engl J Med* 343:1520–1528, 2000.

69. Silverstein FE, Faich G, Goldstein JL, et al: Gastrointestinal toxicity with celecoxib vs nonsteroidal anti-inflammatory drugs for osteoarthritis and rheumatoid arthritis: The CLASS study-randomized controlled trial: Celecoxib Long-term Arthritis Safety Study, *JAMA* 284:1247–1255, 2000.

70. Cheng Y, Austin SC, Rocca B, et al: Role of prostacyclin in the cardiovascular response to thromboxane A2, *Science* 296:539–541, 2002.

71. Mukherjee D, Nissen SE, Topol EJ: Risk of cardiovascular events associated with selective COX-2 inhibitors, *JAMA* 286:954–959, 2001.

73. Boileau C, Martel-Pelletier J, Jouzeau JY, et al: Licofelone (ML-3000), a dual inhibitor of 5-lipoxygenase and cyclooxygenase, reduces the level of cartilage chondrocyte death in vivo in experimental dog osteoarthritis: inhibition of pro-apoptotic factors, *J Rheumatol* 29:1446–1453, 2002.

74. Raffa RB, Friederichs E, Reimann W, et al: Opioid and non-opioid components independently contribute to the mechanism of action of tramadol, an "atypical" opioid analgesic, *J Pharmacol Exp Ther* 260:275–285, 1992.

76. Silverfield JC, Kamin M, Wu SC, et al: Tramadol/acetaminophen combination tablets for the treatment of osteoarthritis flare pain:

a multicenter, outpatient, randomized, double-blind, placebo-controlled, parallel-group, add-on study, *Clin Ther* 24:282–297, 2002.

80. Emkey R, Rosenthal N, Wu SC, et al: Efficacy and safety of tramadol/acetaminophen tablets (Ultracet) as add-on therapy for osteoarthritis pain in subjects receiving a COX-2 nonsteroidal antiinflammatory drug: a multicenter, randomized, double-blind, placebo-controlled trial, *J Rheumatol* 31:150–156, 2004.

81. Gana TJ, Pascual ML, Fleming RR, et al: Extended release tramadol in the treatment of osteoarthritis: a multicenter, randomized, double-blind, placebo-controlled clinical trial, *Curr Med Res Opin* 22:1391–1401, 2006.

82. Kivitz A, Ma C, Ahdieh H, Galer BS: A 2-week, multicenter, randomized, double-blind, placebo-controlled, dose-ranging, phase III trial comparing the efficacy of oxymorphone extended release and placebo in adults with pain associated with osteoarthritis of the hip or knee, *Clin Ther* 28:352–364, 2006.

83. Langford R, McKenna F, Ratcliffe S, et al: Transdermal fentanyl for improvement of pain and functioning in osteoarthritis: a randomized, placebo-controlled trial, *Arthritis Rheum* 54:1829–1837, 2006.

84. Young L, Katrib A, Cuello C, et al: Effects of intraarticular glucocorticoids on macrophage infiltration and mediators of joint damage in osteoarthritis synovial membranes: findings in a double-blind, placebo-controlled study, *Arthritis Rheum* 44:343–350, 2001.

86. Raynauld JP, Buckland-Wright C, Ward R, et al: Safety and efficacy of long term intraarticular steroid injections in osteoarthritis of the knee: a randomized, double-blind, placebo-controlled trial, *Arthritis Rheum* 48:370–377, 2003.

87. Bellamy N, Campbell J, Robinson V, et al: Intraarticular corticosteroid for treatment of osteoarthritis of the knee, *Cochrane Database Syst Rev* 2:CD005328, 2006.

89. Peyron JG: Intraarticular hyaluronan injections in the treatment of osteoarthritis: state-of-the art review, *J Rheumatol* 20(Suppl 39):10–15, 1993.

90. Petrella RJ, DiSilvestro MD, Hildebrand C: Effects of hyaluronate sodium on pain and physical functioning in osteoarthritis of the knee: a randomized, double-blind, placebo-controlled clinical trial, *Arch Intern Med* 162:292–298, 2002.

91. Kuiper-Geertsma DG, Bijlsma JW: Intra-articular injection of hyaluronic acid as an alternative option to corticosteroid injections for arthrosis, *Ned Tijdschr Geneeskd* 144:2188–2192, 2000.

92. Chevalier X, Jerosch J, Goupille P, et al: Single, intra-articular treatment with 6 ml hylan G-F 20 in patients with symptomatic primary osteoarthritis of the knee: a randomized, multicentre, double-blind, placebo controlled trial, *Ann Rheum Dis* 69:113–119, 2010.

93. Leardini G, Mattara L, Franceschini M, Perbellini A: Intra-articular treatment of knee osteoarthritis: a comparative study between hyaluronic acid and 6-methyl prednisolone acetate, *Clin Exp Rheumatol* 9:375–381, 1991.

94. Adams ME, Atkinson MH, Lussier AJ, et al: The role of viscosupplementation with hylan G-F 20 (Synvisc) in the treatment of osteoarthritis of the knee: a Canadian multicenter trial comparing hylan G-F 20 alone, hylan G-F 20 with non-steroidal anti-inflammatory drugs (NSAIDs) and NSAIDs alone, *Osteoarthritis Cartil* 3:213–225, 1995.

95. Altman RD, Moskowitz R: Intraarticular sodium hyaluronate (Hyalgan) in the treatment of patients with osteoarthritis of the knee: a randomized clinical trial. Hyalgan Study Group, *J Rheumatol* 25:2203–2212, 1998.

97. Altman RD, Moskowitz R, Joacobs S, et al: A double-blind randomized trial of intra-articular injection of sodium hyaluronate for the treatment of chronic shoulder pain [abstract 1206], *Arthritis Rheum* 52 Suppl:S461, 2005.

99. Jubb RW, Beinat L, Dacre J, et al: A one-year randomized, placebo (saline) controlled clinical trial of 500-730 kDa sodium hyaluronate (Hyalgan) on the radiological change in osteoarthritis of the knee, *Int J Clin Pract* 57:467–474, 2003.

103. Bassleer C, Reginster JY, Franchimont P: Effects of glucosamine on differentiated human chondrocytes cultivated in clusters [abstract], *Rev Esp Reumatol* 20(Suppl 1):96, 1993.

104. Shikman AR, Kuhn K, Alaaeddine N, Lotz M: N-acetylglucosamine prevents IL-1 beta-mediated activation of human chondrocytes, *J Immunol* 166:5155–5160, 2001.

106. Reichelt A, Forster KK, Fischer M, et al: Efficacy and safety of intramuscular glucosamine sulfate in osteoarthritis of the knee: a randomised, placebo-controlled, double-blind study, *Arzneimittelforschung Drug Res* 44:75–80, 1994.

107. Muller-Fabender H, Bach GL, Haase W, et al: Glucosamine sulfate compared to ibuprofen in osteoarthritis of the knee, *Osteoarthritis Cartil* 2:61–69, 1994.

112. Towheed T, Maxwell L, Anastassiades T, et al: Glucosamine therapy for treating osteoarthritis, *Cochrane Database Syst Rev* 2:CD002946, 2005.

115. Clegg DO, Reda DJ, Harris CL, et al: Glucosamine, chondroitin sulfate, and the two in combination for painful knee osteoarthritis, *N Engl J Med* 354:795–808, 2006.

117. Reginster JY, Deroisy R, Rovati LC, et al: Long-term effects of glucosamine sulphate on osteoarthritis progression: a randomised, placebo-controlled clinical trial, *Lancet* 357:251–256, 2001.

118. Pavelka K, Gatterova J, Olejarova M, et al: Glucosamine sulfate use and delay of progression of knee osteoarthritis: a 3-year, randomized, placebo-controlled, double-blind study, *Arch Intern Med* 162:2113–2123, 2002.

119. Mazzuca SA, Brandt KD, Lane KA, et al: Knee pain reduces joint space width in conventional standing anteroposterior radiographs of osteoarthritic knees, *Arthritis Rheum* 46:1223–1227, 2002.

121. Mazieres B, Loyau G, Menkes CJ, et al: Chondroitin sulfate in the treatment of gonarthrosis and coxarthrosis: 5-month results of a multicenter double-blind controlled prospective study using placebo, *Rev Rhum* 59:466–472, 1992.

123. Michel BA, Stucki G, Frey D, et al: Chondroitins 4 and 6 sulfate in osteoarthritis of the knee: a randomized, controlled trial, *Arthritis Rheum* 52:779–786, 2005.

127. Altman RD, Marcussen KC: Effects of a ginger extract on knee pain in patients with osteoarthritis, *Arthritis Rheum* 44:2531–2538, 2001.

128. Henrotin YE, Sanchez C, Deberg MA, et al: Avocado/soybean unsaponifiables increase aggrecan synthesis and reduce catabolic and proinflammatory mediator production by human osteoarthritic chondrocytes, *J Rheumatol* 30:1825–1834, 2003.

130. Maheu E, Mazieres B, Valat JP, et al: Symptomatic efficacy of avocado/soybean unsaponifiables in the treatment of osteoarthritis of the knee and hip: a prospective, randomized, double-blind, placebo-controlled, multicenter clinical trial with six-month treatment period and two-month follow-up demonstrating a persistent effect, *Arthritis Rheum* 41:81–91, 1998.

132. Piscoya J, Rodriguez Z, Bustamante SA, et al: Efficacy and safety of freeze-dried cat's claw in osteoarthritis of the knee: mechanisms of action of the species *Uncaria guianensis*, *Inflamm Res* 50:442–448, 2001.

133. Nadanaka S, Clement A, Masayama K, et al: Characteristic hexasaccharide sequences in octasaccharides derived from shark cartilage chondroitin sulfate D with a neurite outgrowth promoting activity, *J Biol Chem* 273:3296–3307, 1998.

134. Barcelo HA, Wiemeyer JC, Sagasta CL, et al: Experimental osteoarthritis and its course when treated with S-adenosyl-L-methionine, *Rev Clin Esp* 187:74–78, 1990.

135. Montrone F, Fumagalli M, Sarzi Puttini P, et al: Double-blind study of S-adenosyl-methionine versus placebo in hip and knee arthrosis, *Clin Rheumatol* 4:484–485, 1985.

138. Altman R, Brandt K, Hochberg M, et al: Design and conduct of clinical trials in patients with osteoarthritis: recommendations from a task force of the Osteoarthritis Research Society, *Osteoarthritis Cartil* 4:217–243, 1996.

139. Lozada CJ, Altman RD: Chondroprotection in osteoarthritis, *Bull Rheum Dis* 46:5–7, 1997.

141. Amin AR, Attur MG, Thakker GD, et al: A novel mechanism of action of tetracyclines: effects on nitric oxide synthases, *Proc Natl Acad Sci U S A* 93:14014–14019, 1996.

144. Yu LP Jr, Smith GN Jr, Hasty KA, Brandt KD: Doxycycline inhibits type XI collagenolytic activity of extracts from human osteoarthritic cartilage and of gelatinase, *J Rheumatol* 18:1450–1452, 1991.

146. Brandt KD, Mazzuca SA, Katz BP, et al: Effects of doxycycline on progression of osteoarthritis: results of a randomized, placebo-controlled, double-blind trial, *Arthritis Rheum* 52:2015–2025, 2005.

151. Pavelka K Jr, Sedlackova M, Gatterova J, et al: Glycosaminoglycan polysulfuric acid (GAGPS) in osteoarthritis of the knee, *Osteoarthritis Cartil* 3:15–23, 1995.

152. Moskowitz RW, Reese JH, Young RG, et al: The effects of Rumalon, a glycosaminoglycan peptide complex, in a partial meniscectomy model of osteoarthritis in rabbits, *J Rheumatol* 18:205–209, 1991.

154. Pavelka K, Gatterova J, Gollerova V, et al: A 5-year randomized controlled, double-blind study of glycosaminoglycan polysulphuric acid complex (Rumalon) as a structure modifying therapy in osteoarthritis of the hip and knee, *Osteoarthritis Cartil* 8:335–342, 2000.

160. Martel-Pelletier J, Mineau F, Jolicoeur FC, et al: In vitro effects of diacerhein and rhein on interleukin 1 and tumor necrosis factor-alpha systems in human osteoarthritic synovium and chondrocytes, *J Rheumatol* 25:753–762, 1998.

162. Brun PH: Effect of diacetylrhein on the development of experimental osteoarthritis: a biochemical investigation [letter], *Osteoarthritis Cartil* 5:289–291, 1997.

164. Pelletier JP, Yaron M, Haraoui B, et al: Efficacy and safety of diacerein in osteoarthritis of the knee, *Arthritis Rheum* 43:2339–2348, 2000.

166. Rintelen B, Neumann K, Leeb BF: A meta-analysis of controlled clinical studies with diacerein in the treatment of osteoarthritis, *Arch Intern Med* 166:1899–1906, 2006.

168. Smith MD, Triantafillou S, Parker A, et al: Synovial membrane inflammation and cytokine production in patients with early osteoarthritis, *J Rheumatol* 24:365–371, 1997.

171. Caron JP, Fernandes JC, Martel-Pelletier J, et al: Chondroprotective effect of intraarticular injections of interleukin-1 receptor antagonist in experimental osteoarthritis: suppression of collagenase-1 expression, *Arthritis Rheum* 39:1535–1544, 1996.

173. Fernandes J, Tardif G, Martel-Pelletier J, et al: In vivo transfer of interleukin-1 receptor antagonist gene in osteoarthritic rabbit knee joints: prevention of osteoarthritis progression, *Am J Pathol* 154:1159–1169, 1999.

178. Doherty PJ, Zhang H, Tremblay L, et al: Resurfacing of articular cartilage explants with genetically-modified human chondrocytes in vitro, *Osteoarthritis Cartil* 6:153–159, 1998.

179. Moseley JB, O'Malley K, Petersen NJ, et al: A controlled trial of arthroscopic surgery for osteoarthritis of the knee, *N Engl J Med* 347:81–88, 2002.

Full references for this chapter can be found on www.expertconsult.com.

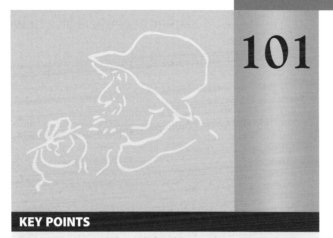

101 Metabolic Bone Disease

NANCY E. LANE

KEY POINTS

Osteoporosis is a disease defined by low bone density and deterioration of microarchitecture, which reduces bone strength and increases fracture risk.

Major clinical risk factors for osteoporotic fractures include older age, low weight, family history of hip fracture, fracture occurring after age 50, glucocorticoid use, and inability to rise from a chair without assistance. More than 50% of osteoporosis in men results from secondary causes.

Postmenopausal and age-related bone loss results from an uncoupling of bone remodeling such that bone resorption is greater than bone formation, resulting in a net loss of bone.

Polymorphisms in antagonists of the wnt/B catenin signaling pathway that result in a gain of function (e.g., LRP5) are associated with a reduced risk of osteoporosis.

Biochemical markers measured in the serum including C and N telopeptide cross-links of type I collagen correlate with osteoclast activity on the bone surface.

Evaluation for risk of osteoporotic fractures with the Fracture Assessment Index (FRAX) for postmenopausal women and men is critical to determine individuals with high enough 10-year fracture risk (hip and major osteoporotic fracture sites) to warrant treatment.

Treatment of high-turnover osteoporosis from estrogen deficiency with antiresorptive agents (estrogen, raloxifene, and bisphosphonates—alendronate, risedronate, zoledronic acid, ibandronate, denosumab) and an anabolic agent (recombinant human parathyroid hormone 1-34) can reduce incident vertebral fractures.

Parathyroid hormone (PTH) increases osteoblast maturation and life span, increases trabecular bone mass and cortical thickness, improves bone strength, and decreases fractures. Antiresorptive therapy is necessary after a full course of PTH to maintain newly formed bone mass.

Glucocorticoid-induced bone loss results from increased osteoclast activity and reduced osteoblast activity and is most severe in the first 6 months of therapy. Bisphosphonate treatment can prevent fractures.

Aromatase inhibitors reduce serum estrogen and result in rapid bone loss in postmenopausal women on adjuvant breast cancer therapy.

Gonadotropin-releasing hormone agonists decrease testosterone and estrogen levels and cause bone loss in men being treated for prostate cancer.

Osteoporosis is characterized by low bone density and a deterioration of bone microarchitecture that reduces bone strength and increases the risk of fracture. The hallmark of osteoporosis is the loss of bone mineral and bone matrix that results in maintenance of a normal mineral-to-matrix ratio. Bone consists of an organic matrix (collagen and noncollagenous proteins) and an inorganic mineral component (calcium and phosphate in hydroxyapatite crystals; see Chapter 4). Normally, bone turnover is tightly coupled with osteoclast-mediated bone resorption followed by osteoblast-stimulated bone formation. This delicate balance in bone remodeling results in no net change in skeletal mass. Osteoblasts synthesize osteoid—bone matrix that subsequently undergoes mineralization and becomes mature bone matrix. The skeleton contains approximately 80% cortical bone, which is concentrated in the appendicular skeleton and femoral neck, and 20% more metabolically active trabecular bone, which is located in the spine, epiphyses, and pelvis. Osteoporosis is characterized by reduced bone strength usually accompanied by a reduction in bone mass. Osteomalacia encompasses disorders in which there is decreased mineralization of bone matrix. Paget's disease is a skeletal disorder characterized by increased rates of bone turnover with the development of disorganized woven bone.

OSTEOPOROSIS

Epidemiology and Clinical Signs

Osteoporosis, the most common metabolic bone disease, affects 200 million individuals worldwide. Approximately 28 million Americans have osteoporosis or are at risk for it. *Osteoporosis*, or "porous bone," is a "disease characterized by low bone mass and structural deterioration of bone tissue, leading to bone fragility and an increased susceptibility to fractures, especially of the hip, spine and wrist."[1] Although usually asymptomatic, osteoporosis can produce loss of height, pain, dowager's hump, and increased risk of fracture. After 50 years of age, there is an exponential rise in fractures, such that 40% of women and 13% of men develop one or more osteoporotic fractures in their lifetimes. In the United States alone, there are more than 1.5 million osteoporotic fractures annually including 250,000 hip, 250,000 wrist, and 500,000 vertebral fractures. Hip fractures are associated with a 12% to 24% mortality rate in women and a 30% mortality rate in men within the first year of fracture, and 50% of patients are unable to ambulate independently and require long-term nursing home care.[2] These numbers will continue to grow exponentially as the elderly population of industrialized nations increases.

Bone accretion occurs during adolescence, when there is a large increment in bone mass. Peak bone density is normally achieved after puberty and into the third decade of life. However, by age 22, most individuals have achieved nearly all of their peak bone mass. At menopause, an acceleration of bone loss usually occurs over approximately 5 to 8 years, with an annual 2% to 3% loss of trabecular bone and a 1% to 2% loss of cortical bone. Both men and women lose bone with age. Over a lifetime, women lose approximately 50% of trabecular and 30% of cortical bone; men generally lose two-thirds of these amounts.[3] Osteoporosis was previously thought to be a silent disease that was part of the normal aging process. However, the advent of bone densitometry has made it possible to accurately and reproducibly identify patients at risk for osteoporosis so that prevention and treatment strategies can be instituted to reduce fractures. With a health care expenditure of $13.8 billion annually for osteoporosis-related fractures and a projected threefold rise in these costs over the next 40 years in the United States, the institution of effective prevention and treatment strategies to reduce fractures is of great importance.[1,4]

Pathophysiology of Menopausal and Age-Related Bone Loss

Bone is constantly undergoing remodeling, whereby areas of bone resorption produced by osteoclastic action are replaced by bone laid down by osteoblasts. Osteoporosis results from an imbalance between bone resorption and formation. The initiation of bone remodeling is still being debated; however, the osteocytes, or terminally differentiated osteoblasts, located within the bone matrix and connected to one another and the bone surface may release chemical mediators that attract osteoclasts to the bone surface (Figure 101-1). Osteoclasts originate from the colony-forming unit granulocyte-monocytes, are attracted to the bone surface, attach to bone matrix, and resorb bone tissue. Generally, bone resorption is rapid, and a resorption pit is formed within 10 to 14 days. After resorption is complete, osteoblasts, derived from the bone marrow stromal cells, attach to the resorbed bone surface and produce osteoid, which is then mineralized. Bone formation can take up to 3 or 4 months. Therefore a normal bone remodeling cycle in adults can last 4 to 6 months (see Figure 101-1A). A number of metabolic changes such as estrogen deficiency, immobilization, metabolic acidosis, hyperparathyroidism, and systemic and local inflammatory diseases can increase osteoclast number and activity, uncoupling bone turnover. This results in greater bone resorption than bone formation and a net loss of bone tissue. New data show that a number of local factors in bone affect the regulation of bone formation and resorption and the coupling of these processes. These include insulin-like growth factors (IGFs), interleukins (IL-1, IL-6, and IL-11), tumor necrosis factor (TNF), receptor activator of nuclear factor κB ligand (RANKL), and transforming growth factor (TGF).[5] Animal studies have shown that IL-1, IL-6, and TNF knockout mice do not lose bone with estrogen deficiency.[6] In addition, inflammatory arthritis animal models find that TNF, IL-1, and IL-6 are all strong stimulators of osteoclastic bone resorption. This link between the immune system and the maintenance

of bone mass is intriguing, but additional work is required before we can understand its significance.

A number of mechanisms underlie primary osteoporosis including a low peak bone mass as a young adult and rapid bone loss during menopause. Factors contributing to age-related bone loss include impaired calcium absorption with age, a compensatory rise in parathyroid hormone (PTH) levels, and greater resorption than formation of bone. Estrogen deficiency is associated with the release of cytokines including RANKL, IL-1, IL-6, and TNF, which leads to the recruitment and stimulation of osteoclasts in the marrow and increased production of bone-resorptive cytokines, which may contribute to menopause-related bone loss.[5] Estrogen therapy, however, inhibits IL-1 release, and in oophorectomized rats and mice, an inhibitor of IL-1 (the IL-1 receptor antagonist) suppresses bone loss.[6] IL-6 levels also increase with age in human marrow cultures[7] and in peripheral monocytes. IL-1 and TNF induce the production of IL-6 from osteoblasts and stromal cells. Further evidence supporting a role of IL-6 in bone turnover includes data showing that oophorectomized IL-6 knockout transgenic mice do not lose bone. Two other proteins have been identified that influence osteoclast activity: osteoprotegerin (OPG) and RANKL, which are produced by osteoblasts.[8] Estrogen deficiency increases osteoblast production of RANKL, which stimulates maturation and activity of osteoclasts by attaching to RANKL on the surface of immature and mature osteoclasts. Simultaneously, estrogen deficiency decreases osteoblast production of OPG, the decoy receptor that reduces RANKL production and activity. Adenoviral delivery of OPG ameliorates bone resorption in a mouse ovariectomy model of osteoporosis.[8] Both preclinical animal models and clinical trials of women with low bone mass have been completed and demonstrate that inhibition of RANKL with a monoclonal antibody (RANKL inhibitor) prevents estrogen-deficiency bone loss.[9]

In addition, a number of genetic, nutritional, and lifestyle risk factors predispose to the development of osteoporosis. Whites and Asians are at risk for low bone mass and osteoporosis, whereas African-Americans have a higher bone density and one-third to one-half the number of fractures.[1,8,9] Some studies show that African-Americans have lower vitamin D and urinary calcium levels, higher PTH levels, and skeletal resistance to the effects of PTH on bone.[10-12] Studies in twins and families show that up to 80% of the variance in bone mass is accounted for by genetic factors.[13] A maternal history of hip fracture, for example, is associated with a twofold increased risk of a hip fracture.[14] Data from Uitterlinden and colleagues[15] show that the gene encoding collagen type IA1 is associated with low bone density with increasing age and an increased risk of fracture. In the ss allele group, bone density was 12% lower at the femoral neck and 20% lower at the lumbar spine than that in the SS group, indicating an increased gene-dose effect with increasing age. However, COLIA1 is associated with a lower baseline bone density and not an increased rate of bone loss. Further, genetically determined architectural features of bone such as a long hip axis length may contribute to increased fracture risk; conversely, a short hip axis length confers some protective effect.[16] Recently, a family has been described whose members have high bone mass but are otherwise phenotypically normal. This family has a

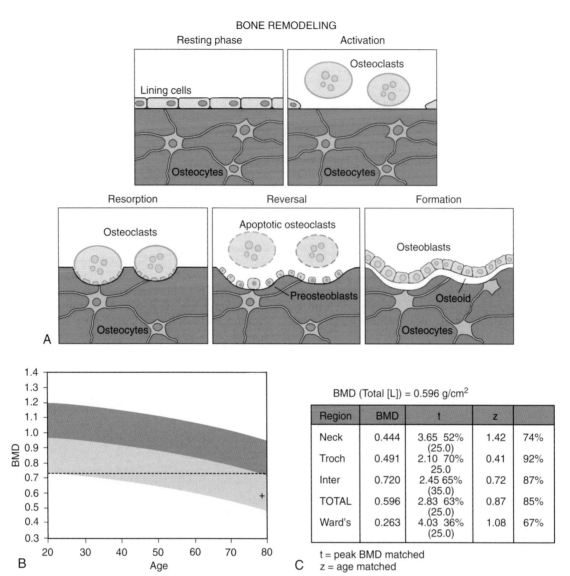

Figure 101-1 **A,** Bone remodeling cycle. Osteocytes most likely release chemicals to the bone surface that attract osteoclasts. Osteoclasts attach to the bone matrix, create a tight ring, and release acid that lowers the pH and dissolves the mineral from the bone matrix. After the mineral is released, the demineralized matrix is broken down. The osteoclast leaves the bone surface, and an osteoblast is attracted to the area of the bone that was resorbed. The resorption phase is about 10 to 14 days. Osteoblasts produce new bone, or osteoid, that fills in the resorption pit. Also, some of the osteoblasts are left within the bone matrix as osteocytes. The osteoid mineralizes over about 3 months, and the bone remodeling cycle is complete. **B** and **C,** The bone density of a postmenopausal woman is compared with that of both young, normal controls and age- and gender-matched controls. The t and z scores represent the number of standard deviations below young, normal controls and age-matched controls, respectively. Because the bone density provides a gradient of fracture risk, therapies can be instituted to prevent the development of osteoporosis or to treat patients at increased risk for fracture. BMD, bone mineral density.

mutation (an amino acid change) in the low-density lipoprotein receptor-related protein 5 (LRP5). Using in situ hybridization to a rat tibia, expression of LRP5 was detected in areas of bone involved in remodeling. Additional studies have reported that this LRP5 mutation increases wnt signaling, which may alter bone mass through a primary defect of bone formation. Individuals with this mutation demonstrate normal levels of bone resorption, but specific markers of bone formation are strikingly elevated. The observation that LRP5 is expressed at high levels in osteoblasts is consistent with its having a role in this area. Further work is now required to determine whether other mutations in the chromosome containing the LRP5 segment are

associated with a variation in bone density in the general population.[17,18]

Recently, genome-wide scans have been performed in a number of cohorts and have found a number of single nucleotide polymorphisms (SNPs) that are associated with osteoporosis (fracture or bone mineral density [BMD] associations). They include VDR, ESR1, ESR2, LRP5, LRP4, SOST, GRP177, OPG, RNAK, RNAKL, COL1A, SPP1, ITGAI, SP7, and SOX6, which can be reasonably assigned as confirmed or replicated, and another 30 or so genes as promising candidates. Of note, confirmed and promising genes are clustered in three biologic pathways: the estrogen endocrine pathway, the wnt/beta-catenin signaling pathway, and the RANKL/RANK/OPG pathway. New biologic pathways will certainly emerge when more osteoporosis genes are identified and validated.[18a] Other risk factors for osteoporosis, as enumerated in Table 101-1, include low body weight and reduced gonadal steroid levels.[13] Lifestyle factors that may contribute to the development of osteoporosis include cigarette smoking, excessive alcohol intake, reduced physical activity, and inadequate calcium intake, according to some reports. Cigarette smokers have poorer health than nonsmokers, impaired calcium absorption, lower estrogen levels, earlier menopause, and more fractures, and they exercise less; smoking cessation reverses this risk of osteoporosis.

In a large, prospective study of 9516 women older than 65 years, the following lifestyle factors significantly increased the risk of hip fracture: no walking for exercise, intake of more than two cups of coffee daily, current use of long-acting benzodiazepines and anticonvulsant drugs, current weight less than weight at age 25 years, height greater than 5 feet 7 inches, age older than 80 years, fracture since age 50 years, inability to stand from a chair without using arms, poor depth perception, and self-evaluation of health as fair to poor.[14] Low bone density in conjunction with a fall or trauma predisposes an individual to a fracture. Poor health and compromise of neuromuscular function increase the risk of osteoporosis and falls, which in turn increase the risk of hip fracture.[14] Importantly, elderly white women with both a low bone mass and more than two risk factors have a nearly 20-fold increased risk for fracture.

Secondary causes of bone loss that can affect women and men of all ages and races are listed in Table 101-2. Glucocorticoid therapy is the most common secondary cause of bone loss. Osteoporotic fractures develop in an estimated 30% to 50% of glucocorticoid-treated patients.[19] Glucocorticoid therapy causes bone loss through a number of different mechanisms such as producing a negative

Table 101-1 Risk Factors for Osteoporosis

Primary
Previous fracture after age 30
Family history of hip fracture
Cigarette smoking
Weight <127 lb
Low bone mineral density

Secondary
Nonmodifiable
White race
Advanced age
Frailty or poor health
Dementia
Modifiable
Low calcium intake
Eating disorder
Low testosterone levels (men)
Premenopausal estrogen deficiency (amenorrhea >1 yr or menopause at age <45 yr)
Excessive alcohol intake
Physical inactivity
Impaired vision
Neurologic disorder
Lack of sunlight exposure

Table 101-2 Medical Disorders and Medications Associated with Bone Loss and Osteoporosis

Primary osteoporosis
  Juvenile osteoporosis
  Postmenopausal osteoporosis
  Involutional osteoporosis
Endocrine abnormalities
  Glucocorticoid excess
  Thyroid hormone excess (supraphysiologic)
  Hypogonadism (including from prolactinoma or anorexia nervosa)
  Hyperparathyroidism
  Hypercalciuria
Processes affecting bone marrow
  Multiple myeloma
  Leukemia
  Gaucher's disease
  Systemic mastocytosis
Immobilization
  Space flight
Gastrointestinal diseases
  Gastrectomy
  Primary biliary cirrhosis
  Celiac disease
Renal insufficiency
Chronic respiratory diseases
Connective tissue disorders
  Osteogenesis imperfecta
  Homocysteinuria
  Ehlers-Danlos syndrome
Rheumatologic disorders
  Ankylosing spondylitis
  Rheumatoid arthritis
  Systemic lupus erythematosus
Medications
  Anticonvulsants
  Heparin
  Methotrexate
  Cyclophosphamide and gonadotropin-releasing hormone agonists (hypogonadism)
  Lithium
  Cyclosporine
  Aluminum
  Excessive alcohol
  Premenopausal tamoxifen
  Aromatase inhibitors

Modified from LeBoff MS: Calcium and metabolic bone disease. In *Medical knowledge self-assessment program*, Philadelphia, 1995, American College of Physicians.

calcium balance through impaired intestinal calcium absorption, increasing urinary calcium excretion, decreasing bone formation, increasing bone resorption by stimulating osteoclast activity by macrophage colony-stimulating factor, and suppressing endogenous gonadal steroid production.[19] Therapy with glucocorticoids leads to an early and, in some instances, dramatic loss of trabecular bone, with less effect on cortical bone. In hyperthyroidism (Graves' disease or toxic nodule) or supraphysiologic therapy with thyroid hormone, the ensuing accelerated bone turnover may produce a reduction in bone mass when the thyroid-stimulating hormone level is suppressed, even when thyroid hormone levels are within the normal range.[20] Athletic amenorrhea, anorexia nervosa, and other hypogonadal states including the use of gonadotropin-releasing hormone agonists[21,22] may result in bone loss. In addition to estrogen deficiency, women with anorexia nervosa have low levels of IGF-I and reduced levels of adrenal androgen dehydroepiandrostenedione, which may contribute to the development of osteoporosis.[23]

Osteoporosis in Men

Osteoporosis in men was not recognized 20 years ago but is now a major public health problem owing to men's longer life spans. The epidemiology of osteoporosis in men is just now being evaluated. Fracture risk occurs in adolescence and young adulthood and then increases after the age of 70. Long bone fractures occur more commonly in young men, while hip and spine fractures are more prevalent in men older than 70 years. The increase in fractures in older men is just as significant as it is in women, but it occurs about 10 years later in life, with an age-adjusted incidence of hip fractures in men of about one-third to one-half of that of women.[24] Elderly men who sustain hip fractures have a greater risk of dying or being permanently disabled compared with women.[24] Risk factors for osteoporosis in men include older age, low BMD, history of a low-trauma fracture as an adult, and a family history of osteoporotic fractures.

There are a number of secondary causes of osteoporosis in men; for instance, hypogonadism causes an increase in bone turnover and rapid bone loss as gonadal function declines with age. At this time, severe hypogonadism from androgen deprivation therapy for prostate cancer is common in elderly men. The exact role of estrogen and androgens in male skeletal health is not yet known. Although estrogen is necessary for the young male skeleton, serum estrogen levels are highly correlated with bone remodeling, BMD, and rate of BMD loss in older men; the associations are stronger than with testosterone. However, serum testosterone levels are also highly correlated with indices of bone resorption and formation. The roles of estrogen and testosterone in the male skeleton need additional investigation.[25] Some of the other common causes of osteoporosis in men that are not as frequent in women are alcoholism, gastrointestinal disorders including hepatic disorders, and malabsorption.[24]

Osteoporosis in Rheumatic Diseases and Other Conditions

Recently, studies have reported significant bone loss in patients with systemic inflammatory diseases such as rheumatoid arthritis, systemic lupus erythematosus (SLE), and ankylosing spondylitis. Patients with rheumatoid arthritis experience periarticular and generalized bone loss, with an increased incidence of fractures compared with the general population.[26] T lymphocytes, tissue macrophages, and synovial-like fibroblasts release inflammatory cytokines (IL-1, TNF, IL-6) and inhibitory wnt signaling proteins such as dkk-1 and RANKL, which stimulate preosteoclasts in the bone marrow and synovium to actively resorb bone; in addition, osteoblast maturation is altered.[27,28] In an animal model of inflammatory arthritis induced with collagen, animals pretreated with OPG did not have bone loss within the periarticular bone or the presence of erosions.[29] Additional factors that may contribute to osteoporosis in patients with rheumatic diseases include decreased mobility, glucocorticoid therapy, and systemic inflammation.[30] Some data,

however, show that low-dose glucocorticoid therapy in women with rheumatoid arthritis does not have adverse skeletal effects, possibly because of a decrease in disease activity in association with the suppression of inflammatory cytokines and improved physical activity and function.[31,32] Ankylosing spondylitis is also associated with fractures and reduced bone density in the spine and proximal femur, even early in the disease.[33] Patients with SLE have a high rate of osteoporotic fractures in the presence of low to normal bone mass, suggesting that systemic inflammation alters bone turnover. Increased serum levels of TNF can reduce osteoblast maturation and increase osteoclast maturation and activity; in addition, other inflammatory factors such as oxidized low-density lipoproteins and inflammatory high-density lipoproteins can direct mesenchymal stem cells to differentiate into adipocytes instead of osteoblasts and impair bone mass.[34] Infiltrative processes in the marrow such as multiple myeloma, mastocytosis, and Gaucher's disease may produce osteoporosis. Patients with Gaucher's disease show an accumulation of glucocerebrosides in macrophages in the spleen, liver, and bone marrow, which causes hepatosplenomegaly, anemia, thrombocytopenia, bone infarcts and infections, fractures, and aseptic necrosis.[35]

The immunosuppressant drug cyclophosphamide (Cytoxan) induces amenorrhea and hypogonadism, which may increase the risk of bone loss. Women who undergo premature menopause from cyclophosphamide therapy can have estrogen-deficiency bone loss in their 30s. Young women with SLE who try to preserve ovarian function while undergoing cyclophosphamide therapy by taking gonadotropin-releasing hormone agonists may also experience estrogen-deficiency bone loss. In rodent models, the immunosuppressive drug cyclosporine produces a time- and dose-dependent bone loss[36]; in contrast, azathioprine (Imuran) and rapamycin (sirolimus) do not appear to adversely affect skeletal homeostasis.[37] Therapy with both cyclosporine and prednisone in transplant recipients is associated with early accelerated bone loss after the initiation of treatment and the development of osteoporosis and fractures with continued exposure.[38]

Vitamin D deficiency may also manifest as osteopenia and fractures, but this condition is both preventable and treatable.[39] Vitamin D insufficiency is common in older patients and in those with SLE who do not get an adequate amount of sunlight or use potent sunscreens. Also, patients with malabsorption syndromes and liver disease can be vitamin D deficient. Unlike the situation in osteoporosis, very low vitamin D levels are often characterized by a mineralization defect and osteomalacia. Vitamin D deficiency is reported to be present in up to 50% of women with hip fractures.[39]

Assessment of Bone Density and Osteoporotic Risk

Osteoporosis may first be diagnosed when a radiograph shows signs of demineralization or a spinal film shows evidence of compression fractures of vertebral bodies. Because an estimated 25% to 50% of bone mass must be lost to show osteopenia on radiographs, conventional radiography is an insensitive technique for diagnosing bone loss. Radiographs may demonstrate signs of secondary causes of osteoporosis such as the presence of subperiosteal resorption in hyperparathyroidism, characteristic lytic changes or bone infarcts in Gaucher's disease, local sites of lytic destruction in malignancy, and pseudofractures in osteomalacia. Bone densitometry makes it possible to measure the amount of bone in the relevant fracture sites of the spine, forearm, and proximal femur, as well as the total body.

Techniques for evaluating bone mass include dual-energy x-ray absorptiometry (DEXA) and quantitative computed tomography (CT) scanning of the spine.[1,2] Bone density evaluations using DEXA incorporate the attenuation of soft tissue and bone by radiographs to calculate the BMD. DEXA is both precise and safe, with a low radiation exposure. With reproducibility errors of approximately 0.6% to 1.5%, this technique can detect small changes over time.[2,40,41] Further, newer DEXA techniques measure bone density rapidly, in 0.5 to 2.5 minutes. Quantitative CT scanning allows for the direct measurements of trabecular bone in the central region of the spine, but the procedure entails a comparatively high radiation exposure and time and precision errors are usually higher than those associated with DEXA.

Figure 101-1B and C show the BMD in a postmenopausal patient compared with that of young, healthy controls to determine whether there is reduction in BMD compared with peak bone mass (percentage of young healthy controls expressed as a t score) and with age-matched controls to assess whether BMD is diminished relative to an age-matched cohort (percentage of age-matched controls expressed as a z score). There is an inverse relationship between bone density and the gradient of risk for fracture.[42] Prospective studies show that bone densitometry identifies patients with an increased gradient of risk for fracture. In 8134 women, a 1–standard deviation (SD) decrement in the bone density of the spine and the femoral neck compared with age-adjusted controls was associated with a 1.6- and 2.6-fold increased risk of hip fracture, respectively.[43] Measurement of bone density in the hip is more predictive of hip fracture than is measurement at another site. Studies show that in women older than 65 years, hip bone density is predictive of spine and hip fracture and that conventional spine density does not add to the diagnostic utility of a single hip bone density test in assessing the risk of fracture.

Although bone densitometry provides a quantitative measure of bone mass, in vitro studies using ultrasonography indicate that this technique also provides information about the mechanical properties of bone including both density and elasticity. These qualities are strong predictors of bone strength. Ultrasound techniques include speed-of-sound and broadband ultrasound attenuation methods; the speed-of-sound technique reflects bone density and elasticity, and broadband ultrasound attenuation is an indicator of bone density, bone structure, and composition. Approved for clinical use by the U.S. Food and Drug Administration (FDA), both ultrasound techniques have been shown to discriminate between normal and osteoporotic patients at increased fracture risk.[44] The t score parameters used by some ultrasound machines do not correspond to t score levels as measured by DEXA. Although ultrasonography is a radiation-free technique that may provide information about the risk of fracture and bone quality, the

reproducibility of this technique and the measurement sites of mainly cortical bone or low-weight-bearing locations may make it unsuitable for monitoring small changes in bone over time. Therefore ultrasound measurements cannot reliably be used to monitor response to osteoporosis therapies. Further data are necessary to validate the clinical utility of ultrasonography.

On the basis of the guidelines of the Scientific Advisory Board of the National Osteoporosis Foundation, bone densitometry is useful in determining which patients might benefit from therapy to protect the skeleton including patients who have a deficiency of gonadal hormones (postmenopausal women younger than 65 years with one or more risk factors or older than 65 years regardless of risk factors), postmenopausal fracture, evidence of osteopenia or a vertebral abnormality on radiographs, hyperparathyroidism, or exposure to supraphysiologic doses of glucocorticoids (Table 101-3). Bone densitometry is also used to decide when to commence therapy for osteoporosis and to assess the clinical response to therapeutic interventions.[40] Screening normal premenopausal women is not cost-effective.

The World Health Organization (WHO) has published criteria for osteoporosis on the basis of bone density[1,45]:

1. Normal bone density if the t score is greater than −1.
2. Osteopenia (low bone mass) is defined as a bone density measurement between 1 and 2.5 SD below the young-adult mean (t score between −1 and −2.5).
3. Osteoporosis is defined as a bone density measurement less than 2.5 SD below that of young, healthy controls (t score < 2.5).

The National Osteoporosis Foundation recommends treatment for all individuals who have a lumbar spine, hip, or femoral neck t score of −2.5 or lower. However, for individuals who have a bone density between −1 and −2.5 the National Osteoporosis Foundation recommends performing a Fracture Risk Assessment or FRAX using a computer program that incorporates clinical risk factors for osteoporosis with and without femoral neck BMD. FRAX also provides a 10-year risk of a hip fracture or a major osteoporotic fracture (hip, proximal humerus, and wrist). The clinical risk factors included in the FRAX program include age, weight, height, history of a fracture as an adult, parental history of a hip fracture, current glucocorticoid use, secondary cause of osteoporosis, alcohol intake of more than two drinks a day, and current smoker.[45,46] These risk factors are added to femoral neck t score for the 10-year fracture risk. In the

Table 101-3 Indications for Bone Densitometry

All postmenopausal women < 65 yr who have one or more additional risk factors for osteoporosis (besides menopause)
All women > 65 yr regardless of additional risk factors
To document reduced bone density in patients with vertebral abnormalities or osteopenia on radiographs
Estrogen-deficient women at risk for low bone density who are considering use of estrogen or an alternative therapy, if bone density would influence the decision
Women who have been on estrogen replacement therapy for prolonged periods or to monitor the efficacy of a therapeutic intervention or interventions for osteoporosis
To diagnose low bone mass in glucocorticoid-treated individuals
To document low bone density in patients with asymptomatic primary or secondary hyperparathyroidism

United States, a 10-year risk of hip fracture of 3% or more or a major osteoporotic fracture of 20% or more is the threshold to recommend treatment. However, the fracture risk threshold for treatment is individualized by treatment, so it is important to enter the country in which you are practicing medicine. FRAX has advantages that include easily determined risk factors, global validation, application in specific regions or nations, and scores that pertain to both men and women. However, there are a number of limitations including that it can lead to underestimates or overestimates of fracture risk in some patients, because it does not include all known risk factors and some risk factors are superficial (e.g., glucocorticoid use is the question, but dose is not evaluated). Such known or suspected risk factors that contribute to fracture risk but are not included in the FRAX algorithm include immobilization, epilepsy, chronic obstructive pulmonary disease, diabetes, and depression. Lastly, the FRAX score is calibrated only for untreated patients and results can be misleading for patients already taking pharmacologic therapy.[45,46]

Markers of Bone Turnover

The development of sensitive biochemical markers of bone turnover makes it possible to analyze changes in bone formation and resorption at a given point in time and obtain additional information about a patient's risk of bone loss and fracture. Only three bone formation markers are currently available. Osteocalcin, a noncollagenous matrix protein in bone, is produced exclusively by osteoblasts; it correlates with histomorphometric bone measurements. In most conditions, bone resorption and formation are tightly coupled and osteocalcin levels reflect bone turnover. The other markers of bone formation are bone-specific alkaline phosphatase (BSAP), an enzyme that is activated as osteoblasts mature, and amino-terminal propeptide of type I procollagen, a protein whose synthesis is high in maturing osteoblasts.[47]

Sensitive indicators of bone resorption derived from the degradation of mature collagen include the urine and serum markers of type I collagen cross-links including aminoterminal telopeptide of type I collagen (N telopeptides, or NTX) or carboxy-terminal telopeptide of type I collagen (C telopeptides, or CTX). Urinary pyridinoline cross-link, NTX, and CTX levels correlate with histomorphometric determinations of bone resorption; these biomarkers increase with menopause and are high in patients with a variety of disorders characterized by accelerated bone turnover including Paget's disease, osteoporosis, and rheumatoid arthritis.[48,49] Urinary excretion of N telopeptides is inversely related to total hip and spinal bone density and, according to some studies, may be a more specific index of bone resorption than urinary pyridinoline levels.[50] Small prospective studies have found high turnover markers, and low BMD has been associated with incident fracture risk but these studies have not been replicated in larger studies.[51,52] In clinical studies, antiresorptive agents such as estrogen, bisphosphonates, and inhibitor of RANKL induce a significant decrease (30% to 80%) first in markers of resorption and then in bone formation markers, often within 3 to 6 months. Resorption markers decrease before formation markers and correlate with either maintenance of or increase

in BMD. A significant change in bone markers can be observed within months of antiresorptive therapy, before there are changes in BMD.[52] Both bone formation and resorption marker changes over 6 to 12 months have been found to predict future fracture risk. In a study of alendronate to reduce osteoporotic fractures, patients who had more than a 30% reduction in bone alkaline phosphatase had the greatest reduction in risk for new vertebral and nonvertebral fractures. Interestingly, studies have found that reductions in markers of bone turnover, either resorption or formation markers, are associated with a reduction in fracture risk. However, long-term, prospective studies of large numbers of women are necessary to determine whether selective biochemical markers of bone turnover can predict changes in BMD or fracture risk and whether these tests should be used in standard clinical practice.

Most bone turnover marker data are derived from large studies of antiresorptive agents. However, a bone-building anabolic agent, PTH, has been approved for the treatment of osteoporosis. PTH's action is to stimulate osteoblast activity; therefore osteocalcin and other markers of bone formation increase rapidly, within a few weeks of the initiation of treatment. However, activation of the osteoblast over time results in RANKL production, which stimulates osteoclast activity. With continued PTH treatment, markers of osteoclast activity also increase, reaching levels equal to those of formation markers. Because the overall result is an increase in bone mass, the bone turnover markers during PTH therapy reflect significant bone remodeling on both trabecular and cortical bone surfaces. A few small studies have found that increases in both bone formation and resorption markers predict an increase in bone mass with PTH treatment.[53-55]

Evaluation for Secondary Bone Loss

The workup for osteoporosis is directed toward excluding secondary causes of bone loss and includes a determination of serum calcium, phosphorus, supersensitive thyroid-stimulating hormone, 25-hydroxyvitamin D (25-OHD), and intact PTH, as well as urine calcium and creatinine levels. Also, a complete blood cell count, alkaline phosphatase and liver function tests, erythrocyte sedimentation rate (in some cases), and serum and urine protein electrophoresis for patients older than 50 years may be necessary (Table 101-4). In men, additional testing for secondary causes of osteoporosis includes serum testosterone and luteinizing hormone.

Further tests to rule out neoplastic or endocrinologic disorders and a bone biopsy (a decalcified bone specimen is obtained after a double tetracycline label with two different fluorescent labels) should be considered in certain patients with progressive bone loss and in those in whom osteoporosis is unlikely. Identification and appropriate therapy for underlying secondary causes of osteoporosis are important. For example, treatment of vitamin D deficiency is best accomplished with vitamin D supplements. Parathyroidectomy in patients with hyperparathyroidism characterized by hypercalcemia, hypercalciuria, nephrolithiasis, age younger than 50 years, or low cortical BMD (z score ≤2) was associated with a large (4% to 12.8%) increase in bone density over 4 years.[56] Bone density was, however, stable for up to

Table 101-4 Evaluation of Osteoporosis

For All Patients
Laboratory tests including SMA, CBC, supersensitive TSH; ± PTH, alkaline phosphatase, 25-hydroxyvitamin D levels, and either measurement or estimate of 24-hr urinary calcium; ± serum and urine protein electrophoresis and ESR

For Selected Patients*
Definitive tests for endocrine, neoplastic, and gastrointestinal disorders
Bone biopsy under calcified sections with double tetracycline label
In some patients, markers of bone turnover to identify those at risk for increased bone loss

*Children, premenopausal women, men younger than 60 yr, black, patients with rapidly progressive disease.

CBC, complete blood cell count; ESR, erythrocyte sedimentation rate; PTH, parathyroid hormone; SMA, sequential multiple analysis; TSH, thyroid-stimulating hormone.

Modified from *Primer on the metabolic bone diseases and disorders of mineral metabolism*, ed 6, Washington, DC, 2006, American Society of Bone and Mineral Research.

6 years in patients with mild hyperparathyroidism.[57] In addition, treatment of hyperthyroidism, hypercortisolism, and a variety of other disorders that may cause osteoporosis can produce increments in bone mass. Reduction in the systemic inflammation associated with rheumatic diseases such as TNF blocking agents for rheumatoid arthritis or ankylosing spondylitis or glucocorticoid-sparing agents for SLE (e.g., azathioprine [Imuran], mycophenolate mofetil [CellCept]) can also produce increments in bone mass.

Treatment

Calcium

The goals of therapy for osteoporosis are to reduce bone resorption and enhance bone formation, if possible. Bone loss occurs when the calcium intake and absorption are insufficient to balance the daily calcium losses. Prospective data show that calcium stabilizes bone mass.[58]

Table 101-5 shows the current recommendations for optimal calcium intake for women and men from the 1997 report of the Institute of Medicine to the National Academy of Sciences.[59] In the absence of kidney stones or an underlying disorder of calcium metabolism, these calcium intakes are safe. To prevent negative calcium balance, premenopausal women require 1000 mg and postmenopausal women 1200 mg of total elemental calcium daily.[60] Children have increasing calcium requirements during adolescence, and data show increased bone accretion with increased calcium intake in prepubescent and pubertal children. Calcium carbonate contains 40% elemental calcium and should be taken with meals because of poor absorption in achlorhydric patients in the absence of food. Calcium citrate, which contains 24% elemental calcium, has better bioavailability and is more readily absorbed.[61] It is also absorbed well on an empty stomach in patients with achlorhydria. Recent studies underscore the fact that only recommended daily allowances of calcium and vitamin D are useful for bone health in postmenopausal women and elderly men. Additional supplementation over the recommended daily allowance has resulted in reports of increased cardiovascular disease.[61a-61c]

Estrogen

Hormone replacement therapy (HRT) was once the mainstay of treatment in osteoporosis because estrogen inhibits bone resorption, produces a small rise in bone density, and reduces the risk of fracture by approximately 50% in retrospective observational studies. Cardiovascular disease is the leading cause of death in postmenopausal women. Previous data from longitudinal observational studies suggested that estrogen replacement had a beneficial effect on reducing primary and secondary cardiac events in postmenopausal women. However, in 1998, data from the 4-year Heart and Estrogen/Progestin Replacement Study were published.[62] In this study, 2763 postmenopausal women with a previous history of heart disease were randomized to receive estrogen (0.625 mg) plus progestin (2.5 mg) or placebo alone. Results showed no reduction in the overall rate of coronary heart disease or cardiac events in the treatment group; in fact, an early increase in risk for cardiac events was noted, possibly related to increased coagulability.[63]

In addition, a large, multicenter, longitudinal study by the Women's Health Initiative (WHI)—in which 162,000 women aged 50 to 79 years were randomized into a placebo group, an HRT group (if the uterus was intact), or an estrogen-only group (if the uterus was absent)—was terminated early due to an increased risk of breast and cardiovascular events. The research goals for the WHI study were to determine the effects of HRT, diet modification, and calcium and vitamin D supplements on heart disease, osteoporosis, and colorectal cancer risk. After a mean follow-up of 5.3 years in an 8.5-year study, the HRT group had an increased risk of seven more cardiac events per 10,000 women taking the drug for a year, eight more invasive breast cancers, eight more strokes, and eight more pulmonary emboli, but six fewer colorectal cancers and five fewer hip fractures.[64]

At this time, the general recommendation is that HRT should be used only for vasomotor symptoms that occur at the time of menopause. When these symptoms abate, it is recommended that estrogen replacement (combined estrogen and progestin for women with an intact uterus) be stopped because the perceived cardiovascular benefits have

Table 101-5 Calcium Requirements Recommended by the National Academy of Sciences (USA)

Age Group	Optimal Daily Calcium Intake (mg)
Infants	
Birth-6 mo	400
6 mo-1 yr	600
Children 1-8 yr	500-800
Adolescents 9-18 yr	
9-10 yr	800-1200
11-18 yr	1200-1500
Pregnant and nursing females	1300
Men and women	
19-50 yr	1000
>50 yr (± hormone replacement therapy)	1200-1500

Modified from Atkinson SA, Abrams SA, Dawson-Hughes B, et al: Calcium. In Young V, editor: *Dietary reference intake for calcium, phosphorus, magnesium, vitamin D and fluoride*, Washington, DC, 1997, National Academy Press, pp 91–143.

not been substantiated, and the cardiovascular disease and breast cancer risk make the benefit-to-risk ratio unacceptable for most women. It is important to acknowledge that the estrogen-only arm of the WHI study in women without a uterus did not show an increased risk of heart disease or breast cancer.

If a woman and her physician decide that she is going to take HRT or estrogen alone for vasomotor symptoms, in those with an increased risk of coagulability, transdermal estrogen replacement should be used.

Selective Estrogen Receptor Modulators

The ideal estrogen replacement therapy would confer the beneficial effects of estrogen on bone and cardiovascular disease without increasing the risk of breast or uterine cancer. Selective estrogen receptor modulators (SERMs) are a nonsteroidal class of drugs that bind to the estrogen receptor and differ from one another in their actions on estrogen-responsive tissues, acting selectively as agonists or antagonists. Tamoxifen, the first available SERM, is an estrogen antagonist that binds to the estrogen receptor and also has estrogen-agonist effects on bone, lipids, clotting factors, and endometrium. Tamoxifen therapy in women with breast cancer produced a small increase in bone density of the spine over 2 years, with no effect on radial bone density, in association with reductions in both low-density lipoprotein and total cholesterol.[65] The Breast Cancer Prevention Trial studied 13,388 women at increased risk for breast cancer, comparing treatment with tamoxifen (20 mg daily) to placebo for 5 years.[66] Tamoxifen reduced the risk of invasive and noninvasive breast cancer by 50%, and a decreased risk of fracture was observed as well: 45% reduction at the hip and 29% at the spine. An increased incidence of low-grade endometrial cancer was noted, but there was no change in the risk of ischemic heart disease.[66]

Raloxifene,[67] now FDA approved for the prevention and treatment of osteoporosis, is a SERM that acts as an estrogen agonist on bone, with antagonist effects on the breast and uterus.[68] Raloxifene (60 mg/day over a 2-year study period) increased BMD in the lumbar spine by 2.4%, in the total hip by 2.4%, and in the total body by 2%, with a reduction in fracture risk at 2 years similar to that seen with estrogen or alendronate (5 mg) treatment. Over the 2-year study period, raloxifene produced a significant reduction in vertebral fractures: Fractures were present in 1.6% of raloxifene-treated women, compared with 2.9% of those in the placebo group; fractures recurred in 7.6% of treated women with a previous fracture, compared with 14.3% of those in the placebo group.[69] Endometrial thickness is not increased by raloxifene, but menopausal symptoms may be made worse. Raloxifene has been shown to decrease low-density lipoprotein cholesterol by 12%, with a nonsignificant increase in high-density lipoprotein cholesterol; cardiovascular protection has not yet been determined.[70] However, raloxifene, unlike estrogen, does not affect C-reactive protein, which is associated with a risk of cardiovascular disease.[71,72] Raloxifene also decreased the incidence of breast cancer by 76% in patients enrolled in a clinical study of osteoporosis, with breast cancer incidence studied as a secondary endpoint.[67] A study that evaluated the effects of raloxifene on cardiovascular disease found no

effect.[73] One study compared tamoxifen and raloxifene, and another study evaluated raloxifene versus placebo, in the prevention of breast cancer. The first study reported that both tamoxifen and raloxifene reduced the risk of developing breast cancer, and the second found that raloxifene reduced the risk of estrogen receptor–positive breast cancer compared with placebo in postmenopausal women.[74,75] At this time, there is little information on the use of raloxifene in men, so it is not recommended for male patients.

Testosterone

Men with osteoporosis, hypogonadism, and symptoms of low libido may benefit from testosterone replacement therapy. This can be administered as testosterone cypionate or enanthate (50 to 400 mg intramuscularly every 2 to 4 weeks) or as a transdermal testosterone replacement patch that is applied to the scrotal area (Testoderm, 4 to 6 mg/day) or elsewhere (Androderm, 2.5 or 5 mg/day).[76] Most studies find that bone mass increases with testosterone replacement when levels of testosterone were low at the initiation of therapy.

Calcitonin

Calcitonin, a 32–amino acid peptide synthesized by the C cells of the thyroid gland, is a potent inhibitor of osteoclast-mediated bone resorption. Although human and salmon calcitonin are commercially available, salmon calcitonin is most commonly used because of its greater potency. On the basis of data showing an increase in total body calcium, parenteral calcitonin was approved by the FDA for the treatment of osteoporosis in 1984, and calcitonin in a nasal spray was approved for the treatment of postmenopausal osteoporosis in 1995. Parenteral calcitonin (100 IU subcutaneously or intramuscularly three times a week or daily) can maintain bone density or produce a small increase in bone mass in the spine and, in some instances, the forearm, particularly in patients with a high bone turnover.[77] Nasal spray calcitonin is absorbed through the nasal mucosa and is approximately 40% as potent as the parenterally administered drug (e.g., 50 to 100 IU of injectable calcitonin is comparable with 200 IU of nasal spray calcitonin).[78] In osteoporotic women more than 5 years past menopause, nasal calcitonin (200 IU/day) increases spinal bone density 2% to 3% compared with placebo, with no effect on proximal femur bone mass; higher doses are necessary in the early menopausal period.[78,79] Nasal spray calcitonin therapy in patients with osteoporosis is associated with a 36% reduction in vertebral fractures over 5 years.[79]

The adverse effects of parenteral calcitonin include nausea, flushing, and local irritation at the injection site. Calcitonin given intranasally is well tolerated, with rhinitis and nasal symptoms such as dryness and crusting being potential side effects. Patients treated with parenteral or intranasal calcitonin may also obtain a beneficial analgesic response in the presence of osteoporotic fractures.

Bisphosphonates

Bisphosphonates are analogues of pyrophosphate, with a P-C-P rather than a P-O-P core; they are absorbed by the

Table 101-6 Inhibition of Metaphyseal Bone Resorption in Vivo by Bisphosphonates

Chemical Modification	Examples	Antiresorptive Potency
First generation: short alkyl or halide side chain	Etidronate	1
	Clodronate	10
Second generation: NH₂-terminal group	Tiludronate*	10
	Pamidronate	100
	Alendronate	100-1000
Third generation: cyclic side chain	Risedronate	1000-10,000
	Ibandronate	1000-10,000
	Zoledronate	10,0000

*Tiludronate has a cyclic side chain, not an NH₂-terminal group, but it is generally classified as a second-generation compound on the basis of its time of development and potency.

Modified from Watts NB: Treatment of osteoporosis with bisphosphonates [review], *Endocrinol Metab Clin North Am* 27:419–439, 1998.

hydroxyapatite of bone and suppress bone resorption. Modification of the side chains can result in the development of a variety of compounds with differing abilities to inhibit bone resorption (Table 101-6). Some bisphosphonates are administered intermittently because of a long skeletal half-life and prolonged retention in bone. These compounds must be taken on an empty stomach because gastrointestinal absorption is less than 10%.

Bisphosphonates have been used for the treatment of patients with Paget's disease of bone, hypercalcemia of malignancy, and osteoporosis and for the prevention and treatment of glucocorticoid-induced osteoporosis. Etidronate (Didronel) administered intermittently (400 mg/day for 2 weeks in 3-month cycles) produced approximately 5% increase in bone density of the spine and a 50% reduction in vertebral fractures at 2 years. Longer follow-up did not reveal a significant reduction in vertebral fractures compared with baseline, except in a post hoc analysis of patients with three or more fractures and low bone density.[80] Etidronate is not approved by the FDA for the treatment of osteoporosis.

Alendronate (Fosamax) is FDA approved for the prevention and treatment of osteoporosis. Data in postmenopausal women with bone density at least 2.5 SD below peak bone mass show that alendronate (10 mg/day) compared with placebo produces an 8.8% and 7.8% increase in bone density in the spine and femoral trochanter, respectively, and a 5.9% increase in the femoral neck after 3 years of therapy[81]; there are smaller rises (2.3% to 4.4%) in bone density in the spine and proximal femur in women within 0.5 to 3 years of menopause. Fosamax treatment in women with osteoporosis (t score < 2.5) yields a significant reduction in spine and hip fractures compared with the placebo-treated patients.[82] Treatment with alendronate (5 mg/day over 2 years) increased BMD in the lumbar spine by 2.9% and in the hip by 1.3%; in contrast, estrogen-progestin therapy increased BMD in these locations by 4% and 1.8%, respectively.[83] Alendronate did not reduce the incidence of clinical fractures in women who had low bone mass but not osteoporosis, although longer studies may be necessary.[84] Alendronate treatment is also effective in increasing bone mass in the spine, hip, and total body and helps prevent vertebral fractures and height loss in men with osteoporosis.[85] Adverse effects of bisphosphonates include

gastrointestinal symptoms such as stomach pain and esophagitis (caution is advised in patients with active symptoms or a history of ulcer disease), myalgias and arthralgias, and, rarely, osteonecrosis of the jaw, and subtrochanteric fractures with long-term use. A once-a-week preparation of alendronate (70 mg) is the most commonly used dose for the treatment of osteoporosis.[86] This preparation increased spinal and hip bone mass similarly to alendronate 10 mg/day over a 2-year study period.

Risedronate, another oral bisphosphonate, administered at a dose of 5 mg/day increased bone mass and reduced the risk of new vertebral fractures 50% better than placebo.[87-89] Another study performed to assess the effect of risedronate on hip fractures found that women with osteoporosis (defined by a femoral neck t score of ≤ –4.0) had a significant reduction in the risk of hip fracture.[90] Risedronate has been approved for the prevention and treatment of osteoporosis (35 mg once a week)[91] and for the treatment of Paget's disease (30 mg/day for 2 months, with retreatment if relapse occurs after 2 months).[92] Studies show that risedronate may be well tolerated even in patients with mild gastrointestinal symptoms. Bisphosphonates may also reduce bone pain.

Ibandronate (Boniva), another aminobisphosphonate, is approved for the treatment and prevention of postmenopausal osteoporosis. In phase III studies of ibandronate (2.5 mg/day) versus placebo in postmenopausal women with osteoporosis, incident vertebral fractures were reduced about 50%. Another study compared ibandronate 150 mg once a month to the daily 2.5-mg dose and found similar gains in lumbar spine and hip BMD. The FDA approved ibandronate 150 mg/month for the treatment of osteoporosis on the basis of this bridging study.[93] Recently, intravenous ibandronate in a dose of 3 mg every 3 months was found to be similar to ibandronate 2.5 mg/day in terms of increasing lumbar spine and hip BMD, and the FDA has approved intravenous ibandronate for this indication. There are no data on hip fractures for this compound.[94]

Zoledronic acid (Reclast) is approved for the treatment and prevention of postmenopausal osteoporosis.[95] In phase III studies in postmenopausal women with osteoporosis treated with zoledronic acid, 5 mg once a year by intravenous infusion, the risk of incident vertebral fractures was reduced by 68%, hip fractures by 40%, and other major osteoporotic fractures by 20% compared with the placebo-treated subjects.[95] Another phase III study of patients who had suffered a hip fracture were randomized to either zoledronic acid 5 mg once a year of placebo and after 3 years found that incident osteoporotic fractures were significantly less in zoledronic-treated patients and the mortality was lowered compared with the placebo-treated patients.[96] Side effects of zoledronic acid include arthralgias and myalagias; however, these adverse events tend to be less frequent with subsequent infusions. Patients undergoing zoledronic acid treatment should have both serum calcium and 25-OHD levels monitored and replaced to normal levels before treatment. Zoledronic acid has been approved for the treatment and prevention of postmenopausal osteoporosis (5 mg once a year), osteoporosis in men (5 mg a year), prevention and treatment of glucocorticoid-induced osteoporosis (5 mg a year), and Paget's disease. Zoledronic acid at a dose of 4 mg intravenously every 4 weeks is currently approved for the prevention and treatment of bone metastases in patients with breast cancer and multiple myeloma.

RANK Ligand Inhibitor

Denosumab (Prolia) is a monoclonal antibody that is directed against RANKL and is approved for the treatment of postmenopausal osteoporosis. In phase III studies in postmenopausal women with osteoporosis treated with denosumab (60 mg subcutaneously every 6 months) for 36 months or 3 years, the incidence of vertebral fractures was reduced by 68%, hip fractures by 40%, and major osteoporotic fractures by 20%.[97] The medication is well tolerated, but adverse events of skin infection requiring hospitalization were higher in denosumab-treated subjects than placebo-treated subjects. Denosumab is a potent inhibitor of bone resorption with suppression of a marker of osteoclast activity.

CTX-1 is suppressed to nearly 90% a few weeks after each injection; however, the suppression of bone turnover is transient and bone turnover and bone density return to baseline levels rapidly if the injections of denosumab are discontinued. Postmenopausal women with low bone mass who were treated with alendronate 70 mg once a week and then switched to denosumab (60 mg every 6 months) had a significant gain of BMD compared with subjects continued on alendronate.[98] Before treatment with denosumab, serum calcium and 25-OHD should be checked and replaced if needed up to normal levels.

Parathyroid Hormone

Small randomized studies have determined that the 1-34 fragment of the PTH protein can significantly increase bone mass in the spine, with small losses or no gain at the skeletal sites rich in cortical bone.[99,99a] In 2001 a recombinant human PTH (rhPTH) composed of the 34 amino acids from the amino-terminal end of the hormone, known as *Fortéo*, was approved for the treatment of postmenopausal osteoporosis. In a large international, multicenter study, osteoporotic women with fracture were randomized to receive rhPTH 20 µg/day, 40 µg/day, or placebo for an average of 21 months. Lumbar spine bone mass increased between 9% and 13% in the rhPTH-treated subjects compared with the placebo-treated ones; hip bone mass also increased slightly. Most important, the risk of new vertebral fractures was reduced nearly 70% in both sets of rhPTH-treated subjects, and nonvertebral low-trauma fractures were reduced nearly 50% compared with placebo-treated patients.[100] This study was initially supposed to continue for 3 years; however, it was stopped at approximately 21 months because of preclinical evidence of malignant bone tumors in animal models. Additional studies of osteoporosis in men treated with rhPTH 1-34 have reported significant gains in bone mass.[100] Fortéo is given as a daily injection. Individuals using this medication may experience headache, nausea, and flushing with initiation of treatment, but these side effects generally become less severe after a few weeks.

A number of recent studies have evaluated whether rhPTH 1-34 or rhPTH 1-84 is more effective in combination with an antiresorptive agent (either bisphosphonates or raloxifene) than rhPTH alone in increasing BMD and reducing fractures.[101,102] Interestingly, two studies found that the combination of PTH and alendronate was less effective in stimulating bone gain at the lumbar spine in both osteopenic women and men over 1 to 1.5 years.[101,102] PTH stimulates new bone formation, increases bone mass, and reduces new vertebral and nonvertebral fractures, but when the medication is discontinued, the bone gained is rapidly lost. Black and colleagues[103] performed a study in which patients were given PTH for 1 year, followed by 1 year of alendronate treatment. Interestingly, the BMD gain after 1 year of PTH was about 6%; when followed by alendronate, nearly 6% BMD was gained at the spine. These data suggest that although PTH is an effective monotherapy for increasing bone mass, especially in the spine, the gain in BMD should be maintained with a potent antiresorptive agent for a number of years. Recent data from Deal and colleagues[104] indicate that lumbar spine BMD gained after PTH therapy is maintained with raloxifene treatment.

PTH is the first bone anabolic agent approved for the treatment of osteoporosis. Patients give themselves a subcutaneous injection daily for 18 to 24 months. Other routes of administration are now being studied including an intranasal route and a skin patch.

Vitamin D

Physiologic doses of vitamin D are important to ensure normal bone mineralization. Individuals 50 years of age and older should take at least 600 to 1000 IU of vitamin D daily as a multivitamin or combined with a calcium supplement. Hypovitaminosis D is common in the elderly population, with one study demonstrating that 57% of patients in a general medical ward were vitamin D deficient.[105] Low vitamin D levels increase the risk of bone loss and fracture. LeBoff and colleagues[39] found that 50% of patients admitted with acute femur fractures had vitamin D deficiency (25-OHD level <12 ng/mL), and 36.7% had secondary hyperparathyroidism. Data show seasonal variations in vitamin D levels; low 25-OHD levels during the winter and spring are associated with decreases in bone density. The importance of vitamin D to skeletal health was shown when elderly women in a nursing home treated with only 800 IU/day of vitamin D had a 40% reduction in incident hip fractures over 18 months, compared with placebo-controlled subjects.[106] Although this dramatic effect on fractures in an elderly population may represent a correction of vitamin D insufficiency, this study underscores that adequate vitamin D replacement can effectively diminish fractures in older individuals. Insufficient calcium and low 25-OHD levels are common in ambulatory patients and should be identified and treated before antiresorptive or other therapies for osteoporosis are initiated.

Although 200 IU of vitamin D prevents bone loss in the spine, data show that a higher daily intake (800 IU) is necessary to diminish bone loss in the hip during the winter and spring. Daily treatment with 700 IU of cholecalciferol and 500 mg of calcium carbonate reduced the rate of bone loss significantly in the femoral neck, spine, and total body and decreased the incidence of nonvertebral fractures by 50%.[107] Therefore to maintain skeletal health, patients require a vitamin D intake that results in a serum 25-OHD level of at least 30 ng/mL. To achieve this level in patients who do not receive regular sunlight, the daily intake of vitamin D needs to be higher. Replacement with 1,25-dihydroxyvitamin D (1,25[OH]$_2$D) is not recommended because hypercalcemia and hypercalciuria are common and require regular and costly monitoring.

Preventive Measures

Because bone loss is not completely reversible with existing therapies, prevention is essential for optimizing skeletal health. Strategies directed at increasing peak bone mass, reducing risk factors for bone loss (e.g., hypogonadism, decreased body fat, cigarette smoking, inactivity, excessive alcohol intake), and reversing the secondary causes of osteoporosis may prevent bone loss. Patients should be advised to consume adequate vitamin D and calcium and participate in a regular weight-bearing exercise program. Weight-bearing exercise increases muscle strength and may stabilize or modestly increase bone density. Emerging data show that increased calcium intake and exercise can add to bone accretion during adolescence and that interventions such as vitamin D and calcium supplementation can reduce fractures in older patients. Thus it is highly recommended that preventive strategies or therapies be instituted at any age to diminish the risk of fractures, which rises exponentially with age.

GLUCOCORTICOID-INDUCED OSTEOPOROSIS

Bone loss is a common sequela of therapy with glucocorticoids,[108] and glucocorticoid use increases the risk of fractures in patients with rheumatic diseases.[19] The severity of the bone loss in glucocorticoid-treated patients varies, with an approximately 3% to 20% decrease in bone density over 1 to 2 years. Glucocorticoid therapy is associated with increased fractures of the ribs and vertebrae, sites that contain predominantly trabecular bone, and it triples the risk of hip fracture in one-third of patients after 5 to 10 years of treatment.[109,110] In adults, alternate-day glucocorticoid therapy does not prevent bone loss. In patients with rheumatic diseases, concerns over the development of glucocorticoid-induced osteoporosis often limit the dose and duration of glucocorticoid therapy.

The lowest possible glucocorticoid dose should be used, along with general preventive strategies such as a regular weight-bearing exercise program, adequate calcium and vitamin D intake, and reduction of other risk factors that might contribute to the development of osteoporosis. However, data show that even patients on prednisone 5 mg/day have accelerated bone loss compared with controls. General prophylactic measures to prevent glucocorticoid-induced osteoporosis are shown in Table 101-7. Intestinal calcium absorption is impaired in glucocorticoid-treated patients, and early studies showed that this could be offset with vitamin D (40 to 100 μg/day two to three times a week) or 25-OHD, which produced an increase in bone density of the forearm. However, the administration of supraphysiologic doses of vitamin D requires careful monitoring of the serum and urinary calcium concentrations in patients at high risk for bone loss (with a normal urinary calcium

Table 101-7 Recommendations for Prevention and Treatment of Glucocorticoid-Induced Osteoporosis

Prevention

Patients starting GC therapy at a dose equivalent to prednisone ≥5 mg/day for 3 mo or longer should:
  Modify risk factors for osteoporosis (stop smoking, decrease excessive alcohol consumption)
  Start regular weight-bearing physical exercise
  Initiate intake of calcium (total 1500 mg/day) and vitamin D (400-800 IU/day)
  Consider BMD testing to predict risk of fracture and bone loss
  Initiate bisphosphonate therapy (alendronate 5 mg/day or 35 mg/wk, or risedronate 5 mg/day or 35 mg/wk)

Treatment

Patients on long-term GC therapy should be tested for osteoporosis using BMD measurement. If the T-score is < −1, consider:
  Risk factor modification including reducing risk of falls
  Regular weight-bearing physical exercises
  Calcium and vitamin D supplementation
  Replacement of gonadal steroids, if deficient
  Bisphosphonate therapy (alendronate 10 mg/day or 70 mg/wk, or risedronate 5 mg/day or 35 mg/wk); if bisphosphonates are contraindicated or not tolerated, consider calcitonin as second-line agent, intravenous bisphosphonate (pamidronate or zolendronate), or parathyroid hormone 1-34
Repeat BMD measurement annually or biannually

BMD, bone mineral density; GC, glucocorticoid.

Modified from Recommendations for the prevention and treatment of glucocorticoid-induced osteoporosis: 2001 update, *Arthritis Rheum* 44:1496–1503, 2001.

level and no history of nephrolithiasis). An alternative approach in patients at risk for osteoporosis and receiving long-term glucocorticoid therapy is to raise the 25-OHD level into the upper-normal range (>30 ng/mL) to ensure adequate intestinal calcium absorption. This can usually be accomplished by administering vitamin D at 800 IU/day.

Because of the enhanced bone resorption in patients treated with glucocorticoids, investigators have examined the effects of inhibitors of bone resorption. The use of bisphosphonates in patients receiving chronic glucocorticoid therapy is beneficial for both the prevention and treatment of osteoporosis. The use of alendronate 5 or 10 mg/day for 1 year in patients receiving glucocorticoid therapy increased lumbar spine BMD by 2.1% and 2.9%, respectively, and increased femoral neck BMD by 1.2% and 1%, respectively ($P < .001$).[110] After 1 year of treatment, there was an insignificant reduction in new vertebral fractures, but after 2 years of treatment, there was a nearly 40% reduction in new vertebral fracture risk. Risedronate 5 mg/day was also effective in the prevention and treatment of glucocorticoid-induced bone loss.[111] Recent studies of zoledronic acid (5 mg IV/year) versus risedronate (5 mg/day) and teriparatide (20 μg/day) versus alendronate (10 mg/day) for 18 months indicated that both zoledronic acid and teriparatide improved bone mass more than the comparator, and teriparatide-treated subjects had a significant vertebral fracture risk reduction[112,113] in glucocorticoid-treated patients. Combination studies of rhPTH 1-34 with HRT were also found to be more effective than HRT alone in glucocorticoid-induced osteoporosis.[114] No difference between treatments in fracture data was observed; however, quantitative CT of the lumbar spine, a measure of only trabecular bone, found a nearly 35% increase in PTH-treated patients compared with the estrogen-only group after 12 months of therapy.[115]

Men on glucocorticoids can have a lowering of testosterone levels.[116] They are generally asymptomatic, but if men on glucocorticoids have evidence of low serum testosterone levels and symptoms of low libido, they can be safely treated with testosterone. Bone mass increases have been observed in men with low testosterone levels on glucocorticoids who were treated with testosterone.[117] However, because of the risks associated with testosterone treatment, it is more prudent to treat these patients with a bisphosphonate medication.

To prevent bone loss in patients with pulmonary diseases requiring glucocorticoid therapy, treatment with inhaled glucocorticoids has been studied.[118] Inhaled glucocorticoids appear to uncouple bone turnover and increase bone loss; however, this is dose dependent. Less than 800 µg/day of inhaled budesonide dipropionate does not increase the risk of osteoporosis, but more than 800 µg/day does. New inhaled steroids are more potent than older ones; for instance, Advair 200 µg/day is equivalent to nearly 5 mg/day of prednisone.[119] Therefore patients on chronic steroid inhalers should be screened for bone loss. Because patients receiving glucocorticoids may lose a dramatic amount of bone, it is important to monitor the efficacy of a treatment intervention, assess the need for further diagnostic evaluation for other causes of bone loss, and consider alternative treatment strategies if a given therapy is ineffective in preventing bone loss or fractures. In patients at increased risk of fracture, therapy with a potent bisphosphonate is highly recommended to slow bone loss and the rate of new fractures. Alendronate, risedronate, and zoledronic acid are available for use, and future studies of more potent bisphosphonates and PTH are expected.[120-122]

OSTEOMALACIA

Osteomalacia is characterized by impaired mineralization of bone matrix. Calcium, phosphate, and vitamin D are necessary for the mineralization of bone. Normally, there is a steep inverse relationship between the serum calcium and PTH concentrations. A small decrease in the serum calcium concentration leads to a rise in PTH release, which promotes distal renal calcium reabsorption, proximal tubulorenal phosphorus excretion, and resorption of calcium from bone. Vitamin D is produced in the skin in the presence of ultraviolet light or absorbed in the intestine from dietary or supplemental sources. Activation of vitamin D to 25-OHD occurs in the liver and to $1,25(OH)_2D$ in the proximal tubules of the kidney. PTH, hypocalcemia, and hypophosphatemia stimulate the renal 1-hydroxylase enzyme that converts 25-OHD to $1,25(OH)_2D$, which in turn indirectly enhances intestinal calcium absorption.[123]

Osteomalacia results from reduced availability of calcium or phosphate for incorporation into the hydroxyapatite of bone or from deficient absorption or activation of vitamin D.[124] The term *rickets* applies to the defective mineralization of bone and the cartilaginous growth plate in growing children. As shown in Table 101-8, osteomalacia or rickets may result from decreased availability of vitamin D as a consequence of insufficient ultraviolet light exposure, insufficient

Table 101-8 Causes of Osteomalacia and Rickets

Vitamin D Deficiency or Dysfunction
Reduced Availability
Nutritional deficit Reduced exposure to ultraviolet light Malabsorption (gastrointestinal or biliary disease, surgical resection)
Alteration in Metabolism
Reduced 25-hydroxyvitamin D from liver or gastrointestinal disease, nephrotic syndrome, anticonvulsant drugs Reduced 1,25-dihydroxyvitamin D from renal disease, vitamin D–dependent rickets type I
Alteration in Action on Target Tissues
Vitamin D–dependent rickets type II
Phosphate Deficiency
Decreased availability—dietary deficiency, phosphate-binding antacids Decreased renotubular phosphate reabsorption Familial—X-linked hypophosphatemic rickets, adult-onset vitamin D–resistant osteomalacia Acquired—hypophosphatemic osteomalacia (phosphate diabetes), oncogenic osteomalacia Generalized renotubular disorders
Acidosis
Renotubular acidosis Ureterosigmoidostomy Carbonic anhydrase inhibitors (acetazolamide)
Miscellaneous Mineralization Defects
Inhibitors of mineralization—fluoride, bisphosphonates (e.g., etidronate), chronic renal failure (aluminum) Hypophosphatasia

Modified from LeBoff MS, Brown EM: Metabolic bone disease. In Hare JW, editor: *Signs and symptoms in endocrine and metabolic disorders*, Philadelphia, 1986, JB Lippincott, pp 239–260.

vitamin intake, or malabsorption in patients with gastrointestinal or biliary disorders. Reduced levels of 25-OHD are caused by severe liver disease, increased renal excretion of vitamin D metabolites due to nephrotic syndrome, or accelerated metabolism of 25-OHD caused by anticonvulsant drugs. Decreased activation of $1,25(OH)_2D$ is seen in patients with renal insufficiency due to increased phosphate levels; the resultant lower ionized calcium levels lead to secondary or tertiary hyperparathyroidism.

A careful history is important in the diagnosis of osteomalacia or vitamin D insufficiency. For example, a history of a malabsorptive process such as gastrectomy, intestinal resection, sprue, primary biliary cirrhosis, or pancreatic deficiency may lead to the identification of vitamin D deficiency and osteomalacia.[124] Patients with osteomalacia may present with generalized pain involving the pelvis, spine, ribs, or lower extremities or with skeletal deformities such as bowing of the long bones, kyphoscoliosis, or pelvic abnormalities. Another clinical sign of osteomalacia in adults is proximal muscle weakness, which may result in an antalgic or waddling gait and difficulty ambulating.

Pain may be elicited by deep palpation of the tibia, ribs, or pubic ramus.[124] One of the radiographic signs of osteomalacia is the presence of pseudofractures, or Looser's zones, which are transverse lines of rarefaction through the cortices, with incomplete healing in the ribs, scapulae, long bones (Figure 101-2), or pubic rami. Pseudofractures,

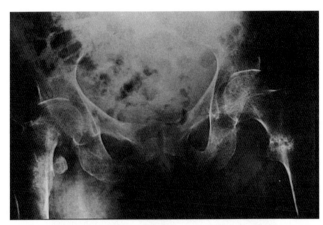

Figure 101-2 Osteomalacia and fractures in a 65-year-old woman with malabsorption. Shown are a pseudofracture of the left lesser trochanter and an avulsion of the right lesser trochanter. This patient also had previous bilateral pubic rami fractures.

however, may be indistinguishable from those associated with osteogenesis imperfecta or Paget's disease. Other radiographic findings in osteomalacia are vertebral fractures or protrusio acetabuli. Vitamin D deficiency may result in irreversible cortical bone loss.[124] In subtle cases of osteomalacia, a bone biopsy with a double tetracycline label may be necessary; characteristic histomorphometric findings in this disorder include increased osteoid and delayed mineralization of bone.

Rickets causes abnormalities of the epiphyseal growth plate, and the clinical signs include an inability to ambulate, growth disturbances, bowing of the long bones, and short stature. Bony deformities of the skull and ribs may develop, with widened cranial sutures (craniotabes), thickened costochondral junctions (rachitic rosary), or indentation of the margins of the ribs (Harrison's grooves).

The biochemical parameters in patients with osteomalacia reflect the underlying pathophysiologic process and the compensatory biologic responses. In vitamin D deficiency states, the serum calcium levels are usually normal or slightly decreased because PTH levels rise rapidly as a compensatory response to impaired calcium absorption.[125] In renal insufficiency phosphate retention, impaired renal production of $1,25(OH)_2D$, hypocalcemia, and skeletal resistance to PTH are thought to lead to the development of hyperparathyroidism and resultant renal osteodystrophy, mixed osteomalacia, and osteitis fibrosa cystica.[126] Also, aluminum intoxication may present with pure osteomalacia or adynamic bone disease.[125,127] Chronic vitamin D deficiency may increase the secretory demands of the parathyroid glands, thereby producing secondary or, in some instances, tertiary hyperparathyroidism. In patients with osteomalacia without hepatobiliary disease, alkaline phosphatase levels are often elevated.[124]

Osteomalacia may be associated with a deficiency of phosphate, principally in patients with decreased renotubular reabsorption of phosphate. Familial hypophosphatemic vitamin D–resistant rickets in children or osteomalacia in adults usually presents with renal phosphate leak, hypophosphatemia, rachitic or osteomalacial changes, and inappropriately normal or low-normal $1,25(OH)_2D$ level for the degree of hypophosphatemia. This X-linked dominant

disorder may present in young children with the inability to walk, followed by progressive bowing and skeletal deformities, without signs of proximal myopathy. The genetic locus for X-linked hypophosphatemic rickets has been mapped to Xp22.1, and the gene is named *PHEX* (phosphate-regulating gene with homology to endopeptidases on the X chromosome).[128]

Oncogenic osteomalacia or rickets is a vitamin D–resistant process associated with certain neoplasias, principally small, benign mesenchymal or endodermal tumors and, infrequently, certain malignant tumors (e.g., multiple myeloma; prostatic, oat cell, breast carcinomas).[129,130] Such patients typically present with decreased renotubular phosphate reabsorption, hypophosphatemia, muscle weakness, diminished $1,25(OH)_2D$ levels, and normocalcemia. The benign tumors tend to be small and difficult to identify on physical examination or radiographs. Surgical removal of these tumors results in a rise in the phosphate and $1,25(OH)_2D$ levels and resolution of the skeletal process. Osteomalacia may also be associated with generalized renotubular disorders and the use of certain drugs that contain inhibitors of mineralization (e.g., fluoride, etidronate, aluminum). The evaluation of a patient suspected of having osteomalacia is outlined in Table 101-9.

Osteomalacia is often a treatable disease, but the diagnosis may be overlooked. Vitamin D deficiency can be treated with physiologic doses of vitamin D, but higher doses (1000 to 2000 IU/day) may hasten the healing of bone. In the presence of intestinal malabsorption, and until the underlying malabsorptive process is corrected, large doses of vitamin D (50,000 IU once a week to three or more times a week) are often required. Careful monitoring of the serum and urinary calcium levels and 25-OHD concentrations is necessary to prevent vitamin D intoxication. Use of the active metabolite of 25-OHD (Calderol) may occasionally be necessary in resistant patients or in those with severe liver disease who cannot achieve activation of this metabolite. The potential advantages of using 25-OHD are more stable bioavailability, shorter half-life, and greater potency than the parent compound,[124] although the cost is greater.

In patients with hypophosphatemia and disorders of renotubular phosphate reabsorption, mineralization of bone occurs with phosphate therapy and moderately high doses of $1,25(OH)_2D$, the latter being necessary to prevent the secondary hyperparathyroidism associated with phosphate therapy. In patients with renal insufficiency or failure, a phosphate binder (calcium acetate or calcium carbonate) should be used after meals to decrease intestinal phosphate absorption. Calcium citrate therapy should not be used because it augments aluminum absorption. In those with

Table 101-9   Evaluation of Osteomalacia

Calcium, phosphorus, alkaline phosphatase, urinary calcium levels; 25-hydroxyvitamin D and intact parathyroid hormone levels
In selected patients:
  1,25-Dihydroxyvitamin D levels (e.g., renal insufficiency, vitamin D–resistant osteomalacia or rickets)
  Vitamin D absorption test: obtain 25-hydroxyvitamin D levels at 0, 4, and 8 hr (e.g., some cases of malabsorption)
  Tubular reabsorption of phosphate (e.g., vitamin D–resistant osteomalacia or rickets)
  Bone biopsy with double tetracycline labels

renal failure, 1,25(OH)$_2$D therapy administered orally[125,131] (or intravenously in some dialysis patients) suppresses parathyroid cell secretion and proliferation; a threefold elevation of the PTH level is advocated by some investigators to prevent adynamic bone disease.[126] Analogues of 1,25(OH)$_2$D that do not produce hypercalcemia but decrease levels of PTH are now available and may be useful in patients with renal insufficiency.

PAGET'S DISEASE OF BONE

Paget's disease of bone affects approximately 2% to 3% of the population older than 50 years and is uncommon in individuals younger than 40 years.[132] Paget's disease is characterized by enhanced resorption of bone by giant, multinucleated osteoclasts, followed by the formation of disorganized woven bone by osteoblasts. The resultant bone is expanded, weak, and vascular, so affected bones may become enlarged and deformed and the overlying skin may feel warm to the touch.[133]

Cause

The cause of Paget's disease is uncertain, although data showing the presence of viral inclusion particles in giant pagetic osteoclasts support a viral cause, possibly associated with measles, respiratory syncytial, or canine distemper virus. Paget's disease tends to aggregate in families in an autosomal dominant pattern, and 40% of patients have at least one other family member affected.[107] Recently, in a family with juvenile Paget's disease, the disease was found to be associated with a polymorphism in the OPG allele.[134] Studies of additional families with this mutation may lead to the discovery of the cause of Paget's disease.

Clinical Features

Many patients with Paget's disease are asymptomatic, and the disease is detected by the incidental finding of an elevated alkaline phosphatase level or characteristic radiographic abnormality. Other patients present with a range of symptoms that include bone pain; skeletal deformities (bowing of long bones, enlarged skull, pelvic alterations); pathologic fractures; increased cardiac output (with extensive disease); and nerve compression. Paget's disease typically includes a lytic phase, a combined lytic and blastic phase, and a sclerotic or "burned out" phase occurring late in the disease process.

Radiographic signs of the three stages of Paget's disease may be present at different sites in the same patient.[132] The skeletal sites commonly involved with Paget's disease include the skull (Figure 101-3), vertebrae, pelvis, sacrum, and lower extremities. Degenerative joint disease may develop adjacent to the bones and cause pain that may obscure the symptoms associated with Paget's disease.[132] Ten percent to 30% of patients with Paget's disease may experience fractures that present initially as asymptomatic or painful short fissure fractures traversing the bony cortex (Figure 101-4). Complete fractures of the bones such as the "chalk stick" fracture also occur; fractures of the long bones may be a serious complication because the increased vascularity of pagetic bone may lead to excessive blood loss.

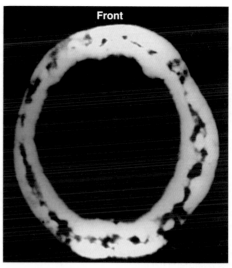

Figure 101-3 Paget's disease of the skull in a woman with signs of increasing head size and progressive hearing loss. The alkaline phosphatase level was 2100 U/L. This computed axial tomogram shows marked thickening of the inner and outer skull tables, with osteoblastic pagetoid changes. Audiologic evaluation revealed bilateral hearing loss.

Healing of fractures in pagetic bone usually occurs normally, although there have been reports of nonunion. A rare complication of Paget's disease of bone is sarcomatous degeneration in less than 1% of patients (with osteogenic sarcomas or, less commonly, fibrosarcomas or chondrosarcomas); these patients generally have a poor prognosis. The development of a sarcoma may be heralded by the presence of a soft tissue mass, localized pain, and rise in the alkaline phosphatase level.

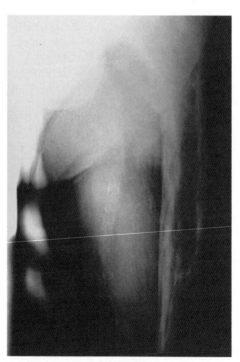

Figure 101-4 Paget's disease of the proximal femur. Note the coarse trabeculae, thickened cortices, lateral fissure fracture, and expanding lytic region characteristic of the "blade-of-grass" lesion.

Neurologic symptoms generally result from compression of the nerves by pagetic bone. Hearing loss is common and is caused by sensory loss and conduction abnormalities due to pagetic involvement of the bones of the inner ear. Paget's disease of the skull may also produce ocular and other cranial nerve palsies. Compression of the base of the skull may lead to basilar invagination, cerebellar dysfunction, or obstructive hydrocephalus, with symptoms of nausea, ataxia, incontinence, gait disturbances, and dementia. Neurologic compromise of the thoracic or lumbar spine may lead to spinal cord compression or, in the latter instance, cauda equina syndrome.

Laboratory Findings

Biochemical indices in patients with Paget's disease usually show normal serum calcium and phosphate levels, although hypercalcemia may develop with immobilization when there is an uncoupling of bone resorption and formation. Patients with Paget's disease may also be hypercalcemic if they coincidentally acquire primary hyperparathyroidism, which can further increase bone remodeling and worsen the disease process. Secondary hyperparathyroidism may develop in approximately 10% to 15% of patients with Paget's disease, presumably because of inadequate calcium intake to meet the skeletal demands of the heightened bone remodeling.[132]

Alkaline phosphatase levels of bone origin (BSAP) are commonly elevated in patients with significant Paget's disease because of the increased osteoblastic activity combined with bone breakdown. In the absence of liver disease, the alkaline phosphatase level typically correlates with the extent of the pagetic involvement of bone, although it may be more elevated in Paget's disease of the skull (see Figure 101-3).

Unexpectedly, circulating osteocalcin levels do not reflect disease activity in patients with Paget's disease as well as bone-specific alkaline phosphatase levels reflect disease activity. Markers of bone resorption such as urinary collagen cross-links like N telopeptides and C telopeptides are also elevated in active Paget's disease. Other laboratory abnormalities in patients with Paget's disease include hypercalciuria, hyperuricuria, and hyperuricemia, possibly related to the increased turnover of osteoclasts. Serum uric acid levels should be measured periodically because of the association of Paget's disease with gouty arthritis.

Diagnosis

Bone scans are valuable tools for assessing the extent of Paget's disease and are therefore useful as part of the initial evaluation.[133] As diagnostic tests, however, bone scans in general are sensitive but not specific for a number of skeletal processes. Radiographs show characteristic radiologic findings such as transverse lucent areas, osteoporosis circumscripta, enlargement of the bones, expanding lytic changes, the "blade-of-grass" lesion shown in Figure 101-4, thickened cortices, a coarse trabecular pattern, or sclerotic changes.

In patients with involvement of the skull and changes in mental status, a skull radiograph, magnetic resonance imaging (MRI), or quantitative computed tomography (QCT) may be useful to diagnose platybasia and flattening of the base of the skull, basilar invagination, or the infrequent complication of hydrocephalus. Audiologic evaluation may reveal hearing loss in patients with pagetic involvement of the skull.

Treatment

The indications for treatment of Paget's disease (Table 101-10) include pain, hypercalcemia, fractures, high-output cardiac failure (rare), and neurologic compromise. Therapy can also be used to prevent the progression of deformity or risk of nerve compression when there is pagetic involvement of the skull, a vertebral body, or a weight-bearing bone (femur) or when disease is present adjacent to a major articular joint.

Treatment of symptomatic Paget's disease is usually directed at suppression of the enhanced bone resorption and skeletal turnover with calcitonin or bisphosphonates.[132,135] Response to therapy is monitored by the reduction of symptoms and maintenance of the alkaline phosphatase level in a mid-normal range, with retreatment once values rise 25% above normal.

Calcitonin

Salmon calcitonin and human calcitonin inhibit the function of osteoclasts, which are active in the pagetic process; both types of calcitonin preparations come in an injectable form and are FDA approved for patients with Paget's disease.[136] Salmon calcitonin therapy is usually initiated at a low dose to ensure patient tolerance and then increased to a daily dose of 100 Medical Research Council units (intramuscularly or subcutaneously). After 6 months of therapy, the patient may be maintained on 50 to 100 Medical Research Council units daily.[132] Approximately two-thirds of patients show a decrease in alkaline phosphatase levels of 50% or more in 2 to 6 months. Some patients experience resistance to the effects of calcitonin, which can be reversed in some instances by switching from salmon calcitonin to human calcitonin. Calcitonin is a safe drug.

Calcitonin is useful in patients with expanding lytic lesions, particularly of a weight-bearing bone, or for preoperative therapy before elective orthopedic procedures. The use of calcitonin nasal spray has few systemic side effects but is not FDA approved for the treatment of Paget's disease.

Bisphosphonates

Several bisphosphonates are currently approved by the FDA for the treatment of Paget's disease; they include

Table 101-10 Indications for Treatment of Paget's Disease of Bone

Pain
Hypercalcemia
Fractures
High-output cardiac failure (rare)
Skull involvement
Neurologic compromise
Periarticular disease
Prevention of progression of Paget's disease

etidronate disodium (Didronel), pamidronate (Aredia), alendronate (Fosamax), tiludronate disodium, risedronate (Actonel), and zoledronic acid (Reclast).

Etidronate disodium is an orally administered drug that produces a clinical and biochemical response similar to that of calcitonin.[136] The therapeutic dose for Paget's disease is 5 mg/kg per day (400 mg/day, or a minimum of 200 mg/day for smaller patients) for 6 months; the drug is then stopped for 6 months before being reinstituted in 6-month cycles of therapy.[137] As mentioned previously, higher doses of etidronate are associated with defective mineralization of bone and osteomalacia, with symptoms of pain and fractures. Measurements of alkaline phosphatase levels at 3- to 6-month intervals are useful to ensure the suppression of bone turnover; an estimated 25% of patients may become resistant to etidronate.[132] However, newer, more potent bisphosphonates are effective for the treatment of Paget's disease.

Parenteral pamidronate is also approved for the treatment of symptomatic Paget's disease of bone in patients with a threefold or greater elevation of alkaline phosphatase concentrations. This more potent bisphosphonate is useful in patients who become resistant to etidronate and in those with more severe disease. An advantage of this therapy is that alkaline phosphatase levels may be reduced to the normal range, with a sustained response for a prolonged period (up to a year or more).[132,138]

The FDA-recommended dose of pamidronate for patients with Paget's disease is 30 mg/day as a 4-hour infusion on 3 sequential days (total dose 90 mg), with retreatment possible if necessary. Other regimens for the treatment of Paget's disease include 60 mg of pamidronate daily (infused over 3 hours) once a week for 1 or 2 weeks in patients with alkaline phosphatase levels between 300 and 400 U/L. For more extensive disease, three or four infusions of pamidronate every 1 to 2 weeks may be necessary. To assess the efficacy of these regimens for Paget's disease, clinical symptoms should be reviewed and alkaline phosphatase levels measured 2 to 3 months later.[138]

Some patients treated with pamidronate may experience a transient fever, musculoskeletal and flulike symptoms, and hypocalcemia; calcium supplementation (500 mg twice daily in vitamin D–replete patients) can offset the hypocalcemia that results from the suppression of bone resorption. Pamidronate is available only as a parenteral drug, which restricts its use.[138]

Oral alendronate has been approved for the treatment of Paget's disease at a dose of 40 mg/day for 6 months. Therapy with alendronate is recommended for patients with at least a twofold elevation in alkaline phosphatase levels or for those with specific indications for therapy (see Table 101-10). The use of alendronate produces a normalization of, or a 60% or greater reduction in, the alkaline phosphatase level in approximately 85% of patients. Studies indicate that this therapy is more effective than etidronate. (All bisphosphonates must be taken correctly to minimize gastrointestinal side effects).[139]

Risedronate is another potent bisphosphonate (see Table 101-6) that is FDA approved for the treatment of Paget's disease. Siris and colleagues[139] treated 162 patients with moderate to severe Paget's disease with oral risedronate (30 mg/day for 84 days, followed by 112 days without

treatment). This cycle was repeated if the serum alkaline phosphatase level did not normalize or increased more than 25% from its nadir value. After the first and second cycles, the serum alkaline phosphatase level decreased 65% and 69%, respectively, and urine markers decreased 50% and 66.9%, respectively. The serum alkaline phosphatase level normalized in 53.8% of patients, and a significant decrease in bone pain was noted. Risedronate is well tolerated and has few adverse effects including a flulike syndrome, gastrointestinal symptoms, and, rarely, iritis. Other groups have shown a decrease in serum alkaline phosphatase levels of 79% and 86%, with an 85% and 100% decrease in urine markers.[140] There is no evidence of osteomalacia in bone biopsies from patients treated with 30 mg of risedronate. Patients who have become resistant to etidronate appear to respond to risedronate. Patients must be instructed to have an adequate intake of calcium and vitamin D while taking risedronate. Recently, zoledronic acid was also found to be effective in the treatment of Paget's disease, and approval is pending from the FDA.[141]

In addition to antiresorptive therapies, nonsteroidal anti-inflammatory drugs (NSAIDs) and aspirin are useful modalities to alleviate the joint pain and other symptoms that result from degenerative joint disease. Finally, surgical intervention is sometimes warranted in patients with Paget's disease and bony deformities, pathologic fractures, nerve compression, or degenerative arthritis. Orthopedic procedures such as total joint replacement and osteotomies are associated with a reduced risk of intraoperative bleeding or other complications if patients are treated medically (e.g., with calcitonin or other bisphosphonates) to reduce the disease activity and vascularity for at least 6 weeks before the procedure.

OTHER MEDICATION-INDUCED OSTEOPOROSIS

Aromatase inhibitors in women undergoing breast cancer treatment are associated with bone loss. Postmenopausal women maintain a low level of circulating estrogen because of aromatization of androgens to estrogen in tissues such as fat and muscle by cytochrome P-450 enzyme. Inhibition of this enzyme is now used in postmenopausal women with breast cancer. There are two classes of aromatase inhibitors: nonsteroidal reversible inhibitors (anastrozole and letrozole) and steroidal reversible inhibitors (exemestane). Because these agents prevent the conversion of androgen to estrogen, this results in low serum estrogen levels and increased bone remodeling. Fracture rates in clinical trials of aromatase inhibitors compared with either tamoxifen or placebo ranged from 3% to 7%.[142] In a 2-year study, significantly higher markers of bone turnover and nearly twice the lumbar spine bone loss and fracture rates were observed with anastrozole compared with tamoxifen.[142] Although the data are just beginning to be collected regarding skeletal health in women treated for breast cancer with aromatase inhibitors, it is important to obtain a history of clinical risk factors for osteoporosis and a BMD measurement of the hip and spine. Preventive treatment should be initiated in women with normal or low bone mass and no history of fractures. Treatment of women with low bone mass (t score ≤ −2) should be initiated with potent antiresorptive agents, and BMD should be monitored at least every 2 years. Recent studies with zoledronic acid and denosumab have been reported to be quite effective in this patient population.[143,144] If a woman continues to lose bone mass on aromatase inhibitors despite compliance with potent antiresorptive agents, and if the patient has not had radiation to the skeleton as part of the breast cancer protocol, rhPTH 1-34 treatment can be used to build up bone mass.

Gonadotropin-releasing hormone antagonists are used to treat women with endometriosis and men with prostate cancer. These compounds induce bone loss by lowering estrogen levels, resulting in accelerated bone turnover. A study of more than 50,000 men with prostate cancer treated with androgen-deprivation therapy consisting of either gonadotropin-releasing hormone agonists or orchiectomy found an increased risk of fracture or hospitalization due to fracture. Although the overall risk of fracture associated with androgen-deprivation therapy was only modestly increased overall, the risk of fracture was significantly associated with the number of doses of gonadotropin-releasing hormone agonists. Other studies have reported that androgen-deprivation therapy increases bone loss at all sites, with a 2% to 8% annual loss in the lumbar spine and a 2% to 6% loss in the hip after 1 year.[145] Given the high incidence of prostate cancer and the increasing use of this treatment, assessment of bone mass and the prevention of additional bone mass loss are probably appropriate. Oncologists currently recommend that BMD be measured at the time of initiation of androgen-deprivation therapy and that clinical risk factors for osteoporosis be reviewed including history of fracture after age 30, family history of hip fracture, smoking history, use of glucocorticoids, low testosterone level, and rheumatoid arthritis. If the patient has a low BMD (t score < −2.5) or a t score between −1 and −2.5 and other risk factors, treatment with calcium and vitamin D supplementation and a bisphosphonate (zoledronic acid, alendronate, risedronate, or denosumab) should be initiated. BMD of the lumbar spine and hip should be measured at least once a year while patients are maintained on androgen-deprivation therapy.[146-149]

Selected References

1. Osteoporosis: review of the evidence for prevention, diagnosis and treatment and cost-effectiveness analysis. Introduction, *Osteoporos Int* 8(Suppl 4):S7–S80, 1998.
2. Riggs BL, Melton LJl: The prevention and treatment of osteoporosis, *N Engl J Med* 327:620–627, 1992.
3. Riggs BL, Wahner HW, Dunn WL, et al: Differential changes in bone mineral density of the appendicular and axial skeleton with aging: relationship to spinal osteoporosis, *J Clin Invest* 67:328, 1981.
4. National Osteoporosis Foundation: *Physician's guide to prevention and treatment of osteoporosis*, Belle Mead, NJ, 1998, Excerpta Medica.
5. Manolagas SC, Jilka RL: Bone marrow, cytokines, and bone remodeling, *N Engl J Med* 332:305–311, 1995.
6. Kimble RB, Kitazawa R, Vannice JL, et al: Persistent bone-sparing effect of interleukin-1 receptor antagonist: a hypothesis on the role of IL-1 in ovariectomy-induced bone loss, *Calcif Tissue Int* 55:260–265, 1996.
7. Cheleuitte D, Mizuno S, Glowacki J: In vitro secretion of cytokines by human bone marrow: effects of age and estrogen status, *J Clin Endocrinol Metab* 83:2043–2051, 1998.
8. Boyce BF, Hughes RD, Wright KR: Recent advances in bone biology provide insights in the pathogenesis of bone disease, *Lab Invest* 79:83–94, 1999.

9. McClung MR, Lewiecki EM, Cohen SB, et al: Denosumab in postmenopausal women with low bone mineral density, *N Engl J Med* 354:821–831, 2006.
10. Nevitt MC: Epidemiology of osteoporosis, *Osteoporosis* 20:535–554, 1994.
11. El-Hajj Fuleihan G, Gundberg CM, Gleason R, et al: Racial differences in parathyroid hormone dynamics, *J Clin Endocrinol Metab* 79:1642–1647, 1994.
12. Bell NH, Shary J, Stevens J: Demonstration that bone mass is greater in black than in white children, *J Bone Miner Res* 6:719–723, 1991.
13. Sambrook PN, Kelly PJ, Morrison NA, et al: Scientific review: genetics of osteoporosis, *Br J Rheumatol* 33:1007–1011, 1994.
14. Cummings SR, Nevitt MC, Browner WS, et al: Risk factors for hip fracture in white women, *N Engl J Med* 332:767–773, 1995.
15. Uitterlinden AG, Burger H, Huang Q, et al: Relation of alleles of the collagen type 1α1 gene to bone density and the risk of osteoporotic fractures in postmenopausal women, *N Engl J Med* 338:1016–1021, 1998.
16. Faulkner KG, Cummings SR, Black D, et al: Simple measurement of femoral geometry predicts hip fracture: the study of osteoporotic fractures, *J Bone Miner Res* 8:1211–1217, 1993.
17. Little RD, Carulli JP, Del Mastro RG, et al: A mutation in the LDL receptor-related protein 5 gene results in the autosomal dominant high-bone mass trait, *Am J Hum Genet* 70:11–19, 2002.
18. Boyden LM, Mao J, Belsky J, et al: High bone density due to a mutation in LDL-receptor protein 5, *N Engl J Med* 346:1513–1521, 2002.
18a. Li W-F, Hou S-X, Yu B, et al: Genetics of osteoporosis: accelerating the pace in gene identification and validation, *Hum Genet* 127:249–285, 2010.
19. Lane NE, Lukert BP: The science and therapy of glucocorticoid-induced osteoporosis, *Endocrinol Metab Clin North Am* 27:465–483, 1998.
20. Ross DS, Neer RM, Ridgway EC: Subclinical hyperthyroidism and reduced bone density as a possible result of prolonged suppression of the pituitary-thyroid axis with L-thyroxine, *Am J Med* 82:1167–1170, 1987.
21. Biller BMK, Saxe V, Herzog DB, et al: Mechanisms of osteoporosis in adult and adolescent women with anorexia nervosa, *J Clin Endocrinol Metab* 68:548–551, 1989.
22. Friedman AJ, Daly M, Juneau-Norcross M, et al: A prospective, randomized trial of gonadotropin-releasing hormone agonist plus estrogen-progestin add-back regimens for women with leiomyomata uteri, *J Clin Endocrinol Metab* 76:1439–1445, 1993.
23. Gordon CM, Grace E, Emans SJ, et al: Changes in bone turnover markers and menstrual function after short-term oral DHEA in young women with anorexia nervosa, *J Bone Miner Res* 14:136–145, 1999.
24. Orwoll ES: *Osteoporosis in men: primer on the metabolic bone diseases and disorders of mineral metabolism*, ed 6, 2006, American Society of Bone and Mineral Research, pp 290-292.
25. Leder BZ, leBlanc A, Schoenfeld DA, et al: Differential effects of androgens and estrogens on bone turnover in normal men, *J Clin Endocrinol Metab* 88:204–210, 2003.
26. Sambrook PN, Ansell BM, Foster S, et al: Bone turnover in early rheumatoid arthritis. II. Longitudinal bone density studies, *Ann Rheum Dis* 44:580–584, 1985.
27. Rehman Q, Lane NE: Therapeutic approaches for preventing bone loss in inflammatory arthritis, *Arthritis Res* 3:221–227, 2001.
28. Gravallese EM, Goldring SR: Cellular mechanisms and the role of cytokines in bone erosions in rheumatoid arthritis, *Arthritis Rheum* 43:2143–2151, 2000.
29. Kong YY, Yoshida H, Sarosi I, et al: OPGL is a key regulator of osteoclastogenesis, lymphocyte development and lymph-node organogenesis, *Nature* 397:316–323, 1999.
30. American College of Rheumatologists Task Force on Osteoporosis Guidelines: Recommendations for the prevention and treatment of glucocorticoid-induced osteoporosis: 2001 update, *Arthritis Rheum* 44:1496–1503, 2001.
31. Hansen M, Florescu A, Stoltenberg M, et al: Bone loss in rheumatoid arthritis: influence of disease activity, duration of the disease, functional capacity, and corticosteroid treatment, *Scand J Rheumatol* 25:367–376, 1996.
32. LeBoff MS, Wade JP, Mackowiak S, et al: Low dose prednisone does not affect calcium homeostasis or bone density in postmenopausal women with rheumatoid arthritis, *J Rheumatol* 18:339–344, 1991.

33. Hunter T, Dubo HI: Spinal fractures complicating ankylosing spondylitis: a longterm follow-up study, *Arthritis Rheum* 26:751–759, 1983.

34. Lane NE: Osteoporosis and osteonecrosis in systemic lupus erythematous, *Nat Clin Pract Rheumatol* 2:562–569, 2006.

35. Stowens DW, Teitelbaum SL, Kahn AJ, et al: Skeletal complications of Gaucher disease, *Medicine* 64:310–322, 1985.

36. Movsowitz C, Epstein S, Fallon M, et al: Cyclosporin-A in vivo produces severe osteopenia in the rat: effect of dose and duration of administration, *Endocrinology* 123:2571–2577, 1988.

37. Bryer HP, Isserow JA, Armstrong EC, et al: Azathioprine alone is bone sparing and does not alter cyclosporin A-induced osteopenia in the rat, *J Bone Miner Res* 10:132–138, 1995.

38. Rich GM, Mudge GH, Laffel GL, et al: Cyclosporine A and prednisone-associated osteoporosis in heart transplant recipients, *J Heart Lung Transplant* 11:950–958, 1992.

39. LeBoff MS, Kohlmeier L, Hurwitz S, et al: Occult vitamin D deficiency in postmenopausal US women with acute hip fracture, *JAMA* 281:1505–1511, 1999.

40. Johnston CC Jr, Slemenda CW, Melton LJ III: Clinical use of bone densitometry, *N Engl J Med* 324:1105–1109, 1991.

41. El-Hajj Fuleihan G, Testa MA, Angell JE, et al: Reproducibility of DXA absorptiometry: a model for bone loss estimates, *J Bone Miner Res* 10:1004–1014, 1995.

42. Melton LJ, Atkinson EJ, O'Fallon WM, et al: Long-term fracture prediction by bone mineral assessed at different skeletal sites, *J Bone Miner Res* 8:1227–1233, 1993.

43. Cummings SR, Black DM, Nevitt MC, et al: Bone density at various sites for prediction of hip fractures: the Study of Osteoporotic Fractures Research Group, *Lancet* 341:72–75, 1993.

44. Stewart A, Reid DM, Porter RW: Broadband ultrasound attenuation and dual energy x-ray absorptiometry in patients with hip fractures: which technique discriminates fracture risk? *Calcif Tissue Int* 54:466, 1994.

45. Kanis JA, Melton LJ III, Christiansen C, et al: Perspective: the diagnosis of osteoporosis, *J Bone Miner Res* 9:1137–1141, 1994.

46. Kanis JA, Borgstrom F, De Laet C, et al: Assessment of fracture risk, *Osteoporos Int* 16:581–589, 2005.

47. Hannon RA, Eastell R: Bone markers and current laboratory assays, *Cancer Treat Rev* 32(Suppl 1):7, 2004.

48. Uebelhart D, Schlemmer A, Johansen JS, et al: Effect of menopause and hormone replacement therapy on the urinary excretion of pyridinium cross-links, *J Clin Endocrinol Metab* 72:367–373, 1991.

49. Delmas PD, Schlemmer A, Gineyts E, et al: Rapid publication: urinary excretion of pyridinoline crosslinks correlates with bone turnover measured on iliac crest biopsy in patients with vertebral osteoporosis, *J Bone Miner Res* 6:639–644, 1991.

50. Rosen HN, Dresner-Pollak R, Moses AC, et al: Specificity of urinary excretion of cross-linked N-telopeptides of type I collagen as a marker of bone turnover, *Calcif Tissue Int* 54:26–29, 1994.

51. Garnero P, Hausherr E, Chapuy MC, et al: Markers of bone resorption predict hip fracture risk in elderly women: the EPIDOS Prospective Study, *J Bone Miner Res* 11:1531–1538, 1996.

52. Seibel MJ, Naganathan V, Barton I, Grauer A: Relationship between pretreatment bone resorption and vertebral fracture incidence in postmenopausal osteoporotic women treated with risedronate, *J Bone Miner Res* 19:323–329, 2004.

53. Lane NE, Sanchez S, Genant HK, et al: Short-term increases in bone turnover markers predict parathyroid hormone-induced spinal bone mineral density gains in postmenopausal women with glucocorticoid-induced osteoporosis, *Osteoporos Int* 11:434–442, 2000.

54. Buxton EC, Yao W, Lane N: Changes in serum receptor activator of nuclear factor-kappaB ligand, osteoprotegerin, and interleukin-6 levels in patients with glucocorticoid-induced osteoporosis treated with human parathyroid hormone (1-34), *J Clin Endocrinol Metab* 89:3332–3336, 2004.

55. Cosman F, Nieves J, Woelfert I: Alendronate does not block the anabolic effect of PTH in postmenopausal osteoporotic women, *J Bone Miner Res* 13:1051–1055, 1998.

56. Silverberg SJ, Gartenberg F, Jacobs TP, et al: Increased bone mineral density after parathyroidectomy in primary hyperparathyroidism, *J Clin Endocrinol Metab* 80:729–734, 1995.

57. Silverberg SJ, Gartenberg F, Jacobs TP, et al: Longitudinal measurements of bone density and biochemical indices in untreated primary hyperparathyroidism, *J Clin Endocrinol Metab* 80:723–728, 1995.

58. Dawson-Hughes B, Dallal GE, Krall EA, et al: A controlled trial of the effect of calcium supplementation on bone density in postmenopausal women, *N Engl J Med* 323:878–883, 1990.

59. Atkinson SA, Abrams SA, Dawson-Hughes B, et al: Calcium. In Young V, editor: *Dietary reference intake for calcium, phosphorus, magnesium, vitamin D and fluoride*, Washington, DC, 1997, National Academy Press, pp 91–143.

60. Optimal calcium intake: NIH Consensus Conference, *JAMA* 272:1942–1947, 1994.

61. Nicar MJ, Pak CYC: Calcium bioavailability from calcium carbonate and calcium citrate, *J Clin Endocrinol Metab* 61:391–393, 1985.

62. Hulley S, Grady D, Bush T, et al: Randomized trial of estrogen plus progestin for secondary prevention of coronary heart disease in postmenopausal women, *JAMA* 280:605–613, 1998.

63. Grady D, Herrington D, Bittner V, et al: Cardiovascular disease outcomes during 6.8 years of hormone therapy: Heart and Estrogen/Progestin Replacement Study follow-up (HERS II), *JAMA* 288:58–66, 2002.

64. Writing Group for the Women's Health Initiative Investigators: Risk and benefits of estrogen plus progestin in healthy postmenopausal women: principal results from the Women's Health Initiative randomized controlled trial, *JAMA* 288:321–333, 2002.

65. Love RR, Mazess RB, Barden HS, et al: Effects of tamoxifen on bone mineral density in postmenopausal women with breast cancer, *N Engl J Med* 326:852–856, 1992.

66. Fisher B, Costantino JP, Wicherham DL, et al: Tamoxifen for prevention of breast cancer: report of the National Surgical Adjuvant Breast and Bowel Project P-1 Study, *J Natl Cancer Inst* 90:1371–1388, 1998.

67. Cummings SR, Eckert S, Krueger KA, et al: The effect of raloxifene on risk of breast cancer in postmenopausal women: results from the MORE randomized trial. Multiple Outcomes of Raloxifene Evaluation, *JAMA* 281:2189–2197, 1999.

68. Delmas P, Bjarnason NH, Mitlak B, et al: Effects of raloxifene on bone mineral density, serum cholesterol concentrations, and uterine endometrium in postmenopausal women, *N Engl J Med* 337:1641–1647, 1997.

69. Ettinger B, Black D, Mitlak B, et al: Reduction of vertebral fracture risk in postmenopausal women with osteoporosis treated with raloxifene: results from 3 year randomized clinical trial (MORE), *JAMA* 282:637–645, 1999.

70. Walsh BW, Kuller LH, Wild RA, et al: Effects of raloxifene on serum lipids and coagulation factors in healthy postmenopausal women, *JAMA* 279:1445–1451, 1998.

71. Walsh BW, Paul S, Wild RA, et al: The effects of hormone replacement therapy and raloxifene on C-reactive protein and homocystein in healthy postmenopausal women: a randomized controlled trial, *J Clin Endocrinol Metab* 85:214–218, 2000.

72. Ridker PM, Buring JE, Shin J, et al: Prospective study of C-reactive protein and the risk of future cardiovascular events among apparently healthy women, *Circulation* 98:731–733, 1998.

73. Barrett-Connor E, Mosca L, Collins P, et al: Raloxifene Use for the Heart (RUTH) Trial Investigators. Effects of raloxifene on cardiovascular events and breast cancer in postmenopausal women, *N Engl J Med* 355:125–137, 2006.

74. Vogel VG, Costantino JP, Wickerham DL, et al: National Surgical Adjuvant Breast and Bowel Project (NSABP). Effects of tamoxifen vs raloxifene on the risk of developing invasive breast cancer and other disease outcomes: the NSABP Study of Tamoxifen and Raloxifene (STAR) P-2 trial, *JAMA* 295:2727–2741, 2006.

75. Bradbury J: CORE breast-cancer prevention trial, *Lancet Oncol* 6:8, 2005.

76. Tenover JL: Male hormone replacement therapy including "Andropause." *Endocrinol Metab Clin North Am* 27:969–988, 1998.

77. Gennari C, Chierichetti SM, Bigazzi S, et al: Comparative effects on bone mineral content of calcium and calcium plus salmon calcitonin given in two different regimens in postmenopausal osteoporosis, *Curr Ther Res* 38:455–464, 1985.

78. Overgaard K, Riis BJ, Christiansen C, et al: Nasal calcitonin for treatment of established osteoporosis, *Clin Endocrinol* 30:435–442, 1989.

79. Chesnut C, Silverman S, Andriono K, et al: A randomized trial of nasal spray salmon calcitonin in postmenopausal women with established osteoporosis: the Prevent Recurrence of Osteoporotic

Fractures Study. PROOF Study Group, *Am J Med* 109:267–276, 2000.

80. Harris ST, Watts NB, Jackson RD, et al: Four-year study of intermittent cyclic etidronate treatment of postmenopausal osteoporosis: three years of blinded therapy followed by one year of open therapy, *Am J Med* 95:557–567, 1993.

81. Liberman UA, Weiss SR, Broll J, et al: Effect of oral alendronate on bone mineral density and the incidence of fractures in postmenopausal osteoporosis, *N Engl J Med* 333:1437–1443, 1995.

82. Black DM, Cummings SR, Karpt DB, et al: Randomized trial of effect of alendronate on risk of fracture in women with existing vertebral fractures, *Lancet* 348:1535–1541, 1996.

83. Hosking D, Chilvers CE, Christiansen C, et al: Prevention of bone loss with alendronate in postmenopausal women under 60 years of age, *N Engl J Med* 338:485–492, 1998.

84. Cummings SR, Black DM, Thompson DE, et al: Effect of alendronate on risk of fracture in women with low bone density but without vertebral fractures, *JAMA* 280:2077–2082, 1998.

85. Orwoll E, Ettinger M, Weiss S, et al: Alendronate for the treatment of osteoporosis in men, *N Engl J Med* 343:604–610, 2000.

86. Schnitzer T, Bone HG, Crepaldi G, et al: Therapeutic equivalence of alendronate 70 mg once-weekly and alendronate 10 mg daily in the treatment of osteoporosis, *Aging* 12:1–12, 2000.

87. Harris ST, Watts NB, Genant HK, et al: Effects of risedronate treatment on vertebral and nonvertebral fractures in women with postmenopausal osteoporosis: a randomized controlled trial. Vertebral Efficacy with Risedronate Therapy (VERT) Study Group, *JAMA* 282:1344, 1999.

88. Heaney RP, Zizic TM, Fogelman I, et al: Risedronate reduces the risk of first vertebral fracture in osteoporotic women, *Osteoporos Int* 13:501–505, 2002.

89. Reginster J.-Y, Minne HW, Sorensen O, et al: Randomized trial of the effects of risedronate on vertebral fractures in women with postmenopausal osteoporosis, *Osteoporos Int* 11:83–91, 2000.

90. McClung MR, Geusens P, Miller PD, et al: Effect of risedronate on the risk of hip fracture in elderly women, *N Engl J Med* 344:333–340, 2001.

91. Delaney M, Harwitz S, Shaw J, LeBoff MS: Bone density changes with once weekly risedronate in postmenopausal women, *J Clin Densitom* 6:45–50, 2003.

92. Miller PD, Brown JP, Siris ES: A randomized double-blind trial of risedronate and etidronate in the treatment of Paget's disease of bone, *Am J Med* 106:513–520, 1999.

93. Reginster JY, Adami S, Lakatos P, et al: Efficacy and tolerability of once-monthly oral ibandronate in postmenopausal osteoporosis: 2 year results from the MOBILE study, *Ann Rheum Dis* 65:654–661, 2006.

94. Delmas PD, Adami S, Strugala C, et al: Intravenous ibandronate injections in postmenopausal women with osteoporosis: one-year results from the dosing intravenous administration study, *Arthritis Rheum* 54:1838–1846, 2006.

95. Black DM, Delmas PD, Eastell R, et al: Once-yearly zoledronic acid for treatment of postmenopausal osteoporosis, *N Engl J Med* 356:1809–1822, 2007.

96. Lyles KW, Colon-Emeric CS, Magaziner JS: Zoledronic acid in reducing clinical fracture and mortality after hip fracture, *N Engl J Med* 357:nihpa40967, 2007.

97. Cummings SR, San Martin J, McClung MR, et al: Denosumab for prevention of fractures in postmenopausal women with osteoporosis, *N Engl J Med* 361:756–765, 2009.

98. Kendler DL, Roux C, Benham CL, et al: Effect of bone mineral density and bone turnover in postmenopausal women transitioning from alendronate therapy, *J Bone Miner Res* 25:72–81, 2010.

99. Finkelstein JS, Klibanski A, Arnold A, et al: Prevention of estrogen deficiency-related bone loss with human parathyroid hormone (1-34), *JAMA* 280:1067–1073, 1998.

99a. Lindsay R, Nieves J, Formica C, et al: Randomized controlled study of effect of parathyroid hormone on vertebral-bone mass and fracture incidence among postmenopausal women on oestrogen with osteoporosis, *Lancet* 350:550–555, 1997.

100. Neer RM, Arnaud CD, Zanchetta JR, et al: Effect of parathyroid hormone (1-34) on fractures and bone mineral density in postmenopausal women with osteoporosis, *N Engl J Med* 344:1434–1441, 2001.

101. Black DM, Greenspan SL, Ensrud KE, et al: The effects of parathyroid hormone and alendronate alone or in combination in postmenopausal osteoporosis, *N Engl J Med* 349:1207–1215, 2003.

102. Finkelstein JS, Hayes A, Hunzelman JL, et al: The effects of parathyroid hormone, alendronate, or both in men with osteoporosis, *N Engl J Med* 349:1216–1226, 2003.

103. Black DM, Bilezikian JP, Ensrud KE, et al: One year of alendronate after one year of parathyroid hormone (1-84) for osteoporosis, *N Engl J Med* 353:555–565, 2005.

104. Deal C, Omizo M, Schwartz EN, et al: Combination teriparatide and raloxifene therapy for postmenopausal osteoporosis: results from a 6-month double-blind placebo-controlled trial, *J Bone Miner Res* 20:1905–1911, 2005.

105. Thomas MK, Lloyd-Jones DM, Thadhani RI, et al: Hypovitaminosis D in medical inpatients, *N Engl J Med* 338:777–783, 1998.

106. Chapay MC, Arlot ME, Duboeuf F, et al: Vitamin D and calcium to prevent hip fractures in elderly women, *N Engl J Med* 327:1637–1642, 1992.

107. Dawson-Hughes B, Harris SS, Krall EA, et al: Effect of calcium and vitamin D supplementation on bone density in men and women 65 years of age or older, *N Engl J Med* 337:670–676, 1997.

108. van Staa TP: The pathogenesis, epidemiology and management of glucocorticoid-induced osteoporosis, *Calcif Tissue Int* 79:129–137, 2006.

109. Adinoff AD, Hollister JR: Steroid-induced fractures and bone loss in patients with asthma, *N Engl J Med* 309:265–268, 1983.

110. Saag HG, Emkey R, Schnitzer TJ, et al: Aledronate for the prevention and treatment of glucocorticoid-induced osteoporosis, *N Engl J Med* 339:292–299, 1998.

111. Cohen S, Levy RM, Keller M, et al: Risedronate therapy prevents corticosteroid-induced bone loss, *Arthritis Rheum* 42:2309–2318, 1999.

112. Reid DM, Devogelaer JP, Saag K, et al: Zoledronic acid and risedronate in the prevention and treatment of glucocorticoid-induced osteoporosis (HORIZON): a multicentre, double-blind, double-dummy, randomised controlled trial, *Lancet* 373:1253–1263, 2009.

113. Saag KM, Shane E, Boonen S, et al: Teriparatide or alendronate for glucocorticoid induced osteoporosis, *N Engl J Med* 357:2028-2039, 2007.

114. Lane NE, Sanchez S, Modin GW, et al: Parathyroid hormone treatment can reverse corticosteroid-induced osteoporosis, *J Clin Invest* 102:1627–1633, 1998.

115. Rehman Q, Lang T, Lane NE: Daily treatment with parathyroid hormone is associated with an increase in vertebral cross-sectional area in postmenopausal women with glucocorticoid-induced osteoporosis, *Osteoporos Int* 41:374–382, 2003.

116. Reid IR, Ibbertson HK, France JT, et al: Plasma testosterone concentrations in asthmatic men treated with glucocorticoids, *Br Med J* 291:574, 1985.

117. Reid IR, Wattie DJ, Evans MC, et al: Testosterone therapy in glucocorticoid-treated men, *Arch Intern Med* 156:1173–1178, 1996.

118. Wang WQ, Ip MS, Tsang KW, Lam KS: Antiresorptive therapy in asthmatic patients receiving high-dose inhaled steroids: a prospective study for 18 months, *J Allergy Clin Immunol* 101:445–450, 1998.

119. Sosa M, Saavedra P, Valero C, et al: Inhaled steroids do not decrease bone mineral density but increase risk of fractures: data from the GIUMO Study Group, *J Clin Densitom* 9:154–158, 2006.

120. Grossman JM, Gordon R, Ranganath VK, et al: American College of Rheumatology 2010 recommendations for the prevention and treatment of glucocorticoid-induced osteoporosis, *Arthritis Care Res* 62:1515–1526, 2010.

Full references for this chapter can be found on www.expertconsult.com.

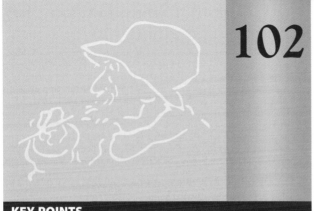

102 Proliferative Bone Diseases

REUVEN MADER

KEY POINTS

Diffuse idiopathic skeletal hyperostosis (DISH) is usually defined by the presence of large flowing osteophytes connecting at least four vertebrae, typically in the thoracic spine. However, the disease often involves the cervical and lumbar spine and peripheral joints, especially entheses.

The etiology of DISH is unclear, but it is associated with a variety of metabolic abnormalities, many of which are also seen in type II diabetes.

Treatment of spinal DISH is mostly symptomatic, but patients and physicians need to be aware of the increased fracture risk of these patients.

Patients with DISH are at increased risk for heterotopic bone formation after joint surgery, and appropriate prophylactic measures should be carried out.

Because of the metabolic abnormalities associated with DISH, many of which are also cardiac risk factors, the discovery of the disease such as an incidental finding on chest x-ray should prompt careful evaluation of known cardiovascular risk factors.

Hypertrophic osteoarthropathy can be seen in many conditions, but growth factors such as platelet-derived growth factor and vascular endothelial growth factor are implicated as the common etiology of most, if not all, cases.

Hypertrophic osteoarthropathy usually responds dramatically to effective treatment of the primary disease such as surgical resection of a lung carcinoma.

SAPHO (synovitis, acne, pustulosis, hyperostosis, and osteitis) syndrome is a chronic inflammatory disorder, often relapsing, of unknown etiology. The most common sites of bone involvement are in the anterior chest wall, mainly the clavicles, sternum, and sternoclavicular joint.

Although the etiology of SAPHO syndrome is unknown, infectious etiology has been proposed on the basis of isolation of *Propionibacterium acnes* from sternal osteosclerotic lesions.

Nonsteroidal anti-inflammatory drugs (NSAIDs) are usually the first line of treatment in SAPHO and may improve the symptoms. However, additional therapy with other modalities is often required. Several empiric therapeutic approaches have been reported in SAPHO including NSAIDs, corticosteroids, bisphosphonates, sulfasalazine, methotrexate, antibiotics, and anti–tumor necrosis factor agents.

Proliferative bone diseases encompass a variety of conditions characterized by exuberant bone and entheseal ossifications and calcifications. New bone formation is the main feature in diffuse idiopathic skeletal hyperostosis (DISH) and hypertrophic osteoarthropathy (HOA) and is a common finding in osteoarthritis. New bone formation may also accompany some spondyloarthropathies such as ankylosing spondylitis, psoriatic arthritis, and sternoclavicular syndrome, also known as SAPHO (synovitis, acne, pustulosis, hyperostosis, and osteomyelitis). New bone formation has also been described in endocrine diseases, however, such as thyroid disorders, acromegaly, and hypoparathyroidism (Table 102-1).[1-3] Osteoarthritis, spondyloarthropathies, and endocrine disorders are discussed elsewhere in this book.

DIFFUSE IDIOPATHIC SKELETAL HYPEROSTOSIS

DISH is a condition characterized by calcification and ossification of soft tissues, mainly ligaments and entheses. This condition was described by Forestier and Rotes-Querol in 1950[4] and was termed *senile ankylosing hyperostosis*. There is a marked predilection to the axial skeleton, particularly the thoracic spine. Recognition that the condition is not limited to the spine and may involve peripheral joints led researchers to coin the name *DISH*, a term now widely used.[5]

DISH is characterized by the production of coarse, flowing osteophytes involving, in particular, the right side of the thoracic spine with preservation of the intervertebral disk space and by ossification of the anterior longitudinal ligament. Calcification and ossification of the posterior longitudinal ligament seem to be additional skeletal manifestations of DISH. Other entheseal regions might be affected such as the peripatellar ligaments, Achilles tendon insertion, plantar fascia, olecranon, and others.[6-8]

The diagnosis is usually based on the definition suggested by Resnick and Niwayama.[5] This radiographic approach requires the presence of flowing, coarse osteophytes on the right side of the thoracic spine, connecting at least four contiguous vertebrae, or ossification of the anterior longitudinal ligament, preserved intervertebral disk height in the involved segment, and the absence of apophyseal joint ankylosis and sacroiliac joint involvement (Table 102-2).[8] Another set of criteria, for epidemiologic purposes, was suggested by Utsinger.[7] These criteria consider also peripheral enthesopathies. A definite diagnosis of DISH is established by criteria similar to those suggested by Resnick and Niwayama. A probable diagnosis of DISH is possible, however, with continuous ossification or calcification, or both, of the anterolateral aspect of at least two contiguous

Table 102-1 Proliferative Bone Diseases

Diffuse idiopathic skeletal hyperostosis
Hypertrophic osteoarthropathy
Thyroid disorders
Acromegaly
Hypoparathyroidism
Seronegative spondyloarthropathies (i.e., psoriatic arthritis, ankylosing spondylitis)
SAPHO
Osteoarthritis

SAPHO, synovitis, acne, pustulosis, hyperostosis, and osteomyelitis.

Table 102-3 Conditions Associated with Diffuse Idiopathic Skeletal Hyperostosis

Non–insulin-dependent diabetes mellitus
Obesity
High waist circumference ratio
Dyslipidemia
Hypertension
Hyperuricemia
Hyperinsulinemia
Elevated insulin-like growth factor-1
Elevated growth hormone
Use of retinoids
Genetic predisposition

vertebral bodies and bilateral well-corticated enthesopathies in the heel, olecranon, and patella. It has also been suggested that peripheral enthesopathies might represent early DISH, which may evolve, over time, to its full radiologic appearance.

Epidemiology

DISH is more common in men than women. An autopsy study reported that in a series of 75 spines studied at autopsy, 28% had DISH.[9] The reported prevalence of DISH varies according to age, ethnic origin, geographic location, and clinical setting (i.e., hospital based versus population based). In a study of a North American metropolitan hospital population, the prevalence in men and women older than 50 years of age was reported to be 25% and 15%, respectively, and the prevalence in men and women older than 70 years was 35% and 26%, respectively.[10] Similar figures were reported for patients from Budapest.[11] Higher figures were reported for Jews older than 40 years living in Jerusalem, reaching a prevalence of 46% for men older than 80.[12] A much smaller prevalence was reported from Korea, barely reaching 9% in the older age group.[13] Native Africans had a prevalence of 13.6% in patients older than 70 years of age with no difference between men and women.[14] In population-based, as opposed to hospital-based, studies, the reported prevalence was slightly greater than 10% in patients older than 70 years of age.[15] Mild DISH was found in human remains dating back 4000 years. In human remains from the 6th to 8th centuries, the prevalence of DISH was higher in men than in women, reaching 3.7%. Although these studies were performed on different and relatively young populations, it seems that the prevalence of DISH is increasing.[16,17]

Etiology and Pathogenesis

The etiology of DISH is unknown. Several metabolic, genetic, and constitutional factors were reported to be associated with this condition, however, including obesity,

Table 102-2 Suggested Diagnostic Criteria for Diffuse Idiopathic Skeletal Hyperostosis

Flowing calcification and ossification along the anterolateral aspect of at least four contiguous vertebral bodies
Preservation of intervertebral disk height in the involved vertebral segment and absence of extensive radiographic changes of degenerative disk disease
Absence of apophyseal joint bony ankylosis and sacroiliac joint erosion, sclerosis, or intra-articular osseous fusion

a high waist circumference ratio, hypertension, diabetes mellitus, hyperinsulinemia, dyslipidemia, elevated growth hormone levels, elevated insulin-like growth factor (IGF)-I, hyperuricemia, use of retinoids, and genetic factors (Table 102-3).[18-26]

The association of DISH with excess body weight has been well known since the early descriptions by Forestier and others.[9,27] This association was reiterated in a study in which patients with DISH were compared with healthy individuals and patients with spondylosis.[28] The association of DISH with diabetes mellitus was reported in several studies.[23,26] It was reported more recently that the prevalence of DISH is no higher in diabetic patients than in nondiabetic subjects, suggesting re-evaluation of diabetes as a risk factor for the development of DISH.[29] More often, DISH was reported to be associated with more complex metabolic and endocrine derangements, with or without overt type II diabetes mellitus, comprising glucose intolerance, hyperinsulinemia, dyslipidemia, hyperuricemia, and elevated levels of growth hormone and IGF-I.[19-20,22] Due to these metabolic abnormalities, patients with DISH have a higher likelihood to be affected by metabolic syndrome and are subjected to a higher coronary artery disease risk.[30]

Hyperinsulinemia has a profound effect on ligaments and entheses, which is independent of age and obesity. The differentiation of mesenchymal cells in ligaments into chondrocytes and the subsequent endochondral ossification is promoted by insulin.[24] The enthesis provides the growth plate for tendons and ligaments in children and persists into adulthood. This particular structure is composed of collagen fibers, fibroblasts, chondrocytes, and calcified matrix, which is probably a target for the ossification process promoted by insulin.[18] Bone morphogenetic protein-2 is a potent osteogenic factor that promotes differentiation of mesenchymal stem cells into osteoblasts and chondroblasts. It stimulates cell proliferation, alkaline phosphatase (ALP) activity, and collagen synthesis.[31] Its ability to promote mineralization is inhibited by matrix Gla protein, which is highly expressed in bone and cartilage. Matrix Gla protein deficiency or its altered carboxylation may cause a high level of bone morphogenetic protein-2 activity that leads to hyperostosis.[26]

The enthesis may also be under the influence of other growth-promoting peptides. Elevated growth hormone levels were reported in DISH. Growth hormone is capable of inducing osteoblast cell proliferation and may promote local production of IGF-I, which mediates the action of growth hormone and can stimulate ALP activity in osteoblasts.[19,26,32,33] ALP promotes the calcification process during bone formation and is considered a good indicator for the maturation stages of osteoblasts.[34,35] There is no explanation yet as to why the new bone formation is localized mainly at the ligamentous and entheseal sites. In male DISH patients, growth hormone serum levels were not elevated in the serum but were much higher in the synovial fluid.[36] In the spine, vertebral blood supply could be a factor in the onset or progression of DISH.[37] Intraerythrocyte growth hormone levels may exceed serum growth hormone levels and could be transported to the vertebral site by the mechanism described by Denko and colleagues.[36]

The expression of various genes involved in cell division and growth is regulated by nuclear factor κB (NFκB), which is capable of regulating the differentiation of multipotential cells. It was shown that activation of environmental factors such as platelet-derived growth factor (PDGF)-BB and transforming growth factor (TGF)-β1 in ligament cells stimulates the activation of NFκB, which influences the osteoblastic differentiation of mesenchymal cells. This event is accompanied by elevation of ALP activity in cells of patients with DISH and serves as an indicator of maturation stages of the osteoblast.[34] Inflammatory cytokines such as PDGF-BB, TGF-β1, and others may be related to the onset of non–insulin-dependent diabetes mellitus and may be the link between this condition and the occurrence of DISH.[38,39]

Vitamin A and its derivatives have been implicated in the pathogenesis of DISH owing to their ability to promote new bone formation. Levels of vitamin A were reported to be higher in patients with DISH compared with controls, and some reports showed DISH-like manifestations in young patients treated with vitamin A or its derivatives.[20,40] The role of vitamin A is unclear, however, because more recent studies did not show an increased prevalence of DISH among patients treated with vitamin A in various dosages and for various lengths of time.[22,25,28] Larger prospective studies are necessary to elucidate the role played by this vitamin in the pathogenesis of DISH.

Familial clustering of DISH or families with early presentation of DISH suggest a genetic background for this disorder.[41,42] Ossification of the posterior longitudinal ligament is closely related to DISH, and the two conditions can coexist. COL6A1, which is the candidate gene for ossification of the posterior longitudinal ligament, was reported to be significantly associated with DISH in Japanese, but not in Czech, patients.[43,44] This finding would suggest that other factors might play an important role in the genetic predisposition for the development of DISH.

There are no convincing explanations for the predilection of the hyperostotic process to affect the anterolateral aspect of the thoracic spine. The limited range of motion of the thoracic spine has been cited as a possible cause for the predilection to this site. This assumption cannot explain the involvement of the extremely mobile cervical spine or the lumbar spine, however. The less frequent involvement of the left side of the thoracic spine was ascribed to the pulsation of the aorta. This assumption was based on a few reports that described left-sided bridging osteophytes in cases with a right-sided aorta, suggesting that the aortic pulsations interfere with the production of the osteophytes.[45] Calcifications, ossification, and subsequent stiffening of

ligaments and joint capsules have important pathogenetic implications.

Osteoarthritis may have pathogenetic features in common with the peripheral joint manifestations of DISH. It was suggested that in the small non–weight-bearing joints in osteoarthritis, the process is caused by an increased intra-articular pressure and subsequent development of "crash" forces.[46] This development was attributed to thickening of the collateral ligaments of these joints that enforce a constraint movement, not to primary damage to the cartilage. It seems reasonable that the joints affected by DISH may develop the same "crash" forces operating in small osteoarthritis joints, as a result of this mechanism. This mechanism might explain the involvement of "atypical" joints, not commonly affected by osteoarthritis, and the hypertrophic osteoarthritic changes in the commonly affected joints.

Clinical Manifestations

The lack of specific symptoms and signs of DISH, as well as the radiographic diagnostic criteria, have raised doubts about DISH as a separate entity.[47] Although the disease may be asymptomatic, it was reported to be associated with morning stiffness, dorsolumbar pain, and reduced range of motion in most patients.[7,8] Patients with DISH may have extremity pain involving peripheral large and small joints and peripheral entheses such as the heel, Achilles tendon, shoulder, patella, and olecranon. Pain in the axial skeleton may involve all three segments of the spine and the costosternal and sternoclavicular joints. The level of pain and disability is significantly higher compared with healthy subjects but is not different from patients with spondylosis.[28] Complaints of pain referable to the thoracic spine are common and are accompanied by a reduced chest expansion.

Although similar in some aspects to osteoarthritis of the spine, DISH is a distinct clinical entity with different characteristics.[48] Classically, the portions of the spine that are involved in osteoarthritis are the lower portions of the cervical spine and the lumbar spine. Thoracic spine involvement is uncommon in osteoarthritis or occurs in late stages of the disease, as opposed to the common involvement of the thoracic spine in DISH. Thoracic spine involvement in DISH is characterized by preserved intervertebral height, whereas in spinal osteoarthritis, reduced intervertebral disk height is common. These differences in the radiologic appearance and anatomic spinal distribution probably have to do with the different pathogenetic mechanisms described earlier. It is presumed that the primary target for the osteoarthritic process is the cartilage represented in the spine by the intervertebral disks and the cartilage of the facet joints.

The wear-and-tear forces operating in the extremely mobile lower cervical and lumbar portions of the spine might explain the frequent involvement of these segments in osteoarthritis, whereas the thoracic spine is the least mobile of the spinal segments. The main targets of the disease in DISH are the spinal ligaments and entheses (Figure 102-1).[5,49] These abnormalities are not limited to the thoracic spine and may involve the lumbar spine and the cervical spine (Figure 102-2). In the lumbar spine, the large bridging osteophytes are not uniformly one-sided.[50]

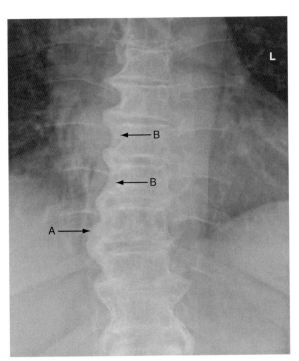

Figure 102-1 Large, flowing, right-sided osteophytes of the thoracic spine *(A)*. Note the translucent area between the vertebral body and the ossified ligamentous tissue *(B)*.

These sites of ossification and the subsequent production of large osteophytes may result in spinal stenosis[51] and spinal stiffening, which increases the risk of fractures.[52] These fractures may be unrecognized, unstable, and associated with treatment delays and permanent neurologic deficits. Severe complications may develop, especially when the cervical

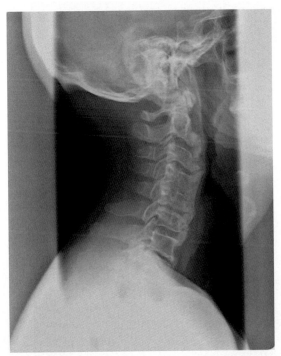

Figure 102-2 Severe bulky ossification of the anterior longitudinal ligament of the cervical spine.

Table 102-4 Clinical Manifestations of Diffuse Idiopathic Skeletal Hyperostosis in the Cervical Spine

Spontaneous
Dysphagia
Hoarseness
Stridor
Ossification of posterior longitudinal ligament
Myelopathy
Aspiration pneumonia
Sleep apnea
Atlantoaxial complications (pseudarthrosis, subluxation)
Thoracic outlet syndrome

Induced
Endoscopic problems
Intubation difficulties
Fractures

From Mader R: Clinical manifestations of diffuse idiopathic skeletal hyperostosis of the cervical spine, *Semin Arthritis Rheum* 32:130–135, 2002.

spine is affected including dysphagia, hoarseness, stridor, ossification of the posterior longitudinal ligament, myelopathy, aspiration pneumonia, sleep apnea, atlantoaxial complications, thoracic outlet syndrome, esophageal obstruction, endoscopic and intubation difficulties, and fractures (Table 102-4).[53] The high prevalence of coexisting intervertebral disk damage in young patients with DISH suggests an important role for DISH in the pathogenesis of spondylosis in this group of patients.[54] At times, patients with DISH may assume the typical postural abnormalities of advanced ankylosing spondylitis such as accentuated kyphosis and reduced mobility of the spine. These two entities, although they may coexist, can usually be distinguished by the different age of onset, clinical presentation, radiographic appearance of the spine and sacroiliac joints, and *HLA-B27* associations.[55,56]

Clinical manifestations similar or identical to those of osteoarthritis are prominent features of DISH in the peripheral joints. The peripheral joints affected by DISH have features that distinguish them from primary osteoarthritis, however. One is the more frequent involvement of joints that are not usually affected in osteoarthritis such as the metacarpophalangeal joints, elbows, and shoulders (Figure 102-3).[57-60] Other features are a more severe hypertrophic disease that may result in a reduced range of motion in the affected joints and calcified and/or ossified prominent enthesopathies.[59,61,62]

As described previously, the primary event in DISH is thickening, calcification, or ossification of ligaments and entheses. In particular, enthesopathy affecting the peripheral joints has been described.[63] The radiographic appearance of peripatellar, cruciate ligament insertion, and pericapsular osseous enthesopathies are some examples of the contribution of DISH to stiffening of the soft tissues surrounding a joint (Figure 102-4).[64] Entheseal ossification at various sites other than joints such as the heel, ribs, and pelvis is a common finding in DISH. These enthesopathies may become symptomatic exhibiting pain and swelling in the affected region. A high probability for the presence of spinal DISH was noted for ossification of the iliolumbar and sacrotuberous ligaments and with bony overgrowth of the inferior acetabular rim.[63,65] The tendency for new bone for-

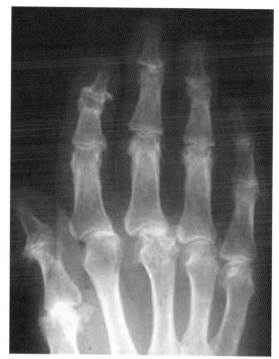

Figure 102-3 Severe hypertrophic osteoarthritis of the proximal and distal interphalangeal joints. Of particular interest is the involvement of the metacarpophalangeal joints with enlarged metacarpal heads, osteophytes, joint space narrowing, and subchondral sclerosis.

Table 102-5 Therapeutic Targets in Diffuse Idiopathic Skeletal Hyperostosis

Symptomatic relief of pain and stiffness
Prevent, retard, or arrest progression
Treatment of associated metabolic disorder
Prevent spontaneous complications
Prevent traumatic complications
Prevent complications that might emerge during diagnostic or therapeutic procedures

From Mader R: Current therapeutic options in the management of diffuse idiopathic skeletal hyperostosis, *Expert Opin Pharmacother* 6:1313–1316, 2005.

described earlier put patients at an increased risk for cardiovascular diseases.[66,67] The diagnosis of DISH should be suspected in patients with osteoarthritis in atypical locations (e.g., elbow), in patients with hypertrophic osteoarthritis, and in patients with large enthesopathies and entrapment neuropathies of uncertain origin. This is particularly true for patients with the associated diseases and metabolic abnormalities discussed earlier. It has been shown that chest radiographs might serve as a screening tool for the diagnosis of DISH with a sensitivity of 77% and specificity of 97%.[68]

Treatment

Treatment of DISH should address several issues. Treatment is expected to alleviate pain and stiffness; prevent, retard, or arrest progression; correct the associated metabolic disorders; and prevent spontaneous or induced complications (Table 102-5).

Specific therapeutic interventions in DISH have not been systematically explored; this is probably related to

mation puts the patient at risk for the development of heterotopic ossification after joint surgery.

Patients with DISH often have higher body weight and body mass index, waist circumference, and systolic blood pressure.[28] These factors and the metabolic abnormalities

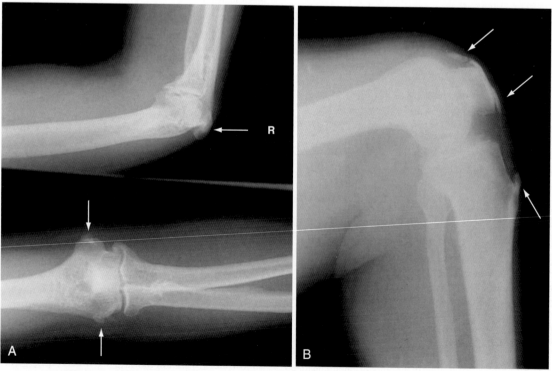

Figure 102-4 **A** and **B,** Ossified enthesopathies in the peripatellar, olecranon, and humeral epicondyles *(arrows).*

the inclusion of DISH in the spectrum of osteoarthritis and the assumption that the same therapeutic interventions for osteoarthritis are suitable for DISH. It was suggested more recently that serum levels of growth hormone and IGF-I might be a useful surrogate marker for assessing DISH progression and remission.[31] It was estimated that a period of at least 10 years is necessary for the pathologic process to evolve completely.[69] This notion implies that a long observation period is necessary to show that a therapeutic intervention prevents the development of the disease, arrest its progression, or, it is hoped, reverses the pathologic changes.

There are few reports about remedies to alleviate the symptoms of the disease, but some investigators have reported on the beneficial effects of light exercise, heat, analgesics, and nonsteroidal anti-inflammatory drugs (NSAIDs).[70] Exercise therapy failed to show a significant improvement in the spinal range of motion except for lumbosacral flexion.[71] More recently, the use of locally acting NSAIDs for the treatment of osteoarthritis was shown to be as effective as the same product by oral route, suggesting that locally acting NSAIDs also might be successfully employed for the symptomatic relief of pain and stiffness in the peripheral joints of patients with DISH.[72] Treatment of symptomatic enthesopathies might be necessary to alleviate local pain and swelling; this can be achieved by local soft applications such as insoles for plantar spurs or protective bandages at other sites. Infiltration of local anesthetic with long-acting corticosteroids might offer at least temporary relief in severely symptomatic cases. When multiple sites are involved, the same therapeutic modalities mentioned for osteoarthritis may be used.

The coexistence of many cardiovascular risk factors places patients with DISH at a higher risk for cardiovascular complications. It seems appropriate to screen these patients for known cardiovascular risk factors and to treat when appropriate. General measures such as weight reduction, adequate physical activity, and a diet low in saturated fat and carbohydrates all might be important in preventing or arresting the progression of DISH. Some of these factors may have pathogenetic implications and may become therapeutic targets. On the basis of present understanding, therapeutic interventions should aim at a reduction of insulin secretion and insulin resistance. In patients with non–insulin-dependent diabetes mellitus, the use of biguanides, which decrease insulin resistance, may offer an advantage over the use of sulfonylureas, which increase insulin secretion. When coexisting hypertension should be treated, medications that might improve insulin resistance such as angiotensin-converting enzyme inhibitors, calcium channel blockers, and α-blockers should be preferred to medications that might worsen insulin resistance such as thiazide diuretics and β-blockers.[73] Some growth factors that might have a role in the development of DISH such as NFκB, PDGF-BB, TGF-β1, growth hormone, and IGF-I may become targets someday for specific therapeutic interventions.

Some complications can be avoided if taken into consideration. Aspiration pneumonia can be partially avoided if instructions in proper deglutition and preservation of an upright position after meals are carefully explained to the patient. Physicians familiar with DISH can avoid or minimize damage to the cervical spine or to soft tissues in

Table 102-6 Future Considerations in Diffuse Idiopathic Skeletal Hyperostosis

Establish and validate diagnostic criteria that consider also the peripheral manifestations of the disease
Clarify the natural course and prognosis
Study the systemic nature and the impact on quality of life and life expectancy
Seek a better understanding of the pathogenetic basis for the disease
Offer a disease-modifying therapeutic approach

patients who might need certain diagnostic or therapeutic interventions such as upper gastrointestinal endoscopy or endotracheal intubation. It is reasonable to adopt the common measures to prevent falls and trauma, especially in elderly patients. Heterotopic ossification after orthopedic surgeries, in particular hip arthroplasty, is common in patients with DISH.[54] Several therapeutic interventions aimed at abolishing heterotopic ossification such as administration of NSAIDs, anti–vitamin K, and irradiation, have been reported with variable success.[74,75] Patients in the high-risk group to develop this complication, such as patients with DISH, should be considered candidates for one of these regimens. The therapeutic options are summarized in Figure 102-5.[76] Many tasks lay ahead to define better, understand the pathogenesis, and delineate effective interventions for this disorder (Table 102-6).

HYPERTROPHIC OSTEOARTHROPATHY

HOA is a well-known entity characterized by skin and bone proliferation. The hallmark and main visual manifestation is a bulbous deformity of the distal end of the digits, also known as *clubbing* or *drumsticks*. Periostosis is a progressive process with predilection for the tubular bones, principally the tibia and fibula. Periostosis is bilateral; is symmetric; and spares the medullary cavity, the axial skeleton, and the skull. The prevalence of the condition is unknown, but it was found in skeletal human remains dating thousands of years ago.[77] It may be primary or secondary to many other diseases.

Etiology

Primary HOA is an autosomal dominant disorder characterized by periostosis, clubbing, thickening of the skin of the face and scalp, seborrhea, and hyperhidrosis. It is also termed *pachydermoperiostosis*. There is a male predominance with a male-to-female ratio of 9 : 1 with one peak of presentation in the first year of life and the other in adolescence.[78]

Secondary forms of HOA may manifest as isolated clubbing or with the full spectrum of the disease. Clubbing may be unilateral or bilateral and has been reported to occur in a variety of diseases including pulmonary (most commonly cancers), cardiac, gastrointestinal, neurologic, infectious, vascular, and other diseases (Table 102-7).[79-85]

Pathogenesis

HOA is characterized by excessive collagen deposition, endothelial hyperplasia, edema, and new bone formation involving mainly the distal extremity and eventually

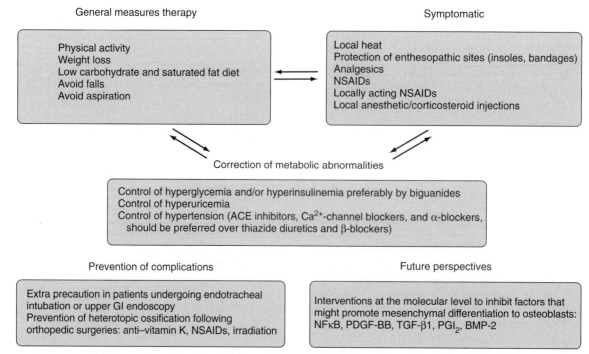

Figure 102-5 Therapeutic options in diffuse idiopathic skeletal hyperostosis. ACE, angiotensin-converting enzyme; BMP-2, bone morphogenetic protein-2; GI, gastrointestinal; NFκB, nuclear factor κB; NSAIDs, nonsteroidal anti-inflammatory drugs; PDGF-BB, platelet-derived growth factor-BB; PGI$_2$, prostaglandin I$_2$; TGF-β1, transforming growth factor-β1. *(From Mader R: Current therapeutic options in the management of diffuse idiopathic skeletal hyperostosis,* Expert Opin Pharmacother *6:1313–1316, 2005.)*

Table 102-7 Etiologies of Hypertrophic Osteoarthropathy

Unilateral
Hemiplegia
Patent ductus arteriosus
Aneurysms
Bilateral
Pulmonary Diseases
Cystic fibrosis
Pulmonary fibrosis
Primary or secondary lung tumors
Lung and pleural infections
Pleural tumors
Heart Diseases
Cyanotic diseases
Infective endocarditis
Gastrointestinal Diseases
Cirrhosis
Hepatic carcinoma
Intestinal and esophageal malignant tumors
Inflammatory bowel diseases
Intestinal polyposis
Other Diseases
Various malignancies
POEMS syndrome
Rheumatic diseases
Thymoma
Acquired immunodeficiency syndrome
Thalassemia

POEMS, polyneuropathy, organomegaly, endocrinopathy, M component, and skin changes.

progressing proximally. Various hypotheses have been generated in an attempt to explain the development of HOA. Most cases with secondary HOA have severe lung or cyanotic heart diseases. It was suggested that megakaryocytes are fragmented into platelets during their passage in the lung capillaries. In severe lung diseases or right-to-left shunts, megakaryocytes or platelet aggregates bypass the pulmonary capillary bed, however, and lodge in the peripheral vasculature of the digits.

It was shown that locally released growth factors such as vascular endothelial growth factor (VEGF) and PDGF were remarkably increased in tissue samples obtained from digits of patients with HOA.[86] It is feasible that these substances might be responsible for the distal overgrowth of collagen and bone. VEGF was found to be produced by a lung tumor in a patient with HOA. In this case, serum levels of VEGF were high and resection of the tumor reversed the digital clubbing and reduced the serum VEGF levels.[87] Activation of platelets and endothelial cells was supported by an increase in circulating von Willebrand factor antigen.[88] Other growth factors have been associated with digital clubbing including hepatocyte growth factor, which was found to be increased in the serum of patients with lung cancer and HOA compared with patients with lung cancer without HOA.[89]

Clinical Manifestations

Often HOA is asymptomatic, and sometimes it is the patient who notes the changes in the shape of the fingers. Symptomatic patients complain about a deep-seated pain in the lower extremity and over the long tubular bones, which is exacerbated by palpation. Large joint effusions are common, and the synovial fluid is thick with few white blood cells.[90] Skin hypertrophy may be confined to the nail beds or involve the face or larger areas overlying the tubular bones or joints.

The most common and apparent clinical manifestation is digital clubbing. The bulbous deformity of the fingertips is accompanied by a convex nail (watch-crystal nail). The skin around the nail bed becomes shiny and thin with disappearance of the creases (Figure 102-6). Palpation of the base of the nail bed yields the sensation of a "floating" nail within the soft tissue. Cases of advanced clubbing can be identified easily. Several methods were developed, however, to diagnose early phases of the condition. Among those techniques, the digital index and the phalangeal depth ratio have been most widely used.[91,92] The digital index measures the ratio between the circumference at the level of the nail bed and the circumference at the distal interphalangeal joint of the 10 fingers. The sum of ratios greater than 10 suggests clubbing. The phalangeal depth ratio measures the ratio between the depth of the distal phalanx and the depth of the distal interphalangeal joint of the index finger. A ratio greater than 1 is considered abnormal.

There are no specific laboratory tests to diagnose HOA. Radiographs of the fingers and toes may show acro-osteolysis, and periostitis manifest by cortical thickening of long bones is often observed. The process may involve few or multiple sites and can be regular or irregular in appearance. Characteristically, there is no reduction in joint space or erosions. Radioisotope bone scanning can be useful for diagnosis and for evaluating the extent of the process. Increased uptake can be seen in the cortex of long bones sometimes in the form of splints (Figure 102-7).

Treatment Considerations

Asymptomatic cases need no treatment. NSAIDs are sometimes useful in symptomatic patients. Case reports have suggested that significant pain relief was observed after treatment with octreotide or pamidronate.[93,94] In secondary cases of HOA, all features and symptoms promptly regress with successful treatment of the primary disease such as correction of a heart malformation, removal of tumors, and therapy of infective endocarditis or inflammatory bowel disease. The role played by VEGF in the pathogenesis of HOA suggests that treatment with VEGF inhibitors might improve the symptoms of this condition.[95]

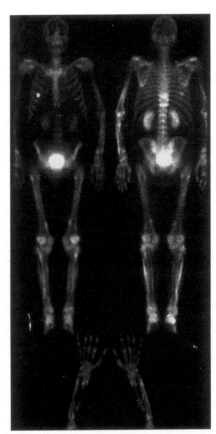

Figure 102-7 Increased non-nodular cortical bone uptake in a patient with bronchogenic carcinoma. *(From Vandemergel X, Blocket D, Decaux G: Periostitis and hypertrophic osteoarthropathy: etiologies and bone scan patterns in 115 cases, Eur J Intern Med 15:375–380, 2004; with permission from the European Federation of Internal Medicine.)*

SAPHO SYNDROME

SAPHO syndrome is a chronic inflammatory disorder, often relapsing, of unknown etiology. The term SAPHO was coined in order to include several associated clinical manifestations: synovitis, acne, pustulosis, hyperostosis, and osteitis.[96] The most common sites of bone involvement are in the anterior chest wall, mainly the clavicles, sternum, and sternoclavicular joint.[97] The syndrome has been associated with a variety of skin lesions such as acne conglobata, acne fulminans, palmoplantar pustulosis, and psoriasis. The condition is uncommon with an estimated prevalence of 1 in 10,000, but the exact prevalence is difficult to establish in the absence of validated diagnostic or classification criteria. Furthermore, it is presumed that the prevalence of SAPHO syndrome is underestimated, in particular with mild or absent skin manifestations.[98]

Etiology and Pathogenesis

The etiology of SAPHO syndrome is unknown. Infectious etiology has been proposed on the basis of the isolation of *Propionibacterium acnes*, a slowly growing anaerobic microorganism often found in acne, from sternal osteosclerotic lesions.[99] It has been postulated that *P. acnes* might act directly inducing bony erosions by chronic indolent inflammation. It has also been suggested that *P. acnes* may trigger complement activation and promote production of

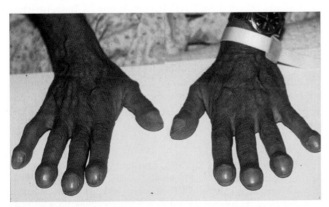

Figure 102-6 Severe clubbing in a patient with advanced lung cancer.

interleukin (IL)-1, IL-8, and tumor necrosis factor (TNF), which contribute to both humoral and cellular proinflammatory responses. An imbalance between proinflammatory and anti-inflammatory mediators has been also suggested to contribute to the inflammatory response and the subsequent damage.[100,101]

Genetic susceptibility has not yet been found. No associations with *HLA-B27*, other alleles often associated with psoriatic arthritis, or other candidate genes have been identified.[97,102,103]

Inconsistencies in the reported prevalence of common autoantibodies encountered in autoimmune diseases, in patients with SAPHO syndrome, preclude at present any firm evidence for their role in the development of this condition.[104] It has been suggested that the increased association of SAPHO syndrome with inflammatory bowel disease might link SAPHO to the seronegative spondyloarthropathies, but this view has not yet been confirmed.[97,105]

Clinical Manifestations and Imaging Findings

SAPHO syndrome is characterized by the combination of skin and osteoarticular manifestations. The skin manifestations include palmoplantar pustulosis, severe acne, suppurative hidradenitis, and at times psoriasis. The skin manifestations can anticipate or follow the osteoarticular manifestations, at times by many years.[97,106,107]

The osteoarticular features of SAPHO syndrome are hyperostosis, aseptic osteitis occasionally involving the adjacent joints, and synovitis. The early histologic findings of the bone lesions are similar to those of osteomyelitis with periosteal bone formation. Subsequently the lesions evolve into chronic inflammation with preponderance of mononuclear infiltrate, and only in the late phases prominent marrow fibrosis, sclerosis, and enlarged bone trabeculae ensue.[108]

The most characteristic clinical manifestation is pain in the anterior chest wall due to common involvement of the clavicles, sternum, and the sternoclavicular joints.[97,107] Other common sites of involvement in the axial skeleton are the vertebral bodies with vertebral sclerosis, hyperostosis, spondylodiskitis, nonmarginal syndesmophytes, at times with anterior bridging; the bone adjacent to the sacroiliac joint; and the pubic symphysis.[105,109] Extraspinal involvement is infrequent but may be observed in the form of osteitis involving the tibia, femur, or mandible and with arthritis involving knees, hips, ankles, or small joints of hands and feet.[97,105,110] The diagnosis is highly suspected in cases with usually sterile, multifocal, recurrent osteomyelitis, with or without cutaneous lesions; arthritis associated with palmoplantar pustulosis, pustular psoriasis, or severe acne; and osteitis associated with severe acne, palmoplantar pustulosis, or pustular psoriasis.[107]

Laboratory investigations may reveal moderately elevated erythrocyte sedimentation rate (ESR) or acute phase reactants such as CRP and C3 and C4. These findings may reflect the inflammatory nature of the condition but are less reliable than in other inflammatory rheumatic disorders.[97,105]

The diagnosis is usually established on the correlation between the clinical presentation and imaging findings. Bone scintigraphy is sensitive to detect the anterior chest

wall involvement demonstrating the characteristic "bull's head" sign.[111] Plain radiographs may detect advanced lesions, but computed tomography (CT) scan enhances the ability to detect these lesions in particular in flat bones. Radiographic studies of the anterior chest lesions show osteitis in the form of osteosclerosis with homogeneous fibrillary pattern, hyperostosis in the form of periosteal reaction, and cortical thickening leading to bone hypertrophy. These lesions with eventual erosive arthritis (due to either primary arthritis or extension of the adjacent osteitis), classically involve the sternoclavicular joint, the upper costosternal and manubriosternal junctions. The spine, being involved in about a third of the patients, presents with similar radiographic appearance with vertebral sclerosis, hyperostosis, spondylodiskitis, nonmarginal asymmetric syndesmophytes, and at times hyperostosis in the form of osseous bridging along the anterior aspect of the spine.[106] In a recent magnetic resonance imaging (MRI) study, corner vertebral erosions were a consistent finding, frequently with involvement of the vertebral end plates and at times adjacent vertebra.[112] The meaning of these findings has not yet been fully elucidated, and further studies are necessary. Entheseal ossifications, osteitis, osteosclerosis, and periosteal new bone formation have all been reported with variable frequency in long bones.

Treatment

Nonsteroidal anti-inflammatory drugs (NSAIDs) are usually the first line of treatment and may improve the symptoms. However, they often fail to control the disease and additional therapy with corticosteroids and other modalities is required.[97,113] Several empiric therapeutic approaches have been reported in SAPHO including NSAIDs, corticosteroids, bisphosphonates, sulfasalazine, methotrexate, antibiotics, and anti-TNF agents.[113] Second-line drugs including methotrexate, cyclosporine, sulfasalazine, and leflunomide have been tried with mixed results.[105,113,114] Treatment with antibiotics, usually azithromycin, has been reported to be beneficial in patients with SAPHO syndrome. However, many patients were also treated with other disease-modifying antirheumatic drugs and the response faded after discontinuation of the antibiotic. It is not clear whether the response to the antibiotic, though transitory, is due to its antibacterial or anti-inflammatory effect.[115] In recent years, bisphosphonates, in particular pamidronate have been reported to elicit a good or partial response in the majority of patients affected by SAPHO syndrome.[116] It seems that beyond their ability to prevent bone resorption, bisphosphonates are capable of suppressing the production of proinflammatory cytokines such as IL-1, TNF, and IL-6.[117] Treatment with TNF blockers has emerged as an effective therapy in SAPHO syndrome. The results appear to be less spectacular than in other seronegative spondyloarthropathies and may be hampered by relapse of the skin manifestations.[118,119]

References

1. Lambert RG, Becker EJ: Diffuse skeletal hyperostosis in idiopathic hypoparathyroidism, *Clin Radiol* 40:212–215, 1989.
2. Fatourechi V, Ahmed DDF, Schwartz KM: Thyroid acropachy: Report of 40 patients treated at a single institution in a 26 years period, *J Clin Endocrinol Metab* 87:5435–5441, 2002.

3. Scarpan R, De Brasi D, Pivonello R, et al: Acromegalic axial arthropathy: a clinical case control study, *J Clin Endocrinol Metab* 89:598–603, 2004.
4. Forestier J, Rotes-Querol J: Senile ankylosing hyperostosis of the spine, *Ann Rheum Dis* 9:321–330, 1950.
5. Resnick D, Niwayama G: Radiographic and pathologic features of spinal involvement in diffuse idiopathic skeletal hyperostosis (DISH), *Radiology* 119:559–568, 1976.
6. Resnick D, Guerra J Jr, Robinson CA, et al: Association of diffuse idiopathic skeletal hyperostosis (DISH) and calcification and ossification of the posterior longitudinal ligament, *AJR Am J Roentgenol* 131:1049–1053, 1978.
7. Utsinger PD: Diffuse idiopathic skeletal hyperostosis, *Clin Rheum Dis* 11:325–351, 1985.
8. Resnick D, Niwayama G: *Diagnosis of bone and joint disorders*, ed 2, Philadelphia, 1988, WB Saunders, pp 1563-1615.
9. Boachie-Adjei O, Bullough PG: Incidence of ankylosing hyperostosis of the spine (Forestier's disease) at autopsy, *Spine* 12:739–743, 1987.
10. Weinfeld RM, Olson PN, Maki DD, et al: The prevalence of diffuse idiopathic skeletal hyperostosis (DISH) in two large American Midwest metropolitan hospital populations, *Skeletal Radiol* 26:222–225, 1997.
11. Kiss C, O'Neill TW, Mituszova M, et al: Prevalence of diffuse idiopathic skeletal hyperostosis in Budapest, Hungary, *Rheumatology (Oxford)* 41:1335–1336, 2002.
12. Bloom RA: The prevalence of ankylosing hyperostosis in a Jerusalem population—with description of a method of grading the extent of the disease, *Scand J Rheumatol* 13:181–189, 1984.
13. Kim SK, Choi BR, Kim CG, et al: The prevalence of diffuse idiopathic skeletal hyperostosis in Korea, *J Rheumatol* 31:2032–2035, 2004.
14. Cassim B, Mody GM, Rubin DL: The prevalence of diffuse idiopathic skeletal hyperostosis in African Blacks, *Br J Rheumatol* 29:131–132, 1990.
15. Julkunen H, Heinonen OP, Knekt P, et al: The epidemiology of hyperostosis of the spine together with its symptoms and related mortality in a general population, *Scand J Rheumatol* 4:23–27, 1975.
16. Arriaza BT: Seronegative spondyloarthropathies and diffuse idiopathic skeletal hyperostosis in ancient northern Chile, *Am J Phys Anthropol* 91:263–278, 1993.
17. Vidal P: A paleoepidemiologic study of diffuse idiopathic skeletal hyperostosis, *Joint Bone Spine* 67:210–214, 2000.
18. Littlejohn GO: Insulin and new bone formation in diffuse idiopathic skeletal hyperostosis, *Clin Rheumatol* 4:294–300, 1985.
19. Denko CW, Boja B, Moskowitz RW: Growth promoting peptides in osteoarthritis and diffuse idiopathic skeletal hyperostosis—insulin, insulin-like growth factor-I, growth hormone, *J Rheumatol* 21:1725–1730, 1994.
20. Nesher G, Zuckner J: Rheumatologic complications of vitamin A and retinoids, *Semin Arthritis Rheum* 24:291–296, 1995.
21. Van Dooren-Greebe RJ, Lemmens JAM, De Boo T, et al: Prolonged treatment of oral retinoids in adults: no influence on the frequency and severity of spinal abnormalities, *Br J Dermatol* 134:71–76, 1996.
22. Vezyroglou G, Mitropoulos A, Kyriazis N, et al: A metabolic syndrome in diffuse idiopathic skeletal hyperostosis: a controlled study, *J Rheumatol* 23:672–676, 1996.
23. Akune T, Ogata N, Seichi A, et al: Insulin secretory response is positively associated with the extent of ossification of the posterior longitudinal ligament of the spine, *J Bone Joint Surg Am* 83:1537–1544, 2001.
24. Ling TC, Parkin G, Islam J, et al: What is the cumulative effect of long term, low dose isotretinoin on the development of DISH? *Br J Dermatol* 144:628–650, 2001.
25. Kiss C, Szilagyi M, Paksy A, et al: Risk factors for diffuse idiopathic skeletal hyperostosis: a case control study, *Rheumatology (Oxford)* 41:27–30, 2002.
26. Sarzi-Puttini P, Atzeni F: New developments in our understanding of DISH (diffuse idiopathic skeletal hyperostosis), *Curr Opin Rheumatol* 16:287–292, 2004.
27. Forestier J, Lagier R: Ankylosing hyperostosis of the spine, *Clin Orthop* 74:65–83, 1971.
28. Mata S, Fortin PR, Fitzcharles MA, et al: A controlled study of diffuse idiopathic skeletal hyperostosis: clinical features and functional status, *Medicine* 76:104–117, 1997.
29. Sencan D, Elden H, Nacitarhan V, et al: The prevalence of diffuse idiopathic skeletal hyperostosis in patients with diabetes mellitus, *Rheumatol Int* 25:518–521, 2005.
30. Mader R, Novofestovsky I, Adawi M, Lavi I: Metabolic syndrome and cardiovascular risk in patients with diffuse idiopathic skeletal hyperostosis, *Semin Arthritis Rheum* 38:361–365, 2009.
31. Kobacz K, Ullrich R, Amoyo L, et al: Stimulatory effects of distinct members of the bone morphogenetic protein family on ligament fibroblasts, *Ann Rheum Dis* 65:169–177, 2006.
32. Denko CW, Malemud CJ: Role of growth hormone/insulin-like growth factor-1 paracrine axis in rheumatic diseases, *Semin Arthritis Rheum* 35:24–34, 2005.
33. Denko CW, Malemud CJ: Body mass index and blood glucose: Correlations with serum insulin, growth hormone, and insulin-like growth factor-1 levels in patients with diffuse idiopathic skeletal hyperostosis (DISH), *Rheumatol Int* 26:292–297, 2006.
34. Kosaka T, Imakiire A, Mizuno F, et al: Activation of nuclear factor κB at the onset of ossification of the spinal ligaments, *J Orthop Sci* 5:572–578, 2000.
35. Denko CW, Boja B, Moskowitz RW: Growth factors, insulin-like growth factor-1 and growth hormone, in synovial fluid and serum of patients with rheumatic disorders, *Osteoarthritis Cartil* 4:245–249, 1996.
36. Denko CW, Boja B, Malemud CJ: Intra-erythrocyte deposition of growth hormone in rheumatic diseases, *Rheumatol Int* 23:11–14, 2003.
37. el Miedany YM, Wassif G, el Baddini M: Diffuse idiopathic skeletal hyperostosis (DISH): is it of vascular etiology? *Clin Exp Rheumatol* 18:193–200, 2000.
38. Inaba T, Ishibashi S, Gotoda T, et al: Enhanced expression of platelet-derived growth factor-beta receptor by high glucose: involvement of platelet-derived growth factor in diabetic angiopathy, *Diabetes* 45:507–512, 1996.
39. Pfeiffer A, Middelberg-Bisping K, Drewes C, et al: Elevated plasma levels of transforming growth factor-beta 1 in NIDDM, *Diabetes Care* 19:1113–1117, 1996.
40. Abiteboul M, Arlet J, Sarrabay MA, et al: Etude du metabolisme de la vitamine A au cours de la maladie hyperostosique de Forestier et Rote's-Querol, *Rev Rhum Ed Fr* 53:143–145, 1986.
41. Gorman C, Jawad ASM, Chikanza I: A family with diffuse idiopathic hyperostosis, *Ann Rheum Dis* 64:1794–1795, 2005.
42. Bruges-Armas J, Couto AM, Timms A, et al: Ectopic calcification among families in the Azores: clinical and radiologic manifestations in families with diffuse idiopathic skeletal hyperostosis and chondrocalcinosis, *Arthritis Rheum* 54:1340–1349, 2006.
43. Havelka S, Vesela M, Pavelkova A, et al: Are DISH and OPLL genetically related? *Ann Rheum Dis* 60:902–903, 2001.
44. Tsukahara S, Miyazawa N, Akagawa H, et al: COL6A1, the candidate gene for ossification of the posterior longitudinal ligament, is associated with diffuse idiopathic skeletal hyperostosis in Japanese, *Spine* 30:2321–2324, 2005.
45. Carile L, Verdone F, Aiello A, et al: Diffuse idiopathic skeletal hyperostosis and situs viscerum inversus, *J Rheumatol* 16:1120–1122, 1989.
46. Smythe HA: The mechanical pathogenesis of generalized osteoarthritis, *J Rheumatol* 10(Suppl 9):11–12, 1983.
47. Hutton C: DISH … a state not a disease? *Br J Rheumatol* 28:277–280, 1989.
48. Mader R: Diffuse idiopathic skeletal hyperostosis: a distinct clinical entity, *Isr Med Assoc J* 5:506–508, 2003.
49. Fornasier VL, Littlejohn GO, Urowitz MB, et al: Spinal entheseal new bone formation: the early changes of spinal diffuse idiopathic skeletal hyperostosis, *J Rheumatol* 10:934–947, 1983.
50. Belanger TA, Rowe DE: Diffuse idiopathic skeletal hyperostosis: musculoskeletal manifestations, *J Am Acad Orthop Surg* 9:258–267, 2001.
51. Laroche M, Moulinier L, Arlet J, et al: Lumbar and cervical stenosis: frequency of the association, role of the ankylosing hyperostosis, *Clin Rheumatol* 11:533–535, 1992.
52. Le Hir PX, Sautet A, Le Gars L, et al: Hyperextension vertebral body fractures in diffuse idiopathic skeletal hyperostosis: a cause of intravertebral fluid-like collections on MR imaging, *AJR Am J Roentgenol* 173:1679–1683, 1999.
53. Mader R: Clinical manifestations of diffuse idiopathic skeletal hyperostosis of the cervical spine, *Semin Arthritis Rheum* 32:130–135, 2002.

54. Di Girolamo C, Pappone N, Rengo C, et al: Intervertebral disc lesions in diffuse idiopathic skeletal hyperostosis (DISH), *Clin Exp Rheumatol* 19:310–312, 2001.

55. Olivieri I, D'angelo S, Cutro MS, et al: Diffuse idiopathic skeletal hyperostosis may give the typical postural abnormalities of advanced ankylosing spondylitis, *Rheumatology (Oxford)* 46: 1709–1711, 2007.

56. Olivieri I, D'angelo S, Palazzi C, et al: Diffuse idiopathic skeletal hyperostosis: differentiation from ankylosing spondylitis, *Curr Rheumatol Rep* 11:321–328, 2009.

57. Littlejohn JO, Urowitz MB, Smythe HA, et al: Radiographic features of the hand in diffuse idiopathic skeletal hyperostosis (DISH), *Diagn Radiol* 140:623–629, 1981.

58. Beyeler C, Schlapbach P, Gerber NJ, et al: Diffuse idiopathic skeletal hyperostosis (DISH) of the shoulder: a cause of shoulder pain? *Br J Rheumatol* 29:349–353, 1990.

59. Utsinger PD, Resnick D, Shapiro R: Diffuse skeletal abnormalities in Forestier's disease, *Arch Intern Med* 136:763–768, 1976.

60. Resnick D, Shapiro RF, Weisner KB, et al: Diffuse idiopathic skeletal hyperostosis (DISH): ankylosing hyperostosis of Forestier and Rotes-Querol, *Semin Arthritis Rheum* 7:153–187, 1978.

61. Schlapbach P, Beyeler C, Gerber NJ, et al: The prevalence of palpable finger joints nodules in diffuse idiopathic skeletal hyperostosis (DISH): a controlled study, *Br J Rheumatol* 31:531–534, 1992.

62. Mader R, Sarzi-Puttini P, Atzeni F, et al: Exstraspinal manifestations of diffuse idiopathic skeletal hyperostosis, *Rheumatology* 48:1478–1481, 2009.

63. Littlejohn JO, Urowitz MB: Peripheral enthesopathy in diffuse idiopathic skeletal hyperostosis (DISH): a radiologic study, *J Rheumatol* 9:568–572, 1982.

64. Resnick D, Shaul SR, Robins JM: Diffuse idiopathic skeletal hyperostosis (DISH): Forestier's disease with extraspinal manifestations, *Radiology* 115:513–524, 1975.

65. Haller J, Resnick D, Miller GW, et al: Diffuse idiopathic skeletal hyperostosis: diagnostic significance of radiographic abnormalities of the pelvis, *Radiology* 172:835–839, 1989.

66. Mader R, Dubenski N, Lavi I: Morbidity and mortality of hospitalized patients with diffuse idiopathic skeletal hyperostosis, *Rheumatol Int* 26:132–136, 2005.

67. Miyazawa N, Akiyama I: Diffuse idiopathic skeletal hyperostosis associated with risk factors for stroke, *Spine* 31:E225–E229, 2006.

68. Mata S, Hill RO, Joseph L, et al: Chest radiographs as a screening tool for diffuse idiopathic skeletal hyperostosis, *J Rheumatol* 20:1905–1910, 1993.

69. Mader R: Diffuse idiopathic skeletal hyperostosis: isolated involvement of cervical spine in a young patient, *J Rheumatol* 31:620–621, 2004.

70. El Garf A, Khater R: Diffuse idiopathic skeletal hyperostosis (DISH): a clinicopathological study of the disease pattern in Middle Eastern populations, *J Rheumatol* 11:804–807, 1984.

71. Al-Herz A, Snip JP, Clark B, et al: Exercise therapy for patients with diffuse idiopathic skeletal hyperostosis, *Clin Rheumatol* 27:207–210, 2008.

72. Roth SH, Shainhouse JZ: Efficacy and safety of a topical diclofenac solution (pennsaid) in the treatment of primary osteoarthritis of the knee: a randomized, double-blind, vehicle-controlled clinical trial, *Arch Intern Med* 164:2017–2023, 2004.

73. Lithell HOL: Effect of antihypertensive drugs on insulin, glucose, and lipid metabolism, *Diabetes Care* 14:203–209, 1991.

74. Guillemin F, Mainard D, Rolland H, et al: Antivitamin K prevents heterotopic ossification after hip arthroplasty in diffuse idiopathic skeletal hyperostosis: a retrospective study in 67 patients, *Acta Orthop Scand* 66:123–126, 1995.

75. Knelles D, Barthel T, Karrer A, et al: Prevention of heterotopic ossification after total hip replacement: a prospective, randomized study using acetylsalicylic acid, indomethacin and fractional or single-dose irradiation, *J Bone Joint Surg Br* 79:596–602, 1997.

76. Mader R: Current therapeutic options in the management of diffuse idiopathic skeletal hyperostosis, *Exp Opin Pharmacother* 6:1313–1316, 2005.

77. Martinez-Lavin M, Mansilla J, Pineda C, et al: Evidence of hypertrophic osteoarthropathy in human skeletal remains from PreHispanic era in Mesoamerica, *Ann Intern Med* 12:238–241, 1994.

78. Martinez-Lavin M, Pineda C, Valdez T, et al: Primary hypertrophic osteoarthropathy, *Semin Arthritis Rheum* 17:156–162, 1988.

79. Spicknall KE, Zirwas MJ, English JC: Clubbing: an update on diagnosis, differential diagnosis, pathophysiology, and clinical relevance, *J Am Acad Dermatol* 52:1020–1028, 2005.

80. Martinez-Lavin M: Hypertrophic osteoarthropathy, *Curr Opin Rheumatol* 9:83–86, 1997.

81. Stridhar KS, Lobo CF, Altman RD: Digital clubbing and lung cancer, *Chest* 114:1535–1537, 1998.

82. Vongpatanasin W, Brickner ME, Hillis LD, et al: The Eisenmenger syndrome in adults, *Ann Intern Med* 128:745–755, 1998.

83. Botton E, Saraux A, Laselve H, et al: Musculoskeletal manifestations in cystic fibrosis, *Joint Bone Spine* 70:327–335, 2003.

84. Dever LL, Matta JS: Digital clubbing in HIV-infected patients: an observational study, *AIDS Patient Care STDS* 23:19–22, 2009.

85. McGuire MM, Demehri S, Kim HB, et al: Hypertrophic osteoarthropathy in intestinal transplant recipients, *J Pediatr Surg* 45:e19–22, 2010.

86. Atkinson S, Fox SB: Vascular endothelial growth factor (VEGF)-A and platelet-derived growth factor (PDGF) play a central role in the pathogenesis of digital clubbing, *J Pathol* 203:721–728, 2004.

87. Olan F, Portela M, Navarro C, et al: Circulating vascular endothelial growth factor concentrations in a case of pulmonary hypertrophic osteoarthropathy: correlation with disease activity, *J Rheumatol* 31:614–616, 2004.

88. Matucci-Cerinic M, Martinez-Lavin M, Rojo F, et al: Von Willebrand factor antigen in hypertrophic osteoarthropathy, *J Rheumatol* 19: 765–767, 1992.

89. Hojo S, Fujita J, Yamadori I, et al: Hepatocyte growth factor and digital clubbing, *Intern Med* 36:44–46, 1997.

90. Schumacher HR Jr: Hypertrophic osteoarthropathy: rheumatologic manifestations, *Clin Exp Rheumatol* 10(Suppl 7):35–40, 1992.

91. Vazquez-Abad D, Pineda C, Martinez-Lavin M: Digital clubbing: a numerical assessment of the deformity, *J Rheumatol* 16:518–520, 1989.

92. Myers KA, Farquhar DRE: Does this patient have clubbing? *JAMA* 286:341–347, 2001.

93. Garske LA, Bell SC: Pamidronate results in symptom control of hypertrophic pulmonary osteoarthropathy in cystic fibrosis, *Chest* 121:1363–1364, 2002.

94. Angel-Moreno Maroto A, Martinez-Quintana E, Suarez-Castellano L, et al: Painful hypertrophic osteoarthropathy successfully treated with ocreotide: the pathogenetic role of vascular endothelial growth factor (VEGF), *Rheumatology (Oxford)* 44:1326–1327, 2005.

95. Martinez-Lavin M, Vargas A, Rivera-Vinas M: Hypertrophic osteoarthropathy: a palindrome with pathogenic connotations, *Curr Opin Rheumatol* 20:88–91, 2008.

96. Chamot AM, Benhamo CL, Khan MF, et al: Acne-pustulosis-hyperostosis-osteitis syndrome. Results of a national survey 85 cases, *Rev Rhum Mal Osteoartic* 54:187–196, 1987.

97. Colina M, Govoni M, Orzincolo C, Trotta F: Clinical and radiologic evolution of synovitis, acne, pustulosis, hyperostosis, and osteitis syndrome: a single center study of a cohort of 71 subjects, *Arthritis Rheum* 61:813–821, 2009.

98. Van Doornum S, Barraclough D, McColl G, Wicks I: SAPHO: rare or just not recognized? *Semin Arthritis Rheum* 30:70–77, 2000.

99. Govoni M, Colina M, Massara A, Trotta F: SAPHO syndrome and infections, *Autoimmun Rev* 8:256–259, 2009.

100. Hurtado-Nedelec M, Chollet-Martin S, Nicaise-Roland P, et al: Characterization of the immune response in the synovitis, acne, pustulosis, hyperostosis, osyeitis (SAPHO) syndrome, *Rheumatology (Oxford)* 47:1160–1167, 2008.

101. Magrey M, Khan MA: New insights into synovitis, acne, pustulosis, hyperostosis, osyeitis (SAPHO) syndrome, *Curr Rheumatol Rep* 11:329–333, 2009.

102. Queiro R, Moreno P, Sarasqueta CL, et al: Synovitis-acne-pustulosis-hyperostosis-osteitis syndrome and psoriatic arthritis exhibit a different immunogenetic profile, *Clin Exp Rheumatol* 26:125–128, 2008.

103. Hurtado-Nedelec M, Chollet-Martin S, Chapeton D, et al: Genetic susceptibility factors in a cohort of 38 patients with SAPHO syndrome: a study of PSTPIP2, NOD2, and LPIN2 genes, *J Rheumatol* 37:401–409, 2010.

104. Grosjean C, Hurtado-Nedelec M, Nicaise-Roland P, et al: Prevalence of autoantibodies in SAPHO syndrome: a single center study of 90 patients, *J Rheumatol* 37:639–643, 2010.

105. Hayem G, Bouchaud-Chabot A, Benali K, et al: SAPHO syndrome: a long-term follow-up study of 120 cases, *Semin Arthritis Rheum* 29:159–171, 1999.
106. Kahn MF, Bouvier M, Palazzo E, et al: Sternoclavicular pustulotic osteitis (SAPHO). 20-year interval between skin and bone lesions, *J Rheumatol* 7:1104–1108, 1991.
107. Kahn MF, Khan MA: The SAPHO syndrome, *Baillieres Clin Rheumatol* 8:333–362, 1994.
108. Reith JD, Bauer TW, Schils JP: Osseous manifestations of SAPHO (synovitis, acne, pustulosis, hyperostosis, osteitis) syndrome, *Am J Surg Pathol* 20:1368–1377, 1996.
109. Cabay JE, Marcelis S, Dondelinger RF: Inflammatory spondylodiscitis as a unique radiological manifestation of the SAPHO syndrome, *J Radiol* 79:337–340, 1998.
110. Boutin RD, Resnick D: The SAPHO syndrome: an evolving concept for unifying several idiopathic disorders of bone and skin, *AJR Am J Roentgenol* 170:585–591, 1998.
111. Freyschmidt J, Sternberg A: The bull's head sign: scintigraphic pattern of sternocostoclavicular hyperostosis and pustulotic arthroosteitis, *Eur Radiol* 8:807–812, 1998.
112. Laredo JD, Vuillemin-Bodaghi V, Boutry N, et al: SAPHO syndrome: MR appearance of vertebral involvement, *Radiology* 242:825–831, 2007.
113. Olivieri I, Padula A, Palazzi C: Pharmacological management of SAPHO syndrome, *Expert Opin Investig Drugs* 15:1229–1233, 2006.
114. Scarppato S, Tirri E: Successful treatment of SAPHO syndrome with leflunomide. Report of two cases, *Clin Exp Rheumatol* 23:731, 2005.
115. Assman G, Kueck O, Kirchhoff T, et al: Efficacy of antibiotic therapy for SAPHO syndrome is lost after its discontinuation: an interventional study, *Arthritis Res Ther* 11:R140, 2009.
116. Amital H, Applebaum YH, Aamar S, et al: SAPHO syndrome treated with pamidronate: an open-label study of 10 patients, *Rheumatology (Oxford)* 43:658–661, 2004.
117. Pennanen N, Lapinjoki S, Urtti A, Monkkonen J: Effect of liposomal and free bisphosphonates on the IL-1β, IL-6 and TNF-α secretion form RAW 264 cells in vitro, *Pharm Res* 12:916–922, 1995.
118. Massara A, Cavazzini PL, Trotta F: In SAPHO syndrome anti-TNF-alpha therapy may induce persistent amelioration of osteoarticular complaints, but may exacerbate cutaneous manifestations, *Rheumatology (Oxford)* 45:730–733, 2006.
119. Ben Abdelghani K, Dran DG, Gottenberg JE, et al: Tumor necrosis factor-alpha blockers in SAPHO syndrome, *J Rheumatol* 37:1699–1704, 2010.

The references for this chapter can also be found on www.expertconsult.com.

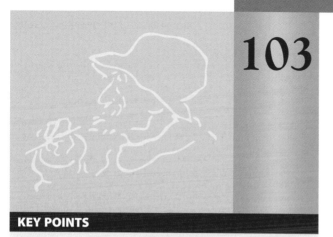

103 Osteonecrosis

CHRISTOPHER CHANG •
ADAM GREENSPAN • M. ERIC GERSHWIN

KEY POINTS

Osteonecrosis affects younger patients more often than osteoarthritis and has significantly greater long-term morbidity.

Corticosteroids constitute the most common cause of nontraumatic osteonecrosis.

The femoral head is the most common site of osteonecrosis.

Bisphosphonate use is associated with osteonecrosis of the jaw.

The final common pathway in the pathogenesis of osteonecrosis is disruption of blood supply to a segment of bone.

Abnormalities in lipid metabolism, bone homeostasis, regulation of apoptosis, coagulopathies, and oxidative stress may play a role in the pathogenesis of osteonecrosis.

Magnetic resonance imaging is currently the optimal test for early diagnosis and identification of the extent of osteonecrosis.

Nonsurgical treatment of osteonecrosis does not change the natural history of the disease.

Although there are many variations on surgical treatment of femoral head osteonecrosis, most patients eventually require total hip arthroplasty.

Knowledge of risk factors and early detection are crucial to the successful management of osteonecrosis.

Due to the lack of successful treatment options, new modes focus on prevention of osteonecrosis.

Osteonecrosis literally means "bone death" (*ossis* [Latin] = bone; *necrosis* = killing or causing to die). Other synonyms include avascular necrosis, ischemic necrosis of bone, aseptic necrosis, and subchondral avascular necrosis. The term *osteonecrosis dissecans* is sometimes used synonymously with osteonecrosis, although, strictly speaking, it is a consequence of osteonecrosis involving dessication of bone leading to fracturing or cracking of bone. The concept of bone death was first described by Hippocrates,[1] but the first clinical description of osteonecrosis was a case of sepsis-induced bone death described by Russell in 1794.[2] It was almost a century later that bone death was described to occur in the absence of infection.[3] The first report of osteonecrosis in a deep sea diver appeared in 1936.[4] The pathogenesis of osteonecrosis is complex, but whatever the mechanism, bone death ultimately occurs as a result of complete or partial disruption of the delivery of oxygen and/or nutrients to the bone and surrounding tissues. It is likely that multiple molecular mechanisms may be simultaneously in play in order for osteonecrosis to occur.[5,6]

EPIDEMIOLOGY

The prevalence of osteonecrosis is unknown, but it is estimated that there are 10,000 to 20,000 new patients diagnosed per year in the United States. Osteonecrosis occurs in 15% to 80% of patients with femoral neck fractures.[7] Ten percent of the 500,000 hip replacements done in the United States each year are thought to be for osteonecrosis.[8] The disease primarily affects men, with a notable exception for osteonecrosis associated with systemic lupus erythematosus, which has a significant female predominance. Osteonecrosis primarily occurs in the third to fifth decade of life.[9] As a result of this age distribution, long-term morbidity can be significant because most hip replacements have a finite period of viability.

ETIOLOGY

Osteonecrosis has been linked to numerous conditions (Table 103-1). The strength of a causal relationship varies greatly, and in some cases only case reports have been published. The most common cause of nontraumatic osteonecrosis is corticosteroid use, which was first described in 1957.[10] Although other adverse effects of corticosteroids are perhaps better known, osteonecrosis of the femoral head is one of the serious complications.

In a 1998 study, in which the investigators reviewed associations in 2500 to 3300 cases of nontraumatic osteonecrosis, corticosteroid use was present in 34.7% of cases. Alcohol use was found in 21.7% of the cases, and the remainder was idiopathic. Although the risk of developing osteonecrosis with corticosteroid use is small, the severity of the adverse event and the high morbidity associated with osteonecrosis make this an important complication to consider when starting a patient on corticosteroids.

Studies have attempted to determine the duration of use and the dosages of corticosteroids necessary to precipitate osteonecrosis. There are several forms of corticosteroids of differing potency and half-life, and dosages and duration of use vary between studies, so any conclusions about a "safe" dose of corticosteroids are wrought with potential confounding variables and errors. In one study of 20 patients diagnosed with stage 1 osteonecrosis by magnetic resonance imaging (MRI), the interval between the use of steroids and diagnosis ranged from 1 to 16 months.[11] The cumulative dose of steroids in this study ranged from 1800 to 15,505 mg (mean, 5928 mg) of prednisolone or the equivalent. In other studies cumulative doses of steroids associated with osteonecrosis ranged from 480[12] to 4320[13] mg of dexamethasone dose equivalence. A recent paper by Powell and colleagues[14] attempted to collectively analyze the available

Table 103-1 Conditions Associated with Osteonecrosis

Dietary, Drugs, and Environmental Factors

Corticosteroids[155-157]
Bisphosphonates[130,158,159]
Alcoholism[22,160]
Cigarette smoking[22]
Dysbaric osteonecrosis[4,161]
Lead poisoning[162,163]
Electric shock[164,165]

Musculoskeletal Conditions: Compromise in Structural Integrity

Trauma[166]
Legg-Calvé-Perthes disease[31,167]
Congenital hip dislocation[168,169]
Slipped femoral capital epiphysis[170,171]

Metabolic Diseases: Abnormality in Fat or Other Metabolic Component

Fat embolism[172,173]
Pancreatitis[69,71,174,175]
Chronic liver disease[176]
Pregnancy[42,177]
Fabry's disease[178,179]
Gaucher's disease[43,180]
Gout[181]
Hyperparathyroidism[182]
Hyperlipidemia[172,173]
Hypercholesterolemia[181]
Diabetes[183]

Hematologic Conditions: Abnormalities in Blood Components

Sickle cell anemia[118,184,185]
Hemophilia[46,47,49]
Hemoglobinopathies
Thalassemia[186]
Disseminated intravascular coagulation[103,187-189]
Thrombophilia[190]
Hypofibrinolysis[190,191]
Marrow infiltrative disorders
Thrombophlebitis/venous thrombosis[192]

Rheumatologic Conditions

Antiphospholipid antibody syndrome[193]
Rheumatoid arthritis[194]
Inflammatory bowel disease[195,196]
Necrotizing arteritis[197]
Mucocutaneous lymph node syndrome[198]
Polymyositis[199]
Sarcoidosis[70]
Mixed connective tissue disease

Infectious Diseases

Human immunodeficiency virus infection[200,201]
Osteomyelitis[202]
Meningococcemia[187,203,204]
Severe acute respiratory syndrome (SARS)[54,106,205]

Oncologic Disorders, Transplantation, and Their Treatment

Organ transplantation (with or without corticosteroid exposure)[206-211]
Radiation exposure[212-217]
Regional deep hyperthermia[218]
Acute lymphoblastic leukemia[219,220]

literature to derive maximum safe levels for duration, maximum daily dose, and average daily dose of corticosteroids. The study confirmed that many other confounding variables affect the development of osteonecrosis, making analysis of dose-response risk for an isolated association difficult. Nonetheless, corticosteroid-induced osteonecrosis is dependent on dosage and the risk factor is higher with the long-acting steroids and with parenteral usage.

Additional host-inherent risk factors also play a role in susceptibility. The incidence of osteonecrosis in a group of patients receiving glucocorticoid replacement therapy for primary or secondary adrenal insufficiency was 2.4%. In a study of renal transplantation patients, the 26 patients who developed osteonecrosis had a higher cumulative oral dose of prednisone after 1 and 3 months compared with 28 control transplant patients who did not develop osteonecrosis.[15] A separate study estimated the incidence of osteonecrosis in renal transplant patients to be 5%.[16] There is no evidence to consistently link the use of topical, inhaled, or nasal corticosteroids to osteonecrosis. The evidence for an association between osteonecrosis and intramuscular or intra-articular corticosteroids is limited to case reports.[17] Parenteral use poses a higher risk because of rapid absorption and longer half-life of the drugs used.

Bisphosphonate-induced osteonecrosis of the jaw is particularly interesting because of the intended use of bisphosphonates on bone diseases.[18-20] There has been a link between cigarette smoking and osteonecrosis, with smokers having a threefold higher relative risk for developing osteonecrosis, independent of all other factors.[21,22]

The association between osteonecrosis and alcohol consumption was first described in 1922.[23] A study of patients with idiopathic osteonecrosis revealed that the risk of osteonecrosis increased with increasing daily consumption of alcohol.[21] The subjects were divided into three groups on the basis of their alcohol consumption of less than 400 mL/week, 400 to 1000 mL/week, and greater than 1000 mL/week, and the relative risk of osteonecrosis, independent of corticosteroid use or smoking, was 3-fold, 10-fold, and 18-fold, respectively, when compared with hospital controls. Liver damage was also found unnecessary for the development of osteonecrosis in alcohol-consuming patients, although elevated liver enzymes may be present.[24] The incidence of osteonecrosis in patients who received treatment for alcoholism was 5.3%. The femoral head was again the most common site (82 of 92 lesions), with the other 10 sites involving the humeral head.[25]

Musculoskeletal conditions can lead to osteonecrosis in children. Legg-Calvé-Perthes disease was first described in children between 3 and 12 years of age in 1910.[26-28] Femoral head osteonecrosis is a feature of this disease and has been linked to trauma,[29,30] congenital hip dislocation,[31] and transient synovitis.[32] Bilateral involvement is common, and associated clinical manifestations include abnormal growth and stature,[33,34] delayed skeletal maturation,[35] disproportionate skeletal growth,[33] congenital anomalies,[36] and abnormal hormone levels.[37,38] Children with acute lymphoblastic leukemia can develop osteonecrosis[39,40] as well, but this may be a result of steroid use. An additional risk factor for this cohort of patients is high body mass index.[41]

Osteonecrosis has also been associated with metabolic disorders and in pregnancy. Diagnosis is often delayed until months after delivery. Women who develop osteonecrosis in pregnancy tended to have a small body frame and a large weight gain.[42]

Hematologic conditions have been associated with osteonecrosis. The long-term morbidity of osteonecrosis in patients with sickle cell anemia is dismal.[43] Common deformities include decreased mobility, abnormal gait, and leg-length discrepancy.[44] Osteonecrosis in hemophilia patients has been reported, but no statistically reliable causal link can be established.[45-50]

Dysbaric osteonecrosis was first described in construction workers in the Elhe tunnel exposed to high-pressure environments.[51] The prevalence of dysbaric osteonecrosis is 4.2% in divers and 17% in compressed air workers.[52] Patients with dysbaric osteonecrosis may have more than one lesion, and common sites besides the femoral head include the tibia and the humeral head and shaft. The condition is not related to decompression sickness, and although proper decompression procedures can reduce "the bends," they do not have any effect on the development of osteonecrosis, which can occur months or years after the last exposure to high-pressure environments.

Osteonecrosis has also been associated with a number of infectious diseases including severe acute respiratory syndrome (SARS). Many patients who contracted SARS in the early 2000s received treatment with corticosteroids, and some subsequently developed osteonecrosis.[53] The incidence of osteonecrosis appears higher in this group of patients compared with patients with other conditions who were treated with corticosteroids.[54] Chan and colleagues[55] reported five children with SARS treated with corticosteroids who developed osteonecrosis.

CLINICAL FEATURES

The primary presenting symptom in osteonecrosis is pain. In osteonecrosis of the femoral hip, the pain is located in the hip joint but may radiate to the groin, anterior thigh, or knee. The severity of the pain can vary, depending on the size of the infarct and whether the onset of disease is insidious or sudden. In trauma, where there is sudden and severe disruption of blood flow, and in Gaucher's disease, dysbarism, or hemoglobinopathy, where the infarcts are large, pain can be intense and sudden. In other conditions where the onset is more insidious, the pain can follow a gradual and slow incremental progression. The pain of osteonecrosis is usually increased with use of the joint, but in advanced disease the pain can be persistent at rest. Limitation of range of motion is progressive and is usually a late symptom, except when resulting from accompanying pain. The risk of developing osteonecrosis of the contralateral hip when one side is affected ranges from 31% to 55%.

In addition to the femoral head, osteonecrosis can affect other sites including the humeral head,[56-59] femoral condyles[60-63] and proximal tibiae,[61,64-66] wrists and ankles,[67] bones of the hands and feet,[68] the vertebrae,[69-71] jaw,[72-75] and bony structures of the face.[76] Osteonecrosis of the humeral head is the second most commonly seen location, and pain is usually in the shoulder and associated with reduced range of motion and weakness. Pain in the ankle is the main presenting symptom in nontraumatic osteonecrosis of the talus, and in some cases, the disease had already progressed to Ficat and Arlet stage 3 by the time of presentation of pain.[67] Kienböck's disease involves osteonecrosis of the lunate. Patients present with pain in the radiolunate joint, along with weakness and limitation of motion. Keinböck's disease appears to be related to manual labor. Soccer players have been reported to develop osteonecrosis of the foot,[77]

Table 103-2 Modified Steinberg Staging Systems for Osteonecrosis

Stage	Radiographic Appearance	Reversible
I	Normal radiographs, but abnormal bone scan or magnetic resonance image	Yes
II	Lucent and sclerotic changes	Yes
III	Subchondral fracture without flattening	No
IV	Subchondral fracture with flattening or segmental depression of femoral head	No
V	Joint space narrowing or acetabular changes	No
VI	Advanced degenerative changes	No

and football players may be prone to developing osteonecrosis of the hip.[78]

The Ficat and Arlet method of staging osteonecrosis consists of four stages. Stages 1 and 2 are reversible, whereas stage 3 (subchondral collapse) and stage 4 (joint space narrowing and destruction of cartilage) are irreversible. The Marcus staging system consists of six stages, in which the first two are reversible and the subsequent four are irreversible. The modified Steinberg staging system is based on the Marcus system and also consists of six stages. Each stage is further divided into three subclasses on the basis of the extent of femoral head involvement. Subclass A involves less than 25%; B involves 26% to 50%, and C involves greater than 50%.

Table 103-2 shows the Modified Steinberg system for staging osteonecrosis. The Association of Research Circulation Osseous (ARCO) has proposed a modification to the Ficat and Arlet system, adding a stage 0 or patients with negative imaging studies but who are at risk for developing osteonecrosis. In addition, stages 1 and 3 are further stratified to take into account lesion size, location, and extent of collapse.[79] In 2001 the Japanese Ministry of Health, Labor and Welfare proposed revising criteria for the diagnosis and staging of osteonecrosis of the femoral head.[80] Diagnostic criteria included the following: (1) collapse of the femoral head without joint space narrowing or acetabular abnormality on plain radiograph, (2) demarcating sclerosis in the femoral head without joint space narrowing or acetabular abnormality, (3) "cold in hot" on bone scans, (4) low-intensity band on T1-weighted MRI, and (5) trabecular and marrow necrosis on histology. If a patient fulfills two of the five criteria, the diagnosis is established. The working group also proposed four types of lesions on the basis of extensiveness and defined stages of disease on the basis of diagnostic imaging.

Bone Marrow Edema

Bone marrow edema is a common observation in osteonecrosis and is frequently accompanied by vascular congestion. Bone marrow edema is not specific for osteonecrosis and may be seen in many musculoskeletal disorders including osteomyelitis, osteoarthritis, occult intraosseous fracture, stress fracture, osteoporosis, and sickle cell crisis.

A specific syndrome known as *bone marrow edema syndrome* has been described and was initially thought to be a precursor to osteonecrosis, but it is now believed to be a separate entity. Bone marrow edema is a transitory, self-limiting condition typically seen in middle-aged men and in women in their third trimester of pregnancy. Patients complain of pain, limited range of motion, and an abnormal gait. Osteopenia is detected on conventional radiographs, and MRI confirms this with a low signal on T1-weighted images and a high signal on T2-weighted images. The three phases of bone marrow edema syndrome include an initial phase lasting about 1 month, followed by a plateau phase lasting 1 or 2 months, and finally a regression phase lasting for an additional 4 to 6 months.[81] Subchondral fractures do not occur. Biopsy specimens obtained in the initial phase show diffuse interstitial edema, fragmentation of fatty marrow cells, and increased new bone formation.[82]

A study of 24 cases of bone marrow edema syndrome of the knee showed that although migrating bone marrow edema occurred in a third of patients at a 5-year follow-up, the patients were asymptomatic and MRI signal alterations had resolved. Biopsy specimens of affected bone were obtained using arthroscopic surgery and core decompression, and histology revealed areas of bone marrow edema and vital trabeculae covered by osteblasts and osteoid seams. None of the cases progressed to osteonecrosis.[83]

Bisphosphonates and Osteonecrosis of the Jaw

Bisphosphonate is a class of drug used to treat osteoporosis and diseases where bone is not formed adequately. Bisphosphonates are composed of two forms, and osteonecrosis appears to occur in association with nitrogen-containing bisphosphonates. The mechanism of action of bisphosphonate-induced osteonecrosis of the jaw appears to parallel that of glucocorticoids, with derangement in lipid metabolism, bone homeostasis, and apoptosis of bone cells. It is interesting that the jawbone seems to be the most vulnerable bone in bisphosphonate-induced disease, as opposed to the femoral head in most other associations or causes of osteonecrosis. This may be because of the high bone turnover rate in the jaw or because bisphosphonates exert their action on not only bone but also many elements of the surrounding tissue including fibroblasts and blood vessels.

PATHOGENESIS

Anatomic Considerations in Trauma-Related Osteonecrosis

The femoral head is the most common site of osteonecrosis. An understanding of the anatomy of the femoral head may help to explain why that is the case. Three arterial networks supply the femoral head and neck. The extracapsular arterial ring consists of the lateral femoral circumflex artery and the medial femoral circumflex artery, which arise from the profunda femoris. The medial femoral circumflex artery and its branches supply most of the blood to the head and neck of the femur. The lateral femoral artery winds anterolaterally, and the medial femoral artery winds posteromedially around the neck of the femur, ultimately anastomosing with each other at the superolateral aspect of the femoral head. The lateral femoral circumflex artery and the medial femoral

circumflex artery further anastomose with the superior and inferior gluteal branches of the internal iliac artery, providing collateral circulation between the femoral artery and the internal iliac artery. Small vessels known as *retinacular arteries,* ascending cervical branches of the extracapsular ring, form an intra-articular ring at the level of the cartilage. Eiphyseal arterial branches arise from this ring and penetrate the head and neck of the femur including the epiphyses. The artery of the ligament of the head of the femur is a branch of the obturator artery and may be the sole supplier of blood to the proximal fragment of the head.

Some of these anatomic features may render the femoral head particularly vulnerable to ischemia. The retinacular arteries are believed to supply 80% of the femoral epiphysis. Compromising this critical vascular system may lead to osteonecrosis originating in the anterosuperior aspect of the femoral head, as indicated by angiographic studies in early osteonecrosis in which these arteries are not visualized. A schematic of the blood supply to the femoral head is shown in Figure 103-1.

Histologically, after an infarct, a rim of bony thickening or sclerosis begins to form at the margins of the infarcted area. If the necrotic lesion is within the weight-bearing region of the femoral head, subchondral fractures follow. With repeated microfractures and continued weight bearing, the original fracture cannot heal completely and new fractures appear. The secondary fracture propagates along the junction between subchondral bone and the necrotic segment. As time goes on, the femoral head becomes flattened and eventually collapses. A nonspherical head articulating with the acetabulum produces friction and erosion and loss of cartilage. The cycle repeats itself, and the structure of the joint deteriorates, leading to degenerative changes and eventual total joint destruction.[84]

Nontraumatic Osteonecrosis

Disruption of the blood supply to the femoral head can occur through a number of different mechanisms. In

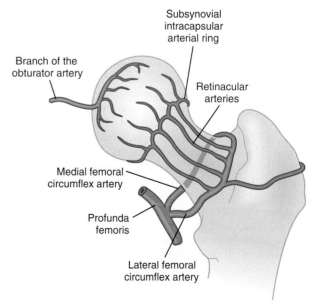

Figure 103-1 Schematic of the blood supply of the femoral head.

Table 103-3 Proposed Mechanism of Disease of Common Conditions Associated with Osteonecrosis

Associated Condition	Mechanism of Osteonecrosis							
	Apoptosis	Osteoblast/ Osteoclast Homeostasis	Lipid Abnormalities	Coagulation Abnormalities	Oxidative Stress	Parathyroid/ Calcium Imbalance	Vascular Plugging	Vasoactive Substances
Corticosteroids	X	X	X	X	X			X
Bisphosphonates	X	X	X					
Alcohol abuse	X	X	X	X	X			
Trauma	X	X						X
Renal transplantation	X	X		X		X		
Dialysis						X		
Sickle cell disease							X	

traumatic osteonecrosis of the femoral head, the cause of this disruption is often viewed as completely mechanical and appears to be easily understood. But there may be an additional component to the disruption that is related to the immunologic and inflammatory changes that occur in damaged bone tissue and surrounding soft tissues.

The immunologic changes occurring in nontraumatic osteonecrosis may help explain why corticosteroids are particularly dangerous to the integrity of the blood supply of the femoral hip. Some have likened osteonecrosis to "coronary disease" of the hip[85,86] and propose that the same mechanisms that cause ischemia of the myocardium may also cause ischemia of the femoral head (Table 103-3).

Mechanical and Vascular Considerations

In Legg-Calvé-Perthes disease, obstruction to venous drainage elevates intraosseous pressure and consequently elevates intra-articular pressures. In a study of patients with Legg-Calvé-Perthes disease, bone scintigraphy using Tc99m methylene diphosphonate (Tc99m MDP) was employed to measure arterial and venous flow in the diseased hip. Although arterial flow was normal, there was significant disruption in venous drainage.[87] This disturbance was reproduced in a dog model in which injection of silicone was used to obstruct venous flow distal to the hip.[88] Ischemia resulted from the obstruction to venous drainage, leading to a cessation of endochondral ossification in the preosseous epiphyseal cartilage and the physeal plate. Widening of the joint space ensued, followed by revascularization of the epiphysis and deposition of new immature bone. A weakened or unstable femoral epiphyseal plate resulted, and the subchondral bone became prone to segmental collapse and fracture.[89]

The pathologic mechanism of dysbaric osteonecrosis is unclear. The most intuitive explanation is that formation of gas bubbles causes arterial occlusion and ischemia. However, the true mechanism may not be quite so simple. Multiple other factors might contribute to the disease including thromboembolic events such as platelet aggregation, erythrocyte clumping, lipid coalescence, intraosseous vessel compression as a result of extravascular gas bubbles, formation of fibrin thrombi, and narrowing of arterial lumina owing to myointimal thickening caused by gas bubbles. The interaction between gas and blood can lead to the formation of vessel-occluding substances. All of these events can lead to redistribution of blood flow.

The increased vulnerability of bone to compression disorders has been explained by several factors including the relative rigidity of bone and inability to absorb increased gas pressure, inherent poor vascularization, and gas supersaturation of fatty marrow.[90] A sheep model of dysbaric osteonecrosis has been developed. Exposure to compressed air at pressures of 2.6 to 2.9 atmospheres for 24 hours results in extensive bone and marrow necrosis. The authors proposed that the initial event involving elevated intramedullary pressures leads to the formation of nitrogen gas bubbles in the fatty marrow of the long bones. Radiography shows medullary opacities and endosteal thickening. Later, neovascularization of previously ischemic fatty marrow occurs, followed by new bone formation. Osteonecrosis occurs in subchondral cortical bone with marrow fibrosis and osteocyte loss.[91]

Changes in the vasculature, through injury or inflammation from other diseases, may in turn lead to a compromise in blood flow. Examples include structural damage to arteriolar walls, degeneration of the tunica media, smooth muscle cell necrosis, and disruption of the internal elastic lamina. These changes can lead to eventual hemorrhagic infarction, which was observed in a study of 24 core biopsy specimens from osteonecrotic femoral heads. The changes did not occur in 11 femoral heads with osteoarthrosis.[92]

Osteoimmunology

Although bone marrow is a critical component of the immune system, bone matrix is often perceived to be static scaffolding that functions primarily to support the musculoskeletal system. It is now known that, in fact, bone matrix is a dynamic tissue that is constantly replacing itself. It is estimated that about 10% of a person's bone is replaced every year. Diseases such as osteopetrosis and osteoporosis are a result of a dysfunction in the balance between bone deposition and bone resorption. The factors that regulate this homeostasis include cells of the bone matrix, immune cells, signaling molecules, cytokines and chemokines, and vitamins. Some of these regulatory factors may be present on both bone cells and immune cells, often serving different functions, thereby providing a link between the immune system and bone. Osteonecrosis, in fact, may be linked to such an imbalance in bone homeostasis. Immune factors may affect surrounding soft tissue as well, contributing to the development of osteonecrosis. The study of immune regulation of bone in osteonecrosis may encompasses many of the previously proposed mechanisms of osteonecrosis including apoptosis, oxidative stress, and genetic predisposition.

Immune factors involved in bone homeostasis include receptor activator of NFκB (RANK) and its ligand (RANKL), IL-1, IL-6, IL-10, TFG-β, TNF, CD80, CD86, CD40, macrophage colony-stimulating factor (M-CSF), NFATc, and vitamin D. (See Table 103-4 for roles and function.) Many of these factors can be categorized into one of two categories, those with the overall effect of inducing osteoclastogenesis and those that inhibit osteoclastogenesis. In addition, factors involved in cell survival and apoptosis such as Blimp-1 and Bcl6 may also play a role. RANKL is expressed on osteoblasts and is critical for the differentiation and proliferation of osteoclasts. Because transcription of factors involved in the regulation of bone homeostasis is often influenced by glucocorticoids, this may begin to explain why steroids may be associated with osteonecrosis.

The action of glucocorticoids is mediated by the glucocorticoid receptor, which is present on many cell types including osteoclasts, osteoblasts, osteocytes, and cartilage. Binding of glucocorticoids to its receptor leads to the anti-inflammatory activity known to be a function of steroids. One mechanism by which this anti-inflammatory effect is mediated is by transcription of genes that inhibit the synthesis of inflammatory mediators.

Osteoblast/Osteoclast Balance

Any disturbance in the normal homeostasis between bone deposition and bone resorption can lead to bone disease. Moreover, defective bone deposition or bone resorption in which new bone is formed in an aberrant manner can lead to disease. Alcohol can affect the ability of mesenchymal stem cells to differentiate into osteogenic lineages. The bone marrow in the proximal head of femurs was isolated during hip replacement surgery from 33 patients with either femoral neck fractures or alcohol-induced osteonecrosis. The cells from femurs of patients with alcohol-induced osteonecrosis showed a reduced ability to differentiate into

Table 103-4 Role and Function of Immune Factors in Osteoimmunology

Immune Factor	Ligand	Cellular Source	Function in Bone Homeostasis	OC	Immune Function
RANK	RANKL	Osteoclasts, dendritic cells	Upon binding to RANKL, signals differentiation into osteoclast	↑	RANKL-RANK binding leads to dendritic cell activation
RANKL	RANK	Osteoblasts, T helper cells	Activation of osteoclasts. Overproduction can result in RA or PA	↑	Dendritic cell maturation
OPG	RANKL		Decoy receptor for RANKL	↓	
M-CSF	CSF-1 receptor	Osteoblasts, macrophages, bone fibroblasts, stromal cells	Stimulates osteoclastogenesis	↑	Influences hematopoietic stem cells to differentiate into macrophages
TNF	TNF receptor	Macrophages, lymphocytes, mast cells, and many others	Stimulates osteoclastogenesis	↑	Influences multiple signaling pathways, including NFκB, death signaling and MAP kinase pathway
TGF-β	TGF-β receptor	Multiple cell lines	Induction of apoptosis	↑	Regulatory role, blocks activation of lymphocyte- and monocyte-derived phagocytosis
Blimp-1	Bcl6 promoter	Plasmablasts, plasma cells	Binds to Bcl6 promoter, suppression expression	↑	Inhibits Tfh cell differentiation in mice[221]
Bcl-6	?	Germinal center B cells	Inhibits osteoclastogenesis	↓	Stimulates Tfh cell differentiation in mice
IL-1	IL-1R	Macrophages, monocytes, fibroblasts, dendritic cells	Directly activates RANK signaling to promote osteoclastogenesis[222]	↑	Proinflammatory cytokine, endogenous pyrogen
IL-6	IL-6R	Osteoblasts	Activation of osteoclastogenesis	↑	Proinflammatory cytokine
IL-10	IL-10Rα	Monocytes, lymphocytes	Suppress bone resorption	↓	Anti-inflammatory cytokine, blocks NFκB activity, regulatory cytokine
Vitamin D	VDR	Osteoblast, monocyte/macrophage	Facilitate adhesion of osteoclast precursor to osteoblast[223]	↑	Cell proliferation and differentiation
Estrogens	Estrogen receptor	Ovarian follicle cells	Reduces osteoclast IL-1 responsiveness and cell survival,[224] stimulates osteoprotegrin	↓	Angiogenesis, endothelial healing
IL-17	IL-17R	T cells	May have opposing roles of bone protection and bone loss[225]	↑↓	Proinflammatory cytokine
IL-18	IL-18R	Macrophages	Inhibits TNF-mediated osteoclastogenesis in a T cell–independent manner	↓	Proinflammatory cytokine, works in synergy with IL-12

Examples of some of the factors involved in bone metabolism. In addition to the factors listed, there are many others that play a role, either by themselves or in conjunction with other factors. The factors listed may have many other functions. Only select functions are listed.

Bcl6, B cell lymphoma 6 protein; Blimp, B lymphocyte–induced maturation protein 1; CSF-1, colony-stimulating factor 1; OC, osteoclastogenic; OPG, osteoprotegrin; PA, psoriatic arthritis; RA, rheumatoid arthritis; RANK, receptor activator for NFκB; RANKL, receptor activator for NFκB ligand; Tfh, T follicular helper cell; TGF-β, transforming growth factor beta; TNF, tumor necrosis factor; VDR, vitamin D receptor.

osteoblasts.[93] A subsequent study compared the mesenchymal stem cells from patients with hip osteoarthritis, idiopathic osteonecrosis, and nontraumatic osteonecrosis associated with steroid or alcohol use. In idiopathic and alcohol-induced osteonecrosis, the ability of mesenchymal stem cells to differentiate into osteoblasts was decreased, but in steroid-induced osteonecrosis, it was elevated, although not to a statistically significant level. The adipogenic differentiation ability was similar in all four groups.[94]

In rats fed a diet of alcohol and glucose, lower bone mineral content and density were detected compared with controls. In hamsters, alcohol led to thinning of the trabeculae of the distal part of the femur. Cytologic effects included mitochondrial swelling in osteoblasts and osteocytes. Partial osteonecrosis of the femoral head was detected in Merino sheep that were injected with ethanol. In humans, alcohol causes increased plasma calcium levels, decreased osteocalcin and circulating parathyroid hormone levels, reduced serum calcitriol, reduced bone volume, and increased osteoclast number.

Alterations in osteoblast function may also contribute to the pathogenesis of osteonecrosis. In one study, osteoblastic cells were obtained from bone biopsy specimens from the intertrochanteric region of the femur and of the iliac crest of 13 patients with osteonecrosis and 8 patients with hip osteoarthritis. Cell replication was measured on the basis of proliferation rate in secondary culture. Levels of alkaline phosphatase activity, collagen synthesis, and the sensitivity to 1,25-dihydroxyvitamin D_3 were measured. The results indicated that although differentiation was not affected, the proliferation rate of osteoblastic cells was reduced in samples obtained from the patients with osteonecrosis compared with patients with osteoarthritic hips.[95]

Apoptosis and Osteonecrosis

Glucocorticoids can also act via its action on apoptosis of immune and bone cells. When mice were administered prednisolone for 27 days, increased metaphyseal apoptotic activity of both osteoblasts and osteoclasts were noted.[96] The result was decreased bone turnover, density, and formation; increased formation of cancellous bone; and decreased trabecular width. The decreased bone turnover can be explained by the reduced osteoclast survival, and the reduction in trabecular width can be explained by a decrease in osteoblasts. An accumulation of apoptotic elements was also found in the region of the "fracture crescent" in the femurs of glucocorticoid-treated patients. On the other hand, glucocorticoids may also increase osteoclast survival, leading to increased bone loss. Clearly, the effect of osteoclast survival on bone disease is more complicated than at first glance, and it involves the interaction of the osteoclast with the osteoblast. Because osteoblasts are also responsible for osteoclast differentiation under the right circumstances, there exists a significant feedback system that maintains bone homeostasis.

Osteocyte death is also a feature of osteonecrosis. In a rat model, ischemia caused an induction in the expression of stress proteins, oxygen-regulated protein (ORP150) and hemoxygenase 1 (HO1). Induction of ischemia in these rates caused DNA fragmentation and the presence of apoptotic bodies in chodrocytes, bone marrow cells, and osteocytes.[97] Both alcohol and corticosteroids can induce osteocyte apoptosis, possibly via lipid abnormalities.

Lipids and Osteonecrosis

The bone marrow of rabbits that were fed alcohol showed fatty infiltration of the liver and adipogenesis in the bone marrow. Increases in fat cell hypertrophy and proliferation, as well as a decrease in hematopoiesis in the subchondral head, were observed. Osteocytes contained triglyceride deposits, and there was an increase in empty osteocyte lacunae. Alcohol also primarily triggered differentiation of bone marrow stromal cells into adipocytes in a dose-dependent manner. Intracellular lipid deposits led to the death of osteocytes.

In corticosteroid-induced osteonecrosis, the alteration in lipid metabolism parallels that of alcohol-induced osteonecrosis. In both cases, fatty infiltration of osteocytes has been postulated to occur.[98-100] Table 103-5 lists lipid-altering effects of corticosteroids and alcohol. In addition, interosseous venous stasis affects the interosseous microcirculation, which can lead to hemodynamic and structural changes in the femoral head. The resulting decrease in blood flow leads to osteonecrosis. In chickens treated with steroids, fatty infiltration of the liver and fat cell hypertrophy and proliferation in the femoral head occurred concurrently 1 week after the initiation of steroids. As in the case of alcohol-induced osteonecrosis, adipocytes contained triglyceride vesicles. In rabbits treated with steroids, it was found that interosseous pressure was increased and the size of bone marrow fat cells was larger than in control rabbits.[101] A histologic study of acetabular and proximal femoral bone in osteonecrosis of the femoral head revealed that osteonecrosis is more extensive in corticosteroid-induced compared with alcohol-induced or idiopathic osteonecrosis.[102] The reason for this is unknown.

In osteonecrosis of the jaw, bisphosphonates inhibit protein prenylation via inhibition of the enzyme farnesyl diphosphate synthase. The normal lipid metabolism of pathways that regulate cytoskeletal integrity and osteoclastogenesis such as Rho, Rac, and Ras is disrupted. This is one of the mechanisms by which bisphosphonates exert their intended action, but their ability to disrupt normal regulation of bone metabolism may instead lead to osteonecrosis.

Coagulation and Osteonecrosis

The hyperlipidemia, increased serum free fatty acids, and increased prostaglandins that are associated with alcohol-induced osteonecrosis may potentially trigger vascular

Table 103-5 Lipid-Altering Effects of Steroids and Alcohol

Fatty liver
Swelling and necrosis of fat cells
Lipid-filled osteocytes
Hyperlipidemia
Adipogenesis of marrow stromal cells
Fatty infiltration of bone marrow
Fat emboli

inflammation and coagulation. Other triggers for intravascular coagulation include atherosclerosis and arteriolar fibroid degeneration. Jones proposed that the progression of osteonecrosis from stage 1A to 1B is linked to an inability to clear procoagulants from blood or tissue.[103] He proposed that decreased clearance of procoagulants leads to persistent levels of tissue thromboplastin, leading to arteriolar thrombosis, vascular stasis, free fatty acid–induced endothelial damage, and hypercoagulability. Studies have shown that patients with osteonecrosis had a much higher frequency of having at least one and at least two abnormal coagulant levels compared with normal controls. Of patients with osteonecrosis, 82% had at least one abnormal procoagulant level, and 47% had at least two. In normal controls, only 30% had one abnormal procoagulant level and only 2.5% had two or more. The procoagulants measured included free protein S, protein C, lipoprotein A, homocysteine, plasminogen activator inhibitor, stimulated tissue plasminogen activator, anticardiolipin antibodies (IgM and IgG), and resistance to activated protein C.[104]

In addition, both thrombophilia and hypofibrinolysis have been associated with osteonecrosis. Hypofibrinolysis leads to an increased likelihood of clot formation, and thrombophilia results in a decreased ability to lyse clots. This is yet another mechanism by which corticosteroids lead to osteonecrosis—high-dose steroids lead to increased plasma plasminogen activator inhibitor, decreased tissue plasminogen activator activity, and inhibition of the fibrinolytic pathway, thus leading to a higher risk for clot formation. There is an early indication that coagulation abnormalities may play a significant role in corticosteroid-induced osteonecrosis in SARS patients.[105,106]

Oxidative Stress and Osteonecrosis

Alcohol consumption is associated with reduced superoxide dismutase activity. Alcohol has deleterious effects on muscle including increased oxygen free radical–related damage, reduced myocardial contractility, defective mitochondrial function, and increased tissue enzymes.[107] When rabbits were injected with methylprednisolone, elevations in 8-hydroxy-2′deoxyguanosine, a marker of DNA oxidative injury, were observed.[108-110] This coincided with the development of osteonecrosis. A polymorphism in nitric oxide synthase, described later, was also associated with the development of osteonecrosis. This relationship between osteonecrosis and oxidative injury leads one to wonder if corticosteroid-induced osteonecrosis can be prevented or lessened in severity by simultaneous or prophylactic administration of antioxidants.

Nitric Oxide Synthase and Osteonecrosis

Glucocorticoids can cause derangements in vascular responsiveness to vasoactive substances such as nitric oxide. Endothelial nitric oxide synthase (eNOS) stimulates the production of nitric oxide. Nitric oxide regulates vascular "tension" by acting as a vasodilator, inhibiting mononuclear adhesion to endothelial cells and preventing platelet aggregation. A defect in this activity can lead to increased vascular resistance and disruption to downstream blood flow, resulting in osteonecrosis.[111]

Multihit Hypothesis

Other proposed mechanisms involve endothelial cell injury,[112] abnormal angiogenesis and repair mechanisms,[113] the effects of vasoactive substances,[114] activity of hepatic cytochrome P450 3A4,[115] and intramedullary hemorrhage.[116] Multiple mechanisms may be simultaneously occurring. Kenzora was the first to introduce the concept of cumulative stress.[117] Corticosteroid-induced osteonecrosis seems to occur with greater frequency in patients who have significant underlying illness such as systemic lupus erythematosus[118] or transplantation and less frequently or never in patients who are not chronically ill but are on steroids for an acute event such as head injury. Recent observations that corticosteroids induce osteonecrosis in SARS patients further support the notion that more than one insult to the bone or surrounding tissue may be necessary to precipitate osteonecrosis. For each of the known associations of osteonecrosis, different mechanisms may predominate such as lipid anomalies and apoptosis of osteoblasts in steroid-induced osteonecrosis, as well as elevated intraosseous pressures and coagulation abnormalities in dysbaric osteonecrosis, but additional factors may be necessary to precipitate osteonecrosis. The accumulated cell stress theory suggests that when the damaging effects of multiple events are added together, the involved bone is unable to recover from the chronic stress and osteonecrosis ensues.

Genetic Considerations

The degree to which genetics and the environment play in the pathogenesis of osteonecrosis is the subject of an ongoing investigation. Certainly, single nucleotide polymorphisms have been noted in a number of genes that may be associated with osteonecrosis. It has been argued that endothelial nitric oxide synthase is an important player in the development of osteonecrosis. Nitric oxide may have beneficial effects on three systems involved in osteonecrosis, namely skeletal, vascular, and thrombotic. Each of these may be targets for proposed mechanisms of pathogenesis of osteonecrosis. A comparative analysis of the 26-base pair repeat polymorphism in intron 4 and the Glu298Asp polymorphism in exon 7 of the eNOS gene in patients with idiopathic, steroid-induced, alcohol-induced, and normal control subjects was performed.[119] The frequency of the homozygous 4a allele was found to be higher in patients with idiopathic osteonecrosis compared with control subjects. The frequency of the 4a/b allele was found to be higher in all types of osteonecrosis when compared with control subjects. The 4a allele is known to be associated with reduced synthesis of endothelial nitric oxide synthase, suggesting that nitric oxide may play a protective role against the development of osteonecrosis.

Forty-one percent of patients with osteonecrosis compared with only 20% of controls were homozygous for the 4G/4G mutation in the plasminogen activator inhibitor-1 gene.[120] This mutation causes increased hypofibrinolytic plasminogen activator inhibitor activity, resulting in decreased stimulated plasminogen activator activity. This observation lends support to the theory that procoagulants may play a significant role in the pathogenesis of osteonecrosis. A polymorphism in the plasminogen activator inihibitor-1 *(PAI-1)* gene has also been reported to be predictive of osteonecrosis in children with acute lymphoblastic leukemia.[121]

Genetic variations in type and levels of lipoprotein (a) have been linked to osteonecrosis. Apo(a) is involved in lipid metabolism and the coagulation systems, and the Apo(a) low-molecular-weight phenotype is associated with an increased risk of osteonecrosis.[122-124] Polymorphisms in the promoter for vascular endothelial growth factor (VEGF) and in the receptor for IL-23 were associated with osteonecrosis in the Korean population,[125,126] reflecting the significance of the association of osteonecrosis with vascular disorders and autoimmune diseases, respectively.

DIAGNOSIS

History and Physical Examination

The diagnosis of osteonecrosis is generally made by history because many patients may not present until they develop hip pain. By the time the patient is clinically symptomatic, the disease may be quite advanced. Therefore a high index of suspicion is necessary for all patients on oral or parenteral steroids. Information that should be elicited from a good history should include any history of trauma; underlying disease; alcohol use; tobacco use; current medications; past medications; history of joint anomalies; presence of pain or limitation of motion; involvement in sports, especially high-impact sports; occupational history; gestational history; and the presence of liver disease or lipid abnormalities.

A good physical examination includes palpating the hip for tenderness, identification of limp, masses, leg-length discrepancy, the presence of masses, abnormal gait, muscle strength, and range of motion.

The Harris hip score is frequently used for evaluation of hip function and is also useful in monitoring the effectiveness of treatment (Figure 103-2).[127-129] The Harris hip score is a multidimensional observational assessment based on eight items that address pain, walking function, daily activity, and range of motion. Scores range from 0 (maximum disability) to 100 (no disability).

Radiologic Imaging

When the diagnosis is suspected clinically, it can be confirmed by radiologic imaging studies. Earlier employed imaging techniques such as conventional radiography were inadequate in establishing the diagnosis because in the early stages of osteonecrosis radiographs may be completely normal. The earliest radiographic sign of osteonecrosis is the presence of a radiolucent crescent-shaped rim along the contour of the femoral head (crescent sign) (Figure 103-3). This appearance on radiographs is the result of structural collapse of a necrotic segment of subchondral trabecular bone. At this stage, the disease is already irreversible. Later, radiographs will begin to show sclerotic changes

Hip joint evaluation system				
Date of assessment:	**Name:**		**Medical record #:**	**DOB:**
Pain	**Distance walked**	**Activities — shoes, socks**	**Public transportation**	**Limp**
☐ Totally disabled, crippled, pain in bed, bedridden ☐ Marked pain, serious limitation of activities ☐ Moderate pain, tolerable but makes concessions to pain. Some limitation of ordinary activity or work. May require occasional pain medication stronger than aspirin ☐ Mild pain, no effect on average activities, rarely moderate pain with unusual activity, may take aspirin ☐ Slight pain, occasional, no compromise in activity ☐ None, or ignores it	☐ Bed and chair only ☐ Two or three blocks ☐ Six blocks ☐ Unlimited	☐ Unable to fit or tie ☐ With difficulty ☐ With ease	☐ Unable to use ☐ Able to use	☐ Severe or unable to walk ☐ Moderate ☐ Slight ☐ None
Support	**Stairs**	**Sitting**	**Limb-length discrepancy**	
☐ Two crutches or not able to walk ☐ Two canes ☐ One crutch ☐ Cane most of the time ☐ Cane for long walks ☐ None	☐ Unable to do stairs in any manner ☐ Normally using a railing ☐ Normally without using a railing	☐ Unable to sit comfortably on any chair ☐ On a high chair for 30 minutes ☐ Comfortably, ordinary chair for 1 hour	_____ cm	**Comments:**
Physician name: _____ Evaluator name: _____	**Motions**			
	Hip flexion: _____	Abduction: _____	Internal rotation: _____	
	Hip extension: _____	Adduction: _____	External rotation: _____	

Figure 103-2 Harris hip score.

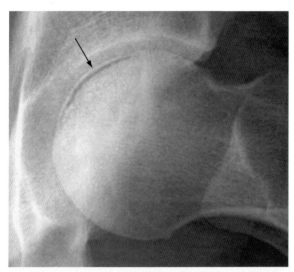

Figure 103-3 A radiolucent crescent in the subchondral region of the left femoral head *(arrow)* is an early radiographic sign of osteonecrosis.

(Figure 103-4). The appearance of radiographic "density" is secondary to compression of bone trabeculae after microfracture of the nonviable bone, calcification of detritic marrow, and repair of the necrotic area by deposition of new bone, the so-called *creeping substitution*. Flattening of the articular surface of bone is the sign of further bone collapse (Figure 103-5). To show best the radiographic appearance of osteonecrosis in the femoral head and better visualize the extent of the necrotic lesion, anteroposterior and frog-leg lateral films of the hip should be obtained.

Skeletal scintigraphy (radionuclide bone scan) using technetium-labeled diphosphonates has also been used to diagnose osteonecrosis. The use of this technique in the

early diagnosis of this condition depends on the fact that osteoblastic activity and blood flow are increased in the early stages of osteonecrosis. In an advanced stage of disease, the appearance may be one of increased activity in a subchondral distribution owing to osteoblastic activity at the reactive interface around the necrotic segment; however, the center of the osteonecrotic lesion may show much less radionuclide uptake (Figure 103-6) or even a complete lack of activity, reflecting decreased metabolism in the necrotic focus as a result of interruption of blood supply.[6]

In addition to bone scintigraphy, single-photon emission computed tomography (SPECT) maximizes sensitivity. A study comparing conventional radiography, MRI, computed tomography (CT), and Tc99m MDP three-phase bone scan in diagnosing bisphosphonate-associated osteonecrosis of the jaw showed that CT and MRI were the best at defining the extent of the disease, but that bone scan was the best at identifying disease at an early stage. Bone scan could be an excellent screening tool for the diagnosis of osteonecrosis before further characterization of the lesions using CT or MRI.[130]

CT allows more detailed examination of the femoral head. A star-shaped structure, formed by weight-bearing bone trabeculae, gives the appearance of an asterisk on CT scan (the asterisk sign).[131-133] This asterisk undergoes a characteristic change in ischemic bone necrosis of the femoral head, and this change was considered important for early detection of osteonecrosis. At a later stage, the collapse of necrotic bone can be well shown (Figure 103-7).

Currently, MRI is the "gold standard" for imaging of osteonecrosis. Most of the staging systems for osteonecrosis are now based on MRI appearance (Table 103-6). MRI of osteonecrosis can show changes earlier than conventional radiography or CT. It can also detect bone marrow edema,

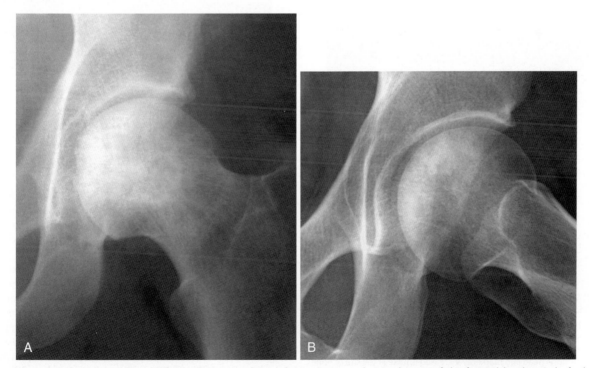

Figure 103-4 Anteroposterior **(A)** and frog-leg **(B)** views of the left hip showing sclerotic changes of the femoral head typical of advanced osteonecrosis.

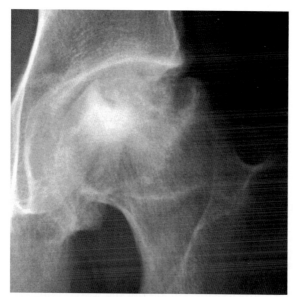

Figure 103-5   Increased density of the femoral head, loss of the normal spherical shape, and flattening of the superior aspect are characteristic radiographic features of osteonecrosis.

a feature sometimes seen in the early phases of osteonecrosis that is not visible on conventional radiography or CT.

The typical MRI findings in osteonecrosis are intermediate or low signal intensity on T1-weighted images and high signal intensity on T2-weighted images (Figure 103-8). As the disease progresses, the subchondral necrotic lesion is surrounded by a low signal line on T1-weighted images. A high signal line is seen on T2-weighted images, central to the low signal line. This produces the "double-line" sign (Figure 103-9). In advanced osteonecrosis, the necrotic segment exhibits low signal intensity on both T1-weighted

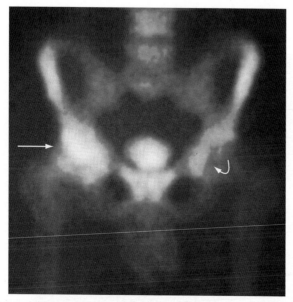

Figure 103-6   Bone scintigraphy of osteonecrosis of both femoral heads using Tc99m methylene diphosphonate showing moderate uptake of radiopharmceutical at the site of the ostenecrotic segment in the right femoral head and markedly increased uptake at the site of bone repair *(straight arrow).* The left femoral head *(curved arrow)* exhibits early-stage disease.

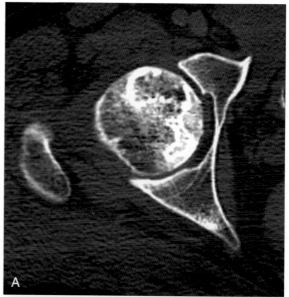

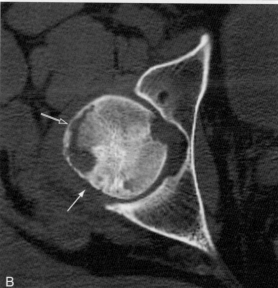

Figure 103-7   **A,** Computed tomography scan shows osteonecrosis of the femoral head. Although there are several sclerotic foci within the trabecular bone, the integrity of the osseous structures is preserved and the femoral head exhibits normal spherical shape. **B,** In more advanced stage of osteonecrosis of the femoral head, note increased sclerosis in the posterior aspect *(solid arrow)* and subchondral collapse of necrotic bone anterolaterally *(open arrow).*

and T2-weighted images (Figure 103-10). MRI is done in the sagittal, coronal, and axial planes and includes T1-weighted and T2-weighted sequences. There is excellent correlation between histologic findings and MRI appearance (see Table 103-6).

MRI is an important tool in determining the extent of femoral head involvement in osteonecrosis. Three techniques are used to evaluate this. The first is estimating head involvement. This method was first proposed by Steinberg and colleagues[134] in 1984, and it is defined by the appearance of abnormal signals on T1-weighted images. The degree of head involvement was classified into three categories: less than 15%, 15% to 30%, and greater than 30%. The second method used to evaluate extent is the index of

Table 103-6 Magnetic Resonance Imaging (MRI) Changes and Their Correlation with Histology in Osteonecrosis

Type of Appearance	Category of Observations	Histology	MRI Appearance
A	Fatlike	Premature fatty marrow development in the femoral neck or intertrochanteric region	Normal fat signal; Sclerotic margin may be seen circumscribing lesion
B	Bloodlike	Bone resorption; replacement by vascular granulation tissue	High signal intensity of inner border; low signal intensity of surrounding rim
C	Fluid-like	Bone marrow edema	Diffusely decreased signal on T1-weighted images; high signal on T2-weighted images
D	Fibrotic	Sclerosis owing to reinforcement of existing trabeculae at margin of live bone (repair tissue interface)	Decreased signal on T1-weighted and T2-weighted images

necrotic extent, which is determined by measuring the angle created by the extent of subchondral involvement. Lesion size was estimated using a "necrotic arc angle," defined by the angle of the arc of the necrotic segment from the center of the femoral head. Two angles are obtained: "A," representing the necrotic arc seen on midcoronal images, and "B," representing the necrotic arc angle seen on midsagittal images. The index is a compilation of these two angles. The third method is a variation of the second, in which the angle is identified not on midcoronal or midsagittal images but on the image that shows the maximum lesion size in the sagittal and coronal planes. It is thought that this method would correct for the underestimation that may be inherent in the second method.

Table 103-7 shows a comparison of various imaging techniques used in the diagnosis and staging of osteonecrosis. Hip arthroscopy is also used in the staging of osteonecrosis. In a study comparing radiography, MRI, and arthroscopy, there was only moderate correlation among the three methods. Arthroscopy was able to detect osteochondral degeneration, not detected by radiography or MRI in 36% of collapsed heads. Figure 103-11 is an algorithm for the diagnosis of osteonecrosis.

Markers of Disease

The ability to find consistent and reliable markers of disease is always a welcome tool, for diagnosis, determination of extent of the disease, or even determination of risk of acquiring the disease. The measurement of serum and urine carboxy-terminal cross-linking telopeptide of type I collagen (CTX-1), a marker of bone resorption, has been proposed as a method of evaluating the risk of osteonecrosis of the jaw secondary to bisphosphonate usage. Serum osteocalcin is another marker for bisphosphonate-related osteonecrosis of the jaw that has been suggested as a risk predictor because levels were significantly lower in the osteonecrosis group compared with a control group.[135]

TREATMENT

Surgical Treatment

Most cases of osteonecrosis ultimately require surgical intervention. There are various surgical techniques ranging from core decompression to total hip replacement. Sometimes surgical procedures can be used in conjunction with

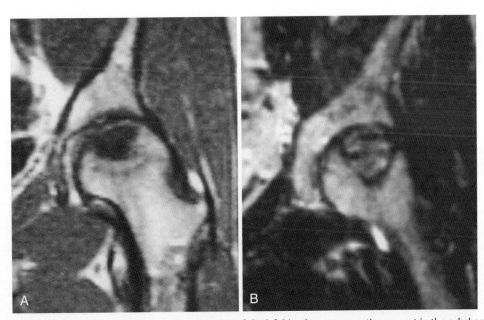

Figure 103-8 **A,** On T1-weighted coronal magnetic resonance image of the left hip, the osteonecrotic segment in the subchondral portion of the femoral head shows low signal intensity. **B,** On T2-weighted coronal image, the necrotic bone exhibits high signal intensity, surrounded by a sclerotic low-signal rim.

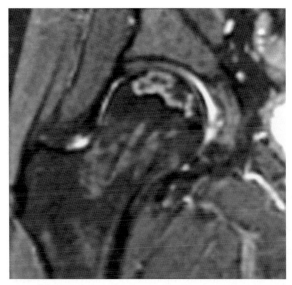

Figure 103-9 Coronal T2-weighted magnetic resonance image of the right femoral head shows the double-line sign, characteristic for osteonecrosis: low signal at periphery of the lesion and high signal band located more centrally.

nonsurgical approaches, as discussed later. The more advanced the disease, the more extensive the surgery.

The various surgical procedures used in the treatment of osteonecrosis include core decompression, structural bone grafting, vascularized fibula grafting, osteotomy, resurfacing arthroplasty, hemiarthroplasty, and total hip replacement. Table 103-8 shows the typical success rates for each of these procedures.

Arthroscopy is a valuable tool used in the treatment of osteonecrosis. It has been used to determine the position of the core decompression tract to the necrotic part of the femoral head, and arthroscopic débridement has been used in the treatment of osteonecrosis of the capitellum of the humerus in adolescents, Kienböck's disease, and osteonecrosis of the scaphoid.

Core decompression, which involves the removal of a core of bone from the femoral neck and head, is indicated in less advanced stages of osteonecrosis. The core acts as a vent to reduce intraosseous pressure and intramedullary pressure, reversing ischemia and improving symptoms. Other benefits of core decompression include stimulation of angiogenesis, which leads to improved vascularization during the repair process. The effectiveness of core decompression in the treatment of nontraumatic osteonecrosis was illustrated in 34 patients with 54 affected hips. Mean age at presentation was 38 years. The patients were monitored for a mean duration of 120 months postsurgery. Success was defined as absence of symptoms, no further progression of disease, and no further surgery. Clinical success was established in 26 hips (48%), and radiographic success was established in 20 hips (37%).

Computer-assisted core decompression has been used to provide greater precision in directing the core into the ischemic area and to minimize the duration of radiation exposure to patients.[136] Because early diagnosis improves outcome and there is a high incidence of developing osteonecrosis in a contralateral hip, core decompression is frequently done on both hips simultaneously. This approach adds little risk over unilateral core decompression with the benefit of better outcomes secondary to early surgical treatment of the contralateral hip.[137]

In structural bone grafting, or bone impaction grafting, the bone graft is inserted into the necrotic segment through the core tract. The bone graft acts in similar fashion to a stent, providing support to overlying subchondral bone. The goal is to prevent collapse. This combination of procedures is frequently used in treating stage 1 or 2 osteonecrotic femoral heads. Allogeneic and autologous bone grafts, mostly harvested from the tibia or fibula, are used. When this technique was attempted in patients with stages 3 and 4 lesions, the outcome was generally poor (100% failure

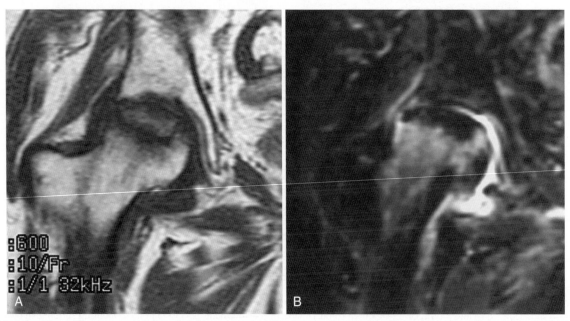

Figure 103-10 Advanced osteonecrosis of the right femoral head exhibits low signal intensity on T1-weighted **(A)** and T2-weighted **(B)** MR images.

Table 103-7 Comparative Sensitivity and Specificity of Diagnostic Radiologic Imaging Modalities in Osteonecrosis

Radiologic Imaging	Earliest Sign Seen	Histologic Correlation	Stage	Degree of Specificity
Conventional radiograph	Crescent sign	Sclerotic rim of reactive bone	2	High
Computed tomography scan	Asterisk sign	Sclerotic rim surrounding a mottled area of osteolysis and sclerosis	2	High
Magnetic resonance image	Low signal intensity on T1-weighted images; high signal intensity on T2-weighted images	Bone marrow edema	1	High
Skeletal scintigraphy	Decreased uptake in subchondral distribution, "cold" spot	Osteonecrosis	1	Low
	Increased uptake in subchondral distribution, "hot spot"	"Creeping substitution"	2	Low

after 2 to 4 years), with progression to collapse and further surgical procedures.[138]

Vascularized structural bone grafting also uses the core tract to insert a corticocancellous bone graft into the femoral neck and head along with its vascular pedicle. The vascular pedicle is anastomosed to a nearby vessel, adding a source of blood to the graft. The results of vascularized fibular grafting in the treatment of hips with osteonecrosis showed a survival of 61% of hips at 5-year follow-up and 42% at a median time of 8 years.[139] In another study, 197 patients with 226 osteonecrotic hips were treated with a combination of autologous cancellous bone impaction and pedicled iliac bone block transfer. The anastomosis was to the ascending branch of the lateral femoral circumflex artery. Fourteen hips required conversion to total hip arthroplasty because of collapse, severe pain, or both. Of the remaining

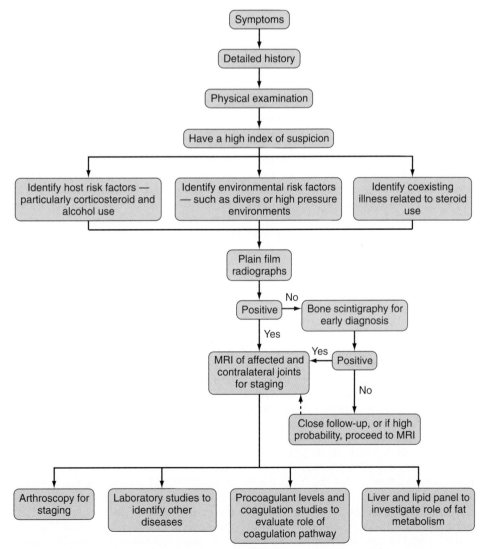

Figure 103-11 Diagnostic algorithm for osteonecrosis. MRI, magnetic resonance image.

Table 103-8   Surgical Treatment of Osteonecrosis

Surgical Procedure	Rationale	Stages of Osteonecrosis	Outcome	Comments
Core decompression	Reduction of intraosseous and intramedullary pressure	Early stages	37% radiographic success, 48% clinical success	Success rate depends on disease stage
Structural bone grafting	Provide support to overlying subchondral bone	1 or 2	Poor in advanced disease	100% failure rate in stages 3 and 4
Vascularized fibula grafting	Increase blood flow to graft	2 to 4	96% success in stage 2, 90% in stage 3, and 57% in stage 4	
Osteotomy	Shifting position of osteonecrotic segment out of weight-bearing region	2 and 3	Not available	
Resurfacing arthroplasty	Preservation of bone and joint mechanics with metallic or ceramic shell over femoral head	Later stages	Mean 7-year success rate is 90%	An alternative to total hip arthroscopy in later stages of disease
Hemiarthroplasty	Replacement of femoral head, preservation of anatomic acetabulum	Later stages	Failure rate for unilateral hemiarthroplasties is 50%-60% at 3 years, for bilateral hemarthroplasties is 44%	Various techniques available, some with better outcome
Total hip replacement	Complete replacement of the hip joint	Late stages	17.4% required revision after 10 years	Eventually most patients will require multiple hip replacements

212 hips, 92% were considered a clinical success and 76% were considered radiographically successful. The success rate declined from stage 2 to stage 4 hips (96% for stage 2 hips, 90% for stage 3 hips, and 57% for stage 4 hips).[140] Free vascularized fibula grafting has been compared favorably with other modes of surgical treatment.[141]

Osteotomy of the femur involves shifting the position of the osteonecrotic segment by making a cut in the proximal femur so that the osteonecrotic segment is rotated or flexed out of the weight-bearing region of the acetabulum and replacing the weight-bearing region with viable bone. Healing of the necrotic region can proceed without the stress of weight bearing. Several different osteotomy techniques have been attempted to salvage hips in stage 2 or 3 osteonecrosis.

Resurfacing arthroplasty uses a metallic or ceramic shell placed over a femoral head that has been débrided of the necrotic area. The potential advantages of resurfacing arthroplasty include preservation of joint mechanics, bone conservation,[142] more physiologic loading of the bone, a lower incidence of perioperative complications, and easier conversion to total hip arthroplasty in case of failure.[143] Complications of this procedure include femoral neck fractures, a secondary osteonecrosis when the procedure is done for other reasons,[144] and increased metal ion levels.[145] Resurfacing arthroplasty has been recommended for patients with later-stage osteonecrosis including those with femoral head collapse.[146] A retrospective study compared the results of limited femoral head resurfacing and total hip arthroplasty in 30 consecutive patients with Steinberg stage 3 or 4 disease. The survival rate at a 7-year mean follow-up period for the resurfacing group was 90%, whereas the survival rate at a mean 8-year follow-up for the total hip arthroplasty group was 93%.[147] A recent level 3 therapeutic study showed that hip resurfacing success rates at a 5-year follow-up were comparable with those of total hip arthroplasty in osteonecrosis patients younger than 25 years of age.[148]

In hemiarthroplasty, only part of the hip joint is replaced. The original acetabulum is preserved, but the femoral head is replaced with a prosthesis. Two kinds of prostheses are used—a unipolar prosthesis and a bipolar prosthesis. In a unipolar prosthesis, the articulation is between the artificial femoral head and the acetabulum. In the bipolar prosthesis, presently the most frequently used, the articulation is within the prosthesis itself. Failure rates for hemiarthroplasties in osteonecrosis are 50% to 60% at 3 years for unipolar prostheses and 44% for bipolar prostheses. Another study evaluated the success rate of Charnley/Bicentric hemiarthroplasty in the treatment of Ficat and Arlet stage 3 osteonecrosis of the femoral head. Failures include three hips that needed to be revised to cementless total hip replacement, two hips with radiographic changes of loosening and imminent failure, and one hip with progressive loss of joint space and secondary degenerative changes. The success rate was 84.2% after a mean of 56 months.

Total hip arthroplasty is complete replacement of the hip joint with a prosthesis including the femoral head and the acetabulum. In a study of 55 consecutive hip arthroplasty procedures, cementless total hip arthroplasty was shown to provide favorable results in advanced-stage osteonecrosis of the femoral head. Although 10 of the 48 hips available for follow-up after a minimum of 5 years required revision, all of these patients had Ficat and Arlet stage 3 or 4 disease. A study of 53 hips in 41 patients treated with cemented total hip replacement showed that at a minimum of 10 years of follow-up, 17.4% required revision. Compared with cemented total hip replacements done for other conditions, osteonecrosis had a greater risk for loosening of acetabular and femoral components. A survivorship analysis of cemented total hip replacements in renal transplant patients with osteonecrosis of the femoral head showed that there was excellent survival after 10 years (98.8%). After 20 years, the survival rate decreased to 63.8%.

In osteonecrosis of the jaw, the most common surgical procedure is resection of the affected bone.[149] Conservative treatment has also been used but carries a higher recurrence rate. A larger extent of surgical excision and a higher number of surgical débridements were associated with a lower recurrence rate. Other modes of surgical therapy for osteonecrosis of the jaw include bone-contouring procedures; fluorescence-guided bone-contouring procedures[150]; and segmental osteotomies, but these are generally reserved for more severe cases. Nonsurgical treatment including hyperbaric oxygen therapy[151] and low-intensity laser therapy are controversial but have been used to treat osteonecrosis of the jaw.

Nonsurgical Approaches

The key to the successful treatment of osteonecrosis is early detection. The choice of conservative nonsurgical versus more aggressive surgical options depends on the clinical and pathologic staging of the disease. Figure 103-12 is an algorithm for the treatment of osteonecrosis.

Nonsurgical treatment of osteonecrosis of the femoral head includes refraining from weight bearing on the affected joint, analgesic and anti-inflammatory medications, and physiotherapy. Conservative medical treatment is effective only in the early stages for symptomatic relief. Nonsurgical

management does not seem to alter the natural course of the disease. Electrical stimulation has been used in the treatment of osteonecrosis, in conjunction with core decompression. Electrical stimulation enhances osteogenesis and neovascularization. It also alters the balance between osteoblast and osteoclast activity, resulting in increased bone deposition and decreased bone resorption. Delivery of electrical stimulation can be done by direct current (DC), pulsed electromagnetic field, and capacitance coupling. The success of electrical stimulation in the treatment of osteonecrosis has been rather mediocre. Eleven hips in eight patients with Ficat stage 2 osteonecrosis who underwent core decompression and placement of an electric stimulating coil within the core in the anterosuperior segment of the femoral head were studied. Of these, five hips required reoperation and six hips had progressive deterioration 13 months after initial placement of the coil. In addition, there was little histologic evidence that the coil did indeed generate new bone deposition around itself.

On the other hand, a study compared the effectiveness of conservative nonsurgical treatment with core decompression with or without direct current electrical stimulation. The clinical symptom scores and the rate of progression to arthroplasty were best in the group with core decompression

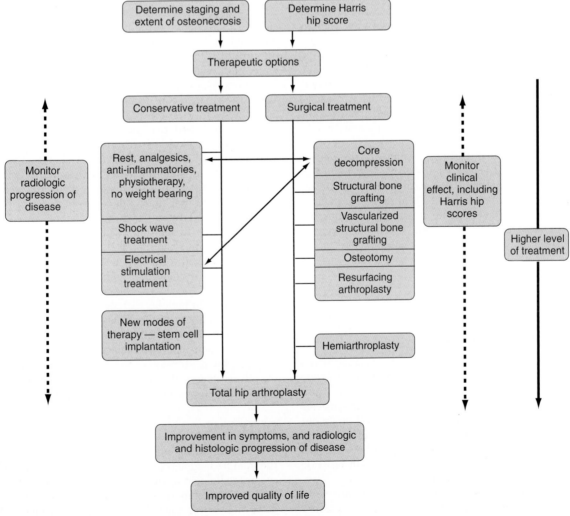

Figure 103-12 Treatment algorithm for osteonecrosis.

and DC electrical stimulation and worst in the nonoperative group. Capacitive coupling can be done with or without core decompression and grafting. Core decompression and grafting were done on 40 patients with stage 1 to 3 osteonecrosis; half of the patients wore active capacitive coupling units with electrodes over the femoral head for 6 months. The control group was 55 patients with osteonecrosis who were treated conservatively. Two- and 4-year follow-up showed that core decompression with or without capacitive coupling provided better clinical and radiologic outcome than conservative treatment. Capacitive coupling did not improve the results further when used with core decompression and grafting.

Extracorporeal shock wave therapy has been used in the treatment of osteonecrosis of the femoral head. A study of 48 patients and 57 hips compared extracorporeal shock wave therapy with core decompression and bone grafting. Twenty-three patients with 29 affected hips were assigned to the shock wave group, and the remaining patients and hips received surgical treatment. The patients in the shock wave group were given treatment of 6000 pulses of shock waves at 28 kV to the affected hip. The patients were evaluated radiographically and by their reports of symptoms (pain), Harris hip scores, and quality of life (daily work activity assessment). Shock wave therapy produced better results than the nonvascularized bone grafting procedure, with comparatively less progression of disease. In 35 patients with 47 osteonecrotic hips, the use of shock wave therapy led to improvements in serum nitric oxide levels, angiogenic factors such as VEGF, and osteogenic factors such as bone morphogenetic protein-2 (BMP-2) and osteocalcin. Levels of inflammatory markers were reduced. It is interesting to note that although these changes did not persist beyond several months, the clinical and radiographic improvement, present in 83% of hips, was present after 12 months.[152]

Conservative treatment of osteonecrosis of the talus is not promising, and the affected ankles generally continue to progress, requiring either core decompression or arthrodesis. Conservative treatment of bisphosphonate-induced osteonecrosis of the jaw includes cessation of bisphosphonate usage or surgical débridement. Good oral hygiene, regular dental assessment, and avoidance of dental procedures during bisphosphonate usage can prevent onset of osteonecrosis.

RECENT DEVELOPMENTS

Prevention versus Treatment

A recent study evaluated the role of antioxidants in the treatment of osteonecrosis. Japanese white rabbits were divided into two groups and fed either a normal diet or a normal diet supplemented with α-tocopherol. Osteonecrosis developed in 14 of 20 rabbits in the control group but only in 5 of 21 rabbits in the experimental group. This suggests that oxidative stress may play a role in the pathogenesis of osteonecrosis and that there may potentially be a role for antioxidants such as vitamin E.[153]

A group of researchers studied the use of adrenocorticotropic hormone (ACTH) in rabbits to prevent corticosteroid-induced osteonecrosis and found that if ACTH is administered along with depot methylprednisolone acetate (DepoMedrol), osteonecrosis is reduced. The authors of this study believe that ACTH enhances osteoblast support and stimulates the production of vascular endothelial growth factor (VEGF), which stimulates the generation of new blood vessels. The result is an increase in blood flow to the vulnerable areas of bone, preventing cell death and reducing the likelihood of osteonecrosis.[154]

Mesenchymal Stem Cells

Corticosteroids interfere with the balance of adipogenesis and osteogenesis in the differentiation of mesenchymal stem cells. Corticosteroids shunt uncommitted osteoprogenitor cells in the bone marrow into the adipocytic pathway, leading to reduced osteoblast formation. Corticosteroids have also been shown to reduce vascular endothelial growth factor, which leads to a reduction in new blood vessel formation and potentially can lead to bone death. Alcohol has a similar effect on the differentiation of progenitor cells.

The balance between adipogenesis and osteogenesis has been targeted as a potential site for the treatment of osteonecrosis. Multipotential mesenchymal stem cells from femoral bone marrow near osteonecrosis sites are able to express messenger RNA aggrecan and type II collagen. Both are deposited into the bone matrix. These features are characteristic of chondrogenic differentiation. The mesenchymal stem cells can be differentiated into osteocytic lineage in vitro.

A pilot study evaluating the effectiveness of implantation of autologous bone marrow cells in the treatment of osteonecrosis used core decompression to implant stem cells into the necrotic lesions of the femoral head. The patients were divided into two groups—one that received core decompression alone as treatment for osteonecrosis (the control group) and one that received autologous bone marrow cell implantation along with core decompression (the treatment group). The patients were followed for 24 months, and at that time, 5 of 8 hips in the control group, but only 1 of 10 in the treatment group, advanced to stage 3 osteonecrosis. In addition, there was greater improvement in pain and joint symptoms in the treatment group and the treatment seemed to be safe. Because of the small number of patients involved, further studies are necessary to confirm these results.

Twenty-eight patients with 44 necrotic hips were treated with percutaneous decompression and autologous bone marrow mononuclear cell infusion. Patients were followed for a minimum of 2 years and evaluated for clinical and radiographic progression of the disease. There seemed to be overall slowing in the progression of the disease stage. The mean Harris hip score improved from 58 to 86.

OUTCOME

The natural history of osteonecrosis depends on the size of the infarcted segment, the site of occurrence, and the clinical and radiologic staging of the disease. At the onset of the disease, range of motion may be well preserved but gradually deteriorates over time. In the early stages of the disease, when it is still reversible, patients may be asymptomatic.

Many patients therefore present with advanced disease. Although spontaneous resolution of femoral head osteonecrosis can occur, it is rare and occurs only when lesion size is small. A study of the prognosis of osteonecrosis of the femoral head as a function of symptoms (pain) and radiographic findings showed that in patients who were asymptomatic and had normal radiographs, progression of the disease was slow, with only 1 of 23 hips progressing to pain and radiographic changes after 5 years. If radiographic changes are already present, disease progresses to pain in 14 of 19 patients after 5 years. In a study of stage 1 osteonecrotic lesions of the hip diagnosed with MRI, 40 patients were followed for an average of 11 years. All patients had stage 1 lesions on the contralateral hip. Overall, 35 of the 40 stage 1 hips became symptomatic and 29 hips showed collapse. The mean interval between diagnosis and collapse was 92 months, whereas the mean interval between symptoms and diagnosis was 80 months. Most stage 1 hips eventually progress to a more advanced stage, requiring surgery, so these hips should be monitored closely.

SUMMARY

Osteonecrosis is a potentially debilitating condition with significant morbidity despite medical interventions or surgery. Corticosteroids are the most common cause of osteonecrosis, and corticosteroid-induced osteonecrosis can be reproduced in animal models. The pathogenesis of osteonecrosis is multifaceted and still not completely understood. Why is it that corticosteroid-induced osteonecrosis is more common in patients with certain underlying diseases and not in others? Is there a genetic basis for osteonecrosis? Common pathogenic mechanisms known to be involved in osteonecrosis include osteoblast/osteoclast survival and apoptosis, lipid metabolism, and coagulation abnormalities. However, it is still unclear how these mechanisms interrelate with each other. In order to better appreciate the risk factors involved in osteonecrosis, a more complete understanding of the pathogenesis is necessary. Until then, the physician should always maintain a high index of suspicion for osteonecrosis whenever known risk factors are present, especially use of corticosteroids and alcohol.

Selected References

1. McCarthy EF: Aseptic necrosis of bone. An historic perspective, *Clin Orthop Relat Res* 168:216–221, 1982.
2. Nixon JE: Avascular necrosis of bone: a review, *J R Soc Med* 76:681–692, 1983.
3. Axhausen G: Uber anamische Infarkte am Knochensystem und ihre Bedeutung fur die Lehre von den primaren Epiphyseonkrosen, *Arch Klin Chir* 151:72–98, 1928.
4. Hutter CD: Dysbaric osteonecrosis: a reassessment and hypothesis, *Med Hypotheses* 54:585–590, 2000.
5. Assouline-Dayan Y, Chang C, Greenspan A, et al: Pathogenesis and natural history of osteonecrosis, *Semin Arthritis Rheum* 32:94–124, 2002.
6. Chang CC, Greenspan A, Gershwin ME: Osteonecrosis: current perspectives on pathogenesis and treatment, *Semin Arthritis Rheum* 23:47–69, 1993.
7. Sevitt S: Avascular necrosis and revascularisation of the femoral head after intracapsular fractures; a combined arteriographic and histological necropsy study, *J Bone Joint Surg Br* 46:270–296, 1964.
8. Mankin HJ: Nontraumatic necrosis of bone (osteonecrosis), *N Engl J Med* 326:1473–1479, 1992.

9. D'Aubigne RM, Frain PG: Theory of osteotomies, *Rev Chir Orthop Reparatrice Appar Mot* 58:159–167, 1972.
10. Peitrogrande V, Mastromarino, R: Osteopatia de prolongato trattamento cortisono, *Ortop Traumatol* 25:793, 1957.
11. Koo KH, Kim R, Kim YS, et al: Risk period for developing osteonecrosis of the femoral head in patients on steroid treatment, *Clin Rheumatol* 21:299–303, 2002.
12. Hurel SJ, Kendall-Taylor P: Avascular necrosis secondary to postoperative steroid therapy, *Br J Neurosurg* 11:356–358, 1997.
13. Gogas H, Fennelly D: Avascular necrosis following extensive chemotherapy and dexamethasone treatment in a patient with advanced ovarian cancer: case report and review of the literature, *Gynecol Oncol* 63:379–381, 1996.
14. Powell C, Chang C, Naguwa SM, et al: Steroid induced osteonecrosis: an analysis of steroid dosing risk, *Autoimmun Rev* 9:721–743, 2010.
15. Vreden SG, Hermus AR, van Liessum PA, et al: Aseptic bone necrosis in patients on glucocorticoid replacement therapy, *Neth J Med* 39:153–157, 1991.
16. Haajanen J, Saarinen O, Laasonen L, et al: Steroid treatment and aseptic necrosis of the femoral head in renal transplant recipients, *Transplant Proc* 16:1316–1319, 1984.
17. Chandler GN, Jones DT, Wright V, Hartfall SJ: Charcot's arthropathy following intra-articular hydrocortisone, *Br Med J* 1:952–953, 1959.
18. Ruggiero SL: Bisphosphonate-related osteonecrosis of the jaw: an overview, *Ann N Y Acad Sci* 1218:38–46, 2011.
21. Matsuo K, Hirohata T, Sugioka Y, et al: Influence of alcohol intake, cigarette smoking, and occupational status on idiopathic osteonecrosis of the femoral head, *Clin Orthop Relat Res* 234:115–123, 1988.
23. Axhausen G: Die Nekrose des proximalen Bruckstuckes beim Schenkelhals bruck und ihre Bedeutung fur das Huftgelenk, *Arch Klin Chir* 120:325–346, 1922.
24. Antti-Poika I, Karaharju E, Vankka E, Paavilainen T: Alcohol-associated femoral head necrosis, *Ann Chir Gynaecol* 76:318–322, 1987.
25. Orlic D, Jovanovic S, Anticevic D, Zecevic J: Frequency of idiopathic aseptic necrosis in medically treated alcoholics, *Int Orthop* 14:383–386, 1990.
26. Calve J: Sur une forme particuliere de pseudocoxalgie greffee sur des deformations caracteristiques de l'extremite superieure du femur, *Rev Chir* 30:48–54, 1910.
29. Bentzon P: Experimental studies on the pathogenesis of coxa plana (Calve-Legg-Perthes-Waldenstrom's disease) and other maniestations of "local dyschondroplasia", *Acad Radiol* 6:155–172, 1926.
31. Goff CW: Legg-Calve-Perthes syndrome (LCPS). An up-to-date critical review, *Clin Orthop* 22:93–107, 1962.
32. Landin LA, Danielsson LG, Wattsgard C: Transient synovitis of the hip. Its incidence, epidemiology and relation to Perthes' disease, *J Bone Joint Surg Br* 69:238–242, 1987.
33. Burwell RG, Dangerfield PH, Hall DJ, et al: Perthes' disease. An anthropometric study revealing impaired and disproportionate growth, *J Bone Joint Surg Br* 60-B:461–477, 1978.
35. Kristmundsdottir F, Burwell RG, Harrison MH: Delayed skeletal maturation in Perthes' disease, *Acta Orthop Scand* 58:277–279, 1987.
36. Hall DJ, Harrison MH, Burwell RG: Congenital abnormalities and Perthes' disease. Clinical evidence that children with Perthes' disease may have a major congenital defect, *J Bone Joint Surg Br* 61:18–25, 1979.
37. Burwell RG, Vernon CL, Dangerfield PH, et al: Raised somatomedin activity in the serum of young boys with Perthes' disease revealed by bioassay. A disease of growth transition? *Clin Orthop Relat Res* 209:129–138, 1986.
38. Rayner PH, Schwalbe SL, Hall DJ: An assessment of endocrine function in boys with Perthes' disease, *Clin Orthop Relat Res* 209:124–128, 1986.
39. Barr RD, Sala A: Osteonecrosis in children and adolescents with cancer, *Pediatr Blood Cancer* 50:483–485; discussion 6, 2008.
41. Niinimaki RA, Harila-Saari AH, Jartti AE, et al: High body mass index increases the risk for osteonecrosis in children with acute lymphoblastic leukemia, *J Clin Oncol* 25:1498–1504, 2007.
42. Montella BJ, Nunley JA, Urbaniak JR: Osteonecrosis of the femoral head associated with pregnancy. A preliminary report, *J Bone Joint Surg Am* 81:790–798, 1999.

43. Hernigou P, Allain J, Bachir D, Galacteros F: Abnormalities of the adult shoulder due to sickle cell osteonecrosis during childhood, *Rev Rhum Engl Ed* 65:27–32, 1998.

44. Hernigou P, Galacteros F, Bachir D, Goutallier D: Deformities of the hip in adults who have sickle-cell disease and had avascular necrosis in childhood. A natural history of fifty-two patients, *J Bone Joint Surg Am* 73:81–92, 1991.

45. Kandzierski G, Gregosiewicz A, Malek U, et al: Femur head necrosis in haemophilia and after prolonged steroid therapy–description of two cases, *Chir Narzadow Ruchu Ortop Pol* 69:269–271, 2004.

51. Twynham G: A case of Caisson disease, *BMJ* 1:190–191, 1888.

52. Davidson JK: Dysbaric disorders: aseptic bone necrosis in tunnel workers and divers, *Baillieres Clin Rheumatol* 3:1–23, 1989.

53. Chan MH, Chan PK, Griffith JF, et al: Steroid-induced osteonecrosis in severe acute respiratory syndrome: a retrospective analysis of biochemical markers of bone metabolism and corticosteroid therapy, *Pathology* 38:229–235, 2006.

54. Lv H, de Vlas SJ, Liu W, et al: Avascular osteonecrosis after treatment of SARS: a 3-year longitudinal study, *Trop Med Int Health* 14(Suppl 1):79–84, 2009.

55. Chan CW, Chiu WK, Chan CC, et al: Osteonecrosis in children with severe acute respiratory syndrome, *Pediatr Infect Dis J* 23:888–890, 2004.

56. Cushner MA, Friedman RJ: Osteonecrosis of the humeral head, *J Am Acad Orthop Surg* 5:339–346, 1997.

60. Baumgarten KM, Mont MA, Rifai A, Hungerford DS: Atraumatic osteonecrosis of the patella, *Clin Orthop Relat Res* 383:191–196, 2001.

61. Berger CE, Kroner A, Kristen KH, et al: Spontaneous osteonecrosis of the knee: biochemical markers of bone turnover and pathohistology, *Osteoarthritis Cartil* 13:716–721, 2005.

62. Kusayama T: Idiopathic osteonecrosis of the femoral condyle after meniscectomy, *Tokai J Exp Clin Med* 28:145–150, 2003.

67. Delanois RE, Mont MA, Yoon TR, et al: Atraumatic osteonecrosis of the talus, *J Bone Joint Surg Am* 80:529–536, 1998.

68. Hirohata S, Ito K: Aseptic necrosis of unilateral scaphoid bone in systemic lupus erythematosus, *Intern Med* 31:794–797, 1992.

71. Sigmundsson FG, Andersen PB, Schroeder HD, Thomsen K: Vertebral osteonecrosis associated with pancreatitis in a woman with pancreas divisum. A case report, *J Bone Joint Surg Am* 86-A:2504–2508, 2004.

75. Van Poznak C: Osteonecrosis of the jaw, *J Oncol Pract* 2:3–4, 2006.

76. Pathak I, Bryce G: Temporal bone necrosis: diagnosis, classification, and management, *Otolaryngol Head Neck Surg* 123:252–257, 2000.

77. Stavinoha RR, Scott W: Osteonecrosis of the tarsal navicular in two adolescent soccer players, *Clin J Sport Med* 8:136–138, 1998.

78. Moorman CT 3rd, Warren RF, Hershman EB, et al: Traumatic posterior hip subluxation in American football, *J Bone Joint Surg Am* 85-A:1190–1196, 2003.

79. Gardeniers J: ARCO international classification of osteonecrosis, *ARCO Newsletter* 5:79, 1993.

80. Sugano N, Atsumi T, Ohzono K, et al: The 2001 revised criteria for diagnosis, classification, and staging of idiopathic osteonecrosis of the femoral head, *J Orthop Sci* 7:601–605, 2002.

81. Schapira D: Transient osteoporosis of the hip, *Semin Arthritis Rheum* 22:98–105, 1992.

82. Plenk H Jr, Hofmann S, Eschberger J, et al: Histomorphology and bone morphometry of the bone marrow edema syndrome of the hip, *Clin Orthop Relat Res* 334:73–84, 1997.

83. Berger CE, Kroner AH, Kristen KH, et al: Transient bone marrow edema syndrome of the knee: clinical and magnetic resonance imaging results at 5 years after core decompression, *Arthroscopy* 22:866–871, 2006.

84. Glimcher MJ, Kenzora JE: The biology of osteonecrosis of the human femoral head and its clinical implications: II. The pathological changes in the femoral head as an organ and in the hip joint, *Clin Orthop Relat Res* 140:273–312, 1979.

85. Chandler FA: Coronary disease of the hip, *J Int Coll Surg* 11:34–36, 1948.

87. Heikkinen ES, Puranen J, Suramo I: The effect of intertrochanteric osteotomy on the venous drainage of the femoral neck in Perthes' disease, *Acta Orthop Scand* 47:89–95, 1976.

88. Liu SL, Ho TC: The role of venous hypertension in the pathogenesis of Legg-Perthes disease. A clinical and experimental study, *J Bone Joint Surg Am* 73:194–200, 1991.

89. Thompson GH, Salter RB: Legg-Calve-Perthes disease. Current concepts and controversies, *Orthop Clin North Am* 18:617–635, 1987.

90. Chryssanthou CP: Dysbaric osteonecrosis. Etiological and pathogenetic concepts, *Clin Orthop Relat Res* 130:94–106, 1978.

91. Lehner CE, Adams WM, Dubielzig RR, et al: Dysbaric osteonecrosis in divers and caisson workers. An animal model, *Clin Orthop Relat Res* 344:320–332, 1997.

92. Ohzono K, Takaoka K, Saito S, et al: Intraosseous arterial architecture in nontraumatic avascular necrosis of the femoral head. Microangiographic and histologic study, *Clin Orthop Relat Res* 277:79–88, 1992.

93. Suh KT, Kim SW, Roh HL, et al: Decreased osteogenic differentiation of mesenchymal stem cells in alcohol-induced osteonecrosis, *Clin Orthop Relat Res* 431:220–225, 2005.

94. Lee JS, Roh HL, Kim CH, et al: Alterations in the differentiation ability of mesenchymal stem cells in patients with nontraumatic osteonecrosis of the femoral head: comparative analysis according to the risk factor, *J Orthop Res* 24:604–609, 2006.

95. Gangji V, Hauzeur JP, Schoutens A, et al: Abnormalities in the replicative capacity of osteoblastic cells in the proximal femur of patients with osteonecrosis of the femoral head, *J Rheumatol* 30:348–351, 2003.

96. Weinstein RS, Nicholas RW, Manolagas SC: Apoptosis of osteocytes in glucocorticoid-induced osteonecrosis of the hip, *J Clin Endocrinol Metab* 85:2907–2912, 2000.

97. Sato M, Sugano N, Ohzono K, et al: Apoptosis and expression of stress protein (ORP150, HO1) during development of ischaemic osteonecrosis in the rat, *J Bone Joint Surg Br* 83:751–759, 2001.

98. Cui Q, Wang GJ, Balian G: Steroid-induced adipogenesis in a pluripotential cell line from bone marrow, *J Bone Joint Surg Am* 79:1054–1063, 1997.

99. Wang GJ, Cui Q, Balian G: The Nicolas Andry award. The pathogenesis and prevention of steroid-induced osteonecrosis, *Clin Orthop Relat Res* 370:295–310, 2000.

100. Yin L, Li YB, Wang YS: Dexamethasone-induced adipogenesis in primary marrow stromal cell cultures: mechanism of steroid-induced osteonecrosis, *Chin Med J (Engl)* 119:581–588, 2006.

101. Miyanishi K, Yamamoto T, Irisa T, et al: Bone marrow fat cell enlargement and a rise in intraosseous pressure in steroid-treated rabbits with osteonecrosis, *Bone* 30:185–190, 2002.

102. Kim YH, Kim JS: Histologic analysis of acetabular and proximal femoral bone in patients with osteonecrosis of the femoral head, *J Bone Joint Surg Am* 86-A:2471–2474, 2004.

103. Jones JP Jr: Intravascular coagulation and osteonecrosis, *Clin Orthop Relat Res* 277:41–53, 1992.

104. Jones LC, Mont MA, Le TB, et al: Procoagulants and osteonecrosis, *J Rheumatol* 30:783–791, 2003.

105. Sun W, Wang BL, Liu BL, et al: Osteonecrosis in patients after severe acute respiratory syndrome (SARS): possible role of anticardiolipin antibodies, *J Clin Rheumatol* 16:61–63, 2010.

107. Preedy VR, Patel VB, Reilly ME, et al: Oxidants, antioxidants and alcohol: implications for skeletal and cardiac muscle, *Front Biosci* 4:e58–66, 1999.

108. Ichiseki T, Matsumoto T: Oxidative stress may underlie the sex differences seen in steroid-induced osteonecrosis models, *Med Hypotheses* 66:1256, 2006.

111. Kerachian MA, Seguin C, Harvey EJ: Glucocorticoids in osteonecrosis of the femoral head: a new understanding of the mechanisms of action, *J Steroid Biochem Mol Biol* 114:121–128, 2009.

112. Kerachian MA, Harvey EJ, Cournoyer D, et al: Avascular necrosis of the femoral head: vascular hypotheses, *Endothelium* 13:237–244, 2006.

113. Feng Y, Yang SH, Xiao BJ, et al: Decreased in the number and function of circulation endothelial progenitor cells in patients with avascular necrosis of the femoral head, *Bone* 46:32–40, 2009.

114. Jones JP Jr, Ramirez S, Doty SB: The pathophysiologic role of fat in dysbaric osteonecrosis, *Clin Orthop Relat Res* 296:256–264, 1993.

115. Tokuhara Y, Wakitani S, Oda Y, et al: Low levels of steroid-metabolizing hepatic enzyme (cytochrome P450 3A) activity may elevate responsiveness to steroids and may increase risk of steroid-induced osteonecrosis even with low glucocorticoid dose, *J Orthop Sci* 14:794–800, 2009.

116. Saito S, Ohzono K, Ono K: Early arteriopathy and postulated pathogenesis of osteonecrosis of the femoral head. The intracapital arterioles, *Clin Orthop Relat Res* 277:98–110, 1992.

117. Kenzora JE, Glimcher MJ: Accumulative cell stress: the multifactorial etiology of idiopathic osteonecrosis, *Orthop Clin North Am* 16:669–679, 1985.

118. Zizic TM, Marcoux C, Hungerford DS, et al: Corticosteroid therapy associated with ischemic necrosis of bone in systemic lupus erythematosus, *Am J Med* 79:596–604, 1985.

119. Koo KH, Lee JS, Lee YJ, et al: Endothelial nitric oxide synthase gene polymorphisms in patients with nontraumatic femoral head osteonecrosis, *J Orthop Res* 24:1722–1728, 2006.

120. Glueck CJ, Fontaine RN, Gruppo R, et al: The plasminogen activator inhibitor-1 gene, hypofibrinolysis, and osteonecrosis, *Clin Orthop Relat Res* 366:133–146, 1999.

121. French D, Hamilton LH, Mattano LA Jr, et al: A PAI-1 (SERPINE1) polymorphism predicts osteonecrosis in children with acute lymphoblastic leukemia: a report from the Children's Oncology Group, *Blood* 111:4496–4499, 2008.

122. Hirata T, Fujioka M, Takahashi KA, et al: ApoB C7623T polymorphism predicts risk for steroid-induced osteonecrosis of the femoral head after renal transplantation, *J Orthop Sci* 12:199–206, 2007.

123. Hirata T, Fujioka M, Takahashi KA, et al: Low molecular weight phenotype of Apo(a) is a risk factor of corticosteroid-induced osteonecrosis of the femoral head after renal transplant, *J Rheumatol* 34:516–522, 2007.

124. Wang XY, Niu XH, Chen WH, et al: [Effects of apolipoprotein A1 and B gene polymorphism on avascular necrosis of the femoral head in Chinese population], *Zhongguo Gu Shang* 21:99–102, 2008.

125. Kim TH, Hong JM, Lee JY, et al: Promoter polymorphisms of the vascular endothelial growth factor gene is associated with an osteonecrosis of the femoral head in the Korean population, *Osteoarthritis Cartil* 16:287–291, 2008.

129. Soderman P, Malchau H: Is the Harris hip score system useful to study the outcome of total hip replacement? *Clin Orthop Relat Res* 384:189–197, 2001.

130. Chiandussi S, Biasotto M, Dore F, et al: Clinical and diagnostic imaging of bisphosphonate-associated osteonecrosis of the jaws, *Dentomaxillofac Radiol* 35:236–243, 2006.

131. Dihlmann W: CT analysis of the upper end of the femur: the asterisk sign and ischaemic bone necrosis of the femoral head, *Skeletal Radiol* 8:251–258, 1982.

134. Steinberg ME, Hayken GD, Steinberg DR: A new method for evaluaton and staging of avascular necrosis of the femoral head. In Arlet J, Ficat RP, Hungerford DS, editors: *Bone circulation.* Baltimore, 1984, Williams & Wilkins, pp 398–403.

135. Kwon YD, Ohe JY, Kim DY, et al: Retrospective study of two biochemical markers for the risk assessment of oral bisphosphonate-related osteonecrosis of the jaws: can they be utilized as risk markers? *Clin Oral Implants Res* 22:100–105, 2011.

136. Beckmann J, Goetz J, Baethis H, et al: Precision of computer-assisted core decompression drilling of the femoral head, *Arch Orthop Trauma Surg* 126:374–379, 2006.

137. Israelite C, Nelson CL, Ziarani CF, et al: Bilateral core decompression for osteonecrosis of the femoral head, *Clin Orthop Relat Res* 441:285–290, 2005.

138. Marcus ND, Enneking WF, Massam RA: The silent hip in idiopathic aseptic necrosis. Treatment by bone-grafting, *J Bone Joint Surg Am* 55:1351–1366, 1973.

139. Marciniak D, Furey C, Shaffer JW: Osteonecrosis of the femoral head. A study of 101 hips treated with vascularized fibular grafting, *J Bone Joint Surg Am* 87:742–747, 2005.

140. Zhao D, Xu D, Wang W, Cui X: Iliac graft vascularization for femoral head osteonecrosis, *Clin Orthop Relat Res* 442:171–179, 2006.

141. Korompilias AV, Beris AE, Lykissas MG, et al: Femoral head osteonecrosis: why choose free vascularized fibula grafting, *Microsurgery* 31:223–228, 2010.

142. Vendittoli PA, Lavigne M, Girard J, Roy AG: A randomised study comparing resection of acetabular bone at resurfacing and total hip replacement, *J Bone Joint Surg Br* 88:997–1002, 2006.

143. Grecula MJ: Resurfacing arthroplasty in osteonecrosis of the hip, *Orthop Clin North Am* 36:231–242, x, 2005.

144. Little CP, Ruiz AL, Harding IJ, et al: Osteonecrosis in retrieved femoral heads after failed resurfacing arthroplasty of the hip, *J Bone Joint Surg Br* 87:320–323, 2005.

145. Shimmin AJ, Bare J, Back DL: Complications associated with hip resurfacing arthroplasty, *Orthop Clin North Am* 36:187–193, ix, 2005.

146. Hungerford MW, Mont MA, Scott R, et al: Surface replacement hemiarthroplasty for the treatment of osteonecrosis of the femoral head, *J Bone Joint Surg Am* 80:1656–1664, 1998.

147. Mont MA, Rajadhyaksha AD, Hungerford DS: Outcomes of limited femoral resurfacing arthroplasty compared with total hip arthroplasty for osteonecrosis of the femoral head, *J Arthroplasty* 16:134–139, 2001.

148. Sayeed SA, Johnson AJ, Stroh DA, et al: Hip resurfacing in patients who have osteonecrosis and are 25 years or under, *Clin Orthop Relat Res* 469:1582–1588, 2011.

149. Carlson ER, Basile JD: The role of surgical resection in the management of bisphosphonate-related osteonecrosis of the jaws, *J Oral Maxillofac Surg* 67:85–95, 2009.

150. Pautke C, Bauer F, Tischer T, et al: Fluorescence-guided bone resection in bisphosphonate-associated osteonecrosis of the jaws, *J Oral Maxillofac Surg* 67:471–476, 2009.

151. Freiberger JJ, Padilla-Burgos R, Chhoeu AH, et al: Hyperbaric oxygen treatment and bisphosphonate-induced osteonecrosis of the jaw: a case series, *J Oral Maxillofac Surg* 65:1321–1327, 2007.

152. Wang CJ, Yang YJ, Huang CC: The effects of shockwave on systemic concentrations of nitric oxide level, angiogenesis and osteogenesis factors in hip necrosis, *Rheumatol Int* 31:871–877, 2011.

153. Kuribayashi M, Fujioka M, Takahashi KA, et al: Vitamin E prevents steroid-induced osteonecrosis in rabbits, *Acta Orthop* 81:154–160, 2010.

154. Zaidi M, Sun L, Robinson LJ, et al: ACTH protects against glucocorticoid-induced osteonecrosis of bone, *Proc Natl Acad Sci U S A* 107:8782–8787, 2010.

Full references for this chapter can be found on www.expertconsult.com.

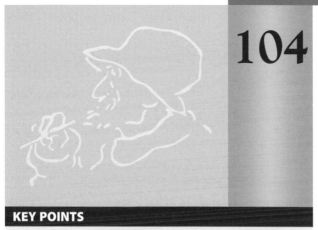

104 Relapsing Polychondritis 📷

GAYE CUNNANE

KEY POINTS

Relapsing polychondritis is a rare disorder that classically affects the cartilaginous structures of the ears and nose, resulting in "cauliflower ear" and "saddle nose" deformities.

It may cause significant pathology of the upper airways, eyes, inner ears, kidneys, and blood vessels with potentially life-threatening consequences.

It may develop in association with other diseases such as myelodysplasia, vasculitis, or other autoimmune/connective tissue disorders.

Due to the multisystem nature of the disease, a broad approach to diagnosis and management is essential.

Treatment is frequently empiric due to the wide variety of disease manifestations and lack of controlled trials. However, immunosuppression is the mainstay of therapy.

Relapsing polychondritis (RPC) is a rare autoimmune disease of unknown etiology, characterized by episodic inflammation of cartilaginous structures throughout the body (e.g., the ears, nose, upper respiratory tract, chest wall, joints). Associated diseases such as vasculitis or myelodysplastic syndromes occur in up to one-third of cases. The severity of the inflammatory process frequently requires the use of immunosuppressive agents. Prognosis is variable with a 5-year survival rate of 45% to 95% depending on organ involvement and disease or treatment complications.

EPIDEMIOLOGY

The worldwide incidence of RPC is unknown, but figures from Rochester, Minnesota, suggest an annual incidence of 3.5 per million in that community.[1] RPC occurs in all racial groups and with similar frequency in men and women. Peak age of onset is 40 to 50 years, but it has been described in children and in people older than 80 years of age. No familial pattern of inheritance has been shown.

PATHOLOGY

Cartilage has a cellular component consisting of chondrocytes and an extracellular matrix made from interlinking fibrils of type II collagen, other collagens, hydrophilic proteoglycan aggregates, and a variety of matrix proteins.[2] One such protein, matrilin-1, is exclusive to the respiratory tract, ears, and xiphisternum in adults and is only found in articular cartilage before skeletal maturity.[3] Cartilage is an avascular structure that derives essential nutrients from adjacent tissue. The composition of cartilage confers resilience to external compressive forces. In normal adults, turnover of cartilage components is slow, with incomplete repair processes.[4] Degradation of collagen fibrils occurs with age resulting from imbalances between naturally occurring proteolytic enzymes and their inhibitors.[5]

In RPC, typical features on hematoxylin-eosin staining include a loss of normal cartilage basophilia and a perichondrial inflammatory infiltrate composed of lymphocytes, neutrophils, eosinophils, and plasma cells.[3,6] Necrosis and a reduction in cartilage components may be observed. The cartilage is subsequently replaced by fibrotic tissue.[6] Immunofluorescence may demonstrate immunoglobulin and complement components in the perichondrial tissue and vessels.[7]

PATHOGENESIS

Although the pathogenesis of RPC is unknown, evidence supports the concept of an autoimmune process. Researchers have observed autoantibodies to types II, IX, and XI collagen in patients with this disease,[3,8-10] while autoantibodies to matrilin-1 have been detected in those with respiratory tract involvement.[11] Specific cytokines such as monocyte chemoattractant protein-1, macrophage inflammatory protein 1β, and interleukin-8 are significantly elevated in active RPC compared with controls.[12] Furthermore, there is a human leukocyte antigen (HLA) class II association with RPC. A twofold increase in HLA-DR4 has been found in RPC, although a specific subtype has not been identified.[13]

Several animal models have helped elucidate some of the pathogenetic mechanisms underlying RPC. Chondritis can be induced in certain rat or mice species following injection of type II collagen.[14,15] In addition, mice expressing HLA-DQ6ab8ab transgenes develop a spontaneous form of polychondritis with auricular, nasal, and joint involvement.[16] Experiments using the matrilin-1-induced rodent model of RPC have demonstrated the importance of T cells, B cells, and complement components in pathogenesis of this disease.[17] Deletion of interleukin (IL)-10 in this model resulted in increased disease severity, suggesting a role for this endogenous cytokine in suppressing episodic inflammation.[18]

The processes involved in the initiation of disease, escalation of the inflammatory response, and subsequent cartilage destruction are poorly understood. In a healthy individual, cartilage is an immunologically privileged site. However, in RPC, cartilage components are exposed and vulnerable to immunologic attack, resulting in a perpetuating process of systemic inflammation and local tissue damage. In genetically susceptible individuals, cartilage

📷 Supplemental image available on the Expert Consult Premium Edition website.

Table 104-1   Diagnostic Criteria

Major Criteria
Proven inflammatory episodes of ear cartilage
Proven inflammatory episodes of nose cartilage
Proven inflammatory episodes of laryngotracheal cartilage

Minor Criteria
Eye inflammation
Hearing loss
Vestibular dysfunction
Seronegative inflammatory arthritis
Diagnosis is made by two major criteria or one major plus two minor criteria.
Histologic examination of affected cartilage is not required.

From Michet CJ Jr, McKenna CH, Luthra HS, et al: Relapsing polychondritis: survival and predictive role of early disease manifestations, *Ann Intern Med* 104:74–78, 1986.

microtrauma or molecular mimicry between an infectious/inciting agent and cartilage structures might instigate a cycle of inflammation similar to other autoimmune disorders.

CLINICAL FEATURES

The diagnostic criteria for RPC are outlined in Table 104-1. Table 104-2 documents the frequency of clinical presentations.

Otorhinologic Disease

The most characteristic manifestation of RPC is auricular chondritis, in which the patient develops acute pain, redness, and swelling of the cartilaginous upper two-thirds of the outer ear, sparing the lobe[19] (Supplemental Figure 104-1 on www.expertconsult.com). It may be unilateral or bilateral and resolves spontaneously over a period of several weeks. Repeated episodes result in visible damage to the ear, with a deformed, flaccid appearance (Figures 104-1A and 104-2). Although classic in RPC, it is the presenting feature in only 40%, whereas up to 85% of patients eventually develop this feature over the course of their disease.[20] Such swelling of the outer ear causes temporary conductive

Table 104-2   Clinical Features of Relapsing Polychondritis

Clinical Feature	Frequency	
	At Presentation	In Total
Auricular chondritis	39	85
Nasal chondritis	24	54
Arthritis	36	52
Eye disease	19	51
Laryngotracheal bronchial disease	26	48
Hearing loss	9	30
Rash	7	28
Systemic vasculitis	3	10
Valvular dysfunction	0	6
Costochondritis	2	2

Modified from Michet CJ, McKenna CH, Luthra HS, et al: Relapsing polychondritis: survival and predictive role of early disease manifestations, *Ann Intern Med* 104:74–78, 1986; and Gergely P, Poór G: Relapsing polychondritis, *Best Pract Res Clin Rheumatol* 18:723–738, 2004.

deafness. However, sensory-neural deafness may result from an associated vasculitis of the internal auditory artery or its branches, leading to additional vertigo in some patients.[6,19] A similar pattern of chondritis in the nose may cause collapse of the nasal bridge and an alteration of the facial appearance—the so-called saddle-nose deformity (Figure 104-1B).

Respiratory Disease

Involvement of the upper respiratory tract may be life threatening and should be investigated at an early stage in the disease course. Approximately 50% of patients with RPC develop respiratory problems, which are associated with a worse prognosis.[21] Hoarseness, dysphonia, a persistent dry cough, or anterior neck tenderness may indicate laryngeal or tracheal disease. Inflammation of the tracheobronchial tree may lead to tracheomalacia, dynamic obstruction, and acute respiratory failure, whereas repeated inflammatory episodes cause subglottic stenosis, chronic dyspnea, and increased susceptibility to infection.[22] Obstruction may be precipitated by attempts at intubation or bronchoscopy.[6] Computed tomography and bronchoscopy appearances of one patient with RPC are demonstrated in Figure 104-1C and D. The development of costochondritis may result in chest pain, leading to additional respiratory symptomatology.

Cardiovascular Disease

Large and small vessel disease can occur during the course of RPC in up to 10% of cases.[23] Inflammation of the aorta, most likely to occur at the level of the root or arch, leads to aneurysm formation and aortic incompetence, which may develop acutely with minimal prior symptoms.[6,24] Aortic valve disease may be due to progressive dilatation of the aortic ring rather than to active local inflammation.[6] Mitral regurgitation may result from valvitis or papillary muscle involvement, whereas myocarditis may lead to cardiac failure and conduction system abnormalities.[1,22,23] Small vessel vasculitis has also been reported and may cause end-organ damage to the skin, kidneys, testes, sclera, cochleovestibular system, or other areas.[6,25] Arterial and venous thromboses have been described in association with RPC.[6]

Eye Disease

Approximately 50% of patients with RPC will develop ocular disease, most commonly episcleritis and scleritis. Uveitis, retinal vasculitis, and optic neuritis are rare complications. Keratoconjunctivitis sicca may occur with associated Sjögren's syndrome. Extraocular muscle palsy, periorbital edema, and proptosis may also occur as part of the RPC symptom complex.[26]

Renal Disease

Proteinuria and/or hematuria may be observed on urinalysis in up to 26% of patients with RPC. Renal pathology has been reported to show mesangial proliferation and segmental necrotizing crescentic glomerulonephritis.[27]

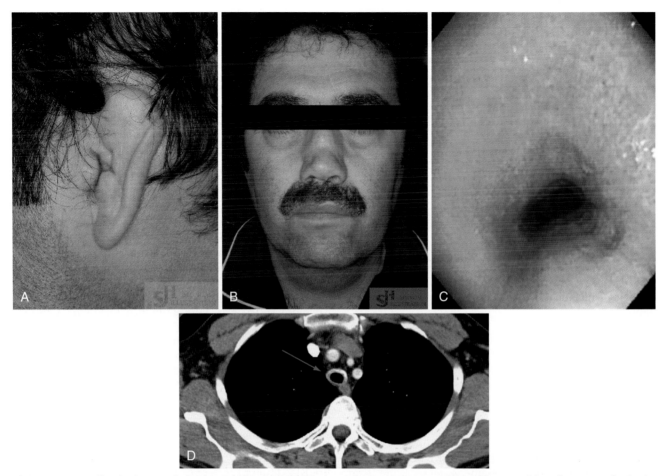

Figure 104-1   A, Chronic changes of relapsing polychondritis (RPC) in the cartilaginous upper two-thirds of the ear, evident after repeated episodes of inflammation in this area. **B,** Saddle nose deformity, developed after episodic nasal chondritis. **C,** Bronchoscopy findings demonstrating mucosal hyperemia, edema with lack of normal detail of tracheal cartilaginous rings, and flattening of the trachea. **D,** Computed tomography thorax with *arrow* demonstrating tracheal flattening and calcification in a patient with RPC. (*A and B, Courtesy Mr. Anthony Edwards, clinical photographer, St. James's Hospital, Dublin 8. C and D, Courtesy Dr. Finbarr O'Connell, consultant pulmonologist, St. James's Hospital, Dublin 8.*)

Electron microscopy may demonstrate immunoglobulin and complement deposits. Renal pathology may also occur in the context of coexisting diseases such as systemic lupus erythematosus or other rheumatic diseases.

Neurologic Disease

Central and peripheral nervous system involvement is rare, affecting less than 5% of patients.[28] Cranial neuropathy is the most common manifestation, but a wide variety of problems including headache, ataxia, hemiplegia, transverse myelitis, mononeuritis multiplex, aseptic meningitis, and encephalopathy have been described. Such lesions may be vasculitic or autoimmune in nature.[1,29]

Skin Disease

Dermatologic manifestations develop in approximately 35% of patients with RCP, relating to the underlying disease or an associated syndrome.[1,30] Skin changes are more likely to occur in patients with concurrent RPC and myelodysplasia.[30] Oral aphthous ulcers are the most common symptom. Peripheral nodules, similar to erythema nodosum, exist in approximately 15% of patients.[30] Rare skin lesions include peripheral limb ulcers, livedo reticularis, panniculitis, superficial thrombophlebitis, urticaria, and angioedema. Leukocytoclastic vasculitis, dermal vessel thrombosis, or septal panniculitis may manifest on biopsy.[30]

Joint Disease

Musculoskeletal manifestations are common and develop in 75% over the course of the disease.[1,23] Involvement of the joints may be oligoarticular or polyarticular, most commonly affecting the ankles, wrists, hands, and feet. However, other joints, including the sacroiliac joints, may also show evidence of disease, although it is possible that the presence of sacroiliitis relates to the coexistence of a spondyloarthropathy.[31] The arthritis associated with RPC is typically episodic and nonerosive, and it does not correlate with activity of RPC.[22,23]

ASSOCIATED DISORDERS

RPC has been described in association with a variety of other disorders including hematologic, rheumatic, and vasculitic syndromes. Its coexistence with Behçet's disease has led to the acronym *MAGIC syndrome:* mouth and genital

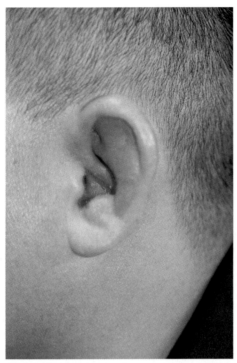

Figure 104-2 Chronic changes of relapsing polychondritis in the cartilaginous upper two-thirds of the ear, evident after repeated episodes of inflammation in this area.

ulcers with inflamed cartilage.[32] In older patients, RPC may be associated with myelodysplasia and a worse prognosis[33,34] (Table 104-3).

DIFFERENTIAL DIAGNOSIS

Auricular chondritis with sparing of the earlobe is characteristic of RPC. Redness and swelling of the whole ear including the earlobe may be the result of trauma or exposure to temperature extremes and should be distinguished

Table 104-3 Diseases Associated with Relapsing Polychondritis

Rheumatic Disorders
Rheumatoid arthritis
Seronegative spondyloarthropathies
Connective tissue disorders
Vasculitides
Hematologic Disorders
Myelodysplasia
Lymphomas
Pernicious anemia
Acute lymphoblastic leukemia
Endocrine Disorders
Type I diabetes mellitus
Thyroid disorders: Hashimoto's/Graves' disease/hypothyroidism
Other Disorders
Inflammatory bowel disease
Primary biliary cirrhosis
Retroperitoneal fibrosis
Myasthenia gravis

from RPC. *Pseudomonas aeruginosa* or *Staphylococcus aureus* are potential causes of unilateral otitis externa, particularly in immunocompromised patients.[35] Other infections associated with chondritis include leprosy and syphilis. Damage to the nose cartilage may be due to trauma, local infections, or granulomatous lesions such as antineutrophil cytoplasmic antibody (ANCA)-associated granulomatosus vasculitis or lethal midline granuloma. Intranasal cocaine use should also be considered. A wide variety of inflammatory, rheumatic, and infectious conditions may mimic some features of RPC, particularly when multiple organs are involved. Cogan's syndrome is an inflammatory autoimmune condition that results in keratitis and vestibulo-auditory symptoms and may be associated with vascular inflammation, although it is not linked with chondritis.[36] Causes of systemic vasculitis (e.g., ANCA-associated vasculitis, polyarteritis nodosa, Behçet's syndrome, rheumatoid arthritis, or those associated with connective tissue disorders) should be taken into consideration, especially when the presentation is atypical. Valvular heart disease, particularly aortic incompetence and aortic root dilatation, may occur in conditions such as Marfan's syndrome, syphilis, and idiopathic medial cystic necrosis and can also develop in relation to diseases that may coincide with RPC (e.g., ankylosing spondylitis).

INVESTIGATIONS

Routine Laboratory Tests

Routine laboratory tests should be performed and may demonstrate nonspecific findings such as anemia or mild thrombocytosis. The acute phase response is typically elevated during periods of inflammation. Urinalysis should always be performed to determine the presence of subclinical renal disease or infection. Autoimmune tests are nonspecific, except where associated diseases are present concurrently.

Tissue Sampling/Histopathology

In typical presentations of RPC, a biopsy is not indicated for diagnosis. However, where the diagnosis is unclear, a biopsy of inflamed cartilage may show evidence of perichondritis, as described earlier.[3,6] Skin rashes may demonstrate leukocytoclastic vasculitis; other frequent findings include panniculitis, neutrophilic dermatoses, or dermal vessel occlusion.[30]

Pulmonary Investigations

Clinicians should conduct pulmonary function tests in all suspected cases of RPC and should be repeated in the event of new respiratory symptoms. If abnormal, computed tomography of the chest is recommended to detect the presence of tracheal or bronchial stenoses or dynamic airway collapse, which may be evident only during the expiratory phase of the respiratory cycle.[37] Extrapulmonary disease from costochondritis may cause a restrictive pattern on pulmonary function testing.

Bronchoscopy is warranted only if specifically indicated in order to avoid inadvertent damage to the upper airways, which poses the risk of precipitating respiratory failure. However, indirect laryngoscopy is helpful to monitor airway involvement. Bronchoscopic ultrasound can also be used to monitor disease.[38]

Cardiac Investigations

Echocardiography is necessary to evaluate the aortic root and heart valves.

Many systemic inflammatory diseases are associated with accelerated atherosclerosis, and this may also be true for patients with RPC, although due to small numbers of cases, this has not been widely described. Nevertheless, other cardiac disease risk factors should be ascertained.

Ocular Investigations

Routine retinoscopy should be performed at diagnosis. Referral to a specialist unit is recommended if abnormalities are detected and/or if symptoms develop.

Musculoskeletal Tests

Plain radiographs of involved joints may show joint space narrowing or periarticular osteopenia. Erosions are not observed, unless there is an associated rheumatic disorder. Dual x-ray absorptiometry may demonstrate osteopenia as a consequence of the underlying inflammation or general debility.

Additional Investigations

At present genetic testing offers little added benefit. Markers of cartilage autoimmunity such as antibodies to types II, IX, or XI collagen or matrilyin-1 are not routinely available, and their role in disease activity monitoring is unclear. A recent report highlighted the relevance of antiglutamate receptor GluR ε2 autoantibodies in the cerebrospinal fluid and sera of a patient with limbic encephalitis.[29] The potential use of other biomarkers such as urinary type II collagen breakdown products has been demonstrated.[39] Additionally, a recent study showed that serum levels of cartilage oligomeric matrix protein (COMP) are elevated during disease flares in RPC.[40]

TREATMENT

Nonsteroidal anti-inflammatory drugs and low-dose corticosteroids may successfully control minor inflammation of the nose, ear, or chest wall. Dapsone may also be used for noncritical cartilaginous inflammation,[1,21] and colchicine is of reported use in auricular chondritis.[41] However, the presence of potentially life-threatening disease or severe chondritis requires high-dose prednisone, typically at a dose of 1 mg/kg, reducing slowly as the inflammation recedes.[1,23] Although the RPC is usually steroid responsive, it can be difficult to withdraw these drugs completely without risking a flare in disease activity and many patients require maintenance doses of prednisone and consideration of alternative immunosuppression. Disease-modifying treatment is indicated in patients who require a steroid-sparing agent and in whom serious manifestations such as vascular or respiratory disease have developed.

Due to the rarity of this disease, there are no controlled trials of therapeutic interventions in RPC. However, methotrexate, cyclophosphamide, mycophenolate mofetil, azathioprine, chlorambucil, and cyclosporine have had successful therapeutic outcomes in some patients.[6,42-49] Varied outcomes have been reported with leflunomide.[50,51] Plasmapheresis has been employed in recalcitrant cases.[6,23] There are several case reports and small case series detailing the use of biologic agents in this disease. However, there have been both positive and negative reports in relation to the anti–tumor necrosis factor agents and anti–B cell drugs.[24,52-57] Interleukin-1 receptor antagonist has demonstrated benefit in a small number of reported cases.[58,59] Tocilizumab, an anti-IL-6 agent, has had beneficial effects in this disease.[60] A successful outcome for autologous stem cell transplantation in treatment-resistant RPC has also been reported.[61] It is not clear, however, if any of these treatments overtly influence the natural history of this disease.

A broad approach to the management of RPC is essential. Awareness of disease complications and recognition of early pathology may be lifesaving. Special consideration should be given to the management of upper airway involvement, and the anesthesia team should be made aware of disease in this region before surgical intervention. Symptomatic airway obstruction might require tracheostomy, tracheal stenting, or nighttime positive pressure ventilation to prevent airway collapse while the patient is asleep. There is limited experience with laryngotracheal reconstruction in patients with this disease, and such interventions should only take place during disease quiescence.[62] Heart surgery to treat aortic root dilatation, aneurysm formation, or valvular disease has a good outcome in most cases, although postoperative dehiscence is a complication in 12%.[63] Most cases require postoperative immunosuppression. For patients with sensorineural deafness, cochlear implantation is usually beneficial with significant restoration of hearing.[64] Neither hormonal activity nor pregnancy is thought to influence disease activity in RPC.[65] However, several case reports have described the treatment of disease flares during pregnancy, typically with corticosteroids, with successful maternal and fetal outcomes.[65-67]

OUTCOME

RPC is an episodic, progressive disease that results in tissue destruction of target organs. Some patients have a mild course, complicated only by recurrent chondritis, whereas others develop potentially life-threatening problems. The most common cause of death is pulmonary infection, arising as a result of the disease or its immunosuppressive treatment.[6] In young patients, adverse prognostic factors at presentation include anemia, hematuria, upper airway disease, arthritis, and saddle nose deformity, whereas in older patients (more than 51 years of age), only anemia at presentation predicts increased mortality.[20] The presence of vasculitis worsens prognosis, with a 5-year survival rate of 45%.[21] In 1986 Michet and and colleagues[20] reported the 10-year survival rate to be 55%, whereas in 1998, perhaps due to improvements in disease monitoring and treatment, Trentham and colleagues[6] described a 94% survival rate.

Future Directions

An international database of RPC, detailing modes of presentation, clinical characteristics, and therapeutic responses, would be a valuable resource in learning more about the epidemiology and treatment of RPC. It would also help clarify some of the discrepancies in the current literature relating to presentation and prognosis of this rare disease. New therapies, with specific cellular or molecular targets, offer promise to patients with chronic inflammatory diseases but should ideally be accompanied by definitive knowledge of their mechanism of action in particular disease subtypes. Increased awareness of the immunogenic precipitants involved in RPC may help to guide future treatments and reduce morbidity and mortality in such patients.

References

1. Kent PD, Michet CJ, Luthra HS: Relapsing polychondritis, *Curr Opin Rheumatol* 16:56–61, 2004.
2. Deleted in proofs.
3. Hansson AS, Holmdahl R: Cartilage-specific autoimmunity in animal models and clinical aspects in patients—focus on relapsing polychondritis, *Arthritis Res* 4:296–301, 2002.
4. Goldring MB: Articular cartilage. In: Klippel JH, editor. *Primer on the rheumatic diseases*, ed 12, Atlanta, 2012, Arthritis Foundation, pp 10–16.
5. Burrage PS, Brinckerhoff CE: Molecular targets in osteoarthritis: metalloproteinases and their inhibitors, *Curr Drug Targets* 8:293–303, 2007.
6. Trentham DE, Le CH: Relapsing polychondritis, *Ann Intern Med* 129:114–122, 1998.
7. Valenzuela R, Cooperrider PA, Gogate P, et al: Relapsing polychondritis: immunomicroscopic findings in cartilage of ear biopsy specimens, *Hum Pathol* 11:19–22, 1980.
8. Foidart JM, Abe S, Martin GR, et al: Antibodies to type II collagen in relapsing polychondritis, *N Engl J Med* 299:1203–1207, 1978.
9. Yang CL, Brinckmann J, Rui HF, et al: Autoantibodies to cartilage collagens in relapsing polychondritis, *Arch Dermatol Res* 285:245–249, 1993.
10. Alsalameh S, Mollenhauer J, Scheuplein F, et al: Preferential cellular and humoral immune reactivities to native and denatured collagen types IX and XI in a patient with fatal relapsing polychondritis, *J Rheumatol* 20:1419–1424, 1993.
11. Hansson AS, Heinegård D, Piette JC, et al: The occurrence of autoantibodies to matrilin 1 reflects a tissue-specific response to cartilage of the respiratory tract in patients with relapsing polychondritis, *Arthritis Rheum* 44:2402–2412, 2001.
12. Stabler T, Piette JC, Chevalier X, et al: Serum cytokine profiles in relapsing polychondritis suggest monocyte/macrophage activation, *Arthritis Rheum* 50:3663–3667, 2004.
13. Lang B, Rothenfusser A, Lanchbury JS, et al: Susceptibility to relapsing polychondritis is associated with HLA-DR4, *Arthritis Rheum* 36:660–664, 1993.
14. Cremer MA, Pitcock JA, Stuart JM, et al: Auricular chondritis in rats: an experimental model of relapsing polychondritis induced with type II collagen, *J Exp Med* 154:535–540, 1981.
15. McCune WJ, Schiller AL, Dynesius-Trentham RA, et al: Type II collagen induced auricular chondritis, *Arthritis Rheum* 25:266–273, 1982.
16. Bradley DS, Das P, Griffiths MM, et al: HLA-DQ6/8 double transgenic mice develop auricular chondritis following type II collagen immunization: a model for human relapsing polychondritis, *J Immunol* 161:5046–5053, 1998.
17. Hansson AS, Heinegård D, Holmdahl R: A new animal model for relapsing polychondritis induced by cartilage matrix protein (matrilin 1), *J Clin Invest* 104:589–598, 1999.
18. Hansson AS, Johansson AC, Holmdahl R: Critical role of the major histocompatibility complex and IL-10 in matrilin-1-induced relapsing polychondritis in mice, *Arthritis Res Ther* 6:R484–491, 2004.
19. McAdam LP, O'Hanlan MA, Bluestone R, et al: Relapsing polychondritis: prospective study of 23 patients and a review of the literature, *Medicine* 55:193–215, 1976.
20. Michet CJ, McKenna CH, Luthra HS, et al Relapsing polychondritis: survival and predictive role of early disease manifestations, *Ann Intern Med* 104:74–78, 1986.
21. Letko E, Zafirakis P, Baltatzis S, et al: Relapsing polychondritis: a clinical review, *Semin Arthritis Rheum* 31:384–395, 2002.
22. Gergely P, Poór G: Relapsing polychondritis, *Best Pract Res Clin Rheumatol* 18:723–738, 2004.
23. Deleted in proofs.
24. McCarthy EM, Cunnane G: Treatment of relapsing polychondritis in the era of biologic agents, *Rheumatol Int* 30:827–828, 2010.
25. Michet CJ: Vasculitis and relapsing polychondritis, *Rheum Dis Clin North Am* 16:441–444, 1990.
26. Isaak BL, Liesegang TJ, Michet CJ: Ocular and systemic findings in relapsing polychondritis, *Ophthalmology* 93:681–689, 1986.
27. Chang-Miller A, Okamura M, Torres VE, et al: Renal involvement in relapsing polychondritis, *Medicine* 66:202–217, 1987.
28. Zeuner M, Straub RH, Rauh G, et al: Relapsing polychondritis: clinical and immunogenetic analysis of 62 patients, *J Rheumatol* 24:96–101, 1997.
29. Kashihara K, Kawada S, Takahashi Y: Autoantibodies to glutamate receptor GluRε2 in a patient with limbic encephalitis associated with relapsing polychondritis, *J Neurol Sci* 287:275–277, 2009.
30. Francès C, el Rassi R, Laporte JL, et al: Dermatologic manifestations of relapsing polychondritis. A study of 200 cases at a single center, *Medicine* 80:173–179, 2001.
31. Pazirandeh M, Ziran BH, Khandelwal BK, et al: Relapsing polychondritis and spondyloarthropathies, *J Rheumatol* 15:630–632, 1988.
32. Firestein GS, Gruber HE, Weisman MH, et al: Mouth and genital ulcers with inflamed cartilage: MAGIC syndrome, *Am J Med* 79:65–72, 1985.
33. Hebbar M, Brouillard M, Wattel E, et al: Association of myelodysplastic syndrome and relapsing polychondritis: further evidence, *Leukemia* 9:731–733, 1995.
34. Myers B, Gould J, Dolan G: Relapsing polychondritis and myelodysplasia: a report of 2 cases and review of the current literature, *Clin Lab Haematol* 22:45–48, 2000.
35. Ninkovic G, Dullo V, Saunders NC: Microbiology of otitis externa in secondary care in the United Kingdom and anti-microbial sensitivity, *Auris nasus larynx* 35:480–484, 2008.
36. Mazlumzadeh M, Matteson EL: Cogan's syndrome: an audiovestibular, ocular and systemic auto-immune disorder, *Rheum Dis Clin North Am* 33:855–874, 2007.
37. Lee KS, Ernst A, Trentham DE, et al: Relapsing polychondritis: prevalence of expiratory CT airway abnormalities, *Radiology* 240:565–573, 2006.
38. Miyazu Y, Miyazawa T, Kurimoto N, et al: Endobronchial ultrasonography in the diagnosis and treatment of relapsing polychondritis with tracheo bronchial malacia, *Chest* 124:2393–2395, 2003.
39. Kraus VB, Stabler T, Le ET, et al: Urinary type II collagen neoepitope as an outcome measure for relapsing polychondritis, *Arthritis Rheum* 48:2942–2948, 2003.
40. Kempta Lekpa F, Piette JC, Bastuji-Garin S, et al: Serum cartilage oligomeric matrix protein (COMP) is a marker of disease activity in relapsing polychondritis, *Clin Exp Rheumatol* 28:553–555, 2010.
41. Mark KA, Franks AG: Colchicine and indomethacin for the treatment of relapsing polychondritis, *J Am Acad Dermatol* 46:S22–S24, 2002.
42. Lahmer T, Treiber M, von Werder A, et al: Relapsing polychondritis: an autoimmune disease with many faces, *Autoimmunity Rev* 9:540–546, 2010.
43. Park J, Gowin KM, Schumacher HR Jr: Steroid sparing effect of methotrexate in relapsing polychondritis, *J Rheumatol* 23:937–938, 1996.
44. Stewart KA, Mazanec DJ: Pulse intravenous cyclophosphamide for kidney disease in relapsing polychondritis, *J Rheumatol* 19:498–500, 1992.
45. Ruhlen JL, Huston KA, Wood WG: Relapsing polychondritis with glomerulonephritis. Improvement with prednisone and cyclophosphamide, *JAMA* 245:847–848, 1981.
46. Goldenberg G, Sangueza OP, Jorizzo JL: Successful treatment of relapsing polychondritis with mycophenolate mofetil, *J Dermatol Treat* 17:158–159, 2006.
47. Michelson JB: Melting corneas with collapsing nose, *Surv Ophthalmol* 29:148–154, 1984.

48. Svenson KL, Holmdahl R, Klareskog L, et al: Cyclosporin A treatment in a case of relapsing polychondritis, *Scand J Rheumatol* 13:329–333, 1984.

49. Priori R, Paroli MP, Luan FL, et al: Cyclosporin A in the treatment of relapsing polychondritis with severe recurrent eye involvement, *Br J Rheumatol* 32:352, 1993.

50. Koenig AS, Abruzzo JL: Leflunomide induced fevers, thrombocytosis and leukocytosis in a patient with relapsing polychondritis, *J Rheumatol* 29:192–194, 2002.

51. Handler RP: Leflunomide for relapsing polychondritis: successful long-term treatment, *J Rheumatol* 33:1916, 2006.

52. Carter JD: Treatment of relapsing polychondritis with a TNF antagonist, *J Rheumatol* 32:1413, 2005.

53. Mpofu S, Estrach C, Curtis J, et al: Treatment of respiratory complications in recalcitrant relapsing polychondritis with infliximab, *Rheumatology (Oxford)* 42:1117–1118, 2003.

54. Cazabon S, Over K, Butcher J: The successful use of infliximab in resistant relapsing polychondritis and associated scleritis, *Eye* 19:222–224, 2005.

55. Saadoun D, Deslandre CJ, Allanore Y, et al: Sustained response to infliximab in 2 patients with refractory relapsing polychondritis, *J Rheumatol* 30:1394–1395, 2003.

56. Lahmer T, Knopf A, Treiber M, et al: Treatment of relapsing polychondritis with the TNF alpha antagonist adalimumab, *Clin Rheumatol* 29:1331–1334, 2010.

57. Leroux G, Costedoat-Chalumeau N, Brihaye B, et al: Treatment of relapsing polychondritis with rituximab: a retrospective study of 9 patients, *Arthritis Rheum* 61:577–582, 2009.

58. Wendling D, Govindaraju S, Prati C, et al: Efficacy of anakinra in a patient with refractory relapsing polychondritis, *Joint Bone Spine* 75:622–624, 2008.

59. Vounotrypidis P, Sakellariou GT, Zisopoulos D, et al: Refractory relapsing polychondritis: rapid and sustained response in the treatment with an IL-1 receptor antagonist (anakinra), *Rheumatology* 45:491–492, 2006.

60. Kawai M, Hagihara K, Hirano T, et al: Sustained response to tocilizumab, anti-interleukin-6 receptor antibody, in two patients with refractory relapsing polychondritis, *Rheumatology* 48:318–319, 2009.

61. Kötter I, Daikeler T, Amberger C, et al: Autologous stem cell transplantation of treatment-resistant systemic vasculitis, *Clin Nephrol* 64:485–489, 2005.

62. Herrington HC, Weber SM, Andersen PE: Modern management of laryngotracheal stenosis, *Laryngoscope* 116:1553–1557, 2006.

63. Dib C, Moustafa SE, Mookadam M, et al: Surgical treatment of the cardiac manifestations of relapsing polychondritis, *Mayo Clin Proc* 81:772–776, 2006.

64. Seo YJ, Choi JY, Kim SH, Kim TJ: Cochlear implantation in a bilateral sensorineural hearing loss patient with relapsing polychondritis, *Rheumatol Int* 2012;32:479–482,

65. Papo T, Wechsler B, Bletry O, et al: Pregnancy in relapsing polychondritis: 25 pregnancies in 11 patients, *Arthritis Rheum* 40:1245–1249, 1997.

66. Krakow D, Greenspoon JS, Firestein GS: Relapsing polychondritis—normal fetal outcomes despite maternal flares, *J Clin Rheumatol* 2:118, 1996.

67. Bellamy N, Dewar CL: Relapsing polychondritis in pregnancy, *J Rheumatol* 17:1525–1526, 1990.

The references for this chapter can also be found on www.expertconsult.com.

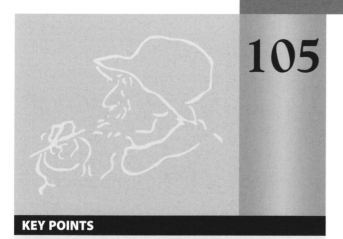

105 Heritable Diseases of Connective Tissue

DEBORAH KRAKOW

KEY POINTS

Heritable disorders of connective tissues are a diverse group of disorders and can be associated with extreme variation in height ranging from very short (dwarfs) to tall stature.

The osteochondrodysplasias or skeletal dysplasias are a heterogeneous group of more than 450 disorders frequently associated with profound short stature and orthopedic complications.

These disorders are diagnosed on the basis of radiographic, morphologic, clinical, and molecular criteria.

The molecular mechanisms have been elucidated in many of these disorders providing for improved clinical diagnosis and reproductive choices for affected individuals and their families.

Mechanism-based treatment options that might improve the quality of life and life span in individuals affected with osteogenesis imperfecta and Marfan syndrome are being investigated. Newer advances in understanding the underpinnings of altered pathways in these disorders are providing potential new targets for treatment.

Heritable disorders of connective tissues are a heterogeneous group of disorders characterized by abnormalities in skeletal tissues including cartilage, bone, tendon, ligament, muscle, and skin. These disorders, originally defined by McKusick,[1] have been classified on the basis of clinical findings and molecular criteria. They are subclassified into disorders that primarily affect cartilage and bone (the skeletal dysplasias) and disorders that have a more profound effect on connective tissue including Ehlers-Danlos syndrome (EDS), Marfan syndrome, and other disorders manifested by abnormal extracellular matrix molecules. The skeletal dysplasias are associated with abnormalities in the size and shape of the appendicular and axial skeleton and frequently result in disproportionate short stature. Until the early 1960s, most individuals with short stature were considered to have pituitary dwarfism, achondroplasia (short-limb dwarfism), or Morquio disease (short-trunked dwarfism). Presently, there are more than 450 well-characterized disorders that are classified primarily on the basis of clinical, radiographic, and molecular criteria.[2] Disorders of connective tissue are genetic defects that result from mutations in genes that encode extracellular matrix proteins, transcription factors, tumor suppressors, signal transducers, enzymes, chaperones, intracellular binding proteins, ribonucleic acid (RNA) processing molecules, and genes of unknown function.

SKELETAL DYSPLASIAS

The skeletal dysplasias, or osteochondrodysplasias, are defined as disorders that are associated with a generalized abnormality in the skeleton. Although each skeletal dysplasia is relatively rare, collectively, the birth incidence of these disorders is almost 1 in 5000.[3] These disorders range in severity from "precocious" arthropathy to perinatal lethality owing to pulmonary insufficiency. Individuals with these disorders can have significant orthopedic, neurologic, and psychological complications. Many of these individuals seek medical attention for orthopedic complaints owing to ongoing pain, arthritic complaints in large joints, and back pain primarily caused by ongoing abnormalities in bone and cartilage frequently leading to spinal stenosis.

Embryology

The human skeleton (from the Greek, *skeletos*, "dried up") is a complex organ consisting of 206 bones (126 appendicular bones, 74 axial bones, and 6 ossicles). The skeleton including tendons, ligaments, and muscles in addition to cartilage and bone has multiple embryonic origins and serves many key functions throughout life such as linear growth, mechanical support for movement, a blood and mineral reservoir, and protection of vital organs.

The patterning and architecture of the skeleton occurs during fetal development (see Chapter 4). During that period, the number, size, and shape of the future skeletal elements are determined, a process that is under complex genetic control.[4] Uncondensed mesenchyme undergoes cellular condensations (cartilage anlagen) at the sites of future bones, and this occurs via two mechanisms.[5] In the process of endochondral ossification, mesenchyme first differentiates into a cartilage model (anlagen), and then the center of the anlagen degrades, mineralizes, and is removed by osteoclast-like cells. This process spreads up and down the bones and allows for vascular invasion and influx of osteoprogenitor cells. The periosteum in the midshaft region of the bone produces osteoblasts, which synthesize the cortex; this is known as the *primary ossification center*.

At the ends of the cartilage anlagen, a similar process leading to the removal of cartilage occurs (secondary center of ossification), leaving a portion of cartilage model "trapped" between the expanding primary and secondary ossification centers. This area is referred to as a *cartilage growth plate* or *epiphysis*. Four chondrocyte cell types exist in the growth plate: reserve, resting, proliferative, and hypertrophic. These growth plate chondrocytes undergo a tightly regulated program of proliferation, hypertrophy, degradation, and replacement by bone (primary spongiosa). This is the major mechanism of skeletogenesis and is the mechanism by which bones increase in length, and the articular surfaces increase in diameter. In contrast, the flat bones of the cranial vault and part of the clavicles and pubis form by intramembranous ossification, whereby fibrous tissue, derived from mesenchymal cells, differentiates directly into osteoblasts, which directly lay down bone.[5] These processes are under specific and direct genetic control, and abnormalities in the genes that encode these pathways frequently lead to skeletal dysplasias.[6-9]

Cartilage Structure

Collagen accounts for two-thirds of the adult weight of adult articular cartilage and provides significant strength and structure to the tissue (see Chapter 3). Collagens are a family of proteins that consist of single molecules (monomers) that combine into three polypeptide chains to form a triple helix structure. In the triple helix, every third amino acid is a glycine residue and the general chain structure is denoted as Gly-X-Y, where X and Y are commonly proline and hydroxyproline. The collagen helix can be composed of identical chains (homotrimeric), as in type II collagen, or can consist of different collagen chains (heterotrimeric), as seen in collagen type XI.[10]

Collagens are widely distributed throughout the body, and 33 collagen gene products are expressed in a tissue-specific manner, leading to 19 triple helical collagens. Collagens are classified further by the structures they form in the extracellular matrix. The most abundant collagens are the fibrillar types (I, II, III, V, and XI), and their extensive cross-linking provides mechanical strength that is necessary for high stress tissue such as cartilage, bone, and skin.[11] Another collagen species is the fibril-associated collagens with interrupted triple helices, which include collagen types IX, XII, XIV, and XVI. These collagens interact with fibrillar collagens and other extracellular molecules including aggrecan, cartilage oligomeric matrix protein, and other sulfated proteoglycans.[11] Collagen types VIII and X are nonfibrillar, short-chain collagens, and type X collagen is the most abundant extracellular matrix molecule expressed by hypertrophic chondrocytes during endochondral ossification.[12] The major collagens of articular cartilage are fibrillar collagen types II, IX, X, and XI. In developing cartilage, the core fibrillar network is a cross-linked copolymer of collagens II, IX, and XI.[13] Mutations in genes that encode these collagens and proteins involved in their processing result in various skeletal dysplasias and highlight the importance of these molecules in skeletal development.

Classification and Nomenclature

As mentioned earlier, in the 1970s, there was recognition of the genetic and clinical heterogeneity of heritable disorders of connective tissue and a new awareness of the complexity of these disorders. As a result, there have been multiple attempts to classify these disorders in a manner that clinicians and scientists could use effectively to diagnose and determine their pathogenicity (International Nomenclature of Constitutional Diseases of Bone, 1970, 1977, 1983, 1992, 2001, 2005, 2010). The initial categories were purely descriptive and clinically based. With the more recent explosion in determining the genetic basis of these

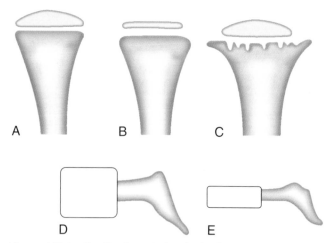

Figure 105-1 Classification of chondrodysplasias based on radiographic involvement of the long bones (**A-C**) and vertebrae (side view of vertebral bodies and spinous processes in **D** and **E**). **A** and **D** are normal, **B** is an epiphyseal abnormality, **C** is a metaphyseal abnormality, and **E** is a "spondylo-" abnormality.

diseases, the classification has evolved into one that combines the older clinical one (including the eponyms and Greek terms) and blends these disorders into families that share a molecular basis or pathway. The most recent updated classification can be found at www.isds.ch. Some of the chondrodysplasia families are listed in Table 105-1.

The most widely used method for differentiating the skeletal disorders has been through the detection of skeletal radiographic abnormalities. Radiographic classifications are based on the different parts of the long bones that are abnormal (epiphyses, metaphyses, and diaphyses) (Figure 105-1). These epiphyseal, metaphyseal, and diaphyseal disorders can be differentiated further depending on whether or not the spine is involved (spondyloepiphyseal, spondylometaphyseal, or spondyloepimetaphyseal dysplasias). The classes of these disorders can be differentiated further into distinct disorders on the basis of other clinical and radiographic findings.

Clinical Evaluation and Features

The skeletal dysplasias are generalized disorders of the skeleton and usually result in disproportionate short stature. Affected individuals usually present because they are disproportionately short. This finding needs to be documented on the appropriate growth curves for gender and ethnicity if possible. As a generalization, most individuals with disproportionate short stature have skeletal dysplasias, and individuals with proportionate short stature have endocrine, nutritional, or prenatal-onset growth deficiency or other disorders. Exceptions to the rule include congenital hypothyroidism, which is associated with disproportionate short stature, and disorders such as osteogenesis imperfecta (OI) and hypophosphatasia can be associated with normal body proportions.

A disproportionate body habitus may not be immediately visible on physical examination. Anthropometric dimensions such as upper-to-lower segment (U/L) ratio, sitting height, and arm span must be measured when considering the possibility of a skeletal dysplasia and should be measured in centimeters. Sitting height is an accurate measurement

Table 105-1 Classification of the Chondrodysplasias

Dysplasia	Inheritance	Gene	Dysplasia	Inheritance	Gene
Achondroplasia Group			Weissenbacher-Zweymuller syndrome	AD	COL11A2
Achondroplasia	AD	FGFR3	Fibrochondrogenesis	AR	COL11A1
Thanatophoric dysplasia, type I	AD	FGFR3			COL11A2
Thanatophoric dysplasia, type II	AD	FGFR3	**Other Spondyloepi-(meta)-physeal [SE(M)D] Dysplasia**		
Achondroplasia	AD	FGFR3	Spondyloepimetaphyseal dysplasia, Pakistani type	AR	ATPSK2
Hypochondroplasia	AD	FGFR3	Spondyloepiphyseal dysplasia tarda	XLR	SEDL
SADDAN	AD	FGFR3	Progressive pseudorheumatoid dysplasia	AR	WISP3
CATSHL	AD	FGFR3	Dyggve-Melchior-Clausen dysplasia	AR	FLJ90130
Osteogleophonic dsyplasia	AD	FGFR1	Wolcott-Rallison dysplasia	AR	EIF2AK3
Severe Spondylodyplastic Dysplasias			Acrocapitofemoral dysplasia	AR	IHH
Achondrogenesis IA	AR	GMAP210	Schimke immuno-osseous dysplasia	AR	SMARCAL1
Opsismodysplasia	AR	Unknown	Sponastrime	AR	Unknown
Schneckenbecken dysplasia	AR	SLC35D1	Spondlyometaphyseal dysplasia, type corner fracture	AD	Unknown
Spondylometaphyseal dysplasia, type Sedaghatian	AR	SBDS	**Multiple Epiphyseal Dysplasia and Pseudoachondroplasia**		
TRPV4/Metatropic Dysplasia Group			Multiple epiphyseal dysplasia	AD	COL9A1
Metatropic dysplasia	AD	TRPV4		COL9A2	COL9A3
Spondyloepiphyseal dysplasia (Kozlowski type)	AD	TRPV4		MATN	COMP
Parastrammetic dysplasia	AD	TRPV4	Pseudoachondroplasia	AD	COMP
Brachyolmia (AD)	AD	TRPV4	**Chondrodysplasia Punctata**		
Short Rib Dysplasia (Polydactyly) Group			Chondrodysplasia punctata, rhizomelic type	AR	PEX7
Short-rib polydactyly type I/III	AR	DYNC2CH1			DHAPAT
		IFT80			AGPS
		WDR35	Chondrodysplasia punctata, Conradi-Hunermann type	XLD	EBP
Short-rib polydactyly type II/IV	AR	NEK1	Hydrops-ectopic calcifications-moth-eaten bones	AR	LBR
Asphyxiating thoracic dysplasia	AR	DYNC2CH1	Chondrodysplasia punctata, brachytelephalangic type	XLR	ARSE
		IFT80	Chondrodysplasia punctata, tibial-metacarpal type	AD	Unknown
Chondroectodermal dysplasia	AR	EVC1, EVC2	**Metaphyseal Dysplasias**		
Thoracolaryngopelvic dysplasia	AD	Unknown	Metaphyseal chondrodysplasia, type Jansen	AD	PTHrP
Filamin-Related Disorders			Eiken dysplasia	AR	PTHrP
Atelosteogenesis I	AD	FLNB	Bloomstrand dysplasia	AR	PTHrP
Atelosteogenesis III	AD	FLNB	Metaphyseal chondrodysplasia, type Schmidt	AD	COL10A1
Larsen syndrome	AD	FLNB	Metaphyseal chondrodysplasia, McKusick type	AR	RMRP
Otopalato-digital syndrome type II	XLR	FLNA	Metaphyseal chondrodysplasia, with pancreatic insufficiency, and cyclin neutropenia	AR	SBDS
Osteodysplasty, Melnick-Needles	XLD	FLNA	Adenosine deaminase deficiency	AR	ADA
Diastrophic Dysplasia Group			**Brachyolmia Spondylodysplasias**		
Achondrogenesis IB	AR	DTDST	Brachyolmia (Hobek type) (Toledo type)	AR	Unknown
Achondrogenesis II	AR	DTDST	Brachyolmia (Maroteaux type)	AR	Unknown
Diastrophic dysplasia	AR	DTDST	**Rhizo- and Mesomelic Dysplasias**		
Recessive multiple epiphyseal dysplasia	AR	DTDST	Omodysplasia	AR	Glypican 6
Dyssegmental Dysplasia Group			Dyschondrosteosis	XLD	SHOX
Dyssegmental dsyplasia	AR	HSPG2	Mesomelic dysplasia, type Lange	XLR	SHOX
Silverman-Handmaker type	AR	HSPG2	Mesomelic dysplasia, type Robinow	AD	
Dyssegmental dsyplasia Rolland-Desbuquois	AR	HSPG2		AR	ROR2
Schwartz-Jampel syndrome	AR	HSPG2	Mesomelic dysplasia, Kantapura type	AD	Duplication in the Hox cluster
Type II Collagenopathies					
Achondrogenesis II	AD	COL2A1			
Kniest dysplasia	AD	COL2A1			
Spondyloepiphyseal dysplasia congenita	AD	COL2A1			
Spondyloepiphyseal dysplasia Strudwick type	AD	COL2A1			
Spondyloperipheral dysplasia	AD	COL2A1			
Arthro-opthamalopathy (Stickler syndrome)	AD	COL2A1			
Type XI Collagenopathies					
Stickler dysplasia	AD	COL11A1			
OSMED	AR	COL11A2			

Continued

Table 105-1   Classification of the Chondrodysplasias—cont'd

Dysplasia	Inheritance	Gene	Dysplasia	Inheritance	Gene
Acromelic and Acromesomelic Dysplasias			**Dysplasia with Prominent Membranous Bone Involvement**		
Acromicric dysplasia	AD	Fibrillin 1	Cleidocranial dysplasia	AD	CBFA1
Geleophysic dysplasia	AD	Fibrillin 1	**Bent Bone Dysplasias**		
	AR	ADAMTSL2			
Trichorhinophalangeal dysplasia, type I	AD	TRPS1	Campomelic dysplasia	AD	SOX9
Trichorhinophalangeal dysplasia, type II	AD	TRPS2	Stüve-Wiedemann dysplasia	AR	LIFR
Acrodysostosis	AD	PRKAR1A	**Multiple Dislocations with Dysplasias**		
Grebe dysplasia	AR	CDMP1	Desbuquois syndrome	AR	CANT1
Acromesomelic dysplasia, Hunter-Thompson	AR	CDMP1	Pseudodiastrophic dysplasia	AR	Unknown
Acromesomelic dysplasia, type Maroteaux	AR	NPRB	Spondyloepimetaphyseal dysplasia with joint laxity	AR	Unknown

AD, autosomal dominant; AR, autosomal recessive; CATSHL, camptodactyly, tall stature, and hearing loss syndrome; OSMED, otospondylometaepiphyseal dysplasia; SADDAN, severe achondroplasia with developmental delay and acanthosis nigricans; TRPV4, transient receptor potential vanilloid 4; XLR, X-linked recessive; XLD, X-linked dominant.

of head and trunk length, but it requires special equipment for precise measurements. U/L ratios are easy to obtain and provide an accurate measurement of proportion. The lower segment is measured from the symphysis pubis to the floor at the inside of the heel. The upper segment is measured by subtracting the lower segment measurement from the total height. McKusick[14] has published standard U/L segment ratios for whites and African-Americans across ages. An average-height white child 8 to 10 years old has a U/L segment ratio of approximately 1 and as an adult has a U/L segment ratio of 0.95. Individuals presenting with disproportionate short stature have altered U/L segment ratios depending on whether they have short limbs, short trunk, or both. An individual with short limbs and normal trunk has an increased U/L segment ratio, and an individual with normal limbs but short trunk has a diminished U/L segment ratio (Figure 105-2). Another means of determining if there is disproportion is based on arm span measurements, which are close to total height in an average-proportioned individual. A short-limbed individual has an arm span considerably shorter than the height.

As in any disorder that has a genetic basis, it is crucial to obtain an accurate family history. This should include any history of previously affected children or parental consanguinity. The skeletal dysplasias are genetically heterogeneous and can be inherited as autosomal dominant, autosomal recessive, X-linked recessive, and X-linked dominant disorders, and rarer genetic mechanisms of disease including germline mosaicism, uniparental disomy, and chromosomal rearrangements have been seen.[15-18] For many patients and families, accurate diagnosis and recurrence risk can have a significant impact on their reproductive decisions. Another consideration for patients with short stature is that there is increased nonrandom mating, which leads to reproductive outcomes that have been previously unknown.[19,20] Homozygous achondroplasia is lethal, and many newborns who inherit two dominant mutations (compound heterozygotes) die early with severe abnormalities of the skeleton.[21] It is also important to obtain an accurate history relative to the onset of short stature and whether it developed immediately in the postnatal period or was noticed at age 2 or 3. Of the 450 skeletal dysplasias, approximately 100 of them have onset in the prenatal period, but

many affected individuals do not develop disproportionate short stature and joint discomfort until childhood.[22,23]

A detailed physical examination may reveal a diagnosis or help differentiate the most likely group of possible diagnoses. It is crucial when disproportion and short stature have been established and the limbs are involved to determine which segment is involved: upper segment (rhizomelic—humerus and femur); middle segment (mesomelic—radius, ulna, tibia, and fibula); and distal segment (acromelic—hands and feet). Numerous head and facial dysmorphisms are seen in the skeletal disorders. Affected individuals frequently have disproportionately large heads. Frontal bossing and flattened nasal bridge are characteristic of achondroplasia, one of the most common skeletal dysplasias.[24] Cleft palate and micrognathia are commonly found in the type II collagen abnormalities, abnormally flattened midface with

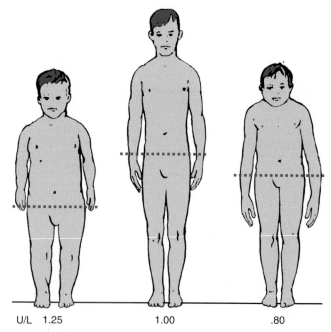

U/L   1.25   1.00   .80

Figure 105-2   Upper segment length/lower segment length (U/L) in 8- to 10-year-old individuals with short limb and short trunk dwarfism. The child on the left has short limbs and an increased U/L ratio; the child on the right has a short trunk and reduced U/L ratio.

a turned-up nose is frequently found in the chondrodysplasia punctata disorders,[25] and abnormal swollen pinnae are seen in diastrophic dysplasia.[26] Individuals with skeletal dysplasias should be screened for ophthalmologic and hearing abnormalities because many of these disorders are associated with eye abnormalities and hearing loss.

Further evaluation of the hands and feet can lead to further differentiation of these disorders. Postaxial polydactyly is characteristically found in chondroectodermal dysplasia and the short-rib polydactyly disorders (see Table 105-1). Short, hypermobile, radially displaced thumbs are seen in diastrophic dysplasia. Nails can be abnormally hypoplastic in chondroectodermal dysplasia and short and broad in cartilage hair hypoplasia. Clubfeet may be seen in many disorders including Kneist dysplasia, spondyloepiphyseal dysplasia congenita, Larsen syndrome, varying forms of osteogenesis imperfecta, and diastrophic dysplasia. Bone fractures occur most commonly in two types of disorders—those that result from undermineralized bone (OI, hypophosphatasia, achondrogenesis IA), or those that result from overmineralized bone (osteopetrosis syndromes and dysosteosclerosis).

Organ systems other than the skeleton can be involved, although rarely. Congenital cardiac defects are seen in chondroectodermal dysplasia (atrial septal defects), the short-rib polydactyly disorders (complex outlet defects including isolated ventricular septal defects), and Larsen syndrome (ventricular septal defects). Gastrointestinal anomalies are rare among the skeletal disorders, but congenital megacolon can be seen in cartilage hair hypoplasia, malabsorption syndrome in Schwachmann-Diamond syndrome, and omphaloceles in otopalatodigital syndrome and atelosteogenesis I.

Diagnosis and Testing

After obtaining a thorough family history and physical examination, the next step is to obtain a full set of skeletal radiographs. A full series of skeletal views includes anterior, lateral, and Towne views of the skull; anterior and lateral views of the entire spine; and anteroposterior views of the pelvis and extremities, with separate views of the hands and feet, especially after the newborn period. Most of the important clues to diagnosis are in skeletal radiographs that are obtained before puberty. When the epiphyses have fused to the metaphyses, determining the precise diagnosis can be extremely challenging. If an adult is evaluated, all attempts should be made to obtain any available childhood radiographs. Many subtle clues in these skeletal radiographs can lead to precise diagnosis. Demonstrating punctate calcifications in the areas of the epiphyses in the chondrodysplasia punctata disorders, multiple ossification centers of the calcaneus in more than 20 disorders,[27] and the type of hand shortening can aid in differentiating many disorders.

After obtaining radiographs, close attention should be paid to the specific parts of the skeleton (spine, limbs, pelvis, skull) involved and to the location of the lesions (epiphyses, metaphyses, and vertebrae) (Figure 105-3). As mentioned earlier, these radiographic abnormalities can change with age, and if available, radiographs across a few years or decades aid in diagnosis. Fractures can be seen in OI (all types) (Figure 105-4; see Table 105-1) and severe hypophosphatasia. In older individuals, fractures may be seen in disorders associated with increased mineralization such as the osteopetrosis syndromes and dysosteosclerosis. When a thorough evaluation of the radiographs reveals abnormalities, but a diagnosis still cannot be made, resources are available. The International Skeletal Dysplasia Registry and European Skeletal Dysplasia Network are available to provide diagnosis for these rare disorders.

Morphologic studies of chondro-osseous tissue have revealed specific abnormalities in many of the skeletal dysplasias.[28-30] In these disorders, histologic evaluation of chondro-osseous morphology can aid in making an accurate diagnosis, and absence of histopathologic alterations can rule out diagnoses. These studies need to be done on cartilage growth plate, and although commonly performed on perinatal lethal skeletal disorders at autopsy, obtaining

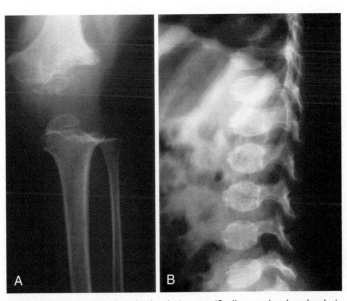

Figure 105-3 Radiographs showing abnormalities in the chondrodysplasias, specifically pseudoachondroplasia. **A,** Irregular metaphyses and small epiphyses. **B,** Small, rounded vertebrae with anterior beaking.

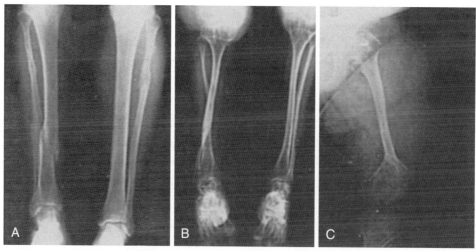

Figure 105-4 Radiographs illustrating skeletal differences among variants of osteogenesis imperfecta (OI). **A,** Dominant OI—mild, with minimal deformity. **B,** Moderate OI—mild epiphyseal dysplasia. **C,** Severe OI—marked diaphyseal narrowing and widening of the metaphysis with severe epiphyseal dysplasia. Lethal OI is not illustrated.

growth plate histology on individuals with nonlethal disorders is difficult. If affected individuals (children) are undergoing surgery, an iliac crest biopsy specimen can be evaluated.

Histomorphology studies done on these disorders have led to important insights on the pathogenesis of these disorders. On morphologic grounds, the chondrodysplasias can be broadly classified into disorders (1) that have a qualitative abnormality in endochondral ossification, (2) that have abnormalities in cellular morphology, (3) that have abnormalities in matrix morphology, and (4) in which the abnormality is primarily localized to the area of chondro-osseous transformation. In thanatophoric dysplasia, there is a defect in endochondral ossification with a short, almost hypertrophic zone; shortened proliferative zone; and overgrowth of the periosteum. In pseudoachondroplasia, there is a distinct lamellar pattern (alternating electron-dense and electron-lucent lamellae) in the rough endoplasmic reticulum of chondrocytes (Figure 105-5) and a grossly abnormal matrix in diastrophic dysplasia, which leads to a characteristic ring around the chondrocytes. All of these findings are characteristic and diagnostic for these disorders and illustrate how

morphology studies can have an integral part in the investigation of these disorders.

There has been significant progress in gene identification in these disorders, which has impact for affected individuals. As illustrated in Table 105-1, for disorders in which the gene is identified, molecular diagnostic testing is potentially available. Molecular diagnosis can be used to confirm a clinical and radiographic diagnosis, predict carrier status in families at risk for a recessive disorder, and, for some individuals, allow for prenatal diagnosis of at-risk fetuses. Because these are rare disorders, commercial testing is not always readily available; however, GeneTests (www.genetests.org) is a publically funded medical genetics website developed for physicians that provides information on diseases and available genetic testing.

Management and Treatment

The optimal management of this diverse set of disorders requires an understanding of the medical, skeletal, and psychosocial consequences.[31] This is often best accomplished by centers that have a multidisciplinary approach, which includes adult and pediatric physicians, orthopedists, rheumatologists, otolaryngologists, neurologists, neurosurgeons, and ophthalmologists who are committed to the care of these patients.

Most medical complications in these disorders result from orthopedic complications, and they vary depending on the specific disorder. In disorders associated with significant odontoid hypoplasia such as Morquio disease, type II collagenopathies, metatropic dysplasia, and Larsen syndrome, flexion-extension films should be monitored at regular intervals to assess for C1-C2 subluxation. Many experts in the field now believe that all individuals with skeletal dysplasias should have evaluation of their cervical spine, regardless of diagnosis. If there is evidence for subluxation, surgery for C1-C2 fixation is indicated. Genu varum—lateral curvature of the lower extremity—is common in many skeletal disorders caused by overgrowth of the fibula; this causes knee or ankle pain in many individuals, especially children, and correction by osteotomy should be

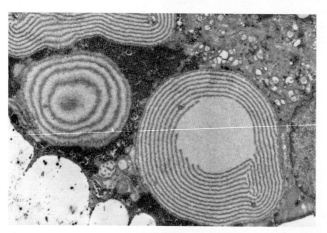

Figure 105-5 Electron micrograph of a chondrocyte from an individual with pseudoachondroplasia. Note the characteristic lamellar pattern in the rough endoplasmic reticulum.

considered. Children and adults with skeletal dysplasias should have regular eye and hearing examinations because they are at increased risk for myopia, retinal degeneration, glaucoma, and hearing loss depending on the disorder.

Frequently, patients with these disorders have significant joint pain and in some cases joint limitations. Because most of these disorders result from mutations in genes crucial to cartilage function, the cartilage at the joint surfaces may not provide adequate support and cushioning function. Many of these patients seek attention for joint pain. Evaluation should include radiographs and magnetic resonance imaging (MRI), when appropriate, to determine the etiology of the pain. In some disorders such as the type II collagenopathies, pseudoachondroplasia, multiple epiphyseal dysplasia, and cartilage hair hypoplasia, by adulthood, so little cartilage remains at the knee or hips that joint replacement is indicated for pain relief. Lastly, overweight in adults with short stature is an ongoing issue and contributes to inactivity, loss of function, adult-onset diabetes, hypertension, and coronary disease.[29]

Achondroplasia

Achondroplasia is the most common of the nonlethal skeletal dysplasias (approximately 1 in 20,000) and serves as an example on how to approach these disorders. Most affected individuals are of normal intelligence, have a normal life span, and lead independent and productive lives. The mean final height in achondroplasia is 130 cm for men and 125 cm for women; specific growth charts have been developed to document and track linear growth, head circumference, and weight in these individuals.[32,33]

In early infancy, there is potentially serious compression of the cervicomedullary spinal cord secondary to a narrow foramen magnum, cervical canal, or both. Clinically, these infants have central apnea, sleep apnea, profound hypotonia, motor delay, emesis while forward positioned in car seats, or excessive sweating. MRI with flow studies is necessary to document the obstruction; if present, obstruction requires decompressive surgery.[34] Other complications include nasal obstruction, venous distention, thoracolumbar kyphosis, and hydrocephalus in a few individuals.[35]

From early childhood, and as children begin to walk around 22 to 24 months, they develop several orthopedic manifestations, which include progressive bowing of the legs owing to fibular overgrowth, lumbar lordosis, and hip flexion contractures. Recurrent ear infections can lead to chronic serous otitis media and deafness. Tympanic membrane tube placement is indicated in many of these patients. Craniofacial abnormalities lead to dental malocclusion, and appropriate treatment is necessary. In adults, the main potential medical complication is impingement of the spinal root canals. This complication can be manifested by lower limb paresthesias, claudication, clonus, or bladder or bowel dysfunction. It is crucial that these complaints are addressed because without appropriate decompression surgery, spinal cord paralysis may result.[36]

Growth hormone has not been effective in increasing height in this disorder.[33] Surgical limb lengthening has been employed successfully to increase limb length by 12 inches,[37] but this technique needs to be done during the teen years and is performed over a 2-year period and is associated with

complications. Recent advances in the molecular understanding underlying achondroplasia have identified molecular targets to potentially treat the disorder, thus improving height and orthopedic complications. Achondroplasia results from heterozygosity for mutations in the gene that encodes fibroblast growth factor receptor 3 (FGFR3). The mutation causes constitutive activation of the receptor leading to increased MAPK signaling with elevated levels of ERK1/2 phosphorylation. Molecules targeted to the tyrosine kinase domain of the receptor and those that diminish ERK signaling have shown efficacy in tissue and animal models. Throughout their lives, individuals with achondroplasia and other skeletal dysplasias and their families experience various psychosocial challenges.[38] These challenges can be addressed by specialized medical and social support systems. Interactions with advocacy groups such as Little People of America (www.lpaonline.org) can provide emotional support and medical information.

Biochemical and Molecular Abnormalities

Similarities in clinical and radiographic findings and histomorphology have placed bone dysplasia into families.[39-41] These families share common pathophysiologic or pathway mechanisms. In recent years, there has been an explosion in understanding of the basic biology of these disorders. This explosion has resulted from the successful human genome project, which improved various methodologies including candidate gene approach, linkage analysis, positional cloning, human/mouse synteny, array comparative genomic hydridization, and massive parallel sequencing (whole exome or whole genome analyses) allowing for identification of the disease genes (see Table 105-1). With gene discovery in the vast number of these osteochondrodysplasias, these genes can be placed into several categories designed to understand their pathogenesis: (1) defects in extracellular proteins; (2) defects in metabolic pathways (enzymes, ion channels, and transporters; (3) defects in folding and degradation of macromolecules; (4) defects in hormones and signal transduction; (5) defects in nuclear proteins; (6) defects in oncogenes and tumor-suppressor genes; (7) defects in RNA and deoxyribonucleic acid (DNA) processing molecules; (8) defects in intracellular structural and organelle proteins; (9) microRNAs; and (10) genes of unknown function.[2] There are still skeletal dysplasias for which the gene and mechanism of disease are unknown. Following are descriptions of some of the molecular mechanisms involved in the skeletal dysplasias.

DEFECTS IN EXTRACELLULAR STRUCTURAL PROTEINS

Type II Collagen and Type XI Collagen

Because type II collagen was found primarily in cartilage, the nucleus pulposus, and the vitreous of the eye, it was hypothesized that skeletal disorders with significant spine and eye abnormalities would result from defects in type II collagen. Type II collagen defects have been identified in a spectrum of disorders ranging from lethal to mild arthropathy, which include achondrogenesis II, hypochondrogenesis, spondyloepiphyseal dysplasia congenita, spondyloepimetaphyseal dysplasia, Strudwick type, Kniest dysplasia, Stickler syndrome, spondyloperipheral dysplasia, and "precocious" familial arthopathy. These disorders are referred to as type II collagenopathies, and they all result from heterozygosity for mutations in *COL2A1*.[42,43] Biochemical analysis of cartilage derived from these individuals shows electrophoretically detectable abnormal type II collagen. Type I collagen is not normally present in cartilage, but in the presence of abnormal type II collagen there is increased type I collagen in the growth plate.

Mutations that result in a substitution for a triple helical glycine residue seem to be the most common type of mutation.[44] There are some correlations between the location of the mutation and the disease phenotype. In spondyloepiphyseal dysplasia, the glycine substitutions are scattered throughout the molecule; however, in Kniest dysplasia, the mutations are in the more amino-terminal end of the molecule.[44-46] Stickler syndrome, a disorder of mild short stature, arthropathy, and high-grade myopia (see Table 105-1), is genetically heterogeneous and results from mutations in *COL2A1* and *COL11A1*, and nonocular forms result from mutations in *COL11A2*.[47,48] In Stickler syndrome, the *COL2A1* and *COL11A1* mutations tend to be nonsense mutations resulting in premature translation stop codons; however, patients with *COL11A1* mutations tend to have a more severe eye phenotype and hearing loss than patients with *COL2A1* mutations.

Individuals heterozygous for various *COL11A2* mutations[49] have a nonocular form of Stickler syndrome, consistent with the absent expression of *COL11A2* in the vitreous humor. Otospondylomegaepiphyseal dysplasia is a rare autosomal recessive disorder caused by loss of function mutations in *COL11A2*.[50] This disorder has radiographic similarities to Kniest dysplasia but is associated with profound sensorineural hearing loss and lack of ocular involvement. Recent discoveries have extended the spectrum of disease for type XI collagen. Autosomal recessive fibrochondrogenesis, a severe skeletal dysplasia, highly associated with lethality, results from mutations in the two genes that encode type XI, *COL11A1* and *COL11A2*.[51,52] Type II and

XI collagens form a heterotypic fibril in the cartilage matrix and not surprisingly, there is significant clinical overlap in the disorders due to mutation in the genes that encode these collagens.

Cartilage Oligomeric Matrix Protein

Heterozygosity for mutations in cartilage oligomeric matrix protein leads to pseudoachondroplasia and multiple epiphyseal dysplasia.[53] Cartilage oligomeric matrix protein is a member of the thrombospondin family of proteins and consists of an epidermal growth factor domain and calcium binding, calmodulin domain.[54] In pseudoachondroplasia and multiple epiphyseal dysplasia, disease-producing mutations occur in the calmodulin domain, with a few in the globular carboxy-terminal domain (Figure 105-6). As opposed to pseudoachondroplasia, multiple epiphyseal dysplasia results from heterozygosity for mutations in numerous genes (*COL9A1*, *COL9A2*, *COL9A3*, and *MATRILIN3*), and there is a recessive form due to mutations in the *DTDST* gene. Both these disorders are associated with significant early destruction of cartilage with many affected individuals undergoing hip and knee replacements at an early age.

Defects in Metabolic Pathways

Defects in metabolic pathways comprise defects in enzymes, ion channels, and transporters essential for cartilage metabolism and homeostasis. An example is the diastrophic dysplasia group (see Table 105-1), a spectrum of disorders (lethal to mild short stature) resulting from mutations in the *DTDST* (*SLC26A2*) gene. These disorders result from a varying defect in the degree of sulfate uptake or transport into chondrocytes.[55] Lack of adequate intracellular sulfate affects the normal post-translational modification of proteoglycans and leads to abnormal chondrogenesis that is proportional to the degree of transporter compromise.[50] Affected individuals suffer from severe degenerative joint disease.

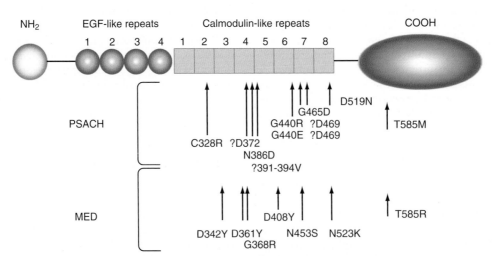

Figure 105-6   Diagram of the cartilage oligomeric matrix protein delineating the domains—NH₂ amino terminus, epidermal growth factor-like (EGF-like), calmodulin-like, carboxy-terminus (COOH), pseudoachondroplasia (PSACH), and multiple epiphyseal dysplasia (MED). Amino acid substitutions are listed below the molecule.

Defects in Intracellular Structural Proteins

Intracellular proteins are ubiquitously expressed proteins; the finding that mutations in the genes encoding filamin A and filamin B produced primarily skeletal disorders was surprising.[56-58] The filamins are cytoskeleton proteins involved in multicellular processes including providing structure to the cell, facilitating signal transduction and transport of small solutes, allowing communication between the intracellular and extracellular environment, and participating in cell division and motility. Defects in these genes have a profound effect on the skeleton ranging from absence of bone formation to significant joint dislocations. The mechanisms by which these mutations produce disease are unclear, though alterations in the cellular and organelle functions are beginning to be elucidated.[59]

Defects in Membrane Channels

Calcium homeostasis is critical for cartilage and bone.[59,60] TRPV4, or transient receptor potential cation channel subfamily V member 4, is a cation channel that mediates calcium influx in response to numerous stimuli. The importance of this channel has been demonstrated because it produces a vast spectrum of autosomal dominant skeletal disorders including lethal metatropic dysplasia, nonlethal metatropic dysplasia, spondyloepiphyseal dysplasia, Kozlowski type, and brachyolmia.[61-63] In addition, heterozygosity for mutations in *TRPV4* also causes neuromuscular diseases without notable boney manifestation that include hereditary motor and sensory neuropathy type IIC, congenital spinal muscular atrophy, and scapuloperoneal spinal muscular atrophy.[64-66] The mechanism by which these mutations scattered throughout the molecule produce such divergent phenotypes is unclear but supports some common pathway in tissues of mesenchymal origin.

Summary

Although these osteochondrodysplasias are rare disorders, affected individuals have significant skeletal complications throughout their lives, first owing to patterning defects, then effects on linear growth, and finally loss of normal structural cartilage as a cushion later in life. The explosion in delineating the molecular defects has shown the complexity of cartilage as a tissue and the large number of cellular processes necessary for a normal skeleton.

OSTEOGENESIS IMPERFECTA

OI is a heritable disorder of bone and was one of the first disorders hypothesized to be a defect in collagen by McKusick.[1] Although an osteochondrodysplasia, OI is discussed separately from the chondrodysplasias delineated previously. OI is a generalized disorder of connective tissue that predominantly affects the skeletal system[67] and affects numerous individuals (estimates at about 1 in 20,000 individuals).

Initially, there were four types of recognized OI in the clinical classification of Sillence.[68] There are now seven well-recognized forms of OI, and through recent gene discoveries it is apparent that a clinical classification system is no longer useful. Because there is enormous clinical variability in these types, the subtypes are discussed separately using historical classifications, but many experts advocate using the terms mild, moderate, and severe (Table 105-2). These disorders all share the same phenotypic finding of hypomineralization of the skeleton.

Mild Osteogenesis Imperfecta (Type I)

Affected individuals with OI type I disease have mild disease in terms of clinical course, the extent of skeletal deformity, and the radiologic appearance of the skeleton (see Figure 105-4A and Table 105-2). They also account for most individuals with OI. Individuals are usually short for their age or their unaffected family members. Many of these individuals experience numerous fractures, especially in childhood; children with OI type I may have 20 fractures by the age of 5.

The disorder is autosomal dominant, and in many cases the individual is the first affected in the family. There is mild facial dysmorphism in OI type I with a mild triangular facial shape. The blue sclerae become gray-to-pale blue in adulthood. Arcus senilis not related to lipid abnormalities may occur in some patients. Other reported ocular defects include scleromalacia, keratoconus, and retinal detachment.[69] Teeth frequently show dentinogenesis imperfecta owing to the effects of mutation on the tooth dentin. The deciduous and permanent teeth have an opalescent and translucent appearance, which tends to darken with age. The enamel is normal, but the dentin is dysplastic; chipping of enamel occurs, and the teeth are subjected to erosion and breakage. Teeth of affected individuals appear discolored or gray. This finding varies in the disorder but does co-segregate in families with OI. During the second and third decades of life, a characteristic high-frequency sensorineural or mixed hearing loss can be detected.[70] The incidence of mitral valve prolapse is not increased in these patients compared with the population at large, but individual kindreds with increased diameter of the aortic root or patients with aortic regurgitation have been reported.[71] Many patients complain of easy bruising, and this may result from the effects of mutation on skin and the vessels below.

Mildly affected patients may not have fractures at birth, although occasionally a fracture of a clavicle or extremity occurs during delivery. Radiographically, affected newborns have wormian bones seen on lateral views of the skull, with significant osteopenia seen through the skeleton, especially the spine. After birth, the frequency of fracture depends on the child's activity, the need for immobilization after lower extremity fractures, and the attitude of the family toward independent activity. Generally, these patients may experience 5 to 15 major fractures before puberty and several minor traumatic fractures of the digits or the small bones of the feet. Characteristically, the fracture rate declines dramatically after puberty, only to increase during later life. Mild scoliosis approximating 20 degrees is common. Osteopenia is observed in vertebral bodies and the peripheral skeleton and progresses with age. In mild OI, the long bones usually heal with no significant deformity. Compared with more severe phenotypes, children with mild OI only infrequently require the insertion of intramedullary rods and almost never experience nonunion at a fracture site.

Table 105-2 Classification and Molecular Basis of Osteogenesis Imperfecta

OI	Clinical Features	Inheritance	Biochemical Abnormality	Gene
Mild (type I)	Normal stature, little or no deformity, blue sclerae, hearing loss, dentinogenesis imperfecta	AD (new mutations are common)	50% reduction in type I collagen synthesis	COL1A1 COL1A2
Lethal (type II)	Lethal; minimal calvarial mineralization, beaded ribs, compressed femurs, long bone deformity	AD (new mutations; gonadal mosaicism) AR	Structural alterations of type I collagen chains—overmodification of type I collagen	COL1A1 COL1A2 CRTAP P3H1 PPBI
Severe (types III and IV)	Progressively deforming bones, dentinogenesis imperfecta, hearing loss, short stature	AD AR	Structural alterations of type I collagen chains—overmodification of type I collagen	COL1A1 COL1A2 CRTAP P3H1 PPBI FKBP10 SERPINH1 SP7
V	Similar to severe OI plus calcification of interosseous membrane of forearm, hyperplastic callus formation	AD	None described	Unknown
VI	Similar to type IV with vertebral compression; mineralization defect	AR	None described	SERPINF1
VII	Moderate to severe, with fractures at birth, early deformity and rhizomelia	AR	None described	CRTAP

AD, autosomal dominant; AR, autosomal recessive; *CRTAP*, cartilage-associated protein; *P3H1*, prolyl-3-hydroxylase 1; *PPBI*, cyclophilin B; *FKBP10*, FK506-binding protein 10; *SERPINH1*, Serpin Peptidase Inhibitor, Clade H, Member1; *SP7*, osterix; *SERPINF1*, Serpin Peptidase Inhibitor, Clade F, Member1.

Although osteopenia with rarefaction of the medullary space and cortical thinning are observed in radiographs, many mild OI cases can be missed on routine radiographic examination and present later in life as individuals with significant osteoporosis. Measurement of bone mineral density by dual-energy x-ray absorptiometry at any age discloses a significant decrease in bone mass.[72] T scores (i.e., standard deviation from the young-adult mean bone mineral density) are frequently in the range of −2.5 to −4.0 at the lumbar spine or proximal femur, consistent with the diagnosis of osteoporosis as defined by the World Health Organization. Low bone mineral density in children with recurrent fractures may assist in identifying children with OI.

Molecular Pathology

As in many other OI phenotypes, OI type I or mild OI is the result of mutations affecting the *COL1A1(I)* and *COL1A2(I)* polypeptide chains of type I collagen. Cultured fibroblasts from individuals with mild OI synthesize low amounts (approximately one-half) of the expected amounts of type I collagen. The molecular basis for the low production of type I collagen seems to be diminished activity of one of the *COL1A1(I)* or *COL1A2(I)* collagen alleles. Many of the reported mutations in OI type I are nonsense and frameshift mutations and are predicted to lead to premature termination codons, although there are some exceptions.[73,74]

Lethal Osteogenesis Imperfecta (Type II)

Approximately 10% of OI patients have the severe neonatal form of the disease, lethal OI. Most cases result from sporadic mutations; however, more recently, recessive forms of the disease have been documented.[75-78] These infants present with severe bone fragility, multiple intrauterine fractures at various stages of healing, deformed extremities, and occasionally hydrops fetalis (Figure 105-7). Radiographic features include wormian bones, multiple fractures, crumbled bones, and characteristic beading of the ribs owing to healing callus formation. There is a subtype of the lethal form, OI type IIC, which is autosomal recessive and is differentiated by the absence of beaded ribs (thin ribs) and a different molecular basis of disease.

Molecular Pathology

Most cases occur de novo, as new dominant mutations; however, autosomal recessive forms have been established, as has recurrence based on germline mosaicism.[79-82] The biochemical abnormality in lethal OI is the inability to synthesize, modify, and secrete normal type I collagen.[83] As a result, the amount of type I collagen in bone is low, much of the secreted collagen is abnormally overmodified, and the quantity of the minor collagen types III and V is high. Bone collagen fibers are thinner than normal, and at the intracellular level, type I collagen is retained within dilated endoplasmic reticulum.

Similar to other forms of OI, mutations in the genes encoding *COL1A1* and *COL1A2A* lead to the dominant form or de novo form of lethal OI.[84] Single glycine substitutions with the Gly-X-Y triplet of either *COL1A1* or *COL1A2* lead to this form of OI, as do some small deletions, all producing severe effects on the triple helix. The recessive form accounts for a few of these cases and results from mutations in the genes encoding either *CRTAP* (cartilage-associated protein), *P3H1* (prolyl-3-hydroxylase 1), and *cyclophilin B (PPBI)*.[75-78] These molecules form a complex that hydroxylates (add an -OH group) to a third position

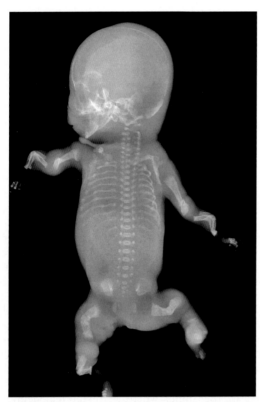

Figure 105-7 Radiograph of lethal osteogenesis imperfecta (type II) showing poorly mineralized calvaria; bent, crumbled bones; and ribs with fractures and callus formation.

residue at proline 986 (Pro986). This modification of a single residue stabilizes the collagen helix.[75-78] Nonsense or frameshift mutations predicted to lead to premature termination codons and absent function of *CRTAP*, *P3H1*, and *PPBI* produce this form of OI.

Severely Deforming Osteogenesis Imperfecta (Including Type III and Type IV)

The deforming variant of OI is the classic form of OI. Similar to lethal OI (OI type II), most cases are inherited as autosomal dominant (or a de novo mutation), although recurrent cases based on autosomal recessive inheritance owing to *CRTAP* or *P3H1* mutations have been described more recently, as well as other recently discovered genes, *FKBP10*, *HSP47*, and *SP7*.[79-81] This variant is characterized by severe deformity of the limbs and marked kyphoscoliosis, thorax deformity, and significant short stature. The extent of growth retardation is remarkable, and in many adults the height may not surpass 3 feet (90 to 100 cm). Abnormal cranial molding occurs in utero and during infancy, producing frontal bossing and a characteristic triangular-shaped facies. Radiographically, wormian bones and delayed closure of the fontanelles may be observed well into the first decade.

Pulmonary function can be diminished because of distortion of the spine and thorax, and this can progress over time and lead to restrictive lung disease and sleep apnea. Because of diminished vital capacity, pulmonary insufficiency is a leading cause of death in patients with OI type III. Many patients with scoliosis greater than 60 degrees develop respiratory compromise and need pulmonary investigations. Many of these individuals need supplemental oxygen.

Platybasia secondary to soft bone at the base of the skull may cause the external ear canals to slant upward as the base of the skull sinks on the cervical vertebrae; this may lead to communicating or obstructive hydrocephalus, cranial nerve palsies, and upper and lower motor neuron lesions. Headache, diplopia, nystagmus, cranial nerve neuralgia, decline in motor function, urinary dysfunction, and respiratory compromise are complications of basilar invagination.[85] As opposed to OI type I, most affected OI type III patients have white sclerae as adults. Approximately 25% of patients with autosomal dominant type III OI have dentinogenesis imperfecta, necessitating constant dental care throughout childhood, though this is not true of the recessive forms of this severe form of OI. Severe hearing impairment occurs in 10% of patients, although milder degrees of hearing loss are more common.

The skeleton in these patients has significant osteopenia, leading to multiple fractures in the upper and lower extremities and vertebral bodies, particularly before puberty. In contrast to OI type I, in which fractures tend to heal without deformity, fractures in OI type III frequently lead to skeletal deformity. Radiographs of the skeleton reveal marked osteopenia, thinning of cortical bone, narrowing of the diaphysis, and widening of the metaphysis, which merges into a dysplastic epiphyseal zone filled with whorls of partially calcified cartilage (i.e., popcorn deformity) (see Figure 105-4C). Osteoporosis leads to collapse of vertebral end plates contributing to worsening kyphoscoliosis. Pectus excavatum or pectus carinatum adds to thoracic deformity. In addition, lack of weight bearing increases the severity of osteoporosis and increases the risk of fracture. Many individuals become wheelchair bound at an early age or walk with mechanical assistance.

Clinically, the phenotype of patients with moderately severe OI (OI type IV) falls between the milder and severe forms of OI. In most cases, this form of OI is inherited in an autosomal dominant fashion. Fractures occur rarely at birth, and some patients may not have an initial fracture until later in the first decade. The extent of skeletal deformity involving the spine, thorax, and extremities is usually intermediate between mild and severe, but these patients have short stature and frequently these patients have scoliosis. Patients may have some mild facial dysmorphisms and hearing loss. Most fractures occur during childhood and may reoccur during the postmenopausal period in women or in men older than age 50 years. Long bone deformity tends to develop after fractures, which may lead to a difficulty in ambulation. Radiographs of the long bones and vertebral bodies show marked osteopenia with vertebral collapse. Although there is marked cortical thinning, bowing, and coarsening of trabeculae, the overall architecture of the bone is normal (see Figure 105-4B).

Molecular Pathology

The molecular basis of OI type III and OI type IV is similar to OI type II. Most cases result from heterozygosity for mutations in *COL1A1(I)* and *COL1A2*.[86,87] These mutations are glycine substitutions scattered throughout the triple helix and in-frame deletions.[68] As in OI type II, familial recurrences result from mutations in *CRTAP, P3H1,* and *PPBI,* which cause autosomal recessive forms of OI. Recently other genes producing autosomal recessive forms of severe OI have been identified including *FKBP10, HSP47,* and *SP7.*[79-81] There may be subtle clinical distinctions between the recessive forms of the disease, though radiographic abnormalities are quite similar. Clinical suspicion of the recessive form of the disease should be considered if there is a family history of recurrence.

Osteogenesis Imperfecta Type V (Moderate to Severe)

OI type V was reported in 2000 as a variant within the heterogeneous group classified under OI type IV.[88] In the initial report of seven OI patients, the phenotype was distinguished by the following criteria: moderate fracture history, hyperplastic callus formation, limitation in forearm pronation and supination as a result of intramembraneous bone formation at the joint, normal sclerae, and no dentinogenesis imperfecta. Bone biopsy specimens showed a meshlike appearance of irregularly spaced lamellae, different from the woven bone seen in OI types II, III, and IV. The etiology of this rare form has not been established.

Osteogenesis Imperfecta Type VI (Moderate to Severe)

The brittle bone phenotype OI type VI was also reported among the heterogeneous OI type IV group of patients. Characteristic among the eight subjects was the occurrence of a first fracture at an early age (4 to 18 months old).[89,90] The bone is severely brittle, and affected patients have white sclerae. All patients had vertebral compression fractures, and patients showed elevated serum alkaline phosphatase levels. The gene for this form of OI has been recently identified, pigment epithelium-derived factor (*PEDF*), also known as serpin F1 (*SERPINF1*), an antiangiogenic protein (unpublished data).

Osteogenesis Imperfecta Type VII (Moderate to Severe)

In addition to OI types V and VI, Glorieux reported on an autosomal recessive form of OI and used the designation OI type VII.[90] This form occurred with a small genetic isolate among the First Nations community in northern Quebec, Canada (S89). The phenotype includes fractures at birth, blue sclerae, osteopenia, rhizomelia, and deformities of the lower extremities. The disorder has been localized to chromosome 3p22-24 and has been shown to result from a hypomorphic allele in *CRTAP.*[63] The identification of the molecular basis of OI type VII changed the molecular view of the basis of disease with the identification of recessively inherited gene defects.

Histopathology of Bone in Osteogenesis Imperfecta

The range of histologic appearances of bone in the different OI phenotypes is as variable as the clinical phenotypes. Undermineralization and overmineralization of bone have been recognized within the same specimen.[91] Bone histomorphology appears relatively normal in OI type I, but osteopenia secondary to thin lamellar plates and diminished cortical width is evident. Immature woven bone and lamellar disarray are characteristic of more severe OI phenotypes.[92]

Treatment

Over the years, there have been multiple attempts to treat OI with a variety of vitamins, hormones, and drugs, none of which has been successful. The list includes administration of mineral supplements, fluoride, androgenic steroids, ascorbic acid, and vitamin D. During the past decade, bisphosphonates administered parenterally or orally to children and adults have shown favorable results. The bisphosphonate pamidronate administered intravenously increased bone mass, decreased skeletal pain, and decreased fracture incidence in children with severe OI.[93] Similar results involving cyclic administration of pamidronate have been reported by other investigators.[94] Dosage regimens in different series for children and adults range from 1 to 3 mg/kg, administered intravenously at 2- to 4-month intervals; lower dosage regimens also have been reported.[94] Generally, reports indicate a significant increase in bone mass in children and a decrease in fracture rate. The effect is most marked in the spine, where vertebral remodeling may improve vertebral height. Metabolic studies have shown a decrease in serum ionized calcium and increase in serum parathyroid hormone.

Urinary excretion of N-telopeptide as an index of bone resorption decreased from 61% to 73%. The major side effects of intravenous bisphosphonate treatment include the acute-phase response (24 hours after infusion) and the occurrence of otitis and vestibular imbalance in a few patients. The currently recommended treatment regimen includes the use of a bisphosphonate, with adequate calcium and vitamin D supplementation to avoid the occurrence of hypercalciuria and to maintain normal serum vitamin D levels. Newer treatments for osteoporosis such as the RANK ligand inhibitor, denosunab, and antisclerostin antibody may hold promise for treatment of patients with OI.

The use of surgery to correct deformities and to facilitate weight bearing has been the subject of several reviews.[95] Multiple osteotomies and realignment of a deformed bone over intramedullary rods is an option for many children with severe bowing.[96] Indications include frequent fractures at the apex of the bow, impaired standing, and limb-length inequality owing to bowing.[97,98] Expanding (telescoping) rods are best for growing children because they require fewer revisions. Spinal deformities are common and usually progressive. Surgical stabilization is most advisable in the teen years or early adulthood when patients can tolerate these complex reconstructions.[99] Early basilar invagination may be halted with prophylactic posterior fusion of the occipital-cervical junction with plate fixation.[100] Patients with severe brain stem compression may require anterior transoral decompression and posterior instrumented fusion. Patients with various types of OI seem to be at increased risk of premature osteoarthritis, the reasons for which are unclear.[101] Total joint arthroplasty is usually successful in these patients, and referral is appropriate if arthroplasty is indicated.

Every child with OI benefits from appropriate rehabilitative therapy.[102,103] Bracing with lightweight plastics as the child begins to walk can minimize microfracture and bowing of the upper femurs. Muscle-strengthening exercises are essential as primary care and after immobilization for fracture. Perhaps the most beneficial programs have been developed around swimming, preferably in heated pools, and as part of continuous rehabilitative medical care.

EHLERS-DANLOS SYNDROME

The heterogeneous group of disorders grouped together as EDS illustrates the genetic and clinical variability characteristic of the heritable disorders of connective tissue. The most cardinal feature of these disorders is the presence of joint hypermobility, associated with an increase in skin elasticity and skin fragility. In 1997, a simplified classification was proposed dividing EDS into six major clinical types. The classification includes the classic, hypermobility, vascular, kyphoscoliosis, arthrochalasia, and dermatosparaxis types, as well as several rarer EDS types grouped into "other forms."[104] Clinically, EDS can be difficult to separate, however, because of considerable overlap in phenotype findings.

Classic Type

The classic type of EDS accounts for about 80% of reported cases[105] and is inherited as an autosomal dominant trait. Originally, EDS was classified as types I and II, and now these types are classified as the classic form, although these subclassifications are still in use. Previously, types I and II EDS were distinguished from each other on the basis of joint laxity and skin fragility, which are less severe in type I than in type II EDS. Most prototypic forms of EDS (Figure 105-8) are characterized by various degrees of hyperextensibility of large and small joints, which are classic findings in EDS. It is crucial that hyperextensibility be defined, and differentiating mild "normal" laxity from hyperextensibility can be challenging. Beighton and colleagues[104] have presented a clinically useful classification of joint laxity (Figure 105-9), as follows:

1. Passive dorsiflexion of the fifth digit beyond 90 degrees = 1 point for each hand
2. Passive apposition of the thumbs to the flexor surface of the radius = 1 point for each hand
3. Hyperextension of the elbows beyond 10 degrees = 1 point for each side
4. Hyperextension of the knees beyond 10 degrees = 1 point for each knee
5. Flexion of the trunk forward so that the palms can be placed flat on the ground = 1 point

A score of 5 or more points is defined as joint hypermobility.

Large joint hyperextensibility is seen in varying degrees in the classic form and decreases with age. Recurrent joint dislocations, periodic joint effusion related to trauma, and the eventual appearance of osteoarthritis pose significant management problems. Bilateral synovial thickening has been observed in EDS, along with the accumulation of small masses of crystalline material in synovial villi. It has been observed that EDS patients constituted 5% of cases in a

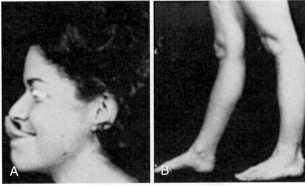

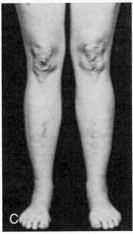

Figure 105-8 Ehlers-Danlos syndrome type I. Tissue elasticity, joint hypermobility, and tissue fragility are shown by the patient's ability to extend her tongue to the tip of the nose (Gorlin's sign) **(A)**, by hyperextensibility at the knee (genu recurvatum) **(B)**, and by characteristic "cigarette paper" or papyraceous scars of the knees and tibial skin **(C)**. *(Courtesy V. McKusick, MD.)*

pediatric arthritis clinic population.[106] There is debate about whether affected infants may be born prematurely to affected mothers because of early rupture of amniotic membranes. Patients with EDS have characteristic facies, with a broad nasal root and epicanthal folds. They may have large, lax ears, and traction on the ears or elbows reveals skin hyperextensibility. Another sign of hypermobility is the ability to touch the tip of the tongue to the nose (Gorlin's sign). In addition, absence of the lingual frenulum is characteristic for this disorder.

In EDS, the skin has a characteristically pleasant soft or "velvety" feel that can be appreciated by stroking the forearms. Thin, atrophic corrugated and hyperpigmented scars are found on the forehead, under the chin, and on the lower extremities (known as cigarette paper or papyraceous scars), although this is not a uniform finding. Typically, skin lesions heal slowly after injury or surgery. Molluscoid pseudotumors (violaceous subcutaneous tumors ranging in size from 0.5 to 3 cm) may be palpated in tissue over pressure points on the forearms and lower extremities and may be seen on radiographs. Although many patients claim to bruise easily, ecchymoses distributed on the extremities are found only in patients with the more severe forms of the disorder. Severe bilateral varicose veins are a common problem.

Associated pulmonary complications of EDS include spontaneous pneumothorax, pneumomediastinum, and

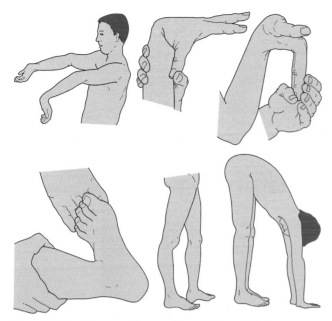

Figure 105-9 Maneuvers that may be used to establish the presence of clinically significant joint laxity found in Ehlers-Danlos syndrome. It is not unusual to find extreme laxity of the small joints and less laxity in large joints. Laxity decreases with age, so the dominant nature of most of these syndromes may not be appreciated when examining older family members. *(Redrawn and modified from Wynne-Davies R: Acetabular dysplasia and familial joint laxity: two etiological factors in congenital dislocation of the hip—a review of 589 patients and their families,* J Bone Joint Surg Br *52:704, 1970.)*

subpleural blebs.[107] Mitral valve prolapse and tricuspid valve insufficiency may complicate classic EDS, and aortic root dilation has been reported, although the rate of progression is unknown.[108,109] Skeletal abnormalities include thoracolumbar kyphoscoliosis; a long, giraffe-like neck; downward sloping of the ribs of the upper part of the thorax; and a tendency toward reversal of the normal cervical, thoracic, and lumbar curves. Anterior wedging of thoracic vertebral bodies is occasionally seen.[110]

Hypermobility Type

The hypermobile type of EDS is a dominantly inherited disorder that manifests as marked joint and spine hypermobility, recurrent joint dislocations, and the typical soft skin that is neither hyperextensible nor velvety. Individuals with EDS type III may have virtually normal skin. Because of the extent of joint laxity affecting large and small joints, these patients experience multiple dislocations and may require surgical repair. The shoulders, patellae, and temporomandibular joints are frequently sites of dislocation. Musculoskeletal pain may mimic that of fibromyalgia syndrome, and patients frequently seek medical attention for symptoms consistent with chronic pain.

One difficulty in this subtype is differentiating it from benign hypermobility syndrome. Benign hypermobility syndrome is used to describe patients with generalized joint laxity, associated musculoskeletal complaints, but normal skin. They do not have the classic stigmata of either EDS or Marfan syndrome. Many of these patients present in their 20s and 30s with rheumatologic symptoms that can pose

problems in diagnosis and treatment. The precise approach and treatment for these patients are unclear.

Structural and Molecular Pathology of the Classic and Hypermobile Types of Ehlers-Danlos Syndrome

Abnormally large, small, or frayed dermal collagen fibrils and disordered elastic fibers have been observed in the classic and hypermobile forms of EDS by electron microscopy.[111] Type V collagen is a heterotrimeric collagen composed of the products of three genes: COL5A1(V), COL5A2(V), and COL5A3(V). Type V collagen may stabilize type I collagen by co-assembling with that protein. Initially, linkage analysis was used to show that some families with the classic form of EDS (originally types I and II) were linked to COL5A1. Subsequently, it has been established that about 50% of patients with either the classic or hypermobility type of EDS have mutations in COL5A1(V) or COL5A2(V). There seems to be no genotype-phenotype correlation in these disorders, and no mutations have been identified in COL5A3(V). In some cases of EDS classic type, heterozyosity for mutations in COL1A1(I) has been shown.[112]

Vascular Type

The vascular type of EDS, an autosomal dominant disorder, is one of the most severe forms of EDS and was formerly referred to as *EDS type IV.* It is associated with arterial rupture, commonly involving iliac, splenic, or renal arteries or the aorta and resulting in either massive hematomas or death.[113] Arterial rupture may lead to stroke or intracompartmental bleeding in a limb. Patients with vascular EDS also are susceptible to rupture of internal viscera and may experience repeated rupture of diverticula on the antimesenteric border of the large bowel. Problems with pregnancy vary from preterm delivery to uterine or vascular rupture, although delivery is uneventful in many instances.[114] Typical causes of death in EDS families have included gastrointestinal rupture, peripartum uterine rupture, rupture of the hepatic artery, and vascular ruptures.

In contrast to the other forms of EDS, EDS type IV is not associated with hyperextensiblity of large joints, although small joints may be minimally hypermobile. These patients have thin, soft, transparent skin, through which a prominent venous pattern is seen, especially on their chest walls. Their skin is not velvety as in the classic form. Excessive bruisability may occur. Vascular EDS includes, as a subgroup, patients who have been described as acrogyric—having characteristically thin faces, prominent eyes, and extremities that lack subcutaneous fat, giving the appearance of premature aging. Peripheral joint contractures and acro-osteolysis have been described.

Spontaneous hemopneumothorax associated with hemoptysis and mitral valve prolapse occurs frequently. Surgical repair of ruptured vessels or internal viscera is extremely difficult because of friable tissues. Anesthetic and surgical difficulties related to intubation, spontaneous arterial bleeding during surgery, and ligation of vessels that tear under pressure complicate surgical maneuvers. Similarly, arteriography may be dangerous in these individuals. These patients can be quite difficult to manage. Imaging studies may reveal normal-appearing aorta or other large vessels that rupture shortly after a "normal study."

Molecular Pathology

Although EDS type IV was clinically recognized as a disorder distinct from the other forms of EDS, the finding that tissues from these individuals were deficient in type III collagen clearly distinguished this as a separate form of EDS. Type III collagen is a homotrimer [1(III)3] found in skin, blood vessels, and the walls of hollow viscera. Heterozygosity for mutations in the gene encoding *COL3A1* leads to EDS vascular type and affects the synthesis and secretion of type III collagen. Various types of mutations have been identified including missense, nonsense, and deletions, and there is no correlation between the clinical phenotype and type III collagen mutation. In this disorder, the biochemical abnormalities include decreased or absent type III collagen or production of an abnormal homotrimer that is retained in the endoplasmic reticulum and, if secreted, contributes to abnormal matrix. Biochemical and mutational analysis for this disorder is available (GeneTests) and should be considered because this is dominantly inherited.

Therapy in Classic, Hypermobility, and Vascular Types of Ehlers-Danlos Syndrome

There are no specific treatments for the classic, hypermobility, and vascular forms of EDS. Supportive therapy is essential, however, for preservation of normal joint function and alleviation of joint pain. Planned exercise programs and muscle strengthening exercises are useful and do much to maintain a positive outlook in these individuals, who may have a poor prognosis if joint stability and articular surfaces are compromised by excessive activity or chronic trauma. Many children and young adults with large joint hypermobility are attracted to activities such as gymnastics and dance, and these activities promote hypermobility and joint damage. The presence of multiple ecchymoses raises concern about a bleeding diathesis, particularly at the time of elective surgery. Although there is no consistent basis for the hemorrhagic tendency in the classic and hyperextensibility forms of EDS, anecdotally, these patients tend to have greater blood losses than expected at surgery. In our center, we discourage pregnancy in patients with the vascular form because the mortality rate is increased.

Arthrochalasia Type

Formerly known as EDS types VIIA and VIIB, the arthrochalasia type of EDS is another autosomal dominant form resulting from mutations that cause faulty processing of type I collagen at the N-terminus. The arthrochalasia type of EDS is characterized by pronounced and generalized joint hypermobility, moderate cutaneous elasticity, moderate bruising, a characteristic round facies with midface hypoplasia, and significant short stature. The skin has a doughy feel and is fragile and hyperelastic. Kyphoscoliosis and muscle hypotonia are frequently present. These patients experience multiple dislocations, particularly involving large joints including the hips, knees, and ankles. These

dislocations manifest in the newborn period, especially hip and ankle dislocations. Patients frequently need orthopedic surgery for joint dislocation, and their tissues are highly friable, which complicates orthopedic procedures.

Molecular Pathology

The two disorders EDS types VIIA and VIIB, now termed *arthrochalasia type*, result from mutations involving the N-terminal propeptide cleavage site of type I collagen.[115-117] The arthrochalasia type of EDS has provided insight into the process of normal type I collagen fiber formation. The initial observation was of an accumulation of unprocessed procollagen within the dermis of affected individuals. With subsequent recognition that procollagen had N-terminal and C-terminal extension propeptides, and that separate enzymes were responsible for their removal, the syndrome became more sharply defined as an accumulation of procollagen with the N-terminal peptides still attached (pN collagen).[100] Of the two distinctly different genetic abnormalities resulting in procollagen accumulation, the more frequent form is the mutational resistance of a procollagen cleavage site to the action of the N-terminal procollagen peptidase. The resistance results from an amino acid substitution or deletion in the proCOL1A1 (EDS type VIIA) or pro2COL2A1 (EDS type VIIB) chain, leading to a portion of the collagen chains containing an abnormal N-terminal extension; this results from mutations in *COL1A1* or *COL1A2* in exon 6 of the molecule, which alters the proteinase cleavage site. Individuals with mutations in exon 6 of *COL1A1* are more severely affected than individuals with similar mutations in *COL1A2*.[116]

Dermatosparaxis Type

The dermatosparaxis type of EDS was formerly known as *EDS type VIIC* and is an autosomal recessive form of EDS. In this type, the skin is extremely fragile, soft, and doughy with easy bruising. The phenotype includes blue sclerae, marked joint hypermobility, micrognathia, large umbilical hernia, epiphyseal delay, and mild hirsutism.[117] The dermatosparaxis type results from a deficiency of the procollagen N-propeptidase, in contrast to the arthrochalasia form, which involves the enzyme cleavage site, and individuals have been identified who are homozygous for mutations in the gene.[103] This defect is homologous to the dermatosparaxis defect in sheep and cattle.[118]

Kyphoscoliosis Type

The kyphoscoliosis type of EDS, formerly known as *EDS type VI*, is inherited as an autosomal recessive disease. The findings in this disorder include severe kyphoscoliosis noted at birth, recurrent joint dislocations, hyperextensible skin and joints, poor tone, and reduced muscle mass.[119] The skin is grossly abnormal and has been described as pale, translucent, and velvety; on trauma, the skin shows gaping wounds that heal poorly. One difference in this form of EDS is that there is significant ocular involvement. Affected individuals have microcornea, retinal detachment, and glaucoma leading to blindness in some individuals. In addition, patients with severe kyphoscoliosis may develop respiratory and cardiac compromise and ultimately cardiorespiratory failure.

Molecular Pathology

The kyphoscoliosis type of EDS results from lysyl hydroxylase deficiency.[119] A variety of mutations within the lysyl hydroxylase gene have been defined and include premature stop codons, amino acid substitutions, internal deletions, and compound heterozygotes.[119] Defective lysyl hydroxylase impairs the conversion of lysyl residues to hydroxylysine on procollagen peptides. The consequence of deficient hydroxylysine content of collagen is the effect it has on crosslinking, which helps stabilize the mature collagen molecule.

Other Ehlers-Danlos Syndrome Types

Numerous other rare forms of EDS have some overlap with other disorders or have been reported only in a small cohort of individuals, and these are not discussed in this chapter.

MARFAN SYNDROME

One of the most common inherited disorders of connective tissue, Marfan syndrome is an autosomal dominant disorder with a reported incidence of 1 in 10,000 to 20,000 individuals.[120] Clinical presentations range from the severe infantile form to individuals who are only mildly affected. Although the most impressive findings in Marfan syndrome are relative to the musculoskeletal, cardiac, and ocular findings, affected individuals also have pulmonary, neurologic, and psychological complications. Marfan syndrome also has become one of the few genetic disorders for which there has been advocacy for treatment to slow the progression of the disease, and physicians need to recognize the phenotype because many affected individuals present with life-threatening emergencies.

Clinical Features

Marfan syndrome can be difficult to diagnose in some individuals and families, and it has been recognized that it has also been overdiagnosed. Stringent criteria for this diagnosis were proposed in 1996.[120] The 1996 criteria rely on the recognition of "major" and "minor" clinical manifestations involving the skeletal, cardiovascular, dura, and ocular systems (excellent review in *GeneReviews*, Marfan syndrome). Major criteria include four of eight typical skeletal manifestations, ectopia lentis, aortic root dilation involving the sinuses of Valsalva or aortic dissection, and lumbosacral dural ectasia by computed tomography or MRI. Major criteria for establishing the diagnosis in a family member include having a parent, child, or sibling who meets major criteria independently, and the presence of a *fibrillin-1* mutation known to cause the syndrome identified in a familial Marfan syndrome patient.

Establishing the diagnosis unequivocally in the absence of a family history requires a major manifestation from two systems and involvement of a third system. If a mutation known to cause Marfan syndrome is identified, the diagnosis requires one major criterion and involvement of a second organ system. The reason is that there is a great deal of intrafamilial variability in this disorder, and there are individuals who harbor heterozygosity for mutations but do not meet criteria for Marfan syndrome and may have different prognoses.[121] Similar to other connective tissue disorders, there is wide variability in phenotypic expression.

Aortic disease leading to the formation of aneurysmal dilation and dissection is the main cause of morbidity and mortality in Marfan syndrome.[122] Dilation of the aorta is found in 50% of children and progresses over time. Echocardiography shows that 60% to 80% of adult patients have dilation of the aortic root that may involve other segments of the thoracic aorta, the abdominal aorta, or even the carotid and intracranial arteries. Dissection usually begins above the coronary ostia and extends the entire length of the aorta. Of Marfan syndrome patients, 60% to 70% have mitral valve prolapse with regurgitation. Heart failure and myocardial infarction may complicate the course of Marfan syndrome patients. Pregnant women are at particular risk for aortic dissection, particularly women who already have aortic root dilation, and this should be taken into consideration when treating a woman of reproductive age with Marfan syndrome.[123]

Arachnodactyly occurs in 90% of patients. Following are techniques that aid in determining arachnodactyly (Figure 105-10):

1. The thumb: The Steinberg test is positive when the thumb, enclosed in the clenched fist, extends beyond the hypothenar border.
2. The wrist: The Walker-Murdoch sign is positive when there is overlap of the thumb and fifth digit as they encircle the opposite wrist.
3. The metacarpal: The metacarpal index is done by radiographic determination and is the mean value of the lengths divided by the midpoint widths of the second, third, and fourth metacarpals. In normal subjects, the metacarpal index ranges from 5.4 to 7.9, whereas this range is 8.4 to 10.4 in patients with Marfan syndrome.

Thoracic kyphosis may be associated with reduced lung capacity and residual volume that may lead to pulmonary insufficiency. Dural ectasia, which may occur in 40% of patients, results from enlargement of the spinal canal owing to progressive ectasia of the dura and neural foramina and erosion of vertebral bone; this usually involves the lower spine.[124] Diminished bone mineral density has been reported in several patients with Marfan syndrome.[125] Ectopia lentis occurs in 50% to 80% of patients with Marfan syndrome. Subluxation of the lens is usually bilateral and appears by age 5 years. Although the lens is typically displaced upward, displacement into any quadrant may occur. Visual acuity is diminished in many patients because of lens subluxation or secondary acute glaucoma. Secondary myopia, retinal detachment, and iritis with loss of vision contribute to most of the ocular-related morbidity.[126]

Marfan syndrome patients have been found to develop large epidural venous plexuses in the lumbar and cervical regions, a major diagnostic criterion for the syndrome. These engorged venous plexuses, which are visualized by MRI myelography, have been associated with the syndrome of spontaneous intracranial hypotension, which is also

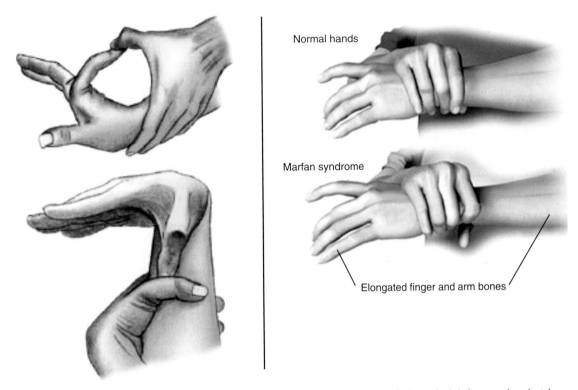

Normal hands

Marfan syndrome

Elongated finger and arm bones

Figure 105-10 Marfan syndrome. The Steinberg test (thumb) and the Walker-Murdoch test (wrist) show arachnodactyly.

associated with dural tears. Clinical signs are severe headache, back and leg pain, radiculopathies, and incontinence secondary to cerebral displacement.[127] Spinal abnormalities in Marfan syndrome include increased interpedicle distance of nonrotated vertebrae, vertebral inversion (flattening of the normal kyphosis at the dorsal level and kyphosis or disappearance of the physiologic lordosis at the lumbar level), and vertebral dysplasia (dolichospondylic, elongated vertebral bodies with increased concavity). Scoliosis constitutes one of the major management problems in Marfan syndrome. In one series, the average age of onset was 10.5 years (range, 3 to 15 years), with rapid progression during adolescence.[128] If mechanical bracing or physical therapy fails to halt progression, spinal fusion should be considered, particularly when the curvature exceeds 45 to 50 degrees.

Differential Diagnosis: Homocystinuria

Homocystinuria, which shares several skeletal and ocular features with Marfan syndrome, is the prime diagnostic consideration. Homocystinuria is an autosomal recessive disease. The characteristic features of this metabolic disorder of sulfur metabolism are marfanoid phenotype with joint laxity, scoliosis, lens dislocation, early-onset osteoporosis, vascular thrombosis affecting arteries and veins owing to increased clotting activity and the cytotoxic effect of homocysteine on vascular endothelial cells, and mild mental retardation.[129]

Cystathionine β-synthase deficiency is the most common cause of homocystinuria.[130] Affected individuals have elevated levels of homocystine and methionine, whereas cystathionine and cysteine levels in blood are decreased. This disorder is differentiated from Marfan syndrome because the direction of ectopia lentis is different than in Marfan syndrome, and there is no progressive aortic root dilation.

Molecular Biology of Marfan Syndrome

Fibrillin-1 protein is an important component of elastic and nonelastic connective tissues throughout the body.[131] It is the main protein of a group of connective tissue microfibrils that are essential for normal elastic fibrillogenesis. In nonelastic tissues, the fibrillin-1-containing microfibril functions as an anchoring fiber. *FBN-1* is a large gene (65 exons) located at chromosome 15q21.1.

Since the first report of an *FBN-1* mutation in Marfan syndrome in 1991, more than 500 different *FBN-1* mutations have been described in Marfan syndrome and related disorders.[132] *FBN-1* mutations occur across a wide range of milder phenotypes that overlap the classic Marfan phenotype including dominantly inherited ectopia lentis, Shprintzen-Goldberg syndrome, and familial or isolated forms of aortic aneurysms.[133] Most of these are private mutations (occur genetically independent with no "hot spot" in the molecule). The one exception is the rare infantile Marfan syndrome mutations that cluster between exons 24 and 26 and exon 32. Heterozygosity for missense, frameshifts, deletions and insertions, splice site alterations, and nonsense mutations all have been seen.[1] Robinson and colleagues[133] stated that at least 337 mainly unique mutations in the *FBN-1* gene had been reported in Marfan syndrome up to that time. The clinical presentation of the fibrillinopathies caused by *FBN-1* mutations ranged from isolated ectopia lentis to neonatal Marfan syndrome, which generally leads to death within the first 2 years of life.

Treatment

In 1972, the life span of untreated patients with classic Marfan syndrome was about 32 years. The early mortality in Marfan syndrome results primarily from complications associated with aortic dilation. This symmetric dilation of the sinuses of Valsalva is progressive throughout life and is often detectable in infancy. In the early 1970s, there was discussion on attempting to reduce the risk of aortic dissection in patients with Marfan syndrome. Shores and colleagues[134] reported on a 10-year open-label trial of propranolol in 70 patients with Marfan syndrome. When compared with the control group, the treated individuals had a significantly slower rate of dilation of the aortic root, improved survival, and fewer treated patients reaching a clinical endpoint (death, congestive heart failure, aortic regurgitation, aortic dissection, or cardiovascular surgery).

More recent data generated from a mouse model of Marfan syndrome suggest excessive signaling by the transforming growth factor transforming growth factor (TGF)-β family of cytokines.[135] There is evidence that aortic aneurysm in the mouse model of Marfan syndrome is associated with increased TGF-β signaling and TGF-β antagonists such as TGF-β-neutralizing antibody or the angiotensin II type 1 receptor blocker, losartan. In this mouse model, losartan (angiotensin II type 1 blockade) fully corrected the abnormalities in the aortic wall. There was some evidence that alveolar septation, which contributes to pulmonary problems in Marfan syndrome, was partially reversed with losartan treatment. Because this drug is in clinical use for hypertension, it could merit further investigation as a preventive treatment in Marfan syndrome. Clinical trials are now under way testing the use of losartan in Marfan syndrome and many individuals with Marfan syndrome are using losartan outside of clinical trials.

Electrocardiogram monitoring is done yearly until the aortic root diameter exceeds 45 mm, at which time monitoring is done every 6 months. Elective repair of aortic root disease before enlargement to 6 cm has occurred is preferable to emergency repair required for marked dilation or dissection. Surgical intervention is considered when the aortic root diameter approaches twice the upper limit of normal for body surface area, or the absolute measurement exceeds 50 to 55 mm. Total aortic root replacement with a composite valve graft (Bentall procedure) and coronary artery implantation have become the surgical procedures of choice and are associated with an 81% 10-year survival rate and a 75% 20-year survival rate.[136,137] Mitral valve replacement and coronary artery implantation may be accomplished during the same procedure. Most importantly, repeated trials have shown that patients who undergo elective repair, as opposed to emergent repair, do substantially better.

Correction of scoliosis may be attempted with bracing; however, surgical repair should be considered when the curve exceeds 40 degrees. Progressive scoliosis in Marfan syndrome may require fixation with rods, and complications of joint laxity may require orthopedic correction. Arthropathy associated with excessive joint mobility may require orthopedic intervention. Dislocated lenses should not be removed surgically, unless more conventional means of correcting vision are ineffective.

LOEYS-DIETZ SYNDROME

In 2005, Loeys and colleagues[138] described individuals with a previously undescribed autosomal dominant aortic aneurysm syndrome. This disorder, now referred to as *Loeys-Dietz syndrome*, also is characterized by hypertelorism, bifid uvula or cleft palate or both, and generalized arterial tortuosity with ascending aortic aneurysm and dissection. Other abnormal findings include craniosynostosis, structural brain abnormalities, mental retardation, congenital heart disease, and aneurysms with dissection throughout the arterial tree.

Some individuals with Loeys-Dietz syndrome had a clinical phenotype that overlapped with Marfan syndrome, but none met diagnostic criteria set forth in 1996.[138] Although Marfan syndrome is associated with progressive arterial disease, in Loeys-Dietz syndrome the aneurysms tended to be particularly aggressive and rupture at an earlier stage and size than seen in Marfan syndrome. Heterozygosity for mutations in *TGFBR1* and *TGFBR* has been identified.[138] From a management perspective, it is important to recognize these individuals because they are managed more aggressively than patients with Marfan syndrome. Aortic aneurysms are corrected at smaller sizes (4 cm), and complaints such as abdominal pain and headache should be thoroughly investigated because they may be associated with aneurysms.

CONGENITAL CONTRACTURAL ARACHNODACTYLY

Congenital contractural arachnodactyly is an autosomal dominant condition that includes tall stature, arachnodactyly, dolichostenomelia, and multiple contractures involving large joints.[139] There is a characteristic "crumpled ear" deformity as a result of a flattened helix with partial obliteration of the concha. Marked deformity of the chest cage also occurs, and scoliosis may be progressive and severe. For unknown reasons, the contractures tend to become less severe with age. Radiographically, osteopenia can be seen. The ocular and typical cardiac lesions of classic Marfan syndrome are absent. This disorder results from heterozygosity for mutation in *fibrillin-2 (FNB-2)*.[140] There are many other extremely rare disorders of connective tissue, especially with profound effects on the skin including the group of disorders termed *cutis laxa* and *pseudoxanthoma elasticum*.[141,142]

SUMMARY

Heritable disorders of connective tissues are a heterogeneous group of disorders characterized by abnormalities in skeletal tissues including cartilage, bone, tendon, ligament, muscle, and skin. The clinical spectrum ranges from extreme short stature to excessively tall individuals, and the types of altered genes span all of the numerous gene families and pathways. Affected individuals usually need medical attention their entire lives and have been victims of appearing different because they cannot mask their abnormalities. Understanding and appreciation for the unique set of medical issues in each disorder would improve these individuals' quality of life and their life span.

Selected References

1. McKusick VA: *Heritable disorders of connective tissue*, St Louis, 1956, CV Mosby.

2. Warman ML, Cormier-Daire V, Hall C, et al: Nosology and classification of genetic skeletal disorders: 2010 revision, *Am J Med Genet A* 155A:943–968, 2011.

3. Orioli IM, Castilla EE, Barbosa-Neto JG: The birth prevalence rates for the skeletal dysplasias, *J Med Genet* 23:328–332, 1986.

4. Kornak U, Mundlos S: Genetic disorders of the skeleton: a developmental approach, *Am J Hum Genet* 73:447–474, 2003.

5. Rosenberg A: Bones and joints and soft tissue tumors. In Cotran RS, Kumar V, Collins T, editors: *Robbins pathologic basis of disease*, ed 6, Philadelphia, 1999, WB Saunders, pp 1215–1221.

6. Karsenty G: Genetics of skeletogenesis, *Dev Genet* 22:301–313, 1998.

7. Dreyer SD, Zhou G, Lee B: The long and the short of it: developmental genetics of the skeletal dysplasias, *Clin Genet* 54:464–473, 1998.

8. Shum L, Nuckolls G: The life cycle of chondrocytes in the developing skeleton, *Arthritis Res* 4:94–106, 2002.

9. Karsenty G: Transcriptional control of skeletogenesis, *Annu Rev Genomics Hum Genet* 9:183–196, 2008.

10. Kuivaniemi H, Tromp G, Prockop DJ: Mutations in fibrillar collagens (types I, II, III, and XI), fibril-associated collagen (type IX), and network-forming collagen (type X) cause a spectrum of diseases of bone, cartilage, and blood vessels, *Hum Mutat* 9:300–315, 1997.

11. Eyre DR: Collagens and cartilage matrix homeostasis, *Clin Orthop* 427(Suppl):S118–S122, 2004.

12. Chan D, Ho MS, Cheah KS: Aberrant signal peptide cleavage of collagen X in Schmid metaphyseal chondrodysplasia: implications for the molecular basis of the disease, *J Biol Chem* 276:7992–7997, 2001.

13. Eyre D: Collagen of articular cartilage, *Arthritis Res* 4:30–35, 2002.

14. McKusick VA: *Heritable disorders of connective tissue*, ed 4, St Louis, 1972, CV Mosby.

15. Rimion DL: Molecular defects in the skeletal chondrodysplasias, *J Med Genet* 63:106–110, 1996.

16. Superti-Furga A, Bonafe L, Rimoin DL: Molecular-pathogenetic classification of the skeleton, *Am J Med Genet* 106:282–293, 2001.

17. Edwards MJ, Wenstrup RJ, Byers PH, et al: Recurrence of lethal osteogenesis imperfecta due to parental mosaicism for a mutation in the COL1A2 gene of type I collagen: the mosaic parent exhibits phenotypic features of a mild form of the disease, *Hum Mutat* 1:47–54, 1992.

18. Stevenson DA, Brothman AR, Chen Z, et al: Paternal uniparental disomy of chromosome 14: confirmation of a clinically-recognizable phenotype, *Am J Med Genet A* 130:88–91, 2004.

19. Unger S, Korkko J, Krakow D, et al: Double heterozygosity for pseudoachondroplasia and spondyloepiphyseal dysplasia congenita, *Am J Med Genet* 101:140–146, 2001.

20. Chitty LS, Tan AW, Nesbit DL, et al: Sonographic diagnosis of SEDC and double heterozygote of SEDC and achondroplasia—a report of six pregnancies, *Prenat Diagn* 26:861–865, 2006.

21. Pauli RM, Conroy MM, Langer LO, et al: Homozygous achondroplasia with survival beyond infancy, *Am J Med Genet* 16:459–473, 1983.

22. Lachman RS: *Radiology of syndromes, skeletal and metabolic disorders*, ed 4, Chicago, 2007, Year Book Medical Publishers.

23. Krakow D, Alanay Y, Rimoin LP, et al: Evaluation of prenatal-onset osteochondrodysplasias by ultrasonography: a retrospective and prospective analysis, *Am J Med Genet A* 146A:1917–1924, 2008.

24. Hunter AG, Bankier A, Rogers JG, et al: Medical complications of achondroplasia: a multicentre patient review, *J Med Genet* 35:705–712, 1998.

25. Sheffield LJ, Danks DM, Mayne V, et al: Chondrodysplasia punctata—23 cases of a mild and relatively common variety, *J Pediatr* 89:916–923, 1976.

26. Lamy M, Maroteaux P: Le nanisme diastrophique, *Presse Med* 68:1977–1980, 1960.

27. Cormier-Daire V, Savarirayan R, Unger S, et al: "Duplicate calcaneus": a rare developmental defect observed in several skeletal dysplasias, *Pediatr Radiol* 31:38–42, 2001.

28. Rimoin DL: The chondrodystrophies, *Adv Hum Genet* 5:1–118, 1975.

29. Sillence DO, Horton WA, Rimoin DL: Morphologic studies in the skeletal dysplasias, *Am J Pathol* 96:813–870, 1979.

30. Rimoin DL, Sillence DO: Chondro-osseous morphology and biochemistry in the skeletal dysplasias, *Birth Defects Orig Artic Ser* 17:249–265, 1981.

31. Krakow D, Rimoin DL: The skeletal dysplasias, *Genet Med* 12(6):327–341, 2010.

32. Hecht JT, Hood OJ, Schwartz RJ, et al: Obesity in achondroplasia, *Am J Med Genet* 31:597–602, 1988.

33. Horton WA, Rotter JI, Rimoin DL, et al: Standard growth curves for achondroplasia, *J Pediatr* 93:435–438, 1978.

34. Hunter AG, Hecht JT, Scott CI Jr: Standard weight for height curves in achondroplasia, *Am J Med Genet* 62:255–261, 1996.

35. Gordon N: The neurological complications of achondroplasia, *Brain Dev* 22:3–7, 2000.

36. Kanaka-Gantenbein C: Present status of the use of growth hormone in short children with bone diseases (diseases of the skeleton), *J Pediatr Endocrinol Metab* 14:17–26, 2001.

37. Yasui N, Kawabata H, Kojimoto H, et al: Lengthening of the lower limbs in patients with achondroplasia and hypochondroplasia, *Clin Orthop* 344:298–306, 1997.

38. Hill V, Sahhar M, Aitken M, et al: Experiences at the time of diagnosis of parents who have a child with a bone dysplasia resulting in short stature, *Am J Med Genet A* 122:100–107, 2003.

39. Spranger J: *Pattern pecognition in bone dysplasias: endocrine and genetics*, New York, 1985, Wiley, pp 315-342.

40. Horton WA: Molecular genetic basis of the human chondrodysplasias, *Endocrinol Metab Clin North Am* 3:683–697, 1996.

41. Francomano CA, McIntosh I, Wilkin DJ: Bone dysplasias in man: molecular insights, *Curr Opin Genet Dev* 3:301–308, 1996.

42. Korkko J, Cohn DH, Ala-Kokko L, et al: Widely distributed mutations in the COL2A1 gene produce achondrogenesis type II/hypochondrogenesis, *Am J Med Genet* 92:95–100, 2000.

43. Lee B, Vissing H, Ramirez F, et al: Identification of the molecular defect in a family with spondyloepiphyseal dysplasia, *Science* 244:978–980, 1998.

44. Nishimura G, Haga N, Kitoh H, et al: The phenotypic spectrum of COL2A1 mutations, *Hum Mutat* 26:36–43, 2005.

45. Wilkin DJ, Artz AS, South S, et al: Small deletions in the type II collagen triple helix produce Kniest dysplasia, *Am J Med Genet* 85:105–112, 1999.

46. Wilkin DJ, Bogaert R, Lachman RS, et al: A single amino acid substitution (G103D) in the type II collagen triple helix produces Kniest dysplasia, *Hum Mol Genet* 3:1999–2003, 1994.

47. Winterpacht A, Hilbert M, Schwarze U, et al: Kniest and Stickler dysplasia phenotypes caused by collagen type II gene (COL2A1) defect, *Nat Genet* 3:323–326, 1994.

48. Williams CJ, Ganguly A, Considine E, et al: A(-2)-to-G transition at the 3-prime acceptor splice site of IVS17 characterizes the COL2A1 gene mutation in the original Stickler syndrome kindred, *Am J Med Genet* 63:461–467, 1996.

49. Annunen S, Korkko J, Czarny M, et al: Splicing mutations of 54-bp exons in the COL11A1 gene cause Marshall syndrome, but other mutations cause overlapping Marshall/Stickler phenotypes, *Am J Hum Genet* 65:974–983, 1999.

50. Vikkula M, Mariman ECM, Lui VCH, et al: Autosomal dominant and recessive osteochondrodysplasias associated with the COL11A2 locus, *Cell* 80:431–437, 1995.

51. Tompson SW, Bacino CA, Safina NP, et al: Fibrochondrogenesis results from mutations in the COL11A1 type XI collagen gene, *Am J Hum Genet* 87:708–712, 2010.

52. Krakow D, personal communication.

53. Briggs MD, Hoffman SMG, King LM, et al: Pseudoachondroplasia and multiple epiphyseal dysplasia due to mutations in the cartilage oligomeric matrix protein gene, *Nat Genet* 10:330–336, 1995.

54. Newton G, Weremowicz S, Morton CC, et al: Characterization of human and mouse cartilage oligomeric matrix protein, *Genomics* 24:435–439, 1994.

55. Karniski LP: Mutations in the diastrophic dysplasia sulfate transporter (DTDST) gene: correlation between sulfate transport activity and chondrodysplasia phenotype, *Hum Mol Genet* 14:1485–1490, 2001.

56. Robertson SP, Twigg SRF, Sutherland-Smith AJ, et al: Localized mutations in the gene encoding the cytoskeletal protein filamin A cause diverse malformations in humans, *Nat Genet* 33:487–491, 2003.

57. Krakow D, Robertson SP, King LM, et al: Mutations in the gene encoding filamin B disrupt vertebral segmentation, joint formation and skeletogenesis, *Nat Genet* 36:405–410, 2004.

58. Farrington-Rock C, Firestein MH, Bicknell LS, et al: Mutations in two regions of FLNB result in atelosteogenesis I and III, *Hum Mutat* 27:705–710, 2006.

59. Gay O, Gilquin B, Nakamura F, et al: RefilinB (FAM101B) targets FilaminA to organize perinuclear actin networks and regulates nuclear shape. *Proc Natl Acad Sci* 108:11464–11469, 2011.

60. Strotmann R, Semtner M, Kepura F, et al: Interdomain interactions control Ca2+-dependent potentiation in the cation channel TRPV4, *PLoS One* 11:e10580, 2010.

61. Camacho N, Krakow D, Johnykutty S, et al: Dominant TRPV4 mutations in nonlethal and lethal metatropic dysplasia, *Am J Med Genet A* 152A:1169–1177, 2010.

62. Krakow D, Vriens J, Camacho N, et al: Mutations in the gene encoding the calcium-permeable ion channel TRPV4 produce spondylometaphyseal dysplasia, Kozlowski type and metatropic dysplasia, *Am J Hum Genet* 84:307–315, 2009.

63. Rock MJ, Prenen J, Funari VA, et al: Gain-of-function mutations in TRPV4 cause autosomal dominant brachyolmia, *Nat Genet* 40:999–1003, 2008.

64. Auer-Grumbach M, Olschewski A, Papić L, et al: Alterations in the ankyrin domain of TRPV4 cause congenital distal SMA, scapuloperoneal SMA and HMSN2C, *Nat Genet* 42:160–164, 2010.

65. Deng HX, Klein CJ, Yan J, et al: Scapuloperoneal spinal muscular atrophy and CMT2C are allelic disorders caused by alterations in TRPV4, *Nat Genet* 42:165–169, 2010.

66. Landouré G, Zdebik AA, Martinez TL, et al: Mutations in TRPV4 cause Charcot-Marie-Tooth disease type 2C, *Nat Genet* 42:170–174, 2010.

67. Rowe D, Shapiro J: Osteogenesis imperfecta. In Avioli I, Krane S, editors: *Metabolic bone disease*, Philadelphia, 1990, WB Saunders.

68. Sillence D: Osteogenesis imperfecta: an expanding panorama of variants, *Clin Orthop* 159:11–25, 1981.

69. Madigan WP, Wertz D, Cockerham GC, et al: Retinal detachment in osteogenesis imperfecta, *J Pediatr Ophthalmol Strabismus* 4:268–269, 1994.

70. Pedersen U: Osteogenesis imperfecta clinical features, hearing loss and stapedectomy: biochemical, osteodensitometric, corneometric and histological aspects in comparison with otosclerosis, *Acta Otolaryngol Suppl* 415:1–36, 1985.

71. Hortop J, Tsipouras P, Hanley JA, et al: Cardiovascular involvement in osteogenesis imperfecta, *Circulation* 73:54–61, 1986.

72. Davie MW, Haddaway MJ: Bone mineral content and density in healthy subjects and in osteogenesis imperfecta, *Arch Dis Child* 70:331–334, 1994.

73. Willing MC, Cohn DH, Byers PH: Frameshift mutation near the 3′ end of the COL1A1 gene of type I collagen predicts an elongated Pro alpha 1(I) chain and results in osteogenesis imperfecta type I, *J Clin Invest* 85:282–290, 1990.

74. Mundlos S, Chan D, Weng YM, et al: Multiexon deletions in the type I collagen COL1A2 gene in osteogenesis imperfecta type IB: molecules containing the shortened alpha2(I) chains show differential incorporation into the bone and skin extracellular matrix, *J Biol Chem* 271:21068–21074, 1996.

75. Cabral WA, Chang W, Barnes AM, et al: Prolyl 3-hydroxylase 1 deficiency causes a recessive metabolic bone disorder resembling lethal/severe osteogenesis imperfecta, *Nat Genet* 39:359–365, 2007.

76. Barnes AM, Chang W, Morello R, et al: Deficiency of cartilage-associated protein in recessive lethal osteogenesis imperfecta, *N Engl J Med* 355:2757–2764, 2006.

77. Morello R, Bertin TK, Chen Y, et al: CRTAP is required for prolyl 3-hydroxylation and mutations cause recessive osteogenesis imperfecta, *Cell* 127:291–304, 2006.

78. van Dijk FS, Nesbitt IM, Zwikstra EH, et al: PPIB mutations cause severe osteogenesis imperfecta, *Am J Hum Genet* 85:521–527, 2009.

79. Alanay Y, Avaygan H, Camacho N, et al: Mutations in the gene encoding the RER protein FKBP65 cause autosomal-recessive osteogenesis imperfecta, *Am J Hum Genet* 86:551–559, 2010.

80. Christiansen HE, Schwarze U, Pyott SM, et al: Homozygosity for a missense mutation in SERPINH1, which encodes the collagen chaperone protein HSP47, results in severe recessive osteogenesis imperfecta, *Am J Hum Genet* 86(3):389–398, 2010.

81. Lapunzina P, Aglan M, Temtamy S, et al: Identification of a frameshift mutation in Osterix in a patient with recessive osteogenesis imperfecta, *Am J Hum Genet* 87:110–114, 2010.

82. Edwards MJ, Wenstrup RJ, Byers PH, et al: Recurrence of lethal osteogenesis imperfecta due to parental mosaicism for a mutation in the COL1A2 gene of type I collagen: the mosaic parent exhibits phenotypic features of a mild form of the disease, *Hum Mutat* 1:47–54, 1992.

83. Byers PH: Brittle bones—fragile molecules: disorders of collagen gene structure and expression, *Trends Genet* 9:293–300, 1990.

84. Marini JC, Forlino A, Cabral WA, et al: Consortium for osteogenesis imperfecta mutations in the helical domain of type I collagen: regions rich in lethal mutations align with collagen binding sites for integrins and proteoglycans, *Hum Mutat* 28:209–221, 2007.

85. Charnas LR, Marini JC: Communicating hydrocephalus, basilar invagination, and other neurologic features in osteogenesis imperfecta, *Neurology* 3:2603–2608, 1993.

86. Cohen-Solal L, Bonaventure J, Maroteaux P: Dominant mutations in familial lethal and severe osteogenesis imperfecta, *Hum Genet* 87:297–301, 1991.

87. Molyneux K, Starman BJ, Byers PH, et al: A single amino acid deletion in the alpha-2(I) chain of type I collagen produces osteogenesis imperfecta type III, *Hum Genet* 90:621–628, 1993.

88. Glorieux FH, Rauch F, Plotkin H: Type V osteogenesis imperfecta: a new form of brittle bone disease, *J Bone Miner Res* 15:1650–1658, 2000.

89. Glorieux FH, Ward LM, Rauch F: Osteogenesis imperfecta type VI: a form of brittle bone disease with a mineralization defect, *J Bone Miner Res* 17:30–38, 2002.

90. Ward LM, Rauch F, Travers R, et al: Osteogenesis imperfecta type VII: an autosomal recessive form of brittle bone disease, *Bone* 31:12–18, 2002.

91. Traub W, Arad T, Vetter U, et al: Ultrastructural studies of bones from patients with osteogenesis imperfecta, *Matrix Biol* 14:337–345, 1994.

92. Glorieux FH: Experience with bisphosphonates in osteogenesis imperfecta, *Pediatrics* 119:S163–S165, 2007.

93. Plotkin H, Rauch F, Bishop NJ, et al: Pamidronate treatment of severe osteogenesis imperfecta in children under 3 years of age, *J Clin Endocrinol Metab* 85:1846–1850, 2000.

94. Gonzalez E, Pavia C, Ros J, et al: Efficacy of low dose schedule pamidronate infusion in children with osteogenesis imperfecta, *J Pediatr Endocrinol Metab* 14:529–533, 2001.

95. Wilkinson JM, Scott BW, Clarke AM, et al: Surgical stabilisation of the lower limb in osteogenesis imperfecta using the Sheffield Telescopic Intramedullary Rod System, *J Bone Joint Surg Br* 80:999–1004, 1998.

96. Zeitlin L, Fassier F, Glorieux FH: Modern approach to children with osteogenesis imperfecta, *J Pediatr Orthop B* 12:77–87, 2003.

97. Naudie D, Hamdy RC, Fassier F, et al: Complications of limb-lengthening in children who have an underlying bone disorder, *J Bone Joint Surg Am* 80:18–24, 1998.

98. Widmann RF, Laplaza FJ, Bitan FD, et al: Quality of life in osteogenesis imperfecta, *Int Orthop* 26:3–6, 2002.

99. Widmann RF, Bitan FD, Laplaza FJ, et al: Spinal deformity, pulmonary compromise, and quality of life in osteogenesis imperfecta, *Spine* 24:1673–1678, 1999.

100. Sawin PD, Menezes AH: Basilar invagination in osteogenesis imperfecta and related osteochondrodysplasias: medical and surgical management, *J Neurosurg* 86:950–960, 1997.

101. Papagelopoulos PJ, Morrey BF: Hip and knee replacement in osteogenesis imperfecta, *J Bone Joint Surg Am* 75:572–580, 1993.

102. Binder H, Conway A, Gerber LH: Rehabilitation approaches to children with osteogenesis imperfecta: a ten-year experience, *Arch Phys Med Rehabil* 74:386–390, 1993.

103. Binder H, Conway A, Hason S, et al: Comprehensive rehabilitation of the child with osteogenesis imperfecta, *Am J Med Genet* 45:265–269, 1993.

104. Beighton P, De Paepe A, Steinmann B, et al: Ehlers-Danlos syndromes: revised nosology, Villefranche, 1997. Ehlers-Danlos National Foundation (USA) and Ehlers-Danlos Support Group (UK), *Am J Med Genet* 77:31–37, 1998.

105. Hollister DW: Heritable disorders of connective tissue: Ehlers-Danlos syndrome, *Pediatr Clin North Am* 3:575–591, 1978.

106. Osborn TG, Lichtenstein JR, Moore TL, et al: Ehlers-Danlos syndrome presenting as rheumatic manifestations in the child, *J Rheumatol* 8:79–85, 1981.

107. Ayres JG, Pope FM, Reidy JF, et al: Abnormalities of the lungs and thoracic cage in the Ehlers-Danlos syndrome, *Thorax* 40:300–305, 1985.

108. Leier CV, Call TD, Fulkerson PK, et al: The spectrum of cardiac defects in the Ehlers-Danlos syndrome, types I and III, *Ann Intern Med* 92:171–178, 1980.

109. Bethea BT, Fitton TP, Alejo DE, et al: Results of aortic valve–sparing operations: experience with remodeling and reimplantation procedures in 65 patients, *Ann Thorac Surg* 78:767–772, 2004.

110. Tiller GE, Cassidy SB, Wensel C, et al: Aortic root dilatation in Ehlers-Danlos syndrome types I, II and III: a report of five cases, *Clin Genet* 53:460–465, 1998.

111. Holbrook KA, Byers PH: Skin is a window on heritable disorders of connective tissue, *Am J Med Genet* 34:105–121, 1989.

112. Malfait F, Symoens S, .DeBacker J, et al: Three arginine to cysteine substitutions in the pro-alpha (I)-collagen chain cause Ehlers-Danlos syndrome with a propensity to arterial rupture in early adulthood, *Hum Mutat* 28(4):387–395, 2007.

113. Hamel BC, Pals G, Engels CH, et al: Ehlers-Danlos syndrome and type III collagen abnormalities: a variable clinical spectrum, *Clin Genet* 53:440–446, 1998.

114. Rudd NL, Nimrod C, Holbrook KA, et al: Pregnancy complications in type IV Ehlers-Danlos syndrome, *Lancet* 1:50–53, 1983.

115. Byers PH, Duvic M, Atkinson M, et al: Ehlers-Danlos syndrome type VIIA and VIIB result from splice-junction mutations or genomic deletions that involve exon 6 in the COL1A1 and COL1A2 genes of type I collagen, *Am J Med Genet* 72:94–105, 1997.

116. D'Alessio M, Ramirez F, Blumberg BD, et al: Characterization of a COL1A1 splicing defect in a case of Ehlers-Danlos syndrome type VII: further evidence of molecular homogeneity, *Am J Hum Genet* 49:400–406, 1991.

117. Colige A, Sieron AL, Li SW, et al: Human Ehlers-Danlos syndrome type VII C and bovine dermatosparaxis are caused by mutations in the procollagen I N-proteinase gene, *Am J Hum Genet* 65:308–317, 1999.

118. Nusgens BV, Verellen-Dumoulin C, Hermanns-Le T, et al: Evidence for a relationship between Ehlers-Danlos type VII C in humans and bovine dermatosparaxis, *Nat Genet* 1:214–217, 1992.

119. Yeowell HN, Walker LC: Mutations in the lysyl hydroxylase 1 gene that result in enzyme deficiency and the clinical phenotype of Ehlers-Danlos syndrome type VI, *Mol Genet Metab* 71:212–220, 2000.

120. De Paepe A, Devereux RB, Dietz HC, et al: Revised diagnostic criteria for the Marfan syndrome, *Am J Med Genet* 62:417–426, 1996.

Full references for this chapter can be found on www.expertconsult.com.

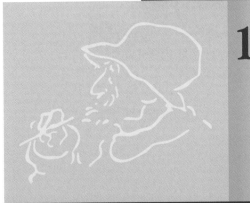

106 Etiology and Pathogenesis of Juvenile Idiopathic Arthritis

LUCY R. WEDDERBURN • KIRAN NISTALA

KEY POINTS

Juvenile idiopathic arthritis (JIA) is a group of conditions with distinct clinical phenotypes and likely differing underlying pathogenic mechanisms.

The heterogeneity of JIA at pathologic and immunologic levels is informative in driving the understanding of these diseases.

An increasing number of genes, outside of the major histocompatibility complex (MHC) locus, have been linked to JIA, but taken together these still account for relatively little of the heritability of JIA.

In JIA, there is evidence to support abnormalities in both innate and adaptive immune systems. Successful treatments may require targeting of multiple cytokine pathways in a single patient.

Strong links with MHC loci and the presence of inflammatory T cells within the inflamed synovium support a role for adaptive immunity in the pathogenesis of JIA.

Systemic arthritis has an immune profile distinct from other types of JIA. Inflammatory mediators of the innate immune system including interleukin (IL)-1β, IL-6, and myeloid related protein play a major role in disease pathogenesis.

Juvenile idiopathic arthritis (JIA) comprises a heterogeneous group of diseases that lead to a final common pathway, namely thickening and inflammation of the joint lining with characteristic onset in children. Infiltrating inflammatory cells interact with each other and resident synovial fibroblasts, promoting a chronic inflammatory process in the synovial membrane and secreted synovial fluid (Figure 106-1). In this chapter, we discuss the genetic factors that predispose to JIA and the abnormalities that underlie synovial and systemic inflammation. In addition to the established association between the major histocompatibility complex (MHC) loci and JIA, more recent studies have detected links to genes that regulate cellular activation or cytokine responses.[1] The fact that immune-related genes make up the major risk alleles in JIA strongly supports the concept of JIA as a disease of disordered immunity. Highly

activated T cells, monocytes, and neutrophils are attracted to joint and secrete mediators that perpetuate inflammation and also attenuate immune regulation. The relative importance of individual cytokines varies between disease subtypes. Results from therapeutic trials support a role for tumor necrosis factor (TNF) in the pathology of polyarthritis forms of JIA and for interleukin (IL)-1β and IL-6 in systemic JIA (sJIA) (Table 106-1). The past decade has seen a step change in the quality of treatments in JIA. To build on this success, researchers need to be able to interrogate the vast array of biologic data that is emerging in the field of JIA and translate this knowledge into novel therapies and a more tailored treatment approach for our patients.

The term *juvenile idiopathic arthritis* refers to a group of conditions, defined under the International League of Associations for Rheumatology (ILAR) classification as conditions starting before the sixteenth birthday that are characterized by arthritis of at least one joint that persists for 6 weeks or more, as a common feature.[2] Although this classification has proven highly valuable for both clinical and basic research and enables more precisely defined subgroups and comparison of data from different studies, it does not encompass all aspects of the heterogeneity of childhood arthritis (e.g., use of the classification criteria by strict exclusion rules may lead to up to 30% of cases being designated as "unclassified"). In addition, certain common features may occur across several subtypes (e.g., factors associated with risk of autoimmune uveitis of JIA include positivity of the antinuclear antibody [ANA], early age at onset, and female sex). Girls with young-age onset of arthritis and ANA positivity represent a group of patients who have been proposed to represent a relatively homogeneous group, yet they currently fall into several subtypes within the ILAR classification. Similarly, genes and immunologic processes that influence the likelihood of mild oligoarthritis to extend to more severe arthritis may well overlap with etiopathologic factors involved in polyarticular JIA.[3,4] Thus in the future a full molecular and genetic analysis of the heterogeneity of childhood arthritis may permit the development of a more mechanism-driven classification, which could help inform

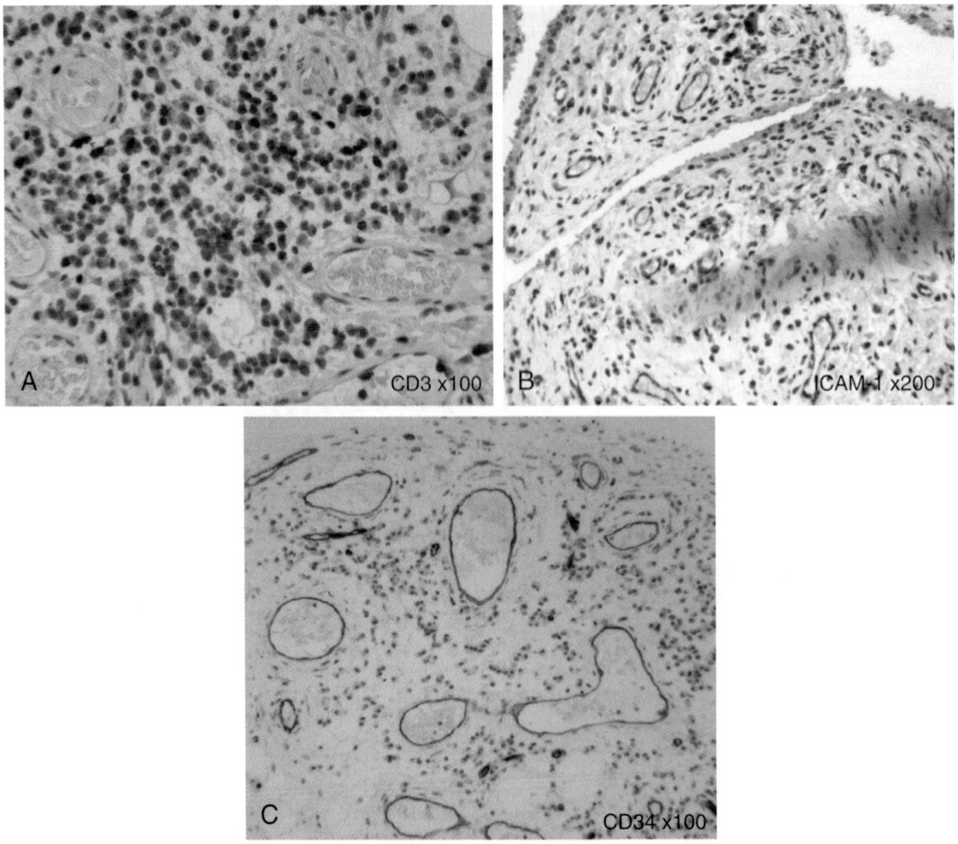

Figure 106-1 Sections of synovium from the knee of a child with oligoarticular juvenile idiopathic arthritis showing intense inflammatory infiltrate and highly vascular hypertrophied tissue. **A,** Stained for CD3 (surface protein on T lymphocytes) (magnification, ×100). **B,** Stained for intracellular adhesion molecule 1, which is expressed on the endothelium and a proportion of the infiltrating cells (magnification, ×200). **C,** Stained for CD34, expressed on vascular endothelium (and hematopoietic stem cells) (magnification, ×100).

on likely disease course, complications, or response to treatment.

Both genetic and environmental factors, as well as the manifestations of their interactions through inflammatory and immunologic mechanisms, are clearly implicated in the pathogenesis of JIA. Recent advances in the understanding of some clinical subtypes, most notably sJIA, have led to recognition of specific and distinct features and novel treatment options. However, it is also increasingly clear that some underlying genetic risk associations and immune

Table 106-1   Summary of Cytokines and Inflammatory Mediators Implicated in Juvenile Idiopathic Arthritis

Cytokine/Mediator	Cell	Pathology
TNF	Monocytes, T, B cells, PMN, mast cells, fibroblasts	Activates monocytes and neutrophils Damages cartilage ↑Endothelial cell adhesion molecules Inhibits regulatory T cells
IL-1β	Monocytes, B cells, fibroblasts	Activates osteoclasts (bone damage) Fibroblast cytokine, chemokine release ↑Endothelial cell adhesion molecules
IL-17	T cells (Th17), mast cells	Chemokine release (recruit PMN) Cartilage damage Activates osteoclasts Synergizes with TNF and IL-1β
IL-6	Monocytes, fibroblasts, B cells	B cell activation Inhibits regulatory T cells Growth retardation Acute-phase response and anemia
IFN-γ	T cells (CD4+ Th1, CD8+, NK cells)	Activates monocytes ↑Endothelial cell adhesion molecules May assist recruitment of Th17 cells
MRP 8/14	Monocytes, PMN	Activates monocytes Promotes pathologic CD8+ T cells Secretion of IL-1β ↑Endothelial cell adhesion molecules

IFN-γ, interferon-gamma; IL, interleukin; MRP, myeloid related protein; NK, natural killer; PMN, polymorphonuclear neutrophil; TNF, tumor necrosis factor.

abnormalities may have effects across several types of childhood arthritis and indeed across many forms of autoimmune disease.

HISTOLOGIC FEATURES OF JUVENILE IDIOPATHIC ARTHRITIS INFLAMED SYNOVIUM

The pathologic hallmark of juvenile idiopathic arthritis is the inflamed synovium. Histology of this tissue shows thickened synovium that is highly vascular and shows marked hyperplasia of synoviocytes in the lining layer, as well as a dense infiltrate of inflammatory cells, comprising T cells, macrophages, dendritic cells, and in some cases B cells and natural killer (NK) cells[5,6] (see Figure 106-1). The hypertrophied synovial layer is highly vascular, with endothelium expressing markers of activation such as human leukocyte antigen (HLA)-DR and intracellular adhesion molecule 1 (ICAM-1). The vascularity is likely related to the increased production of proangiogenic factors such as vascular endothelial growth factor (VEGF), osteopontin, and the angiogenic chemokines,[7-9] while recruitment of this inflammatory infiltrate is likely mediated by multiple chemokines shown to be increased in JIA including CCL5, CXCL10, CCL20, IL-8, and MCP-1 among others.[10,11] The proteolytic enzymes matrix metalloproteinases MMP-1 and MMP-3 are abundantly expressed in synovial lining, and their levels correlate with degree of infiltration, in particular by myeloid CD68[+] cells.[11] The T cells that infiltrate the inflamed synovium, like those in the excess synovial fluid, are highly activated memory cells[12-14] of both CD4 and CD8 populations.[15-17]

GENETICS OF JUVENILE IDIOPATHIC ARTHRITIS

KEY POINTS

There is strong evidence for a genetic component to the etiology of JIA.

The strongest genetic associations of JIA are with genes of the MHC.

Specific MHC class I alleles are associated with enthesitis-related arthritis (ERA).

Distinct MHC class II alleles are associated with oligoarthritis and polyarthritis subtypes.

Several genes that alter the threshold of T cell activation, or relate to cytokines and their receptors, are linked with JIA.

There is strong evidence for a genetic component to the etiology of the JIA diseases. Twin studies have shown concordance rates in monozygotic twins of between 20% and 40%.[18] A study of 164 affected sibling pairs (ASPs) with JIA showed a 70% concordance for gender, 73% for age at disease onset, and 66% for disease course.[19] Estimates suggest that the recurrence risk for siblings of a proband with JIA are between 15 and 30 times that of the general pediatric population, a figure that is as high as for insulin-dependent diabetes mellitus (IDDM) or multiple sclerosis.[20] In addition, first-degree relatives of children with JIA have a higher

rate of other autoimmune disease than controls.[21] Despite this evidence, families of multiple affected siblings are still relatively rare. One caveat in comparing early studies is that some were performed using the American College of Rheumatology (ACR) classification criteria (at that time called *juvenile rheumatoid arthritis*), so they may not be directly comparable with studies that have used the current ILAR classification of JIA. However, there is now a growing body of data that has been analyzed using the ILAR criteria, making comparisons feasible.

Genetic influences on JIA susceptibility and phenotype are polygenic, such that JIA is thought of as a complex genetic trait.[20] Although some studies have analyzed all forms of JIA together, the heterogeneity of childhood arthritis would lead to the prediction of different genetic risk associations for different disease phenotypes, and this has been confirmed in recent adequately powered studies. The unique features of different subtypes of JIA mean that it is perhaps unsurprising that there are also genetic associations with specific subtypes.

The strongest genetic associations with JIA are of genes that lie within the MHC, or HLA; these were the first to be documented as associated with childhood arthritis.[22] The MHC region, located on chromosome 6 of the human genome, includes more than 200 genes, many of which are central to functions of the immune system. Numerous associations between HLA genes and JIA have been reported, and these involve many different populations (reviewed by Prahalad and Glass[1]). The best characterized associations are with genes of the so-called MHC class I and class II loci, genes that code for heterodimeric proteins that present peptide antigen to the specific antigen receptor of T cells (the TCR).

Class I loci include HLA-A, HLA-B, and HLA-C, of which the earliest report was of the association between HLA-B27 and the form of JIA known as *enthesitis-related arthritis* (ERA), which includes children whose disease has parallels with adult ankylosing spondylitis (see Chapters 74 and 75). The HLA-A2 allele HLA-A*0201 is increased in several types of JIA, especially oligoarthritis and children with early-age onset.[23,24] A recent study has also implicated HLA-C*0202 in association with persistent oligoarticular JIA.[25]

Multiple studies have revealed associations of class II MHC loci (HLA-DR, HLA-DP, and HLA-DQ) with JIA, of which the strongest are DRB1*0801 and 11 with oligoarticular JIA, as well as DRB1*1301, in particular in *ANA-positive* cases.[26] Because of inheritance of genes in the MHC region together in so-called haplotypes due to linkage disequilibrium (LD), observed associations may in fact be due to genes within the haplotype, distinct from the locus first implicated. Several haplotypes across the MHC confer an increased risk for all types of JIA such as DRB1*08-DQA1*0401-DQB1*0402, which confers an odds ratio of 6.1 and 10.3 for persistent and extended oligoarticular JIA, respectively. Frequency of the DRB1*1301-DQA1*01-DQB1*06 haplotype distinguishes persistent from extended oligoarticular JIA, whereas DRB1*0801 and DRB1*1401 are associated with polyarticular JIA.[26] Together, these effects may be large: In one study the presence of the combination of the HLA-DRB1*0801, HLA-DRB1*1101, and DPB1*0201 alleles conferred a relative risk of 236.[27] Some associations closely mirror those of the corresponding adult disease such as the strong association of the HLA-B27 allele with spondyloarthropathy and the HLA-DRB1*0401 with rheumatoid factor (RF)-positive polyarticular JIA. Although sJIA shows less strong associations with HLA alleles, even in this subtype, specific haplotypes (such as DRB1*11-DQA1*05-DQB1*03) are increased compared with control subjects. A recent study that used fine allele-specific typing across eight HLA loci in a large cohort and analysis by haplotype has confirmed that within class II loci, HLA-DR is the driving association, rather than HLA-DP.[25] Remarkably, some HLA allele/JIA subtype associations show age-specific effects, in that they confer risk over a specific age range only.[24] Another recent study confirmed both age- and gender-specific effects.[25] Thus, for example, in polyarticular JIA the HLA-DRB1*0801 allele has risk effect in those whose arthritis starts after the age of 6, whereas in younger-onset polyarticular JIA the risk alleles are more closely related to those of patients with oligoarticular JIA, HLAB1*1103/1104.[25] In addition to these risk alleles, some alleles, notably DRB1*0401, *0701 and *1501, are consistently reduced in frequency in JIA cases compared with controls, suggesting a protective effect, for some or even all subtypes. These associations between genes that code for proteins whose central function is the presentation of antigenic peptides to T cells implicate a T cell–driven process in at least part of the etiopathogenesis of JIA.

In addition to the genes coding for MHC proteins, a large number of other candidate genes (now totaling more than 100) have been the focus in different studies of JIA.[28] Inflammatory cytokines have been an important target for drug development in JIA over the past decade, and similarly their gene polymorphisms have been a key area of scrutiny. Genes studied have included cytokine and chemokine genes such as IL-1, IL-6, TNF, MIF, and IL-10; their receptors (including IL-1R, IL-2RA, and CCR5); and key signaling molecules including CTLA4 and PTPN22. However, only a few of these loci have been independently validated: PTPN22, MIF, SLC11A6, WISP3, TNF,[1,29] and in a recent meta-analysis, CCR5.[30]

Genetic association at the TNF locus is complex to study given the position of the TNF gene within the MHC, but some data suggest that several HLA-independent TNF haplotypes are significantly associated with JIA, although the functional consequences of these alleles are not yet clear.[31] The hypothesis suggesting a link between sJIA and IL-6 was proposed many years ago because several clinical features in sJIA resembled the phenotype of IL-6 overexpression (e.g., fevers, stunted growth, anemia).[32,33] A polymorphism (−174G/C) in the regulatory region of the IL-6 gene alters transcription of IL-6 in response to IL-1 and LPS; sJIA patients have significantly lower frequency of the protective CC genotype,[34] and the IL-6 −174G allele has been confirmed as a susceptibility gene for sJIA.[35] Macrophage inhibitory factor (MIF) gene is associated with JIA.[36] This polymorphism (MIF −173*C) results in higher MIF production in the serum and synovium of JIA patients and has been suggested to be predictive of outcome of intra-articular steroid injections in sJIA.[37]

The apparently conflicting studies on several of these candidate gene loci reflect two problems that have hindered progress: the heterogeneity of JIA, which means that combining all JIA into one study may lead to loss of detection of effects specific for a subtype, and opposing this, the difficulty of reaching adequate power for genetic studies, if stratification by subtype is preferred. Recently, new insights have come from the application of new knowledge from other diseases to the understanding of JIA genetics. Thus the highly successful Wellcome Trust case control Consortium performed genome-wide association studies in seven major common diseases including rheumatoid arthritis (RA).[38] Extrapolation of new loci implicated in RA to JIA has been fruitful and has suggested that other key loci that show association with JIA are IL-2/IL-21 and IL-2RA, the α chain of the IL-2 receptor, also known as CD25.[39,40] A recent study focused on specific subtypes of JIA and comparison with their adult disease counterparts. The genetic loci IL-23R and endoplasmic reticulum (ER) aminopeptidase-1 (ERAP1) have been identified as carrying risk associations with ankylosing spondylitis (AS) and psoriatic arthritis in adults.[41] Genotyping of these genes in a large cohort of JIA cases has shown associations of both with the ERA subtype of JIA but no association with JIA as a whole, again emphasizing subtype-specific genetic features and likely pathogenesis.[42] ERAP1 is of particular interest given its functional role in trimming of peptides within the ER, for presentation of peptide on, and folding of, MHC class I molecules, and given the strong evidence for MHC class I folding abnormalities in patients with the HLA-B27 risk alleles (HLA-B*2705 and *2702 among others[41]); see also section on enthesitis-related arthritis (and Chapter 74). ERAP1 is also thought to have a role in trimming of cytokine receptors at the cell surface. IL-23 is of great functional interest because of the central role of IL-23 in the Th17 pathways, as well as the demonstration that Th17 cells may play a role in both JIA and adult AS/psoriatic arthritis.

New insights into the pathogenesis of childhood arthritis are eagerly awaited from large international efforts to perform genome-wide association studies (GWASs) in JIA, of which several are in progress, some targeting specific subtypes or specific research questions such as response to medication.

ADAPTIVE IMMUNE SYSTEM

KEY POINTS

Effector T cells secreting proinflammatory cytokines are enriched in the joint membrane and synovial fluid.

T cells with a regulatory phenotype have been detected within the joints of JIA patients and are enriched in persistent oligoarthritis patients.

A B cell gene expression signature has been detected in the peripheral blood of patients with early-age onset of JIA.

T Cells

The strong association of many JIA subtypes with genetic variants at HLA loci, as well as the central role of HLA proteins in presenting peptide antigens to T cells for recognition, which is central to T cell function, led to intense investigation of the role of T cells in the pathology of JIA. Highly activated memory T cells make up a significant proportion of the inflammatory infiltrate in JIA and express an "oligoclonal" or restricted set of T cell receptors (TCRs).[14,16,17] Specific T cell clones can be long-lived and are detectable in different inflamed joints.[17] Nevertheless, it is still unclear whether these clones represent autoreactive T cells specific for an "arthritogenic" epitope, akin to islet cell antigens in type I diabetes. Although immune activation leads to tissue damage in JIA, the role of self-antigen recognition in this process remains unclear. However, the association of JIA with genetic loci that influence the threshold of T cell activation such as PTPN22, as well as those central to recognition of antigen by T cells, supports the concept of JIA as a disease of dysregulated adaptive immunity.

Early work examining animal models of arthritis led to the hypothesis that cells of the T helper 1 (Th1) lineage, secreting interferon-γ (IFN-γ), were central to pathogenesis. Th1 cells are recruited to the joint by high levels of chemokines CCL5, macrophage inflammatory protein (MIP)-1α, and IP-10[43] and make up the majority of T cells in the JIA joint.[12] However, in both mouse models of arthritis and early adult clinical trials, blocking IFN-γ has offered little clinical benefit, which suggests that other players may be important to pathogenicity. TNF, the prototypic inflammatory cytokine in arthritis, is secreted by T cells and macrophages within the joint and is detectable within inflamed synovial tissue,[44] and to a lesser extent in synovial fluid.[45] The success of TNF blockade in polyarthritis and extended oligoarthritis subtypes implicates TNF in JIA pathology.[46] Still, up to a third of patients fail to respond adequately or relapse on anti-TNF therapy and a recently discovered T cell population, "Th17" secreting IL-17 and IL-22, may account for this recalcitrant disease.[47] IL-17 causes significant bony and cartilage damage in the joint by promoting neutrophil influx via the secretion of IL-8 and synergizing with IL-1β and TNF to drive metalloproteinase secretion and osteoclast activation.[48] Th17 cells are enriched in the joints of JIA patients, and Th17 numbers correlate with the severity of disease course in oligoarthritis.[11] Recent evidence suggests that a significant proportion of the inflammatory T cells in the joint have a Th17 ancestry, raising the hope that Th17 blockade will be an effective treatment in some subtypes of JIA.[49]

In addition to proinflammatory processes, there is strong evidence for ongoing immune regulation in JIA. Children with persistent oligoarticular JIA have high numbers of a regulatory subset of T cells (Treg) within the joint that express CD25 and Foxp3, and the number of Tregs is significantly higher in the children with persistent oligoarticular JIA than those with the more severe extended oligoarticular disease.[50,51] In addition, T cells specific for the conserved self-antigen heat shock proteins (HSPs) play a similar regulatory role.[52] Although synovial Treg suppress effector T cell functions in vitro, inflammatory cytokines such as IL-6 and TNF, present in the arthritic joint,[10,53] may attenuate Treg function in vivo. Treatment strategies that expand Treg numbers and augment function are currently under investigation.[54-56]

Antigen-Presenting Cells

Dendritic cells are specialized antigen-presenting cells (APCs) that activate T cells, as well as promote the differentiation of effector T cell functions. Comparatively little is known about their role in JIA. In the inflamed joint, myeloid dendritic cells (mDCs) are localized to the synovial lining layer, whereas interferon-α–secreting plasmacytoid dendritic cells (pDCs) are in T and B cell–rich aggregates.[45] Both subsets are found in high numbers within synovial fluid when compared with peripheral blood. Synovial mDCs express high levels of co-stimulatory molecules including CD80, CD86, and RANK,[57,58] which augment T cell activation and lead to the secretion of proinflammatory cytokines and chemokines. A triggering receptor expressed on myeloid cells (Trem-1) may play a role in activating mDCs in response to local hypoxia.[59] In contrast to mDCs, some studies suggest that synovial pDCs may provide a regulatory function. pDCs within the joint also do express markers of activation[60] but secrete high levels of Granzyme B, which limits T cell proliferation.[61]

B Cells

There has been a renewed interest in B cell effector function in adult arthritis following the efficacy of the anti-CD20 agent, rituximab, in RA. In JIA, the exact role of B cells as effector or regulatory players is still unclear. B cell–derived autoantibodies, antinuclear antibodies (ANAs), RF, and anticitrullinated protein antibodies (ACPAs) are common in some JIA subtypes, but none are considered to be directly pathogenic (see Chapter 107). Interestingly, patients that are ANA positive are more likely to have T–B cell aggregates in their synovial membrane, suggesting a link between lymphoid neogenesis and autoantibody production.[62] Although lymphoid aggregates are seen in JIA synovium, mature germinal centers are rare when compared with RA.[63] Total B cell numbers do not vary between JIA patients and healthy controls, but oligoarthritis patients have higher numbers of transitional type B cells in the synovial fluid exudate (CD38high, CD24high) in peripheral blood than controls.[63] Patients with an early onset of disease also have expression of B cell– and immunoglobulin-related genes in peripheral blood.[64] The B cell signature, as well as frequent ANA positivity in oligoarthritis patients, has led some authors to suggest a major role for B cells in the pathogenesis of this subtype.[64]

INNATE IMMUNE SYSTEM

> **KEY POINTS**
>
> Defects in the innate immune system have been most closely associated with systemic JIA.
>
> Neutrophils and monocytes secrete myeloid-related protein 8/14, IL-6, IL-1β, and TNF, which drive systemic inflammation.

Many cytokines detectable in the inflamed joint are the products of the innate immune system. The successful targeting of these cytokines with biologic agents (e.g., IL-1β and IL-6) heavily implicates the innate immune system in the pathology of JIA, particularly the sJIA subtype.

Macrophages/Monocytes

Monocytes and their tissue counterparts, macrophages, are key effector cells of the innate immune system and have been linked to the pathogenesis of autoimmune arthritis for several decades.[65] In JIA, analysis of gene expression has detected an activated macrophage gene expression signature in the cells within synovial fluid of early oligoarthritis patients at risk of extension[66] and a monocyte signature in the peripheral blood of patients with an older-onset oligoarthritis,[64] as well as RF-positive polyarthritis patients.[67] Monocytes typically make up equivalent proportions of synovial fluid and peripheral blood mononuclear cells (≈10%), but they have a highly activated phenotype, secreting high levels of IL-6, IL-1β, and TNF, within the joint.[66,68] Synovial monocytes also secrete vascular endothelial growth factor (VEGF) and osteopontin (OPN), which contribute to the vascularity of inflamed pannus,[69] and the chemokine CCL20, which drives Th17 cell recruitment to the joint.[11,70]

Neutrophils

Neutrophils may make up the major fraction of the synovial infiltrate but have remained an infrequent research interest in JIA. sJIA patients have high levels of the heterodimeric myeloid related protein (MRP) 8/14 secreted by activated monocytes and neutrophils.[71] Roth and colleagues[72] have shown that MRP 8/14, although secreted by cells of the innate immune system, induces autoreactive CD8+ T cells, illustrating how cross-talk between the innate and adaptive immune system can lead to chronic inflammation.

Examination of neutrophils from JIA has found more than 700 genes that are differentially expressed in patients' blood compared to controls.[73] Genes linked to IL-8 and IFN-γ were prominent among these differences but failed to return to baseline levels after clinical remission. Rather, disease quiescence was associated with an increase in regulatory genes, such as transforming growth factor-β (TGF-β) and retinoic acid, suggesting that remission reflects a balanced state of inflammation and regulation rather than true immunologic resetting.

Stromal Cells

Resident tissue stromal cells are important targets of both the innate and adaptive immune system and may play an important role in defining the anatomic location of inflammation after systemic immune dysregulation. Synovial fibroblasts from JIA patients secrete metalloproteinases and chemokines in response to locally secreted proinflammatory cytokines[74] and may be an important therapeutic target of the future.[75]

DISEASE SUBTYPE–SPECIFIC PATHOGENESIS

KEY POINTS

Excessive secretion of IL-1β and IL-6 contributes to many of the clinical features seen in patients with sJIA.

The balance between inflammatory and regulatory T cell populations may determine the severity of clinical course in oligoarticular forms of JIA.

RF-negative polyarthritis shares immunopathologic features with oligoarthritis subtype, whereas RF-positive polyarthritis patients are more closely aligned with RA.

In ERA, HLA-B27 protein is prone to misfolding generating an unfolded protein response within cells, which leads to inflammation and arthritis.

Psoriasis and psoriatic arthritis have been strongly linked to pathogenic T cells secreting IL-22 and IL-17.

Systemic Juvenile Idiopathic Arthritis

A key role for IL-1β, IL-6, and IL-18, cytokines of the innate immune system, as well as the absence of autoantibodies or a strong association with MHC, have led many to propose sJIA as an autoinflammatory disease. This hypothesis is supported by the close mirroring of these cytokines with the characteristic fever of sJIA,[76] the high levels of IL-6 and IL-18 in serum from active sJIA patients,[43,77] and enrichment of monocytes in sJIA blood,[78] secreting high levels of IL-1β after activation. Early studies reported a significantly higher ratio of IL-1 receptor antagonist (IL-1ra) to IL-1 in these sJIA patients,[76,79] although this may be difficult to interpret because IL-1α and IL-1β are highly labile in serum. Early evidence of successful treatment with a soluble IL-1, anakinra, at least for some patients with sJIA supports a role for IL-1.[80,81] Interestingly, IL-1β secretion in sJIA may be mediated by MRP 8/14 because once this protein is removed from JIA serum, the potential to induce IL-1β is almost completely attenuated.[82] This study confirmed that levels of serum MRP 8/14 are high in active sJIA and that this measure is both sensitive and specific in distinguishing sJIA from other important diagnoses such as infection or hematopoietic malignancy.

IL-18, a macrophage-derived proinflammatory cytokine with a similar signal transduction pathway to IL-1β, is also grossly elevated in JIA with serum levels correlating with disease activity.[83] High IL-18 levels may account for the defective NK cytotoxic function found in sJIA. Follow-up studies of anakinra have cast doubt on the primacy of IL-1β in sJIA because more than 50% of patients are either nonresponders or relapse on treatment. Even in responders, it is likely that other inflammatory mediators are involved because treatment response to anakinra fails to correlate with either pretreatment IL-1β or IL-18 secretion[84] or changes in gene expression of the IL-1β pathway.[85]

IL-6 is another key player in the pathogenesis of sJIA, secreted by a range of cells including monocytes. IL-6 levels are elevated in the serum and synovial fluid of sJIA patients, and levels correlate with disease activity.[33] Spikes and falls in fever are secondary to the circadian rhythm of IL-6,[76] and many clinical features including growth failure and osteoporosis can be explained by high levels of IL-6.[86] Trial data show efficacy of IL-6 blockade with the monoclonal antibody to soluble IL-6 receptor, tocilizumab. A trial of tocilizumab demonstrated impressive results with 86% of patients achieving an ACR50 response[87] (see Chapter 107). IL-6 expression is upregulated by IL-1β, so the success of IL-6 blockade may represent its role as the final common pathway for inflammation, both IL-1 dependent and independent.

Gene expression profiling from sJIA patients has confirmed pathways that involve IL-6 and IL-1 and that can distinguish active from inactive patients.[88] In addition to these roles for monocytes in sJIA, defects of NK cell function, in particular perforin function, are well recognized.[89] The defect in perforin function in active sJIA has been seen to reverse on successful treatment with autologous stem cell transplantation.[90]

Macrophage Activation Syndrome

MAS is a potentially life-threatening complication of sJIA (as well as sometimes complicating other rheumatologic conditions such as JSLE) that results from immune activation of pathogenic T cells and hemophagocytotic macrophages.[91] These macrophages express CD163, a scavenger receptor that recognizes haptoglobin-hemoglobin (HP-Hb) complexes. Increased uptake of these complexes within the macrophage leads to production of ferritin, explaining the hyperferritinemia associated with MAS. Soluble forms of CD25, the α chain of the IL-2 receptor expressed on T cells, and CD163 are useful biomarkers for MAS in JIA.[92]

MAS shares many similarities with a group of inherited disorders called hemophagocytic lymphocytic histiocytosis (HLH). Defects in the perforin gene and related genes involved its cytosolic secretory pathway (MUNC13-4, Rab27a, and SH2D1A) have been identified as causes of HLH. When examined in JIA, polymorphisms in MUNC13-4 and perforin have been associated with MAS in some studies[93,94] but not others.[95] How defects in cytotoxic function lead to MAS is still unclear, but it has been proposed that appropriate clearance of microbial antigens or activated macrophages is prevented, leading to chronic immune stimulation.

A recent gene expression profiling study of active sJIA showed that patients with active sJIA, and in particular those with MAS, have a signature in PBMC that is similar to patients with familial HLH and characteristic of immature erythropoeisis.[96]

Oligoarthritis

There is increasing evidence that the balance between inflammation and regulation plays a role in driving the clinical phenotype of oligoarthritis patients.[97] The dominance of Treg within the joints of patients with persistent oligoarthritis may explain the relatively benign prognosis of this subgroup, in contrast to the extended subgroup that has a low ratio of Treg to Th17 cells. Those who remain in the mild prognosis group have higher numbers of regulatory T cells in the joint, both as defined by CD25 or Foxp3 expression,[11,50] as well as of CD30+ Treg cells, which are specific to the human self-antigen hsp60,[98] and these CD30+ regulatory cells have recently been shown to reside within the Foxp3+ population.[52]

Although oligoarthritis JIA patients all present with few joints involved and apparently mild disease, evidence suggests that underlying differences between the groups that remain mild and those that go on to extend are present even early in disease. Thus genetic differences between persistent and extended oligoarticular phenotypes include

variation in the MHC class I allele associations[26] and IL-10.[99] A recent study using gene expression, cellular and cytokine profiling showed that those children destined to go on to extend had a more heavily IFN-γ-driven and activated macrophage signature in synovial cells, as well as differences in levels of the chemokine RANTES (CCL5), from the start of disease even before extension occurs.[66] Similarly, proteomic profiles have been shown to be distinct, early in disease, in those who go on to extended disease.[100] These data have led to the concept of a separate group of patients with oligoarthritis who are destined to progress to more severe disease, the so-called extended-to-be group.[66] There is strong evidence to link Th17 cells with autoimmune uveitis, and so agents targeting IL-17, currently under trial in RA, may ameliorate both joint and eye disease in extended oligoarticular JIA.

Rheumatoid Factor–Positive Polyarthritis

The presence of RF and a severe erosive disease course suggests that children in this subgroup represent an early presentation of adult-onset RA. Indeed, this subtype of JIA shares genetic associations with adult rheumatoid arthritis, including the HLA DRB1 locus, in particular the association with the DRB1*0401 allele at this locus.[101] However, few studies have directly compared immunology between adult and childhood onset of disease. Studies of ACPA positivity in children with JIA have shown association with RF-positive polyarticular disease,[102] and there is evidence to support a pathogenic role for RF and associated autoantibodies against citrullinated peptides by fixation of complement on synovial endothelium.[103] In animals, transfer of ACPAs does not lead to arthritis but enhances tissue injury when there is a background of low-grade joint inflammation.[72] Children with RF-positive polyarthritis may share histologic features with adult RA patients, with lymphoid follicles and germinal centers that may be more abundant than in RF-negative patients.[62,104]

Rheumatoid Factor–Negative Polyarthritis

RF-negative polyarthritis represents a more heterogeneous group than RF-positive polyarthritis, with several studies suggesting clinically distinct subgroups (see Chapter 107). Analysis of gene expression data from polyarthritis patients showed three separate signatures.[67] The first was associated with monocyte-related genes and had the highest proportion of RF-positive patients. The third signature found in RF-negative patients was associated with reduced CD8+ T cells and increased plasmacytoid DC. Interestingly, patients did not have overlap between signatures 1 and 3, suggesting distinct immunopathology. It is noteworthy that a significant proportion of patients (24 out of a total of 61) who were younger and had a higher rate of ANA positivity did not fall in a clearly distinct category. A further gene expression study suggested these patients may overlap with ANA-positive oligoarthritis patients and that age of onset of disease is a more important distinguishing factor than the number of involved joints.[64] These data are consistent with results of cytokine levels in plasma and synovial fluid from oligoarthritis and polyarthritis.[105] Both subtypes clustered together and were distinct from sJIA and RA patients. As discussed, there are similar immune pathways in RF-negative polyarthritis and oligoarthritis patients, and overall disease expression may depend on the balance between immune regulation and inflammation.

Enthesitis-Related Arthritis

The HLA-B27 allele, recognized many years ago for its association with autoimmune arthritis, appears to play a particular role in pathogenesis through its molecular properties. The presence of a cysteine residue at position 67 of the HLA-B27 α1 helix heavy chain makes possible a disulfide bond that promotes the formation of homodimers of the B27 chain.[106] These homodimers, which can form in the absence of antigenic peptide and can induce ER stress,[107] have been shown to be proinflammatory and to be ligands for NK cell receptors such as KIR3DL1 and KIR3DL2[108] (see also Chapter 74).

Cells expressing HLA-B27, which is prone to this abnormal folding of the HLA molecule, and which in the context of microbial antigens drives high expression of IL-23, may contribute to factors promoting Th17 cells.[109] This hypothesis may also explain the association between ERA and inflammatory bowel disease because Th17 cells also drive pathology in the latter condition and pathogenic cells readily recirculate from gut to joint. Patients with ERA may be particularly prone to disease induction by bacterial pathogens because cells from patients have high expression of pathogen recognition molecules TLR2 and TLR4 when compared with healthy controls.[110] Along with putative misfolding in the ER by HLA-B27, this allele may alter the antigenic peptides available for T cell recognition.[111] It is interesting that ERAP1, which is strongly associated with adult ankylosing spondylitis (AS), is also associated with pediatric-onset ERA.[42] This protein is thought to affect the repertoire of peptides available to bind class I MHC, by cleavage of N-terminal amino acids from peptide precursors in the ER.[112]

Psoriatic Arthritis

The etiology of psoriatic arthritis shares features with enthesitis-related arthritis, having a genetic association with MHC class I loci, a clonal expansion of CD8 T cells in inflamed joints,[113] and a putative role for Th17 cells. Certainly in adult psoriasis and psoriatic arthritis there is strong evidence that Th17 cytokines IL-22 and IL-17 contribute to the disease process.[114,115] The receptor for IL-23, a key cytokine that induces Th17 cells, is linked to the juvenile form of the disease and IL-23 blockade appears promising in trials of skin and joint disease in adult patients.[116] The innate immune system may also play a role because a recent study found genetic associations with autoinflammatory genes in juvenile psoriatic arthritis patients.[117]

TRANSLATION FROM UNDERSTANDING PATHOGENESIS TO CLINICAL PRACTICE

The heterogeneity of childhood arthritis is complex but is gradually being characterized and harnessed, through the application of novel methods including gene expression profiling, proteomics, and high-throughput genetics. Major progress in the understanding of immunologic processes involved has occurred. In this chapter, cellular processes at play in JIA have been considered. The immune system acts in concert to create vastly complex networks. The challenge is to understand the functional hierarchy of these networks and discover checkpoints that will be amenable to therapeutic targeting in the future.

In addition to new treatments, better biomarkers are required for use in the clinic. For example, in the case of MAS, as knowledge of pathogenesis improves, more biomarkers will become available to predict adverse outcomes.[118] The task in coming years will be to integrate the vast body of data that will be generated through these novel approaches in order to allow the development of more precise classification definitions and, perhaps more importantly, predictive tools and algorithms with which to drive treatment choices for patients and so allow accurate stratification for those who should receive novel biologic agents (e.g., TNF or IL-6 blockade) early in their disease, to achieve early remission.

References

1. Prahalad S, Glass DN: A comprehensive review of the genetics of juvenile idiopathic arthritis, *Pediatr Rheumatol Online J* 6:11, 2008.
2. Petty RE, Southwood TR, Manners P, et al: International League of Associations for Rheumatology classification of juvenile idiopathic arthritis: second revision, Edmonton, 2001, *J Rheumatol* 31:390–392, 2004.
3. Hunter PJ, Wedderburn LR: Pediatric rheumatic disease: can molecular profiling predict the future in JIA? *Nat Rev Rheumatol* 5:593–594, 2009.
4. Barnes MG, Grom AA, Thompson SD, et al: Subtype-specific peripheral blood gene expression profiles in recent-onset juvenile idiopathic arthritis, *Arthritis Rheum* 60:2102–2112, 2009.
5. Bywaters EG: Pathologic aspects of juvenile chronic polyarthritis, *Arthritis Rheum* 20:271–276, 1977.
6. Murray KJ, Luyrink L, Grom AA, et al: Immunohistological characteristics of T cell infiltrates in different forms of childhood onset chronic arthritis, *J Rheumatol* 23:2116–2124, 1996.
7. Vignola S, Picco P, Falcini F, et al: Serum and synovial fluid concentration of vascular endothelial growth factor in juvenile idiopathic arthritides, *Rheumatology (Oxford)* 41:691–696, 2002.
8. Gattorno M, Gregorio A, Ferlito F, et al: Synovial expression of osteopontin correlates with angiogenesis in juvenile idiopathic arthritis, *Rheumatology (Oxford)* 43:1091–1096, 2004.
9. Barnes MG, Aronow BJ, Luyrink LK, et al: Gene expression in juvenile arthritis and spondyloarthropathy: pro-angiogenic ELR+ chemokine genes relate to course of arthritis, *Rheumatology (Oxford)* 43:973–979, 2004.
10. de Jager W, Hoppenreijs EP, Wulffraat NM, et al: Blood and synovial fluid cytokine signatures in patients with juvenile idiopathic arthritis: a cross-sectional study, *Ann Rheum Dis* 66:589–598, 2007.
11. Nistala K, Moncrieffe H, Newton KR, et al: Interleukin-17-producing T cells are enriched in the joints of children with arthritis, but have a reciprocal relationship to regulatory T cell numbers, *Arthritis Rheum* 58:875–887, 2008.
12. Wedderburn LR, Robinson N, Patel A, et al: Selective recruitment of polarized T cells expressing CCR5 and CXCR3 to the inflamed joints of children with juvenile idiopathic arthritis, *Arthritis Rheum* 43:765–774, 2000.
13. Gattorno M, Prigione I, Morandi F, et al: Phenotypic and functional characterisation of CCR7+ and CCR7- CD4+ memory T cells homing to the joints in juvenile idiopathic arthritis, *Arthritis Res Ther* 7:R256–R267, 2005.
14. Black AP, Bhayani H, Ryder CA, et al: T-cell activation without proliferation in juvenile idiopathic arthritis, *Arthritis Res* 4:177–183, 2002.

15. Thompson SD, Murray KJ, Grom AA, et al: Comparative sequence analysis of the human T cell receptor b chain in juvenile rheumatoid arthritis and juvenile spondyloarthropathies, *Arthritis Rheum* 41:482–497, 1998.

16. Wedderburn LR, Patel A, Varsani H, et al: Divergence in the degree of clonal expansions in inflammatory T cell subpopulations mirrors HLA-associated risk alleles in genetically and clinically distinct subtypes of childhood arthritis, *Int Immunol* 13:1541–1550, 2001.

17. Wedderburn LR, Maini MK, Patel A, et al: Molecular fingerprinting reveals non-overlapping T cell oligoclonality between an inflamed site and peripheral blood, *Int Immunol* 11:535–543, 1999.

18. Prahalad S, Ryan MH, Shear ES, et al: Twins concordant for juvenile rheumatoid arthritis, *Arthritis Rheum* 43:2611–2612, 2000.

19. Moroldo MB, Chaudhari M, Shear E, et al: Juvenile rheumatoid arthritis affected sibpairs: extent of clinical phenotype concordance, *Arthritis Rheum* 50:1928–1934, 2004.

20. Glass DN, Giannini EH: Juvenile rheumatoid arthritis as a complex genetic trait, *Arthritis Rheum* 42:2261–2268, 1999.

21. Prahalad S, Shear ES, Thompson SD, et al: Increased prevalence of familial autoimmunity in simplex and multiplex families with juvenile rheumatoid arthritis, *Arthritis Rheum* 46:1851–1856, 2002.

22. Edmonds J, Metzger A, Terasaki P, et al: Proceedings: HL-A antigen W27 in juvenile chronic polyarthritis, *Ann Rheum Dis* 33:576, 1974.

23. Brunner HI, Ivaskova E, Haas JP, et al: Class I associations and frequencies of class II HLA-DRB alleles by RFLP analysis in children with rheumatoid-factor-negative juvenile chronic arthritis, *Rheumatol Int* 13:83–88, 1993.

24. Murray KJ, Moroldo MB, Donnelly P, et al: Age specific (susceptibilty and protection) for JRA-associated HLA alleles, *Arthritis Rheum* 42:1843–1853, 1999.

25. Hollenbach JA, Thompson SD, Bugawan TL, et al: Juvenile idiopathic arthritis and HLA class I and class II interactions and age-at-onset effects, *Arthritis Rheum* 62:1781–1791, 2010.

26. Thomson W, Barrett JH, Donn R, et al: Juvenile idiopathic arthritis classified by the ILAR criteria: HLA associations in UK patients, *Rheumatology (Oxford)* 41:1183–1189, 2002.

27. Paul C, Schoenwald U, Truckenbrodt H, et al: HLA-DP/DR interaction in early onset pauciarticular juvenile chronic arthritis, *Immunogenetics* 37:442–448, 1993.

28. Phelan JD, Thompson SD, Glass DN: Susceptibility to JRA/JIA: complementing general autoimmune and arthritis traits, *Genes Immun* 7:1–10, 2006.

29. Woo P, Colbert RA: An overview of genetics of paediatric rheumatic diseases, *Best Pract Res Clin Rheumatol* 23:589–597, 2009.

30. Hinks A, Martin P, Flynn E, et al: Association of the CCR5 gene with juvenile idiopathic arthritis, *Genes Immun* 11:584–589, 2010.

31. Zeggini E, Thomson W, Kwiatkowski D, et al: Linkage and association studies of single-nucleotide polymorphism-tagged tumor necrosis factor haplotypes in juvenile oligoarthritis, *Arthritis Rheum* 46:3304–3311, 2002.

32. Woo P: Cytokines in childhood rheumatic diseases, *Arch Dis Child* 69:547–549, 1993.

33. de Benedetti F, Massa M, Robbioni P, et al: Correlation of serum interleukin-6 levels with joint involvement and thrombocytosis in systemic juvenile rheumatoid arthritis, *Arthritis Rheum* 34:1158–1163, 1991.

34. Fishman D, Faulds G, Jeffery R, et al: The effect of novel polymorphisms in the interleukin-6 (IL-6) gene on IL-6 transcription and plasma IL-6 levels, and an association with systemic-onset juvenile chronic arthritis, *J Clin Invest* 102:1369–1376, 1998.

35. Ogilvie EM, Fife MS, Thompson SD, et al: The -174G allele of the interleukin-6 gene confers susceptibility to systemic arthritis in children: a multicenter study using simplex and multiplex juvenile idiopathic arthritis families, *Arthritis Rheum* 48:3202–3206, 2003.

36. Donn R, Alourfi Z, Zeggini E, et al: A functional promoter haplotype of macrophage migration inhibitory factor is linked and associated with juvenile idiopathic arthritis, *Arthritis Rheum* 50:1604–1610, 2004.

37. De Benedetti F, Meazza C, Vivarelli M, et al: Functional and prognostic relevance of the -173 polymorphism of the macrophage migration inhibitory factor gene in systemic-onset juvenile idiopathic arthritis, *Arthritis Rheum* 48:1398–1407, 2003.

38. Craddock N, Hurles ME, Cardin N, et al: Genome-wide association study of CNVs in 16,000 cases of eight common diseases and 3,000 shared controls, *Nature* 464:713–720, 2010.

39. Hinks A, Eyre S, Ke X, et al: Association of the AFF3 gene and IL2/IL21 gene region with juvenile idiopathic arthritis, *Genes Immun* 11:194–198, 2010.

40. Hinks A, Ke X, Barton A, et al: Association of the IL2RA/CD25 gene with juvenile idiopathic arthritis, *Arthritis Rheum* 60:251–257, 2009.

41. Brown MA: Genetics of ankylosing spondylitis, *Curr Opin Rheumatol* 22:249–257, 2010.

42. Hinks A, Martin P, Flynn E, et al: Subtype specific genetic associations for juvenile idiopathic arthritis: ERAP1 with the enthesitis related arthritis subtype and IL23R with juvenile psoriatic arthritis, *Arthritis Res Ther* 13:R12, 2011.

43. Pharoah DS, Varsani H, Tatham RW, et al: Expression of the inflammatory chemokines CCL5, CCL3 and CXCL10 in juvenile idiopathic arthritis, and demonstration of CCL5 production by an atypical subset of CD8+ T cells, *Arthritis Res Ther* 8:R50, 2006.

44. Grom AA, Murray KJ, Luyrink L, et al: Patterns of expression of tumor necrosis factor alpha, tumor necrosis factor beta, and their receptors in synovia of patients with juvenile rheumatoid arthritis and juvenile spondylarthropathy, *Arthritis Rheum* 39:1703–1710, 1996.

45. Gattorno M, Chicha L, Gregorio A, et al: Distinct expression pattern of IFN-alpha and TNF-alpha in juvenile idiopathic arthritis synovial tissue, *Rheumatology (Oxford)* 46:657–665, 2007.

46. Lovell DJ, Giannini EH, Reiff A, et al: Etanercept in children with polyarticular juvenile rheumatoid arthritis. Pediatric Rheumatology Collaborative Study Group, *N Engl J Med* 342:763–769, 2000.

47. Miossec P, Korn T, Kuchroo VK: Interleukin-17 and type 17 helper T cells, *N Engl J Med* 361:888–898, 2009.

48. van Hamburg JP, Asmawidjaja PS, Davelaar N, et al: Th17 cells, but not Th1 cells, from patients with early rheumatoid arthritis are potent inducers of matrix metalloproteinases and proinflammatory cytokines upon synovial fibroblast interaction, including autocrine interleukin-17A production, *Arthritis Rheum* 63:73–83, 2011.

49. Nistala K, Adams S, Cambrook H, et al: Th17 plasticity in human autoimmune arthritis is driven by the inflammatory environment, *Proc Natl Acad Sci U S A* 107:14751–14756, 2010.

50. de Kleer IM, Wedderburn LR, Taams LS, et al: CD4+CD25bright regulatory T cells actively regulate inflammation in the joints of patients with the remitting form of juvenile idiopathic arthritis, *J Immunol* 172:6435–6443, 2004.

51. Ruprecht CR, Gattorno M, Ferlito F, et al: Coexpression of CD25 and CD27 identifies FoxP3+ regulatory T cells in inflamed synovia, *J Exp Med* 201:1793–1803, 2005.

52. de Kleer I, Vercoulen Y, Klein M, et al: CD30 discriminates heat shock protein 60-induced FOXP3+ CD4+ T cells with a regulatory phenotype, *J Immunol* 185:2071–2079, 2010.

53. Valencia X, Stephens G, Goldbach-Mansky R, et al: TNF downmodulates the function of human CD4+ CD25hi T-regulatory cells, *Blood* 108:253–261, 2006.

54. Pahwa R, Jaggaiahgari S, Pahwa S, et al: Isolation and expansion of human natural T regulatory cells for cellular therapy, *J Immunol Methods* 363:67–79, 2010.

55. Golovina TN, Mikheeva T, Brusko TM, et al: Retinoic acid and rapamycin differentially affect and synergistically promote the ex vivo expansion of natural human T regulatory cells, *PLoS One* 6:e15868, 2011.

56. Brusko TM, Putnam AL, Bluestone JA: Human regulatory T cells: role in autoimmune disease and therapeutic opportunities, *Immunol Rev* 223:371–390, 2008.

57. Smolewska E, Stanczyk J, Brozik H, et al: Distribution and clinical significance of blood dendritic cells in children with juvenile idiopathic arthritis, *Ann Rheum Dis* 67:762–768, 2008.

58. Varsani H, Patel A, van Kooyk Y, et al: Synovial dendritic cells in juvenile idiopathic arthritis (JIA) express receptor activator of NF-kappaB (RANK), *Rheumatology (Oxford)* 42:583–590, 2003.

59. Bosco MC, Pierobon D, Blengio F, et al: Hypoxia modulates the gene expression profile of immunoregulatory receptors in human mature dendritic cells: identification of TREM-1 as a novel hypoxic marker in vitro and in vivo, *Blood* 117:2625–2639, 2011.

60. Gattorno M, Chicha L, Gregorio A, et al: Enrichment of plasmacytoid dendritic cells in synovial fluid of juvenile idiopathic arthritis, *Arthritis Rheum* 48:S101, 2003.

61. Jahrsdorfer B, Vollmer A, Blackwell SE, et al: Granzyme B produced by human plasmacytoid dendritic cells suppresses T-cell expansion, *Blood* 115:1156–1165, 2010.

62. Gregorio A, Gambini C, Gerloni V, et al: Lymphoid neogenesis in juvenile idiopathic arthritis correlates with ANA positivity and plasma cells infiltration, *Rheumatology (Oxford)* 46:308–313, 2007.

63. Corcione A, Ferlito F, Gattorno M, et al: Phenotypic and functional characterization of switch memory B cells from patients with oligo-articular juvenile idiopathic arthritis, *Arthritis Res Ther* 11:R150, 2009.

64. Barnes MG, Grom AA, Thompson SD, et al: Biologic similarities based on age at onset in oligoarticular and polyarticular subtypes of juvenile idiopathic arthritis, *Arthritis Rheum* 62:3249–3258, 2010.

65. Saklatvala J: Tumour necrosis factor alpha stimulates resorption and inhibits synthesis of proteoglycan in cartilage, *Nature* 322:547–549, 1986.

66. Hunter PJ, Nistala K, Jina N, et al: Biologic predictors of extension of oligoarticular juvenile idiopathic arthritis as determined from synovial fluid cellular composition and gene expression, *Arthritis Rheum* 62:896–907, 2010.

67. Griffin TA, Barnes MG, Ilowite NT, et al: Gene expression signatures in polyarticular juvenile idiopathic arthritis demonstrate disease heterogeneity and offer a molecular classification of disease subsets, *Arthritis Rheum* 60:2113–2123, 2009.

68. Saxena N, Aggarwal A, Misra R: Elevated concentrations of monocyte derived cytokines in synovial fluid of children with enthesitis related arthritis and polyarticular types of juvenile idiopathic arthritis, *J Rheumatol* 32:1349–1353, 2005.

69. Bosco MC, Delfino S, Ferlito F, et al: The hypoxic synovial environment regulates expression of vascular endothelial growth factor and osteopontin in juvenile idiopathic arthritis, *J Rheumatol* 36:1318–1329, 2009.

70. Hirota K, Yoshitomi H, Hashimoto M, et al: Preferential recruitment of CCR6-expressing Th17 cells to inflamed joints via CCL20 in rheumatoid arthritis and its animal model, *J Exp Med* 204:2803–2812, 2007.

71. Wittkowski H, Frosch M, Wulffraat N, et al: S100A12 is a novel molecular marker differentiating systemic-onset juvenile idiopathic arthritis from other causes of fever of unknown origin, *Arthritis Rheum* 58:3924–3931, 2008.

72. Loser K, Vogl T, Voskort M, et al: The Toll-like receptor 4 ligands Mrp8 and Mrp14 are crucial in the development of autoreactive CD8+ T cells, *Nat Med* 16:713–717, 2010.

73. Jarvis JN, Petty HR, Tang Y, et al: Evidence for chronic, peripheral activation of neutrophils in polyarticular juvenile rheumatoid arthritis, *Arthritis Res Ther* 8:R154, 2006.

74. Agarwal S, Misra R, Aggarwal A: Interleukin 17 levels are increased in juvenile idiopathic arthritis synovial fluid and induce synovial fibroblasts to produce proinflammatory cytokines and matrix metalloproteinases, *J Rheumatol* 35:515–519, 2008.

75. Niedermeier M, Pap T, Korb A: Therapeutic opportunities in fibroblasts in inflammatory arthritis, *Best Pract Res Clin Rheumatol* 24:527–540, 2010.

76. Rooney M, David J, Symons J, et al: Inflammatory cytokine responses in juvenile chronic arthritis, *Br J Rheumatol* 34:454–460, 1995.

77. De Benedetti F, Massa M, Pignatti P, et al: Serum soluble interleukin 6 (IL-6) receptor and IL-6/soluble IL-6 receptor complex in systemic juvenile rheumatoid arthritis, *J Clin Invest* 93:2114–2119, 1994.

78. Macaubas C, Nguyen K, Deshpande C, et al: Distribution of circulating cells in systemic juvenile idiopathic arthritis across disease activity states, *Clin Immunol* 134:206–216, 2010.

79. De Benedetti F, Pignatti P, Massa M, et al: Circulating levels of interleukin 1 beta and of interleukin 1 receptor antagonist in systemic juvenile chronic arthritis, *Clin Exp Rheumatol* 13:779–784, 1995.

80. Pascual V, Allantaz F, Arce E, et al: Role of interleukin-1 (IL-1) in the pathogenesis of systemic onset juvenile idiopathic arthritis and clinical response to IL-1 blockade, *J Exp Med* 201:1479–1486, 2005.

81. De Kleer IM, Brinkman DM, Ferster A, et al: Autologous stem cell transplantation for refractory juvenile idiopathic arthritis: analysis of clinical effects, mortality, and transplant related morbidity, *Ann Rheum Dis* 63:1318–1326, 2004.

82. Frosch M, Ahlmann M, Vogl T, et al: The myeloid-related proteins 8 and 14 complex, a novel ligand of toll-like receptor 4, and interleukin-1beta form a positive feedback mechanism in systemic-onset juvenile idiopathic arthritis, *Arthritis Rheum* 60:883–891, 2009.

83. Maeno N, Takei S, Imanaka H, et al: Increased interleukin-18 expression in bone marrow of a patient with systemic juvenile idiopathic arthritis and unrecognized macrophage-activation syndrome, *Arthritis Rheum* 50:1935–1938, 2004.

84. Bosco MC, Delfino S, Ferlito F, et al: Hypoxic synovial environment and expression of macrophage inflammatory protein 3gamma/CCL20 in juvenile idiopathic arthritis, *Arthritis Rheum* 58:1833–1838, 2008.

85. Allantaz F, Chaussabel D, Stichweh D, et al: Blood leukocyte microarrays to diagnose systemic onset juvenile idiopathic arthritis and follow the response to IL-1 blockade, *J Exp Med* 204:2131, 2007.

86. De BF, Alonzi T, Moretta A, et al: Interleukin 6 causes growth impairment in transgenic mice through a decrease in insulin-like growth factor-I. A model for stunted growth in children with chronic inflammation, *J Clin Invest* 99:643–650, 1997.

87. Yokota S, Imagawa T, Mori M, et al: Efficacy and safety of tocilizumab in patients with systemic-onset juvenile idiopathic arthritis: a randomised, double-blind, placebo-controlled, withdrawal phase III trial, *Lancet* 371:998–1006, 2008.

88. Ogilvie EM, Khan A, Hubank M, et al: Specific gene expression profiles in systemic juvenile idiopathic arthritis, *Arthritis Rheum* 56:1954–1965, 2007.

89. Grom AA, Villanueva J, Lee S, et al: Natural killer cell dysfunction in patients with systemic-onset juvenile rheumatoid arthritis and macrophage activation syndrome, *J Pediatr* 142:292–296, 2003.

90. Wulffraat NM, Rijkers GT, Elst E, et al: Reduced perforin expression in systemic juvenile idiopathic arthritis is restored by autologous stem-cell transplantation, *Rheumatology (Oxford)* 42:375–379, 2003.

91. Grom AA, Mellins ED: Macrophage activation syndrome: advances towards understanding pathogenesis, *Curr Opin Rheumatol* 22:561–566, 2010.

92. Bleesing J, Prada A, Siegel DM, et al: The diagnostic significance of soluble CD163 and soluble interleukin-2 receptor alpha-chain in macrophage activation syndrome and untreated new-onset systemic juvenile idiopathic arthritis, *Arthritis Rheum* 56:965–971, 2007.

93. de Kleer I, Vastert B, Klein M, et al: Autologous stem cell transplantation for autoimmunity induces immunologic self-tolerance by reprogramming autoreactive T cells and restoring the CD4+CD25+ immune regulatory network, *Blood* 107:1696–1702, 2006.

94. Zhang K, Biroschak J, Glass DN, et al: Macrophage activation syndrome in patients with systemic juvenile idiopathic arthritis is associated with MUNC13-4 polymorphisms, *Arthritis Rheum* 58:2892–2896, 2008.

95. Donn R, Ellison S, Lamb R, et al: Genetic loci contributing to hemophagocytic lymphohistiocytosis do not confer susceptibility to systemic-onset juvenile idiopathic arthritis, *Arthritis Rheum* 58:869–874, 2008.

96. Hinze CH, Fall N, Thornton S, et al: Immature cell populations and an erythropoiesis gene-expression signature in systemic juvenile idiopathic arthritis: implications for pathogenesis, *Arthritis Res Ther* 12:R123, 2010.

97. Nistala K, Wedderburn LR: Th17 and regulatory T cells: rebalancing pro- and anti-inflammatory forces in autoimmune arthritis, *Rheumatology (Oxford)* 60:2113–2123, 2009.

98. de Kleer IM, Kamphuis SM, Rijkers GT, et al: The spontaneous remission of juvenile idiopathic arthritis is characterized by CD30+ T cells directed to human heat-shock protein 60 capable of producing the regulatory cytokine interleukin-10, *Arthritis Rheum* 48:2001, 2010, 2003.

99. Crawley E, Kon S, Woo P: Hereditary predisposition to low interleukin-10 production in children with extended oligoarticular juvenile idiopathic arthritis, *Rheumatology (Oxford)* 40:574–578, 2001.

100. Gibson DS, Finnegan S, Jordan G, et al: Stratification and monitoring of juvenile idiopathic arthritis patients by synovial proteome analysis, *J Proteome Res* 8:5601–5609, 2009.

101. Zeggini E, Packham J, Donn R, et al: Association of HLA-DRB1*13 with susceptibility to uveitis in juvenile idiopathic arthritis in two independent data sets, *Rheumatology (Oxford)* 45:972–974, 2006.

102. Kasapcopur O, Altun S, Aslan M, et al: Diagnostic accuracy of anti-cyclic citrullinated peptide antibodies in juvenile idiopathic arthritis, *Ann Rheum Dis* 63:1687–1689, 2004.

103. Zvaifler NJ: Breakdown products of C 3 in human synovial fluids, *J Clin Invest* 48:1532–1542, 1969.

104. Randen I, Mellbye OJ, Forre O, et al: The identification of germinal centres and follicular dendritic cell networks in rheumatoid synovial tissue, *Scand J Immunol* 41:481–486, 1995.
105. van den Ham HJ, de JW, Bijlsma JW, et al: Differential cytokine profiles in juvenile idiopathic arthritis subtypes revealed by cluster analysis, *Rheumatology (Oxford)* 48:899–905, 2009.
106. Allen RL, O'Callaghan CA, McMichael AJ, et al: Cutting edge: HLA-B27 can form a novel beta 2-microglobulin-free heavy chain homodimer structure, *J Immunol* 162:5045–5048, 1999.
107. Turner MJ, Sowders DP, DeLay ML, et al: HLA-B27 misfolding in transgenic rats is associated with activation of the unfolded protein response, *J Immunol* 175:2438–2448, 2005.
108. Kollnberger S, Chan A, Sun MY, et al: Interaction of HLA-B27 homodimers with KIR3DL1 and KIR3DL2, unlike HLA-B27 hetero-trimers, is independent of the sequence of bound peptide, *Eur J Immunol* 37:1313–1322, 2007.
109. Goodall JC, Wu C, Zhang Y, et al: Endoplasmic reticulum stress-induced transcription factor, CHOP, is crucial for dendritic cell IL-23 expression, *Proc Natl Acad Sci U S A* 107:17698–17703, 2010.
110. Myles A, Aggarwal A: Expression of Toll-like receptors 2 and 4 is increased in peripheral blood and synovial fluid monocytes of patients with enthesitis-related arthritis subtype of juvenile idiopathic arthritis, *Rheumatology (Oxford)* 50:481–488, 2011.
111. Bowness P, Zaccai N, Bird L, et al: HLA-B27 and disease pathogenesis: new structural and functional insights, *Expert Rev Mol Med* Oct 26:1–10, 1999.
112. Hearn A, York IA, Rock KL: The specificity of trimming of MHC class I-presented peptides in the endoplasmic reticulum, *J Immunol* 183:5526–5536, 2009.
113. Costello PJ, Winchester RJ, Curran SA, et al: Psoriatic arthritis joint fluids are characterized by CD8 and CD4 T cell clonal expansions appear antigen driven, *J Immunol* 166:2878–2886, 2001.
114. Jandus C, Bioley G, Rivals JP, et al: Increased numbers of circulating polyfunctional Th17 memory cells in patients with seronegative spondylarthritides, *Arthritis Rheum* 58:2307–2317, 2008.
115. Wilson NJ, Boniface K, Chan JR, et al: Development, cytokine profile and function of human interleukin 17 producing helper T cells, *Nat Immunol* 8:950–957, 2007.
116. Gottlieb A, Menter A, Mendelsohn A, et al: Ustekinumab, a human interleukin 12/23 monoclonal antibody, for psoriatic arthritis: randomised, double-blind, placebo-controlled, crossover trial, *Lancet* 373:633–640, 2009.
117. Day TG, Ramanan AV, Hinks A, et al: Autoinflammatory genes and susceptibility to psoriatic juvenile idiopathic arthritis, *Arthritis Rheum* 58:2142–2146, 2008.
118. Fall N, Barnes M, Thornton S, et al: Gene expression profiling of peripheral blood from patients with untreated new-onset systemic juvenile idiopathic arthritis reveals molecular heterogeneity that may predict macrophage activation syndrome, *Arthritis Rheum* 56:3793–3804, 2007.

The references for this chapter can also be found on www.expertconsult.com.

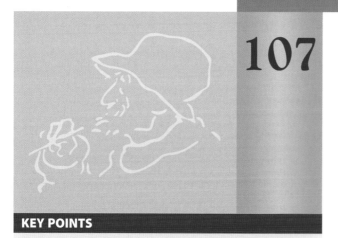

107

Treatment of Juvenile Idiopathic Arthritis

JOYCE J. HSU • TZIELAN CHANG LEE • CHRISTY I. SANDBORG

KEY POINTS

Juvenile idiopathic arthritis (JIA) is the umbrella term for the family of childhood arthritides of unknown cause.

JIA affects at least 1 in 1000 children.

Before wide use of methotrexate and biologic therapies, 50% of children with JIA would reach adulthood with significant disabilities.

The goals of treatment in JIA are complete suppression of inflammation on medications and remission when possible.

Oligoarticular JIA, characterized by early age of onset, female predominance, antinuclear antibody positivity, and frequent subacute anterior uveitis, occurs only in childhood.

Systemic JIA is distinct from other subgroups of JIA in its equal sex distribution, lack of autoantibodies and human leukocyte antigen associations, and increased responsiveness to interleukin (IL)-1 and IL-6 inhibition compared with tumor necrosis factor inhibition.

Enthesitis-related arthritis typically occurs in children greater than 6 years of age, but sacroiliitis may not develop until adolescence.

Arthritis in a child can result in overgrowth (in the knee causing length discrepancy) and undergrowth (in the temporomandibular joint causing micrognathia) of joints.

Because bone erosions on conventional radiographs are late radiographic findings in growing children, early joint damage may require different imaging modalities.

Considerable progress in understanding the genetics and pathogenesis of JIA has revealed subtype-specific associations, as well as some common mechanisms of disease that will translate to more effective and targeted therapies.

Juvenile idiopathic arthritis (JIA) is the most common rheumatic disease in childhood, but actual estimates of prevalence and incidence vary remarkably in different geographic regions, ranging from 7 to 400 per 100,000 children, reflecting variations in disease reporting, classification, and ethnic and environmental differences in disease expression.[1] Reasonable working estimates are 150 per 100,000 children, which makes JIA one of the most common chronic diseases of childhood. There are significant differences in the disease manifestations in children compared with adults, with some types occurring exclusively in children. This chapter discusses the current understanding of the key clinical features of the various forms of JIA, differential diagnoses, treatment approaches, prognosis, and outcomes. The rapid growth in understanding the biologic basis for JIA and

the ongoing development of targeted therapies for rheumatic diseases are likely to lead to enhancements in these recommendations. Data concerning long-term disease course and outcome in children with JIA in this modern treatment era remain limited, and there are international prospective inception cohorts of children with arthritis designed to address these gaps in knowledge.[2,3]

CLASSIFICATION CRITERIA FOR JUVENILE IDIOPATHIC ARTHRITIS

Differential Diagnosis

In the past, different groups had used various types of nomenclature to classify children with persistent arthritis including "juvenile rheumatoid arthritis" (American College of Rheumatology [ACR]) and "juvenile chronic arthritis" (European League Against Rheumatism), which created problems in comparing research studies and outcomes. The goal of the International League of Associations for Rheumatology (ILAR) is to identify subtypes of JIA for research purposes that are homogeneous and mutually exclusive. JIA classification is currently based on predominant clinical and laboratory features and the number of involved joints at disease onset.[4] There is a continual renewal process, with the second revision occurring in Edmonton in 2001, which is presented in Table 107-1. However, classification systems are ever evolving, and categorization may evolve to more biologically and genetically similar subgrouping, especially with recent advances in etiology and pathogenesis. For example, age of onset may be a more biologically relevant parameter to distinguish between subtypes of JIA than classification based on number of involved joints. PBMC gene expression analysis reveals biologic differences between patients with early-onset (<6 years) and late-onset (>6 years) JIA, which was independent of oligoarthritis or polyarthritis subtype.[5] Ravelli and colleagues[6] provided clinical support for this approach, showing that antinuclear antibody (ANA)-positive patients with oligoarthritis and rheumatoid factor (RF)-negative polyarthritis were similar in terms of early age at onset, female predilection, increased frequency of asymmetric arthritis, and increased frequency of uveitis.

Pattern recognition is perhaps the most significant skill needed by clinicians in the diagnostic evaluation of patients. The usual patterns in children with rheumatic diseases often overlap with malignancies, infection, and trauma (especially nonaccidental). Therefore it is crucial to evaluate these diagnostic possibilities first before accepting the diagnosis of JIA. The ILAR categories are meant to simplify classification and are useful for typical presentations of

Table 107-1 International League of Associations for Rheumatology Classification Criteria for Juvenile Idiopathic Arthritis (JIA)[4]

General definition of JIA: arthritis of unknown etiology that begins before the sixteenth birthday and persists for at least 6 wk; other known conditions are excluded

Subcategory	Definition	Exclusions
Oligoarthritis 1. Persistent oligoarthritis: Affecting ≤4 joints throughout the disease course 2. Extended oligoarthritis: affecting a total of >4 joints after the first 6 mo of disease	Arthritis affecting 1-4 joints during the first 6 mo of disease	a. Psoriasis or a history of psoriasis in the patient or first-degree relative b. Arthritis in an HLA-B27–positive male beginning after the sixth birthday c. Ankylosing spondylitis, ERA, sacroiliitis with inflammatory bowel disease, reactive arthritis, acute anterior uveitis, or a history of one of these disorders in a first-degree relative d. The presence of IgM RF on at least 2 occasions at least 3 mo apart e. The presence of systemic JIA in the patient
RF-Negative Polyarthritis	1. Arthritis affecting ≥5 joints during the first 6 mo of disease and 2. Test for RF is negative	a, b, c, d, e
RF-Positive Polyarthritis	1. Arthritis affecting ≥5 joints during the first 6 mo of disease, and 2. ≥2 positive RF tests (as routinely defined in an accredited laboratory), at least 3 mo apart during the first 6 mo of disease	a, b, c, e

Psoriatic Arthritis	1. Arthritis and psoriasis, or
	2. Arthritis and at least 2 of the following:
	  1. Dactylitis
	  2. Nail pitting (minimum of 2 pits on 1 or more nails at any time) or onycholysis
	  3. Psoriasis in a first-degree relative
		b, c, d, e

Enthesitis-Related Arthritis	1. Arthritis *and* enthesitis, or
	2. Arthritis *or* enthesitis, with at least 2 of the following:
	  a. The presence of or a history of sacroiliac joint tenderness and/or inflammatory lumbosacral pain
	  b. The presence of HLA-B27
	  c. Onset of arthritis in a male >6 yr of age
	  d. Acute (symptomatic) anterior uveitis
	  e. History of ankylosing spondylitis, ERA, sacroiliitis with inflammatory bowel disease, reactive arthritis, or acute anterior uveitis in a first-degree relative
		a, d, e

Systemic JIA	Arthritis in 1 or more joints with, or preceded by, fever of at least 2 weeks' duration that is documented to be daily and quotidian (fever that rises to ≥39° C once a day and returns to ≤37° C between fever peaks) for at least 3 days, and accompanied by 1 or more of the following: 1. Evanescent (nonfixed) erythematous rash 2. Generalized lymph node enlargement 3. Hepatomegaly and/or splenomegaly 4. Serositis	a, b, c, d
Undifferentiated Arthritis	Arthritis that fulfills criteria in no category or in ≥2 of the above categories	

ERA, enthesitis-related arthritis; RF, rheumatoid factor.

disease. However, if a patient does not easily fit into the ILAR classification system, clinicians must carefully consider all other possibilities, rheumatologic and nonrheumatologic. To this end, ILAR recommends the following descriptors in order to obtain more clinical information: age at onset; characteristics of articular involvement; serologies (ANA, RF, anticitrullinated protein antibody [ACPA]); uveitis; and the human leukocyte antigen (HLA) allelic associations. For example, a 2-year-old girl who wakes up crying at night from back or hip pain should immediately trigger alarms of infection or malignancy rather

than a rheumatic condition. This case is different from a 12-year-old boy with back stiffness and hip and entheseal pain, which would be a classic presentation of enthesitis-related arthritis (ERA) in this age group.

Among patients with acute lymphocytic leukemia (ALL), 15% to 30% present with musculoskeletal symptoms and may be misdiagnosed as JIA.[7] Up to 75% of children ultimately diagnosed with ALL presenting with musculoskeletal complaints did not have blasts in the peripheral blood at the time of evaluation by pediatric rheumatologists, although low white blood cell count, mild thrombocytopenia, and nighttime pain were early indicators of ALL. ANA status, rash, radiographic abnormalities, and objective signs of arthritis were not helpful in distinguishing between ALL and JIA because they occurred at similar rates in both groups.[8]

Each subcategory is discussed later, focusing on clinical manifestations, diagnostic features, treatment, outcome, and prognosis. Treatment recommendations are discussed later for each of the subtypes of JIA on the basis of current available evidence including the recently developed ACR recommendations for the treatment of JIA.[9]

RHEUMATOID FACTOR–NEGATIVE POLYARTHRITIS

Clinical Manifestations and Diagnostic Features

RF-negative polyarthritis makes up 10% to 30% of all JIA cases, with a bimodal distribution of age of onset with the first peak at 1 to 4 years of age and the second peak at 10 to 12 years. Girls are more commonly affected than boys with a ratio of 3.2:1, and subacute anterior uveitis occurs in 4% to 25%.[10] Any joint may be affected in RF-negative polyarthritis JIA, with more involvement of hip, shoulder, cervical spine, and distal interphalangeal joints than in adults. The arthritis is often usually insidious and can be symmetric or asymmetric, affecting both large and small joints. Some authors distinguish between two clinical subgroups on the basis of ANA status: (1) an ANA-positive form that resembles oligoarthritis, except for the number of joints affected in the first 6 months of disease, consisting of young girls (younger than age 6) with an asymmetric-onset arthritis and at a high risk of uveitis, and (2) an ANA-negative form that is similar to adult-onset RF-negative rheumatoid arthritis (RA), characterized by symmetric synovitis of large and small joints, with onset in a slightly older age group (ages 7 to 9). The similarities between ANA-positive, RF-negative polyarthritis and oligoarthritis have led to the hypothesis that these two entities are actually in the same disease spectrum.[6]

RF-negative polyarthritis may be associated with elevated acute phase reactants, mild anemia, and ANA positivity in up to 40%. Even though RF is negative, 50% to 80% of patients are ACPA positive,[10] using high-sensitivity (but low-specificity) testing methods.[11]

Differential Diagnosis

The differential diagnosis of RF-negative polyarthritis includes the other JIA subtypes including ERA, which should be considered particularly in boys older than 6 years of age because sacroiliac involvement may not occur until adolescence. Other major diagnostic considerations include other rheumatic conditions such as lupus, especially in an older girl who is ANA positive; lymphoma; and leukemia. *Neisseria gonorrhoeae* and Lyme disease can present as an acute polyarthritis.

Treatment

With the current development of increasingly more effective biologic treatment for arthritis, pediatric rheumatologists now aim to achieve complete disease remission as early as possible in the disease course. Several studies support the paradigm of treating aggressively to reach inactive disease as early as possible, which may ultimately lead to better outcome such as improved quality of life, shorter periods of time spent in active disease, and less long-term joint damage. Active disease in the first 2 years was significantly associated with the duration of active disease in the following 3 years,[12] and conversely, improved disease control with disease-modifying antirheumatic drugs (DMARDs) and/or biologics was associated with improved outcomes.[13] To this end, children with polyarthritis require a disease-modifying agent as soon as practically possible after the diagnosis has been confirmed. If nonsteroidal anti-inflammatory drugs (NSAIDs) are initially used as monotherapy, with or without intra-articular steroids (IASs), continued disease activity at no more than 2 months should prompt escalation of therapy.[9] As shown in Figure 107-1, methotrexate (MTX) is the first DMARD of choice, but if there is an inadequate response to MTX by 2 months, anti–tumor necrosis factor (TNF) agents should be initiated.[14,15] The different TNF inhibitors have not been directly compared against each other, so it is not possible to determine which might be most effective and safe in a given patient. Switching between TNF inhibitors in children has not been well studied. Sulfasalazine and leflunomide can still be used before an anti-TNF agent in mild disease, although evidence suggests that leflunomide may be slightly less effective than MTX.[16] Polyarticular disease course of any type, which does not respond well to MTX or anti-TNF agents, is now increasingly being treated with a range of newer biologics. Physiotherapy (PT) is important for all children with JIA, for stretching, muscle building, and consequent joint protection. Children with hand involvement need occupational therapy (OT) assessment and input regarding writing and school accommodations. The following paragraphs summarize specific information about different therapies used in children and may be applied to all types of JIA as appropriate. (See Table 107-2 for medications, dosing, route, and safety monitoring recommendations.)

Nonsteroidal Anti-inflammatory Drug Use in Children

NSAIDs may help control symptoms but do not alter the natural history of JIA. In general, NSAIDs should only be considered as monotherapy in initial therapy in low disease activity. If control is not achieved in 1 to 2 months, additional therapy should be considered.[9] NSAIDs are frequently used for symptom control as an adjunctive therapy to more definitive therapies. Gastric protection with H_2 blockers or proton pump inhibitors may be required.

Intra-articular Steroid Injections

The use of intra-articular triamcinolone hexacetonide (THA), 1 mg/kg in large joints such as the knee and 0.5 mg/kg in smaller joints such as the ankle, has been found to be superior to triamcinalone acetonide, betamethasone, and methylprednisolone acetate in randomized controlled trials.[17-22] Early treatment is associated with better outcome,[23] and IASs are expected to result in clinical improvement of

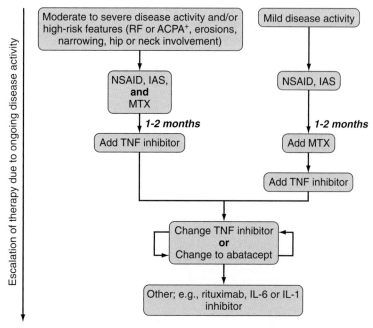

Figure 107-1 Polyarticular-course juvenile idiopathic arthritis treatment algorithm including rheumatoid factor (RF)-negative, RF-positive, extended oligoarticular, and psoriatic arthritis treatment. The treatment goal is remission of disease activity and is stratified by severity of disease. More disease activity or high-risk features should prompt disease-modifying antirheumatic drug use as initial therapy, whereas nonsteroidal anti-inflammatory drug (NSAID) monotherapy could be used initially for 1 to 2 months. If NSAID monotherapy is ineffective, treatment should be escalated. ACPA, anticitrullinated protein antibody; IAS, intra-articular steroid; IL, interleukin; MTX, methotrexate; TNF, tumor necrosis factor.

arthritis for at least 4 months. Therefore if arthritis recurs, joint injections can be repeated up to three times in a 12-month period. Difficult-to-reach joints such as the hip, sacroiliac (SI) joint, temporomandibular joint (TMJ), and subtalar joint may be injected using ultrasound or fluoroscopy. IASs should be administered under sedation or general anesthesia for the young. The use of IASs for active arthritis has been recommended by the ACR guidelines regardless of concurrent therapy, JIA subtype, disease activity, prognostic features, or joint contracture. If the duration of clinical improvement is shorter than 4 months, systemic treatment (e.g., MTX) may be indicated.[9]

Corticosteroid Use in Children with Juvenile Idiopathic Arthritis

In general, systemic corticosteroids should be used sparingly in the treatment of any subgroup of JIA because of the severe morbidity associated with chronic use, even at low doses. Newer therapeutic modalities such as biologics reduce the dependence for any corticosteroids and/or limit the doses needed. The evidence for use of corticosteroids for the synovitis of JIA is controversial and conflicting, and the ACR recommendations for JIA treatment were unable to make any recommendations for corticosteroid use, except in systemic juvenile idiopathic arthritis (sJIA) for severe systemic features.[9] However, in some cases, low doses of corticosteroids (<0.1 mg prednisone equivalent/kg/day) or brief high-dose regimens (intravenous methylprednisolone 30 mg/kg/day for 1 to 3 days) may be used in polyarticular JIA, in order to bridge constitutional features of pain and fatigue while waiting for DMARDs or biologic therapies to reach their therapeutic effect. Local use of corticosteroids for uveitis is discussed later in "Uveitis."

Methotrexate

MTX is the most commonly used DMARD in JIA.[24] In a retrospective cohort study involving all JIA subtypes, the strongest predictor of response to MTX at 6 months of treatment was the time from diagnosis to start of MTX, suggesting that starting MTX early will lead to a better response.[25] The ACR guidelines support a maximum dose of 0.6 mg/kg once weekly (equivalent to 15 mg/m^2/week, maximal 25 mg/week) of parenteral MTX.[9] In patients with lower disease severity, lower doses (8 to 12.5 mg/m^2/week oral or parenteral) may be effective, and these doses are similar in safety.[15] Most pediatric rheumatologists start folic acid at 1 mg/day, but daily folate supplementation remains controversial. Routine monitoring of liver enzyme tests should be done as noted in Table 107-2, but liver biopsies are not indicated except in unusual circumstances. Some children develop an intolerance to MTX, and leflunomide may be used as an alternative.[16,26] Both MTX and leflunomide are associated with teratogenic effects.

Tumor Necrosis Factor Inhibitors

Anti-TNF agents are effective in many children with polyarticular-course JIA of any onset type who fail to respond fully to MTX. The first TNF inhibitor to be studied in JIA, etanercept, demonstrated efficacy and safety in a novel randomized withdrawal trial design in patients with polyarticular JIA, in which the study design was based on an open-label period, followed by randomization of responders to placebo or study drug with the primary endpoint being time to flare.[14] Since that initial randomized control study in 2000, long-term studies and registries have continued to demonstrate the safety and efficacy of etanercept in children

Table 107-2 Commonly Used Medications in Juvenile Idiopathic Arthritis[9,176]

Medication	Typical Maximum Dose	Typical Frequency
Abatacept	10 mg/kg (max 1000 mg) IV	Load at 0, 2, 4 wk, then every 4 wk
Adalimumab	24 mg/m^2	Every 2 wk
	<30 kg: 20 mg SQ	
	>30 kg: 40 mg SQ	
Anakinra	2 mg/kg (max 100 mg) SQ	Daily
Cyclosporine	6 mg/kg/day orally	Divided twice a day
Diclofenac (SR preparation available)	1-3 mg/kg/day (max 150 mg/day)	Divided 1-3 times a day
Etanercept	0.8 mg/kg/wk (max 50 mg)* SQ	Once weekly
	0.4 mg/kg/dose (max 25 mg) SQ	2×/wk
Ibuprofen	≥6 mo of age: 30-40 mg/kg/day	Divided 3-4 times a day
Indomethacin (SR preparation available)	>1 mo of age: 1-2 mg/kg/day (max 50 mg/day)	Divided 1-2 times a day
Infliximab	10 mg/kg/dose IV	Load at 0, 2, 6 wk, then every 4 wk
Intravenous immunoglobulin	2 g/kg/dose IV	Every 2 wk
Leflunomide	<40 kg: 10 mg orally	Daily
	>40 kg: 20 mg orally	
Methotrexate	15 mg/m^2/dose SQ	Weekly
	(0.6 mg/kg; max 25 mg)	
Naproxen	>2 yr of age: 20-30 mg/kg/day (max 1 g/day)	Divided twice a day
Piroxicam	<15 kg: 5 mg orally	Daily
	16-25 kg: 10 mg orally	
	26-45 kg: 15 mg orally	
	>46 kg: 20 mg orally	
Rilonacept	2.2-4.4 mg/kg SQ	Once weekly
Rituximab	750 mg/m^2 (max 1000 mg) IV	Twice 2 wk apart
Sulfasalazine	50 mg/kg/day (max 2 g) orally	Divided twice a day
Tacrolimus	0.2 mg/kg/day orally	Divided twice a day
Thalidomide	5 mg/kg/dose orally	Daily
Tocilizumab	<30 kg: 12 mg/kg IV	Every 2 wk
	>30 kg: 8 mg/kg IV	

*The effectiveness of the 0.8 mg/kg/wk dose has been evaluated in JIA patients.[177,178]

IV, intravenous; SQ, subcutaneous; SR, sustained release.

Summary of Recommendations for Medication Safety Monitoring
Nonsteroidal Anti-inflammatory Drugs
Complete blood count, liver enzymes, serum creatinine
Before or soon after initiation of routine use
Repeat approximately twice yearly for chronic daily use
Repeat approximately once yearly for routine use (3-4 days/wk)
Methotrexate
Complete blood count, liver enzymes, serum creatinine
Before initiation
Approximately 1 mo after initiation
Approximately 1-2 mo after increase in dose
Repeat approximately every 3-4 mo if prior results normal and dose stable
Tumor Necrosis Factor Inhibitors
Complete blood count, liver enzymes, serum creatinine
Before initiation
Repeat approximately every 3-6 mo
Tuberculosis screening
Before initiation
Repeat approximately once yearly

with polyarthritis, with and without MTX.[27-32] The frequency of major serious adverse events (SAEs) have been low, with adjusted rates of 0.12 events per patient year and 0.03 medically important infections per patient year in open-label extensions.[30] Importantly, no cases of lupus, demyelinating disorders, malignancies, opportunistic infections, or tuberculosis were seen. Although there have been several long-term studies of etanercept with international registries, the total number of patient-years available for evaluation is still too small to be able to detect rare long-term SAEs such as malignancy or demyelinating diseases.

A 1-year prospective, observational study to compare combination etanercept and MTX with etanercept monotherapy demonstrated that the likelihood of achieving 70% disease control (ACR Pedi 70) was increased with combination therapy (odds ratio of 2.1, 95% CI 1.2 to 3.5) as compared with etanercept monotherapy.[27] In this cohort, there were 24 infectious SAEs and 23 noninfectious SAEs including three malignancies in 496 patients over 12 months. Growth delay in JIA was improved and reversed with the use of etanercept.[33]

An international, multicenter, randomized, double-blind, placebo-controlled trial of infliximab provided important lessons regarding dosing in children.[34] The initial dose of 3 mg/kg/infusion based on adult studies did not demonstrate efficacy at 3 months compared with placebo; however, a separate arm suggested that 6 mg/kg/infusion had better pharmacokinetics leading to better effectiveness. In a 4-year, long-term, open-label extension, 14% of patients discontinued infliximab due to SAEs including six infectious SAEs in 120 patients over 52 weeks.[35] Significant infusion reactions associated with infliximab antibodies and asymptomatic development of antinuclear antibodies were observed.

Adalimumab was shown to be efficacious and safe in a randomized placebo-controlled withdrawal trial in patients with moderately to severely active polyarticular JIA with or without MTX, and there was a trend toward more improvement with combination therapy, although the study was not statistically powered to measure this difference.[36] The dose used was adalimumab 24 mg/m^2 (maximum dose, 40 mg) subcutaneously every other week. SAEs possibly related to adalimumab occurred in 14 patients (total 177), seven of which were serious infections.

In August 2009, the U.S. Food and Drug Administration issued a black box warning on the increased risk of cancer, particularly lymphoma, in children and adolescents receiving TNF inhibitors for arthritis or inflammatory bowel disease (IBD).[37] The other adverse events involved with TNF inhibitors are similar to that of adults and have been reported in children as well including serious infections, demyelinating processes, optic neuritis, injection site reactions or infusion reactions, and development of autoimmune conditions. Because of the voluntary nature of reporting rare adverse drug events in the United States, the actual risk of any of these rare events is not known.

Abatacept

The T cell co-stimulatory inhibitor, CTLA4-Ig (abatacept), was studied in an international placebo-controlled randomized withdrawal trial in 190 patients with active polyarthritis regardless of onset type who had inadequate response or intolerance to one DMARD in the past including TNF inhibitors.[38] Concurrent MTX was allowed. Thirty-percent improvement (ACR Pedi 30) response rates were 76% in biologic-naïve patients and 39% in patients with prior biologic therapy. Abatacept continued to be clinically significant with durable efficacy in patients with JIA, and some patients require longer periods for optimal response (>3 to 4 months) compared with TNF inhibitors.[39] No cases of tuberculosis or malignancy were detected, but patient numbers were small and follow-up time was limited.

Other Biologics

The ACR guidelines recommend consideration of rituximab as a treatment option for patients who have received TNF inhibitor and abatacept sequentially and have high disease activity.[9] IL-6 and IL-1 inhibition are discussed in more detail later in "Systemic Juvenile Idiopathic Arthritis" but have not been specifically studied in polyarticular disease. The use of nonbiologic DMARD combinations (such as MTX plus sulfasalazine and/or hydroxychloroquine) has not been studied in children.

Outcome

Early response to treatment was an important predictor of long-term outcome.[13] Symmetric arthritis and early hand involvement predicted future disability and poorer overall well-being.[40] The ACR guidelines for JIA treatment also consider the following as poor prognostic factors in patients with RF-negative polyarthritis: arthritis of hip or cervical spine; positive ACPAs; and radiographic damage (erosions or joint space narrowing by radiograph).[9]

RF-negative polyarthritis has a variable outcome, which shows the heterogeneity of the subtype,[41] but the overall prognosis appears to be better than RF-positive polyarticular JIA.[42] Approximately 30% of children will go into long-term remission off medication, with the chance of remission being highest in the first 5 years of disease.[43,44] However, flare of disease 2 years after reaching clinical remission off medication had occurred in 69% of patients.[43]

RHEUMATOID FACTOR–POSITIVE POLYARTHRITIS

Clinical Manifestations and Diagnostic Features

RF-positive polyarthritis is a well-characterized JIA subcategory and is part of the same disease spectrum as adult RF-positive RA,[45] sharing immunogenetic and serologic factors. This subcategory makes up 5% to 10% of cases of JIA[10] and is more common in girls, with reported female-to-male ratios between 5.7 and 12.8 : 1.0.[46,47] Age of onset occurs in late childhood or adolescence and typically is an aggressive, symmetric polyarthritis affecting the small joints of the hands, as well as large joint involvement in a pattern that resembles RA. These children frequently have more than 30 joints with arthritis. Hip involvement is common and may be debilitating. The arthritis can be quite severe, often resulting in bony erosions and joint destruction. Radiologic changes tend to take place early,[42] especially in hands and feet. With active disease, patients may occasionally have mild systemic signs and symptoms such as weight loss, low-grade fever, malaise, mild hepatosplenomegaly, or lymphadenopathy. Rheumatoid nodules occur in up to 10% of cases, most frequently around the elbow. Other extra-articular manifestations are reported less often than in adults. Uveitis is an unusual feature of this subtype, occurring in only about 0% to 2% of patients.[10]

Polyarthritis may be associated with mild to moderate inflammation such as elevated acute-phase reactants and a normocytic, normochromic anemia. By definition, all patients have IgM-anti-IgG RF. The ANA test is positive in about 55% of patients,[10] and ACPAs have been reported in 57% to 73%.[48,49]

Differential Diagnosis

The differential diagnosis of RF-positive polyarthritis includes other JIA subcategories, especially when there is no confirmed RF-positive test on two occasions. Such cases are frequently unclassified in the JIA system; however, management and therapy remain similar.

Treatment

Treatment algorithms and ACR guidelines for patients with all types of polyarthritis are discussed in Figure 107-1. However, because children with RF-positive polyarthritis are at higher risk of prolonged erosive arthritis compared with other types of JIA, these children should be considered to be in the more severe disease category, requiring rapid escalation of treatment if even mild disease activity persists. Rather than an initial period of NSAID monotherapy, RF-positive polyarthritis patients should receive MTX, at the time of diagnosis, with rapid addition of a TNF inhibitor if response is not adequate.[9] Some children benefit from multiple joint injections to maintain control of the arthritis.

Outcome

Children with RF-positive polyarthritis have a poorer long-term prognosis than the other JIA subcategories.[42,50] Inactive disease is difficult to achieve with 84% of the disease course consisting of active disease, and only 5% of patients were able to maintain remission after cessation of therapy.[43]

OLIGOARTICULAR JUVENILE IDIOPATHIC ARTHRITIS

Clinical and Diagnostic Features

Oligoarticular JIA accounts for up to 20% of all new rheumatic diagnoses in the general pediatric rheumatology clinic[47] and is the most prevalent of all the JIA subcategories, comprising 30% to 60% of all JIA patients in North America and Europe.[41] Oligoarticular JIA has no adult equivalent. The peak age of onset occurs in Caucasian children ages 2 to 4 years from the United States and Europe.[10] Females are affected more commonly than males, 3:1.[10] Two general subgroups are recognized within oligoarticular JIA: extended oligoarticular involvement, in which many additional joints develop arthritis after the initial 6 months, as contrasted to persistent oligoarticular JIA, in which the number of joints affected remains less than 5. Currently,

there is no single reliable predictor of extension, but symmetric disease, ankle and/or wrist involvement, and an elevated erythrocyte sedimentation rate (ESR) in the first 6 months of disease may indicate likelihood of extension.[51,52] Disease extension to the extended subtype has been reported to be 30% to 50% at 4 to 6 years after disease onset.[51,53]

Oligoarticular JIA usually presents as an asymmetric arthritis affecting one or two large joints, especially of the lower extremities, with the knee being the most commonly affected, followed by the ankle, wrist, and digits. Hand involvement is the third most commonly affected location, but this pattern may portend the later onset of psoriatic arthritis.[54] Involvement of the hip and back, especially in young children, is so unusual that extensive evaluation is warranted to rule out other conditions such as infection or tumors.

Significant constitutional and systemic symptoms are unusual in oligoarticular JIA and, if present, should raise concern regarding the accuracy of the initial diagnosis. Pain in an obviously inflamed joint is surprisingly minimal compared with septic arthritis, and in up to 25% of cases the symptoms may be subtle with parents only noticing a limp and joint swelling. In a young child there is reluctance to walk and bear weight with a return to crawling. There is a high risk for developing a relatively asymptomatic chronic uveitis, especially in ANA-positive individuals, requiring regular ophthalmology examinations to detect early changes. (See Table 107-3 for guidelines and "Uveitis" later for treatment.) Other complications that can be prevented in most patients with proper treatment include growth discrepancies in muscle tone and bulk, leg length, and the development of micrognathia and joint contractures.

Among children with oligoarthritis, 75% to 85% have a positive ANA (70% to 80% in persistent oligoarticular JIA and 80% to 95% in extended oligoarticular JIA),[10] with low to moderate titers (1:40 to 1:320). The rate of ANA positivity is even higher in girls with an early onset.[55] Patients are RF negative, although ACPAs have been detected in some patients with oligoarticular JIA, depending on the enzyme-linked immunoreceptor assay (ELISA) method used for screening.[11] Some suggest that ANA serology should delineate a homogeneous group of arthritis patients, independent of the course of arthritis and number of joints involved.[6]

Table 107-3 American Academy of Pediatrics Recommended Ophthalmologic Screening Frequency for Asymptomatic Uveitis in Juvenile Idiopathic Arthritis (JIA) Patients*[67]

JIA Subtype	Antinuclear Antibody Status	Age of JIA Onset (yr)	Duration of Disease (yr)	Uveitis Risk Category	Eye Examination Frequency (mo)
Oligoarthritis or polyarthritis	+	≤6	≤4	High	3
	+	≤6	>4	Moderate	6
	+	≤6	>7	Low	12
	+	>6	≤4	Moderate	6
	+	>6	>4	Low	12
	−	≤6	≤4	Moderate	6
	−	≤6	>4	Low	12
	−	>6	NA	Low	12
Systemic JIA	NA	NA	NA	Low	12

*Several investigators have recommended the most intensive screening ophthalmologic exams in ANA-positive girls with JIA onset <7 yr of age independent of JIA subtype. Patients with JIA onset <5 yr should have eye exams every 3 mo until 7 yr after JIA diagnosis.[64] On the other hand, in a large, German, population-based study using the International League of Associations for Rheumatology classification system of JIA, certain modifications were proposed that were less conservative than the American Academy of Pediatrics in terms of frequency of eye exams, so the timing of screening exams remains unclear.[65]

NA, not applicable.

The typical child with oligoarticular JIA will have normal white blood counts, normal or mild to moderately elevated acute-phase reactants, and in some cases, mild anemia. Elevated acute-phase reactants may suggest other conditions with inflammatory features such as IBD or malignancy.

Differential Diagnosis

The differential diagnosis of oligoarticular JIA includes other JIA subtypes, especially ERA and psoriatic JIA; other rheumatic diseases of childhood; and nonrheumatic causes of joint pain and swelling such as septic arthritis, benign or malignant tumors, reactive arthritis, foreign body synovitis, pigmented villonodular synovitis, arterial-venous malformation, bleeding disorders (such as hemophilia), or severe trauma including nonaccidental injury. Mild trauma such as from a fall does not cause persistent joint swelling, and trauma is rarely a cause of joint swelling unless there is an internal derangement seen in older, not younger, children. Children with hypermobility can develop transient joint effusions after exercise,[56] but this should not be long-lasting swelling. Lyme disease (in an endemic area) can cause recurrent monoarticular arthritis (typically involving the knee and often popliteal cysts), usually for less than 6 weeks. As described earlier, ALL may present with bone and joint pain and swelling, often monoarticular. If there is any concern of malignancy or infection, a complete blood count with manual differential and peripheral smear is crucial and bone marrow examination should be performed if indicated.

A common initial response by general pediatricians when evaluating children with joint pain or swelling is to believe the problem is mechanical. However, in young children and toddlers, orthopedic problems such as meniscal tears or ligamentous injury are exceedingly rare because of the nature of pediatric musculoskeletal development and anatomy. In general, ligaments and tendons are stronger than growing bone in children, and the bone-ligament or bone-tendon junction is the weakest link. Therefore fractures are more common in children than adults, but nonaccidental trauma should always be considered, especially in children younger than 3 years.

Treatment

The treatment strategies for extended versus persistent oligoarticular JIA differ in both the approach to therapy and the intensity of escalating treatment on the basis of the number of joints at risk for significant damage. For *extended oligoarticular JIA*, treatment approaches are similar to RF-positive or RF-negative polyarticular JIA because these subtypes all have polyarticular involvement (see Figure 107-1). Treatment of *persistent oligoarticular JIA* is usually approached in a stepwise fashion (Figure 107-2). For these patients with a history of arthritis in four or fewer joints, the initial treatment is an NSAID, with or without an adjunctive IAS, followed by MTX if there is an inadequate response to one or more IASs. Initiation of MTX was recommended in the ACR guidelines for JIA as initial treatment for children with oligoarticular JIA with high disease activity and poor prognostic features, defined as involvement of hip, cervical spine, ankle or wrist, high inflammatory markers, or radiologic changes.[9] Partial or complete remission on MTX can be induced in 60% to 70% with extended oligoarticular JIA.[15,57,58] TNF inhibition should be considered in resistant cases, often in combination with MTX.

Concurrent sulfasalazine and hydroxychloroquine have been used with variable success. Sulfasalazine is more typically used with HLA-B27–associated arthritis and ERA.

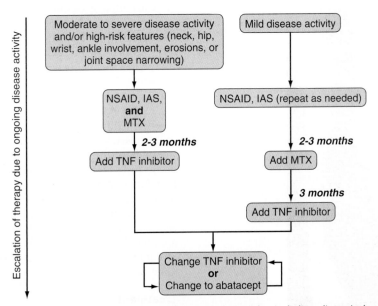

Figure 107-2 Persistent oligoarticular juvenile idiopathic arthritis (JIA) treatment algorithm including oligoarticular course psoriatic JIA. The treatment goal is remission of disease activity and is stratified by severity of disease. More disease activity or high-risk features should prompt disease-modifying antirheumatic drug use as initial therapy, whereas nonsteroidal anti-inflammatory drug (NSAID) monotherapy could be used initially for 2 to 3 months. If NSAID monotherapy is ineffective, therapy should be escalated. IAS, intra-articular steroid; MTX, methotrexate; TNF, tumor necrosis factor.

Special Considerations: Knee Monoarthritis

Because knee monoarthritis is the most common presentation of oligoarticular JIA, specific management is discussed here. The two treatments to be considered are NSAIDs and IASs, with evidence that IASs may be more effective even though most pediatric rheumatologists use NSAIDs before IASs.[59] An initial trial of NSAIDs may be conducted with the hopes of avoiding IASs in some patients, but the risk of IASs must be weighed against the cost of continued active arthritis. Choosing among treatment strategies involves a tradeoff between several different outcomes including duration of active arthritis, potential for long-term complications, adverse effects of therapies, discomfort of daily medications or potentially painful procedures and anesthesia, as well as parental preferences. Synovectomy is not indicated in oligoarticular JIA.

Outcome

Long-term studies of adults treated before the use of biologic agents have shown that up to 50% of adults who had oligoarticular JIA may have ongoing active disease or functional problems in adulthood,[60] and the rate of remission after 6 to 10 years from onset of disease ranges only from 23% to 47%.[51,61] Ongoing disease activity and extension of joint involvement is related to a poor outcome and radiographic damage,[62] and therefore emphasis on control of disease activity is critical. Morbidity from long-term inflammation can cause problems as well such as leg-length discrepancy with knee arthritis, muscle atrophy, bony overgrowth, and joint contractions (Figure 107-3), as well as other growth abnormalities such as micrognathia.

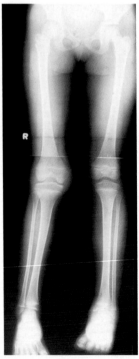

Figure 107-3 Radiograph of a young girl with oligoarticular juvenile idiopathic arthritis involving the right knee, demonstrating bony hypertrophy of the affected knee, with leg-length discrepancy and flexion contracture.

Patients with persistent oligoarthritis generally have the best outcome with 68% of patients achieving clinical remission off medication.[43,51] Patients with an extended oligoarticular JIA have higher cumulative duration of active arthritis,[43] more erosive disease, and a higher risk of chronic disability.[51] Only 31% of children with extended oligoarticular JIA achieved remission after discontinuing their medication.[43] Relapses occur, and within 2 years after clinical remission off medication, flares occurred in 47% of patients with persistent oligoarthritis and 67% of patients with extended oligoarthritis.[43] Diligence regarding ophthalmologic screening for asymptomatic uveitis needs to continue as described in "Uveitis."

UVEITIS

Clinical Manifestations and Diagnostic Features

Chronic anterior uveitis, defined as inflammation involving the anterior uveal tract including the iris and ciliary body, is the most frequent extra-articular manifestation of JIA. Uveitis is most common in oligoarticular JIA and RF-negative polyarticular JIA, with a prevalence ranging from 17% to 26% and 4% to 25%, respectively. It is rare in RF-positive polyarticular JIA and sJIA.[10] Risk factors for uveitis include ANA positivity, being younger than 6 years of age at JIA onset, female sex, and oligoarticular subtype.[63] These risk factors of developing uveitis are larger influences in girls but not boys.[64] The interval from diagnosis of JIA to the development of uveitis is longer the younger the age at onset of JIA, especially in ANA-positive patients.[64] Overall, uveitis is observed in 30% of ANA-positive patients with JIA.[65]

Chronic anterior uveitis is typically nongranulomatous and asymptomatic at onset, and if unrecognized it can lead to serious visual deficits. Because of its insidious onset, regularly scheduled screening by an experienced ophthalmologist with slit lamp examination is required for early diagnosis and treatment. Newly diagnosed patients are ideally screened within 6 weeks of diagnosis[66] because in 5% of cases, uveitis occurs before diagnosis of JIA.[67] The highest risk period for uveitis development is the first 4 years after arthritis onset, although the risk is never completely eliminated.[67] The frequency of ophthalmologic screening according to the American Academy of Pediatrics guidelines is determined by the degree of risk such as ANA status, age of JIA onset, and duration of disease shown in Table 107-3.[67] In children with HLA-B27–related disease, anterior uveitis occurs in 10% to 15% but is usually highly symptomatic and therefore does not require routine screening.[63] The severity of chronic anterior uveitis associated with JIA is unrelated to the severity of the underlying joint disease, and the clinical course of the uveitis and arthritis may not parallel one another. Disease is eventually bilateral in nearly two-thirds of patients, but both eyes are not always inflamed at the same time.[68]

Treatment

Differential Diagnosis

When evaluating the etiology of uveitis, it is important to consider infectious causes, such as tuberculosis, toxoplasmosis, cytomegalovirus, herpes simplex virus, syphilis, human immunodeficiency virus, Lyme disease, cat scratch disease, and fungus. Uveitis can be confined primarily to the eye or occur secondary to a systemic illness, such as in Behçet's disease, sarcoidosis, autoinflammatory syndromes, multiple sclerosis, TINU (tubulointerstitial nephritis and uveitis syndrome), and Vogt-Koyanagi-Harada syndrome. Although the cause of uveitis often remains idiopathic, it is important to not miss a malignancy such as lymphoma or retinoblastoma.[63]

Uveitis is initially treated with topical corticosteroids and mydriatics, although in approximately 30% of patients the uveitis remains active even with topical or local treatment with subtenon corticosteroid injections, and immunosuppressive medications are indicated to attempt to aggressively control the inflammation and prevent poor visual outcomes. Although there are no prospective randomized controlled studies on the use of immunosuppressive medications in children with uveitis, several observational studies suggest the effectiveness of these treatments. MTX, either oral or parenteral, is usually the first choice of treatment and is also used as a steroid-sparing agent.[69-71] Other effective immunosuppressives include mycophenolate mofetil[72] and azathioprine, while cyclosporine has limited value.[73] Treatment of uveitis requires close collaboration between the affected child's rheumatologist and ophthalmologist.

In cases of refractory inflammation, biologic agents should be considered. TNF inhibitors are the most commonly used, specifically infliximab and adalimumab, which appear to be more effective than etanercept.[74-81] The dosing range and frequency of infliximab varies widely when used for uveitis, and up to 10 mg/kg/month are often required for control and should be used with MTX to prevent development of anti-infliximab antibodies. Adalimumab is given 20 to 40 mg subcutaneously every 2 weeks, and when ineffective, it can be administered weekly.[78] A case series reported remission with the administration of abatacept 10 mg/kg intravenously monthly in six of seven patients refractory to immunosuppressives and TNF inhibition.[82] High-dose intravenous daclizumab, a humanized monoclonal antibody against IL-2 receptor, has been reported to be effective but is no longer available in the United States.[83]

In the past, ophthalmologists were concerned about primary placement of intraocular lens in JIA patients with history of uveitis with subsequent formation of cataracts.[84] Now, with the more widespread practice of strict control of uveitis, good visual outcomes with cataract surgery and intraocular lens placement can be achieved using aggressive systemic immunomodulatory therapy perioperatively.[85] The general expert opinion among uveitis specialists is to try to taper immunomodulatory therapy after 12 to 24 months of quiescence of uveitis; however, this has not been studied.[86]

Outcome

Complications resulting from uveitis include posterior synechiae, cataract, band keratopathy, glaucoma, papillitis, or cystoid macular edema. Posterior synechiae (fibrous bands adhering the iris to the lens, Figure 107-4) result in a distorted papillary border. Band keratopathy (a layer of calcium deposited in Bowman's membrane of the cornea), is not

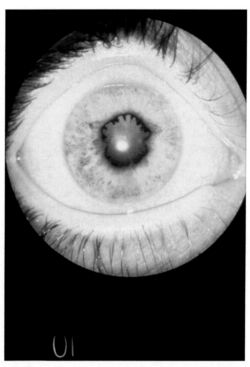

Figure 107-4 Chronic anterior uveitis associated with oligoarticular and polyarticular rheumatoid factor–negative juvenile idiopathic arthritis, demonstrating posterior synechiae and absence of significant sclera inflammation.

uncommon. Cataracts and glaucoma may develop as a complication of the uveitis or its treatment, so chronic monotherapy with topical corticosteroids should be avoided.

The reported rate of visual loss due to JIA-related uveitis has decreased from 22% to 66% in studies before 1990 to 3% to 25% in newer studies, suggesting that newer and more aggressive approaches are effective.[87] Ongoing active intraocular inflammation with greater than or equal to 0.5+ cells was associated with increased risk of visual impairment and blindness.

Prognostic factors in JIA-associated uveitis are not clearly identified, and the results of the studies are often controversial. Different studies have revealed the following as potential factors associated with poor prognosis: short intervals between the diagnosis of arthritis and uveitis,[88-90] severity of uveitis at first examination,[91,92] signs of anterior chamber involvement (cells and flare),[92] and male gender.[89-93]

JUVENILE PSORIATIC ARTHRITIS

Clinical Manifestations and Diagnostic Features

Juvenile psoriatic arthritis (JPsA) was initially defined as juvenile-onset arthritis associated with psoriasis occurring at some point during the disease course. This definition has been expanded to include not only patients with overt psoriatic lesions but also arthritis who only have nail abnormalities or a first-degree relative with overt psoriasis.[94,95] JPsA represents 2% to 15% of all JIA with slight female preponderance and a bimodal pattern of onset (2 to 4 years and 7 to 10 years).[94,96,97] The psoriasis typically occurs within

2 years of the onset of arthritis, and for the majority of children the skin symptoms follow the arthritis symptoms.[98] Up to 80% of children have a classic psoriatic vulgaris or plaque psoriasis characterized by well-demarcated erythematous scaly lesions occurring over extensor surfaces (elbows and knees), scalp, and trunk.[98-100] However, in small children younger than the age of 2, the most common finding is psoriatic diaper rash.[100] Additional areas that should be evaluated include the hairline behind the ears, the navel, the groin region, and superior to the gluteal cleft.[98]

Because JPsA shares similar manifestations with multiple subtypes of juvenile arthritis, there is not one specific articular presentation. Patterns of joint involvement can be similar to both oligoarticular or polyarticular JIA with 60% to 70% of JPsA patients having an oligoarticular onset (<5 joints).[101] There were no differences in ANA or HLA-B27 positivity, or frequency of uveitis between oligoarticular JIA and JPsA with fewer than 5 joints at onset, although dactylitis was more frequent, reported in 15% to 37% of JPsA.[54,94,102] When JPsA subjects who had a polyarticular type course were compared with polyarticular JIA subjects, there was also no difference seen in ANA positivity, HLA-B27 positivity, and dactylitis. JPsA is associated with subacute anterior uveitis and ANA positivity in 15% to 20% of children with JPsA.[102] A recent study of childhood psoriatic arthritis argued for two distinct subpopulations: (1) a younger group (median age, 2.7 years), ANA positive, with a female preponderance, all of whom had dactylitis and more persistent disease, and (2) an older group (median age 9.5 years), more likely to be oligoarticular, have axial disease and enthesitis, and have higher remission rates.[94]

Children with psoriatic arthritis may have mild elevated acute-phase reactants (ESR, C-reactive protein [CRP], and platelets) and a mild anemia of chronic disease. However, up to one-third have no laboratory evidence of inflammation. Serologies and HLA associations are noted earlier.

Treatment

To date there have been no controlled studies examining the efficacy of antirheumatic medications in JPsA. A recent study compared treatment regimens of JPsA patients versus olgioarticular and polyarticular JIA patients and found no difference in use of NSAIDs, MTX, and TNF inhibitors.[102] In general, the treatment of JPsA should follow the treatment approaches for oligoarticular or RF-negative polyarticular JIA (see Figures 107-1 and 107-2) depending on the patient's pattern of joint involvement. MTX is of benefit for both the skin psoriasis and arthritis and, when used in children, is recommended as a single weekly dose rather than split doses.[99] In children with more aggressive disease, TNF inhibitors (which have also been successful in treating psoriasis) are indicated and may significantly limit bony destruction.[100,103,104] Regular screening for uveitis is required, especially in ANA-positive patients with both oligoarticular and polyarticular courses, with monitoring and management as described later in "Uveitis."

Outcome

Because of the heterogeneity in the patterns of arthritis in JPsA, the outcomes are variable and tend to track with the pattern of joint involvement. Although in one study erosions were less common in JPsA compared with polyarticular JIA (23% vs. 46%, respectively), there appears to be more persistent disease activity and more evidence of physical limitations and ongoing disease activity continuing into adulthood in patients with JPsA compared with oligoarticular and polyarticular JIA patients.[95,105] The uveitis of psoriatic arthritis, like that of oligoarticular disease, can lead to blindness if untreated.

ENTHESITIS-RELATED ARTHRITIS/ JUVENILE SPONDYLOARTHROPATHY

Clinical Manifestations and Diagnostic Features

The current ILAR category of ERA is a spectrum that includes spondyloarthropathies, juvenile ankylosing spondylitis, and SEA (spondylitis enthesitis and arthritis). ERA accounts for about 20% of JIA in one U.S. study,[47] but previous classification schemas have included JPsA within spondyloarthropathies resulting in variability in incidence and prevalence data.[106] In some cases, patients are first diagnosed as oligoarticular JIA, but characteristics of ERA later evolve. ERA occurs after age 6 and is more common in boys (male-to-female ratio of 7:1), although it may be under-recognized in symptomatic girls who can have milder disease with less axial skeleton involvement.[107]

The typical feature of ERA is the presence of enthesitis, or inflammation of the tendons and ligaments where they attach to bone (or enthesis). It is an early manifestation and occurs more frequently in children than in adult-onset ankylosing spondylitis (AS).[98] The typical enthesitis sites are around the patella (at the 2, 6, and 10 o'clock positions); Achilles' tendon; plantar fascia insertions into the calcaneus and metatarsal heads, greater trochanter, tibial tuberosity, and the base of the fifth metatarsal. Children may report vague buttock pain, groin pain, or heel pain, and a classic finding is of tarsitis with inflammation of the subtalar joint and surrounding tendon sheaths. At onset spinal symptoms are rare, but a subgroup of children with ERA will progress to features more typical of adult AS with SI joint and spinal inflammation during adolescence. This progression is more likely in boys who are HLA-B27 positive and have spinal or sacroiliac pain within 1 year of diagnosis.[108] The modified Schober's test can be used to evaluate lower lumbar flexibility with a change less than 6 cm being abnormal.[109] Because thoracic excursion varies greatly in a growing child, only performing sequential measurements are helpful. In the adolescent, any thoracic excursion less than 5 cm should be regarded as abnormal.[98]

ERA is associated with an acute anterior uveitis (AAU) in 6% to 27% of children, which typically presents as an acutely red, painful eye that needs immediate medical attention to avoid blindness.[98,110,111] Cardiovascular disease, although uncommon, can be severe in patients with ERA that has evolved into juvenile ankylosing spondylitis, with inflammatory aortic regurgitation reported in up to 10% of patients.[112] Restrictive pulmonary disease has been seen in juvenile spondyloarthritis without clinical or radiologic findings.

Reactive arthritis is categorized under ERA, following infection with organisms from the gastrointestinal tract (e.g., *Salmonella*, *Shigella*, *Yersinia*, *Campylobacter*, *Clostridium difficile*) or genitourinary tract (i.e., *Chlamydia* or *Ureaplasma*) without actual infection in the joint tissues. Usually self-limited, the arthritis can persist and transform into a more chronic arthropathy.[113] In addition to the arthritis, urethritis and uveitis have been documented in children to complete the classic triad for reactive arthritis. The clinical infection usually precedes the arthritis, enthesitis, or extra-articular disease by 1 to 4 weeks. Arthritis associated with IBD (Crohn's disease or ulcerative colitis) is seen in children, and two distinct patterns of joint involvement are noted: (1) peripheral arthritis and (2) sacroiliitis and spondylitis, with the former more common than the latter. Additional clinical manifestations unique to arthritis associated with IBD include clubbing, periostitis, erythema nodosum, pyoderma gangrenosum, osteoporosis, and rarely hypertrophic osteoarthropathy. The peripheral arthritis activity has been shown to correlate with gut disease activity unlike the SI joint activity, which tends not to correlate.[109]

Compared with adults, in whom radiologic evidence of sacroiliitis is the diagnostic hallmark of ankylosing spondylitis, radiologic evaluation in children with ERA is less often diagnostic because sacroiliitis is rare as a presenting symptom. Magnetic resonance imaging (MRI) with contrast is being increasingly used to detect evidence of acute sacroiliitis without chronic changes in children. MRI has also been used to evaluate enthesitis.[114] HLA-B27 is present in 80% to 90% of cases depending on ethnicity. The ESR may be mildly or markedly raised, and there may be a mild anemia, but these should also raise the suspicion that the child may have subclinical IBD. RF is negative, and ANA may be positive.

Differential Diagnosis

Children with true infectious arthritides (viral, rheumatic fever, poststreptococcal, Lyme) can present with similar manifestations as ERA patients. More benign entities such as toxic synovitis and benign limb pains of childhood (growing pains), as well as more concerning entities such as malignancies and solid tumors, should be considered. Orthopedic diagnoses such as Legg-Calvé-Perthes disease, slipped capital femoral epiphyses disease, and Osgood-Schlatter disease and less common rheumatologic diseases such as SAPHO (synovitis, acne, pustulosis, hyperostosis, and osteomyelitis), Kawasaki's syndrome, and vasculitis can share similar articular and extra-articular manifestations with ERA. Lastly, children with widespread amplified musculoskeletal pain may have tender entheses that can be mistaken for enthesitis.

Treatment

Treatment of ERA ranges from NSAIDs to DMARDs with the use of biologics in the most aggressive cases. To date there have been few randomized controlled trials in this population. One study of sulfasalazine showed no significant effects in juvenile spondyloarthropathy, whereas another showed good response in oligoarticular- and polyarticular-onset JIA patients.[115,116] Most respond well to intra-articular corticosteroid injections, but many may need a DMARD. For severe symptoms or evidence of potential joint damage

(such as erosive sacroiliitis), the use of TNF inhibitors has been effective on the basis of small pediatric studies.[117,118]

Outcome

Long-term outcome of ERA is unknown, but a proportion of these children may progress to the adult form of AS. Predictors of sacroiliitis were HLA-B27 positivity, absence of DPB1*02, hip joint involvement within the first 6 months, and disease onset after age 8 years.[119] When compared with adult-onset ankylosing spondylitis, juvenile-onset ankylosing spondylitis had less severe axial involvement but worse hip involvement, and in some studies, worse functional impairment.[120,121] The probability of remission remains low with remission rates reported ranging from 17% to 44%. Predictors for failure to achieve remission include family history of AS in first-degree relative, female sex, younger age at disease onset, arthritis in ankle joint within 6 months of disease onset, and HLA-DRB1*08.[122] Minden and colleagues[50] showed that if ERA persisted for more than 5 years, the chance of remission was only 17%.

SYSTEMIC JUVENILE IDIOPATHIC ARTHRITIS

Clinical Manifestations and Diagnostic Features

sJIA, which makes up 10% of all JIA, has unique characteristics that include fever, specific rash, and significantly elevated inflammatory markers in addition to arthritis. Recent research has identified biologic differences between sJIA and the other subcategories including prominent involvement of components of the innate immune system (in particular, inflammatory cytokines IL-1, IL-6, IL-18, neutrophils, and monocytes/macrophages), suggesting that sJIA may be in the autoinflammatory disease spectrum.[123]

sJIA occurs at any age with a tendency toward younger than 5 years peaking around 2 years of age.[124,125] Rarely it occurs in adults and is called adult-onset Still's disease. The gender predilection has stayed neutral, and some studies have suggested that sJIA may be relatively more frequent in Asian countries.[125] The systemic features of this disease are striking and are always present at onset, often predominating the clinical presentation. The arthritis may not be clinically present at onset, although arthralgias and myalgias are almost universally present at onset.[98] The fever is typically spiking in character with a peak of at least 39° C daily, occurring once or twice a day. Interestingly, the temperatures can become subnormal between fevers. The child is usually unwell and irritable during the fever but often recovers in between. In 80% of patients, the fevers are accompanied by an evanescent, migratory, salmon pink, and sometimes urticarial macular rash (Figure 107-5).[124] The rash typically spares the face and can occur without specific pattern on any part of the trunk or extremities. It can be subtle and scattered or diffuse and almost confluent. A helpful diagnostic feature is that the rash can be elicited by the Koebner phenomenon in which rubbing or scratching the skin elicits the rash.

Other systemic features include lymphadenopathy, hepatosplenomegaly, serositis (pleural/pericardial involvement/

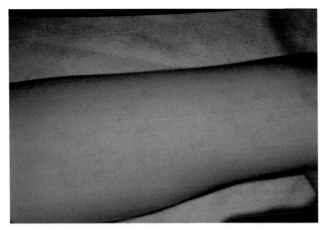

Figure 107-5 Typical rash of systemic juvenile idiopathic arthritis, with small 1- to 5-mm flat or slightly raised salmon pink macules.

abdominal pain), headaches, and sore throat. sJIA has the most common and severe cardiac presentations of all the subtypes of JIA. Pericarditis and pericardial effusions are the most common organ system manifestations, occurring in up to 10% of the presentations.[124] A serious life-threatening systemic manifestation called *macrophage activation syndrome* (MAS) is discussed in more detail later. The arthritis in sJIA can be varied from minimal to oligoarticular to polyarticular presentation[124] and typically does not correlate with the severity of the systemic manifestations.[126] Tenosynvositis and synovial cyst formation can also be seen. Although the systemic manifestations can be serious initially, the long-term morbidity is due to articular disease and adverse effects of medications, especially chronic corticosteroids.

There are no diagnostic tests for sJIA, but there are characteristic patterns of laboratory abnormalities including high inflammatory markers (CRP, ESR), significant leukocytosis with neutrophilia and bandemia, thrombocytosis, and anemia. Liver transaminases, aldolase, ferritin, fibrin split products, and coagulation screen may be abnormal in severe cases and can be signs of early or impending macrophage activation syndrome (MAS). ANA or other autoantibodies are rarely present. Inflammatory cytokine gene expression profiles have been shown to distinguish sJIA from other febrile inflammatory diseases seen in children and may lead to more specific tests in the future.[127]

Differential Diagnosis

Due to the nonspecific nature of the characteristics of sJIA, the diagnosis can be difficult and should be approached as a diagnosis of exclusion. Infections, Kawasaki's syndrome, malignancy, and other autoimmune diseases can present with similar symptoms; therefore it is necessary to screen for infectious agents and neoplasia, especially leukemia and neuroblastoma with appropriate tests including cultures, bone marrow aspiration and biopsy, and urinary vanillylmandelic acids. Some physicians do these tests routinely because malignancies are often close mimics to the early stages of sJIA. The recurrent fever syndromes are often mistaken for sJIA, but the character of the fevers and the fixed rashes associated with these syndromes should alert

the clinician to a different diagnosis. Other childhood rheumatic diseases should be considered such as systemic lupus erythematosus, Behçet's syndrome, and others.

Special Considerations: Macrophage Activation Syndrome

About 10% of the sJIA patients will develop overt life-threatening MAS, and up to 30% will develop a milder form, which if inadequately treated could lead to full-blown MAS.[128-130] MAS is a form of secondary or acquired hemophagocytic lymphohistiocytosis (HLH) seen within rheumatic disease. Two-thirds of the mortality seen in all patients with JIA are due to this entity.[131] The main manifestations include unrelenting high fevers, hepatosplenomegaly, lymphadenopathy, severe cytopenias, liver dysfunction, central nervous system (CNS) involvement (seizures/coma), and coagulopathy (Table 107-4). The ferritin often exceeds 10,000 ng/mL, and coagulopathy can be impressive with elevated prothrombin and partial thrombin times, hypofibrinogenemia, petechiae, mucosal bleeding, epistaxis,

Table 107-4 Preliminary Diagnostic Guidelines for Macrophage Activation Syndrome (MAS) Complicating Systemic Juvenile Idiopathic Arthritis (sJIA)[179]

Laboratory Criteria
Decreased platelet count ($\leq$262 × 10⁹/L)
Elevated levels of aspartate aminotransferase (>59 U/L)
Decreased white blood cell count ($\leq$4 × 10⁹/L)
Hypofibrinogenemia ($\leq$2.5 g/L)

Clinical Criteria
Central nervous system dysfunction (irritability, disorientation, lethargy, headache, seizures, coma)
Hemorrhages (purpura, easy bruising, mucosal bleeding)
Hepatomegaly ($\geq$3 cm below the costal arch)

Histopathologic Criterion
Evidence of macrophage hemophagocytosis in the bone marrow aspirate

Diagnostic Rule
The diagnosis of MAS requires the presence of any 2 or more laboratory criteria or of any 2 or 3 or more clinical and/or laboratory criteria. A bone marrow aspirate for the demonstration of hemophagocytosis may be required only in doubtful cases.

Recommendations
The aforementioned criteria are of value only in patients with active sJIA. The thresholds of laboratory criteria are provided by way of example only.

Comments
The clinical criteria are probably more useful as classification criteria rather than as diagnostic criteria because they often occur late in the course of MAS and therefore may be of limited value for the early suspicion of the syndrome.
Other abnormal clinical features in sJIA-associated MAS, not aforementioned, may include nonremitting high fever, splenomegaly, generalized lymphadenopathy, and paradoxical improvement of signs and symptoms of arthritis.
Other abnormal laboratory findings in sJIA-associated MAS, not aforementioned, may include anemia, erythrocyte sedimentation rate fall, elevated levels of alanine aminotransferase, increased bilirubin, presence of fibrin degradation products, elevated lactate dehydrogenase, hypertriglyceridemia, low sodium levels, decreased albumin, and hyperferritinemia.

and hematemesis. Often MAS is heralded by a decrease of the ESR, leukocyte and platelet counts, and liver dysfunction.[132] Histologically, patients with MAS show expansion of well-differentiated macrophages exhibiting hemophagocytosis in the bone marrow, lymph nodes, and other organs such as the liver and lungs. There is no gender, age, or race predilection for MAS in sJIA.[132] It often occurs during active systemic disease but has also been seen in the quiescence phase of the disease (no clinical symptoms but still on medications).[133] Triggers for MAS in sJIA include bacterial, fungal, and parasitic infections. Epstein-Barr virus, varicella, coxsackie, parvovirus B19, hepatitis A, *Salmonella*, and *Pneumocystis* infections have been implicated. Drugs have also been implicated including aspirin, NSAIDs, sulfasalazine, MTX, etanercept, anakinra, and gold salts. One must be cautious to quickly lay blame because many patients who are receiving these medications have active disease and may have been developing MAS despite the medications.[132,134] Most of the time, the trigger is unknown. Poor natural killer cell cytolytic activity leading to low levels of perforin expression has been reported in sJIA, a unique finding compared with the other subtypes of JIA.[128,132,135] Soluble IL-2Rα receptors and soluble CD163 are increased severalfold in MAS.[128,136]

Treatment

sJIA is an active area of research with increasing understanding of the autoinflammatory biology and the potential therapeutic roles for targeted biologics. Therapies such as MTX and TNF inhibition are less helpful in sJIA compared with other forms of JIA.[45,125,137,138] An approach to treating sJIA is shown in Figure 107-6, separating this complex disease into different severities and manifestations. This algorithm is consistent with the recently published ACR guidelines for JIA.[9] Mild sJIA, defined as mild systemic symptoms without organ system involvement and synovitis, can be successfully treated with anti-inflammatory doses of NSAIDs. Certain NSAIDs are helpful for different aspects of the disease (e.g., indomethacin can be used for fever control and serositis symptoms). In addition, if there are only a few large joints involved, intra-articular steroid injections are an additional option.

In the more severe cases with persistent fevers, cardiopulmonary symptoms, significant anemia, and significantly elevated inflammatory markers, corticosteroids may be used, often given as pulsed intravenous high-dose methylprednisolone (30 mg/kg/dose) daily for 3 days in a row followed by tapering doses of oral prednisolone.[139] Increasingly, as shown in Figure 107-6, IL-1 or IL-6 inhibition is instituted to avoid steroid toxicity and in some recent studies is being used as initial therapy before corticosteroids.[140] Use of DMARDs and TNF inhibitors may be more helpful for more significant articular disease. TNF inhibition has been shown to be effective in some patients with sJIA, though to a lesser extent than in other types of JIA.[137] Similarly, MTX may be helpful in sJIA with prominence of articular symptoms over systemic features.[9] Cyclosporine as

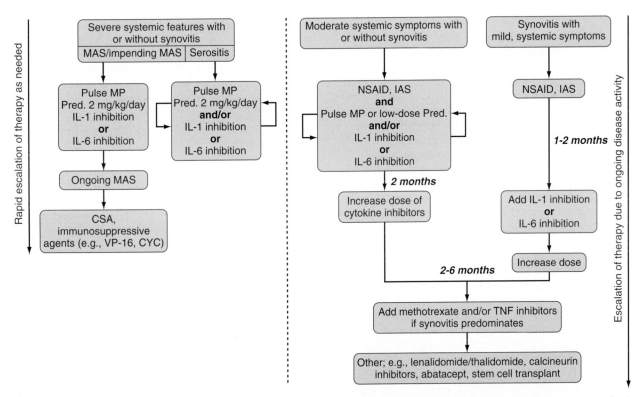

Figure 107-6 Systemic juvenile idiopathic arthritis treatment algorithm. The treatment goal is remission of disease activity, both systemic and articular, and is stratified by severity of disease. Algorithm is divided into severe systemic disease manifestations (macrophage activation syndrome [MAS], serositis) or synovitis with milder systemic disease. Currently there is significant variability in practice regarding using corticosteroid as initial systemic therapy or moving directly to inflammatory cytokine inhibitors. At the time of this writing, interleukin (IL)-1 inhibition and IL-6 inhibition are currently in trials, and more information is likely to be available in the future. CSA, cyclosporine A; CYC, cyclophosphamide; IAS, intra-articular steroid; MP, methylprednisolone; NSAID, nonsteroidal anti-inflammatory drug; Pred., prednisone; TNF, tumor necrosis factor.

well as monthly intravenous immunoglobulin have shown some benefit in systemic symptoms and can be used for steroid-sparing effects.[140,141] Unfortunately, effectiveness of these DMARDS is much less than in other subtypes of JIA with cyclosporine less than MTX.

The newer biologics that block IL-6 and IL-1 signaling are promising according to the recent elucidations in the pathophysiology of sJIA, as well as recent clinical trials and studies. Initial reports on IL-1 blockade using anakinra showed rapid and sustained remission within a few days in sJIA patients with chronic disease activity resistant to conventional therapy.[142] However, more recently reports have called into question the sustainability of the response using these medications.[140,143,144] Newer IL-1 inhibitors such as rilonacept (currently being studied in a clinical trial, NCT00534495) and anti-IL-1β monoclonal antibody (canakinumab) may shed more light on the effectiveness of these therapies and the biology of the responses. Two phase III placebo-controlled, double-blind trials using the IL-6 receptor antagonist tocilizumab showed significant improvement of ACR Pedi 30, 50, and 70 responses.[145,146] In the TENDER trial, the tocilizumab dose for patients less than 30 kg was 12 mg/kg/dose and for greater than 30 kg was 8 mg/kg/dose every 2 weeks.[145]

Thalidomide has also been reported to improve symptoms in refractory sJIA patients.[147] The teratogenic potential of thalidomide and its newer analogue lenalidomide limits the usefulness of these medications.[148]

Abatacept has been used in sJIA patients who have failed previous treatments. In the open-label portion of a double-blind placebo-controlled trial of abatacept therapy in JIA patients, 24 of 37 (65%) of sJIA patients had an ACR Pedi 30 response. This was comparable with the other JIA subtypes evaluated in that study.[38]

The 2010 ACR guidelines for JIA treatment divided sJIA treatment into two groups: active systemic features and active arthritis. But the guidelines did not include patients with MAS, impending MAS, or life-threatening manifestations (e.g., cardiac tamponade).[9] The algorithm shown in Figure 107-6 incorporates some of the principles from the guidelines, expanding the area's severe systemic disease and MAS. One difference is that the guideline supports earlier use of methotrexate and TNF inhibition in patients with active sJIA with primarily articular manifestations.

The optimal treatment for MAS continues to be controversial. Therapy should be aggressive and usually starts with high-dose steroids and disease-modifying agents such as cyclosporine and IL-1 blockade.[149,150] Almost 50% of patients in one study showed response to steroids alone.[134] A consensus treatment protocol for HLH has been published and uses a combination of VP-16 (etoposide), dexamethasone, with or without intrathecal methotrexate, followed by a maintenance with cyclosporine A.[151] This protocol or parts of it have been used with MAS in sJIA patients with success.[152] However, the new use of the powerful IL-1 and IL-6 inhibitors may preclude the need for the HLH approach with its potential serious bone marrow suppression.[151]

For the severe refractory cases, stem cell transplantation has been done. A recent review of the experience showed favorable response with more than 50% sustained drug-free remission. Early experience demonstrated cases of induction of MAS during transplant conditioning and immediately post-transplant. This early morbidity has improved with less intense conditioning regimen.[153] A follow-up study reported that late relapses were noted with lower percentages for drug-free long-term outcome. The late relapses were often less severe and treated successfully with conventional drugs.[154-156]

Outcome

sJIA is heterogeneous in severity, disease course, and outcome. Studies of the natural history of sJIA before biologic therapies demonstrate that the course can be monocyclic, with remission within 2 to 4 years; relapsing, characterized by flares of systemic features with mild arthritis; or continuous with persistent destructive arthritis, often more prominent after the regression of systemic features.[125,157] Patients with severe disease can have flares of extra-articular features at any time and may have active arthritis into adult life despite standard therapies.[157] Emerging evidence suggests that IL-1 and IL-6 inhibitors have permitted significant disease control with no or much lower doses of corticosteroids, which were one of the major causes of morbidity in sJIA in the past.

Predictors of poor articular outcome in sJIA include the systemic features 6 months after onset, thrombocytosis, and the presence of polyarthritis with hip involvement.[126,158,159] The mortality rate for sJIA is still perceived to be higher than the mortality rate associated with other subtypes of JIA in clinical practice now, although no formal figures are available. As a result of the inadequate control of the disease with the available therapies, growth failure and osteoporosis are serious and lasting complications. The use of growth hormone (GH) is now more accepted with recent reviews outlining the safety of its use in sJIA. Growth hormone therapy can improve linear growth even during active phase of the disease, resulting in an ultimate higher final height.[160]

Amyloidosis was previously a major cause of death in sJIA but is now less common, most likely due to the use of more aggressive therapy to better control inflammation. Recently MEFV mutations seen in familial Mediterranean fever have been identified in sJIA patients, and these patients were noted to have the most resistant disease.[161] Pulmonary hypertension has also been reported in a few case reports and one case series.[162]

IMAGING

Imaging is important in JIA to confirm the diagnosis; to exclude other diseases such as infection, malignancy, osteoid osteoma, or avascular necrosis; and to monitor therapy. Determining the presence of cartilage loss and erosions are complicated by the anatomically changing joints during the normal growth process. Because children have a large amount of cartilage in their joints, a significant amount of destruction can occur before erosions are identified on plain radiographs (Figure 107-7). Local growth disturbances can also be seen in children including bony overgrowth, particularly in the small joints of the hands and feet and in the knees, likely due to chronic hyperemia. Bony hypertrophy around the knee joints can lead to leg-length discrepancies,

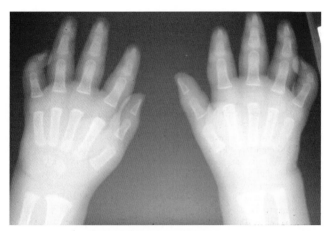

Figure 107-7   Plain radiograph of a young child with active polyarticular juvenile idiopathic arthritis, demonstrating the challenge in evaluating joint damage in the growing child. Periarticular osteoporosis and early periostitis of the metacarpals are noted.

permanent gait disturbances, and secondary scoliosis (see Figure 107-3). In contrast, premature fusion of the epiphyses can lead to shortening of certain joints, most notably the TMJs, leading to micrognathia.[163-165] Interestingly, the articular cartilage of growing children has been shown to have unique regenerative qualities and studies have shown that children with JIA can have improvement in their radiographic joint damage.[165]

Plain radiographs in patients with JIA show soft tissue swelling as an early but nonspecific finding. The most common form of radiographic damage in JIA is joint space narrowing due to erosion, thinning, and loss of articular cartilage.[163,165] Periarticular osteopenia due to hyperemia of inflamed joints is frequently seen. Erosions and ankylosis can be seen as late findings in radiographs.[163] Lastly, periostitis along the shafts of the phalanges, metacarpals, and metatarsals and calcifications from steroid joint injections can be seen. The trend toward early aggressive treatment to prevent erosive disease shifts the imaging need away from plain radiographs and toward other imaging modalities that are more sensitive in detecting early disease activity.[164] Therefore MRI and ultrasound (US) are becoming more popular.

US is reliable, safe, and relatively inexpensive but not as well standardized in children as in adults. It has been shown to be more sensitive than plain radiography in the detection of effusion, synovial thickening, and synovial cysts. In more experienced hands, cartilage thinning and bone erosions can also be seen. Inflammatory involvement of the hip, shoulder, and elbow is more frequently accurately detected by US compared with clinical examination.[166,167] Color and power Doppler US can facilitate the evaluation of hyperemia and vascular abnormalities in affected joints and tendon involvement.[168]

MRI is the most sensitive imaging modality currently available for detecting synovial inflammation; however, its use is limited by expense and the need for anesthesia in young children. With the use of contrast, accurate differentiation between active and inactive states can be established. Synovial enhancement and thickening can easily be seen,[169] and pannus volume measurements can be tracked.[170] MRI is the only technique available to visualize bone

marrow edema, which has been shown to be an important predictor of erosive joint damage in RA patients, but the connection is not established in JIA patients. For evaluating bony erosions, MRI was found to be the most sensitive imaging modality in wrists of JIA patients, revealing more than twice as many erosions compared with plain radiography and US.[171] Pilot MRI grading scores of hip and knee disease activity and damage in JIA have been proposed but not validated.[164] A recent systematic review of the literature assessed that the overall quality of the reporting of methods in studies on the MRI assessment of JIA is heterogeneous and fair overall.[172]

SPECIAL CONSIDERATIONS: REHABILITATION IN CHILDREN

PT and OT play a crucial role in JIA patients. PT and OT can consult for stretches, range-of-motion evaluation, joint protection, muscle building and strengthening, as well as endurance and graduated aerobic activity. Children who present late in the course of oligoarthritis may already have flexion contractures, which require splinting and serial casting. Serial casting is done two or three times a week for up to a month if necessary and is probably most effective when started just after joint injections. Some children with marked leg-length discrepancy (resulting from overgrowth of the affected knee) may require a shoe lift/raise. Strict limitations from physical education at school and sports are generally not encouraged because physical activity plays an important role in rehabilitation and therapy; however, impact sports should be limited in the presence of joint effusions or when there is a concern for joint instability (e.g., C1/C2 atlantoaxial subluxation). A modified physical education program and sports activities to the patients' own tolerance are recommended instead. Orthotics can be helpful in foot involvement in ERA, as well as other types of JIA.

Although there is a wide within-patient and between-patient variability, children with early-disease onset and a greater number of restricted joints have the highest risk of developing long-term functional physical disability.[173] In addition, health-related quality of life was significantly lower in patients with JIA than in healthy children, and patients with persistent oligoarthritis were less severely affected compared with the other JIA subcategories.[174] Total energy and activity-related energy expenditure, as well as physical activity levels, were significantly lower in JIA patients compared with controls, and only 23% of the JIA patients met the public health guidelines on physical activity compared with 66% in controls.[175]

SUMMARY

The modern treatment of JIA has significantly decreased the long-term burden of disease but requires early recognition and diagnosis. It also requires aggressive treatment to extinguish disease activity and multidisciplinary approaches to maintain and improve function and quality of life. Pediatric rheumatologists have in their favor the remarkable capacity for childhood growth and development to allow repair and restoration of function, in contrast to adults with inflammatory arthritis. The advent of new biologic therapies and rapid translation of basic research into therapeutic strategies and an increased willingness on the part of regulatory bodies to make new therapies available to children should combine to continue to improve the outlook for children with arthritis.

Selected References

1. Helmick CG, Felson DT, Lawrence RC, et al: Estimates of the prevalence of arthritis and other rheumatic conditions in the United States: part I, *Arthritis Rheum* 58(1):15–25, 2008.
2. Oen K, Duffy CM, Tse SML, et al: Early outcomes and improvement of patients with juvenile idiopathic arthritis enrolled in a Canadian multicenter inception cohort, *Arthritis Care Res (Hoboken)* 62(4):527–536, 2010.
3. Hyrich KL, Lal SD, Foster HE, et al: Disease activity and disability in children with juvenile idiopathic arthritis one year following presentation to paediatric rheumatology. Results from the Childhood Arthritis Prospective Study, *Rheumatology (Oxford)* 49(1):116–122, 2010.
4. Petty RE, Southwood TR, Manners P, et al: International League of Associations for Rheumatology classification of juvenile idiopathic arthritis: second revision, Edmonton, 2001, *J Rheumatol* 31(2):390–392, 2004.
5. Barnes MG, Grom AA, Thompson SD, et al: Biologic similarities based on age at onset in oligoarticular and polyarticular subtypes of juvenile idiopathic arthritis, *Arthritis Rheum* 62(11):3249–3258, 2010.
6. Ravelli A, Felici E, Magni-Manzoni S, et al: Patients with antinuclear antibody-positive juvenile idiopathic arthritis constitute a homogeneous subgroup irrespective of the course of joint disease, *Arthritis Rheum* 52(3):826–832, 2005.
8. Jones OY, Spencer CH, Bowyer SL, et al: A multicenter case-control study on predictive factors distinguishing childhood leukemia from juvenile rheumatoid arthritis, *Pediatrics* 117(5):e840–844, 2006.
9. Beukelman T, Patkar N, Saag K, et al: 2010 American College of Rheumatology recommendations for the treatment of juvenile idiopathic arthritis: initiation and safety monitoring of therapeutic agents for the treatment of arthritis and systemic features, *Arthritis Care Res* 62:1515–1526, 2010.
10. Macaubas C, Nguyen K, Milojevic D, et al: Oligoarticular and polyarticular JIA: epidemiology and pathogenesis, *Nat Rev Rheumatol* 5(11):616–626, 2009.
12. Albers HM, Brinkman DMC, Kamphuis SSM, et al: Clinical course and prognostic value of disease activity in the first two years in different subtypes of juvenile idiopathic arthritis, *Arthritis Care Res (Hoboken)* 62(2):204–212, 2010.
13. Bartoli M, Tarò M, Magni-Manzoni S, et al: The magnitude of early response to methotrexate therapy predicts long-term outcome of patients with juvenile idiopathic arthritis, *Ann Rheum Dis* 67(3):370–374, 2008.
14. Lovell D, Giannini E, Reiff A, et al: Etanercept in children with polyarticular juvenile rheumatoid arthritis, *N Engl J Med* 342(11):763–769, 2000.
15. Ruperto N, Murray KJ, Gerloni V, et al: A randomized trial of parenteral methotrexate comparing an intermediate dose with a higher dose in children with juvenile idiopathic arthritis who failed to respond to standard doses of methotrexate, *Arthritis Rheum* 50(7):2191–2201, 2004.
25. Albers HM, Wessels JAM, van der Straaten RJHM, et al: Time to treatment as an important factor for the response to methotrexate in juvenile idiopathic arthritis, *Arthritis Rheum* 61(1):46–51, 2009.
27. Horneff G, De Bock F, Foeldvari I, et al: Safety and efficacy of combination of etanercept and methotrexate compared to treatment with etanercept only in patients with juvenile idiopathic arthritis (JIA): preliminary data from the German JIA Registry, *Ann Rheum Dis* 68(4):519–525, 2009.
28. Lovell DJ, Giannini EH, Reiff A, et al: Long-term efficacy and safety of etanercept in children with polyarticular-course juvenile rheumatoid arthritis: interim results from an ongoing multicenter, open-label, extended-treatment trial, *Arthritis Rheum* 48(1):218–226, 2003.
29. Lovell DJ, Reiff A, Jones OY, et al: Long-term safety and efficacy of etanercept in children with polyarticular-course juvenile rheumatoid arthritis, *Arthritis Rheum* 54(6):1987–1994, 2006.
30. Lovell DJ, Reiff A, Ilowite NT, et al: Safety and efficacy of up to eight years of continuous etanercept therapy in patients with juvenile rheumatoid arthritis, *Arthritis Rheum* 58(5):1496–1504, 2008.
31. Southwood TR, Foster HE, Davidson JE, et al: Duration of etanercept treatment and reasons for discontinuation in a cohort of juvenile idiopathic arthritis patients, *Rheumatology (Oxford)* 50:189–195, 2011.
32. Giannini EH, Ilowite NT, Lovell DJ, et al: Long-term safety and effectiveness of etanercept in children with selected categories of juvenile idiopathic arthritis, *Arthritis Rheum* 60(9):2794–2804, 2009.
33. Vojvodich PF, Hansen JB, Andersson U, et al: Etanercept treatment improves longitudinal growth in prepubertal children with juvenile idiopathic arthritis, *J Rheumatol* 34(12):2481–2485, 2007.
34. Ruperto N, Lovell DJ, Cuttica R, et al: A randomized, placebo-controlled trial of infliximab plus methotrexate for the treatment of polyarticular-course juvenile rheumatoid arthritis, *Arthritis Rheum* 56(9):3096–3106, 2007.
35. Ruperto N, Lovell DJ, Cuttica R, et al: Long-term efficacy and safety of infliximab plus methotrexate for the treatment of polyarticular-course juvenile rheumatoid arthritis: findings from an open-label treatment extension, *Ann Rheum Dis* 69(4):718–722, 2010.
36. Lovell D, Ruperto N, Goodman S, et al: Adalimumab with or without methotrexate in juvenile rheumatoid arthritis, *N Engl J Med* 359(8):810–820, 2008.
38. Ruperto N, Lovell DJ, Quartier P, et al: Abatacept in children with juvenile idiopathic arthritis: a randomised, double-blind, placebo-controlled withdrawal trial, *Lancet* 372(9636):383–391, 2008.
39. Ruperto N, Lovell DJ, Quartier P, et al: Long-term safety and efficacy of abatacept in children with juvenile idiopathic arthritis, *Arthritis Rheum* 62(6):1792–1802, 2010.
41. Ravelli A, Martini A: Juvenile idiopathic arthritis, *Lancet* 369(9563):767–778, 2007.
42. Ringold S, Seidel KD, Koepsell TD, Wallace CA: Inactive disease in polyarticular juvenile idiopathic arthritis: current patterns and associations, *Rheumatology (Oxford)* 48(8):972–977, 2009.
43. Wallace CA, Huang B, Bandeira M, et al: Patterns of clinical remission in select categories of juvenile idiopathic arthritis, *Arthritis Rheum* 52(11):3554–3562, 2005.
45. Martini A, Lovell DJ: Juvenile idiopathic arthritis: state of the art and future perspectives, *Ann Rheum Dis* 69(7):1260–1263, 2010.
47. Bowyer S, Roettcher P: Pediatric rheumatology clinic populations in the United States: results of a 3 year survey. Pediatric Rheumatology Database Research Group, *J Rheumatol* 23(11):1968–1974, 1996.
50. Minden K, Kiessling U, Listing J, et al: Prognosis of patients with juvenile chronic arthritis and juvenile spondyloarthropathy, *J Rheumatol* 27(9):2256–2263, 2000.
51. Guillaume S, Prieur A, Coste J, Job-Deslandre C: Long-term outcome and prognosis in oligoarticular-onset juvenile idiopathic arthritis, *Arthritis Rheum* 43(8):1858–1865, 2000.
52. Al-Matar MJ, Petty RE, Tucker LB, et al: The early pattern of joint involvement predicts disease progression in children with oligoarticular (pauciarticular) juvenile rheumatoid arthritis, *Arthritis Rheum* 46(10):2708–2715, 2002.
54. Huemer C, Malleson PN, Cabral DA, et al: Patterns of joint involvement at onset differentiate oligoarticular juvenile psoriatic arthritis from pauciarticular juvenile rheumatoid arthritis, *J Rheumatol* 29(7):1531–1535, 2002.
57. Woo P, Southwood TR, Prieur AM, et al: Randomized, placebo-controlled, crossover trial of low-dose oral methotrexate in children with extended oligoarticular or systemic arthritis, *Arthritis Rheum* 43(8):1849–1857, 2000.
58. Ravelli A, Viola S, Migliavacca D, et al: The extended oligoarticular subtype is the best predictor of methotrexate efficacy in juvenile idiopathic arthritis, *J Pediatr* 135(3):316–320, 1999.
60. Packham JC, Hall MA: Long-term follow-up of 246 adults with juvenile idiopathic arthritis: functional outcome, *Rheumatology (Oxford)* 41(12):1428–1435, 2002.
61. Oen K, Malleson PN, Cabral DA, et al: Disease course and outcome of juvenile rheumatoid arthritis in a multicenter cohort, *J Rheumatol* 29(9):1989–1999, 2002.

62. Oen K, Reed M, Malleson PN, et al: Radiologic outcome and its relationship to functional disability in juvenile rheumatoid arthritis, *J Rheumatol* 30(4):832–840, 2003.

63. Wright T, Cron RQ: Pediatric rheumatology for the adult rheumatologist, II: uveitis in juvenile idiopathic arthritis, *J Clin Rheumatol* 13(4):205–210, 2007.

64. Saurenmann RK, Levin AV, Feldman BM, et al: Risk factors for development of uveitis differ between girls and boys with juvenile idiopathic arthritis, *Arthritis Rheum* 62(6):1824–1828, 2010.

65. Heiligenhaus A, Niewerth M, Ganser G, et al; German Uveitis in Childhood Study Group: Prevalence and complications of uveitis in juvenile idiopathic arthritis in a population-based nation-wide study in Germany: suggested modification of the current screening guidelines, *Rheumatology (Oxford)* 46(6):1015–1019, 2007.

66. Davies K, Cleary G, Foster H, et al: BSPAR Standards of Care for children and young people with juvenile idiopathic arthritis, *Rheumatology* 49(7):1406–1408, 2010.

67. Cassidy J, Kivlin J, Lindsley C, Nocton J, the Section on Rheumatology, and the Section on Ophthalmology: Ophthalmologic examinations in children with juvenile rheumatoid arthritis, *Pediatrics* 117(5):1843–1845, 2006.

78. Biester S, Deuter C, Michels H, et al: Adalimumab in the therapy of uveitis in childhood, *Br J Ophthalmol* 91(3):319–324, 2007.

82. Zulian F, Balzarin M, Falcini F, et al: Abatacept for severe anti-tumor necrosis factor alpha refractory juvenile idiopathic arthritis-related uveitis, *Arthritis Care Res (Hoboken)* 62(6):821–825, 2010.

87. Saurenmann RK, Levin AV, Feldman BM, et al: Prevalence, risk factors, and outcome of uveitis in juvenile idiopathic arthritis: a long-term followup study, *Arthritis Rheum* 56(2):647–657, 2007.

88. Sabri K, Saurenmann RK, Silverman ED, Levin AV: Course, complications, and outcome of juvenile arthritis-related uveitis, *J AAPOS* 12(6):539–545, 2008.

89. Chia A, Lee V, Graham EM, Edelsten C: Factors related to severe uveitis at diagnosis in children with juvenile idiopathic arthritis in a screening program, *Am J Ophthalmol* 135(6):757–762, 2003.

90. Zulian F, Martini G, Falcini F, et al: Early predictors of severe course of uveitis in oligoarticular juvenile idiopathic arthritis, *J Rheumatol* 29(11):2446–2453, 2002.

91. Edelsten C, Lee V, Bentley CR, et al: An evaluation of baseline risk factors predicting severity in juvenile idiopathic arthritis associated uveitis and other chronic anterior uveitis in early childhood, *Br J Ophthalmol* 86(1):51–56, 2002.

92. Holland GN, Denove CS, Yu F: Chronic anterior uveitis in children: clinical characteristics and complications, *Am J Ophthalmol* 147(4):667–678.e5, 2009.

93. Ayuso VK, Ten Cate HAT, van der Does P, et al: Male gender and poor visual outcome in uveitis associated with juvenile idiopathic arthritis, *Am J Ophthalmol* 149(6):987–993, 2010.

94. Stoll ML, Zurakowski D, Nigrovic LE, et al: Patients with juvenile psoriatic arthritis comprise two distinct populations, *Arthritis Rheum* 54(11):3564–3572, 2006.

95. Flatø B, Lien G, Smerdel-Ramoya A, Vinje O: Juvenile psoriatic arthritis: longterm outcome and differentiation from other subtypes of juvenile idiopathic arthritis, *J Rheumatol* 36(3):642–650, 2009.

98. Cassidy CJ, Petty RE, Laxer RM, Lindsley C: *Textbook of pediatric rheumatology*, ed 5, Philadelphia, 2005, Elsevier Saunders.

99. Lewkowicz D, Gottlieb AB: Pediatric psoriasis and psoriatic arthritis, *Dermatol Ther* 17(5):364–375, 2004.

101. Southwood TR, Petty RE, Malleson PN, et al: Psoriatic arthritis in children, *Arthritis Rheum* 32(8):1007–1013, 1989.

102. Butbul YA, Tyrrell PN, Schneider R, et al: Comparison of patients with juvenile psoriatic arthritis and nonpsoriatic juvenile idiopathic arthritis: how different are they? *J Rheumatol* 36(9):2033–2041, 2009.

106. Hofer M: Spondylarthropathies in children—are they different from those in adults? *Best Pract Res Clin Rheumatol* 20(2):315–328, 2006.

107. Burgos-Vargas R, Pacheco-Tena C, Vázquez-Mellado J: Juvenile-onset spondyloarthropathies, *Rheum Dis Clin North Am* 23(3):569–598, 1997.

108. Burgos-Vargas R, Vázquez-Mellado J, Cassis N, et al: Genuine ankylosing spondylitis in children: a case-control study of patients with early definite disease according to adult onset criteria, *J Rheumatol* 23(12):2140–2147, 1996.

109. Burgos-Vargas R, Lardizabal-Sanabria J, Katona G: Anterior spinal flexion in healthy Mexican children, *J Rheumatol* 12(1):123–125, 1985.

111. Kotaniemi K, Arkela-Kautiainen M, Haapasaari J, Leirisalo-Repo M: Uveitis in young adults with juvenile idiopathic arthritis: a clinical evaluation of 123 patients, *Ann Rheum Dis* 64(6):871–874, 2005.

112. Huppertz H, Voigt I, Müller-Scholden J, Sandhage K: Cardiac manifestations in patients with HLA B27-associated juvenile arthritis, *Pediatr Cardiol* 21(2):141–147, 2000.

113. Azouz EM, Duffy CM: Juvenile spondyloarthropathies: clinical manifestations and medical imaging, *Skeletal Radiol* 24(6):399–408, 1995.

115. Burgos-Vargas R, Vázquez-Mellado J, Pacheco-Tena C, et al: A 26 week randomised, double blind, placebo controlled exploratory study of sulfasalazine in juvenile onset spondyloarthropathies, *Ann Rheum Dis* 61(10):941–942, 2002.

116. van Rossum MA, Fiselier TJ, Franssen MJ, et al: Sulfasalazine in the treatment of juvenile chronic arthritis: a randomized, double-blind, placebo-controlled, multicenter study. Dutch Juvenile Chronic Arthritis Study Group, *Arthritis Rheum* 41(5):808–816, 1998.

117. Henrickson M, Reiff A: Prolonged efficacy of etanercept in refractory enthesitis-related arthritis, *J Rheumatol* 31(10):2055–2061, 2004.

118. Tse SML, Burgos-Vargas R, Laxer RM: Anti-tumor necrosis factor alpha blockade in the treatment of juvenile spondylarthropathy, *Arthritis Rheum* 52(7):2103–2108, 2005.

119. Flatø B, Smerdel A, Johnston V, et al: The influence of patient characteristics, disease variables, and HLA alleles on the development of radiographically evident sacroiliitis in juvenile idiopathic arthritis, *Arthritis Rheum* 46(4):986–994, 2002.

121. Gensler LS, Ward MM, Reveille JD, et al: Clinical, radiographic and functional differences between juvenile-onset and adult-onset ankylosing spondylitis: results from the PSOAS cohort, *Ann Rheum Dis* 67(2):233–237, 2008.

122. Flatø B, Hoffmann-Vold A, Reiff A, et al: Long-term outcome and prognostic factors in enthesitis-related arthritis: a case-control study, *Arthritis Rheum* 54(11):3573–3582, 2006.

123. Thompson SD, Barnes MG, Griffin TA, et al: Heterogeneity in juvenile idiopathic arthritis: impact of molecular profiling based on DNA polymorphism and gene expression patterns, *Arthritis Rheum* 62(9):2611–2615, 2010.

124. Behrens EM, Beukelman T, Gallo L, et al: Evaluation of the presentation of systemic onset juvenile rheumatoid arthritis: data from the Pennsylvania Systemic Onset Juvenile Arthritis Registry (PASOJAR), *J Rheumatol* 35(2):343–348, 2008.

125. Woo P: Systemic juvenile idiopathic arthritis: diagnosis, management, and outcome, *Nat Clin Pract Rheumatol* 2(1):28–34, 2006.

126. Sandborg C, Holmes TH, Lee T, et al: Candidate early predictors for progression to joint damage in systemic juvenile idiopathic arthritis, *J Rheumatol* 33(11):2322–2329, 2006.

127. Allantaz F, Chaussabel D, Stichweh D, et al: Blood leukocyte microarrays to diagnose systemic onset juvenile idiopathic arthritis and follow the response to IL-1 blockade, *J Exp Med* 204(9):2131–2144, 2007.

128. Grom AA, Mellins ED: Macrophage activation syndrome: advances towards understanding pathogenesis, *Curr Opin Rheumatol* 22(5):561–566, 2010.

129. Sawhney S, Woo P, Murray KJ: Macrophage activation syndrome: a potentially fatal complication of rheumatic disorders, *Arch Dis Child* 85(5):421–426, 2001.

130. Behrens EM, Beukelman T, Paessler M, Cron RQ: Occult macrophage activation syndrome in patients with systemic juvenile idiopathic arthritis, *J Rheumatol* 34(5):1133–1138, 2007.

133. Behrens EM: Macrophage activation syndrome in rheumatic disease: what is the role of the antigen presenting cell? *Autoimmun Rev* 7(4):305–308, 2008.

134. Kelly A, Ramanan AV: Recognition and management of macrophage activation syndrome in juvenile arthritis, *Curr Opin Rheumatol* 19(5):477–481, 2007.

135. Wulffraat NM, Rijkers GT, Elst E, et al: Reduced perforin expression in systemic juvenile idiopathic arthritis is restored by autologous stem-cell transplantation, *Rheumatology (Oxford)* 42(2):375–379, 2003.

137. Kimura Y, Pinho P, Walco G, et al: Etanercept treatment in patients with refractory systemic onset juvenile rheumatoid arthritis, *J Rheumatol* 32(5):935–942, 2005.

138. Ruperto N, Ravelli A, Castell E, et al: Cyclosporine A in juvenile idiopathic arthritis. Results of the PRCSG/PRINTO phase IV post marketing surveillance study, *Clin Exp Rheumatol* 24(5):599–605, 2006.

139. Adebajo AO, Hall MA: The use of intravenous pulsed methylprednisolone in the treatment of systemic-onset juvenile chronic arthritis, *Br J Rheumatol* 37(11):1240–1242, 1998.

140. Nigrovic PA, Mannion M, Prince FHM, et al: Anakinra as first-line disease modifying therapy in systemic juvenile idiopathic arthritis, *Arthritis Rheum* 63:545–555, 2011.

142. Pascual V, Allantaz F, Arce E, et al: Role of interleukin-1 (IL-1) in the pathogenesis of systemic onset juvenile idiopathic arthritis and clinical response to IL-1 blockade, *J Exp Med* 201(9):1479–1486, 2005.

143. Lequerré T, Quartier P, Rosellini D, et al: Interleukin-1 receptor antagonist (anakinra) treatment in patients with systemic-onset juvenile idiopathic arthritis or adult onset Still disease: preliminary experience in France, *Ann Rheum Dis* 67(3):302–308, 2008.

144. Woo P: Anakinra treatment for systemic juvenile idiopathic arthritis and adult onset Still disease, *Ann Rheum Dis* 67(3):281–282, 2008.

145. Benedetti F, Brunner HI, Ruperto N, et al: Tocilizumab in patients with systemic juvenile idiopathic arthritis: efficacy data from the placebo-controlled 12 week part of the phase 3 TENDER trial, *Arthritis Rheum* 62(Suppl 10):1434, 2010.

146. Yokota S, Imagawa T, Mori M, et al: Efficacy and safety of tocilizumab in patients with systemic-onset juvenile idiopathic arthritis: a randomised, double-blind, placebo-controlled, withdrawal phase III trial, *Lancet* 371(9617):998–1006, 2008.

147. Lehman TJA, Schechter SJ, Sundel RP, et al: Thalidomide for severe systemic onset juvenile rheumatoid arthritis: a multicenter study, *J Pediatr* 145(6):856–857, 2004.

148. Hayward K, Wallace CA: Recent developments in anti-rheumatic drugs in pediatrics: treatment of juvenile idiopathic arthritis, *Arthritis Res Ther* 11(1):216, 2009.

149. Vastert SJ, Kuis W, Grom AA: Systemic JIA: new developments in the understanding of the pathophysiology and therapy, *Best Pract Res Clin Rheumatol* 23(5):655–664, 2009.

150. Miettunen P, Narendran A, Jayanthan A, et al: Successful treatment of severe paediatric rheumatic disease-associated macrophage activation syndrome with interleukin-1 inhibition following conventional immunosuppressive therapy: case series with 12 patients, *Rheumatology (Oxford)* 50:417–419, 2011.

151. Henter J, Samuelsson-Horne A, Aricò M, et al: Treatment of hemophagocytic lymphohistiocytosis with HLH-94 immunochemotherapy and bone marrow transplantation, *Blood* 100(7):2367–2373, 2002.

152. Filipovich A: Hemophagocytic lymphohistiocytosis and related disorders, *Curr Opin Allergy Clin Immunol* 6:410–415, 2006.

156. Wulffraat NM, van Rooijen EM, Tewarie R, et al: Current perspectives of autologous stem cell transplantation for severe juvenile idiopathic arthritis, *Autoimmunity* 41(8):632–638, 2008.

157. Lomater C, Gerloni V, Gattinara M, et al: Systemic onset juvenile idiopathic arthritis: a retrospective study of 80 consecutive patients followed for 10 years, *J Rheumatol* 27(2):491–496, 2000.

158. Singh-Grewal D, Schneider R, Bayer N, Feldman BM: Predictors of disease course and remission in systemic juvenile idiopathic arthritis: significance of early clinical and laboratory features, *Arthritis Rheum* 54(5):1595–1601, 2006.

159. Spiegel LR, Schneider R, Lang BA, et al: Early predictors of poor functional outcome in systemic-onset juvenile rheumatoid arthritis: a multicenter cohort study, *Arthritis Rheum* 43(11):2402–2409, 2000.

160. Simon D, Bechtold S: Effects of growth hormone treatment on growth in children with juvenile idiopathic arthritis, *Horm Res* 72(Suppl 1):55–59, 2009.

161. Ayaz NA, Ozen S, Bilginer Y, et al: MEFV mutations in systemic onset juvenile idiopathic arthritis, *Rheumatology (Oxford)* 48(1):23–25, 2009.

163. Azouz EM: Juvenile idiopathic arthritis: how can the radiologist help the clinician? *Pediatr Radiol* 38(Suppl 3):S403–S408, 2008.

164. Damasio MB, Malattia C, Martini A, Tomà P: Synovial and inflammatory diseases in childhood: role of new imaging modalities in the assessment of patients with juvenile idiopathic arthritis, *Pediatr Radiol* 40(6):985–998, 2010.

165. Ravelli A: The time has come to include assessment of radiographic progression in juvenile idiopathic arthritis clinical trials, *J Rheumatol* 35(4):553–557, 2008.

167. Magni-Manzoni S, Epis O, Ravelli A, et al: Comparison of clinical versus ultrasound-determined synovitis in juvenile idiopathic arthritis, *Arthritis Rheum* 61(11):1497–1504, 2009.

168. Rooney ME, McAllister C, Burns JFT: Ankle disease in juvenile idiopathic arthritis: ultrasound findings in clinically swollen ankles, *J Rheumatol* 36(8):1725–1729, 2009.

169. Graham TB, Laor T, Dardzinski BJ: Quantitative magnetic resonance imaging of the hands and wrists of children with juvenile rheumatoid arthritis, *J Rheumatol* 32(9):1811–1820, 2005.

170. Lamer S, Sebag GH: MRI and ultrasound in children with juvenile chronic arthritis, *Eur J Radiol* 33(2):85–93, 2000.

171. Malattia C, Damasio MB, Magnaguagno F, et al: Magnetic resonance imaging, ultrasonography, and conventional radiography in the assessment of bone erosions in juvenile idiopathic arthritis, *Arthritis Rheum* 59(12):1764–1772, 2008.

172. Miller E, Roposch A, Uleryk E, Doria AS: Juvenile idiopathic arthritis of peripheral joints: quality of reporting of diagnostic accuracy of conventional MRI, *Acad Radiol* 16(6):739–757, 2009.

173. Magni-Manzoni S, Pistorio A, Labò E, et al: A longitudinal analysis of physical functional disability over the course of juvenile idiopathic arthritis, *Ann Rheum Dis* 67(8):1159–1164, 2008.

174. Oliveira S, Ravelli A, Pistorio A, et al: Proxy-reported health-related quality of life of patients with juvenile idiopathic arthritis: the Pediatric Rheumatology International Trials Organization multinational quality of life cohort study, *Arthritis Rheum* 57(1):35–43, 2007.

176. Gartlehner G, Hansen RA, Jonas BL, et al: Biologics for the treatment of juvenile idiopathic arthritis: a systematic review and critical analysis of the evidence, *Clin Rheumatol* 27(1):67–76, 2008.

179. Ravelli A, Magni-Manzoni S, Pistorio A, et al: Preliminary diagnostic guidelines for macrophage activation syndrome complicating systemic juvenile idiopathic arthritis, *J Pediatr* 146(5):598–604, 2005.

Full references for this chapter can be found on www.expertconsult.com.

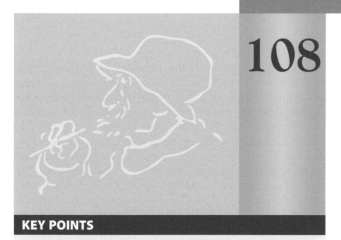

108

Pediatric Systemic Lupus Erythematosus, Dermatomyositis, Scleroderma, and Vasculitis

RONALD M. LAXER • SUSANNE M. BENSELER

KEY POINTS

Pediatric systemic lupus erythematosus (SLE) accounts for 11% of patients referred to pediatric rheumatology clinics and approximately 20% of all cases of SLE.

Children with SLE appear to have more severe disease than adults, with an especially high incidence of renal involvement.

Thrombocytopenic purpura and autoimmune hemolytic anemia may be presenting manifestations of SLE in children.

With the use of aggressive treatment regimens, including intravenous cyclophosphamide and (presumably) mycophenolate mofetil, the prognosis for children with lupus nephritis has improved considerably, with greater than 90% survival and good renal function at 5 years.

Neonatal lupus, characterized by rash, fever, and other systemic manifestations, with or without congenital complete heart block, is caused by maternal anti-Ro antibodies in association with other factors, one of which is maternal HLA-DR3.

Inflammatory muscle disease in children almost always takes the form of juvenile dermatomyositis, with childhood polymyositis being very rare. Unlike in adults with dermatomyositis, an immune complex vasculitis is often present in childhood dermatomyositis and may be a major cause of morbidity and mortality. It has a predilection to involve the skin and the gastrointestinal tract.

Myositis is present in as many as 25% of children with systemic sclerosis and may be the presenting manifestation.

Localized scleroderma, including linear scleroderma and morphea, is three times more common than diffuse systemic sclerosis in children. In most cases, the disease remains localized and does not progress to diffuse disease.

Although the cause of Kawasaki disease is still unknown, treatment with intravenous IgG has been shown to improve mortality results by decreasing the number and severity of coronary atery aneurysms.

Henoch-Schönlein purpura, an IgA-mediated vasculitis, is the most common cause of vasculitis in children. It usually has a good prognosis, even in children with nephritis.

This chapter focuses on some of the most common systemic rheumatic diseases of childhood: pediatric systemic lupus erythematosus (SLE), juvenile dermatomyositis (JDM), scleroderma and its distinct subtypes, and the diseases in the spectrum of childhood vasculitis. Recent international collaborative efforts have substantially increased our understanding of these diseases and enabled us to recognize novel inflammatory diseases and their mimics.

SYSTEMIC LUPUS ERYTHEMATOSUS

Definition and Classification

Pediatric SLE (pSLE) is a chronic multisystem autoimmune disease with remitting, relapsing course and onset of symptoms before age 18 years, accounting for approximately 20% of all SLE.[1] This clinically heterogeneous disease is characterized by a distinct spectrum of autoantibodies including antinuclear antibody (ANA), double-stranded deoxyribonucleic acid (dsDNA), and antibodies against extractable nuclear antigens (ENAs). In genetically susceptible hosts B cell–mediated autoimmune processes lead to a variable combination and severity of clinical symptoms including antibody-mediated vasculitis, direct antibody binding to target cells, and thrombotic organ dysfunction.

The American College of Rheumatology (ACR) classification criteria for adults with SLE are commonly applied to children with pSLE.[2] The classification of neuropsychiatric SLE (NPSLE) in children and adolescents remains a challenge.[3,4] The 1990 ACR NPSLE nomenclature and case definitions appear to have limited applicability for children in certain domains.[5-7]

Epidemiology

Pediatric SLE affects children and adolescents around the world.[8-10] On average, 60% of patients develop pSLE after age 10, 35% between 5 and 10 years, and only 5% before age 5. In studies from Asia, the mean ages at diagnosis were reported to be 8.6 to 13.5 years.[8,9] The incidence and prevalence of pSLE varies between populations. Similar to adults, SLE more commonly affects non-Caucasian populations.[8,9,11] Overall, incidence rates of pSLE have been reported to be 0.28 to 0.48 per 100,000 children with prevalence rates of 6.3 to 24 per 100,000 depending on the ethnic background of the population.[9] The prevalence of pSLE is consistently higher in girls than boys: Canadian and Taiwan studies estimated a factor of 6.[12,13] Female predominance increases with age. This observation strongly supports the suggested role of female hormones.[14] Although pSLE is less common than adult SLE, childhood onset was recently found to be a strong, independent predictor of overall lupus mortality.[15]

Children with pSLE are likely to have relatives with SLE. The pattern of familial aggregation for siblings with SLE suggests a polygenic inheritance.[16] In addition, pSLE patients often have asymptomatic relatives with evidence of autoantibodies.[17]

Causes

Genes

Enabled by large international collaborations, susceptibility genes have been identified suggesting a dysregulated immune phenotype in lupus patients partially overlapping with other autoimmune diseases.[18] These include genetic variants in the cytokine interferon-α pathway and their functional impact,[19] the contribution of signal transduction *STAT4* gene variations on lupus susceptibility,[20] and the association of the interleukin-1 receptor-associated kinase-1 (*IRAK1*), an X chromosome gene, and disease susceptibility in pSLE.[21]

Beyond the type of gene variant (mutation, polymorphisms), altered copy number variations reflecting "gene dose" and epigenetic modifications of key lupus genes are reported in pediatric lupus patients: Garcia-Ortiz demonstrated an association of the lupus gene Toll-like receptor 7 (*TLR7*) copy number variation with susceptibility to pSLE in Mexican populations.[22] Drug-induced SLE and incomplete monozygotic twin concordance rates suggest an important role of epigenetic factors such as histone modification or altered DNA methylation in pSLE.[23] Finally, mitochondrial DNA polymorphisms may also be important in the pathogenesis of SLE.[24] Children with inherited complement deficiencies including C2, C4A/C4B, C1q, and C1s can present with pSLE.[25] These single gene defects are more commonly seen in familial cases of lupus.

Environment

Beyond genes and epigenetics, other potential contributing factors have been intensely studied in pSLE including environmental factors such as parental smoking[26] and organic dust exposure.[27] As a link between genetic and environmental factors, endogenous and external viruses are currently being studied in pSLE.[28] The presence of an interferon signature pattern had raised suspicion for a potential viral contribution and discovery of the genetic basis of chilblain lupus.[29] This focused the researchers' attention to DNA repair of endogenous virus as a potential pathogenetic factor in pSLE.

Pathology

Similar to adult SLE, the inflammatory processes leading to organ dysfunction are heterogeneous between and within organs (see Chapter 79). Immunoglobulin deposition in small vessels such as glomerulus or lung capillaries, complement activation, antibody-binding to single cells, and microthrombotic or macrothrombotic vessel disease are the hallmarks of lupus. Hematologic manifestations of lupus are often related to direct antibody-binding and complement activation.[30] In contrast, the histology of pediatric lupus nephritis is more variable and includes the distinct subtypes of mesangial, focal, or diffuse proliferative and membranous nephritis, which can coexist.[31] Renal biopsies are required to distinguish subtypes and define treatment regimens. In children, severity of the glomerulonephritis on renal biopsy was shown to be associated with treatment choice and response and long-term outcome.[31-34] Confounding risk factors for severe lupus nephritis and adverse renal outcome include evidence of thrombotic microangiopathy, antiphospholipid antibodies, tubulointerstitial disease, hypertension, nephrotic syndrome, and access to health care.[31-35]

Clinical Features

The clinical presentation of pSLE was reported in large series from many countries, allowing a better understanding of the clinical diversity, impact of ethnicity, confounding factors including infections, and access to health care[8,11,36-47] (Table 108-1).

Systemic features including fever and fatigue are found in more than 90% of children at diagnosis of pSLE. Arthritis is the most frequently reported organ manifestation in pSLE. Typically pSLE arthritis is a nonerosive, painful polyarthritis. Mucocutaneous involvement includes the typical "butterfly" or malar rash, an erythematous rash in the malar distribution sparing the nasolabial folds (Figure 108-1). Diffuse hair loss is commonly seen in children with active disease. In addition, children with lupus can present with a photosensitive rash, exacerbated in sun-exposed areas including upper arms, neckline, and face; Raynaud's phenomenon of fingers and toes; a vasculitic skin rash, which is often raised and painful affecting the fingers and toes; and oral and/or nasal ulcers. Oral ulcers are typically located on the hard palate and are painless (Figure 108-2). Uncommon skin manifestations include discoid lupus lesions, which heal with scarring.[48]

Nephritis is the most common major organ manifestation and occurs in more than 50% of children with pSLE, most commonly at diagnosis. Children with lupus nephritis present with peripheral edema, proteinuria, active urine sediment, and hypertension. Focal or diffuse proliferative

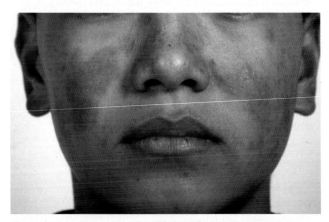

Figure 108-1 Malar rash of a 14-year-old patient with pediatric systemic lupus erythematosus. The disease's typical "butterfly" or malar rash is an erythematous rash in the malar distribution, which includes the cheeks and crosses the nasal bridge but spares the nasolabial folds.

Table 108-1 Clinical Characteristics of Children at Diagnosis of Pediatric Systemic Lupus Erythematosus (pSLE): Comparison of Four Recent Cohorts

	Vachvanichsanong 2010[43]	Agrawal 2009[44]	Hiraki 2008[41]	Ramirez Gomez 2008[11]
Country	Thailand	India	Canada	Latin America
Time frame of study	1985-2007	1987-2006	1982-2005	1996-2007
Number of pediatric SLE patients	213	70	258	230
Age at diagnosis	11.6 (±2.6)	10.5 (4-15)	13.1 (±3.2)	15.3 (13.2-16.7)
Female-to-male ratio	4.2:1	6:1	4.7:1	9:01
Median follow-up	3.6 yr	NR	3.5 yr	1.7 yr
Generalized symptoms				
Fatigue	NR	NR	50%	NR
Fever	NR	92%	39%	NR
Weight loss	NR	30%	29%	63%
Lymphadenopathy/hepatosplenomegaly	NR	42%/47%	19%	NR
Organ manifestations				
Hematologic disease	NR	NR	55%	NR
Thrombocytopenia	NR	24%	29%	25%
Lymphopenia	NR	NR	29%	60%
Coombs-positive hemolytic anemia	NR	58%	23%	16%
Mucocutaneous disease				
Malar rash	NR	57%	61%	70%
Photosensitivity	NR	51%	17%	53%
Oral ulcers	NR	NR	21%	49%
Nasal ulcers	NR	NR	8%	NR
Arthritis	NR	66%	61%	83%
Nephritis	81% total	77% total	37% total	49% total
Mesangial—WHO Class II	47%	NR	15%	NR
Focal proliferative—WHO Class III	2%	NR	28%	NR
Diffuse proliferative—WHO Class IV	37%	NR	47%	NR
Membranous—WHO Class V	8%	NR	16%	NR
Neuropsychiatric disease	NR	21%	16%	NR
Serositis				
Pericarditis	NR	3%	12%	17%
Pleuritis	NR	3%	12%	17%
Cardiac disease				
Myocarditis	NR	NR	1%	NR
Endocarditis	NR	NR	0%	NR
Pneumonitis	NR	NR	0.4%	NR
Gastrointestinal disease	NR	NR	NR	NR

NR, not reported; WHO, World Health Organization.

glomerulonephritis accounts for more than 50% of all pediatric lupus nephritis in most series. Acute renal failure can occur in a third of children presenting with proliferative lupus nephritis.[33] Mesangial and membranous nephritis are less common and can occur in conjunction with

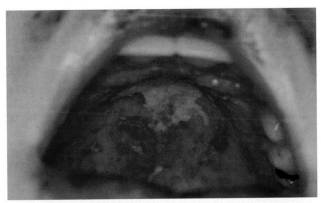

Figure 108-2 Oral ulcers in a 16-year-old girl with active pediatric systemic lupus erythematosus. Characteristic oral ulcers and hyperemia in children with lupus can be found on the hard palate. These ulcers are typically painless.

proliferative lupus nephritis. Posterior reversible encephalopathy (PRES) is an increasingly recognized central nervous system (CNS) complication of lupus nephritis and hypertension.[49]

Neuropsychiatric disease affects about a quarter of children with pSLE. Headaches in conjunction with psychosis or cerebrovascular disease presenting as seizures or severe cognitive dysfunction are the most common clinical phenotypes. Isolated lupus headache is uncommon.[7] Psychosis in pSLE is characterized by optic and acoustic hallucinations and visual distortions. Many patients have overlapping features of cognitive dysfunction, headaches, and mood disorder.[5] Isolated mood disorders such as depression are uncommon in pSLE. CNS vasculitis in pSLE more commonly affects the small vessels. Angiography-positive disease and strokes are uncommon.[7] Transverse myelitis is an uncommon, serious manifestation of pSLE.[50] Peripheral neuropathies are uncommon in children with lupus.

The diagnosis of NPSLE in children is based on clinical assessment including comprehensive neurocognitive testing,[51] inflammatory markers, and neuroimaging. Children with neuropsychiatric disease commonly have antiphospholipid antibodies, in particular anti–β_2-glycoprotein I (anti-β_2GPI).[52] A positive lupus anticoagulant is often detectable in children with cerebrovascular disease including sinus vein thrombosis (SVT) and chorea. Neuroimaging demonstrates only subtle abnormalities in half of patients[5] including the majority of children presenting with psychosis.

Hematologic disease is common in pSLE and affects a quarter of children. Treatment-refractory idiopathic thrombocytopenic purpura (ITP) or severe autoimmune hemolytic anemia can be the presenting features of pSLE. A positive ANA and older age were found to be risk factors of pSLE in ITP.[53] Serositis including pleuritis, pericarditis, and less commonly peritonitis affects about 20% of children with pSLE. Chest pain is the most common presenting feature. Inflammatory lung lesions including capillaritis and alveolar hemorrhage are uncommon. Although cardiomegaly due to pericarditis and arrhythmia/conduction anomaly occur frequently, myocarditis and coronary arteritis are serious yet uncommon lupus features in children.[54,55] The most common gastrointestinal (GI) manifestation of pSLE is lupus hepatitis. Inflammatory bowel manifestations are rare. Overall atypical presentations can be found in up to a quarter of children ultimately diagnosed with pSLE and, when present, were found to correlate with poor outcome.[56] Endocrinopathies of pSLE include hypothyroidism or hyperthyroidism and diabetes mellitus.[57] Menstrual cycle disturbances and transient amenorrhea are common in girls with pSLE and may be associated with pituitary dysfunction or treatment with cyclophosphamide, leading to a decreased progesterone production.[58]

Diagnosis and Diagnostic Tests

The diagnosis of pSLE is based on clinical findings, laboratory test results including inflammatory markers, complement levels, markers of organ involvement, and specific autoantibodies. Tissue biopsies and imaging studies can further support and/or classify pSLE subtypes. The presence of 4 of 11 ACR classification criteria was found to have a sensitivity of 96% and a specificity of 100%.[2] A careful evaluation of potential organ involvement of pSLE is mandatory. Characteristic abnormal laboratory markers of active pSLE may include a raised erythrocyte sedimentation rate (ESR), anemia, which may be Coombs positive and hemolytic, a low white blood count with predominant lymphopenia, low platelets, and low C3 and/or C4 complement levels. Paradoxically, the C-reactive protein (CRP) is normal in the vast majority of children with active lupus, except for those presenting with serositis or concurrent infections. An abnormal urinalysis including microscopic evidence of casts indicated renal involvement. Renal function impairment is best evaluated by serum creatinine, albumin, and urine protein–to-creatinine ratio. Lupus anticoagulant and specific lupus autoantibody testing including ANA, dsDNA, ENA, and antiphospholipid antibodies is mandatory. ANA is found is almost every child with pSLE, while dsDNA is detected in more than 80%.[41,59] Novel antibodies have been proposed and require prospective validation in pSLE.[60] Children may have frank hypothyroidism or hyperthyroidism or solely raised titers of thyroid antibodies.[41]

Lipid abnormalities are increasingly recognized in children with pSLE.[61] Dyslipidemia may contribute to a risk of premature arteriosclerosis in pSLE patients.[62,63] Cytokines derived from adipocytes including leptin, adiponectin, and ghrelin were recently shown to correlate with disease activity in pSLE.[64] Markers of bone health and fracture risk have been extensively evaluated in children with pSLE.[65] A comprehensive assessment may include these markers in conjunction with bone density measurement.

The differential diagnosis of pSLE is wide and includes infections such as cytomegalovirus (CMV), Epstein-Barr virus, and tuberculosis, malignancies such as lymphomas, endocrinopathies, primary inflammatory or idiopathic organ diseases such as membranoproliferative nephritis, or idiopathic psychosis and pediatric autoimmune diseases including JDM, systemic sclerosis, Sjögren's syndrome, overlap syndromes, and polyarticular and systemic juvenile idiopathic arthritis.[66,67] Children with a recent diagnosis of pSLE can present with concurrent infections such as CMV, which may confound the clinical presentation and response to therapy.[68] Uncommon infections may be present.[69] Macrophage activation syndrome (MAS, a secondary hemophagocytic lymphohistiocytosis [HLH] syndrome) is a newly recognized inflammatory emergency and can present in pSLE patients.[70] MAS has to be considered in a child with pSLE and unexplained fever and cytopenia, when associated with marked hyperferritinemia.

Treatment

The care for children with lupus, similar to other multiorgan rheumatic diseases, mandates a multidisciplinary approach of different subspecialty physicians including pediatric rheumatologists, nephrologists, psychiatrists, and adolescent medicine, allied health care specialists, social workers, and teachers.

Immunosuppression

The choice and dosing of immunosuppressive therapy regimen must be tailored to the extent and severity of the child's organ disease. A thorough diagnostic evaluation is mandatory before initiating therapy. Immunosuppressive treatment protocols are commonly adopted from adult trials and meta-analyses.[71] Treatment response criteria for pSLE were recently developed and validated.[72]

Corticosteroids are the mainstay of lupus therapy. The general approach for major organ disease includes initial high-dose treatment with 2 mg/kg prednisone equivalent in two to three divided doses followed by a slow taper. This includes treatment of proliferative lupus nephritis, neuropsychiatric lupus except for chorea and SVT, myocarditis, and lung disease. Pulse intravenous (IV) methylprednisolone is frequently used for emergent situations including acute psychosis, MAS, and myocarditis. Arthritis, serositis, nonproliferative lupus nephritis, and mucocutaneous disease may require smaller initial doses of corticosteroids. The efficacy of corticosteroids in pSLE is well established. However, the significant toxicity limits its long-term use at high doses. Short-term side effects include weight gain, sleep disturbances, emotional instability, increased hair growth, and impaired glucose metabolism. Long-term effects include cataracts, growth arrest, vertebral fractures, and avascular necrosis.[57]

Combination immunosuppressive regimens are commonly used in children with major organ involvement. Cyclophosphamide, mycophenolate mofetil (MMF), and azathioprine have been studied in observational cohorts of pSLE patients. IV cyclophosphamide was considered the gold standard for severe organ disease such as proliferative lupus nephritis and neuropsychiatric disease. In accordance to adult SLE protocols, cyclophosphamide is commonly used for induction over 6 months, followed by either azathioprine or MMF.[73] Induction therapy with MMF was found to be safe, well tolerated, and effective in a small cohort of renal and nonrenal pSLE patients.[74-77] Complete renal remission is achieved in 40% to 50% of children at 6 months and 75% at 12 months.[78] Commonly reported side effects that led to discontinuation of MMF therapy included severe diarrhea and abdominal pain.[75] In children, optimal dosing may require pharmacokinetic evaluation on a stable dose.[79,80] Efficacy and safety of MMF as maintenance drug is well established in pSLE.[73,81,82] Induction therapy with azathioprine was found to be equally efficacious as cyclophosphamide in children with proliferative lupus nephritis and renal failure.[33] Azathioprine has a good efficacy and safety profile.[83] Routine monitoring of blood counts and liver function is required. Significant toxicity may occur in children with mutations in the gene encoding thiopurine methyltransferase or thiopurine S-methyltransferase (TPMT); however, the role of genotyping remains controversial.[84] Azathioprine is also used as a maintenance drug following induction with cyclophosphamide.[73]

Dialysis is required in children with end-stage renal disease.[33] Plasmapheresis is indicated for specific disease manifestations such as thrombotic-thrombocytopenic purpura (TTP),[85] transverse myelitis, and steroid-resistant nephritis.[86] B cell depletion with the anti-CD20 antibody rituximab is the main biologic therapy currently used in pSLE.[87-91] It was shown to be effective as a single agent in hematologic disease and in addition to standard therapy in refractory, difficult-to-treat pSLE. The safety profile remains to be systematically studied in pSLE. Autologous stem cell transplantation is rarely performed in pSLE.[92]

MAS therapy in pSLE may include IV immunoglobulin, IV methylprednisolone pulse therapy, cyclosporine, or even chemotherapy according to HLH protocol.[93]

Antimalarials

Antimalarials are strongly recommended for children and adults with SLE.[94] On the basis of predominantly adult studies and meta-analysis, antimalarials are thought to decrease overall mortality and improve long-term outcome,[95] modify lipid profiles,[96] and control joint and skin disease, in particular discoid lupus lesions.[97,98]

Adjunctive Therapy

Supportive medical therapies include angiotensin-converting inhibitors for renal protection and hypertension, contraception when applicable, organ dysfunction therapies including anticonvulsants and antipsychotic medication, and anticoagulation when applicable. High-factor

sunscreen for sunburn protection is important. Educational efforts have to include disease and treatment, medication side effects, infection risk, and impact on social life and school.

Vitamin D is known to be a strong factor of bone protection in pSLE.[99,100] Sufficient vitamin D doses in addition to calcium intake and physical activity are required to maintain good bone health. More recently a novel role of vitamin D in maintaining immune homeostasis was recognized. This is supported by studies demonstrating an inverse correlation between vitamin D levels and disease activity,[101,102] in particular in overweight children with pSLE.

Outcome

Lupus in children and adults is a relapsing/remitting disease. The burden of pSLE is complex to determine because many factors such as access to health care, individual patient characteristics, disease activity, confounding diseases such as infections, and responsiveness to treatment all contribute to overall mortality and morbidity.[1]

The overall mortality as captured by standard mortality rate (SMR) for all SLE in the United States between 1992 and 2001 was 3.06 deaths per million inhabitants per year,[103] in Brazil between 1985 and 2004 it was 3.8 (2601 deaths, 90% female),[104] and in Denmark it was 4.6.[105] With improved therapies, mortality rates were shown to decrease in Canada (SMR, 10.1 in 1970-1977; 4.8 in 1978-1985, and 3.3 in 1986-1994).[106] When comparing childhood- with adult-onset SLE, childhood-onset SLE was found to be independently associated with an increased mortality risk (hazard ratio [HR], 3.1), as was low socioeconomic status measured by education (HR, 1.9), and end-stage renal disease (HR, 2.1).[15]

Young age at disease onset was repeatedly shown to be a predictor of adverse outcome.[47,107] Children with pSLE in poor countries clearly have a higher mortality: In a small study from Nigeria the mortality was 30%.[108] The Latin American LUMINA cohort had an 81% survival at last follow-up, the recent 5-year patient survival rate in Iran was 82.5%,[32] and in Canada it was 100%.[41,109] Infections continue to be the main cause of death in developing countries with limited access to health care.[34,110] Nephritis has been consistently identified as a predictor of poor outcome in pSLE. Histologic subtype of proliferative disease, evidence of disease relapse, certain ethnicities, and poor response to therapy were strong predictors of end-stage renal disease in pSLE.[111] Gibson demonstrated that treatment resistance portended a high risk of end-stage kidney disease and disproportionately affected African-American children with lupus nephritis.[111]

Children with pSLE accrue disease- and treatment-related damage as captured in the domains of the Systemic Lupus International Collaborative Clinics (SLICC) Damage Index (see Chapter 80), constantly adding to the overall disease burden.[1,57] Osteoporosis, cataracts, and osteonecrosis/avascular necrosis (AVN) are the leading domains of damage accrual. Individual patient characteristics, disease activity, corticosteroid therapy, calcium/vitamin D deficiency, and immobility contribute to impaired bone health in pSLE.[112,113] AVN occurs in 6% to 10% of pSLE patients overall and is associated with corticosteroid therapy.[41] Nakamura[114] recently observed the complete absence of AVN in children younger than 14 years of age and suggested that age at the time of the initial corticosteroid therapy affects AVN occurrence. Neurocognitive deficits secondary to disease and treatment are increasingly recognized and significantly affect school performance and overall health-related quality of life.[115,116] Early cardiovascular events including myocardial infarctions and strokes have become a major cause of morbidity and mortality.[1]

Drug-Induced Lupus Erythematosus

Several medications can cause systemic and subacute or chronic cutaneous lupus phenotypes in children.[117] The cutaneous manifestations of systemic drug-induced lupus (DIL) include malar rash, purpura, erythema nodosum, urticaria, and photosensitivity. Systemic symptoms include arthritis, oral ulcers, pleuritis, hematologic manifestations, and less commonly renal disease. Characteristic laboratory findings of DIL are positive ANA and antihistone antibodies. Drugs implicated are minocycline, anticonvulsive drugs, hydralazine, procainamide, and isoniazid.[118]

Management of drug-induced lupus is based on the withdrawal of the offending drug. Topical and/or systemic corticosteroids and other immunosuppressive agents may be required in resistant cases.

Neonatal Lupus Erythematosus

Neonatal lupus erythematosus (NLE) is an acquired disease of the newborn caused by placental transfer of maternal anti-SSA/Ro and anti-SSB/La IgG antibodies. These can be present in mothers with SLE, Sjögren's syndrome, and other autoimmune connective disorders, as well as clinically healthy women. Antibody transfer can lead to inflammation of the cardiac conducting system and subsequent fibrosis resulting in congenital heart block (CHB), which may be detected as early as 20 weeks of gestation. A prolonged PR interval is the first electrocardiographic sign of conduction system abnormality in NLE. The degree of heart block can vary, and rapid clinical progression from normal sinus rhythm to complete CHB over 2 weeks may be observed, causing life-threatening cardiomyopathy and fetal hydrops in the most severe cases. Isolated endocardial fibroelastosis can be found in some infants.[119] Interestingly, infants with prenatal exposure to high-titer anti-SSB/La antibody levels are more likely to have noncardiac features of NLE, whereas cardiac disease tends to be associated with moderate or high maternal anti-SSA/Ro levels, independent of anti-SSB/La titers in CHB.[120] The overall risk of CHB in anti-SSA/Ro–positive women is estimated to be 2% to 5%,[120] but this risk may be increased by 10-fold in women with a previous child with CHB.[121] A recent study suggests an overall recurrence rate of cardiac NLE of 17%, independent of maternal health, antenatal use of steroids, antibody status, severity of cardiac disease in the first affected child, or sex of the subsequent child.[122]

In addition to heart block, newborns with NLE can present with a characteristic NLE rash, hepatic dysfunction, and hematologic abnormalities including significant thrombocytopenia. Typically the NLE rash is located around the eyes but may present elsewhere on the body.[123]

Hepatobiliary disease can have three distinct presentations: (1) transient conjugated hyperbilirubinemia with mildly raised liver function tests (LFTs) in the first weeks of life; (2) mild elevations of LFTs at 2 to 3 months of life; and (3) severe liver failure during gestation or in the neonatal period.[124] NLE neurologic involvement can include magnetic resonance imaging (MRI) findings of nonspecific white matter changes and calcification of the basal ganglia. NLE "vasculopathy" is reported. Recently, an association of NLE and hydrocephalus has been recognized.[125] Chondrodysplasia punctata, a stippling of the epiphyses, and pulmonary capillaritis are rare clinical presentations of NLE.[123,126]

In a prospective multicenter study of 128 infants whose mothers had been referred for the presence of anti-SSA/Ro antibodies, regardless of their diagnosis, hematologic abnormalities and raised liver enzymes were seen in 27% and 26%, respectively.[127] Cutaneous NLE manifestations were present in 16%. Only 2 of the 128 infants (1.6%) presented with complete CHB. In a recent Japanese review, 193 infants with NLE were described reporting CHB in 23%.[128]

Treatment of CHB in NLE remains controversial. Prevention of progression to complete CHB may be achieved by treating the mother with fluorinated steroids (dexamethasone or betamethasone), which are not metabolized by the placenta and are available to the fetus in an active form. IV immunoglobulin had been used to prevent the development of CHB in the index patient and in subsequent pregnancies.[129] The current recommendation is to screen anti-Ro/SSA antibody–positive mothers with serial echocardiograms and obstetric sonograms biweekly starting from week 16 of gestation. Early detection of cardiac manifestations of NLE including premature atrial contractions or moderate pericardial effusion preceding CHB may potentially be targeted with preventive therapy.[129-131] First-degree heart blocks can be reversed by dexamethasone treatment of the mother.[132] Once third-degree block is unequivocally identified, reversal is unlikely to be achieved. The majority of children with CHB require pacemakers.[121]

The treatment approach to extracardiac manifestations of NLE is conservative. Skin disease may require topical corticosteroids and sun protection.[133] Transient elevations of LFTs and cytopenias commonly do not require therapy.[124]

The morbidity of cardiac neonatal lupus is estimated to be 20%.[121] Mortality is particularly high in patients with CHB and concurrent cardiomyopathy. Children with NLE can develop SLE later in life. Concerns of potential long-term neurocognitive deficits of NLE patients need further evaluation.[134]

JUVENILE DERMATOMYOSITIS

Definition and Criteria

Juvenile dermatomyositis (JDM) is an inflammatory, immune-mediated vasculopathy with predominant involvement of muscle and skin that may involve other organs as well. JDM is by far the most common form of idiopathic inflammatory myopathy (IIM) in children and adolescents; therefore other types (such as juvenile polymyositis) are not addressed in this chapter.

Epidemiology

The incidence of JDM has been reported at approximately two to three cases per million children[135-137] with a mean age of onset of JDM of 6 to 9 years of age.[136,138-141] JDM may begin before 4 years of age in approximately 25% of cases.[139] Females are affected more commonly than males in a ratio of approximately 2 : 1.[136,138-141] Birth distributions for some subgroups of JDM patients have been noted and suggest that perinatal exposures may influence the onset of disease.[142]

Genetics, Etiology, and Pathogenesis

It is thought that JDM is an autoimmune disorder in which environmental factors trigger an immune vasculopathy in genetically susceptible individuals. There is circumstantial evidence supporting the possible role of infection in the pathogenesis of JDM.[139,143] Gene expression profiling in newly diagnosed JDM patients demonstrated interferon signature patterns in affected muscle tissue, suggesting preceding viral infection.[144] Electron microscopic studies of affected muscle demonstrate tubuloreticular inclusions, which can also indicate a type I interferon response. Many different infections have been associated with JDM.

Both human leukocyte antigen (HLA) and non-HLA genetic relationships have been reported to be disease associated or protective. In Caucasians, the HLA allele HLA DRB1*0301 is the strongest HLA risk factor (odds ratio [OR], 3.9). The HLA associations do not seem to affect disease course or complications.[145] Similarly, the presence of polymorphisms of cytokine genes may confer an increased risk on the development of JDM or may be protective.[146] Polymorphisms at these and other alleles may also be associated with disease complications and course.

The central events of the immune angiopathy of JDM include an overexpression of major histocompatibility complex (MHC) type I molecules on the surface of myofibers and a type I interferon response.[147] An immune complex–mediated vasculopathy with the presence of the C5-9 membrane attack complex, as well as immunoglobulins and C3 complement with complement activation, is evident. There is also a perivascular and perimysial infiltration of plasmacytoid dendritic cells, leading eventually to infiltration by CD4+ T cells, B cells, macrophages, proinflammatory cytokines, and chemokines. This leads to vascular damage, capillary dropout, and muscle ischemia. Upregulation of MHC class I molecules on myofibers is associated with the activation of nuclear factor κβ (NFκB), which can lead to muscle damage. Maternal microchimerism has been noted in the majority of patients with JDM and in frequencies much greater than siblings or healthy controls,[147] suggesting that mechanisms similar to graft-versus-host disease may also play a role in the pathogenesis of JDM.

Clinical Features

Patients usually present with an insidious onset of fatigue, decreased functional ability, stiffness, and weakness. Irritability may result from muscle pain and an inability to participate in routine activities, especially in young children. A more acute onset, with fever, may occur in about half of patients. Weakness with rash is the presenting problem in about 50% of cases, weakness alone in about 25%, and the remainder present with predominantly skin symptoms. The clinical features at presentation are shown in Table 108-2.[136,140,148-151]

Symmetric proximal muscle weakness typically presents first in the lower extremities, manifesting as difficulty climbing stairs and running. Patients may demonstrate a Gower sign reflecting weakness of the lower limb and trunk muscles. Reaching for objects above the head and hair brushing are difficult because of weakness of the shoulder girdle. An increased lumbar lordosis results from weakness of the trunk muscles, which also makes it difficult to roll in bed and get out of bed. Neck flexor weakness makes it difficult to hold the head upright. The muscles may be painful and tender to touch due to edema. Weakness of the distal musculature is unusual but may be present late in disease. Weakness of the palatal musculature results in dysphonia, dysphagia, and nasal regurgitation.[152] Rarely, patients may be so weak as to be bedbound.

Skin rashes are present in approximately 75% of patients at presentation. Rash may be the presenting feature and in fact the only symptom (clinically amyopathic dermatomyositis), although subtle abnormalities may be detected on muscle MRI. Some skin features are predictive of poor outcome such as calcinosis and severe nail-fold capillary abnormalities.

The cutaneous features of JDM have been well summarized in a comprehensive review.[153] It is important to note that activity of the skin disease frequently does not correlate with activity of the muscle disease, and cutaneous abnormalities may have a significant impact on the patient's quality of life.

Gottron papules occur over the extensor surfaces of the metacarpophalangeal (MCP) and interphalangeal (IP) joints, as well as the knees, elbows, and medial malleoli (Figure 108-3A). They are erythematous to violaceous papules and may have associated scaling, crusting, erosions, ulcerations, or pigmentary change. This is differentiated from Gottron sign, which involves macular lesions occurring in the same distribution.

The pathognomonic heliotrope rash consists of violaceous to erythematous discrete or confluent macules confined to the upper eyelids (Figure 108-3B). This can extend periorbitally and often presents with generalized periorbital edema with discoloration.

Other cutaneous lesions include erythematous lesions in both sun-exposed and non–sun-exposed areas. Common

Table 108-2 Clinical Features at Presentation of Juvenile Dermatomyositis[136,140,148-151,418]

Clinical Feature	% Patients Affected
Proximal muscle weakness	82-100
Characteristic rash (Gottron papule ± heliotrope)	66-95
Calcinosis	5-30
Dysphagia	18-44
Dyspnea	5-43
Arthritis	23-61

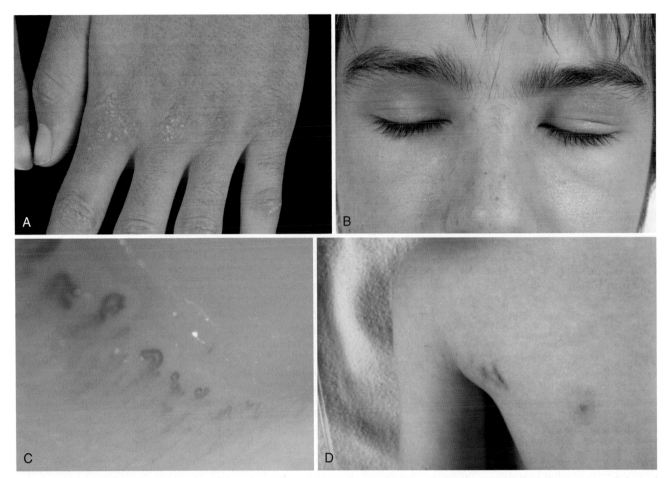

Figure 108-3 Fifteen-year-old boy with newly diagnosed juvenile dermatomyositis demonstrating Gottron papules over the metacarpophalangeal and proximal interphalangeal joints **(A)**, helitrope rash with periorbital swelling **(B)**, and nail-fold capillary dropout, dilatation, and tortuosity **(C)**. **D** shows a 4-year-old boy with juvenile dermatomyositis with a cutaneous ulcer adjacent to his right axilla. He died 3 months after presentation.

areas of involvement include the cheeks, the shawl area of the shoulders, and the "V" area of the lower anterior neck and chest wall. As opposed to SLE, the malar rash of JDM often involves the nasolabial folds and may involve the chin and forehead as well. Both the shawl sign and "V" rash are associated with anti-synthetase antibodies. Linear erythematous lesions may occur over extensor surfaces including the tendons of the hands and feet.

Vasculopathy is the characteristic pathologic feature of JDM. Cutaneous manifestations of vasculopathy include livedo reticularis and ulceration (Figure 108-3D). Ulcerative lesions are more common over extensor surfaces and the inner canthi of the eye. Erythema and capillary dilatation of the gingiva are a part of the vasculopathic manifestations. Capillary nail-fold changes are a major manifestation of JDM and are often visible to the naked eye. These are best observed under a microscope, but excellent resolution may be obtained by placing a drop of oil or water at the nail bed and magnifying this with a dermatoscope, otoscope, or ophthalmoscope at plus 40 diopters (Figure 108-3C). Characteristic changes include dilatation of the vessels, tortuosity, bushy capillaries, dropout, hemorrhage, and thrombosis. The severity of the capillary change may reflect the degree of disease activity and may also correlate with damage.

Calcinosis cutis can occur in up to 40% of patients with JDM; occasionally it may be present at the time of diagnosis.

It is a dystrophic calcification and occurs more often in patients who have been "undertreated" or had a delay in the start of treatment. Calcinosis may take several forms: superficial plaques and nodules; tumoral; fascial plane deposition; and an exoskeleton (Figure 108-4A,D). Patients may have more than one pattern. The superficial lesions are often subject to minor trauma and can lead to skin breakdown. They may also extrude a chalklike material (see Figure 108-4A). Tumoral deposits can impair function and lead to skin breakdown, especially when they involve flexural areas. Occasionally the calcinosis in these areas leads to an intense inflammatory reaction resembling cellulitis. Fascial plane calcinosis may impair function when crossing joint lines (see Figure 108-4B). An exoskeleton may give a scleroderma-like picture. Contrary to old beliefs that calcinosis was purely a healing process indicating that JDM was inactive, these lesions are often associated with ongoing active disease requiring more aggressive systemic treatment.

Lipodystrophy is a late manifestation reported in up to 40% of patients, developing a median of 4.6 years after diagnosis.[154] It may be localized, partial, or generalized and frequently occurs with metabolic syndrome, which includes hyperglycemia, hypertriglyceridemia, insulin resistance, hepatomegaly, transaminitis, and premature organ failure. Acanthosis nigricans may occur as well.

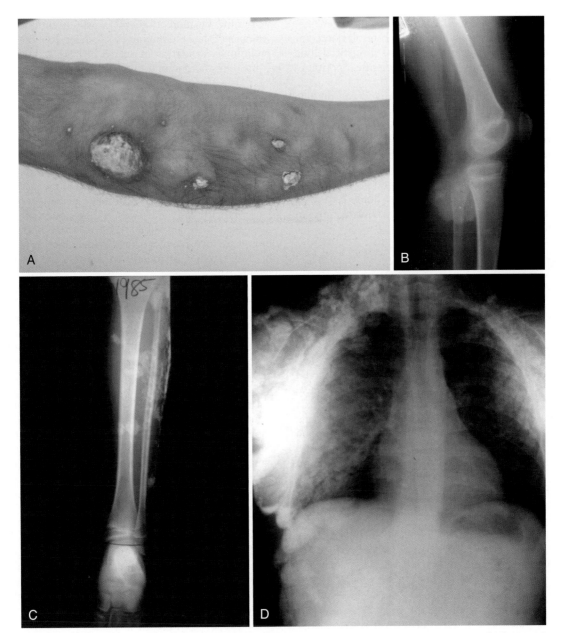

Figure 108-4 **A,** Elbow and forearm of a 14-year-old girl with chronic continuous juvenile dermatomyositis showing multiple sites of tumoral calcinosis. Several of these, particularly over pressure points, have ulcerated extruding a chalklike material. **B,** Solitary site of tumoral calcinosis posterior to the knee resulted in limited range of motion. **C,** Fascial and tumoral calcinosis affecting the lower extremity. **D,** Same patient as in **A** demonstrating marked calcification giving an exoskeleton-like appearance across the chest wall.

Clinically amyopathic JDM (CAJDM) is a unique form of JDM in which patients have a characteristic skin rash in the absence of any abnormalities of muscle including MRI changes for at least 6 months.[155] Some patients have cutaneous changes and no weakness but abnormal muscle tests and may be categorized as "hypopathic JDM."[156] In a systematic review, 26% of 68 patients with CAJDM developed classic JDM, with weakness developing a mean interval of 1.9 years after the onset of cutaneous symptoms; calcinosis developed in 4%. No laboratory or ancillary muscle testing was predictive of the development of muscle disease. Therefore immunosuppressive treatment is generally not indicated (other than required for the skin disease), but close follow-up is essential.

GI manifestations include dysphagia from both palatal muscle weakness and involvement of the distal esophagus. Intestinal vasculopathy can result in diffuse abdominal pain, lower GI bleeding, or bowel perforation with peritoneal free air.

Arthritis occurred in 61% of patients in one cohort, reported a median of 4.5 months after the JDM onset.[157] Osteopenia may result from disuse and treatment, and pathologic fractures may develop. Rhabdomyolysis is a rare complication that may follow infection.

Multiple respiratory manifestations may occur and are often subclinical. In one large case series followed for a mean of 16.8 years,[158] a low total lung capacity (TLC) was found in about 25% and a low diffusing capacity for carbon monoxide (DLco) in about 50% of patients. Just over one-third of patients had abnormalities on high-resolution computed tomography (CT) scanning such as interstitial lung disease, chest wall calcinosis, and airway disease. Spontaneous pneumothorax has been reported.

Cardiac manifestations are uncommon and can include pericarditis, myocarditis, and arrhythmias. However, subclinical left ventricular diastolic dysfunction, systolic hypertension, and electrocardiogram abnormalities occurred in 22% of one series of patients and were associated with cumulative organ damage.[159] Hypertension is usually associated with high-dose glucocorticoid therapy.

The association with malignancy is limited to case reports such that a search for malignancy is not required in children with JDM.

Disease Monitoring

Muscle enzyme levels are frequently normal soon after treatment and are therefore unreliable indicators of disease activity. Several tools have been developed and validated to monitor the course and outcome of children with JDM. These include the 0- to 10-point Manual Muscle Test,[160] the Childhood Health Assessment Questionnaire (CHAQ),[161] the Childhood Myositis Assessment Scale (CMAS),[162] the Disease Activity Score (DAS),[163] the Myositis Damage Index (MDI), and the Intention to Treat Index (MITAX). The Myositis Disease Activity Assessment Visual Analogue Scale (MYOACT) consists of a series of 10 visual analogue scales in different organ systems.[164] In 2008 a prospective validation study of a core set for the evaluation of response to therapy in JDM was published under the auspices of the Paediatric Rheumatology International Trials Organization, the ACR, and the European League Against Rheumatism (EULAR) (Table 108-3).[165] Provisional criteria for the evaluation of response to therapy in JDM include at least 20% improvement from baseline in three of six core set variables with no more than one of the remaining

Table 108-3 Domains and Suggested Variables Included in the Final Core Set for the Evaluation of Response to Therapy in Juvenile Dermatomyositis (JDM)

Domain	Suggested Variables
Physician's global assessment of patient's overall disease activity	10-cm VAS
Muscle strength	CMAS (or MMT)
Global JDM disease activity tool	DAS (or MYOACT or MITAX)
Parent's global assessment of patient's overall well-being	10-cm VAS
Functional ability assessment	CHAQ
Health-related quality of life assessment	CHQ physical summary score

CHAQ, Childhood Health Assessment Questionnaire; CHQ, Child Health Questionnaire; CMAS, Childhood Myositis Assessment Scale; MITAX, Myositis Intention to Treat Index; MMT, Manual Muscle Test; MYOACT, Myositis Disease Activity Assessment; VAS, Visual Analogue Scale.
From Ruperto N, Mistorio A, Rivelli A, et al: The Paediatric Rheumatology International Trials Organisation provisional criteria for the evaluation of response to therapy in juvenile dermatomyositis, *Arthritis Care Res (Hoboken)* 62:1533–1541, 2010.

worsening by more than 30%, which cannot be muscle strength.[166] The Cutaneous Assessment Tool has undergone preliminary validation in a series of 113 children with JDM. It measures both skin activity and skin damage.[167,168]

Diagnosis and Diagnostic Tests

The diagnostic criteria published by Bohan and Peter[169,170] require that patients have a characteristic skin rash plus three of the following four to meet the definition of "definite" JDM: symmetric proximal muscle weakness, elevated serum levels of muscle-derived enzymes, myopathic electromyogram (EMG), and histologic evidence of myositis. Patients with rash and two of these four criteria may be diagnosed with "probable" JDM. Because both EMG and biopsy are invasive procedures, many practitioners now rely on MRI studies of muscle to support the diagnosis (see later).

Laboratory evaluation in children with JDM helps to support the diagnosis and exclude other causes of muscle weakness. Systemic markers of inflammation such as the ESR and CRP generally reflect the degree of disease activity. Serum levels of neopterin and elevated levels of CD19[+] B lymphocytes have been suggested as good markers of disease activity, as has von Willebrand factor.[171]

Elevated serum levels of muscle enzymes form one of the diagnostic criteria of JDM. Measurements of creatine kinase, lactate dehydrogenase, aspartate transaminase, and aldolase should all be obtained. However, their degree of elevation does not necessarily correlate with active disease and they can occasionally be normal, even at presentation, particularly with long-standing disease. Serum levels of muscle enzymes drop dramatically with treatment, often before a clinical improvement is seen.

Electromyography has generally fallen out of favor despite still being part of the diagnostic criteria, especially if MRI is available. Characteristic EMG changes include spontaneous fibrillations, increased insertional activity, decreased amplitude, and duration of action potentials.

Although abnormal muscle biopsy is one of the criteria proposed by Bohan and Peter in the diagnostic criteria for juvenile dermatomyositis, many clinicians elect not to do muscle biopsies when patients present with classic clinical features of JDM. This is because the procedure is invasive, painful, may not add to the diagnostic accuracy in individual patients, and may be normal in up to 20% of patients. Normal results may occur because of sampling error or patchy muscle involvement. Better yield might be afforded through the use of MRI to determine best sites for biopsy. Care should be taken not to biopsy a site that has previously undergone electromyography.

The characteristic light microscopic features are suggestive of an inflammatory vasculopathy. This includes endothelial cell swelling, capillary dropout with a reduced capillary-to-muscle fiber ratio, microthrombosis, and infarction. There is a relatively sparse inflammatory infiltrate consisting mainly of T cells, but there may be myeloid cells present as well. Muscle fibers demonstrate perifascicular atrophy, overexpression of class I major histocompatibility complex, deposition of immunoglobulin, and the membrane attack complex C5-9. There are also areas of degenerating and regenerating muscle fibers. Chronic changes include an increase in the perimysial and endomysial connective tissue, thought to reflect muscle fiber damage and loss. Histopathologic changes have been shown to correlate with both ulcerative disease and poor prognosis.[172]

Recently, an international group has developed a scoring system that can be used in routine laboratories. The scoring tool uses four domains to reflect the degree of pathology: inflammatory, vascular, muscle fiber, and connective tissue. It also includes a visual analogue scale from 0 to 10 to reflect overall damage.[173]

Currently the diagnosis of JDM is made on the basis of Bohan and Peter criteria. However, many pediatric rheumatologists now have turned to MRI to assist with the diagnosis and avoid more invasive tests such as EMG and muscle biopsy.[174] Inflammation characteristic of JDM is seen as high-signal intensity on fat-suppressed weighted and short tau inversion recovery (STIR) images.[175] STIR sequences can also reveal fasciitis and panniculitis. Muscle atrophy is best appreciated on T1-weighted sequences as increased signal between muscle planes. An increase in mean T2 relaxation time correlates with increased muscle disease activity and muscle strength.[176]

ANA positivity is seen in 10% to 85% of patients with JDM. Myositis-associated (MAA) and myositis-specific antibodies (MSA) are uncommon unless the JDM is part of an overlap syndrome.[177,178] In those patients who are positive for MAAs and MSAs (anti–signal-recognition particle, anti-synthetase, and anti-Mi2), the clinical associations are the same as in adult disease. The newly described autoantibody anti-p155/140 has been identified in up to 29% of one series of JDM patients,[179] and anti-p140 has been identified in 23% of JDM patients, associated with calcinosis in one series.[180]

Differential Diagnosis

The most important differential diagnosis for patients presenting with rash and muscle weakness is SLE, particularly for those patients presenting with significant arthritis and a malar rash. Characteristic autoantibodies of SLE, cytopenias, renal disease, and hypocomplementemia help to differentiate these disorders. Patients with systemic sclerosis and prominent myositis may be difficult to differentiate from patients with JDM. Patients with mixed connective tissue disease and other overlap syndromes may have features of JDM in addition to those of other autoimmune connective tissue diseases.

Other idiopathic inflammatory myopathies are extremely rare in children. These include inclusion body myositis, granulomatous myositis, and macrophagic myositis.

Patients who present with either no rash or mild rash and predominant muscle weakness may need to be differentiated from patients with primary myopathies. Patients with muscular dystrophies often have positive family histories and an insidious onset of disease with characteristic muscle groups involved. Congenital myopathies usually present in infancy with hypotonia. Metabolic myopathies may be associated with developmental delay. Cramping and weakness after exertion may also be signs of metabolic myopathy.

Various infections may lead to an acute myositis. Perhaps the best recognized is influenza B, presenting with acute calf pain, weakness, and raised muscle enzyme levels. *Trichinella* infection may be associated with periorbital edema and significant peripheral eosinophilia. Many other bacteria, viruses, and parasites may cause myositis; they should be suspected in the appropriate clinical circumstance.

Treatment

The management of patients with JDM requires a multidisciplinary team approach with medical specialists (rheumatologists, dermatologists, neurologists); nurses; rehabilitation specialists; social workers; and nutrition specialists.

Early aggressive treatment has been shown to result in better long-term outcomes and prevent disease-related complications.[139,141,181,182] The cornerstone of treatment is high-dose, daily corticosteroid, usually combined with a second-line agent, typically methotrexate (MTX). Some practitioners advise the early use of high-dose, IV pulse methylprednisolone to ensure appropriate absorption when there may be a concern of intestinal vasculitis,[183] when there is a flare of disease, or when a patient seems unresponsive to standard steroid therapy. The usual course has been to start at 2 mg/kg/day in one to three divided doses and to begin to taper when muscle enzymes have normalized and strength has improved, with a subsequent slow taper over 18 to 24 months in uncomplicated cases. With steroid treatment alone, a significant number of patients do not respond fully and have complications, and some patients may be overtreated and have steroid-related complications. As a result, other agents are commonly prescribed.

MTX has been used for decades in children with steroid-resistant JDM and has recently been incorporated into many treatment protocols. In addition to its anti-inflammatory effect, it allows for a lower cumulative dose of corticosteroids.[184] A recent survey of North American pediatric rheumatologists documented that the most common treatment approach to patients with JDM is a combination of prednisone and MTX.[185]

In patients who do not respond adequately, there are several options. IV immunoglobulin (IVIG) has been shown in a randomized controlled trial in adults with dermatomyositis to be effective,[186] as well as in case series in childhood JDM.[187] Several different protocols have been described. Generally, if there is no improvement within 2 months, it is unlikely that additional IVIG will be effective.

Mycophenolate mofetil at an initial dose of 20 mg/kg in two divided doses was studied in 50 patients who had not responded to prednisone and MTX.[188] A significant improvement in muscle and skin DAS was noted at 12 months, with a significant reduction on steroid dose and no serious adverse events. There was an increase in mean height and weight as well.

Cyclosporine A is used frequently in Europe as a second-line agent with good results.[189] A trial is currently under way in Europe for newly diagnosed patients with JDM comparing prednisone alone with prednisone plus MTX with prednisone plus cyclosporine A.

Cyclophosphamide has generally been reserved for patients with treatment-resistant disease, severe ulcerative disease, or lung involvement. Major clinical benefit was noted in a small cohort of patients without serious toxicity.[190]

The results with anti–tumor necrosis factor (TNF) treatment with both etanercept and infliximab have been reported in several small case series, with both positive and negative outcomes.[191] There are reports of several cases of myositis developing while on etanercept treatment. The use of rituximab has been reported in only a small number of patients with good results.[192] The results of the rituximab in myositis trial are awaited. Nevertheless, a trial may be warranted in patients with severe unresponsive disease. It is possible that patients who have myositis-specific autoantibodies would respond better. A few patients have undergone successful autologous stem cell transplantation.[193]

One approach to the treatment of patients with JDM has been to use a step-wise addition of medications if patients fail to improve according to a predetermined outcome (similar to "treat-to-target" approach in rheumatoid arthritis). Using this approach, Kim and colleagues[182] reported excellent outcomes in a series of patients who were treated, progressively, with prednisone (98%), MTX (78%), IV methylprednisolone (84%), cyclosporine A (27%), IVIG (20%), plasma exchange (8%), and cyclophosphamide (4%).

Recently, the Childhood Arthritis and Rheumatology Research Alliance (CARRA), using consensus building techniques, proposed three protocols for the treatment of moderately severe JDM. All include corticosteroids in one to two doses per day (maximum 60 mg) plus MTX, preferably given by the subcutaneous route at the lower dose. Clinicians may also add either pulse steroids or IVIG of 15 mg/m² or 1 mg/kg, maximum 40 mg/wk.[194] One approach to the pharmacologic management of JDM is listed in Table 108-4.

Cutaneous disease occasionally requires specific treatment irrespective of the treatment of the muscle disease. Sun protection with broad-spectrum sunscreens with an SPF of 30 or higher should be used daily. Topical emollients are helpful for dry and pruritic skin. Antihistamines may be helpful in reducing pruritus. Topical corticosteroids and tacrolimus may be indicated for the very inflamed lesions in patients who either do not respond to, or do not require, systemic therapy. Hydroxychloroquine was associated with a significant improvement of skin disease in a small cohort of patients who had an incomplete response to systemic corticosteroids.[195]

Physiotherapy and occupational therapy are important to all children with JDM. Early in the disease, attention must be paid to stretching joints to prevent muscle contractures. Occasionally, contracted joints should be splinted. As the muscles heal, a more vigorous active exercise program can be initiated to strengthen muscles that may have atrophied from the combined effects of the inflammatory myopathy, disuse, and high-dose corticosteroid treatment. Active exercise may in fact exert anti-inflammatory effects in exercised skeletal muscle.[196]

Treatment for calcinosis has been disappointing. Case reports with positive results have included bisphosphonates and calcium channel inhibitors, but most patients do not respond. Surgical excision may be necessary for particularly troublesome individual lesions and can have excellent results.

Table 108-4 An Approach to the Management of a Patient with Juvenile Dermatomyositis

For Muscle Weakness
Initial Treatment
Prednisone Methotrexate subcutaneously ± IV pulse methylprednisolone ± IVIG
If Failure to Respond to Initial Treatment, Consider Adding:
IV pulse methylprednisolone IVIG monthly Azathioprine Mycophenolate mofetil Cyclosporine A
If Failure to Respond to Second-Line Treatment, Consider Adding:
Cyclophosphamide Tacrolimus Infliximab Rituximab
For Skin
Initial Treatment
Hydration Sun protection
If Failure to Respond to Second-Line Treatment, Consider Adding:
Hydroxychloroquine Topical tacrolimus

IV, intravenous; IVIG, intravenous immunoglobulin.

Outcome

In the precorticosteroid era, approximately one-third of patients with JDM went into a complete clinical remission, one-third had a chronic course, and one-third died.[197] Advances in medical therapy, earlier diagnosis, and more aggressive treatment protocols have led to significantly improved outcomes; however, there is still significant morbidity and a small mortality associated. Current mortality is less than 5%.[198,199]

Patients may follow one of three disease courses: monocyclic, polycyclic (flares of disease while off treatment), or chronic continuous courses. Delayed recognition of disease and initial undertreatment may result in more prolonged disease course. In the "modern era," two large series showed that approximately 40% of patients pursued a monophasic course and the remainder had either a polycyclic or a chronic continuous course.[141,199] Using an aggressive early stepwise treatment approach, only 4% had a chronic disease course, suggesting that early control of muscle inflammation prevents long-term morbidity.[182]

The largest follow-up study included 490 patients from Europe and Latin America followed for a mean of 7.7 years seen between January 1980 and December 2004.[199] Reduced muscle strength and/or endurance were documented in 40% to 50%, although it was severe in less than 10% of patients. Persistent disease activity was noted in 40% to 60%. Cumulative damage occurred in 70%, primarily cutaneous. Decreased functional ability was reported in 40% and major impairment in 7%. A chronic course was the strongest predictor of poor prognosis.

There are a number of factors considered to predict a poor outcome including a delay in treatment or undertreatment,[181] chronic continuous course,[199] presence of rash and capillary nail-fold dropout at 6 months of treatment,[141] ulcerative skin disease, and abnormalities on initial muscle biopsy.[172] In addition, the presence of myositis-specific antibodies, unique HLA types, and the TNF polymorphism 308 may also determine a poorer outcome.

SCLERODERMA

The scleroderma disorders in children can be classified into systemic, localized, and others (Table 108-5). The systemic scleroses are rare in the pediatric age group and are outnumbered by the localized forms by approximately 10:1.

Systemic Sclerosis

Epidemiology

Juvenile systemic sclerosis (JSSc) makes up approximately 10% of all cases of systemic sclerosis[200]; the incidence rate in a recent U.K. study was reported as 0.27 per million children. Females outnumber males anywhere from 4:1[201] to 10:1.[202] The incidence seems to increase with increasing age,[200,203] although in one large multicenter review the mean age of onset was 8.1 years.[201] Diffuse disease is much more common than limited disease. An increased family history of autoimmune disease including scleroderma has been noted in some series.

Little work on etiology and pathogenesis has been done specifically in juvenile systemic sclerosis, and it is assumed to be identical to adult disease. The interested reader is referred to Chapter 83.

Clinical Features

The onset of diffuse systemic sclerosis is often insidious, and delay in diagnosis ranged from a median of 1 to 2.8 years in three large series.[200-202] The most common presenting features are Raynaud's phenomenon, skin edema, and sclerodactyly (Table 108-6). The diagnosis should be considered suspect in the absence of Raynaud's phenomenon.

Although skin edema is the earliest cutaneous abnormality, it is followed fairly quickly by induration, sclerodactyly, and loss of facial creases.

Table 108-5 Classification of Scleroderma in Childhood

Systemic Sclerosis
Diffuse
Limited
Overlap Syndromes
Mixed connective tissue disease
Overlap with features of SLE, JDM, and JIA
Localized Scleroderma*
Circumscribed morphea
Linear morphea
Generalized morphea
Pansclerotic morphea
Mixed morphea

*Proposed Pavia criteria.[215]
   JDM, juvenile dermatomyositis; JIA, juvenile idiopathic arthritis; SLE, systemic lupus erythematosus.

Table 108-6 Clinical Features at Diagnosis and during Course in 153 Patients with Juvenile Systemic Sclerosis from 55 Centers

Feature	% At Diagnosis	% During Course
Skin		
Edema	35	46
Sclerodactyly	46	66
Skin induration	74	76
Calcinosis	9	19
Peripheral Vascular		
Raynaud's phenomenon	75	84
Digital infarcts	19	29
Digital pitting	28	38
Abnormal capillaroscopy	25	52
Respiratory		
Dyspnea	10	18
Abnormal chest radiograph	12	29
Abnormal chest CT scan	5	23
Reduced DLco	8	27
Reduced FVC	11	42
Cardiac		
Pericarditis/arrhythmia	5	10
Heart failure	2	7
Pulmonary hypertension	1	7
Musculoskeletal		
Muscle weakness	12	24
Arthritis	17	27
Arthralgia	26	36
Tendon friction rubs	6	11
Gastrointestinal		
Dysphagia	10	24
Reflux	8	30
Diarrhea	2	10
Weight loss	18	27
Renal		
Raised creatinine/proteinuria	3	5
Renal crisis	0	1
Hypertension	1	3
Nervous System		
Seizures	1	3
Peripheral neuropathy	1	1
Abnormal brain MRI	2	3

CT, computed tomography; DLco, diffusing capacity for carbon monoxide; FVC, forced vital capacity.
   Modified from Martini G, Foeldvari I, Russo R: Systemic sclerosis in childhood: clinical and immunologic features of 153 patients in an international database, *Arthritis Rheum* 54:3971–3978, 2006.

Raynaud's phenomenon involves the distal extremities and rarely other acral areas such as the earlobes and tip of the nose. Occasionally it may lead to digital infarcts resulting in pitting or more significant gangrenous change. Capillary nail-fold abnormalities, visible either to the naked eye or by capillary microscopy, have been reported in at least 50% of patients and include areas of dropout and abnormal capillaries with dilatation and tortuosity.

Abnormalities of the musculoskeletal system include mild inflammatory synovitis, which is nonerosive; joint contractures most commonly resulting from skin and subcutaneous tightness around the joints; and myositis. In patients with overlap syndromes the muscle involvement is more significant. Otherwise scleroderma myositis is generally quite mild. Tendon friction rubs may be felt or heard in a minority of patients.

Involvement of the respiratory system has become the most significant cause of morbidity and mortality in patients with systemic sclerosis. Early changes may be documented by high-resolution computed tomography, although this may not offer much greater benefit than well-performed pulmonary function tests (PFTs).[204] It is important to document the pulmonary status early in the disease process because it is only then, before irreversible fibrosis occurs, that reversal of abnormalities may be possible. Pulmonary function abnormalities include a reduced forced vital capacity, a reduced FEV_1-to–forced vital capacity (FVC), and a reduced DLco. Severe chest wall involvement with restriction of movement may also lead to abnormal PFTs. Early CT changes include a ground-glass appearance suggestive of alveolitis.[205] Rarely, pleural effusions may occur. Cardiac involvement includes pericarditis (which may be asymptomatic), arrhythmia, and congestive heart failure (CHF). Pulmonary arterial hypertension may develop in the face of severe lung disease. Cardiac disease (resulting primarily from CHF) was the most common cause of mortality in one series of 135 patients with juvenile systemic sclerosis.[206]

Involvement of the GI system is common with symptoms of dysphagia and gastroesophageal reflux. More diffuse involvement can lead to reduced GI motility with bacterial overgrowth resulting in malabsorption. Severe constipation may occasionally occur. Renal involvement is much less common in juvenile than adult scleroderma and can include proteinuria, hypertension, and the eventual development of renal crisis. Neurologic involvement is unusual but can include seizure, stroke, and peripheral neuropathy.

Diagnosis and Diagnostic Tests

The diagnosis of systemic sclerosis rests on the presenting signs and symptoms and the investigation of organs that may be affected by the process. Seventy-five to 97% of patients were antinuclear antibody positive in three series.[200-202] Specific autoantibodies include anti-topoisomerase in approximately 33%, anticentromere antibody in less than 10%, and autoantibodies associated with overlap syndromes (anti-PM-Scl, anti-U1-RNP, anti-Ro) in a smaller number depending on the series. Rheumatoid factor may be present in up to 20% of patients.

Skin biopsy is rarely performed. Pathologic findings include dense collagenization and loss of adnexal structures. An inflammatory infiltrate composed primarily of mononuclear and mast cells is seen early in the course.

It is important to investigate the various organ systems that may be involved by systemic sclerosis in order to help prognosticate and develop an appropriate management plan. Investigations should include, at a minimum, PFTs with a DLco, an electrocardiogram, an echocardiogram, and a chest radiograph. For patients unable to perform PFTs, high-resolution CT scan is indicated. This is also indicated in patients with abnormal PFTs to detect early alveolitis. Serum KL-6 is a mucin-like glycoprotein strongly expressed in type II pneumocytes and may be a useful noninvasive marker of pulmonary fibrosis in children with JSSc.[207]

It can be assumed that most patients have GI involvement and that an upper GI series will be abnormal. This test is indicated for patients with severe pain unresponsive to standard agents and severe dysphagia. Hydrogen breath test and measuring fat-soluble vitamins may be helpful in patients with suspected malabsorption. Radiographs of the hands may be helpful in showing distal acro-osteolysis in patients with severe Raynaud's phenomenon and occasionally may show calcinosis.

When patients present with Raynaud's phenomenon, capillary nail-fold abnormalities, and edematous or indurated skin, the diagnosis is clear and the differential diagnosis is limited. However, patients are often seen early in the course with just Raynaud's phenomenon and a positive ANA. In those situations the most important differential diagnoses to consider are systemic lupus erythematosus, overlap syndrome/mixed connective tissue disease, and juvenile dermatomyositis. Although many other diseases are associated with skin fibrosis, they are not associated with the characteristic multisystem involvement as systemic sclerosis and should not pose a diagnostic challenge.

Provisional classification criteria have been developed and accepted by the Pediatric Rheumatology European Society (PReS), ACR, and EULAR on the basis of a Delphi survey and nominal group techniques.[208] These were proposed because current criteria had not been studied in children and are not sensitive enough to detect early disease. Furthermore, they do not include key features of early disease such as Raynaud's phenomenon, ANA positivity, and capillary nail-fold changes. The proposed criteria are listed in Table 108-7. The presence of the one major and at least two minor criteria in a patient younger than 16 years classifies the patient as having juvenile systemic sclerosis, with a sensitivity of 90% and a specificity of 96%.

Treatment

The approach to the management of patients with systemic sclerosis should include treating the basic disease process itself, as well as the various organ manifestations. No controlled studies exist in children, and data must be extrapolated from the adult literature. The EULAR Scleroderma Trials and Research Group has made recommendations regarding management of patients with systemic sclerosis, and they should be considered for all patients.[209] Because no specific treatment studies have been reported in children and adolescents, the reader is referred to Chapter 84 for a discussion of treatment where the same principles hold. It should be noted that for patients with rapidly progressive disease and progressive lung disease, autologous stem cell transplantation may provide the only opportunity for survival and has been successful in a number of patients with juvenile systemic sclerosis.[210]

Outcome

Very little long-term outcome data are available for JSSc. Morbidity is substantial from the multisystem involvement with marked impact on the quality of life. The survival rates in juvenile systemic sclerosis are better than adult disease. Mortality in three large series varied from 12% to 30%.[200,201,203] The most common causes of death include

Table 108-7 Provisional Criteria for the Classification of Juvenile Systemic Sclerosis (SSc)

Major Criterion (Required)
Proximal skin sclerosis/induration of the skin
Minor Criteria (At Least 2 Required)
Cutaneous
Sclerodactyly
Peripheral Vascular
Raynaud's phenomenon
Nail-fold capillary abnormalities
Digital tip ulcers
Gastrointestinal
Dysphagia
Gastroesophageal reflux
Cardiac
Arrhythmias
Heart failure
Renal
Renal crisis
New-onset arterial hypertension
Respiratory
Pulmonary fibrosis (HRCT/radiography)
Decreased DLco
Pulmonary arterial hypertension
Neurologic
Neuropathy
Carpal tunnel syndrome
Musculoskeletal
Tendon friction rubs
Arthritis
Myositis
Serologic
Antinuclear antibodies
SSc-selective autoantibodies (anticentromere, anti-topoisomerase I [Scl-70], antifibrillarin, anti-PM-Scl, antifibrillin or anti-RNA polymerase I or III)

DLco, diffusing capacity for carbon monoxide; HRCT, high-resolution computed tomography.

The presence of the 1 major and at least 2 minor criteria in a patient younger than 16 years classifies the patient as having juvenile systemic sclerosis, with a sensitivity of 90% and a specificity of 96%.

From Zulian F, Woo P, Athreya BH, et al: The Pediatric Rheumatology European Society/American College of Rheumatology/European League Against Rheumatism provisional classification criteria for juvenile systemic sclerosis, *Arthritis Rheum* 57:203–212, 2007.

cardiac (including pulmonary arterial hypertension) and respiratory failure. Factors considered to be significant predictors of mortality include fibrosis on chest radiograph, raised creatinine levels, and pericarditis, whereas a short disease duration at diagnosis may confer protection.[211]

Localized Scleroderma

Epidemiology

Localized scleroderma (LSc), also known as *morphea*, had a reported incidence of 2.7 per 100,000 of the general population in the Mayo Clinic series,[212] and 3.4 per million children in the United Kingdom,[213] making it much more common than systemic sclerosis in the pediatric age group. The female-to-male ratio is approximately 2:1, and the average age of onset is approximately 7 years. Mild lesions may never get to medical attention, so the incidence may be even higher. Congenital morphea has been reported.[214] Several classification schemes have been developed; the proposed Pavia criteria are listed in Table 108-5.[215]

Linear lesions are more common in the pediatric age group.[213,216-218]

Etiology and Pathogenesis

Like systemic sclerosis, it is likely that environmental factors trigger immune activation leading ultimately to fibrosis. There have been no genetic studies to date to suggest that the HLA or non-HLA systems play a role, although those studies are under way. Familial occurrence is uncommon, but there is a strong family history of other autoimmune disorders.[216,219] Trauma has been considered as a possible inciting feature.[220] *Borrelia* infections have been implicated in Europe but not in North America. The presence of elevated levels of serum cytokines (such as TNF and interleukin [IL]-1) that may influence fibroblast proliferation provide strong evidence for the role of immune activation in disease pathogenesis.[221] Microchimerism has been reported, and as with other connective tissue diseases it suggests that mechanisms similar to graft-versus-host disease also may play a role. Several drugs and toxins may lead to cutaneous fibrosis, although none has been consistently identified in patients with LSc.

Clinical Features

There is usually a delay in presentation of several months because the lesions themselves are typically not symptomatic. Active circumscribed (Figure 108-5A) and linear lesions (Figure 108-5B) usually have a shiny, waxy appearance surrounded by a violaceous, erythematous border. They may be warmer than the surrounding and contralateral skin. Rarely there may be local itching or tingling. The lesions are indurated, and they may be either superficial or can extend to muscle and bone. Occasionally with linear lesions, extensive fascial involvement may occur. Lesions heal with hyperpigmentation or hypopigmentation and generally soften with time. Atrophy of the subcutaneous tissues is common. Linear lesions, if untreated, may result in growth deformity, joint contracture, loss of muscle bulk, and marked extremity weakness.

Lesions on the face and head can take the form of either a "saber-cut"–like lesion (en coup de sabre) or progressive hemifacial atrophy (also known as *Parry-Romberg syndrome*), where the epidermal changes are minimal but there is marked dermal and subcutaneous atrophy (Figure 108-5C). These may coexist in the same patient. With time, as the unaffected side of the face grows normally, there is progression of the facial asymmetry even though the disease may be inactive. Facial lesions may be associated with hemiatrophy of the tongue (Figure 108-5D), dental abnormalities, and ocular abnormalities. A small number of children develop seizures.[222]

Pansclerotic morphea is rare but can be life threatening. There is marked thickening of the skin and deeper tissues involving the extremities and trunk, sparing the distal extremities. Although it is similar to systemic sclerosis in the extent of the fibrosis, internal organ involvement does not occur and Raynaud's phenomenon is not common.

Extracutaneous signs and symptoms have been reported in up to 20% of patients.[216] They are more common in patients with linear lesions. The most common is arthritis,

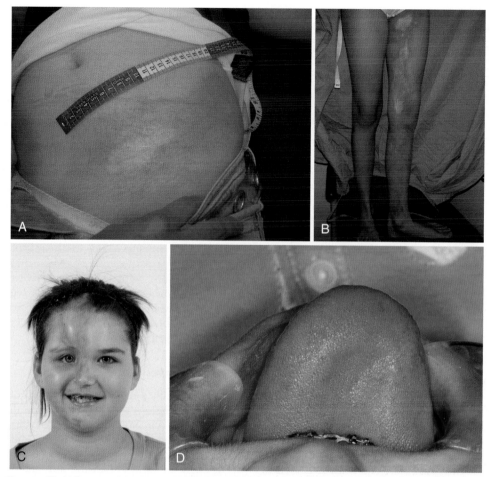

Figure 108-5 **A,** Circumscribed/plaque morphea on the abdomen of a 5-year-old girl with localized scleroderma. Note the central ivory-colored area of induration surrounded by intense erythema indicative of an active lesion. **B,** Linear localized scleroderma involving the inner aspect of the left leg of an 11-year-old girl. Note areas of porcelain-white lesions surrounded by erythema. **C,** A 10-year-old girl with a history of linear scleroderma of the face with both en coup de sabre and Parry-Romberg lesions of 7 years' duration. Note frontal alopecia and two bands of linear scleroderma on the right side of the forehead and face. There is hyperpigmentation and marked subcutaneous atrophy. Note also the loss of eyebrow and eyelashes on the right, small right nares, and thin lips on the right. **D,** Same patient as in **C** showing atrophy of the tongue.

not necessarily associated in the area of skin involvement. It is seen more commonly in patients with a positive rheumatoid factor. Neurologic manifestations of seizure and headache occur almost exclusively in patients with facial lesions. Ocular abnormalities including asymptomatic anterior uveitis were reported in 3% of one large series.[223]

Diagnosis and Diagnostic Tests

The diagnosis of LSc is usually made on the basis of characteristic cutaneous features. A skin biopsy can be of assistance when the diagnosis is not clear. Abnormalities consist of edema, an early infiltration by mononuclear cells, and excessive deposition of collagen. With time there is loss of skin appendages and rete pegs. Other skin diseases that may have a similar clinical presentation include lichen sclerosis et atrophicus, connective tissue nevus, collagenoma, and localized fibrotic disorders. The absence of significant internal organ involvement and Raynaud's phenomenon help differentiate LSc from systemic sclerosis and other autoimmune conditions.

Laboratory investigations are nonspecific and show mild or no systemic inflammation (ESR, CRP). Eosinophilia and

hypergammaglobulinemia have been reported to correlate with active lesions,[224] but this is not always the case. Rheumatoid factor is present in 10% to 25% and ANA positivity in approximately 50% of cases. Multiple specific autoantibodies have been reported, but antibodies to topoisomerase-I and centromere are distinctly unusual.[221,225]

Treatment

The treatment of localized scleroderma depends on the stage of the lesion, as well as the extent of involvement. Few controlled studies have been done; therefore treatment recommendations have relied on general experience. Plaque lesions can generally be treated topically with either corticosteroids and/or calcipotriene.[226] Markedly indurated lesions may respond better to imiquimod.[227] Topical tacrolimus may also be used. Systemic treatment is usually indicated for rapidly progressive lesions, for lesions crossing joint lines, and for lesions that are potentially cosmetically deforming. A combination of corticosteroids and MTX is generally recommended.[228-231] Corticosteroids may be administered as monthly pulses or orally in a dose of 1 to 2 mg/kg with a taper over 3 to 6 months. MTX is administered at a dose of up to 1 mg/kg or 15 mg/m² weekly. At higher doses, the subcutaneous route is probably more effective. Treatment should be administered for at least 2 years, and 1 year after all activity has disappeared because there is about a 30% chance of recurrence if treatment is stopped too early. MMF may be used for patients who have not responded to this combination.[232] Imatininb, cyclosporine A, and tacrolimus have also been effective in a small number of cases. Ultraviolet A therapy is used more frequently in Europe with good success.[233] Autologous stem cell transplantation may be required for patients with pansclerotic morphea.

Patients with facial lesions have undergone cosmetic repair with generally good outcomes.[234] Surgery may also be required to lengthen Achilles tendons.

In addition to medical and surgical treatment, a combined team approach is often required for patients with more extensive disease. Physical and occupational therapy are essential in improving and maintaining muscle strength, range of motion, and function. Psychosocial support is especially helpful for patients with facial lesions. Other medical personnel whose involvement may be required are neurologists, ophthalmologists, craniofacial surgeons, orthopedic surgeons, dentists, and orthodontists.

Disease Monitoring

To date, it has been difficult to monitor the course of the disease as clinicians have relied on insensitive measures such as warmth, color change, and change in size over time. Recently, some more objective measures have been studied including ultrasound,[235] computerized skin score,[236] and laser Doppler flow.[237] A disease activity score has recently been developed,[238] and initial validation of a disease damage score has been undertaken.[239] CARRA is currently establishing scores for activity and damage.

Outcome

Lesions tend to soften spontaneously over several years and to heal with pigmentary change (usually hyperpigmentation) and subcutaneous atrophy. Linear limb lesions may lead to marked atrophy and joint contracture. Lesions may recur after many years of apparent inactivity. Neither self-esteem nor health-related quality of life appear to be diminished compared with controls, although not many patients with more disfiguring lesions were studied.[240-242] Rarely patients have developed other autoimmune connective tissue disorders including systemic sclerosis and SLE. Patients with pediatric onset of LSc have a higher incidence of autoimmune disorders as adults.[243]

Eosinophilic Fasciitis

Eosinophilic fasciitis (EF) is included by some within the classification of localized scleroderma,[212] and several authors have reported that children with EF have a disease evolution to morphea.[244,245] EF is extremely rare in the pediatric population. Affected children present with marked induration of cutaneous and subcutaneous tissues of the upper or lower extremities and occasionally the trunk or face. Its onset may be preceded by intense exercise. Raynaud's phenomenon, internal organ involvement, and nail-fold capillary abnormalities are rare but may occur.[246]

Mixed Connective Tissue Disease

Mixed connective tissue disease (MCTD) was initially reported as a disorder associated with a favorable prognosis and an excellent initial response to low-dose glucocorticoid therapy. It had a frequency of 0.3% in the U.S. Pediatric Rheumatology Database. Children present with arthritis, myositis, and cutaneous disease characteristic of scleroderma, SLE, or JDM.[247] A decrease in aerobic capacity may occur from reduced muscle strength.[248] Progression to a more scleroderma-like disease has occurred, with sclerodactyly and GI involvement, or an SLE-like disease may evolve.[249-251] Nephritis may be more frequent and more severe in children than in adults. Children often have less pulmonary disease (hypertension) and more hematologic complications (thrombocytopenia) than adults. ANAs are present in high titers, often in a speckled pattern, to an extractable nuclear antigen and ribonuclear protein (RNP).

VASCULITIS

Vasculitis is a common clinical phenomenon in children. Vasculitis can occur in association with infections, medications, hypersensitivity reactions, and in the context of childhood systemic rheumatic diseases such as lupus. The most common primary or idiopathic vasculitis types are Henoch-Schönlein purpura (HSP)[252] and Kawasaki disease (KD).[253] Incidences of vasculitis subtype vary widely depending on characteristics of populations such as ethnicity and the method of ascertainment.

Similar to adults, childhood vasculitis is categorized by predominantly affected vessel size as small, medium, or large vessel vasculitis.[254] The histopathologic characteristics vary between diseases and include karyorhexis, neutrophilic infiltration and necrosis, giant cell formation, and lymphocyte infiltrates. In 2005 a classification system for childhood vasculitis was proposed.[255] In 2008 the so-called "EULAR/PReS endorsed consensus criteria for childhood vasculitis" were validated.[256,257]

Small Vessel Vasculitis

Inflammation of the small vessels is the most common vasculitis subtype in children. Typically exposure to infectious agents, medications, hypersensitivity such as serum sickness, or systemic illness can cause migration of neutrophils through the vessel wall, leukocytoclasis, and fibrinoid necroses. The resulting histologic diagnosis of leukocytoclastic vasculitis is a common result found on superficial punch biopsies done for suspected vasculitis. Additional immunofluorescence studies may reveal immunoglobulin (Ig) deposits along the vessel wall, evidence of immune complexes and/or complement activation. Deposition of IgA is the hallmark of HSP.

Henoch-Schönlein Purpura

HSP (or anaphylactoid purpura) is an IgA-mediated small vessel vasculitis predominantly affecting the skin and causing a palpable purpura. Histologically, a leukocytoclastic vasculitis with extravasation of leukocytes and red cells, vessel wall damage, fibrinoid necrosis, and IgA1 deposition at the vessel wall and in the mesangium of the kidney can be found.[258] Preceding upper respiratory tract infections are reported in more than 50% of children. A variety of bacterial and viral triggers, environmental stimuli, and host susceptibility factors such as autoinflammatory disease genes have been reported.[259-262] HSP can occur before or during the course of systemic diseases such as antineutrophil cytoplasm antibody (ANCA) vasculitis or Crohn's disease.[263]

IgA appears to play a pivotal role in the pathogenesis of HSP. Abnormal glycosylation of the hinge region O-linked glycan of IgA1 has been implicated in the etiopathology of HSP: Abnormal IgA1 molecules were found to have a higher tendency to aggregate, interact with IgG, and form IgA-IgG complexes and deposits in the kidney.[258,264] Similarly, serum levels of galactose-deficient IgA1 are elevated in Caucasian and Asian patients with IgA nephropathy.[265] Schmitt demonstrated deposits of IgA-binding streptococcal M protein in the skin and kidney of HSP patients directly linking infection and vasculitis.[266] Wu studied the role of leukotrienes and suggested that abnormally high levels of leukotriene B$_4$ and lipoxin A4, potent activators of neutrophils, found in HSP patients with nephritis differentiate them from those without nephritis.[267]

Definition and Classification. HSP is the most common defined childhood small vessel vasculitis characterized by the classic triad of palpable purpura, arthritis, and abdominal pain. In 2006 EULAR/PReS-endorsed consensus criteria for HSP were proposed (Table 108-8). The sensitivity of these criteria was found to be 100%, the specificity 87%.[257]

Epidemiology. Overall the incidence of HSP is estimated at 10 to 20 per 100,000 children younger than 17 years old.[268-271] Boys are more commonly affected than girls; the male-to-female ratio was recently reported at 1.8:1.[272] Gardner-Medwin reported an annual incidence of 70.3 per 100,000 between the ages of 4 and 6 years in a population-based study.[269] In contrast, HSP is a rare disease in adults but may have a severe course and poor renal outcome.[273]

Clinical Presentation. Purpura is the leading symptom of HSP. In a recent Italian study purpura was present in all

Table 108-8 European League Against Rheumatism/Pediatric Rheumatology European Society Endorsed Consensus Criteria for the Classification of Childhood Vasculitides[257]

Vasculitis Type	Classification Criteria
Predominant Small Vessel Vasculitis	

Henoch-Schönlein purpura	Palpable purpura (mandatory criterion) plus at least one of:
	  Diffuse abdominal pain
	  Any biopsy showing predominant IgA deposition
	  Arthritis or arthralgia (acute, any joint)
	  Renal involvement (any hematuria and/or proteinuria)

Childhood granulomatosis with polyangiitis[296]	At least 3 of the following 6 criteria must be present:
	  Abnormal urinalysis (hematuria and/or significant proteinuria)
	  Granulomatous inflammation on biopsy (if a kidney biopsy is done it
	    characteristically shows pauci-immune necrotizing glomerulonephritis)
	  Nasal sinus inflammation
	  Subglottic, tracheal, or endobronchial stenosis
	  Abnormal chest radiograph or computed tomography
	  Proteinase 3 ANCAs or c-ANCA staining (sensitivity/specificity calculated for *any*
	    positive ANCA)

Childhood microscopic polyangiitis	No proposed criteria; for description see text
Childhood Churg-Strauss syndrome	No proposed criteria; for description see text
Predominant Medium Vessel Vasculitis	

Childhood (systemic) polyarteritis nodosa	Biopsy evidence of necrotizing vasculitis *or* angiographic abnormalities (mandatory
	    criterion) plus at least one of:
	  Skin involvement (livedo reticularis, tender subcutaneous nodules, other vasculitic
	    lesions, superficial or deep infarctions)
	  Myalgia or muscle tenderness
	  Systolic/diastolic hypertension (>95th percentile)
	  Mononeuropathy or polyneuropathy
	  Renal involvement (proteinuria, hematuria, impaired renal function)

Childhood cutaneous polyarteritis nodosa	No proposed criteria; for description see text
Predominant Large Vessel Vasculitis	

Childhood Takayasu's arteritis	Angiography of the aorta or its main branches and pulmonary arteries showing
	    aneurysms/dilatation, occlusion or thickened arterial wall not due to
	    fibromuscular dysplasia (mandatory criterion) plus at least 1 of:
	  Pulse deficit or claudication
	  Blood pressure discrepancy (>10 mm Hg)
	  Bruits
	  Hypertension
	  Acute-phase reactant (erythrocyte sedimentation rate >20 mm/hr, C-reactive
	    protein abnormal)

ANCA, antineutrophil cytoplasm antibody; c-ANCA, cytoplasmic antineutrophil cytoplasm antibody.

cases, arthritis/arthralgias in 74%, abdominal symptoms in 51% including intussusception in 0.6%, renal disease in 54% including severe nephropathy in 7%, and acute renal failure in 2%.[272] Scrotal edema was reported in 13%. Correspondingly, Dolezalova and colleagues[270] described purpura present in 100% of Czech HSP patients; arthritis/arthralgia in 52%; abdominal pain and/or GI bleeding in 40%; hematuria/proteinuria in 15%; and genital involvement in 2.8%. Eye findings including anterior uveitis can be seen in HSP patients.[274]

Skin disease in HSP has a characteristic appearance: Petechial or palpable purpuric lesions are located on dependent areas including lower legs and feet, buttocks, and arms. Lesions can have different sizes and stages ranging from fresh petechial rashes to confluent bruises. An associated edema is commonly found, hands and feet appear puffy, and scrotal edema may be present in boys. Children younger than 2 years have been reported to have more significant edema. Lesions occur in waves, and skin disease in HSP is reported to last from 4 to 8 weeks.[272]

HSP arthritis is often painful, nonerosive, and nonmigratory. Ankles, knees, hands, and wrists are most commonly inflamed. Arthralgias are found in a similar distribution. GI symptoms are common in HSP patients including intermittent abdominal discomfort, pain, and vomiting. Abdominal complications including intussusception are rare; however, they always have to be considered when a child presents with HSP features and complains of abdominal pain and possibly associated bloody stools. Oftentimes bowel wall thickening on ultrasound is detected.

Overall renal disease in HSP occurs in 40% to 50% of children and manifests itself as microscopic hematuria or low-grade proteinuria, which completely resolves in the vast majority.[275] Older children may be at higher risk for nephritis.[276] Overall progression to end-stage renal disease occurs in 1% to 3% of children.[277] Renal biopsies are done in children with renal compromise and histologically demonstrate IgA nephropathy.[275] The degree of damage on renal biopsy and the degree of proteinuria predicts poor outcome.[278] Reported 10-year renal survival rates for children undergoing renal biopsies for HSP ranged from 73% to 90%.[279,280] Though uncommon in HSP, overall IgA nephropathy and HSP nephritis represent the most common chronic glomerulonephritis in childhood.[277]

Diagnosis and Diagnostic Tests. Children with HSP may have a raised erythrocyte sedimentation rate (ESR) (57%), elevated serum IgA (37%), and proteinuria (42%).[272] All children require serial urinalyses. Jauhola and colleagues[276] demonstrated that HSP nephritis occurred on average 14 days after HSP diagnosis, and within 1 month in the majority of cases. The risk of developing HSP nephritis after 2 months was 2%. Laboratory tests or blood pressure measurement at onset did not predict the occurrence of nephritis. Overall specific diagnostic markers of HSP are not readily available. Alternative complement pathway markers including activated C3 and C4 were reported in children and adults and may be associated with disease progression.[275] Urinary proteomic patterns and serum levels of galactose-deficient IgA1 are promising and are currently being studied.[281]

Skin biopsies are done to confirm the diagnosis of HSP and to exclude differential diagnoses. Overlapping clinical features may be found in infection, inflammation or medication associated leukocytoclastic vasculitis, rheumatic fever, poststreptococcal glomerulonephritis, lupus, and systemic vasculitis.[282,283] Renal biopsies are performed in a select group of HSP patients.[275]

Treatment. In most children HSP is a benign disease and does not require specific therapy. There is significant variation demonstrated for inpatient therapy and evaluation of children with HSP, which may contribute to varying clinical outcomes.[284] Immunosuppressive therapy of HSP targets severe disease presentations including nephritis and gastrointestinal vasculitis. In 2006, Ronkainen and co-workers published a randomized placebo-controlled trial demonstrating that prednisone reduces the severitiy of joint and abdominal pain, while having no effect on purpura, prevention of nephritis, or recurrence of HSP.[285] A recent retrospective cohort study of 1895 children discharged with HSP between 2000 and 2007 from 36 tertiary care children's hospitals in the United States determined that early corticosteroid treatment was associated with significantly less abdominal surgery, endoscopy, and abdominal imaging during hospitalization suggesting a protective effect of corticosteroid therapy for abdominal complications of HSP.[286] In contrast, a prospective study from Finland reported that corticosteroids although alleviating clinical symptoms, did not alter the clinical course of HSP during 6 months of follow-up. Prednisone prophylaxis did not affect the timing of the appearance of nephritis.[276] The addition of cyclophosphamide did not show a benefit in adults with HSP nephritis in a small trial.[287] A stepwise approach is often used, including the use of nonsteroidal anti-inflammatory medication for mild HSP, corticosteroids for moderate to severe HSP, and addition of angiotensin-converting enzyme (ACE) inhibitors for nephritis. Evidence is emerging that treatment with high-dose IV pulse methylprednisolone coupled with azathioprine or cyclophosphamide may be beneficial in patients with severe nephritis.[288] Cyclosporine also has been successfully used for severe nephritis.[289]

Outcome. In the majority of children HSP is a self-limiting disease, which resolves within 4 to 6 weeks.[258] Patients with microscopic hematuria and trivial proteinuria have an excellent prognosis.[290] In contrast, 30% of pediatric HSP patient with nephritis will have renal impairment and 5% will develop end-stage renal disease.[291] Recurrence of HSP is seen in a third of patients; symptoms resolve within 4 to 6 weeks in the majority of patients. Children older than 8 years of age and those with nephritis are significantly more likely to experience recurrences.[292]

Antineutrophil Cytoplasm Antibody Vasculitis

The group of childhood systemic vasculitides associated with ANCA include granulomatosis with polyangiitis (GPA; formerly known as Wegener's granulomatosis), microscopic polyangiitis (mPA), and Churg-Strauss syndrome (CSS). The conceptual framework provided by the Chapel Hill Consensus Conference on the Nomenclature of Systemic Vasculitis is commonly accepted for childhood ANCA vasculitis. Necrotizing small vessel vasculitis of venules, capillaries, arterioles, and small arteries is the hallmark of ANCA vasculitis. Pathogenetic studies were not primarily done in children and are therefore not covered here. Pauci-immune necrotizing and crescentic glomerulonephritis, as well as hemorrhagic pulmonary capillaritis, frequently present as pulmonary-renal syndrome. Limited phenotypes including pauci-immune glomerulonephritis with ANCA and nonrenal, upper respiratory tract, or limited GPA are commonly included in the group of ANCA vasculitides of children and adults.[293] These diseases are rare in childhood. However, recent collaborative efforts such as "A Registry for Childhood Vasculitis (ARChiVe)" have substantially increased the knowledge and understanding of childhood ANCA vasculitis.[257,294,295]

Definition and Classification

Granulomatosis with Polyangiitis. The proposed EULAR/PReS-endorsed consensus criteria for GPA are shown in Table 108-8.[296] The sensitivity as determined in the validation process described earlier was found to be 93.3%, and the specificity was 99.2%, when including evidence of *any* ANCA. Cabral and colleagues[294] have recently validated the proposed criteria in a large multicenter cohort of children with systemic vasculitis (no HSP) and determined a diagnostic sensitivity of 73.6% and specificity of 73.2%.

Microscopic Polyangiitis. In children, MPA is a rare diagnosis.[294] No formal classification criteria were proposed for MPA in children by the "EULAR conference expert group." Instead, the existing Chapel Hill description was modified by formally adding ANCA.[296]

Churg-Strauss Syndrome. CSS (allergic granulomatosis) is even less common than MPA in children. No pediatric classification criteria exist, and therefore adult ACR criteria are commonly applied.[297] The pediatric literature is limited to case reports and small series.[298,299] A recent literature review identified a total of 33 children with a female predominance (male-to-female ratio, 0.74) with a mean age of 12 years.[300] All patients had significant asthma and histologic evidence of eosinophilia and/or vasculitis. ANCAs were only found in 25%. Children with CSS typically present with a necrotizing vasculitis affecting the lungs, GI system, peripheral nerves, heart, skin, and kidneys along with a history of severe asthma, other allergic symptoms, and peripheral and tissue eosinophilia.[301]

Epidemiology

Childhood ANCA vasculitis is a rare group of diseases.[302] In Southern Alberta, Canada, the average annual incidence of GPA in children was estimated at 2.75 cases per million per year, with a steep increase over the past 5 years to 6.39 cases per million per year.[303] A recent study from Japan reported the adult MPA incidence at 14.8 per million, whereas GPA was present in 2 per million adult patients.[304] Within the group of ANCA vasculitis, MPA may be more common than GPA in adults, while it is definitely less common in children.[294,305] However, Reinhold-Keller and associates suggested that the incidence of GPA of all age groups was two to three times greater than those of MPA and CSS. There was no regional difference in incidence rates found.[306] Girls are consistently more commonly affected than boys; the male-to-female ratio is reported to be 1:3 to 4.[307]

Clinical Presentation

The clinical presentation of ANCA vasculitis is widely overlapping.[308] In children, GPA and MPA patients are commonly reported in combined series. In the largest single-center cohort of 25 children,[309] the median duration of symptoms before establishing the diagnosis was 2 months. Children presented most frequently with constitutional symptoms (96%) and glomerulonephritis (88%) with renal failure in half. Recovery from renal failure was uncommon (1/11). Upper airway disease was present in 84% including one child with subglottic stenosis. Overall, 80% had pulmonary involvement at diagnosis, most commonly nodules (44%) and pulmonary hemorrhage (44%). Five children with pulmonary hemorrhage required ventilation, and four children had venous thrombotic events.[309] The ARChiVe group reported 117 pediatric patients including GPA (n = 76), microscopic polyangiitis (n = 17), ANCA-positive pauci-immune glomerulonephritis (n = 5), CSS (n = 2), and unclassified vasculitis (n = 17). In the 65 of 76 who met ACR criteria for GPA, the median interval from symptom onset to diagnosis was 2.7 months (range, 0 to 49 months). The most frequently presenting features by organ system were constitutional (89%); pulmonary (80%); ear, nose, and throat (80%); and renal (75%).[294] Zwerina and co-workers suggested that children compared with adults with CSS had a predominance of cardiopulmonary disease manifestations, less peripheral nerve involvement, and higher mortality.[300]

Diagnosis and Diagnostic Tests

Raised inflammatory markers including ESR and CRP, leukocytosis, and positive ANCAs are commonly found at diagnosis of ANCA vasculitis.[294,309] Akikusa and colleagues[309] documented ANCA positivity in 22 of 25 children. Cabral and co-workers identified cytoplasmic ANCA (c-ANCA) positivity in 66% of pediatric GPA patients, 93% of whom were anti-PR3 positive on enzyme-linked immunosorbent assay. Accordingly, 22% were perinuclear ANCA (p-ANCA) positive, of which 21% had anti-PR3 and 57% anti-MPO specificity.[294]

Endothelial cell markers including von Willebrand factor antigen, antiendothelial cell antibodies, and circulating endothelial cells are potential biomarkers.[310-312] Disease activity and damage tools are currently being developed based on modifications of the available adult vasculitis measures.

Treatment

The treatment of ANCA vasculitis in children is grounded in knowledge gained from studies in adults. No randomized trials or prospective observational studies are available in children. The recently reported EULAR recommendations for management of vasculitis synthesize the available evidence.[313,314] Children commonly receive induction therapy with cyclophosphamide and high-dose corticosteroids for severe disease, followed by a combination maintenance regimen with either MTX or azathioprine plus low-dose corticosteroids.[294,309] Children with limited disease may be primarily treated with MTX and corticosteroids.[294] In contrast, the initial treatment of CSS in children was corticosteroid monotherapy in 76% (n = 33), while only 24% received combination immunosuppressive therapy. In a retrospective series, Wright and Dillon[315] reported that therapeutic plasma exchange may be of benefit during the acute phase of childhood systemic vasculitis. New drugs including rituximab and other biologic therapies are increasingly used in children.[316] Supportive therapy regimens such as ACE inhibitors and antibiotic prophylaxis vary and have not been systematically studied in children with ANCA vasculitis.[317]

Outcome

ANCA vasculitis is a relapsing/remitting chronic disease in children and adults. Phillip and Luqmani[318] calculated overall 5-year survival rates for GPA of all ages at 75%, MPA at 45% to 75%, and CSS at 68% to 100% at 5 years. The pediatric CSS literature review captured six deaths (18%), all related to the underlying disease, occurring after a mean disease duration of 14 months.[300] Mortality rates may be falling as a result of more effective intervention, but they remain elevated substantially in severe disease. Early deaths were attributed to active disease (multiorgan failure, infection). Late deaths reflected the cumulative burden of disease and treatment in addition to comorbidities.[318]

Disease activity has consistently been reported to be high at diagnosis of ANCA vasculitis in children.[294,309] Risk factors associated with mortality or morbidity remain to be identified in children.

Medium-Sized Vessel Vasculitis

KD, polyarteritis nodosa (PAN), and cutaneous PAN are characterized by medium-sized muscular artery inflammation. KD is the most common cause of acquired heart disease in Western countries. Vessel wall histology on autopsies was recently reported to demonstrate a proliferative, granulomatous process with accumulation of monocytes/macrophages and rare occurrence of fibrinoid necrosis.[319] KD is a monophasic inflammatory disease that leads to transient coronary artery lesions in 20% to 25% of children, while coronary artery damage (e.g., aneurysms, stenoses) is found in 5 to 8% of treated patients.[253,320] In contrast, PAN is a rare disease, with difficult-to-control chronic disease activity, and high morbidity and mortality rates.[321] Biopsy specimens demonstrate systemic transmural necrotizing vasculitis. Cutaneous PAN has a similar histology; however, in general it has a less severe disease course.[322]

Kawasaki Disease

Kawasaki disease (KD) is better classified as an inflammatory "syndrome." Infectious triggers and possibly other environmental factors lead to a stereotypical inflammatory process in a susceptible host.[323,324] Host susceptibility clearly differs between ethnic groups. This may be related to genetic polymorphisms of proinflammatory genes such as the signal transduction caspase-3 gene *CASP3* or the *ITPKC* gene, which encodes a regulator of T cell activation.[325,326]

Genes involved in vascular remodeling such as matrix metalloproteinases may confer an increased risk of vessel damage and aneurysm formation.[327]

Definition and Classification. The diagnosis of KD remains grounded in recognition of a clinical pattern: Children, in whom the diagnosis of typical KD is made, present with a minimum of 5 days of fever plus at least four of five criteria including oral changes of cracked lips/strawberry tongue (as seen in 94%), bilateral nonpurulent conjunctivitis (92%), rash (90%), erythema and/or swelling of hands and/or feet (77%), and cervical lymphadenopathy (64%).[328]

The diagnosis of KD is more challenging in children with incomplete clinical features. In 2004 the American Heart Association (AHA) proposed an algorithm for diagnosing and treating suspected incomplete KD.[329] Yellen and coworkers tested the performance in a retrospective multicenter series of 195 patients with KD and coronary artery aneurysms. The authors demonstrated that applying the AHA algorithm would have significantly increased the rate of IVIG treatment from 70% (classic KD criteria) to 97%[330] and possibly prevented aneurysms. Similarly, Heuclin and colleagues recently demonstrated a significantly increased detection rate of KD—in particular incomplete KD with coronary lesion—when applying the AHA algorithm.[331]

Epidemiology. KD primarily affects young children; 80% of cases occur in children younger than 5 years of age.[332] Boys are more commonly affected than girls; the male-to-female ratio is reported to be 1.4 to 1.9 : 1.[333] Recurrence rates of KD are estimated at 3%.[334] Atypical KD is more common in children younger than 1 year or older than 9 years of age, accounting for one-third of KD diagnoses in these age groups.[328]

Incidence rates clearly vary between ethnic groups. Asian children are at highest risk: In 2010, Park and colleagues recently reported an average annual incidence rate of KD in Korea of 113.1 per 100,000 in children younger than 5 years.[334] In Japan, the annual incidence rate was even higher at 218.6 per 100,000 children younger than 5 years of age.[332] Around the same time, in the rest of the world annual KD incidence rates were reported between 5 and 13 per 100,000 children younger than 5 years.[328,335-338]

Clinical Presentation. Fever in KD patients is typically continuous. It is reported to be either absent or less prominent or consistent in children younger than 1 year of age and older than 9 years of age. Eye findings include bilateral nonpurulent conjunctivitis, which is particularly prominent with fever. Other inflammatory eye findings including asymptomatic uveitis have been reported. Rash of all types can be associated with KD. The rash is also more prominent with fever. Frequently it is confluent in the diaper area and axilla in the acute phase. Skin peeling classically starts on the fingertips in the subacute phase. Blisters are uncommon. Oral changes include dry, red, and cracked lips; prominent follicles of the tongue (strawberry tongue); and an oral anathema. Aphthous ulcers can be present, primarily when associated with a triggering herpes-group virus infection. Cervical lymphadenopathy is frequently asymmetric. The criteria state they should be 1.5 cm or greater. Nodes can be tender, and a secondary lymphadenitis can occur, which may require additional therapy. Hands and feet frequently appear puffy and erythematous.

Neurologic symptoms are common in children with KD: The majority of toddlers are extremely irritable. Often children are withdrawn, lethargic, and clingy or complain of headaches, in particular with fever. Transient hearing loss can be present in a significant number of patients, most commonly sensorineural hearing loss (20 to 35 dB). It may be related to salicylate toxicity in some children. Persistent hearing loss is rare.[339]

Other organ manifestations include acute arthritis,[340] hepatitis,[341] gallbladder hydrops, intussusception, or pseudo-obstruction presenting as acute abdomen,[342] dysuria with sterile pyuria, genital swelling, and muscle pain and weakness.

Diagnosis and Diagnostic Tests. Inflammatory markers are commonly raised in children with KD. ESR and CRP, leukocytosis, anemia, mildly raised liver function tests, and low albumin levels are expected in children with acute KD.[343,344] Laboratory markers are included in the AHA algorithm[329] and have been used to predict adverse outcome.[344]

Because infections are commonly found in children with KD, an infectious workup is mandatory to detect concurrent ongoing infections that may require additional therapy. Cardiac evaluation in KD patients includes a chest radiograph, electrocardiogram, and echocardiography. DeZorzi and associates defined body-surface area–adjusted standards (z scores) for coronary artery abnormalities on echocardiography.[345] These scores have subsequently been used to establish a classification system for the entire spectrum of coronary artery abnormalities including aneurysms.[346] Follow-up echocardiography is required at 2 weeks in children with evidence of coronary damage and at 6 weeks in all children because vascular disease commonly peaks at 2 to 4 weeks.[347]

A severe complication of KD is increasingly recognized: macrophage activation syndrome (MAS).[348] Latino and co-workers reported 12 of 638 KD patients who developed clinical and laboratory features of MAS including hepatosplenomegaly, cytopenia in two or more cell lines, hyperferritinemia and elevated hepatic enzymes, hypertriglyceridemia and/or hypofibrinogenemia, increased D-dimers, and evidence of hemophagocytosis on biopsy (4/12). Early recognition of MAS and increased immunosuppression are crucial.

Treatment. The first-line treatment for children with KD is IVIG at a dose of 2 g/kg.[349] In addition, high-dose acetylsalicylic acid (ASA) at 30 to 50 mg/kg or 80 to 100 mg/kg is frequently used as an antipyretic and anti-inflammatory drug while the child is febrile. However, a metaanalysis did not find sufficient evidence for ASA treatment in KD.[350] Conceptually, there is strong support for the use of ASA in KD because IVIG and ASA were found to differentially modulate the expression of TNF and its downstream effects in the KD animal model.[351] Importantly, low-dose ASA has an antithrombotic effect by inhibiting the production of thromboxane A_2 and prostacyclin in platelets.

Recurrence of fever after a dose of IVIG is commonly treated with a repeat dose of IVIG.[352] Children with refractory KD, defined as failure to respond to IVIG retreatment commonly receive corticosteroid therapy. A trial exploring the efficacy of early corticosteroids for primary KD therapy in addition to IVIG did not demonstrate a significant benefit.[349] In nonresponders TNF inhibitors have been used.[353,354] Son and co-workers reported that patients treated with infliximab had a faster resolution of fever and fewer days of hospitalization.[355] Abciximab is a monoclonal antibody against glycoprotein (GP)IIb-IIIa on platelets. A small study of 18 children with KD and large coronary artery aneurysms suggested that abciximab treatment may be associated with improved vascular remodeling.[356]

Children with KD require cardiology follow-up at 6 weeks including clinical assessment and echocardiography. Commonly, low-dose ASA treatment is discontinued in all patients in whom the coronary artery lesions have resolved. Children with evidence of coronary disease at 6 weeks require long-term care. In many centers asymptomatic KD patients are reassessed at 12 months and then discharged.

Outcome. The 5-year survival of children with KD is excellent at greater than 99%.[318] However, one in 20 children with KD will develop permanent damage to their coronary arteries.[357,358] Children may develop vascular aneurysms and stenoses beyond the coronary arteries (Figure 108-6). Early interventions including stenting or coronary bypass operations may be required.[359] Even asymptomatic children with KD and aneurysms are at high risk of myocardial lesions.[360] The long-term impact of "transient" coronary artery dilatations/ectasia remains to be determined.[361] KD may lead to endothelial dysfunction and premature arteriosclerosis.[362] The psychosocial impact of KD was recently explored: Parents of KD patients report significant distress and anxiety even years after the acute illness.[363]

Polyarteritis Nodosa

Polyartertis nodosa (PAN) is a rare necrotizing vasculitis of medium-sized vessels.[321,364] The focal/segmental, transmural necrosis can lead to aneurysm formation. Classically lesions heal and scar with a palpable fibrotic nodule (nodosa). The

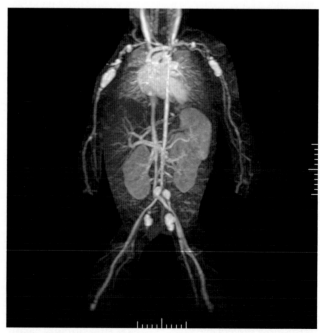

Figure 108-6 Giant aneurysms in a 6-month-old girl with Kawasaki disease. Gadolinium-enhanced, reconstructed magnetic resonance imaging angiography demonstrates multiple irregular aneurysms of the coronary arteries, the brachial and subclavian arteries, and both common iliac arteries and internal iliac arteries.

classic or systemic form can affect medium-sized arteries in multiple organs and typically presents with clinical and laboratory features of severe systemic inflammation. In contrast, cutaneous PAN is limited to the medium-sized arteries of the skin. It is more common and is characterized by periodic exacerbations often associated with *Streptococcus* infection.[321]

Definition and Classification. The proposed EULAR/PReS-endorsed consensus criteria for (systemic) childhood PAN are shown in Table 108-8.[296] The group modified the adult ACR PAN criteria by making biopsy evidence of necrotizing vasculitis *or* angiographic abnormalities a mandatory criterion.

The sensitivity as determined in the validation process described earlier was 89.6%, and the specificity was 99.6%. The mandatory criterion of biopsy evidence had the highest sensitivity and specificity (>80%). Peripheral neuropathy was the least sensitive (26%), and renal involvement was the least specific (37%) criterion.[296] The consensus conference did not propose criteria for cutaneous PAN but recognized the need for a separate category.[255] The disease characteristics were described as presence of subcutaneous nodular, painful, nonpruritic lesions with or without livedo reticularis with no systemic involvement except for myalgia, arthralgia, and nonerosive arthritis; biopsy evidence of necrotizing, nongranulomatous vasculitis; negative tests for ANCAs; and an association with streptococcal infections.[255]

Epidemiology. Systemic PAN is a rare disease. The overall incidence is estimated at 2 to 9 per million[365] and varies among ethnicities.[321] In a recent 5-year survey of all childhood vasculitis at 15 Turkish centers, PAN accounted for only 6% of cases. An association of systemic PAN with familial Mediterranean fever (FMF) was suggested.[366] Associations with hepatitis B and other viruses with childhood PAN have been reported.[321]

In 2004 an international PAN survey of 22 pediatric centers identified 110 children, of whom 63 children (57%) had systemic PAN and only 33 (30%) had cutaneous PAN.[364] However, in many centers the number of children with cutaneous PAN is significantly higher than with systemic PAN. The association of cutaneous PAN with medications and systemic inflammatory/autoimmune diseases has been reported.[367-369]

Clinical Presentation. Systemic inflammation often presents as fevers, fatigue, and weight loss in children with systemic PAN.[321] Decreased perfusion through medium-sized vessels can cause focal organ ischemia including severe abdominal pain,[370] cardiac ischemia, muscle pain, skin infarction with gangrene, livedo reticularis, and renal hypertension. The severe focal vessel inflammation can present as cutaneous painful nodules often located on the calves or feet, focal muscle pain, peripheral or cranial neuropathy, and inflammatory CNS lesions among others.[321,371] Necrotizing vascular inflammation in systemic PAN can lead to fragility of the medium-sized arterial vessel wall and significant hemorrhage.[372] Renal disease in systemic PAN is classically renal hypertension due to segmental artery disease; however, small vessel involvement presenting as isolated proteinuria, nephritic or nephrotic syndrome, and renal failure are reported in a series of 26 children from Turkey.[373]

Cutaneous PAN is characterized by the presence of deep skin nodules predominantly on the lower legs, which are frequently found at different stages of development. Most commonly a violaceous color or pigmentation with retiform appearance persists for months (Figure 108-7A-C). Ulceration can be a complication. Pain, arthralgias/arthritis, malaise, and moderate fever are associated symptoms in children with cutaneous PAN.[374]

Diagnosis and Diagnostic Tests. Inflammatory markers including ESR and CRP are commonly raised in children with active systemic and cutaneous PAN.[321] Organ function parameter may be abnormal. Specific diagnostic markers for PAN are not available. Characteristic PAN skin biopsy features are identical to adult PAN (see Chapter 90). Characteristic angiography findings include aneurysms and stenoses of the medium-sized arteries.[321]

Treatment. The treatment of childhood systemic PAN is based on adult studies and recommendations and is summarized in Chapter 90.[313] Pediatric case reports and series supported the efficacy of corticosteroids, combination immunosuppression, and biologic therapies including TNF inhibitors and B cell depletion using rituximab.[316,321,371,373] Addition of antiplatelet agents may be required. Children with cutaneous PAN are commonly treated with nonsteroidal anti-inflammatory medication or corticosteroids. Refractory patients require immunosuppressive combination therapy. Prophylactic antibiotics are considered in children with evidence of *Streptococcus* infections.[321]

Outcome. The 1-year and 5-year survival rates of 26 Turkish children with systemic PAN was only 72.5% and 60%, respectively.[373] This is significantly worse than outcomes described by Ribi and colleagues of adult PAN 1-year and 5-year survival rates at 99% and 92%, respectively.[375] However, Phillip and Luqmani reported a 5-year survival rate of 75% to 80% in a recent systematic review.[318] Relapses are common in adults with PAN: Pagnoux reported 5-year relapse-free survival rates of only 59%; 86 patients (25%) died during the study interval of almost 6 years. In contrast, cutaneous PAN appears to have a good prognosis. No prospective long-term data are available for childhood PAN.

Large Vessel Vasculitis

Takayasu's arteritis (TA) is the most common childhood large vessel vasculitis.[376] Histologically, TA is indistinguishable from giant cell arteritis (GCA) in adults. TA and GCA may represent a disease spectrum rather than different entities.[377,378] Both diseases are characterized by giant cells, which represent multinuclear cells formed by fusion of monocytes/macrophages and in TA can be found in the wall of large vessels including the aorta and its major branches.

Definition and Classification

The proposed EULAR/PReS-endorsed consensus criteria for TA are shown in Table 108-8.[296] Angiographic abnormalities are a mandatory criterion. In addition, at least one of five criteria including pulse deficit or claudication, blood pressure discrepancy of greater than 10 mm Hg, bruits, hypertension, or elevated acute-phase reactant has to be present. The sensitivity and specificity as determined in the

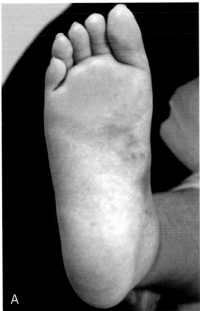

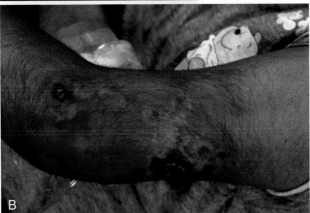

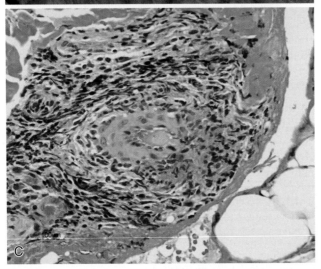

Figure 108-7 Nodular skin lesions in a 16-year-old girl with cutaneous polyarteritis nodosa. Painful subcutaneous nodules on the sole of the foot of a child with active cutaneous polyarteritis nodosa. Some nodules have evolved into purple lesions appearing like bruises. New lesions are pink and tender **(A).** Healed and crusted lesions on the elbow at a later stage of illness **(B).** Hematoxylin-eosin staining of a skin nodule demonstrating the segmental necrotizing inflammation, with fibrin deposits and disruption of the arterial vessel wall integrity **(C).**

validation process described earlier were 100% and 99.9%, respectively.[257]

Epidemiology

The incidence of adult TA was recently reported at 0.8 per million in the United Kingdom.[379] It may vary between ethnicities with higher incidences in Asia,[380,381] Africa,[382] and Latin America.[383] No population-based pediatric data are available; however, children may account for up to 30% of patients in some studies.[384-386] Most commonly, childhood TA is diagnosed in adolescence. All series have a female predominance ranging from 14:1 to 1.4:1. Recent case series reported a total of 99 children with TA.[382,387-389] Associations of *Mycobacterium tuberculosis* and TA have consistently been suggested.[390]

Clinical Presentation

Children with TA often present with clinical signs of organ ischemia and systemic inflammation. Most commonly, headache or associated neurologic deficits such as strokes, seizures or syncope, chest or abdominal pain, claudication of extremities, fever, and weight loss are the presenting symptoms.[387,388] Examination frequently reveals hypertension, absent pulses, and bruits.

Diagnosis and Diagnostic Tests

The diagnosis of TA is based on clinical pattern recognition and confirmation by angiography. Inflammatory markers including CRP and ESR have limited sensitivity for active TA[391]; no disease-specific markers have been identified. Hoffman and Ahmed demonstrated that there is a poor correlation between serum markers and vascular histopathology in adult TA.[392] Angiography is the cornerstone of diagnosing and monitoring TA (see Figure 108-8A,B). Inflammatory arterial wall disease presents as arterial wall thickening, vessel stenosis, occlusion, or rarely aneurysms.[393] Different vascular imaging modalities are used in TA, each with distinct advantages and limitations.[394,395] Conventional angiography provides information about blood flow, perfusion pattern, collateralization, and degree of vessel stenosis. It reliably identifies clots or low-flow vessel segments posing a risk for subsequent artery to artery embolisms. Magnetic resonance angiography (MRA) is noninvasive and provides information about the characteristics of the vessel wall including thickening, contrast enhancement, and surrounding soft tissue inflammation.[396] CT angiography may provide similar information as MRA; however, the associated radiation exposure often limits its use in children. Recent studies highlighted the utility of 18F-fluorodeoxyglucose (18FDG) positron emission tomography scan.[397] Doppler ultrasound correlates well with angiography in delineating homogenous wall thickening in the aorta and its branches. It may be a promising tool for childhood TA.[398]

Treatment

Corticosteroids are the cornerstone of medical TA treatment in adults and children.[314] Combination

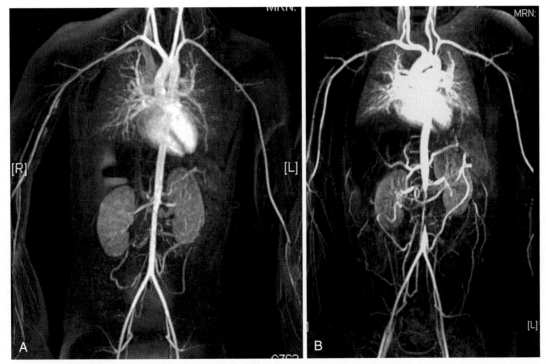

Figure 108-8 Angiographic progression of Takayasu arteritis in a 6-year-old girl. Gadolinium-enhanced, reconstructed magnetic resonance angiography (MRA) demonstrates a critical superior mesenteric artery stenosis at diagnosis of Takayasu arteritis in a 6-year-old girl **(A).** Nine months later the repeat MRA demonstrates significant progression despite high-dose immunosuppressive treatment **(B).**

immunosuppression with cyclophosphamide was found to be effective in controlling disease activity in childhood TA.[388,399] MTX was suggested in adult TA studies. Refractory childhood TA has been successfully treated with biologic therapies, primarily TNF inhibitors.[400]

Surgical treatment includes stenting, dilatation, and bypass surgery.[388] Corresponding to adult TA recommendations, the best time for vascular intervention in children is in inactive disease.[401] A close collaboration between all treating subspecialties is mandatory.

Outcome

The overall outcome of TA is poor. The 5-year survival rate was reported to be 70% to 93%.[318] Maksimowicz-McKinnon and colleagues gave a guarded prognosis of 93% attaining remission but only 28% having sustained remission of at least 6 months' duration after prednisone was tapered to less than 10 mg daily. Angioplasty and vascular surgery were initially successful. Restenosis occurred in 78% of angioplasty and 36% of bypass/reconstruction procedures. More than two-thirds of TA patients had difficulty performing routine daily activities, and one-fourth were unable to work.[402] Jales-Neto and co-workers recently determined that patients with childhood-onset TA had a significantly lower frequency of disease remission compared with adult-onset TA (24% vs. 56%) and more aneurysms (41% vs. 11%).[403]

Central Nervous System Vasculitis

Childhood CNS vasculitis is an increasingly recognized inflammatory brain disease.[404] CNS vasculitis is classified as secondary, when it occurs in association with a systemic illness including infection, malignancy, or rheumatic disease such as a systemic vasculitis (Table 108-9). Childhood primary CNS vasculitis solely affects the vessels of the brain and spinal cord.

Definition and Classification

The diagnosis of childhood primary CNS vasculitis is based on the modified Calabrese criteria for primary angiitis of the CNS (PACNS), which mandate (1) a newly acquired focal or diffuse neurologic deficit or a psychiatric manifestation in a patient 18 years of age or younger <u>and</u> (2) angiography and/or brain biopsy evidence of CNS vasculitis *in the absence* of a systemic underlying condition known to cause or mimic CNS vasculitis.[404,405] Childhood PACNS (cPACNS) is further subdivided into angiography-positive cPACNS and angiography-negative, small vessel cPACNS (SVcPACNS), with the latter being confirmed on elective brain biopsies.[404,406]

Epidemiology

The incidence of childhood CNS vasculitis is unknown. New clinical phenotypes continue to be recognized: Angiography-positive CNS vasculitis was found to be the underlying process in a large subgroup of vascular strokes, a condition neurologists may diagnose as transient cerebral arteriopathy (TCA).[406,407] Recently, new clinical phenotypes of cPACNS have been described including refractory seizure status, movement disorder, and optic neuritis.[408,409] Children with cPACNS may be diagnosed as "atypical" demyelinating disease.

Table 108-9 Classification of Childhood Primary and Secondary Central Nervous System (CNS) Vasculitis

Childhood Primary CNS Vasculitis (cPACNS)
Angiography-positive, nonprogressive cPACNS (NPcPACNS)
Angiography-positive, progressive cPACNS (PcPACNS)
Angiography-negative, small vessel cPACNS (SVcPACNS)
Secondary CNS Vasculitis in Children
Infection or postinfectious
Bacterial infection
Mycobacterium tuberculosis
Mycoplasma pneumoniae
Streptococcus pneumoniae
Treponema pallidum
Spirochete infection
Borrelia burgdorferi
Viral infection
Cytomegalovirus
Enterovirus
Epstein-Barr virus
Hepatitis C virus
Human immunodeficiency virus
Influenza virus
JC virus (progressive multifocal leukoencephalopathy)
Parvovirus B19 virus
Varicella zoster virus
West Nile virus
Fungal infection
Actinomycosis
Aspergillus
Candida albicans
Rheumatic disease
Collagen vascular diseases
Behçet's disease
Juvenile dermatomyositis
Morphea (en coup de sabre)
Sjögren syndrome
Systemic lupus erythematosus
Systemic vasculitides
Kawasaki disease
Henoch-Schönlein purpura
Microscopic polyarteritis
Granulomatosis with polyangiitis
Inflammatory bowel disease
Hemophagocytic
Lymphohistiocytosis
Mitochondrial diseases
Drug-induced central nervous system vasculitis
Hemoglobinopathies
Malignancy
Radiation

Clinical Presentation

Children with cPACNS can present with *any* focal or diffuse neurologic deficits or psychiatric symptoms. Children with angiography-positive disease typically present with headaches and strokes including acute hemiparesis, facial droop, hemisensory deficits, fine motor deficits, or dysphasia. Additional seizures and severe cognitive dysfunction are more commonly seen in progressive cPACNS.[406]

Children with angiography-negative small vessel cPACNS may present with systemic features including fever, malaise, and flulike symptoms, associated with headache, neurocognitive dysfunction, behavior changes, or intractable seizures. Focal neurologic deficits, optic neuritis, and myelitis can be presenting features. Previously healthy children may have developed a rapid neurologic

deterioration and present with an acute encephalitis or may have had subacute progression of symptoms such as worsening seizures or behavior changes over weeks to months.[404]

Diagnosis and Diagnostic Tests

The suspected diagnosis of cPACNS mandates a thorough evaluation. Systemic illnesses and other inflammatory and noninflammatory brain diseases have to be considered.[404] A diagnostic algorithm was recently proposed (Figure 108-9). Inflammatory markers can be elevated in children with cPACNS, most commonly in the small vessel subtype. Von Willebrand factor antigen appears to correlate with clinical disease activity. Cerebrospinal fluid (CSF) analysis frequently reveals a mild pleocytosis with predominantly lymphocytes and occasionally elevated CSF protein. Frequently the opening pressure is raised.

The absence of laboratory markers does not exclude cPACNS. In fact, children with angiography-positive, nonprogressive cPACNS frequently have normal inflammatory markers. In contrast, angiography-positive progressive cPACNS and small vessel cPACNS patients commonly present with laboratory signs of inflammation. Serial testing may be required. Oligoclonal banding is found in children with confirmed small vessel cPACNS.[409]

MRI studies identify ischemic, diffusion-restricted lesions and inflammatory, fluid-attenuated inversion recovery (FLAIR)-positive parenchymal lesions.[410] MRA and conventional angiography characterize vascular stenoses[411,412] (Figure 108-10A,B). Gadolinium-enhanced MRA sequences can demonstrate vessel wall enhancement and thickening in more than 85% of adult and pediatric patients with active cPACNS.[413]

Brain biopsies confirm the diagnosis of angiography-negative cPACNS[409] (Figure 108-11). In contrast to adults, biopsies are not required in children with angiography-positive disease because the diagnosis is not confounded by arteriosclerosis. Elective brain biopsies can be lesional as determined by MRI or nonlesional in the nondominant hemisphere.[409] The diagnostic yield is greater than 90% in

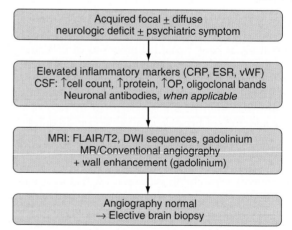

Figure 108-9 Proposed diagnostic algorithm for children with suspected central nervous system vasculitis. CSF, cerebrospinal fluid; CRP, C-reactive protein; DWI, diffusion-weighted imaging; ESR, erythrocyte sedimentation rate; FLAIR, fluid-attenuated inversion recovery; MR, magnetic resonance; MRI, magnetic resonance image; OP, opening pressure; vWF, von Willebrand factor.

children. Nondiagnostic biopsies are most commonly found when inadequate specimens are obtained.[409]

The differential diagnosis of childhood CNS vasculitis includes nonvasculitic inflammatory brain diseases such as neuronal autoantibody-mediated disease and demyelinating diseases. Neuronal autoantibodies should be tested when clinically indicated. In addition, noninflammatory vasculopathies have to be considered.[404]

Treatment

No randomized controlled trials are available for CNS vasculitis in adults and children. A recent prospective observational cohort study evaluated the efficacy and safety of a

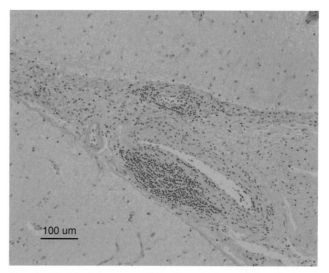

Figure 108-11 Primary, angiography-negative childhood central nervous system vasculitis in a 6-year-old girl. The elective, nonlesional brain biopsy demonstrates a lymphocytic vasculitis of the small muscular arteries. The intramural lymphocytic infiltrate consists of predominantly helper T cells (hematoxylin-eosin staining, magnification ×400).

24-month induction-maintenance protocol for small vessel cPACNS,[414] demonstrating a full neurologic recovery in two-thirds of children. Case reports and series describe the efficacy of other immunosuppressive treatments for different types of cPACNS.[415-417] In children with nonprogressive cPACNS, adjunctive corticosteroids may prevent recurrent ischemic events and improve neurologic outcome.

Outcome

There is limited information about the long-term outcome of children with CNS vasculitis. In angiography-positive cPACNS, two-thirds have a monophasic, nonprogressive course. These children often present with large ischemic lesions due to proximal large vessel stenosis and ischemia in the vascular territory. Although progression of inflammation and involvement of other vascular beds is limited in this group, the associated neurologic deficit often exceeds the other subtypes characterized by progression of inflammation. Inflammation is reversible when recognized and treated early, as recently demonstrated in the small vessel cPACNS study.[414] Disease flares are seen in a significant number of patients. Prospective collaborative studies are ongoing to further characterize the long-term outcome of children with CNS vasculitis worldwide.

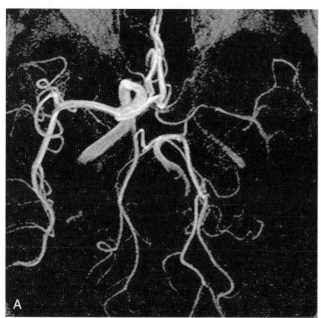

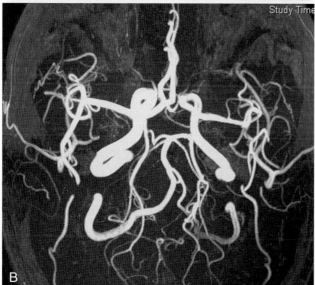

Figure 108-10 Primary, angiography-positive childhood central nervous system (CNS) vasculitis in an 8-year-old boy. Serial magnetic resonance angiography demonstrates severe stenosis of the right middle cerebral artery at diagnosis of CNS vasculitis **(A)**. Immunosuppressive therapy led to excellent revascularization of the stenosed vessel and neurologic recovery of the child at the 12-month follow-up **(B)**.

Selected References

1. Kamphuis S, Silverman ED: Prevalence and burden of pediatric-onset systemic lupus erythematosus, *Nat Rev Rheumatol* 6:538–546, 2010.
2. Ferraz MB, Goldenberg J, Hilario MO, et al: Evaluation of the 1982 ARA lupus criteria data set in pediatric patients, *Clin Exp Rheumatol* 12:83–87, 1994.
5. Muscal E, Bloom DR, Hunter JV, Myones BL: Neurocognitive deficits and neuroimaging abnormalities are prevalent in children with lupus: clinical and research experiences at a US pediatric institution, *Lupus* 19:268–279, 2010.
9. Hiraki LT, Benseler SM, Tyrrell PN, et al: Ethnic differences in pediatric systemic lupus erythematosus, *J Rheumatol* 36:2539–2546, 2009.

11. Ramirez Gomez LA, Uribe Uribe O, Osio Uribe O, et al: Childhood systemic lupus erythematosus in Latin America. The GLADEL experience in 230 children, *Lupus* 17:596–604, 2008.

12. Huang JL, Yao TC, See LC: Prevalence of pediatric systemic lupus erythematosus and juvenile chronic arthritis in a Chinese population: a nation-wide prospective population-based study in Taiwan, *Clin Exp Rheumatol* 22:776–780, 2004.

15. Hersh AO, Trupin L, Yazdany J, et al: Childhood-onset disease as a predictor of mortality in an adult cohort of patients with systemic lupus erythematosus, *Arthritis Care Res (Hoboken)* 62:1152–1159, 2010.

18. Harley IT, Kaufman KM, Langefeld CD, et al: Genetic susceptibility to SLE: new insights from fine mapping and genome-wide association studies, *Nat Rev Genet* 10:285–290, 2009.

21. Jacob CO, Zhu J, Armstrong DL, et al: Identification of *IRAK1* as a risk gene with critical role in the pathogenesis of systemic lupus erythematosus, *Proc Natl Acad Sci U S A* 106:6256–6261, 2009.

29. Lee-Kirsch MA, Gong M, Schulz H, et al: Familial chilblain lupus, a monogenic form of cutaneous lupus erythematosus, maps to chromosome 3p, *Am J Hum Genet* 79:731–737, 2006.

31. Hobbs DJ, Barletta GM, Raipal JS, et al: Severe paediatric systemic lupus erythematosus nephritis—a single-centre experience, *Nephrol Dial Transplant* 25:457–463, 2010.

33. Benseler SM, Bargman M, Feldman BM, et al: Acute renal failure in paediatric systemic lupus erythematosus: treatment and outcome, *Rheumatology (Oxford)* 48:176–182, 2009.

37. Gutierrez-Suarez R, Ruperto M, Gastaldi R, et al: A proposal for a pediatric version of the Systemic Lupus International Collaborating Clinics/American College of Rheumatology Damage Index based on the analysis of 1,015 patients with juvenile-onset systemic lupus erythematosus, *Arthritis Rheum* 54:2989–2996, 2006.

40. Bader-Meunier B, Armangaud JB, Haddad E, et al: Initial presentation of childhood-onset systemic lupus erythematosus: a French multicenter study, *J Pediatr* 146:648–653, 2005.

41. Hiraki LT, Benseler SM, Tyrrell PN, et al: Clinical and laboratory characteristics and long-term outcome of pediatric systemic lupus erythematosus: a longitudinal study, *J Pediatr* 152:550–556, 2008.

43. Vachvanichsanong P, Dissaneewate P, McNeil E: Twenty-two years' experience with childhood-onset SLE in a developing country: are outcomes similar to developed countries? *Arch Dis Child* 96:44–49, 2010.

49. Muscal E, Traipe E, de Guzman MM, et al: MR imaging findings suggestive of posterior reversible encephalopathy syndrome in adolescents with systemic lupus erythematosus, *Pediatr Radiol* 40:1241–1245, 2010.

52. Avcin T, Benseler SM, Tyrrell PN, et al: A followup study of antiphospholipid antibodies and associated neuropsychiatric manifestations in 137 children with systemic lupus erythematosus, *Arthritis Rheum* 59:206–213, 2008.

57. Hiraki LT, Hamilton J, Silverman ED: Measuring permanent damage in pediatric systemic lupus erythematosus, *Lupus* 16:657–662, 2007.

63. Schanberg LE, Sandborg C, Barnhart HX, et al: Premature atherosclerosis in pediatric systemic lupus erythematosus: risk factors for increased carotid intima-media thickness in the atherosclerosis prevention in pediatric lupus erythematosus cohort, *Arthritis Rheum* 60:1496–1507, 2009.

66. Tucker LB: Making the diagnosis of systemic lupus erythematosus in children and adolescents, *Lupus* 16:546–549, 2007.

70. Parodi A, Davi S, Pringe AB, et al: Macrophage activation syndrome in juvenile systemic lupus erythematosus: a multinational multicenter study of thirty-eight patients, *Arthritis Rheum* 60:3388–3399, 2009.

72. Brunner HI, Higgins GC, Wiers K, et al: Prospective validation of the provisional criteria for the evaluation of response to therapy in childhood-onset systemic lupus erythematosus, *Arthritis Care Res (Hoboken)* 62:335–344, 2010.

79. Sagcal-Gironella AC, Fukuda T, Wiers K, et al: Pharmacokinetics and pharmacodynamics of mycophenolic acid and their relation to response to therapy of childhood-onset systemic lupus erythematosus, *Semin Arthritis Rheum* 40:307–313, 2011.

87. Kumar S, Benseler SM, Kirby-Allen M, Silverman ED: B-cell depletion for autoimmune thrombocytopenia and autoimmune hemolytic anemia in pediatric systemic lupus erythematosus, *Pediatrics* 123: e159–163, 2009.

94. Shinjo SK, Bonfa E, Wojdyla D, et al: Antimalarial treatment may have a time-dependent effect on lupus survival: data from a multinational Latin American inception cohort, *Arthritis Rheum* 62:855–862, 2010.

96. Ardoin SP, Sandborg C, Schanberg LE: Management of dyslipidemia in children and adolescents with systemic lupus erythematosus, *Lupus* 16:618–626, 2007.

99. Panopalis P, Yazdany J: Bone health in systemic lupus erythematosus, *Curr Rheumatol Rep* 11:177–184, 2009.

100. Huber AM, Gaboury I, Cabral DA, et al: Prevalent vertebral fractures among children initiating glucocorticoid therapy for the treatment of rheumatic disorders, *Arthritis Care Res (Hoboken)* 62:516–526, 2010.

103. Hashkes PJ, Wright BM, Lauer MS, et al: Mortality outcomes in pediatric rheumatology in the US, *Arthritis Rheum* 62:599–608, 2010.

107. Brunner HI, Gladman DD, Ibanez D, et al: Difference in disease features between childhood-onset and adult-onset systemic lupus erythematosus, *Arthritis Rheum* 58:556–562, 2008.

109. Miettunen PM, Ortiz-Alvarez O, Petty RE, et al: Gender and ethnic origin have no effect on longterm outcome of childhood-onset systemic lupus erythematosus, *J Rheumatol* 31:1650–1654, 2004.

110. Laoprasopwattana K, Dissaneewate P, Vachvanichsanong P: Fatal infection in children with lupus nephritis treated with intravenous cyclophosphamide, *Pediatr Nephrol* 24:1337–1343, 2009.

112. Compeyrot-Lacassagne S, Tyrell PM, Atenafu E, et al: Prevalence and etiology of low bone mineral density in juvenile systemic lupus erythematosus, *Arthritis Rheum* 56:1966–1973, 2007.

115. Moorthy LN, Peterson MG, Hassett A, et al: Impact of lupus on school attendance and performance, *Lupus* 19:620–627, 2010.

116. Klein-Gitelman M, Brunner HI: The impact and implications of neuropsychiatric systemic lupus erythematosus in adolescents, *Curr Rheumatol Rep* 11:212–217, 2009.

120. Jaeggi E, Laskin C, Hamilton R, et al: The importance of the level of maternal anti-Ro/SSA antibodies as a prognostic marker of the development of cardiac neonatal lupus erythematosus: a prospective study of 186 antibody-exposed fetuses and infants, *J Am Coll Cardiol* 55:2778–2784, 2010.

121. Buyon JP, Clancy RM, Friedman DM: Cardiac manifestations of neonatal lupus erythematosus: guidelines to management, integrating clues from the bench and bedside, *Nat Clin Pract Rheumatol* 5:139–148, 2009.

123. Silverman E, Jaeggi E: Non-cardiac manifestations of neonatal lupus erythematosus, *Scand J Immunol* 72:223–225, 2010.

127. Cimaz R, Spence DL, Hornberger L, Silverman ED: Incidence and spectrum of neonatal lupus erythematosus: a prospective study of infants born to mothers with anti-Ro autoantibodies, *J Pediatr* 142:678–683, 2003.

130. Friedman DM, Llanos C, Izmirly PM, et al: Evaluation of fetuses in a study of intravenous immunoglobulin as preventive therapy for congenital heart block: results of a multicenter, prospective, open-label clinical trial, *Arthritis Rheum* 62:1138–1146, 2010.

132. Rein AJ, Mevorach D, Perles Z, et al: Early diagnosis and treatment of atrioventricular block in the fetus exposed to maternal anti-SSA/Ro-SSB/La antibodies: a prospective, observational, fetal kinetocardiogram-based study, *Circulation* 119:1867–1872, 2009.

136. Sanner H, Gran JT, Sjaastad I, Flato B: Cumulative organ damage and prognostic factors in juvenile dermatomyositis: a cross-sectional study median 16.8 years after symptom onset, *Rheumatology (Oxford)* 48:1541–1547, 2009.

141. Stringer E, Singh-Grewal D, Feldman BM: Predicting the course of juvenile dermatomyositis: significance of early clinical and laboratory features, *Arthritis Rheum* 58:3585–3592, 2008.

144. Tezak Z, Hoffman EP, Lutz JL, et al: Gene expression profiling in DQA10501+ children with untreated dermatomyositis: a novel model of pathogenesis, *J Immunol* 168:4154–4163, 2002.

147. Khanna S, Reed AM: Immunopathogenesis of juvenile dermatomyositis, *Muscle Nerve* 41:581–592, 2010.

153. Dugan EM, Huber AM, Miller FW, et al: Review of the classification and assessment of the cutaneous manifestations of the idiopathic inflammatory myopathies, *Dermatol Online J* 15:2, 2009.

154. Bingham A, Mamyrova G, Rother KI, et al: Predictors of acquired lipodystrophy in juvenile-onset dermatomyositis and a gradient of severity, *Medicine (Baltimore)* 87:70–86, 2008.

158. Sanner H, Kirkhus E, Merckoll E, et al: Long-term muscular outcome and predisposing and prognostic factors in juvenile dermatomyositis:

a case-control study, *Arthritis Care Res (Hoboken)* 62:1103–1111, 2010.

166. Ruperto N, Pistorio A, Ravelli A, et al: The Paediatric Rheumatology International Trials Organisation provisional criteria for the evaluation of response to therapy in juvenile dermatomyositis, *Arthritis Care Res (Hoboken)* 62:1533–1541, 2010.

168. Huber AM, Dugan EM, Lachenbruch PA, et al: Preliminary validation and clinical meaning of the Cutaneous Assessment Tool in juvenile dermatomyositis, *Arthritis Rheum* 59:214–221, 2008.

173. Wedderburn LR, Varsani H, Li CK, et al: International consensus on a proposed score system for muscle biopsy evaluation in patients with juvenile dermatomyositis: a tool for potential use in clinical trials, *Arthritis Rheum* 57:1192–1201, 2007.

181. Bowyer SL, Blane CE, Sullivan DB, Cassidy JT: Childhood dermatomyositis: factors predicting functional outcome and development of dystrophic calcification, *J Pediatr* 103:882–888, 1983.

182. Kim S, El-Hallak M, Dedeoglu F, et al: Complete and sustained remission of juvenile dermatomyositis resulting from aggressive treatment, *Arthritis Rheum* 60:1825–1830, 2009.

184. Ramanan AV, Campbell-Wester N, Ota S, et al: The effectiveness of treating juvenile dermatomyositis with methotrexate and aggressively tapered corticosteroids, *Arthritis Rheum* 52:3570–3578, 2005.

186. Dalakas MC, Illa I, Dambrosia JM, et al: A controlled trial of high-dose intravenous immune globulin infusions as treatment for dermatomyositis, *N Engl J Med* 329:1993–2000, 1993.

198. Huber AM, Lang BA, LeBlanc CM, et al: Medium- and long-term functional outcomes in a multicenter cohort of children with juvenile dermatomyositis, *Arthritis Rheum* 43:541–549, 2000.

199. Ravelli A, Trail L, Ferrari C, et al: Long-term outcome and prognostic factors of juvenile dermatomyositis: a multinational, multicenter study of 490 patients, *Arthritis Care Res (Hoboken)* 62:63–72, 2010.

201. Martini G, Foeldvari I, Russo R, et al: Systemic sclerosis in childhood: clinical and immunologic features of 153 patients in an international database, *Arthritis Rheum* 54:3971–3978, 2006.

208. Zulian F, Woo P, Athreya BH, et al: The Pediatric Rheumatology European Society/American College of Rheumatology/European League against Rheumatism provisional classification criteria for juvenile systemic sclerosis, *Arthritis Rheum* 57:203–212, 2007.

209. Kowal-Bielecka O, Landewe R, Avouac J, et al: EULAR recommendations for the treatment of systemic sclerosis: a report from the EULAR Scleroderma Trials and Research group (EUSTAR), *Ann Rheum Dis* 68:620–628, 2009.

210. Martini A, Maccario R, Ravelli A, et al: Marked and sustained improvement two years after autologous stem cell transplantation in a girl with systemic sclerosis, *Arthritis Rheum* 42:807–811, 1999.

214. Zulian F, Vallongo C, de Oliveira SK, et al: Congenital localized scleroderma, *J Pediatr* 149:248–251, 2006.

215. Laxer RM, Zulian F: Localized scleroderma, *Curr Opin Rheumatol* 18:606–613, 2006.

220. Vancheeswaran R, Black CM, David J, et al: Childhood-onset scleroderma: is it different from adult-onset disease, *Arthritis Rheum* 39:1041–1049, 1996.

221. Takehara K, Sato S: Localized scleroderma is an autoimmune disorder, *Rheumatology (Oxford)* 44:274–279, 2005.

222. Kister I, Inglese M, Laxer RM, Herbert J: Neurologic manifestations of localized scleroderma: a case report and literature review, *Neurology* 71:1538–1545, 2008.

223. Zulian F, Vallongo C, Woo P, et al: Localized scleroderma in childhood is not just a skin disease, *Arthritis Rheum* 52:2873–2881, 2005.

228. Uziel Y, Feldman BM, Krafchik BR, et al: Methotrexate and corticosteroid therapy for pediatric localized scleroderma, *J Pediatr* 136:91–95, 2000.

230. Weibel L, Sampaio MC, Vinsentin MT, et al: Evaluation of methotrexate and corticosteroids for the treatment of localized scleroderma (morphoea) in children, *Br J Dermatol* 155:1013–1020, 2006.

233. Kreuter A, Hyun J, Stucker M, et al: A randomized controlled study of low-dose UVA1, medium-dose UVA1, and narrowband UVB phototherapy in the treatment of localized scleroderma, *J Am Acad Dermatol* 54:440–447, 2006.

234. Palmero ML, Uziel Y, Laxer RM, et al: En coup de sabre scleroderma and Parry-Romberg syndrome in adolescents: surgical options and patient-related outcomes, *J Rheumatol* 37:2174–2179, 2010.

239. Arkachaisri T, Vilaiyuk S, Torok KS, Medsger TA Jr: Development and initial validation of the localized scleroderma skin damage index and physician global assessment of disease damage: a proof-of-concept study, *Rheumatology (Oxford)* 49:373–381, 2010.

243. Saxton-Daniels S, Jacobe HT: An evaluation of long-term outcomes in adults with pediatric-onset morphea, *Arch Dermatol* 146:1044–1045, 2010.

253. Yeung RS: Kawasaki disease: update on pathogenesis, *Curr Opin Rheumatol* 22:551–560, 2010.

254. Dillon MJ, Ozen S: A new international classification of childhood vasculitis, *Pediatr Nephrol* 21:1219–1222, 2006.

255. Ozen S, Ruperto N, Dillon MJ, et al: EULAR/PRES Endorsed Consensus Criteria for the Classification of Childhood Vasculitides under review by the ACR, *Ann Rheum Dis* 65:936–941, 2006.

256. Ruperto N, Ozen S, Pistorio A, et al: EULAR/PRINTO/PRES criteria for Henoch-Schonlein purpura, childhood polyarteritis nodosa, childhood Wegener granulomatosis and childhood Takayasu arteritis: Ankara 2008. Part I: Overall methodology and clinical characterisation, *Ann Rheum Dis* 69:790–797, 2010.

257. Ozen S, Pistorio A, Iusan SM, et al: EULAR/PRINTO/PRES criteria for Henoch-Schonlein purpura, childhood polyarteritis nodosa, childhood Wegener granulomatosis and childhood Takayasu arteritis: Ankara 2008. Part II: Final classification criteria, *Ann Rheum Dis* 69:798–806, 2010.

264. Lau KK, Suzuki H, Novak J, Wyatt RJ: Pathogenesis of Henoch-Schonlein purpura nephritis, *Pediatr Nephrol* 25:19–26, 2010.

269. Gardner-Medwin JM, Dolezalova P, Cummins C, Southwood TR: Incidence of Henoch-Schonlein purpura, Kawasaki disease, and rare vasculitides in children of different ethnic origins, *Lancet* 360:1197–1202, 2002.

271. Watts RA, Scott DG: Epidemiology of the vasculitides, *Semin Respir Crit Care Med* 25:455–464, 2004.

276. Jauhola O, Ronkainen J, Koskimies O, et al: Renal manifestations of Henoch-Schonlein purpura in a 6-month prospective study of 223 children, *Arch Dis Child* 95:877–882, 2010.

279. Scharer K, Krmar R, Querfeld U, et al: Clinical outcome of Schonlein-Henoch purpura nephritis in children, *Pediatr Nephrol* 13:816–823, 1999.

284. Weiss PF, Klink AJ, et al: Hexem K, Variation in inpatient therapy and diagnostic evaluation of children with Henoch-Schonlein purpura, *J Pediatr* 155:812–818 e811, 2009.

285. Ronkainen J, Koskimies O, Ala-Houhala M, et al: Early prednisone therapy in Henoch-Schonlein purpura: a randomized, double-blind, placebo-controlled trial, *J Pediatr* 149:241–247, 2006.

286. Weiss PF, Klink AJ, Localio R, et al: Corticosteroids may improve clinical outcomes during hospitalization for Henoch-Schonlein purpura, *Pediatrics* 126:674–681, 2010.

294. Cabral DA, Uribe AG, Benseler S, et al: Classification, presentation, and initial treatment of Wegener's granulomatosis in childhood, *Arthritis Rheum* 60:3413–3424, 2009.

296. Ozen S, Ruperto N, Dillon MJ, et al: EULAR/PReS endorsed consensus criteria for the classification of childhood vasculitides, *Ann Rheum Dis* 65:936–941, 2006.

302. Lane SE, Watts R, Scott DG: Epidemiology of systemic vasculitis, *Curr Rheumatol Rep* 7:270–275, 2005.

307. Belostotsky VM, Shah V, Dillon MJ: Clinical features in 17 paediatric patients with Wegener granulomatosis, *Pediatr Nephrol* 17:754–761, 2002.

309. Akikusa JD, Schneider R, Harvey EA, et al: Clinical features and outcome of pediatric Wegener's granulomatosis, *Arthritis Rheum* 57:837–844, 2007.

312. Clarke LA, Hong Y, Eleftheriou D, et al: Endothelial injury and repair in systemic vasculitis of the young, *Arthritis Rheum* 62:1770–1780, 2010.

313. Mukhtyar C, Guillevin L, Cid MC, et al: EULAR recommendations for the management of primary small and medium vessel vasculitis, *Ann Rheum Dis* 68:310–317, 2009.

314. Mukhtyar C, Guillevin L, Cid MC, et al: EULAR recommendations for the management of large vessel vasculitis, *Ann Rheum Dis* 68:318–323, 2009.

315. Wright E, Dillon MJ, Tullus K: Childhood vasculitis and plasma exchange, *Eur J Pediatr* 166:145–151, 2007.

316. Eleftheriou D, Melo M, Marks SD, et al: Biologic therapy in primary systemic vasculitis of the young, *Rheumatology (Oxford)* 48:978–986, 2009.

317. Hugle B, Solomon M, Harvey E, et al: *Pneumocystis jiroveci* pneumonia following rituximab treatment in Wegener's granulomatosis, *Arthritis Care Res (Hoboken)* 62:1661–1664, 2010.

320. McCrindle BW: Kawasaki disease: a childhood disease with important consequences into adulthood, *Circulation* 120:6–8, 2009.

324. Benseler SM, McCrindle BW, Silverman ED, et al: Infections and Kawasaki disease: implications for coronary artery outcome, *Pediatrics* 116:e760–766, 2005.

329. Newburger JW, Takahashi M, Gerber MA, et al: Diagnosis, treatment, and long-term management of Kawasaki disease: a statement for health professionals from the Committee on Rheumatic Fever, Endocarditis, and Kawasaki Disease, Council on Cardiovascular Disease in the Young, American Heart Association, *Pediatrics* 114:1708–1733, 2004.

330. Yellen ES, Gauvreau K, Takahashi M, et al: Performance of 2004 American Heart Association recommendations for treatment of Kawasaki disease, *Pediatrics* 125:e234–241, 2010.

339. Knott PD, Orloff LA, Harris JP, et al: Sensorineural hearing loss and Kawasaki disease: a prospective study, *Am J Otolaryngol* 22:343–348, 2001.

342. Akikusa JD, Laxer RM, Friedman JN: Intestinal pseudoobstruction in Kawasaki disease, *Pediatrics* 113:e504–506, 2004.

345. de Zorzi A, Colan SD, Gauvreau K, et al: Coronary artery dimensions may be misclassified as normal in Kawasaki disease, *J Pediatr* 133:254–258, 1998.

346. Manlhiot C, Millar K, Golding F, McCrindle BW: Improved classification of coronary artery abnormalities based only on coronary artery z-scores after Kawasaki disease, *Pediatr Cardiol* 31:242–249, 2010.

348. Latino GA, Manlhiot C, Yeung RS, et al: Macrophage activation syndrome in the acute phase of Kawasaki disease, *J Pediatr Hematol Oncol* 32:527–531, 2010.

349. Newburger JW, Sleeper LA, McCrindle BW, et al: Randomized trial of pulsed corticosteroid therapy for primary treatment of Kawasaki disease, *N Engl J Med* 356:663–675, 2007.

350. Baumer JH, Love SJ, Gupta A, et al: Salicylate for the treatment of Kawasaki disease in children, *Cochrane Database Syst Rev* 4:CD004175, 2006.

353. Burns JC, Best BM, Mejias A, et al: Infliximab treatment of intravenous immunoglobulin-resistant Kawasaki disease, *J Pediatr* 153:833–838, 2008.

355. Son MB, Gauvreau K, Burns JC, et al: Infliximab for intravenous immunoglobulin resistance in Kawasaki disease: a retrospective study, *J Pediatr* 158:644–649, 2010.

362. Noto N, Okada T, Karasawa K, et al: Age-related acceleration of endothelial dysfunction and subclinical atherosclerosis in subjects with coronary artery lesions after Kawasaki disease, *Pediatr Cardiol* 30:262–268, 2009.

364. Ozen S, Anton J, Arisoy N, et al: Juvenile polyarteritis: results of a multicenter survey of 110 children, *J Pediatr* 145:517–522, 2004.

376. Brunner J, Feldman BM, Tyrell PN, et al: Takayasu arteritis in children and adolescents, *Rheumatology (Oxford)* 49:1806–1814, 2010.

379. Watts R, Al-Taiar A, Mooney J, Scott D, Macgregor A: The epidemiology of Takayasu arteritis in the UK, *Rheumatology (Oxford)* 48:1008–1011, 2009.

382. Hahn D, Thomson PD, Kala U, et al: A review of Takayasu's arteritis in children in Gauteng, South Africa, *Pediatr Nephrol (Berlin)* 12:668–675, 1998.

385. Al Abrawi S, Fouillet-Desjonqueres M, David L, et al: Takayasu arteritis in children, *Pediatr Rheumatol Online J* 6:17, 2008.

386. Ruige JB, Van Geet C, Nevelsteen A, Verhaeghe R: A 16-year survey of Takayasu's arteritis in a tertiary Belgian center, *Int Angiol* 22:414–420, 2003.

387. Jain S, Sharma N, Singh S, et al: Takayasu arteritis in children and young Indians, *Int J Cardiol* 75 S:153–S157, 2000.

388. Cakar N, Yalcinkaya F, Duzova A, et al: Takayasu arteritis in children, *J Rheumatol* 35:913–919, 2008.

399. Ozen S, Duzova A, Bakkaloglu A, et al: Takayasu arteritis in children: preliminary experience with cyclophosphamide induction and corticosteroids followed by methotrexate, *J Pediatr* 150:72–76, 2007.

404. Cellucci T, Benseler SM: Central nervous system vasculitis in children, *Curr Opin Rheumatol* 22:590–597, 2010.

407. Braun KP, Bulder MM, Chabrier S, et al: The course and outcome of unilateral intracranial arteriopathy in 79 children with ischaemic stroke, *Brain* 132:544–557, 2009.

408. Benseler SM, deVeber G, Hawkins C, et al: Angiography-negative primary central nervous system vasculitis in children: a newly recognized inflammatory central nervous system disease, *Arthritis Rheum* 52:2159–2167, 2005.

409. Elbers J, Halliday W, Hawkins C, et al: Brain biopsy in children with primary small-vessel central nervous system vasculitis, *Ann Neurol* 68:602–610, 2010.

413. Kuker W, Gaertner S, Nagale T, et al: Vessel wall contrast enhancement: a diagnostic sign of cerebral vasculitis, *Cerebrovasc Dis* 26:23–29, 2008.

414. Hutchinson C, Elbers J, Halliday W, et al: Treatment of small vessel primary CNS vasculitis in children: an open-label cohort study, *Lancet Neurol* 9:1078–1084, 2010.

416. Sen ES, Leone V, Abinum M, et al: Treatment of primary angiitis of the central nervous system in childhood with mycophenolate mofetil, *Rheumatology (Oxford)* 49:806–811, 2010.

Full references for this chapter can be found on www.expertconsult.com.

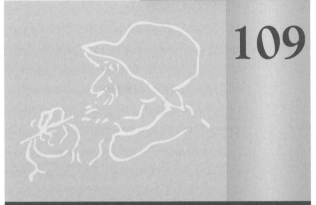

109 Bacterial Arthritis

PAUL P. COOK • DAWD S. SIRAJ

EPIDEMIOLOGY

Bacterial infections of the joint are usually curable with treatment, but morbidity and mortality are still significant in patients with underlying rheumatoid arthritis (RA), patients with prosthetic joints, elderly patients, and patients who have severe and multiple comorbidities. Goldenberg[1] wrote in 1994, "Treatment and outcome [of septic arthritis] have not improved substantially over the past 20 years." This statement is probably still true today. Incremental knowledge of the pathogenesis of septic arthritis caused by two common organisms, *Neisseria gonorrhoeae* and *Staphylococcus aureus*, and understanding of the pathobiology of prosthetic devices may lead to innovations in the management and prevention of bacterial joint infections.

The normal diarthrodial joint is resistant to bacterial infection because of local and systemic host defenses. Bacteria can reach the synovial-lined joint, however, via the hematogenous route and result in septic arthritis. The large joints are affected more commonly than the small joints, and monoarticular infection is the rule, with polyarticular infection (more than one joint involved) in less than 20% of cases. A prospective series from a community-based population in the Netherlands reflected a representative distribution of joint involvement: knee 55%, ankle 10%, wrist 9%, shoulder 7%, hip 5%, elbow 5%, sternoclavicular joint 5%, sacroiliac joint 2%, and foot joint 2%.[2]

The incidence of septic arthritis ranges from 2 to 5/100,000/year in the general population, 5.5 to 12/100,000/year in children, 28 to 38/100,000/year in patients with RA, and 40 to 68/100,000/year in patients with joint prostheses.[3,4] The incidence appears to be increasing, probably related to orthopedic procedures, an aging population, and the increased use of immunosuppressive therapy.[5] The organisms causing bacterial arthritis depend on the epidemiologic circumstances (Table 109-1). Monoarthritis of a prosthetic joint in an elderly man is likely due to *Staphylococcus*, whereas a migratory arthritis in a sexually active woman with skin lesions is likely due to disseminated gonococcal infection. Septic arthritis caused by methicillin-resistant *S. aureus* (MRSA) is common in the elderly, in persons who use intravenous drugs, and in individuals with prosthetic joints.[6]

Table 109-1 Organisms Causing Joint Infection in Various Hosts

Adults	Children ≤5 yr old	Children >5 yr old	Neonates	Prosthetic
Common	**Common**	**Common**	**Common**	**Common**
Staphylococcus aureus	*S. aureus*	*S. aureus*	*S. aureus*	Coagulase-negative
Streptococcus pneumoniae	*Haemophilus influenzae**	Group A streptococci	Group B streptococci	staphylococci
β-Hemolytic streptococci	Group A streptococci		Enterobacteriaceae	*S. aureus*
(mainly Lancefield groups	*S. pneumoniae*			
A, G, and B)				
Neisseria gonorrhoeae (adult				
and sexually active				
adolescent)				
Enterobacteriaceae (age > 60				
or predisposing condition)				
Salmonella				
Rare	**Rare**	**Rare**	**Rare**	**Less Common**
Pseudomonas	*Salmonella*	*N. meningitidis*	*Pseudomonas*	*Corynebacterium*
Mycobacterium tuberculosis	*H. influenzae*	*N. gonorrhoeae*	*H. influenzae*	Enterococci and
H. influenzae	*N. meningitidis*	*K. kingae*	*N. gonorrhoeae*	streptococci
Neisseria meningitidis	*N. gonorrhoeae*	*M. tuberculosis*		*Pseudomonas aeruginosa*
Pasteurella	*Kingella kingae*	*B. burgdorferi*		Enterobacteriaceae
Anaerobes	*M. tuberculosis*			*Propionibacterium*
Mycoplasma/Ureaplasma	*B. burgdorferi*			Other anaerobes
Fungi (*Sporothrix*, dimorphic				*Candida*
fungi, *Cryptococcus*)				*M. tuberculosis*
Borrelia burgdorferi				

*Rare in children immunized with Hib vaccine.
Modified from Atkins BL, Bowler IC: The diagnosis of large joint sepsis, *J Hosp Infect* 40:263–274, 1998.

ETIOLOGY

Most cases of septic arthritis result from hematogenous seeding of the synovial membrane. The abundant vascular supply of the synovium and the lack of a limiting basement membrane allow organisms to target joints during bacteremia. Less common causes of septic arthritis include direct inoculation after joint aspiration or corticosteroid injection of a joint; animal or human bites; nail puncture wounds or plant thorn injury; joint surgery, especially hip and knee arthroplasties; and spread by contiguous osteomyelitis, cellulitis, or septic bursitis.

Table 109-1 lists the common organisms that cause joint infections according to the age of the patient and whether the joint is native or prosthetic.[5] Overall, *S. aureus* is the most common etiologic agent among children of all age groups, followed by group A streptococci and *Streptococcus pneumoniae*.[7] Neonates and infants younger than 2 months old are more susceptible to group B streptococci and gram-negative enteric bacilli than older children. Rarely, *Pseudomonas*, *N. gonorrhoeae*, and *Candida albicans* may be responsible in very young children. Since the introduction of the *Haemophilus influenzae* type B vaccine, the incidence of septic arthritis caused by *H. influenzae* has declined dramatically.[8] In sexually active adolescents, *N. gonorrhoeae* must be considered. *Pseudomonas aeruginosa* and *Candida* are potential pathogens in adolescent intravenous drug abusers. Patients with sickle cell anemia are prone to develop *Salmonella* arthritis, and immunocompromised children are at higher risk for infection with gram-negative bacilli. Other unusual joint pathogens in children include *Neisseria meningitidis*, anaerobes, *Brucella*, and *Kingella kingae*.

The organisms causing nongonococcal septic arthritis in adults are 75% to 80% gram-positive cocci and 15% to 20% gram-negative bacilli.[9] *S. aureus* is the most common organism in native and prosthetic joint infections.

Staphylococcus epidermidis is common in prosthetic joint infections but is a rare cause of native joint infections. The streptococci including *Streptococcus pneumoniae* are the next most common group of gram-positive aerobes. *Streptococcus pyogenes* is followed by groups B, G, C, and F in frequency. Patients with non–group A streptococcal disease often have comorbidities such as immunosuppression, diabetes mellitus, malignancy, and severe genitourinary or gastrointestinal infections.[10] Group B streptococcal arthritis in adults is uncommon, but it can be a serious infection in adult diabetics and patients with late prosthetic hip infections.[11] Aggressive polyarthritis caused by group B streptococci may result in serious functional damage and permanent morbidity.[12] Patients predisposed to gram-negative bacillary infections include patients with a history of intravenous drug abuse, very young and very old patients, and immunocompromised patients.[13] The most common gram-negative organisms are *Escherichia coli* and *P. aeruginosa*.

Anaerobes account for 5% to 7% of septic arthritis.[2,3,14] Common anaerobes include *Bacteroides*, *Propionibacterium acnes*, and various anaerobic gram-positive cocci. Predisposing factors include wound infections, joint arthroplasty, and immunocompromised hosts. Foul-smelling synovial fluid or air in the joint space should raise the suspicion of anaerobic infection, and appropriate cultures should be obtained and held for at least 2 weeks. Anaerobes and coagulase-negative staphylococci are more common in prosthetic joint infections.

Polyarticular septic arthritis is much less common than monoarticular infection.[15] Many of the patients have one or more comorbidities, and some have been intravenous drug abusers. Occurrence of polyarticular septic arthritis is high in patients with RA and averages 25% (range, 18% to 35%).[16] Although *S. aureus* is the most common pathogen, group G streptococci, *H. influenzae*, *S. pneumoniae*, or mixed aerobic and anaerobic bacteria have been responsible for polyarticular infections. Involvement of more than one joint also can occur in certain patient populations such as neonates and patients with sickle cell anemia, or with certain organisms, such as *N. gonorrhoeae*, *N. meningitidis*, and *Salmonella*.[17]

Polymicrobial (two or more bacterial species), polyarticular (two or more joints) septic arthritis is a rare clinical entity.[18] Large joints are usually affected. Among five reported cases, the knee was affected in four cases (bilaterally in two); the elbow and wrist were affected in three cases, and the shoulder was affected in two cases. The mean number of joints infected was three. Bacteremia was present in all but one case (80%) and always involved the same organisms that were in the synovial fluids. Most bacterial species isolated were the usual organisms seen in septic arthritis. Combinations of gram-positive aerobic and anaerobic organisms were common. A characteristic of most cases (80%) was the extension of locally destructive processes as a result of the contiguous spread of infection from the affected joints such as osteomyelitis, fasciitis with compartment syndrome, and abscess or sinus tract formation. Systemic complications including septic shock, multiorgan failure, and toxic shock syndrome were noted in 60% of cases. The mortality rate of polymicrobial, polyarticular septic arthritis in this small series was 60%.[18]

Arthrocentesis is a common procedure frequently used in conjunction with corticosteroid administration in patients with various forms of joint diseases. Septic arthritis after joint aspiration and injection is extremely rare, occurring in 0.0002% of patients.[19] Arthroscopic surgery is also a common procedure that is complicated by a low incidence of septic arthritis (<0.5% of procedures).[20] Coagulase-positive and coagulase-negative staphylococci account for more than 87% of these infections. In rare cases of septic arthritis of the knee related to anterior cruciate ligament repair, the tissue allografts were identified as the source of the infection.[21] Cultures yielded gram-negative organisms such as *Pseudomonas aeruginosa*, *Citrobacter*, *Klebsiella oxytoca*, and mixed infection with *S. aureus*, *Enterococcus faecalis*, and *P. aeruginosa*.

PATHOGENESIS

Acute bacterial arthritis is usually designated gonococcal or nongonococcal. In the case of gonococcal arthritis, *N. gonorrhoeae* possesses a variety of virulence factors on the cell surface. *N. gonorrhoeae* is able to attach to cell surfaces via filamentous outer-membrane appendages, or pili. Another outer membrane protein, protein I, has forms IA and IB. Protein IA binds the host factor H and inactivates complement component, C3b, circumventing the host's complement system.[22] Protein IA also prevents phagolysosomal fusion in neutrophils, enabling survival of the organism within the phagocytes. Lipo-oligosaccharide is a gonococcal molecule similar to lipopolysaccharide of other gram-negative bacteria and possesses endotoxin activity, which contributes to the joint damage seen in gonococcal arthritis.[23]

S. aureus is the most common organism that causes nongonococcal arthritis. The virulence of *S. aureus* is associated with its ability to attach to host tissue within the joint, evade host defenses, and cause damage to the joint.

Table 109-2 Virulence Factors of *Staphylococcus aureus* and Their Mechanisms of Action

Virulence Factor	Mechanism of Action
Collagen-binding protein	Binds collagen
Clumping factor A and B	Binds fibrinogen
Fibronectin-binding protein A and B	Binds fibronectin
Capsular polysaccharide	Antiphagocytic
Protein A	Binds fragment crystallizable portion of IgG
Toxic shock syndrome toxin-1	Superantigen
Enterotoxins	Superantigens

Table 109-2 lists some of these virulence factors and their mechanisms of action. The attachment of *S. aureus* to the joint tissues is facilitated by microbial surface components recognizing adhesive matrix molecules (MSCRAMMs). MSCRAMMs are embedded in the cell wall peptidoglycan of *S. aureus* (Figure 109-1).[24] They bind to host matrix proteins including collagen, fibrinogen, elastin, vitronectin, laminin, and fibronectin. Gene knockout experiments in animal models showed that the gene coding for the protein that binds collagen is an important virulence factor for *S. aureus* joint infections.[25] Most *S. aureus* isolates also express the fibronectin-binding proteins, FnbpA and FnbpB. Disruption of the respective genes, *fnbpA* and *fnbpB*, by knockout gene experiments completely obliterates adherence of *S. aureus* to fibronectin-coated surfaces (e.g., prosthetic joints).[26]

The genes of several *S. aureus* cell surface proteins (e.g., protein A, fibronectin-binding proteins, coagulase) and

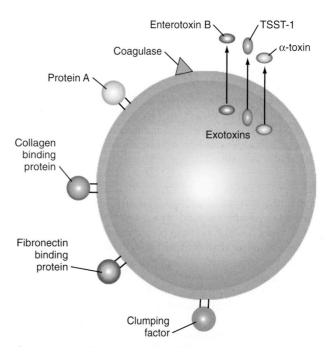

Figure 109-1 Schematic diagram of *Staphylococcus aureus*. Many of the cell surface proteins are regulated by the agr locus (see text). At low cell concentrations, agr facilitates the production of the cell-surface proteins, which facilitate attachment to tissue. At higher cell concentrations, as occurs with establishment of infection, agr downregulates production of the cell surface proteins and activates genes coding for exotoxins. TSST-1, toxic shock syndrome toxin-1.

exotoxins (e.g., toxic shock syndrome toxin-1 [TSST-1], enterotoxin B, proteases, and hemolysins) are regulated by the accessory gene regulator *agr*.[27] At low cell numbers such as at the time of infection, production of cell surface proteins for attachment to host tissues is facilitated by the *agr* gene. When the cells have attached to tissue or an orthopedic device and have passed from exponential to stationary phase of growth, *agr* represses the expression of genes coding for cell surface proteins and activates genes coding for exotoxins and tissue-destroying exoenzymes. Because of this complex effect on the different stages of infection, inhibitors of *agr* may reduce tissue destruction but enhance tissue colonization. This effect could have implications for chronic infections such as occur with prosthetic joints.

Adherence receptors may allow intracellular movement of *S. aureus* into host cells (e.g., osteoblasts, endothelial cells, neutrophils).[28] When internalized, the organism is protected from the host's immune system and from antimicrobial agents. After adherence to the joint tissue, the bacteria activate the host immune response. Opsonization and phagocytosis are key defenses to eradicate the organism. *S. aureus* possesses two virulence factors, protein A and capsular polysaccharide, which interfere with these defenses. Protein A interferes with binding of complement by binding to the fragment crystallizable (Fc) portion of IgG. Protein A has been termed a *superantigen* for B cells because 30% of human B cells show Fab-mediated binding of the protein A molecule.[29] Binding of protein A by B cells leads to activation and subsequently to depletion of B cells through apoptosis.[30] This process may have implications regarding the ability of the immune system to control infection with *S. aureus*. The gene coding for protein A had been experimentally disrupted, and joint infection caused by the altered strain in a mouse model resulted in less joint destruction than infection caused by the wild-type strain.[31]

Capsular polysaccharide interferes with opsonization and phagocytosis. Of the 11 reported capsule serotypes of *S. aureus*, types 5 and 8 account for 85% of clinical infections.[32] The capsule of these two serotypes is thinner, which facilitates the attachment to host fibronectin and fibrin.[33] When attached to these host proteins, capsule production is upregulated to form a thicker capsule, which makes the bacteria more resistant to opsonization and phagocytosis. The thicker capsule can also conceal the highly immunogenic adherence proteins (MSCRAMMs).[34] A mutant of the type 5 capsule in a murine model had a lower rate of infection and resulted in less severe arthritis compared with mice infected with the wild-type strain.[35] A vaccine consisting of types 5 and 8 polysaccharide reduced *S. aureus* bacteremia by more than half in hemodialysis patients.[36] The duration of protection was approximately 40 weeks after a single vaccination.

S. aureus exotoxins (e.g., TSST-1 and enterotoxins) act as superantigens that bind to host major histocompatibility complex (MHC) class II molecules and T cell receptors, resulting in clonal expansion and activation of some T cells. This activation triggers the release of numerous cytokines including interleukin (IL)-2, interferon-γ, and tumor necrosis factor (TNF).[37] Induction of these cytokines results in systemic toxicity and joint damage. The stimulated T cells initially proliferate but later disappear, likely due to apoptosis, and result in immunosuppression.[38] Internalized

organisms that had been protected from this inflammatory response may cause fulminant or persistent infection. Mice injected with strains of *S. aureus* lacking TSST-1 and enterotoxins rarely develop arthritis; when arthritis is induced, it is much milder compared with arthritis in animals injected with the wild-type strain.[37] Vaccination of mice with a mutated, recombinant form of enterotoxin A devoid of superantigen function was associated with a significant reduction in mortality.[39]

In response to bacterial infection of the joint space, the host releases a variety of cytokines and inflammatory mediators. Initially, IL-1β and IL-6 are released into the joint space, leading to an influx of inflammatory cells. These neutrophils and macrophages engulf invading bacteria and release additional cytokines including TNF, IL-1, IL-6, and IL-8. Blocking TNF with a monoclonal antibody and IL-1 with an IL-1 receptor antagonist inhibited leukocyte infiltration into the joint by 80% in a rabbit model of *S. aureus*–induced arthritis when the cytokine inhibitors were given simultaneously with *S. aureus*.[40] When the same inhibitors were given 24 hours after infection, however, there was no effect on leukocyte infiltration, suggesting the crucial roles of TNF and IL-1 in the early stages of *S. aureus*–induced arthritis. Release of interferon-γ is associated with the influx of T cells, which occurs a few days after infection. In a mouse model of *S. aureus* septic arthritis, interferon-γ has been associated with a worsening of the severity of arthritis while protecting the animals from septicemia.[41] The host's early cytokine response may aid the clearance of organisms and limit infection in the host. A late cytokine response may amplify the destructiveness of an established infection.

CLINICAL FEATURES

Acute bacterial arthritis is most commonly monoarticular. Polyarticular infection occurs in 5% to 8% of pediatric cases and in 10% to 19% of adult nongonococcal cases.[42] The differential diagnosis of acute monoarthritis overlaps with many causes of polyarthritis because virtually any form of arthritis can initially manifest as a single swollen joint. The three main etiologies to consider when a patient presents with acute monoarticular arthritis are trauma, infection, and crystal-induced synovitis such as gout or pseudogout. Polyarticular septic arthritis is usually seen in patients with systemic inflammatory disorders such as the spondyloarthropathies, RA, systemic lupus erythematosus, and other connective tissue diseases or patients with overwhelming sepsis.[15,43]

Disseminated gonococcal infection occurs in 1% to 3% of patients infected with *N. gonorrhoeae*. Gonococcal arthritis is the most common cause of acute monoarthritis in sexually active young adults. In the preantibiotic era, gonococcal arthritis was a well-recognized illness in neonates. Disseminated gonococcal infection is three times more common in women than men. Women are more commonly affected because they are more likely to have asymptomatic and untreated primary infections. Bacterial dissemination has been associated with intrauterine devices and has occurred during menstruation, pregnancy, and pelvic operation.[44]

Table 109-3 Risk Factors for Development of Septic Arthritis

Age >80 yr[3]
Diabetes mellitus[3]
Presence of a prosthetic joint in the knee or the hip[3]
Recent joint surgery[3]
Skin infection[3]
Previous septic arthritis[43]
Recent intra-articular injection[6]
HIV or AIDS
Intravenous drug abuse
End-stage renal disease on hemodialysis
Advanced hepatic disease
Hemophilia with or without AIDS
Sickle cell disease
Underlying malignancy
Hypogammaglobulinemia (susceptible to *Mycoplasma* infections)[45]
Late complement-component deficiency (susceptible to *Neisseria* infections)[44]
Low socioeconomic status with high rate of comorbidities[43]

AIDS, acquired immunodeficiency syndrome; HIV, human immunodeficiency virus.

Patients with gonococcal joint disease typically present with one of two forms. The first form is characterized by fever, shaking chills, vesiculopustular skin lesions, tenosynovitis, and polyarthralgias. Blood cultures are frequently positive, whereas synovial fluid cultures are rarely positive. *N. gonorrhoeae* can be cultured from genital, rectal, and pharyngeal sites. Tenosynovitis of multiple tendons of the wrist, fingers, ankle, and toes is a unique feature of this form of disseminated gonococcal infection and distinguishes it from other forms of infectious arthritis. In the second form of gonococcal infection, patients have purulent arthritis, most commonly of the knee, wrist, or ankle, and more than one joint can be infected simultaneously. *N. gonorrhoeae* can frequently be cultured from the synovial fluid.[45]

The classic presentation of nongonococcal septic arthritis is the acute onset of pain, swelling, and decreased range of motion in a single joint. Large joints are affected most commonly. In adults, the knee is involved in more than 50% of cases; hip, ankle, and shoulder infections are less common.[41] In infants and small children, the hip is more often involved.[46] Patients with septic arthritis often have underlying illnesses and predispositions to infections. Many are immunocompromised; are intravenous drug abusers; have prosthetic joints; and have diseases such as neoplasia, renal failure, and RA. Table 109-3 lists the risk factors that predispose to septic arthritis.[3,5,47]

Most patients with bacterial arthritis are febrile, although chills are unusual. Fever may be absent in elderly patients. In children, septic arthritis usually is accompanied by fever, malaise, poor appetite, irritability, and progressive reluctance to use the affected limb. Physical examination typically reveals warmth and tenderness of the affected joint, joint effusion, and limited active and passive range of motion. Septic arthritis among patients with RA has been a special challenge to clinicians because of the high incidence of infection and the poor outcome. Septic arthritis in patients with RA is associated with poor joint outcome and high mortality.[42,48] In many cases, it is difficult to differentiate septic arthritis in a joint already affected by RA from rheumatoid flare. Whenever bacterial arthritis is suspected, the most important diagnostic procedure is arthrocentesis

and examination of the synovial fluid. For joints that are deep and more difficult to aspirate, ultrasound-guided or fluoroscopy-guided needle aspiration should be done.

DIAGNOSIS AND DIAGNOSTIC TESTS

Arthrocentesis and synovial fluid analysis should be performed for all patients who present with an inflamed joint. Normal joints contain a small amount of synovial fluid that is clear, is highly viscous, and has few white blood cells (WBCs). The protein concentration is approximately one-third that of plasma, and the glucose concentration is similar to that of plasma. Infected synovial fluid is usually purulent with an elevated leukocyte count typically greater than 50,000 WBC/mm^3 and often exceeding 100,000 WBC/mm^3 with polymorphonuclear cell predominance. Synovial fluid levels of glucose, lactate dehydrogenase, and total protein have limited value in the diagnosis of septic arthritis. Although a low synovial fluid glucose (<40 mg/dL or less than half the serum glucose concentration) and an elevated lactate dehydrogenase suggest bacterial infection, they are not sufficiently sensitive or specific for the diagnosis.[49] Figure 109-2 is an algorithm for synovial fluid analysis; Table 109-4 lists the differential diagnoses of septic arthritis and the known causes of pseudoseptic arthritis.[50]

A definite diagnosis of bacterial arthritis can be made only by visualizing bacteria on a gram-stained smear or by culturing bacteria from the synovial fluid. In patients not previously treated with antibiotics, synovial fluid cultures are positive in 70% to 90% of cases of nongonococcal bacterial arthritis.[5,51] Blood cultures are positive in 40% to 50% of cases of septic arthritis and are the only method of identifying the pathogen in about 10% of cases.[52,53] Occasionally, an extra-articular site of infection offers a clue to the etiologic organism infecting the joint. Examples include septic arthritis in association with pneumococcal pneumonia, *E. coli* urinary tract infection, and cellulitis caused by staphylococci or streptococci. Gram-positive

Table 109-4 Differential Diagnosis of Septic Arthritis and Reported Causes of Pseudoseptic Arthritis*

Partially treated septic arthritis
Rheumatoid arthritis
Juvenile rheumatoid arthritis
Gout
Pseudogout
Apatite-related arthropathy
Reactive arthritis
Psoriatic arthritis
Systemic lupus erythematosus
Sickle cell disease
Dialysis-related amyloidosis
Transient synovitis of the hip
Plant thorn synovitis
Metastatic carcinoma
Pigmented villonodular synovitis
Hemarthrosis
Neuropathic arthropathy
Synovitis after injection of hylan

*Extremely inflammatory synovitis with negative culture is referred to as *pseudoseptic arthritis*. Typically, synovial fluid analysis shows ≥50,000 white blood cells (WBC)/mm^3. Often the WBC count is >100,000 WBC/mm^3.
Data from references 6, 52, 53.

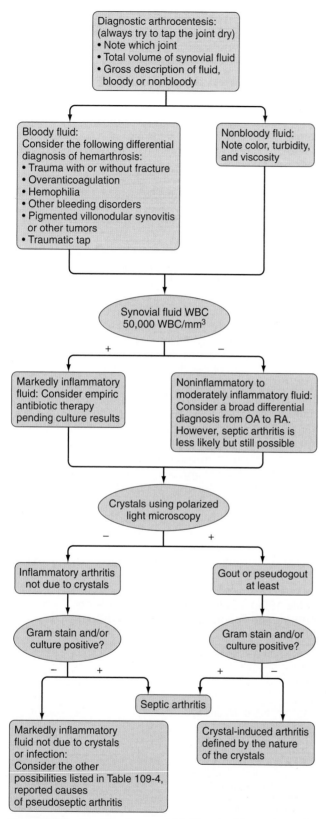

Figure 109-2　Algorithm for synovial fluid analysis in septic arthritis. OA, osteoarthritis; RA, rheumatoid arthritis; WBC, white blood cells.

cocci are identified in 50% to 75% of synovial fluid gram-stained smears, but gram-negative bacilli are identified less than 50% of the time in culture-proven cases.[51]

Inflammatory markers such as erythrocyte sedimentation rate (ESR), C-reactive protein (CRP), and WBC are usually raised, but the sensitivity is low and their absence does not exclude the diagnosis of septic arthritis.[47,54] Serum and joint fluid procalcitonin levels as a marker of septic arthritis have been studied, but the results are inconclusive.[55] A study that evaluated neutrophil-derived circulating free deoxyribonucleic acid (j-cf-DNA) in synovial fluid of 42 patients found out that at a cutoff of 300 ng/mL, j-cf-DNA had a sensitivity of 89%, a specificity of 100%, a positive predictive value of 100%, and a negative predictive value of 97%.[56] If validated and standardized, this could be a valuable additional test to diagnose septic arthritis.

Culture for *N. gonorrhoeae* is almost always negative in skin lesions and is positive in less than 50% of synovial fluid samples and in less than one-third of blood cultures; this may be the result of the fastidious growth requirements of *N. gonorrhoeae*. The organism can often be easily recovered from other sites such as urethral, cervical, rectal, or pharyngeal specimens (i.e., the genitourinary tract). In culture-negative septic arthritis where *N. gonorrhoeae* is suspected, polymerase chain reaction techniques can be used to detect gonococcal DNA in the synovial fluid. Unfortunately, the technique is not standardized and is not widely avilable.[57]

When culturing the synovial fluid, it should be brought directly to the laboratory and placed on conventional broth and solid media or into aerobic and anaerobic blood culture bottles. Inoculating blood culture bottles with 5 to 10 mL of joint fluid or smaller volumes into isolator tubes may increase the yield of positive cultures beyond that of standard techniques.[58,59] Synovial fluid culture using the BACTEC Peds Plus/F bottle and the BACTEC 9240 instrument (Becton Dickinson Diagnostic Systems, Sparks, Md) detected significantly more pathogens and fewer contaminants than culture by the agar-plate method.[60]

Plain radiographs in septic arthritis are usually normal early in the course of the infection, but baseline films should be obtained to look for evidence of other disease and contiguous osteomyelitis. Radiographs often show nonspecific changes of inflammatory arthritis including periarticular osteopenia, joint effusion, soft tissue swelling, and joint space loss. In more advanced infection, periosteal reaction, marginal or central erosions, and destruction of subchondral bone may be seen. Bony ankylosis is a late sequela of septic arthritis. Dislocation or subluxation of the femoral head is unique to hip infection of neonates.[61]

Ultrasound of the hip is the modality of choice to detect fluid collections in this deep joint and can serve as a guide in its aspiration. Ultrasound can be similarly used in other joints such as the popliteal cyst of the knee, shoulder, acromioclavicular, or sternoclavicular joints. Triple-phase bone scan using technetium 99m is often done in children to identify an associated metaphyseal osteomyelitis or avascular necrosis of the femoral head. Whole-body bone scan is preferred in young children because, despite focal symptoms, septic arthritis and osteomyelitis may be multifocal in this age group.[62] In septic arthritis of all age groups, the periarticular distribution of increased uptake is seen on the early "blood-pool" phase and the delayed images of the joint. Bone scans provide only nonspecific information, however, and cannot differentiate septic from noninfectious causes of joint inflammation. Bone scans are more sensitive than standard radiography in the diagnosis of arthritis because radionuclide uptake precedes morphologic bone changes that are seen on radiograph. A suggestive bone scan must be interpreted in the proper clinical context and supported by microbiologic data for a definitive diagnosis of joint or bone infection.

In joints that are difficult to evaluate otherwise or that have complex anatomic structures, computed tomography (CT) and magnetic resonance imaging (MRI) can provide useful images to delineate the extent of the infection.[63] MRI is highly sensitive in early detection of joint fluid and is superior to CT in the delineation of soft tissue structures and soft tissue abscess. These images can show early bone erosion; reveal soft tissue extension; and facilitate arthrocentesis of joints such as shoulders, hips, acromioclavicular,[64] sternoclavicular, sacroiliac, and facet joints of the spine. MRI findings such as reactive bone marrow can suggest presence of secondary osteomyelitis, which can complicate septic arthritis. When multiple joint involvement is suspected, triple-phase bone scintigraphy is the preferred modality of investigation.

TREATMENT

Treatment of septic arthritis must begin immediately after the clinical evaluation is complete and all appropriate cultures are taken. A serious clinical suspicion of a joint infection warrants the initiation of antibiotic therapy before culture confirmation is available. Delays in treatment allow the infection to become more established in the joint and permanently damage the articular cartilage. Untreated, there is the opportunity for the joint infection to spread to other body sites via the hematogenous route and become more widespread and more difficult to cure.

The principles of treatment of an infected joint, whether natural or prosthetic, follow those of treatment of an infected body cavity in which antibiotics must be used in conjunction with adequate drainage of the infected closed space. The clinical circumstances and the preliminary laboratory data aid the selection of antibiotic agents. Host factors, any extra-articular sites of infection, and the gram-stained smear of the synovial fluid are the best early guides for the antibiotic agents with which to start. Table 109-5 lists current antibiotic agents for adults,[53] and Table 109-6 lists agents for children.[65]

Narrow antibiotic coverage is indicated if gram-positive cocci are found in the synovial fluid, and the clinician suspects a primary source of staphylococcal infection from the skin. Appropriate monotherapy in this case may be a penicillinase-resistant penicillin or vancomycin if methicillin resistance is likely. If gram-negative bacilli are noted in the synovial fluid and the patient has a kidney infection, specific agents (e.g., ampicillin or a cephalosporin) against E. coli and other common urinary tract pathogens may be used. In healthy, young, sexually active individuals with community-acquired septic arthritis and a negative synovial fluid gram-stained smear, ceftriaxone is a reasonable option to cover N. gonorrhoeae. If synovial fluid gram stain shows gram-positive cocci, vancomycin should be the empiric therapeutic option considering the fact that a significant proportion of community-acquired S. aureus infections are now methicillin resistant.[66] A reasonable initial empiric therapy to cover gonococci, S. aureus, and streptococci is ceftriaxone plus vancomycin pending final culture results. In elderly debilitated patients or adults with low risk for sexually transmitted disease, as well as a negative gram-stained smear of synovial fluid, broad antibiotic coverage against a wide variety of organisms including S. aureus, streptococci, and gram-negative bacilli should be given initially. A typical regimen includes an antistaphylococcal agent (e.g., vancomycin) plus a third-generation cephalosporin (e.g., ceftriaxone).

When the identity and the sensitivities of the organism are known, antibiotic therapy should continue with the most efficacious agent that has the best safety profile and narrowest spectrum. The parenteral route of antibiotic administration is the preferred initial treatment. Continued antibiotic therapy may be switched to oral agents if adequate blood levels can be achieved and maintained by this route. There is no evidence that the direct intra-articular instillation of drugs is necessary or preferable in septic arthritis because there is no barrier against the free diffusion of antibiotic agents from the blood to the synovial fluid. In cases in which uncertainty exists, serum and synovial fluid levels of antibiotic drugs can be measured to ensure that therapeutic levels are reached.

Although some clinicians feel that patients with native-joint septic arthritis need urgent surgical drainage, the medical literature suggests otherwise. Most individuals with septic arthritis respond adequately to appropriate antimicrobial agents after initial joint aspiration for fluid analysis. In experimental infectious arthritis cases, early antibiotic therapy was shown to reduce the loss of collagen and erosion of articular surface, which minimizes the need for open surgical drainage.[67] It is generally accepted that prompt and adequate drainage of the septic joint is essential to decrease the risks of substantial loss of articular function; however, the best approach to drain the joint remains controversial.[68]

From retrospective studies, daily aspiration of an infected joint showed better functional outcome than open surgical drainage, although the former had higher overall mortality.[69,70] An explanation for higher mortality could be the higher comorbid conditions of patients who had daily aspirations than the ones who were more fit and underwent open surgical drainage.[69] If the synovial fluid cell count and polymorphonuclear percentage decrease with successive aspiration, the antimicrobial therapy is probably effective.[14,71] If needle aspiration is technically difficult (as in the hip or the shoulder) or does not provide thorough drainage of the joint, if the joint effusion does not resolve promptly, if sterilization of the joint fluid is delayed, if the infected joint is already damaged by pre-existing rheumatoid disease, or if infected synovial tissue or bone needs débridement, surgical drainage should be considered sooner rather than later.[14,51,72] Arthroscopy is emerging as an alternative to arthrotomy with the advantage of reduced surgical morbidity. Wound healing is faster, and rehabilitation time is shortened.[73] A recent retrospective analysis from the United Kingdom suggested that most patients can be treated

Table 109-5 Antibiotic Agents Used in Adults

Synovial Fluid Gram Stain	Organism	Antibiotic	Dose
Gram-positive cocci (clusters)	*Staphylococcus aureus* (methicillin-sensitive)	Nafcillin/oxacillin or	2 g IV q4h
		Cefazolin	1-2 g IV q8h
	S. aureus (methicillin-resistant)	Vancomycin or	1 g IV q12h
		Clindamycin or	900 mg IV q8h
		Linezolid	600 mg IV q12h
Gram-positive cocci (chains)	*Streptococcus*	Nafcillin or	2 g IV q4h
		Penicillin or	2 million U IV q4h
		Cefazolin	1-2 g IV q8h
Gram-negative diplococci	*Neisseria gonorrhoeae*	Ceftriaxone or	2 g IV q24h
		Cefotaxime or	1 g IV q8h
		Ciprofloxacin	400 mg IV q12h
Gram-negative bacilli	Enterobacteriaceae (*Escherichia coli, Proteus, Serratia*)	Ceftriaxone or	2 g IV q24h
		Cefotaxime	2 g IV q8h
	Pseudomonas	Cefepime or	2 g IV q12h
		Piperacillin or	3 g IV q6h
		Imipenem plus	500 mg IV q6h
		Gentamicin	7 mg/kg IV q24h
Polymicrobial infection	*S. aureus, Streptococcus*, gram-negative bacilli	Nafcillin/oxacillin* plus	2 g IV q4h
		Ceftriaxone or	2 g IV q24h
		Cefotaxime or	2 g IV q8h
		Ciprofloxacin	400 mg IV q12h

*If penicillin allergic, vancomycin plus third-generation cephalosporin or ciprofloxacin.
IV, intravenously; q4h, every 4 hours; q6h, every 6 hours; q8h, every 8 hours; q12h, every 12 hours; q24h, every 24 hours.
Data from references 76-80.

Table 109-6 Antibiotic Agents Used in Children

Age	Likely Pathogen	Antibiotic	Dosage (mg/kg/day)	Doses/day
Neonate	*Staphylococcus aureus*; group B streptococci; gram-negative bacilli	Nafcillin plus	100	4
		Cefotaxime or	150	3
		Gentamicin	5-7.5	3
Child <5 yr old	*S. aureus; Haemophilus influenzae**; group A streptococci; *Streptococcus pneumoniae*	Nafcillin† plus	150	4
		Cefotaxime or	100-150	3-4
		Ceftriaxone or	50	1-2
		Cefuroxime	150-200	3-4
Child >5 yr old	*S. aureus*; group A streptococci	Nafcillin† or	150	4
		Cefazolin	50	3-4
Adolescent (sexually active)	Previous organisms; *Neisseria gonorrhoeae*	Ceftriaxone	50	1-2

*Decreased incidence in children fully immunized with Hib vaccine.
†If patient is penicillin allergic, alternatives include vancomycin (40 mg/kg/day divided into four doses) or clindamycin (20-40 mg/kg/day divided into four doses).
Modified from Gutierrez KM: Infectious and inflammatory arthritis. In Long SS, Pickering LK, Prober CG, editors: *Principles and practice of pediatric infectious diseases*, ed 2, New York, 2002, Churchill Livingstone, pp 475–481.

medically (with repeated aspirations) and do not require surgical drainage (either by arthroscopy or arthrotomy).[74] Though statistically not significant, medical therapy resulted in more complete cure and less deterioration of functional status at time of discharge. Another study, which included 20 adults with native hip joint septic arthritis, concluded that symptom duration, especially if it is longer than 3 weeks before presentation, was a statistically significant predictor of the need for excision arthroplasty.[75] These results highlight the need for careful case selection for surgical intervention.

The optimal duration of antibiotic treatment has not been prospectively studied. For native joint infections caused by *N. gonorrhoeae*, a 1-week course of ceftriaxone should be adequate. For septic arthritis caused by organisms other than *N. gonorrhoeae*, therapy ranging from 2 weeks to 6 weeks is recommended depending on type, sensitivity of microorganism, and presence of osteomyelitis. If long-term antibiotics are chosen (4 to 6 weeks' duration), parenteral antibiotics may be switched to oral antibiotics after 2 weeks provided that there is clinical improvement, inflammatory markers are trending down, and oral antibiotics are available to which the microorganism is susceptible.[53] The duration of antibiotic administration can be 2 weeks for uncomplicated infection by susceptible microorganisms or 4 to 6 weeks for more extensive infection in an immunocompromised host. For septic arthritis caused by *H. influenzae*, streptococci, or gram-negative cocci, 2 weeks of antibiotic therapy is usually adequate. Staphylococcal septic arthritis usually requires 3 to 4 weeks of therapy, and for pneumococcal or gram-negative bacillary infections, therapy should be continued for at least 4 weeks.[72,76]

During the first few days of management, immobilization of the infected joint by external splinting and adequate analgesic administration ensure patient comfort. Physical therapy, starting with passive then graduating to active motion, should be instituted as soon as the patient can tolerate mobilization of the inflamed joint because early active range-of-motion exercises are beneficial for ultimate functional recovery. Involving the orthopedic surgeon and the physical therapist early on in the course of treatment facilitates the best choice of drainage procedure and results in the best functional outcome.[77]

PROSTHETIC JOINT INFECTIONS

Total joint replacement for advanced arthritis is one of the major advances in medicine in the 20th century and continues to improve in the 21st century. Infection of prosthetic joints is an uncommon but devastating complication of joint replacement surgery. Nearly 800,000 total knee and total hip replacements were done in the United States in 2006 (www.cdc.gov/nchs/fastats/insurg.htm), with an infection rate of 1% to 3%.[78] The infection rate is higher for knee arthroplasty (1% to 2%) compared with hip and shoulder arthroplasty (0.3% to 1.3%) and is much higher in patients undergoing reimplantation because of infection of the initial prosthesis (3% for hips and 6% for knees).[79,80] The risk of infection is about twofold higher in patients with RA compared with patients with osteoarthritis.[81]

The risk of infection is related to many factors. In a retrospective study of 462 infected orthopedic implants, the most important risks for infection included (1) a surgical site infection at a site other than the prosthesis (odds ratio [OR], 35.9), (2) a score of 2 on the National Nosocomial Infections Surveillance System surgical patient risk index (OR, 3.9), (3) the presence of a malignancy (OR, 3.1), and (4) a history of joint arthroplasty (OR, 2.0).[82] Certain patient populations are at increased risk of infection because of comorbid conditions (e.g., diabetes mellitus and RA). Other surgical risk factors include simultaneous bilateral arthroplasty, long operative time (>2.5 hours), blood transfusion, urinary tract infection, and *Staphylococcus aureus* bacteremia.[83,84]

Orthopedic implants adversely affect host defenses. Prosthetic devices impair opsonic activity and diminish the ability of neutrophils to kill bacteria.[85] Polymorphonuclear leukocytes release lysosomal enzymes and superoxide into the area surrounding the prosthesis, resulting in tissue damage and local devascularization.[86] Phagocytes may be focused on removal of the foreign body such that fewer cells are available to fight infection.[87] Finally, polymethyl methacrylate bone cement can inhibit neutrophil and complement functions, and the heat produced by the polymerization of polymethyl methacrylate can damage adjacent cortical bone and result in a devascularized necrotic area, which is ideal for bacterial growth. After implantation, prosthetic joints are immediately coated by host proteins including albumin, fibrinogen, and fibronectin. *S. aureus*, which possesses numerous host protein binding receptors (MSCRAMMs), is a common pathogen in infection of prosthetic joints. Patients with a prosthetic joint who develop *S. aureus* bacteremia have an approximate one in three chance of developing an infection of the implant.[88]

Another phenomenon crucial to development of infection is the ability of organisms to form biofilms on the surface of the prosthetic device. A biofilm is defined as "an assemblage of microbial cells that is irreversibly associated with a surface and enclosed in a matrix of primarily polysaccharide material."[89] Biofilm formation is a natural process. Organisms grow on indwelling medical devices, potable water system pipes, and living tissues. *S. epidermidis* is particularly adept at attaching to and forming biofilms on foreign bodies such as prosthetic joints. Small numbers of these organisms from the patient's skin or mucous membranes, or from the hands of the surgeons or clinical staff, contaminate and colonize the orthopedic device at the time of implantation. Staphylococcal surface proteins, SSP-1 and SSP-2, are fimbria-like polymers that facilitate adherence of *S. epidermidis* to polystyrene.[90] *S. epidermidis* produces a polysaccharide/adhesin substance crucial to the formation of this extracellular matrix known as slime. Polysaccharide/adhesin mutants have been shown to be less virulent than the wild-type strain in a rabbit model of endocarditis.[91]

Prosthetic joint infections are divided into early onset (<3 months after placement), delayed (3 to 24 months postsurgery), and late onset (>24 months after placement).[92] Early and delayed infections are usually related to surgical contamination at the time of the implantation, whereas late infections usually result from hematogenous seeding of the joint. Owing to its high virulence, *S. aureus* accounts for most early and late infections (see Table 109-1). So-called small colony variants of *S. aureus* may be responsible for persistent and recurrent infections of prosthetic implants.[93]

These subspecies of S. *aureus* are difficult to treat because they grow slowly and are relatively resistant to cell-wall active antimicrobial agents and aminoglycosides. Delayed infections are usually caused by less virulent microorganisms such as coagulase-negative staphylococci and P. *acnes*. Because these low-virulence organisms are common skin contaminants, it is important to interpret culture results carefully.

Clinically, the most common symptom in patients with prosthetic joint infection is pain of the affected joint. Differentiating pain from mechanical loosening of the prosthesis from pain related to infection can be difficult. Typically, a patient with mechanical loosening but no infection has pain only with motion, whereas a patient with infection experiences pain at rest and with motion. Warmth at the implant site, effusion, erythema, and fever are frequently associated with early and late, but not delayed, infections. This difference in clinical presentation likely represents the virulence of the most common organisms associated with the three categories of infection. The presence of a sinus tract with purulent discharge suggests involvement of the implant and is an indication for removal of the prosthesis.

Inflammatory blood laboratory markers have variable sensitivity and specificity in the diagnosis of prosthetic joint infection. In a recent meta-analysis, elevated levels of interleukin-6 (IL-6) and CRP had a much higher sensitivity (97% and 88%, respectively) than an elevation of the WBC count or ESR (45% and 75%, respectively).[94] The specificity of an elevated level of IL-6 (91%) was the highest of these markers with elevation of WBC (87%), CRP (74%), and ESR (70%) somewhat lower. Inflammatory markers increase following arthroplasty, and the return to normal levels is quite variable. IL-6 will return to normal within a matter of a few days following surgery, whereas the CRP level may remain elevated for up to 3 weeks and the ESR for several months following arthroplasy.[94] Therefore a low or normal CRP or IL-6 level in a patient with suspected prosthetic joint infection has a good negative-predictive value. Serial plain radiographs may be helpful; the presence of subperiosteal bone growth and transcortical sinus tracts is specific for infection.[95] Bone scans using technetium 99m–labeled methylene diphosphonate are sensitive but lack specificity because the bone scan is typically positive for 6 to 12 months after the original implantation.[96] Bone scans may be a useful screening test for patients with suspected late prosthetic joint infection. CT has limitations because of the imaging artifacts caused by the metal implant. MRI can be performed only in patients with titanium or tantalum implants.

Aspiration of the joint may be helpful in differentiating infection from noninfectious causes of joint pain, particularly in patients without RA. In one study, a synovial fluid leukocyte count of greater than 1700/mm³ had a sensitivity of 94% for determining infection, whereas a differential count of greater than 65% neutrophils had a sensitivity of 97%.[97] The specificities of these two measurements were 88% and 98% in patients without underlying inflammatory diseases such as RA. Gram-stained smear of the synovial fluid has a low sensitivity (<20%) but a high specificity (>97%).[98] Cultures of drainage from a sinus tract are not helpful, unless the culture grows S. *aureus*.[99]

Generally, at least three tissue specimens should be taken at the time of surgery including tissue from the joint capsule, synovial lining, bone-cement interface, and samples from purulent material or sequestrum.[84,98] Swabs of the joint have a low sensitivity and should be avoided. Unless the patient is septic or otherwise systemically ill, antimicrobial therapy should be discontinued a minimum of 2 weeks before the revision surgery and perioperative antibiotics should not be administered until all of the tissue cultures have been obtained. Using this methodical approach, there is a direct correlation between the number of tissue specimens positive for a particular microorganism and the probability of infection. The probability of infection has been estimated to be less than 5% if all tissue specimens are negative and greater than 94% if three or more tissue specimens are positive for growth.[98] Finally, the location of the prosthesis is helpful in the interpretation of the positive culture. The isolation of P. *acnes* from a single tissue culture from a knee prosthesis is more likely to be a contaminant than if the same organism is obtained from a shoulder prosthesis.[100]

For patients who have received recent antibiotics, there may be a role for sonication of the prosthesis at the time of explantation. A recent study determined that culturing of the explanted prosthesis that has been sonicated to remove adherent bacteria had a higher sensitivity (75%) as compared with culture of periprosthetic tissue (45%) in patients who had received antibiotics in the past 14 days.[101]

Medical therapy of patients with prosthetic joint infections is challenging. Organisms existing in biofilms are much more resistant to antimicrobial agents for several reasons. First, the drugs have difficulty penetrating the biofilm layer. The biofilm-associated organisms also grow much slower than organisms in suspension. As a result, antimicrobial agents such as vancomycin, penicillins, and cephalosporins, which act on rapidly dividing organisms, are not effective in treating device-related infections.[102,103] Rifampin and fluoroquinolones may be more effective because they are active against organisms in the stationary phase of growth.[103,104] Although most experts recommend rifampin in combination with another agent for the treatment of rifampin-susceptible strains of S. *aureus*, there are little clinical data to support the benefit of combination therapy versus monotherapy in the treatment of prosthetic joint infections.[105] The role of newer antibiotics such as linezolid, daptomycin, and tigecycline is unclear at this time.[106] In a rabbit experimental model of S. *aureus* osteomyelitis, the combination of tigecycline and rifampin eradicated infection in 100% of 14 rabbits.[107]

Treatment of late prosthetic joint infections is complex. In most patients, effective therapy requires a combination of antibiotics with the removal of the orthopedic device. Failure to remove the infected prosthesis is frequently associated with an unacceptably high rate of relapse, probably related to biofilm formation on the orthopedic implant. Removal of the joint prosthesis, débridement of infected bone, and placement of a new prosthesis during the same operation has been associated with a high rate of recurrence of infection,[108] but studies indicate that single-stage revision or débridement with retention of the prosthesis may be effective in certain situations.[109] Patients whose symptoms of pain and swelling of the joint have been less than 8 days[109] or less than 3 weeks[110] and who have a stable

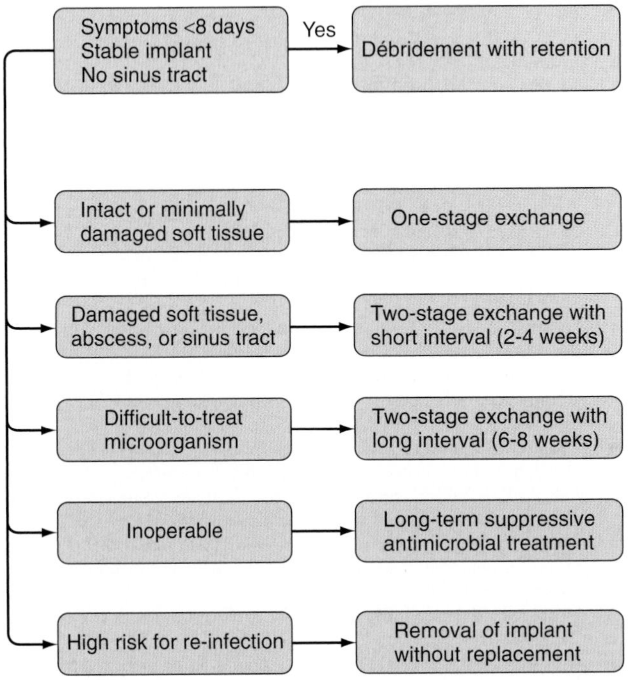

Figure 109-3 Algorithm for the management of an infected joint prosthesis. *(Modified from Trampuz A, Zimmerli W: Prosthetic joint infections: update in diagnosis and treatment,* Swiss Med Wkly *135:243–251, 2005.)*

prosthesis with little soft tissue damage and no sinus tract are candidates for débridement, antibiotics, and implant retention (DAIR) if the preoperative synovial fluid cultures are negative or if the cultures grow an easily treatable organism (Figure 109-3).[109,111] The treatment of choice for most patients is a two-stage process involving removal of the infected prosthesis and débridement of infected bone, stabilization of the joint using an antibiotic-impregnated methyl methacrylate spacer, and 6 weeks of intravenous antibiotics (first stage), followed by reimplantation of a second orthopedic implant (second stage).[112] Using this approach, the success rate is approximately 80% to 90%. Rarely, antibiotic treatment is continued indefinitely in a patient in whom the risk of removing the infected prosthesis is too great, the prosthesis is not loose, and the organism responsible for the infection can be reasonably suppressed by the use of an oral antibiotic agent.[113]

The pathogenesis of bacterial infection in prosthetic joints is complex. Anatomic, virulence, and host factors affect prognosis and approach to therapy. An understanding of these interactions may lead to novel therapeutic and preventive strategies such as vaccines against capsule antigens or surface adhesins in patients undergoing elective joint replacements.

PREVENTION OF PROSTHETIC JOINT INFECTIONS

There is consensus that preoperative evaluation of a patient for occult infection such as periodontal disease or bacteriuria is warranted, and corrective steps to eradicate any infection are essential before joint replacement. There is also consensus that perioperative antibiotic prophylaxis significantly reduces the rate of early postoperative infection, and this practice is routine. The role of antibiotic prophylaxis to prevent late prosthetic joint infection before diagnostic or therapeutic procedures that lead to transient bacteremia, especially dental treatment, is controversial.

A position paper of the American Academy of Oral Medicine in 2010 stated that "the risk of patients' experiencing drug reactions or drug-resistant bacterial infections and the cost of antibiotic medications alone do not justify the practice of using antibiotic prophylaxis in patients with prosthetic joints."[114] Many orthopedic and oral and maxillofacial surgeons have argued that there is "no scientific evidence to support the view that patients with arthroplasties, even in the high-risk groups, require antibiotic prophylaxis during dental treatment."[115]

The incidence of late infection of a prosthetic joint as a result of procedure-related bacteremia is extremely low—10 to 100 cases per 100,000 patients with total joint replacement per year. The cost of providing antibiotic prophylaxis to all patients with prosthetic joints before all procedures that are associated with transient bacteremia is substantial. The efficacy of such antibiotic prophylaxis is unknown. Cost-effective analyses have shown mixed results.[116,117] These discrepancies are due to the lack of reliable data and the different assumptions used in the calculations. In the patient with the greatest risk of infection, an invasive procedure that leads to bacteremia sometimes can result in an infected total joint replacement. Counseling these patients on the risks and benefits of antibiotic prophylaxis would lead to an informed decision on which the patient and the physician can agree.

As we gain experience with the use of biologic agents in the management of RA and other inflammatory arthritides, there remains the conundrum of whether the increased risk of infection from TNF inhibitor and methotrexate warrants holding them before an elective orthopedic procedure. A retrospective analysis of 10 cases of postoperative infections showed the use of a TNF inhibitor was significantly associated with the development of a serious infection (OR, 4.4).[118] A meta-analysis of the clinical literature on TNF inhibitors through 2005 found an increased risk of serious infection.[119] The risks and benefits must be weighed carefully, and the patients must be fully informed on how these agents should be used on a case-by-case basis.

OUTCOME

In the 21st century, patients with septic arthritis as a group are becoming older, with more risk factors for infection and more comorbidities. The number of patients with prosthetic joints is increasing as the population of older patients grows and people live longer. It is not surprising to see more cases of infection in total joint replacements. The organisms have not changed significantly, however. Staphylococci (44% to 66%) are still the dominant organisms followed by streptococci (18% to 28%) and gram-negative bacilli (9% to 19%).[6] The emerging challenges in the treatment of septic arthritis are how to improve outcome, how to deal with resistant organisms, and how to overcome host factors that portend a poor prognosis.

The outcome of treated septic arthritis can be measured as mortality, as the functional outcome of the infected joint,

Table 109-7 Factors That Might Portend a Poor Outcome in Septic Arthritis

Older age
Pre-existing arthritis, especially rheumatoid arthritis, but also osteoarthritis and tophaceous gout
Presence of synthetic material (e.g., total joint replacement)
Delay in diagnosis or long duration of symptoms before seeking medical attention
Polyarticular infection, especially if >3 joints and small hand joints are affected
Presence of bacteremia
Infection caused by virulent or difficult-to-treat organisms (e.g., *Staphylococcus aureus, Pseudomonas aeruginosa,* or some gram-negative bacilli)
Patients receiving immunosuppressive therapy
Serious underlying comorbidities (e.g., liver, kidney, or heart diseases)
Peripheral leukocytosis at presentation
Worsening renal function

Data from references 36, 43, 49, 120.

or as short-term and long-term outcomes. Among the survivors, loss of articular cartilage, loss of motion, or increase in pain in the affected joint would be considered poor functional outcomes. Loss of the limb to infection and need for surgery to fuse the joint or restore function are also poor outcomes. Most studies report the outcome at the time of hospital discharge, and long-term data on adults with septic arthritis are unavailable. The rate of development of degenerative joint disease, the rate of relapse or recurrence of infection, and the rate of progression of functional impairment in the affected joint over time have not been well studied.

Many retrospective studies have characterized features that may increase the chance of a poor outcome at the time of hospital discharge (Table 109-7).[15,47,120] One prospective community-based study of adults and children found poor joint outcome in 33% of survivors among 154 patients with bacterial arthritis and noted older age, pre-existing joint disease, and an infected joint containing synthetic material as negative prognostic factors by univariate analysis.[120] These investigators noted no association between poor outcome and young age, comorbidity, immunosuppressive medication, functional class, multiple infected joints, type of organism, or treatment delay. In a large retrospective study from the United Kingdom on the outcome of 243 patients, 11.5% died secondary to septic arthritis and additional morbidity was noted in 31.6% of patients. Multivariate analysis suggests that important predictors of death are confusion at presentation, age 65 years or older, multiple joint sepsis, and involvement of the elbow joint. Predictors of morbidity were age 65 years or older, diabetes mellitus, open surgical drainage, and gram-positive infections other than *S. aureus.*[52]

References

1. Goldenberg DL: Bacterial arthritis, *Curr Opin Rheumatol* 6:394–400, 1994.
2. Kaandorp CJE, Dinant HJ, van de Laar MAFJ, et al: Incidence and sources of native and prosthetic joint infection: a community based prospective survey, *Ann Rheum Dis* 56:470–475, 1997.
3. Kaandorp CJ, Van Schaardenburg D, Krijnen P, et al: Risk factors for septic arthritis in patients with joint disease: a prospective study, *Arthritis Rheum* 38:1819–1825, 1995.
4. Geirsson AJ, Statkevicius S, Vikingsson A: Septic arthritis in Iceland 1990–2002: increasing incidence due to iatrogenic infections, *Ann Rheum Dis* 67:638–643, 2008.
5. Mathews CJ, Weston VC, Jones A, et al: Bacterial septic arthritis in adults, *Lancet* 375:846–855, 2010.
6. Dubost JJ, Soubrier M, De Champs C, et al: No changes in the distribution of organisms responsible for septic arthritis over a 20 year period, *Ann Rheum Dis* 61:267–269, 2002.
7. Al Saadi MM, Al Zamil FA, Bokhary NA, et al: Acute septic arthritis in children, *Pediatr Int* 51:377–380, 2009.
8. Adams WG, Deaver KA, Cochi SL, et al: Decline of childhood *Haemophilus influenzae* type b Hib disease in the Hib vaccine era, *JAMA* 269:221–226,1993.
9. Goldenberg DL, Cohen AS: Acute infectious arthritis, *Am J Med* 60:369–377, 1976.
10. Schattner A, Vosti KL: Bacterial arthritis due to beta-hemolytic streptococci of serogroups A, B, C, F, and G: analysis of 23 cases and review of the literature, *Medicine* 77:122–139, 1998.
11. Duggan JM, Georgiadis G, VanGorp C, et al: Group B streptococcal prosthetic joint infections, *J South Orthop Assoc* 10:209–214, 2001.
12. Pischel KD, Weisman MH, Cone RO: Unique features of group B streptococcal arthritis in adults, *Arch Intern Med* 145:97–102, 1985.
13. Goldenberg DL, Brandt K, Cathcart E, et al: Acute arthritis caused by gram-negative bacilli: a clinical characterization, *Medicine* 53:197–208, 1974.
14. Pioro MH, Mandell BF: Septic arthritis, *Rheum Dis Clin N Am* 23:239–258, 1997.
15. Dubost J, Fis I, Denis P, et al: Polyarticular septic arthritis, *Medicine* 72:296–310, 1993.
16. Ho G Jr: Bacterial arthritis. In McCarty DJ, Koopman WJ, editors: *Arthritis and allied conditions,* ed 12, Philadelphia, 1993, Lea & Febiger, pp 2003–2023.
17. Gutierrez KM: Infectious and inflammatory arthritis. In Long SS, Pickering LK, Prober CG, editors: *Principles and practice of pediatric infectious diseases,* ed 2, New York, 2002, Churchill Livingstone, pp 475–481.
18. Gilad J, Borer A, Riesenberg K, et al: Polymicrobial polyarticular septic arthritis: a rare clinical entity, *Scand J Infect Dis* 33:381–383, 2001.
19. Esterhai JL Jr, Gelb I: Adult septic arthritis, *Orthop Clin North Am* 22:503–514, 1991.
20. Armstrong RW, Bolding F, Joseph R: Septic arthritis following arthroscopy: clinical syndromes and analysis of risk factors, *Arthroscopy* 8:213–223, 1992.
21. Centers for Disease Control and Prevention: Septic arthritis following anterior cruciate ligament reconstruction using tendon allografts—Florida and Louisiana, 2000, *MMWR Morb Mortal Wkly Rep* 50:1081–1083, 2001.
22. Ram S, Mackinnon FG, Gulati S, et al: The contrasting mechanisms of serum resistance of *Neisseria gonorrhoeae* and group B *Neisseria meningitidis, Mol Immunol* 36:915–928, 1999.
23. Goldenberg DL, Reed JI, Rice PA: Arthritis in rabbits induced by killed *Neisseria gonorrhoeae* and gonococcal lipopolysaccharide, *J Rheumatol* 11:3–8, 1984.
24. Patti JM, Allen BL, McGavin MJ, et al: MSCRAMM-mediated adherence of microorganisms to host tissues, *Annu Rev Microbiol* 48:585–617, 1994.
25. Patti JM, Bremell T, Krajewska-Pietrasik D, et al: The *Staphylococcus aureus* collagen adhesin is a virulence determinant in experimental septic arthritis, *Infect Immun* 62:152–161, 1994.
26. Greene C, McDevitt D, Francois P, et al: Adhesion properties of mutants of *Staphylococcus aureus* defective in fibronectin-binding proteins and studies on the expression of fnb genes, *Mol Microbiol* 17:1143–1152, 1995.
27. Winzer K, Williams P: Quorum sensing and the regulation of virulence gene expression in pathogenic bacteria, *Int J Med Microbiol* 291:131–143, 2001.
28. Hudson MC, Ramp WK, Nicholson NC, et al: Internalization of *Staphylococcus aureus* by cultured osteoblasts, *Microb Pathog* 19:409–419, 1995.
29. Silverman GJ, Sasano M, Wormsley SB: Age-associated changes in binding of human B lymphocytes to a VH3-restricted unconventional bacterial antigen, *J Immunol* 151:5840–5855, 1993.
30. Palmqvist N, Silverman GJ, Josefsson E, et al: Bacterial cell wall-expressed protein A triggers supraclonal B-cell responses upon in vivo

infection with *Staphylococcus aureus*, *Microb Infect* 7:1501–1511, 2005.

31. Gemmell CG, Goutcher SC, Reid R, et al: Role of certain virulence factors in a murine model of *Staphylococcus aureus* arthritis, *J Med Microbiol* 46:208–213, 1997.

32. Albus A, Arbeit RD, Lee JC: Virulence of *Staphylococcus aureus* mutants altered in type 5 capsule production, *Infect Immun* 59:1008–1014, 1991.

33. Buxton TB, Rissing JP, Horner JA, et al: Binding of a *Staphylococcus aureus* bone pathogen to type I collagen, *Microb Pathog* 8:441–448, 1990.

34. Vandenesch F, Projan SJ, Kreiswirth B, et al: Agr-related sequences in *Staphylococcus lugdunensis*, *FEMS Microbiol Lett* 111:115–122, 1993.

35. Nilsson IM, Lee JC, Bremell T, et al: The role of staphylococcal polysaccharide microcapsule expression in septicemia and septic arthritis, *Infect Immun* 65:4216–4221, 1997.

36. Shinefield H, Black S, Fattom A, et al: Use of a *Staphylococcus aureus* conjugate vaccine in patients receiving hemodialysis, *N Engl J Med* 346:491–496, 2002.

37. Bremell T, Tarkowski A: Preferential induction of septic arthritis and mortality by superantigen-producing staphylococci, *Infect Immun* 63:4185–4187, 1995.

38. Renno T, Hahne M, MacDonald HR: Proliferation is a prerequisite for bacterial superantigen-induced T cell apoptosis in vivo, *J Exp Med* 181:2283–2287, 1995.

39. Nilsson IM, Verdrengh M, Ulrich RG, et al: Protection against *Staphylococcus aureus* sepsis by vaccination with recombinant staphylococcal enterotoxin A devoid of superantigenicity, *J Infect Dis* 180:1370–1373, 1999.

40. Kimura M, Matsukawa A, Ohkawara S, et al: Blocking of TNF-alpha and IL-1 inhibits leukocyte infiltration at early, but not at late stage of *S. aureus*-induced arthritis and the concomitant cartilage destruction in rabbits, *Clin Immunol Immunopathol* 82:18–25, 1997.

41. Zhao YX, Nilsson IM, Tarkowski A: The dual role of interferon-gamma in experimental *Staphylococcus aureus* septicemia versus arthritis, *Immunology* 93:80–85, 1998.

42. Epstein JH, Zimmermann B III, Ho G Jr: Polyarticular septic arthritis, *J Rheumatol* 13:1105–1107, 1986.

43. Christodoulou C, Gordon P, Coakley G: Polyarticular septic arthritis, *BMJ* 333:1107–1108, 2006.

44. Cucurull E, Espinoza LR: Gonococcal arthritis, *Rheum Dis Clin N Am* 24:305–322, 1998.

45. O'Brien JP, Goldenberg DL, Rice PA: Disseminated gonococcal infection: a prospective analysis of 49 patients and a review of pathophysiology and immune mechanisms, *Medicine* 62:395–406, 1983.

46. Goldenberg DL: Septic arthritis and other infections of rheumatologic significance, *Rheum Dis Clin N Am* 17:149–156, 1991.

47. Gupta MN, Sturrock RD, Field M: A prospective 2-year study of 75 patients with adult-onset septic arthritis, *Rheumatology (Oxford)* 40:24–30, 2001.

48. Nolla JM, Gomez-Vaquero C, Fiter J, et al: Pyarthrosis in patients with rheumatoid arthritis: a detailed analysis of 10 cases and literature review, *Semin Arthritis Rheum* 30:121–126, 2000.

49. Shmerling RH, Delbanco TL, Tosteson ANA, et al: Synovial fluid tests: what should be ordered? *JAMA* 264:1009–1014, 1990.

50. Perez-Ruiz F, Testillano M, Gastaca MA, et al: Pseudoseptic pseudogout associated with hypomagnesemia in liver transplant patients, *Transplantation* 71:696–698, 2001.

51. Goldenberg DL: Septic arthritis, *Lancet* 351:197–202, 1998.

52. Weston VC, Jones AC, Bradbury N, et al: Clinical features and outcome of septic arthritis in a single UK health district 1982–1991, *Ann Rheum Dis* 58:214–219, 1999.

53. Coakley G, Mathews C, Field M, et al, on behalf of the British Society for Rheumatology Standards, Guidelines and Audit Working Group: BSR & BHPR, BOA, RCGP and BSAC guidelines for management of the hot swollen joint in adults, *Rheumatology (Oxford)* 45:1039–1041, 2006.

54. Li SF, Henderson J, Dickman E, et al: Laboratory tests in adults with monoarticular arthritis: can they rule out a septic joint? *Acad Emerg Med* 11:276–280, 2004.

55. Martinot M, Sordet C, Soubrier M, et al: Diagnostic value of serum and synovial procalcitonin in acute arthritis: a prospective study of 42 patients, *Clin Exp Rheumatol* 23:303–310, 2005.

56. Logters T, Paunel-Gorgulu A, Zilkens C, et al. Diagnostic accuracy of neutrophil-derived circulating free DNA (cf-DNA/NETs) for septic arthritis, *J Orthop Res* 27:1401–1407, 2009.

57. Muralidhar B, Rumore PM, Steinman CR: Use of the polymerase chain reaction to study arthritis due to *Neisseria gonorrhoeae*, *Arthritis Rheum* 37:710–717, 1994.

58. von Essen R: Culture of joint specimens in bacterial arthritis: impact of blood culture bottle utilization, *Scand J Rheumatol* 26:293–300, 1997.

59. Yagupsky P, Press J: Use of the isolator 1.5 microbial tube for culture of synovial fluid from patients with septic arthritis, *J Clin Microbiol* 35:2410–2412, 1997.

60. Hughes JG, Vetter EA, Patel R, et al: Culture with BACTEC Peds Plus/F bottle compared with conventional methods for detection of bacteria in synovial fluid, *J Clin Microbiol* 39:4468–4471, 2001.

61. Bennett OM, Namnyak SS: Acute septic arthritis of the hip joint in infancy and childhood, *Clin Orthop* 281:123–132, 1992.

62. Mandell GA: Imaging in the diagnosis of musculoskeletal infections in children, *Curr Probl Pediatr* 26:218–237, 1996.

63. Sanchez RB, Quinn SF: MRI of inflammatory synovial processes, *Magn Reson Imaging* 7:529–540, 1989.

64. Widman DS, Craig JG, Van Holsbeeck MT: Sonographic detection, evaluation and aspiration of infected acromioclavicular joints, *Skeletal Radiol* 30:388–392, 2001.

65. Gutierrez KM: Infectious and inflammatory arthritis. In Long SS, Pickering LK, Prober CG, editors: *Principles and practice of pediatric infectious diseases*, ed 2, New York, 2002, Churchill Livingstone, pp 475–481.

66. Fridkin SK, Hageman JC, Morrison M, et al. Methicillin-resistant *Staphylococcus aureus* disease in three communities, *N Engl J Med* 352:1436–1444, 2005.

67. Smith RL, Schurman DJ, Kajiyama G, et al: The effect of antibiotics on the destruction of cartilage in experimental infectious arthritis, *J Bone Joint Surg Am* 69:1063–1068, 1987.

68. Manadan AM, Block JA: Daily needle aspiration versus surgical lavage for the treatment of bacterial septic arthritis in adults, *Am J Ther* 11:412–415, 2004.

69. Goldenberg D, Brandt K, Cohen A, et al: Treatment of septic arthritis: Comparison of needle aspiration and surgery as initial modes of joint drainage, *Arthritis Rheum* 18:83–90, 1975.

70. Broy S, Schmid F: A comparison of medical drainage (needle aspiration) and surgical drainage in the initial treatment of infected joints, *Clin Rheum Dis* 12:501–521, 1986.

71. Goldenberg DL, Reed JI: Bacterial arthritis, *N Engl J Med* 312:764–771, 1985.

72. Smith JW, Piercy EA: Infectious arthritis, *Clin Infect Dis* 20:225–231, 1995.

73. Parisien JS, Shafer B: Arthroscopic management of pyoarthrosis, *Clin Orthop* 275:243–247, 1992.

74. Ravindran V, Logan I, Bourke BE: Medical vs surgical treatment for the native joint in septic arthritis: a 6-year, single UK academic centre experience, *Rheumatology (Oxford)* 48:1320–1322, 2009.

75. Matthews PC, Dean BJF, Medagoda K, et al. Native hip joint septic arthritis in 20 adults: delayed presentation beyond three weeks predicts need for excision arthroplasty, *J Infect* 57:185–190, 2008.

76. Ross JJ, Saltzman CL, Carling P, et al: Pneumococcal septic arthritis: review of 190 cases, *Clin Infect Dis* 36:319–327, 2003.

77. Ho G Jr: How best to drain an infected joint: will we ever know for certain? *J Rheumatol* 20:2001–2003, 1993.

78. Darouiche RO: Device-associated infections: a macroproblem that starts with microadherence, *Clin Infect Dis* 33:1567–1572, 2001.

79. Lidgren L, Knutson K, Stefansdottir A: Infection and arthritis: infection of prosthetic joints, *Best Pract Res Clin Rheumatol* 17:209–218, 2003.

80. Sperling JW, Kozak TK, Hanssen AD, et al: Infection after shoulder arthroplasty, *Clin Orthop* 382:206–216, 2001.

81. Robertsson O, Knutson K, Lewold S, et al: The Swedish Knee Arthroplasty Register 1975-1997: an update with special emphasis on 41,223 knees operated on in 1988-1997, *Acta Orthop Scand* 72:503–513, 2001.

82. Berbari EF, Hanssen AD, Duffy MC, et al: Risk factors for prosthetic joint infection: case-control study, *Clin Infect Dis* 27:1247–1254, 1998.

83. Jämsen E, Huhtala H, Puolakka T, Moilanen T: Risk factors for infection after knee arthroplasty: a register-based analysis of 43,149 cases, *J Bone Joint Surg Am* 91:38–47,2009.

84. Del Pozo JL, Patel R: Infection associated with prosthetic joints, *N Engl J Med* 361:787–794, 2009.

85. Zimmerli W, Waldvogel FA, Vaudaux P, et al: Pathogenesis of foreign body infection: description and characteristics of an animal model, *J Infect Dis* 146:487–497, 1982.

86. Roisman FR, Walz DT, Finkelstein AE: Superoxide radical production by human leukocytes exposed to immune complexes: inhibitory action of gold compounds, *Inflammation* 7:355–362, 1983.

87. Wang JY, Wicklund BH, Gustilo RB, et al: Prosthetic metals impair murine immune response and cytokine release in vivo and in vitro, *J Orthop Res* 15:688–697, 1997.

88. Murdoch DR, Roberts SA, Fowler VG, et al: Infection of orthopedic prostheses after *Staphylococcus aureus* bacteremia, *Clin Infect Dis* 32:647–649, 2001.

89. Donlan RM: Biofilms: Microbial life on surfaces, *Emerg Infect Dis* 8:881–890, 2002.

90. Veenstra GJ, Cremers FF, van Dijk H, et al: Ultrastructural organization and regulation of a biomaterial adhesin of *Staphylococcus epidermidis*, *J Bacteriol* 178:537–541, 1996.

91. Shiro H, Muller E, Gutierrez N, et al: Transposon mutants of *Staphylococcus epidermidis* deficient in elaboration of capsular polysaccharide/adhesin and slime are avirulent in a rabbit model of endocarditis, *J Infect Dis* 169:1042–1049, 1994.

92. Zimmerli W, Trampuz A, Ochsner PE: Prosthetic-joint infections, *N Engl J Med* 351:1645–1654, 2004.

93. Sendi P, Rohrbach M, Graber P, et al: *Staphylococcus aureus* small colony variants in prosthetic joint infection, *Clin Infect Dis* 43:961–967, 2006.

94. Berbari E, Mabry T, Tsaras G, et al: Inflammatory blood laboratory levels as markers of prosthetic joint infection: a systematic review and meta-analysis, *J Bone Joint Surg Am* 92:2102–2109, 2010.

95. Tigges S, Stiles RG, Roberson JR: Appearance of septic hip prosthesis on plain radiographs, *AJR Am J Roentgenol* 163:377–380, 1994.

96. Smith SL, Wastie ML, Forster I: Radionuclide bone scintigraphy in the detection of significant complications after total knee joint replacement, *Clin Radiol* 56:221–224, 2001.

97. Trampuz A, Hanssen AD, Osmon DR, et al: Synovial fluid leukocyte count and differential for the diagnosis of prosthetic knee infection, *Am J Med* 117:556–562, 2004.

98. Atkins BL, Athanasou N, Deeks JJ, et al: Prospective evaluation of criteria for microbiological diagnosis of prosthetic-joint infection at revision arthroplasty. The OSIRIS Collaborative Study Group, *J Clin Microbiol* 36:2932–2939, 1998.

99. Mackowiak PA, Jones SR, Smith JW: Diagnostic value of sinus-tract cultures in chronic osteomyelitis, *JAMA* 239:2772–2775, 1978.

100. Steckelberg J, Osmon D: Prosthetic joint infections. In Waldvogel F, Bisno A, editors: *Infections associated with indwelling medical devices*, ed 3, Washington, DC, 2000, American Society for Microbiology Press.

101. Trampuz A, Piper KE, Jacobson MJ, et al: Sonication of removed hip and knee prostheses for diagnosis of infection, *N Engl J Med* 357:654–663, 2007.

102. Stewart PS, Costerton JW: Antibiotic resistance of bacteria in biofilms, *Lancet* 358:135–138, 2001.

103. Rose WE, Poppens PT: Impact of biofilm on the in vitro activity of vancomycin alone and in combination with tigecycline and rifampicin against *Staphylococcus aureus*, *J Antimicrob Chemother* 63:485–488, 2009.

104. Widmer AF, Frei R, Rajacic Z, et al: Correlation between in vivo and in vitro efficacy of antimicrobial agents against foreign body infections, *J Infect Dis* 162:96–102, 1990.

105. Samuel JR, Gould FK: Prosthetic joint infections: single versus combination therapy, *J Antimicrob Chemother* 65:18–23, 2010.

106. Trampuz A, Widmer AF: Infections associated with orthopedic implants, *Curr Opin Infect Dis* 19:349–356, 2006.

107. Yin LY, Lazzarini L, Fan L, et al: Comparative evaluation of tigecycline and vancomycin, with and without rifampicin, in the treatment of methicillin-resistant *Staphylococcus aureus* experimental osteomyelitis in a rabbit model, *J Antimicrob Chemother* 55:995–1002, 2005.

108. Brandt CM, Sistrunk WW, Duffy MC, et al: *Staphylococcus aureus* prosthetic joint infection treated with debridement and prosthesis retention, *Clin Infect Dis* 24:914–919, 1997.

109. Marculescu CE, Berberi EF, Hanssen AD, et al: Outcome of prosthetic joint infections treated with debridement and retention of components, *Clin Infect Dis* 42:471–478, 2006.

110. Trampuz A, Zimmerli W: Prosthetic joint infections: update in diagnosis and treatment, *Swiss Med Wkly* 135:243–251, 2005.

111. Byren I, Bejon P, Atkins BL, et al: One hundred and twelve infected arthroplasties treated with 'DAIR' (debridement, antibiotics and implant retention): antibiotic duration and outcome, *J Antimicrob Chemother* 63:1264–1271, 2009.

112. Brandt CM, Duffy MCT, Berbari EF, et al: *Staphylococcus aureus* prosthetic joint infection treated with prosthesis removed and delayed reimplantation arthroplasty, *Mayo Clin Proc* 74:553–558, 1999.

113. Stein A, Bataille JF, Drancourt M, et al: Ambulatory treatment of multi-drug resistant *Staphylococcus*-infected orthopedic implants with high-dose oral co-trimoxazole, *Antimicrob Agents Chemother* 42:3086–3091, 1998.

114. Little JW, Jacobson JJ, Lockhart PB: The dental treatment of patients with joint replacements: a position paper from the American Academy of Oral Medicine, *J Am Dent Assoc*141:667–671, 2010.

115. Sandhu SS, Lowry JC, Morton ME, et al: Antibiotic prophylaxis, dental treatment and arthroplasty: time to explode a myth, *J Bone Joint Surg Br* 79:521–522, 1997.

116. Krijnen P, Kaandorp CJE, Steyerberg EW, et al: Antibiotic prophylaxis for haematogenous bacterial arthritis in patients with joint disease: a cost effective analysis, *Ann Rheum Dis* 60:359–366, 2001.

117. Jacobson JJ, Schweitzer SO, Kowalski CJ: Chemoprophylaxis of prosthetic joint patients during dental treatment: a decision-utility analysis, *Oral Surg Oral Med Oral Pathol* 72:167–177, 1991.

118. Giles JT, Bartlett SJ, Gelber AC, et al: Tumor necrosis factor inhibitor therapy and risk of serious postoperative orthopedic infection in rheumatoid arthritis, *Arthritis Care Res* 55:333–337, 2006.

119. Bongartz T, Sutton AJ, Sweeting MJ, et al: Anti-TNF antibody therapy in rheumatoid arthritis and the risk of serious infections and malignancies: systematic review and meta-analysis of rare harmful effects in randomized controlled trials, *JAMA* 295:2275–2285, 2006.

120. Kaandorp CJE, Krijnen P, Moens HJB, et al: The outcome of bacterial arthritis: a prospective community-based study, *Arthritis Rheum* 40:884–892, 1997.

The references for this chapter can also be found on www.expertconsult.com.

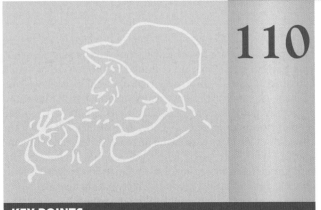

110

Lyme Disease

LINDA K. BOCKENSTEDT

KEY POINTS

Lyme disease is caused by infection with tick-transmitted spirochetes of the genus *Borrelia burgdorferi sensu lato* and has a worldwide distribution.

Lyme disease has a characteristic pattern of signs and symptoms and usually begins with the expanding macular skin lesion erythema migrans.

Earlier recognition and treatment has led to a decline in the incidence of carditis, acute neurologic disease, and late disease manifestations.

Musculoskeletal manifestations occur in more than 50% of patients and at all stages of infection, but frank arthritis is a sign of late disease and is uncommon (<10% of patients).

The diagnosis of Lyme disease should be suspected when a patient who lives, works, or vacations in an endemic area presents with signs and symptoms of *B. burgdorferi* infection.

Two-tiered serologic tests (enzyme-linked immunosorbent assay and immunoblot) can be negative with early infection but become positive in most patients with infection of greater than 1 month's duration.

Most patients are cured with 2 to 4 weeks of antibiotic therapy, although the time to disease resolution may extend beyond the duration of therapy and irreversible tissue damage may occur.

Antibiotic-refractory arthritis occurs in less than 10% of patients with Lyme arthritis, responds to disease-modifying antirheumatic drugs, and typically resolves within 4 to 5 years.

Post-Lyme disease syndrome (persistent debilitating complaints of fatigue, mild cognitive dysfunction, and musculoskeletal pain) after antibiotic treatment for Lyme disease occurs in a minority of patients. *B. burgdorferi* cannot be detected in these patients, and controlled treatment trials show no benefit of prolonged antibiotic therapy over placebo.

Lyme disease is a multisystem disorder caused by the tick-borne spirochete *Borrelia burgdorferi*.[1] The disease first came to medical attention in the United States in the late 1970s with the investigation of a clustering of cases of juvenile arthritis in the region of Lyme, Connecticut.[2] A characteristic skin rash described as single or multiple expanding red macules often heralded the onset of arthritis.[2] This rash, termed *erythema migrans* (EM), had been linked in Europe to the bite of *Ixodes* ticks and the subsequent development of neurologic abnormalities.[3,4] Further investigation revealed that arthritis was one manifestation of a systemic disorder affecting the skin, heart, joints, and nervous system. In 1982 Burgdorfer isolated the causative agent, the spirochete *B. burgdorferi*, from *Ixodes* ticks.[5] Demonstration that patients with Lyme disease developed antibodies to this organism and its eventual culture from skin, cerebrospinal fluid (CSF), and synovial tissue confirmed the infectious etiology of the disorder.[6] It is now the most common vector-borne disease in the United States.[1]

ECOLOGY AND EPIDEMIOLOGY OF LYME DISEASE

Lyme disease has a worldwide distribution, with most cases reported in North America, Europe, and Asia.[7] On each of these continents, hard-shelled ticks of the *Ixodes* family are the only known vectors for the disease. Other arthropods and blood-sucking insects such as mosquitos cannot transmit the infection. The incidence of Lyme disease varies geographically and is determined by the prevalence of *B. burgdorferi*–infected ticks. In the United States, cases of Lyme disease have been reported in all 50 states and the District of Columbia, but most are clustered in the Northeast and mid-Atlantic region, upper Midwest, and northern California. In 2009, 29,959 confirmed and 8509 probable cases were reported to the Centers for Disease Control and Prevention, with 93% of confirmed cases originating from 11 states: Pennsylvania, New Jersey, New York, Massachusetts, Connecticut, Wisconsin, Maryland, Minnesota, New Hampshire, Delaware, and Maine.[8]

The spirochetes associated with Lyme disease reside within the genus *B. burgdorferi sensu lato* (*sl*), and the vast majority of cases are caused by *B. burgdorferi sensu stricto* (*ss*), *Borrelia garinii*, and *Borrelia afzelii*.[7] All three genospecies can be found in Europe, whereas *B. burgdorferi ss* is the main species found in North America. Variation among the genospecies may account for the differences in clinical expression of Lyme disease between the two continents, with *B. garinii* associated with neurologic disease, *B. afzelii* associated with late skin involvement, and *B. burgdorferi ss* associated with arthritis.[7,9] Because of the prominence of musculoskeletal manifestations with *B. burgdorferi ss* infection, this chapter focuses mainly on Lyme disease in North America.

TICKS AND LYME DISEASE

Lyme disease is found primarily in temperate climates where humans can have incidental exposure to questing ticks. *Ixodes* ticks have a 2-year life span in which they pass through three developmental stages—larva, nymph, and adult—feeding only once per stage.[10] B. burgdorferi is not passed transovarially and is maintained by passage between reservoir hosts and ticks. Small rodents are the main reservoirs for B. burgdorferi ss and B. afzelii, whereas birds are the principal haven for B. garinii.[7] In the southern United States, ticks feed preferentially on lizards, which are not competent reservoirs for B. burgdorferi; this may explain in part the rarity of Lyme disease in this region.

Larvae acquire B. burgdorferi after feeding on an infected reservoir host in early spring and then molt to nymphs, which lay dormant until the following late spring and summer. The peak incidence of Lyme disease is in the summer months, when humans come in contact with questing nymphs, which have more promiscuous feeding patterns.[10] Engorged nymphs molt into adult ticks, which feed almost exclusively on deer. B. burgdorferi does not persist in deer, which serve to maintain and propagate the tick population.

PATHOGENESIS

Borrelia burgdorferi Invasion of the Mammalian Host

During tick feeding, B. burgdorferi migrate from the tick midgut to the salivary glands, where they are deposited with saliva into the blood meal host.[11,12] Migration takes about 24 hours, during which time spirochetes multiply and undergo phenotypic changes that permit their survival in mammals. Spirochetes multiply first at the tick bite site in the skin, and if not eliminated by the cutaneous immune response, they can disseminate through tissues and the bloodstream to infect any organ system at least transiently. The degree to which B. burgdorferi cause disease in tissues depends on spirochete virulence, growth conditions that allow persistence at a particular site, and host factors that modulate the inflammatory response.

Analysis of the B. burgdorferi genome has revealed no known virulence factors common to other bacterial pathogens to help explain the pathogenesis of Lyme disease.[13,14] Instead, the genome is remarkably rich in genes encoding putative lipoproteins, only a handful of which have been studied in detail. Outer surface protein (Osp) A is a midgut adhesin required for spirochete infection of ticks.[15] Osp C is essential for initial infection of the mammal but is dispensable after spirochetes have disseminated and colonized other tissue.[16] To do so, B. burgdorferi harnesses host plasmin to move through tissues[17,18] and expresses adhesins including decorin binding proteins A and B, BBK32, and p66, which allow it to bind to extracellular matrix proteins and integrins on cells.[19-22] Expression of VlsE, an Osp that undergoes antigenic variation, is required for infection to persist in immunocompetent hosts.[23,24]

Pathology of Lyme Disease

Because intact spirochetes are seen only rarely in tissue specimens and the spirochete genome reveals no known toxins, the pathology of Lyme disease is believed to be due to the host inflammatory response to B. burgdorferi components rather than tissue destruction by the spirochete itself.

Histopathologic studies of EM lesions, cardiac tissue, synovial biopsy specimens, and limited nervous system tissue (meninges, spinal cord, and nerve roots) reveal varying degrees of monocytic and lymphoplasmacytic infiltrates, especially perivascular, that stain positively for cell surface markers for macrophages, T cells, and B cells.[25,26] The joint effusions of patients with Lyme arthritis reveal acute inflammation with elevated leukocyte counts, whereas the synovium resembles that of rheumatoid arthritis, with chronic inflammation mediated by mononuclear cell infiltration and pseudolymphoid follicles formed by T cells, B cells, and plasma cells. In the synovium and less commonly the epineural area, perivascular infiltrates can be associated with endarteritis obliterans.

Immune Response to Borrelia burgdorferi

Innate immune cells respond to B. burgdorferi through engagement of the Toll-like receptor (TLR) family of pattern recognition receptors, especially TLR2/TLR1 heterodimers (lipoproteins), TLR5 (flagellin), and TLR9 (spirochete DNA).[26] As a consequence, proinflammatory cytokines (including interleukin-1β [IL-1β] and tumor necrosis factor), chemokines (IL-8), nitric oxide, and prostaglandins that recruit inflammatory cells to the site of infection are produced.[26-30] B. burgdorferi also induces matrix metalloproteinase expression in tissues through TLR-dependent and non–TLR-dependent pathways that contribute to pathology.[30] Other pattern recognition receptors may be engaged by B. burgdorferi after its ingestion by phagocytes, including the intracellular NOD2 receptors, which respond to peptidoglycan and have been shown to potentiate the inflammatory response in vitro.[31]

Humoral immunity is a key host defense against B. burgdorferi infection. B. burgdorferi lipoproteins are B cell mitogens, and antibodies that arise in the absence of T cell help are sufficient to resolve inflammation and prevent challenge infection in the mouse model of Lyme borreliosis.[32,33] With the induction of adaptive immunity, IgG-containing immune complexes and cryoglobulins can be found in the serum of patients with Lyme disease and are concentrated in the joints of patients who develop Lyme arthritis.[34] B cell–recruiting chemokines such as CXCL13 and pathogen-specific antibody production can be found in the CSF of patients with neuroborreliosis[35,36]; some of these antibodies can also bind neural antigens.[37-40]

B. burgdorferi infection primes CD4+ and CD8+ T cells, and the predominance of T helper type 1 responses correlates with more severe arthritis and neuroborreliosis.[42,43] Th17 cells are also involved, as demonstrated by the finding that the B. burgdorferi neutrophil-activing protein A (NapA) can elicit IL-17 from synovial fluid T cells ex vivo.[44] There is an association between T cell and B cell responses to Osp A and the development of antibiotic-refractory Lyme arthritis.[45,46] Although evidence has been presented to suggest an autoimmune etiology (see later section on antibiotic-refractory arthritis), the self-limited nature of Lyme arthritis also raises the possibility that the immune responses detected are appropriate and directed toward eliminating persisting antigens rather than viable organisms. Alternatively, prolonged arthritis may be due to abnormal or delayed regulation of the host immune response when the pathogen and its inflammatory products have been eliminated. Deficiency in CD25[+] T regulatory cells prolongs murine Lyme arthritis,[47] and synovial fluid γδ T cells isolated from patients with Lyme arthritis can modulate *B. burgdorferi*–specific CD4[+] T cell responses by inducing apoptosis in a Fas-dependent fashion.[48]

Mechanisms of Spirochete Persistence

When visualized in vivo, *B. burgdorferi* resides primarily in the extracellular matrix in connective tissue.[25] Despite occasional sightings of spirochetes inside cells,[49] an intracellular phase of the *B. burgdorferi* life cycle has not been shown. *B. burgdorferi* employs immune evasion strategies of an extracellular pathogen, which are directed toward deterring phagocyte ingestion and antibody- and complement-mediated lysis.[4] *B. burgdorferi* expresses Erp and complement regulator–acquiring surface proteins that bind host factor H to prevent complement-mediated lysis.[50-52] To impede antibody-mediated clearance, *B. burgdorferi* undergoes antigenic variation[23] and reduces expression of lipoproteins as infection progresses.[53] The *vlsE* gene undergoes random rearrangement of its expression locus, producing antigenically distinct variants of VlsE, a protein essential for spirochete survival in vivo.[23] In the chronic phase of *B. burgdorferi* infection in mice, spirochetes can be visualized in the extracellular matrix of connective tissue, especially in the skin, without an associated inflammatory response.[54]

CLINICAL FEATURES OF LYME DISEASE

Lyme disease occurs in stages that reflect the immune response to the spirochete as it establishes infection in the skin and later disseminates to distant organ sites (Table 110-1). Presenting clinical manifestations depend on the stage of the illness in which patients first seek medical attention. A characteristic feature of Lyme disease is that clinical signs can resolve without specific therapy, and patients may present in later stages of the illness without exhibiting signs of early disease.

Early Localized Infection

The hallmark of Lyme disease is the skin lesion EM, which is present in about 80% of patients (Figure 110-1).[55] The lesion arises within 1 month (median, 7 to 10 days) at the tick bite site, especially in skin folds or where clothes bind in adults and around the hairline in children. EM begins as a red macule that expands at the rate of 2 to 3 cm/day, enlarging to more than 70 cm in diameter. Characteristic lesions greater than 5 cm in diameter in an appropriate clinical setting are sufficient for establishing the diagnosis of Lyme disease.[56] EM most often manifests with uniform erythema, but central clearing can occur in larger lesions, producing a classic "bull's eye" appearance (see Figure 110-1B). Vesicular or necrotic centers are rarer (see Figure 110-1D), but even these EM lesions have relatively few symptoms other than a tingling or burning sensation. Intense pruritus or pain is unusual and should raise concern for alternative diagnoses.

EM may be accompanied by systemic flulike symptoms including low-grade fever, malaise, neck pain or stiffness,

Table 110-1 Clinical Manifestations of Lyme Disease

Early Localized Infection
Occurs 3 to 30 days after tick bite
EM in 80%-90% of patients; single lesion, occasionally associated with fever, malaise, neck pain or stiffness, arthralgias and myalgias
Systemic symptoms noted above in the absence of EM during summer months
Borrelial lymphocytoma (rare, seen primarily in Europe)

Early Disseminated Infection
Occurs weeks to months after tick bite
Profound malaise and fatigue common
Multiple EM lesions with systemic symptoms similar to early localized infection
Musculoskeletal
Migratory polyarthralgias and myalgias
Carditis (<3% of untreated patients)
Varying degrees of atrioventricular nodal block
Mild myopericarditis
Neurologic (<10% of untreated patients)
Cranial neuropathies (especially facial nerve palsy)
Lymphocytic meningitis
Radiculoneuropathies
Encephalomyelitis

Late Disease
Occurs months to years after tick bite
Arthritis (<10% of patients)
Acute monoarticular or migratory pauciarticular inflammatory arthritis, usually involving the knee
Chronic antibiotic-refractory arthritis (<10% of patients with arthritis)
Neurologic (rare)
Peripheral neuropathies
Mild encephalopathy
Encephalomyelitis (primarily seen in Europe)
Skin
Acrodermatitis chronica atrophicans (primarily seen in Europe)

EM, erythema migrans.

arthralgias, and myalgias.[57,58] Particularly severe systemic symptoms should alert the physician to possible co-infection with another tick-borne pathogen such as *Babesia microti* or *Anaplasma phagocytophilum* (the agent of human granulocytic anaplasmosis, formerly known as *human granulocytic erhlichiosis*). Lyme disease can also manifest with systemic symptoms alone.[59,60] Absence of upper respiratory or gastrointestinal symptoms may help distinguish Lyme disease from common viral infections. Musculoskeletal complaints and debilitating fatigue associated with Lyme disease should be distinguished from fibromyalgia and chronic fatigue syndrome, which are typically more insidious in onset and are not associated with objective findings or laboratory abnormalities.

A newly recognized southern tick–associated rash illness (STARI) can produce a skin lesion similar to the bull's eye form of EM.[61] The rash is associated with the bite of the Lone Star tick, *Amblyomma americanum*, which is endemic to the southeastern and south-central states, but which also can be found as far north as Maine or west as central Texas and Oklahoma. Similar to EM, systemic symptoms can accompany the rash of STARI, but disease in organs other than the skin does not occur. The etiology of STARI is unknown. Although a noncultivable spirochete named *Borrelia lonestari* has been found in *A. americanum*, STARI

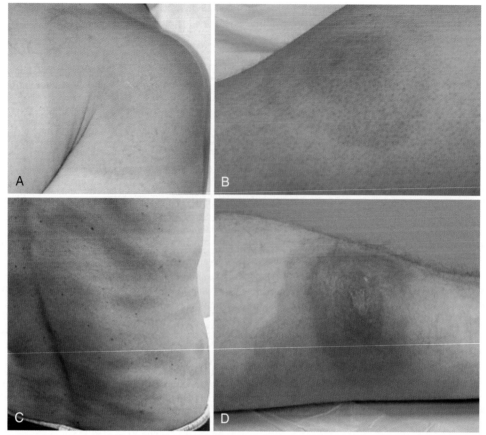

Figure 110-1   Erythema migrans rash of Lyme disease. **A,** Typical macular lesion on left shoulder. **B,** Bull's eye lesion on lateral thigh with central punctum. **C,** Multiple lesions on back. **D,** Lesion with vesicular center on posterior thigh. *(Courtesy Juan Salazar, MD, University of Connecticut Health Center.)*

patients do not develop positive Lyme serologies and the organism has not been found in skin biopsy specimens of the STARI lesions.[62] Antibiotics resolve EM and STARI, but STARI patients recover more quickly from systemic symptoms than do patients with EM.

Early Disseminated Infection

Within weeks of the onset of infection, *B. burgdorferi* can disseminate through the skin, blood, and lymphatics to infect multiple tissues. Clinically apparent disease at this stage, however, is usually seen in the skin, heart, or nervous system. Patients with disseminated infection have debilitating fatigue and appear ill. Specific localizing signs and symptoms may fluctuate, but profound fatigue is a consistent complaint.

Skin Disease

Fifty percent of patients with untreated Lyme disease develop multiple EM lesions, a sign of disseminated infection (see Figure 110-1C).[55] Secondary lesions are typically smaller and can occur anywhere on the body, but they are most noticeable on the trunk. The lesions usually appear as flat macules and can develop partial central clearing. EM lesions may be accompanied by migratory muscle, joint, and periarticular pain that lasts hours to days, but frank arthritis is now considered a late manifestation of the disease.

Cardiac Disease

The incidence of cardiac involvement has declined to 1% in recent years, possibly owing to earlier recognition and treatment of *B. burgdorferi* infection. It most often occurs within the first 2 months of infection and manifests as varying degrees of atrioventricular block, occasionally accompanied by mild myopericarditis.[63] Electrophysiologic studies have mapped the conduction defect to the area above the bundle of His and involving the atrioventricular node, although multiple levels can be affected. Overt congestive heart failure is rare, and chronic cardiomyopathy, reported in Europe, has not been documented to occur in the United States.[64] Patients with Lyme carditis often have a history of EM and may have concomitant arthralgia and myalgia at the time of presentation. Absence of valvular heart disease helps distinguish Lyme carditis from acute rheumatic fever, and prominent myocardial dysfunction or pericardial involvement should suggest other infectious etiologies.

Nervous System Involvement

Acute neurologic Lyme disease occurs in less than 10% of patients and most commonly manifests as cranial nerve palsy or meningitis, although radiculopathy and encephalomyelitis are also occasionally seen.[65-69] Cranial palsy occurs in 8% of cases and usually affects the seventh nerve, resulting in unilateral or bilateral facial palsy. Even in endemic areas, however, onset of seventh nerve palsy in the nonwinter months is due to *B. burgdorferi* infection in only 25% of cases.[70] Bilateral facial palsy is seen in only a few other conditions—Guillain-Barré syndrome, human immunodeficiency virus infection, sarcoidosis, and other causes of chronic meningitis—all of which are readily distinguished from Lyme disease. Rarely, other cranial nerves (III, IV, V, VI, or VIII) may be involved. Lyme meningitis manifests with fever, headache, and stiff neck similar to viral meningitis, along with a CSF lymphocytosis and elevated protein.[68] In children, meningitis may occur with EM, cranial nerve involvement, and increased intracranial pressure (papilledema), which is rare in adults.[68,69,71] Lyme radiculopathy typically manifests as pain, weakness, numbness, and reflex loss in a dermatomal distribution, resembling mechanical radiculopathies.[67] Lyme disease should be considered when there is no obvious precipitating factor for disk-related symptoms, and imaging studies do not delineate pathology at the appropriate root level. Untreated Lyme radiculopathy can progress to become bilateral, which helps distinguish it from mechanical disease. When truncal involvement causes unilateral chest or abdominal pain, Lyme radiculopathy is often mistaken for visceral disease or early herpes zoster before the development of vesicular lesions.

Other Organ System Involvement

A variety of other organs can exhibit pathology with disseminated *B. burgdorferi* infection including the eye (keratitis), the ear (sensorineural hearing loss), the liver (hepatitis), the spleen (necrosis), skeletal muscle (myositis), and subcutaneous tissue (panniculitis).[72] In general, other, more classic manifestations of Lyme disease are present concurrently or have been present in the recent past to suggest the diagnosis.

Late Disease

Months after the onset of infection, untreated patients can develop late manifestations of Lyme disease, usually involving the joints (discussed separately later), nervous system, and the skin. At this stage of infection, two-tier (enzyme-linked immunosorbent assay [ELISA] and IgG immunoblot) serologic testing for *B. burgdorferi* should be positive.

Late Neurologic Disease

Late neurologic Lyme disease is now rare; patients may present with encephalomyelitis, peripheral neuropathy, or encephalopathy.[73,74] Encephalomyelitis, seen predominantly in Europe with *B. garinii* infection, is a slowly progressive, unifocal or multifocal inflammatory disease of the central nervous system, with increased T2 signals in the white matter on magnetic resonance imaging (MRI). CSF examination often reveals a lymphocytic pleocytosis, elevated protein, and normal glucose, and serum IgG to *B. burgdorferi* and intrathecal antibody production can be found. These findings help distinguish Lyme encephalomyelitis from multiple sclerosis, which may rarely be associated with positive IgG reactivity to *B. burgdorferi* in serum and CSF samples, but there is no intrathecal antibody production.[75,76]

Multiple sclerosis patients with positive Lyme serologies do not respond to antibiotics used for neurologic Lyme disease.

Late peripheral nervous system involvement manifests as a mild sensorimotor neuropathy in a "stocking and glove" distribution, with evidence of a mild confluent mononeuritis multiplex on electrophysiologic studies.[77] Patients may have intermittent limb paresthesias and occasionally radicular pain. The most common finding on physical examination is reduced vibratory sensation in the lower extremities. Serum IgG to *B. burgdorferi* should be present, but CSF examination is normal, consistent with disease confined to the peripheral nervous system. Patients with this form of neuropathy should be evaluated for other infectious diseases (syphilis, human immunodeficiency virus, and hepatitis C virus); metabolic disorders (especially vitamin B_{12} deficiency, diabetes mellitus, and thyroid disease); and autoimmune diseases (antinuclear antibody [ANA] or rheumatoid factor associated).

Patients with Lyme encephalopathy complain of memory impairment and cognitive dysfunction that are best shown by formal neuropsychological testing.[78,79] Occasionally, patients may have CSF abnormalities with elevated protein, lymphocytic pleocytosis, and intrathecal antibody to *B. burgdorferi*, but CSF examination can also be normal. Serum IgG to *B. burgdorferi* should be present, however, to consider the diagnosis. The mild cognitive dysfunction seen in patients with Lyme encephalopathy must be distinguished from neurocognitive deficits secondary to chronic stress, sleep deprivation, fibromyalgia, chronic fatigue syndrome, or aging. As for any chronic encephalopathy, toxic-metabolic causes should be excluded. Brain imaging studies are generally normal or show only nonspecific abnormalities and are not useful in establishing a diagnosis of encephalopathy associated with Lyme disease.

Late Skin Disease

The late skin lesion acrodermatitis chronica atrophicans is found mainly in Europe because of its association with *B. afzelii* infection, although any *B. burgdorferi* species can cause the lesion.[80] Acrodermatitis chronica atrophicans develops insidiously over years and is most often found on the dorsum of the hands or feet.[81] It begins as a unilateral bluish red discoloration and swelling, which evolves to atrophic, cellophane-like skin with prominent appearance of the blood vessels. About 60% of patients also have a peripheral sensory neuropathy affecting the involved extremity. A prominent lymphoplasmacytic infiltrate is shown on the skin biopsy specimen. Antibiotics can lead to improvement in pain and swelling, but atrophic skin remains.

LYME ARTHRITIS AND OTHER MUSCULOSKELETAL MANIFESTATIONS OF LYME DISEASE

Musculoskeletal symptoms are common in all stages of Lyme disease and include migratory pain in joints, tendons, bursae, and muscles.[82] Typically, musculoskeletal pain affects one or two sites at a time, lasts only hours to a few days at any one location, and is associated with significant fatigue.

The incidence of frank arthritis has declined from 50% in early studies to less than 10% in more recent years.[26] ELISA and IgG immunoblot for *B. burgdorferi* are positive when arthritis appears, and *B. burgdorferi* DNA can be detected by polymerase chain reaction (PCR) in synovium and synovial fluid even though cultures are usually negative. Although Lyme arthritis can resemble pauciarticular juvenile arthritis or reactive arthritis, patients generally test negative for ANA, rheumatoid factor, and anticitrullinated protein antibodies (ACPAs) and do not have an increased frequency of HLA-B27 alleles. Joint fluid analysis and synovial histopathology cannot distinguish these entities. Axial and sacroiliac joint involvement is not a feature of Lyme disease, but enthesitis can be seen. Most patients with Lyme arthritis have positive two-tier serologic tests for *B. burgdorferi* infection.

Arthritis usually begins months or years after *B. burgdorferi* infection and is predated by migratory arthralgias in half of patients.[82] The most typical pattern is a monoarticular or oligoarticular arthritis involving one or a few large joints (fewer than five total), with the knee affected in 80% of cases. Joints are warm with large effusions, often greater than 100 mL in the knee, but comparatively little pain. Synovial fluid is inflammatory with white blood cell counts ranging from approximately 2000 to 70,000/mm^3 (median ≈ 24,000/mm^3), with a predominance of neutrophils.[83] Depending on the chronicity of the arthritis, synovial biopsy specimens reveal only mononuclear cell infiltration or more advanced changes consistent with rheumatoid synovium.[25] Large effusions can lead to Baker's cyst formation and rupture. The temporomandibular joint is also frequently involved and in one study was the first joint to be affected in 25% of patients with arthritis.[82] Other joints commonly affected include the shoulder, ankle, elbow, wrist, and hip. Lyme arthritis is often intermittent, with episodes lasting a few weeks to months. Recurrent episodes are notable for smaller effusions and progressive synovial hypertrophy, bony erosion, and cartilage destruction. A small percentage (<10%) of patients with intermittent arthritis settle into a pattern of chronic arthritis, generally affecting only a single joint and often the knee. Inflammation of a single joint that persists for more than 12 months would be an unusual presenting manifestation of Lyme arthritis, as is the prominent involvement of small joints.

The natural history of Lyme arthritis suggests that it is a self-limited disorder. In the late 1970s, before the use of antibiotics for Lyme disease, 21 patients who presented with EM and later developed Lyme arthritis were followed for 1 to 8 years without antimicrobial therapy.[82] Six patients had only a single episode of arthritis, and the remaining 15 had recurrent episodes that decreased in frequency over the study period. On average, the number of patients who continued to experience episodes of arthritis decreased by 10% to 20% each year. Similar results were found in children in whom antibiotic treatment for arthritis was delayed 4 years.[84]

Antibiotic-Refractory Lyme Arthritis

A few patients treated with standard antibiotic regimens for Lyme arthritis have persistent joint inflammation and proliferative synovitis that does not respond to further antimicrobial therapy.[26,85] The pathogenesis of "antibiotic-refractory" Lyme arthritis is unknown but may be due to persistent spirochetes or their antigens, infection-induced autoimmunity, or inadequate regulation of the inflammatory response.[25] Spirochete virulence may play a role as a retrospective study of archived tissue samples obtained before treatment revealed that patients who went on to develop antibiotic-refractory arthritis had a higher prevalence of infection with the more invasive RST1 *B. burgdorferi* strains.[86,87] Although patients with antibiotic-refractory Lyme arthritis no longer have PCR evidence for spirochete DNA in tissues,[85] experiments in the mouse model of Lyme borreliosis suggest that spirochete debris, including *B. burgdorferi* DNA, can persist near cartilage and in the entheses for extended periods after infectious spirochetes have been killed with antibiotics, particularly when the initial pathogen burden was high.[88] Recently, a single nucleotide polymorphism in TLR1 (TLR1 1805 GG) that impairs the innate immune response to *B. burgdorferi* was found to be more prevalent among patients who developed antibiotic-refractory Lyme arthritis.[89] A genetic predisposition had been suggested in earlier studies that found an increased frequency of the rheumatoid arthritis–related alleles HLA-DRB1*0401, HLA-DRB1*0101, and HLA-DRB1*0404 in patients with antibiotic-refractory Lyme arthritis.[90] Because of the high prevalence of B cell and T cell responses to *B. burgdorferi* Osp A in patients with antibiotic-refractory arthritis, it had been proposed that immune responses to Osp A triggered by infection may be perpetuated by a self-antigen after the pathogen has been eliminated.[26,90] An Osp A peptide corresponding to amino acids 163 through 175 (Osp A$_{163-175}$) was found to share an epitope with human leukocyte function–associated antigen 1α, an adhesion molecule expressed on inflamed tissues.[91] The leukocyte function–associated antigen 1α peptide stimulated Osp A$_{163-175}$-specific T cells only weakly, however, and did not promote production of the T helper (Th)1 cytokine interferon-γ normally found in antibiotic-refractory arthritis.[92] Antibodies to cytokeratin 10, a constituent of synovial capillaries, have been found in the blood and synovial tissue of patients with antibiotic-refractory Lyme arthritis.[93] These antibodies also react with Osp A and may contribute to ongoing inflammation when infection is cleared. Linked T and B cell responses to peptides of epidermal cell growth factor have been found in about 50% of patients with antibiotic-refractory Lyme arthritis, but their role in perpetuating the inflammatory response is unclear.[94] If autoimmunity is responsible for antibiotic-refractory Lyme arthritis, it must eventually succumb to immune regulation because even this form of Lyme arthritis generally resolves within 4 to 5 years.[82,85] In this regard, the presence of a higher percentage of T regulatory cells correlates with more rapid resolution of joint inflammation after treatment for antibiotic-refractory Lyme arthritis.[95]

DIAGNOSIS

The diagnosis of Lyme disease should be considered in individuals who present with an appropriate clinical history and who have a reasonable risk of exposure to *B. burgdorferi*–infected ticks (Figure 110-2).[36] Supporting serologic evidence is necessary to secure the diagnosis for all stages of

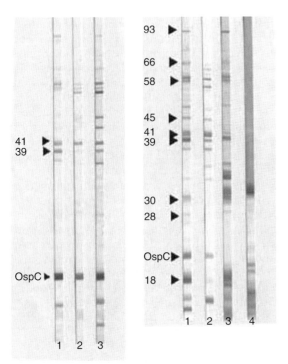

Figure 110-2 *Left,* Selected IgM immunoblot reactivities. *Lane 1,* Serum band locator control showing several bands including the significant 41-kD protein, 39-kD protein, and OspC *(arrowheads). Lane 2,* Serum sample from a patient with early Lyme borreliosis with erythema migrans. *Lane 3,* Serum sample from a patient with early disseminated Lyme borreliosis with multiple erythema migrans lesions. Note the larger number of bands observed in a serum sample of the patient with early disseminated Lyme borreliosis. *Right,* Selected IgG immunoblot reactivities. *Lane 1,* Serum band locator control showing several immunoreactive bands including those considered significant in the IgG blot criteria *(arrowheads). Lane 2,* Serum sample from a patient with early disseminated Lyme borreliosis with neurologic involvement. *Lane 3,* Serum sample from a patient with Lyme arthritis. *Lane 4,* Serum sample from an individual who received three doses of OspA vaccine; note the strong reactivity with OspA (31 kD) and other antigens below OspC. *(From Aguero-Rosenfeld ME, Wang G, Schwartz I, et al: Diagnosis of Lyme borreliosis,* Clin Microbiol Rev *18:484, 2005.)*

infection except for early localized disease in which EM can be recognized by morphologic features alone. Routine laboratory tests are nonspecific, with some patients exhibiting mildly elevated white blood cell (neutrophil) counts, erythrocyte sedimentation rates, and liver function tests. Culture or microscopic visualization of spirochetes in clinical samples is not sensitive enough for routine use in diagnosis. Culture of a skin biopsy specimen taken from the leading margin of an EM lesion is an exception, with *B. burgdorferi* detected in more than 40% of samples, but is rarely necessary to identify EM.

Serologic Testing

Detection of antibodies to *B. burgdorferi* is the mainstay of laboratory testing for Lyme disease.[36] Presence of antibodies to *B. burgdorferi* at best indicates previous exposure to the organism, however, and should not be considered evidence of active infection. In nonendemic areas, about 5% of normal human serum samples yield positive results on serologic tests for Lyme disease.[96] In endemic areas,

asymptomatic IgG seroconversion to *B. burgdorferi* has been found in about 7% of subjects.[97]

A two-tiered approach is recommended for detection of *B. burgdorferi*–specific antibodies.[98] An ELISA or an indirect immunofluorescence assay to detect IgM and IgG reactivity to *B. burgdorferi* should be used as an initial screening test, followed by an immunoblot (Western blot) to confirm that positive or equivocal results are due to antibodies that bind *B. burgdorferi* antigens. ELISA and immunofluorescence assays are highly sensitive tests but lack specificity because of cross-reactivity of antibodies to *B. burgdorferi* with other bacterial pathogens.[36] A positive or equivocal ELISA or immunofluorescence assay should be confirmed by immunoblot analysis of *B. burgdorferi* proteins (Table 110-2). Banding patterns characteristic of early infection include antibodies to the 41-kD flagellin protein and Osp C, which has a molecular weight ranging from 21 to 24 kD depending on the *B. burgdorferi* strain used (see Figure 110-2). With disseminated infection and especially with late Lyme disease, IgG reactivity to an expanding array of *B. burgdorferi* proteins can be seen (see Figure 110-2).

Some commercial laboratories have developed assays using recombinant antigens or employ criteria for the interpretation of immunoblots that have not been validated and published in peer-reviewed literature.[99] For this reason, the Centers for Disease Control and Prevention advises using only validated tests approved by the U.S. Food and Drug Administration (FDA) for serologic diagnosis of Lyme disease.

Two-tier testing for IgM and IgG should be performed for individuals with suspected Lyme disease and signs and symptoms of less than 1 month's duration, whereas only IgG results should be considered for illnesses of longer duration.[98] Positive IgM serologies alone after 1 month of illness are most often false-positive tests, which occur in the setting of other infectious diseases (especially infectious mononucleosis and other spirochetal and tick-borne infections), rheumatoid arthritis (with or without rheumatoid factor), and conditions associated with a positive ANA (systemic lupus erythematosus).[100] No further testing is recommended if ELISA or immunofluorescence assay results are negative. Two-tier testing has overall sensitivities of 29% to 40% in EM during the acute phase; 29% to 78% for EM in the

Table 110-2 Criteria for Western Blot Interpretation in the Serologic Confirmation of Lyme Disease

Duration of Disease	Isotype Tested	Criteria for Positive Test
First month of infection	IgM	2 of the following 3 bands are present: 23 kD (OspC), 39 kD (BmpA), and 41 kD (Fla)
After first month of infection	IgG	5 of 10 bands are present: 18 kD, 21 kD, 28 kD, 30 kD, 39 kD, 41 kD, 45 kD, 58 kD (not GroEL), 66 kD, and 93 kD

Modified from Centers for Disease Control and Prevention: Recommendations for test performance and interpretation from the Second National Conference on Serologic Diagnosis of Lyme Disease, *MMWR Morb Mortal Wkly Rep* 44:590–591, 1995.

convalescent phase; and greater than 95% in neurologic, arthritis, and other manifestations of late disease.[36]

A peptide-based ELISA that uses a highly conserved invariant region of the VlsE protein, termed C6 (IR6), is now commercially available.[101,102] The C6 peptide ELISA has a high degree of sensitivity and specificity in all stages of Lyme disease and may be particularly useful in early Lyme disease.[102] A positive or equivocal test should be confirmed with IgM and IgG immunoblots.

After antibiotic therapy, IgM and IgG titers to *B. burgdorferi* measured by either whole cell ELISA or the C6 peptide ELISA (IgG only) generally decrease slowly but can remain positive for years.[103,104] Repeat serologic testing is not recommended as a means for assessing response to treatment.

Detection of Antibodies to *Borrelia burgdorferi* in Cerebrospinal Fluid

In suspected cases of neuroborreliosis, intrathecal antibody production is usually assessed by measuring the ratio of IgG to *B. burgdorferi* in CSF and serum.[36,105] Intrathecal antibody production is more commonly found in European neuroborreliosis than in North American Lyme disease, which may be due to the higher prevalence of *B. garinii* in central nervous system (CNS) infection than *B. burgdorferi ss.* Antibodies to *B. burgdorferi* may persist in CSF after treatment for Lyme disease and should not be used to assess efficacy of therapy.

Polymerase Chain Reaction

PCR has been used to detect *B. burgdorferi* DNA in a variety of clinical specimens with variable success.[106] The greatest utility of PCR clinically is in Lyme arthritis, in which the sensitivity of PCR for detection of *B. burgdorferi* DNA is 85%.[107] In contrast, the sensitivity of PCR for detecting *B. burgdorferi* DNA in CSF is low (<40%) and most often positive in patients with a CSF pleocytosis. PCR of urine specimens is not recommended because of inconsistent sensitivity and documented nonspecific amplification of non–*B. burgdorferi* DNA targets.[36] Although certain commercial laboratories currently offer PCR tests for *B. burgdorferi* DNA in blood or urine specimens, these have not been validated.[99] There are no FDA-approved tests for PCR-based molecular techniques for detecting *B. burgdorferi* DNA in patient specimens.

Other Tests for Lyme Disease

A urine antigen test, immunofluorescent staining for cell wall–deficient forms of *B. burgdorferi*, and lymphocyte transformation assays are offered by some commercial laboratories to aid in the diagnosis of Lyme disease. These tests have not been adequately validated for accuracy or clinical usefulness, and the Centers for Disease Control and Prevention cautions against their use.[99]

Diagnostic Imaging

Imaging studies have a limited role in the evaluation of patients with Lyme disease because no feature is sufficiently distinctive to confirm the diagnosis. Plain radiographs of arthritic joints show changes consistent with an inflammatory arthropathy including joint effusions, synovial hypertrophy, periarticular osteoporosis, cartilage loss, bony erosions, and calcified entheses.[108] MRI of arthritic joints can confirm the radiographic findings and reveal associated myositis and adenopathy, which may be useful in distinguishing Lyme arthritis from septic arthritis in children.[109]

Cranial and spinal MRI findings in neuroborreliosis can reveal focal nodular lesions or patchy white matter lesions on T2-weighted images, consistent with inflammatory or demyelinating processes.[110,111] These lesions typically resolve after treatment for Lyme disease,[111] in some cases only after several years.[112] In patients with post–Lyme disease syndrome, cerebral MRI and the more sensitive technique of fluid-attenuated inversion recovery are normal in about 50% of cases or show nonspecific findings of small white matter lesions.[113] Positron emission tomography and single-photon emission computed tomography studies are often normal or show only nonspecific changes with subcortical and cortical hypoperfusion.[114,115]

TREATMENT AND OUTCOME

Updated guidelines for the clinical assessment (Figure 110-3) and treatment (Table 110-3) of Lyme disease have been published.[116] Because many of the manifestations of Lyme disease resolve without specific therapy, the goal of antibiotic treatment is to hasten resolution of signs and symptoms and to prevent later clinical manifestations. Generally, oral antibiotics are sufficient therapy for EM, disseminated EM, uncomplicated facial palsy, mild carditis (first-degree atrioventricular block), and arthritis. Disseminated infection and late manifestations of Lyme disease may require longer courses of antibiotics, and there is often a greater lag time to symptom resolution compared with early disease. Doxycycline is the antibiotic of choice in nonpregnant adults and children 8 years old and older because it is also effective against *A. phagocytophilum*, which may occur with early Lyme disease.[116] Amoxicillin and cefuroxime axetil are acceptable alternatives for the treatment of EM, facial palsy, and other non-neurologic manifestations of Lyme disease. Macrolide antibiotics are less effective than other antimicrobials and should be used only in individuals who cannot take doxycycline, amoxicillin, or cefuroxime axetil. First-generation cephalosporins are not effective therapy for Lyme disease.

Documented nervous system involvement (other than isolated facial palsy) and symptomatic cardiac involvement are the two main indications for intravenous antibiotic therapy.[116] Ceftriaxone administered intravenously for 2 to 4 weeks is the preferred antimicrobial, with parenteral cefotaxime or penicillin G acceptable alternatives. There is increasing evidence, however, that oral doxycycline, which is well absorbed and has a high CNS penetration, may be effective for meningitis or radiculopathy.[117-119] Lumbar puncture is recommended in individuals with cranial nerve palsies who have symptoms of meningeal irritation because a CSF pleocytosis would be an indication to treat with intravenous therapy. Asymptomatic CSF pleocytosis can occur in the setting of facial palsy and is not an indication

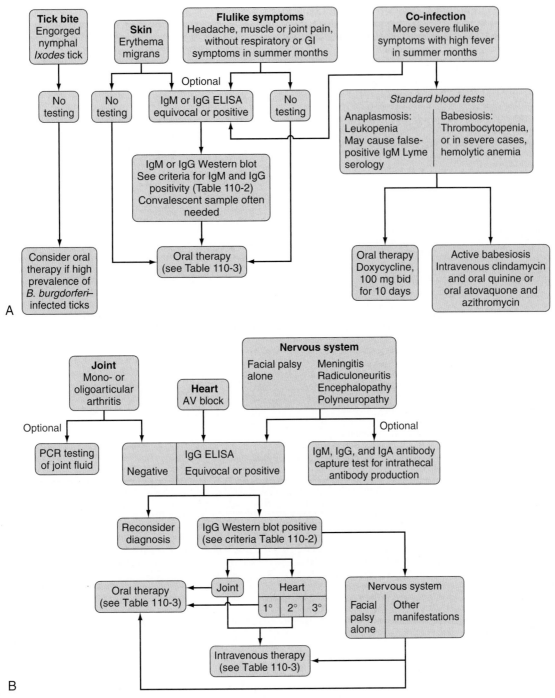

Figure 110-3 **A,** Algorithm for evaluation and management of early Lyme disease. **B,** Algorithm for evaluation and management of later organ involvement in Lyme disease. AV, atrioventricular; ELISA, enzyme-linked immunosorbent assay; GI, gastrointestinal; PCR, polymerase chain reaction. *(From Steere AC, Coburn J, Glickstein L: The emergence of Lyme disease, J Clin Invest 113:1093–1101, 2004.)*

for intravenous therapy. Repeat treatment is not recommended for chronic neurologic abnormalities, unless objective signs of relapse are present.

Patients with symptomatic cardiac involvement (chest pain, shortness of breath, syncope) or with significant conduction system disease (first-degree atrioventricular block with P-R intervals ≥0.3 msec, or second-degree or third-degree block) should be hospitalized for cardiac monitoring and intravenous antibiotic therapy. Consultation with a cardiologist is recommended, and placement of a temporary pacemaker may be necessary. Oral antibiotics can be

substituted for intravenous antibiotics at the time of hospital discharge to complete the course of therapy.[116]

For arthritis, a 1-month course of oral doxycycline or amoxicillin is recommended, with a repeat course of oral therapy if inflammation does not resolve within 3 months of treatment.[116] For patients with moderate-to-severe joint swelling after a 1-month course of oral antibiotics, intravenous ceftriaxone for 2 to 4 weeks can be used[120]; when inflammation is mild, an additional 1-month course of oral antibiotics can be considered, although arthritis usually resolves without additional therapy. Longer courses of

Table 110-3   Recommended Treatment of Lyme Disease*

Manifestation	Drug	Adult Dosage	Pediatric Dosage	Duration (Range)
Erythema migrans (recommended)	Doxycycline[†]	100 mg orally (PO) bid	<8 yr—not recommended ≥8 yr—4 mg/kg/day in 2 divided doses (max 100 mg/dose)	14 days (10-21 days)
	Amoxicillin	500 mg PO tid	50 mg/kg/day in 3 divided doses	14 days (14-21 days)
	Cefuroxime axetil	500 mg PO bid	30 mg/kg/day in 2 divided doses	14 days (14-21 days)
Erythema migrans (alternative)[‡]	Azithromycin	500 mg PO qd	10 mg/kg qd (max 500 mg/day)	7-10 days
	Clarithromycin	500 mg PO bid (if patient is nonpregnant)	7.5 mg/kg bid (max 500 mg/dose)	14-21 days
	Erythromycin	500 mg PO qid	12.5 mg/kg qid (max 500 mg/dose)	14-21 days
Acute neurologic disease Cranial nerve palsy[§]	Same as oral regimens for erythema migrans			14 days (14-21 days)
Meningitis or radiculopathy[‖]	Ceftriaxone	2 g IV qd	50-75 mg/kg IV qd in single dose (max 2 g/day)	14 days (10-28 days)
(Alternative IV)	Cefotaxime	2 g IV q8h	150-200 mg/kg/day IV in 3-4 divided doses (max 6 g/day)	
	Penicillin G	18-24 million U/day, divided q4h	200,000-400,000 U/kg/day divided q4h (max 18-24 million U/day)	
Cardiac disease[¶]	Same as for erythema migrans OR			14 days (14-21 days)
	IV regimen as for neurologic disease			14 days (14-21 days)
Late disease Arthritis without neurologic involvement	Same as for erythema migrans			28 days (28 days)
Recurrent arthritis after oral regimen	Repeat oral regimen OR IV regimen as for neurologic disease			14 days (14-28 days)
Central or peripheral nervous system disease	IV regimen as for acute neurologic disease			14 days (14-28 days)

*Complete response to treatment may be delayed beyond the treatment period, regardless of the clinical manifestation, and relapse may recur. Patients with objective signs of relapse may need a second course of treatment.

†Tetracyclines are relatively contraindicated in pregnant or lactating women and in children younger than 8 yr of age.

‡Due to their lower efficacy, macrolides are reserved for patients who are unable to take or who are intolerant of tetracyclines, penicillins, and cephalosporins.

§Patients without clinical evidence of meningitis may be treated with an oral regimen. The recommendation is based on experience with seventh cranial nerve palsy. Whether oral therapy would be as effective for patients with other cranial neuropathies is unknown; the decision between oral and parenteral therapy should be individualized.

‖For nonpregnant adult patients intolerant of β-lactam agents, doxycycline 200-400 mg/day orally (or IV if unable to take oral medications) in 2 divided doses may be adequate. For children 8 yr of age and older, the dosage of doxycycline for this indication is 4-8 mg/kg/day in two divided doses (maximum daily dosage of 200-400 mg).

¶A parenteral antibiotic regimen is recommended at the start of therapy for patients who have been hospitalized for cardiac monitoring; an oral regimen may be substituted to complete a course of therapy or to treat outpatients. A temporary pacemaker may be required for patients with advanced heart block.

antibiotics provide no additional benefit when PCR for B. burgdorferi in joint fluid is negative.[85] In this situation, nonsteroidal anti-inflammatory drugs and hydroxychloroquine are recommended for treatment of antibiotic-refractory Lyme arthritis. In rare patients who fail to respond to this approach, other disease-modifying antirheumatic drugs such as methotrexate and tumor necrosis factor inhibitors have been used anecdotally with success. Arthroscopic synovectomy is curative in most patients who fail to respond to medical management.[121] Intra-articular corticosteroids may be associated with a higher rate of antibiotic unresponsiveness and are rarely used.[85]

Pregnancy and Lyme Disease

Pregnant and lactating women with Lyme disease can be treated with the same antibiotic regimens recommended for nonpregnant patients except that doxycycline should be avoided.[116] Maternal-fetal transmission of B. burgdorferi does occur,[122] but in contrast to syphilis in pregnancy, there is no evidence that the organism causes a congenital syndrome.[123,124] Pregnant patients should be reassured that with recommended therapy for Lyme disease, B. burgdorferi infection in the mother should not cause harm to the fetus.[124]

Expected Outcomes

Most patients treated for Lyme disease with recommended courses of antibiotics experience resolution of all signs and symptoms of the disorder.[68,125,126] About 15% of patients treated for Lyme disease may experience a Jarisch-Herxheimer reaction, a self-limited worsening of symptoms within 24 to 48 hours of initiation of antibiotic therapy.[4] Within the first week of treatment, patients may rarely show evolution of disease such as the development of new EM lesions or facial nerve palsy, but these signs should improve as therapy progresses. Most patients with Lyme arthritis experience resolution of joint inflammation after a 1-month course of oral antibiotics, and less than 10% of patients progress to antibiotic-refractory arthritis, which nevertheless resolves within 4 years.[85]

Subjective complaints of fatigue and musculoskeletal pain may persist for months after treatment for Lyme disease.[127] When patients complain of persistent pain and fatigue, evaluation for co-infection with *B. microti* or *A. phagocytophilum* should be performed.[128] Patients with coinfection tend to be more symptomatic at presentation and can have a delayed resolution of symptoms compared with patients with Lyme disease alone. Objective, nonprogressive signs such as mild facial weakness after facial palsy are likely due to irreversible tissue damage, and further antibiotic therapy does not seem to be beneficial.[129-132]

Chronic Lyme Disease and Post–Lyme Disease Syndrome

There is a great deal of controversy over the potential for Lyme disease to cause life-altering chronic morbidity in patients. It is unusual to have objective signs after recommended antibiotic regimens for Lyme disease diagnosed according to the guidelines discussed earlier, and when such signs (e.g., Lyme arthritis) are present, further antibiotic therapy does not alter outcome.[85] Even when objective signs are present, they are usually nonprogressive (e.g., residual facial weakness after facial palsy) or resolve over time (as is the case for Lyme arthritis). Use of the term *chronic Lyme disease*, which implies ongoing infection, for nonprogressive signs and symptoms after Lyme disease is not valid.

A few patients treated for Lyme disease may have fatigue, musculoskeletal pain, and complaints of memory impairment despite conventional or prolonged courses of antibiotic therapy, a condition referred to as *post–Lyme disease syndrome*.[129,133] In several controlled, population-based cohort studies that used validated standardized measures of outcomes (e.g., SF-36), patients with Lyme disease had more joint pain, symptoms of memory impairment, and worse functional status because of pain compared with controls.[126,134,135] These complaints could not be documented by abnormalities on physical examination or by neurocognitive testing, however, and a follow-up study showed that quality-of-life measures improved with time.[136] Psychological factors and the presence of psychiatric comorbidity in patients with Lyme disease correlate with poor functional outcomes after treatment.[137] More recently, a European study demonstrated that the frequency of nonspecific symptoms at 6 and 12 months after treatment for early Lyme disease was no greater than that of the control group, which included family members without a history of Lyme disease.[138] Children are less likely than adults to have persistent complaints after treatment for Lyme disease.[135]

Two randomized, double-blind, placebo-controlled trials of antibiotic therapy were conducted on seropositive and seronegative patients with chronic symptoms (>6 months) after treatment for Lyme disease.[130] Patients were randomly assigned to receive either intravenous ceftriaxone for 1 month followed by 2 months of oral doxycycline or matched intravenous and oral placebos. An interim analysis of the first 129 subjects enrolled (78 seropositive, 51 seronegative) resulted in termination of the study because no differences in outcome between groups receiving antibiotics or placebo were found, and evidence of ongoing infection could not be documented. Another trial of antibiotics for post-treatment Lyme disease symptoms found that fatigue, as assessed by the Fatigue Severity Scale–11, improved in the group receiving intravenous ceftriaxone, but cognitive dysfunction did not.[131] Individuals who had positive IgG immunoblots for Lyme disease and who had not received prior treatment with intravenous antibiotics were more likely to have improvement in fatigue. Subsequently, a randomized, placebo-controlled trial of a 10-week course of intravenous ceftriaxone for memory impairment after treatment for Lyme disease did not show sustained improvement in cognitive function.[132] An open pilot study provided evidence that gabapentin may be effective in the treatment of chronic pain syndromes after Lyme disease.[139]

A growing number of patients with similar subjective complaints are being treated for months or years with antibiotics for presumed *B. burgdorferi* infection.[140-144] These patients are diagnosed with *chronic Lyme disease* even though they often have no serologic evidence of *B. burgdorferi* exposure or are considered as testing positive on the basis of IgM reactivity on immunoblot despite years of not feeling well. They typically experience only partial resolution of their symptoms with antibiotics. Occasionally, patients may have other conditions such as rheumatoid arthritis or fibromyalgia, for which therapy has been delayed because of a misdiagnosis of Lyme disease.[140] Musculoskeletal pain is common in the general population; 20% to 30% of adults complain of chronic fatigue.[145] In the absence of a clinical history with objective manifestations of Lyme disease or positive two-tiered serologic tests, definitive attribution of symptoms to *B. burgdorferi* infection cannot be made. Caution should be exercised when attributing the response of symptoms to the antimicrobial effects of antibiotics. Ceftriaxone and other β-lactam antibiotics can modulate neurotransmitter activity,[146] and tetracyclines inhibit matrix metalloproteinases.[147,148] Prolonged antibiotic use is not without risk. Minor side effects are common, and serious adverse events such as biliary complications from ceftriaxone therapy or indwelling catheter–related infections occur at high enough rates to warrant only judicious use of antibiotics.[130,132,142]

PREVENTION

The most effective way to prevent Lyme disease is to reduce exposure risk to *B. burgdorferi*–infected ticks through personal protective measures and environmental controls.[149] These measures include avoidance of tick habitats such as wooded areas, stone fences, woodpiles, and tall grass; wearing protective clothing; and performing daily surveillance and prompt removal of ticks (within 24 hours of feeding). Other effective measures include use of DEET-containing insecticide sprays, yearly application of acaricides to property to kill ticks, construction of four-poster bait stations that apply acaricides onto deer as they feed, and tall fences to prevent deer from incidentally transporting ticks to an area.

A single 200-mg dose of doxycycline (or 4 mg/kg up to 200 mg for children 8 years old and older) has been shown to reduce the incidence of Lyme disease after a recognized tick bite[150] but is not routinely recommended because of the low rate of infection.[116] An FDA-approved recombinant Osp A–based vaccine to prevent Lyme disease was withdrawn because of low market demand and concern for potential vaccine-related side effects.[151,152]

SUMMARY

Lyme disease is a localized or systemic infection that usually manifests with skin and musculoskeletal signs and symptoms, but it can involve other organ systems, especially the heart and nervous system. The diagnosis should be based on objective clinical findings consistent with Lyme disease and supporting serologic tests. Most patients are cured with 2 to 4 weeks of antibiotic therapy, although the time to disease resolution may be prolonged, especially for individuals in whom therapy was delayed; irreversible tissue damage may occur. A poor response to antibiotic therapy should raise concern for alternative diagnoses or co-infection with other tick-borne pathogens. Arthritis becomes refractory to antibiotics in less than 10% of patients with Lyme disease. Treatment with nonsteroidal anti-inflammatory drugs and hydroxychloroquine usually resolves arthritis within 4 to 5 years. Some patients treated for Lyme disease develop a post–Lyme disease syndrome of fatigue, headaches, mild memory impairment, and musculoskeletal pain. Ongoing infection cannot be shown, and controlled treatment trials show no benefit of prolonged antibiotic therapy over placebo. Referral to an academic medical center with experience in the diagnosis and treatment of Lyme disease should be considered when patients do not respond as expected to therapy.

Selected References

1. Bockenstedt LK, Malawista SE: Lyme disease. In Cecil RL, Goldman L, Bennett JC, editors: *The Cecil textbook of medicine*, ed 23. Philadelphia, 2008, WB Saunders, pp 2289–2294.
2. Steere AC, Malawista SE, Snydman DR, et al: Lyme arthritis: an epidemic of oligoarticular arthritis in children and adults in three Connecticut communities, *Arthritis Rheum* 20(1):7–17, 1977.
5. Burgdorfer W, Barbour AG, Hayes SF, et al: Lyme disease—a tick-borne spirochetosis? *Science* 216(4552):1317–1319, 1982.
6. Steere AC, Grodzicki RL, Kornblatt AN, et al: The spirochetal etiology of Lyme disease, *N Engl J Med* 308(13):733–740, 1983.
7. Piesman J, Gern L: Lyme borreliosis in Europe and North America, *Parasitology* 129(Suppl):S191–S220, 2004.
8. Centers for Disease Control and Prevention: *Reported Lyme disease cases by state, 1995-2009* (website). www.cdc.gov/ncidod/dvbid/lyme/ld_rptdLymeCasesbyState.htm. Accessed 2010.
10. Steere AC, Coburn J, Glickstein L: The emergence of Lyme disease, *J Clin Invest* 113(8):1093–1101, 2004.
12. Dunham-Ems SM, Caimano MJ, Pal U, et al: Live imaging reveals a biphasic mode of dissemination of *Borrelia burgdorferi* within ticks, *J Clin Invest* 119(12):3652–3665, 2009.
13. Fraser CM, Casjens S, Huang WM, et al: Genomic sequence of a Lyme disease spirochaete, *Borrelia burgdorferi*, *Nature* 390(6660):580–586, 1997.
15. Pal U, de Silva AM, Montgomery RR, et al: Attachment of *Borrelia burgdorferi* within *Ixodes scapularis* mediated by outer surface protein A, *J Clin Invest* 106(4):561–569, 2000.
16. Tilly K, Krum JG, Bestor A, et al: *Borrelia burgdorferi* OspC protein required exclusively in a crucial early stage of mammalian infection, *Infect Immun* 74(6):3554–3564, 2006.

18. Lagal V, Pornoi D, Faure G, et al: *Borrelia burgdorferi sensu stricto* invasiveness is correlated with OspC-plasminogen affinity, *Microbes Infect* 8(3):645–652, 2006.
23. Norris SJ: Antigenic variation with a twist—the *Borrelia* story, *Mol Microbiol* 60(6):1319–1322, 2006.
25. Duray PH: Histopathology of clinical phases of human Lyme disease, *Rheum Dis Clin North Am* 15(4):691–710, 1989.
26. Steere AC, Glickstein L: Elucidation of Lyme arthritis, *Nat Rev Immunol* 4(2):143–152, 2004.
29. Kawai T, Akira S: Pathogen recognition with Toll-like receptors, *Curr Opin Immunol* 17(4):338–344, 2005.
30. Behera AK, Hildebrand E, Uematsu S, et al: Identification of a TLR-independent pathway for *Borrelia burgdorferi*-induced expression of matrix metalloproteinases and inflammatory mediators through binding to integrin alpha 3 beta 1, *J Immunol* 177(1):657–664, 2006.
31. Oosting M, Berende A, Sturm P, et al: Recognition of *Borrelia burgdorferi* by NOD2 is central for the induction of an inflammatory reaction, *J Infect Dis* 201(12):1849–1858, 2010.
32. Fikrig E, Barthold SW, Chen M, et al: Protective antibodies in murine Lyme disease arise independently of CD40 ligand, *J Immunol* 157(1):1–3, 1996.
33. McKisic MD, Barthold SW: T-cell-independent responses to *Borrelia burgdorferi* are critical for protective immunity and resolution of Lyme disease, *Infect Immun* 68(9):5190–5197, 2000.
34. Hardin JA, Steere AC, Malawista SE: Immune complexes and the evolution of Lyme arthritis: dissemination and localization of abnormal C1q binding activity, *N Engl J Med* 301(25):1358–1363, 1979.
35. Senel M, Rupprecht TA, Tumani H, et al: The chemokine CXCL13 in acute neuroborreliosis, *J Neurol Neurosurg Psychiatry* 81(8):929–933, 2010. Correction 81(10):1177, 2010.
36. Aguero-Rosenfeld ME, Wang G, Schwartz I, et al: Diagnosis of Lyme borreliosis, *Clin Microbiol Rev* 18(3):484–509, 2005.
37. Dai Z, Lackland H, Stein S, et al: Molecular mimicry in Lyme disease: monoclonal antibody H9724 to *Borrelia burgdorferi* flagellin specifically detects chaperonin-HSP60, *Biochim Biophys Acta* 1181(1):97–100, 1993.
39. Alaedini A, Latov N: Antibodies against OspA epitopes of *Borrelia burgdorferi* cross-react with neural tissue, *J Neuroimmunol* 159(1-2):192–195, 2005.
40. Chandra A, Wormser GP, Klempner MS, et al: Anti-neural antibody reactivity in patients with a history of Lyme borreliosis and persistent symptoms, *Brain Behavior Autoimm* 24(6):1018–1024, 2010.
42. Gross DM, Steere AC, Huber BT: T helper 1 response is dominant and localized to the synovial fluid in patients with Lyme arthritis, *J Immunol* 160(2):1022–1028, 1998.
43. Widhe M, Jarefors S, Ekerfelt C, et al: *Borrelia*-specific interferon-gamma and interleukin-4 secretion in cerebrospinal fluid and blood during Lyme borreliosis in humans: association with clinical outcome, *J Infect Dis* 189(10):1881–1891, 2004.
44. Codolo G, Amedei A, Steere AC, et al: *Borrelia burgdorferi* NapA-driven Th17 cell inflammation in Lyme arthritis, *Arthritis Rheum* 58(11):3609–3617, 2008.
45. Kalish RA, Leong JM, Steere AC: Association of treatment-resistant chronic Lyme arthritis with HLA-DR4 and antibody reactivity to OspA and OspB of *Borrelia burgdorferi*, *Infect Immun* 61(7):2774–2779, 1993.
46. Lengl-Janssen B, Strauss AF, Steere AC, et al: The T helper cell response in Lyme arthritis: differential recognition of *Borrelia burgdorferi* outer surface protein A in patients with treatment-resistant or treatment-responsive Lyme arthritis, *J Exp Med* 180(6):2069–2078, 1994.
47. Iliopoulou BP, Alroy J, Huber BT: CD28 deficiency exacerbates joint inflammation upon *Borrelia burgdorferi* infection, resulting in the development of chronic Lyme arthritis, *J Immunol* 179(12):8076–8082, 2007.
48. Vincent MS, Roessner K, Lynch D, et al: Apoptosis of Fas(high) CD4⁺ synovial T cells by Borrelia-reactive Fas-ligand(high) gamma delta T cells in Lyme arthritis, *J Exp Med* 184(6):2109–2117, 1996.
49. Chary-Valckenaere I, Jaulhac B, Champigneulle J, et al: Ultrastructural demonstration of intracellular localization of *Borrelia burgdorferi* in Lyme arthritis, *Br J Rheumatol* 37(4):468–470, 1998.
51. Kraiczy P, Skerka C, Kirschfink M, et al: Immune evasion of *Borrelia burgdorferi* by acquisition of human complement regulators FHL-1/reconectin and factor H, *Eur J Immunol* 31(6):1674–1684, 2001.

52. Stevenson B, El-Hage N, Hines MA, et al: Differential binding of host complement inhibitor factor H by *Borrelia burgdorferi* Erp surface proteins: a possible mechanism underlying the expansive host range of Lyme disease spirochetes, *Infect Immun* 70(2):491–497, 2002.

53. Liang FT, Nelson FK, Fikrig E: Molecular adaptation of *Borrelia burgdorferi* in the murine host, *J Exp Med* 196(2):275–280, 2002.

54. Barthold SW, de Souza MS, Janotka JL, et al: Chronic Lyme borreliosis in the laboratory mouse, *Am J Pathol* 143(3):959–971, 1993.

55. Edlow JA: Erythema migrans, *Med Clin North Am* 86(2):239–260, 2002.

56. Centers for Disease Control and Prevention: *Lyme disease* (Borrelia burgdorferi) *2008 case definition* (website). www.cdc.gov/ncphi/disss/nndss/casedef/lyme_disease_2008.htm. Accessed 2010.

59. Feder HM Jr, Gerber MA, Krause PJ, et al: Early Lyme disease. A flu-like illness without erythema migrans, *Pediatrics* 91(2):456–459, 1993.

60. Steere AC, Dhar A, Hernandez J, et al: Systemic symptoms without erythema migrans as the presenting picture of early Lyme disease, *Am J Med* 114(1):58–62, 2003.

61. Centers for Disease Control and Prevention: *Southern tick-associated rash illness* (website). www.cdc.gov/ncidod/dvbid/stari/. Accessed 2010.

63. Steere AC, Batsford WP, Weinberg M, et al: Lyme carditis: cardiac abnormalities of Lyme disease, *Ann Intern Med* 93(1):8–16, 1980.

64. Sangha O, Phillips CB, Fleischmann KE, et al: Lack of cardiac manifestations among patients with previously treated Lyme disease, *Ann Intern Med* 128(5):346–353, 1998.

65. Reik L, Steere AC, Bartenhagen NH, et al: Neurologic abnormalities of Lyme disease, *Medicine (Baltimore)* 58(4):281–294, 1979.

66. Halperin JJ, Pass HL, Anand AK, et al: Nervous system abnormalities in Lyme disease, *Ann N Y Acad Sci* 539(1):24–34, 1988.

67. Halperin JJ: Lyme disease and the peripheral nervous system, *Muscle Nerve* 28(2):133–143, 2003.

68. Nachman SA, Pontrelli L: Central nervous system Lyme disease, *Semin Pediatr Infect Dis* 14(2):123–130, 2003.

71. Eppes SC, Nelson DK, Lewis LL, et al: Characterization of Lyme meningitis and comparison with viral meningitis in children, *Pediatrics* 103(5):957–960, 1999.

72. Steere AC: Lyme disease, *N Engl J Med* 321(9):586–596, 1989.

73. Logigian EL, Kaplan RF, Steere AC: Chronic neurologic manifestations of Lyme disease, *N Engl J Med* 323(21):1438–1444, 1990.

74. Halperin JJ: Central nervous system Lyme disease, *Curr Neurol Neurosci Rep* 5(6):446–452, 2005.

76. Coyle PK, Krupp LB, Doscher C: Significance of reactive Lyme serology in multiple sclerosis, *Ann Neurol* 34(5):745–747, 1993.

77. Halperin JJ, Little BW, Coyle PK, et al: Lyme disease: cause of a treatable peripheral neuropathy, *Neurology* 37(11):1700–1706, 1987.

78. Halperin JJ, Krupp LB, Golightly MG, et al: Lyme borreliosis-associated encephalopathy, *Neurology* 40(9):1340–1343, 1990.

79. Logigian EL, Kaplan RF, Steere AC: Successful treatment of Lyme encephalopathy with intravenous ceftriaxone, *J Infect Dis* 180(2):377–383, 1999.

81. Asbrink E, Hovmark A, Olsson I: Clinical manifestations of acrodermatitis chronica atrophicans in 50 Swedish patients, *Zentralbl Bakteriol Mikrobiol Hyg [A]* 263(1-2):253–261, 1986.

82. Steere AC, Schoen RT, Taylor E: The clinical evolution of Lyme arthritis, *Ann Intern Med* 107(5):725–731, 1987.

83. Steere AC, Malawista SE, Hardin JA, et al: Erythema chronicum migrans and Lyme arthritis: the enlarging clinical spectrum, *Ann Intern Med* 86(6):685–698, 1977.

84. Szer IS, Taylor E, Steere AC: The long-term course of Lyme arthritis in children, *N Engl J Med* 325(3):159–163, 1991.

85. Steere AC, Angelis SM: Therapy for Lyme arthritis: strategies for the treatment of antibiotic-refractory arthritis, *Arthritis Rheum* 54(10):3079–3086, 2006.

86. Jones KL, McHugh GA, Glickstein LJ, et al: Analysis of *Borrelia burgdorferi* genotypes in patients with Lyme arthritis: high frequency of RST1 strains in antibiotic-refractory arthritis, *Arthritis Rheum* 60(7):2174–2182, 2009.

88. Bockenstedt LK, Gonzalez D, Haberman A, et al: Spirochete antigens persist near cartilage after murine Lyme borreliosis therapy, *J Clin Invest* 122(7):2652–2660, 2012.

89. Strle K, Shin JJ, Glickstein L, et al: Toll-like receptor 1 polymorphism (1805GG) is a risk factor for antibiotic-refractory Lyme arthritis [abstract 12]. In: *Programs and abstracts of the XIIth International Conference on Lyme Borreliosis and Other Tick-Borne Diseases*, Ljubljana, Slovenia, 2010, p 12.

90. Steere AC, Klitz W, Drouin EE, et al: Antibiotic-refractory Lyme arthritis is associated with HLA-DR molecules that bind a *Borrelia burgdorferi* peptide, *J Exp Med* 203(4):961–971, 2006.

91. Gross DM, Forsthuber T, Tary-Lehmann M, et al: Identification of LFA-1 as a candidate autoantigen in treatment-resistant Lyme arthritis, *Science* 281(5377):703–706, 1998.

92. Trollmo C, Meyer AL, Steere AC, et al: Molecular mimicry in Lyme arthritis demonstrated at the single cell level: LFA-1 alpha L is a partial agonist for outer surface protein A-reactive T cells, *J Immunol* 166(8):5286–5291, 2001.

93. Ghosh S, Seward R, Costello CE, et al: Autoantibodies from synovial lesions in chronic, antibiotic treatment-resistant Lyme arthritis bind cytokeratin-10, *J Immunol* 177(4):2486–2494, 2006.

94. Drouin EE, Seward RJ, Yao C, et al: A novel human autoantigen endothelial cell growth factor induces linked T and B cell responses in patients with antibiotic-refractory Lyme arthritis [abstract 13]. In: *Programs and abstracts of the XIIth International Conference on Lyme Borreliosis and Other Tick-Borne Diseases*, Ljubljana, Slovenia, 2010, p 13.

95. Shen S, Shin JJ, Strle K, et al: Treg cell numbers and function in patients with antibiotic-refractory or antibiotic-responsive Lyme arthritis, *Arthritis Rheum* 62(7):2127–2137, 2010.

97. Steere AC, Sikand VK, Schoen RT, et al: Asymptomatic infection with *Borrelia burgdorferi*, *Clin Infect Dis* 37(4):528–532, 2003.

98. Centers for Disease Control and Prevention: Recommendations for test performance and interpretation from the Second National Conference on Serologic Diagnosis of Lyme Disease, *MMWR Morb Mortal Wkly Rep* 44(31):590–591, 1995.

99. Centers for Disease Control and Prevention: Notice to readers: caution regarding testing for Lyme disease, *MMWR Morb Mortal Wkly Rep* 54(05):125, 2005.

100. Aguero-Rosenfeld ME, Nowakowski J, Bittker S, et al: Evolution of the serologic response to *Borrelia burgdorferi* in treated patients with culture-confirmed erythema migrans, *J Clin Microbiol* 34(1):1–9, 1996.

101. Bacon RM, Biggerstaff BJ, Schriefer ME, et al: Serodiagnosis of Lyme disease by kinetic enzyme-linked immunosorbent assay using recombinant VlsE1 or peptide antigens of *Borrelia burgdorferi* compared with 2-tiered testing using whole-cell lysates, *J Infect Dis* 187(8):1187–1199, 2003.

103. Kalish RA, McHugh G, Granquist J, et al: Persistence of immunoglobulin M or immunoglobulin G antibody responses to *Borrelia burgdorferi* 10-20 years after active Lyme disease, *Clin Infect Dis* 33(6):780–785, 2001.

104. Peltomaa M, McHugh G, Steere AC: Persistence of the antibody response to the VlsE sixth invariant region (IR6) peptide of *Borrelia burgdorferi* after successful antibiotic treatment of Lyme disease, *J Infect Dis* 187(8):1178–1186, 2003.

105. Wilske B, Schierz G, Preac-Mursic V, et al: Intrathecal production of specific antibodies against *Borrelia burgdorferi* in patients with lymphocytic meningoradiculitis (Bannwarth's syndrome), *J Infect Dis* 153(2):304–314, 1986.

106. Schmidt BL: PCR in laboratory diagnosis of human *Borrelia burgdorferi* infections, *Clin Microbiol Rev* 10(1):185–201, 1997.

108. Lawson JP, Rahn DW: Lyme disease and radiologic findings in Lyme arthritis, *AJR Am J Roentgenol* 158(5):1065–1069, 1992.

109. Ecklund K, Vargas S, Zurakowski D, et al: MRI features of Lyme arthritis in children, *AJR Am J Roentgenol* 184(6):1904–1909, 2005.

110. Kalina P, Decker A, Kornel E, et al: Lyme disease of the brainstem, *Neuroradiology* 47(12):903–907, 2005.

111. Agosta F, Rocca MA, Benedetti B, et al: MR imaging assessment of brain and cervical cord damage in patients with neuroborreliosis, *Am J Neuroradiol* 27(4):892–894, 2006.

112. Steinbach JP, Melms A, Skalej M, et al: Delayed resolution of white matter changes following therapy of B. *burgdorferi* encephalitis, *Neurology* 64:758–759, 2005.

113. Morgen K, Martin R, Stone RD, et al: FLAIR and magnetization transfer imaging of patients with post-treatment Lyme disease syndrome, *Neurology* 57(11):1980–1985, 2001.

114. Logigian EL, Johnson KA, Kijewski MF, et al: Reversible cerebral hypoperfusion in Lyme encephalopathy, *Neurology* 49(6):1661–1670, 1997.

115. Fallon BA, Keilp J, Prohovnik I, et al: Regional cerebral blood flow and cognitive deficits in chronic Lyme disease, *J Neuropsychiatry Clin Neurosci* 15(3):326–332, 2003.

116. Wormser GP, Dattwyler RJ, Shapiro ED, et al: The clinical assessment, treatment, and prevention of Lyme disease, human granulocytic anaplasmosis, and babesiosis: clinical practice guidelines by the Infectious Diseases Society of America, *Clin Infect Dis* 43(9):1089–1134, 2006.

121. Schoen RT, Aversa JM, Rahn DW, et al: Treatment of refractory chronic Lyme arthritis with arthroscopic synovectomy, *Arthritis Rheum* 34(8):1056–1060, 1991.

122. Schlesinger PA, Duray PH, Burke BA, et al: Maternal-fetal transmission of the Lyme disease spirochete, *Borrelia burgdorferi*, *Ann Intern Med* 103(1):67–68, 1985.

123. Williams CL, Strobino B, Weinstein A, et al: Maternal Lyme disease and congenital malformations: a cord blood serosurvey in endemic and control areas, *Paediatr Perinat Epidemiol* 9(3):320–330, 1995.

124. Strobino BA, Williams CL, Abid S, et al: Lyme disease and pregnancy outcome: a prospective study of two thousand prenatal patients, *Am J Obstet Gynecol* 169(2 Pt 1):367–374, 1993.

125. Shapiro ED: Long-term outcomes of persons with Lyme disease, *Vector Borne Zoonotic Dis* 2(4):279–281, 2002.

126. Shadick NA, Phillips CB, Sangha O, et al: Musculoskeletal and neurologic outcomes in patients with previously treated Lyme disease, *Ann Intern Med* 131(12):919–926, 1999.

127. Wormser GP, Ramanathan R, Nowakowski J, et al: Duration of antibiotic therapy for early Lyme disease: a randomized, double-blind, placebo-controlled trial, *Ann Intern Med* 138(9):697–704, 2003.

128. Krause PJ, McKay K, Thompson CA, et al: Disease-specific diagnosis of coinfection tickborne zoonoses: babesiosis, human granulocytic ehrlichiosis, and Lyme disease, *Clin Infect Dis* 34(9):1184–1191, 2002.

129. Asch ES, Bujak DI, Weiss M, et al: Lyme disease: an infectious and postinfectious syndrome, *J Rheumatol* 21(3):454–461, 1994.

130. Klempner MS, Hu LT, Evans J, et al: Two controlled trials of antibiotic treatment in patients with persistent symptoms and a history of Lyme disease, *N Engl J Med* 345(2):85–92, 2001.

131. Krupp LB, Hyman LG, Grimson R, et al: Study and treatment of post Lyme disease (STOP-LD). A randomized double masked clinical trial, *Neurology* 60(12):1923–1930, 2003.

132. Fallon BA, Keilp JG, Corbera KM, et al: A randomized, placebo-controlled trial of repeated IV antibiotic therapy for Lyme encephalopathy, *Neurology* 70(13):992–1003, 2008.

134. Shadick NA, Phillips CB, Logigian EL, et al: The long-term clinical outcomes of Lyme disease. A population-based retrospective cohort study, *Ann Intern Med* 121(8):560–567, 1994.

135. Seltzer EG, Gerber MA, Cartter ML, et al: Long-term outcomes of persons with Lyme disease, *JAMA* 283(5):609–616, 2000.

136. Shadick NA, Phillips CB, Sangha O, et al: Diminished health-related quality-of-life improves over time in Lyme disease: the 12 yr followup from the Nantucket Lyme disease cohort study [abstract O-36]. In: *Programs and abstracts of the IX International Conference on Lyme Borreliosis and Other Tick-borne Diseases*, New York, 2002, p 36.

137. Hassett AL, Radvanski DC, Buyske S, et al: Role of psychiatric comorbidity in chronic Lyme disease, *Arthritis Rheum* 59(12):1742–1749, 2008.

138. Cerar D, Cerar T, Ruzic-Sabljic E, et al: Subjective symptoms after treatment of early Lyme disease, *Am J Med* 123(1):79–86, 2010.

139. Weissenbacher S, Ring J, Hofmann H: Gabapentin for the symptomatic treatment of chronic neuropathic pain in patients with late-stage Lyme borreliosis: a pilot study, *Dermatology* 211(2):123–127, 2005.

142. Reid MC, Schoen RT, Evans J, et al: The consequences of overdiagnosis and overtreatment of Lyme disease: an observational study, *Ann Intern Med* 128(5):354–362, 1998.

144. Feder HM Jr, Johnson BJB, O'Connell S, et al: A critical appraisal of "chronic Lyme disease", *N Engl J Med* 357(14):1422–1430, 2007.

146. Rothstein JD, Patel S, Regan MR, et al: Beta-lactam antibiotics offer neuroprotection by increasing glutamate transporter expression, *Nature* 433(7021):73–77, 2005.

147. Sadowski T, Steinmeyer J: Effects of tetracyclines on the production of matrix metalloproteinases and plasminogen activators as well as of their natural inhibitors, tissue inhibitor of metalloproteinase-1 and plasminogen activator inhibitor-1, *Inflamm Res* 50(3):175–182, 2001.

148. Bernardino L, Kaushal D, Philipp MT: The antibiotics doxycycline and minocycline inhibit the inflammatory responses to the Lyme disease spirochete *Borrelia burgdorferi*, *J Infect Dis* 199(9):1379–1388, 2009.

149. Hayes EB, Piesman J: How can we prevent Lyme disease? *N Engl J Med* 348(24):2424–2430, 2003.

150. Nadelman RB, Nowakowski J, Fish D, et al: Prophylaxis with single-dose doxycycline for the prevention of Lyme disease after an *Ixodes scapularis* tick bite, *N Engl J Med* 345(2):79–84, 2001.

151. Steere AC, Sikand VK, Meurice F, et al: Vaccination against Lyme disease with recombinant *Borrelia burgdorferi* outer-surface lipoprotein A with adjuvant. Lyme Disease Vaccine Study Group, *N Engl J Med* 339(4):209–215, 1998.

152. Hanson MS, Edelman R: Progress and controversy surrounding vaccines against Lyme disease, *Expert Rev Vaccines* 2(5):683–703, 2003.

Full references for this chapter can be found on www.expertconsult.com.

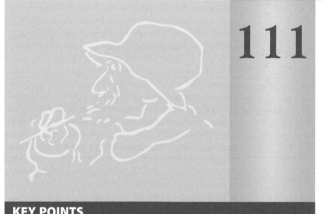

111 Mycobacterial Infections of Bones and Joints

ERIC M. RUDERMAN • JOHN P. FLAHERTY

KEY POINTS

Global rates of tuberculosis disease have increased due to the expanding human immunodeficiency virus pandemic and the growing problem of antituberculous drug resistance; rheumatologists have seen an increase in tuberculosis disease in response to the expanded use of anti–tumor necrosis factor (TNF) agents.

Musculoskeletal tuberculosis typically presents as a chronic localized infection, most commonly involving the spine, less often the hip or knee.

Diagnosis may be very difficult and often requires biopsy for histopathology and culture of the bone or synovium; rapid diagnostic test techniques have not yet proven reliable in bone and joint specimens.

The tuberculin skin test can be helpful in identifying latent tuberculosis before treatment with anti-TNF agents, but it is limited by false-positive and false-negative results; the availability of interferon-γ release assays, when available, may be a useful alternative screening procedure.

Treatment requires multiple agents selected on the basis of susceptibility testing for 6 to 9 months and has been complicated by the increasing incidence of drug resistance.

Nontuberculous mycobacteria are becoming important pathogens to recognize in the face of biologic therapy for rheumatic diseases.

Recognition of tuberculosis (TB) and other mycobacterial infections of the musculoskeletal system has become a major challenge for rheumatologists in the United States and in other developed countries. Before 1999, most rheumatologists could easily go an entire year without seeing a single case of mycobacterial infection. Such cases were rare even at academic centers, where they would likely be presented as unusual teaching cases at clinical conferences.

However, 1999 introduced the routine clinical use of anti–tumor necrosis factor (TNF) therapy in the United States, and with it came an unexpected increase in TB cases seen by rheumatologists. Fortunately, the initiation of routine screening with tuberculin skin tests (TSTs) and other methods has led to a sharp decline in the number of new cases, particularly those associated with reactivation of latent infection. However, the risk of primary infection with new exposure mandates continued vigilance in these patients and potentially in patients on other biologic therapies. Moreover, for non-TB mycobacterial infections, no screening tests are available, making vigilance on immunosuppressive therapy even more important.

Another major force driving the increase in mycobacterial infection is the human immunodeficiency virus (HIV) epidemic that continues to be a worldwide problem. By 1991, 21% of extrapulmonary TB cases in the United States were associated with acquired immunodeficiency syndrome (AIDS). In developing countries, the HIV pandemic has led to marked increases in osteoarticular TB co-infection.[1] These cases are distinguished by disseminated multifocal disease suggestive of hematogenous spread, rapid progression, and more common coexistence with pulmonary infection.[2,3] HIV testing should be a routine part of the workup of any patient presenting with a musculoskeletal infection secondary to *Mycobacterium tuberculosis*. Since the introduction of effective antiretroviral therapy, the incidence of TB and nontuberculous mycobacterial infection in patients co-infected with HIV has sharply declined in the United States.

Although TB is uncommon among the non–HIV-infected population in the developed world (in the United States, TB is steadily declining among the general population), it remains a major problem in developing countries. There, TB continues to ravage the population, with 9 million new cases of active disease and 1.6 million deaths each year.[4] Worldwide, it is the number two infectious disease killer after HIV/AIDS. Someone in the world is newly infected with TB bacilli every second. About one-third of the world's population is infected with TB, providing a reservoir that will continue to complicate its global control.[5] More alarming is the emergence of extensively drug-resistant TB (XDR-TB).[6] These strains fail to respond to all first-line and most second-line TB agents. An outbreak of XDR-TB in South Africa was associated with a mortality rate of 100%, with a median survival of only 16 days after diagnosis. Globalization of the world economy is encouraging increased contact between populations of the developed and developing worlds. Recent immigrants to the United States from endemic areas constitute an expanding reservoir of patients with latent TB.

The challenge of diagnosing musculoskeletal mycobacterial infection reaches beyond the rarity of the disease. Such infections are often indolent and may lack the pain, fevers, chills, and other prominent symptoms that typically accompany bacterial infections of the musculoskeletal system. In addition, unless the diagnosis of TB is a consideration from the outset, routine culture techniques will not isolate the organism. Delay in the diagnosis of mycobacterial infection of the musculoskeletal system is common and will continue without a heightened index of suspicion for these types of infections.

For all these reasons, 21st century rheumatologists need to be well informed about a group of diseases with which they may have had little or no experience during their formal medical training.

CLINICAL SCENARIOS

To appreciate the entire spectrum of clinical problems that a rheumatologist may encounter in dealing with mycobacterial infection, it is useful to think in terms of several distinct categories. Franco-Paredes[7] and colleagues provided a clinically useful division of mycobacterial infections into four major categories. The following sections reflect that division.

Direct Involvement of the Musculoskeletal System

Musculoskeletal infections caused by mycobacteria typically present as chronic, indolent, localized involvement of the bones, spine, peripheral joints, or soft tissues that produces a focus of nonspecific pain and, less often, swelling. In infections initiated by direct tissue inoculation, the traumatic event is often trivial or remote in time from the onset of clinical disease. Diagnosis may be delayed for months to years, in part because of minimal early symptoms and attribution of those symptoms to a noninfectious disorder until disease progression and disability prompt a more aggressive diagnostic investigation.

Constitutional symptoms are typically subtle or absent, and laboratory indicators of inflammation are often normal. Synovial effusion is frequently minimal, and the fluid, if it is attainable, shows nonspecific inflammation. Radiographic abnormalities may be delayed, although newer imaging techniques have allowed the earlier detection of abnormalities and the distinction of TB from other infections and neoplasm.[8,9] Characteristic pulmonary or extrapulmonary findings are not always present; for example, less than 50% of osteoarticular TB presents with evidence of active or past pulmonary disease. Tuberculin skin tests (TSTs) and interferon-γ release assay (IGRA) testing may provide useful clues to the cause, but results are not invariably positive, especially in debilitated or immunosuppressed patients. Correct diagnosis is highly dependent, in most cases, on demonstration of the infectious agent by microscopic examination and culture of affected tissue.

In HIV-infected patients, mycobacterial infections are often diagnosed before patients' HIV-positive status is known, sometimes leading to its recognition.[10] Atypical pulmonary TB and extrapulmonary (often multifocal) infection are common; extrapulmonary infection occurs in 60% to 70% of such cases, compared with 16% of all TB patients.

The clinical patterns of musculoskeletal TB include spondylitis, osteomyelitis, peripheral joint infection, and soft tissue abscess. In a series of 230 consecutive cases of TB from the preantibiotic era, 5.2% had skeletal involvement; the spine was affected in 60% of these cases.[11] TB of the bones and joints is spread hematogenously. The sites most commonly affected are the spine and hips, followed by the knees and wrists; other joint involvement is rare. Constitutional symptoms are unusual in musculoskeletal TB and, when present, suggest TB in other organs. Vertebral collapse due to spinal TB may initially be attributed to the more common osteoporosis-caused spinal compression fracture. TB only rarely involves skeletal muscle but must be considered in the differential diagnosis of an enlarging muscle

Table 111-1 Causes of False-Negative Purified Protein Derivative Test

Increased age (>70 yr)
Steroid use (prednisone ≥15 mg/day)
Hypoalbuminemia (<2 g/dL)
Azotemia
Impaired cellular immunity
Human immunodeficiency virus infection

lesion.[12-16] Isolated cases involving tendons, trochanteric bursae, and fasciae latae illustrate the variety of possibilities.[17-19] Biopsy and culture are required for diagnosis. Imaging studies do not reliably distinguish TB from neoplasm.

In nonendemic areas, skeletal TB usually occurs in elderly, debilitated patients, most often in the form of solitary osteolytic lesions in the axial skeleton. The development of skeletal disease is often remote from the initial infection, which strongly implies reactivation of previous subclinical disease. Patients may have false-negative TSTs for several reasons, including long-term corticosteroid use or coexisting debilitating disease, such as rheumatoid arthritis or chronic renal failure, which compromises resistance and produces anergy (Table 111-1).[20,21] Spinal disease in children in nonendemic regions has largely been eliminated by effective medical therapy of pulmonary infection.

In contrast, in endemic areas with high infectivity rates, those infected are more commonly children and young to middle-aged adults. These individuals have a higher incidence of multifocal skeletal involvement in the ribs, pelvis, vertebral appendages, cervical spine, feet, and long bone diaphyses, and they show positive TST reactivity.[22] Bone seeding occurs through hematogenous spread, sometimes secondarily from another extrapulmonary site. When pulmonary findings are present, a miliary pattern is typical. Spread to bone may also occur from infected nodes, by direct extension or through draining lymph channels.[23]

Spondylitis

The spine is the dominant site of involvement in skeletal TB, accounting for 50% to 60% of cases.[24] Between 48% and 67% of lesions occur in the lower thoracic and thoracolumbar spine in HIV-negative patients, whereas the lumbar spine is most commonly involved in HIV-positive patients.[3] Infection usually begins in the anterior subchondral bone of a single vertebra adjacent to the intervertebral disk (Figures 111-1 and 111-2). Progression to bone takes 2 to 5 months and begins with extension from cancellous to cortical bone, and then across the disk space to adjacent vertebrae (Figure 111-3). Bone destruction may lead to vertebral collapse, which typically occurs anteriorly, resulting in gibbus deformity. Isolated neural arch involvement and intraspinal abscess may also occur.

Paravertebral abscess begins with extension of infection under the anterior longitudinal ligament. In the thoracic spine, it may extend into the pleural space and the lung parenchyma. In the cervical region, it may present in the posterior cervical triangle or the retropharyngeal space. In the lumbar spine, a cold abscess characteristically produces lateral displacement of the psoas muscle and may dissect

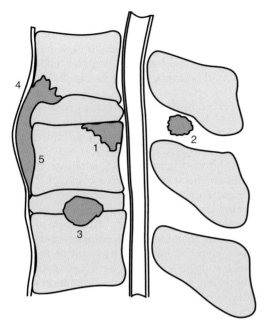

Figure 111-1 Tuberculous spondylitis: sites of involvement. Tuberculous lesions can localize in the vertebral body *(1)* or, more rarely, in posterior osseous or ligamentous structures *(2)* . Extension to the intervertebral disk *(3)* or prevertebral tissues *(4)* is not infrequent; subligamentous spread *(5)* can lead to erosion of the anterior vertebral surface. *(From Resnick D: Diagnosis of bone and joint disorders, ed 3, Philadelphia, 1995, WB Saunders, p 2464.)*

along its length to present as a mass in the inguinal triangle, gluteal muscle, or upper thigh. In isolated cases, a cold abscess occurs without apparent bone involvement.

A particular variant of this presentation is subligamentous TB, in which infection spreads up and down the spine beneath the longitudinal ligament, producing scalloping of multiple anterior vertebral bodies without disk involvement. This pattern is more common in the cervical spine.[25]

The clinical presentation of spinal TB usually consists of localized pain, which may be accompanied by low-grade fever, weight loss, chills, and nonspecific constitutional

symptoms. Paraparesis and paraplegia have been reported in 1% to 27% of patients in various series. In comparison with pyogenic vertebral osteomyelitis, spinal TB more often presents with a prolonged clinical course, thoracic segment involvement, absence of fever, spinal deformity, neurologic deficit, and paravertebral or epidural masses.[25] On occasion, tuberculous spondylitis may present with chronic inflammatory-type back pain more typical of a spondyloarthropathy.[26]

Mycobacterial colony counts in bone biopsy specimens are relatively low. Only 40% of smears and cultures from psoas abscesses are positive. Among patients meeting strict clinical and radiographic criteria in one series, between 73% and 82% had compatible histologic features on biopsy; of these, 80% to 95% had positive cultures.[23] The differential diagnosis, which is extensive, includes pyogenic and fungal osteomyelitis, primary and metastatic tumors, sarcoidosis, multiple myeloma, and eosinophilic granuloma.

Cervical spine involvement is relatively rare, accounting for only 0.4% to 1.2% of cases of extrapulmonary TB in the United States.[27] The most common presenting symptoms are neck pain and stiffness, although hoarseness, dysphagia, torticollis, fever, anorexia, and neurologic disorders may also occur. Spinal involvement can progress to myelopathy because of delays in diagnosis. Radiographs may show characteristic osteolysis of the anterior vertebral body with sparing of the posterior portion, gibbus deformity, disk involvement, and a partially calcified paraspinous mass. Computed tomography (CT) or magnetic resonance imaging (MRI) is useful for assessing compromise of the spinal canal. Retropharyngeal infection may extend into the craniocervical junction and, if not promptly recognized, may cause atlantoaxial dislocation and neurologic complications.[28,29]

The sacroiliac joint is involved in up to 10% of cases of skeletal TB, often without other evidence of disease.[30] Infection, TB in particular, should be considered in all cases of unilateral sacroiliitis, particularly when other features of a spondyloarthropathy are absent. Emigration from an endemic area and a past history of TB increase the likeli-

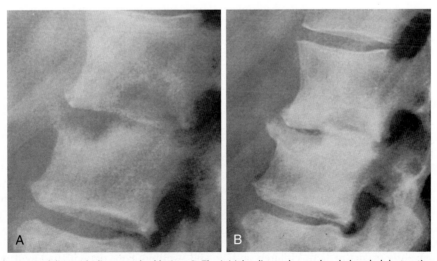

Figure 111-2 Tuberculous spondylitis with discovertebral lesion. **A,** The initial radiograph reveals subchondral destruction of two vertebral bodies, with mild surrounding eburnation and loss of intervertebral disk height. The appearance is identical to that in pyogenic spondylitis. **B,** Several months later, an osseous response is evident. Note the increased sclerosis. Osteophytosis and improved definition of the osseous margins can be seen. *(From Resnick D: Diagnosis of bone and joint disorders, ed 3, Philadelphia, 1995, WB Saunders, p 2465.)*

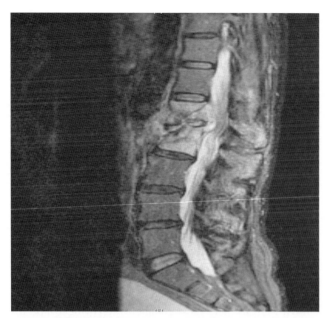

Figure 111-3 Tuberculous spondylitis with spinal cord compression. Magnetic resonance image of the lumbar spine shows destruction of contiguous vertebral bodies and an inflammatory mass pressing on the spinal cord. This patient was successfully treated with medical therapy alone.

hood of this cause. Buttock pain on the involved side is the presenting symptom and is often accompanied by proximal leg or radicular pain. Examination reveals sacroiliac tenderness to palpation and stress maneuvers. Sacroiliac films show joint widening and erosion. An elevated erythrocyte sedimentation rate (ESR) and anemia are common, and a positive tuberculin reaction is typical. Biopsy of the sacroiliac joint shows granulomatous histologic features or nonspecific inflammation and a positive culture in most cases.

Atypical spinal lesions, which occur in about 10% of cases, may lead to delayed diagnosis and treatment. Atypical radiographic presentations in a single vertebra include concentric collapse, sclerotic foci, and selective involvement of the vertebral arches and costotransverse joints. Multiple vertebrae may be involved in continuity or as skipped lesions. Atypical clinical presentations may suggest a herniated intervertebral disk, failed back syndrome, spinal tumor, or a meningeal granuloma.[24,31]

Tuberculous Osteomyelitis

Bone lesions begin with hematogenous implantation of organisms in the medullary area. Metaphyseal involvement is most common, and lesions may spread through the growth plate to involve the adjacent joint, usually late in the disease course. Lesions are typically destructive. Lytic lesions in unusual areas, such as the pubic symphysis, sacroiliac joint, and elbow, can be misdiagnosed as malignancy.[32] Osteomyelitis may develop in a bone or a joint that has been previously exposed to trauma.

Tuberculous osteomyelitis occurs in both children and adults.[33] Although any bone can be involved, the femur and the tibia are most commonly affected. Dactylitis may also occur in children. In one large series from an endemic area,

such cases represented 19% of bone and joint TB and 15% of cases of osteomyelitis of hematogenous origin.[34] Bone pain was the most common presentation; a draining sinus, abscess formation, and local swelling and tenderness were also common. The average delay before diagnosis was 28 months.

Multifocal osteoarticular TB is a less common variant of the disease,[34,35] but TB should be considered in all patients from endemic areas who present with multiple destructive skeletal lesions.

For a definitive diagnosis of osteoarticular TB, a biopsy specimen of an affected site must be obtained.[18] Soft tissue lesions characteristically demonstrate rim enhancement on CT examination. CT may also facilitate percutaneous needle biopsy or abscess drainage.[36] Histologic examination generally reveals granulomatous inflammation. In one series of 121 cases, biopsy showed a positive culture in 33%, granulomatous histologic features in 46%, and both in 21%.[37] Radiographic findings include cavity formation with a thin adjacent layer of sclerosis in about 50% of cases, sometimes containing a sequestrum. The true extent of bone involvement may be difficult to detect because of clinically silent lesions. Bone imaging with technetium 99, although more sensitive than conventional radiographs, may provide false-negative information in early, indolent, or highly destructive disease. Tuberculin test reactions are positive in more than 80% of cases.[38]

Treatment with chemotherapy is generally effective. In a minority of cases, surgical débridement is required for healing. Initiation of therapy on the basis of histologic findings is appropriate pending culture results. Sinus cultures are commonly positive for pyogenic bacteria both before and after antituberculous therapy, but these are presumed to be contaminants. Healing is associated with sclerosis at the margin of lesions. Misdiagnosis of the condition as pyogenic osteomyelitis may lead to unnecessary surgery or to delayed antituberculous treatment, resulting in extension of infection into the joint and chronic disability.

Septic Arthritis

Tuberculous joint involvement is second in frequency to vertebral infection.[24] The typical pattern is a monoarticular arthritis involving the large joints, most commonly the hip and knee (Figures 111-4 and 111-5).[39,40] Other joints less commonly involved include the sacroiliac, shoulder, elbow, ankle, carpal, and tarsal joints. Infection begins in the synovium, with slower progression of destructive changes than in pyogenic septic arthritis. Prosthetic joint infection with M. tuberculosis has been reported and usually is caused by local reactivation of latent disease.[41]

The diagnosis of tuberculous arthritis is often missed. A consecutive series spanning the years 1970 to 1984 emphasized typical features.[42] Of 23 cases of musculoskeletal TB, 9 involved the spine, 1 the hip, and the remaining 13 the peripheral joints. Most patients were men older than 50 years. The history of TB or exposure was generally forgotten. In all cases, presenting symptoms included joint pain and swelling. Four patients had evidence of active pulmonary TB, and in two patients with sterile pyuria, M. tuberculosis grew from the urine. Only 5 of 10 patients tested had a positive TST. Radiographs showed changes of erosive

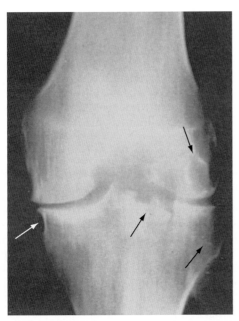

Figure 111-4 Tuberculous arthritis of the knee. On conventional computed tomography, typical marginal and central osseous erosions *(arrows)* accompany tuberculous arthritis. Osteoporosis is not prominent. *(From Resnick D: Diagnosis of bone and joint disorders, ed 3, Philadelphia, 1995, WB Saunders, p 2480.)*

arthritis in 7 and no changes in 4 of 11 joints studied. The median delay in diagnosis was 8 months.

Arriving at a correct diagnosis requires vigorous pursuit and usually a synovial biopsy and culture. Initial studies are often misleading and may contribute to delayed diagnosis or misdiagnosis. Synovial fluid findings are variable and do not distinguish this arthropathy from other inflammatory or

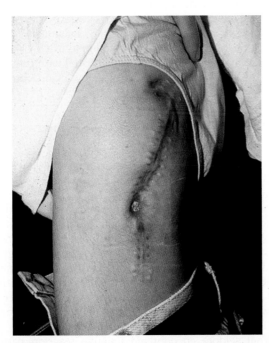

Figure 111-5 Tuberculous arthritis following total hip replacement. A sinus tract emerges from the scar following total hip arthroplasty for childhood destructive arthritis of unknown cause. The young man was originally from Vietnam.

septic arthritides.[43] Cell counts more often suggest bland inflammatory, rather than septic, arthritis and may contain a preponderance of neutrophils. The diagnosis may be facilitated if the organism is observed on an acid-fast smear of synovial fluid, but only 10% to 20% of reported cases are positive. In contrast, synovial fluid cultures are frequently positive. Radiographic changes are similar to those seen in other septic arthritides, beginning with juxta-articular bone demineralization and progressing to marginal bone erosion and articular cartilage destruction (see Figure 111-4).

With the open biopsy technique, granulomatous histologic features and positive cultures are present in more than 90% of cases.[43] No data are available for direct amplification tests in mycobacterial arthritis, but their use can be considered in suspected cases to arrive at an earlier diagnosis. The histologic examination alone may be confusing, because granulomatous synovitis can also be found in nontuberculous mycobacterial infection, sarcoidosis, erythema nodosum, brucellosis, Crohn's disease, and foreign body reaction. As noted, synovial acid-fast smear is of limited value. Tuberculous arthritis is also reported in children, sometimes early in the disease course; synovial biopsy and culture are recommended in children with monoarthritis and a positive tuberculin reaction.[44]

TB must be considered among the possible causes of septic arthritis in patients with pre-existing rheumatoid arthritis, although it is not widely seen in developed countries.[45,46] Conversely, rheumatoid factor may be present in TB, leading to diagnostic confusion in the presence of chronic monoarthritis.[45]

Emergence of Tuberculosis during Treatment of Rheumatic Disease

Many patients with systemic rheumatic disease have dysregulated immune systems that are treated with immunosuppressive drugs. Such an impaired immune response may permit the reactivation of latent TB. TNF plays a key role in granuloma formation and stabilization, which promotes the containment of M. *tuberculosis*. The rate of TB among patients with rheumatoid arthritis before the widespread use of anti-TNF drugs was approximately 6 cases per 100,000,[47] although some studies have suggested that the rate in rheumatoid arthritis is higher than in the general population.[48] In one large patient registry, the estimated incidence of TB associated with infliximab in rheumatoid arthritis patients was in excess of 1000 per 100,000 person-years of exposure during the years 2000-2001.[49] In the United States, the rate was 52 per 100,000 person-years during the same time period.[47] Etanercept may be associated with a lower risk for TB reactivation than infliximab: 10 cases per 100,000 person-years of exposure with etanercept, versus 41 per 100,000 person-years with infliximab, according to an analysis of Food and Drug Administration data.[50] More recently, both British and French registries of biologic use have identified a greater risk for TB associated with the use of adalimumab and infliximab than with etanercept.[51,52] Fewer data are available for the newer TNF antagonists, and comparisons are complicated by the widespread use of pretreatment screening instituted after the first agents in this class were approved for use. Monoclonal antibodies to TNF may play a greater role in destabilizing granulomata than

TNF receptors. Nonetheless, similar precautions should be taken with any TNF antagonist, and all should be presumed to increase risk of new infection and reactivation of latent infection.

Other biologic agents may pose a lower risk for reactivation of TB because the mechanisms of action are not intimately involved with host defenses related to intracellular organisms. Animal studies have suggested that abatacept does not impair the ability of mice to respond to M. tuberculosis, but this has not been confirmed in humans.[53] Patients treated with abatacept and tocilizumab in clinical trials were prescreened with a TST and excluded if positive, thus making a direct comparison difficult. Little or no evidence indicates that B cells play a major role in containing TB, and no recommendation for TB screening is included in the labeling for rituximab.

Glucocorticoid use poses a significant hazard for patients with latent TB. Many mechanisms account for this effect, such as impairment of cellular immune responses and monocyte chemotaxis and function, including the monocyte's production of TNF. The use of glucocorticoids has been associated with a five times increased risk for the development of TB in a case-control study based on a large general practice database in the United Kingdom.[54] The risk appeared to be dose related but was seen even at the physiologic dose of prednisone 7.5 mg/day. Just as with anti-TNF therapy, the risk for TB was greatest early in the course of treatment. In a more recent study from France, prednisone given at 10 mg or more per day, but not at lower doses, was associated with an increased risk for developing TB.[52]

Reactivation of TB in the face of anti-TNF therapy typically occurs within 6 months of treatment and often presents as extrapulmonary disease. Institution of a TB screening protocol in rheumatoid arthritis patients and treatment of latent TB before TNF antagonist administration resulted in a 78% decrease in active TB.[55] Strategies to treat latent TB infection that are tailored to the at-risk population can effectively and safely lessen the likelihood of active TB in patients treated with TNF antagonists. Indeed, it has been suggested that much of the blame for the development of active TB in this situation can be attributed to incomplete compliance with screening protocols.[56] Conversely, in a report of 84 patients at a single center treated with etanercept after demonstrating a positive purified protein derivative (PPD), no cases of active TB were seen during a mean of 2 years of follow-up, despite the fact that only 78 patients received prophylaxis, and 26 of those failed to complete the prescribed course.[57] Although screening for latent TB infection has reduced the incidence of active disease, false-negative TSTs can undermine such good intentions (see Table 111-1).

The approach to a patient with latent TB who needs anti-TNF therapy has not been standardized. Many authorities recommend that patients with positive TSTs and normal chest radiographs who have never been treated for TB receive at least 1 to 2 months of therapy before beginning an anti-TNF drug, if for no other reason than to be certain that they will be able to tolerate the full course of latent TB therapy. Appropriate regimens include 9 months of isoniazid or 4 months of rifampin. Patients discovered to have active TB should receive a complete course of standard antituberculous therapy before any consideration is given to using an anti-TNF drug.

Although anti-TNF therapy and steroids stand out as particular risk factors for the development of TB, all rheumatic disease patients treated with immunosuppressive therapy that impairs cellular immunity should be considered at risk. This is especially true for the elderly, the malnourished, and immigrants from countries with high endemic rates of TB.

Rheumatic Disorders Precipitated by Treatment of Tuberculosis

A variety of rheumatic conditions may be precipitated by drugs used in the treatment of TB. These include drug-induced lupus caused by isoniazid (INH) and rifampin (RIF). As with other cases of drug-induced lupus, they are associated with positive antinuclear antibodies and the presence of antihistone antibodies. Typically, these patients follow a benign course, with reversal of disease after the drug is discontinued.

Arthropathy and tendinopathy have been described with the use of fluoroquinolones, especially ciprofloxacin and levofloxacin. Risk of tendon rupture (usually the Achilles tendon) is greatest in patients older than 50 years and increases with concomitant use of corticosteroids.

Pyrazinamide interferes with the renal tubular excretion of uric acid and has been associated with the development of hyperuricemia and gout in adults.

Some patients develop a paradoxical worsening of their condition upon initiation of antituberculous therapy. Such a development may raise questions about a flare of the underlying disease, especially if immunosuppressive therapy has been withdrawn in the face of infection. Symptoms include fever, malaise, weight loss, and increasing respiratory symptoms. The mechanism for such reactions is not completely understood but has been categorized within the spectrum of immune reconstitution inflammatory syndromes. Such reactions are more common in HIV patients and have also been seen in patients treated with infliximab following cessation of anti-TNF therapy.[58] Corticosteroids may ameliorate this response.

Reactive Immunologic Phenomenon in the Setting of Tuberculosis

A variety of reactive immunologic phenomena have been associated with M. tuberculosis infection. These are uncommonly found in clinical practice.

Poncet's disease is an aseptic inflammatory polyarthritis that occurs in the presence of active TB. Although any joints can be involved, the most commonly affected are the knees, ankles, and elbows.[59] The mechanism is thought to be similar to other forms of reactive arthritis secondary to remote infection. Most cases resolve after satisfactory treatment of the TB. A reactive arthritis has been described following intravesicular instillation of bacille Calmette-Guérin (BCG) vaccine for bladder cancer.[60]

Other seldom encountered immune reaction patterns described with M. tuberculosis include erythema nodosum, erythema induratum, and amyloidosis (AA type).

DIAGNOSIS

Tuberculin Skin Test

The TST—also called the purified protein derivative (PPD)—has been in use for nearly a century and remains the most widely used screening test for TB. It is routinely administered in rheumatology offices that prescribe anti-TNF therapy. The test represents a crude mix of antigens from M. *tuberculosis* and is plagued by both false-positive and false-negative results. It is unable to distinguish latent infection from active disease and may be negative in the face of severe active TB. Corticosteroids (≥15 mg/day prednisone) may render the PPD negative in the face of latent TB. Elderly and malnourished patients may not exhibit a positive TST. Table 111-1 provides a partial list of causes of a false-negative TST that are of special interest to rheumatologists.

False-positive results may likewise occur in the case of infection with nontuberculous mycobacteria or previous BCG vaccine. PPD positivity degrades over time in BCG-vaccinated patients at a variable rate. The degree of positivity is influenced by a number of factors, including the number of BCG vaccinations and the number of subsequent PPD tests performed. Some patients may retain a response as long as 15 years after BCG vaccine. However, a PPD result of 20 mm or greater is rarely due to BCG. In addition, if faced with a high-risk situation, such as initiation of anti-TNF therapy, one probably should make a presumption of latent TB even if the diameter of induration measures as little as 5 mm.

The important message for rheumatologists is that the TST is an important but imperfect screening tool for latent TB infection, with sensitivity and specificity in the range of 70%. A negative TST should not eliminate the clinician's vigilance in monitoring patients who are being treated with anti-TNF therapy for reactivated or new-onset TB, especially in high-risk populations.

Imaging

Although imaging patterns suggestive of TB have been discussed, no pathognomonic skeletal radiographic features can establish the diagnosis. Early features on radiographs may be equivocal or nonexistent. Chest radiographs often are normal or fail to show features characteristic of TB.

Conventional radiography is generally a useful approach for defining bone destruction, extent of disease, and adjacent soft tissue lesions.[52] MRI is more effective in identifying early disease; it may help distinguish TB from other infections and neoplasms and can aid in evaluating the extent of disease.[9,61] Scintiscans with technetium and gallium may also be helpful in localizing bone and soft tissue lesions, but early false-negative findings are not uncommon.[62] CT can be helpful in guiding diagnostic needle biopsy. Fine-needle biopsy is an acceptable alternative to core-needle biopsy and open biopsy for the diagnosis of osteoarticular TB in both the axial and the peripheral skeleton, and it has the advantage of obviating general anesthesia.[63,64] Both CT and MRI may be helpful in monitoring therapy.[65]

Culture

Nearly all species of *Mycobacteria* are slow growing, with M. *tuberculosis* being the slowest. Other bacteria may rapidly outgrow mycobacteria if the specimen is not inoculated on special isolation media. The small number of mycobacteria found in clinically infected areas further challenges the ability to confirm mycobacterial infection and accounts for the low yield of positive Ziehl-Neelsen staining (10% to 20%) in synovial fluid and other biologic fluids.

Synovial fluid and other bodily fluids are less likely than tissue to yield a positive culture. If a joint is suspected of harboring TB, a synovial biopsy should be obtained. Arthroscopically derived tissue yields higher positive cultures than needle biopsies do. CT-guided needle aspiration and biopsy can provide invaluable information in the case of spinal involvement. Characteristic features on tissue pathology, including caseating and noncaseating granulomata, may allow an early presumptive diagnosis of TB pending culture results, which may take 4 to 6 weeks to be finalized.

Advanced Diagnostic Testing

Interferon-γ Release Assays

The limitations of the traditional PPD skin test in terms of specificity and sensitivity in identifying latent TB have led to the development of new T cell–based testing. These assays measure the production of interferon-γ by whole blood mononuclear cells stimulated by specific M. *tuberculosis* antigens. The interferon-γ release assays (IGRAs) have become a useful test for latent TB and have good sensitivity and specificity for latent TB infection.[66,67] These assays may prove particularly helpful in distinguishing TB from nontuberculous mycobacteria and in assessing patients who have had recent BCG vaccines. They also offer the opportunity to circumvent operator error with TST administration and do not require patients to return for a reading. IGRAs have replaced the TST in some centers for routine screening for latent TB infection.

The role of IGRAs in the diagnosis of latent TB infection in patients with immune-mediated inflammatory disorders before initiation of anti-TNF therapy remains unsettled.[68-73] The weight of evidence suggests that IGRAs are more sensitive and more specific than TSTs in this patient population. Indeterminate results from IGRAs in this setting have ranged from 1.2% to 28.6%, raising concerns about the performance of the assay from center to center.[74,75] Overall, agreement of IGRAs with the TST is poor owing to a lower proportion of positive TSTs. Positive IGRAs are more closely related to TB risk factors than are positive TSTs. Discordant IGRA-negative/TST-positive results are associated with prior BCG vaccination, and discordant IGRA-positive/TST-negative results are associated with corticosteroid therapy, suggesting that the former represents a false-positive TST and the latter represents a false-negative TST. Nevertheless, the meaning of a discordant result is uncertain enough that patients with a positive test result with IGRA or TST should be considered for therapy of possible latent TB infection.[76] Additional experience will be required to provide confidence that a negative IGRA in the setting of a positive TST reliably excludes latent TB infection. If only one testing modality is utilized, one recent analysis found that use of an IGRA was more cost effective than use of the TST for patients being screened before receiving anti-TNF therapy.[77]

IGRAs have also been studied in patients receiving anti-TNF therapy to identify previously undiagnosed ("hidden") latent TB infection or newly acquired TB infection. However, currently no guidelines are available for monitoring for tuberculosis infection in patients on anti-TNF therapy. Rates of TST conversion in patients on anti-TNF therapy have been reported to be 33% and 37% from centers in Korea and Taiwan; corresponding rates of IGRA conversion were 14% and 11%, respectively, and appeared to better correlate with the risk of active tuberculosis.[78,79] Pending formal guidelines, in regions where ongoing exposure to infectious tuberculosis may occur, routine monitoring of patients with TB on therapy—perhaps annually—is probably wise.

Nucleic Acid Amplification

Molecular diagnostics using nucleic acid amplification may be helpful in patients with low mycobacterial loads and may provide more rapid diagnosis. The presence of polymerase chain reaction (PCR) inhibitors, especially in extrapulmonary specimens, can lead to false-negative results. Despite more than a decade of experience, the role of nucleic acid amplification tests in diagnosing TB infection is still being defined. These assays must be interpreted with caution in extrapulmonary tissue specimens, and when the clinical suspicion of infection is low.[80-82] In a small cohort of patients with vertebral osteomyelitis, multiplex PCR testing of bone biopsy specimens demonstrated 90% sensitivity and 100% specificity for tuberculous infection, illustrating the potential for this technology to provide rapid and accurate diagnosis.[83]

TREATMENT

Appropriate management of tuberculous infection of bones and joints is a complex and evolving process. Proper selection of antibiotic regimens and ongoing disease monitoring should involve co-management with an infectious disease consultant. Nonetheless, rheumatologists should be familiar with the basic treatment principles.

Treatment of M. *tuberculosis* infections that involve the musculoskeletal system consists of the same combination chemotherapy regimens that are effective in pulmonary TB. Treatment regimens for infections of the bone and spine are longer than those recommended for lung disease and other extrapulmonary sites. The longer courses for musculoskeletal disease have been based on poor tissue penetration into osseous tissues and higher rates of relapse.

Current guidelines on the treatment of TB published jointly by the Centers for Disease Control and Prevention, the American Thoracic Society, and the Infectious Diseases Society of America recommend a 6-month course of therapy for all sites except the bone (6 to 9 months) and the central nervous system (9 to 12 months).[84] Rifampin is the critical component that allows shorter-course therapy.

The standard approach to TB therapy (both pulmonary and extrapulmonary) in the United States currently includes four drugs to start: isoniazid, rifampin, ethambutol, and pyrazinamide—known as IREZ therapy. Once the bacillus is confirmed to be sensitive to INH, ethambutol can be discontinued. Pyrazinamide is administered for 2 months, and rifampin and INH are continued for the duration of therapy.

Longer courses of therapy are required for patients who are slow to respond. Radiographic features of mycobacterial disease may not change much after 6 months of treatment, and response to treatment is based mainly on clinical features, including reduction in pain, resolution of constitutional symptoms, and emergence of increased mobility. Longer courses are advised for cases of relapse and for resistant organisms.

Surgical intervention is seldom indicated for the initial management of osteoarticular TB. Possible exceptions at presentation include patients with advanced or progressive disease or spinal kyphosis of 40 degrees or greater. Multidrug-resistant tuberculosis may also provide a relative indication for surgical débridement. Patients who have extensive joint destruction and immobility after an adequate course of chemotherapy may be candidates for surgery.

Following successful antibiotic therapy, arthroplasty of the hip and knee may be undertaken and is usually successful. Recurrence of disease in the prosthetic joint is less likely if the surgery is performed years after the infection, and if the tissue obtained at surgery is culture negative. This may be impractical, however, when a patient is unable to ambulate following an adequate course of therapy. In such cases, TB therapy is continued through surgery and for at least 3 months postoperatively. If TB recurs in the prosthetic joint, it can sometimes be managed with antibiotic therapy alone. However, in many cases, removal of the prosthesis is necessary for complete resolution of infection.

The increasing incidence of drug-resistant TB complicates the selection of appropriate drugs.[85,86] Primary monoresistance to isoniazid occurs in about 7% of TB isolates in the United States. When identified, this does not substantially impact the treatment outcome. Multidrug-resistant TB (MDR-TB) refers to isolates that are resistant to isoniazid and rifampin. The rate of MDR-TB in the United States has been relatively stable for the past decade, at less than 1%. In other parts of the world, MDR-TB rates may exceed 6% for new cases and 30% in previously treated individuals. The treatment of MDR-TB is complex and often requires the use of multiple (often toxic) second-line agents for 18 to 24 months or longer. XDR-TB—that is, strains resistant to all first-line TB drugs and to at least three second-line agents—has been reported in at least 17 countries, with particularly high rates in Kazakhstan, Iran, and South Africa.[87] Options for treatment of XDR-TB are very limited, and risks of treatment failure and death are high.[88]

Incomplete adherence to treatment is a particularly important risk factor for secondary drug resistance, and the likelihood of drug resistance increases following relapse after treatment. Directly observed therapy is strongly advocated to reduce the spread of infection and the frequency of drug-resistant TB.[89]

OSTEOARTICULAR INFECTIONS CAUSED BY NONTUBERCULOUS MYCOBACTERIA

Nontuberculous mycobacteria (NTM) are ubiquitous in the environment, including soil, water, and animal reservoirs. They are not typically spread from human to human, and infections with these organisms have been reported with increasing frequency.[90] Although a vast majority of infections caused by these organisms are pulmonary, skin and soft tissue infections may be seen in normal hosts; children may develop a localized lymphadenitis.[91] Osteoarticular infections are usually caused by direct inoculation of the organism or by spread of contiguous infection.[91] Blunt trauma has been implicated as a risk factor in cases of vertebral osteomyelitis due to NTM.[92] Immunosuppressed hosts may develop nontuberculous mycobacterial infections of the musculoskeletal system, but these infections are much less common than TB. In contrast to TB, nontuberculous infection is more likely to cause tenosynovitis, synovitis, or osteomyelitis and is less likely to cause spinal infection. A review identified only 31 cases of vertebral osteomyelitis due to NTM reported between 1965 and 2003.[93] Although more than 120 species of nontuberculous mycobacteria are known, most musculoskeletal infections are caused by *Mycobacterium marinum*, *Mycobacterium kansasii*, and *Mycobacterium avium-intracellulare* (also called M. *avium* complex, or MAC), but cases of musculoskeletal infection with *Mycobacterium haemophilum*, *Mycobacterium chelonae*, and *Mycobacterium xenopi* have also been reported.[94-97]

Three distinct patterns of musculoskeletal involvement have been reported: tenosynovitis, synovitis, and osteomyelitis.[98,99] Tenosynovitis typically presents as chronic unilateral hand and wrist swelling (Figure 116A-C).[100] Synovitis typically presents as chronic indolent asymmetric swelling in a knee, hand, or wrist. A number of species have been associated with these syndromes, and the number isolated from immunosuppressed patients is growing.[10] Predisposing factors, in addition to immunosuppression and direct inoculation, include environmental exposure and pre-existing joint disease.[101]

Musculoskeletal infections with atypical mycobacteria may be indistinguishable from M. *tuberculosis* infections, so that correct diagnosis usually requires tissue biopsy and culture. Synovial fluid, when attainable, is typically inflammatory, and a culture may be helpful only if specific mycobacterial cultures are requested. Identification of acid-fast bacilli on smear and granulomatous inflammation from a tissue biopsy specimen often provides direction for an appropriate microbiologic investigation, but histologic features do not consistently demonstrate granuloma formation. With a compatible clinical presentation and histologic findings, mycobacterial culture, including special techniques for M. *marinum*, should be requested. Direct amplification testing may be useful for more rapid identification of mycobacterial species in tissue specimens, but data from musculoskeletal cases are limited.[81,102] In addition to mycobacteria, causes of granulomatous synovitis include fungi, brucellosis, sarcoidosis, inflammatory bowel disease, and nonmetallic foreign bodies. *Mycobacteria* other than M. *tuberculosis* are responsible for a significant proportion of these cases.[103]

MAC has become the most common mycobacterial infectious agent affecting patients with HIV/AIDS, in

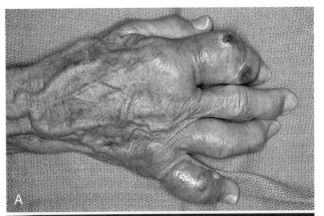

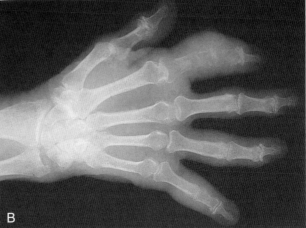

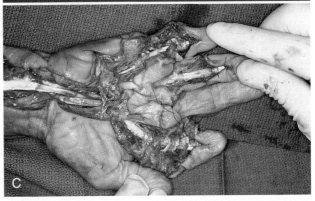

Figure 111-6 A, Hand demonstrating tenosynovitis and synovitis secondary to *Mycobacterium marinum*. **B,** Radiograph of the hand in **A** demonstrates joint destruction secondary to M. *marinum*. **C,** Hand depicted in **A** and **B** shows extensive tenosynovitis at the time of synovectomy.

whom it has a tendency to cause disseminated disease.[10] Fortunately, a sharp decline in the incidence of MAC has been noted following the introduction of effective antiretroviral therapy and MAC prophylaxis.

Isolation of M. *tuberculosis* is always clinically significant. In contrast, when dealing with a nontuberculous mycobacterial isolate, the clinician must judge whether it is a contaminant, represents insignificant colonization, or is the cause of disease. Certain guidelines have proved useful in this respect[43,101,104,105]:

- The illness should be consistent with one or more syndromes associated with mycobacterial infection.

- Other causes of disease, such as TB and fungal infection, should be excluded.
- The mycobacterial species isolated is one associated with human disease, the most significant being those that are not common environmental contaminants (M. kansasii, M. marinum, M. simiae, M. szulgai, and M. ulcerans).
- The site of isolation of the organism should favor true infection over contamination or colonization. (Isolation from bone biopsy, synovial tissue, or synovial fluid strongly suggests infection; isolation from the respiratory tract may represent infection or colonization.)
- Heavier growth suggests significant infection.
- Repeatedly positive cultures suggest significant infection.

Because laboratory identification of the organism and sensitivity testing may take weeks to months, initial therapy often includes multiple drugs to cover both TB and other mycobacteria. One common approach to initial empiric therapy is to link standard IREZ therapy for TB with clarithromycin until final culture results are available. The most recent American Thoracic Society guidelines for the treatment of nontuberculous mycobacteria were published in 2007.[106] Surgical débridement of infected tissue may play an important role in the treatment of selected patients, especially for resistant organisms. The most efficacious drugs remain controversial, prolonged treatment is often necessary, and relapses are not uncommon. As with TB, therapy customized to the individual patient is crucial with nontuberculous mycobacterial infection. The key to effective therapy lies in the unique characteristics of the culture and in the sensitivity of the particular isolate.

EMERGENCE OF NONTUBERCULOUS MYCOBACTERIAL INFECTION DURING THE TREATMENT OF RHEUMATIC DISEASE

No published data exist on the risk of nontuberculous mycobacterial infection in the setting of therapy with nonbiologic disease-modifying antirheumatic drugs, including methotrexate. The decision to interrupt or continue therapy in such instances should be made on a case-by-case basis and should involve an infectious disease specialist, with recognition that alternative treatments, such as steroids and biologics, may carry an even greater risk.

Nontuberculous mycobacteria are increasingly recognized as important pathogens in patients receiving anti-TNF therapy. Indeed, these infections now occur twice as frequently as TB in the United States, presumably because of the use of screening tests for the latter.[107] The complexity of these infections was illustrated by a recent review of 239 cases of nontuberculous mycobacterial infection reported to the MedWatch database, in which only 105 were established to be probable or confirmed according to established disease criteria.[108] The most commonly reported presentation was seen in elderly women with rheumatoid arthritis (RA), possibly because both nontuberculous mycobacterial infection and RA are common in this group; most patients were also taking concomitant steroids and/or methotrexate. Infections with several different species within this group

have been reported, with MAC being the most common. As with TB, the risk appears to be associated with all drugs in the class, rather than with a specific agent, although more infections have been reported with infliximab.[108] Extrapulmonary disease is a common finding and is unusual for these organisms. A paradoxical response to therapy, similar to that seen with TB, has been reported with treatment of MAC following infliximab.[109] Although cessation of anti-TNF therapy is appropriate following the development of an atypical mycobacterial infection, the safe reintroduction of etanercept during treatment of M. marinum has been reported.[110]

Managing the risk of nontuberculous mycobacterial infection in the setting of anti-TNF therapy can be challenging. Although screening has been helpful in reducing the risk of TB infection in this setting, no method of screening for atypical mycobacteria is currently available. Because these infections are more common in individuals with pre-existing pulmonary disease, clinicians may wish to consider more extensive evaluation of RA patients with bronchiectasis about to initiate anti-TNF therapy. Although MAC prophylaxis is recommended for HIV-positive patients with CD4 counts of 50 or lower, no experience with and no guidelines for such prophylaxis with anti-TNF therapy have been put forth. The complex nature of these infections has been further demonstrated by a case of M. marinum mimicking RA, with synovitis and subcutaneous nodules developing during infliximab therapy.[111]

References

1. Shafer RW, Kim DS, Weiss JP, Quale JM: Extrapulmonary tuberculosis in patients with human immunodeficiency virus infection, *Medicine* 70:384–397, 1991.
2. Havlir DV, Barnes PF: Tuberculosis in patients with human immunodeficiency virus infection, *N Engl J Med* 340:367–373, 1999.
3. Jellis JE: Human immunodeficiency virus and osteoarticular tuberculosis, *Clin Orthop Relat Res* 398:27–31, 2002.
4. Global Tuberculosis Control: *Surveillance, planning, financing, WHO report WHO/HTM/TB/2007.376*, Geneva, 2007, World Health Organization.
5. Bloom BR: Tuberculosis—the global view, *N Engl J Med* 346:1434–1435, 2002.
6. Gandhi NR, Moll A, Sturm AW, et al: Extensively drug-resistant tuberculosis as a cause of death in patients co-infected with tuberculosis and HIV in a rural area of South Africa, *Lancet* 368:1575–1580, 2006.
7. Franco-Paredes C, Diaz-Borjon A, Senger MA, et al: The ever-expanding association between rheumatologic diseases and tuberculosis, *Am J Med* 119:470–477, 2006.
8. Griffith JF, Kumta SM, Leung PC, et al: Imaging of musculoskeletal tuberculosis: a new look at an old disease, *Clin Orthop Relat Res* 398:32–39, 2002.
9. Moore SL, Rafii M: Imaging of musculoskeletal and spinal tuberculosis, *Radiol Clin North Am* 39:329–342, 2001.
10. Mycobacterioses and the acquired immunodeficiency syndrome: joint position paper of the American Thoracic Society and the Centers for Disease Control, *Am Rev Respir Dis* 136:492–496, 1987.
11. Lafond EM: An analysis of adult skeletal tuberculosis, *J Bone Joint Surg Am* 40:346–364, 1958.
12. Abdelwahab IF, Kenan S, Hermann G, Klein MJ: Tuberculous gluteal abscess without bone involvement, *Skeletal Radiol* 27:36–39, 1998.
13. Ashworth MJ, Meadows TH: Isolated tuberculosis of a skeletal muscle, *J Hand Surg Br* 17:235, 1992.
14. George JC, Buckwalter KA, Braunstein EM: Case report 824: tuberculosis presenting as a soft tissue forearm mass in a patient with a negative tuberculin skin test, *Skeletal Radiol* 23:79–81, 1994.
15. Hasan N, Baithun S, Swash M, Wagg A: Tuberculosis of striated muscle, *Muscle Nerve* 16:984–985, 1993.

16. Indudhara R, Singh SK, Minz M, et al: Tuberculous pyomyositis in a renal transplant recipient, *Tuber Lung Dis* 73:239–241, 1992.
17. Albornoz MA, Mezgarzedeh M, Neumann CH, Myers AR: Granulomatous tenosynovitis: a rare musculoskeletal manifestation of tuberculosis, *Clin Rheumatol* 17:166–169, 1998.
18. Chen WS: Tuberculosis of the fascia lata, *Clin Rheumatol* 17:77–78, 1998.
19. King AD, Griffith J, Rushton A, Metreweli C: Tuberculosis of the greater trochanter and the trochanteric bursa, *J Rheumatol* 25:391–393, 1998.
20. Alvarez S, McCabe WR: Extrapulmonary tuberculosis revisited: a review of experience at Boston City and other hospitals, *Medicine (Baltimore)* 63:25–55, 1984.
21. el-Shahawy MA, Gadallah MF, Campese VM: Tuberculosis of the spine (Pott's disease) in patients with end-stage renal disease, *Am J Nephrol* 14:55–59, 1994.
22. Jacobs P: Osteo-articular tuberculosis in coloured immigrants: a radiological study, *Clin Radiol* 15:59–69, 1964.
23. Gorse GJ, Pais MJ, Kusske JA, Cesario TC: Tuberculous spondylitis: a report of six cases and a review of the literature, *Medicine (Baltimore)* 62:178–193, 1983.
24. Chapman M, Murray RO, Stoker DJ: Tuberculosis of the bones and joints, *Semin Roentgenol* 14:266–282, 1979.
25. Colmenero JD, Jimenez-Mejias ME, Sanchez-Lora FJ, et al: Pyogenic, tuberculous, and brucellar vertebral osteomyelitis: a descriptive and comparative study of 219 cases, *Ann Rheum Dis* 56:709–715, 1997.
26. Cantini F, Salvarani C, Olivieri I, et al: Tuberculous spondylitis as a cause of inflammatory spinal pain: a report of 4 cases, *Clin Exp Rheumatol* 16:305–308, 1998.
27. Slater RR Jr, Beale RW, Bullitt E: Pott's disease of the cervical spine, *South Med J* 84:521–523, 1991.
28. Bhojraj SY, Shetty N, Shah PJ: Tuberculosis of the craniocervical junction, *J Bone Joint Surg Br* 83:222–225, 2001.
29. Krishnan A, Patkar D, Patankar T, et al: Craniovertebral junction tuberculosis: a review of 29 cases, *J Comput Assist Tomogr* 25:171–176, 2001.
30. Pouchot J, Vinceneux P, Barge J, et al: Tuberculosis of the sacroiliac joint: clinical features, outcome, and evaluation of closed needle biopsy in 11 consecutive cases, *Am J Med* 84(3 Pt 2):622–628, 1988.
31. Pande KC, Babhulkar SS: Atypical spinal tuberculosis, *Clin Orthop Relat Res* 398:67–74, 2002.
32. Tsay MH, Chen MC, Jaung GY, et al: Atypical skeletal tuberculosis mimicking tumor metastases: report of a case, *J Formos Med Assoc* 94:428–431, 1995.
33. Shih HN, Hsu RW, Lin TY: Tuberculosis of the long bone in children, *Clin Orthop Relat Res* 335:246–252, 1997.
34. Babhulkar SS, Pande SK: Unusual manifestations of osteoarticular tuberculosis, *Clin Orthop Relat Res* 398:114–120, 2002.
35. Muradali D, Gold WL, Vellend H, Becker E: Multifocal osteoarticular tuberculosis: report of four cases and review of management, *Clin Infect Dis* 17:204–209, 1993.
36. Coppola J, Muller NL, Connell DG: Computed tomography of musculoskeletal tuberculosis, *Can Assoc Radiol J* 38:199–203, 1987.
37. Martini M, Adjrad A, Boudjemaa A: Tuberculous osteomyelitis: a review of 125 cases, *Int Orthop* 10:201–207, 1986.
38. Ruiz G, Garcia Rodriguez J, Guerri ML, Gonzalez A: Osteoarticular tuberculosis in a general hospital during the last decade, *Clin Microbiol Infect* 9:919–923, 2003.
39. Babhulkar S, Pande S: Tuberculosis of the hip, *Clin Orthop Relat Res* 398:93–99, 2002.
40. Hoffman EB, Allin J, Campbell JA, Leisegang FM: Tuberculosis of the knee, *Clin Orthop Relat Res* 398:100–106, 2002.
41. Khater FJ, Samnani IQ, Mehta JB, et al: Prosthetic joint infection by *Mycobacterium tuberculosis*: an unusual case report with literature review, *South Med J* 100:66–69, 2007.
42. Evanchick CC, Davis DE, Harrington TM: Tuberculosis of peripheral joints: an often missed diagnosis, *J Rheumatol* 13:187–189, 1986.
43. Wallace R, Cohen AS: Tuberculous arthritis: a report of two cases with review of biopsy and synovial fluid findings, *Am J Med* 61:277–282, 1976.
44. Jacobs JC, Li SC, Ruzal-Shapiro C, et al: Tuberculous arthritis in children: diagnosis by needle biopsy of the synovium, *Clin Pediatr* 33:344–348, 1994.
45. Davidson PT, Horowitz I: Skeletal tuberculosis: a review with patient presentations and discussion, *Am J Med* 48:77–84, 1970.
46. Mateo Soria L, Miquel Nolla Sole J, Rozadilla Sacanell A, et al: Infectious arthritis in patients with rheumatoid arthritis, *Ann Rheum Dis* 51:402–403, 1992.
47. Wolfe F, Michaud K, Anderson J, Urbansky K: Tuberculosis infection in patients with rheumatoid arthritis and the effect of infliximab therapy, *Arthritis Rheum* 50:372–379, 2004.
48. Carmona L, Hernandez-Garcia C, Vadillo C, et al: Increased risk of tuberculosis in patients with rheumatoid arthritis, *J Rheumatol* 30:1436–1439, 2003.
49. Gomez-Reino JJ, Carmona L, Valverde VR, et al: Treatment of rheumatoid arthritis with tumor necrosis factor inhibitors may predispose to significant increase in tuberculosis risk: a multicenter active-surveillance report, *Arthritis Rheum* 48:2122–2127, 2003.
50. Mohan AK, Cote TR, Block JA, et al: Tuberculosis following the use of etanercept, a tumor necrosis factor inhibitor, *Clin Infect Dis* 39:295–299, 2004.
51. Dixon WG, Hyrich KL, Watson KD, et al: Drug-specific risk of tuberculosis in patients with rheumatoid arthritis treated with anti-TNF therapy: results from the British Society for Rheumatology Biologics Register (BSRBR), *Ann Rheum Dis* 69:522–528, 2010.
52. Tubach F, Salmon D, Ravaud P, et al: Risk of tuberculosis is higher with anti-tumor necrosis factor monoclonal antibody therapy than with soluble tumor necrosis factor receptor therapy: the three-year prospective French Research Axed on Tolerance of Biotherapies registry, *Arthritis Rheum* 60:1884–1894, 2009.
53. Bigbee CL, Gonchoroff DG, Vratsanos G, et al: Abatacept treatment does not exacerbate chronic *Mycobacterium tuberculosis* infection in mice, *Arthritis Rheum* 56:2557–2565, 2007.
54. Jick SS, Lieberman ES, Rahman MU, Choi HK: Glucocorticoid use, other associated factors, and the risk of tuberculosis, *Arthritis Rheum* 55:19–26, 2006.
55. Carmona L, Gomez-Reino JJ, Rodriguez-Valverde V, et al: Effectiveness of recommendations to prevent reactivation of latent tuberculosis infection in patients treated with tumor necrosis factor antagonists, *Arthritis Rheum* 52:1766–1772, 2005.
56. Gomez-Reino JJ, Carmona L, Angel Descalzo M: Risk of tuberculosis in patients treated with tumor necrosis factor antagonists due to incomplete prevention of reactivation of latent infection, *Arthritis Rheum* 57:756–761, 2007.
57. Aggarwal R, Manadan AM, Poliyedath A, et al: Safety of etanercept in patients at high risk for mycobacterial tuberculosis infections, *J Rheumatol* 36:914–917, 2009.
58. Garcia Vidal C, Rodriguez Fernandez S, Martinez Lacasa J, et al: Paradoxical response to antituberculous therapy in infliximab-treated patients with disseminated tuberculosis, *Clin Infect Dis* 40:756–759, 2005.
59. Dall L, Long L, Stanford J: Poncet's disease: tuberculous rheumatism, *Rev Infect Dis* 11:105–107, 1989.
60. Pancaldi P, Van Linthoudt D, Alborino D, et al: Reiter's syndrome after intravesical bacillus Calmette-Guerin treatment for superficial bladder carcinoma, *Br J Rheumatol* 32:1096–1098, 1993.
61. Gupta RK, Gupta S, Kumar S, et al: MRI in intraspinal tuberculosis, *Neuroradiology* 36:39–43, 1994.
62. Lifeso RM, Weaver P, Harder EH: Tuberculous spondylitis in adults, *J Bone Joint Surg Am* 67:1405–1413, 1985.
63. Masood S: Diagnosis of tuberculosis of bone and soft tissue by fine-needle aspiration biopsy, *Diagn Cytopathol* 8:451–455, 1982.
64. Mondal A: Cytological diagnosis of vertebral tuberculosis with fine-needle aspiration biopsy, *J Bone Joint Surg Am* 76:181–184, 1994.
65. Omari B, Robertson JM, Nelson RJ, Chiu LC: Pott's disease: a resurgent challenge to the thoracic surgeon, *Chest* 95:145–150, 1989.
66. Updated guidelines for using interferon gamma release assays to detect *Mycobacterium tuberculosis* infection—United States, 2010, *MMWR Morb Mortal Wkly Rep* 59:1–24, 2010.
67. Menzies D, Pai M, Comstock G: Meta-analysis: new tests for the diagnosis of latent tuberculosis infection: areas of uncertainty and recommendations for research, *Ann Intern Med* 146:340–354, 2007.
68. Bocchino M, Matarese A, Bellofiore B, et al: Performance of two commercial blood IFN-gamma release assays for the detection of *Mycobacterium tuberculosis* infection in patient candidates for anti-TNF-alpha treatment, *Eur J Clin Microbiol Infect Dis* 27:907–913, 2008.
69. Dinser R, Fousse M, Sester U, et al: Evaluation of latent tuberculosis infection in patients with inflammatory arthropathies before treatment with TNF-alpha blocking drugs using a novel flow-cytometric

interferon-gamma release assay, *Rheumatology (Oxford)* 47:212–218, 2008.

70. Greenberg JD, Reddy SM, Schloss SG, et al: Comparison of an in vitro tuberculosis interferon-gamma assay with delayed-type hypersensitivity testing for detection of latent *Mycobacterium tuberculosis:* a pilot study in rheumatoid arthritis, *J Rheumatol* 35:770–775, 2008.

71. Hanta I, Ozbek S, Kuleci S, Kocabas A: The evaluation of latent tuberculosis in rheumatologic diseases for anti-TNF therapy: experience with 192 patients, *Clin Rheumatol* 27:1083–1086, 2008.

72. Murakami S, Takeno M, Kirino Y, et al: Screening of tuberculosis by interferon-gamma assay before biologic therapy for rheumatoid arthritis, *Tuberculosis* 89:136–141, 2009.

73. Ponce de Leon D, Acevedo-Vasquez E, Alvizuri S, et al: Comparison of an interferon-gamma assay with tuberculin skin testing for detection of tuberculosis (TB) infection in patients with rheumatoid arthritis in a TB-endemic population, *J Rheumatol* 35:776–781, 2008.

74. Bartalesi F, Vicidomini S, Goletti D, et al: QuantiFERON-TB Gold and the TST are both useful for latent tuberculosis infection screening in autoimmune diseases, *Eur Respir J* 33:586–593, 2009.

75. Shovman O, Anouk M, Vinnitsky N, et al: QuantiFERON-TB Gold in the identification of latent tuberculosis infection in rheumatoid arthritis: a pilot study, *Int J Tuberc Lung Dis* 13:1427–1432, 2009.

76. Lalvani A, Millington KA: Screening for tuberculosis infection prior to initiation of anti-TNF therapy, *Autoimmun Rev* 8:147–152, 2008.

77. Kowada A: Cost effectiveness of interferon-gamma release assay for tuberculosis screening of rheumatoid arthritis patients prior to initiation of tumor necrosis factor-α antagonist therapy, *Mol Diagn Ther* 14:367–373, 2010.

78. Chen DY, Shen GH, Hsieh TY, et al: Effectiveness of the combination of a whole-blood interferon-gamma assay and the tuberculin skin test in detecting latent tuberculosis infection in rheumatoid arthritis patients receiving adalimumab therapy, *Arthritis Rheum* 59:800–806, 2008.

79. Park JH, Seo GY, Lee JS, et al: Positive conversion of tuberculin skin test and performance of interferon release assay to detect hidden tuberculosis infection during anti-tumor necrosis factor agent trial, *J Rheumatol* 36:2158–2163, 2009.

80. Catanzaro A, Perry S, Clarridge JE, et al: The role of clinical suspicion in evaluating a new diagnostic test for active tuberculosis: results of a multicenter prospective trial, *JAMA* 283:639–645, 2000.

81. Harrington JT: The evolving role of direct amplification tests in diagnosing osteoarticular infections caused by mycobacteria and fungi, *Curr Opin Rheumatol* 11:289–292, 1999.

82. Woods GL: Molecular techniques in mycobacterial detection, *Arch Pathol Lab Med* 125:122–126, 2001.

83. Colmenero JD, Morata P, Ruiz-Mesa JD, et al: Multiplex real-time polymerase chain reaction: a practical approach for rapid diagnosis of tuberculous and brucellar vertebral osteomyelitis, *Spine* 35:E1392–E1396, 2010.

84. Recommendations for the treatment of tuberculosis, *MMWR Morb Mortal Wkly Rep* 52:1–77, 2003.

85. Bradford WZ, Daley CL: Multiple drug-resistant tuberculosis, *Infect Dis Clin North Am* 12:157–172, 1998.

86. Parsons LM, Driscoll JR, Taber HW, Salfinger M: Drug resistance in tuberculosis, *Infect Dis Clin North Am* 11:905–928, 1997.

87. Raviglione MC, Smith IM: XDR tuberculosis—implications for global public health, *N Engl J Med* 356:656–659, 2007.

88. Mitnick C, Bayona J, Palacios E, et al: Community-based therapy for multidrug-resistant tuberculosis in Lima, Peru, *N Engl J Med* 348:119–128, 2003.

89. Chaulk CP, Kazandjian VA: Directly observed therapy for treatment completion of pulmonary tuberculosis: consensus statement of the Public Health Tuberculosis Guidelines Panel, *JAMA* 279:943–948, 1998.

90. Lai CC, Tan CK, Chou CH, et al: Increasing incidence of nontuberculous mycobacteria, Taiwan, 2000-2008, *Emerg Infect Dis* 16:294–296, 2010.

91. Piersimoni C, Scarparo C: Extrapulmonary infections associated with nontuberculous mycobacteria in immunocompetent persons, *Emerg Infect Dis* 15:1351–1358, quiz 1544, 2009.

92. Chan ED, Kong PM, Fennelly K, et al: Vertebral osteomyelitis due to infection with nontuberculous *Mycobacterium* species after blunt trauma to the back: 3 examples of the principle of locus minoris resistentiae, *Clin Infect Dis* 32:1506–1510, 2001.

93. Petitjean G, Fluckiger U, Scharen S, Laifer G: Vertebral osteomyelitis caused by non-tuberculous mycobacteria, *Clin Microbiol Infect* 10:951–953, 2004.

94. Plemmons RM, McAllister CK, Garces MC, Ward RL: Osteomyelitis due to *Mycobacterium haemophilum* in a cardiac transplant patient: case report and analysis of interactions among clarithromycin, rifampin, and cyclosporine, *Clin Infect Dis* 24:995–997, 1997.

95. Rahman I, Bhatt H, Chillag S, Duffus W: *Mycobacterium chelonae* vertebral osteomyelitis, *South Med J* 102:1167–1169, 2009.

96. Salliot C, Desplaces N, Boisrenoult P, et al: Arthritis due to *Mycobacterium xenopi:* a retrospective study of 7 cases in France, *Clin Infect Dis* 43:987–993, 2006.

97. Wallace RJ Jr, Brown BA, Onyi GO: Skin, soft tissue, and bone infections due to *Mycobacterium chelonae chelonae:* importance of prior corticosteroid therapy, frequency of disseminated infections, and resistance to oral antimicrobials other than clarithromycin, *J Infect Dis* 166:405–412, 1992.

98. Kelly PJ, Karlson AG, Weed LA, Lipscomb PR: Infection of synovial tissues by mycobacteria other than *Mycobacterium tuberculosis, J Bone Joint Surg Am* 49:1521–1530, 1967.

99. Marchevsky AM, Damsker B, Green S, Tepper S: The clinicopathological spectrum of non-tuberculous mycobacterial osteoarticular infections, *J Bone Joint Surg Am* 67:925–929, 1985.

100. Zenone T, Boibieux A, Tigaud S, et al: Non-tuberculous mycobacterial tenosynovitis: a review, *Scand J Infect Dis* 31:221–228, 1999.

101. Glickstein SL, Nashel DJ: *Mycobacterium kansasii* septic arthritis complicating rheumatic disease: case report and review of the literature, *Semin Arthritis Rheum* 16:231–235, 1987.

102. Weigl JA, Haas WH: Postoperative *Mycobacterium avium* osteomyelitis confirmed by polymerase chain reaction, *Eur J Pediatr* 159:64–69, 2000.

103. Sutker WL, Lankford LL, Tompsett R: Granulomatous synovitis: the role of atypical mycobacteria, *Rev Infect Dis* 1:729–735, 1979.

104. Ahn CH, McLarty JW, Ahn SS, et al: Diagnostic criteria for pulmonary disease caused by *Mycobacterium kansasii* and *Mycobacterium intracellulare, Am Rev Respir Dis* 125:388–391, 1982.

105. Wolinsky E: When is an infection disease? *Rev Infect Dis* 3:1025–1027, 1981.

106. Griffith DE, Aksamit T, Brown-Elliott BA, et al: An official ATS/IDSA statement: diagnosis, treatment, and prevention of nontuberculous mycobacterial diseases, *Am J Respir Crit Care Med* 175:367–416, 2007.

107. Winthrop KL, Yamashita S, Beekmann SE, Polgreen PM: Mycobacterial and other serious infections in patients receiving anti-tumor necrosis factor and other newly approved biologic therapies: case finding through the Emerging Infections Network, *Clin Infect Dis* 46:1738–1740, 2008.

108. Winthrop KL, Chang E, Yamashita S, et al: Nontuberculous mycobacteria infections and anti-tumor necrosis factor-alpha therapy, *Emerg Infect Dis* 15:1556–1561, 2009.

109. Salvana EM, Cooper GS, Salata RA: Mycobacterium other than tuberculosis (MOTT) infection: an emerging disease in infliximab-treated patients, *J Infect* 55:484–487, 2007.

110. Dare JA, Jahan S, Hiatt K, Torralba KD: Reintroduction of etanercept during treatment of cutaneous *Mycobacterium marinum* infection in a patient with ankylosing spondylitis, *Arthritis Rheum* 61:583–586, 2009.

111. Lam A, Toma W, Schlesinger N: *Mycobacterium marinum* arthritis mimicking rheumatoid arthritis, *J Rheumatol* 33:817–819, 2006.

The references for this chapter can also be found on www.expertconsult.com.

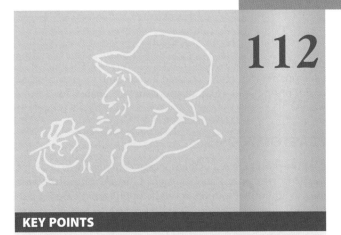

112 Fungal Infections of Bones and Joints

ERIC M. RUDERMAN • JOHN P. FLAHERTY

KEY POINTS

Fungi are an infrequent but clinically important cause of bone and joint infections.

These infections are often indolent in onset and may masquerade as other disorders.

Travel and immigration have affected the geographic localization of several important fungal infections, which may be seen in nonendemic areas.

Although diagnosis may be assisted by clinical presentation and serologic testing, examination and culture of infected tissue are critical.

New antifungal therapies have broadened the effective options, but choice of drugs, duration of treatment, and combined surgical débridement must be carefully considered to achieve optimal outcomes.

Immunocompromise including antirheumatic biologic therapies predisposes to fungal infections, often resulting in more acute and widely disseminated disease.

Screening and/or prophylactic therapy have not proven useful for patients on immunosuppressive therapy, so a high index of suspicion should be maintained when such patients present with an acute febrile illness.

Fungal infection is a relatively infrequent but important cause of osteomyelitis and arthritis. Fungal diseases that commonly cause osteomyelitis include coccidioidomycosis, blastomycosis, cryptococcosis, candidiasis, and sporotrichosis (Table 112-1). Fungal arthritis is less common and is most often associated with sporotrichosis, cryptococcosis, coccidioidomycosis, blastomycosis, candidiasis, and, occasionally, other species. The epidemiology of these fungal infections, their musculoskeletal presentations, and their treatment are considered in this chapter.

The epidemiology and clinical features of individual deep mycoses may suggest the diagnosis in some cases, but their indolent presentation, which often resembles that of other noninfectious diseases, may be misleading. Travel and immigration have blurred their geographic localization. Infection may be acute and overwhelming in immunocompromised patients, for whom disseminated fungal infections are a major risk. Anticytokine and other immunosuppressive treatments for rheumatic diseases, particularly those targeting tumor necrosis factor (TNF), are associated with disseminated fungal infection,[1,2] as are acquired immunodeficiency syndrome (AIDS), pregnancy, and treatments for transplantation and malignancies,[3] in some cases. For rheumatologists, disseminated fungal infections are an important diagnostic consideration in some patients and must be considered before starting biologic treatments in those at risk; they may also complicate the clinical course of other arthritides. The presentation of fungal infections as a consequence of rheumatic disease therapy will also be considered in this chapter.

Fungal infections are generally diagnosed by histologic examination or culture of involved tissues. Improved biopsy techniques may assist the diagnosis, provided the possibility of fungal infection is considered and proper studies are requested. Synovial fluid leukocyte counts and culture results vary among fungal infections and in individual cases and may be misleading. Serologic testing may also assist in diagnosing and staging several fungal infections. Detecting fungal antigens and DNA in blood and tissue is now possible in some cases, but the clinical use of these methods is still under investigation.[4]

COCCIDIOIDOMYCOSIS

The soil fungi *Coccidioides immitis* and *Coccidioides posadasii* generally cause a primary respiratory illness after spores are inhaled. A self-limited acute pneumonia may result, associated with systemic manifestations such as arthralgia and erythema nodosum (valley fever), but infection is often unapparent and only infrequently becomes chronic or disseminated.[5] Coccidioidomycosis is endemic to the southwestern United States and areas of Central and South America, but cases are increasingly diagnosed in nonendemic areas because of travel, infection from fomites, and reactivation of remote infection. Cases increase when soil is disturbed and in windy conditions. Direct human-to-human transmission is rare. Extrapulmonary infection is almost always caused by hematogenous spread from an initial pulmonary focus. The bones and joints are frequent sites of dissemination, particularly in immunocompromised hosts.

Septic arthritis of the knee is common, generally arising from direct infection of the synovium. Other joint infections are caused by spread from a contiguous osteomyelitis involving the vertebrae, wrists, hands, ankles, feet, pelvis, and long bones.[6] The onset is characterized by gradually increasing pain and joint stiffness, with little swelling but early radiographic changes. In one series, arthritis was the only manifestation of disseminated coccidioidomycosis in 51 of 57 patients and was an aspect of more generalized disease in the remaining 6 patients.[7]

Diagnostic confusion is common in osteoarticular coccidioidomycosis because of the delayed dissemination (months to years) after primary infection and because of atypical clinical presentations. The criteria for diagnosis

Table 112-1 Disseminated Fungal Infections Reported with Tumor Necrosis Factor Antagonist Therapy

Organism	References
Aspergillosis	1, 49, 101
Candidiasis	1
Coccidioidomycosis	99, 100
Cryptococcosis	29, 102
Histoplasmosis	69, 72
Pneumocystosis	110, 119
Scedosporiosis	103
Sporotrichosis	49

include compatible clinical features, serologic studies, histologic examination, and culture. Early infections, often before systemic spread, are associated with a positive antibody precipitin test that detects immunoglobulin (Ig) M antibody. Complement fixation serologic values detecting IgG antibodies are in a range indicative of disseminated disease in a majority of patients and show a significant decrease with effective treatment. Serologic testing for *Coccidioides* may have negative results early in the infection and in immunosuppressed patients. A specific enzyme immunoassay (EIA) to *Coccidioides* galactomannan antigen in urine has shown promise in the diagnosis of severe coccidioidomycosis infection.[8,9] The definitive diagnosis is most commonly made by the demonstration of granulomatous synovitis and typical spherules in a biopsy specimen, confirmed in some cases by positive culture and direct amplification testing. Synovial fluid, when obtainable, does not necessarily demonstrate septic leukocyte counts and may have a lymphocyte predominance. Synovial fluid is rarely culture positive; culture of synovial tissue may be more helpful. Radioisotope bone scans may be helpful to identify areas of infection.[10]

With early diagnosis of effusive synovitis, antifungal treatment alone is appropriate. Treatment is usually initiated with oral azole antifungal agents, most commonly fluconazole or itraconazole.[11] Amphotericin B is recommended for alternative therapy, especially if lesions are appearing to worsen rapidly and are in particularly critical locations such as in vertebral osteomyelitis. Lipid formulations of amphotericin B have demonstrated less nephrotoxicity and infusion-related side effects than conventional deoxycholate amphotericin B and may be given at doses higher than those tolerated with conventional amphotericin, but they have never been formally studied in clinical trials. With more widely disseminated infection or involvement of critical areas such as the spine, as well as in high-risk hosts, the choice and duration of treatments are often complicated. Factors that favor surgical intervention are large size of abscesses, progressive enlargement of abscesses or destructive lesions, presence of bony sequestrations, instability of the spine, or impingement on critical organs or tissues (e.g., epidural abscess compressing the spinal cord).[7,12,13] Newer antifungal agents such as voriconazole and posaconazole show promise as alternative therapy.[11,14-16] Long-term prophylaxis with fluconazole can limit the risk for reactivation in immunosuppressed patients.

Coccidioidal synovitis may also occur as a consequence of immune complex–mediated inflammation, a presentation that may complicate either primary pulmonary or disseminated disease and is typically polyarticular. It is accompanied by fever, erythema nodosum or multiforme, eosinophilia, and hilar adenopathy. It abates in 2 to 4 weeks.[5,17]

BLASTOMYCOSIS

Blastomycosis, caused by *Blastomyces dermatitidis*, is endemic in the north-central and southern United States. Infection most commonly produces sporadic or clustered cases of pulmonary disease and is induced by exposure to soil or dust containing decomposed wood and, presumably, contaminated with the organism.[18] Affected individuals do not appear to have any distinguishing or predisposing characteristics except for exposure to the organism during work or recreation. Clinical presentation includes high fever and other constitutional symptoms, pulmonary and skin involvement, and a significant mortality rate; leukocytosis and an elevated sedimentation rate are frequently seen.[19] Bone pain, swelling, and soft tissue abscesses are the most common manifestations of osteoarticular disease.[20] Hematogenous dissemination is common; skin disease and osteoarticular disease occur most frequently. Bone involvement occurs in 25% to 60% of disseminated cases, and arthritis is estimated to occur in 3% to 5%.[19] In a study of 45 patients with skeletal blastomycosis, 41 had osteomyelitis while 12 presented with septic arthritis.[20] The skeletal areas most commonly affected are the long bones, vertebrae, and ribs (Figure 112-1).[21-23]

Arthritis is usually monoarticular in the knee, ankle, or elbow but may rarely be polyarticular.[19,24] Joint infection is an isolated skeletal disorder in only a few cases; joint radiographs more commonly show punched-out bone lesions (Figure 112-2A). Synovial fluid is commonly purulent, and organisms are evident on microscopic examination, as well as by culture. The synovial histologic examination shows epithelioid granulomas with budding yeast forms (Figure 112-2B). The diagnosis is also commonly made from involved nonarticular sites. Urinary antigen testing appears to be sensitive but may be falsely positive in patients with other endemic fungal infections.[25] For moderately severe or severe disease, treatment with amphotericin B for 1 to 2 weeks or until improvement is noted, followed by oral itraconazole for a total of at least 12 months, is recommended. For mild to moderate disease, oral itraconazole for 12 months is recommended. Serum levels of itraconazole should be determined after the patient has been on treatment for at least 2 weeks, to ensure adequate drug exposure.[18,26-28]

CRYPTOCOCCOSIS

Cryptococcus neoformans, the fungus causing cryptococcosis, is geographically ubiquitous and is found in pigeon feces; a related species, *Cryptococcus gattii*, is associated with certain types of eucalyptus trees in tropical climates and has been associated with an ongoing outbreak of disease on Vancouver Island and surrounding areas of Canada and the northwestern United States. It is a common pathogen only in association with defects in cell-mediated host defense including human immunodeficiency virus (HIV) infection, transplantation, lymphoreticular malignant

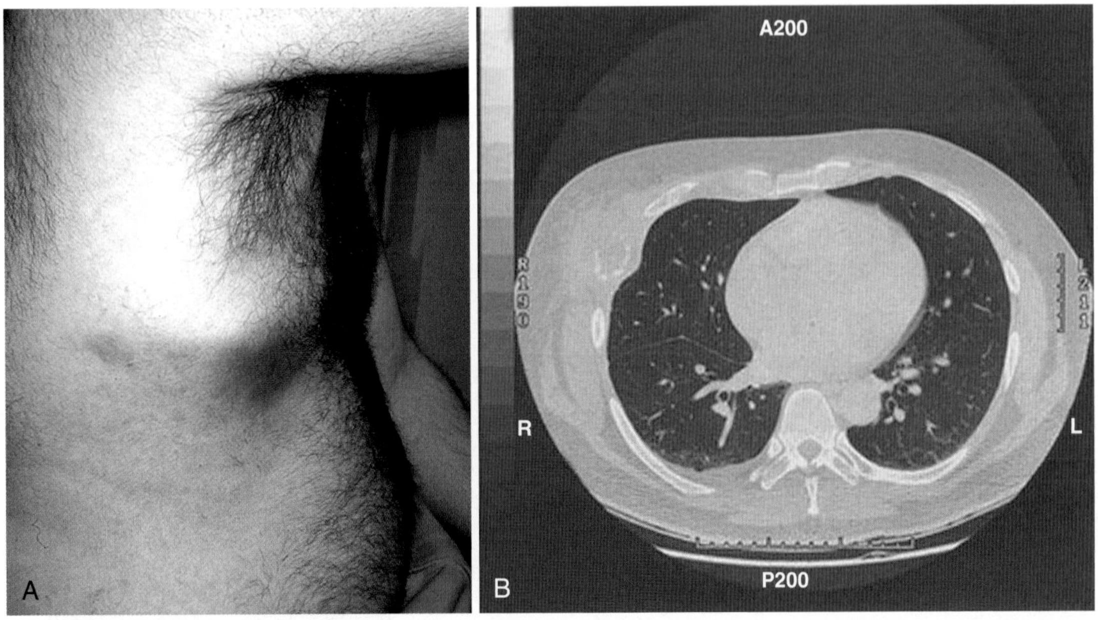

Figure 112-1 A, Blastomycosis osteomyelitis of a rib and chest wall. **B,** Computed tomography scan appearance. Primary infection in the blood may spread to the skeleton.

neoplasms, TNF antagonist treatment,[29,30] and corticosteroid therapy.

Cryptococcosis varies in acuity, usually affecting the lungs in its primary form, but it sometimes disseminates hematogenously to a wide variety of sites including the central nervous system and skin. Although bone infection is common, causing osteolytic lesions in 5% to 10% of cases, articular involvement is rarely reported.[31,32] Bone lesions may be confused with metastatic neoplasm (Figure 112-3).

Cryptococcal arthritis is an indolent monoarticular arthritis in about 60% of reported cases and a polyarthritis in the remainder.[33,34] The knee is most commonly involved. A single case of tenosynovitis with carpal tunnel syndrome has been recognized. The majority of cases reported from the pre-AIDS era also demonstrated radiographic evidence of periarticular osteomyelitis. These patients were young adults, did not have debilitating disease or other evidence of dissemination, and had pulmonary involvement in only 50% of cases. Synovial tissue showed acute and chronic synovitis, multinucleate giant cells, prominent granuloma formation, and large numbers of budding yeast with special stains. Most recently reported cases are associated with immunosuppression and disseminated infection. Interestingly, osteoarticular cryptococcal infections have been linked to sarcoidosis, although it is unclear whether this association relates to the immunologic impact of the sarcoidosis or to the immunosuppressive therapies used to treat it.[35] Serum cryptococcal antigen testing appears to be sensitive, in part because osteoarticular infection results from hematogenous dissemination. The choice of treatment for cryptococcal disease depends on both the anatomic sites of involvement and the host's immune status, with amphotericin B and fluconazole being considered most effective.[34,36] 5-Flucytosine is typically added to amphotericin B or fluconazole for the first 2 to 4 weeks (induction therapy) in cases of severe cryptococcal infection.[37]

CANDIDIASIS

Candida species are widely distributed yeasts. *Candida albicans* is a normal commensal of humans, and other species can probably live in nonanimate environments such as soil. Since the advent of antibiotic therapy in the 1940s, and related to the common use of immunosuppression and parenteral lines, candidiasis has been responsible for an increasing incidence of mucocutaneous and deep-organ infections.[38] Osteomyelitis, though rarely reported, is a potentially serious complication of hematogenous dissemination in both adults and children.[39,40] It may also occur from direct tissue inoculation during surgery or by injection of contaminated heroin,[41] and bone infection may emerge after successful amphotericin B treatment of other sites. Infection is commonly located in two adjacent vertebrae or in a single long bone. Surgical inoculation has occurred in the sternum, spine, and mandible. A few patients have had multiple sites of involvement. Candidal prosthetic joint infections may also occur as a late consequence of total joint replacement.[42]

The clinical presentation is localized pain. Other symptoms and laboratory abnormalities vary. Bone changes of osteomyelitis are commonly demonstrated in radiographs of the symptomatic site. The diagnosis is established when culture of involved bone obtained by either open or needle biopsy has identified a variety of *Candida* species. Use of direct amplification testing has been reported.[43] Treatment with azoles (fluconazole, itraconazole, voriconazole, or posaconazole); echinocandins (caspofungin, micafungin, or anidulafungin); or amphotericin B formulations may be effective.[44,45] Species identification and susceptibility testing assist antifungal therapy selection. For example, *Candida glabrata* frequently demonstrate reduced susceptibility to azole antifungal agents and amphotericin but remain susceptible to echinocandins; *Candida krusei* are often resistant to azoles and may show reduced susceptibility to amphotericin but also remain susceptible to echinocandins; *Candida lusitaniae* are often resistant to amphotericin; and *Candida parapsilosis* may demonstrate reduced susceptibility to echinocandins.[45] The use of surgical débridement must be individualized. With vertebral involvement but no neurologic complications, medication alone has been effective.

Candidiasis is an uncommon cause of monoarticular arthritis.[46] *C. albicans* is the most common pathogen, although septic arthritis due to other candidal species has been reported.[47] Reported cases commonly involve a knee, occur in the context of multifocal extra-articular *Candida* infection, and are accompanied by constitutional symptoms. Both children and adults have been affected. Predisposing conditions include gastrointestinal and pulmonary disorders, narcotic addiction, intravenous catheters, leukopenia, immunosuppressive treatment (including TNF antagonists), broad-spectrum antibiotics, and corticosteroids. Some involved joints were previously affected by arthritis, and infection has followed arthrocentesis in isolated cases. In most cases, radiographs reveal coincident

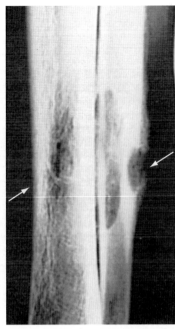

Figure 112-3 Cryptococcosis (torulosis). Discrete osteolytic foci with surrounding sclerosis and, in some places, periosteal reaction are seen *(arrows)*. This involvement of bone protuberances such as the calcaneus is not unexpected in this disease. The resulting appearance simulates that of other fungal diseases, especially coccidioidomycosis, as well as neoplastic disorders. *(From Resnick D: Diagnosis of bone and joint disorders, ed 3, Philadelphia, 1995, WB Saunders, p 2507.)*

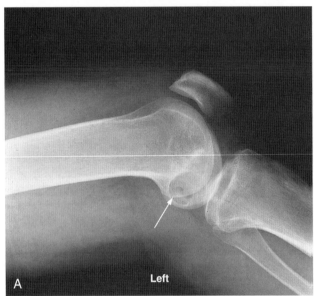

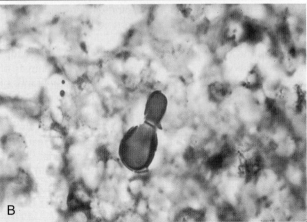

Figure 112-2 Blastomycosis joint infection. **A,** Radiographs commonly show punched-out bone lesions. **B,** Synovial histology shows epithelioid granulomas with budding yeast forms.

osteomyelitis. Synovial fluid leukocyte counts may vary; *Candida* species have been cultured from synovial fluid in all cases but are not commonly identified on smear. Histologic studies of synovium show nonspecific chronic inflammation rather than granulomas.

SPOROTRICHOSIS

Sporotrichosis is caused by *Sporothrix schenckii*, a saprophyte found widely in soil and plants. Infection in humans occurs through inoculation of the skin or, rarely, inhalation into the respiratory tract; it is a source of infection among agricultural workers in tropical and subtropical areas. It most commonly involves the skin and lymphatics but may disseminate from the lungs to the central nervous system, eyes, bones, and joints.[48] In immunocompetent hosts, a single site is typically involved; in immunocompromised hosts including patients on anticytokine therapy, multifocal disease may occur.[49]

In contrast to the relatively common occurrence of skin infection, articular sporotrichosis is a rare disorder.[50,51] In 84% of patients in one series, there was no accompanying skin involvement, suggesting entry through the lungs. Sporotrichosis most often occurs in individuals with a chronic illness that alters host defense such as alcoholism or a myeloproliferative disorder. *Sporothrix* arthritis is most often indolent and infects a single joint or multiple joints in equal proportions. The knee, hand, wrist, elbow, and shoulder are most frequently involved; hand and wrist involvement distinguishes this from other fungal arthritides. Articular infection shows a propensity to spread to adjacent soft tissues, forming draining sinuses. Constitutional symptoms are unusual.

Radiographic changes vary from juxta-articular osteopenia to the commonly observed punched-out bone lesions. When it can be obtained, synovial fluid is inflammatory. Synovitis is characterized on gross evaluation by destructive pannus and on microscopic examination by granulomatous histologic features or, less frequently, by nonspecific inflammation. Organisms are difficult to identify in tissue, and the diagnosis is often made by positive culture of joint fluid or involved tissue. Incubation at room temperature assists growth of the mycelial phase of *S. schenckii*. Serologic testing is not useful in the diagnosis of sporotrichosis. In a small number of cases, sporotrichosis may disseminate to cause a potentially fatal infection characterized by low-grade fever, weight loss, anemia, osteolytic bone lesions, arthritis, skin lesions, and involvement of the eyes and central nervous system.[52-55] These infections occur in immunosuppressed patients with either hematologic malignancies or HIV infection.

In 44 cases reported in 1979, treatment was optimal with combined joint débridement and high-dose intravenous amphotericin B (11 of 11 cured) and slightly less effective with amphotericin alone (14 of 19 cured).[50] More recently, itraconazole has proven effective for initial therapy of most patients,[56] with amphotericin B being reserved for those with extensive involvement and for itraconazole failures. In contrast, fluconazole has demonstrated only modest success in osteoarticular sporotrichosis.[57,58] Long-term suppressive therapy with itraconazole may be required for patients with AIDS.[56]

ASPERGILLOSIS

Aspergillus species are ubiquitous, but infection occurs only rarely in immunocompetent individuals. In contrast, invasive infection is an important life-threatening complication in immunocompromised adults and children.[59-61] It may spread directly from the lung to adjacent vertebrae, disk spaces, and ribs (more often in children) or through the bloodstream (Figure 112-4).[62-64] Rare cases of monoarthritis with adjacent osteomyelitis are also reported. The knee is the most commonly involved joint. The organism may be observed in infected tissue (see Figure 112-4B). The galactomannan EIA has been validated as a surrogate marker for invasive aspergillosis and the $(1\rightarrow3)$-β-D-glucan assay may similarly provide support for the diagnosis of invasive fungal infection. Treatment with combined surgical débridement and antifungal therapy is an ongoing challenge.[60,63,65] Voriconazole has proven superior to amphotericin for the treatment of invasive aspergillosis and is now recommended for initial therapy.[65,66] Liposomal amphotericin B, posaconazole, caspofungin, and micafungin have demonstrated efficacy in salvage situations.[67] Combination therapy has not demonstrated clear improvement in outcomes over monotherapy.

HISTOPLASMOSIS

Histoplasma capsulatum is a soil fungus that causes endemic disease in the midwestern and southeastern United States.[33,68] Bone and joint involvement is rare but has been reported in the knee, wrist, and ankle. Immunosuppression

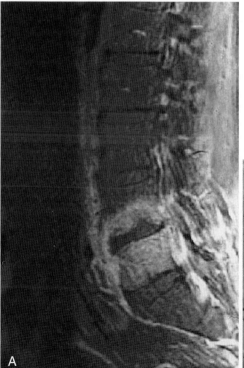
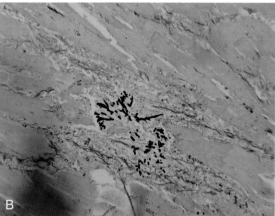

Figure 112-4 Aspergillosis vertebral osteomyelitis and diskitis. **A,** *Aspergillus* may spread directly from the lung to adjacent vertebrae, disk spaces, and ribs (more often in children) or through the bloodstream. **B,** Infected tissue may show characteristic organisms.

including the use of TNF antagonists predisposes to disseminated histoplasmosis in adults and children, which may be confused clinically with sarcoidosis, tuberculosis, and reactive inflammatory conditions.[69-72] Diagnosis depends on appropriate use of fungal staining and culture methods, antigen detection, and serologic antibody testing.[73] A case report emphasizes the rare occurrence of fungal prosthetic joint arthritis.[74] The more common osteoarticular involvement with histoplasmosis is a hypersensitivity syndrome accompanying acute pulmonary infection; it is characterized by self-limited polyarthritis, erythema nodosum, and erythema multiforme. Liposomal amphotericin B followed by itraconazole is the preferred treatment for severe infection and itraconazole for less severe cases.[68,75,76]

SCEDOSPORIOSIS

Scedosporium species are environmental molds that have recently been identified as fungal pathogens in both immunocompetent and immunocompromised hosts. They may cause focally invasive and disseminated infection after cutaneous inoculation. *Scedosporium prolificans* has a predilection for bone and cartilage, leading to both septic arthritis and osteomyelitis. Infections are difficult to eradicate with surgery and antifungal agents, and the organism is resistant to amphotericin.[77,78] Case reports suggest improved infection control with voriconazole or voriconazole combined with terbenafine.[79-81]

TREATMENT OF FUNGAL INFECTION

Antifungal chemotherapy has improved over the past several decades, first with the introduction of amphotericin B and then with the oral antifungal agents flucytosine, ketoconazole, fluconazole, and itraconazole. More recent advances include the development of less toxic formulations of amphotericin B, liposomal amphotericin B, and amphotericin B lipid complex. Voriconazole and posaconazole, which are broad-spectrum azole antifungals, have demonstrated improved activity against aspergillosis and mucormycosis, respectively. The echinocandin antifungal agents caspofungin, micafungin, and anidulafungin have emerged as alternative therapies for aspergillosis and as the treatments of choice for some *Candida* infections. For detailed treatment guidelines, several excellent reviews are available.[82-91] In choosing an appropriate drug (Table 112-2) and course of treatment, the clinician must consider the infecting agent, clinical manifestations of the disease,

immune status of the host, antimicrobial resistance, drug side effect profile, and direct and indirect costs of treatment. Treatment has become more complex because of immune system compromise in infected patients being treated for transplant rejection, autoimmune disorders, malignant disease, and AIDS.[92]

Itraconazole has become the first choice for treatment of the endemic mycoses—blastomycosis, histoplasmosis, and sporotrichosis. A loading dose of itraconazole of 200 mg three times a day for 3 days is recommended, followed by 200 mg to 400 mg daily. Absorption of itraconazole is unpredictable, and blood levels of itraconazole should be measured to ensure adequate drug exposure. Absorption of itraconazole requires stomach acid, so concurrent administration of drugs that reduce the acidity of the stomach such as proton pump inhibitors and H_2 blockers should be avoided. At least 6 months of treatment is required, and some patients may need up to a year of therapy. For cryptococcosis, fluconazole is the recommended azole.[34,36] Amphotericin B is the preferred drug for meningeal and life-threatening infections. Specific treatment protocols and detailed side effect profiles are presented in reviews,[82-91] Infectious Diseases Society of America guidelines,[11,28,37,45,67,76] and infection-specific references (see Table 112-2).

FUNGAL INFECTION AS A CONSEQUENCE OF ANTIRHEUMATIC THERAPY

Many of the same fungal infections associated with osteoarticular disease may cause infection in patients treated with antirheumatic therapy, particularly biologic therapy. Animal models of infection point to an important role for TNF in host defense against many of these organisms including *Aspergillus*,[93] *Candida*,[94] *Cryptococcus*,[95,96] *Coccidioides*,[97] and *Sporothrix*.[98]

Coccidioidomycosis infection following TNF antagonist therapy has been reported in endemic areas in the southwestern United States. In the largest published series, 12 of 13 cases followed therapy with infliximab and 1 was associated with etanercept.[99] All but two of these cases were believed to represent new infection rather than reactivation. In one medical center included in this series, the relative risk of coccidioidomycosis infection was 5.23 with infliximab therapy compared with other antirheumatic therapy. In all cases, coccidioidomycosis infection developed in the absence of other known risk factors including diabetes, pregnancy, and HIV infection. Coccidioidomycosis infection has also been reported in nonendemic areas, presumably as a consequence of fomite exposure.[100]

Disseminated histoplasmosis infections have been reported following TNF antagonist therapy in endemic areas in the Ohio-Mississippi River valley regions of the central United States; as with coccidioidomycosis infections, these have been reported more frequently following infliximab therapy than with the other agents.[69] The reason for the larger number of cases with infliximab is unclear; possibilities include a unique mechanism of action for infliximab, larger numbers of patients treated, patient selection, concomitant immunosuppressive therapy, or some combination of all of these. In most cases, patients

Table 112-2 Drug Treatment of Osteoarticular Mycotic Infections

Infection	Drug Recommended	Infection-Specific References
Coccidioidomycosis	Itraconazole	3, 7, 12, 13
Blastomycosis	Itraconazole	18, 27, 117
Cryptococcosis	Fluconazole	34, 36, 117
Candidiasis	Fluconazole	44-46, 117, 118
Sporotrichosis	Itraconazole	50, 57, 58
Aspergillosis	Voriconazole	61, 64, 117
Histoplasmosis	Itraconazole	68, 75
Scedosporiosis	Voriconazole	77, 80, 81

developing disseminated histoplasmosis with TNF antagonist therapy have been taking additional immunosuppressive therapy. Patients typically present with cough, dyspnea, fever, and malaise and can rapidly become quite ill. Histoplasma antigen may be identified in the urine in 92% of cases with disseminated histoplasmosis, and this test may assist rapid diagnosis.[71] Exposure to *Histoplasma* may result in asymptomatic latent infection; it has been difficult, however, to determine whether symptomatic infections following TNF antagonist therapy represent reactivation or new infection. Both pulmonary and disseminated infections with cryptococcal infections have been reported with TNF antagonist therapy, as have infections with *Aspergillus, Candida, Scedosporium,* and *Sporothrix.*[1,29,49,101-104] Fungal infections have not been reported as a consequence of abatacept or rituximab therapy in rheumatic diseases. Whether this relates to decreased risk with these agents or smaller numbers of patients treated remains to be seen.

Pneumocystis jiroveci pneumonia (PCP) is caused by a fungus originally classified as a protozoan (*Pneumocystis carinii*). PCP, an opportunistic infection seen in association with HIV infection, has been reported with a number of antirheumatic therapies including cyclophosphamide and low-dose methotrexate, often in combination with corticosteroid therapy.[105,106] Interestingly, PCP as a consequence of low-dose methotrexate therapy has been reported as a particular concern in Japan, where the prevalence of asymptomatic carriage of *Pneumocystis* has been reported to be as high as 18.8% in the elderly.[107] These same authors have suggested that polymerase chain reactive (PCR) testing may identify carriers at increased risk for PCP during therapy.[108] The use of biologic therapy including rituximab[109] and TNF antagonists[110] has been associated with the development of PCP. PCP presents as fever, dry cough, and dyspnea. The clinical presentation in patients receiving immunosuppressive therapy is typically more acute than in HIV-associated cases. Organisms may be identified in sputum from HIV patients but are seen less commonly in rheumatologic patients; presumptive diagnosis may be made on the basis of PCR testing for *P. jiroveci* DNA. Elevated serum levels of β-D-glucan, a common component of fungal cell walls, may aid in the diagnosis. One series of 21 patients identified older age, pre-existing pulmonary disease, higher corticosteroid doses, and low serum albumin and IgG levels as potential risk factors for PCP in patients treated with infliximab.[110] Chest radiographs may show diffuse infiltrates, while CT scans demonstrate ground-glass opacities (Figures 112-5 and 112-6); radiographic findings may be difficult to distinguish from methotrexate pneumonitis. Treatment includes supplemental oxygen and trimethoprim/sulfamethoxazole (TMP/SMX) or pentamidine isethionate. High-dose corticosteroids are commonly used as adjunctive therapy in the treatment of HIV patients with PCP but are less well studied in patients taking immunosuppressives.

PCP infection is also of concern with nonbiologic immunosuppressive therapy. In particular, the use of cyclophosphamide to treat systemic lupus, vasculitis, and other autoimmune diseases has been associated with a risk of developing PCP, although the overall risk appears to be low. In a recent review of published data on 76,156 cases of systemic lupus erythematosus treated with cyclophosphamide, the risk of PCP was 15.88 per 10,000 patients, or

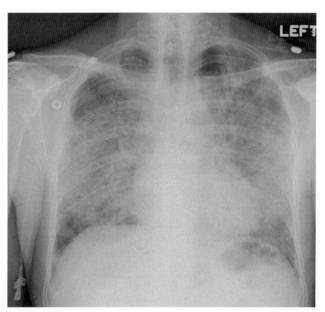

Figure 112-5   Chest radiograph showing diffuse interstitial infiltrate in a patient with *Pneumocystis jiroveci* pneumonia,

0.158%.[105] Potential risk factors include high-dose corticosteroid use, lymphopenia (especially low CD4 counts), renal disease, and overall high disease activity.[105,111] Vasculitis patients with pulmonary involvement may be at increased risk, and diagnosis may be difficult in both these patients and lupus patients with pulmonary disease. Unfortunately, there are no published guidelines to address the use of PCP prophylaxis in autoimmune diseases or a clear consensus regarding the standard of care in this situation. Recent clinical trials in vasculitis have routinely employed PCP prophylaxis as part of the protocol, suggesting it is becoming the standard of care.[112] Two recent surveys of U.S. rheumatologists, however, found that just 50.4% and 69.5%, respectively, routinely prescribed prophylactic antibiotics.[105,113] Academic rheumatologists and more recent graduates are more likely to prescribe prophylactic therapy. TMP/SMX appears to be more effective than dapsone or aerosolized

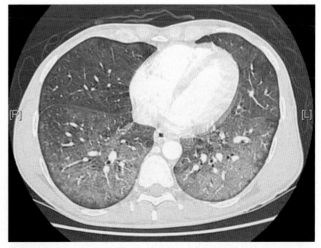

Figure 112-6   Computed tomography scan of the chest demonstrating ground-glass opacity in a patient with *Pneumocystis jiroveci* pneumonia.

pentamidine, despite an apparent increased risk of sulfon-amide allergy in the lupus population.[114,115] There are no consistent standards, or recommendations, for the use of prophylaxis for fungal infection other than *Pneumocystis*.

Given the risk of fungal infection with biologic therapy, careful patient selection for these compounds is understandably important. Patients with a history of fungal infection or those with significant exposure to these organisms should receive these drugs only when alternatives are not available or appropriate. Patients should be cautioned to minimize exposure to sources of infection during therapy (e.g., avoid exposure to histoplasmosis in old buildings [demolition, remodeling, cleaning], chicken coops, bird roosts, wood piles, or caves [spelunking]) and avoid exposure to outdoor dust in regions endemic for coccidioidomycosis. There is, as yet, no practical role for screening for latent infection or for prophylactic therapy.[116] Serum IgG and IgM antibody titers may be elevated in patients who have had exposure to *Coccidioides*. Antibody titers normalize 3 to 6 months after initial exposure, however, rendering these tests unsuitable for identifying distant infections. Delayed-type hypersensitivity testing, which may help identify older infections, is not readily available in the United States. Moreover, most coccidioidomycosis infections seen in this situation appear to represent acute infection rather than reactivation. Chest radiographs may identify calcified granulomas consistent with prior histoplasmosis infection, but this is a nonspecific finding. In Japan, it has been suggested that TMP/SMX therapy may normalize PCR testing in asymptomatic *P. jiroveci* carriers treated with methotrexate and that this might reduce the risk of developing pneumonia, but this has not been studied in a U.S. population.[108] The lack of useful screening tests makes early recognition of infection and institution of therapy critical. Indeed, the U.S. Food and Drug Administration has mandated a "black box" warning regarding the risk of fungal infections on the product labels of TNF antagonists, reflecting the potentially fatal consequences of delayed recognition of such infections.

References

1. Filler SG, Yeaman MR, Sheppard DC: Tumor necrosis factor inhibition and invasive fungal infections, *Clin Infect Dis* 41(Suppl 3):S208–S212, 2005.
2. Giles JT, Bathon JM: Serious infections associated with anticytokine therapies in the rheumatic diseases, *J Intensive Care Med* 19(6):320–334, 2004.
3. Blair JE, Smilack JD, Caples SM: Coccidioidomycosis in patients with hematologic malignancies, *Arch Intern Med* 165(1):113–117, 2005.
4. Bialek R, Gonzalez GM, Begerow D, Zelck UE: Coccidioidomycosis and blastomycosis: advances in molecular diagnosis, *FEMS Immunol Med Microbiol* 45(3):355–360, 2005.
5. Chiller TM, Galgiani JN, Stevens DA: Coccidioidomycosis, *Infect Dis Clin North Am* 17(1):41–57, viii, 2003.
6. Holley K, Muldoon M, Tasker S: *Coccidioides immitis* osteomyelitis: a case series review, *Orthopedics* 25(8):827–831, 831–832, 2002.
7. Bayer AS, Guze LB: Fungal arthritis. II. Coccidioidal synovitis: clinical, diagnostic, therapeutic, and prognostic considerations, *Semin Arthritis Rheum* 8(3):200–211, 1979.
8. Durkin M, Estok L, Hospenthal D, et al: Detection of *Coccidioides* antigenemia following dissociation of immune complexes, *Clin Vaccine Immunol* 16(10):1453–1456, 2009.
9. Durkin M, Connolly P, Kuberski T, et al: Diagnosis of coccidioidomycosis with use of the *Coccidioides* antigen enzyme immunoassay, *Clin Infect Dis* 47(8):e69–73, 2008.
10. Stadalnik RC, Goldstein E, Hoeprich PD, et al: Diagnostic value of gallium and bone scans in evaluation of extrapulmonary coccidioidal lesions, *Am Rev Respir Dis* 121(4):673–676, 1980.
11. Galgiani JN, Ampel NM, Blair JE, et al: Coccidioidomycosis, *Clin Infect Dis* 41(9):1217–1223, 2005.
12. Bried JM, Galgiani JN: Coccidioides immitis infections in bones and joints, *Clin Orthop Relat Res* 211:235–243, 1986.
13. Galgiani JN, Catanzaro A, Cloud GA, et al: Comparison of oral fluconazole and itraconazole for progressive, nonmeningeal coccidioidomycosis. A randomized, double-blind trial. Mycoses Study Group, *Ann Intern Med* 133(9):676–686, 2000.
14. Catanzaro A, Cloud GA, Stevens DA, et al: Safety, tolerance, and efficacy of posaconazole therapy in patients with nonmeningeal disseminated or chronic pulmonary coccidioidomycosis, *Clin Infect Dis* 45(5):562–568, 2007.
15. Freifeld A, Proia L, Andes D, et al: Voriconazole use for endemic fungal infections, *Antimicrob Agents Chemother* 53(4):1648–1651, 2009.
16. Stevens DA, Rendon A, Gaona-Flores V, et al: Posaconazole therapy for chronic refractory coccidioidomycosis, *Chest* 132(3):952–958, 2007.
17. Smith CE: Coccidioidomycosis, *Pediatr Clin North Am* Feb:109–125, 1955.
18. Bradsher RW, Chapman SW, Pappas PG: Blastomycosis, *Infect Dis Clin North Am* 17(1):21–40, vii, 2003.
19. Bayer AS, Scott VJ, Guze LB: Fungal arthritis. IV. Blastomycotic arthritis, *Semin Arthritis Rheum* 9(2):145–151, 1979.
20. Oppenheimer M, Embil JM, Black B, et al: Blastomycosis of bones and joints, *South Med J* 100(6):570–578, 2007.
21. MacDonald PB, Black GB, MacKenzie R: Orthopaedic manifestations of blastomycosis, *J Bone Joint Surg Am* 72(6):860–864, 1990.
22. Pritchard DJ: Granulomatous infections of bones and joints, *Orthop Clin North Am* 6(4):1029–1047, 1975.
23. Saccente M, Abernathy RS, Pappas PG, et al: Vertebral blastomycosis with paravertebral abscess: report of eight cases and review of the literature, *Clin Infect Dis* 26(2):413–418, 1998.
24. Abril A, Campbell MD, Cotten VR Jr, et al: Polyarticular blastomycotic arthritis, *J Rheumatol* 25(5):1019–1021, 1998.
25. Durkin M, Witt J, Lemonte A, et al: Antigen assay with the potential to aid in diagnosis of blastomycosis, *J Clin Microbiol* 42(10):4873–4875, 2004.
26. Bradsher RW: Therapy of blastomycosis, *Semin Respir Infect* 12(3):263–267, 1997.
27. Chapman SW, Bradsher RW Jr, Campbell GD Jr, et al: Practice guidelines for the management of patients with blastomycosis. Infectious Diseases Society of America, *Clin Infect Dis* 30(4):679–683, 2000.
28. Chapman SW, Dismukes WE, Proia LA, et al: Clinical practice guidelines for the management of blastomycosis: 2008 update by the Infectious Diseases Society of America, *Clin Infect Dis* 46(12):1801–1812, 2008.
29. Horcajada JP, Pena JL, Martinez-Taboada VM, et al: Invasive cryptococcosis and adalimumab treatment, *Emerg Infect Dis* 13(6):953–955, 2007.
30. True DG, Penmetcha M, Peckham SJ: Disseminated cryptococcal infection in rheumatoid arthritis treated with methotrexate and infliximab, *J Rheumatol* 29(7):1561–1563, 2002.
31. Behrman RE, Masci JR, Nicholas P: Cryptococcal skeletal infections: case report and review, *Rev Infect Dis* 12(2):181–190, 1990.
32. Ortiz M, Gonzalez E, Munoz MA, Andres A: Cryptococcal monoarthritis without systemic involvement in a renal transplant patient, *Transplantation* 78(2):301–302, 2004.
33. Bayer AS, Choi C, Tillman DB, Guze LB: Fungal arthritis. V. Cryptococcal and histoplasmal arthritis, *Semin Arthritis Rheum* 9(3):218–227, 1980.
34. Bruno KM, Farhoomand L, Libman BS, et al: Cryptococcal arthritis, tendinitis, tenosynovitis, and carpal tunnel syndrome: report of a case and review of the literature, *Arthritis Rheum* 47(1):104–108, 2002.
35. Geller DS, Pope JB, Thornhill BA, Dorfman HD: Cryptococcal pyarthrosis and sarcoidosis, *Skeletal Radiol* 38(7):721–727, 2009.
36. Saag MS, Graybill RJ, Larsen RA, et al: Practice guidelines for the management of cryptococcal disease. Infectious Diseases Society of America, *Clin Infect Dis* 30(4):710–718, 2000.
37. Perfect JR, Dismukes WE, Dromer F, et al: Clinical practice guidelines for the management of cryptococcal disease: 2010 update by the

Infectious Diseases Society of America, *Clin Infect Dis* 50(3):291–322, 2010.

38. Edwards JEJ: Candida species. In Mandell GL, Bennett JE, Dolin R, editors. *Mandell, Douglas, and Bennett's principles and practice of infectious diseases.* Philadelphia, 2000, Churchill Livingstone, pp 2656–2674.

39. Arias F, Mata-Essayag S, Landaeta ME, et al: *Candida albicans* osteomyelitis: case report and literature review, *Int J Infect Dis* 8(5):307–314, 2004.

40. McCullers JA, Flynn PM: *Candida tropicalis* osteomyelitis: case report and review, *Clin Infect Dis* 26(4):1000–1001, 1998.

41. Lafont A, Olive A, Gelman M, et al: *Candida albicans* spondylodiscitis and vertebral osteomyelitis in patients with intravenous heroin drug addiction. Report of 3 new cases, *J Rheumatol* 21(5):953–956, 1994.

42. Lerch K, Kalteis T, Schubert T, et al: Prosthetic joint infections with osteomyelitis due to *Candida albicans*, *Mycoses* 46(11–12):462–466, 2003.

43. Harrington JT: The evolving role of direct amplification tests in diagnosing osteoarticular infections caused by mycobacteria and fungi, *Curr Opin Rheumatol* 11(4):289–292, 1999.

44. Martin MV: The use of fluconazole and itraconazole in the treatment of *Candida albicans* infections: a review, *J Antimicrob Chemother* 44(4):429–437, 1999.

45. Pappas PG, Rex JH, Sobel JD, et al: Guidelines for treatment of candidiasis, *Clin Infect Dis* 38(2):161–189, 2004.

46. Bayer AS, Guze LB: Fungal arthritis. I. *Candida* arthritis: diagnostic and prognostic implications and therapeutic considerations, *Semin Arthritis Rheum* 8(2):142–150, 1978.

47. Bariola JR, Saccente M: *Candida lusitaniae* septic arthritis: case report and review of the literature, *Diagn Microbiol Infect Dis* 61(1):61–63, 2008.

48. Morris-Jones R: Sporotrichosis, *Clin Exp Dermatol* 27(6):427–431, 2002.

49. Gottlieb GS, Lesser CF, Holmes KK, Wald A: Disseminated sporotrichosis associated with treatment with immunosuppressants and tumor necrosis factor-alpha antagonists, *Clin Infect Dis* 37(6):838–840, 2003.

50. Bayer AS, Scott VJ, Guze LB: Fungal arthritis. III. Sporotrichal arthritis, *Semin Arthritis Rheum* 9(1):66–74, 1979.

51. Crout JE, Brewer NS, Tompkins RB: Sporotrichosis arthritis: clinical features in seven patients, *Ann Intern Med* 86(3):294–297, 1977.

52. al-Tawfiq JA, Wools KK: Disseminated sporotrichosis and *Sporothrix schenckii* fungemia as the initial presentation of human immunodeficiency virus infection, *Clin Infect Dis* 26(6):1403–1406, 1998.

53. Lynch PJ, Voorhees JJ, Harrell ER: Systemic sporotrichosis, *Ann Intern Med* 73(1):23–30, 1970.

54. Oscherwitz SL, Rinaldi MG: Disseminated sporotrichosis in a patient infected with human immunodeficiency virus, *Clin Infect Dis* 15(3):568–569, 1992.

55. Wilson DE, Mann JJ, Bennett JE, Utz JP: Clinical features of extracutaneous sporotrichosis, *Medicine (Baltimore)* 46(3):265–279, 1967.

56. Appenzeller S, Amaral TN, Amstalden EM, et al: *Sporothrix schenckii* infection presented as monoarthritis: report of two cases and review of the literature, *Clin Rheumatol* 25(6):926–928, 2006.

57. Kauffman CA, Hajjeh R, Chapman SW: Practice guidelines for the management of patients with sporotrichosis. For the Mycoses Study Group. Infectious Diseases Society of America, *Clin Infect Dis* 30(4):684–687, 2000.

58. Sharkey-Mathis PK, Kauffman CA, Graybill JR, et al: Treatment of sporotrichosis with itraconazole. NIAID Mycoses Study Group, *Am J Med* 95(3):279–285, 1993.

59. Cuellar ML, Silveira LH, Espinoza LR: Fungal arthritis, *Ann Rheum Dis* 51(5):690–697, 1992.

60. Dotis J, Roilides E: Osteomyelitis due to *Aspergillus* spp. in patients with chronic granulomatous disease: comparison of *Aspergillus nidulans* and *Aspergillus fumigatus*, *Int J Infect Dis* 8(2):103–110, 2004.

61. Kontoyiannis DP, Bodey GP: Invasive aspergillosis in 2002: an update, *Eur J Clin Microbiol Infect Dis* 21(3):161–172, 2002.

62. Pasic S, Abinun M, Pistignjat B, et al: *Aspergillus* osteomyelitis in chronic granulomatous disease: treatment with recombinant gamma-interferon and itraconazole, *Pediatr Infect Dis J* 15(9):833–834, 1996.

63. Paterson DL: New clinical presentations of invasive aspergillosis in non-conventional hosts, *Clin Microbiol Infect* 10(Suppl 1):24–30, 2004.

64. Vinas FC, King PK, Diaz FG: Spinal aspergillus osteomyelitis, *Clin Infect Dis* 28(6):1223–1229, 1999.

65. Kirby A, Hassan I, Burnie J: Recommendations for managing *Aspergillus* osteomyelitis and joint infections based on a review of the literature, *J Infect* 52(6):405–414, 2006.

66. Golmia R, Bello I, Marra A, et al: *Aspergillus fumigatus* joint infection: a review, *Semin Arthritis Rheum* 40:580–584, 2010.

67. Walsh TJ, Anaissie EJ, Denning DW, et al: Treatment of aspergillosis: clinical practice guidelines of the Infectious Diseases Society of America, *Clin Infect Dis* 46(3):327–360, 2008.

68. Wheat J, Sarosi G, McKinsey D, et al: Practice guidelines for the management of patients with histoplasmosis. Infectious Diseases Society of America, *Clin Infect Dis* 30(4):688–695, 2000.

69. Lee JH, Slifman NR, Gershon SK, et al: Life-threatening histoplasmosis complicating immunotherapy with tumor necrosis factor alpha antagonists infliximab and etanercept, *Arthritis Rheum* 46(10):2565–2570, 2002.

70. Weinberg JM, Ali R, Badve S, Pelker RR: Musculoskeletal histoplasmosis. A case report and review of the literature, *J Bone Joint Surg Am* 83-A(11):1718–1722, 2001.

71. Wood KL, Hage CA, Knox KS, et al: Histoplasmosis after treatment with anti-tumor necrosis factor-alpha therapy, *Am J Respir Crit Care Med* 167(9):1279–1282, 2003.

72. Hage CA, Bowyer S, Tarvin SE, et al: Recognition, diagnosis, and treatment of histoplasmosis complicating tumor necrosis factor blocker therapy, *Clin Infect Dis* 50(1):85–92, 2010.

73. Wheat LJ: Laboratory diagnosis of histoplasmosis: update 2000, *Semin Respir Infect* 16(2):131–140, 2001.

74. Fowler VG Jr, Nacinovich FM, Alspaugh JA, Corey GR: Prosthetic joint infection due to *Histoplasma capsulatum*: case report and review, *Clin Infect Dis* 26(4):1017, 1998.

75. Mocherla S, Wheat LJ: Treatment of histoplasmosis, *Semin Respir Infect* 16(2):141–148, 2001.

76. Wheat LJ, Freifeld AG, Kleiman MB, et al: Clinical practice guidelines for the management of patients with histoplasmosis: 2007 update by the Infectious Diseases Society of America, *Clin Infect Dis* 45(7):807–825, 2007.

77. Levine NB, Kurokawa R, Fichtenbaum CJ, et al: An immunocompetent patient with primary *Scedosporium apiospermum* vertebral osteomyelitis, *J Spinal Disord Tech* 15(5):425–430, 2002.

78. Wilson CM, O'Rourke EJ, McGinnis MR, Salkin IF: *Scedosporium inflatum*: clinical spectrum of a newly recognized pathogen, *J Infect Dis* 161(1):102–107, 1990.

79. Dalton PA, Munckhof WJ, Walters DW: Scedosporium prolificans: an uncommon cause of septic arthritis, *Austr N Z J Surg* 76(7):661–663, 2006.

80. Steinbach WJ, Schell WA, Miller JL, Perfect JR: Scedosporium prolificans osteomyelitis in an immunocompetent child treated with voriconazole and caspofungin, as well as locally applied polyhexamethylene biguanide, *J Clin Microbiol* 41(8):3981–3985, 2003.

81. Studahl M, Backteman T, Stalhammar F, et al: Bone and joint infection after traumatic implantation of *Scedosporium prolificans* treated with voriconazole and surgery, *Acta Paediatr* 92(8):980–982, 2003.

82. Alexander BD, Perfect JR: Antifungal resistance trends towards the year 2000. Implications for therapy and new approaches, *Drugs* 54(5):657–678, 1997.

83. Espinel-Ingroff A: Clinical relevance of antifungal resistance, *Infect Dis Clin North Am* 11(4):929–944, 1997.

84. Martino P, Girmenia C: Are we making progress in antifungal therapy? *Curr Opin Oncol* 9(4):314–320, 1997.

85. Meier JL: Mycobacterial and fungal infections of bone and joints, *Curr Opin Rheumatol* 6(4):408–414, 1994.

86. Mora-Duarte J, Betts R, Rotstein C, et al: Comparison of caspofungin and amphotericin B for invasive candidiasis, *N Engl J Med* 347(25):2020–2029, 2002.

87. Perez-Gomez A, Prieto A, Torresano M, et al: Role of the new azoles in the treatment of fungal osteoarticular infections, *Semin Arthritis Rheum* 27(4):226–244, 1998.

88. Rapp RP, Gubbins PO, Evans ME: Amphotericin B lipid complex, *Ann Pharmacother* 31(10):1174–1186, 1997.

89. Sarosi GA, Davies SF: Therapy for fungal infections, *Mayo Clin Proc* 69(11):1111–1117, 1994.

90. Summers KK, Hardin TC, Gore SJ, Graybill JR: Therapeutic drug monitoring of systemic antifungal therapy, *J Antimicrob Chemother* 40(6):753–764, 1997.

91. Terrell CL, Hughes CE: Antifungal agents used for deep-seated mycotic infections, *Mayo Clin Proc* 67(1):69–91, 1992.

92. Currier JS, Williams PL, Koletar SL, et al: Discontinuation of *Mycobacterium avium* complex prophylaxis in patients with antiretroviral therapy–induced increases in CD4+ cell count. A randomized, double-blind, placebo-controlled trial. AIDS Clinical Trials Group 362 Study Team, *Ann Intern Med* 133(7):493–503, 2000.

93. Cenci E, Mencacci A, Fe d'Ostiani C, et al: Cytokine- and T helper–dependent lung mucosal immunity in mice with invasive pulmonary aspergillosis, *J Infect Dis* 178(6):1750–1760, 1998.

94. Marino MW, Dunn A, Grail D, Inglese M, et al: Characterization of tumor necrosis factor–deficient mice, *Proc Natl Acad Sci U S A* 94(15):8093–8098, 1997.

95. Bauman SK, Huffnagle GB, Murphy JW: Effects of tumor necrosis factor alpha on dendritic cell accumulation in lymph nodes draining the immunization site and the impact on the anticryptococcal cell-mediated immune response, *Infect Immun* 71(1):68–74, 2003.

96. Huffnagle GB, Toews GB, Burdick MD, et al: Afferent phase production of TNF-alpha is required for the development of protective T cell immunity to *Cryptococcus neoformans*, *J Immunol* 157(10):4529–4536, 1996.

97. Cox RA, Magee DM: Production of tumor necrosis factor alpha, interleukin-1 alpha, and interleukin-6 during murine coccidioidomycosis, *Infect Immun* 63(10):4178–4180, 1995.

98. Tachibana T, Matsuyama T, Mitsuyama M: Involvement of CD4+ T cells and macrophages in acquired protection against infection with *Sporothrix schenckii* in mice, *Med Mycol* 37(6):397–404, 1999.

99. Bergstrom L, Yocum DE, Ampel NM, et al: Increased risk of coccidioidomycosis in patients treated with tumor necrosis factor alpha antagonists, *Arthritis Rheum* 50(6):1959–1966, 2004.

100. Dweik M, Baethge BA, Duarte AG: Coccidioidomycosis pneumonia in a nonendemic area associated with infliximab, *South Med J* 100(5):517–518, 2007.

101. De Rosa FG, Shaz D, Campagna AC, et al: Invasive pulmonary aspergillosis soon after therapy with infliximab, a tumor necrosis factor-alpha-neutralizing antibody: a possible healthcare-associated case? *Infect Control Hosp Epidemiol* 24(7):477–482, 2003.

102. Hage CA, Wood KL, Winer-Muram HT, et al: Pulmonary cryptococcosis after initiation of anti-tumor necrosis factor-alpha therapy, *Chest* 124(6):2395–2397, 2003.

103. Ngai JC, Lam R, Ko FW, et al: Pulmonary scedosporium infection as a complication of infliximab therapy for ankylosing spondylitis, *Thorax* 64(2):184, 2009.

104. van der Klooster JM, Bosman RJ, Oudemans-van Straaten HM, et al: Disseminated tuberculosis, pulmonary aspergillosis and cutaneous herpes simplex infection in a patient with infliximab and methotrexate, *Intensive Care Med* 29(12):2327–2329, 2003.

105. Gupta D, Zachariah A, Roppelt H, et al: Prophylactic antibiotic usage for *Pneumocystis jirovecii* pneumonia in patients with systemic lupus erythematosus on cyclophosphamide: a survey of US rheumatologists and the review of literature, *J Clin Rheumatol* 14(5):267–272, 2008.

106. Kaneko Y, Suwa A, Ikeda Y, Hirakata M: *Pneumocystis jiroveci* pneumonia associated with low-dose methotrexate treatment for rheumatoid arthritis: report of two cases and review of the literature, *Mod Rheumatol* 16(1):36–38, 2006.

107. Mori S, Cho I, Ichiyasu H, Sugimoto M: Asymptomatic carriage of *Pneumocystis jiroveci* in elderly patients with rheumatoid arthritis in Japan: a possible association between colonization and development of *Pneumocystis jiroveci* pneumonia during low-dose MTX therapy, *Mod Rheumatol* 18(3):240–246, 2008.

108. Mori S, Cho I, Sugimoto M: A followup study of asymptomatic carriers of *Pneumocystis jiroveci* during immunosuppressive therapy for rheumatoid arthritis, *J Rheumatol* 36(8):1600–1605, 2009.

109. Teichmann LL, Woenckhaus M, Vogel C, et al: Fatal *Pneumocystis pneumonia* following rituximab administration for rheumatoid arthritis, *Rheumatology (Oxford)* 47(8):1256–1257, 2008.

110. Komano Y, Harigai M, Koike R, et al: *Pneumocystis jiroveci* pneumonia in patients with rheumatoid arthritis treated with infliximab: a retrospective review and case-control study of 21 patients, *Arthritis Rheum* 61(3):305–312, 2009.

111. Lertnawapan R, Totemchokchyakarn K, Nantiruj K, Janwityanujit S: Risk factors of *Pneumocystis jeroveci* pneumonia in patients with systemic lupus erythematosus, *Rheumatol Int* 29(5):491–496, 2009.

112. Moosig F, Holle JU, Gross WL: Value of anti-infective chemoprophylaxis in primary systemic vasculitis: what is the evidence? *Arthritis Res Ther* 11(5):253, 2009.

113. Cettomai D, Gelber AC, Christopher-Stine L: A survey of rheumatologists' practice for prescribing pneumocystis prophylaxis, *J Rheumatol* 37(4):792–799, 2010.

114. Kimura M, Tanaka S, Ishikawa A, et al: Comparison of trimethoprim-sulfamethoxazole and aerosolized pentamidine for primary prophylaxis of *Pneumocystis jiroveci* pneumonia in immunocompromised patients with connective tissue disease, *Rheumatol Int* 28(7):673–676, 2008.

115. Thomas CF Jr, Limper AH: Pneumocystis pneumonia, *N Engl J Med* 350(24):2487–2498, 2004.

116. Winthrop KL: Risk and prevention of tuberculosis and other serious opportunistic infections associated with the inhibition of tumor necrosis factor, *Nat Clin Pract Rheumatol* 2(11):602–610, 2006.

117. Kohli R, Hadley S: Fungal arthritis and osteomyelitis, *Infect Dis Clin North Am* 19(4):831–851, 2005.

118. Barson WJ, Marcon MJ: Successful therapy of *Candida albicans* arthritis with a sequential intravenous amphotericin B and oral fluconazole regimen, *Pediatr Infect Dis J* 15(12):1119–1122, 1996.

119. Kaur N, Mahl TC: *Pneumocystis jiroveci (carinii)* pneumonia after infliximab therapy: a review of 84 cases, *Dig Dis Sci* 52(6):1481–1484, 2007.

The references for this chapter can also be found on www.expertconsult.com.

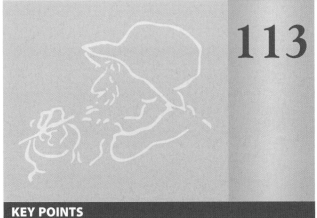

113 Rheumatic Manifestations of Human Immunodeficiency Virus Infection

JOHN D. REVEILLE • EMILY W. HUNG

KEY POINTS

With patients with human immunodeficiency virus (HIV) living longer as a result of more effective and available treatments, the challenges of HIV-associated rheumatic manifestations are growing.

Certain diseases seem to be particular to HIV infection (i.e., HIV-associated arthritis, diffuse infiltrative lymphocytosis syndrome [DILS], HIV-associated polymyositis).

Other diseases, specifically CD4-mediated diseases such as rheumatoid arthritis and systemic lupus erythematosus, tend to go into remission with disease activity and to flare with antiretroviral treatment.

Effective antiretroviral therapy has resulted in certain diseases (i.e., DILS, late opportunistic infections) decreasing in prevalence but also is associated with new side effects (e.g., osteonecrosis, myopathy, rhabdomyolysis).

With immune reconstitution after antiretroviral therapy, a new spectrum of autoimmune and autoinflammatory disease has emerged requiring special attention.

In the years since acquired immunodeficiency syndrome (AIDS) was initially described in 1981, the human immunodeficiency virus (HIV) pandemic has become one of the leading global health crises. According to new data in the Joint United Programme on HIV/AIDS (UNAIDS) 2008 report, the AIDS epidemic seems to be slowing down globally, but new cases are continuing to increase at alarming rates in certain regions, such as southern Africa, eastern Europe, and central and eastern Asia. An estimated 33 million people worldwide are living with HIV (Figure 113-1). Approximately 2.7 million people became newly infected with HIV in 2007, and 2 million people died.

Progress in dealing with the HIV epidemic, including progress in education and in public health awareness, has undoubtedly influenced the decrease in prevalence seen among young people in some countries in recent years. As availability of newer treatment strategies and better access to health care result in increased life expectancy in the next decade, it is expected that HIV infection will be managed increasingly as a chronic illness, and complications such as musculoskeletal and rheumatic conditions associated with HIV infection and its treatment are expected to increase (Tables 113-1 and 113-2).

Among the rheumatologic disorders, clinicians face the challenge of treating potentially disabling inflammatory disorders with immunosuppressive therapy in the face of ongoing viral-induced immunocompromise. Diagnosing infection is especially important in an immunocompromised patient because the probability of an opportunistic infection as a cause for a musculoskeletal complaint increases with advancing stages of the patient's HIV disease. At early stages (CD4$^+$ count >300/μL), opportunistic infections are unlikely, although bacterial infections (especially tuberculosis) still can occur. There should be a very high threshold for using immunosuppressive drugs in this population.

HIV-ASSOCIATED BONE AND JOINT DISEASE

HIV-Associated Arthralgia

More than 5% of HIV-positive patients may have otherwise unexplained arthralgia. Arthralgias and myalgias also form a part of the constitutional symptoms of HIV seroconversion. Whether arthralgia can be attributed to circulating viral and host immune complexes owing to HIV infection per se or to other infections (e.g., hepatitis C) has not been determined. The pathogenesis is unclear but may involve cytokines or transient bone ischemia.[1] However, patients presenting with arthralgia alone rarely progress to inflammatory joint disease. The most appropriate treatment consists of non-narcotic analgesics and reassurance.

Painful Articular Syndrome

Painful articular syndrome is a self-limited syndrome lasting less than 24 hours, associated with few objective clinical findings, and characterized by severe bone and joint pain.[2] It occurs predominantly in the late stages of HIV infection. Its cause is unknown, and no evidence of synovitis has been found in these patients. The knee is most commonly affected, but the elbow and shoulders also can be involved. Radiographic features are nonspecific; occasionally, periarticular osteopenia is seen. Treatment is symptomatic.

HIV-Associated Arthritis

The first reports of a seronegative arthritis associated with HIV infection appeared in 1988, with frequencies of 12%. HIV-associated arthritis seems to be most common in sub-Saharan Africa, where HIV infection is pandemic. In the Congo, where the seroprevalence of HIV infection is 7% to 8%, AIDS is the leading cause of aseptic arthritis (60% of cases).[3] This is usually an oligoarthritis (Table 113-3),

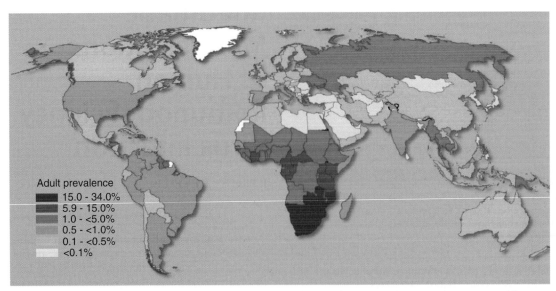

Figure 113-1   A global view of human immunodeficiency virus (HIV) infection—33 million living with HIV in 2007. *(Extracted from* 2008 Report on the Global AIDS Epidemic, *UNAIDS, 2008.)*

predominantly involving the lower extremities, and tends to be self-limited, lasting less than 6 weeks.[2,4] Most commonly involved are the knees (84%), ankles (59%), and metatarsophalangeal joints (23%) in the lower limbs, and the wrists (41%), elbows (29%), and metacarpophalangeal and interphalangeal joints (25%) in the upper limbs, similar to other viral arthritides. Some patients have been reported as having a longer course, with joint destruction.[5,6]

The origin is unclear; no association has been noted with HLA-B27 or any other known genetic factor. Synovial fluid cultures are typically sterile, although one report described the presence of tubuloreticular inclusions, suggesting a viral origin, possibly HIV itself.[2,4] Radiographs of affected joints are usually normal, except in uncommon cases with prolonged symptoms, in which joint space narrowing and destruction can occur. Treatment includes nonsteroidal anti-inflammatory drugs (NSAIDs) and, in more severe cases, low-dose glucocorticoids. Hydroxychloroquine and sulfasalazine also have been used.[7]

Reactive Arthritis Occurring in HIV Infection

Early reports in the United States suggested that reactive arthritis occurred more commonly in the setting of HIV infection; however, later studies showed that this may be reflective of the sexually active nature of the population at highest risk for HIV infection.[8] This contention is not borne out in studies from sub-Saharan Africa, where HLA-B27 is rare, as were reports of spondyloarthritis before the HIV epidemic. With the arrival of AIDS, a dramatic upsurge in the prevalence of reactive arthritis and undifferentiated spondyloarthritis, and less often psoriatic arthritis,[6,9] was seen, suggesting a pathogenic role of HIV infection.

The typical presentation is a seronegative lower extremity peripheral arthritis, usually accompanied by enthesitis (dactylitis, Achilles tendinitis, and plantar fasciitis). Mucocutaneous features are common, especially keratoderma blennorrhagicum (Figure 113-2) and circinate balanitis. Extensive psoriasiform skin rashes can occur. The clinical overlap makes it difficult sometimes to distinguish HIV-associated reactive arthritis from psoriatic arthritis.[10]

Table 113-1   Rheumatic Diseases Associated with or Occurring in Patients with Human Immunodeficiency Virus (HIV) Infection

Unique to HIV Infection	Encountered in HIV-Infected Patients	Ameliorated by HIV Infection but Worsening or Reappearing with IRIS
Diffuse infiltrative lymphocytosis syndrome	HIV-associated reactive arthritis	Rheumatoid arthritis
HIV-associated arthritis	Polymyositis	Systemic lupus erythematosus
Zidovudine-associated myopathy	Psoriatic arthritis	
	Polyarteritis nodosa	
	Giant cell arteritis	
Painful articular syndrome	Hypersensitivity angiitis	
	Granulomatosis with polyangiitis	
	Henoch-Schönlein purpura	
	Behçet's syndrome	
	Infectious arthritis (bacterial, fungal)	

IRIS, immune reconstitution inflammatory syndrome.

Table 113-2   Distribution of Various Rheumatic Diseases from Various Sites

Feature	Cincinnati, Ohio	Houston, Texas	Madrid, Spain
No. of patients	1100	4467	556
HIV-associated arthralgia	NA	0.7%	1.6%
Myalgia	0.7%	0.6%	4.5%
PsA/Reactive arthritis	0.5%	0.6%	0.5%
HIV-associated arthritis	0%	0.5%	0.4%
DILS/Sjögren's syndrome	NR	3%-4%	NR

DILS, diffuse infiltrative lymphocytosis syndrome; HIV, human immunodeficiency virus; NA, not applicable; NR, not reported; PsA, psoriatic arthritis.

Table 113-3 Contrasting Features of Human Immunodeficiency Virus (HIV)–Associated Arthritis and Reactive Arthritis

Feature	HIV-Associated Arthritis	HIV-Associated Reactive Arthritis
Joint involvement	Asymmetric oligoarthritis/ polyarthritis	Asymmetric oligoarthritis/ polyarthritis
Mucocutaneous involvement	Absent	Present
Enthesopathy	Absent	Frequent
Synovial fluid white blood cell count	500-2000/μL	2000-10,000/μL
Synovial fluid cultures	Negative	Negative
Microorganisms in synovial membranes	HIV virus (?)	Chlamydia*
HLA-B27 association	Absent	70%-90%†

*Shown in non–HIV-associated reactive arthritis. Reports of such infections in patients with HIV-associated reactive arthritis are lacking.
†In whites.

Urethritis occurs in similar frequency as in HIV-negative reactive arthritis. Axial involvement and uveitis seem to be less common but do occur. Longitudinal studies from Africa have described an aggressive course with a poor prognosis.[11,12]

HLA-B27 is found in 80% to 90% of patients with HIV-associated reactive arthritis, at least among whites.[10] Studies from Africa have found most patients to be HLA-B27 negative, however.[6,9] Some studies suggest that the presence of HLA-B27 antigen may slow the progression to AIDS.[11,12] In asymptomatic HIV-infected, HLA-B27–positive individuals, cytotoxic T lymphocyte response is dominated by recognition of a gag-encoded p24 protein epitope that is not seen in HIV-positive, HLA-B27–negative individuals.[13,14] Other human leukocyte antigen (HLA) class I antigens that have been associated with a better outcome in HIV

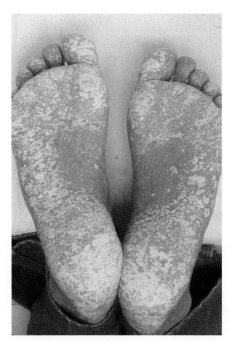

Figure 113-2 Keratoderma blennorrhagicum in a patient with reactive arthritis and human immunodeficiency virus infection.

infection have been implicated in psoriasis and psoriatic arthritis and include HLA-B13 and HLA-B17 (B57, B58).[12,13] HLA-B*5703 was protective against HIV progression in a Zambian population but conferred susceptibility to spondyloarthritis.[15]

Treatment

Treatment is similar to that for HIV-negative patients with reactive arthritis. NSAIDs are the mainstay; in particular, indomethacin is recommended, not only for its efficacy, but also for its inhibition of HIV replication that has been observed in vitro, which seems to be unique to this NSAID.[16] Patients frequently have an inadequate response to NSAIDs alone. Sulfasalazine has been shown to be effective in some studies at doses of 2 g/day, and one study suggested that it ameliorated HIV infection.[17,18] Methotrexate was initially believed to be contraindicated because of its immunosuppressive effect, but with careful monitoring of HIV viral loads, CD4+ counts, and the patient's clinical status, more recent studies have suggested a place for methotrexate in the treatment of reactive arthritis and psoriatic arthritis occurring in HIV infection.[19]

Hydroxychloroquine has been reported to be efficacious not only in treating HIV-associated reactive arthritis, but also in reducing HIV replication in vitro and in reducing HIV viral loads in vivo.[20] Arthritis and the cutaneous lesions of HIV-associated reactive arthritis and psoriatic arthritis have been found to respond to etretinate (0.5 to 1 mg/kg/day),[21] although because of the side effects of this drug, its use should be reserved for patients unresponsive to other treatments. Tumor necrosis factor blockers have been used,[22,23] although these agents should be used with extreme caution and only in patients with CD4+ counts greater than 200/μL and HIV viral load less than 60,000 copies/mm³.[24,25] One prospective study of eight HIV patients with spondyloarthritis or rheumatoid arthritis found tumor necrosis factor blockers effective and safe for up to 5 years when these precautions were followed at initiation of therapy.[25]

Psoriasis and Psoriatic Arthritis

The extent of skin involvement with psoriasis can be extensive (Figure 113-3) in HIV-positive patients, especially in patients not on antiretroviral treatment. Of note, cutaneous T cell lymphoma can resemble psoriasis and should be considered in the differential diagnosis of psoriasis in HIV-positive individuals.[26] A report from Zambia found 27 of 28 African patients with psoriatic arthritis to be HIV positive.[27] The arthritis was predominantly polyarticular, lower limb, and progressive. Psoriasis was commonly an extensive guttate-plaque admixture and, in contrast to the articular disease, was nonremittive with the onset of AIDS.[28] Antiretroviral treatment has been shown to be effective in treating HIV-associated psoriasis and its associated arthritis.[29] Phototherapy may improve the skin rash but also may enhance viral replication, worsen HIV disease, and increase the risk of skin cancer. Other agents reported to be efficacious include cyclosporine (although renal function must be monitored carefully) and etretinate. Methotrexate also can be used, albeit with caution.[19] Tumor necrosis factor blockers can be used in patients with refractory disease, and a

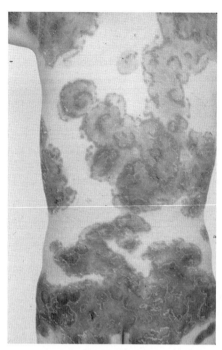

Figure 113-3 Disseminated psoriasis vulgaris in a patient with human immunodeficiency virus–associated psoriasis.

number of patients have shown dramatic improvement in skin lesions and in arthritis,[24,25] although with the usual precautions (see earlier) because frequent polymicrobial infections while on the drug resulted in its discontinuation in some patients.[30]

Undifferentiated Spondyloarthritis

Symptoms of reactive arthritis or psoriatic arthritis such as enthesopathy (plantar fasciitis, Achilles tendinitis) are observed in patients who do not otherwise develop full-blown disease.[31] Treatment is symptomatic (NSAIDs, intralesional corticosteroid injections), although sulfasalazine should be considered in patients with more extensive disease.

Avascular Necrosis of Bone

Most cases of osteonecrosis have occurred after the introduction of highly active antiretroviral therapy (HAART).[32] Dyslipidemia associated with protease inhibitors has been implicated most frequently, although no controlled studies have been performed to establish whether antiretroviral drugs per se predispose to this.[33] Other contributing factors include alcohol abuse and use of corticosteroids, megestrol acetate, antiphospholipid antibodies,[34] and intravenous drug abuse,[35] as well as HIV itself. The most common presenting symptom of osteonecrosis is pain on weight bearing and activity. Some patients may be asymptomatic, and the diagnosis is made based on incidental findings in radiologic studies. Most patients tend to present when subchondral collapse already has occurred. Radiographs, computed tomography (CT), magnetic resonance imaging (MRI), and nuclear medicine studies have been used successfully to diagnose osteonecrosis, as in HIV-negative patients.

Hypertrophic Pulmonary Osteoarthropathy

Hypertrophic pulmonary osteoarthropathy affects bones, joints, and soft tissues and can develop in HIV-infected patients with *Pneumocystis jiroveci* pneumonia. It is characterized by severe pain in the lower extremity; digital clubbing; arthralgia; nonpitting edema; and periarticular soft tissue involvement of the ankles, knees, and elbows. The skin over the affected areas is glistening, edematous, and warm. Radiography reveals extensive periosteal reaction and subperiosteal proliferative changes in the long bones of the lower extremity. A bone scan shows increased uptake along the cortical surfaces. Treatment of *P. jiroveci* pneumonia usually alleviates this condition.[36]

Osteopenia and Osteoporosis

Osteopenia and osteoporosis occur more than three times as commonly in HIV-infected patients regardless of antiretroviral treatment[37] and can result in pathologic fractures. One meta-analysis found 15% of HIV-positive patients to have osteoporosis, and 52% to have osteopenia.[38] Abnormal bone metabolism was attributed to the HIV infection itself by some authors.[38] Risk factors for the development of osteopenia include use of protease inhibitors, longer duration of HIV infection, high viral load, high lactate levels, low bicarbonate levels, increased alkaline phosphatase levels, and lower body weight before antiretroviral therapy.[39] Vitamin D deficiency is also common in HIV patients, with reported frequency of 47% for moderate to severe vitamin D deficiency in one cohort.[40] A retrospective review of 211 HIV-positive patients found vitamin D deficiency to be associated with concomitant hepatitis C infection, previous AIDS, and higher CD4+ counts.[41] Clinicians should have a low threshold to screen for vitamin D deficiency and should provide adequate repletion as necessary. Bisphosphonates and, in patients with HIV wasting syndrome, testosterone, have been used to preserve bone density.[42]

HIV-ASSOCIATED MUSCLE DISEASE

Muscle involvement in HIV infection varies from uncomplicated myalgias or asymptomatic creatine kinase elevation to severe, disabling, HIV-associated polymyositis or pyomyositis (Table 113-4). HIV seroconversion also can coincide with myoglobinuria and acute myalgia, suggesting that myotropism for HIV may be present early in the infection.

Myalgia and Fibromyalgia

One-third of HIV-positive outpatients report myalgias,[43] and 11% describe fibromyalgia.[44] Fibromyalgia is associated with longer disease duration and a history of depression. Treatment is similar to that for fibromyalgia in the non-HIV setting.

Noninflammatory Necrotizing Myopathy and HIV-Related Wasting Syndrome

Severe wasting from chronic infection, malignancy, malabsorption, and nutritional deficiency often accounts for

Table 113-4   Myopathies Associated with Human Immunodeficiency Virus (HIV) Infection

HIV-Associated Myopathies	Myopathies Secondary to Antiretrovirals	Others
HIV polymyositis	Zidovudine myopathy	Opportunistic infections involving
Inclusion body myositis	Toxic mitochondrial myopathies related	muscle (toxoplasmosis)
Nemaline myopathy	to other NRTIs	Tumor infiltrations of skeletal muscle
Diffuse infiltrative lymphocytosis syndrome	HIV-associated lipodystrophy syndrome	Rhabdomyolysis
HIV wasting syndrome	Immune reconstitution syndrome related	
Vasculitic processes	to HAART	
Myasthenia gravis and other myasthenic syndromes		
Chronic fatigue and fibromyalgia		

HAART, highly active antiretroviral therapy; NRTIs, nucleoside reverse transcriptase inhibitors.

weakness and disability in patients with AIDS. This wasting leads to loss of lean body and muscle mass. Cachexia and muscle wasting associated with HIV constitute slim disease in Africa. A noninflammatory necrotizing myopathy of unclear pathogenesis has been described, accounting for 42% of patients diagnosed with myopathy.[45] Even in patients without significant wasting, muscle biopsy specimens have shown diffuse atrophy, mild neurogenic atrophy, or thick filament loss without conspicuous inflammation. Whether this condition is immune mediated, as some have suggested,[46] or whether it is due to metabolic or nutritional factors remains unclear. Corticosteroids have been reported to restore muscle strength and mass.[47]

Nemaline Myopathy

Nemaline myopathy is a rare disorder that has been described in some HIV-positive patients, in addition to its occurrence as a congenital disorder. Nemaline myopathy represents a nonspecific myofibril alteration resulting from Z band disruption.[48] Muscle biopsy specimens disclose prominent, randomly distributed atrophic type 1 fibers with numerous intracytoplasmic rod bodies in the centers of the fibers, corresponding to nemaline rods at electron microscopy. Necrotic fibers and inflammatory infiltrates usually are not found. Some patients have been described to have associated monoclonal gammopathy.[49] Although no inflammation is noted, corticosteroids may be useful. In addition, two cases of successful treatment with intravenous immunoglobulin (IVIG) have been reported.[50]

HIV-Associated Polymyositis

HIV-associated polymyositis most typically manifests early in the course of HIV infection and may be the presenting feature. In one large series of HIV-positive outpatients from a county clinic in Texas, the frequency was 2.2 per 1000.[51] The pathogenesis of HIV-associated polymyositis is unclear—possibly stemming from direct viral invasion (leading to a cytopathic effect and subsequent muscle necrosis), as suggested in one pathologic study,[52] or from an autoimmune response of the HIV host, as suggested by another study.[53]

The most common manifestation is a subacute, progressive proximal muscle weakness occurring in the setting of an elevated creatine kinase. Myalgia is not a prominent presenting feature. Skin involvement is unusual, as is involvement of extraocular muscles and facial muscles. On the other hand, only a handful of cases of dermatomyositis

in HIV have been reported, usually in the setting of advanced immunodeficiency.[54]

It has been suggested that creatine kinase levels may be less elevated or even normal in some HIV-associated polymyositis patients. One retrospective report from sub-Saharan Africa found that creatine kinase elevations were fourfold lower in those with HIV-associated polymyositis than in patients with polymyositis without HIV infection.[55]

On MRI, T2-weighted studies with or without fat saturation show high signal intensity without rim enhancement, in contrast to pyomyositis, in which rim enhancement is seen.[56] MRI also is helpful in guiding muscle biopsy—the definitive diagnostic test. Electromyographic studies reveal myopathic motor unit potentials with early recruitment and full interference patterns and fibrillation potentials, positive sharp waves, and complex repetitive discharges indicative of an irritative process. Light microscopy of muscle biopsy specimens shows interstitial inflammatory infiltrates of variable intensity accompanied by degenerating and regenerating myofibrils, similar to those seen in polymyositis without HIV (Figure 113-4). Concomitant vasculitis rarely occurs. In specimens from HIV-positive and HIV-negative patients with myositis, the predominant cell populations were CD8+ T cells and macrophages invading or surrounding healthy muscle fibers that express major histocompatibility complex (MHC) class I antigens on their cell surfaces.[57] Endomysial infiltrates in specimens from HIV-positive patients differed from those of patients with polymyositis without HIV infection only by a significant reduction of CD4+ cells.[53]

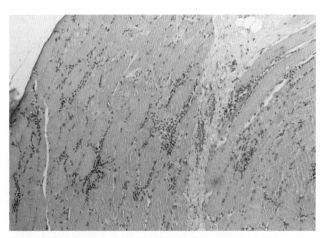

Figure 113-4   Muscle biopsy specimen from a patient with human immunodeficiency virus–associated polymyositis.

Treatment is similar to that provided for other inflammatory myopathies. Creatine kinase elevation and muscle weakness respond to moderate-dose glucocorticoids.[51] Refractory cases may require immunosuppressive agents, such as methotrexate, azathioprine, or mycophenolate mofetil. Intravenous immunoglobulin has been used with some success. These agents should be used with caution, however, with careful monitoring of the patient's clinical status, CD4+ counts, and HIV mRNA levels.

Creatine kinase elevation is commonly encountered in outpatients with HIV infection, secondary to HIV per se, behaviors associated with higher risk for HIV infection (e.g., cocaine use), or HIV treatment.[51] In most patients, these elevations are transient and are of little consequence, but they require careful follow-up for any sign of clinical deterioration before electrodiagnostic and biopsy studies are undertaken.

Inclusion Body Myositis

Inclusion body myositis has been recognized as a complication of HIV infection.[58] This condition is clinically, histologically, and immunologically identical to sporadic inclusion body myositis. Muscle biopsy specimens suggest two concurrently ongoing processes—an autoimmune process mediated by cytotoxic T cells and a degenerative process manifested by vacuolated muscle fibers and deposits of amyloid-related proteins. Of particular interest has been the finding of elevated mRNA levels and constitutive expression of Toll-like receptor 3, which is known to mediate inflammatory stimuli from pathogens and endogenous danger signals, and to link the innate and adaptive immune systems, in muscle fibers of patients with HIV-associated inclusion body myositis in close proximity with infiltrating mononuclear cells.[59] One review of four cases of HIV-associated inclusion body myositis found that involved CD8+ cells surrounding muscle fibers were virus-specific and may cross-react with antigens on the surface of muscle fibers, suggesting that HIV may trigger a viral-specific inflammatory response that can lead to inclusion body myositis.[60]

Myopathy Associated with Treatment

A reversible toxic mitochondrial myopathy occurring in patients who received high doses of zidovudine has been described, which manifests as myalgias, muscle tenderness, and proximal muscle weakness mimicking HIV polymyositis.[61] Reports have also described mitochondrial toxicity presenting as ptosis or ophthalmoplegia in HIV-positive patients on zidovudine and other nucleoside reverse transcriptase inhibitors (NRTIs) such as didanosine.[62,63] Histologically, it is characterized by the presence of *ragged red fibers,* a term coined to designate atrophic ragged red fibers with marked myofibril alterations, including thick myofilament loss and cytoplasmic body formation,[64] and minimal inflammatory infiltrates. Symptoms tend to improve as the drug is discontinued, with creatine kinase levels returning to normal within 4 weeks of discontinuing the drug, and muscle strength returning within 8 weeks. In any HIV-infected patient presenting with an elevated creatine kinase, especially when symptoms of myalgia or muscle weakness

are present, zidovudine should be discontinued for 4 weeks and the patient re-evaluated before electromyography or muscle biopsies are undertaken.

Rhabdomyolysis

Rhabdomyolysis can occur at all stages of HIV infection and may be separated into three groups: (1) HIV-associated rhabdomyolysis, including rhabdomyolysis in primary HIV infection, recurrent rhabdomyolysis, and isolated rhabdomyolysis; (2) drug-induced rhabdomyolysis; and (3) rhabdomyolysis at the end stage of AIDS, associated or not with opportunistic infection of muscle. Drugs implicated in rhabdomyolysis in HIV patients include didanosine, lamivudine, trimethoprim-sulfamethoxazole, ritonavir, indinavir, and raltegravir.[65,66]

DIFFUSE INFILTRATIVE LYMPHOCYTOSIS SYNDROME

Diffuse infiltrative lymphocytosis syndrome (DILS), found exclusively in HIV-positive patients, is characterized by salivary gland enlargement and peripheral CD8+ lymphocytosis often accompanied by sicca symptoms and other extraglandular features. The prevalence of DILS is declining since the introduction of HAART.[67] Using parotid enlargement as a criterion, the prevalence in Houston, Texas, was 4% in the pre-HAART era, declining to 0.8% after the introduction of aggressive HIV therapy.[67,68] In another study from Greece, using xerophthalmia and xerostomia as the defining criteria (and requiring confirmatory minor salivary gland biopsy specimen and technetium scintigraphy),[69] the prevalence of DILS was 7.8% and decreased dramatically after the introduction of HAART.

The primary immunogenetic association has been with HLA-DRB1 alleles expressing the ILEDE amino acid sequence in the third diversity region—usually HLA-DRB1*1102, DRB1*1301, and DRB1*1302.[67,70] Delayed progression to AIDS in patients with DILS has been attributed to delay in the evolution of the HIV virus from the less aggressive M-tropic strain to the more rapidly replicating T-tropic strain by a more effective CD8+ lymphocyte response.[70] This response has been attributed in part to the finding of sequence homology of a six-residue epitope shared by HLA-DRB1 alleles associated with DILS with a V3 loop on M-tropic HIV strains. Studies of immunophenotypes of circulating and tissue-infiltrating lymphocytes and salivary gland T cell receptor sequence analysis suggested that DILS represents an MHC-restricted, antigen-driven, oligoclonal selection of CD8+, CD29− lymphocytes that express selective homing receptors and infiltrate the salivary glands, lungs, and other organs, where they are postulated to suppress HIV replication.[71]

Minor salivary gland biopsy specimens show a focal sialadenitis, similar to that observed in Sjögren's syndrome, although destruction of the salivary glands tends to be lessened (Figure 113-5). CD8+ lymphocytes constitute most of the inflammatory infiltrate,[72,73] in contrast to that seen in primary (non–HIV-associated) Sjögren's syndrome. Lymphoepithelial cysts are seen frequently in the parotid glands of patients with DILS, leading to inspissated salivary secretions that may be painful.

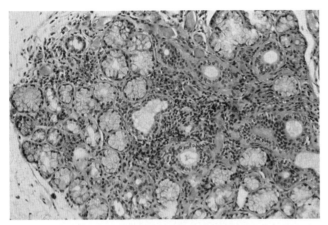

Figure 113-5 Minor salivary gland biopsy specimen from a patient with diffuse infiltrative lymphocytosis syndrome. Note the relative preservation of the glandular architecture, even with significant interstitial inflammation.

The characteristic, if not defining, presentation of DILS consists of painless parotid enlargement, often massive (Figure 113-6). This enlargement is accompanied by sicca symptoms in more than 60% of patients. Although parotid and submandibular enlargement is nearly universal in this disorder, certain extraglandular features also are prominent (Table 113-5). DILS and Sjögren's syndrome share some similarities and differences (Table 113-6).

Diagnostic criteria have been proposed for DILS as follows:

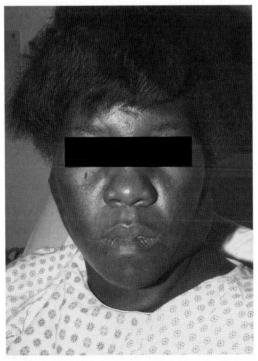

Figure 113-6 Massive bilateral asymmetric salivary gland enlargement in a patient with diffuse infiltrative lymphocytosis syndrome. This was the presenting feature of human immunodeficiency virus infection in this patient. Computed tomography revealed this to be a solid mass. At follow-up 2 years after this photograph was taken, the gland had not changed in size.

Table 113-5 Extraglandular Features of Diffuse Infiltrative Lymphocytosis Syndrome

Pulmonary
Lymphocytic interstitial pneumonitis*
Neurologic
Cranial nerve VII palsy[†] Aseptic lymphocytic meningitis Peripheral neuropathy
Gastrointestinal
Lymphocytic hepatitis
Renal
Renal tubular acidosis Interstitial nephritis
Musculoskeletal
Peripheral arthritis Polymyositis
Hematologic
Lymphoma[‡]

*25% to 50%, but decreasing.
 †Due to mechanical compression by inflamed parotid tissue.
 ‡Poor prognostic indicator.

1. HIV seropositive by enzyme-linked immunosorbent assay and Western blot analysis.
2. Bilateral salivary gland enlargement or xerostomia persisting for longer than 6 months.
3. Histologic confirmation of salivary or lacrimal gland lymphocytic infiltration in the absence of granulomatous or neoplastic enlargement.

Minor salivary gland biopsy specimens are usually positive (see Figure 113-5). Gallium-67 scintigraphy (Figure 113-7) of the salivary glands has been used when lip biopsy was not feasible or equivocal. Tc99m pertechnetate scanning offers little diagnostic help. Scintigraphy is used as a primary diagnostic aid in patients on protease inhibitors because minor salivary gland biopsy specimens are rarely positive in patients on these drugs. CT also has been used to determine the extent of glandular swelling and to evaluate parotid cysts and possible salivary glandular malignancy.

Patients with asymptomatic glandular swelling and mild, if any, sicca symptoms can be observed over time (Table 113-7). Antiretroviral treatment is effective in treating the glandular swelling and sicca symptoms associated with DILS

Table 113-6 Similarities and Differences between Diffuse Infiltrative Lymphocytosis Syndrome (DILS) and Sjögren's Syndrome

Feature	DILS	Sjögren's Syndrome
Parotid swelling	Ubiquitous	Uncommon
Sicca symptoms	Common	Very common
Extraglandular symptoms	Common	Uncommon
Autoantibodies (antinuclear antibodies, anti-Ro/La)	Rare	Common
HLA class II association	DRB1*1102, DRB1*1301, DRB1*1302	DRB1*0301, DQA1*0501, DQB1*0201

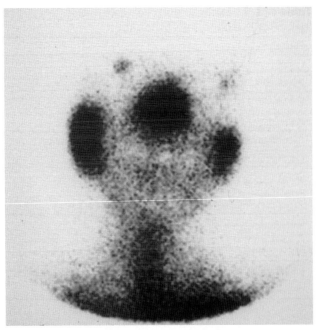

Figure 113-7 The "snowman" sign. Gallium-67 scintigraphy of the parotid glands of a patient with diffuse infiltrative lymphocytosis syndrome occurring in the setting of hemophilia.

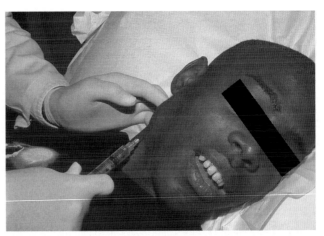

Figure 113-8 Aspiration of a parotid epithelial cyst in a patient with diffuse infiltrative lymphocytosis syndrome.

and complications such as neuropathy.[67] We have found also that moderate doses of corticosteroids (30 to 40 mg/day of prednisone) are effective in treating the glandular swelling and sicca symptoms of DILS without adversely affecting the frequency of opportunistic infections, increasing the viral loads, or depressing the CD4[+] counts, although the effect is transient. Lymphocytic interstitial pneumonitis may require higher doses of corticosteroids (60 mg/day of prednisone), sometimes for extended periods. Radiation therapy should be avoided. Cranial nerve VII palsy tends to respond poorly to any treatment. Combination antiretroviral therapy has been reported to be effective in resolving parotid epithelial cysts, although when refractory, the cysts can be managed by aspiration and instillation of 1 mL (40 mg) of either methylprednisolone or triamcinolone suspension into the cyst (Figure 113-8). Frequent recurrence may necessitate surgical excision.

VASCULITIS ASSOCIATED WITH HIV INFECTION

A wide spectrum of vasculitis has been described in patients with HIV infection.[74,75] Fever, malaise, weakness, rash,

Table 113-7 Treatment of Diffuse Infiltrative Lymphocytosis Syndrome

Reassurance and education
Regular dental care
No specific treatment for asymptomatic individuals
Effective antiretroviral treatment
Pilocarpine or cevimeline for sicca symptoms
Systemic glucocorticoids
Drainage and instillation of corticosteroids into parotid
  lymphoepithelial cysts
Radiation of parotid cysts

headaches, and neurologic symptoms are common in HIV-positive patients, and triggers of vasculitis range from specific infectious agents and drugs to idiopathic causes. Among infectious causes, cytomegalovirus and tuberculosis are probably the most common. Inflammatory vasculitides are less common rheumatologic diseases that occur in less than 1% of HIV patients.

One series found 34 (23%) of 148 "symptomatic" HIV-positive patients to have vasculitis.[76] Of these patients, 11 met American College of Rheumatology criteria for a distinct category of vasculitis, including hypersensitivity vasculitis in 6, polyarteritis nodosa in 4, and Henoch-Schönlein purpura in 1. Another series of 98 Chinese patients found that 20% had vasculitis, including 15 with Behçet's-like disease, 2 cases of Henoch-Schönlein purpura, 2 cases of digital gangrene, and 1 case of central nervous system vasculitis.[77] Granulomatosis with polyangiitis (formerly Wegener's granulomatosis) and pulmonary microscopic polyangiitis can occur in patients with high CD4[+] counts and during immune reconstitution. Churg-Strauss vasculitis has also been described.[78] Behçet's syndrome and relapsing polychondritis occur in HIV infection[79] and respond to HAART.[80] Rapidly progressive focal necrotizing vasculitis of the aorta and large arteries with aneurysm formation and rupture has been described in Africans with HIV infection.[81] Giant cell arteritis likewise has been described in patients with HIV infection with aortic root dilation.[82] Kawasaki disease has been reported in HIV-positive children and adults.[83] Cryoglobulinemic vasculitis with associated lymphocytic interstitial pneumonia occurs with and without hepatitis C co-infection.

Patients with isolated central nervous system angiitis usually present with organic brain syndromes and neurologic deficit.[84] In children and in one case report in an adult, HIV-associated cerebral aneurysmal arteriopathy was described as causing multiple fusiform aneurysms in the circle of Willis.[85] Central nervous system vasculitis may manifest as recurrent strokes. Although imaging studies (MRI, angiography) may be helpful, brain biopsy may be necessary to establish the diagnosis. Necrotizing granulomatous vasculitis not limited to the central nervous system has been reported in patients with low CD4[+] counts that respond to antiretroviral therapy.[74] More recently, a case report has described leukocytoclastic cerebral vasculitis treated with anti-CD25 antibody.[86]

Diagnosis is based on a high degree of suspicion and on angiography and biopsy of specific organ beds. Similar to immunocompetent patients, perinuclear antineutrophil cytoplasmic antigen (pANCA) and cytoplasmic antineutrophil cytoplasmic antigen (cANCA) may be useful with granulomatosis with polyangiitis or microscopic polyangiitis. However, biopsy with cultures is important to rule out infectious mimics.

Corticosteroids are the mainstay of treatment for HIV-associated vasculitis, although cytotoxic agents such as cyclophosphamide, intravenous immunoglobulin, and plasmapheresis have been used in refractory cases. Painful neuropathy secondary to vasculitis responds well to high-dose glucocorticoids, in contrast to HIV-associated peripheral neuropathy.[87]

PRIMARY PULMONARY HYPERTENSION

Pulmonary hypertension is a severe life-limiting disease that often affects younger patients. Patients with AIDS and primary pulmonary hypertension present with a higher degree of pulmonary hypertension than non-AIDS patients.[88,89] The predominant histopathologic finding has been a plexogenic pulmonary arteriopathy, although thromboembolic changes also have been reported. One group found an association with HLA-DRB1*1301 and HLA-DRB1*1302 and with the linked allele HLA-DRB3*0301.[90]

Symptoms include progressive shortness of breath, pedal edema, nonproductive cough, fatigue, syncope or near-syncope, and chest pain. Pulmonary function tests show mild restrictive patterns with variably reduced diffusing capacities. In a review of 131 cases of pulmonary hypertension associated with HIV infection, the interval between the diagnosis of HIV disease and the diagnosis of pulmonary hypertension was 33 months. The median length of time from diagnosis to death was 6 months.[91] Responses to vasodilator agents—calcium channel blockers, sildenafil, intravenous and inhaled prostanoids, and endothelin antagonists—and to HAART vary, and some studies show improved mortality.[92]

HIV-ASSOCIATED MUSCULOSKELETAL INFECTION

Pyomyositis

Pyomyositis is a primary infection of skeletal muscle that does not arise from contiguous infection; it is presumably hematogenous in origin and often is associated with abscess formation. Rarely seen in developed countries, infectious myositis nonetheless is an important complication of HIV infection in areas most endemic for HIV, such as Africa and India. It tends to occur in later stages of the infection, with CD4+ counts less than 200/µL. *Staphylococcus aureus* is the most common pathogen.[93] Other organisms that have been implicated include *Streptococcus pyogenes, Cryptococcus neoformans, Mycobacterium tuberculosis, Mycobacterium avium-intracellulare, Nocardia asteroides, Salmonella enteritidis,*

Escherichia coli, Citrobacter freundii, Morganella morganii, Pseudomonas aeruginosa, and group A streptococci.

The clinical course of pyomyositis can be roughly divided into three stages: invasive, suppurative, and late. The first stage, which typically lasts 1 to 3 weeks, is characterized by localized cramp-like pain and induration in conjunction with a low-grade fever. Large muscle groups, particularly those of the lower extremities, are most often affected. The degrees of pain and fever increase in the second stage, which is characterized further by the development of edema and pus in the affected muscle. Untreated, the disease progresses to the third stage; within 3 weeks of onset, sepsis and death can occur.[94] The mortality rate associated with pyomyositis has been estimated to range from 1% to 20%. Ultrasound and MRI with contrast enhancement are effective in localizing infection, although sometimes, tagged white blood cell scans may be needed. Oral and intravenous antibiotics in conjunction with surgical drainage are often required.

Bacterial Arthritis and Osteomyelitis

No data suggest that bacterial infection of bones or joints occurs more frequently in patients with HIV infection. *S. aureus* is the most common infectious agent encountered, but parenteral drug use and not HIV infection per se may account for this. Many other organisms have been reported to cause osteomyelitis in HIV-infected patients, including *Mycobacterium tuberculosis, Salmonella, Nocardia asteroides, Streptococcus pneumoniae, Neisseria gonorrhoeae,* cytomegalovirus, invasive *Aspergillus, Toxoplasma gondii, Torulopsis glabrata, Cryptococcus neoformans,* and *Coccidioides immitis.* Osteomyelitis is associated with mortality rates of greater than 20% in HIV-infected patients. The most frequently involved bones are the wrist, tibia, femoral heads, and thoracic cage, but other rare sites, such as the patella and the mandible, have been reported.

Musculoskeletal Tuberculosis

Musculoskeletal involvement, the fourth most common extrapulmonary manifestation of tuberculosis, is found in about 1% to 5% of patients with tuberculosis. It can mimic many skeletal diseases and can manifest in various locations. Less than 50% of reported patients with musculoskeletal tuberculosis have radiographic evidence of pulmonary tuberculosis. M. *tuberculosis* disseminates hematogenously after an acute or reactivated pulmonary infection. Usually, skeletal tuberculosis lesions in immunocompetent patients are solitary, but in AIDS patients, they may have a multicentric distribution in about 30% of cases.[95] The vertebrae are the most common site involved, mostly the lower thoracic or upper lumbar segments. The frequency of tuberculous spondylitis is 50% to 66%, peripheral arthritis 20% to 30%, osteomyelitis 10% to 20%, and tenosynovitis and bursitis about 1% to 3%. Treatment includes four-drug antitubercular therapy and often surgical intervention.

Atypical Mycobacterial Infection

Musculoskeletal infection caused by atypical mycobacterial species is unusual in immunocompetent individuals.[96]

Atypical mycobacterial species most commonly implicated in causing septic arthritis or osteomyelitis in HIV include *M. avium-intracellulare* complex, *Mycobacterium kansasii*, *Mycobacterium haemophilum*, *Mycobacterium terrae*, and *Mycobacterium fortuitum*. *M. haemophilum* has been most frequently implicated in skeletal infection, accounting for more than half of cases, and *M. kansasii* is second, accounting for an additional 25%. These are systemic infections that have involved several joints or skeletal sites. Cutaneous lesions, such as nodules, ulcers, and draining sinus tracts, occur in approximately 50% of patients.[96] These infections tend to occur late in the course of HIV, usually when the CD4+ T lymphocyte count is less than 100/μL. *M. avium-intracellulare* complex osteomyelitis has also been associated with immune reconstitution inflammatory syndrome after initiation of HAART.[97] Along with standard antituberculosis therapy, clarithromycin is effective.[96]

Bacillary Angiomatosis Osteomyelitis

Bacillary angiomatosis is a multisystem infectious disease caused by two closely related organisms—*Bartonella henselae* and *Bartonella quintana*—initially described in patients with AIDS by Stoler and colleagues in 1983.[98] It seems to be a disease unique to HIV-infected patients and to a lesser degree to other immunocompromised patients.[1]

The name *bacillary angiomatosis* came from descriptions of vascular proliferation as seen on histologic examination of clinical specimens, and from the bacilli identified on Warthin-Starry silver stain. Bacterial infection results in a vascular proliferative response ensuing in lesions in the skin (resembling Kaposi's sarcoma), lymph nodes (adenitis), central nervous system (aseptic meningitis or intracranial masses), bone (osteomyelitis), and liver (peliosis hepatis). Osteomyelitis is found in about one-third of patients in association with skin disease. These lesions usually are characterized by extensive destruction of the cortical bone, periostitis, medullary invasion, and an overlying soft tissue mass that might resemble cellulitis. Complete remission of bacillary angiomatosis after doxycycline or erythromycin therapy occurs, although bone lesions may need surgical drainage.

Fungal Infections

In addition to bacterial infection, patients with advanced HIV infection (CD4+ T lymphocyte count <100/μL) are at high risk for fungal musculoskeletal infections, particularly infections caused by *Candida albicans*[99] and *Sporothrix schenckii*.[100] *S. schenckii* can manifest with oligoarticular or even polyarticular involvement and tenosynovitis (Figure 113-9), and can be particularly difficult to eradicate, requiring long-term suppressive antifungal therapy. Various disseminated fungal infections, such as histoplasmosis, cryptococcosis, and blastomycosis, occur in HIV and often cause osteomyelitis.

Parasitic Infections

Muscle toxoplasmosis is found in profoundly immunodepressed patients, typically presenting with a painful subacute myopathy and concurrent multivisceral toxoplasmosis.[101] *Toxoplasma* cysts are observed mainly in muscle fibers in muscle biopsy specimens, and identification of cysts as *Toxoplasma* may be easier when specific antibodies or electron microscopy is used. Muscle weakness such as in polymyositis can occur in muscle toxoplasmosis. Treatment is based on a combination of drugs acting synergistically against *T. gondii*, including pyrimethamine and sulfadiazine or trisulfapyrimidines.

RESPONSE OF OTHER RHEUMATIC DISEASES TO HIV INFECTION

Early reports suggested that rheumatoid arthritis went into remission in the face of HIV infection. Early reports likewise suggested that HIV infection might reduce the activity of

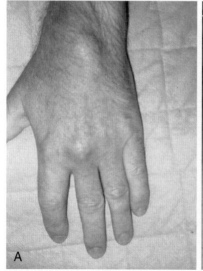 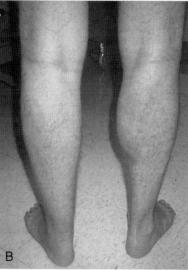

Figure 113-9 A, Third metacarpophalangeal synovitis and common extensor digitorum longus tendon sheath effusion at the dorsal surface of the wrist. **B,** Dissecting Baker's cyst in the same patient with disseminated *Sporothrix schenckii* infection (organism cultured from synovial fluid obtained from both sites).

systemic lupus erythematosus, particularly at times of low CD4[+] T cell counts. With emergence of the immune reconstitution syndrome, most autoimmune diseases appear de novo or recur with institution of HAART and increased CD4[+] counts.[5,102]

HAART-RELATED IMMUNE RECONSTITUTION SYNDROME

Coverage of antiretroviral therapy has increased from 7% in 2003 to 20% in 2005. Immune reconstitution inflammatory syndrome (IRIS) is a paradoxical clinical deterioration that occurs in patients with HIV who receive HAART as a result of improvement in cellular immunity. It was initially described with recrudescence of infections, but now, autoinflammatory and autoimmune phenomena are being described. A meta-analysis of more than 13,000 HIV patients starting HAART found that 13% developed IRIS.[103] The mean time of onset of IRIS from the time of HAART initiation is approximately 9 months.[102]

Shelburne and co-workers[104] put forth four criteria required for the diagnosis of immune reconstitution inflammatory syndrome, as follows:

1. Patient has been diagnosed with AIDS.
2. Treatment with anti-HIV therapy results in increased CD4[+] counts and decreased HIV viral load.
3. Infectious and inflammatory symptoms appear during therapy.
4. Symptoms cannot be explained by a new cause.

Improved understanding of the immunology of IRIS has helped elucidate how atypical, hyperaccentuated inflammatory host responses to pre-existing or coexisting infection can occur in HIV patients taking HAART. HIV infection causes a relentless decline in CD4[+] memory and naïve cells, an increase in activated T cells in the peripheral blood, and thymic dysfunction. HAART can lead to sustained suppression of HIV and concomitant repopulation of T cell counts in a biphasic mode.[105] The first phase represents the release of predominantly memory CD4[+] cells and lasts a few weeks to months. The second phase, from approximately 6 months on, represents the main phase of naïve T cell proliferation and is accompanied by changes in T helper cytokine production profiles.[106,107] IRIS can occur during both phases of immune recovery, and different infections and autoimmune phenomena occur in phase 1 compared with phase 2.

Organ-specific autoimmune phenomena have been described more often than generalized systemic autoimmune disease and tend to occur later during reconstitution. These phenomena may be a manifestation of naïve T cell release as opposed to memory T cell reconstitution. Graves' thyroiditis occurring about 21 months after initiation of HAART has been described in about 17 cases.[108] Terminal ileitis, alopecia universalis, cerebral CD8[+] lymphocytosis, and Guillain-Barré syndrome[105,109] have been reported. Polymyositis,[110] rheumatoid arthritis,[102] systemic lupus erythematosus,[111] Kawasaki-like febrile illness,[83] autoimmune hepatitis, adult Still's disease, and sarcoidosis[112] newly developing after initiation of HAART also have been described. These conditions tend to occur earlier during reconstitution compared with organ-specific autoimmunity. In addition, IRIS has been reported in the setting of tumor necrosis factor (TNF) blocker discontinuation, with cryptococcal pneumonia occurring in an HIV-positive patient after stopping adalimumab.[113]

If a diagnosis of IRIS is made, HAART is continued and most symptoms resolve with little or no therapy. If inflammatory symptoms involve areas where significant damage secondary to uncontrolled inflammation is likely to occur, such as in the central nervous system or eye, HAART should be stopped, and careful use of corticosteroids should be considered. IRIS is less likely to occur if the CD4[+] count is greater than 200/μL when HAART is initiated. Other risk factors for IRIS include being HAART naïve and the presence of a high antigenic burden with opportunistic infection when HAART is begun.[114,115] Continued systematic analysis is needed, however, and guidelines need to be established for defining the autoimmunity associated with immune reconstitution. The prognosis for most IRIS cases is favorable because a robust inflammatory response may predict an excellent response to HAART in terms of immune reconstitution and, perhaps, improved survival.

RHEUMATOLOGIC COMPLICATIONS OF HIV TREATMENT

The myopathy associated with nucleoside transcriptase inhibitors such as zidovudine and the osteonecrosis and parotid lipomatosis associated with the use of protease inhibitors have been discussed previously. In addition to these conditions, cases of adhesive capsulitis, Dupuytren's contracture, tenosynovitis, and temporomandibular joint dysfunction have been reported as a consequence of indinavir treatment.[116]

LABORATORY ABNORMALITIES ASSOCIATED WITH HIV INFECTION

Humoral immunologic abnormalities are frequent in patients with HIV but are rarely associated with severe clinical signs. The most common laboratory abnormality is polyclonal hyperglobulinemia, found in 45% of HIV-positive individuals.[117] Rheumatoid factor and antinuclear antibodies, usually in low titer, have been described in 17% of patients with HIV infection in some series,[117] although anti-dsDNA antibodies and hypocomplementemia are rare. IgG anticardiolipin antibodies are found in 95% of untreated patients with AIDS, particularly in patients with advanced disease, and overall in 20% to 30% of HIV-positive individuals.[118] They are rarely associated with thrombotic events. cANCAs and pANCAs have been described in the serum of HIV-positive individuals, as have anti–glomerular basement membrane antibodies.[119] Cryoglobulinemia is decreasing in this population since the introduction of HAART.[120] Indeed with HAART, many of these serologic abnormalities tend to decrease or resolve.

CONCLUSION

The impact of the global HIV pandemic continues to grow, and rheumatologists need to be aware of the wide spectrum of rheumatic diseases that occur in HIV-positive patients.

HAART has changed the natural history of HIV infection. It has modified the frequency and expression of some HIV-related clinical syndromes and has been associated directly (toxicity) and indirectly (immune reconstitution) with the development of new ones. With longer survival and newer refinements in treatment, the spectrum of rheumatic disease seen in HIV-positive patients is very much a moving target for rheumatologists and is likely to continue to evolve.

References

1. Biviji AA, Paiement GD, Steinbach LS: Musculoskeletal manifestations of human immunodeficiency virus infection, *J Am Acad Orthop Surg* 10:312–320, 2002.
2. Rynes RI, Goldenberg DL, DiGiacomo R, et al: Acquired immunodeficiency syndrome-associated arthritis, *Am J Med* 84:810–816, 1988.
3. Bileckot R, Mouaya A, Makuwa M: Prevalence and clinical presentations of arthritis in HIV-positive patients seen at a rheumatology department in Congo-Brazzaville, *Rev Rhum Engl Ed* 65:549–554, 1998.
4. Berman A, Cahn P, Perez H, et al: Human immunodeficiency virus infection associated arthritis: clinical characteristics, *J Rheumatol* 26:1158–1162, 1999.
5. Reveille JD: The changing spectrum of rheumatic disease in human immunodeficiency virus infection, *Semin Arthritis Rheum* 30:147–166, 2000.
6. Mody GM, Parke FA, Reveille JD: Articular manifestations of human immunodeficiency virus infection, *Best Pract Res Clin Rheumatol* 17:265–287, 2003.
7. Ornstein MH, Sperber K: The antiinflammatory and antiviral effects of hydroxychloroquine in two patients with acquired immunodeficiency syndrome and active inflammatory arthritis, *Arthritis Rheum* 39:157–161, 1996.
8. Clark MR, Solinger AM, Hochberg MC: Human immunodeficiency virus infection is not associated with Reiter's syndrome: data from three large cohort studies, *Rheum Dis Clin N Am* 18:267–276, 1992.
9. Njobvu P, McGill P: Human immunodeficiency virus related reactive arthritis in Zambia, *J Rheumatol* 32:1299–1304, 2005.
10. Reveille JD, Conant MA, Duvic M: Human immunodeficiency virus-associated psoriasis, psoriatic arthritis, and Reiter's syndrome: a disease continuum? *Arthritis Rheum* 33:1574–1578, 1990.
11. Kaslow RA, Carrington M, Apple R, et al: Influence of combinations of human major histocompatibility complex genes on the course of HIV-1 infection, *Nat Med* 2:405–411, 1996.
12. Carrington M, O'Brien SJ: The influence of HLA genotype on AIDS, *Annu Rev Med* 54:535–551, 2003.
13. Altfeld M, Kalife ET, Qi Y, et al: HLA alleles associated with delayed progression to AIDS contribute strongly to the initial CD8(+) T cell response against HIV-1, *PLoS Med* 3:e403, 2006.
14. Frahm N, Kiepiela P, Adams S, et al: Control of human immunodeficiency virus replication by cytotoxic T lymphocytes targeting subdominant epitopes, *Nat Immunol* 7:173–178, 2006.
15. Lopez-Larrea C, Njobvu PD, Gonzalez S, et al: The HLA-B*5703 allele confers susceptibility to the development of spondylarthropathies in Zambian human immunodeficiency virus-infected patients with slow progression to acquired immunodeficiency syndrome, *Arthritis Rheum* 52:275–279, 2005.
16. Bourinbaiar AS, Lee-Huang S: The non-steroidal anti-inflammatory drug, indomethacin, as an inhibitor of HIV replication, *FEBS Lett* 360:85–88, 1995.
17. Njobvu PD, McGill PE: Sulphasalazine in the treatment of HIV-related spondyloarthropathy, *Br J Rheumatol* 36:403–404, 1997.
18. Disla E, Rhim HR, Reddy A, et al: Improvement in CD4 lymphocyte count in HIV-Reiter's syndrome after treatment with sulfasalazine, *J Rheumatol* 21:662–664, 1994.
19. Maurer TA, Zackheim HS, Tuffanelli L, et al: The use of methotrexate for treatment of psoriasis in patients with HIV infection, *J Am Acad Dermatol* 31:372–375, 1994.
20. Chiang G, Sassaroli M, Louie M, et al: Inhibition of HIV-1 replication by hydroxychloroquine: mechanism of action and comparison with zidovudine, *Clin Ther* 18:1080–1092, 1996.
21. Louthrenoo W: Successful treatment of severe Reiter's syndrome associated with human immunodeficiency virus infection with etretinate: report of 2 cases, *J Rheumatol* 20:1243–1246, 1993.
22. Gill H, Majithia V: Successful use of infliximab in the treatment of Reiter's syndrome: a case report and discussion, *Clin Rheumatol* 27:121–123, 2008.
23. Kim SY, Solomon DH: Tumor necrosis factor blockade and the risk of viral infection, *Nat Rev Rheumatol* 6:165–174, 2010.
24. Filippi J, Roger PM, Schneider SM, et al: Infliximab and human immunodeficiency virus infection: viral load reduction and CD4+ T-cell loss related to apoptosis, *Arch Intern Med* 166:1783–1784, 2006.
25. Cepeda EJ, Williams FM, Ishimori ML, et al: The use of anti-tumor necrosis factor therapy in HIV-positive individuals with rheumatic disease, *Ann Rheum Dis* 67:710–712, 2008.
26. Morar N, Willis-Owen SA, Maurer T, Bunker CB: HIV-associated psoriasis: pathogenesis, clinical features and management, *Lancet Infect Dis* 10:470–478, 2010.
27. Njobvu P, McGill P: Psoriatic arthritis and human immunodeficiency virus infection in Zambia, *J Rheumatol* 27:1699–1702, 2000.
28. Espinoza LR, Berman A, Vasey FB, et al: Psoriatic arthritis and acquired immunodeficiency syndrome, *Arthritis Rheum* 31:1034–1040, 1988.
29. Duvic M, Crane MM, Conant M, et al: Zidovudine improves psoriasis in human immunodeficiency virus-positive males, *Arch Dermatol* 130:447–451, 1994.
30. Bartke U, Venten I, Kreuter A, et al: Human immunodeficiency virus-associated psoriasis and psoriatic arthritis treated with infliximab, *Br J Dermatol* 150:784–786, 2004.
31. McGonagle D, Reade S, Marzo-Ortega H, et al: Human immunodeficiency virus associated spondyloarthropathy: pathogenic insights based on imaging findings and response to highly active antiretroviral treatment, *Ann Rheum Dis* 60:696–698, 2001.
32. Gerster JC, Camus JP, Chave JP, et al: Multiple site avascular necrosis in HIV infected patients, *J Rheumatol* 18:300–302, 1991.
33. Allison GT, Bostrom MP, Glesby MJ: Osteonecrosis in HIV disease: epidemiology, etiologies, and clinical management, *AIDS* 17:1–9, 2003.
34. Gutierrez F, Padilla S, Masia M, et al: Osteonecrosis in patients infected with HIV: clinical epidemiology and natural history in a large case series from Spain, *J Acquir Immune Defic Syndr* 42:286–292, 2006.
35. Matos MA, Alencar RW, Matos SS: Avascular necrosis of the femoral head in HIV infected patients, *Braz J Infect Dis* 11:31–34, 2008.
36. Gunnarsson G, Karchmer AW: Hypertrophic osteoarthropathy associated with *Pneumocystis carinii* pneumonia and human immunodeficiency virus infection, *Clin Infect Dis* 22:590–591, 1996.
37. Brown TT, Qaqish RB: Antiretroviral therapy and the prevalence of osteopenia and osteoporosis: a meta-analytic review, *AIDS* 20:2165–2174, 2006.
38. Paccou J, Viget N, Legrout-Gerot I, et al: Bone loss in patients with HIV infection, *J Bone Spine* 76:637–641, 2009.
39. Amorosa V, Tebas P: Bone disease and HIV infection, *Clin Infect Dis* 42:108–114, 2006.
40. Rodriguez M, Daniels B, Gunawardene S, Robbins GK: High frequency of vitamin D deficiency in ambulatory HIV-positive patients, *AIDS Hum Retroviruses* 25:9–14, 2009.
41. Mueller J, Fux CA, Ledergerber B, et al: High prevalence of severe vitamin D deficiency in combined antiretroviral therapy-naïve and successfully treated Swiss HIV patients, *AIDS* 24:1127–1134, 2010.
42. Lin D, Rieder M: Interventions for the treatment of decreased bone mineral density associated with HIV infection, *Cochrane Database Syst Rev* (2):CD005645, 2007.
43. Buskila D, Gladman D: Musculoskeletal manifestations of infection with human immunodeficiency virus, *Rev Infect Dis* 12:223–235, 1990.
44. Simms RW, Zerbini CA, Ferrante N, et al: Fibromyalgia syndrome in patients infected with human immunodeficiency virus. The Boston City Hospital Clinical AIDS Team, *Am J Med* 92:368–374, 1992.
45. Miro O, Pedrol E, Cebrian M, et al: Skeletal muscle studies in patients with HIV-related wasting syndrome, *J Neurol Sci* 150:153–159, 1997.
46. Gherardi R, Chariot P, Authier FJ: [Muscular involvement in HIV infection], *Rev Neurol (Paris)* 151:603–607, 1995.

47. Simpson DM, Bender AN, Farraye J, et al: Human immunodeficiency virus wasting syndrome may represent a treatable myopathy, *Neurology* 40:535–538, 1990.
48. Miro O, Masanes F, Pedrol E, et al: [A comparative study of the clinical and histological characteristics between classic nemaline myopathy and that associated with the human immunodeficiency virus], *Med Clin (Barc)* 105:500–503, 1995.
49. Nakagawa M, Hirata K: [Adult onset nemaline myopathy and monoclonal gammopathy], *Ryoikibetsu Shokogun Shirizu* 35:406–413, 2001.
50. de Sanctis JT, Cumbo-Nacheli G, Dobbie D, Baumgartner D: HIV-associated nemaline rod myopathy: role of intravenous immunoglobulin therapy in two persons with HIV/AIDS, *AIDS Read* 18:90–94, 2008.
51. Johnson RW, Williams FM, Kazi S, et al: Human immunodeficiency virus-associated polymyositis: a longitudinal study of outcome, *Arthritis Rheum* 49:172–178, 2003.
52. Seidman R, Peress NS, Nuovo GJ: In situ detection of polymerase chain reaction-amplified HIV-1 nucleic acids in skeletal muscle in patients with myopathy, *Mod Pathol* 7:369–375, 1994.
53. Leon-Monzon M, Lamperth L, Dalakas MC: Search for HIV proviral DNA and amplified sequences in the muscle biopsies of patients with HIV polymyositis, *Muscle Nerve* 16:408–413, 1993.
54. Carroll MB, Holmes R: Dermatomyositis and HIV infection: case report and review of the literature, *Rheumatol Int* 31:673–679, 2011.
55. Heckmann JM, Pillay K, Hearn AP, Kenyon C: Polymyositis in African HIV-infected subjects, *Neuromuscul Disord* 20:735–739, 2010.
56. Tehranzadeh J, Ter-Oganesyan RR, Steinbach LS: Musculoskeletal disorders associated with HIV infection and AIDS, Part I. Infectious musculoskeletal conditions, *Skeletal Radiol* 33:249–259, 2004.
57. Illa I, Nath A, Dalakas M: Immunocytochemical and virological characteristics of HIV-associated inflammatory myopathies: similarities with seronegative polymyositis, *Ann Neurol* 29:474–481, 1991.
58. Cupler EJ, Leon-Monzon M, Miller J, et al: Inclusion body myositis in HIV-1 and HTLV-1 infected patients, *Brain* 119(Pt 6):1887–1893, 1996.
59. Schreiner B, Voss J, Wischhusen J, et al: Expression of toll-like receptors by human muscle cells in vitro and in vivo: TLR3 is highly expressed in inflammatory and HIV myopathies, mediates IL-8 release and up-regulation of NKG2D-ligands, *FASEB J* 20:118–120, 2006.
60. Dalakas MC, Rakocevic G, Shatunov A, et al: Inclusion body myositis with human immunodeficiency virus infection: four cases with clonal expansion of viral-specific T cells, *Ann Neurol* 61:466–475, 2007.
61. Walsh K, Kaye K, Demaerschalk B, et al: AZT myopathy and HIV-1 polymyositis: one disease or two? *Can J Neurol Sci* 29:390–393, 2002.
62. Zannou DM, Azon-Kouanou A, Bashi BJ, et al: Mitochondrial toxicity: a case of palpebral ptosis in a woman infected by HIV and treated with HAART including zidovudine, *Bull Soc Pathol Exot* 102:97–98, 2009.
63. Pfeffer G, Cote HCF, Montaner JS, et al: Ophthalmoplegia and ptosis: mitochondrial toxicity in patients receiving HIV therapy, *Neurology* 73:71–72, 2009.
64. Dalakas MC, Illa I, Pezeshkpour GH, et al: Mitochondrial myopathy caused by long-term zidovudine therapy, *N Engl J Med* 322:1098–1105, 1990.
65. Authier FJ, Gherardi RK: [Muscular complications of human immunodeficiency virus (HIV) infection in the era of effective antiretroviral therapy], *Rev Neurol (Paris)* 162:71–81, 2006.
66. Zembower TR, Gerzenshtein L, Coleman K, Palella FJ Jr: Severe rhabdomyolysis associated with raltegravir use, *AIDS* 22:1382–1384, 2008.
67. Basu D, Williams FM, Ahn CW, et al: Changing spectrum of the diffuse infiltrative lymphocytosis syndrome, *Arthritis Rheum* 55:466–472, 2006.
68. Williams FM, Cohen PR, Jumshyd J, et al: Prevalence of the diffuse infiltrative lymphocytosis syndrome among human immunodeficiency virus type 1-positive outpatients, *Arthritis Rheum* 41:863–868, 1998.
69. Kordossis T, Paikos S, Aroni K, et al: Prevalence of Sjogren's-like syndrome in a cohort of HIV-1-positive patients: descriptive pathology and immunopathology, *Br J Rheumatol* 37:691–695, 1998.
70. Itescu S, Rose S, Dwyer E, et al: Certain HLA-DR5 and -DR6 major histocompatibility complex class II alleles are associated with a CD8

lymphocytic host response to human immunodeficiency virus type 1 characterized by low lymphocyte viral strain heterogeneity and slow disease progression, *Proc Natl Acad Sci U S A* 91:11472–11476, 1994.
71. Itescu S, Dalton J, Zhang HZ, et al: Tissue infiltration in a CD8 lymphocytosis syndrome associated with human immunodeficiency virus-1 infection has the phenotypic appearance of an antigenically driven response, *J Clin Invest* 91:2216–2225, 1993.
72. Kazi S, Cohen PR, Williams F, et al: The diffuse infiltrative lymphocytosis syndrome: clinical and immunogenetic features in 35 patients, *AIDS* 10:385–391, 1996.
73. Itescu S, Winchester R: Diffuse infiltrative lymphocytosis syndrome: a disorder occurring in human immunodeficiency virus-1 infection that may present as a sicca syndrome, *Rheum Dis Clin N Am* 18:683–697, 1992.
74. Garcia-Garcia JA, Macias J, Castellanos V, et al: Necrotizing granulomatous vasculitis in advanced HIV infection, *J Infect* 47:333–335, 2003.
75. Guillevin L: Vasculitides in the context of HIV infection, *AIDS* 22(Suppl 3):S27–S33, 2008.
76. Gherardi R, Belec L, Mhiri C, et al: The spectrum of vasculitis in human immunodeficiency virus-infected patients: a clinicopathologic evaluation, *Arthritis Rheum* 36:1164–1174, 1993.
77. Zhang X, Li H, Li T, et al: Distinctive rheumatic manifestations in 98 patients with human immunodeficiency virus infection in China, *J Rheumatol* 34:1760–1764, 2007.
78. Nguyen H, Ferentz K, Patel A, Le C: Churg-Strauss syndrome associated with HIV infection, *J Am Board Fam Pract* 18:140–142, 2005.
79. Belzunegui J, Cancio J, Pego JM, et al: Relapsing polychondritis and Behcet's syndrome in a patient with HIV infection, *Ann Rheum Dis* 54:780, 1995.
80. Cicalini S, Gigli B, Palmieri F, et al: Remission of Behcet's disease and keratoconjunctivitis sicca in an HIV-infected patient treated with HAART, *Int J STD AIDS* 15:139–140, 2004.
81. Chetty R, Batitang S, Nair R: Large artery vasculopathy in HIV-positive patients: another vasculitic enigma, *Hum Pathol* 31:374–379, 2000.
82. Javed MA, Sheppard MN, Pepper J: Aortic root dilation secondary to giant cell aortitis in a human immunodeficiency virus-positive patient, *Eur J Cardiothorac Surg* 30:400–401, 2006.
83. Stankovic K, Miailhes P, Bessis D, et al: Kawasaki-like syndromes in HIV-infected adults, *J Infect* 55:488–494, 2007.
84. Brannagan TH III: Retroviral-associated vasculitis of the nervous system, *Neurol Clin* 15:927–944, 1997.
85. Ake JA, Erickson JC, Lowry KJ: Cerebral aneurysmal arteriopathy associated with HIV infection in an adult, *Clin Infect Dis* 43:e46–e50, 2006.
86. Nieuwhof CM, Damoiseaux J, Cohen Tervaert JW: Successful treatment of cerebral vasculitis in an HIV-positive patient with anti-CD25 treatment, *Ann Rheum Dis* 65:1677–1678, 2006.
87. Bradley WG, Verma A: Painful vasculitic neuropathy in HIV-1 infection: relief of pain with prednisone therapy, *Neurology* 47:1446–1451, 1996.
88. Coplan NL, Shimony RY, Ioachim HL, et al: Primary pulmonary hypertension associated with human immunodeficiency viral infection, *Am J Med* 89:96–99, 1990.
89. Morse JH, Barst RJ, Itescu S, et al: Primary pulmonary hypertension in HIV infection: an outcome determined by particular HLA class II alleles, *Am J Respir Crit Care Med* 153:1299–1301, 1996.
90. Gutierrez F, Masia M, Padilla S, et al: Occult lymphadenopathic Kaposi's sarcoma associated with severe pulmonary hypertension: a clinical hint about the potential role of HHV-8 in HIV-related pulmonary hypertension? *J Clin Virol* 37:79–82, 2006.
91. Mehta NJ, Khan IA, Mehta RN, et al: HIV-related pulmonary hypertension: analytic review of 131 cases, *Chest* 118:1133–1141, 2000.
92. Nunes H, Humbert M, Sitbon O, et al: Prognostic factors for survival in human immunodeficiency virus-associated pulmonary arterial hypertension, *Am J Respir Crit Care Med* 167:1433–1439, 2003.
93. Ansaloni L: Tropical pyomyositis, *World J Surg* 20:613–617, 1996.
94. Scharschmidt TJ, Weiner SD, Myers JP: Bacterial pyomyositis, *Curr Infect Dis Rep* 6:393–396, 2004.
95. Jellis JE: Human immunodeficiency virus and osteoarticular tuberculosis, *Clin Orthop Relat Res* 398:27–31, 2002.
96. Hirsch R, Miller SM, Kazi S, et al: Human immunodeficiency virus-associated atypical mycobacterial skeletal infections, *Semin Arthritis Rheum* 25:347–356, 1996.

97. Kahlon SS, East JW, Sarria JC: Mycobacterium-avium-intracellulare complex immune reconstitution inflammatory syndrome in HIV/AIDS presenting as osteomyelitis, AIDS Read 18:515–518, 2008.

98. Stoler MH, Bonfiglio TA, Steigbigel RT, et al: An atypical subcutaneous infection associated with acquired immune deficiency syndrome, Am J Clin Pathol 80:714–718, 1983.

99. Edelstein H, McCabe R: Candida albicans septic arthritis and osteomyelitis of the sternoclavicular joint in a patient with human immunodeficiency virus infection, J Rheumatol 18:110–111, 1991.

100. Heller HM, Fuhrer J: Disseminated sporotrichosis in patients with AIDS: case report and review of the literature, AIDS 5:1243–1246, 1991.

101. Gherardi R, Baudrimont M, Lionnet F, et al: Skeletal muscle toxoplasmosis in patients with acquired immunodeficiency syndrome: a clinical and pathological study, Ann Neurol 32:535–542, 1992.

102. Calabrese LH, Kirchner E, Shrestha R: Rheumatic complications of human immunodeficiency virus infection in the era of highly active antiretroviral therapy: emergence of a new syndrome of immune reconstitution and changing patterns of disease, Semin Arthritis Rheum 35:166–174, 2005.

103. Muller M, Wandel S, Colebunders R, et al: Immune reconstitution inflammatory syndrome in patients starting antiretroviral therapy for HIV infection: a systematic review and meta-analysis, Lancet Infect Dis 10:251–261, 2010.

104. Shelburne SA III, Hamill RJ, Rodriguez-Barradas MC, et al: Immune reconstitution inflammatory syndrome: emergence of a unique syndrome during highly active antiretroviral therapy, Medicine (Baltimore) 81:213–227, 2002.

105. DeSimone JA, Pomerantz RJ, Babinchak TJ: Inflammatory reactions in HIV-1-infected persons after initiation of highly active antiretroviral therapy, Ann Intern Med 133:447–454, 2000.

106. Hardy G, Worrell S, Hayes P, et al: Evidence of thymic reconstitution after highly active antiretroviral therapy in HIV-1 infection, HIV Med 5:67–73, 2004.

107. Lederman MM, Connick E, Landay A, et al: Immunologic responses associated with 12 weeks of combination antiretroviral therapy consisting of zidovudine, lamivudine, and ritonavir: results of AIDS Clinical Trials Group Protocol 315, J Infect Dis 178:70–79, 1998.

108. Chen F, Day SL, Metcalfe RA, et al: Characteristics of autoimmune thyroid disease occurring as a late complication of immune reconstitution in patients with advanced human immunodeficiency virus (HIV) disease, Medicine (Baltimore) 84:98–106, 2005.

109. Gray F, Bazille C, dle-Biassette H, et al: Central nervous system immune reconstitution disease in acquired immunodeficiency syndrome patients receiving highly active antiretroviral treatment, J Neurovirol 11(Suppl 3):16–22, 2005.

110. Calza L, Manfredi R, Colangeli V, et al: Polymyositis associated with HIV infection during immune restoration induced by highly active anti-retroviral therapy, Clin Exp Rheumatol 22:651–652, 2004.

111. Schneider J, Zatarain E: IRIS and SLE, Clin Immunol 118:152–153, 2006.

112. Ferrand RA, Cartledge JD, Connolly J, et al: Immune reconstitution sarcoidosis presenting with hypercalcaemia and renal failure in HIV infection, Int J STD AIDS 18:138–139, 2007.

113. Cadena J, Thompson GR 3rd, Ho TT, et al: Immune reconstitution inflammatory syndrome after cessation of the tumor necrosis factor alpha blocker adalimumab in cryptococcal pneumonia, Diagn Microbiol Infect Dis 64:327–330, 2009.

114. McIlleron H, Meintjes G, Burman WJ, Maartens G: Complications of antiretroviral therapy in patients with tuberculosis: drug interactions, toxicity, and immune reconstitution inflammatory syndrome, J Infect Dis 196(Suppl 1):S63–S75, 2007.

115. Shelburne SA, Montes M, Hamill RJ: Immune reconstitution inflammatory syndrome: more answers, more questions, J Antimicrob Chemother 57:167–170, 2006.

116. Florence E, Schrooten W, Verdonck K, et al: Rheumatological complications associated with the use of indinavir and other protease inhibitors, Ann Rheum Dis 61:82–84, 2002.

117. Kaye BR: Rheumatologic manifestations of infection with human immunodeficiency virus (HIV), Ann Intern Med 111:158–167, 1989.

118. Petrovas C, Vlachoyiannopoulos PG, Kordossis T, et al: Antiphospholipid antibodies in HIV infection and SLE with or without anti-phospholipid syndrome: comparisons of phospholipid specificity, avidity and reactivity with beta2-GPI, J Autoimmun 13:347–355, 1999.

119. Savige JA, Chang L, Horn S, Crowe SM: Anti-nuclear, anti-neutrophil cytoplasmic and anti-glomerular basement membrane antibodies in HIV-infected individuals, Autoimmunity 18:205–211, 1994.

120. Bonnet F, Pineau JJ, Taupin JL, et al: Prevalence of cryoglobulinemia and serological markers of autoimmunity in human immunodeficiency virus infected individuals: a cross-sectional study of 97 patients, J Rheumatol 30:2005–2010, 2003.

The references for this chapter can also be found on www.expertconsult.com.

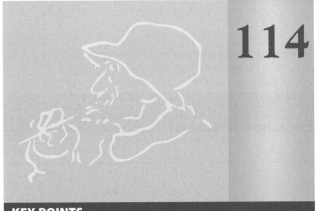

114 Viral Arthritis

STANLEY J. NAIDES

KEY POINTS

Acute-onset, symmetric polyarthritis can be caused by viral infection, especially when accompanied by rash.

Always take exposure, travel, occupation, and vaccination histories.

Parvovirus B19 is the most common viral arthritis in the United States.

In adults with parvovirus B19 infection, rash may be subtle or absent.

Rubella arthritis occurs in young adults. Rubella vaccination has reduced the overall incidence of rubella infection but has shifted the peak age to young adults.

Arthralgia, arthritis, or neuropathic pain may occur after rubella vaccination; these conditions are usually self-limited in duration.

Alphaviruses are mosquito-borne causes of arthritis and rash. Outbreaks occur in endemic areas associated with rising mosquito populations and should be considered in travelers entering the United States.

Hepatitis B virus infection presents as an arthritis-urticaria syndrome.

Hepatitis C virus infection causes cryoglobulinemia and vasculitis. Cryoglobulinemic vasculitis often presents as palpable purpura of the lower legs.

The history of risk behaviors associated with hepatitis C virus infection may be remote.

Viruses are candidate causative agents for various rheumatic diseases in part because arthralgia and arthritis are prominent features of certain viral infections. Understanding how viruses cause arthritis and the nature of virus–host cell interactions may suggest how viruses precipitate, establish, or maintain chronic inflammatory arthritis such as rheumatoid arthritis.

Viral effects in a given host may depend on host factors such as age, gender, genetic background, infection history, and immune response. The ability of a given virus to infect a host may also depend on the viral mode of host entry, tissue tropism, replication strategy, cytopathologic effects, ability to establish persistent infection, viral expression of host-like antigens, and ability to alter host antigens. Viral modification of the regulation of cellular gene expression may contribute to autoimmunity. Infected cells may die by classic cell necrosis, programmed cell death (apoptosis), or autophagy. Initiation of an immune response to virally encoded antigens on the cell surface may target that cell for destruction and alter cell-cell interactions. The antibody response may generate immune complexes that are deposited locally at the site of viral infection or systemically in synovium. Alternatively, cells may survive, but their behavior may be altered by the expression of viral genes. Transactivation of cellular genes by viral gene products may induce the cell cycle or cytokines that elicit or perpetuate an immune response targeting host cells. Molecular mimicry of host autoantigens by viral proteins may break immune tolerance. Viral components may elicit "danger signals" that trigger an immune response.[1,2]

PARVOVIRUS B19

Human parvovirus B19 is a member of the family Parvoviridae, subfamily Parvoviridae, genus *Erythrovirus*. It consists of the small, single-stranded DNA viruses that autonomously replicate in erythroid precursors (hence the genus name). B19 has no envelope and is approximately 23 nm in diameter. Productive infection occurs in erythroid precursors; infection of nonerythroid tissues occurs but is restricted, which means that if assembly of virions occurs, it is inefficient, or that nonstructural but not capsid structural viral genes are expressed, preventing virion assembly. Parvoviruses are species specific and are not known to readily cross species barriers. The common canine parvovirus does not infect humans.

Epidemiology

B19 infection is common and occurs worldwide. B19 typically is transmitted by respiratory secretions but may also be transmitted via pooled blood products. Outbreaks commonly occur in late winter and spring, when close contact is most common, although epidemics may also occur in summer and fall. Most B19 infections, especially in children, remain asymptomatic or are diagnosed as nonspecific viral illnesses. Outbreaks tend to occur in 3- to 5-year cycles, representing the time required for a new cohort of susceptible children to enter school. Up to 60% of adults have serologic evidence of past B19 infection.[3,4] Susceptible adults in occupations with multiple exposures to children, such as schoolteachers and pediatric nurses, are at greatest risk (up to 50%) of acquiring infection during outbreaks.[4,5] Sporadic cases do occur during nonepidemic periods. The diagnosis should be entertained even in the absence of surveillance data suggesting an outbreak.

Pathogenesis

The onset of joint symptoms and rash is associated temporally with the appearance of serum anti-B19 immunoglobulin (Ig)M antibody, suggesting a role for circulating immune complexes during the acute phase of the illness.[6] Although little evidence of circulating virus has been noted in patients who have chronic joint symptoms, B19 DNA may be found in the bone marrow and synovium of patients with chronic B19 arthropathy. Persistence in chronic B19 arthropathy may be facilitated by failure to develop IgG antibodies to the N-terminal region of the minor capsid protein VP1, known to encode neutralizing epitopes.[6] The presence of antibody to the B19 nonstructural protein NS1 in some cases of chronic B19 arthropathy probably reflects the immune response to NS1 on the surface of B19 virions or NS1 spilled during cell death.[7] NS1 protein itself, however, may play a pathogenic role in perpetuating chronic B19 arthropathy through its interaction with cellular genes.[8] NS1 protein upregulates in vitro transcription from the interleukin (IL)-6 promoter and from human immunodeficiency virus (HIV) long terminal repeats in the presence of *tat* and an intact *tar* element.[9,10] A high prevalence of B19 DNA and proteins in synovium from rheumatoid arthritis patients was reported in association with enhanced synovial production of IL-6 and tumor necrosis factor.[8] These findings remain controversial.[11] B19 may induce apoptosis through NS1, which is known to be toxic to cells.[12,13] Production of NS1 in nonpermissive synoviocytes could theoretically induce autoimmunity by disrupting normal patterns of cell interactions and intercellular regulation.

Diagnosis

Clinical Features

The incubation period from B19 infection to symptom onset is 7 to 18 days. B19 causes transient aplastic crisis in the setting of chronic hemolytic anemia.[6] In otherwise healthy children, B19 causes erythema infectiosum, or fifth disease, characterized by bright red "slapped cheeks" and a macular or maculopapular eruption on the torso and extremities. Up to 70% of infected children may be asymptomatic; others may have mild flu-like symptoms, including fever, headache, sore throat, cough, anorexia, vomiting, diarrhea, and arthralgia. In adults, the rash tends to be subtler, and the slapped-cheek rash is usually absent. Uncommon dermatologic manifestations include vesicular or hemorrhagic vesiculopustular eruptions, purpura with or without thrombocytopenia, Henoch-Schönlein purpura, and a "socks and gloves" acral erythema. B19 infection may be associated with paresthesias in the fingers and, rarely, with numbness of the toes. Progressive arm weakness has been associated with mild nerve conduction slowing and decreased motor and sensory potential amplitudes. B19 may cross the placenta to infect the fetus, which may develop hydrops fetalis on the basis of B19-induced anemia or viral cardiomyopathy. Less commonly, B19 may cause pancytopenia, isolated anemia, thrombocytopenia, leukopenia, myocarditis, neuropathy, or hepatitis.[14] Reports suggest that B19 may be associated with vasculitis, including giant cell arteritis.[15,16] Patients with congenital or acquired immunodeficiencies, including prior chemotherapy or acquired immunodeficiency syndrome (AIDS) due to HIV infection, may

Table 114-1 Prevalence of Joint Symptoms in Fifth Disease by Age: Port Angeles, Washington, 1961-1962

Symptom	Prevalence (%) by Age		
	0-9 yr	10-19 yr	>20 yr
Pain	5.1	11.5	77.2
Swelling	2.8	5.3	59.6

Data from Ager EA, Chin TDY, Poland JD: Epidemic erythema infectiosum, *N Engl J Med* 275:1326, 1966.

develop persistent B19 infection with chronic or recurrent anemia, thrombocytopenia, or leukopenia. B19 infection is the leading cause of pure red cell aplasia in patients with AIDS.[17,18]

In a study of an erythema infectiosum outbreak in Port Angeles, Washington, in which subjects were identified on the basis of rash, the incidence of arthralgia and joint swelling increased with age (Table 114-1).[19] In adults, a severe flu-like illness consisting of fever, chills, malaise, and myalgias may precede or accompany sudden-onset, moderately severe, symmetric polyarthritis in a rheumatoid-like distribution. The arthritis is characterized by prominent involvement of the finger proximal interphalangeal, metacarpophalangeal, wrist, knee, and ankle joints. Within 24 to 48 hours of onset, all affected joints become involved. Axial skeleton involvement is uncommon. Joint symptoms are usually self-limited.

After the initial infection, objective joint swelling, heat, and erythema, when present, tend to resolve over several weeks. A minority of patients have prolonged symptoms that fall into one of two patterns. Approximately two-thirds have continuous morning stiffness and arthralgias with intermittent flares. The remaining patients are symptom free between flares. Chronic B19 arthropathy may last months to years. Pain remains a prominent feature during flares; patients commonly report morning stiffness. Approximately 12% of patients presenting with "early synovitis" have B19 infection; most are women.[6]

Laboratory Tests

Viremia lasts 5 to 6 days and is associated with an absence of reticulocytosis and, in otherwise normal individuals, a minimal decrease in the concentrations of hemoglobin, neutrophils, and lymphocytes. Flu-like symptoms may occur during viremia. An IgM antibody response follows the initial viremia in 4 to 6 days and is associated with clearing of viremia and cessation of nasal shedding of virus.

The antibody response is associated with the second phase of clinical illness, characterized by rash and joint symptoms. Onset of the anti-B19 IgG antibody response occurs almost concurrently with the IgM response. The two clinical phases of illness often overlap. Low to moderate titers of rheumatoid factor and anti-DNA, antilymphocyte, antinuclear, and antiphospholipid antibodies may be present initially.[20-24]

During viremia, immune electron microscopy may detect virions in serum. However, this method is not readily available to clinicians. B19 DNA may be detected during viremia. However, because adult patients usually present after the onset of joint symptoms, the most useful diagnostic test is anti-B19 IgM serology. Radioimmunoassays and enzyme-linked immunosorbent assays have been used to detect B19 antigen and specific antibody to B19 capsid.[6,25,26] The anti-B19 IgM antibody response is usually positive for 2 months after the acute illness and may wane shortly thereafter. In some patients, anti-B19 IgM may be detected for 6 months or longer. A positive anti-B19 IgG antibody test in the absence of anti-B19 IgM usually is not diagnostically helpful because of the high seroprevalence of anti-B19 IgG in the adult population. Reports of B19 DNA in normal synovium suggest that testing for B19 DNA in these tissues is of little clinical utility in the absence of anti-B19 IgM.[27]

Differential Diagnosis

Many patients with B19 arthropathy meet the American Rheumatism Association criteria for a diagnosis of rheumatoid arthritis: morning stiffness lasting longer than an hour; symmetric involvement; involvement of at least three joints; and involvement of the finger proximal interphalangeal, metacarpophalangeal, and wrist joints. Rheumatoid factor may be present at low to moderate titers. Absence of both rheumatoid nodules and joint destruction differentiate B19 arthropathy from classic, erosive rheumatoid arthritis.

Occasionally, B19 infection may present with features of systemic lupus erythematosus (SLE). Whether this represents a clinical mimic or indicates that B19 plays a role in initiating or precipitating SLE in these patients remains to be determined.[6]

Rubella in adults may present with rash and symmetric polyarthralgia or polyarthritis that is clinically indistinguishable from B19 infection. A history of prenatal rubella testing, prior rubella vaccination, or rubella exposure may aid the clinician in choosing the appropriate diagnostic serologies.

Treatment and Outcome

No specific treatment or vaccine has been identified for B19 infection. Therefore, treatment is symptomatic and consists of nonsteroidal anti-inflammatory drugs. Intravenous immunoglobulin has been successful in the treatment of bone marrow suppression and B19 persistence in immunocompromised patients,[18] but initial studies suggest that this is not applicable to patients with chronic arthropathy. Long-term prognosis is good. Although subjective arthralgias and morning stiffness may be prolonged, joint destruction is not a feature of chronic B19 arthropathy. The role of B19 as a cofactor in the development of classic erosive rheumatoid arthritis has not been confirmed.

TOGAVIRUSES

The family Togaviridae includes the *Rubivirus* and *Alphavirus* genera.

Rubella Virus

Rubella virus is the sole member of the genus *Rubivirus*. It consists of enveloped, single-stranded RNA viruses. The rubella virion is spherical and measures 50 to 70 nm in diameter, with a 30-nm dense core. Envelope glycoproteins form 5- to 6-nm spike-like projections that contain hemagglutination activity.[28]

Epidemiology

Transmission is by nasopharyngeal secretions, with a peak incidence in late winter and spring. Vaccination has reduced the incidence of rubella outbreaks and has shifted the demographic profile from children to college students and adults. The incubation period from infection to rash is 14 to 21 days. Viremia precedes rash by 6 to 7 days, peaks just before the onset of rash, and clears within 48 hours after the onset of rash. Nasopharyngeal shedding of virus is detectable from 7 days before the appearance of rash until 14 days afterward, but it is maximal from just before the rash until 5 to 6 days later.[29]

Pathogenesis

Rubella virus can persistently infect synoviocytes and chondrocytes in vitro. An inadequate humoral immune response to specific rubella envelope glycoprotein epitopes may allow rubella virus to persistently infect synovium and lymphocytes in patients with chronic rubella arthritis. The onset of rash and arthritis is concurrent with antibody production, suggesting a role for antibody or immune complexes.[29] Concentrations of rubella antibody are higher in synovial fluid than in serum. Synovial lymphocytes from infected individuals spontaneously secrete rubella antibody in vitro, suggesting that an immune response to rubella infection occurs in the joint.[30]

Diagnosis

Clinical Features. Asymptomatic infection occurs in children and adults. Low-grade fever, malaise, coryza, and prominent lymphadenopathy involving posterior cervical, postauricular, and occipital nodes may precede rash by 5 days. A morbilliform rash may initially appear on the face and then spread to the torso, upper extremities, and lower extremities over 2 to 3 days. The facial rash may coalesce and clear as the extremities become involved. In some cases, the rash is only a transient blush.

Joint symptoms commonly occur in women beginning 1 week before or 1 week after the appearance of the rash. Symmetric or migratory arthralgias are more common than synovitis. Morning stiffness is prominent. Joint symptoms usually resolve over a few days to 2 weeks. Proximal interphalangeal, metacarpophalangeal, wrist, elbow, ankle, and knee joints are most frequently affected. Periarthritis, tenosynovitis, and carpal tunnel syndrome may be seen. In some patients, symptoms may persist for months to years.[31,32]

Live attenuated rubella vaccines have caused a high frequency of postvaccination myalgia, arthralgia, arthritis, and paresthesia—symptoms similar to those seen in natural infection—beginning 2 weeks after inoculation and lasting less than a week. However, in some patients, symptoms may persist for longer than a year. RA27/3, the vaccine strain in current use, may cause postvaccination joint symptoms in 15% or more of recipients.[31,32]

Two rheumatologic syndromes may complicate natural infection or vaccination in children. In the catcher's crouch syndrome, a lumbar radiculoneuropathy causes popliteal fossa pain on arising in the morning. Exacerbation of the pain by knee extension encourages the assumption of a baseball catcher's crouch position. The pain gradually subsides through the day but recurs the next morning. In the arm syndrome, brachial neuropathy causes arm and hand pain and dysesthesias that are worse at night. Both syndromes may occur beginning 1 to 2 months after infection or vaccination, with the initial episode lasting up to 2 months. Episodes recur for up to 1 year but eventually resolve without long-term sequelae.[33]

Laboratory Tests. Although rubella may be cultured from tissues and body fluids, including throat swabs, detecting antirubella IgM antibody usually establishes the diagnosis of acute rubella infection. Diagnosis by anti-IgG antibody seroconversion requires paired acute and convalescent sera. IgM and IgG are usually present at the onset of joint symptoms. IgM antibody levels peak 8 to 21 days after symptom onset and wane by 5 weeks. Antirubella IgG rises rapidly over a period of 1 to 3 weeks and is long lived. A single positive IgG serum sample or a set of untitered IgG-positive screens documents only immunity.[29]

Differential Diagnosis. Rubella arthritis needs to be differentiated from other viral arthritides and from inflammatory arthritides, including rheumatoid arthritis. It may be confused with parvovirus B19 infection.

Treatment and Outcome

Nonsteroidal anti-inflammatory drugs are useful to control symptoms. Some investigators have suggested the use of low to moderate doses of steroids to control symptoms and viremia.[34] Long-term prognosis is good.

Alphaviruses

Members of the genus *Alphavirus* are enveloped, single-stranded RNA viruses transmitted by mosquitoes.[35] Several cause acute febrile arthropathy, and their names reflect local appreciation of their clinical impact. For example, *chikungunya* means "that which twists or bends up" (Tanzania). The related *o'nyong-nyong* virus means "joint breaker" in the Acholi (Uganda) dialect. *Igbo-ora* is "the disease that breaks your wings."

Epidemiology

Chikungunya, o'nyong-nyong, and igbo-ora viruses form a serologically related group. Chikungunya virus was isolated during an epidemic of febrile arthritis in Tanzania between 1952 and 1953. Similar epidemics probably occurred in Africa, Asia, India, Indonesia, and possibly the southern United States as early as 1779.[35] Mosquitoes responsible for transmission to humans define its geographic distribution (Table 114-2). A feared consequence of global warming is spread of the geographic range of infected mosquitoes.[36-39]

Chikungunya fever occurs endemically and in epidemics.[40] Outbreaks have been described in the Indian Ocean islands, Malaysia, and Hong Kong.[41-44] An outbreak occurred in Italy in 2007. A large-scale outbreak of the serologically related o'nyong-nyong virus occurred in the Acholi province of northwestern Uganda in February 1959; this outbreak spread through Uganda and the surrounding region at a rate of 2 to 3 kilometers daily, affecting more than 2 million people within 2 years.[45] After the initial o'nyong-nyong epidemic, clinical disease was not detected again until it re-emerged in the Acholi region in 1996.[46] Despite the absence of outbreaks in the intervening years, serologic surveys have demonstrated that o'nyong-nyong virus is endemic.[47]

Weber's line is a hypothetical demarcation separating the Australian and Asiatic geographic zones. Antibodies to chikungunya virus are found west of Weber's line, and Ross River virus antibodies are found only east of it. Ross River virus causes epidemics of fever and rash in Australia, New Zealand, and the western Pacific islands.[48] In the Fiji Islands from 1979 to 1980, Ross River virus caused febrile polyarthritis in more than 40,000 individuals.[49] In Australia, endemic cases and epidemics occur in tropical and

Table 114-2 Mosquito Vectors and Reservoirs of Alphaviruses

Virus	Mosquito	Reservoir	Region
Chikungunya virus	*Aedes* species *Mansonia africana*	Baboons, monkeys, *Scotophilus* bat species	Africa, Asia
O'nyong-nyong virus	*Anopheles funestus* *Anopheles gambiae*	Unknown	Africa
Igbo-ora virus	*Anopheles funestus* *Anopheles gambiae*	Unknown	Ivory Coast
Ross River virus	*Aedes vigilax* *Aedes camptorhynchus* *Culex annulirostris* *Mansonia uniformis* *Aedes polynesiensis* *Aedes aegypti*	Rodents, marsupials, domestic animals	Australia, New Zealand, Papua New Guinea, Pacific Islands
Barmah forest virus	*Aedes* species *Anopheles* species *Culex* species	Unknown	Australia
Sindbis virus	*Aedes* species *Culex* species *Culiseta* species	Unknown	Sweden, Finland, Karelian Isthmus of Russia
Mayaro virus	*Haemagogus janthinomys*	Marmosets	Bolivia, Brazil, Peru

temperate regions annually.[50] Most cases occur in Queensland and New South Wales territories, where high rainfall and subsequent increases in mosquito populations usually precede epidemic periods. Infection rates in Australia range from 0.2% to 3.5% per year. Male and female infection rates are similar, but a female predominance has been noted in presenting cases. Most infected adults are symptomatic; the case rate for children is lower. Barmah Forest virus, another alphavirus with an increasing incidence in Australia, may manifest in a fashion similar to Ross River virus.[51-56]

Individuals involved in outdoor activities or occupations in forested areas in Sweden, Finland, and the neighboring Karelian isthmus of Russia are at greatest risk for infection with Sindbis virus; in those regions, it is known as Okelbo disease, Pogosta disease, and Karelian fever, respectively. Birds are the intermediate host.[57] It has also been reported in central Africa, Zimbabwe, South Africa, and Australia in sporadic cases or small outbreaks.[35]

Mayaro virus, first recognized in Trinidad in 1954, is endemic in the tropical rain forests of Bolivia, Brazil, and Peru. Cases have been imported into the United States in individuals traveling from endemic areas.[58]

Diagnosis

Clinical Features. Chikungunya fever presents with an explosive onset of high fever and severe arthralgia after a 1- to 12-day incubation period. The fever lasts 1 to 7 days. Typically, a macular or maculopapular, sometimes pruritic, rash on the torso, extremities, and occasionally the face, palms, and soles occurs on day 2 to 5 of illness as the patient defervesces. The rash may last 1 to 5 days and may recur with fever. Isolated petechiae and mucosal bleeding may occur. In some patients, involved skin desquamates.[59,60] Chemosis is prominent. Headache, photophobia, retro-orbital pain, pharyngitis, anorexia, nausea, vomiting, and abdominal pain may be present. Diffuse myalgia and back and shoulder pain are common. Migratory polyarthralgia, stiffness, and swelling affect predominantly the small joints of the hands, wrists, feet, and ankles. Large joints are less severely affected. Previously injured joints may be disproportionately affected. Large effusions are uncommon. Symptoms in children tend to be milder. Low-titer rheumatoid factor may be found in those with long-standing symptoms.

O'nyong-nyong fever is clinically similar to chikungunya fever.[61,62] In 1984, igbo-ora caused an epidemic of fever, myalgias, arthralgias, and rash in four Ivory Coast villages. Sequencing of isolates from the 1996 outbreak of o'nyong-nyong fever suggested that igbo-ora virus is a variant of o'nyong-nyong virus.[46]

Ross River virus polyarthralgia is severe, incapacitating, and often migratory and asymmetric.[63] Symptoms follow a 7- to 11-day incubation period. Finger interphalangeal and metacarpophalangeal joints, wrists, knees, ankles, shoulders, elbows, and toes are often involved. Polyarticular swelling and tenosynovitis are common. Arthralgias are worse in the morning and after inactivity. Rash is macular, papular, or maculopapular and may be pruritic. Vesicles, papules, or petechiae are typically seen on the trunk and extremities. The palms, soles, and face may be involved. Rash typically appears 1 to 2 days before joint symptoms,

but it may occur anywhere from 11 days before to 15 days after the onset of arthralgias, and it resolves by fading to a brownish discoloration or by desquamation. Half of patients have no fever, and those who do may have only modest fever lasting 1 to 3 days. Nausea, headache, and myalgia are common. Respiratory symptoms, mild photophobia, and lymphadenopathy may occur. Up to a third of patients have paresthesias and palm or sole pain. Carpal tunnel syndrome may be seen. Arthritis is less common and less prominent in Barmah Forest virus infection than in Ross River virus infection, but the rash is more common and florid.[64,65]

Rash and arthralgia are the presenting symptoms in Sindbis virus infection, although one may precede the other by a few days. Constitutional symptoms are usually mild and include low-grade fever, headache, fatigue, malaise, nausea, vomiting, pharyngitis, and paresthesias. A macular rash typically begins on the torso and then spreads to arms and legs, palms, soles, and occasionally the head. Macules evolve to form papules that tend to vesiculate. Vesiculation is prominent on pressure points, including the palms and soles. As the rash fades, a brownish discoloration is left. Vesicles on the palms and soles may become hemorrhagic. The rash may recur during convalescence.[66]

A Mayaro virus outbreak in Belterra, Brazil, in 1988 was characterized by sudden onset of fever, headache, dizziness, chills, and arthralgias in the wrists, fingers, ankles, and toes. The clinical attack rate was 80%. Joint swelling, unilateral inguinal lymphadenopathy, and leukopenia may be present. A maculopapular rash on the trunk and extremities lasts about 3 days.[67]

Laboratory Tests. The diagnosis of alphavirus infection requires laboratory confirmation. Any febrile patient residing in or returning from an endemic area should undergo a laboratory investigation. Chikungunya virus may be isolated from serum on days 2 through 4 of illness.[68] Neutralizing antibody, hemagglutination inhibition activity, and complement fixation tests may be used to detect antibodies. Chikungunya virus–specific IgM antibodies may be found for 6 months or longer.[69] O'nyong-nyong virus may be isolated by intracerebral injection into suckling mice, in which it produces alopecia, rash, and runting. Hemagglutination inhibition or complement fixation tests identify o'nyong-nyong virus.[70,71] Because chikungunya and o'nyong-nyong viruses are closely related serologically, mouse antisera raised to chikungunya virus or o'nyong-nyong virus react equally well with o'nyong-nyong virus, but o'nyong-nyong antisera do not react well with chikungunya virus. Molecular detection methods have improved diagnostic specificity.[72-75] Specific reverse transcriptase polymerase chain reaction–based assays have been developed for viral RNA detection.[73,76]

In chikungunya fever, synovial fluid shows decreased viscosity, poor mucin clot, and 2000 to 5000 white blood cells/mm³. Ross River virus has been isolated only from antibody-negative sera. In Australian epidemics before 1979, patients were antibody positive at the time of presentation. In contrast, patients during the Pacific island epidemics of 1979 to 1980 remained viremic and seronegative for up to 1 week after the onset of symptoms. Synovial fluid cell counts range from 1500 to 13,800 cells/mm³, predominantly monocytes and vacuolated macrophages.[77] Barmah Forest virus infection is confirmed by rising titers of specific

IgG.[64] Diagnosis of Sindbis virus infection is confirmed by specific serology.

Pathogenesis

Little is known about the pathogenesis of chikungunya fever or arthritis. Involved skin shows erythrocyte extravasation from superficial capillaries and perivascular cuffing. The virus adsorbs to human platelets, causing aggregation, suggesting a mechanism for bleeding. Synovitis probably results from direct viral infection of synovium. In one patient with chronic arthropathy, the synovium appeared atrophic on arthroscopy and was histologically normal.[78] The mechanisms of o'nyong-nyong virus pathogenesis are unknown. However, the virus was isolated from peripheral blood mononuclear cells in a patient in Chad.[79]

Ross River virus antigen may be detected early in monocytes and macrophages by immunofluorescence, but intact virus is not identifiable by electron microscopy or cell culture.[80] Erythematous and purpuric rashes show mild dermal perivascular mononuclear cell infiltrates, mostly T lymphocytes. Purpuric areas also show erythrocyte extravasation. Viral antigen may be detected in epithelial cells in erythematous and purpuric skin lesions and in perivascular zones in erythematous lesions.[81]

Sindbis virus has been isolated from a skin vesicle in the absence of viremia. Skin lesions show perivascular edema, hemorrhage, lymphocytic infiltrates, and areas of necrosis. Anti–Sindbis virus IgM may persist for years, raising the possibility that Sindbis virus arthritis is associated with viral persistence.[82]

Treatment and Outcome

Management is supportive. Nonsteroidal anti-inflammatory agents are useful, but aspirin should be avoided in view of the tendency for alphavirus rashes to develop a hemorrhagic component. Chloroquine has been used in chikungunya fever when nonsteroidal anti-inflammatory agents failed.[83] During the acute attack, range-of-motion exercises may decrease stiffness. In general, management of alphavirus infection is symptomatic; patients recover without sequelae. After acute chikungunya fever, symptoms may persist for months before resolution. Approximately 10% of patients still have joint symptoms 1 year after infection.[78] A few patients may develop chronic arthralgia. Case reports suggest that a few patients with chronic arthropathy develop destructive joint lesions, but a second process cannot be ruled out.

For persons with Ross River virus arthritis, mild exercise tends to improve joint symptoms. Half of all patients are able to resume their daily activities within 4 weeks, although residual polyarthralgia may be present. Joint symptoms may recur.[84] Arthralgia, myalgia, and lethargy may continue for at least 6 months in up to half of patients.[64] Relapsing episodes gradually resolve, but joint symptoms have been reported in a few patients for up to 3 years.[63,85]

Nonerosive chronic arthropathy is common after Sindbis virus infection, with up to one-third of patients having arthropathy 2 years or longer after onset. A smaller number have symptoms for as long as 5 to 6 years.[82] Mayaro virus–infected patients have persistent arthralgias for months.

HEPATITIS B VIRUS

Hepatitis B virus (HBV), a member of the family Hepadnaviridae, genus *Orthohepadnavirus*, is an enveloped, double-stranded, icosahedral DNA virus measuring 42 nm in diameter.[86,87]

Epidemiology

HBV occurs worldwide and is transmitted by parenteral and sexual routes. Prevalence is highest in Asia, the Middle East, and sub-Saharan Africa. In China, the prevalence is as high as 10%, compared with 0.01% in the United States. In endemic regions, infection occurs at an early age, frequently perinatally. Early HBV infection is usually asymptomatic. Rates of HBV carriage and specific antibody positivity decline with age. In the West, most infections are acquired during adulthood through sexual or needle exposure, leading to acute hepatitis. Of those with hepatitis, 5% to 10% develop persistent infection. In endemic regions, HBV is a common cause of chronic liver disease and a leading cause of hepatocellular carcinoma.[86]

Clinical Features

The time from infection to clinical hepatitis is usually 45 to 120 days. A preicteric prodromal period lasts several days to a month and may be associated with fever, myalgia, malaise, anorexia, nausea, and vomiting. Joint involvement is usually sudden in onset and often severe, with symmetric and simultaneous involvement of several joints. Alternatively, arthritis may be migratory or additive.[88,89] The joints of the hand and knee are most often affected, but wrists, ankles, elbows, shoulders, and other large joints may be involved as well. Fusiform swelling occurs in the small joints of the hand. Morning stiffness is common. Arthritis and urticaria may precede jaundice by days to weeks and may persist for several weeks, but they usually subside soon after the onset of clinical jaundice. Arthritis is usually limited to the preicteric prodrome. Those who develop chronic active hepatitis or chronic HBV viremia may have recurrent polyarthralgia or polyarthritis.[90] Polyarteritis nodosa may be associated with chronic hepatitis B viremia.[91]

Diagnosis

Urticaria in the presence of polyarthritis should suggest the possibility of HBV infection. Acute hepatitis may be asymptomatic, but elevated bilirubin and transaminases are usually present when arthritis appears. At the onset of arthritis, peak levels of serum hepatitis B surface antigen (HBsAg) are detectable. Virions, viral DNA, polymerase, and hepatitis B antigen may be detectable in serum. Anti–hepatitis B core antigen IgM antibodies indicate acute HBV infection rather than past or chronic infection.[92]

Pathogenesis

Significant viremia occurs early in infection. Soluble immune complexes with circulating HBsAg form as anti-HBsAg antibodies are produced. An immune complex–mediated arthritis usually results, with immune complex deposition in synovium. Immune complexes containing HBsAg, antibody, and complement components may be detected.

HEPATITIS C VIRUS

Hepatitis C virus (HCV), a member of the family Flaviviridae, is an enveloped, single-stranded, spherical RNA virus measuring 38 to 50 nm in diameter.[93,94]

Epidemiology

HCV infection occurs worldwide. Like HBV infection, seroprevalence is higher in Africa and Asia, where it may cause one-fourth of acute and chronic hepatitis cases. In Japan, up to 50% of hepatitides may be caused by HCV.[95] In the United States, an estimated 2.7 million individuals are infected.[96,97]

HCV is transmitted by the parenteral route. Sexual transmission may occur but is uncommon.[98] More than half of all cases of non-A, non-B hepatitis are attributable to HCV infection.[99] Multiple HCV genotypes and quasispecies are organized into six major groups. They differ in pathogenicity, severity of disease, and response to interferon.[99-103]

Clinical Features

Acute HCV infection is usually benign. Up to 80% of post-transfusion infections are anicteric and asymptomatic. Liver enzyme elevations, when present, are usually minimal. Normal transaminase levels do not exclude HCV infection. Community-acquired cases may present more symptomatically and with significant transaminase elevations. Acute fulminant HCV hepatitis is rare. Acute HCV infection may be accompanied by acute-onset polyarthritis in a rheumatoid distribution, including the small joints of the hand, wrists, shoulders, knees, and hips.[104]

HCV is often associated with mixed (type II and III) cryoglobulinemia. Essential mixed cryoglobulinemia—a triad of arthritis, palpable purpura, and cryoglobulinemia—is associated with HCV infection in most cases. Cryoglobulinemia in HCV infection is also seen in the absence of arthritis and purpura.[105] Cryoglobulinemia may be associated with necrotizing vasculitis. The presence of anti-HCV antibodies in essential mixed cryoglobulinemia is associated with more severe cutaneous involvement, such as Raynaud's phenomena, purpura, livedo, distal ulcers, and gangrene.[106] HCV RNA may be found in 75% of cryoprecipitates from patients with essential mixed cryoglobulinemia and anti-HCV antibodies.[107]

Diagnosis

Serologic tests use an array of antigens in an enzyme immunoassay. A recombinant antigen strip immunoblot assay is confirmatory.[108] Polymerase chain reaction–based diagnostics allow confirmation of HCV viremia, viral load, and genotype.[100,101] A minority of patients may have HCV RNA detectable by polymerase chain reaction amplification methods in the absence of positive serologic findings.[108-113] Liver biopsy for staging of liver disease is usually indicated in patients who have serum anti-HCV antibody or RNA, even in the setting of normal liver enzymes, because liver enzymes do not reflect liver histology. A number of algorithms based on blood measures of liver involvement have been proposed to aid in staging.[114-118]

Pathogenesis

HCV infection persists despite antibody response to viral epitopes. Increased CD4+CD25+ regulatory T lymphocytes may blunt the immune response to HCV.[118] A high rate of mutation in the envelope protein is responsible for the emergence of neutralization-escape mutants and quasispecies.[119] HCV may contain an IgG Fc binding region on its surface; humoral immune response to HCV would, by epitope spreading, also target bound immunoglobulin Fc structures.[120] Chronic HCV infection leads to cirrhosis, end-stage liver failure, and hepatocellular carcinoma after a period of up to 20 years, but the frequency of these sequelae is debated, and the mechanisms by which they occur are unknown.[121]

Treatment

Initially, interferon-alfa2b was used to suppress viral titers and ameliorate HCV liver disease in about half of patients and may have benefited HCV-associated cryoglobulinemia.[122] Relapse after completion of the initial course of therapy was common. The current use of pegylated interferons that increase drug half-life and decrease clearance, and the addition of ribavirin, have improved outcomes.[123] Controversy continues regarding whether interferon therapy precipitates autoimmune diseases such as autoimmune thyroiditis.[124,125] Those with cryoglobulinemia who fail interferon therapy require immunosuppressive therapy when vasculitis is present.

HUMAN T-LYMPHOTROPIC VIRUS TYPE 1

Human T-lymphotropic virus type 1 (HTLV-1), a retrovirus, is endemic in southern Japan, where it has been associated with oligoarthritis and a nodular rash (Figure 114-1). Anti-HTLV serology is positive. Type C viral particles are found in skin nodules. Synovial tissue is infiltrated by leukemic T lymphocytes with lobulated nuclei.[126-128]

OTHER VIRUSES

Joint involvement occasionally occurs in numerous other commonly encountered viral syndromes. Children with varicella rarely develop brief monoarticular or pauciarticular arthritis.[129] Mumps in adults is occasionally associated with small or large joint synovitis preceding or following the onset of parotitis by up to 4 weeks. Mumps arthritis may last several weeks.[130] Infection with adenovirus and with coxsackieviruses A9, B2, B3, B4, and B6 has been associated with recurrent episodes of polyarthritis, pleuritis, myalgia, rash, pharyngitis, myocarditis, and leukocytosis.[131] Epstein-Barr virus–induced mononucleosis is frequently accompanied by polyarthralgia, but monoarticular knee arthritis sometimes occurs. A few cases of polyarthritis, fever, and myalgia due to echovirus 9 infection have been reported.[132]

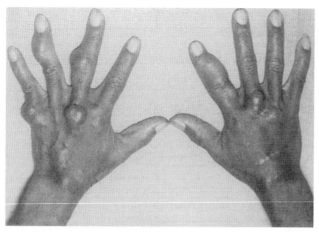

Figure 114-1 Nodular synovitis associated with human T-lymphotropic virus type 1 infection. *(From Yancey WB Jr, Dolson LH, Oblon D, et al: HTLV-I-associated adult T-cell leukemia/lymphoma presenting with nodular synovial masses, Am J Med 89:676, 1990.)*

Arthritis associated with herpes simplex virus or cytomegalovirus infection is rare, but a severe cytomegalovirus polyarthritis has been described in several immunocompromised bone marrow transplant recipients.[133] *Herpes hominis* occasionally causes arthritis of the knee in wrestlers, a condition referred to as *herpes gladiatorum*.[134] Knee arthritis has been reported as a rare complication after vaccinia inoculation.[135]

Selected References

1. Pennisi E: Teetering on the brink of danger, *Science* 271:1665, 1996.
2. Albert LJ, Inman RD: Molecular mimicry and autoimmunity, *N Engl J Med* 341:2068, 1999.
3. Gillespie SM, Cartter ML, Asch S, et al: Occupational risk of human parvovirus B19 infection for school and day-care personnel during an outbreak of erythema infectiosum, *JAMA* 263:2061, 1990.
4. Bell LM, Naides SJ, Stoffman P, et al: Human parvovirus B19 infection among hospital staff members after contact with infected patients, *N Engl J Med* 321:485, 1989.
5. Anderson MJ, Higgins PG, Davis LR, et al: Experimental parvoviral infection in humans, *J Infect Dis* 152:257, 1985.
6. Naides SJ: Rheumatic manifestations of parvovirus B19 infection, *Rheum Dis Clin North Am* 24:375, 1998.
7. Von Poblotzki A, Hemauer A, Gigler A, et al: Antibodies to the nonstructural protein of parvovirus B19 in persistently infected patients: implications for pathogenesis, *J Infect Dis* 172:1356, 1995.
8. Takahashi Y, Murai C, Shibata S, et al: Human parvovirus B19 as a causative agent for rheumatoid arthritis, *Proc Natl Acad Sci U S A* 95:8227, 1998.
9. Hsu TC, Tzang BS, Huang CN, et al: Increased expression and secretion of interleukin-6 in human parvovirus B19 non-structural protein (NS1) transfected COS-7 epithelial cells, *Clin Exp Immunol* 144:152, 2006.
10. Sol N, Morinet F, Alizon M, et al: Trans-activation of the long terminal repeat of human immunodeficiency virus type 1 by the parvovirus B19 NS1 gene product, *J Gen Virol* 74:2011, 1993.
11. Peterlana D, Puccetti A, Beri R, et al: The presence of parvovirus B19 VP and NS1 genes in the synovium is not correlated with rheumatoid arthritis, *J Rheumatol* 30:1907, 2003.
12. Poole BD, Karetnyi YV, Naides SJ: Parvovirus B19-induced apoptosis of hepatocytes, *J Virol* 78:7775, 2004.
13. Poole BD, Zhou J, Grote A, et al: Apoptosis of liver-derived cells induced by parvovirus B19 nonstructural protein, *J Virol* 80:4114, 2006.
14. Karetnyi YV, Beck PR, Markin RS, et al: Human parvovirus B19 infection in acute fulminant liver failure, *Arch Virol* 144:1713, 1999.
15. Gabriel SE, Espy M, Erdman DD, et al: The role of parvovirus B19 in the pathogenesis of giant cell arteritis: a preliminary evaluation, *Arthritis Rheum* 42:1255, 1999.
16. Veraldi S, Mancuso R, Rizzitelli E, et al: Henoch-Schönlein syndrome associated with human parvovirus B19 primary infection, *Eur J Dermatol* 9:232, 1999.
17. Heegaard ED, Rosthoj S, Petersen B, et al: Role of parvovirus B19 infection in childhood idiopathic thrombocytopenic purpura, *Acta Paediatr* 88:614, 1999.
18. Frickhofen N, Abkowitz JL, Safford M, et al: Persistent B19 parvovirus infection in patients infected with human immunodeficiency virus type 1 (HIV-1): a treatable cause of anemia in AIDS, *Ann Intern Med* 113:926, 1990.
19. Ager EA, Chin TDY, Poland JD: Epidemic erythema infectiosum, *N Engl J Med* 275:1326, 1966.
20. Naides SJ, Field EH: Transient rheumatoid factor positivity in acute parvovirus B19 infection, *Arch Intern Med* 148:2587, 1988.
21. Kerr JR, Boyd N: Autoantibodies following parvovirus B19 infection, *J Infect* 32:41, 1996.
22. Lunardi C, Tiso M, Borgato L, et al: Chronic parvovirus B19 infection induces the production of anti-virus antibodies with autoantigen binding properties, *Eur J Immunol* 28:936, 1998.
24. von Landenberg P, Lehmann HW, Knöll A, et al: Antiphospholipid antibodies in pediatric and adult patients with rheumatic disease are associated with parvovirus B19 infection, *Arthritis Rheum* 48:1939, 2003.
25. Anderson LJ, Tsou C, Parker RA, et al: Detection of antibodies and antigens of human parvovirus B19 by enzyme-linked immunosorbent assay, *J Clin Microbiol* 24:522, 1986.
27. Soderlund M, von Essen R, Haapasaari J, et al: Persistence of parvovirus B19 DNA in synovial membranes of young patients with and without chronic arthropathy, *Lancet* 349:1063, 1997.
29. Chantler J, Wolinsky JS, Tingle A: Rubella. In Knipe DM, Howley PM, editors: *Fields virology*, ed 4, Philadelphia, 2001, Lippincott Williams & Wilkins, pp 963–990.
30. Mims CA, Stokes A, Grahame R: Synthesis of antibodies, including antiviral antibodies, in the knee joints of patients with arthritis, *Ann Rheum Dis* 44:734, 1985.
31. Tingle AJ, Allen M, Petty RE, et al: Rubella-associated arthritis. I. Comparative study of joint manifestations associated with natural rubella infection and RA 27/3 rubella immunization, *Ann Rheum Dis* 45:110, 1986.
32. Howson CP, Katz M, Johnston RB Jr, et al: Chronic arthritis after rubella vaccination, *Clin Infect Dis* 15:307, 1992.
33. Schaffner W, Fleet WF, Kilroy AW, et al: Polyneuropathy following rubella immunization: a follow-up study and review of the problem, *Am J Dis Child* 127:684, 1974.
34. Mitchell LA, Tingle AJ, Shukin R, et al: Chronic rubella vaccine-associated arthropathy, *Arch Intern Med* 153:2268, 1993.
35. Griffin DE: Alphaviruses. In Knipe DM, Howley PM, editors: *Fields virology*, ed 4, Philadelphia, 2001, Lippincott Williams & Wilkins, pp 917–962.
37. Jetten TH, Focks DA: Potential changes in the distribution of dengue transmission under climate warming, *Am J Trop Med Hyg* 57:285, 1997.
38. Reiter P: Climate change and mosquito-borne disease, *Environ Health Perspect* 109(Suppl 1):141, 2001.
40. Halstead SB, Nimmannitya S, Margiotta MR: Dengue and chikungunya virus infection in man in Thailand, 1962-1964. II. Observations on disease in outpatients, *Am J Trop Med Hyg* 18:972, 1969.
41. Sam IC, AbuBakar S: Chikungunya virus infection, *Med J Malaysia* 61:264, 2006.
42. Schuffenecker I, Iteman I, Michault A, et al: Genome microevolution of chikungunya viruses causing the Indian Ocean outbreak, *PLoS Med* 3:e263, 2006.
43. Lee N, Wong CK, Lam WY, et al: Chikungunya fever, Hong Kong, *Emerg Infect Dis* 12:1790, 2006.
44. AbuBakar S, Sam JC, Wong PF, et al: Reemergence of endemic Chikungunya, Malaysia, *Emerg Infect Dis* 13:147, 2007.
45. Williams MC, Woodall JP, Gillett JD: O'nyong-nyong fever: an epidemic in East Africa. VII. Virus isolations from man and serological studies up to July 1961, *Trans R Soc Trop Med Hyg* 59:186, 1965.
46. Lanciotti RS, Ludwig ML, Rwaguma EB, et al: Emergence of epidemic o'nyong-nyong fever in Uganda, after a 35 year absence, *Virology* 252:258, 1998.

48. Harley D, Sleigh A, Ritchie S: Ross River virus transmission, infection, and disease: a cross-disciplinary review, *Clin Microbiol Rev* 14:909, 2001.

49. Bennett NM, Cunningham AL, Fraser JR, et al: Epidemic polyarthritis acquired in Fiji, *Med J Aust* 1:316, 1980.

50. Mudge PR, Aaskov JG: Epidemic polyarthritis in Australia, 1980-1981, *Med J Aust* 2:269, 1983.

51. Lindsay MDA, Johansen CA, Broom AK, et al: Emergence of Barmah Forest virus in Western Australia, *Emerg Infect Dis* 1:22, 1995.

52. Harvey L, Dwyer D: Recent increases in the notification of Barmah Forest virus infections in New South Wales, *N S W Public Health Bull* 15:199, 2004.

53. Liu C, Broom AK, Kurcz N, et al: Communicable Diseases Network Australia: National Arbovirus and Malaria Advisory Committee annual report 2004-2005, *Commun Dis Intell* 29:341, 2005.

54. Quinn HE, Gatton ML, Hall G, et al: Analysis of Barmah Forest virus disease activity in Queensland, Australia, 1993-2003: identification of a large, isolated outbreak of disease, *J Med Entomol* 42:882, 2005.

55. Liu C, Johansen C, Kurucz N, et al: Communicable Diseases Network Australia: National Arbovirus and Malaria Advisory Committee annual report, 2005-06, *Commun Dis Intell* 30:411, 2006.

56. Kelly-Hope LA, Kay BH, Purdie DM, et al: The risk of Ross River and Barmah Forest virus disease in Queensland: implications for New Zealand, *Aust N Z J Public Health* 26:69, 2002.

57. Brummer-Korvenkontio M, Vapalahti O, Kuusisto P, et al: Epidemiology of Sindbis virus infections in Finland 1981-96: possible factors explaining a peculiar disease pattern, *Epidemiol Infect* 129:335, 2002.

58. Tesh RB, Watts DM, Russell KL, et al: Mayaro virus disease: an emerging mosquito-borne zoonosis in tropical South America, *Clin Infect Dis* 28:67, 1999.

59. Moore CG: *Aedes albopictus* in the United States: current status and prospects for further spread, *J Am Mosq Control Assoc* 15:221, 1999.

60. Halstead SB, Udomsakdi S, Singharaj P, et al: Dengue and chikungunya virus infection in man in Thailand, 1962-1964. III. Clinical, epidemiologic, and virologic observations on disease in non-indigenous white persons, *Am J Trop Med Hyg* 18:984, 1969.

61. Sanders EJ, Rwaguma EB, Kawamata J, et al: O'nyong-nyong fever in south-central Uganda, 1996-1997: description of the epidemic and results of a household-based seroprevalence survey, *J Infect Dis* 180:1436, 1999.

62. Kiwanuka N, Sanders EJ, Rwaguma EB, et al: O'nyong-nyong fever in south-central Uganda, 1996-1997: clinical features and validation of a clinical case definition for surveillance purposes, *Clin Infect Dis* 29:1243, 1999.

64. Flexman JP, Smith DW, Mackenzie JS, et al: A comparison of the diseases caused by Ross River virus and Barmah Forest virus, *Med J Aust* 169:159, 1998.

65. Passmore J, O'Grady KA, Moran R, et al: An outbreak of Barmah Forest virus disease in Victoria, *Commun Dis Intell* 26:600, 2002.

66. Julkunen I, Brummer-Korvenkontio M, Hautanen A, et al: Elevated serum immune complex levels in Pogosta disease, an acute alphavirus infection with rash and arthritis, *J Clin Lab Immunol* 21:77, 1986.

67. Pinheiro FP, Freitas RB, Travassos da Rosa JF, et al: An outbreak of Mayaro virus disease in Belterra, Brazil. I. Clinical and virological findings, *Am J Trop Med Hyg* 30:674, 1981.

68. Nimmannitya S, Halstead SB, Cohen SN, et al: Dengue and chikungunya virus infection in man in Thailand, 1962-1964. I. Observations on hospitalized patients with hemorrhagic fever, *Am J Trop Med Hyg* 18:954, 1969.

71. Williams MC, Woodall JP, Porterfield JS: O'nyong-nyong fever: an epidemic virus disease in East Africa, *Trans R Soc Trop Med Hyg* 59:186, 1965.

72. Hasebe F, Parquet MC, Pandey BD, et al: Combined detection and genotyping of chikungunya virus by a specific reverse transcription-polymerase chain reaction, *J Med Virol* 67:370, 2002.

73. Pfeffer M, Linssen B, Parke MD, et al: Specific detection of chikungunya virus using a RT-PCR/nested PCR combination, *J Vet Med B Infect Dis Vet Public Health* 49:49, 2002.

74. Corwin A, Simanjuntak CH, Ansari A: Emerging disease surveillance in Southeast Asia, *Ann Acad Med Singapore* 26:628, 1997.

75. Junt T, Heraud JM, Lelarge J, et al: Determination of natural versus laboratory human infection with Mayaro virus by molecular analysis, *Epidemiol Infect* 123:511, 1999.

76. Pastorino B, Bessaud M, Grandadam M, et al: Development of a TaqMan RT-PCR assay without RNA extraction step for the detection and quantification of African chikungunya viruses, *J Virol Methods* 124:65, 2005.

77. Aaskov JG, Mataika JU, Lawrence GW, et al: An epidemic of Ross River virus infection in Fiji, 1979, *Am J Trop Med Hyg* 30:1053, 1981.

78. Brighton SW, Prozesky OW, De la Harpe AL: Chikungunya virus infection: a retrospective study of 107 cases, *S Afr Med J* 63:313, 1983.

79. Bessaud M, Peyrefitte CN, Pastorino BA, et al: O'nyong-nyong virus, Chad, *Emerg Infect Dis* 12:1248, 2006.

80. Fraser JR, Cunningham AL, Clarris BJ, et al: Cytology of synovial effusions in epidemic polyarthritis, *Aust N Z J Med* 11:168, 1981.

81. Fraser JR, Ratnamohan VM, Dowling JP, et al: The exanthem of Ross River virus infection: histology, location of virus antigen and nature of inflammatory infiltrate, *J Clin Pathol* 36:1256, 1983.

82. Niklasson B, Espmark A, Lundstrom J: Occurrence of arthralgia and specific IgM antibodies three to four years after Ockelbo disease, *J Infect Dis* 157:832, 1988.

84. Mylonas AD, Brown AM, Carthew TL, et al: Natural history of Ross River virus-induced epidemic polyarthritis, *Med J Aust* 177:356, 2002.

85. Laine M, Luukkainen R, Jalava J, et al: Prolonged arthritis associated with Sindbis-related (Pogosta) virus infection, *Rheumatology (Oxford)* 41:829, 2002.

86. Robinson WS: Hepatitis B viruses: general features (human). In Webster RG, Granoff A, editors: *Encyclopedia of virology*, San Diego, 1994, Academic Press, pp 554–559.

87. Bendinelli M, Pistello M, Maggi F, et al: Blood-borne hepatitis viruses: hepatitis B, C, D, and G viruses and TT virus. In Specter S, Hodinka RL, Young SA, editors: *Clinical virology manual*, Washington, DC, 2000, ASM Press, pp 306–337.

88. Hollinger FB, Liang TJ: Hepatitis B virus. In Knipe DM, Howley PM, Griffin DE, et al, editors: *Fields virology*, Philadelphia, 2001, Lippincott Williams & Wilkins, pp 2971–3036.

89. Alarcon GS, Townes AS: Arthritis in viral hepatitis: report of two cases and review of the literature, *Johns Hopkins Med J* 132:1, 1973.

90. Csepregi A, Rojkovich B, Nemesanszky E, et al: Chronic seropositive polyarthritis associated with hepatitis B virus-induced chronic liver disease: a sequel of virus persistence, *Arthritis Rheum* 43:232, 2000.

91. Guillevin L, Lhote F, Cohen P, et al: Polyarteritis nodosa related to hepatitis B virus: a prospective study with long-term observation of 41 patients, *Medicine (Baltimore)* 74:238, 1995.

92. Hoofnagle JH: Serologic markers of hepatitis B virus infection, *Annu Rev Med* 32:1, 1981.

93. Gronboek KE, Jensen OJ, Krarup HB, et al: Biochemical, virological and histopathological changes in Danish blood donors with antibodies to hepatitis C virus, *Dan Med Bull* 43:186, 1996.

94. Lindebach BD, Rice CM: Flaviviridae: the viruses and their replication. In Knipe DM, Howley PM, Griffin DE, et al, editors: *Fields virology*, Philadelphia, 2001, Lippincott Williams & Wilkins, pp 991–1041.

95. Kuboki M, Shinzawa H, Shao L, et al: A cohort study of hepatitis C virus (HCV) infection in an HCV epidemic area of Japan: age- and sex-related seroprevalence of anti-HCV antibody, frequency of viremia, biochemical abnormality and histological changes, *Liver* 19:88, 1999.

97. Williams I: Epidemiology of hepatitis C in the United States, *Am J Med* 107:2S, 1999.

98. Neumayr G, Propst A, Schwaighofer H, et al: Lack of evidence for the heterosexual transmission of hepatitis C, *QJM* 92:505, 1999.

99. Bhandari BN, Wright TL: Hepatitis C: an overview, *Annu Rev Med* 46:309, 1995.

100. Pawlotsky JM: Hepatitis C virus genetic variability: pathogenic and clinical implications, *Clin Liver Dis* 7:45, 2003.

101. Pawlotsky JM: Use and interpretation of hepatitis C virus diagnostic assays, *Clin Liver Dis* 7:127, 2003.

102. Davis GL: Hepatitis C virus genotypes and quasispecies, *Am J Med* 107:21S, 1999.

104. Siegel LB, Cohn L, Nashel D: Rheumatic manifestations of hepatitis C infection, *Semin Arthritis Rheum* 23:149, 1993.

105. Arranz FR, Diaz RD, Diez LI, et al: Cryoglobulinemic vasculitis associated with hepatitis C virus infection: a report of eight cases, *Acta Derm Venereol (Stockh)* 75:234, 1995.

106. Sansonno D, Cornacchiulo V, Iacobelli AR, et al: Localization of hepatitis C virus antigens in liver and skin tissues of chronic hepatitis

C virus-infected patients with mixed cryoglobulinemia, *Hepatology* 21:305, 1995.

107. Munoz-Fernandez S, Barbado FJ, Martin Mola E, et al: Evidence of hepatitis C virus antibodies in the cryoprecipitate of patients with mixed cryoglobulinemia, *J Rheumatol* 21:229, 1994.

108. van der Poel CL: Hepatitis C virus: into the fourth generation, *Vox Sang* 67(Suppl 3):95, 1994.

109. Schmidt WN, Klinzman D, LaBrecque DR, et al: Direct detection of hepatitis C virus (HCV) RNA from whole blood, and comparison with HCV RNA in plasma and peripheral blood mononuclear cells, *J Med Virol* 47:153, 1995.

110. Schmidt WN, Wu P, Cederna J, et al: Surreptitious hepatitis C virus (HCV) infection detected in the majority of patients with cryptogenic chronic hepatitis and negative HCV antibody tests, *J Infect Dis* 176:27, 1997.

111. Stapleton JT, Klinzman D, Schmidt WN, et al: Prospective comparison of whole-blood- and plasma-based hepatitis C virus RNA detection systems: improved detection using whole blood as the source of viral RNA, *J Clin Microbiol* 37:484, 1999.

112. Schmidt W, Stapleton JT: Whole-blood hepatitis C virus RNA extraction methods, *J Clin Microbiol* 39:3812, 2001.

113. George SL, Gebhardt J, Klinzman D, et al: Hepatitis C virus viremia in HIV-infected individuals with negative HCV antibody tests, *J Acquir Immune Defic Syndr* 31:154, 2002.

114. Colletta C, Smirne C, Fabris C, et al: Value of two noninvasive methods to detect progression of fibrosis among HCV carriers with normal aminotransferases, *Hepatology* 42:838, 2005.

115. Wilson LE, Torbenson M, Astemborski J, et al: Progression of liver fibrosis among injection drug users with chronic hepatitis C, *Hepatology* 43:788, 2006.

116. Zaman A, Rosen HR, Ingram K, et al: Assessment of FIBROSpect II to detect hepatic fibrosis in chronic hepatitis C patients, *Am J Med* 120:e9, 2007.

117. Adams LA, Bulsara M, Rossi E, et al: Hepascore: an accurate validated predictor of liver fibrosis in chronic hepatitis C infection, *Clin Chem* 51:1867, 2005.

119. Shimizu YK, Hijikata M, Iwamoto A, et al: Neutralizing antibodies against hepatitis C virus and the emergence of neutralization escape mutant viruses, *J Virol* 68:1494, 1994.

120. Wunschmann S, Medh JD, Klinzmann D, et al: Characterization of hepatitis C virus (HCV) and HCV E2 interaction with CD81 and the low density lipoprotein receptor, *J Virol* 74:10055, 2000.

123. Baker DE: Pegylated interferon plus ribavirin for the treatment of chronic hepatitis C, *Rev Gastroenterol Disord* 3:93, 2003.

124. Morisco F, Mazziotti G, Rotondi M, et al: Interferon-related thyroid autoimmunity and long-term clinical outcome of chronic hepatitis C, *Dig Liver Dis* 33:247, 2001.

125. Rocco A, Gargano S, Provenzano A, et al: Incidence of autoimmune thyroiditis in interferon-alpha treated and untreated patients with chronic hepatitis C virus infection, *Neuroendocrinol Lett* 22:39, 2001.

126. Yancey WB Jr, Dolson LH, Oblon D, et al: HTLV-I-associated adult T-cell leukemia/lymphoma presenting with nodular synovial masses, *Am J Med* 89:676, 1990.

127. Masuko-Hongo K, Nishioka K: HTLV-I associated arthropathy (HAAP)—a review, *Ryoikibetsu Shokogun Shirizu* 32:525, 2000.

128. Nishioka K, Nakajima T, Hasunuma T, et al: Rheumatic manifestation of human leukemia virus infection, *Rheum Dis Clin North Am* 19:489, 1993.

129. Chen MK, Wang CC, Lu JJ, et al: Varicella arthritis diagnosed by polymerase chain reaction, *J Formos Med Assoc* 98:519, 1999.

130. Gordon SC, Lauter CB: Mumps arthritis: a review of the literature, *Rev Infect Dis* 6:338, 1984.

131. Bayer AS: Arthritis associated with common viral infections: mumps, coxsackievirus, and adenovirus, *Postgrad Med* 68:55, 1980.

132. Blotzer JW, Myers AR: Echovirus-associated polyarthritis: report of a case with synovial fluid and synovial histologic characterization, *Arthritis Rheum* 21:978, 1978.

133. Burns LJ, Gingrich RD: Cytomegalovirus infection presenting as polyarticular arthritis following autologous BMT, *Bone Marrow Transplant* 11:77, 1993.

134. Shelley WB: Herpetic arthritis associated with disseminated herpes simplex in a wrestler, *Br J Dermatol* 103:209, 1980.

135. Silby HM, Farber R, O'Connell CJ, et al: Acute monarticular arthritis after vaccination: report of a case with isolation of vaccinia virus from synovial fluid, *Ann Intern Med* 62:347, 1965.

Full references for this chapter can be found on www.expertconsult.com.

115 Poststreptococcal Arthritis and Rheumatic Fever

ALLAN GIBOFSKY • JOHN B. ZABRISKIE

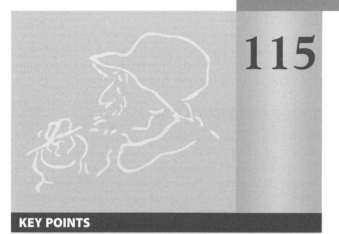

KEY POINTS

Acute rheumatic fever (ARF) is a delayed, nonsuppurative sequel of a pharyngeal infection with group A streptococci. Although a dramatic decline in the severity and the mortality of the disease has been noted, reports have described its resurgence in the United States.

Adequate treatment of documented streptococcal pharyngitis markedly reduces the incidence of subsequent ARF. Appropriate antimicrobial prophylaxis prevents recurrence of disease in known patients with ARF.

The clinical presentation of ARF varies. The lack of a single pathognomonic feature led to the development of the revised Jones criteria, which should be used to establish a diagnosis.

The terms *migrating* and *migratory* are often used to describe the polyarthritis of ARF, but these designations do not signify that the inflammation disappears in one joint when it appears in another. Rather, the various localizations usually overlap in time, and the onset, as opposed to the full course of arthritis, "migrates" from joint to joint.

Many investigators have suggested that poststreptococcal migratory arthritis (in adults and children) in the absence of carditis might be an entity distinct from ARF. Although these features may be seen (admittedly rarely), migratory arthritis without evidence of other major Jones criteria but supported by two minor manifestations still should be considered ARF, especially in children.

Antibiotic prophylaxis with penicillin should be started immediately after resolution of the acute episode. The optimal regimen consists of oral penicillin VK, 250,000 U twice a day, or parenteral penicillin G, 1.2 million U intramuscularly every 4 weeks.

Acute rheumatic fever (ARF) is a delayed, nonsuppurative sequel of pharyngeal infection with group A streptococci. After the initial streptococcal pharyngitis, a latent period of 2 to 3 weeks occurs. The onset of disease usually is characterized by an acute febrile illness, which may manifest in one of three classic ways: (1) The patient may present with migratory arthritis predominantly involving the large joints of the body; (2) concomitant clinical and laboratory signs of carditis and valvulitis may be noted; or (3) involvement of the central nervous system may manifest as Sydenham's chorea. The clinical episodes are self-limiting, but damage to the valves may be chronic and progressive, resulting in cardiac decompensation and death.

Although a dramatic decline in severity and mortality of the disease has been observed since the turn of the 20th century, reports in recent years have described its resurgence in the United States[1] and in many military installations throughout the world—a reminder that the disease remains a public health problem even in developed countries. In addition, the disease continues essentially unabated in many developing countries. Estimates suggest that 10 to 20 million new cases will be reported per year in countries where two-thirds of the world population lives. For all of these reasons, it is important to keep rheumatic fever in the differential diagnosis of acute febrile illnesses, as well as acute inflammatory arthritis, in both children and adults.

EPIDEMIOLOGY

The incidence of ARF began to decline long before the introduction of antibiotics into clinical practice, decreasing from 250 to 100 patients per 100,000 population from 1862 to 1962 in Denmark.[2] The introduction of antibiotics in 1950 rapidly accelerated this decline, until by 1980, the incidence ranged from 0.23 to 1.88 patients per 100,000, with disease occurring primarily in children and teenagers. A notable exception has been in the native Hawaiian and Maori populations (both of Polynesian ancestry), among whom the incidence continues to be 13.4 per 100,000 hospitalized children per year.[3]

Only a few M serotypes (types 5, 14, 18, and 24) have been identified with outbreaks of ARF, suggesting that certain strains of group A streptococci may be more "rheumatogenic" than others.[4] In Trinidad, types 41 and 11 have been the most common strains isolated from the oropharynx of patients with ARF. In our own series, conducted over a 20-year period (Table 115-1), many different M serotypes were isolated, including six strains that could not be typed. Kaplan and colleagues[5] isolated several M types from patients seen during an outbreak of ARF in Utah, and these strains were mucoid and nonmucoid in character. Whether or not certain strains are more "rheumatogenic" than others remains unresolved. What is true, however, is that a streptococcal strain capable of causing well-documented pharyngitis is generally capable of causing ARF, although some notable exceptions have been recorded.[6]

PATHOGENESIS

Although little evidence suggests the direct involvement of group A streptococci in the affected tissues of ARF patients, a large body of epidemiologic and immunologic evidence indirectly implicates group A streptococci in initiation of the disease process: (1) It is well known that outbreaks of ARF closely follow epidemics of streptococcal sore throat or scarlet fever[6]; (2) adequate treatment of documented

Table 115-1   Positive Throat Cultures for Group A β-Hemolytic Streptococci among Rockefeller University Hospital Rheumatic Fever Patients ($n = 87$)

M Type	RHD	No RHD	Total
Nontypable	1	5	6
1	1	1	2
2	0	1	1
5	1	1	2
6	1	1	2
12	0	2	2
18	2	2	4
19	2	1	3
28	1	0	1
TOTAL	9	14	23

No RHD, patients without rheumatic heart disease; RHD, patients with rheumatic heart disease.

streptococcal pharyngitis markedly reduces the incidence of subsequent ARF[7]; (3) appropriate antimicrobial prophylaxis prevents recurrence of disease in known patients with ARF[8]; and (4) if one tests the sera of ARF patients for three antistreptococcal antibodies (streptolysin O, hyaluronidase, and streptokinase), most ARF patients (whether or not they recall an antecedent streptococcal sore throat) are found to have elevated antibody titers to these antigens.[9]

A note of caution is necessary concerning documentation (clinical or microbiologic) of an antecedent streptococcal infection. The frequency of isolation of group A streptococci from the oropharynx is extremely low, even in populations with limited access to antibiotics. An age-related discrepancy in the clinical documentation of an antecedent sore throat has been noted. In older children and young adults, the recollection of a streptococcal sore throat approaches 70%; in younger children, this rate approaches only 20%.[1] It is important to have a high index of suspicion of ARF in children or young adults presenting with signs of arthritis or carditis or both, even in the absence of a clinically documented sore throat.

Another intriguing, and as yet unexplained, observation has been the invariable association of ARF only with streptococcal pharyngitis. Although many outbreaks of impetigo have occurred, ARF almost never occurs after infection with these strains. In Trinidad, where impetigo and ARF are common infections, the strains colonizing the skin are different from those associated with ARF, and this does not influence the incidence of ARF.[10] The explanation for these observations remains obscure.

Group A streptococci fall into two main classes based on differences in the C-repeat regions of the M protein.[11] One class is associated with streptococcal pharyngeal infection, and the other (with some exceptions) is commonly associated with impetigo. The particular strain of streptococci may be crucial in initiating the disease process. The pharyngeal site of infection with its large repository of lymphoid tissue also may be important in initiation of the abnormal humoral response by host to antigens cross-reactive with target organs. Finally, although impetigo strains do colonize the pharynx, they do not seem to elicit as strong an immunologic response to the M protein moiety as do the pharyngeal strains.[12,13] This may prove to be an important factor,

especially in light of known cross-reactions between various streptococcal structures and mammalian proteins.

GROUP A STREPTOCOCCI

Figure 115-1 shows a schematic cross-section of group A streptococci. The capsule is composed of equimolar concentrations of N-acetyl glucosamine and glucuronic acid and is structurally identical to hyaluronic acid of mammalian tissues.[14] Although numerous attempts to produce antibodies to this capsule have been unsuccessful,[15,16] Fillet and colleagues[17] were able to show high antibody titers to hyaluronic acid using techniques designed to detect nonprecipitating antibodies in the sera of immunized animals. Similar antibodies have been noted in humans.[18] Data establishing the importance of this capsule in human infection have been almost nonexistent, although Stollerman[19] commented on the presence of a large mucoid capsule as one of the more important characteristics of certain "rheumatogenic" strains.

With respect to the M protein moiety, investigations by Lancefield and others spanning almost 70 years[20] have established that the M protein molecule (at least 80 distinct serologic types) is perhaps the most important virulence factor in group A streptococcal infection of humans. The protein is a helical, coiled-coil structure that bears a striking structural homology to the cardiac cytoskeletal proteins, tropomyosin and myosin, and to many other coiled-coil structures, including keratin, DNA, lamin, and vimentin. When the amino acid sequence of many M proteins was delineated, it was possible to localize specifically the cross-reactive areas of the molecules. Studies of Dale and Beachey[21] showed that the segment of the M protein involved in the opsonic reaction cross-reacted with human sarcolemma antigens. Sargent and co-workers[22] more precisely localized this cross-reaction to the M protein amino acid residues 164 through 197.

Evidence implicating these cross-reactions in the pathogenesis of ARF remains scant. Antibodies to myosin have

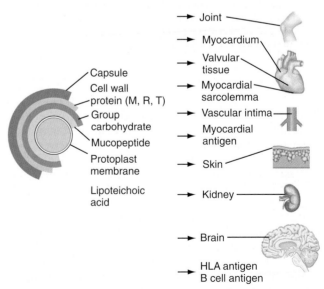

Figure 115-1   Schematic representation of various structures of group A streptococci. Note the wide variety of cross-reactions between antigens and mammalian tissues.

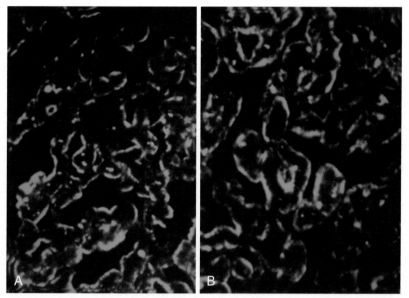

Figure 115-2 Photomicrographs of immunofluorescent staining of heart sections with rabbit serum immunized with group A streptococcal membranes **(A)** and human serum obtained from a patient with acute rheumatic fever **(B).** Note the identical sarcolemmal staining patterns of these sera.

been detected in the sera of ARF patients, but they also are present in a high percentage of the sera obtained from individuals who had a streptococcal infection but did not subsequently develop ARF.[23] The significance of this observation is unclear because myosin is an internal protein of cardiac muscle cells and is not easily exposed to M protein cross-reacting antibodies. The group-specific carbohydrate of the streptococcus is a polysaccharide chain consisting of repeating units of rhamnose capped by N-acetyl glucosamine molecules. The N-acetyl glucosamine is immunodominant and gives rise to the serologic group specificity of group A streptococci.[24]

Goldstein and associates[25] first described the cross-reaction between group A carbohydrate and valvular glycoproteins, and this reactivity was related to the N-acetyl glucosamine moiety present in both structures. Goldstein and Caravano[26] noted that rheumatic fever (RF) sera reacted to the heart valve glycoprotein. Fillet (unpublished data) observed strong reactivity of RF sera with purified proteoglycan material. These cross-reactions could involve the sugar moiety present in the proteoglycan portion of the glycoprotein and the carbohydrate.

It generally has been assumed that group A anticarbohydrate antibodies do not play a role in phagocytosis of group A streptococci. Salvadori and co-workers[27] showed, however, that human sera containing high titers of anti–group A carbohydrate antibody promoted opsonization and phagocytosis of many different M protein–specific strains, and the opsonophagocytic antibodies were directed to the N-acetyl glucosamine moiety of the group A carbohydrate. The mucopeptide portion of the cell wall is the "backbone" of the organism and is quite rigid in structure. It is composed of repeating units of muramic acid and N-acetyl glucosamine, cross-linked by peptide bridges.[28] It is particularly difficult to degrade and induces a wide variety of lesions when injected into various species, including arthritis in rats[29] and myocardial granulomas in mice resembling (but not identical to) RF Aschoff lesions.[30]

The relationship of cell wall mucopeptides to the pathogenesis of ARF remains obscure. Elevated levels of antimucopeptide antibody have been detected not only in the sera of patients with ARF, but also in the sera of patients with rheumatoid arthritis and juvenile rheumatoid arthritis[31]; however, its pathogenetic relationship to clinical disease has been difficult to establish. No evidence indicates that cell wall antigens are present in the Aschoff lesion or in the myocardial tissue obtained from patients with ARF. Perhaps the most significant cross-reactions lie in the streptococcal membrane structure. We have shown that immunization with membrane material[32] elicited antibodies that were bound to heart sections in a pattern similar to that observed with acute RF sera (Figure 115-2).

Kingston and Glynn[33] were the first to show that animals immunized with streptococcal antigens developed antibodies in their sera that stained astrocytes. Husby and associates[34] showed that sera from ARF patients with chorea exhibited antibodies that were specific for caudate cells. Absorption of the sera with streptococcal membrane antigens eliminated reactivity with caudate cells. Numerous other cross-reactions between streptococcal membranes and other organs have been reported (e.g., renal basement membranes, basement membrane proteoglycans, skin [particularly keratin]). In the context of this chapter, space does not permit an exhaustive discussion of these cross-reactions, and the reader is referred to other studies[35,36] for a more detailed discussion. Whether or not these cross-reactions (especially the cross-reactions seen with basement membranes and skin) play a role in the disease awaits further study.

GENETICS

The concept that ARF might be the result of a host genetic predisposition has intrigued investigators for more than a century.[37] It has been variously suggested that the disease gene is transmitted in an autosomal dominant fashion[38] or in an autosomal recessive fashion with limited penetrance,[39] or that it is possibly related to the genes conferring blood group secretor status.[40] Renewed interest in the genetics of ARF occurred with recognition that gene products of the human major histocompatibility complex (MHC) were associated with certain clinical disease states. Using an alloserum from a multiparous donor, an increased frequency of a B cell alloantigen was reported in several genetically distinct and ethnically diverse populations of ARF patients and was not MHC related.[41]

More recently, a monoclonal antibody (D8/17) was prepared by immunizing mice with B cells from an ARF patient.[42] A B cell antigen identified by this antibody was found to be expressed on increased numbers of B cells in 100% of rheumatic patients of diverse ethnic origins, and in only 10% of normal individuals. The antigen defined by this monoclonal antibody showed no association with or linkage to any of the known MHC haplotypes, and it did not seem to be related to B cell activation antigens. Studies with D8/17 have been expanded to a larger number of patients with RF (see Table 115-1) of diverse ethnic origins with essentially the same results. As discussed subsequently, the presence or absence of elevated levels of D8/17[+] B cells in cases of questionable RF has been helpful in establishing or ruling out the diagnosis.

These studies contrast with other reports in which an increased frequency of HLA-DR4 and HLA-DR2 has been seen in white and black patients with rheumatic heart disease (RHD).[43] Other studies have implicated HLA-DR1 and HLA-DRW6 as susceptibility factors in South African black patients with RHD.[44] Guilherme and associates[45] have reported an increased frequency of HLA-DR7 and HLA-DW53 in RF patients in Brazil.

These seemingly conflicting results concerning HLA antigens and RF susceptibility prompt speculation that these reported associations might be of class II genes close to (or in linkage disequilibrium with), but not identical to, the putative RF susceptibility gene. Alternatively, and more likely, susceptibility to ARF is polygenic, and the D8/17 antigen might be associated with only one of the genes (i.e., genes of the MHC complex encoding for DR antigens) conferring susceptibility. Although the explanation remains to be determined, the presence of the D8/17 antigen does seem to identify a population at special risk of contracting ARF (Table 115-2).

ETIOLOGIC CONSIDERATIONS

Although a large body of immunologic and epidemiologic evidence has implicated group A streptococci in the induction of the disease process, the precise pathologic mechanisms involved remain obscure. At least three main theories have been proposed. The first theory is concerned with the question of whether persistence of the organism is important. Despite several controversial reports, no investigators have been able to show consistently and reproducibly live organisms in RF cardiac tissues or valves.[46]

The second theory revolves around the question of whether deposition of toxic products is required. Although an attractive hypothesis, little or no experimental evidence has been obtained to support this concept. Halbert and colleagues[47] have suggested that streptolysin O (an

Table 115-2 Frequency of the D8/17 Marker in Patients with Rheumatic Fever, Patients with Other Diseases, and Controls in Various Geographic Populations

	Number	% Positive
Rheumatic Fever Patients		
New York	43/45	93
New Mexico	30/31	97
Utah*	18/18	100
Russia (Georgia)	27/30	90
Russia (Moscow)	50/52	96
Mexico	35/39	89
Chile	45/50	90
Normals		
Russia	4/78	5
New York	6/68	8
Chile	8/50	16
Mexico	6/72	8
Other Diseases		
Rheumatoid arthritis	2/42	4
Ischemic heart disease	0/10	0
Multiple sclerosis	1/25	4
Systemic lupus erythematosus	1/12	9

*Acute patients.

extracellular product of group A streptococci) is cardiotoxic and might be carried to the site by circulating complexes containing streptolysin O and antibody. Despite an intensive search for these products, no such complexes in situ have been identified, however.[48,49] Renewed interest in these extracellular toxins has emerged more recently with the observation by Schlievert and co-workers[50] that certain streptococcal pyrogenic toxins (A and C) may act as superantigens. These antigens may stimulate large numbers of T cells through their unique bridging interaction with T cell receptors of specific Vβ types and class II MHC molecules. This interaction is distinct from conventional antigen presentation in the context of the MHC complex. When activated, these cells elaborate tumor necrosis factor, interferon-γ, and numerous interleukin moieties, contributing to the initiation of pathologic damage. It has been suggested[51] that in certain disease states, such as rheumatoid arthritis, autoreactive cells of specific Vβ lineage may "home" to the target organ.

Although an attractive hypothesis, no data concerning the role of these superantigens in ARF have yet been forthcoming. Perhaps the best evidence to date favors a third theory of an abnormal host immune response (humoral and cellular) in a genetically susceptible individual to the streptococcal antigens cross-reactive with mammalian tissues. Evidence supporting this theory may be divided into three broad categories:

1. Employing a wide variety of methods, numerous investigators have documented the presence of heart-reactive antibodies in ARF sera. The prevalence of these antibodies has ranged from 33% to 85% in various series. Although these antibodies are seen in other individuals (notably individuals with uncomplicated streptococcal infections that do not progress to RF and patients with poststreptococcal glomerulonephritis), the titers are always lower than those seen in RF and decrease with time during the convalescent

Table 115-3 Heart-Reactive Antibody Titers in Sera of Patients with Acute Rheumatic Fever Compared with Uncomplicated Streptococcal Infections

| Clinical Disorder | No. Patients | Serum Dilutions | | | Average ASO Titer |
		1:5	1:10	1:20	
Acute rheumatic fever (grade I)	34	4+	2+	+*	700
Uncomplicated streptococcal infection (grade II)	40	1+	0	0	561
APSGN	20	+/−	0	0	520
Rheumatoid arthritis	10	0	0	0†	ND
Systemic lupus erythematosus	10	0	0	0	ND

*Serum samples obtained at onset of rheumatic fever and at a comparable time in the group with uncomplicated scarlet fever.
†Serum samples obtained during active disease.
APSGN, acute poststreptococcal glomerulonephritis; ASO, antistreptolysin O; ND, not determined.

period (Table 115-3). An important point in terms of diagnosis and prognosis has been the observation by Zabriskie and associates[52] that these heart-reactive antibody titers decline over time. By the end of 3 years, these titers are essentially undetectable in patients who had only a single attack (Figure 115-3). This pattern is consistent with the well-known clinical observation that recurrences of RF most often occur within the first 2 to 3 years after the initial attack and become rarer 5 years after an initial episode.

As illustrated in Figure 115-4, this pattern of titers also has prognostic value. During the 2- to 5-year period after the initial attack, a patient's titers decreased to undetectable levels. With a known break in prophylaxis starting in year 6, at least two streptococcal infections occurred, as evidenced by an increase in antistreptolysin O (ASO) titers during that period. The concomitant increase in heart-reactive antibody titers was notable. The final infection was followed by a clinical recurrence of classic rheumatic carditis complete with isolation of the organism, elevated heart-reactive antibodies, and acute phase reactants 11 years after the initial attack.

2. Sera from patients with ARF also contain increased levels of antibodies to myosin and tropomyosin compared with sera from patients with pharyngeal streptococcal infections that do not progress to ARF. These myosin affinity purified antibodies also cross-react

with M protein moieties, suggesting that this molecule could be the antigenic stimulus for the production of myosin antibodies in these sera.[23,53]

3. Finally, as indicated earlier, autoimmune antibodies are a prominent finding in chorea, another major clinical manifestation of ARF, and these antibodies are directed against the cells of the caudate nucleus. The titer of this antibody corresponds with clinical disease activity.[34] Although not autoimmune in nature, the presence of elevated levels of immune complexes in ARF has been well documented in the sera and in the joints of ARF patients.[54] Elevated levels of immune complexes, which may be as high as the levels seen in classic poststreptococcal glomerulonephritis, may be responsible for the immune complex vasculitis seen in ARF tissues and may provide the initial impetus for vascular damage, followed by the secondary penetration of autoreactive antibodies. Support for this concept is the close clinical similarity of RF arthritis to experimentally induced serum sickness in animals or the arthritis seen secondary to drug hypersensitivity.

Deposition of host immunoglobulin and complement also is seen in the cardiac tissues of ARF patients, suggesting autoimmune deposition of immunoglobulins in or near the Aschoff lesions. At a cellular level, ample evidence has been found for the presence of lymphocytes and macrophages at the site of pathologic damage in the heart in patients with ARF.[55] The cells are predominantly CD4+ helper lymphocytes during acute stages of the disease (4:1). The ratio of CD4+ to CD8+ lymphocytes (2:1) more closely approximates the normal ratio in chronic valvular specimens. Most of these cells express DR antigens. A potentially important finding has been the observation that macrophage-like fibroblasts present in the diseased valves express DR antigens[56] and might be the antigen-presenting cells for the CD4+ lymphocytes. Increased cellular reactivity to streptococcal antigens also has been noted in the peripheral blood mononuclear cell preparations of ARF patients compared with these cells isolated from nephritis patients.[57]

This abnormal reactivity peaks at 6 months after the attack, but may persist for 2 years after the initial episode. The reactivity was specific only for the strains associated with ARF, suggesting an abnormal humoral and cellular response to streptococcal antigens unique to RF-associated streptococci. Support for the potential pathologic importance of these T cells is strengthened further by the observation that lymphocytes obtained from experimental animals

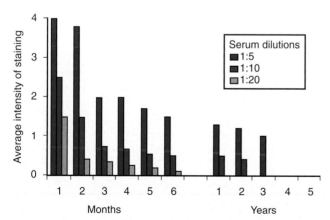

Figure 115-3 Serial heart-reactive antibody titers in 40 patients with documented acute rheumatic fever. Note the slow decline of these titers over the first 2 years after the initial episode and the absence of these antibodies 5 years after the initial attack.

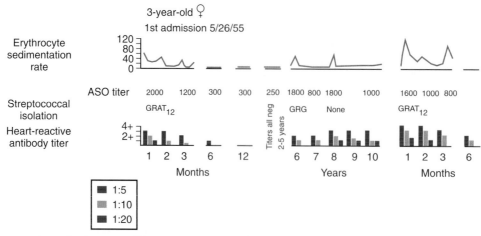

Figure 115-4 Heart-reactive antibody titers and laboratory data obtained from a patient with rheumatic fever who had two well-documented acute attacks 11 years apart. Note absence of the heart-reactive antibody during years 2 to 5 and its reappearance during years 6 to 10 after evidence of two intercurrent streptococcal infections secondary to breaks in penicillin prophylaxis (see antistreptolysin O [ASO] titers). High titers of heart-reactive antibody appeared with the second attack. CRP, C-reactive protein.

sensitized to cell membranes, but not to cell walls, are specifically cytotoxic for syngeneic embryonic cardiac myofibers in vitro.[58] In humans, normal mononuclear cells primed in vitro by M protein molecules from an RF-associated strain also are cytotoxic for myofibers, but specificity solely for cardiac cells was lacking in human studies.[59] Similar studies have not been performed yet using lymphocytes from active ARF patients (Table 115-4).

CLINICAL FEATURES

The clinical presentation of ARF varies, and the lack of a single pathognomonic feature has resulted in the development of revised Jones criteria (Table 115-5),[60] which are used to establish a diagnosis. These criteria were established only as guidelines for the diagnosis and were never intended to be "etched in stone." Depending on the age, geographic location, and ethnic population, emphasis on one criterion for the diagnosis of ARF may be more important than others. Manifestations of RF that are not clearly expressed pose a dilemma because of the importance of identifying a first rheumatic attack definitively to establish the need for prophylaxis of recurrences (see later). Some of the isolated manifestations, particularly polyarthritis, may be difficult or impossible to distinguish from other diseases, especially at their onset. The diagnosis can be made, however, when "pure" chorea is the sole manifestation

Table 115-4 Composition of Mononuclear Cellular Infiltrates in Acute and Chronic Active Rheumatic Valvulitis

Patient	Type of Valve	Type of Valvulitis*	Composition of Infiltrate (%)						CD4/CD8 Ratio
			HLA-DR+	CD14+†	CD20+‡	CD3+§	CD4+ ‖	CD8+¶	
Acute Valvulitis									
1	Mitral	Acute	58.9	42.6	5.1	49.5	75.6	23.9	3.1
2	Mitral	Acute	49.8	43.1	6.9	43.1	58.7	34.3	1.9
	Aortic	Acute	52.7	51	3.9	38.1	65.9	26.5	2.3
3	Mitral	Acute	63.9	42	5.5	52.4	75.4	18.9	4
4	Aortic	Acute	68.1	56	7.4	33.7	71.6	22	1.9
Chronic Valvulitis									
4	Mitral	Chronic active	49.4	47.4	7.4	44.3	53.7	38.8	1.4
5	Mitral	Chronic active	48.8	39.1	1.4	53.9	45.2	51.5	0.9
	Aortic	Chronic active	67.8	35	4	36.8	47.5	49.1	1
6	Mitral	Chronic active	41.8	23.4	8	65.9	57.3	33.3	1.7
	Aortic	Chronic active	69.6	48.7	6.2	30.1	58.2	32.6	1.8
7	Mitral	Chronic active	55.4	24.2	8.1	59.8	64.9	24.7	2.6
8	Mitral	Chronic active	80.4	34.1	13.4	44.4	44.8	50.9	0.9
9	Mitral	Chronic active	46.1	29.6	0.8	65.6	61.6	33.3	1.8

*Determined in the frozen valve samples studied.
†CD14+ monocytes/macrophages.
‡B cells.
§Pan T cells.
‖Helper T cells.
¶Suppressor cells.

Table 115-5 Revised Jones Criteria for Diagnosis of Acute Rheumatic Fever*

Major Manifestations
Polyarthritis
Chorea
Subcutaneous nodules
Erythema marginatum
Carditis

Minor Manifestations
Arthralgia
Fever
Previous rheumatic fever or rheumatic heart disease

Supporting Evidence of Preceding Streptococcal Infection
Positive throat culture for group A beta-hemolytic streptococci
Increased antistreptolysin O or other streptococcal antibodies
Recent scarlet fever

Other Findings
Elevated acute phase reactants (C-reactive protein or erythrocyte sedimentation rate)
Prolonged P-R interval

*The diagnosis is made if the patient has two major criteria OR one major and two minor criteria if the history includes a preceding streptococcal infection.

Data from Jones criteria 1992 update: guidelines for diagnosis of rheumatic fever, *JAMA* 268:2069–2070, 1992.

because of the rarity with which this syndrome is due to any other cause. More recently, the World Health Organization updated the Jones criteria to allow for the diagnosis of recurrent ARF in patients with established RHD and chronic RHD (Table 115-6).

Table 115-6 Summary of 2002 World Health Organization Criteria for the Diagnosis of Rheumatic Fever (RF) and Rheumatic Heart Disease (RHD)

Diagnostic Categories	Criteria
Primary episode of RF	Two major or one major and two minor manifestations plus evidence of a preceding group A streptococcal infection
Recurrent attack of RF in patients without established RHD	Two major or one major and two minor manifestations plus evidence of a preceding group A streptococcal infection
Recurrent attack of RF in patients with established RHD	Two minor manifestations plus evidence of a preceding group A streptococcal infection
Rheumatic chorea, insidious onset of rheumatic carditis	One major manifestation or evidence of a preceding group A streptococcal infection
Chronic valve lesions of RHD (i.e., patients presenting for the first time with pure mitral stenosis, mixed mitral valve disease, and aortic valve disease)	No other criteria required for diagnosis of RHD

From *Rheumatic fever and rheumatic heart diseases: report of a WHO expert consultation*, WHO technical report series no. 923, Geneva, Switzerland, 2004, World Health Organization.

Arthritis

In classic, untreated cases, the arthritis of ARF affects several joints in quick succession, each for a short time. The legs usually are affected first, and the arms are affected later. The terms *migrating* and *migratory* are often used to describe the polyarthritis of ARF, but these designations are not meant to signify that the inflammation disappears in one joint when it appears in another. Rather, the various localizations usually overlap in time, and onset, as opposed to the full course of arthritis, "migrates" from joint to joint.

Joint involvement is more common, and also is more severe, in teenagers and young adults than in children. Arthritis is usually the earliest symptomatic manifestation of the disease, although asymptomatic carditis may precede it. Rheumatic polyarthritis may be excruciatingly painful but is almost always transient. The pain is usually more prominent than the objective signs of inflammation. When the disease is allowed to express itself fully, unmodified by anti-inflammatory treatment, more than half of patients studied show a true polyarthritis, with inflammation in 6 to 16 joints. Classically, each joint is maximally inflamed for only a few days, or a week at the most; the inflammation decreases, perhaps lingering for another week or so, and then disappears completely. Radiographs at this point may show a slight effusion but most likely are unremarkable.

In routine practice, many patients with arthritis or arthralgias are treated empirically with salicylates or other nonsteroidal anti-inflammatory drugs; arthritis subsides quickly in the joints already affected and does not migrate to new joints. Therapy may deprive the diagnostician of a useful sign. In a large series of patients with ARF and associated arthritis, most of whom had been treated, involvement of only a single large joint was common (25%). One or both knees were affected in 76%, and one or both ankles were affected in 50%. Elbows, wrists, hips, or small joints of the feet were involved in 12% to 15% of patients, and shoulders or small joints of the hand were affected in 7% to 8%. Rarely affected joints included the lumbosacral (2%), cervical (1%), sternoclavicular (0.5%), and temporomandibular (0.5%). Involvement of the small joints of the hands or feet alone occurred in only 1% of patients.[61] Analysis of the synovial fluid in well-documented cases of ARF with arthritis generally reveals a sterile, inflammatory fluid. The complement components C1q, C3, and C4 may be decreased, indicating their consumption by immune complexes in the joint fluid.[9]

Poststreptococcal Reactive Arthritis

Numerous investigators[62-64] have suggested that poststreptococcal migratory arthritis (in adults and children) in the absence of carditis might be a distinct entity from ARF for the following reasons: (1) The latent period between the antecedent streptococcal infection and the onset of poststreptococcal reactive arthritis is shorter (1 to 2 weeks) than the 3 to 4 weeks usually seen in classic ARF; (2) the response of the poststreptococcal reactive arthritis to aspirin and other nonsteroidal medications is poor compared with the dramatic response seen in classic ARF; (3) evidence of carditis is not usually seen in these patients, and the severity of the arthritis is marked; and (4) extra-articular manifestations (e.g., tenosynovitis, renal abnormalities) are often seen in these patients.

Although these features may be seen (admittedly rarely), migratory arthritis without evidence of other major Jones criteria, if supported by two minor manifestations (see Table 115-5), still must be considered ARF, especially in children. Variations in the response to aspirin in these children often are not documented with serum salicylate levels, and an unusual clinical course is insufficient to exclude the diagnosis of ARF. Appropriate prophylactic measures should be taken.[65] Support for this concept may be found in the work of Crea and Mortimer.[66] In their series of patients with ARF, 50% of the children who presented solely with signs of migratory arthritis went on to develop significant valvular damage. RF also occurs in adults. Although migratory arthritis is a common presenting symptom, an outbreak in San Diego Naval Training Camp[67] revealed a 30% incidence of valvular damage in these patients. The importance of clearly defining this reactive arthritis as an RF variant has obvious implications for secondary prophylactic treatment. As suggested by some investigators, poststreptococcal reactive arthritis is a benign condition without the need for prophylaxis. Because most patients fulfill the Jones criteria (one major, two minor), they should be considered as having RF and, in our opinion, should be treated accordingly.

Carditis

Cardiac valvular and muscle damage can manifest in a variety of signs or symptoms. These manifestations include organic heart murmurs, cardiomegaly, congestive heart failure, and pericarditis. Mild to moderate chest discomfort, pleuritic chest pain, and a pericardial friction rub are indications of pericarditis. On clinical examination, the patient can have new or changing organic murmurs, most commonly mitral regurgitant murmurs and occasionally aortic regurgitant murmurs and systolic ejection murmurs, caused by acute valvular inflammation and deformity. Rarely, a Carey Coombs mid-diastolic murmur caused by rapid flow over the mitral valve is heard. If the valvular damage is severe, and concurrent cardiac dysfunction is present, congestive heart failure may occur. Congestive heart failure is the most life-threatening clinical syndrome of ARF and must be treated aggressively and early with a combination of anti-inflammatory drugs, diuretics, and, occasionally, steroids to decrease cardiac inflammation acutely.

Electrocardiogram abnormalities may include all degrees of heart block, including atrioventricular dissociation,

but first-degree heart block is not associated with a poor prognosis. Second-degree or third-degree heart block occasionally can be symptomatic. If heart block is associated with congestive heart failure, temporary pacemaker placement may be required. The most common manifestation of carditis is cardiomegaly, as seen on radiograph. Among patients at the Rockefeller University Hospital who were diagnosed with ARF between 1950 and 1970 with an average of 20 years of follow-up, 90% had evidence of carditis at diagnosis (Table 115-7). In Bland and Jones'[68] classic review of 1000 patients with ARF, only 65% of patients were diagnosed with carditis. However, when Doppler sonography was employed in the clinical evaluation of patients during the Utah outbreak, 91% of patients had carditis,[1] indicating that, with more sensitive measurements of cardiac dysfunction, almost all ARF patients have signs of acute carditis.

Rheumatic Heart Disease

RHD is the most severe sequel of ARF. Usually occurring 10 to 20 years after the original attack, it is the major cause of acquired valvular disease in the world. The mitral valve is mainly involved, and aortic valve involvement occurs less often. Mitral stenosis is a classic RHD finding and can manifest as a combination of mitral insufficiency and stenosis, secondary to severe calcification of the mitral valve. When symptoms of left atrial enlargement are present, mitral valve replacement may become necessary.

In various studies, the incidence of RHD in patients with a history of ARF has varied. In Bland and Jones'[67] classic follow-up study of patients with ARF, after 20 years, one-third of patients had no murmur, another one-third had died, and the remaining one-third were alive with RHD. Most of the patients who died had RHD. Although the classic dogma is that patients with RHD invariably have had more than one attack of ARF, analysis of our patients at the Rockefeller University Hospital disproves this notion. The population studied consisted of 87 patients who had only one documented attack of ARF with no evidence (clinical or laboratory) of recurrence during a 20-year follow-up under close supervision. More than 80% had carditis at admission, and approximately 50% now have organic murmurs (see Table 115-7). Valvular damage manifesting as organic murmurs later in life is still likely to occur in 50% of patients, particularly if they presented with evidence of carditis at initial diagnosis. All of the patients in our population who ended up with RHD had presented with carditis at diagnosis.

Table 115-7 Signs and Symptoms of Acute Rheumatic Fever: Rockefeller University Hospital, 1950 to 1970

	RHD (n = 40) (%)	No RHD (n = 47) (%)	Total (N = 87) (%)	Bland and Jones (%)
Carditis	100	83	90.1	65.3
Arthritis	67.5	68.1	67.8	41
Epistaxis	0	10.6	5.7	27.4
Chorea	5	2.1	3.4	51.8
Pericarditis	2.5	4.3	3.4	13
Subcutaneous nodules	7.5	0	3.4	8.8
Erythema marginatum	0	4.3	2.3	7.1

RHD, rheumatic heart disease.

Chorea

Sydenham's chorea (chorea minor, or St. Vitus' dance) is a neurologic disorder consisting of abrupt, purposeless, nonrhythmic involuntary movements, muscular weakness, and emotional disturbances. Involuntary movements disappear during sleep but may occur at rest and may interfere with voluntary activity. Initially, it may be possible to suppress these movements, which may affect all voluntary muscles, with the hands and face usually the most obviously affected. Grimaces and inappropriate smiles are common. Handwriting usually becomes clumsy and provides a convenient way of following the patient's course. Speech is often slurred.

Movements are commonly more marked on one side and occasionally are completely unilateral (hemichorea). Muscular weakness is best revealed by asking the patient to squeeze the examiner's hands: The pressure of the patient's grip increases and decreases continuously and capriciously—a phenomenon known as *relapsing grip*, or the *milking sign*. Emotional changes manifest as outbursts of inappropriate behavior, including crying and restlessness. In rare cases, psychological manifestations may be severe, possibly resulting in transient psychosis. The neurologic examination fails to reveal sensory losses or pyramidal tract involvement. Diffuse hypotonia may be present.

Chorea may follow streptococcal infection after a latent period, which is longer, on average, than the latent period of other rheumatic manifestations. Some patients with chorea have no other symptoms, but other patients develop chorea weeks or months after arthritis. In both cases, examination of the heart may reveal murmurs.

It has been known for years that the early symptoms of chorea often manifest as emotional or behavioral changes in the patient,[69] and only later do the choreiform motor symptoms appear. It also has been noted that many chorea patients years after choreiform symptoms had subsided would present with behavioral disorders, such as tics or obsessive-compulsive disorders. These earlier observations, combined with the known presence of antibrain antibodies in the sera of Sydenham's chorea patients, raised the question of whether a prior streptococcal infection (or infection with other microbes) might induce antibodies cross-reactive with brain antigen involved in neural pathways associated with behavior. Two more recent articles[70,71] suggest a strong association of the D8/17 B cell marker (described earlier) with children with obsessive-compulsive disorder (see Table 115-6). Although Swedo and co-workers[70] selected patients on the basis of a strong history of prior streptococcal infection, Murphy and colleagues[71] noted a strong association of the marker in patients with obsessive-compulsive disorder without a history of streptococcal infection. These preliminary studies suggest that streptococci and probably other microbes may induce antibodies that functionally disrupt the basal ganglia pathways, leading not only to classic chorea, but also to behavioral disorders without evidence of classic chorea.

Subcutaneous Nodules

The subcutaneous nodules of ARF are firm and painless. The overlying skin is not inflamed and usually can be moved over the nodules. The diameter of these round lesions varies from a few millimeters to 1 or 2 cm. They are located over bony surfaces or prominences or near tendons. Their number varies from a single nodule to a few dozen and averages three or four; when numerous, they are usually symmetric. Nodules are rarely present for longer than 1 month. They are smaller and more short-lived than the nodules of rheumatoid arthritis. Although in both diseases, the elbows are most frequently involved, rheumatic nodules are more common on the olecranon, whereas nodules of rheumatoid arthritis are usually found 3 or 4 cm distal to it. Rheumatic subcutaneous nodules generally appear only after the first few weeks of illness, usually only in patients with carditis.

Erythema Marginatum

Erythema marginatum is an evanescent, nonpruritic skin rash, pink or faintly red, that affects usually the trunk and sometimes the proximal parts or the limbs, but not the face. This lesion extends centrifugally, while the skin in the center returns gradually to normal—hence the name *erythema marginatum*. The outer edge of the lesion is sharp, whereas the inner edge is diffuse. Because the margin of the lesion is usually continuous, making a ring, it is also termed *erythema annulare*. Individual lesions may appear and disappear in a matter of hours, usually to return. A hot bath or shower may make them more evident or may reveal them for the first time. Erythema marginatum usually occurs in the early phase of the disease. It often persists or recurs, even when all other manifestations of disease have disappeared. Occasionally, the lesions appear for the first time or, more likely, are noticed for the first time late in the course of the illness or even during convalescence. This disorder usually occurs only in patients with carditis.

Minor Manifestations

Fever

Temperature is increased in almost all ARF attacks and ranges from 38.4° C to 40° C. Usually, fever decreases in approximately 1 week without antipyretic treatment and may become low grade for another 1 or 2 weeks. Fever rarely lasts for longer than 3 to 4 weeks.

Abdominal Pain

The abdominal pain of RF resembles that of other conditions associated with acute microvascular mesenteric inflammation and is nonspecific. It usually occurs at or near the onset of the RF attack, so that other manifestations may not yet be present to clarify the diagnosis. In many cases, abdominal pain may mimic acute appendicitis.

Epistaxis

In the past, epistaxis occurred most prominently and severely in patients with severe and protracted rheumatic carditis. Early clinical studies reported a frequency of 48%, but it probably occurs even less frequently now (see Table 115-6). Although epistaxis has been correlated in the past with the severity of rheumatic inflammation, it is difficult to assess retrospectively the possible thrombasthenic effect of large doses of salicylates, administered for prolonged periods in protracted attacks.

Rheumatic Pneumonia

Pneumonia may appear during the course of severe rheumatic carditis. This inflammatory process is difficult or impossible to distinguish from pulmonary edema or the alveolitis associated with respiratory distress syndromes owing to a variety of pathophysiologic states.

LABORATORY FINDINGS

The diagnosis of ARF cannot readily be established by laboratory tests. Nevertheless, such tests may be helpful in two ways: first, in showing that an antecedent streptococcal infection has occurred, and second, in documenting the presence or persistence of an inflammatory process. Serial chest radiographs may be helpful in following the course of carditis, and an electrocardiogram may reflect the inflammatory process on the conduction system. Throat cultures are usually negative by the time ARF appears, but an attempt should be made to isolate the organism. It is our practice to take three throat cultures during the first 24 hours, before administration of antibiotics. Streptococcal antibodies are more useful because (1) they reach a peak titer at about the time of onset of ARF; (2) they indicate true infection, rather than transient carriage; and (3) when several tests for different antibodies are performed, any significant recent streptococcal infection can be detected.

To show a rising titer, it is useful to take a serum specimen when the patient is first seen and to take another 2 weeks later for comparison. The specific antibody tests that have been used most frequently to diagnose streptococcal infection are those directed against extracellular products, including ASO, anti-DNAse B, antihyaluronidase (anti–diphosphopyridine nucleotide [anti-DNAse]), and anti-streptokinase. ASO has been the most widely used test and is generally available in U.S. hospitals. ASO titers vary with age, season, and geography. They reach peak levels in elementary school–aged children; titers of 200 to 300 Todd units/mL are common in healthy children. After streptococcal pharyngitis, the antibody response peaks at about 4 to 5 weeks, which is usually during the second or third week of ARF (depending on how early it is detected). Antibody titers decrease rapidly over the next several months, and after 6 months, they decline more slowly.

Because only 80% of cases of documented ARF exhibit an increase in the ASO titer, it is recommended that other antistreptococcal antibody tests be done in the absence of a positive ASO titer. These include anti-DNAse B, antihyaluronidase, and anti-streptozyme (a combination of various streptococcal antigens). Streptococcal antibodies, when increased, support but do not prove the diagnosis of ARF, and they are not a measure of rheumatic activity. Even in the absence of intercurrent streptococcal infection, titers decline during the rheumatic attack despite the persistence or severity of rheumatic activity.

Acute Phase Reactants

Acute phase reactants are elevated during ARF, just as they are during other inflammatory conditions. C-reactive protein and erythrocyte sedimentation rates are almost invariably elevated during the active rheumatic process, if they are not suppressed by antirheumatic drugs. These values may be normal, however, during episodes of pure chorea or persistent erythema marginatum. Particularly when treatment has been discontinued or is being tapered off, C-reactive protein and erythrocyte sedimentation rates are useful in monitoring "rebounds" of rheumatic inflammation, which indicate that the rheumatic process is still active. If C-reactive protein or erythrocyte sedimentation rate remains normal a few weeks after antirheumatic therapy is discontinued, the attack may be considered ended unless chorea appears. Usually, no exacerbation of systemic inflammation occurs, and chorea is present as an isolated manifestation.

Anemia

A mild, normochromic, normocytic anemia of chronic infection or inflammation may be seen during ARF. Suppressing the inflammation usually improves the anemia; hematinic therapy usually is not indicated.

Other Supporting Findings

As noted in Figures 115-3 and 115-4 and Table 115-2, two other tests have been helpful in our experience in confirming the diagnosis of ARF, especially when the diagnosis is in doubt. First, one can detect elevated titers of heart-reactive antibodies directed against sarcolemmal antigens in most ARF patients. Elevated levels of these antibodies are not seen in uncomplicated streptococcal infection or acute poststreptococcal glomerulonephritis. With the use of enzyme-linked immunosorbent assay, antibodies directed against cytoskeletal constituents such as myosin and tropomyosin also are seen to be elevated in ARF patients; this observation might be helpful in determining whether or not cross-reactive antibodies unique to ARF exist.[51] Second, use of the D8/17 monoclonal antibody mentioned earlier also has proved helpful in the differential diagnosis of ARF from other disorders. In our hands, all RF patients express abnormal levels of D8/17+ B cells, especially during the acute attack. In cases in which the diagnosis of ARF has been doubtful, the presence of elevated levels of D8/17+ B cells has proved very helpful in establishing the correct diagnosis.[41]

CLINICAL COURSE AND TREATMENT

The mainstay of treatment for ARF has always been anti-inflammatory agents, most commonly aspirin. Dramatic improvement in symptoms usually is seen after initiation of therapy. Usually, 80 to 100 mg/kg/day in children and 4 to 8 g/day in adults is required for an effect to be seen. Aspirin levels can be measured; 20 to 30 mg/dL is the therapeutic range. Duration of anti-inflammatory therapy can vary, but treatment needs to be maintained until all symptoms are absent and laboratory values are normal. If severe carditis also is present (as indicated by significant cardiomegaly, congestive heart failure, or third-degree heart block), steroid therapy can be instituted. The usual dosage is 2 mg/kg/day of oral prednisone during the first 1 to 2 weeks. Depending on clinical and laboratory improvement, the dosage is tapered over the next 2 weeks, and during the last week, aspirin may be added in the above recommended dose, sufficient to achieve 20 to 30 mg/dL.

As noted by Cillers[72] in a clinical review, studies have shown no difference in the risk of cardiac disease at 1 year in groups treated with aspirin or corticosteroids. Similarly, although nonsteroidal anti-inflammatory drugs also have been used to treat acute inflammation, none have been the subject of randomized controlled trials. Whether or not signs of pharyngitis are present at the time of diagnosis, antibiotic therapy with penicillin should be started and maintained for at least 10 days, given in doses recommended for the eradication of streptococcal pharyngitis. Additionally, all family contacts should be cultured and treated for streptococcal infection if positive. If compliance is an issue, depot penicillins (i.e., benzathine penicillin G, 600,000 U in children and 1.2 million U in adults) should be given. Recurrence of ARF is most common within 2 years of the original attack but can occur at any time. The risk of recurrence decreases with age. Recurrence rates have been decreasing, from 20% in past years to 2% to 4% in more recent outbreaks. This decrease might be due to better surveillance and treatment.

PROPHYLAXIS

Antibiotic prophylaxis with penicillin should be started immediately after resolution of the acute episode. The optimal regimen consists of oral penicillin V potassium, 250,000 U twice a day, or parenteral penicillin G, 1.2 million U intramuscularly every 4 weeks. One study suggests, however, that injections every 3 weeks are more effective than every-4-week injections in preventing ARF recurrence.[73] If the patient is allergic to penicillin, erythromycin, 250 mg/day, can be substituted. If the patient is allergic to penicillin, a narrow-spectrum oral cephalosporin (e.g., cefadroxil, cephalexin) or an oral macrolide (e.g., erythromycin 250 mg per day) can be substituted. Because some penicillin-allergic persons (up to 10%) are also allergic to cephalosporins, these agents should not be used in patients with immediate (anaphylactic-type) hypersensitivity to penicillin.[74]

The endpoint of prophylaxis is unclear; most authors believe it should continue at least until the patient is a young adult, which is usually 10 years from an acute attack with no recurrence. In our opinion, individuals with documented evidence of RHD should be on continuous prophylaxis indefinitely because our experience has been that ARF recurrences can occur even in the fifth or sixth decade. A potential problem for ARF recurrence involves young children in the household, who could transmit new group A streptococcal infection to RF-susceptible individuals. The alternative to long-term prophylaxis in an individual with ARF would be the introduction of streptococcal vaccines designed not only to prevent recurrent infection in susceptible individuals with previous ARF, but also to prevent streptococcal disease in general.

STREPTOCOCCAL VACCINES

Difficulties associated with developing a streptococcal vaccine have been related mainly to the numerous reports that streptococcal antigens are known to cross-react with mammalian tissues.[65] Despite these caveats, more recent work indicates progress in this area. Perhaps the most advanced has been the work of Dale and colleagues,[75] in which investigators synthesized short peptides (20 to 30 amino acids) of many different M proteins, linked them together, and showed that they can develop type-specific antibodies that also are opsonic. Little toxicity or cross-reactivity to human tissues has been noted with the antigen or the antibodies.

A second approach revolves around the C-repeat region of the M protein moiety, which is common to all group A streptococci. Bessen and Fischetti[76] used a commensural organism commonly found in the oral mucosa of humans in which by genetic engineering they inserted the C-repeat of the M protein, which is preferentially displayed on the surface of the organism. This induces immunoglobulin (Ig) A antibodies, preventing oral colonization of mice by live group A streptococci. Bronze and colleagues[77] have confirmed these results using a different M-type organism. Golbus and Golbus[78] used similar methods, except that they inserted additional amino acids, making their antibodies opsonic.

Based on the observation by Ellis and colleagues[36] that human sera rarely, if ever, contain more than one type-specific M protein antibody, Salvadori and co-workers[27] examined other possible streptococcal antigens that might explain the broad-based immunity to streptococcal infection that occurs with increasing age. Their studies indicate that the streptococcal group A carbohydrate (GRA-CHO) might be a good immunogen for the following reasons. Antibodies to GRA-CHO are present in human sera, increase with age, and are opsonic for several distinct M+-type strains. Active and passive immunization with GRA-CHO in mice provided protection against a live lethal challenge in mice. No cross-reactive antibodies have been detected.

Two other candidates also are under consideration. Gerber and associates[74] described a surface antigen present on group A streptococci called *C5a peptidase*. This enzyme specifically cleaves the human serum chemotoxin C5a at the polymorphonuclear binding site. These observations led to experiments in which intranasal inoculation with C5a peptidase resulted in the appearance of antibodies that clearly reduced the potential of several different M+ strains to colonize mice.[74] Finally, Lukomski and colleagues[79] showed that the presence of SPEB markedly increases the virulence of a given group A streptococcal strain. Inactivation of the SPEB gene markedly decreases the lethality (IP challenge) of at least two strains—type 49 and S43 type 6. The mechanism whereby SPEB⁻ strains decrease the lethality of the strain seems to be related to the fact that polymorphonuclear neutrophils were able to clear the mutant strain from the circulation and tissues much more rapidly than the wild-type strain.[79]

CONCLUSION

Despite its disappearance in many areas of the world, ARF continues to be a serious problem in the geographic areas inhabited by two-thirds of the population. In developed countries with full access to medical care, better nutrition, and housing, resurgence of the disease emphasizes the need for continued vigilance of physicians and other health officials in diagnosing and treating ARF. Whether this resurgence represents a change in the virulence of the organism or failure to recognize the importance and adequate treatment of an antecedent streptococcal infection remains an area of intense debate and requires careful and controlled epidemiologic surveillance.

The importance of early diagnosis and therapy cannot be overemphasized. Joint manifestations may be transient and self-limited; however, cardiac sequelae may be chronic and life threatening. Nevertheless, ARF remains one of the few autoimmune disorders known to occur as a result of infection with a specific organism. The confirmed observation of increased frequency of a B cell alloantigen in several populations of rheumatic patients suggests that it might be possible to identify at birth individuals who are susceptible to ARF. If so, from a public health standpoint, (1) these individuals would be prime candidates for immunization with any streptococcal vaccine that might be developed in the future; (2) careful monitoring of streptococcal disease in the susceptible population could lead to early and effective antibiotic strategies, resulting in disease prevention; and (3) in individuals previously infected, who later present with subtle or nonspecific manifestations of the disease, the presence or absence of the marker could be valuable in arriving at a diagnosis.

Continued study of ARF as a paradigm for microbial-host interactions has important implications for the study of autoimmune diseases in general, and rheumatic diseases in particular. Further insight into this intriguing host-parasite relationship may shed additional light on diseases in which infection is presumed but has not yet been identified.

References

1. Veasy LG, Wiedmeier SE, Orsmond GS, et al: Resurgence of acute rheumatic fever in the intermountain area of the United States, *N Engl J Med* 316:421–427, 1987.
2. Gordis L: The virtual disappearance of rheumatic fever in the United States: lessons in the rise and fall of disease, *Circulation* 72:1155–1162, 1985.
3. Pope RM: Rheumatic fever in the 1980s, *Bull Rheum Dis Arthritis Foundation* 38:1–8, 1989.
4. Markowitz M, Gordis L: *Rheumatic fever*, ed 2, Philadelphia, 1972, WB Saunders.
5. Kaplan EL, Anthony BF, Chapman SS, et al: The influence of the site of infection on the immune response to group A streptococci, *J Clin Invest* 49:1405–1414, 1970.
6. Whitnack E, Bisno AL: Rheumatic fever and other immunologically mediated cardiac diseases. In Parker C, editor: *Clinical immunology*, vol II, Philadelphia, 1980, WB Saunders, pp 894–929.
7. Denny FW Jr, Wannamaker LW, Brink WR, et al: Prevention of rheumatic fever: treatment of the preceding streptococcal infection, *JAMA* 143:151–153, 1950.
8. Markowitz M: Rheumatic fever: recent outbreaks of an old disease, *Conn Med* 51:229–233, 1987.
9. Stollerman GH, Lewis AJ, Schultz I, et al: Relationship of the immune response to group A streptococci to the cause of acute, chronic and recurrent rheumatic fever, *Am J Med* 20:163–169, 1956.
10. Potter EV, Svartman M, Mohammed I, et al: Tropical acute rheumatic fever and associated streptococcal infections compared with concurrent acute glomerulonephritis, *J Pediatr* 92:325–333, 1978.
11. Bessen D, Jones KF, Fischetti VA: Evidence for the distinct classes of streptococcal M protein and their relationship to rheumatic fever, *J Exp Med* 169:269–283, 1989.
12. Kaplan EL, Johnson DR, Cleary PP.: Group A streptococcal serotypes isolated from patients and sibling contacts during the resurgence of rheumatic fever in the United States in the mid 1980's, *J Infect Dis* 159:101–103, 1989.
13. Bisno AL, Nelson KE: Type-specific opsonic antibodies in streptococcal pyoderma, *Infect Immun* 10:1356–1361, 1975.
14. Kendall F, Heidelberger M, Dawson M: A serologically inactive polysaccharide elaborated by mucoid strains of group A hemolytic streptococcus, *J Biol Chem* 118:61–82, 1937.
15. Seastone CV: The virulence of group C hemolytic streptococci of animal origin, *J Exp Med* 70:361–378, 1939.
16. Quinn RW, Singh KP: Antigenicity of hyaluronic acid, *Biochem J* 95:290–301, 1957.
17. Fillet HM, McCarty M, Blake M: Induction of antibodies to hyaluronic acid by immunization of rabbits with encapsulated streptococci, *J Exp Med* 164:762–776, 1986.
18. Faarber P, Capel PJ, Rigke PM, et al: Cross reactivity of anti DNA antibodies with proteoglycans, *Clin Exp Immunol* 55:402–412, 1984.
19. Stollerman GH: Rheumatic fever and heritable connective tissue disease of the cardiovascular system. In Stollerman GH, editor: *Rheumatic fever and streptococcal infection*, New York, 1975, Grune & Stratton, p 70.
20. Fischetti VA: Streptococcal M protein: molecular design and biological behavior, *Clin Microbiol Rev* 2:285–314, 1989.
21. Dale JB, Beachey EH: Multiple cross reactive epitopes of streptococcal M proteins, *J Exp Med* 161:113–122, 1985.
22. Sargent SJ, Beachey EH, Corbett CE, et al: Sequence of protective epitopes of streptococcal M proteins shared with cardiac sarcolemmal membranes, *J Immunol* 139:1285–1290, 1987.
23. Cunningham MW, McCormack JM, Talaber LR, et al: Human monoclonal antibodies reactive with antigens of the group A streptococcus and human heart, *J Immunol* 141:2760–2766, 1988.
24. McCarty M: The streptococcal cell wall, *The Harvey Lectures Series* 65:73–96, 1970.
25. Goldstein I, Rebeyrotte P, Parlebas J, et al: Isolation from heart valves of glycopeptides which share immunological properties with streptococcus haemolyticus group A polysaccharides, *Nature* 219:866–868, 1968.
26. Goldstein I, Caravano R: Determination of anti-group A streptococcal polysaccharide antibodies in human sera by a hemagglutination technique, *Proc Soc Exp Biol Med* 124:1209–1212, 1967.
27. Salvadori LG, Blake MS, McCarty M, et al: Group A streptococcus-liposome ELISA antibody titers to group A polysaccharide and opsonophagocytic capabilities of the antibodies, *J Infect Dis* 171:593–600, 1995.
28. Chetty C, Schwab JH: Chemistry of endotoxins. In Rietschel ET, editor: *Handbook of endotoxin*, vol 1, Amsterdam, 1984, Elsevier Science, pp 376–410.
29. Cromartie WJ, Craddock JB, Schwab JH, et al: Arthritis in rats after systemic injection of streptococcal cells or cell walls, *J Exp Med* 146:1585–1602, 1977.
30. Cromartie WJ, Craddock JB: Rheumatic-like cardiac lesions in mice, *Science* 154:285–287, 1966.
31. Heymer B, Schleifer KH, Read SE, et al: Detection of antibodies to bacterial cell wall peptidoglycan in human sera, *J Immunol* 117:23–26, 1976.
32. Zabriskie JB: Rheumatic fever: the interplay between host genetics and microbe, *Circulation* 71:1077–1086, 1985.
33. Kingston D, Glynn LE: A cross-reaction between *Streptococcus pyogenes* and human fibroblasts, endothelial cells and astrocytes, *Immunology* 21:1003–1016, 1971.
34. Husby G, van de Rijn I, Zabriskie JB, et al: Antibodies reacting with cytoplasm of subthalamic and caudate nuclei neurons in chorea and acute rheumatic fever, *J Exp Med* 144:1094–1110, 1976.

35. Froude J, Gibofsky A, Buskirk DR, et al: Cross reactivity between streptococcus and human tissue: a model of molecular mimicry and autoimmunity, *Curr Top Microbiol Immunol* 145:5–26, 1989.

36. Ellis NM, Kurahara DK, Vohra H, et al: Priming the immune system for heart disease: a perspective on group A streptococci, *J Infect Dis* 202:1059–1067, 2010.

37. Cheadle WB: Harvean lectures on the various manifestations of the rheumatic state as exemplified in childhood and early life, *Lancet* 1:821–832, 1889.

38. Wilson MG, Schweitzer MD, Lubschez R: The familial epidemiology of rheumatic fever, *J Pediatr* 22:468–482, 1943.

39. Taranta A, Torosdag S, Metrakos JD, et al: Rheumatic fever in monozygotic and dizygotic twins, *Circulation* 20:778–792, 1959.

40. Glynn LE, Halborrow EJ: Relationship between blood groups, secretion status and susceptibility to rheumatic fever, *Arthritis Rheum* 4:203, 1961.

41. Patarroyo ME, Winchester RJ, Vejerano A, et al: Association of a B cell alloantigen with susceptibility to rheumatic fever, *Nature* 278:173–174, 1979.

42. Khanna AK, Buskirk DR, Williams RC Jr, et al: Presence of a non-HLA B cell antigen in rheumatic fever patients and their families as defined by a monoclonal antibody, *J Clin Invest* 83:1710–1716, 1989.

43. Ayoub EA, Barrett DJ, Maclaren NK, et al: Association of class II human histocompatibility leucocyte antigens with rheumatic fever, *J Clin Invest* 77:2019–2026, 1986.

44. Maharaj B, Hammond MG, Appadoo B, et al: HLA-A, B, DR and DQ antigens in black patients with severe chronic rheumatic heart disease, *Circulation* 765:259–261, 1987.

45. Guilherme L, Weidenbach W, Kiss MH, et al: Association of human leucocyte class II antigens with rheumatic fever or rheumatic heart disease in a Brazilian population, *Circulation* 83:1995–1998, 1991.

46. Watson RF, Hirst GK, Lancefield RC: Bacteriological studies of cardiac tissues obtained at autopsy from eleven patients dying with rheumatic fever, *Arthritis Rheum* 4:74–85, 1961.

47. Halbert SP, Bircher R, Dahle E: The analysis of streptococcal infections. V: Cardiotoxicity of streptolysin O for rabbits in vivo, *J Exp Med* 113:759–784, 1961.

48. Wagner BM: Studies in rheumatic fever. III: Histochemical reactivity of the Aschoff body, *Ann N Y Acad Sci* 86:992–1008, 1960.

49. Zabriskie JB: Unpublished data, 1959.

50. Schlievert PM, Johnson LP, Tomai MA, et al: Characterization and genetics of group A streptococcal pyrogenic exotoxins. In Ferretti J, Curtis R, editors: *Streptococcal genetics*, Washington, DC, 1987, ASM, pp 136–142.

51. Paliard X, West SG, Lafferty JA, et al: Evidence for the effects of superantigen in rheumatoid arthritis, *Science* 253:325–329, 1991.

52. Zabriskie JB, Hsu KC, Seegal BC: Heart-reactive antibody associated with rheumatic fever: characterization and diagnostic significance, *Clin Exp Immunol* 7:147–159, 1970.

53. Khanna AK, Nomura Y, Fischetti VA, et al: Antibodies in the sera of acute rheumatic fever patients bind to human cardiac tropomyosin, *J Autoimmun* 10:99–106, 1997.

54. van de Rijn I, Fillit H, Brandis WE, et al: Serial studies on circulating immune complexes in post-streptococcal sequelae, *Clin Exp Immunol* 34:318–325, 1978.

55. Kemeny E, Grieve T, Marcus R, et al: Identification of mononuclear cells and T cell subsets in rheumatic valvulitis, *Clin Immunol Immunopathol* 52:225–237, 1989.

56. Amoils B, Morrison RC, Wadee AA, et al: Aberrant expression of HLA-DR antigen on valvular fibroblasts from patients with acute rheumatic carditis, *Clin Exp Immunol* 66:84–94, 1986.

57. Read SE, Reid HFM, Fischetti V, et al: Serial studies on the cellular immune response to streptococcal antigens in acute and convalescent rheumatic fever patients in Trinidad, *J Clin Immunol* 6:433–441, 1986.

58. Yang LC, Soprey PR, Wittner MK, et al: Streptococcal induced cell mediated immune destruction of cardiac myofibers in vitro, *J Exp Med* 146:344–360, 1977.

59. Dale JB, Beachey EH: Human cytotoxic T lymphocytes evoked by group A streptococcal M proteins, *J Exp Med* 166:1825–1835, 1987.

60. Jones criteria 1992 update: guidelines for diagnosis of rheumatic fever, *JAMA* 268:2069–2070, 1992.

61. Feinstein AR, Spagnulo M: The clinical patterns of rheumatic fever: a reappraisal, *Medicine (Baltimore)* 41:279–305, 1962.

62. Goldsmith DP, Long SS: Poststreptococcal disease of childhood—a changing syndrome, *Arthritis Rheum* 25:S18, 1982 (abstract).

63. Arnold MH, Tyndall A: Post-streptococcal reactive arthritis, *Ann Rheum Dis* 48:681–688, 1989.

64. Fink CW: The role of streptococcus in post streptococcal reactive arthritis and childhood polyarteritis nodosa, *J Rheumatol* 18:14–20, 1991.

65. Gibofsky A, Zabriskie JB: Rheumatic fever: new insights into an old disease, *Bull Rheum Dis Arthritis Foundation* 42:5–7, 1994.

66. Crea MA, Mortimer EA: The nature of scarlatinal arthritis, *Pediatrics* 23:879–884, 1959.

67. Wallace MR, Garst PD, Papadimos TJ, et al: The return of acute rheumatic fever in young adults, *JAMA* 262:2557–2561, 1989.

68. Bland EF, Jones TD: Rheumatic fever and rheumatic heart disease: a twenty year report on 1,000 patients followed since childhood, *Circulation* 4:836–843, 1951.

69. Osler W: *On chorea and choreiform movements*, London, 1894, HK Lewis & Co.

70. Swedo SE, Leonard HL, Mittleman BB, et al: Children with PANDAS (pediatric autoimmune neuropsychiatric disorders associated with strep infections) are identified by a marker associated with rheumatic fever, *Am J Psychiatry* 154:110–112, 1997.

71. Murphy T, Goodman W: D8/17 reactivity as an immunologic marker of susceptibility to nonpsychiatric disorders, *J Am Acad Child Adolesc Psychiatry* 41:98–100, 2002.

72. Cillers AM: Rheumatic fever and its management, *BMJ* 333:1153–1156, 2006.

73. Lue HC, Mil-Wham W, Hsieh KH, et al: Rheumatic fever recurrences: controlled study of 3 week versus 4 week benzathine penicillin prevention programs, *J Pediatr* 108:299–304, 1986.

74. Gerber MA, Baltimore RS, Eaton CB, et al: Prevention of rheumatic fever and diagnosis of acute streptococcal pharyngitis: a scientific statement from the American Heart Association Rheumatic Fever, Endocarditis, and Kawasaki Disease Committee of the Council on Cardiovascular Disease in the Young, the Interdisciplinary Council on Functional Genomics and Translational Biology, and the Interdisciplinary Council on Quality of Care and Outcomes Research: endorsed by the American Academy of Pediatrics, *Circulation* 119:1541–1551, 2009.

75. Dale JB, Simmons M, Chiang EC, et al: Recombinant, octavalent group A streptococcal M protein vaccine, *Vaccine* 14:944–948, 1996.

76. Bessen D, Fischetti VA: Influence of intranasal immunization with synthetic peptides corresponding to conserved epitopes of M protein on mucosal colonization by group A streptococci, *Infect Immun* 56:2666–2672, 1988.

77. Bronze MS, Courtney HS, Dale JB: Epitopes of group A streptococcal M protein that evoke cross protection local immune responses, *J Immunol* 148:888–893, 1992.

78. Golbus JR, Golbus J: Keeping rheumatic fever in the differential, *J Musculoskel Med* 26:10–19, 2009.

79. Lukomski S, Burns EH, Wyde PR, et al: Genetic inactivation of an extracellular cysteine protease (SPEB) expression by *Streptococcus pyogenes* decreases resistance to phagocytosis and dissemination to organs, *Infect Immun* 66:771–776, 1998.

The references for this chapter can also be found on www.expertconsult.com.

116 Amyloidosis

DAVID C. SELDIN • MARTHA SKINNER

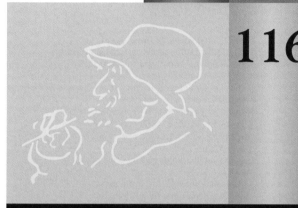

KEY POINTS

Amyloidosis is the term for systemic disease in which aggregated proteins form extracellular fibrils in tissues of the body, eventually leading to organ failure and death if not effectively treated.

Patients with amyloidosis can present with joint symptoms and soft tissue deposits that mimic rheumatologic disorders, and inadequately controlled rheumatologic disease or chronic infection can lead to secondary AA amyloidosis.

The diagnosis of amyloidosis requires a tissue biopsy that demonstrates green birefringence of deposits using polarization microscopy after staining with Congo red.

Appropriate treatment depends upon accurate biochemical or immunochemical identification of amyloid type, distinguishing hereditary from acquired forms of amyloidosis.

The term *amyloidosis* includes diseases that have in common the extracellular deposition of insoluble fibrillar proteins in tissues and organs. These diseases are a subset of a growing group of disorders recognized to be caused by misfolding of proteins; they include Alzheimer's and other neurodegenerative diseases, prion diseases, serpinopathies, some of the cystic fibroses, and others. A unifying feature of the amyloidoses is that the deposits share a common β-pleated sheet structural conformation that confers unique staining properties. The name "amyloid" is attributed to the pathologist Virchow, who in 1854 thought such deposits in autopsy livers were cellulose because of their peculiar staining reaction with iodine and sulfuric acid.[1] In the 20th century, amyloid was found to be a proteinaceous fibrillar deposit in tissues.[2] Biochemical characterization of fibril proteins from clinical cases proved the amyloidoses to be diverse diseases, many with a potentially fatal outcome owing to progressive deposition of amyloid fibrils in major organs. A growing number of treatments are available to target the source of the abnormal protein and, for some types, to inhibit the amyloidogenic protein misfolding process.

CLASSIFICATION AND EPIDEMIOLOGY

Amyloid diseases are defined by the biochemical nature of the protein in the deposited fibril. The proteins are diverse and are unrelated in primary amino acid sequence, resulting in classification of amyloid diseases according to whether they are systemic or localized, acquired or inherited; their recognized clinical patterns also determine how they are classified (Table 116-1).[3] Each amyloid disease has a shorthand nomenclature, expressed as A for amyloidosis and an abbreviation for the biochemical nature of the fibrils; for example, *AL* is amyloid of immunoglobulin *light chain* origin. The discussion in this chapter is limited to the systemic amyloidoses because these are the diseases that can involve the joints and are potentially confused with autoimmune rheumatologic disorders.

The acquired systemic amyloidoses are AL (immunoglobulin light chain, or primary), AA (reactive, secondary), and $A\beta_2M$ (β_2-microglobulin, dialysis-associated) types. The AL type is most common, although epidemiologic data are limited. One study based on National Center for Health Statistics data estimated the incidence as 4.5 per 100,000.[4] AL amyloidosis usually manifests after age 40 years and is associated with rapid progression, multisystem involvement, and short survival. AA amyloidosis is rare, occurring in less than 1% of patients with chronic inflammatory diseases in the United States and Europe, but it is more common in Turkey and the Middle East, where it occurs in association with familial Mediterranean fever.[5] As treatments for chronic inflammation and infection improve, the origin of AA amyloidosis appears to be shifting toward rare hereditary periodic fever syndromes or hematologic disorders associated with production of inflammatory cytokines such as Castleman's disease; workup should include genetic testing and imaging to screen for these conditions.[6] The onset of AA amyloidosis is variable and can occur as soon as 1 year after the onset of an inflammatory disease or many years later, often corresponding to the degree of inflammation. It is the only type of amyloidosis that occurs in children, such as children with juvenile rheumatoid arthritis.[7] $A\beta_2M$ amyloidosis is a chronic rheumatologic complication that occurs in a few patients on long-term dialysis and is related to a high concentration of β_2-microglobulin.[8]

Table 116-1 Classification of Amyloidosis

Term	Fibril Composition	Systemic (S) or Localized (L)	Clinical Syndrome
AL	Immunoglobulin light chains (κ or λ)	S, L	Primary; myeloma-associated; systemic or localized in skin, lymph nodes, bladder, tracheobronchial tree
AA	Amyloid A protein	S	Secondary; reactive; familial Mediterranean fever
Aβ₂M	β₂-Microglobulin	S	Long-term hemodialysis or ambulatory peritoneal dialysis
ATTR	Transthyretin (106 familial variants); wild-type TTR in senile systemic amyloidosis	S	Familial amyloidotic polyneuropathy and cardiomyopathy; senile systemic amyloidosis
AApoA	Apolipoprotein A-I (16 familial variants) or apolipoprotein A-II (4 familial variants)	S	Familial polyneuropathy with nephropathy
AGel	Gelsolin (variant Asn 187, Tyr 187)	S	Familial polyneuropathy with lattice corneal dystrophy, cranial neuropathy, nephropathy
AFib	Fibrinogen A alpha (9 familial variants)	S	Familial amyloidosis with nephropathy
ALys	Lysozyme (5 familial variants)	S	Familial amyloidosis with nephropathy
Aβ	Amyloid β protein	L	Alzheimer's disease; Down syndrome; cerebral amyloid angiopathy (Dutch)
ACys	Cystatin C (variant with N-terminal deletion and Glu 68)	S	Cerebral amyloid angiopathy (Icelandic)
AIAPP	Islet amyloid polypeptide	L	Type 2 diabetes mellitus; insulinoma
ACal	Calcitonin	L	Medullary carcinoma of the thyroid
AANF	Atrial natriuretic factor	L	Atrial amyloid, localized

The inherited amyloidoses are rare autosomal dominant diseases in which a variant plasma protein forms amyloid deposits beginning in midlife.[9] The most common form is caused by variant transthyretins (TTRs), of which more than 100 types are known to be associated with amyloidosis.[10] One variant, with a substitution of isoleucine for valine at position 122 (V122I), has a carrier frequency that may be 4% in the black population and is associated with late-onset cardiac amyloidosis. Among a large cohort of African-Americans over age 65, the frequency of congestive heart failure and mortality was higher among those carrying the *V122I* gene than in age, gender, and ethnically matched controls.[11] In an amyloidosis referral population, African-Americans over age 60 who presented with amyloid cardiomyopathy were twice as likely to have TTR amyloidosis (ATTR) due to *V122I* as to have the more common AL type of amyloidosis.[12] Even wild-type TTRs can form fibrils, leading to senile systemic amyloidosis, which predominantly affects the heart, in older patients.[13]

PATHOLOGY AND PATHOGENESIS OF AMYLOID FIBRIL FORMATION

Pathologic Features

Amyloid deposits are widespread in AL amyloidosis and can be present in the extracellular spaces and blood vessels of all organs. Deposits in AA amyloidosis usually develop in the kidneys, liver, and spleen, although widespread deposits can be found late in the course of the disease. In Aβ₂M amyloidosis, deposits tend to occur in synovial membrane, cartilage, and bone, but visceral organs are sometimes affected. In ATTR amyloidosis, the nervous system, heart, and thyroid are frequently affected organs, and only small deposits are found elsewhere.

All amyloid deposits stain with Congo red dye and exhibit a unique green birefringence by polarized light microscopy,[14] although the deposits also can be recognized on routine hematoxylin and eosin–stained sections. By electron microscopy, amyloid fibrils are 8 to 10 nm wide and of varying lengths, with a 2.5- to 3.5-nm filamentous subunit arranged along the long axis of the fibril in a slow twist.[15] Typing of amyloid deposits can be done with conventional immunohistochemical staining. False-positive results can occur, however, owing to the presence of nonamyloid serum proteins, and immunoelectron microscopy can provide more definitive immunologic identification of the protein in the fibril, or the composition of extracted fibrils can be identified by mass spectrometric proteomic analysis.[16,17]

Pathogenesis of Amyloid Fibril Formation

The exact mechanism of fibril formation is unknown and may differ among the various types of amyloid.[18] Studies suggest a common underlying mechanism, however, in which a partially unfolded protein intermediate forms multimers and then higher-order polymers. Factors that contribute to fibrillogenesis include variant or unstable protein structure, extensive β-conformation of the precursor protein, proteolytic processing of the precursor protein, association with components of the serum or extracellular matrix (e.g., serum amyloid P [SAP] component, amyloid enhancing factor, apolipoprotein E, glycosaminoglycans), and physical properties such as pH of the tissue site.

AL amyloidosis is a plasma cell dyscrasia with an excess of clonal plasma cells in the bone marrow; it can occur in isolation or in combination with multiple myeloma. Similar cytogenetic changes have been identified in these plasma cell diseases, suggesting that they may have a common molecular pathogenesis.[19,20] By two-dimensional gel electrophoresis and mass spectrometry, it can be seen that the amyloid fibril deposits are composed of intact 23-kD monoclonal immunoglobulin light chains and C-terminal truncated fragments.[16] Although all κ and λ light chain subtypes have been identified in amyloid fibrils, λ subtypes predominate, and the λ 6 subtype seems to have unique structural properties that predispose it to fibril formation,[21] often in the kidney.[22] AL amyloidosis is usually a rapidly progressive disease with amyloid deposits in multiple tissue sites.

The AA type of amyloidosis is a complication of severe, long-standing inflammation, as occurs in chronic inflammatory disorders or infections. AA amyloid fibrils usually are composed of an 8-kD, 76 amino acid amino-terminal portion of the 12-kD precursor, serum amyloid A (SAA).[23] SAA is a polymorphic protein encoded by a family of SAA genes, which are acute phase apoproteins synthesized in the liver and transported by a high-density lipoprotein, HDL3, in the plasma.[24] An underlying inflammatory disease of several years' duration causing an elevated SAA usually precedes fibril formation, although infection can produce AA deposition more quickly. AA fibril formation can be accelerated by an amyloid enhancing factor present in high concentration in the spleen (which may be early SAA aggregates or deposits), by basement membrane heparan sulfate proteoglycan, or by seeding with AA or heterologous fibrils.[25,26]

Factors related to β_2-microglobulin fibril formation are under investigation. The high prevalence of Aβ_2M disease in patients undergoing long-term dialysis argues against an amyloidogenic variant β_2-microglobulin molecule. The permeability of dialysis membranes may be a factor because the molecular weight of β_2-microglobulin is 11.8 kD—above the porosity of standard membranes. It has been hypothesized that dialysis membranes may be bioincompatible and may induce proinflammatory mediators that stimulate β_2-microglobulin and contribute to fibril formation.[27]

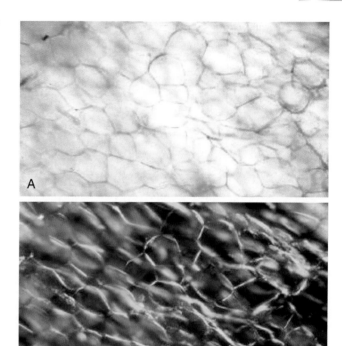

Figure 116-2 Subcutaneous fat aspirate stained with Congo red viewed by light microscopy **(A)** and polarized light **(B)** (×200). Staining and birefringence are evident in the walls and connective tissues surrounding the adipose cells.

In ATTR (also called *familial amyloidotic polyneuropathy*) and all other forms of familial amyloidosis, inherited mutations or polymorphisms in the genes encoding large serum proteins produce amyloid-prone variants. The process of fibrillogenesis has been best studied for TTR, in which variant TTR molecules seem to be prone to dissociation from stable tetramers and to unfolding, leading to misfolding, polymerization, and fibril formation.[28] The role of aging is intriguing because patients with variant proteins do not have clinically apparent disease until midlife or later, despite the lifelong presence of the abnormal protein.[29] Further evidence of an age-related trigger is that senile cardiac amyloidosis, caused by the deposition of fibrils derived from normal TTR, is exclusively a disease of elderly individuals.[13]

DIAGNOSIS

A tissue biopsy specimen showing amyloid fibrils is necessary for the diagnosis of amyloidosis (Figure 116-1). The least invasive biopsy is the abdominal fat aspirate, which is positive in 80% to 90% of patients with AL or ATTR amyloidosis and in 60% to 70% of patients with AA amyloidosis.[30,31] It is easy to perform after local injection of anesthetic and has a low rate of infectious or hemorrhagic complications (Figure 116-2). If the aspirate is negative, but clinical suspicion for disease persists, a more invasive tissue biopsy should be done. Although a biopsy specimen of a clinically involved organ is recommended, almost any tissue biopsy specimen is likely to be positive if the patient has systemic amyloidosis: In a series of 100 patients with AL amyloidosis, 85% of 249 tissue biopsy specimens were positive, including

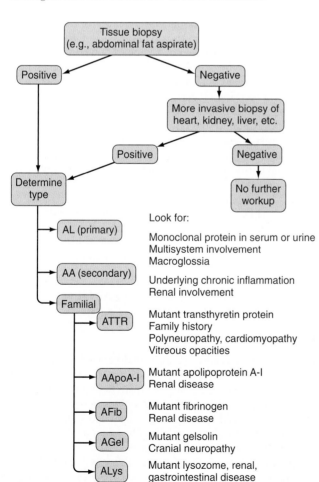

Figure 116-1 Algorithm for the diagnosis of amyloidosis and determination of type.

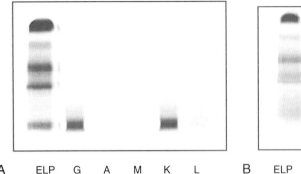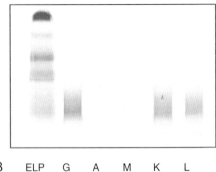

A   ELP G A M K L   B   ELP G A M K L

Figure 116-3 **A,** Pretreatment serum immunofixation electrophoresis (ELP) shows an IgG (G) κ monoclonal protein. **B,** Post-treatment serum immunofixation electrophoresis shows absence of the monoclonal protein. A, IgA; K, kappa chain; L, lambda chain; M, IgM.

all samples from the kidney, heart, and liver.[32] When the diagnosis of amyloidosis is made, careful evaluation of the entire clinical picture, including manner of presentation, organ system involvement, underlying disease, and family history, should provide a clue to the type of amyloid.

Identification of a plasma cell dyscrasia distinguishes AL from other types of amyloidosis (Figure 116-3). More than 90% of patients have a serum or urine monoclonal immunoglobulin protein or a free light chain on testing by immunofixation electrophoresis or by a recently available nephelometric assay for free light chains.[33,34] In addition, the percentage of plasma cells in the bone marrow is often increased; these are monoclonal on immunohistochemical staining (Figure 116-4).[35] A monoclonal serum protein by itself is not diagnostic of amyloidosis because monoclonal gammopathy of uncertain significance is common in older patients. When monoclonal gammopathy of uncertain significance is present in a patient with biopsy-proven amyloidosis, however, the AL type is strongly suspected. Immunohistochemical staining by light or electron

microscopy should be done by a laboratory familiar with the techniques and able to perform appropriate controls. Mass spectrometry–based microsequencing of small amounts of protein extracted from fibril deposits ultimately may be the most reliable way to identify the components of the fibrils.[16,17] AA amyloidosis is suspected in patients with renal amyloidosis and a chronic inflammatory condition or infection. AL and ATTR amyloidosis must be ruled out. AA amyloidosis must be confirmed by immunohistochemical staining for AA protein.

Familial amyloidosis must be excluded in every patient who does not have a plasma cell dyscrasia or the AA type of amyloidosis. Although the disease has a dominant inheritance, family history may not be apparent when the disease occurs later in life; also, some cases occur through new mutations. Variant TTR proteins usually can be detected by isoelectric focusing (Figure 116-5).[36] Abnormal isoelectric focusing should prompt genetic testing to determine the precise TTR mutation. Genetic testing should be employed when screening tests fail to identify the fibril protein. With the use of polymerase chain reaction–based sequencing, abnormal fibrinogens and apolipoproteins and variant TTRs can be detected.[37]

A novel renal amyloid protein, leukocyte chemotactic factor 2 (LECT2), has been found in glomeruli, renal vessels, and interstitium in patients with isolated renal amyloidosis and should be considered in patients who are negative for the more common types of amyloidosis.[38]

CLINICAL FEATURES AND TREATMENT OF THE SYSTEMIC AMYLOIDOSES

AL Amyloidosis

AL amyloidosis usually occurs in middle-aged or older individuals but also can occur in the third or fourth decade of life. It has a wide spectrum of organ system involvement, and presenting features reflect the organs most prominently affected.[39,40] Initial symptoms of fatigue and weight loss are frequent, but the diagnosis is rarely made until symptoms referable to a specific organ appear.

The kidneys are commonly affected; renal amyloidosis is manifested by proteinuria, sometimes massive, with edema and hypoalbuminemia. Mild renal dysfunction is frequent, but rapidly progressing renal failure is rare. Cardiac

Figure 116-4 Bone marrow biopsy specimen stained with antibody to λ light chain shows predominance of λ plasma cells and staining of amyloid deposit around a blood vessel (×400).

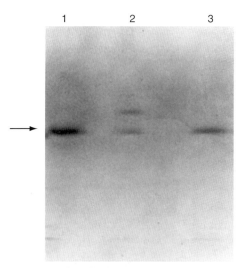

Figure 116-5 Isoelectric focusing of serum samples shows two bands of variant and wild-type transthyretin (TTR) protein from a patient with TTR amyloidosis *(lane 2)* and a single band of wild-type TTR in normal subjects *(lanes 1 and 3, indicated with an arrow).*

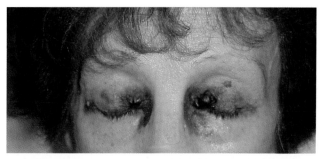

Figure 116-7 Periorbital ecchymoses in a patient with AL amyloidosis.

involvement, often with congestive heart failure, is a common presentation.[41] The electrocardiogram may show low voltage with a pattern of myocardial infarction. The echocardiogram frequently shows concentrically thickened ventricles and a normal or mildly reduced ejection fraction. Nervous system features include peripheral sensory neuropathy, carpal tunnel syndrome, and autonomic dysfunction with gastrointestinal motility disturbances (early satiety, diarrhea, constipation) and orthostatic hypotension. Macroglossia, a classic feature pathognomonic of AL amyloidosis, is found in 10% of patients (Figure 116-6). Hepatomegaly may be massive with mild cholestatic abnormalities of liver function, although liver failure is uncommon, even when hepatomegaly is massive. The spleen is frequently involved, and functional hyposplenism may occur, even in the absence of significant splenomegaly. Cutaneous ecchymoses are common, particularly around the eyes, giving the "raccoon-eyes" sign, and appear spontaneously or when provoked by minor trauma (Figure 116-7). Other findings include nail dystrophy (Figure 116-8), alopecia, and amyloid arthropathy with thickening of synovial membranes. We

have reviewed the soft tissue and joint manifestations of AL amyloidosis in a series of almost 200 patients.[42] Symptoms and signs mimicking rheumatologic diseases, with arthropathy, subcutaneous tissue deposits, muscle pseudohypertrophy, adenopathy, carpal tunnel syndrome, submandibular gland enlargement, and macroglossia, occur in more than 40% of patients with AL amyloidosis.

Timely diagnosis of AL amyloidosis is crucial. Patients with any of these clinical syndromes should be screened for amyloid deposition and for a plasma cell disorder as previously described. Note that the sensitivity of serum or urine protein electrophoresis (SPEP and UPEP) without immunofixation is poor; these tests alone are not useful for excluding or diagnosing AL amyloidosis.

Extensive multisystem involvement typifies AL amyloidosis, and median survival with no treatment is usually only about 1 year from diagnosis. Current therapies target clonal bone marrow plasma cells using chemotherapy approaches employed for multiple myeloma (Table 116-2). Oral melphalan and prednisone constituted the first regimen tried for AL amyloidosis; it was minimally effective[32,43] and is rarely used today because recent studies show that substitution of high-dose dexamethasone for prednisone seems to increase response rates significantly.[44]

High-dose intravenous melphalan followed by autologous stem cell transplantation is highly effective. Of more than 500 patients treated on such protocols at Boston Medical Center, approximately 40% of evaluable patients had achieved a hematologic complete response when assessed at 1 year post treatment; most experienced significant improvement or stabilization of organ function.[45] Median survival in treated patients exceeds 4.5 years and

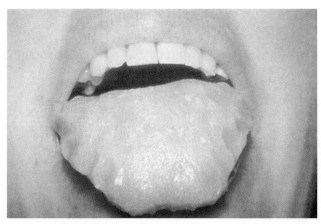

Figure 116-6 Enlarged tongue of a patient with AL amyloidosis.

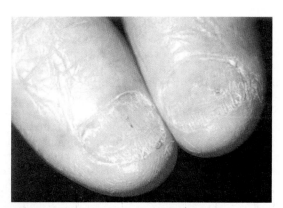

Figure 116-8 Fingernail dystrophy in a patient with AL amyloidosis.

Table 116-2 Major Treatment Options for Amyloidosis

AL Amyloidosis
Intravenous melphalan with autologous stem cell rescue
Granulocyte colony-stimulating factor–mobilized peripheral
blood stem cell collection
Intravenous melphalan 140-200 mg/m²
Autologous stem cell reinfusion
Cyclic oral melphalan and dexamethasone
Melphalan 0.22 mg/kg/day × 4 days
Dexamethasone 20-40 mg/day × 4 days, or weekly
Repeat administration every 4 weeks
Immunomodulators
Lenalidomide 5-15 mg/day × 21 days
Dexamethasone 20-40 mg/day weekly
Repeat administration every 4 weeks
Proteasome inhibitors
Intravenous bortezomib, 0.7-1.6 mg/m² 1-2 times per week
Repeat every 3-5 weeks
AA Amyloidosis
Aggressive treatment of underlying inflammatory disease
Medical or surgical treatment of underlying infection
Colchicine 1.2-1.8 mg/day for AA amyloidosis secondary to familial
Mediterranean fever
Antifibril drug, eprosidate (investigational)
ATTR Amyloidosis
Orthotopic liver transplantation
Transthyretin stabilizers: tafamadis, diflunisal (investigational)

is durable.[46] Other referral centers have found similar results.[47-49] However, patients with amyloidosis and organ impairment have high rates of treatment-related morbidity and mortality with aggressive treatment. Factors that contribute to mortality include amyloid cardiomyopathy, poor performance or nutritional status, reduced pulmonary function, and amyloid-associated bleeding disorders. The only randomized multicenter study comparing oral melphalan chemotherapy with intravenous (IV) melphalan chemotherapy with stem cell support was plagued by high treatment-related mortality and failed to show benefit for the high-dose regimen.[50] At experienced centers, this treatment is still considered first-line in low-risk patients. Age alone[51] or renal failure[52] does not exclude patients from such treatment. Cardiac biomarkers have been used to stratify risk for high-dose therapy.[53]

For patients with significantly impaired cardiac function or arrhythmias resulting from amyloid involvement of the myocardium, median survival is only about 6 months without treatment, and stem cell mobilization and high-dose chemotherapy are associated with great morbidity. In such patients, orthotopic cardiac transplantation followed by intravenous melphalan and stem cell rescue to prevent fibrillogenesis in the transplanted heart or other organs can be effective.[54]

New agents that are efficacious in reducing the plasma cell burden in multiple myeloma are being tested for AL amyloidosis. These include immunomodulators such as lenalidomide[55-57] that affect the bone marrow microenvironment, as well as proteasome inhibitors to which plasma cells are particularly sensitive, such as bortezomib.[58-60] These agents generally have been tested for use in patients for whom alkylator chemotherapy has failed; current clinical trials are examining these novel agents in combination with alkylators, as induction before transplant, and for maintenance. Weekly rather than bi-weekly dosing of bortezomib appears to reduce the incidence of peripheral neuropathy and may be safer in AL amyloidosis patients. Innovative approaches target the amyloid fibrils themselves or accessory binding proteins. The anthracycline derivative 4′-iodo-4′-deoxydoxorubicin (IDOX) was noted to cause resorption of amyloid deposits in model systems, but clinical trials have failed to show any clinical benefit.[61] The agent R-1-[6-[R-2-carboxy-pyrrolidin-1-yl]-6-oxo-hexanoyl]pyrrolidine-2-carboxylic acid (CPHPC) binds serum amyloid P protein and accelerates clearance from the circulation and from amyloid fibrils in animal models,[62] but it has not been proven to provide any clinical benefit on its own. In animal models, the addition of component antibody against SAP appears to further accelerate clearance, and clinical trials with this combination are being planned.[63] Supportive treatment is recommended for patients with all types of amyloidosis (Table 116-3). At times, supportive treatment may be lifesaving (e.g., heart or kidney transplantation, renal dialysis, cardiac pacemaker, nutritional support). Digitalis, calcium channel blockers, and β-blockers are relatively contraindicated because toxicity has been observed at therapeutic levels.

AA Amyloidosis

AA amyloidosis can occur at any age. The primary clinical manifestation is proteinuria or renal insufficiency or both.[5] A study from Finland found AA amyloidosis to be the most common cause of nephrotic syndrome in patients with rheumatoid arthritis.[64] Hepatomegaly, splenomegaly, and autonomic neuropathy frequently occur as the disease progresses; cardiomyopathy occurs rarely. With chronic inflammatory diseases, amyloid progression is slow, and survival is often longer than 10 years, particularly with treatment for end-stage renal disease. In contrast, untreated infections, such as osteomyelitis, tuberculosis, or leprosy, can produce a more rapidly progressive amyloid syndrome, which remits with effective medical or surgical treatment of the infection.

The major therapy in AA amyloidosis is treatment of the underlying inflammatory or infectious disease. Treatment that suppresses or eliminates the inflammation or infection also decreases the SAA protein. For familial Mediterranean fever, colchicine, 1.2 to 1.8 mg/day, is the appropriate treatment. Colchicine has not been helpful for AA amyloidosis of other causes or for other amyloidoses. A multicenter randomized trial using a new antiamyloid drug, eprodisate, has been completed; the drug was found to significantly delay worsening of renal function in patients with AA amyloidosis.[65] A second multicenter trial requested by the Food and Drug Administration (FDA) is now underway. Eprodisate interferes with the interaction of AA amyloid protein and glycosaminoglycans in tissues and prevents fibril formation and deposition.

Aβ₂M Amyloidosis

Several distinct rheumatologic conditions are observed in Aβ₂M amyloidosis, including carpal tunnel syndrome, persistent joint effusions, spondyloarthropathy, and cystic bone

Table 116-3 Supportive Treatment for All Types of Amyloidosis

Organ System	Symptom	Treatment Options
Cardiac	Congestive failure	Salt restriction of 1-2 g/day
		Diuretics: furosemide, spironolactone, metolazone
	Arrhythmia	Pacemaker
		Automatic implantable cardiac defibrillator
		Antiarrhythmics
Renal	Nephrotic syndrome	Salt restriction of 1-2 g/day
		Elastic stockings, leg elevation
		Maintaining dietary protein
		Angiotensin-converting enzyme inhibitor, if blood pressure tolerates
	Renal failure	Dialysis (long-term ambulatory peritoneal dialysis or hemodialysis)
Autonomic nervous	Orthostatic hypotension	Midodrine
		Increased dietary salt or added fludrocortisone, depending on edema
		Elastic stockings
	Gastric atony or ileus	Small frequent feedings (6/day) low in fat
		Oral nutritional supplements
		Jejunostomy tube feeding
		Parenteral nutrition
Gastrointestinal	Diarrhea	Low-fat diet (≤40 g)
		Psyllium hydrophilic mucilloid (Metamucil)
		Loperamide hydrochloride (Imodium)
		Tincture of opium
		Parenteral nutrition
	Macroglossia	Soft solid diet
		Partial glossectomy (rarely effective)
Peripheral nervous	Sensory neuropathy	Avoiding trauma
		Gabapentin (Neurontin) 100-300 mg 3 times daily
		Amitriptyline 25-50 mg at bedtime
		Pregabalin (Lyrica) 50-100 mg 3 times daily
	Motor neuropathy	Ankle-foot orthotics for footdrop
		Physical therapy
Hematologic	Intracutaneous bleeding	Avoiding trauma, antiplatelet agents
	Factor X deficiency	Factor replacement (recombinant factor VIIa, prothrombin complex concentrates)
		Splenectomy for splenomegaly

lesions. Carpal tunnel syndrome is usually the first symptom of disease. Persistent joint effusions accompanied by mild discomfort occur in 50% of patients on dialysis for longer than 12 years. Involvement is bilateral, and large joints (shoulders, knees, wrists, and hips) are more frequently affected. The synovial fluid is noninflammatory, and β_2-microglobulin amyloid deposits can be found if the sediment is examined with Congo red staining. Spondyloarthropathy with destructive changes in the intervertebral disks and paravertebral erosions have occurred in association with β_2-microglobulin amyloid deposits. Cystic bone lesions sometimes leading to pathologic fractures have been described in the femoral head, acetabulum, humerus, tibial plateau, vertebral bodies, and carpal bones. Although less common, visceral β_2-microglobulin amyloid deposits occasionally occur in the gastrointestinal tract, heart, tendons, and subcutaneous tissues of the buttocks.

Treatment for $A\beta_2M$ amyloidosis is difficult to provide because the 11-kD β_2-microglobulin molecule is too large to pass through a dialysis membrane. Consistent with a postulated role of copper in initiating $A\beta_2M$ fibrillogenesis,[66] copper-free dialysis membranes seem to reduce the incidence of disease. Patients on continuous ambulatory peritoneal dialysis usually have lower plasma levels of β_2-microglobulin than patients on hemodialysis and may not develop amyloid deposits as quickly. Symptoms of arthropathy are common, and prevalence may approach 100% of individuals on dialysis for longer than 15 years. Patients who have received kidney transplants after developing $A\beta_2M$ report improvement in symptoms.

ATTR Amyloidosis

The clinical features of ATTR amyloidosis overlap AL amyloidosis such that the diseases cannot be reliably distinguished on clinical grounds alone. A family history makes ATTR more likely, but many patients seem to present sporadically with new mutations. Within each family, disease begins at nearly the same age, and symptoms usually include neuropathy or cardiomyopathy or both. Peripheral neuropathy begins as a lower extremity sensory and motor neuropathy and progresses to the upper extremities. Autonomic neuropathy is manifested by gastrointestinal symptoms of diarrhea with weight loss and orthostatic hypotension. Cardiomyopathy and conduction system defects are similar to those caused by AL amyloidosis, although in ATTR, heart failure is less common, and the prognosis is better.[67] Vitreous opacities caused by amyloid deposits are pathognomonic of ATTR amyloidosis.

The TTR variant, V122I, is a common allele in African-Americans and is associated with cardiomyopathy. In a large referral population, 25% of African-American patients with amyloidosis had this TTR variant.[11,12] ATTR due to V122I is likely underdiagnosed because of lack of physician awareness and the difficulty of distinguishing amyloid and hypertensive cardiomyopathy without an endomyocardial biopsy.

Without intervention, survival after ATTR disease onset is 5 to 15 years. Orthotopic liver transplantation, which removes the major source of variant TTR production and replaces it with normal TTR, is the major treatment for ATTR amyloidosis.[68,69] Liver transplantation arrests disease progression, and some improvement in autonomic and peripheral neuropathy may occur.[70] Cardiomyopathy does not improve and in some patients seems to worsen after liver transplantation.[71] A beneficial long-term outcome depends on transplantation early in the disease course.[72] Two international multicenter randomized placebo-controlled clinical trials have been conducted to test the efficacy of the nonsteroidal anti-inflammatory drug, diflunisal, and its analog tafamidis, for the treatment of ATTR amyloidosis (www.bu.edu/amyloid/doctors/trials/html) based on laboratory studies showing that these agents stabilize TTR and prevent unfolding and aggregation.[73] Antisense and small interfering RNA approaches are also being developed.

SUMMARY

Timely and accurate diagnosis of amyloidosis is essential because effective treatments for some forms of amyloidosis are available or are undergoing clinical trials. The first step is recognition of a clinical syndrome consistent with amyloidosis; this is followed by an appropriate biopsy or fat aspirate to identify tissue fibrils. The next priority should be to determine whether an associated plasma cell disorder can be identified, because AL is the most rapidly progressive type of systemic amyloidosis, and therapy should be initiated before heart, kidney, or liver failure occurs. Definitive identification of the amyloid precursor protein is essential for appropriate therapy, and amyloid referral centers can provide specialized diagnostic techniques and access to clinical trials. An understanding of the biophysical properties of amyloid proteins and of the mechanisms of protein misfolding and tissue damage will enable the further development of more specific and less toxic anti-amyloid therapeutics.

Acknowledgments

This chapter was supported by grants from the National Institutes of Health (HL 68705), the Gerry, Gruss, and Wildflower Foundations; the Young Family Amyloid Research Fund; and the Amyloid Research Fund at Boston University.

References

1. Virchow VR: Ueber einem Gehirn and Rueckenmark des Menchen auf gefundene Substanz mit chemischen reaction der Cellulose, Virchows Arch Pathol Anat 6:135–138, 1854.
2. Cohen AS, Calkins E: Electron microscopic observations on a fibrous component in amyloid of diverse origins, Nature 183:1202–1203, 1959.
3. Westermark P, Benson MD, Buxbaum JN, et al: Amyloid: towards terminology clarification. Report from the Nomenclature Committee of the International Society of Amyloidosis, Amyloid J Protein Folding Disorders 12:1–4, 2005.
4. Simms RW, Prout MN, Cohen AS: The epidemiology of AL and AA amyloidosis, Baillieres Clin Rheumatol 8:627–634, 1994.
5. Livneh A, Langevitz P, Shinar Y, et al: MEFV mutation analysis in patients suffering from amyloidosis of familial Mediterranean fever, Amyloid 6:1–6, 1999.
6. Girnius S, Dember L, Doros G, et al: The changing face of AA amyloidosis: a single center experience, Amyloid 18 Suppl 1:221–223, 2011.
7. David J, Vouyiouka O, Ansell BM, et al: Amyloidosis in juvenile chronic arthritis: a morbidity and mortality study, Clin Exp Rheumatol 11:85–90, 1993.
8. Drueke TB: Beta 2-microglobulin and amyloidosis, Nephrol Dial Transplant 15(Suppl 1):17–24, 2000.
9. Benson MD, Kincaid JC: The molecular biology and clinical features of amyloid neuropathy, Muscle Nerve 36:411–423, 2007.
10. Connors LH, Lim A, Prokaeva T, et al: Tabulation of human transthyretin (TTR) variants, 2003, Amyloid J Protein Folding Disorders 10:160–184, 2003.
11. Connors LH, Prokaeva T, Lim A, et al: Cardiac amyloidosis in African Americans: comparison of clinical and laboratory features of transthyretin V122I amyloidosis and immunoglobulin light chain amyloidosis, Am Heart J 158:607–614, 2009.
12. Buxbaum J, Alexander A, Kaziol J, et al: Significance of the amyloidogenic transthyretin Val 122 Ile allele in African Americans in the Arteriosclerosis Risk in Communities (ARIC) and Cardiovascular Health (CHS) studies, Am Heart J 159:864–870, 2010.
13. Ng B, Connors LH, Davidoff R, et al: Senile systemic amyloidosis presenting with heart failure: a comparison with light chain-associated amyloidosis, Arch Intern Med 165:1425–1429, 2005.
14. Bennhold H: Eine spezifische Amyloidfarbung mit Kongorot, Munch Med Wochenschr 69:1537–1538, 1922.
15. Shirahama T, Cohen AS: High-resolution electron microscopic analysis of the amyloid fibril, J Cell Biol 33:679–708, 1967.
16. Lavatelli F, Perlman DH, Spencer B, et al: Amyloidogenic and associated proteins in systemic amyloidosis proteome of adipose tissue, Mol Cell Proteomics 7:1570–1583, 2008.
17. Vrana JA, Gamez JD, Madden BJ, et al: Classification of amyloidosis by laser microdissection and mass spectrometry-based proteomic analysis in clinical biopsy specimens, Blood 114:4957–4959, 2009.
18. Merlini G, Bellotti V: Molecular mechanisms of amyloidosis, N Engl J Med 349:583–596, 2003.
19. Hayman SR, Bailey RJ, Jalal SM, et al: Translocations involving the immunoglobulin heavy-chain locus are possibly early genetic events in patients with primary systemic amyloidosis, Blood 98:2266–2268, 2001.
20. Perfetti V, Coluccia AM, Intini D, et al: Translocation T(4;14) (p16.3;q32) is a recurrent genetic lesion in primary amyloidosis, Am J Pathol 158:1599–1603, 2001.
21. Solomon A, Frangione B, Franklin EC: Bence Jones proteins and light chains of immunoglobulins: preferential association of the V lambda VI subgroup of human light chains with amyloidosis AL (lambda), J Clin Invest 70:453–460, 1982.
22. Teng J, Russell WJ, Gu X, et al: Different types of glomerulopathic light chains interact with mesangial cells using a common receptor but exhibit different intracellular trafficking patterns, Lab Invest 84:440–451, 2004.
23. Husby G, Marhung G, Dowton B, et al: Serum amyloid A (SAA): biochemistry, genetics, and the pathogenesis of AA amyloidosis, Amyloid Int J Exp Clin Invest 1:119–137, 1994.
24. Kluve-Beckerman B, Dwulet FE, Benson MD: Human serum amyloid A, J Clin Invest 82:1670–1675, 1988.
25. Johan K, Westermark G, Engstrom U, et al: Acceleration of amyloid protein A amyloidosis by amyloid-like synthetic fibrils, Proc Natl Acad Sci U S A 95:2558–2563, 1998.
26. Kluve-Beckerman B, Manaloor J, Liepnieks J: A pulse-chase study tracking the conversion of macrophage-endocytosed serum amyloid A into extracellular amyloid, Arthritis Rheum 46:1905–1913, 2002.
27. Zingraff J, Drueke T: Beta2-microglobulin amyloidosis: past and future, Artif Organs 22:581–584, 1998.
28. Hammarstrom P, Wiseman RL, Powers ET, et al: Prevention of transthyretin amyloid disease by changing protein misfolding energetics, Science 299:713–716, 2003.
29. Suhr OE, Svendsen IH, Ohlsson P, et al: Impact of age and amyloidosis on thiol conjugation of transthyretin in hereditary transthyretin amyloidosis, Amyloid Int J Exp Clin Invest 6:187–191, 1999.
30. Libbey CA, Skinner M, Cohen AS: Use of abdominal fat tissue aspirate in the diagnosis of systemic amyloidosis, Arch Intern Med 143:1549–1552, 1983.
31. Duston MA, Skinner M, Shirahama T, et al: Diagnosis of amyloidosis by abdominal fat aspiration: analysis of four years' experience, Am J Med 82:412–414, 1987.
32. Skinner M, Anderson J, Simms R, et al: Treatment of 100 patients with primary amyloidosis: a randomized trial of melphalan, prednisone, and colchicine versus colchicine only, Am J Med 100:290–298, 1996.
33. Abraham RS, Clark RJ, Bryant SC, et al: Correlation of serum immunoglobulin free light chain quantification with urinary Bence Jones protein in light chain myeloma, Clin Chem 48:655–657, 2002.

34. Akar H, Seldin DC, Magnani B, et al: Quantitative serum free light-chain assay in the diagnostic evaluation of AL amyloidosis, *Amyloid J Protein Folding Disorders* 12:210–215, 2005.

35. Swan N, Skinner M, O'Hara C: Bone marrow core biopsy specimens in AL (primary) amyloidosis: a morphologic and immunohistochemical study of 100 cases, *Am J Clin Pathol* 120:610–616, 2003.

36. Connors LH, Ericsson T, Skare J, et al: A simple screening test for variant transthyretins associated with familial transthyretin amyloidosis using isoelectric focusing, *Biochim Biophys Acta* 1407:185–192, 1998.

37. Benson MD: Amyloidosis. In Scriver CR, Beaudet AL, Sly WS, et al, editors: *The metabolic and molecular bases of inherited disease*, ed 7, New York, 1999, McGraw-Hill, pp 4159–4191.

38. Benson MD: LECT2 amyloidosis, *Kidney Int* 77:757–759, 2010.

39. Falk RH, Comenzo RL, Skinner M: The systemic amyloidoses, *N Engl J Med* 337:898–909, 1997.

40. Merlini G, Bellotti V: Molecular mechanisms of amyloidosis, *N Engl J Med* 349:583–596, 2003.

41. Dubrey SW, Cha K, Anderson J, et al: The clinical features of immunoglobulin light-chain (AL) amyloidosis with heart involvement, *QJM* 91:141–157, 1998.

42. Prokaeva T, Spencer B, Kaut M, et al: Soft tissue, joint, and bone manifestations of AL amyloidosis: clinical presentation, molecular features, and survival, *Arthritis Rheum* 56:3858–3868, 2007.

43. Kyle RA, Gertz MA, Greipp PR, et al: A trial of three regimens for primary amyloidosis: colchicine alone, melphalan and prednisone, and melphalan, prednisone, and colchicine, *N Engl J Med* 336:1202–1207, 1997.

44. Pallidini G, Perfetti V, Obici L, et al: Association of melphalan and high-dose dexamethasone is effective and well tolerated in patients with AL (primary) amyloidosis who are ineligible for stem cell transplantation, *Blood* 103:2936–2938, 2004.

45. Skinner M, Sanchorawala V, Seldin DC, et al: High-dose melphalan and autologous stem-cell transplantation in patients with AL amyloidosis: an 8-year study, *Ann Intern Med* 140:85–93, 2004.

46. Sanchorawala V, Skinner M, Quillen K, et al: Long-term outcome of patients with AL amyloidosis treated with high-dose melphalan and stem-cell transplantation, *Blood* 110:3561–3563, 2007.

47. Dispenzieri A, Kyle RA, Lacy MQ, et al: Superior survival in primary systemic amyloidosis patients undergoing peripheral blood stem cell transplantation: a case-control study, *Blood* 103:3960–3963, 2004.

48. Schonland SO, Lokhorst H, Buzyn A, et al: Allogeneic and syngeneic hematopoietic cell transplantation in patients with amyloid light-chain amyloidosis: a report from the European Group for Blood and Marrow Transplantation, *Blood* 107:2578–2584, 2006.

49. Perfetti V, Siena S, Palladini G, et al: Long-term results of a risk-adapted approach to melphalan conditioning in autologous peripheral blood stem cell transplantation for primary (AL) amyloidosis, *Haematologica* 91:1635–1643, 2006.

50. Jaccard A, Moreau P, Leblond V, et al: High-dose melphalan versus melphalan plus dexamethasone for AL amyloidosis, *N Engl J Med* 357:1083–1093, 2007.

51. Seldin DC, Anderson JJ, Skinner M, et al: Successful treatment of AL amyloidosis with high-dose melphalan and autologous stem cell transplantation in patients over age 65, *Blood* 108:3945–3947, 2006.

52. Casserly LF, Fadia A, Sanchorawala V, et al: High-dose intravenous melphalan with autologous stem cell transplantation in AL amyloidosis-associated end-stage renal disease, *Kidney Int* 63:1051–1057, 2003.

53. Dispenzieri A, Gertz MA, Kyle RA, et al: Prognostication of survival using cardiac troponins and N-terminal pro-brain natriuretic peptide in patients with primary systemic amyloidosis undergoing peripheral blood stem cell transplantation, *Blood* 104:1881–1887, 2004.

54. Dey BR, Chung SS, Spitzer TR, et al: Cardiac transplantation followed by dose-intensive melphalan and autologous stem-cell transplantation for light chain amyloidosis and heart failure, *Transplantation* 90:905–911, 2010.

55. Sanchorawala V, Wright DG, Rosenzweig M, et al: Lenalidomide and dexamethasone in the treatment of AL amyloidosis: results of a phase 2 trial, *Blood* 109:492–496, 2007.

56. Dispenzieri A, Lacy MQ, Zeldenrust SR, et al: The activity of lenalidomide with or without dexamethasone in patients with primary systemic amyloidosis, *Blood* 109:465–470, 2007.

57. Dimopoulos MA, Kastritis E, Rajkumar SV: Treatment of plasma cell dyscrasias with lenalidomide, *Leukemia* 22:1343–1353, 2008.

58. Kastritis E, Anagnostopoulos A, Roussou M, et al: Treatment of light chain (AL) amyloidosis with the combination of bortezomib and dexamethasone, *Haematologica* 92:1351–1358, 2007.

59. Wechalekar AD, Lachmann HJ, Offer M, et al: Efficacy of bortezomib in systemic AL amyloidosis with relapsed/refractory clonal disease, *Haematologica* 93:295–298, 2008.

60. Reece DE, Sanchorawala V, Hegenbart U, et al: Weekly and twice-weekly bortezomib in patients with systemic AL amyloidosis: results of a phase 1 dose-escalation study, *Blood* 114:1489–1497, 2009.

61. Gertz MA, Lacy MQ, Dispenzieri A, et al: A multicenter phase II trial of 4′-iodo-4′-deoxydoxorubicin (IDOX) in primary amyloidosis (AL), *Amyloid J Protein Folding Disorders* 9:24–30, 2002.

62. Pepys MB, Herbert J, Hutchinson WL, et al: Targeted pharmacological depletion of serum amyloid P component (SAP) for treatment of human amyloidosis, *Nature* 417:254–259, 2002.

63. Bodin K, Ellmerich S, Kahan MC, et al: Antibodies to human serum amyloid P component eliminate visceral amyloid deposits, *Nature* 468:93–97, 2010.

64. Helin HJ, Korpela MM, Mustonen JT, et al: Renal biopsy findings and clinicopathologic correlations in rheumatoid arthritis, *Arthritis Rheum* 38:242–247, 1995.

65. Dember LM, Hawkins PN, Hazenberg BPC, et al: Eprodisate for the treatment of AA amyloidosis, *N Engl J Med* 356:2349–2360, 2007.

66. Morgan CJ, Gelfand M, Atreya C, et al: Kidney dialysis-associated amyloidosis: a molecular role for copper in fiber formation, *J Mol Biol* 309:339–345, 2001.

67. Rapezzi C, Merlini G, Quarta CC, et al: Systemic cardiac amyloidosis: disease profiles and clinical courses of the 3 main types, *Circulation* 120:1203–1212, 2009.

68. Holmgren G, Steen L, Ekstedt J, et al: Biochemical effect of liver transplantation in two Swedish patients with familial amyloidotic polyneuropathy (FAP-met30), *Clin Genet* 40:242–246, 1991.

69. Lewis WD, Skinner M, Simms RW, et al: Orthotopic liver transplantation for familial amyloidotic polyneuropathy, *Clin Transplant* 8:107–110, 1994.

70. Bergethon P, Sabin T, Lewis D, et al: Improvement in the polyneuropathy associated with familial amyloid polyneuropathy after liver transplantation, *Neurology* 47:944–951, 1996.

71. Dubrey SW, Davidoff R, Skinner M, et al: Progression of ventricular wall thickening after liver transplantation for familial amyloidosis, *Transplantation* 64:74–80, 1997.

72. de Carvalho M, Conceicao I, Bentes C, et al: Long-term quantitative evaluation of liver transplantation in familial amyloid polyneuropathy (Portuguese V30M), *Amyloid J Protein Folding Disorders* 9:126–133, 2002.

73. Sekijima Y, Dendle MA, Kelly JW: Orally administered diflunisal stabilizes transthyretin against dissociation required for amyloidogenesis, *Amyloid J Protein Folding Disorders* 13:236–249, 2006.

The references for this chapter can also be found on www.expert.consult.com.

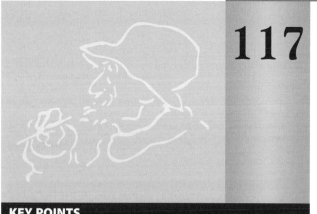

117

Sarcoidosis 📷

NADERA J. SWEISS • ROBERT P. BAUGHMAN

KEY POINTS

Sarcoidosis is a heterogeneous multisystem inflammatory disease of unknown cause characterized by the development and accumulation of noncaseating granulomata in any organ system.

Sarcoidosis occurs worldwide and affects people of all racial and ethnic backgrounds.

The pathogenesis of sarcoidosis likely involves the interplay of different cells, cytokines, and other inflammatory mediators.

Rheumatologic manifestations are common in sarcoidosis and are often overlooked or misdiagnosed.

No treatments have been FDA-approved for sarcoidosis or for any of its manifestations, including sarcoid arthritis.

New treatment modalities, including tumor necrosis factor (TNF) inhibitors, appear to be promising for the treatment of extrathoracic sarcoidosis based on case series, although randomized controlled trials have shown limited benefit in cases of pulmonary involvement.

Sarcoidosis is an orphan, systemic, clinically heterogeneous disorder. Its cause has yet to be identified, but environmental, genetic, and infectious causes have been suggested. The hallmark of sarcoidosis is the development and accumulation of noncaseating granulomas in any organ system. Organ system involvement, which is unpredictable and varies between patients, is the major determinant of morbidity and mortality in sarcoidosis. Although any organ system can be involved, the lungs are affected in most cases. Lymphatic, skin, and ocular findings are also common. Given the variability of sarcoidosis manifestations, diagnosing this disorder is often difficult. Patients may be asymptomatic or may present with a range of nonspecific symptoms, but specific symptoms such as cough, dyspnea, burning of eyes, or rash may suggest the diagnosis.[1] When extrapulmonary symptoms develop, they sometimes result in rheumatologic manifestations including but not limited to arthritis, skin lesions, arthralgias, and neuropathy.[2]

EPIDEMIOLOGY

Sarcoidosis is a global disease. Because of its clinical heterogeneity and its variable diagnostic criteria in different countries, the worldwide prevalence and incidence of sarcoidosis have been difficult to calculate. In Northern Europe, up to 40 cases per 100,000 people have been reported.[3,4] A study from Eastern Europe found only 3.68 cases of sarcoidosis per 100,000 people.[5] The incidence of sarcoidosis in Japan is also low, with one study estimating it at 3.7 cases per 100,000 individuals.[6] Within countries, incidence rates may vary between races. In the United States, the annual incidence of sarcoidosis is more than three times higher in black individuals (35.5 per 100,000) than in white people (10.9 per 100,000).[7] Furthermore, the disease course of sarcoidosis is more progressive and may be more fatal in black Americans.[8,9] Despite numerous epidemiologic studies of sarcoidosis, many clinicians and researchers believe that estimates of prevalence and incidence are lower than actual rates of the disease owing to inaccurate diagnoses or asymptomatic cases that are never diagnosed.

Although sarcoidosis affects men and women of all ages and from diverse ethnic backgrounds,[4,10] some disparities in how it affects these groups have been noted. The fact that it affects slightly more women than men has been confirmed in studies from around the world; estimates indicate that 57% of patients with sarcoidosis are women.[4] Relative to men, women with sarcoidosis have a greater number of ocular and neurologic manifestations. People of any age may acquire the disease, but the median age of onset is around 40.[4] A second peak of incidence has been reported around age 65, especially in women.[8,11]

IMMUNOPATHOGENESIS

The pathogenesis of sarcoidosis likely involves the interplay of many different cells, cytokines, and other inflammatory mediators. Granuloma development is the characteristic pathologic feature of tissue involvement in sarcoidosis. Physiologically, granulomas act as shields, protecting tissues from pathogens, thereby pre-empting inflammatory reactions. Their formation is the end product of a coordinated effort involving T cell activation, antigen-presenting cell (APC) activation, and cell signaling. Granulomas consist of a core of mononuclear phagocytes, such as epithelioid cells, multinucleated giant cells, and macrophages, which are encased by lymphocytes, including B cells, CD4+ T cells, and CD8+ T cells.[12]

Innate Immunity

T cell activation is required for granulomas to form. Early in the course of sarcoidosis, an unknown antigen or multiple antigens activate T cells and macrophages, thereby triggering downstream signaling from both cell types. Locally activated CD4+ T helper cells differentiate into T helper type 1 (Th1)-like cells, causing subsequent elevations in Th1-associated inflammatory mediators, such as interleukin (IL)-2, interferon (IFN)-α, IFN-γ, monocyte chemotactic

📷 Supplemental image available on the Expert Consult Premium Edition website.

protein-1 (MCP-1), macrophage inflammatory protein-1 (MIP-1), and granulocyte-macrophage colony-stimulating factor (GM-CSF). CD4$^+$ T helper cells also interact with APCs to initiate the development of and preserve granulomas.[3] Thus, T cells undergo oligoclonal proliferation in areas of immune system activity. At this point in the disease process, lymphocyte levels are typically increased, and the ratio of CD4/CD8 cells becomes elevated in the lungs and other affected organs.

Acquired Immunity

In sarcoidosis, uptake of antigens is the most likely trigger for activation of macrophages, which are then able to produce IL-12, IL-15, IL-18, and tumor necrosis factor (TNF). Macrophage-derived cytokines contribute to the external signaling milieu that selectively pressures toward Th1 differentiation of CD4$^+$ cells.[12,13] Ultimately, a feedback loop from downstream-produced cytokine cascade induces macrophages to differentiate into epithelioid cells, which gain secretory capability, lose phagocytic capacity, and fuse to form multinucleated giant cells.[3] These epithelioid cells form the cellular basis of granulomas. Also contributing to granuloma formation are Th2 cells. These cells synthesize fibronectin and CC motif ligand 18 (CCL18). Release of these mediators results in a positive feedback loop of CCL18-activated and macrophage-mediated collagen formation. Although granulomas spontaneously resolve without causing damage in most cases, this cycle leads to fibrosis in up to 25% of patients with sarcoidosis.[3] As patients' fibrosis becomes more extensive, their prognosis worsens. Although the mechanisms responsible for granuloma fibrosis have not been fully characterized, patterns of cytokines change, and Th2 cells may pressure toward an increased ratio of CD8 to CD4 cells. Less than 5% of patients die from sarcoidosis, but fibrosis leading to respiratory failure is a contributing factor in many sarcoidosis deaths.

In summary, the essential immunologic events in granuloma formation can be summarized as follows[13,14]: (1) antigen exposure, (2) antigen processing and presentation by macrophages, resulting in T cell immunity against the antigen, (3) T-effector cell production, (4) macrophage activation, and (5) granuloma formation.

ETIOLOGY

Sarcoidosis has yet to be attributed to a single factor. The heterogeneity of the disease suggests that multiple causative agents may be responsible for the variable disease manifestations of sarcoidosis. Given the immunopathogenic mechanisms that underlie sarcoidosis, such a disease trigger might be a T cell antigen that stimulates the cascade of events leading to granuloma formation. Because the lungs are affected in more than 90% of cases of sarcoidosis, it is likely that an environmental agent (including an infectious agent, potentially exposed via the pulmonary route) might contribute to onset of sarcoidosis.

Both inorganic and organic environmental factors with antigenic capabilities have been implicated in the pathogenesis of sarcoidosis. Early studies on the causes of sarcoidosis suggested a link between sarcoidosis and agents

associated with a rural lifestyle, such as the lumber industry and burning wood.[15,16] These data have been extended in the ACCESS study, which found that agricultural debris and wood burning are associated particularly with pulmonary sarcoidosis but not with systemic sarcoidosis.[17] In a different analysis of the ACCESS trial, radiation, insecticides, mildew, and mold were environmental factors associated with systemic sarcoidosis phenotype.[18] These findings may indicate that each of these unique sarcoidosis subtypes has its own causes.

Numerous methods have been used to look for an infectious agent as a cause of sarcoidosis. When in situ hybridization was used, *Mycobacterium tuberculosis* catalase-peroxidase protein (mKatG) was found in nearly 40% of tissue samples from patients with sarcoidosis. Recombinant mKatG protein was then used to measure mKatG antibodies in patients with sarcoidosis, which were present in 50% of patients studied.[19] Others have found evidence of an immunologic reaction to additional mycobacterial antigens.[20,21] *Propionibacterium acnes* has been found more frequently in granulomas from sarcoidosis patients but can also be found in individuals without sarcoidosis, so its primary role in pathogenesis remains unclear.[22-24] These studies suggest that sarcoidosis may represent overexposure of the patient to a commonly encountered microorganism associated with dysregulated resultant immune responses. Because several types of bacteria have been associated with sarcoidosis, some clinicians have attempted to use antibiotics to manage the disease. Although skin sarcoidosis has, on occasion, responded to antibiotics,[25] their usefulness in other forms of sarcoidosis appears minimal.[22]

GENETICS

Compelling studies of familial clustering and incidence of sarcoidosis among different racial groups indicate that sarcoidosis susceptibility is influenced by the interplay of genetic factors. In the ACCESS study, first-degree relatives were reported to have a fivefold increase in risk of developing the disease.[26] Associations have been found between risk of sarcoidosis and class I and II human leukocyte antigen (HLA) gene products, which have essential roles in antigen presentation. It is considered likely that a susceptibility locus for sarcoidosis exists within the HLA gene region, as is the case with other autoimmune diseases and cancers such as Hodgkin's lymphoma. An intriguing analysis of data from the ACCESS study identified associations between genetic factors (HLA alleles), environmental factors, and sarcoidosis phenotypes. In considering together several of the factors postulated to cause sarcoidosis, a compelling argument can be made for a genetic factor that predisposes individuals to the disease and a subsequent environmental exposure that triggers onset of sarcoidosis. Specifically, Rossman and colleagues found that HLA-DRB1*1101 and insecticide exposure at work are significantly associated with cardiac sarcoidosis and hypercalcemia.[27] A similar relationship between HLA-DRB1*1101, mold and musty odors, and pulmonary sarcoidosis was described.[27]

HLA polymorphisms have also been linked to Löfgren's syndrome, an acute form of sarcoidosis characterized by bilateral hilar lymphadenopathy (BHL), erythema nodosum (EN), fever, and periarticular ankle inflammation or arthritis of the ankle. In patients with Löfgren's syndrome, HLA-DRB1*03 is four times more common than in healthy individuals[28] and has been associated with EN and ankle arthritis, which are favorable prognostic factors. A more recent study found that DRB1*03-positive and DRB1*03-negative patients have different disease courses. For example, most DRB1*03-positive patients experienced resolution of Löfgren's syndrome within 2 years after diagnosis. By contrast, nearly half of patients without this allele had resolving disease.[29] The mechanism underlying this difference in disease course remains unknown. A relationship between HLA-DRB1*03 and interferon-γ-3,3 homozygosity has been suggested in sarcoidosis. Wysoczanska and colleagues reported that when combined, these two genetic factors increase the risk of Löfgren's syndrome, and this may be indicative of a complex gene-gene interaction underlying this sarcoidosis phenotype.[30]

Genetic studies of non-HLA genes have been inconclusive. Loci coding for TNF, co-stimulatory molecules on antigen-presenting cells such as CD80 and CD86, chemokine receptors CCR2 and CCR5, and many others have been suggested as possible susceptibility factors, but their roles have not been fully characterized.[22,31] Of these, chemokine receptor genes have been associated with particular sarcoidosis phenotypes. For example, the C-C chemokine receptor 2 (CCR2) haplotype 2 has been linked to Löfgren's syndrome.[32] In this study, the association between CCR2 haplotype 2 and Löfgren's syndrome remained significant even after adjustment for the presence of DRB1*03.[32]

Ongoing genome-wide association studies (GWASs) are seeking to identify additional genes that may be linked to sarcoidosis onset and susceptibility. To date, these studies have identified several novel gene candidates.[33] In family clusters with sarcoidosis, GWASs have identified areas of interest in a German population.[34] A similar analysis of African-American familial sarcoidosis did not have identical findings but did find the same linkage at chromosomes 1p and 9q.[35]

DIAGNOSING SARCOIDOSIS

The diagnosis of musculoskeletal disease related to sarcoidosis must be examined on the basis of two different presentations. The first is a patient with known sarcoidosis who presents with musculoskeletal complaints. The other is a patient with musculoskeletal disease in whom sarcoidosis is a possibility. Although the evaluations may be similar, crucial differences in approach are required.

One can never be sure of the diagnosis of sarcoidosis. The American Thoracic Society (ATS), the European Respiratory Society (ERS), and the World Association of Sarcoidosis and Other Granulomatous Disorders (WASOG) have developed diagnostic criteria. The patient with appropriate clinical presentation and multiple organ involvement who has granulomas identified in one or more organs, and who has no other cause for the granulomatous reaction, is considered to have sarcoidosis.[1] Figure 117-1 presents some features consistent with the disease.[36] Diagnosis relies

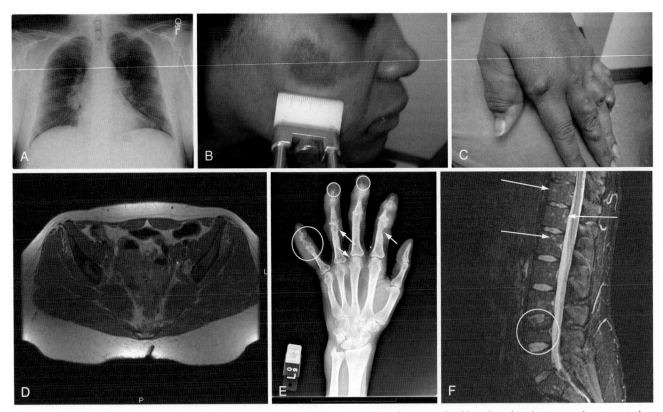

Figure 117-1 Various manifestations of sarcoidosis. **A,** Bilateral hilar adenopathy and right paratracheal lymph node enlargement demonstrated on a posterior anterior chest roentgenogram, Scadding stage 1.[38] **B,** Facial lesion consistent with lupus pernio.[60] **C,** Hand changes consistent with sarcoidosis in the fingers. **D,** Noncontrast magnetic resonance image of the pelvis demonstrating bone marrow replacement by granulomatous tissue. **E,** Cystic changes (arrows) within the bones of the fingers of a patient with sarcoidosis. **F,** Gadolinium enhancement of lesions of the spine seen on magnetic resonance image of a sarcoidosis patient. (**B,** Reproduced with permission from the patient.)

Table 117-1 Major Causes of Granulomatous Reaction besides Sarcoidosis

Infection	Environmental	Miscellaneous
Mycobacterium tuberculosis	Berylliosis	ANCA-associated vasculitis
Fungal	Hard metal	Necrotizing sarcoid
Mycoplasma	Zirconium	granuloma
Pneumocystis jiroveci	Tattoo	Lymphoma
Brucellosis	Hypersensitivity pneumonitis	Cancer
Cat-scratch fever	Drugs (e.g., methotrexate)	Granulomatous lesions of unknown significance
Atypical mycobacteria		Crohn's disease
Toxoplasmosis		Lymphocytic interstitial pneumonia
		Behçet's disease
		Rheumatoid nodules

ANCA, antineutrophil cytoplasm antibody.

Adapted from American Thoracic Society: Statement on sarcoidosis: joint statement of the American Thoracic Society (ATS), the European Respiratory Society (ERS) and the World Association of Sarcoidosis and Other Granulomatous Disorders (WASOG) adopted by the ATS Board of Directors and by the ERS Executive Committee, February 1999, *Am J Respir Crit Care Med* 160:736–755, 1999.

heavily on the finding of granulomas in the biopsy. However, many other conditions can lead to a granulomatous reaction, as is summarized in Table 117-1. Although sarcoidosis granulomas tend to be noncaseating and non-necrotizing, a significant number of sarcoidosis patients exhibit evidence of some necrosis in part of their granulomatous response. Certain features such as erythema nodosum, BHL, gallium scan showing increased activity in the parotids and lacrimal glands, an elevated angiotensin-converting enzyme (ACE) level, and bronchoalveolar lavage with increased lymphocytes with a CD4/CD8 ratio greater than 3.5 are strongly suggestive of sarcoidosis, even in a patient in whom a biopsy has not been performed.

The heterogeneity of the disease leads to varied clinical presentations, which may result in delayed diagnosis. One study of 189 patients with sarcoidosis found that only 15.3% of patients receive a diagnosis during their first visit to a physician.[37] Moreover, sarcoidosis can affect any organ, and this may cause a patient to be referred to a specialist who may not commonly manage sarcoidosis.[37] Complicating

further the diagnosis of sarcoidosis is its similarity of presentation to or concurrent existence with a variety of other conditions, most notably autoimmune disorders. Thus, sarcoidosis sometimes is diagnosed after other potential diagnoses have been excluded.

For the patient who presents with musculoskeletal disease and possible sarcoidosis, a vigilant approach is mandatory. A comprehensive multisystem evaluation as is commonly performed in rheumatology practice should prove informative. Table 117-2 lists some of the common manifestations that support or refute the diagnosis. For example, hilar adenopathy on a posterior chest roentgenogram is seen in about two-thirds of patients. Scadding proposed a staging system of the chest roentgenogram[38]: stage 1 disease consists of hilar adenopathy alone (see Figure 117-1A); stage 2 disease is hilar adenopathy plus infiltrates; stage 3 is infiltrates alone; and stage 4 is fibrosis. Although this scoring is commonly used, differences may be noted in staging of the roentgenogram, even among sarcoidosis experts.[39] Patients may have evidence of pathology on chest computed tomography (CT) scan. Table 117-2 lists some less common features, which, when present, support the diagnosis.[36] These include erythema nodosum, lupus pernio (see Figure 117-1B), cranial seventh nerve paralysis, and hypercalcemia.

For patients with sarcoidosis, several tests (summarized in Table 117-3) have been proposed to serve as a minimal evaluation.[40] These tests reflect the fact that sarcoidosis is a multiple-organ disease, and one needs to look for evidence of specific organ involvement. Figure 117-1 demonstrates some of the features associated with sarcoidosis. Magnetic resonance imaging (MRI) with gadolinium may identify involvement of sarcoidosis in the brain[41] or in the heart.[42] MRI findings may also be useful in bone sarcoidosis or sarcoid arthritis.

Several lines of evidence have indicated that 18F-fluorodeoxyglucose positron-emission tomography (18F-FDG/PET) may be useful in extrapulmonary sarcoidosis, but it usually is not recommended as a first diagnostic tool. 18F-FDG/PET can be used to determine which organs are affected, particularly when no evidence of lung involvement is found. This includes cardiac sarcoidosis.[42] Furthermore, this test can point investigators to appropriate organs

Table 117-2 Features Characteristic of Sarcoidosis

	More Likely Sarcoidosis	Less Likely Sarcoidosis
Chest roentgenogram	Bilateral hilar adenopathy	Pleural effusion
	Upper lobe disease	
Computed tomography of chest	Subpleural reticulonodular infiltrates	Subpleural honeycombing
	Mediastinal adenopathy	
	Peribronchial thickening	
	Traction bronchiectasis of upper lobe	
Skin lesions	Erythema nodosum	
	Lupus pernio	
	Maculopapular lesions	
Ocular disease	Uveitis	Episcleritis
	Optic neuritis	
Neurologic disease	Cranial seventh nerve paralysis	
Renal disease	Nephrocalcinosis	
Laboratory data	Elevated angiotensin-converting enzyme	Positive antineutrophil cytoplasm antibody
	Elevated serum calcium	
	Elevated alkaline phosphatase	

Table 117-3 Evaluation of Patient with Sarcoidosis

Initial Evaluation Suggested for All Patients
History, including occupational and environmental exposures
Physical examination
Posterior-anterior chest roentgenogram
Spirometry
Complete blood count
Liver function studies and serum calcium
Routine ophthalmic examination

Evaluation Considered in Selected Patients
Computed tomography scan of chest
Holter monitor and/or electrocardiogram
Urine analysis
Diffusion capacity of lung of carbon monoxide
X-ray of involved joints and/or ultrasound/magnetic resonance imaging

Follow-up Every 6-12 Months
Any abnormality noted on initial evaluation
Chest roentgenogram
Liver function studies and serum calcium
Spirometry

Modified from American Thoracic Society: Statement on sarcoidosis: joint statement of the American Thoracic Society (ATS), the European Respiratory Society (ERS) and the World Association of Sarcoidosis and Other Granulomatous Disorders (WASOG) adopted by the ATS Board of Directors and by the ERS Executive Committee, February 1999, *Am J Respir Crit Care Med* 160:736–755, 1999.

to biopsy when no distinct organ system involvement is obvious.[43]

Criteria for specific organ involvement in patients with known sarcoidosis have been proposed.[44] Definitive organ involvement may be obvious or can be established by a positive granuloma biopsy from the affected tissue. For example, it is possible that arthritis with no other cause may be attributed to underlying sarcoidosis. However, patients with phalangeal cystic changes almost definitely can consider their arthritis to be a manifestation of their sarcoidosis[44] (Table 117-4).

Sarcoid Arthritis

Between 15% and 25% of patients with sarcoidosis have arthritis, which is the most frequently observed rheumatologic symptom of sarcoidosis. In patients with sarcoidosis, arthritis can be acute or chronic; the acute form is most common. Chronic arthritis is typically associated with multisystem sarcoidosis.[45]

Acute Sarcoid Arthritis

Febrile arthropathy is the most frequently observed joint involvement in sarcoidosis. Although any joint may be involved, the condition usually is symmetric, involving ankles, knees, wrists, and elbows, and exists with BHL and erythema nodosum. Patients with acute sarcoid arthritis exhibit pain and stiffness, and their joints may be swollen or tender (Supplemental Figure 117-1 on www.expertconsult.com). Acute sarcoid arthritis sometimes resolves within weeks of onset, but occasionally symptoms last for several months. Once it resolves, this condition usually does not recur.

In a study of patients with acute sarcoid arthritis, Visser and colleagues prospectively evaluated patients and published criteria to assist in diagnosis.[45] Of 579 participants, 55 (9%) patients were eventually diagnosed with sarcoid arthritis. Diagnoses were made after it was established that patients had a combination of arthritis and BHL, as determined by chest radiography. From the findings of their study, investigators established criteria with 93% sensitivity and 99% specificity to guide physicians in differentiating between sarcoid and other causes of arthritis. Of the following criteria, patients must have three out of four characteristics to establish a diagnosis of sarcoid arthritis: younger than 40 years of age, EN, symmetric ankle arthritis, and symptoms lasting less than 2 months.[45]

In addition to Visser's criteria, most symptoms of sarcoid arthritis vary among patients. Patients with sarcoid arthritis frequently have elevated erythrocyte sedimentation rates,[45,46] but other symptoms, such as fever, are observed only in up to 66% of patients.[45-48] Of note, a small minority of patients with acute sarcoid arthritis may develop abnormal alterations in their bones that can be seen on radiographs of the hands or feet. In some patients, sarcoid dactylitis may be the presenting symptom (see Figure 117-1C and E), characterized by swollen soft tissues surrounding affected fingers, erythematous skin, or tenderness. Individuals with dactylitis may also have nail abnormalities, such as dystrophy. Therefore, it is important to rule out other conditions that affect the nails, such as psoriatic arthritis, when making sarcoid arthritis diagnoses.

Other bone areas that may be affected by sarcoidosis include nasal bones, pelvic girdle structures, ribs, and skull. Patients with lupus pernio may be particularly at risk for developing abnormalities in their nasal bones. Because of similarities between a patient with sarcoidosis who has nasal bone involvement and a patient with granulomatosis with polyangiitis (GPA) (formerly Wegener's granulomatosis), it is important to distinguish between these conditions.[49] Serology may be useful because most patients with GPA will have a positive antineutrophil cytoplasm antibody (ANCA), but sarcoidosis does not lead to a positive ANCA.[50] On the other hand, about 60% of sarcoidosis patients will have an elevated ACE level at presentation; this is not seen in the presence of vasculitis.[49] Lesions in the pelvic bones (see Figure 117-1D) or in the spine (see Figure 117-1F) may, at first, lead one to suspect cancer metastases. Therefore, a comprehensive assessment is warranted in patients who present with changes in their skeletal bones, even if they exhibit other symptoms reminiscent of sarcoidosis.

Chronic Sarcoid Arthritis

The chronic form of sarcoid arthritis is less common than the acute form, and it affects more African-American than Caucasian individuals. It most often affects individuals with systemic sarcoidosis and multiorgan involvement. In some patients, joint symptoms manifest early in the course of sarcoidosis, whereas other patients develop sarcoid arthritis several years after onset of the disorder. Lupus pernio and chronic uveitis may manifest concomitantly with the chronic form of arthritis.

As is the case with other organ system manifestations, several conditions may mimic sarcoid arthritis and should

Table 117-4 Features Comparing Sarcoidosis with Other Rheumatologic Diseases

	Sarcoidosis	SLE	RA	PsA	Systemic Vasculitis
Clinical Findings	Lungs, eyes, and skin most common; any other organ (heart, brain, skin, bone, liver, etc.) may also be affected	Joints, kidneys (nephritis), mucous membranes, circulatory system, nervous system, lymph nodes, spleen	Joints (most common), lungs, blood vessels	Joints (oligoarthritis, polyarthritis), skin (psoriatic lesions), nails (dystrophy, dactylitis)	Blood vessels (wall thickening), skin (purpura, infarct ulcers), nervous system (headache, meningitis, seizures), joints (arthritis), kidneys (hypertension), heart, GI system
Radiographic Findings	Bilateral and mediastinal hilar adenopathy, reticulonodular opacities	Bilateral, diffuse air space opacity; diaphragm elevation ("shrinking lung syndrome")	Joint space narrowing, joint erosions, inflammation	Joint space narrowing, erosions, ossification near joints	Granulomatous lesions; multiple bilateral nodules; patchy areas of consolidation
Pathologic Findings	Noncaseating granulomas	Inflammation, blood vessel abnormalities such as vasculitis, immune complex deposits	Swollen synovium; presence of fibroblast-like and macrophage-like synoviocytes, macrophages, T and B cells	Increased synovial vascularity, dilated blood vessels, neutrophil infiltration	ANCA staining pattern on neutrophils and monocytes; patchy infiltrates, vessel wall granulomas, fibrous tissue
Laboratory Findings	Elevated ACE; hypercalcemia; presence of ANAs, ANCAs, and anti-dsDNA	Anti-dsDNA, anti-Smith, ANAs, RNP, antithrombin, anti-Ro/SSA, anti-La/SSB, anti-topoisomerase, aPL	Rheumatoid factor, ACPA, aPL	ANA (common), anti-dsDNA, rheumatoid factor, anti-Ro, anti-RNP (rare), aPL	ANCA, aPL, inflammatory markers (CRP)

	MCTD	Scleroderma	Antiphospholipid Syndrome	Sjögren's Syndrome	Ankylosing Spondylitis	Reactive Arthritis
Clinical Findings	Raynaud's phenomenon; joints, muscles, lungs, heart, kidneys, and nervous system may be affected	Skin (tightening, thickening, induration), joints, GI system, lung, heart, kidney	Blood vessels (arterial/venous thrombosis, thrombocytopenia, fetal loss	Eyes, mouth, and mucous membrane dryness; joints (arthritis), skin, kidneys, nervous system, lymph nodes may be affected	Vertebral arthritis, back pain, stiffness, synovitis, peripheral arthritis, pulmonary symptoms, iritis	Arthritis, conjunctivitis; urethritis; usually following genitourinary or gastrointestinal infection
Radiographic Findings	Diffuse periarticular osteopenia; swelling of soft tissue; joint erosions, joint space narrowing, tuft resorption, and soft tissue atrophy	Pulmonary fibrosis, diffuse reticulonodular pattern	Patchy infiltrates	Mild joint space narrowing	Vertebral inflammation; sacroiliitis; bone erosions, syndesmophytes	Proliferation at tendon insertion; sacroiliitis; syndesmophytes
Pathologic Findings	Autoantigen modifications, B and T cell activation	Excess matrix deposition, fibrosis; endothelial cell dysfunction and death; destruction of small vessels	Structural glomerular changes	B cell infiltration	Capsular fibrosis; ossification	Bacterial infection (Shigella, Salmonella, Campylobacter)
Laboratory Findings	ANA, RNP, aPL	ANA (anti-topoisomerase), aPL, ACAs	Lupus anticoagulant, aPL, anti-protein C, anti-prothrombin, anti-protein S, anti-annexin	ANA, anti-Ro/SSA, rheumatoid factor, aPL	Elevated ESR, leukocytosis, HLA-B27	ANCA, HLA-B27; elevated ESR, CRP

ACA, anticardiolipin antibody; ACE, angiotensin-converting enzyme; ACPA, anticitrullinated protein antibody; ANA, antinuclear antibody; ANCA, antineutrophil cytoplasm antibody; aPL, antiphospholipid antibody; CRP, C-reactive protein; dsDNA, double-stranded DNA; ESR, erythrocyte sedimentation rate; GI, gastrointestinal; MCTD, mixed connective tissue disease; PsA, prostate-specific antigen; RA, rheumatoid arthritis; RNP, ribonucleotide protein; SLE, systemic lupus erythematosus; TNF, tumor necrosis factor.

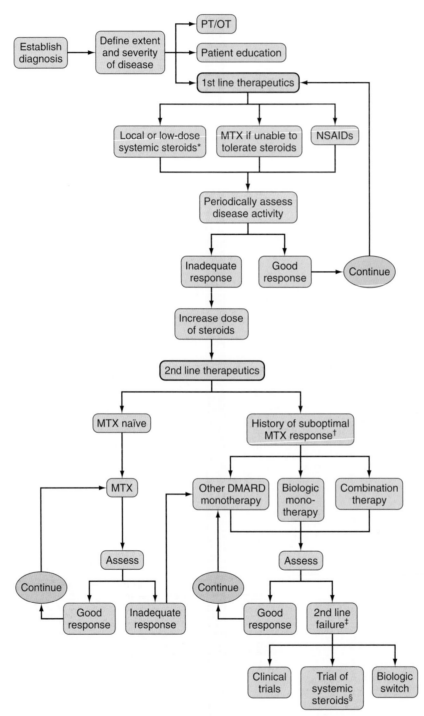

Figure 117-2 Algorithm describing an approach to treating sarcoidosis arthritis. *, Low dose steroids: <10 to 20 mg prednisone daily. †, Suboptimal response to MTX: intolerance to drug, lack of satisfactory efficacy on dosage up to 25 mg/wk, or a contraindication to medication use. ‡, DMARD failure: progressive disease or drug intolerance. §, Methylprednisone preferred over prednisone if prednisone has been used previously. DMARD, disease-modifying antirheumatic drug; MTX, methotrexate; NSAIDs, nonsteroidal anti-inflammatory drugs; OT, occupational therapy; PT, physical therapy. *(Reproduced with permission from Sweiss NJ, Patterson K, Sawaqed R, et al: Rheumatologic manifestations of sarcoidosis,* Semin Respir Crit Care Med *31:463–473, 2010.)*

be excluded. For example, symmetric oligoarthritis or polyarthritis and an elevated rheumatoid factor are common features of sarcoid arthritis, but they may also result from reactive arthritis or rheumatoid arthritis (RA). Furthermore, a subset of patients with RA may develop some lung dysfunction, which can cause confusion in differentiating RA from sarcoidosis. In addition, some patients with RA have been reported to eventually develop coincident sarcoidosis, although sarcoidosis coexisting with connective disease disorders is rare. Therefore, it is crucial for physicians to distinguish between the two conditions, or to determine whether the two diseases are comorbid within the same patient.

In patients with migratory polyarthritis, rheumatic fever may be suspected, particularly when joint symptoms manifest before additional sarcoidosis-related symptoms are noted. A biopsy of the synovium or tendon sheaths may be helpful with characteristic granulomas appearing at pathology. Differential diagnoses for patients with monarthritis include gout, septic arthritis, and calcium pyrophosphate dihydrate (CPPD)-positive arthritis (see Tables 117-3, 117-4, and supportive content for detailed consideration of the diagnostic approach).[2]

MANAGING SARCOIDOSIS: FOCUSING ON SARCOID ARTHRITIS

No treatments have been U.S. Food and Drug Administration (FDA)-approved for sarcoidosis or for any of its manifestations, including sarcoid arthritis. Furthermore, no randomized trials have been conducted that can guide clinical decision making. To help guide clinicians in management, we have proposed a treatment algorithm, which is shown in Figure 117-2.[2] Nonsteroidal anti-inflammatory drugs, methotrexate, and local or low-dose systemic corticosteroids are our preferred first-line therapies. Alternatively, hydroxychloroquine may be used. Using information obtained from the diagnostic evaluation, the clinician usually makes treatment decisions after carefully considering the disease severity and its probable clinical course, as revealed by its radiographic progression.

The proposed algorithm requires regular patient visits to monitor disease activity and therapeutic efficacy and tolerability. Responders remain on first-line agents until disease resolution or, alternatively, treatment failure. Before nonresponders are prescribed second-line therapies, higher doses of corticosteroids may be used, depending on tolerability and manifest toxicity. If patients do require second-line medications, two options are available: (1) methotrexate may be given to methotrexate-naïve patients, or (2) biologic therapies consisting of nonmethotrexate disease-modifying antirheumatic drugs (e.g., sulfasalazine, hydroxychloroquine, azathioprine), monotherapy, or combinations thereof may be prescribed to patients who inadequately respond to first-line methotrexate.

For patients for whom this treatment approach fails, one can consider an alternative biologic therapy or an aggressive course of systemic corticosteroids with careful toxicity monitoring. Alternatively, participating in a clinical trial may be appropriate for some patients.

Vitamin D metabolism represents a complex issue in sarcoidosis. Up to 10% of sarcoidosis patients will have hypercalcemia or hypercalciuria.[52] The mechanism usually attributed has been increased production of 1,25-dihydroxyvitamin D (1,25-OH$_2$D) by epithelioid cells in the granuloma. In one study, elevated 1,25-OH$_2$D was associated with prolonged need for treatment.[53] However, this same group of patients often requires treatment for osteoporosis.[54] Bisphosphonates alone may be adequate to treat corticosteroid-induced osteoporosis.[55] Because of the disassociation between 25-hydroxyvitamin D (25-OHD) and 1,25-OH$_2$D in sarcoidosis, it seems reasonable to measure both levels to ascertain which patients should receive vitamin D supplements.

Future Directions

Much remains to be learned about sarcoidosis. Its causes remain unclear, and no medications have been FDA-approved for its treatment. Although increasing attention has been paid to the underlying mechanisms of granuloma formation, full details of sarcoidosis immunopathogenesis have yet to be determined. Appropriate animal models and candidate genes are needed to help advance our understanding of this disease.

Large clinical trials are warranted. We have presented an algorithm for use in treating patients with an established diagnosis of sarcoidosis. However, treatment approaches vary by institution and by individual clinician owing to a myriad of conflicting studies that have been published about sarcoidosis management. Furthermore, therapeutic choices will likely differ according to the type and extent of organ system involvement observed in individual patients.

For relapsed and refractory disease, steroid-sparing agents including cytotoxic drugs and novel biologic therapies such as anti-TNF treatments have been used increasingly. Anti-TNF agents have been investigated in numerous sarcoidosis studies because of the potential role of TNF and other proinflammatory factors in sarcoidosis pathogenesis. Limiting their usefulness in this setting are mounting reports of granulomatous reactions to anti-TNF therapies in patients treated with these agents for nonsarcoidosis indications. Simply put, TNF inhibitors may help treat *and may cause* sarcoidosis.[56-59] With this point in mind, it is relevant to our discussion that the presentation of anti-TNF–induced sarcoidosis, similar to all phenotypes of sarcoidosis, is a unique entity, but it does overlap with that of other autoimmune diseases. Furthermore, anti-TNF agents have been reported to induce autoimmune diseases other than sarcoidosis, including systemic lupus erythematosus (SLE), vasculitis, and interstitial lung disease. Diagnosing these conditions in patients with anti-TNF–induced sequelae is critical.

References

1. American Thoracic Society: Statement on sarcoidosis: joint statement of the American Thoracic Society (ATS), the European Respiratory Society (ERS) and the World Association of Sarcoidosis and Other Granulomatous Disorders (WASOG) adopted by the ATS Board of Directors and by the ERS Executive Committee, February 1999, *Am J Respir Crit Care Med* 160:736–755, 1999.
2. Sweiss NJ, Patterson K, Sawaqed R, et al: Rheumatologic manifestations of sarcoidosis, *Semin Respir Crit Care Med* 31:463–473, 2010.
3. Iannuzzi MC, Rybicki BA, Teirstein AS: Sarcoidosis, *N Engl J Med* 357:2153–2165, 2007.
4. Sharma OP: Sarcoidosis around the world, *Clin Chest Med* 29:357–363, vii, 2008.

5. Kolek V: Epidemiological study on sarcoidosis in Moravia and Silesia, *Sarcoidosis* 11:110–112, 1994.

6. Pietinalho A, Hiraga Y, Hosoda Y, et al: The frequency of sarcoidosis in Finland and Hokkaido, Japan: a comparative epidemiological study, *Sarcoidosis* 12:61–67, 1995.

7. Rybicki BA, Major M, Popovich J Jr, et al: Racial differences in sarcoidosis incidence: a 5-year study in a health maintenance organization, *Am J Epidemiol* 145:234–241, 1997.

8. Baughman RP, Teirstein AS, Judson MA, et al: Clinical characteristics of patients in a case control study of sarcoidosis, *Am J Respir Crit Care Med* 164:1885–1889, 2001.

9. Westney GE, Judson MA: Racial and ethnic disparities in sarcoidosis: from genetics to socioeconomics, *Clin Chest Med* 27:453–462, vi, 2006.

10. Jones N, Mochizuki M: Sarcoidosis: epidemiology and clinical features, *Ocul Immunol Inflamm* 18:72–79, 2010.

11. Hillerdal G, Nou E, Osterman K, Schmekel B: Sarcoidosis: epidemiology and prognosis. A 15-year European study, *Am Rev Respir Dis* 130:29–32, 1984.

12. Gerke AK, Hunninghake G: The immunology of sarcoidosis, *Clin Chest Med* 29:379–390, vii, 2008.

13. Zissel G, Prasse A, Muller-Quernheim J: Sarcoidosis—immunopathogenetic concepts, *Semin Respir Crit Care Med* 28:3–14, 2007.

14. Baughman RP, Culver DA, Judson MA: A concise review of pulmonary sarcoidosis, *Am J Respir Crit Care Med* 173:573–581, 2010.

15. Gentry JT, Nitowsky HM, Michael M Jr: Studies on the epidemiology of sarcoidosis in the United States: the relationship to soil areas and to urban-rural residence, *J Clin Invest* 34:1839–1856, 1955.

16. Kajdasz DK, Lackland DT, Mohr LC, Judson MA: A current assessment of rurally linked exposures as potential risk factors for sarcoidosis, *Ann Epidemiol* 11:111–117, 2001.

17. Kreider ME, Christie JD, Thompson B, et al: Relationship of environmental exposures to the clinical phenotype of sarcoidosis, *Chest* 128:207–215, 2005.

18. Newman LS, Rose CS, Bresnitz EA, et al: A case control etiologic study of sarcoidosis: environmental and occupational risk factors, *Am J Respir Crit Care Med* 170:1324–1330, 2004.

19. Song Z, Marzilli L, Greenlee BM, et al: Mycobacterial catalase-peroxidase is a tissue antigen and target of the adaptive immune response in systemic sarcoidosis, *J Exp Med* 201:755–767, 2005.

20. Drake WP, Dhason MS, Nadaf M, et al: Cellular recognition of Mycobacterium tuberculosis ESAT-6 and KatG peptides in systemic sarcoidosis, *Infect Immun* 75:527–530, 2007.

21. Oswald-Richter KA, Culver DA, Hawkins C, et al: Cellular responses to mycobacterial antigens are present in bronchoalveolar lavage fluid used in the diagnosis of sarcoidosis, *Infect Immun* 77:3740–3748, 2009.

22. Chen ES, Moller DR: Etiology of sarcoidosis, *Clin Chest Med* 29:365–377, vii, 2008.

23. Drake WP, Newman LS: Mycobacterial antigens may be important in sarcoidosis pathogenesis, *Curr Opin Pulm Med* 12:359–363, 2006.

24. Ezzie ME, Crouser ED: Considering an infectious etiology of sarcoidosis, *Clin Dermatol* 25:259–266, 2007.

25. Bachelez H, Senet P, Cadranel J, et al: The use of tetracyclines for the treatment of sarcoidosis, *Arch Dermatol* 137:69–73, 2001.

26. Rybicki BA, Iannuzzi MC, Frederick MM, et al: Familial aggregation of sarcoidosis: a case-control etiologic study of sarcoidosis (ACCESS), *Am J Respir Crit Care Med* 164:2085–2091, 2001.

27. Rossman MD, Thompson B, Frederick M, et al: HLA and environmental interactions in sarcoidosis, *Sarcoidosis Vasc Diffuse Lung Dis* 25:125–132, 2008.

28. Berlin M, Fogdell-Hahn A, Olerup O, et al: HLA-DR predicts the prognosis in Scandinavian patients with pulmonary sarcoidosis, *Am J Respir Crit Care Med* 156:1601–1605, 1997.

29. Grunewald J, Eklund A: Lofgren's syndrome: human leukocyte antigen strongly influences the disease course, *Am J Respir Crit Care Med* 179:307–312, 2009.

30. Wysoczanska B, Bogunia-Kubik K, Suchnicki K, et al: Combined association between IFN-gamma 3,3 homozygosity and DRB1*03 in Lofgren's syndrome patients, *Immunol Lett* 91:127–131, 2004.

31. Smith G, Brownell I, Sanchez M, Prystowsky S: Advances in the genetics of sarcoidosis, *Clin Genet* 73:401–412, 2008.

32. Spagnolo P, Renzoni EA, Wells AU, et al: C-C chemokine receptor 2 and sarcoidosis: association with Lofgren's syndrome, *Am J Respir Crit Care Med* 168:1162–1166, 2003.

33. Hofmann S, Franke A, Fischer A, et al: Genome-wide association study identifies ANXA11 as a new susceptibility locus for sarcoidosis, *Nat Genet* 40:1103–1106, 2008.

34. Schurmann M, Reichel P, Muller-Myhsok B, et al: Results from a genome-wide search for predisposing genes in sarcoidosis, *Am J Respir Crit Care Med* 164:840–846, 2001.

35. Iannuzzi MC, Iyengar SK, Gray-McGuire C, et al: Genome-wide search for sarcoidosis susceptibility genes in African Americans, *Genes Immun* 6:509–518, 2005.

36. Judson MA: The diagnosis of sarcoidosis, *Clin Chest Med* 29:415–427, viii, 2008.

37. Judson MA, Thompson BW, Rabin DL, et al: The diagnostic pathway to sarcoidosis, *Chest* 123:406–412, 2003.

38. Scadding JG: Prognosis of intrathoracic sarcoidosis in England: a review of 136 cases after five years' observation, *Br Med J* 2:1165–1172, 1961.

39. Baughman RP, Shipley R, Desai S, et al: Changes in chest roentgenogram of sarcoidosis patients during a clinical trial of infliximab therapy: comparison of different methods of evaluation, *Chest* 136:526–535, 2009.

40. Hunninghake GW, Costabel U, Ando M, et al: ATS/ERS/WASOG statement on sarcoidosis: American Thoracic Society/European Respiratory Society/World Association of Sarcoidosis and other Granulomatous Disorders, *Sarcoidosis Vasc Diffuse Lung Dis* 16:149–173, 1999.

41. Lower EE, Weiss KL: Neurosarcoidosis, *Clin Chest Med* 29:475–492, ix, 2008.

42. Ohira H, Tsujino I, Ishimaru S, et al: Myocardial imaging with 18F-fluoro-2-deoxyglucose positron emission tomography and magnetic resonance imaging in sarcoidosis, *Eur J Nucl Med Mol Imaging* 35:933–941, 2008.

43. Nunes H, Brillet PY, Valeyre D, et al: Imaging in sarcoidosis, *Semin Respir Crit Care Med* 28:102–120, 2007.

44. Judson MA, Baughman RP, Teirstein AS, et al: Defining organ involvement in sarcoidosis: the ACCESS proposed instrument. ACCESS Research Group. A case control etiologic study of sarcoidosis, *Sarcoidosis Vasc Diffuse Lung Dis* 16:75–86, 1999.

45. Visser H, Vos K, Zanelli E, et al: Sarcoid arthritis: clinical characteristics, diagnostic aspects, and risk factors, *Ann Rheum Dis* 61:499–504, 2002.

46. Gran JT, Bohmer E: Acute sarcoid arthritis: a favourable outcome? A retrospective survey of 49 patients with review of the literature, *Scand J Rheumatol* 25:70–73, 1996.

47. Glennas A, Kvien TK, Melby K, et al: Acute sarcoid arthritis: occurrence, seasonal onset, clinical features and outcome, *Br J Rheumatol* 34:45–50, 1995.

48. Spilberg I, Siltzbach LE, McEwen C: The arthritis of sarcoidosis, *Arthritis Rheum* 12:126–137, 1969.

49. Baughman RP, Lower EE, Tami T: Upper airway. 4: Sarcoidosis of the upper respiratory tract (SURT), *Thorax* 65:181–186, 2010.

50. Baughman RP, Iannuzzi MC: Diagnosis of sarcoidosis: when is a peek good enough? *Chest* 117:931–932, 2000.

51. Deleted in proofs.

52. Adams JS: Hypercalcemia and hypercalciuria, *Semin Respir Med* 13:402–410, 1992.

53. Zissel G, Ernst M, Schlaak M, Muller-Quernheim J: Accessory function of alveolar macrophages from patients with sarcoidosis and other granulomatous and nongranulomatous lung diseases, *J Investig Med* 45:75–86, 1997.

54. Rizzato G, Montemurro L: Reversibility of exogenous corticosteroid-induced bone loss, *Eur Respir J* 6:116–119, 1993.

55. Gonnelli S, Rottoli P, Cepollaro C, et al: Prevention of corticosteroid-induced osteoporosis with alendronate in sarcoid patients, *Calcif Tissue Int* 61:382–385, 1997.

56. Sweiss NJ, Baughman RP: Tumor necrosis factor inhibition in the treatment of refractory sarcoidosis: slaying the dragon? *J Rheumatol* 34:2129–2131, 2007.

57. Sweiss NJ, Curran J, Baughman RP: Sarcoidosis, role of tumor necrosis factor inhibitors and other biologic agents: past, present, and future concepts, *Clin Dermatol* 25:341–346, 2007.

58. Sweiss NJ, Hushaw LL: Biologic agents for rheumatoid arthritis: 2008 and beyond, *J Infus Nurs* 32:S4–S17; quiz S9-S24, 2009.

59. Sweiss NJ, Welsch MJ, Curran JJ, Ellman MH: Tumor necrosis factor inhibition as a novel treatment for refractory sarcoidosis, *Arthritis Rheum* 53:788–791, 2005.

60. Baughman RP, Judson MA, Teirstein A, et al: Chronic facial sarcoidosis including lupus pernio: clinical description and proposed scoring systems, *Am J Clin Dermatol* 9:155–156, 2008.

The references for this chapter can also be found on www.expert.consult.com.

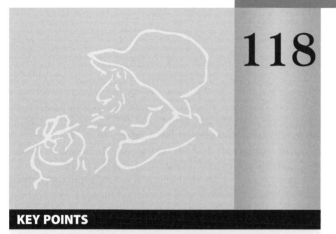

118 Hemochromatosis

GAYE CUNNANE

KEY POINTS

Elevated ferritin (>200 µg/L) and transferrin saturation (>45%) in the absence of other causes are useful screening measures for hereditary hemochromatosis (HHC).

Genetic testing should be reserved for patients with suggestive biochemical abnormalities or a positive family history of HHC or both.

Disease phenotype varies greatly among individuals with similar genotypes of the key gene associated with this disease, including genes encoding HFE, hepcidin, hemojuvelin transferrin receptor 2, and ferroportin.

Diet, alcohol intake, and other risk factors for chronic liver disease all influence the clinical expression of HHC.

Phlebotomy is an effective treatment for decreasing iron stores.

Some clinical manifestations of disease improve with treatment (constitutional symptoms, diabetes mellitus, liver enzyme abnormalities), whereas others are unaltered (arthritis, hypogonadism, cirrhosis).

Atypical osteoarthritis or chondrocalcinosis should trigger a search for an underlying metabolic disorder.

The earlier the diagnosis, the better is the prognosis.

Hemochromatosis refers to the presence of excess iron in body tissues because of increased iron absorption. Primary or hereditary hemochromatosis (HHC) is an autosomal recessive disease, whereas *secondary hemochromatosis* refers to iron overload as a result of increased iron availability, ineffective erythropoiesis, or inherited abnormalities of iron metabolism.

Hemochromatosis was first recognized in the 1880s in a series of case reports that described "bronze diabetes" and "pigmented cirrhosis," but von Recklinghausen is credited with the first use of the term in 1889.[1] In 1935, the familial pattern of HHC was described by Sheldon,[2] who suggested that the disease was due to an inborn error of metabolism. Finch and Finch in 1955[3] showed that HHC was caused by abnormal iron absorption in the presence of a normal diet. At that time, premorbid recognition of the problem was uncommon, however, and most cases were diagnosed at autopsy. In 1972, serum ferritin became available as a measure of iron stores. Three years later, Simon and colleagues[4] discovered that the HHC gene was present on chromosome 6, close to the HLA-A locus. It took 21 more years for the mutated gene, *HFE*, to be described, and in the last decade, it has been recognized that other gene mutations also can cause iron overload.[5] Genetic testing has revolutionized the diagnosis of HHC, although the phenotype of any given mutation may vary greatly.[6,7] Nevertheless, the detection of such genes has greatly enhanced the overall prognosis of this condition by allowing the disease to be diagnosed at a preclinical stage in high-risk individuals. This discovery has helped many patients with HHC achieve a normal life expectancy. Improved knowledge at a molecular level has further aided our understanding of the pathogenesis and therapeutic implications of hemochromatosis, permitting many patients with this disease to achieve a normal life expectancy.

NORMAL IRON METABOLISM

The average total body iron content in adults is 3 to 4 g, mostly contained within hemoglobin, but also present in myoglobin and cytochromes, in addition to the storage proteins ferritin and hemosiderin (Table 118-1). Of a typical daily Western diet of 10 to 20 mg of iron, 1 to 2 mg is absorbed by duodenal enterocytes each day.[8,9] Heme dietary sources from fish and meat have a higher bioavailability than nonheme sources, such as vegetables. The addition of ascorbic acid to the meal increases absorption of nonheme iron, whereas tannins, bran, and phytates inhibit iron absorption.[10,11]

Iron homeostasis is tightly controlled at cellular and molecular levels, influenced by numerous mechanisms, including recent dietary iron intake, the extent of iron stores in the body, and key regulatory peptides. Communication between sites of iron uptake (enterocytes), storage (liver and macrophages), and utilization (erythroid cells) is essential, and an antimicrobial peptide, hepcidin, plays a key role in this regard.[12] Hepatic synthesis of hepcidin is stimulated by increases in the body's iron requirements, as in situations of anemia, hypoxia, or inflammation.[13,14] Hepcidin prevents iron loss by reducing the entry of iron into the bloodstream via inhibition of ferroportin, a membrane-bound iron exporter protein found on macrophages, hepatocytes, and enterocytes.[14,15] Hepcidin production is downregulated when iron requirements return to normal. In the presence of normal iron stores, iron is retained in the intestinal cells by the protein, mobilferritin, and is subsequently excreted when these cells are shed.

When body iron stores reach an adequate level, ferritin production is increased to facilitate storage, and the transferrin receptor is downregulated to minimize the entry of iron into the cells. The iron responsive element binding protein mediates this process by detaching from ferritin mRNA so that more ferritin can be produced.[16] With increasing iron stores, circulating transferrin becomes saturated, and iron is preferentially offloaded to tissue sites

Table 118-1 Definitions of Terms Used in Iron Metabolism

Term	Definitions
Ferritin	Major iron storage protein in iron storage diseases and inflammation
	Markedly increased in adult-onset Still's disease
	Plasma levels reflect iron stores (e.g., 1 ng/mL ferritin = 10 mg iron)
Transferrin	Transporter protein for iron in plasma
	Synthesized in liver
	Increased in iron deficiency states
Transferrin saturation	Serum iron (μg/dL) ÷ total iron-binding capacity (μg/dL) × 100 in iron deficiency anemia/chronic disease/ferroportin mutation in hemochromatosis/ineffective erythropoiesis/iron overload states/severe liver failure
Iron regulatory proteins	Maintain iron homeostasis by modulating synthesis of transferrin receptors/ferritin/duodenal iron transporter
HFE protein	Identified in cells of deep crypts of duodenum and in Kupffer cells
	Modulates uptake of transferrin-bound iron into duodenal crypt cells
Iron exporter proteins	Ferroportin/hephaestin/divalent metal transporter 1 (DMT1)
Hepcidin	Acute phase reactant produced by liver
	Intrinsic antimicrobial activity
	Negative regulator of iron absorption
	Reduces iron release from macrophages
	Prevents iron loss by reducing entry of iron into bloodstream via inhibition of ferroportin
	Mutations found in some families with juvenile hereditary hemochromatosis
Hemojuvelin	Modulates hepcidin expression
Hemosiderin	Histologic identification of iron stain in tissues

that contain cells with high levels of transferrin receptors, such as liver, heart, thyroid, gonads, and pancreatic islet cells.[17]

GENETICS OF HEMOCHROMATOSIS

Four types of HHC have now been described, all linked to gene mutations (Table 118-2).[18,19] Classic HHC (type 1) is

Table 118-2 Hereditary Hemochromatosis (HHC)

Name	Gene	Gene Product	Pattern of Inheritance
HFE-Related HHC			
Type 1	*HFE*, 6p21.3	HFE	Autosomal recessive
Juvenile-Type HHC			
Type 2A	*HJV*, 1q21	Hemojuvelin	Autosomal recessive
Type 2B	*HAMP*, 19q13.1	Hepcidin	
TfR2-Related HHC			
Type 3	*TfR2*, 7q22	Transferrin receptor 2	Autosomal recessive
Ferroportin-Related HHC			
Type 4	*SLC40A1*, 2q32	Ferroportin	Autosomal dominant

an autosomal recessive disorder, with a mutation of the *HFE* gene, located on chromosome 6 (*HFE*-related HHC). Although numerous such mutations have been described, the most common is a single amino acid substitution of tyrosine for cysteine at position 282 (C282Y). This particular mutation is thought to have arisen in a Celtic/Viking ancestor more than 2000 years ago and is now one of the most common genetic defects in individuals of Northern European origin. This anomaly had no reproductive implications, but may have had survival advantages by protecting against iron deficiency in a susceptible population. Homozygosity for this mutation is a risk factor for organ damage secondary to iron deposition, although phenotypic expression varies widely. Other mutations of the *HFE* gene include the replacement of histidine with aspartic acid at position 63 (H63D) and the substitution of serine for cysteine at position 65 (S65C). Clinical manifestations of the latter mutations seem to be less serious, although compound heterozygosity of such defects may be associated with evidence of iron overload.

Unlike mutations of the *HFE* gene that may become clinically obvious in middle age, hemojuvelin (HJV-related HHC, type 1A) or hepcidin (HAMP-related HHC, type 2B) mutations result in juvenile HHC (type 2), which may manifest in the teens or twenties. The rate of iron accumulation seems to be greater than in adult HHC and is often associated with widespread organ involvement and early mortality.[20] In contrast to the Northern European inheritance of HFE mutations, juvenile HHC has been most commonly reported in Italy.[21] Clinical manifestations of transferrin receptor mutations (TfR2-related HHC, type 3) seem to resemble manifestations of the classic *HFE*-related HHC. Such mutations are rare, and few cases have been described.[22,23]

Type 4 or ferroportin-related HHC is an autosomal dominant condition, described in European and Australian families.[24,25] Two types of ferroportin mutations have been reported. In the first, loss of surface localization of ferroportin results in a decreased ability of cells to export iron, causing iron to build up predominantly in macrophages. In the second, hepcidin-induced ferroportin dysfunction leads to iron accumulation in parenchymal cells of the liver and other tissues. Phenotypic expression varies, with some patients manifesting the effects of iron overload in a similar manner to classic HHC, and others showing minimal evidence of organ damage.[26]

EPIDEMIOLOGY

Although HHC previously was thought to be a rare condition, genetic testing has revealed that it is one of the most common heritable disorders. Although 5 out of every 1000 individuals of Northern European origin are homozygous for the *HFE* mutation, phenotypic expression varies, and clinical cases are much fewer in number. In a study of nearly 100,000 individuals from primary care practices in the United States, the prevalence of C282Y homozygosity was as follows: white, 0.44%; Native American, 0.11%; Hispanic, 0.027%; African-American, 0.014%; Pacific Islander, 0.012%; and Asian, 0.0004%.[27] Peak age at the time of diagnosis is 40 to 60 years for classic HHC.

PHENOTYPIC DISEASE EXPRESSION

Clinical manifestations of HHC vary greatly between individuals with similar mutations, suggesting that other factors influence disease expression. One study demonstrated that among C282Y homozygotes, up to 82% have hyperferritinemia, while approximately 28% of male and 1% of females ultimately develop clinical manifestations of HHC—defined as the presence of liver disease, hepatocellular carcinoma, and arthritis of the second and third metacarpophalangeal joints—by the age of 65.[28] In contrast, compound heterozygotes with *C282Y/H63D* mutations exhibit higher serum ferritin and transferrin saturation levels compared with normal controls, but are at very low risk of clinical HHC.[29]

Other genes may play a role in modifying the phenotypic expression of iron overload. The presence of the gene *CYBRD1*, which encodes duodenal reductase DCYTB, has been shown to be associated with lower serum ferritin levels in C282Y homozygotes.[30] Furthermore, mutations of other iron-related genes, such as hepcidin, hemojuvelin, haptoglobin, and bone morphogenetic protein, may influence disease manifestations.[31-35] In addition, profibrotic genes (e.g., TGF) may accelerate the onset of cirrhosis in susceptible individuals.[36]

Why HHC disease penetrance is more evident in C282Y homozygote males than females may be explained by recurrent menstrual blood loss and consequent slower accumulation of iron stores in women. However, genetically determined sex differences in ferritin levels may occur, as distinct HLA A*03B*07 and A*03B*14 haplotypes have been reported in men and women with clinical evidence of HHC.[37]

Environmental factors, including diet, smoking, alcohol intake, and comorbid diseases, also influence clinical expression of HHC. The metabolic syndrome is associated with insulin resistance–associated iron overload, which, in the presence of HHC, may have a synergistic effect on liver damage.[14] Concurrent liver disease, due to hepatitis or steatosis, may exacerbate the process of fibrogenesis.[38] Excess alcohol, meat consumption, and high citrus fruit intake also contribute to increased iron loading. However, ingestion of noncitrus fruits may have a protective effect.[39]

PATHOGENESIS

Hepcidin is a key regulatory peptide in the pathogenesis of HHC. Produced by the liver, it acts by binding to ferroportin on enterocytes and macrophages, thereby restricting dietary iron absorption from the gut and inhibiting release of iron recycled by macrophages from aging red cells.[12,15] In HHC, inadequate hepcidin synthesis leads to increased intestinal iron absorption and the subsequent deposition of iron in tissues. Absence of hepcidin results in early, severe iron loading, and overexpression of this protein can significantly improve iron deposition in a mouse model of HHC.[12,40-42]

Chronic iron overload is thought to cause tissue damage via several mechanisms, including weakening of lysosomal membranes and consequent discharge of enzymes into the cytoplasm. Increased free radical formation contributes to lipid peroxidation of cell membranes. The extent and duration of iron deposition correlate with the development of fibrosis, and it is thought that substantial hepatocyte and Kupffer cell iron accumulation precedes organ damage.[14] In HHC, iron first accumulates in parenchymal cells, with reticuloendothelial (RE) involvement a late feature, in contrast to transfusional iron overload, in which RE cells are primarily targeted. Values of serum ferritin exceeding 1000 µg/L are associated with significantly increased risks of liver fibrosis and cirrhosis.[7,43]

CLINICAL FEATURES

Extra-articular Manifestations

HHC is more common in men than in women and typically manifests in middle-aged adults as iron stores gradually accumulate, often reaching 20 to 30 g. Organ involvement varies and is unpredictable, although the liver, as the major site of iron storage, is typically affected. Commonly, abnormalities of the liver enzymes, checked as part of a routine health screen, are the initial indication of disease. The degree of iron overload has a direct impact on the life expectancy of the affected individual. Without an early diagnosis, progressive fibrosis leading to cirrhosis may occur.[44,45] The risk of hepatocellular carcinoma is greatly increased in patients with established cirrhosis.[46]

Glucose intolerance tends to be a late finding in HHC and is due to progressive iron accumulation in pancreatic beta cells causing low C-peptide and insulin levels. Alpha cell function is usually preserved, however, and serum glucagon levels are normal or increased.[47] The risk of diabetes mellitus also is higher in C282Y heterozygotes with no clinical evidence of HHC compared with controls.[48]

Iron deposition in the heart can result in conduction system abnormalities and heart failure. Several large population studies of HHC and atherosclerosis have failed to find a link. However, elevated ferritin levels, particularly in the setting of nonalcoholic fatty liver disease, may be associated with vascular damage via hepcidin upregulation.[49-51]

Pituitary involvement in HHC is due to iron deposition, resulting in reduced serum levels of secreted hormones from this gland. Low levels of gonadotropic hormone cause loss of libido and erectile dysfunction.[44,52] Hypothyroidism in HHC is thought to be due to a direct toxic effect of iron on thyroid cells and is associated with low thyroxine and elevated thyroid-stimulating hormone.[53] Such endocrine abnormalities may contribute to the development of osteoporosis in these individuals.

Skin discoloration occurs as a result of extra melanin and iron in the epidermis. It is a late finding, and the development of "bronze diabetes" represents the end stage of years of iron accumulation in the tissues.

Patients with HHC have increased susceptibility to certain infections. High serum iron concentrations may increase bacterial virulence, whereas excess iron in macrophages is thought to reduce phagocytosis.[54] Particular caution is advised with uncooked seafood because of the risk of septicemia from *Vibrio vulnificus*. In addition, *Yersinia enterocolitica*, *Listeria monocytogenes*, *Salmonella enteritidis* serotype *typhimurium*, *Klebsiella pneumoniae*, *Escherichia coli*,

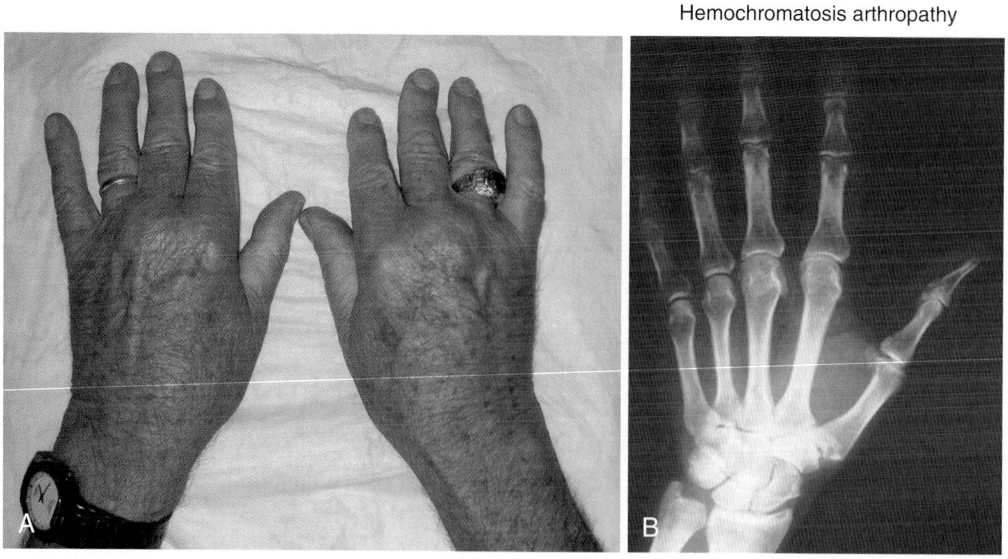

Hemochromatosis arthropathy

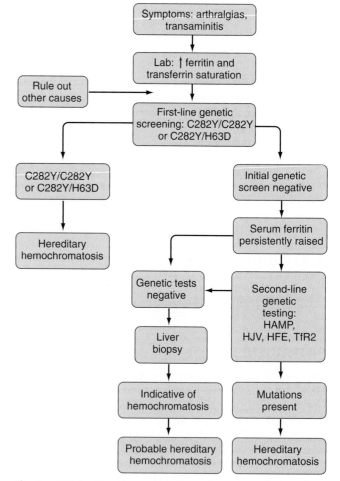

Figure 118-1 **A** and **B,** Arthritis of the second and third metacarpophalangeal joints, characteristic of hereditary hemochromatosis.

Rhizopus arrhizus, and *Mucor* species all have been reported to cause severe illness in patients with iron overload.[8]

Apart from the increased risk of malignant hepatoma in patients with established cirrhosis is an independent association of nonhepatic cancers, particularly breast and colorectal tumors, in HFE C282Y homozygotes.[55] H63D homozygosity confers a threefold increased risk of colorectal cancer in carriers of the *MMR* gene mutation.[56] Iron is potentially carcinogenic via several mechanisms, including its immunosuppressive properties and its role as an essential cofactor for tumor cell growth and in catalyzing the formation of hydroxyl radicals.[55] Furthermore, cancer risk is lower with reduced iron stores.[57]

Articular Features

Arthralgia/arthritis is a common presentation in HHC, affecting 50% to 80% of patients and significantly interfering with quality of life.[58-63] Although it tends to be a late feature, joint pain may nevertheless be the presenting symptom of HHC, alerting a diligent physician to the presence of an underlying metabolic disorder. Articular involvement may be widespread, but changes to the second and third metacarpophalangeal joints are most characteristic[64] (Figures 118-1 and 118-2). Arthritis may be present in the proximal interphalangeal joints, wrists, shoulders, hips, knees, and ankles.[63] Patients notice pain and stiffness of the involved joints, but evidence of synovitis is usually absent. Hip damage develops in approximately 25% of individuals with HHC, and after hip arthroplasty, the risk of aseptic loosening of the prosthesis is increased.[65,66] The differential diagnosis of HHC-related arthropathy includes severe osteoarthritis, rheumatoid arthritis, other forms of inflammatory arthritis, and crystal arthritis. Rheumatoid factor is typically negative, however, and radiographs, in established cases, show distinctive findings, such as joint space narrowing of the second and third metacarpophalangeal joints, hook-like osteophytes on the radial aspect of the metacarpal heads, and chondrocalcinosis, particularly of the triangular

Symptoms: arthralgias, transaminitis

Lab: ↑ ferritin and transferrin saturation

Rule out other causes

First-line genetic screening: C282Y/C282Y or C282Y/H63D

C282Y/C282Y or C282Y/H63D

Initial genetic screen negative

Hereditary hemochromatosis

Serum ferritin persistently raised

Genetic tests negative

Second-line genetic testing: HAMP, HJV, HFE, TfR2

Liver biopsy

Indicative of hemochromatosis

Mutations present

Probable hereditary hemochromatosis

Hereditary hemochromatosis

Figure 118-2 Algorithm for the diagnosis of hereditary hemochromatosis.

fibrocartilage adjacent to the ulnar styloid. HHC-related arthritis is more common in male C282Y homozygotes than in other genotypes.[7]

The pathogenetic mechanisms underlying HHC-related arthritis are unknown, and the prevalence of joint pain in this condition has not been found to correlate with body iron stores. Toxic effects from local iron deposition, acceleration of cartilage defects, and immunologic mechanisms have been implicated.[60,61,67] Under light microscopy, the involved synovium demonstrates iron deposits, particularly in the lining cells, but inflammatory cell infiltration is not typical.[68-70] Neutrophil infiltration of the synovial sublining layer has been described.[71] Apatite and calcium pyrophosphate dihydrate crystals may be observed, but why they are preferentially expressed in HHC is unknown. In association with the increased incidence of calcium pyrophosphate dihydrate deposition disease in HHC, a putative role for a parathyroid hormone fragment (PTH 44-68) has been suggested.[72]

DIFFERENTIAL DIAGNOSIS

Because no physiologic mechanism is in place to increase iron excretion, the inevitable result of increased iron entry into the body is iron overload. Excess iron may accumulate because of high intake of iron by oral or parenteral means. A full history of medication use, including over-the-counter iron tablets, and a review of any blood transfusions should be elicited. Ineffective erythropoiesis in conditions such as the thalassemias or sideroblastic anemia also results in the buildup of iron stores. Porphyria cutanea tarda is associated with hyperferritinemia, high transferrin saturation levels, and an increased incidence of *HFE* mutations.[73] However, the clinical findings, particularly dermatologic, distinguish this disease from HHC. Elevated ferritin levels may result from severe inflammation. Interleukin-6 is a potent stimulator of hepcidin via the STAT3 pathway, resulting in reduced iron absorption and elevation of tissue and serum ferritin levels.[74] However, these changes are accompanied by low transferrin saturation. Chronic liver disease resulting from hepatitis, alcohol excess, or fatty infiltration is associated with hyperferritinemia and normal or elevated transferrin saturation values. Alcohol, independent of liver damage, induces ferritin synthesis.[46,75]

Genetic factors not related to HHC have been linked to other iron overload syndromes. The African iron overload syndrome occurs in a few Africans who drink locally brewed beer containing extremely high levels of iron (80 mg/L). Not all Africans who drink this beer develop hemochromatosis, leading to suggestions that additional genetic factors contribute to the development of disease. It is thought that a polymorphism of the ferroportin 1 gene is involved.[76] Separately, a familial association has been noted with a syndrome of very high ferritin levels (>1000 ng/mL) and bilateral congenital cataracts. This hereditary hyperferritinemia-cataract syndrome involves several mutations in the iron responsive element of L-ferritin and is inherited in an autosomal dominant fashion. The cataracts are thought to be due to excessive ferritin production within the lens fibers.[77]

INVESTIGATIONS

A high index of suspicion is helpful when a patient presents with joint pain and abnormal liver enzymes. Although the differential diagnosis is wide, the presence of elevated ferritin and transferrin saturation levels (serum iron × 100/ total iron-binding capacity) strongly points to the answer. Serum iron should be measured with the patient fasting because concentrations may be increased after a meal.[44] High ferritin levels also may be caused by systemic inflammation or malignancy, but these conditions tend to be associated with reduced transferrin saturation. Other causes of elevated transferrin saturation include high serum iron secondary to hepatic cytolysis or low transferrin levels secondary to liver failure, and these possibilities should be excluded. If ferritin measures greater than 200 µg/L, and transferrin saturation is greater than 45%, genetic screening is recommended.[14,19,27] The finding of homozygosity for the C282Y mutation or compound heterozygosity for C282Y/H63D confirms the diagnosis.

Liver biopsy may be considered for prognostic purposes in established cases.[6,18,44,78] HHC can be distinguished histologically from alcoholic cirrhosis by the preferential distribution of iron in the hepatocytes in the former and in the Kupffer cells in the latter.[44] Magnetic resonance imaging of the abdomen also can be used to determine iron overload in the internal organs. Gradient T2-weighted sequences show decreased signal intensity and correlate highly with liver iron concentrations. This imaging method also can identify other locations of iron deposition (e.g., in the spleen, pancreas, lymph nodes, and heart).[44,79] Because HHC is a systemic condition, other investigations should include a search for diabetes, thyroid disease, hypogonadism, osteoporosis, and cardiomyopathy. Disease mimickers, such as porphyria cutanea tarda, ineffective erythropoiesis, and chronic alcohol excess, should be excluded.

SCREENING

Greater disease awareness and the availability of genetic screening have meant that HHC is increasingly likely to be diagnosed before the classic triad of cirrhosis, diabetes, and skin hyperpigmentation develops. Late presentation with evidence of end-organ damage does occur, however, particularly in patients with additional risk factors for iron overload or liver disease.

HHC is an attractive clinical target for population screening because of its high prevalence, potential disease severity, availability of effective treatment, and impact of early diagnosis on the morbidity and mortality of affected individuals. Certain groups are more at risk than others, however, and the disease prevalence is higher in white than in nonwhite individuals.[6,7,27,80,81] Biochemical measures, such as serum ferritin, may serve as a cost-effective method of screening in whites during routine health checks and in individuals who complain of nonspecific symptoms, such as excessive fatigue and arthralgias. Elevation of serum ferritin in the absence of other causes should prompt measurement of transferrin saturation. Levels greater than 45% in men and greater than 35% in premenopausal women, without adequate explanation, warrant further investigation.

Genetic testing should be reserved for patients with suggestive biochemical abnormalities or a family history of HHC. Routine population screening for *C282Y* or *H63D* mutations is not recommended because of the variable clinical penetrance of these genes and the potential negative consequences of a positive result in asymptomatic patients, such as financial, legal, insurance, and psychological implications.[19] When a case of HHC is diagnosed, however, and two gene mutations are identified (i.e., *C282Y/C282Y* or *C282Y/H63D*), siblings also should be tested for these mutations. *H63D/H63D* homozygotes are not thought to be at risk of clinical disease. Children of a patient with HHC or of an individual with *C282Y/H63D* heterozygosity are at risk only if the other parent also carries hemochromatosis gene mutations.

For individuals in whom genetic testing has identified a risk of HHC, but with no clinical evidence of disease, yearly biochemical screening should be done, with measures of ferritin, transferrin saturation, and liver enzymes. Such monitoring allows early detection of organ compromise and timely initiation of treatment (see Figure 118-2).

MANAGEMENT

Removing excess iron before the development of organ damage significantly abrogates the adverse consequences of HHC. Target groups for treatment include asymptomatic individuals with biochemical evidence of high iron stores, in addition to patients with overt clinical disease. Some features of HHC improve with bloodletting, including constitutional symptoms, diabetes, and liver enzyme abnormalities. Phlebotomy has no effect, however, on arthritis, hypogonadism, and liver fibrosis.[18] When cirrhosis is established, the risk of hepatocellular carcinoma is greatly increased, even after a satisfactory reduction in iron stores.[18,46]

Phlebotomy is an effective method of removing excess iron. The use of chelating agents is rarely necessary. Every 500 mL of whole blood contains 200 to 250 mg of iron, depending on the hematocrit. Phlebotomy can be arranged once or twice weekly, as tolerated by the patient, aiming for serum ferritin of 50 ng/mL. It can take longer than 1 year for iron stores to normalize with this regimen. Iron deficiency anemia should always be avoided, and when ferritin levels reach their target, the frequency of bloodletting may be reduced. Transferrin saturation levels are not an accurate measure of therapeutic efficacy because they are relatively resistant to changes in iron stores in C282Y homozygotes.[14] Phlebotomy continues for life, and the maintenance schedule depends on the patient's ability to sustain the ferritin level in the low-normal range. It is important to avoid very low ferritin levels because this situation may increase iron absorption via further reduction in hepcidin levels or increased erythropoiesis in C282Y homozygotes.[14] Blood removal in HHC is not without risks. In particular, life-threatening cardiac arrhythmias may develop during rapid mobilization of iron stores. Vitamin C supplementation may precipitate such problems by facilitating iron release and increasing pro-oxidant and free radical activity.[18] Patients undergoing phlebotomy for HHC should not take extra vitamin C, but can continue to eat fresh produce containing this vitamin.

Other dietary recommendations include reduction or avoidance of food containing high doses of iron, such as red meat and internal organs. Uncooked shellfish is a particular hazard because of the risk of contamination with *V. vulnificus*. Some alcoholic drinks contain iron, and all are potentially hepatotoxic. Alcohol should be consumed only occasionally because it seems to have a synergistic effect in the presence of iron overload on the development of cirrhosis and hepatocellular carcinoma.[82,83] Maintenance of normal body weight is important to avoid the hepatic damage associated with steatosis.[38]

Just as the pathogenesis of joint pain in HHC is unclear, treatment of arthritis in this condition is unsatisfactory, and joint symptoms may progress despite effective phlebotomy. Nonsteroidal anti-inflammatory drugs, colchicine, and intra-articular corticosteroids may be helpful in some cases. Osteoporosis is a potential disease complication, particularly in the setting of hypogonadism or reduced thyroid function. Hormone replacement, if indicated, should be instituted, although some patients may require additional treatment with calcium and bisphosphonates. Screening for malignancy, particularly for carcinoma of the breast and colon, should be considered in the holistic care of patients with HHC.

OUTCOME

The earlier HHC is diagnosed, the better the prognosis, because morbidity and mortality are directly related to the extent of iron overload and consequent organ damage. The development of cirrhosis is a serious indicator of reduced longevity. For patients with HHC-related hepatic failure who undergo liver transplantation, survival rates are lower compared with individuals who receive liver transplants for other reasons. Postoperative death in these circumstances is typically due to cardiac complications or infection.[18,84]

In the absence of cirrhosis or diabetes, patients with HHC have a normal life expectancy. Given the importance of timely recognition of this common metabolic problem, a vigilant physician can make an enormous difference in the lives of patients who present with early symptoms of this disease. In this context, the rheumatologist has a particularly relevant role in keeping a high index of suspicion for the diagnosis of HHC in patients with atypical osteoarthritis or chondrocalcinosis.

Future Directions

Cost-effective screening focused on those at greatest risk of clinical disease, in association with a high level of diagnostic suspicion in patients with relevant symptoms and signs, should reduce the number of patients presenting with irreversible organ damage from HHC. In addition, greater understanding of the genetic and environmental modifiers of clinical disease expression may help to delay or mitigate the consequences of iron overload in susceptible individuals. How comorbid disease influences the onset and extent of disease is particularly relevant in the context of the growing numbers of patients with obesity, metabolic syndrome, and hepatic steatosis. Although phlebotomy has been the mainstay of treatment for many years, exact targets for iron stores and ferritin levels warrant further investigation. Other commonly used medications, such as proton pump inhibitors, which inhibit absorption of nonheme iron, or calcium channel blockers, which may have a role in reducing iron overload via divalent metal transporter-1, have a potentially therapeutic benefit in HHC.[85,86] Currently at the experimental stage is the concept of hepcidin peptides or hepcidin agonists, aimed at correcting the physiologic deficit linked to increased iron absorption and deposition.[12]

References

1. von Recklinghausen FD: Uber Haemochromatose: Tageblatt Versammlung Dtsche Naturforscher, *Artzte Heidelberg* 62:324–325, 1889.
2. Sheldon JH: *Haemochromatosis*, London, 1935, Oxford University Press.
3. Finch SC, Finch CA: Idiopathic hemochromatosis, an iron storage disease, *Medicine (Baltimore)* 34:381–430, 1955.
4. Simon M, Pawlotsky Y, Bourel M, et al: Hémochromatose idiopathique maladie associée à l'antigene tissulaire HLA-3, *Nouv Presse Med* 4:1432, 1975.
5. Feder JN, Gnirke A, Thomas W, et al: A novel MHC class 1-like gene is mutated in patients with hereditary hemochromatosis, *Nat Genet* 13:399–408, 1996.
6. Olynyk JK, Cullen DJ, Sina Aquilia BA, et al: A population based study of the clinical expression of the hemochromatosis gene, *N Engl J Med* 341:718–724, 1999.
7. Gan EK, Ayonrinde OT, Trinder D, et al: Phenotypic expression of hereditary hemochromatosis: what have we learned from population studies? *Curr Gastroenterol Rep* 12:7–12, 2010.
8. Andrews NC: Disorders of iron metabolism, *N Engl J Med* 341:1986–1995, 1999.
9. Finch CA, Huebers H: Perspectives in iron metabolism, *N Engl J Med* 306:1520–1528, 1982.
10. Hallberg L, Brune M, Rossander L: The role of vitamin C in iron absorption, *Int J Vitam Nutr Res Suppl* 30:103–108, 1989.
11. Hallberg L, Rossander L, Skanberg AB: Phytates and the inhibitory effect of bran on iron absorption in man, *Am J Clin Nutr* 45:988–996, 1987.
12. Pietrangelo A: Hepcidin in human iron disorders: therapeutic implications, *J Hepatol* 54:173–181, 2011.
13. Nicolas G, Chauvet C, Viatte L, et al: The gene encoding the iron regulatory peptide hepcidin is regulated by anemia, hypoxia and inflammation, *J Clin Invest* 110:1037–1044, 2002.
14. Janssen MC, Swinkels DW: Hereditary hemochromatosis, *Best Pract Res Clin Gastroenterol* 23:171–183, 2009.
15. Roy CN: Anemia of inflammation, *Hematology Am Soc Hematol Educ Program* 2010:276–280, 2010.
16. Fleming RE, Bacon BR: Orchestration of iron homeostasis, *N Engl J Med* 352:1741–1744, 2005.
17. Dix DJ, Lin PN, Kimata Y, et al: The iron regulatory region of ferritin mRNA is also a positive control element for iron-dependent translation, *Biochemistry* 31:2818–2822, 1992.
18. Tavill AS: Diagnosis and management of hemochromatosis, *Hepatology* 33:1321–1328, 2001.
19. Pietrangelo A: Hereditary hemochromatosis—a new look at an old disease, *N Engl J Med* 350:2383–2397, 2004.
20. Cazzola M, Cerani P, Rovati A, et al: Juvenile genetic hemochromatosis is clinically and genetically distinct from the classical HLA-related disorder, *Blood* 92:2979–2981, 1998.
21. Lanzara C, Roetto A, Daraio F, et al: Spectrum of hemojuvelin gene mutations in 1q-linked juvenile hemochromatosis, *Blood* 103:4317–4321, 2004.
22. Roetto A, Totaro A, Piperno A, et al: New mutations inactivating transferrin receptor 2 in hemochromatosis type 3, *Blood* 97:2555–2560, 2001.
23. Girelli D, Bozzini C, Roetto A, et al: Clinical and pathologic findings in hemochromatosis type 3 due to a novel mutation in transferrin receptor 2 gene, *Gastroenterology* 122:1295–1302, 2002.
24. Njajou OT, Vaessen N, Joosse M, et al: A mutation in *SLC11A3* is associated with autosomal dominant hemochromatosis, *Nat Genet* 28:213–214, 2001.
25. Montosi G, Donovan A, Totaro A, et al: Autosomal dominant hemochromatosis is associated with a mutation in the ferroportin (*SLC11A3*) gene, *J Clin Invest* 108:619–623, 2001.
26. Cremonesi L, Forni GL, Soriani N, et al: Genetic and clinical heterogeneity of ferroportin disease, *Br J Haematol* 131:663–670, 2005.
27. Adams PC, Reboussin DM, Barton JC, et al: Hemochromatosis and iron-overload screening in a racially diverse population, *N Engl J Med* 352:1769–1778, 2005.
28. Allen KJ, Gurrin LC, Constantine CC, et al: Iron-overload-related disease in HFE hereditary hemochromatosis, *N Engl J Med* 358:221–230, 2008.
29. Gurrin LC, Bertalli NA, Dalton GW, et al: HFE C282Y/H63D compound heterozygotes are at low risk of hemochromatosis-related morbidity, *Hepatology* 50:94–101, 2009.
30. Constantine CC, Anderson GJ, Vulpe CD, et al: A novel association between a SNP in CYBRD1 and serum ferritin levels in a cohort study of HFE hereditary haemochromatosis, *Br J Haematol* 147:140–149, 2009.
31. Rochette J, Le Gac G, Lassoued K, et al: Factors influencing disease phenotype and penetrance in HFE haemochromatosis, *Hum Genet* 128:233–248, 2010.
32. Jacolot S, Le Gac G, Scotet V, et al: HAMP as a modifier gene that increases the phenotypic expression of the HFE pC282Y homozygous genotype, *Blood* 103:2835–2840, 2004.
33. Le Gac G, Scotet V, Ka C, et al: The recently identified type 2A juvenile haemochromatosis gene (HJV), a second candidate modifier of the C282Y homozygous phenotype, *Hum Mol Genet* 13:1913–1918, 2004.
34. Milet J, Dehais V, Bourgain C, et al: Common variants in the BMP2, BMP4, and HJV genes of the hepcidin regulation pathway modulate HFE hemochromatosis penetrance, *Am J Hum Genet* 81:799–807, 2007.
35. Van Vlierberghe H, Langlois M, Delanghe J, et al: Haptoglobin phenotype 2-2 overrepresentation in Cys282Tyr hemochromatotic patients, *J Hepatol* 35:707–711, 2001.
36. Osterreicher CH, Datz C, Stickel F, et al: TGF-beta1 codon 25 gene polymorphism is associated with cirrhosis in patients with hereditary hemochromatosis, *Cytokine* 31:142–148, 2005.
37. Barton JC, Wiener HW, Acton RT, et al: HLA haplotype A*03-B*07 in hemochromatosis probands with HFE C282Y homozygosity: frequency disparity in men and women and lack of association with severity of iron overload, *Blood Cells Mol Dis* 34:38–47, 2005.
38. Powell EE, Ali A, Clouston AD, et al: Steatosis is a cofactor in liver injury in hemochromatosis, *Gastroenterology* 129:1937–1943, 2005.
39. Milward EA, Baines SK, Knuiman MW, et al: Noncitrus fruits as novel dietary environmental modifiers of iron stores in people with or without *HFE* gene mutations, *Mayo Clin Proc* 83:543–549, 2008.
40. Ludwiczek S, Theurl I, Bahram S, et al: Regulatory networks for the control of body iron homeostasis and their dysregulation in HFE mediated hemochromatosis, *J Cell Physiol* 204:489–499, 2005.
41. Nicolas G, Viatte L, Lou DQ, et al: Constitutive hepcidin expression prevents iron overload in a mouse model of hemochromatosis, *Nat Genet* 34:97–101, 2003.
42. Bridle KR, Frazer DM, Wilkins SJ, et al: Disrupted hepcidin regulation in HFE-associated haemochromatosis and the liver as a regulator of body iron homeostasis, *Lancet* 361:669–673, 2003.
43. Guyader D, Jacquelinet C, Moirand R, et al: Noninvasive prediction of fibrosis in C282Y homozygous hemochromatosis, *Gastroenterology* 115:929–936, 1998.
44. Chung RT, Misdraji J, Sahani DV: Case 33-2006. A 43-year-old man with diabetes, hypogonadism, cirrhosis, arthralgias and fatigue, *N Engl J Med* 355:1812–1819, 2006.
45. Adams PC, Deugnier Y, Moirand R, et al: The relationship between iron overload, clinical symptoms and age in 410 patients with genetic hemochromatosis, *Hepatology* 25:162–166, 1997.
46. Elmberg M, Hultcrantz R, Ekbom A, et al: Cancer risk in patients with hereditary hemochromatosis and in their first-degree relatives, *Gastroenterology* 125:1733–1741, 2003.
47. Yaouanq JM: Diabetes and hemochromatosis: current concepts, management and prevention, *Diabetes Metab* 21:319–329, 1995.

48. Salonen JT, Tuomainen TP, Kontula K: Role of C282Y mutation in haemochromatosis gene in the development of type 2 diabetes in healthy men, *BMJ* 320:1706–1707, 2000.

49. Ellervik C, Tybjaerg-Hansen A, Grande P, et al: Hereditary hemochromatosis and risk of ischemic heart disease, *Circulation* 112:185–193, 2005.

50. Engberink MF, Povel CM, Durga J, et al: Hemochromatosis (HFE) genotype and atherosclerosis: increased susceptibility to iron-induced vascular damage in C282Y carriers? *Atherosclerosis* 211:520–525, 2010.

51. Valenti L, Swinkels DW, Burdick L, et al: Serum ferritin levels are associated with vascular damage in patients with non-alcoholic fatty liver disease, *Nutr Metab Cardiovasc Dis* 21:568–575, 2011.

52. Cundy T, Butler J, Bomford A, et al: Reversibility of hypogonadotropic hypogonadism associated with genetic haemochromatosis, *Clin Endocrinol* 38:617–620, 1993.

53. Edwards CQ, Kelly TM, Ellwein G, et al: Thyroid disease in hemochromatosis, *Arch Intern Med* 143:1890–1893, 1983.

54. van Asbeck BS, Verbrugh HA, van Oost VA, et al: *Listeria monocytogenes* meningitis and decreased phagocytosis associated with iron overload, *BMJ* 284:542–544, 1982.

55. Osborne NJ, Gurrin LC, Allen KJ, et al: HFE C282Y homozygotes are at increased risk of breast and colorectal cancer, *Hepatology* 51:1311–1318, 2010.

56. Shi Z, Johnstone D, Talseth-Palmer BA, et al: Haemochromatosis HFE gene polymorphisms as potential modifiers of hereditary nonpolyposis colorectal cancer risk and onset age, *Int J Cancer* 125:78–83, 2009.

57. Zacharski LR, Chow BK, Howes PS, et al: Decreased cancer risk after iron reduction in patients with peripheral arterial disease: results from a randomized trial, *J Natl Cancer Inst* 100:996–1002, 2008.

58. Ross JM, Kowalchuk RM, Shaulinsky J, et al: Association of heterozygous hemochromatosis C282Y gene mutation with hand osteoarthritis, *J Rheumatol* 30:121–125, 2003.

59. von Kempis J: Arthropathy in hereditary hemochromatosis, *Curr Opin Rheumatol* 13:80–83, 2001.

60. Schumacher HR: Haemochromatosis, *Baillieres Best Pract Res Clin Rheumatol* 14:277–284, 2000.

61. Ines LS, da Silva JA, Malcata AB, et al: Arthropathy of genetic hemochromatosis: a major and distinctive manifestation of disease, *Clin Exp Rheumatol* 19:98–102, 2001.

62. Adams PC, Speechley M: The effect of arthritis on the quality of life in hereditary hemochromatosis, *J Rheumatol* 23:707–710, 1996.

63. Sahinbegovic E, Dallos T, Aigner E, et al: Musculoskeletal disease burden of hereditary hemochromatosis, *Arthritis Rheum* 62:3792–3798, 2010.

64. Cunnane G, O'Duffy JD: The iron salute sign of haemochromatosis, *Arthritis Rheum* 38:558, 1995.

65. Axford JS, Bomford A, Revell P, et al: Hip arthropathy in genetic hemochromatosis: radiographic and histologic features, *Arthritis Rheum* 34:357–361, 1991.

66. Lunn JV, Gallagher PM, Hegarty S, et al: The role of hereditary hemochromatosis in aseptic loosening following primary total hip arthroplasty, *J Orthop Res* 23:542–548, 2005.

67. Arosa FA, Oliveira L, Porto G, et al: Anomalies of the CD8+ T cell pool in haemochromatosis, *Clin Exp Immunol* 107:548–554, 1997.

68. Schumacher HR: Ultrastructural characteristics of the synovial membrane in idiopathic hemochromatosis, *Ann Rheum Dis* 31:465–473, 1972.

69. Walker RJ, Dymock IW, Ansell ID, et al: Synovial biopsy in hemochromatosis arthropathy, *Ann Rheum Dis* 31:98–102, 1972.

70. Bomers MK, Terpstra V: Arthritis caused by hereditary hemochromatosis, *Arthritis Rheum* 62:3791, 2010.

71. Heiland GR, Aigner E, Dallos T, et al: Synovial immunopathology in haemochromatosis arthropathy, *Ann Rheum Dis* 69:1214–1219, 2010.

72. Pawlotsky Y, Le Dantec P, Moirand R, et al: Elevated parathyroid hormone 44-68 and osteoarticular changes in patients with genetic hemochromatosis, *Arthritis Rheum* 42:799–806, 1999.

73. Ellervik C, Birgens H, Tybjaerg-Hansen A, et al: Hemochromatosis genotypes and risk of 31 disease endpoints: meta-analyses including 66,000 cases and 226,000 controls, *Hepatology* 46:1071–1080, 2007.

74. Wrighting DM, Andrews NC: Interleukin-6 induces hepcidin expression through STAT3, *Blood* 108:3204–3209, 2006.

75. Lieb M, Palm U, Hock B, et al: Effects of alcohol consumption on iron metabolism, *Am J Drug Alcohol Abuse* 37:68–73, 2011.

76. Gordeuk VR, Caleffi A, Corradini E, et al: Iron overload in Africans and African-Americans and a common mutation in the *SLC40A1* (ferroportin 1) gene, *Blood Cells Mol Dis* 31:299–304, 2003.

77. Cazzola M: Role of ferritin and ferroportin genes in unexplained hyperferritinaemia, *Best Pract Res Clin Haematol* 18:251–263, 2005.

78. Tavill AS, Adams PC: A diagnostic approach to hemochromatosis, *Can J Gastroenterol* 20:535–540, 2006.

79. Beddy P, McCann J, Ahern M, et al: MRI assessment of changes in liver iron deposition post-venesection, *Eur J Radiol* 80:204–207, 2011.

80. Tavill AS: Clinical implications of the hemochromatosis gene, *N Engl J Med* 341:755–757, 1999.

81. Niederau C, Fischer R, Purschel A, et al: Long term survival in patients with hereditary hemochromatosis, *Gastroenterology* 110:1107–1119, 1996.

82. Stal P, Olsson J, Svoboda P, et al: Studies on genotoxic effects of iron overload and alcohol in an animal model of hepatocarcinogenesis, *J Hepatol* 27:562–571, 1997.

83. Britton RS, Bacon BR: Hereditary hemochromatosis and alcohol: a fibrogenic cocktail, *Gastroenterology* 122:563–565, 2002.

84. Kowdley KV, Brandhagen DJ, Gish RG, et al: Survival after liver transplantation in patients with hepatic iron overload: the National Hemochromatosis Transplant Registry, *Gastroenterology* 129:494–503, 2005.

85. Hutchinson C, Geissler CA, Powell JJ, et al: Proton pump inhibitors suppress absorption of dietary non-haem iron in hereditary hemochromatosis, *Gut* 56:1291–1295, 2007.

86. Ludwiczek S, Theurl I, Muckenthaler MU, et al: Ca²⁺ channel blockers reverse iron overload by a new mechanism via divalent metal transporter-1, *Nat Med* 13:448–454, 2007.

The references for this chapter can also be found on www.expertconsult.com.

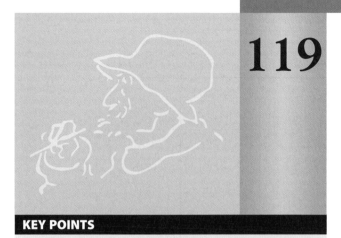

119

Hemophilic Arthropathy

KATHERINE S. UPCHURCH •
DOREEN B. BRETTLER

KEY POINTS

Severe hemophilia, if not aggressively treated, is often complicated by recurrent hemarthrosis.

Recurrent hemarthrosis causes chronic arthropathy with overlapping clinical and pathologic features of osteoarthritis and rheumatoid arthritis.

Septic arthritis should be considered in hemophilic patients with risk factors (previous arthrocentesis, intravenous drug use, human immunodeficiency virus infection) and acute monoarticular arthritis.

Soft tissue and muscle hemorrhage are frequent complications of hemophilia.

With continuous factor infusion, surgical procedures, including total joint replacements, can be done safely in hemophilic patients.

The best treatment for hemophilic arthropathy is prevention of recurrent hemarthrosis through regular prophylactic factor replacement.

Although spontaneous joint hemorrhage has been described in a variety of inherited disorders of coagulation[1-3] and in the setting of anticoagulation therapy,[4] it occurs most frequently in hemophilia. Bleeding into the joints is the complication of hemophilia that most often requires therapeutic intervention and, when it is recurrent, can lead to chronic, deforming arthritis that is independent of bleeding episodes.

Hemophilia refers to a group of inherited diseases characterized by functional deficiency of a specific clotting factor. The most common are hemophilia A (classic hemophilia) and hemophilia B (Christmas disease); the deficient factors are factor VIII (hemophilia A) and factor IX (hemophilia B). The incidence and severity of hemorrhagic complications of hemophilia are directly related to the severity of the underlying coagulation defect.

Although the intrinsic pathway of coagulation is severely impaired in hemophilia, the extrinsic tissue–dependent pathway remains intact and is probably the major hemostatic regulatory system. Normal synovial tissue and cultures of synovial fibroblasts have been found to be deficient in tissue factor,[5] which suggests that in synovium-lined joints, hemophiliacs have functional inactivity of intrinsic and extrinsic coagulation pathways. This observation may explain the marked propensity toward hemorrhage in joints compared with other tissue sites in these patients.

CLINICAL FEATURES

The spectrum of articular disease in hemophilic patients has been the subject of numerous comprehensive reviews[6-10] and includes acute hemarthrosis, subacute or chronic arthritis, and end-stage hemophilic arthropathy. The usual distribution of joint involvement is shown in Figure 119-1. Involvement of the small joints of the hands and feet also may occur, although infrequently.

Acute Hemarthrosis

Nearly all patients with severe hemophilia A or B (<1% activity of the deficient factor) and half of patients with moderate disease activity experience hemarthrosis. Acute hemarthroses generally first occur when a child begins to walk, and they continue, usually cyclically, into adulthood, when the frequency diminishes. Patients frequently have premonitory symptoms, such as stiffness or warmth in the affected joint, followed by intense pain, which may be due in part to rapid joint capsule distention.

Pain is accompanied by objective clinical findings of warmth, a tense effusion, tenderness, limitation of motion, and a joint that is often held in a flexed position. Joint pain responds rapidly to replacement of the deficient clotting factor. If hemostasis is achieved early after onset of hemarthrosis, full joint function may be regained within 12 to 24 hours. If the hemorrhage is more advanced, however, blood is resorbed slowly over 5 to 7 days, and full joint function is regained within 10 to 14 days.

Subacute or Chronic Arthritis

Recurrent hemarthroses, particularly in patients with severe factor deficiency, may lead to a self-perpetuating condition in which joint abnormalities persist in intervals between bleeding episodes. The involved joint is chronically swollen, although painless and only slightly warm. Chronic synovitis, including prominent synovial proliferation with or without effusion, may be present. Mild limitation of motion may be noted, often with a flexion deformity. Factor replacement does not modify these findings.

End-Stage Hemophilic Arthropathy

Long-standing end-stage hemophilic arthropathy has features in common with degenerative joint disease and advanced rheumatoid arthritis. The joint appears enlarged and "knobby," owing to osteophytic bone overgrowth. Synovial thickening and effusion are not prominent, however. Range of motion is severely restricted, and fibrous

Percentage of joints with:

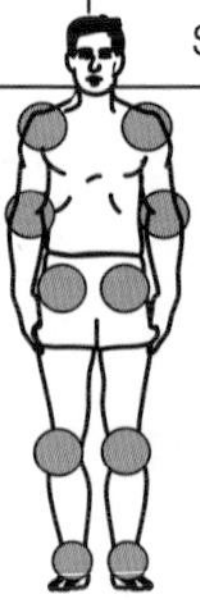

Any hemarthrosis	Many hemarthroses	Chronic pain	Synovitis	Limitation of motion	Any radiologic abnormality
34.5	13.3	13.9	—	16.9	21.6
54.0	38.5	13.8	9.8	27.0	52.6
28.6	8.0	5.4	—	19.8	18.8
63.1	50.9	26.8	11.6	27.0	50.2
60.8	42.8	15.2	2.2	34.2	52.4

Figure 119-1 Distribution of acute hemarthrosis based on a study of 139 patients with hemophilia. Clinical and radiologic features of chronic arthritis in hemophilia. *(Adapted from Steven MM, Yogarojah S, Madhok R, et al: Haemophilic arthritis, QJM 58:181, 1986.)*

ankylosis is common. Subluxation, joint laxity, and malalignment are frequently present. Hemarthroses decrease in frequency, however.

Septic Arthritis

Until the early 1980s, septic arthritis rarely occurred in hemophilic patients. With widespread occurrence of human immunodeficiency virus (HIV) infection as a result of contaminated factor concentrates, the incidence of this complication has increased significantly.[11,12] Septic arthritis is seen more often in adult than in pediatric hemophilic patients and is most commonly monoarticular, usually involving the knee. In contrast to spontaneous hemarthrosis, septic arthritis is significantly associated with a temperature greater than 38° C within 12 hours of presentation and articular pain that does not improve with replacement therapy.[11] Peripheral leukocyte count may not be elevated, particularly in HIV-positive patients.[13] A predisposing factor other than hemophilic arthropathy is often identifiable, including previous arthrocentesis or arthroplasty, intravenous drug use, and an infected indwelling venous access catheter. *Staphylococcus aureus* is the most frequently identified organism even in HIV-infected patients, followed by *Streptococcus pneumoniae*.[13]

Muscle and Soft Tissue Hemorrhage

Bleeding into muscles and soft tissue is common in hemophilic patients and may be more insidious than hemarthrosis because of the lack of premonitory symptoms. Bleeding into the iliopsoas and gastrocnemius muscles and the forearm results in well-described syndromes with which the rheumatologist should be familiar. Iliopsoas hemorrhage produces acute groin pain with marked pain on hip extension and a hip flexion contracture. Rotation is preserved, in contrast to intra-articular hemorrhage. If untreated, the expanding soft tissue mass may compress the femoral nerve, causing signs and symptoms of femoral neuropathy.[6,14] Bleeding into the gastrocnemius muscle can cause an equinus deformity from heel cord contracture.[6] Finally, hemorrhage into closed compartments can cause acute muscle necrosis and nerve compression.[15] Of particular importance is bleeding into the volar compartment of the forearm, which can cause flexion deformities of the wrist and fingers. If a compartment syndrome is suspected, compartment pressures should be measured to confirm the diagnosis.

A large intramuscular hemorrhage uncommonly results in the formation of a simple muscle cyst, which clinically appears to be an encapsulated soft tissue area of swelling overlying muscle. Cyst formation in this setting is confined by the muscular fascial plane and most likely results from inadequate resorption of blood and clot. Subperiosteal or intraosseous hemorrhage, in contrast, may lead to a pseudotumor, a rare skeletal complication of hemophilia. Hemophilic pseudotumors are of two types: the adult type, which occurs proximally, usually in the pelvis or femur; and the childhood type, which occurs distal to the elbows or knees and carries a better prognosis.[16,17]

Conservative early management of muscle cysts and childhood-type pseudotumors is indicated, including immobilization and factor replacement. In adult-type pseudotumors, which usually are refractory to conservative therapy, and in progressive childhood pseudotumors, surgical removal is indicated[16] to prevent serious complications, such as spontaneous rupture, fistula formation, neurologic or vascular entrapment, and fracture of adjacent bone. Aspiration of a pseudotumor or cyst is contraindicated.

DIAGNOSTIC IMAGING

Radiographs

The earliest radiographic changes in hemophilic arthropathy are confined to the soft tissue and reflect acute hemarthrosis. The joint capsule is distended with displacement of fat pads, and an increased hazy density caused by intra-articular blood is noted. Hemarthrosis before epiphyseal plate closure may result in epiphyseal overgrowth and irregularity. Occasionally, premature epiphyseal closure is seen.

With progression of chronic proliferative synovitis, irreversible radiologic changes appear.[18] These changes reflect the inflammatory and degenerative nature of chronic hemophilic arthropathy (Table 119-1 and Figure 119-2A). Certain changes unique to hemophilic arthropathy occur as well (see Table 119-1 and Figure 119-2B). Radiographic findings in hemophilic arthropathy have been recently reviewed.[18a]

Table 119-1 Radiologic Manifestations of Chronic Hemophilic Arthropathy

Characteristic	Also Seen in
Periarticular soft tissue swelling	RA
Periarticular demineralization	RA
Marginal erosions	RA
Subchondral irregularity and cyst formation	RA, OA
Decreased joint space	OA
Osteophyte formation	OA*
Chondrocalcinosis	CPPD
Specific	
Femoral intercondylar notch widening	
Squaring of distal patellar margin (lateral view)	
Proximal radial enlargement (see Figure 119-2B)	
Talar flattening ± ankle ankylosis†	

CPPD, calcium pyrophosphate deposition disease; OA, osteoarthritis; RA, rheumatoid arthritis.

*From Jensen PS, Putnam CE: Chondrocalcinosis and hemophilia, *Clin Radiol* 28:401, 1977.

†From Schreiber RR: Musculoskeletal system: radiologic findings. In Brinkhous KM, Hemker HC, editors: *Handbook of hemophilia I*, New York, 1975, Elsevier.

A study of serial radiographs of symptomatic joints in hemophilic patients suggests that serial scoring with conventionally accepted techniques may be a cost-effective alternative to magnetic resonance imaging (MRI) in predicting progressive synovial hypertrophy.[19]

Other Imaging Methods

MRI is now routinely used to stage hemophilic arthritis accurately to determine optimal treatment and to follow response to therapy.[20] A scoring system based on MRI has been proposed.[21] MRI has been demonstrated to be superior to conventional radiography and computed tomography in the detection of erosions and cysts, bone marrow edema and hemorrhage, and synovial hypertrophy and torn ligaments

(the latter in patients whose radiographs showed widened intercondylar notches).[22] As preventive measures improve, it will continue to be important to use the most advanced techniques, including MRI, both to stage hemophilic arthropathy and to assess the benefits of new therapies such as prophylactic infusion.[23] Additionally, MRI and ultrasonography are useful in the detection and quantitation of soft tissue bleeding, cysts, and pseudotumors.[24,25]

PATHOLOGIC FEATURES AND PATHOGENESIS

Pathologic studies of human hemophilic arthropathy have been limited to synovial specimens obtained at surgery[26,27] or at postmortem examination and reflect changes of advanced disease only. Studies of experimentally produced hemarthrosis in animals,[28,29] post-traumatic hemarthrosis in nonhemophilic humans,[30] and canine and murine models of hemophilia A[31-33] have provided an understanding of the earliest changes induced by acute hemarthrosis and their evolution to chronic arthritis.

As reviewed more recently,[34] the process most likely includes catabolic activation of synovial cells by exposure to blood components with subsequent cartilage destruction and a direct destructive effect of intra-articular blood on cartilage. A single synovial hemorrhage induces serial changes in the synovial membrane, including early focal villous synovial proliferation and subsynovial diapedesis of erythrocytes, followed by the appearance of perivascular inflammatory cells, patchy subsynovial fibrosis, and intracellular iron accumulation in synovial cells and subsynovial macrophages. With repeated hemarthroses, the synovium becomes grossly hypertrophied and hyperpigmented, with eventual organization into a pannus that invades and erodes marginal cartilage. On histologic examination, villous

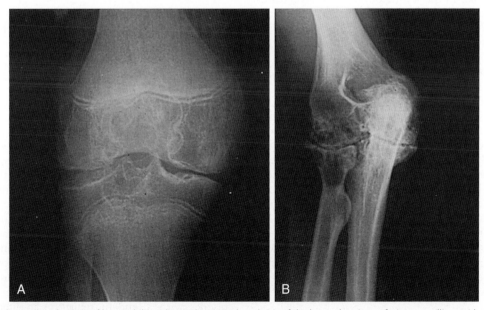

Figure 119-2 Radiographic changes of hemophilic arthropathy. **A,** Early arthritis of the knee, showing soft tissue swelling, widening of the femoral condyles and tibial plateau, irregularity of the distal femoral epiphysis, and a few subchondral bone cysts. **B,** More advanced arthritis involving the elbow, showing almost complete loss of joint space and extensive subchondral cyst formation. Widening of the proximal radius is characteristic of hemophilic arthropathy.

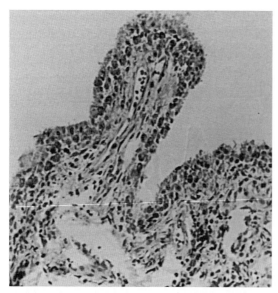

Figure 119-3 Proliferative synovitis of hemophilia. Villous hypertrophy of the synovium with pigment deposition in superficial cells. The reaction is mainly synovial cell hyperplasia. Infiltrating inflammatory cells are scarce. (Hematoxylin and eosin, ×2500.)

hypertrophy and subsynovial fibrosis progress, but inflammatory cells are scarce (Figure 119-3).[27] Seventy-five percent of synoviocytes contain siderosomes (electron-dense, iron-filled deposits within lysosomes), in contrast to 10% in normal synovium and 25% in rheumatoid synovium.[35] Iron deposits are associated with the production of proinflammatory cytokines and synovial inhibition of the formation of human cartilage matrix. Although the inflammatory synovial changes are mild, the synovial production of proinflammatory mediators, including interleukin-1 and interleukin-6 and tumor necrosis factor, approaches that of rheumatoid synovium.[34] The articular cartilage is grossly and microscopically abnormal in the setting of recurrent hemarthrosis.[28] Areas of cartilaginous fissuring and rarefaction expose sclerotic bone. The remaining cartilage is thin and unevenly distributed, often freely protruding into the joint cavity. Bone erosions appear at weight-bearing surfaces. Loss of matrix glycosaminoglycan occurs and is also seen in degenerative arthritis.[27,36]

Current studies suggest that recurrent hemarthrosis induces joint destruction in hemophilic arthropathy through direct and indirect effects of iron on the synovium[35,37] and cartilage,[36,38] by the degradative effect of proliferative synovium,[39] and through an alteration in cartilage biochemical composition similar to that seen in degenerative arthritis. A relationship between hemarthrosis-induced overexpression of oncogenes (e.g., c-myc and mdm-2) and the dysregulated, tumor-like proliferation of hemophilic synovium has been noted.[40-42] Angiogenesis induced by growth factors such as vascular-derived endothelial growth factor may be important in inducing and sustaining a synovial proliferative response to hemarthrosis.[42]

DIAGNOSIS

In most cases of congenital coagulopathy, the diagnosis has been made before presentation to a rheumatologist. In the case of hemophilia, if an affected family member is identified, prenatal diagnosis is possible. Because the spontaneous mutation rate in hemophilia is significant, the diagnosis may not be suspected until infancy, when recurrent, large ecchymoses or sustained oral hemorrhages commonly develop in most affected patients. In the case of hemophilia A or hemophilia B, hemarthrosis is usually a later manifestation, but it may be the initial symptom of other, less severe coagulopathies, even in adulthood. When a coagulopathy is suspected, baseline screening tests, including prothrombin time, activated partial thromboplastin time, and platelet count, should be performed. In patients with hemophilia, prothrombin time and platelet count are normal, and activated partial thromboplastin time is prolonged, denoting a defect in the intrinsic clotting cascade. Referral to a hematologist, who obtains the appropriate factor assays, is the next step.

Individuals with factor VIII or IX levels of 1% or less of the normal level have joint and muscle hemorrhages requiring therapy an average four or five times per month. Such patients are classified as having severe hemophilia. Individuals with factor VIII or IX levels greater than 5% of normal are considered to have mild hemophilia and usually bleed only with trauma or at surgery. Occasional "spontaneous" hemarthrosis may occur in such patients, especially in joints damaged by previously undertreated hemorrhage.

Patients whose factor VIII or IX levels fall between these two ranges are considered to have moderately severe hemophilia, and their clinical picture falls somewhere between the extremes. If such patients have had multiple untreated or suboptimally treated hemarthroses with subsequent joint damage, the anatomic instability of these joints will cause frequent and severe bleeding, and the condition will appear clinically more severe than the factor VIII or IX assay might suggest.

TREATMENT OF HEMOPHILIA

Until recent years, factor replacement therapy has been given on demand in most hemophilia centers, that is, factor concentrate has been infused at the earliest sign of a hemorrhage. Because of the introduction of highly purified, safe concentrates, prophylactic treatment is now much more common in countries where this product is available, especially in pediatric patients.[43,44] Instead of providing infusion when a hemorrhage has occurred, factor concentrate is given regularly three times per week to prevent bleeds. Prophylaxis is started before any joint damage has occurred, usually at approximately 2 years of age, with the goal of minimizing bleeding episodes to no more than four to six per year. Indwelling catheters, such as Port-A-Cath and Hickman lines, are required for factor administration because frequent venipunctures are painful and cumbersome. A recent multicenter prospective randomized controlled trial[45] confirmed earlier work[46-48] and showed that regular prophylactic factor infusion as opposed to episodic factor replacement at the time of hemarthrosis was associated with significantly less joint damage from bleeding episodes with attendant reduction in lifetime disability. Unfortunately, the cost of treatment was enormous, and specifics such as the optimum time to initiate prophylaxis were not addressed. At present, these issues remain unanswered[49] and act as "a barrier to widespread acceptance of prophylaxis,"[45] even in the United States, but especially in the developing world.

With adequate factor replacement, all types of surgery, including joint replacements, can be done. Surgical intervention should be provided for patients with hemophilia, but only at specialized centers with blood bank and coagulation laboratory support and with the participation of a hematologist who specializes in clotting disorders. A surgeon who feels comfortable operating on patients with clotting disorders also is essential. Constant-infusion techniques for administering factor concentrate during and after surgery have made adequate factor levels easier to maintain and have decreased overall perioperative use of factor concentrates.[50] Many types of commercial factor VIII concentrate are available, most of which are manufactured with recombinant technology.

Factor VIII Replacement

All plasma-derived factor concentrates are virally inactivated by various methods, including exposure to solvent detergent, heat, and pasteurization. Recombinant factor VIII concentrates, manufactured by inserting the human factor VIII gene into a mammalian cell line, are widely available and are used almost exclusively, especially in developed countries.[51,52] Because human plasma is not used in their production, transfusion-transmitted diseases, such as hepatitis and HIV, are no longer a risk. Recombinant concentrates at doses similar to those of plasma-derived concentrates have been efficacious in the treatment of hemorrhage. Half-life and recovery times for infused factor VIII are similar to those for plasma-derived concentrates. Current prices range from $0.35 to $0.90 per unit for factor VIII plasma-derived concentrates and from $1.00 to $1.20 per unit for recombinant factor VIII. In most hemophilia centers in the United States, recombinant factor concentrates are the only concentrates used, although high-purity, plasma-derived concentrates are still available. Because these concentrates have made early and intensive home therapy possible, overall costs of health care have greatly declined for patients treated with these materials.

Arginine vasopressin (desmopressin), a vasopressin analogue, can be used in the treatment of mild hemophilia A to increase the endogenous factor VIII level. Desmopressin increases the baseline factor VIII level about threefold, so a baseline level of at least 10% is required for efficacy.[53] Because this is not a blood product, it poses no danger of transmitting blood-borne viruses. Although cryoprecipitate contains factor VIII, its use has been discouraged because it is not virally inactivated. It is less safe than concentrates.

Factor IX Replacement

Factor IX is not found in cryoprecipitate or factor VIII concentrate; these two materials are totally ineffective for the treatment of hemophilia B. Fresh-frozen plasma does contain factor IX and has been used in the past. Most fresh-frozen plasma products are not virally inactivated, however, and are less safe than factor IX concentrates.

The principles of treatment are similar to those for factor VIII replacement. Because the half-life of factor IX is longer,

however, it can be given less frequently. Demand therapy is still commonly used; as for factor VIII deficiency, however, prophylaxis is beginning to be used in pediatric patients. Several plasma-derived factor IX concentrates are available, all virally inactivated. In the past, all such concentrates also contained factors II, VII, and X (prothrombin complex concentrates). Currently, only pure factor IX concentrates are used to treat factor IX deficiency. As with factor VIII concentrates, a recombinant factor IX concentrate is available and is widely used. Recovery is less than that of its plasma-derived counterpart, however, and higher doses (approximately 1.5 times calculated levels) must be infused to reach appropriate levels.

Complications of Factor Replacement Therapy

Inhibitor Antibodies

Inhibitor antibodies may develop after exposure to factor concentrate. They occur most often in patients with severe hemophilia after 9 to 30 exposures of replacement therapy, usually before the age of 5 years. A familial predisposition to the development of this complication may be noted. Because bleeding cannot be reliably controlled in patients with inhibitor antibodies, elective surgery in these patients should be done only after careful deliberation.

Inhibitor antibodies in factor VIII–deficient hemophilic patients are immunoglobulin (Ig)G antibodies (usually IgG4) and may have an unpredictable natural history. Low titer and clinically weak antibodies sometimes are easily neutralized by factor VIII and do not undergo anamnestic increases in titer after multiple factor VIII challenges. Such antibodies may rarely become high in titer. In other patients, antibody titers increase after each exposure to factor VIII. Still other patients seem to lose antibody spontaneously despite multiple subsequent factor VIII challenges. The type of antibody response to factor VIII infusion and the patient's clinical response dictate therapy.

Therapy for patients with inhibitor antibodies has been reviewed more recently.[54] Induction of immune tolerance through frequent administration of factor VIII successfully eliminates inhibitors in 80% of patients. In patients in whom immune tolerance therapy is unsuccessful, several approaches are available for management of acute bleeding episodes, including administration of activated prothrombin complex concentrate or, more recently, recombinant activated factor VIIa (rVIIa, Novo-Seven; Novo Nordisk, Bagsvaerd, Denmark). rVIIa is thought to function directly at the site of injury, causing activation of factor IX and the extrinsic clotting system locally. Porcine factor VIII, which has limited cross-reactivity with the human antibody, was used previously, but has been removed from the market because of contamination with porcine parvovirus. A recombinant form of this protein is being investigated.[55]

Use of immunosuppressives or glucocorticoids has been abandoned in most centers owing to lack of efficacy in this condition and serious side effects. Regimens of regular factor VIII infusions for induction of tolerance have been successful in eliminating the antibody. It has been suggested by some groups that an immune tolerance regimen should be started as early as possible after an inhibitor develops.

Rituximab may be useful for suppressing inhibitor titers in refractory patients.[56]

Inhibitor antibodies against factor IX are exceedingly rare. No efficacious therapy has been generally accepted. Treatment usually includes large and frequent doses of factor IX concentrate. Induction of immune tolerance with elimination of the antibody also has been done, but with less success than with antibodies to factor VIII. Use of large doses of purified factor IX concentrate in some patients with inhibitor antibodies to factor IX has resulted in anaphylactic reactions and nephrotic syndrome secondary to immune complex formation and deposition in the kidney.[57,58]

Human Immunodeficiency Virus

HIV was introduced into the U.S. blood supply in the 1970s. By the late 1970s, factor concentrate was widely contaminated. By 1982, approximately 50% of patients with hemophilia were infected with HIV.[59] Currently, approximately 10% to 20% of American hemophilic patients are infected with HIV. As with other infected individuals, CD4+ lymphocyte counts and HIV titers are used to guide treatment regimens. Since 1985, in the manufacture of plasma-derived concentrates, a triple barrier to viral contamination of plasma-derived concentrates has been applied: (1) self-exclusion for donors, (2) donor screening with serologic tests for HIV, and (3) viral inactivation during concentrate production. Recombinant concentrates also are now widely available. Acquisition of HIV through factor concentrate in patients with hemophilia has been virtually nonexistent since 1985.

Viral Hepatitis

A second infectious side effect of cryoprecipitate or factor concentrate is hepatitis, which may result from parenterally transmitted hepatitis A, B, C, or G virus; cytomegalovirus; or another as yet unidentified pathogens. In most series, most patients with hemophilia treated before the 1980s have plasma levels of hepatitis B virus surface antibody, and a few (2% to 5%) carry hepatitis B virus surface antigen. Approximately 80% of hemophilic patients transfused before 1990 have antibody to hepatitis C virus,[60] which, in contrast to hepatitis B virus antibody, is a marker for ongoing infection. Virucidal concentrate treatment methods have reduced, but not eliminated, parenteral transmission of hepatitis B and C viruses. Transmission of hepatitis A and G viruses has been reported with the use of plasma-derived concentrates. Vaccination against hepatitis B and hepatitis A is now recommended for infants born in the United States, and vaccination against hepatitis A is recommended for infants with hemophilia. Transmission of hepatitis has decreased dramatically because almost all pediatric patients are treated with recombinant products.

Therapy for Musculoskeletal Complications of Hemophilia

Acute Hemarthrosis

The most important measure in therapy for acute hemarthrosis is prompt correction of the clotting abnormality by

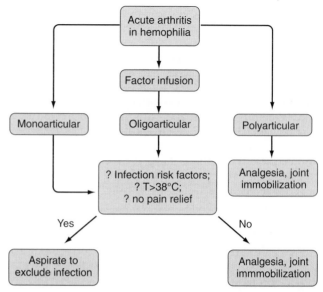

Figure 119-4   Algorithm for acute arthritis in hemophilia.

administration of the deficient factor. Arthrocentesis, if it is accomplished within 24 hours of the onset of symptoms (but after factor replacement), may be symptomatically beneficial in advanced acute hemarthrosis; however, for diagnostic and potentially therapeutic purposes, it should be considered mandatory at any time if suspicion of infection is high.[12,14] Analgesia and brief joint immobilization for no longer than 2 days often aid in pain control. Subsequently, passive range-of-motion isometric exercise should be initiated to reduce the likelihood of joint contracture (Figure 119-4).

Chronic Hemophilic Arthropathy

Nonsurgical management of hemophilic arthropathy has been reviewed.[61]

Conservative. A variety of conservative measures can bring remarkable benefit in the setting of chronic hemophilic arthropathy,[62-65] including the following:
- Prophylactic factor infusions
- Intensive physical therapy for muscle building and increased joint stability
- Periods of avoidance of weight bearing to allow regression of synovitis
- Correction of flexion contractures with wedging casts, night splints, or the judicious use of traction
- Training in sports to allow future maintenance of muscle mass

In modern treatment programs, aspiration of joints with chronic synovial effusions is rarely necessary or of lasting benefit. Failure of these conservative modalities to relieve symptoms or produce regression of synovitis should prompt consideration of other options, including local corticosteroid injections (which have been described as useful),[66] use of nonsteroidal anti-inflammatory drugs (NSAIDs), synovectomy, and joint replacement in the end stage.

Despite the obvious theoretical contraindications to the use of NSAIDs in hemophilia (i.e., the antiplatelet effects), several NSAIDs may be used safely for short periods as adjuncts to the conservative regimen. Ibuprofen, salsalate, and magnesium salicylate have been shown in a few patients to be safe and efficacious in reducing joint pain and analgesic dependence,[67,68] although long-term regression of synovitis and modification of the course of chronic hemophilic arthropathy have not been shown with any NSAID. Selective cyclooxygenase-2 inhibitors of NSAIDs do not have significant antiplatelet effects and theoretically should be safer than conventional NSAIDs in patients with hemophilia. Rofecoxib and valdecoxib have been withdrawn from the market because of a causative link to increased risk of cardiovascular events. Although others are in development, celecoxib, the only remaining cyclooxygenase-2 inhibitor on the market, has not been specifically tested in hemophilic patients and, similar to other NSAIDs, should be used with caution.

Synovectomy. Synovectomy in the setting of hemophilic arthritis has been shown to reduce the incidence of recurrent hemarthrosis and the severity of synovitis. This procedure can be accomplished surgically, arthroscopically, or through intra-articular injection of radioactive colloids or chemical substances. Patients should be considered for synovectomy if, despite aggressive conservative measures as outlined previously, persistent hemarthroses continue with ongoing chronic synovitis. At our center, specific indications for synovectomy include persistence of at least two hemarthroses per month in the same joint accompanied by symptoms and signs of chronic synovitis despite at least 4 months of conservative therapy, including intensive factor replacement. The major drawback to surgical synovectomy remains the observation, confirmed in most series,[69,70] that joint motion is reduced postoperatively compared with preoperative baseline joint motion, despite intensive rehabilitation.

To overcome this finding and the high cost of hospitalization and factor replacement therapy attendant with surgical synovectomy, arthroscopic synovectomy has been used for chronic hemophilic arthritis in recent years. Most follow-up series report that this technique is as successful as surgical synovectomy and results in less loss of motion,[71-73] particularly when continuous passive motion is used in the postoperative period.[74] The total cost of the procedure is less than that of surgical synovectomy, as is the rehabilitation period. Postoperative bleeding after arthroscopic synovectomy has been associated with poor results.

An alternative to surgical or arthroscopic synovectomy is ablation of the synovium using radioisotopic or chemical agents, as reviewed more recently.[44,75-77] Such a nonoperative approach has been successful in reducing bleeding episodes by 70% to 80% in patients with hemophilia[78] and is especially useful in patients with circulating factor inhibitors, in whom surgery is relatively contraindicated. Commonly used radioisotopes in the United States have included colloidal ^{32}P chromic phosphate, yttrium (^{90}Y), and radioactive colloidal gold (^{198}Au). Rhenium (^{186}Re) and erbium (^{169}Er) have also been used with success. Theoretical long-term carcinogenic and teratogenic effects remain major concerns associated with this technique in patients who may have long life expectancies and are still of reproductive age; these effects have limited the use of radioisotopes in the United States, but less so in Europe. Chemical synovectomies using osmic acid, rifampicin, and hyaluronic acid

have been attempted in some European centers with modest success, especially in children.[75] Short-term results of radioactive and chemical synovectomies are similar, although long-term outcomes may be superior in radioisotopic synovectomy.[44] Radioactive and chemical synovectomies remain experimental in the United States. Both offer the advantages of being minimally invasive, requiring little factor replacement, and resulting in little morbidity, and both are much less expensive than operative procedures.

Total Joint Replacement. Major orthopedic procedures, including total joint replacement,[79-82] have been performed safely and successfully in end-stage hemophilic arthropathy, including in patients with inhibitor antibodies.[83] The primary indication for total joint replacement is pain in an involved joint that is refractory to all conservative measures. Careful preoperative planning is imperative, including assessment for the presence of inhibitors, planning for factor replacement, and planning for a multidisciplinary rehabilitative program.[84] It is a matter of concern, however, that most hemophilic patients in need of total joint replacement are young and may, if they are not infected with HIV, have a long life expectancy. If the procedure is performed at a young age, this virtually ensures the need for one or more revisions during the patient's lifetime. Long-term follow-up studies of total knee replacement in hemophilic patients have shown improved functional scores but conflicting results with regard to prosthetic survival and the incidence of postoperative infection. Although an increased incidence of prosthetic infection and loosening has been noted in hemophilic patients in one large series[85] (in keeping with many previous smaller reports), a recent 25-year follow-up study encouragingly suggests that the outcome of total knee replacement can approach that of nonhemophilic patients.[86] This was believed to be due in large part to the use of continuous factor infusions in the perioperative period, in addition to a coordinated multidisciplinary approach by specialists within a hemophilia center. In this setting, total knee replacement has been suggested to be the treatment of choice for advanced hemophilic arthropathy.[86] Despite this, however, concerns with regard to perioperative complications (paradoxically including deep venous thrombosis),[87] infection, and late loosening in this population of patients remain. A comprehensive review details the many orthopedic procedures that are now available for alleviating the pain and deformity resulting from hemophilic arthropathy.[88]

CONCLUSION

Gene therapy or repair to cure hemophilia may someday be a reality, although this approach currently is still fraught with serious safety concerns.[89,90] Until that time, the best therapy for hemophilic arthropathy remains its prevention, and prevention is now achievable in many patients. With improvements in the safety and availability of factor concentrates, prophylactic infusion, although expensive, is now feasible, has been shown to reduce hemarthrosis and improve long-term joint outcomes,[45] and at some time in the future may be widely available at an affordable cost. In the meantime, through a combination of prevention of hemarthrosis or correction of the hemostatic defect at the earliest symptom of joint hemorrhage, education of the patient, application of comprehensive care, and emphasis on the importance of physical activity to maintain muscle mass, the incidence of new or progressive arthropathy can be significantly reduced.[91]

References

1. Roberts HR, Escobar M, White GC: Hemophilia A and hemophilia B. In Lichtman MA, Beutler E, Kaushansky K, et al, editors: *Williams hematology*, ed 7, New York, 2005, McGraw-Hill, pp 1867–1886.
2. Larrieu MJ, Caen JP, Meyer DO, et al: Congenital bleeding disorders with long bleeding time and normal platelet count, II: Von Willebrand's disease (report of thirty-seven patients), *Am J Med* 45:354–372, 1968.
3. Ahlberg A, Silwer J: Arthropathy in von Willebrand's disease, *Acta Orthop Scand* 41:539–544, 1970.
4. Wild JH, Zvaifler NJ: Hemarthrosis associated with sodium warfarin therapy, *Arthritis Rheum* 19:98–102, 1976.
5. Green D, Ryan C, Malandruccuolo N, et al: Characterization of the coagulant activity of cultured human fibroblasts, *Blood* 37:47–51, 1971.
6. Hilgartner MW: Hemophilic arthropathy, *Adv Pediatr* 21:165–193, 1975.
7. Arnold WD, Hilgartner MW: Hemophilic arthropathy: current concepts of pathogenesis and management, *J Bone Joint Surg Am* 59:287–305, 1977.
8. Gilbert MS: Musculoskeletal manifestations of hemophilia, *Mt Sinai J Med* 44:339–358, 1977.
9. Steven MM, Yogarajah S, Madhok SY, et al: Hemophilic arthritis, *QJM* 58:181–197, 1986.
10. Rodriguez-Merchan EC: Pathogenesis, early diagnosis, and prophylaxis for chronic hemophilic synovitis, *Clin Orthop Relat Res* 343:6–11, 1997.
11. Ellison RT, Reller LB: Differentiating pyogenic arthritis from spontaneous hemarthrosis in patients with hemophilia, *West J Med* 144:42–45, 1986.
12. Gilbert MS, Aledort LM, Seremetis S, et al: Long term evaluation of septic arthritis in hemophilic patients, *Clin Orthop Relat Res* 338:54–59, 1996.
13. Merchan EC, Magallon M, Manso F, et al: Septic arthritis in HIV positive haemophiliacs, *Int Orthop* 16:302–306, 1992.
14. Helm M, Horoszowski H, Seligsohn U, et al: Iliopsoas hematoma: its detection, and treatment with special reference to hemophilia, *Arch Orthop Trauma Surg* 99:195–197, 1982.
15. Madigan RP, Hanna WT, Wallace SL: Acute compartment syndrome in hemophilia, *J Bone Joint Surg Am* 63:1327–1329, 1981.
16. Gilbert MS, Kreel I, Hermann G: The hemophilic pseudotumor. In Hilgartner MW, Pochedly C, editors: *Hemophilia in the child and adult*, New York, 1989, Raven Press.
17. Kilcoyne RF, Nuss R: Radiological evaluation of hemophilic arthropathy, *Semin Thromb Hemost* 29:43–48, 2003.
18. Ng WH, Chu WCW, Shing MK, et al: Role of imaging in management of hemophilic patients, *AJR Am J Roentgenol* 184:1619–1623, 2005.
18a. Jaganathan S, Gamanagatti S, Goyal A: Musculoskeletal manifestations of hemophilia: imaging features, *Curr Probl Diagn Radiol* 40:191–197, 2011.
19. Kilcoyne RF, Nuss R: Radiological assessment of haemophilic arthropathy with emphasis on MRI findings, *Haemophilia* 9(Suppl 1):57–64, 2003.
20. Soler R, Lopez-Fernandez F, Rodriguez E, et al: Hemophilic arthropathy: a scoring system for magnetic resonance imaging, *Eur Radiol* 12:836–843, 2002.
21. Yu W, Lin Q, Guermazi A: Comparison of radiography, CT and MR imaging in detection of arthropathies in patients with haemophilia, *Haemophilia* 15:1090–1096, 2009.
22. Thomason HC, Wilson FC, Lachiewicz PF, et al: Knee arthroplasty in hemophilic arthropathy, *Clin Orthop Relat Res* 360:169–173, 1999.
23. Norian JM, Ries MD, Karp S, et al: Total knee arthroplasty in hemophilic arthropathy, *J Bone Joint Surg Am* 84:1138–1141, 2002.
24. Jelbert A, Vaidya S, Fotiadis N: Imaging and staging of haemophilic arthropathy, *Clin Radiol* 64:1119–1128, 2009.
25. Wilson DA, Prince JR: MR imaging of hemophilic pseudotumors, *AJR Am J Roentgenol* 150:349–350, 1988.
26. Wilson DJ, McLardy-Smith PD, Woodham CH, et al: Diagnostic ultrasound in haemophilia, *J Bone Joint Surg Br* 69:103–107, 1987.
27. Ghadially FN, Ailsby RL, Yong NK: Ultrastructure of the hemophilic synovial membrane and electron-probe x-ray analysis of hemosiderin, *J Pathol* 120:201–208, 1976.
28. Roosendaal G, Mauser-Bunschoten EP, De Kleijn P, et al: Synovium in hemophilic arthropathy, *Haemophilia* 4:502–505, 1998.
29. Roy S, Ghadially FN: Pathology of experimental hemarthrosis, *Ann Rheum Dis* 25:402–415, 1966.
30. Hoaglund FT: Experimental hemarthrosis, *J Bone Joint Surg Am* 49:285–298, 1967.
31. Roy S, Ghadially FN: Ultrastructure of synovial membrane in human hemarthrosis, *J Bone Joint Surg Am* 49:1636–1646, 1967.
32. Swanton MC, Wysocki GP: Pathology of joints in canine hemophilia A. In Brinkhous KM, Hemker HC, editors: *Handbook of hemophilia*, I, New York, 1975, American Elsevier.
33. Bi L, Lawler AM, Antonarakis SE, et al: Targeted disruption of the mouse factor VIII gene produces a model of haemophilia A, *Nat Genet* 10:119–121, 1995.
34. Valentino LA, Hakobyan N, Kazarian T, et al: Experimental synovitis in a murine model of human haemophilia, *Haemophilia* 10:280–287, 2004.
35. Hoots WK: Pathogenesis of hemophilic arthropathy, *Semin Hematol* 43(1 Suppl 1):S18–S22, 2006.
36. Hooiveld M, Roosendaal G, Vianen M, et al: Blood-induced joint damage: longterm effects in vitro and in vivo, *J Rheumatol* 30:339–344, 2003.
37. Morris CJ, Blake DR, Wainwright AC, et al: Relationship between iron deposits and tissue damage in the synovium: an ultrastructural study, *Ann Rheum Dis* 45:21–26, 1986.
38. Hough AJ, Banfield WG, Sokoloff L: Cartilage in hemophilic arthropathy, *Arch Pathol Lab Med* 100:91–96, 1976.
39. Okazaki I, Brinckerhoff CE, Sinclair JF, et al: Iron increases collagenase production by rabbit synovial fibroblasts, *J Lab Clin Med* 97:396–402, 1981.
40. Choi YC, Hough AJ, Morris GM, et al: Experimental siderosis of articular chondrocytes cultured in vitro, *Arthritis Rheum* 24:809–823, 1981.
41. Mainardi CL, Levine PH, Werb Z, et al: Proliferative synovitis in hemophilia: biochemical and morphologic observations, *Arthritis Rheum* 21:137–144, 1978.
42. Rodriguez-Merchan EC, Wiedel JD, Wallny T, et al: Elective orthopedic procedures for hemophilia patients with inhibitors, *Semin Hematol* 41(Suppl 1):109–116, 2004.
43. Wen FQ, Jabbar AA, Chen YX, et al: C-myc protooncogene expression in hemophilic synovitis: in vitro studies of the effects of iron and ceramide, *Blood* 100:912–916, 2002.
44. Hakobyan N, Kazarian T, Jabbar AA, et al: Pathobiology of hemophilic synovitis, I: overexpression of mdm2 oncogene, *Blood* 104:2060–2064, 2004.
45. Valentino LA, Hakobyan N, Enockson C: Blood-induced joint disease: the confluence of dysregulated oncogenes, inflammatory signals, and angiogenic cues, *Semin Hematol* 45(2 Suppl 1):S50–S57, 2008.
46. Berntorp E, Michiels J: A healthy hemophilic patient without arthropathy: from concept to clinical reality, *Semin Thromb Hemost* 29:5–10, 2003.
47. Hilgartner MW: Current treatment of hemophilic arthropathy, *Curr Opin Pediatr* 14:46–49, 2002.
48. Ingerslev J, Hvid I: Surgery in hemophilia: the general view. Patient selection, timing, and preoperative assessment, *Semin Hematol* 43(Suppl 1):S23–S26, 2006.
49. Silva M, Luck JV Jr: Long-term results of primary total knee replacement in patients with hemophilia, *J Bone Joint Surg Am* 87:85–91, 2005.
50. Manco-Johnson MJ, Abshire TC, Shapiro AD, et al: Prophylaxis versus episodic treatment to prevent joint disease in boys with severe hemophilia, *N Engl J Med* 357:535–544, 2007.
51. Nilsson IM, Berntorp E, Lofqvist T, et al: Twenty-five years' experience of prophylactic treatment in severe haemophilia A and B, *J Intern Med* 232:25–32, 1992.

52. Astermark J, Petrini P, Tengborn L, et al: Primary prophylaxis in severe haemophilia should be started at an early age but can be individualized, *Br J Haematol* 105:1109–1113, 1999.

53. Fischer K, van der Bom J, Mauser-Bunschoten EP, et al: The effects of postponing prophylactic treatment on long-term outcome in patients with severe hemophilia, *Blood* 99:2337–2341, 2002.

54. Roosendaal G, Lafeber F: Comment: prophylactic treatment for prevention of joint disease in hemophilia—cost versus benefit, *N Engl J Med* 357:603–605, 2007.

55. Goddard NJ, Mann HA, Lee CA: 25-Year results: total knee replacement in patients with endstage haemophilic arthropathy, *J Bone Joint Surg Br* 92:1085–1089, 2010.

56. Varon D, Martinowitz U: Continuous infusion therapy in hemophilia, *Haemophilia* 4:431–435, 1998.

57. White GC, MacMillan CW, Kingdon HS, et al: Use of recombinant hemophilic factor in the treatment of two patients with classic hemophilia, *N Engl J Med* 320:166–170, 1989.

58. Schwartz RS, Agilgaard CF, Aledort LM, et al: Human recombinant DNA derived antihemophilic factor (factor VIII) in the treatment of hemophilia A, *N Engl J Med* 323:1800–1805, 1990.

59. Mannucci PM, Ruggeri ZM, Pareti FI, et al: DDAVP in haemophilia, *Lancet* 2:1171–1172, 1977.

60. Young G: New approaches in the management of inhibitor patients, *Acta Haematol* 115:172–179, 2006.

61. Zakarija A, Aledort L: How we treat: venous thromboembolism prevention in haemophilia patients undergoing major orthopaedic surgery, *Haemophilia* 15:1308–1310, 2009.

62. Den UI, Mauser-Bunschoten EP, Roosendaal G, et al: Efficacy assessment of a new clotting factor concentrate in haemophilia A patients, including prophylactic treatment, *Haemophilia* 15:1215–1218, 2009.

63. Mathias M, Khair K, Hann I, et al: Rituximab in the treatment of alloimmune factor VIII and IX antibodies in two children with severe haemophilia, *Br J Haematol* 125:366–368, 2004.

64. Warrier I: Factor IX antibody and immune tolerance, *Vox Sang* 77(Suppl 1):70–71, 1999.

65. Ewenstein B, Takemoto C, Warrier I, et al: Nephrotic syndrome as a complication of immune tolerance in hemophilia B, *Blood* 89:1115–1116, 1997 (letter).

66. Levine PH: The acquired immune deficiency syndrome in persons with hemophilia, *Ann Intern Med* 103:723–726, 1985.

67. Brettler DB, Alter HJ, Dienstag JL, et al: Prevalence of hepatitis C virus antibody in a cohort of hemophilia patients, *Blood* 76:254–256, 1990.

68. Bossard D, Carrillon Y, Stieltjes N, et al: Management of haemophilic arthropathy, *Haemophilia* 14(Suppl 4):11–19, 2008.

69. Miser AW, Miser JS, Newton WA: Intensive factor replacement for management of chronic synovitis in hemophilic children, *Am J Pediatr Hematol Oncol* 8:66–69, 1986.

70. Buzzard BM: Physiotherapy for prevention and treatment of chronic hemophilic synovitis, *Clin Orthop Relat Res* 343:42–46, 1997.

71. Schumacher P: Discussion paper: orthotic management in hemophilia, *Ann N Y Acad Sci* 240:344, 1975.

72. Atkins RM, Henderson NJ, Duthie RB: Joint contractures in the hemophilias, *Clin Orthop Relat Res* 219:97–106, 1987.

73. Fernandez-Palazzi F, Caviglia HA, Salazar JR, et al: Intraarticular dexamethasone in advanced chronic synovitis in hemophilia, *Clin Orthop Relat Res* 343:25–29, 1997.

74. Thomas P, Hepburn B, Kim HC, et al: Non-steroidal anti-inflammatory drugs in the treatment of haemophilic arthropathy, *Am J Hematol* 12:131–137, 1982.

75. Inwood MJ, Killackey B, Startup SJ: The use and safety of ibuprofen in the haemophiliac, *Blood* 61:709–711, 1983.

76. Montane I, McCollough NC, Lian EC-Y: Synovectomy of the knee for hemophilic arthropathy, *J Bone Joint Surg Am* 68:210–216, 1986.

77. Rodriguez-Merchan EC: Orthopedic surgery of haemophilia in the 21st century: an overview, *Haemophilia* 8:360–368, 2002.

78. Post M, Watts G, Telfer M: Synovectomy in hemophilic arthropathy: a retrospective review of 17 cases, *Clin Orthop Relat Res* 202:139–146, 1986.

79. Weidel JD: Arthroscopic synovectomy for chronic hemophilic synovitis of the knee, *Arthroscopy* 1:205–209, 1985.

80. Weidel JD: Arthroscopic synovectomy of the knee in hemophilia: 10- to 15-year follow-up, *Clin Orthop Relat Res* 328:46–53, 1996.

81. Verma N, Valentino LA, Chawla A: Arthroscopic synovectomy in haemophilia: indications, technique and results, *Haemophilia* 13(Suppl 3):38–44, 2007.

82. Limbird TJ, Dennis SC: Synovectomy and continuous passive motion (CPM) in hemophiliac patients, *Arthroscopy* 3:74–79, 1987.

83. Heim M: The treatment of intra-articular synovitis by the use of chemical and radioactive substances, *Haemophilia* 8:369–371, 2002.

84. Schneider P, Farahati J, Reiners C: Radiosynovectomy in rheumatology, orthopedics and hemophilia, *J Nucl Med* 46(Suppl 1):48S–54S, 2005.

85. Lozier J: Gene therapy of the hemophilias, *Semin Hematol* 41:287–296, 2004.

86. Gan SU, Kon OL, Calne RY: Genetic engineering for haemophilia A, *Exp Opin Biol Ther* 6:1023–1030, 2006.

87. Berntorp E: Joint outcomes in patients with haemophilia: the importance of adherence to preventive regimens, *Haemophilia* 15:1219–1227, 2009.

88. Pasta G, Mancuso ME, Perfetto OS, Solimeno LP: Synoviorthesis in haemophilia patients with inhibitors, *Haemophilia* 14(Suppl 6):52–55, 2008.

89. Siegel HJ, Luck JV Jr, Siegel ME, et al: Phosphate-32 colloid radiosynovectomy in hemophilia: outcome in 125 patients, *Clin Orthop Relat Res* 392:409–417, 2001.

90. Birch NC, Ribbans WJ, Goldman E, et al: Knee replacement in haemophilia, *J Bone Joint Surg Br* 76:165–166, 1994.

91. Rodriguez-Merchan EC: Total joint arthroplasty: the final solution for knee and hip when synovitis could not be controlled, *Haemophilia* 13(Suppl 3):49–58, 2007.

The references for this chapter can also be found on www.expertconsult.com.

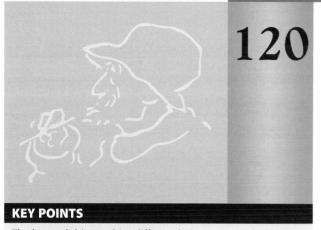

120 Rheumatologic Manifestations of Hemoglobinopathies

BRIAN MANDELL

KEY POINTS

The hemoglobinopathies differ in their pattern and severity of musculoskeletal manifestations.

Sickle cell disease is characterized by painful vaso-occlusive crises, which stem in part from bone and muscle ischemia.

Patients with sickle cell disease (rarely sickle trait) suffer frequent bone infarctions in the long bone shafts, especially in the humeral and femoral heads.

Sickle cell synovial infarctions may mimic acute septic or gouty arthritis.

Salmonella osteomyelitis is a rare complication of sickle cell disease; septic arthritis is usually due to *Staphylococcus* (a significant minority of patients have gram-negative infections).

The thalassemias rarely cause arthritis; however, the iron chelator deferiprone has been associated with severe joint pain.

CLINICAL BIOLOGY OF THE HEMOGLOBINOPATHIES

The hemoglobinopathies comprise a group of genetic disorders characterized by the presence of variant hemoglobins in circulating erythrocytes. Clinical manifestations differ dramatically based on the physicochemical behavior of the abnormal hemoglobin, and how the variant protein chains interact with other hemoglobin chains, the erythrocyte membrane, ion transporters, and oxygen. Some variant hemoglobins exhibit abnormal oxygen-dissociation curves or erythrocyte fragility resulting in dyspnea, fatigue, or hemolysis. Relevant to rheumatologic manifestations, the red cells of patients with sickle cell variants are structurally rigid, and as they traverse the microvasculature are unable to deform in small vessels; they occlude the vascular lumina and abnormally adhere to endothelial cells. As a result, patients with homozygous hemoglobin S disorder (sickle cell anemia, Hgb SS) exhibit a broad range of clinical syndromes caused by variable intensity of the intracellular sickling process and resultant vaso-occlusion. The degree of hemoglobin sickling dictates the complications and is affected by several factors, including the presence and amount of alternative hemoglobin forms (e.g., fetal hemoglobin, Hgb F). Our molecular understanding of this process has grown over the past 30 years,[1] and greater understanding has contributed to the development of management strategies for treating and limiting these vaso-occlusive episodes.

Sickling and vaso-occlusion occur more in tissues with low oxygen tension and lower pH. Ischemic phenomena, sometimes with lasting sequelae, seem to be particularly common in kidney, eye, bone, synovium, muscle, and skin. Other striking organ involvement may include stroke, mitral valve damage, splenic infarction with hypofunction, and acute pulmonary syndromes. Under certain conditions, these complications may mimic systemic inflammatory, autoimmune, or primary thrombotic disorders.

As a result of chronic hemolysis, some of the hemoglobinopathies such as the thalassemias (imbalanced synthesis of normal globin chains) result in hyperplastic marrow with skeletal abnormalities.[2] Patients may require frequent transfusions, which can lead to syndromes associated with iron overload, or painful joint complications from the required use of iron chelators.

CLINICAL FEATURES OF MUSCULOSKELETAL SYNDROMES LINKED TO HEMOGLOBINOPATHIES

The recurrent painful crisis is the hallmark of sickle disease, with marked pain in the muscles and joints, as well as in the abdomen and chest. These episodes involve muscles and joints and are sometimes difficult to localize; frequently, the pattern of pain is repeated in recurrent crises. Pain that is clearly localized to an isolated area, such as a single shoulder, right upper quadrant, buttock, or groin, warrants aggressive and rapid evaluation. The pain may be severe enough to require narcotics, but extreme diligence must be paid to the development of individualized pain control care plans to limit the expectation and delivery of escalating narcotics in all patients. Painful crises may begin as early as 6 months of age as the concentration of fetal hemoglobin F wanes, permitting sickling to occur more readily.

Avascular necrosis (AVN; osteonecrosis) and ischemic bone syndromes are common in both adults and children with sickle cell anemia (but are not usually seen in patients with heterozygous Hgb S disease—sickle trait[3]). In very young children, repeated vaso-occlusive crises involving growing small bones of the hands and feet cause the *hand-foot syndrome*, characterized by diffuse painful hand/foot swelling, which may be accompanied by low-grade fever. Radiographic changes may be seen approximately 10 days after the onset of symptoms; these consist of subperiosteal new bone formation in the hands and feet. Cortical thinning, multiple irregular intramedullary deposits, and areas of spotty destruction and formation of periosteal new bone may appear later. These changes can lead to a "moth-eaten" appearance.[4] AVN is often multifocal but characteristically affects the femoral heads.[5] The pain may be of acute onset or may progress insidiously from intermittent pain to pain with use, and finally to constant discomfort or severe pain at rest. Frequently, this condition is diagnosed in young to middle-aged patients who have experienced years of vaso-occlusive crises. Presumably, it occurs as the result of multiple ischemic and occlusive episodes, resulting in bone death as well as progressively increased intraosseous pressure. The prevalence of femoral head AVN is likely greater than 40%. Humeral heads are frequently affected. AVN can mimic a true arthritis with the presence of significant synovial effusion. The pathogenesis of these noninflammatory effusions is not certain, but they may result from hydrostatic pressure increases in vessels draining into the necrotic bone.

Noninfectious arthritis is well described in the setting of acute vaso-occlusive crisis.[6-8] Most patients have homozygous SS disease, but a few may have hemoglobin SC (Hgb SC) disease or hemoglobin S-beta thalassemia (β-thalassemia). Crystal-induced arthritis and infection should be excluded by synovial fluid analysis and culture as appropriate. Some of the effusions (monoarticular or oligoarticular) accompany painful crises and joint examination may reveal that adjacent bone is more tender than the joint capsule itself. Almost all synovial fluids are noninflammatory, hence the possibility that bone infarction with a "sympathetic" or transudative effusion offers a pathologic explanation for these effusions. Polyarthritis with minimal or mildly inflammatory fluid has been described in the setting of crisis.[7] In a series of 70 patients with sickle disease (including Hgb SC disease and Hgb S-thalassemia) followed prospectively, 32 had joint manifestations (30 with Hgb SS disease),[6] indicating that if carefully looked for, articular involvement is fairly common. Most cases of acute monoarticular and oligoarticular arthritis happened in the setting of a painful crisis, but a very significant subgroup (44%) exhibited arthritis and fever as major symptoms (infection was excluded). In this series, synovial fluid analyses were striking. Sickle cells were seen in many of the synovial fluid samples—an observation that has been noted by others. Whereas cultures were negative and no crystals were observed, many of the synovial fluid samples were inflammatory in cellular appearance with neutrophilic predominance. Nonetheless, arthritis lasted only a mean of 5 days.[6] An ankle arthritis associated with new or worsening distal leg ulcers has also been described[8]; both may result from occlusive small vessel disease. The synovial histopathology in sickle cell–associated arthritis is generally fairly bland—minimal inflammation with some intimal proliferation and vascular congestion with occasional thrombosis has been reported.[9]

Joint and bone infections are well-recognized complications in patients with sickle cell disease, although they are not particularly common. *Salmonella* is an unusual cause of musculoskeletal infection associated with sickle disease.[10] It is more frequent in children than in adults, and more frequently will result in osteomyelitis rather than septic arthritis. Reasons for susceptibility to this specific organism remain unclear. Patients with sickle cell anemia exhibit potentially altered gut mucosal integrity due to small vessel ischemic injury, splenic infarction with dysfunction, and decreased complement activation, all of which may render patients at increased relative risk. Moreover, damage to joints from repetitive ischemic injury provides a nidus for bacterial "seeding." The diaphysis is most commonly involved in osteomyelitis, although infection may involve the epiphysis, and bacteria may thereby migrate to the joint space.

In a recent retrospective study of 2000 consecutive adults with sickle cell disease, 59 (3%) were found to have had septic arthritis.[11] The hip was involved in 61% of recorded cases—a disturbing observation in that this is a joint that physicians are often reluctant to aspirate and for which it is often tempting on clinical grounds to attribute acute pain to hip AVN. Also of note, in this study from France, no cases of *Salmonella* were reported. Most infections were due to *Staphylococcus aureus*, as observed in other series of patients with septic arthritis without sickle disease. A relatively large proportion of gram-negative infections theoretically could be due to increased bacterial translocation across the bowel mucosa. The authors documented a strong association in these adults with the presence of previous childhood osteomyelitis or AVN. Overall, *Salmonella* infection seems to be more strongly associated with osteomyelitis in patients with sickle cell disease[10] than in those with arthritis. It is important to note that osteomyelitis may be multifocal.

Sickle cell disease is associated with hyperuricemia, likely due to increased uric acid generation associated with hemolysis and erythroid proliferation. Gout has been described in young patients with sickle disease. Although an infrequent occurrence in young patients, it is generally unexpected and can be confused with other more common causes of acute joint pain in these patients.[12]

Patients with thalassemias have rarely been described as having arthritis or joint pain associated with their dysregulated hemoglobin synthesis. However, chelation therapy with deferiprone, which is often needed to reverse the iron load from frequent transfusions, has been associated with multiple musculoskeletal complications.[13] Arthralgias seem to be particularly common, perhaps in 20% of patients, although arthritis has been described. Whether some of these patients may have been experiencing a reaction to periarticular and synovial iron overload, and not directly to the drug, is difficult to ascertain given short-term follow-up after drug withdrawal. Successful response to nonsteroidal anti-inflammatory therapy has been suggested by several authors to indicate a useful palliative therapy.[14]

DIFFERENTIAL DIAGNOSIS AND DIAGNOSTIC TESTS

The approach to patients with hemoglobinopathies who experience acute monoarticular or oligoarticular arthritis should be no different than that taken with other patients. However, as noted previously, concern about and therefore vigilance concerning infection, AVN, and "true" sickle cell arthritis should be greater. Thus, arthrocentesis should be performed early in the diagnostic process. Patients with sickle cell disease and ongoing hemolysis often have a leukocytosis, and older literature suggests that some patients may exhibit a blunted erythrocyte sedimentation rate (ESR) response to inflammatory stimuli; however, C-reactive protein (CRP) should be reasonably reliable. Note that not all patients with septic arthritis have markedly elevated acute phase reactants; hence no reliable substitute for arthrocentesis has been found with fluid culture performed to diagnose or exclude an infected joint. Indirect serologic studies, such as rheumatoid factor, anticyclic citrullinated protein antibodies, and antinuclear antibodies, generally should be avoided in the initial workup of acute monoarticular and oligoarticular arthritis; this is no different in the patient with a hemoglobinopathy. No imaging test will reliably distinguish infection from crystalline arthritis or sickle cell arthritis (synovial infarction).

In patients experiencing diffuse crisis pain, careful examination must performed to find specifically affected joints. Infection can trigger a generalized crisis. It should be remembered that joint pain not worsened by provocative physical examination may be due to referred pain, and such causes as splenic infarction (left shoulder), necrotic gallbladder or pulmonary infarction with effusion (right shoulder), and periarticular osteomyelitis or bone infarction should be considered in the differential diagnosis.

AVN is diagnosed as in other patients with suspected necrosis. Synovial fluid, if present, is bland. Radiographs are insensitive (flattening and the "crescent sign" are not early findings). Magnetic resonance imaging (MRI) is much more sensitive in demonstrating the necrotic process and marrow edema.

TREATMENT

Treatment is generally supportive and analgesic based, once infection and gout have been excluded. Advances have been made in limiting the number of vaso-occlusive crises, but in general, most patients continue to experience painful attacks.[1] For most patients with transient arthritis associated with crises, treatment usually involves analgesics and hydration. Intra-articular corticosteroids are not useful, and as noted, the risk of AVN is already heightened. If infection is suspected by detection of inflammatory synovial fluid, empiric antibiotics should be instituted until culture results have been returned; it should not be assumed that the inflammatory fluid is due to sickle arthritis until cultures are found to be negative. It is far more critical to adequately cover for staph species (including methicillin-resistant Staphylococcus aureus [MRSA]) than to cover for salmonella alone, although a recent study[11] suggests the need for broad gram-negative coverage as well. In the setting of osteomyelitis, every effort should be made to obtain culture definition of the infecting organism before a prolonged course of antibiotic therapy is initiated.

No "proven" treatment approaches for AVN are known (see Chapter 103); conservative methods, such as avoidance of weight bearing with crutches and bed rest, have been used widely, but without proven success.[15] Core decompression is a procedure that is commonly used to treat AVN at early stages; however, its use is based mainly on orthopedic case series, and formal trial-based evidence for this approach is lacking. Moreover, use of non–weight-bearing crutches may be problematic because AVN of the humeral heads may also be present, making the use of crutches difficult. Nonetheless, given the young age of patients with AVN, delaying the initial total hip arthroplasty is believed by many to be rational; core decompression may relieve some of the pain, at least temporarily. Authors have expressed concern that the failure rate for total hip arthroplasty is especially high among patients with sickle disease—another reason why some surgeons prefer to delay this procedure in younger patients with sickle disease. Ultimately, explanation, patient education, and early involvement of the multidisciplinary team will offer additional support for this patient group, given the paucity of clinical evidence supporting therapeutic decisions.

References

1. Prabhakar H, Haywood C Jr, Molokie R: Sickle cell disease in the United States: looking back and forward at 100 years of progress in management and survival, *Am J Hematol* 85:346–353, 2010.
2. Angastiniotis M, Eleftheriou A: Thalassaemic bone disease, *Pediatr Endocrinol Rev* 6(Suppl 1):73–80, 2008.
3. Tsaras G, Owusu-Ansah A, Boateng FO, Amoateng-Adjepong Y: Complications associated with sickle cell trait: a brief narrative review, *Am J Med* 122:507–512, 2009.
4. Babhulkar SS, Pande K, Babhulkar B: The hand-foot syndrome in sickle-cell haemoglobinopathy, *J Bone Joint Surg Br* 77:310–312, 1995.
5. Mukisi-Mukaza M, Elbaz A, Samuel-Leborgne Y, et al: Prevalence, clinical features, and risk factors of osteonecrosis of the femoral head among adults with sickle cell disease, *Orthopedics* 23:357–363, 2000.
6. Espinoza LR, Spilberg I, Osterland CK, et al: Joint manifestations of sickle cell disease, *Medicine (Baltimore)* 53:295–305, 1971.
7. Hanissian AS, Silverman A: Arthritis of sickle cell anemia, *South Med J* 67:28–32, 1974.
8. de Ceulaer K, Forbes M, Roper D, Serjeant GR: Non-gouty arthritis in sickle cell disease: report of 37 consecutive cases, *Ann Rheum Dis* 43:599–603, 1984.
9. Schumacher HR, Andrews R, McLaughin G: Arthropathy in sickle cell disease, *Ann Intern Med* 78:203–211, 1973.
10. Anand AJ, Glatt AI: *Salmonella* osteomyelitis and arthritis in sickle cell disease, *Semin Arthritis Rheum* 24:211–221, 1994.
11. Hernigou P, Daltro G, Flouzat-Lachaniette CH, et al: Septic arthritis in adults with sickle cell disease is associated with osteomyelitis or osteonecrosis, *Clin Orthop Relat Res* 468:1676–1681, 2010.
12. Reynolds MD: Gout and hyperuricemia associated with sickle cell anemia, *Semin Arthritis Rheum* 12:404–413, 1983.
13. Kellenberger CJ, Schmugge M, Saurenmann T: Radiographic and MRI features of deferiprone-related arthropathy of the knees in patients with β-thalassemia, *Am J Radiol* 183:989–994, 2004.
14. Vlachaki E, Tselios K, Perifanis V, et al: Deferiprone-related arthropathy of the knee in a thalassemic patient: report of a case and review of the literature, *Clin Rheumatol* 27:1459–1461, 2008.
15. Garino JP, Steinberg ME: Total hip arthroplasty in patients with avascular necrosis of the femoral head: a 2- to 10-year follow-up, *Clin Orthop Relat Res* 334:108–115, 1997.

The references for this chapter can also be found on www.expertconsult.com.

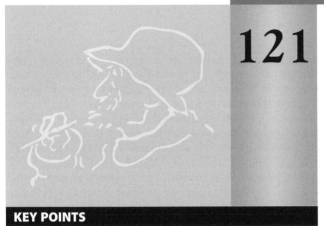

121 Endocrine Diseases and the Musculoskeletal System

MAURIZIO CUTOLO

KEY POINTS

Both hypothyroidism and hyperthyroidism are characterized by frequent symptomatic involvement of the musculoskeletal system.

Diseases of the parathyroid gland can manifest in bone and muscle presentations. The most important joint manifestation of primary hyperparathyroidism is calcium pyrophosphate deposition (CPPD) disease.

Cushing's disease, a subtype (80%) of Cushing's syndrome, is caused by a pituitary adenoma, which is a benign tumor resulting in excess adrenocorticotropic hormone (ACTH), whereas iatrogenic Cushing's syndrome is secondary to exogenous high-dosage long-term glucocorticoid therapy. Varied musculoskeletal manifestations may arise, which may be indolent and require high levels of clinical vigilance for detection.

Diabetes mellitus can manifest a variety of musculoskeletal presentations in joints, in long bones, and in connective tissues. Several manifestations are characterized by tissue fibrosis. Abnormal tendon biology may contribute to these presentations. Charcot's diabetic osteoarthropathy is a severe, destructive form of degenerative arthritis resulting from underlying diabetic neuropathy.

Musculoskeletal manifestations are a common presenting feature of endocrine disease; therefore, a high level of vigilance should be maintained during initial and ongoing assessment of patients with bone, muscle, and soft tissue complaints. Similarly, endocrine disease can arise in the treatment of rheumatic diseases, especially with the use of glucocorticoids. Whereas the underlying mechanisms of many such presentations remain uncertain, their association is sufficiently common as to merit detailed consideration in the history and examination of all new rheumatic disease presentations, and superficial endocrine assessment should form a part of the routine early investigation of new-onset arthralgia and myalgia patients. This chapter addresses some of the more common musculoskeletal elements of endocrine syndromes.

HYPOTHYROIDISM

Deficiency of thyroid hormone leads to the state of hypothyroidism. The most common cause is Hashimoto's thyroiditis, an autoimmune process in which lymphocytic infiltration and fibrous tissue accumulation cause replacement of normal thyroid tissue and thereby gland dysfunction.[1] The incidence of autoimmune hypothyroidism (Hashimoto's thyroiditis) is increased in patients with systemic sclerosis, as well as with systemic lupus erythematosus (SLE), rheumatoid arthritis (RA), mixed connective tissue disease, Sjögren's syndrome, and polymyositis.[2] Most patients develop antibodies against thyroid peroxidase and/or thyroglobulin.[3] Hashimoto's thyroiditis is associated with HLA-B8, HLA-DR3, HLA-Aw30, and HLA-DR5.[4] Some patients with Hashimoto's thyroiditis also exhibit antinuclear antibodies, and many have anti-DNA antibodies; despite this, overt SLE is uncommon. Other potential causes of thyroid gland dysfunction include treatment with radioactive iodine (^{131}I) for Graves' disease and drug-induced hypothyroidism, for example, associated with amiodarone, iodine (i.e., Wolff-Chaikoff effect), or other drugs.[5-8] In addition, hereditary disorders of the iodothyronine synthesis pathway (thyroxine [T_4] and triiodothyronine [T_3]), as well as pituitary tumors and related surgical resections, are possible causes.[9,10]

Hypothyroidism can cause a broad range of symptoms associated with mild (e.g., fatigue, weight gain, cold intolerance, mental slowing, muscle cramping, bradycardia) to severe complications (e.g., heart enlargement, myxedema coma [rare]). Neuromuscular and musculoskeletal manifestations are observed in many patients. These manifestations can occur at any time in the disease process and include weakness, joint and muscle pain, aching, and stiffness.[11] Overall, 30% to 80% of hypothyroid patients manifest neuromuscular symptoms, depending on the severity of hypothyroidism, whereas weakness is observed in almost 30% of patients.[12] More rarely, hypothyroid myopathy manifests as a polymyositis-like illness with proximal muscle weakness and an increased creatinine phosphokinase level. It may also present as muscle enlargement (pseudohypertrophy); in adults, this condition is called *Hoffmann's syndrome*.[13] In children with hypothyroid disease (cretinism), a pattern of proximal weakness and diffuse muscle enlargement is known as *Kocher-Debre-Semelaigne syndrome*.[14] Several case reports describe rhabdomyolysis associated with hypothyroidism; in these cases, hypothyroidism is thought to have been causative.[15] Myxedema represents a phenomenon in which thickening of muscle tissue occurs after light percussion in approximately 30% of patients; however, it is not entirely specific for the latter.[16] Myxedema is likely caused by delayed calcium reuptake by the sarcoplasmic reticulum, which thereby prolongs muscle contraction. This prolongation of muscle contraction is thought to be related to the development of muscle hypertrophy. A further neuromuscular manifestation concerns peripheral neuropathy. In particular, carpal tunnel syndrome is found in 15% to 30% of patients with hypothyroidism.[17]

HYPERTHYROIDISM

Hyperthyroidism (Graves' disease) may affect the musculoskeletal system in several ways; the most common manifestation is osteopenia and potentially osteoporosis. The latter may occur in patients with idiopathic Graves' disease but also in those with iatrogenic hyperthyroidism.[18] Failure to recognize the declining need for thyroid replacement with age is a further important cause of iatrogenic hyperthyroidism in older women. For this reason, patients with hypothyroidism who are on thyroid hormone and estrogen therapy should have thyroid-stimulating hormone levels monitored and the dose readjusted to keep the thyroid-stimulating hormone level within the normal range.[19] Bone density has been shown to increase after correction of the hyperthyroid state.[20]

Pretibial myxedema is a syndrome of painless nodules that occur over the pretibial areas; virtually all affected patients have concomitant Graves' ophthalmopathy.[21] Cutaneous lesions vary in size, ranging from nodules with a diameter of 1 cm to very large lesions covering most of the pretibial surface.[22] The lesions are colored differently—from pink to a light purple hue—and can be misdiagnosed as erythema nodosum. In contrast to erythema nodosum, however, the lesions are painless. They are caused by the accumulation of hyaluronic acid in the skin and in some cases exhibit a shiny appearance resembling systemic sclerosis or morphea.[23]

Hyperthyroidism may be associated with changes in the nails, including onycholysis, or elevation of the nail from the nail bed, and clubbing.[24] Clubbing usually is part of the condition known as *thyroid acropachy*, a rare manifestation of hyperthyroidism associated with periostitis around the metacarpal joints and distal soft tissue swelling of the digits.[25] This condition is not clearly related to levels of thyroid hormone, and it may be seen after the patient has reverted to the euthyroid state.

Proximal muscle weakness, a common complication of hyperthyroidism, is present in most patients. Most patients have lost weight and have other evidence of loss of muscle mass.[26] Proximal muscle weakness reverts rapidly with correction of the hyperthyroid state, suggesting a direct metabolic link to thyroxine effector function. Perhaps related to the proximal myopathy, adhesive capsulitis of the shoulder seems to be increased in patients with hyperthyroidism.[27] In these patients, the condition can be insidious and difficult to treat, with frozen-shoulder syndrome often the initial manifestation.

Strong relationships have been noted between Graves' disease and Hashimoto's thyroiditis and other rheumatic diseases. Seventy-five percent to 90% of patients with Graves' disease have antinuclear antibodies, and a proportion also express anti-DNA antibodies, despite the fact that overt SLE is uncommon.[3] Graves' disease is associated with HLA-B8, HLA-A1, HLA-Cw7, and HLA-DR3, and combinations of these antigens correlate with persistent disease.[28]

HYPOPARATHYROIDISM

Hypoparathyroidism is usually secondary to surgical removal of the parathyroid glands and commonly is characterized by proximal muscle weakness related to the degree of hypocalcemia.[29] This condition responds rapidly to treatment with vitamin D and calcium. Other common musculoskeletal manifestations of hypoparathyroidism include osteomalacia and rickets, which are discussed elsewhere. Idiopathic hypoparathyroidism is a rare disorder, seen as part of DiGeorge's syndrome with thymic hypoplasia.[30] Pseudohypoparathyroidism, known as *Albright's hereditary osteodystrophy*, is caused by end-organ resistance to the effects of parathyroid hormone.[31] Pseudohypoparathyroidism is due to a defect in GNAS1 (guanine nucleotide binding protein, alpha-stimulating activity polypeptide 1).[32] Patients show persistent hypocalcemia and hyperphosphatemia, but parathyroid hormone levels are consistently elevated. Type Ia pseudohypoparathyroidism, which is autosomal dominant, is characterized by short stature, calcification of perispinal ligaments, and, usually, mental retardation.[33] Patients may present with shortening of the fourth metacarpal and metatarsal bones, and instead of the usual knuckle appearance over the fourth metacarpal head, these individuals have a dimple. Patients affected by type Ib pseudohypoparathyroidism also show resistance to parathyroid hormone but have normal phenotype.[34] Type Ia pseudohypoparathyroidism is almost always inherited maternally, and type Ib is inherited paternally.

HYPERPARATHYROIDISM

Primary hyperparathyroidism results from hyperfunction of the parathyroid glands themselves. The condition is characterized by hypersecretion of parathyroid hormone (PTH) caused by adenoma, hyperplasia, or, rarely, carcinoma of the parathyroid glands.[35] Secondary hyperparathyroidism comprises the reaction of the parathyroid glands to hypocalcemia caused by pathologic conditions other than parathyroid pathology (e.g., chronic kidney disease).[36] The most important joint manifestation of primary hyperparathyroidism is calcium pyrophosphate deposition (CPPD) disease, a disorder with varied clinical manifestations attributed to precipitation of calcium pyrophosphate dihydrate crystals in the connective tissues.[37,38] *Chondrocalcinosis* refers to radiographic evidence of calcification in hyaline and/or fibrocartilage.[39] *Pseudogout* refers to clinically evident acute synovitis that results from shedding of crystals in the joint space after rupture of a CPPD deposit; it is characterized by red, tender, and swollen joints that may resemble gouty arthritis[40] (see Chapter 96). CPPD crystal deposition disease is a polyarticular arthritis (i.e., it leads to inflammation of several joints), although it can initially present as monoarthritis.[41] Diffuse idiopathic skeletal hyperostosis (DISH) and pseudo-ankylosing spondylitis are considered additional possible forms of calcium pyrophosphate dehydrate crystal deposition disease (CPPD CDD).[42] These syndromes are considered in detail in Chapter 96.

Some patients with long-standing hyperparathyroidism report proximal muscle weakness—a condition rapidly reversed by removal of the parathyroid adenoma.[43] In these patients, the muscle enzymes are normal, and electromyography and muscle biopsy reveal a picture most consistent with denervation. In secondary hyperparathyroidism associated with advanced renal disease, numerous bone and articular abnormalities are described.[44] The musculoskeletal changes of renal osteodystrophy resulting from secondary hyperparathyroidism include erosive arthritis in the hands, resorption of the distal clavicle, and erosions in the axial skeleton.[45] In children, widespread bone deformities of osteitis fibrosa cystica can be very disabling.[46] Other musculoskeletal manifestations of advanced renal failure include aluminum-induced osteomalacia[33] and β2-microglobulin amyloidosis.[47,48]

ADRENAL GLAND DISORDERS

Primary Cushing's disease is caused by a pituitary adenoma, which is a benign tumor resulting in excess adrenocorticotropic hormone (ACTH).[49,50] It may also arise from adrenal adenomas. Iatrogenic Cushing's syndrome (hypercortisolism/hyperadrenalism) secondary to exogenous high-dose long-term glucocorticoid therapy is the most common condition involving adrenal hormones that mediates adverse effects on the musculoskeletal system.[51] Osteonecrosis, a common late complication of high-dose glucocorticoid therapy, may first become evident months or years after glucocorticoid therapy has been discontinued.[52] It is observed less commonly after short courses of therapy, however, or after intermittent high-dose intravenous therapy, although clinical vigilance is required. Because rheumatic patients receiving high-dosage glucocorticoid therapy have associated diseases characterized by joint pain, the risk of osteonecrosis should be considered, particularly in the differential diagnosis. Use of the lowest acceptable dose of glucocorticoids has reduced the risk of osteonecrosis.[53,54]

Steroid-induced myopathy may be difficult to recognize in patients being treated for primary or secondary inflammatory rheumatic conditions, particularly myopathies.[55] However, steroid myopathy is characteristically more severe in the pelvic girdle. It may come on gradually or abruptly, starting with weakness and muscle aching, and can be sufficiently severe to render patients bedbound.[56] Biopsy specimens or T2 relaxation times are compatible with muscle fiber atrophy, whereas muscle enzymes are normal.[57] Long-acting and fluorinated glucocorticoids are more likely to induce myopathy, and treatment usually requires ultimate discontinuation of glucocorticoids before any improvement is seen; weeks or months may pass before muscle strength begins to return.[58]

Osteopenia as a secondary effect of hypercortisolism (primary or secondary) is independent of degree or duration of hypercortisolism (adenoma) but may be related to the total dose and duration of glucocorticoid therapy and is more frequent with dosages greater than the equivalent of 7.5 mg/day of prednisone.[59,60] Prophylaxis is recommended, and regimens shown to be effective in preventing or treating glucocorticoid-induced osteoporosis must include calcium, vitamin D$_3$, and bisphosphonates.[61]

Cushing's disease may be confused with primary musculoskeletal disease, including polymyalgia rheumatica, polymyositis, or statin myopathy, or it may be mistaken for back pain that may arise from osteoporotic fractures or other pathologies.[62] In Cushing's syndrome secondary to ectopic adrenocorticotropic hormone production, glucocorticoid serum levels may be extremely high, inducing severe myopathy and additional complications such as steroid psychosis.[63] Several other side effects of glucocorticoids on the musculoskeletal system are less well understood. Some patients describe intense joint pain, frequently most severe in the knees, when high doses of glucocorticoids are started. This pain typically resolves even if the dose is left unchanged.

Adrenal insufficiency is classified into three subtypes based on where the abnormality is based in the hypothalamic-pituitary-adrenal (HPA) axis.[62] Primary insufficiency is caused by adrenal gland damage (Addison's disease). The secondary form is related to insufficient corticotropin (ACTH) from the pituitary gland. The tertiary form is related to insufficient corticotropin-releasing hormone (CRH) generated from the hypothalamus. Acute adrenal insufficiency, or adrenal crisis, is severe and is characterized by shock. Primary adrenal insufficiency (Addison's disease) is almost exclusively autoimmune (now only rarely related to tuberculosis) and is characterized by weakness, weight loss, abdominal pain, hyperpigmentation, nausea, and hypotension.[64] Secondary adrenal insufficiency can be related to destruction of the pituitary gland or to deficiency of ACTH. Classically, it is associated with hemorrhage of the pituitary gland, or thrombosis, or it may be noted during infiltrative processes such as those seen when sarcoidosis affects the pituitary gland. Glucocorticoid use and subsequent withdrawal can cause secondary or tertiary adrenal insufficiency. Iatrogenic Addison's disease can be subtle because mineralocorticoids are still being produced; salt wasting, hyperkalemia, and postural hypotension are usually less impressive; and hyperpigmentation is not seen because the pituitary is suppressed. Adrenal insufficiency, particularly in such circumstances, can mimic fibromyalgia syndrome.[65] Tertiary adrenal insufficiency is most commonly related to withdrawal of glucocorticoids.[66] Glucocorticoid-induced adrenal insufficiency can be caused by several mechanisms, including decreased hypothalamic synthesis of CRH, blockade of the actions of CRH on the anterior pituitary, and, after prolonged or profound deficiency of ACTH, adrenal atrophy. As in idiopathic Addison's disease, features may not be evident unless the individual undergoes a new exogenous stressful condition, such as surgery or infection. Adrenal insufficiency (adrenal crisis) is a rare disorder that usually manifests with gradually evolving clinical symptoms and signs.[67] Occasionally, acute adrenal insufficiency (crisis) can become a life-threatening condition as the result of acute interruption of a normal or hyperfunctioning adrenal or pituitary gland, or sudden interruption of adrenal replacement therapy. Addisonian crisis has been seen even in individuals still receiving physiologic or "replacement" doses of glucocorticoids. It should be assumed that individuals taking glucocorticoids at greater than the equivalent of 5 mg/day of prednisone have a pituitary-adrenal axis unable to respond to severe stress (medical and surgical stress, concomitant use of certain medications); consequently, increases in the glucocorticoid dose should be considered in the acute setting.

Musculoskeletal Manifestations and Steroid Deficiency

The so-called steroid withdrawal syndrome consists of widespread arthralgias, myalgias, malaise, and sometimes low-grade fever.[68] It may be seen when high-dose glucocorticoids have been used for nonrheumatic conditions, such as asthma or inflammatory bowel disease, and it arises from suppression of the pituitary-adrenal axis. Moreover, abrupt reduction of the dose of glucocorticoid can cause a severe rebound flare of the underlying disease, at least in rheumatic diseases.[69] This condition may arise even though the dose of glucocorticoid remains in the pharmacologic range. It is important to recall that treatment with glucocorticoids should not be stopped until endogenous synthesis of glucocorticoids is fully efficient. Administration of low-dose "modified-release" glucocorticoids, which addresses appropriate timing of administration (at night, reflecting HPA circadian rhythms), has been shown to reduce the severity of this syndrome.[70-72]

Subclinical hypoadrenalism associated with insufficient production of cortisol may arise in conditions of chronic stress (e.g., interpersonal conflict, chronic inflammatory disease state), especially in the elderly.[73,74] In this circumstance, a new stressor may induce the development of polymyalgia rheumatica[75,76] (see Chapter 88).

DIABETES MELLITUS

Diabetes mellitus (DM) may affect the musculoskeletal system in myriad ways. Many rheumatologic disorders have been observed more frequently among individuals with DM than in the general population.[77] The metabolic perturbation characterized by diabetes (including glycosylation of proteins; microvascular abnormalities with damage to blood vessels and nerves; and accumulation of extracellular matrix proteins in skin and periarticular structures) results in overall changes in the connective tissue.[78] Musculoskeletal complications are most commonly seen in patients with a long-standing history of type 1 diabetes, but they also may be observed in patients with type 2 diabetes.[79] Some of these complications have a direct association with diabetes, whereas others have a suggested but unproven association (Table 121-1).

Table 121-1 Rheumatic Complications of Diabetes Mellitus (DM)

Conditions Limited to DM
Diabetic muscle infarction
Conditions Occurring More Frequently in DM
Diabetic cheiroarthropathy, or limited joint mobility, or stiff hand syndrome
Flexor tenosynovitis, or trigger finger
Dupuytren's contracture
Carpal tunnel syndrome
Adhesive shoulder capsulitis, or frozen shoulder
Calcific shoulder periarthritis (tendinitis)
Reflex sympathetic dystrophy, or shoulder-hand syndrome, or complex regional pain syndrome
Diabetic osteoarthropathy, or Charcot's arthropathy, or neuropathic arthropathy
Conditions Sharing Risk Factors of DM
Diffuse idiopathic skeletal hyperostosis
Gout/Pseudogout
Osteoarthritis

Hands

Diabetic cheiroarthropathy, also known as *diabetic stiff hand syndrome* or *limited joint mobility syndrome*, has been reported in 8% to 50% of all patients with type 1 diabetes and is also seen in type 2 diabetic patients.[80] Prevalence increases with the duration of diabetes, and the disorder is associated with and is predictive of other diabetic complications. Diabetic cheiroarthropathy is characterized by thick, tight, waxy skin reminiscent of systemic sclerosis with limited joint range of motion (inability to fully flex or extend the fingers) and possible sclerosis of tendon sheaths. Once again, the underlying causes are thought to be multifactorial and include increased glycosylation of collagen in the skin and periarticular tissue, decreased collagen degradation, and diabetic microangiopathy.[81] As a consequence, flexion contractures of the fingers may develop at advanced stages, and the classic indication of the presence of this condition is known as the "prayer sign,"[80] which is seen as a patient's inability to press the palms together completely without a gap remaining between opposed palms and fingers.

Another frequent complication affecting the hands is *flexor tenosynovitis* (or trigger finger); patients describe a catching sensation or a locking phenomenon that may be associated with pain in the affected fingers.[82] Physical examination reveals a palpable nodule, usually in the area overlying the metacarpophalangeal joint, and thickening along the affected flexor tendon sheath on the palmar aspects of the finger and hand. Flexor tenosynovitis is thought to have the same pathogenesis as diabetic cheiroarthropathy; its prevalence is similarly related to the duration of diabetes.[82] Abnormalities of matrix metalloproteinases and their tissue inhibitors have been demonstrated in diabetic fibroblast culture systems ex vivo (Brown I and McInnes IB, personal communication). *Dupuytren's contracture* results from thickening, shortening, and fibrosis of the palmar fascia; nodule formation along the fascia is often detected.[83] Flexion contractures of the fingers may result, usually at the fourth finger but sometimes involving any of the second through fifth digits. Dupuytren's contracture has been reported in 16% to 42% of diabetic patients, with pathogenesis that is thought to be the same as that for cheiroarthropathy. Once again, the prevalence of this condition increases with disease duration, but Dupuytren's contracture also may be seen early in the course of the disease.

Another frequent complication of DM is *carpal tunnel syndrome* (CTS), which is observed in up to 20% of diabetic patients; the specific relationship to diabetes is thought to be median nerve entrapment caused by diabetes-induced connective tissue alterations, as previously mentioned.[84] CTS usually is diagnosed on the basis of patient history and classic clinical findings, such as Tinel's sign (tapping over the median nerve on the volar aspect of the wrist) and results of Phalen's test (the wrist flexion test).[84] It is important to examine patients for possible motor weakness caused by median nerve compression; electromyography/nerve conduction velocity (EMG/NCV) testing can confirm the diagnosis of CTS in uncertain cases, helping to localize the site of nerve entrapment. In any case, management of CTS is the same for diabetic patients as for nondiabetic patients.

Shoulder

The most common shoulder involvement in diabetes occurs as adhesive capsulitis, or frozen shoulder, which has been reported in 19% of diabetic patients.[85] *Adhesive capsulitis* refers to a stiffened glenohumeral joint, usually caused by a reversible contraction of the joint capsule; patients report shoulder stiffness, along with decreased range of motion.[85] *Calcific shoulder periarthritis (tendinitis)* occurs at least three times more frequently than in people without DM and most commonly affects the shoulder in which calcium hydroxyapatite crystals deposit, predominantly in periarticular areas.[86] Shoulder radiographs show calcium deposits outside of the joint, often in the area of the rotator cuff tendons; however, in up to 60% of cases, this condition is asymptomatic in DM.

Reflex sympathetic dystrophy, also known as *shoulder-hand syndrome* or *complex regional pain syndrome* (CRPS), has been reported in diabetic patients, although whether it occurs with increased frequency is controversial, and it may be associated with adhesive capsulitis (with or without calcific periarthritis).[87] Patients describe pain from shoulder to hand in the affected limb, and classic symptoms include swelling of the affected limb/area, skin changes (changes in hair growth, shiny skin, color and temperature changes), increased sensitivity to temperature and touch (hyperesthesia), and vasomotor instability. Transient, patchy osteoporosis may be seen.[87]

Feet

Diabetic osteoarthropathy (also known as *Charcot's* or *neuropathic arthropathy*) is a condition involving destructive, lytic joint changes that most commonly affect the pedal bones.[88] It presents as a severe, destructive form of degenerative arthritis caused by loss of sensation (brought on by underlying diabetic neuropathy) in involved joints, leading to inadvertent (often unappreciated) repeated microtrauma to the joints with consecutive degenerative changes. Diabetic osteoarthropathy is rare, affecting only 0.1% to 0.4% of diabetic patients, and is seen in both type 1 and type 2 diabetes.[89] The average duration of Charcot's arthropathy in affected patients is 15 years, and physical examination reveals peripheral neuropathy. Additional symptoms include skin changes such as erythema, swelling, hyperpigmentation, or purpura and soft tissue ulcers over the affected area, as well as joint loosening or instability and joint deformities. The diagnosis is made on the basis of radiographic findings, with symptoms often milder than would be expected from a view of the radiographs. Usually, no history of overt trauma is reported. Depending on the stage and severity of Charcot's arthropathy, radiographs can show degenerative changes with subluxation, bone fragments, osteolysis, periosteal reaction, deformity, and/or ankylosis.

Computed tomography (CT) scans are insensitive in evaluating disease activity, whereas magnetic resonance imaging (MRI) and bone scintigraphy studies are valuable adjuncts to plain films in this regard. Diabetic peripheral neuropathy is thought to play the greatest pathogenic role in diabetic osteoarthropathy. Differential diagnosis includes inflammatory and degenerative processes, infections, tumors, deep venous thrombosis or thrombophlebitis, and neuropathic arthropathies secondary to other conditions.

Muscles

Diabetic muscle infarction is a rare condition characterized by spontaneous infarction with no history of trauma that tends to affect patients with a long history of poorly controlled DM.[90] It is seen more frequently in patients with insulin-requiring diabetes, and most affected patients show multiple microvascular complications (e.g., neuropathy, nephropathy, retinopathy). The condition is characterized by an acute onset of pain and swelling over days to weeks in affected muscle groups (usually the thigh or calf), along with varying degrees of tenderness; creatinine phosphokinase levels may be normal or elevated.[90] However, laboratory investigations need to exclude other conditions such as tumor, muscle infection/abscess, thrombophlebitis/thrombosis, localized myositis, and osteomyelitis. CT scans are nonspecific, and MRI may show high signals of the involved muscle on T2-weighted images.[91]

Incisional muscle biopsy may be needed to confirm the diagnosis; primary findings on biopsy include muscle edema and necrosis. Because excisional muscle biopsy may worsen the muscle lesion, this procedure should be done only to rule out infection or malignancy. If such a biopsy is performed, it is important that tissue is sent for culture, and that consideration is given to the presence of atypical organisms and of mycobacteria.

Diffuse Skeletal Disease

Diffuse idiopathic skeletal hyperostosis (DISH) is characterized by metaplastic calcification of spinal ligaments (diagnosed on lateral spine radiographs), along with osteophyte formation.[92] However, disk spaces, apophyseal joints, and sacroiliac joints are spared, and the thoracic spine is most commonly affected. DISH may be accompanied by more generalized calcification of other extra-axial ligaments and tendons[92] (Figure 121-1). The underlying pathophysiology

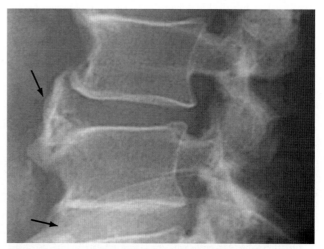

Figure 121-1 Diffuse idiopathic skeletal hyperostosis (DISH): lumbar spine. This lateral radiograph of the lumbar spine shows early changes of DISH. Calcifications of the anterior longitudinal spinal ligament *(arrows)* are evident and will eventually evolve into flowing osteophytes extending across multiple spinal levels.

is unclear; however, DISH clearly has greater prevalence among diabetic patients than among people without diabetes, particularly in association with type 2 diabetes, and in obese patients.[92] Classically, patients complain of stiffness in the neck and back with decreased range of motion, and pain generally is not a prominent symptom.

References

1. Boelaert K, Newby PR, Simmonds MJ, et al: Prevalence and relative risk of other autoimmune diseases in subjects with autoimmune thyroid disease, *Am J Med* 123:183–189, 2010.
2. Antonelli A, Ferri C, Fallahi P, et al: Clinical and subclinical autoimmune thyroid disorders in systemic sclerosis, *Eur J Endocrinol* 156:431–437, 2007.
3. Nakamura H, Usa T, Motomura M, et al: Prevalence of interrelated autoantibodies in thyroid diseases and autoimmune disorders, *J Endocrinol Invest* 31:861–865, 2008.
4. Jacobson EM, Huber A, Tomer Y: The HLA gene complex in thyroid autoimmunity: from epidemiology to etiology, *J Autoimmun* 30:58–62, 2008.
5. Anolik JR: Hypothyroid symptoms following radioiodine therapy for Graves' disease, *Clin Cornerstone* 7(Suppl 2):S25–S27, 2005.
6. Eskes SA, Wiersinga WM: Amiodarone and thyroid, *Best Pract Res Clin Endocrinol Metab* 23:735–751, 2009.
7. Markou K, Georgopoulos N, Kyriazopoulou V, et al: Iodine-induced hypothyroidism, *Thyroid* 11:501–510, 2001.
8. Barbesino G: Drugs affecting thyroid function, *Thyroid* 20:763–770, 2010.
9. Dumitrescu AM, Di Cosmo C, Liao XH, et al: The syndrome of inherited partial SBP2 deficiency in humans, *Antioxid Redox Signal* 12:905–920, 2010.
10. De Marinis L, Fusco A, Bianchi A, et al: Hypopituitarism findings in patients with primary brain tumors 1 year after neurosurgical treatment: preliminary report, *Endocrinol Invest* 29:516–522, 2006.
11. Punzi L, Betterle C: Chronic autoimmune thyroiditis and rheumatic manifestations, *Joint Bone Spine* 71:275–283, 2004.
12. McDermott MT: In the clinic: hypothyroidism, *Ann Intern Med* 151:ITC61, 2009.
13. Udayakumar N, Rameshkumar AC, Srinivasan AV: Hoffmann syndrome: presentation in hypothyroidism, *J Postgrad Med* 51:332–334, 2005.
14. Salaria M, Parmar VR: Kocher-Debre-Semelaigne syndrome—a case report and review of literature, *J Indian Med Assoc* 102:645–646, 2004.
15. Chowta MN, Chowta NK: Hypothyroidism-associated rhabdomyolysis, *Indian J Med Sci* 62:496–577, 2008.
16. Bhansali A, Chandran V, Ramesh J, et al: Acute myoedema: an unusual presenting manifestation of hypothyroid myopathy, *Postgrad Med J* 76:99–100, 2000.
17. Palumbo CF, Szabo RM, Olmsted SL: The effects of hypothyroidism and thyroid replacement on the development of carpal tunnel syndrome, *J Hand Surg Am* 25:734–739, 2000.
18. Belaya ZE, Melnichenko GA, Rozhinskaya LY, et al: Subclinical hyperthyroidism of variable etiology and its influence on bone in postmenopausal women, *Hormones (Athens)* 6:62–70, 2007.
19. Flynn RW, Bonellie SR, Jung RT, et al: Serum thyroid-stimulating hormone concentration and morbidity from cardiovascular disease and fractures in patients on long-term thyroxine therapy, *J Clin Endocrinol Metab* 95:186–193, 2010.
20. Zaidi M, Davies TF, Zallone A, et al: Thyroid-stimulating hormone, thyroid hormones, and bone loss, *Curr Osteoporos Rep* 7:47–52, 2009.
21. Khalilzadeh O, Mojazi Amiri H, Tahvildari M, et al: Pretibial myxedema is associated with polymorphism in exon 1 of CTLA-4 gene in patients with Graves' ophthalmopathy, *Arch Dermatol Res* 301:719–723, 2009.
22. Hunzeker CM, Kamino H, Walters RF, et al: Nodular pretibial myxedema, *Dermatol Online J* 14:8–10, 2008.
23. Kerns MJ, Mutasim DF: Focal cutaneous mucinosis in Graves disease: relation to pretibial myxedema, *Am J Dermatopathol* 32:196–197, 2010.
24. Fatourechi V, Ahmed DD, Schwartz KM: Thyroid acropachy: report of 40 patients treated at a single institution in a 26-year period, *J Clin Endocrinol Metab* 87:5435–5441, 2002.
25. Tran HA: Thyroid acropachy, *Intern Med J* 34:513–514, 2004.
26. Brennan MD, Powell C, Kaufman KR, et al: The impact of overt and subclinical hyperthyroidism on skeletal muscle, *Thyroid* 16:375–380, 2006.
27. Wohlgethan JR: Frozen shoulder in hyperthyroidism, *Arthritis Rheum* 30:936–939, 1987.
28. Zeitlin AA, Heward JM, Newby PR, et al: Analysis of HLA class II genes in Hashimoto's thyroiditis reveals differences compared to Graves' disease, *Genes Immun* 9:358–363, 2008.
29. Khan MI, Waguespack SG, Hu MI: Medical management of postsurgical hypoparathyroidism, *Endocr Pract* 6:1–19, 2010.
30. Sullivan KE: DiGeorge syndrome/velocardiofacial syndrome: the chromosome 22q11.2 deletion syndrome, *Adv Exp Med Biol* 601:37–49, 2007.
31. Wémeau JL, Balavoine AS, Ladsous M, et al: Multihormonal resistance to parathyroid hormone, thyroid stimulating hormone, and other hormonal and neurosensory stimuli in patients with pseudohypoparathyroidism, *J Pediatr Endocrinol Metab* 19(Suppl 2):653–661, 2006.
32. Mariot V, Maupetit-Méhouas S, Sinding C, et al: A maternal epimutation of GNAS leads to Albright osteodystrophy and parathyroid hormone resistance, *J Clin Endocrinol Metab* 93:661–665, 2008.
33. Semiz S, Duzcan F, Candemir M, et al: Pseudohypoparathyroidism type IA (PHP-Ia): maternally inherited GNAS gene mutation, *J Pediatr Endocrinol Metab* 22:107–108, 2009.
34. Weinhaeusel A, Thiele S, Hofner M, et al: PCR-based analysis of differentially methylated regions of GNAS enables convenient diagnostic testing of pseudohypoparathyroidism type Ib, *Clin Chem* 54:1537–1545, 2008.
35. Carlson D: Parathyroid pathology: hyperparathyroidism and parathyroid tumors, *Arch Pathol Lab Med* 134:1639–1644, 2010.
36. Goto S, Fukagawa M: Clinical aspect of recent progress in phosphate metabolism: pathophysiology of secondary hyperparathyroidism in chronic kidney disease, *Clin Calcium* 19:809–814, 2009.
37. Sekijima Y, Yoshida T, Ikeda S: CPPD crystal deposition disease of the cervical spine: a common cause of acute neck pain encountered in the neurology department, *J Neurol Sci* 296:79–82, 2010.
38. Viriyavejkul P, Wilairatana V, Tanavalee A, et al: Comparison of characteristics of patients with and without calcium pyrophosphate dihydrate crystal deposition disease who underwent total knee replacement surgery for osteoarthritis, *Osteoarthritis Cartil* 15:232–235, 2007.
39. Foldes K: Knee chondrocalcinosis: an ultrasonographic study of the hyalin cartilage, *Clin Imaging* 26:194–196, 2002.
40. Cassetta M, Gorevic PD: Crystal arthritis: gout and pseudogout in the geriatric patient, *Geriatrics* 59:25–30, 2004.
41. Molloy ES, McCarthy GM: Calcium crystal deposition diseases: update on pathogenesis and manifestations, *Rheum Dis Clin North Am* 32:383–400, 2006.
42. Armas JB, Couto AR, Bettencourt BF: Spondyloarthritis, diffuse idiopathic skeletal hyperostosis (DISH) and chondrocalcinosis, *Adv Exp Med Biol* 649:37–56, 2009.
43. Chou FF, Chee EC, Lee CH, et al: Muscle force, motor nerve conduction velocity and compound muscle action potentials after parathyroidectomy for secondary hyperparathyroidism, *Acta Neurol Scand* 106:218–221, 2002.
44. Llach F, Velasquez Forero F: Secondary hyperparathyroidism in chronic renal failure: pathogenic and clinical aspects, *Am J Kidney Dis* 38(5 Suppl 5):S20–S33, 2001.
45. Griffin CN Jr: Severe erosive arthritis of large joints in chronic renal failure, *Skeletal Radiol* 12:29–33, 1984.
46. Triantafillidou K, Zouloumis L, Karakinaris G, et al: Brown tumors of the jaws associated with primary or secondary hyperparathyroidism: a clinical study and review of the literature, *Am J Otolaryngol* 27:281–286, 2006.
47. Malluche HH: Aluminium and bone disease in chronic renal failure, *Nephrol Dial Transplant* 17(Suppl 2):21–24, 2002.
48. Yamamoto S, Kazama JJ, Narita I, et al: Recent progress in understanding dialysis-related amyloidosis, *Bone* 45(Suppl 1):S39–S42, 2009.
49. Bertagna X, Guignat L, Groussin L, et al: Cushing's disease, *Best Pract Res Clin Endocrinol Metab* 23:607–623, 2009.
50. Dias RP, Kumaran A, Chan LF, et al: Diagnosis, management and therapeutic outcome in prepubertal Cushing's disease, *Eur J Endocrinol* 162:603–609, 2010.
51. Hopkins RL, Leinung MC: Exogenous Cushing's syndrome and glucocorticoid withdrawal, *Endocrinol Metab Clin North Am* 34:371–384, 2005.

52. Kerachian MA, Séguin C, Harvey EJ: Glucocorticoids in osteonecrosis of the femoral head: a new understanding of the mechanisms of action, *J Steroid Biochem Mol Biol* 114:121–128, 2009.

53. Da Silva JA, Jacobs JW, Kirwan JR, et al: Safety of low dose glucocorticoid treatment in rheumatoid arthritis: published evidence and prospective trial data, *Ann Rheum Dis* 65:285–293, 2006.

54. van der Goes MC, Jacobs JW, Boers M, et al: Monitoring adverse events of low-dose glucocorticoid therapy: EULAR recommendations for clinical trials and daily practice, *Ann Rheum Dis* 69:1913–1919, 2010.

55. Lee HJ, Oran B, Saliba RM, et al: Steroid myopathy in patients with acute graft-versus-host disease treated with high-dose steroid therapy, *Bone Marrow Transplant* 38:299–303, 2006.

56. Bae JS, Go SM, Kim BJ: Clinical predictors of steroid-induced exacerbation in myasthenia gravis, *J Clin Neurosci* 13:1006–1010, 2006.

57. Hatakenaka M, Soeda H, Okafuji T, et al: Steroid myopathy: evaluation of fiber atrophy with T2 relaxation time—rabbit and human study, *Radiology* 238:650–657, 2006.

58. Pereira RM, Freire de Carvalho J: Glucocorticoid-induced myopathy, *Joint Bone Spine* 78:41–44, 2011.

59. Lodish MB, Hsiao HP, Serbis A, et al: Effects of Cushing disease on bone mineral density in a pediatric population, *J Pediatr* 156:1001–1005, 2010.

60. Chiodini I, Francucci CM, Scillitani A: Densitometry in glucocorticoid-induced osteoporosis, *J Endocrinol Invest* 31(7 Suppl):33–37, 2008.

61. Tauchmanova L, Guerra E, Pivonello R, et al: Weekly clodronate treatment prevents bone loss and vertebral fractures in women with subclinical Cushing's syndrome, *J Endocrinol Invest* 32:390–394, 2009.

62. Ormseth MJ, Sergent JS: Adrenal disorders in rheumatology, *Rheum Dis Clin North Am* 36:701–712, 2010.

63. Coe SG, Tan WW, Fox TP: Cushing's syndrome due to ectopic adrenocorticotropic hormone production secondary to hepatic carcinoid: diagnosis, treatment, and improved quality of life, *J Gen Intern Med* 23:875–878, 2008.

64. Erichsen MM, Løvås K, Skinningsrud B, et al: Clinical, immunological, and genetic features of autoimmune primary adrenal insufficiency: observations from a Norwegian registry, *J Clin Endocrinol Metab* 94:4882–4890, 2009.

65. Boomershine C, Crofford L: A symptom-based approach to pharmacologic management of fibromyalgia, *Nat Rev Rheumatol* 5:191–219, 2009.

66. Goichot B: Is corticosteroid-induced adrenal insufficiency predictable? *Rev Med Interne* 31:329–331, 2010.

67. Bouillon R: Acute adrenal insufficiency, *Endocrinol Metab Clin North Am* 35:767–775, 2006.

68. Margolin L, Cope DK, Bakst-Sisser R, et al: The steroid withdrawal syndrome: a review of the implications, etiology, and treatments, *J Pain Symptom Manage* 33:224–228, 2007.

69. Cutolo M, Straub RH, Bijlsma JW: Neuroendocrine-immune interactions in synovitis, *Nat Clin Pract Rheumatol* 3:627–634, 2007.

70. Cutolo M, Sulli A, Pizzorni C, et al: Circadian rhythms: glucocorticoids and arthritis, *Ann N Y Acad Sci* 1069:289–299, 2006.

71. Gorter SL, Bijlsma JW, Cutolo M, et al: Current evidence for the management of rheumatoid arthritis with glucocorticoids: a systematic literature review informing the EULAR recommendations for the management of rheumatoid arthritis, *Ann Rheum Dis* 69:1010–1014, 2010.

72. Buttgereit F, Doering G, Schaeffler A, et al: Efficacy of modified-release versus standard prednisone to reduce duration of morning stiffness of the joints in rheumatoid arthritis (CAPRA-1): a double-blind, randomised controlled trial, *Lancet* 371:205–214, 2008.

73. Cutolo M, Straub RH: Stress as a risk factor in the pathogenesis of rheumatoid arthritis, *Neuroimmunomodulation* 13:277–282, 2006.

74. Straub RH, Cutolo M: Does stress influence the course of rheumatic diseases? *Clin Exp Rheumatol* 24:225–228, 2006.

75. Cutolo M, Straub RH: Polymyalgia rheumatica: evidence for a hypothalamic-pituitary-adrenal axis–driven disease, *Clin Exp Rheumatol* 18:655–658, 2010.

76. Straub RH, Cutolo M: Further evidence for insufficient hypothalamic-pituitary-glandular axes in polymyalgia rheumatica, *J Rheumatol* 33:1219–1223, 2006.

77. Crispin JC, Alcocer-Varela J: Rheumatologic manifestations of diabetes mellitus, *Am J Med* 114:753–757, 2003.

78. Lebiedz-Odrobina D, Kay J: Rheumatic manifestations of diabetes mellitus, *Rheum Dis Clin North Am* 36:681–699, 2010.

79. Burner TW, Rosenthal AK: Diabetes and rheumatic diseases, *Curr Opin Rheumatol* 21:50–54, 2009.

80. Arkkila PE, Kantola IM, Viikari JS: Limited joint mobility in type 1 diabetic patients: correlation to other diabetic complications, *J Intern Med* 236:215–223, 1994.

81. Rosenbloom AL, Silverstein JH: Connective tissue and joint disease in diabetes mellitus, *Endocrinol Metab Clin North Am* 25:473–483, 1996.

82. Ryzewicz M, Wolf JM: Trigger digits: principles, management, and complications, *J Hand Surg Am* 31:135–146, 2006.

83. Arkkila PE, Kantola IM, Viikari JS: Dupuytren's disease in type 1 diabetic patients: a five-year prospective study, *Clin Exp Rheumatol* 14:59–65, 1996.

84. Perkins BA, Olaleye D, Bril V: Carpal tunnel syndrome in patients with diabetic polyneuropathy, *Diabetes Care* 25:565–569, 2002.

85. Balci N, Balci MK, Tuzuner S: Shoulder adhesive capsulitis and shoulder range of motion in type II diabetes mellitus: association with diabetic complications, *J Diabetes Complications* 13:135–140, 1999.

86. Mavrikakis ME, Drimis S, Kontoyannis DA: Calcific shoulder periarthritis (tendinitis) in adult onset diabetes mellitus: a controlled study, *Ann Rheum Dis* 48:211–214, 1998.

87. Garcilazo C, Cavallasca JA, Musuruana JL: Shoulder manifestations of diabetes mellitus, *Curr Diabetes Rev* 6:334–340, 2010.

88. Lee L, Blume PA, Sumpio B: Charcot joint disease in diabetes mellitus, *Ann Vasc Surg* 17:571–580, 2003.

89. Jeffcoate WJ: Charcot neuro-osteoarthropathy, *Diabetes Metab Res Rev* 24:S62–S65, 2008.

90. Trujillo-Santos AJ: Diabetic muscle infarction: an underdiagnosed complication of long-standing diabetes, *Diabetes Care* 26:211–215, 2003.

91. Kattapuram TM, Suri R, Rosol MS: Idiopathic and diabetic skeletal muscle necrosis: evaluation by magnetic resonance imaging, *Skeletal Radiol* 34:203–220, 2005.

92. Sencan D, Elden H, Nacitarhan V: The prevalence of diffuse idiopathic skeletal hyperostosis in patients with diabetes mellitus, *Rheumatol Int* 25:518–521, 2005.

The references for this chapter can also be found on www.expertconsult.com.

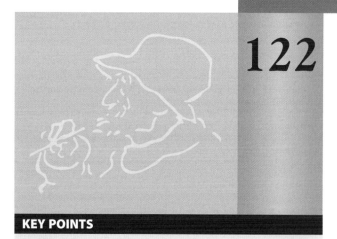

122 Musculoskeletal Syndromes in Malignancy

ELIZA F. CHAKRAVARTY

KEY POINTS

Musculoskeletal and rheumatic syndromes can occasionally be the first presentation of an underlying malignancy. Older age of onset, prominent constitutional symptoms, atypical features of rheumatic disease, and absence of response to glucocorticoids or other conventional therapy may be suggestive of a paraneoplastic process.

Data from numerous cohorts have confirmed an elevated (>threefold) incidence of malignancy associated with dermatomyositis, including clinically amyopathic dermatomyositis and, to a lesser extent, polymyositis. Solid organ tumors, including lung, colon, and ovarian tumors in European populations and nasopharyngeal tumors in Asian populations, are among the most commonly found tumors in dermatomyositis patients; most malignancies are diagnosed within 1 year of diagnosis of myopathy.

Although to a lesser magnitude than dermatomyositis, investigators in several large population-based studies have found polymyositis to be associated with an increased incidence of malignancy.

Chronic autoimmune conditions such as Sjögren's syndrome, rheumatoid arthritis, and systemic lupus erythematosus are associated with increased risk for the development of lymphoid malignancies compared with the general population. This is believed to be due, at least in part, to chronic inflammation and immune stimulation.

Patients with systemic sclerosis are at increased risk for the development of solid organ tumors primarily involving tissues affected by the fibrotic process.

Musculoskeletal syndromes may be associated with malignancy in a variety of ways. Cause and effect are difficult to define clearly in many situations, however. Certain chronic rheumatic diseases have been associated with increased risk of the subsequent development of malignancy; one example is lymphoma in an individual with primary Sjögren's syndrome. The converse situation also exists, in that certain rheumatic diseases, such as dermatomyositis, are seen more frequently in the presence of an underlying malignancy. Little is understood regarding the pathogenesis of connective tissue disease in association with neoplastic disease. Other factors can contribute to the association of musculoskeletal syndromes and malignancy. Many of the medications used to treat rheumatic diseases modulate the immune system and may be associated directly or indirectly with increased risk for the subsequent development of malignancy. In unusual circumstances, musculoskeletal involvement occurs as a paraneoplastic process, defined as a hormonal, neurologic, hematologic, or biochemical disturbance associated with malignancy, but not directly related to invasion by the neoplasm or its metastases.[1]

PARANEOPLASTIC SYNDROMES

Musculoskeletal syndromes can develop as a manifestation of a paraneoplastic process and occasionally can be the first presentation of an underlying malignancy. Hematologic malignancies, lymphoproliferative disorders, and solid tumors are associated with a wide variety of paraneoplastic rheumatic syndromes. Older age of onset, atypical features of rheumatic disease, and absence of response to glucocorticoids or other conventional therapy may suggest a paraneoplastic process. Knowledge of the associations with rheumatic syndromes and underlying malignancy is crucial when caring for these patients. Hypertrophic osteoarthropathy, amyloidosis, and secondary gout are reviewed in Chapters 102, 116, 94, and 95. Table 122-1 lists common paraneoplastic associations.

Carcinomatous Polyarthritis

The term *carcinomatous polyarthritis* is used to describe the development of arthritis in association with malignancy, but it is distinct from arthritis associated with metastasis or direct tumor invasion. Table 122-2 lists common features of carcinomatous polyarthritis. It generally occurs in patients who are older; it has an explosive onset and often develops in close temporal correlation with discovery of the malignancy. Although it can have various presentations and may mimic the appearance of rheumatoid arthritis (RA)[2] or asymptomatic migratory polyarthritis,[3] carcinomatous polyarthritis is more often a seronegative asymmetric disease with predominant involvement of the lower extremities and some sparing of the small joints of the hands. No evidence of direct tumor extension or metastasis has been found, and no specific histologic or radiographic appearance has been identified. Carcinomatous polyarthritis can occur in association with many types of malignancy, but has been reported in greatest frequency in association with breast, colon, lung, and ovarian cancers and with lymphoproliferative disorders.[4] The underlying pathogenesis of this process has not been elucidated; however, the arthritic symptoms may be improved with successful treatment of the malignancy.[5]

Vasculitis

Vasculitis in association with malignancy is uncommon and has a reported prevalence of only 8% among patients with malignancy.[6] The association seems to be significantly

Table 122-1 Paraneoplastic Syndromes

Connective Tissue Disease	Malignancy	Clinical Setting	Clinical Alert
Carcinomatous polyarthritis	Multiple types of solid tumors, including breast; lymphoproliferative disorders	See Table 122-2	See Table 122-2
Vasculitis	Lymphopoietic and hematopoietic malignancies	Cutaneous vasculitis most common; systemic vasculitis rare	Vasculitis not related to infections, medications, or autoimmune disease
Mixed cryoglobulinemia	Non-Hodgkin's lymphoma	Immune complex–mediated disease with cutaneous vasculitis, neuropathy, fatigue, and visceral organ involvement	Usually appears 5-10 yr after diagnosis of cryoglobulinemia
Panniculitis	Hematologic malignancies; pancreatic, breast, and prostate cancers	Induration of skin and deeper tissues; eosinophilia often present	Usually refractory to prednisone
Fasciitis	Ovarian, breast, gastric, and pancreatic cancers	Palmar fasciitis with inflammatory polyarthritis; similar in presentation to reflex sympathetic dystrophy	Bilateral presentation; severe fibrosis and contractures; aggressive course
Reflex sympathetic dystrophy syndrome	Multiple cancer types; Pancoast tumors	Tumors may invade stellate ganglion or brachial plexus on affected side	Absence of typical antecedent factors; failure to respond to conventional therapies
Erythromelalgia	Myeloproliferative disorders	Often seen in setting of thrombocytosis	—
Atypical polymyalgia rheumatica	Renal, lung, and colon cancer; multiple myeloma	—	Age <50 yr; asymmetric involvement; poor response to prednisone
Digital necrosis	Gastrointestinal and pulmonary tumors	Severe Raynaud's phenomenon with onset >50 yr old	Asymmetric features; digital necrosis
Remitting seronegative symmetric synovitis with pitting edema	Several tumor types	Abrupt onset of arthritis and edema surrounding wrists and small joints of hands	Presence of fever, weight loss; poor response to prednisone
Multicentric reticulohistiocytosis	Lung, stomach, breast, cervix, colon, and ovarian carcinomas	—	—
Lupus-like syndromes	Variety of solid tumors and lymphoproliferative disorders	—	Rare associations with malignancy limited to case reports
Antiphospholipid antibodies	Multiple cancer types	Association between antibodies, cancer, and risk of thrombosis unclear	Higher presence of antibodies found in patients with malignancy
Osteogenic osteomalacia	Solid tumors and tumors of mesenchymal origin	Bone pain and muscle weakness	Diligent search is indicated in all patients with late-onset apparent idiopathic osteomalacia
Sarcoidosis	Cervical, bladder, gastric, lung, breast, and renal cancers and cutaneous and pulmonary squamous cell carcinomas	Highest incidence of "malignancy" during first 4 yr after detection of granulomata	Malignant tumors can cause sarcoid-like tissue reactions leading to mistaken diagnosis of sarcoidosis before recognition of malignancy
Lymphomatoid granulomatosis	Lymphoma	Unusual granulomatous form of vasculitis with angiodestructive infiltration of various tissues	—

Table 122-2 Features of Carcinomatous Polyarthritis

Close temporal relationship between onset of arthritis and discovery of malignancy
Late age of onset of arthritis
Asymmetric joint involvement
Explosive onset
Predominant lower extremity involvement with sparing of wrists and small joints of hands
Absence of rheumatoid nodules
Absence of rheumatoid factor
No family history of rheumatoid disease
Nonspecific histopathologic appearance of synovial lining
No periosteal reaction

higher with lymphoproliferative and myeloproliferative disorders than with solid tumors, and vasculitis commonly predates the identification of malignancy. The vasculitic process is most often small vessel and cutaneous and only rarely involves significant organs. Up to 5% of patients with cutaneous vasculitis have an underlying neoplasm.[7] Treatment often requires the use of glucocorticoids and therapy directed against the underlying malignancy, although it seems that this is often ineffective. Table 122-1 shows malignancies associated with vasculitis. In the setting of malignancy, it is believed that persistent antigen stimulation from the tumor results in T cell activation or immune complex formation and deposition.

The development of small vessel vasculitis has been reported to antedate and postdate the development of lymphoproliferative and myeloproliferative diseases. One group looked retrospectively at 222 patients with vasculitis and identified 11 who had developed an associated malignancy.[8] Of these 11 patients, 7 had hematologic neoplasia, and 4 had malignant solid tumors. Nine of the patients manifested cutaneous vasculitis, and the remaining 2 had vasculitic involvement in the bowel. In 4 patients, the development of vasculitis antedated the diagnosis of malignancy.[8] Similar findings were reported by investigators, who found an underlying malignancy in 8 of 192 patients with cutaneous vasculitis. Most malignancies were hematologic (6 of 8) and predated (5 of 8) the diagnosis of cancer.[9] In a retrospective analysis of 23 patients with cutaneous vasculitis and hematologic malignancies, the authors were able to attribute the presence of vasculitis to the malignancy itself in 61% of cases.[10]

Systemic vasculitis is much less commonly associated with underlying malignancy. Case reports and small series have found antineutrophil cytoplasmic antibody (ANCA)–negative and ANCA-positive vasculitis associated with hematologic malignancies.[11-13] Granulomatosis with polyangiitis (GPA) (formerly Wegener's granulomatosis) has likewise been associated with the development of several types of malignancies, including lymphoproliferative disorders, bladder cancer, and renal cell carcinoma.[14,15] In some cases, the malignancy was diagnosed within months of the diagnosis of GPA,[14] and in other reports, cancer developed many years after diagnosis and treatment of vasculitis,[15] making it unclear whether the malignancies were a result of the vasculitis or possibly the treatment. A group from the Cleveland Clinic did a retrospective study to assess directly the temporal relationship between vasculitis and cancer.[16] During an 18-year study period, the authors found only 12 cases of vasculitis and cancer diagnosed within the same 12-month period: Six patients had lymphoproliferative disorders, and 6 had solid tumors. In most cases, the vasculitis responded partially to immunosuppressive therapy, but investigators observed a more impressive improvement in vasculitis with definitive treatment for the underlying malignancy. A more recent study found 20 cases of malignancy among 200 patients with ANCA-positive vasculitis; 6 were diagnosed concurrently with a diagnosis of vasculitis, and 14 predated vasculitis by a median of 96 months.[17] Only 4 of 20 malignancies in this series were lymphoproliferative; the remaining malignancies were solid organ tumors.

Vasculitis associated with underlying malignancy is often poorly responsive to conventional therapy directed against the vasculitis. In one series of 13 patients with cutaneous vasculitis and lymphoproliferative or myeloproliferative disorder, symptoms of vasculitis were poorly responsive to therapy with nonsteroidal anti-inflammatory drugs (NSAIDs), glucocorticoids, antihistamines, and antiserotonin agents. Although investigators described lessening of the severity of vasculitis after chemotherapy directed against the malignancy, they generally found chemotherapy to be ineffective. Of 13 patients identified, 10 died as a direct result of the malignancy.[18] Similarly, Hutson and Hoffman[16] found general concurrence between improvement in vasculitic syndrome and definitive treatment for the associated underlying malignancy. More recently, a study of cutaneous small vessel vasculitis associated with solid tumors (most commonly lung, breast, and prostate) found a significant response to immunosuppressive therapy directed against the vasculitis, although concurrent treatments for the underlying malignancy were undertaken.[19]

Cryoglobulinema

Cryoglobulins are immunoglobulins that precipitate at reduced temperature. Cryoglobulinemia can be characterized by hyperviscosity symptoms or by vasculitis. Patients often have fatigue, arthralgia or arthritis, cutaneous vasculitis or purpura, neuropathy, digital ischemia, and visceral organ involvement (renal or pulmonary). Three types of cryoglobulins have been identified:

Type I: Monoclonal immunoglobulin, either IgG or IgM; this type is associated with lymphoproliferative disorders.

Type II: Monoclonal IgM directed against polyclonal IgG; type II cryoglobulins were initially thought to be idiopathic and were known as mixed essential cryoglobulinemia. With the identification of hepatitis C virus (HCV), it has been discovered that most of these patients have HCV infection that is directly involved in the pathogenesis of the cryoglobulins. Specific epitopes of HCV antigens are recognized by IgG components of immune complexes, and viral particles are found in the cryoprecipitate.[20] One study found clonal B cell populations in the peripheral blood of 48% of HCV-positive patients with type II cryoglobulinemia, many of whom were eventually diagnosed with a B cell malignancy.[21] Overall, it is estimated that approximately 5% to 8% of patients with mixed cryoglobulinemia may go on to develop non-Hodgkin's lymphoma, usually after 5 to 10 years of cryoglobulinemia.[22,23] The risk of developing non-Hodgkin's lymphoma among HCV-positive cryoglobulinemic patients may be 35 times higher than in the general population.[24] Other data suggest that HCV infection may be associated with other hematologic malignancies.[25,26] At this time, the subset of patients with mixed cryoglobulinemia who will develop lymphoma cannot be predicted.

Type III: Mixed polyclonal IgG and IgM; type III cryoglobulins are commonly seen with a variety of illnesses, including connective tissue diseases (systemic lupus erythematosus [SLE] and RA) and infections. In one study of 607 patients diagnosed with mixed cryoglobulinemia, 27 cases of hematologic malignancy were identified. Of these, systemic autoimmune diseases were detected in 56% of cases of non-Hodgkin's lymphoma.[26]

Panniculitis

The fasciitis-panniculitis syndrome, which includes eosinophilic fasciitis, is characterized by swelling and induration of the skin that extends into deeper subcutaneous tissues and is associated with fibrosis and chronic inflammation. Patients may develop arthritis and subcutaneous nodules similar to those seen in erythema nodosum. The arthropathy seems to be secondary to periarticular fat necrosis, can be monoarticular or polyarticular,[27] and may mimic RA or juvenile RA.[28] Blood and tissue eosinophilia is commonly, but not always, present.[29] This syndrome can be idiopathic and have a benign course, or it can be secondary to a variety of infectious, vascular, or traumatic events. In a few patients, the fasciitis-panniculitis syndrome is associated with an underlying malignancy. Hematologic malignancies are most often associated with this syndrome and are usually diagnosed concurrently or within the first year.[30,31] Pancreatic cancer and pancreatitis also can be associated with this syndrome.[27,28] Patients with cancer-associated fasciitis-panniculitis syndrome are predominantly female and are generally refractory to prednisone.[29]

Palmar Fasciitis

Palmar fasciitis with arthritis is a syndrome characterized by progressive bilateral contractures of the digits, fibrosis of the palmar fascia, and inflammatory polyarthritis.[32,33] The metacarpophalangeal and proximal interphalangeal joints are most commonly affected; other affected joints include the elbows, wrists, knees, ankles, and feet. Indurated reticulate palmar erythema can also be seen as part of the palmar fasciitis spectrum.[34] Palmar fasciitis is almost uniformly associated with the presence of an underlying malignancy, most often ovarian, breast, gastric, and pancreatic tumors.[33,35,36] Although initially thought to be an atypical variant of reflex sympathetic dystrophy, the severity of manifestations, bilateral presentation, and strong association with occult malignancy suggest that, in these cases, palmar fasciitis is a distinct entity that behaves as a paraneoplastic syndrome. Glucocorticoids, chemotherapy, or both do not seem to result in improvement, although fasciitis occasionally regresses with treatment of the underlying malignancy.[32]

Reflex Sympathetic Dystrophy

Reflex sympathetic dystrophy and a variant, shoulder-hand syndrome, are characterized by regional pain, swelling, vasomotor instability, and focal osteoporosis in a given limb; this condition is thought to be caused by sympathetic dysfunction. Absence of associated antecedent factors, such as stroke, myocardial infarction, or trauma, and failure to respond to conventional therapy warrant a search for an underlying malignancy. A variety of malignancies have been associated with the development of reflex sympathetic dystrophy or its variants.[37,38] Pancoast tumor of the lung apices and other malignancies that infiltrate the stellate ganglion or brachial plexus have been described in patients with reflex sympathetic dystrophy.[39-41] Therapy directed against the underlying malignancy may lead to some amelioration of symptoms associated with reflex sympathetic dystrophy.

Erythromelalgia

Erythromelalgia is an enigmatic condition characterized by attacks of severe burning, erythema, and warmth of the extremities with symptoms predominantly involving the feet.[42,43] Symptoms are often exacerbated when the extremities are placed in a dependent position, during ambulation, or during exposure to increased temperatures. Partial relief can be obtained through elevation or cooling of the extremity. This disorder can occur idiopathically (60%) or secondary to another disease (40%).[42,44] Myeloproliferative disorders, including polycythemia vera and essential thrombocytosis, are common primary causes and have been found to precede the diagnosis of erythromelalgia by several years.[7,43,45] The underlying pathophysiology of this disease is unknown; however, it is often associated with thrombocythemia. In the largest published retrospective cohort, 168 patients at the Mayo Clinic were identified with this diagnosis between 1970 and 1994.[46] The authors found that after a mean follow-up of 8.7 years, 31.9% of patients reported worsening of disease, 26.6% reported no change, 30.9% reported improvement, and 10.6% reported complete resolution of symptoms. Kaplan-Meier survival curves revealed a significant decrease in survival compared with controls. A history of myeloproliferative disease was found in 15 of 168 patients. The exact cause of the symptoms is unclear, but microvascular arteriovenous shunting has been hypothesized.[47] In cases of secondary erythromelalgia, platelet breakdown products and platelet microthrombi may underlie disease pathogenesis.[7] The most effective therapy seems to be the use of daily aspirin, leading to significant relief of symptoms, which is believed to be related to inhibition of cyclooxygenase-1. A host of other therapies have been tried with varying success.[48] Because of the association with myeloproliferative diseases, routine monitoring with complete blood counts is prudent.

Polymyalgia Rheumatica

Polymyalgia rheumatica is a disorder affecting older adults that manifests with discomfort and stiffness in the shoulder and hip girdle, fatigue, anemia of chronic disease, and elevated erythrocyte sedimentation rate (ESR). Classically, this condition responds to moderate doses of prednisone within 48 hours. A variety of other conditions can have presentations that mimic polymyalgia rheumatica, including other rheumatic disorders, systemic infections, and malignancy.[49] Although the association between polymyalgia rheumatica and malignancy has been controversial, atypical features of polymyalgia rheumatica may suggest the presence of occult malignancy, including age younger than 50 years, limited or asymmetric involvement of typical sites, ESR less than 40 mm/hr or greater than 100 mm/hr, severe anemia, proteinuria, and poor or delayed response to 20 mg daily of prednisone. Kidney, lung, and colon cancer and multiple myeloma are most often found in patients presenting with atypical polymyalgia rheumatica.[50-52] One study of patients undergoing evaluation for possible polymyalgia rheumatica found 10% to have a diagnosis of malignant neoplasms.[53] In contrast, several prospective studies have shown that patients who present with classic polymyalgia rheumatica or temporal arteritis do not seem to have an increased risk of developing malignancy over age-matched controls.[54-58]

Raynaud's Phenomenon and Digital Necrosis

The development of digital necrosis or profound Raynaud's phenomenon may suggest the presence of infection, inflammatory disease, or an underlying malignancy. In patients older than 50 years, the development of Raynaud's phenomenon, particularly in an asymmetric fashion or in association with digital necrosis, should raise the possibility that this is a paraneoplastic process. These features often antedate the diagnosis of the malignancy by an average of 7 to 9 months.[59,60] A variety of solid tumors and lymphoproliferative disorders have been associated with this syndrome.[59-65] Certainly, the presence of digital necrosis in patients with dermatomyositis is highly suggestive of the presence of an underlying malignancy. Mechanisms proposed include cryoglobulinemia, immune complex–induced vasospasm, hypercoagulability, marantic endocarditis with emboli, and necrotizing vasculitis.[65] Therapy with interferon-α also has been reported in association with the development of Raynaud's phenomenon and digital necrosis.[66-68]

Remitting Seronegative Symmetric Synovitis with Pitting Edema

Remitting seronegative symmetric synovitis with pitting edema (RS₃PE) is an uncommon disorder primarily affecting the metacarpophalangeal joints and the wrists. Although the underlying cause and pathogenesis of this illness are unclear, lymphoma, myelodysplastic syndromes, and several solid tumors, mostly adenocarcinoma, all have been reported in association with it.[69-73] One retrospective study from a single center in the United States found that 3 of 14 patients with RS₃PE developed cancer.[74] Characteristics that suggest possible underlying malignancy include the presence of systemic features, such as fever or weight loss, and a poor response to glucocorticoids.[71,72]

Multicentric Reticulohistiocytosis

Multicentric reticulohistiocytosis is a rare condition characterized by the presence of cutaneous papules often associated with a destructive arthritis of the interphalangeal joints of the hands. The papules are flesh-colored to brown-yellow and are classically present in the periungual region and on the dorsal hands and face. Arthritis mutilans may develop in 50% of cases. The characteristic histologic appearance of tissue infiltration with histiocytes and multinucleated giant cells can be found in affected skin, joints, and occasionally internal organs.[75] Multicentric reticulohistiocytosis has been reported in association with hyperlipidemia, malignancies, and autoimmune diseases. Malignancy has been associated in 25% to 31% of cases, although most literature consists of individual case reports.[76,77] The most frequently seen malignancies include carcinoma of the lung, stomach, breast, cervix, colon, and ovary.[75]

Lupus-like Syndromes

Lupus-like syndromes are rarely associated with underlying malignancy. Isolated case reports have described lupus-like syndromes with ovarian carcinoma[78,79] and hairy cell leukemia[80]; subacute cutaneous lupus was reported in a patient with breast carcinoma.[81] Studies on the presence of antinuclear antibodies (ANAs) in patients with cancer have yielded mixed results. Two studies were unable to find a

significantly increased prevalence of ANAs in patients with solid tumor or lymphoma compared with healthy controls.[82,83] In contrast, one smaller study found an increased prevalence in patients with non-Hodgkin's lymphoma compared with controls (21% vs. 0),[84] and another study found a prevalence of ANAs of 27.7% in 274 patients with various malignancies compared with 6.45% of 140 healthy controls.[85] No predictive features seem to suggest occult malignancy in patients presenting with lupus-like syndromes or positive ANAs.

Antiphospholipid Antibodies

Antiphospholipid antibodies and their association with thromboses have been described as a primary syndrome and a secondary phenomenon in autoimmune diseases, primarily SLE. More recently, antiphospholipid antibodies have been associated with a variety of malignancies. Correlations between antiphospholipid antibodies in cancer patients and thromboembolic events have been less clear, however.

Several studies have shown the presence of antiphospholipid antibodies in patients with solid tumors and lymphoproliferative disorders at a higher frequency than the 1% to 5% seen in the general population.[86,87] An early study of 216 consecutive patients with cancer found 22% positive for anticardiolipin antibodies compared with 3.4% in controls. This study found a two-fold increase in the development of thromboembolism in patients with positive antibodies compared with patients with negative serologies; it also indicated that most thromboembolic events occurred in patients with higher antibody titers.[88] Other studies have confirmed the association between malignancy and antiphospholipid antibodies (12.5% to 68%), but have been unable to show a correlation with thromboembolic events.[84,86,89-93] A correlation between antibody titer and disease activity has been shown in some studies,[81,83] and decreased survival in others.[93,94] A review of the literature concluded that antiphospholipid antibodies resolve in one-third of cancer patients after treatment for the underlying malignancy.[95]

Studies of the prevalence of antiphospholipid antibodies in unselected patient populations have shown an association with underlying malignancy. A prospective study in France found that 7% of 1014 consecutive patients admitted to a medical ward had antiphospholipid antibodies.[96] In antibody-positive patients, cancer was the most frequently associated disease. A more recent study in patients presenting with a first ischemic stroke found a significantly higher rate of development of cancer within 12 months in patients who had anticardiolipin antibodies (19% vs. 5%).[97]

Osteomalacia

Osteomalacia is the softening of bones often associated with failure of adequate calcification secondary to renal dysfunction or to lack of vitamin D. Osteomalacia has been associated with benign and malignant solid tissue and mesenchymal tumors.[98] Tumors causing oncogenic osteomalacia have been shown to overproduce fibroblast growth factor 23 (FGF-23), and elevated serum levels of FGF-23 can be detected in patients with this paraneoplastic condition.[99,100] Octreotide scintigraphy may be a useful tool for identifying occult tumors.[101] With removal of the tumor, there often seems to be resolution of the osteomalacia and normalization of serum FGF-23 levels.[100]

Sarcoidosis

Noncaseating granulomata can occur in numerous settings and are not pathognomonic for sarcoidosis. Granulomata resembling those of sarcoidosis may be found in lymph nodes that drain sites of malignancy. These tumor-related tissue reactions resulting in granuloma formation have been described with many types of malignant lesions, including solid tumors and lymphomas.[102,103] The clinical and radiographic presentation of sarcoidosis and cancer can be virtually indistinguishable, making it important to pursue aggressive evaluation in a patient with sarcoidosis.[104,105]

The risk of malignancy developing in patients with an established diagnosis of sarcoidosis is controversial. Some studies have shown an increased risk of developing lung cancer and lymphoma,[106-108] whereas others have shown no increased risk of cancer over the general population.[104,109,110]

Lymphomatoid Granulomatosis

Lymphomatoid granulomatosis is a rare disorder with angiodestructive and lymphoproliferative features involving the lung and, less often, the skin and central nervous system. Although lymphocytic infiltration of vessels is a hallmark of the disease, lymphomatoid granulomatosis now seems to fall within the spectrum of lymphoproliferative disorders.[111] Despite the predominance of T cells within inflammatory infiltrates, studies have suggested that an Epstein-Barr virus (EBV)-associated B cell proliferation may underlie the pathogenesis of the disease.[112,113] Prognosis is generally poor, with a median survival from diagnosis of 14 months,[114] although more recent reports suggest some response to rituximab therapy.[115,116] Frank lymphomas evolve in 25% of cases.[117]

INFLAMMATORY MYOPATHIES

The inflammatory myopathies in adult populations encompass a group of illnesses characterized by an idiopathic immune-mediated attack on skeletal muscle resulting in muscle weakness. Many associations between the inflammatory myopathies and the presence of malignancy have been noted, but the reason for the association remains unknown.[118] Dermatomyositis has classically been associated with occult malignancies, whereas associations between polymyositis and inclusion body myositis are becoming increasingly recognized. A further issue is whether the inflammatory myopathy predates the malignancy and can be considered a primary rheumatic disease with known risks of developing malignancy, or whether it simply represents a manifestation of a paraneoplastic process.

On average, the prevalence of malignancy in association with inflammatory myopathies has been approximately 15% to 25%, which appears to be consistent across populations studied. The frequency of malignancy has ranged, however, from 6% to 60% in patients with dermatomyositis, and from 0 to 28% in patients with polymyositis.[118,119] Other estimates have placed the incidence of cancer in patients with inflammatory myopathies at five to seven times that of the general population.[118]

Dermatomyositis has been associated with a wide range of malignancies; solid tumors are most often seen in cancer-associated myositis as opposed to lymphoid malignancies. Ovarian, lung, and gastric tumors are most common in European populations, and nasopharyngeal malignancies in Asian populations. Studies have confirmed a strong association between dermatomyositis and malignancy. Hill and colleagues[120] studied a pooled cohort of patients from Sweden, Denmark, and Finland and found 198 cases of cancer in 618 patients with dermatomyositis. The standardized incidence ratio (SIR) for malignancy with dermatomyositis was 3. Similar results were found in a Scottish cohort of 286 patients with dermatomyositis.[121] Of these patients, 77 were found to have underlying malignancies, with an SIR of 3.3 to 7.7. Buchbinder and co-workers[122] used strict histopathologic criteria to classify myositis in patients from Victoria, Australia. This group found 36 cases of cancer in 85 patients diagnosed with dermatomyositis and an SIR of 4.3 to 6.2. All of these studies have suggested that cancers are most commonly diagnosed within 1 to 2 years of diagnosis of dermatomyositis.

In contrast to previous work, studies of Asian populations have shown a higher association of nasopharyngeal carcinomas with dermatomyositis. In a nationwide Taiwanese study, 9.4% of 1012 patients with dermatomyositis were found to have an underlying malignancy, the most common of which was nasopharyngeal cancer, followed by lung cancer.[123,124] In a smaller study, 66.6% of 15 dermatomyositis patients in Singapore had malignancies, most of which were nasopharyngeal carcinoma.[125] Eight white patients with nasopharyngeal carcinoma within 1 year of diagnosis of dermatomyositis were reported more recently in Tunisia.[126] A similar study from Japan found that cancer was diagnosed in 24% of dermatomyositis patients; most cases involved gastric cancer, a common malignancy in the Japanese population.[127]

In polymyositis, the relative risk for developing internal malignancies seems to be lower than that for dermatomyositis, but it is consistently increased over that expected in the general population. Studies have found a 14% to 30% prevalence of cancer among patients with polymyositis, with SIRs increased to 1.2 to 2.1.[120-123] The nationwide Taiwanese study found a 4.4% incidence of cancer among 643 patients with polymyositis, with an SIR of 2.15 compared with the general population.[124] Small numbers of many types of cancers were found. These studies confirm results reported in previous large studies of Swedish and Finnish populations and a 1994 meta-analysis of all published case-control and cohort studies of malignancy and myositis, which identified an odds ratio for the association of cancer with dermatomyositis of 4.4, and of cancer with polymyositis of 2.1.[128]

In amyopathic dermatomyositis, a variant of dermatomyositis in which typical cutaneous manifestations are present with subclinical or no identifiable muscle disease, the association with underlying malignancy is now becoming clear. Whereas previous published reports were limited to small groups of patients,[125,129-131] recently published cohort studies and a systematic review of the amyopathic dermatomyositis literature have suggested similar associations between amyopathic dermatomyositis and internal malignancies.[127,132,133]

Far less is known about the association of inclusion body myositis with underlying malignancy. In Buchbinder's study from Northern Europe, 52 patients were identified with inclusion body myositis.[122] Of these patients, 12 were found to have internal malignancies, with an SIR of 2.4. The numbers of each type of cancer seen are too small to reveal specific associations.[107]

Not all studies concur regarding the association between the inflammatory myopathies and malignancy.[134,135] In a study done at the Mayo Clinic, patients with myositis did not seem to be at statistically significant risk for the development of malignancy. No clinical differences were seen between patients who developed a malignancy and patients who did not.[135]

Despite the negative results of some studies, it seems that most work supports the notion of an increased risk of malignancy in association with dermatomyositis and polymyositis. For patients in whom an inflammatory myopathy has been diagnosed, a workup for the presence of malignancy should be done. The extent of this workup has been debated, however, because extensive undirected searches often result in a very low yield. It is probably rare for an undirected workup to yield evidence of malignancy in polymyositis and dermatomyositis patients[136]; any workup should be tailored to the individual patient's age, symptoms, and signs. Studies have suggested that imaging of the chest, abdomen, and pelvis may increase the potential for discovery of underlying malignancy.[137,138] Other studies have suggested the use of serum tumor markers (CA125 and CA19-9) to augment detection of patients with dermatomyositis or polymyositis at highest risk for associated malignancy.[139] More recently, a prospective study of whole body positron emission tomography (PET)/computed tomography (CT) was found to be comparable with broad conventional screening (including chest, abdominal, and pelvic CT scans, among other tests).[140] Malignancies associated with inflammatory myopathies have been known to develop many years after the diagnosis of muscle disease, so continued vigilance and repeated screening for malignancy are warranted.

In certain cohorts, the risk of malignancy may be higher, including those with older age at diagnosis,[141] evidence of distal extremity weakness,[142] and prominent pharyngeal and diaphragmatic involvement.[142] Patients with myositis-associated autoantibodies may be at less risk for the development of malignancy.[142-144] More recent work has suggested that the presence of leukocytoclastic vasculitis[145] and cutaneous ulceration,[142] as well as the absence of pulmonary involvement,[141] increases further the possibility that an underlying malignancy is present.

Although the pathogenesis is unknown, the types of malignancy associated with inflammatory myopathies have been varied, including adenocarcinomas of the breast, ovaries, and stomach. Most cases of dermatomyositis and malignancy seem to occur within 1 year of each other, with myositis diagnosed first in most cases.[118] When identified, removal of the malignancy may result in improvement of the myopathic process, which further supports the paraneoplastic nature of myositis in some cases.[146]

RISKS OF DEVELOPING LYMPHOPROLIFERATIVE DISORDERS IN RHEUMATIC DISEASES

Since the 1960s, increasing numbers of reports have described the association between rheumatic disease and the development of malignancy, particularly lymphoproliferative disorder. Table 122-3 shows pre-existing connective tissue diseases that have been associated with malignancy. Much of what is known about associations between rheumatic disease and malignancy is drawn from retrospective and prospective cohort studies, registry linkage studies, small series, and case reports. This is thought to be mediated, at least in part, by chronic immune stimulation and hyperactivity that may lead to malignant transformation. In addition, certain confounding factors need to be considered when the risk of development of malignancy is assessed, including the potential oncogenic properties of many of the immunosuppressive and cytotoxic medications prescribed to treat autoimmune diseases. Lymphoproliferative disorders have developed in patients with rheumatic diseases and in recipients of solid organ transplantations treated with immunosuppressive agents. EBV has been implicated in the development of lymphoid neoplasia in immunosuppressed patients. In the following sections, many of the rheumatic diseases and the therapies used to treat them are discussed.

Sjögren's Syndrome

Sjögren's syndrome, an autoimmune exocrinopathy, is characterized by a benign lymphocytic infiltrate of salivary and lacrimal glands that leads to the development of sicca syndrome (keratoconjunctivitis and xerostomia).[147] The development of lymphoproliferative disorders in the setting of Sjögren's syndrome is perhaps the prototypic example of chronic autoimmune disease with increased risk of malignancy. In 1964, investigators first reported the development of four cases of lymphoproliferative disorders in a cohort of 58 patients with Sjögren's syndrome.[148] In 1978, 7 of 136 patients with sicca syndrome were identified as having developed non-Hodgkin's lymphoma. Compared with the expected incidence of cancer among women of the same age range, a 44-fold increased risk of developing non-Hodgkin's lymphoma was noted.[149] These findings have been reproduced numerous times in other cohorts. Lymphoproliferative disorders complicate approximately 4% to 10% of cases of primary Sjögren's syndrome.[150-157] The relative risk for development of lymphoproliferative disorders in patients with primary Sjögren's syndrome ranges from 6 to 44,[149,158-163] and a meta-analysis of cohort studies has found a pooled SIR of 18.8.[160] Most lymphoproliferative disorders were non-Hodgkin's lymphoma, specifically mucosa-associated lymphoid tissue (MALT) lymphoma, other marginal-zone lymphomas, and diffuse large B cell lymphoma.[155,156] Waldenström's macroglobulinemia, chronic lymphocytic leukemia, and multiple myeloma were more rarely reported.[149,153,154,159]

Table 122-3 Pre-existing Connective Tissue Diseases Associated with Malignancy

Connective Tissue Disease	Malignancy	Associated Factors	Clinical Alert
Sjögren's syndrome	Lymphoproliferative disorders	Glandular features: lymphadenopathy, parotid or salivary enlargement	Clues to progression from pseudolymphoma to lymphoma include worsening of clinical features, disappearance of rheumatoid factor, and decline of IgM
		Extraglandular features: purpura, vasculitis, splenomegaly, lymphopenia, low C4 cryoglobulins	
Rheumatoid arthritis	Lymphoproliferative disorders	Presence of paraproteinemia, greater disease severity, longer disease duration, immunosuppression, Felty's syndrome	Rapidly progressive, refractory flare in long-standing rheumatoid disease may suggest an underlying malignancy
SLE	Lymphoproliferative disorders	—	Non-Hodgkin's lymphoma should be considered in SLE patients who develop adenopathy or masses; lymphoma of the spleen is another cause of splenic enlargement in SLE
Discoid lupus erythematosus	Squamous cell epithelioma	Found in oldest plaques, ≥20 yr after onset of discoid lesion, primarily in men 30-60 yr old	Poorly healing skin lesion within discoid plaques should be evaluated
Systemic sclerosis (scleroderma)	Alveolar cell carcinoma	Pulmonary fibrosis, interstitial lung disease	Annual chest radiograph after fibrosis is detected
	Nonmelanoma skin cancer	Areas of scleroderma and fibrosis in the skin	Changes in skin features or poorly healing lesions should be evaluated
	Adenocarcinoma of the esophagus	Barrett's metaplasia	Esophagoscopy and biopsy, if indicated, of distal esophageal constricting lesions
Paget's disease of bone	Osteogenic sarcoma	Development of severe pain; increasing incidence with age	Swelling and bone destruction in pre-existing Paget's disease may be sarcoma; diagnosis may require biopsy
Dermatomyositis	Ovarian, lung, and gastric cancer in Western populations; nasopharyngeal carcinoma in Asian populations	Older age, presence of cutaneous vasculitis; less likely in setting of myositis-specific antibodies or interstitial lung disease	Malignancy evaluation needs to be tailored to individual patient's age, symptoms, and signs

SLE, systemic lupus erythematosus.

Generally, the development of lymphoma is a late manifestation of Sjögren's syndrome, often seen after 6.5 years of disease.[151,152,164] Clinical and laboratory features seem to be associated with or predictive of development of lymphoproliferative disorders, including palpable purpura,[148,153,154,163] cutaneous ulcerations,[150] cryoglobulinemia,[154,155] low serum complement levels,[153-155,165] monoclonal gammopathies,[166,167] cytopenias,[148,155,163] splenomegaly,[148,155] and adenopathy.[150] Progression to high-grade lymphoma portends a poor prognosis.* In contrast, the incidence of other malignancies or all-cause mortality was not increased in patients with Sjögren's syndrome compared with the general population.[159,163,164,168] It is believed that chronic B cell stimulation may lead to the malignant transformation of clonal lines characteristic of Sjögren's syndrome.[147] The presence of a viral trigger accounting for malignant transformation is one possible theory. EBV, among other viruses, has been implicated, but studies have failed to find EBV or other viral particles in lymphoma specimens associated with Sjögren's syndrome.[169]

Other reports have described the presence of chromosomal translocations with increased frequency in patients with Sjögren's syndrome who have developed lymphoma. One group of investigators identified the presence of translocations of the proto-oncogene *bcl-2*[170] in 5 of 7 patients with Sjögren's syndrome and lymphoma by the use of polymerase chain reaction. Such translocations were found in peripheral blood or bone marrow in 5% of unselected patients with Sjögren's syndrome without evidence of lymphoma in another study.[171] Conversely, no evidence of *bcl-2* translocations was present in 50 salivary gland biopsy specimens of patients with Sjögren's syndrome without evidence of lymphoma.[172] Analysis of biopsy specimens taken before the development of lymphoma from the 7 patients previously mentioned revealed no evidence of *bcl-2* translocation. Translocation seemed to correlate with the development of lymphoma in at least a subset of patients with Sjögren's syndrome, and the use of polymerase chain reaction technology may allow early detection of malignant transformation.[171-173]

Rheumatoid Arthritis

Data from numerous studies since the 1970s are persuasive that RA is associated with a twofold to threefold increased risk for the development of lymphoproliferative disorders,

---

*References 30, 132, 133, 140, 151, 153, 154, 163.

the magnitude of which has remained constant despite dramatic changes in therapy. Many factors, including chronic inflammation and immune dysregulation, in addition to potential oncogenic properties of immunosuppressive therapies for the treatment of RA, must be considered when the risk of development of hematologic malignancies is evaluated. It is often difficult to separate the effects of medication use from the underlying severity of inflammation that makes medication use necessary or indicated, a concept termed *confounding by indication*.[174] This association has been highlighted further by widespread use of tumor necrosis factor (TNF) inhibitors for patients with refractory disease and the potential for these medications to interfere with innate immune tumor surveillance.

In 1978, an SIR of 2.7 for lymphoma was reported in a group of 46,101 Finnish RA patients compared with the general population.[175] A similarly increased risk of 2.4 for lymphoma was seen later in a group of 20,699 Danish patients,[176] and an SIR of 1.9 to 2 was reported in a large cohort of 76,527 Swedish patients.[177,178] In the United States, an increased risk of 1.9 was found in a cohort of 18,527 patients,[179] and an SIR of 2.2 was noted in a separate cohort of 8458 patients 65 years old and older.[180] In the United Kingdom, an SIR of 2 to 2.4 for lymphoma was observed in an inception cohort of 2015 patients with inflammatory arthritis compared with the general population,[181] and an SIR of 2.04 to 2.39 was seen for non-Hodgkin's lymphoma in a cohort of 26,623 RA patients in Scotland.[182] A meta-analysis of nine cohort studies of RA patients found a pooled SIR of 3.9 for lymphoma using a random effects model.[161] Canadian investigators found an increased risk of leukemia (SIR, 2.47) among RA patients, but were unable to confirm elevated rates of lymphomas compared with the general population.[183] Data from case-control studies of patients with non-Hodgkin's lymphoma have shown similar results: Odds ratios of 1.3 to 1.5 were found for underlying RA.[160,162] These associations have been recently confirmed in other populations, including patients from Japan,[184] Taiwan,[185] California,[186] and Spain.[187] In general, lymphomas in patients with RA seem to be predominately diffuse large B cell type and recently have been shown to favor nongerminal center subtypes.[188]

Most studies have suggested that the risk for development of lymphoma is related to the degree of inflammation. The Swedish group identified high inflammatory activity (defined by ESR, swollen and tender joint counts, and the physician's global assessment of disease activity) as a significant risk factor, with an odds ratio of 25.8 compared with low disease activity.[189] No association between any specific drug and the development of lymphoma was identified; however, the cohort examined was treated between 1965 and 1983, and few of these patients were apparently treated with immunosuppressive drugs, making the lack of association less certain. In a follow-up case-control study of 378 lymphomas in a Swedish group of RA patients published more recently, a 71-fold increased risk of lymphoma was reported in patients with high cumulative disease activity compared with low disease activity.[190] Immunosuppressive therapy did not seem to modify risk for lymphoma in this study. Patients did not have increased rates of lymphoma development before disease onset.[191] Patients with Felty's

syndrome (a variant of RA associated with neutropenia and splenomegaly) were found in a Veterans Affairs study of 906 men to have a twofold increase in total cancer incidence, but a 12-fold increase in risk of non-Hodgkin's lymphoma.[192]

Disease-Modifying Antirheumatic Drug Therapy

Several studies have looked at the contribution of disease-modifying antirheumatic drug (DMARD) therapy to the elevated risk of malignancy in RA patients. A prospective, observational study was performed in a group of Canadian RA patients enrolled in a DMARD registry.[193] Although this study found an increased rate of lymphoproliferative disorders in this cohort compared with the general Canadian population (SIR, 8.05), no significant differences in DMARD exposure were noted between patients who developed malignancy and patients who did not. A second group of Canadian investigators similarly identified an increased risk for the development of lymphoma and myeloma in RA patients overall compared with control groups.[194] In this study, the risk of lymphoma and myeloma seemed to be fourfold greater in the RA group when DMARD use was not controlled for and 3.4-fold greater when individual DMARD use was controlled for. Despite the low level of DMARD exposure in this population, no strong effect of DMARD use was seen.

Similar effects of DMARD use were seen in the study of Swedish patients with RA and lymphoma: Treatment with any DMARD (odds ratio [OR], 0.9) or specific use of methotrexate (OR, 0.8) did not seem to be associated with increased risk of lymphoma compared with DMARD-naïve RA patients; however, no patients had been treated with TNF inhibition.[177] In contrast, a European cohort of RA patients enrolled in a DMARD registry was evaluated longitudinally for the development of malignancies.[195] Investigators found an increased risk of lymphoproliferative disorders in patients with the highest cumulative exposure to DMARDs compared with patients with less than 1 year of exposure (SIR, 4.82).

Although inconclusive, data from these studies when taken together suggest a possible increased risk for the development of lymphoproliferative disorders in RA patients treated with DMARDs. More recent studies have suggested, however, that this increased risk may be due to the duration and severity of the underlying disorder, rather than to specific medication use. Associations of specific immunosuppressive therapy for the treatment of autoimmune diseases are discussed further in Chapters 61 and 62.

Risk of Solid Tumor in Patients with Rheumatoid Arthritis

Despite persuasive evidence of increased risks of lymphoproliferative disorders associated with underlying RA, overall rates of all-site malignancies do not seem to be higher compared with the general population.[175-177,182,183,196,197] The overall "null" result of all malignancies is due to the combination of increased risk of lymphoproliferative disorders offset by an apparently decreased risk of colorectal malignancies.[175-177,182,183,198] The decreased risk of colorectal cancer has been attributed to long-term use of NSAIDs among RA patients. Aside from lymphoproliferative disorders, only a few solid tumors, including lung cancer and skin cancer, have been associated with RA.

Increased risk of lung cancer in RA patients has been seen in multiple studies.[175-177,182-187,196-198] A study evaluating three separate RA cohorts (an inpatient registry of 53,067 prevalent cases of RA, an inception cohort of 3703 incident RA cases, and a registry of 4160 RA patients treated with TNF inhibitors) found a consistently increased risk of lung cancer in all cohorts (SIR, 1.48 to 2.4) compared with the general population.[81,198] This association may be related to tobacco use, which seems to be a common risk factor for the development of RA, in addition to its well-known association with lung cancer,[199] although the particular association of lung cancer among RA patients who smoke is unknown. Similarly, a study of lung cancer in a cohort of 8768 U.S. veterans (92% male) with RA found an increased risk of lung cancer (OR, 1.43; 95% confidence interval [CI], 1.23 to 1.65) after adjustment for covariates such as age, gender, and tobacco exposure.[200]

A slightly increased risk for the development of non-melanoma skin cancer (most commonly basal cell carcinoma and squamous cell carcinoma) has been noted in several studies,[175,176,198,201,202] although the significance of these tumors, which carry a low probability of metastasis, is unclear. Unfortunately, nonmelanoma skin cancer is rarely captured in national cancer registries, so its incidence among the general population or subpopulations such as RA is difficult to quantify or compare. Furthermore, important risk factors for nonmelanoma skin cancer, including ultraviolet light exposure, are almost impossible to quantitate in observational studies. What is of greater concern, however, are newer data suggesting an increased rate of melanoma among patients with RA.[180,185,202-204] Because of the suggestion of increased risk of skin cancer, whether attributed to underlying disease or immunosuppressive therapies, it is reasonable to suggest periodic skin examinations in RA patients, particularly those with other risk factors, including smoking and increased ultraviolet light exposure. Certainly, all suspicious lesions should be evaluated by a dermatologist and biopsy strongly considered.

Systemic Lupus Erythematosus

The risks of developing malignancy in association with SLE have been difficult to estimate in the past. Small series and cohort studies have noted that patients with SLE might be at increased risk for malignancy, including non-Hodgkin's lymphoma, sarcoma, and breast carcinoma.[205-209] Other small series have not found differences,[210] however, or have found infrequent associations[211] in number or type of malignancy between patients with lupus and the general population.[210] Conflicting results also are seen in case-control studies of larger groups of patients, with some cohorts showing an increased overall risk of malignancy,[212-214] although others have failed to do so.[215-218] Some studies that did not find increased risk of overall malignancies in patients with SLE have shown increased risk of lymphoproliferative disorders, however.[160,162,216-218] Confounding factors complicating interpretation of these studies include possible incomplete ascertainment of malignancies, inclusion of

nonrepresentative cohorts of patients with SLE, and selection of inappropriate control populations.[219]

To determine more adequately whether individuals with SLE are at increased risk, studies of large multinational cohorts, systematic reviews, and meta-analyses of pooled data are necessary. The SIR of individual studies has ranged from 1.1 to 2.6.[220] A meta-analysis of six of the clinical cohort studies found a slightly increased risk of overall malignancies in cohorts of patients with SLE, with an SIR of 1.58.[221] This analysis showed an increased risk of lymphoma in these cohorts, with an SIR of 3.57 for non-Hodgkin's lymphoma and 2.35 for Hodgkin's disease. A separately performed meta-analysis of the incidence of lymphoma in patients with SLE found an SIR of 7.4.[161] Individual hospital discharge database studies have shown a consistently higher risk of non-Hodgkin's lymphoma (SIR, 3.72 to 6.7), but these studies examined only hospitalized patients with SLE.[200] Pooled analysis showed a slightly elevated risk for the development of breast cancer, with an SIR of 1.53, but they did not find an increased risk of lung or colorectal cancer in these patients.[221] The same confounding factors influencing individual studies are a factor in interpreting these pooled data.

A more recent series of studies analyzing nearly 9500 lupus patients (≈77,000 patient-years of observation) in a multinational cohort study has helped to define better potential associations with malignancy.[222,223] The authors found a slightly increased risk of malignancies overall (SIR, 1.15) with higher risks for the development of hematologic malignancies (SIR, 2.75), particularly non-Hodgkin's lymphoma (SIR, 3.64).[222] Forty-two cases of non-Hodgkin's lymphoma were identified, most of which were of aggressive histologic subtypes.[224] The incidence of lymphoma in this study was evident early in the course of SLE, rather than after many years of chronic disease activity or use of multiple immunosuppressive medications.[223,225] The elevated risk of non-Hodgkin's lymphoma in this cohort seemed to be independent of race or ethnicity, although white patients seemed to have higher rates of malignancy in general compared with patients of other ethnicities.[226] In a case-control study within the multisite international SLE cohort, age, disease-related damage, and smoking were found to be associated with increased risk of malignancy; use of immunosuppressant medications (particularly lagged 5 years) may contribute to increased risk of hematologic malignancy.[227]

Although the exact cause of the association is unknown, several theories have arisen to explain the possible connection between SLE and malignancy, especially B cell lymphoma. Some authors have postulated that certain immunologic defects may predispose patients to SLE and B cell lymphoma, including apoptosis dysfunction, chronic antigenic stimulation, and overexpression of *bcl-2* oncogene.[220,228] Viruses, EBV in particular, also have been postulated as part of the development of SLE and lymphoma.[220,228] Studies have not conclusively validated any of these theories to date, however.

The relative prevalence of cervical cancer in SLE patients is difficult to estimate because national cancer registries often do not record malignancies in situ. Cervical cancer remains an important issue for women with SLE, and an increased risk may come about for different reasons, including (1) reduced clearance of human papillomavirus (HPV), the causal agent in most cases of cervical cancer; (2) increased risks of cervical cancer associated with immunosuppressive medications; and (3) reduced rates of routine Pap smears and other screening procedures in a population of patients with chronic illnesses. In the large multinational study performed more recently, the SIR for invasive cervical cancer was found to be elevated at 1.26, albeit with confidence intervals that cross the null.[222] Other studies have confirmed increased risks of abnormal Pap smears and cervical dysplasia in women with SLE.[229,230] Different studies have implicated increased prevalence of HPV infection and other sexually transmitted diseases,[230-233] and immunosuppression[232-235] may partly explain this association. As with mammography, women with SLE seem less likely to undergo routine Pap testing than women in the general population.[236,237]

Several studies have identified a link between SLE and the development of lung cancer.[225] Indeed, the largest multinational cohort of SLE subjects found an increased incidence of lung cancer compared with the general population (SIR, 1.37; 95% CI, 1.05 to 1.76).[222] Further analyses of the cases of lung cancer in this cohort revealed a variety of tumor types, including adenocarcinoma, bronchoalveolar carcinoma, squamous cell carcinoma, small cell carcinoma, large cell carcinoma, and carcinoid tumor.[238] Most cases (71%) occurred in smokers, 25% of cases were in men, and few (20%) had previous exposure to immunosuppressive agents.[238] To date, no particular demographic or clinical features have been found to explain this apparently increased risk.

Overall, the presence of SLE seems to carry a small increased risk for the development of cancer, particularly lymphoproliferative disorders such as non-Hodgkin's lymphoma, lung cancer, and cervical cancer. The underlying causes of these associations are unknown, but they do not seem to be exclusively related to the use of immunosuppressive or cytotoxic agents.* Data suggest that lupus patients may be less likely to receive recommended cancer screening.

Systemic Sclerosis

Although data are conflicting, most evidence suggests that individuals with systemic sclerosis seem to have an increased risk of developing malignancy.[240,241] Estimates of the prevalence of cancer among scleroderma patients range from 3.6% to 10.7%.[241,242] However, 13% of deaths are reported among patients with systemic sclerosis.[243] The malignancies that have been implicated are often observed in organs affected by inflammation and fibrosis, including the lung, breast, esophagus, and skin. The SIR of malignancy in the scleroderma population is 1.5 to 5.1 compared with that of the general population.[244-249] An apparent increase has been reported in the observed number of cases of lung cancer that occur in the setting of pulmonary fibrosis, but not in association with tobacco use.[248,250] A different study evaluating 20 lung cancers among 632 scleroderma patients in Australia found that cigarette smoking, but not underlying pulmonary

fibrosis, was associated with increased risk of lung cancer.[251] Studies have been mixed regarding increased risk or a temporal relationship between scleroderma and breast cancer.[241,244,252] Older age at the time of diagnosis of systemic sclerosis seems to be a significant risk factor for the development of cancer.[245] Data are mixed regarding associations between systemic sclerosis–specific autoantibodies and the development of cancer: Selected studies support potential associations,[247,253] whereas others do not.[248,254] A recent study found a close temporal relationship to cancer (within 1 to 2 years of scleroderma diagnosis) in scleroderma patients with positive antibodies for RNA polymerase I/III.[255] Expression of RNA polymerase I and RNA polymerase III was detected in the tumors of affected individuals.[255]

Although the SIR for all malignancies is 1.5 to 2.4, the incidence ratio for lung cancer can be as high as 7.8, and for non-Hodgkin's lymphoma, 9.6. Cases of non-Hodgkin's lymphoma seem to be more likely to occur within the first year of diagnosis of systemic sclerosis.[253] Elevations in incidence have been found for other specific cancers as well, including nonmelanoma skin cancers (4.2), primary liver cancers (3.3), and hematopoietic cancers (2.3)—all having a higher incidence than is seen in the general population. The greatest risk seems to correspond to areas commonly affected by fibrosis, particularly the lung and skin. Esophageal involvement, common to limited and diffuse systemic sclerosis, is the likely cause for an increased incidence of Barrett's esophagus (12.7%)[256] and development of esophageal cancer (SIR, 9.6).[257] In contrast to the data previously described, one study found no increase in overall or specific malignancies in patients with systemic sclerosis (SIR, 0.91 overall).[254] Localized scleroderma, including morphea or linear scleroderma, does not seem to convey an increased risk of malignancy.[258] Several reports have described the development of postirradiation morphea in patients treated for breast cancer.[259]

PRIMARY TUMORS AND METASTATIC DISEASE

Primary Musculoskeletal Tumors

This section does not provide in-depth knowledge of the primary tumors of the musculoskeletal system. Rather, it provides a reference to the most common primary malignant musculoskeletal tumors and symptoms that may arise in association with them. Primary tumors of bone, including benign and malignant tumors, are discussed in greater detail in Chapter 123.

A primary malignant bone cancer is any neoplasm that develops from the tissues or cells found within bone that has the ability to metastasize. Neoplasms may develop or arise from any of the types of cells present within the bone—osteoblasts, chondrocytes, adipose and fibrous tissue, vascular cells, hematopoietic cells, and neural tissue.[260] A neoplasm developing from any of these tissues is called a *sarcoma*, which signifies that it is derived from mesenchymal tissue. The bone sarcomas are named for the predominant differentiated tissue type, such as osteosarcomas, chondrosarcomas, liposarcomas, and angiosarcomas.[260]

The most common manifestation of these tumors is the development of pain in the area of the lesion, which may

---

*References 205, 216, 218, 220, 227, 239.

Table 122-4 Primary Bone Tumors

Nonosseous Tumors
Multiple myeloma
Round cell tumors

Osseous Tumors
Osteosarcoma
Chondrosarcoma
Giant cell tumors
Fibrosarcoma

be accompanied by a sympathetic effusion or stiffness in the surrounding joint. This discomfort does not seem to be activity related and is often worse at night. These tumors can manifest, however, as painless masses or as pathologic fractures. Systemic features, such as fatigue, malaise, weight loss, fevers, and night sweats, are rare with all of these tumors except for Ewing's sarcoma.[260] Primary malignant bone tumors are uncommon, particularly compared with other types of cancer. They have their highest incidence in childhood and adolescence and constitute 3.2% of childhood malignancies that occur before age 15 years. The incidence has been reported in this age group as 3 per 100,000 individuals.[261] These tumors commonly arise out of areas of rapid growth, with the most common site of primary bone sarcomas being the metaphysis near the growth plate.[262]

Table 122-4 lists the most common types of primary malignant bone tumors. Osteosarcoma is the most common of the tumors and generally occurs in individuals in the second decade of life or in elderly individuals.[263] Osteosarcoma can occur secondary to radiation therapy delivered as treatment for other malignancies. Paget's disease of bone can rarely (<1% of cases) proceed to malignant transformation.[264] Severe pain in the setting of Paget's disease may signal transformation to osteogenic sarcoma. Tumors most frequently affect the femur, humerus, skull, and pelvis and can result in pathologic fractures. Survival is usually less than 1 year. Differentiating malignancy from Paget's disease may require a biopsy.[265,266]

Chondrosarcoma has been reported as the second most common of the malignant bone tumors. This tumor may occur as a primary tumor or as a malignant transformation in the setting of benign lesions, such as enchondromas or osteochondromas.[267] Fibrosarcoma is significantly less common than the previously mentioned tumors and accounts for less than 4% of primary malignant bone tumors.[268]

As a group, round cell tumors include primary lymphoma of bone, Ewing's sarcoma, and metastatic neuroblastoma. Ewing's sarcoma is a common primary bone tumor of childhood. Giant cell tumors as a group account for 4.5% of bone tumors. They usually arise from the metaphysis or epiphysis of long bones, generally around the knee. Most are benign, but a few are malignant lesions, usually arising out of a previously irradiated benign giant cell tumor.[260]

In addition to the primary malignancies of bone, a plethora of malignant tumors can arise from mesenchymal connective tissue; these are also known as *sarcomas*.[268,269] They can result in joint complaints, but more often result in soft tissue complaints. They are very rare. Rhabdomyosarcoma is a malignant tumor arising from muscle tissue. It is the fourth most common solid tumor in children and is responsible for more than half of all soft tissue sarcomas in children. Rhabdomyosarcoma rarely occurs in adults. It can appear at any site, and the symptoms most often are referable to the site involved. Most commonly, rhabdomyosarcoma affects the orbits, genitourinary tract, limbs, head and neck, and parameningeal areas. It commonly metastasizes to lymph nodes, lungs, and bone.[262,270]

Metastatic Disease

When bone lesions are identified, primary tumors need to be considered, although most malignant lesions in bone are metastatic. Metastasis rarely affects muscles, joints, or adjacent connective tissue. More commonly, it affects bone. The most common sites of metastasis are the spine and pelvis. It is uncommon to find metastatic lesions distal to the elbow, and, although rare, metastasis to the foot is more common than to the hand.[271] When distal or acral metastasis is identified, it is often associated with lung cancer.[272] Primary tumors generally associated with metastases to bone include tumors in the prostate, thyroid, lung, breast, and kidney.[273] Although most skeletal metastases do not produce pain, one of the most common causes of cancer pain is infiltration of bone. The pain can be intense and stabbing or dull. It is often constant rather than intermittent, is worse at night, and often is worse with weight bearing and movement.[274] Rheumatic or arthritic complaints often occur before lesions are easily identified on radiographs. Arthritis associated with metastatic carcinoma is most commonly monoarticular and most commonly affects the knee. Metastases to the hip, ankle, wrist, hand, and foot have been reported, but occur less frequently. Breast and lung carcinomas are present in most patients.[275] Metastases to the extremities can simulate gout, osteomyelitis, tenosynovitis, or acro-osteolysis. Joint involvement can be related to direct synovial implantation or involvement of the juxta-articular or subchondral bone.[276] Table 122-5 presents the clinical features suggestive of underlying metastases.

Radiographic features of bone tumors can be significant when the duration of disease and the type of malignancy are interpreted. Lesions may be lytic or blastic, and patterns of destruction often reflect the aggressiveness of tumors. Well-circumscribed lesions may be indicative of slower growth, whereas a "moth-eaten" pattern with evidence of cortical destruction typically signifies a more rapid rate of growth. What has been described as a permeative pattern suggests an extremely rapid rate of destruction and is often associated with an extraosseous soft tissue mass.[260] Computed tomography, magnetic resonance imaging, and radionucleotide imaging can provide significant information for diagnosis, staging, prognosis, and therapy.

Table 122-5 Frequent Features of Arthritis Resulting from Metastatic Carcinoma

Presence of constitutional symptoms
Prior history of malignancy
Protracted clinical course
Negative culture results, negative crystal analysis
Medical therapeutic failure
Rapid reaccumulation of hemorrhagic noninflammatory effusion
Radiologic evidence of destructive process

Postchemotherapy Rheumatism

Several rheumatic or musculoskeletal manifestations can develop in patients after administration of chemotherapy for the treatment of malignancy. Postchemotherapy rheumatism has been best described in patients treated for breast cancer, but has also been described in other malignancies, including ovarian cancer and non-Hodgkin's lymphoma.[277-279] The phenomenon has been described as a noninflammatory, self-limited, migratory arthropathy. Typically, symptoms develop several weeks to several months after the completion of chemotherapy and often include myalgia, stiffness, arthralgia, and arthritis involving the small joints of the hands, ankles, and knees.[278] It can be mistaken for RA based on its symptoms; however, most patients have little or no evidence of synovial thickening and have no radiographic or serologic evidence to suggest RA. The pathogenesis of this process is unknown; however, it is self-limited, usually lasting less than 1 year, and is best treated in a conservative fashion. Evaluation should be performed to exclude recurrent carcinoma or another inflammatory condition. The medications most frequently implicated in this phenomenon include cyclophosphamide, 5-fluorouracil, methotrexate, and tamoxifen.[279-281]

Other immunomodulatory agents also have been linked to the development of musculoskeletal findings. Tamoxifen use has been associated with the development of an acute inflammatory arthritis similar to RA[281]; however, a randomized controlled trial of tamoxifen or placebo in 7145 women at high risk for breast cancer (but without a diagnosis of cancer) did not find an increased prevalence of arthralgia or arthritis symptoms in the tamoxifen arm.[282] More recently, aromatase inhibitors have been used widely for hormone receptor–positive breast cancer, with increasing reports of associated arthralgia and arthritis. A retrospective, exploratory analysis of the Arimidex Tamoxifen Alone or in Combination (ATAC) trial evaluated the development of joint symptoms in 5433 women with early breast cancer randomized to receive anastrozole alone or tamoxifen alone.[283] When analysis was limited to women who entered the study without joint symptoms at randomization, 35.2% developed joint symptoms on anastrozole compared with 30.3% on tamoxifen (P < .0001). However, intensity of symptoms was not different between groups. A prospective, nonrandomized study evaluated the prevalence of musculoskeletal symptoms in women who switched from anastrozole to letrozole because of articular symptoms.[284] Most (61%) were able to continue with letrozole, with 28.5% discontinuing the second aromatase inhibitor owing to severe musculoskeletal symptoms. Therefore, switching of aromatase inhibitors may be a reasonable strategy when an initial agent is intolerable because of arthralgia or arthritis; many women continue to be intolerant to more than one agent.

Biologic agents used for the treatment of chronic viruses or a variety of malignancies can similarly lead to autoimmune phenomenon. Use of interleukin-2 can result in spondyloarthritis or inflammatory arthritis. Interferon-α administration can result in seropositive nodular RA and myalgia and arthralgia.[285,286] Use of interferon can also result in autoantibody formation and features suggestive of SLE and autoimmune thyroid disease.[286-288]

LYMPHOPROLIFERATIVE AND MYELOPROLIFERATIVE DISEASES

Leukemia

Leukemia can result in the development of musculoskeletal complaints. Bone pain, the most common musculoskeletal manifestation, has been reported to occur in 50% of adults with leukemia.[289] Long bone pain is more common in children, whereas axial pain is more common in adults. Generally, bone pain is more common in the lower than the upper extremities.[290] Overt synovitis can develop in association with acute and chronic leukemia and can lead to the development of monoarticular or polyarticular arthritis.[291] The pathogenesis seems to be leukemic infiltration of the synovium and subperiosteal tissue. Bleeding or hemorrhage in the joint also may be associated with the process. Most cases of arthritis associated with leukemia are seen in children—14% to 50% compared with 4% to 16.5% in adults.[292-294]

In a series of adult patients with acute leukemia studied over a 10-year period, 5.8% (8 of 139) of patients presented with rheumatic manifestations. On average, symptoms of arthritis preceded the diagnosis of leukemia by 3.25 months.[295] The most common patterns of presentation included asymmetric large joint involvement in association with low back pain, followed by symmetric polyarthritis mimicking early RA. Rheumatic manifestations included morning stiffness, low back pain, nonarticular bone pain, pain out of proportion to objective findings, low-grade fever, and elevation of the ESR. The response to NSAIDs, glucocorticoids, and conventional antirheumatic therapy was reportedly poor, but tumor-directed chemotherapy resulted in substantial improvement of rheumatic manifestations. Patients with these manifestations were more likely to exhibit early osteopenia or lytic bone lesions. Ultimately, prognosis and mortality rates were no different between patients presenting with or without rheumatic manifestations.[295]

In contrast, a large retrospective study of children with leukemia found that 21.4% (36 of 168) with acute lymphoblastic leukemia and 10.5% (6 of 57) with acute nonlymphoblastic leukemia developed symptoms associated with bones and joints. Thirteen of these patients with acute lymphoblastic leukemia had evidence of bony lesions on radiographs.[296] Many of these children had been incorrectly treated for juvenile RA or osteomyelitis before the diagnosis of leukemia. The group with bone lesions seemed to do very well; their condition might fall into a subgroup of childhood leukemia that has a better prognosis.[291,296] A more recent study found that the presence of subtle blood count changes and nighttime pain may help distinguish leukemia from juvenile RA.[294]

Multiple Myeloma

Multiple myeloma is a neoplastic proliferation of plasma cells, causing a nonosseous malignant tumor to arise in the marrow. In contrast to the other primary tumors of bone, which have their highest incidence in children and adolescents, myeloma is a tumor of adults, occurring most commonly in the fifth and sixth decades of life. The most common musculoskeletal feature of this disease is the development of bone pain. Other hallmark features are diffuse pain and stiffness. Patients characteristically develop osteopenia, and osteolytic lesions are seen on radiographs. Lytic lesions, which can occur in any area of the skeleton, are produced by focal accumulations of plasma cells. Osteosclerotic lesions also have been reported.[297] True arthritis is rare, but cases of arthritis secondary to articular and periarticular invasion with malignant cells have been reported in multiple myeloma and in Waldenström's macroglobulinemia.[298] A secondary feature of the disease, which can often lead to additional musculoskeletal complaints, is the development of hyperuricemia and secondary gout. Sjögren's syndrome and other autoimmune phenomena have also been described in association with multiple myeloma.[299]

Lymphoma

Musculoskeletal symptoms have been reported in 25% of cases of non-Hodgkin's lymphoma.[300] The most common musculoskeletal problem associated with lymphoma is the development of bone pain associated with metastasis or lymphoma in the bone. By report, more than 50% of patients have evidence of bone lesions at autopsy; however, few patients actually present with arthritis or bone pain.[291,301] Nonetheless, non-Hodgkin's lymphoma has been reported to manifest as a seronegative arthritis with or without other features, such as lymphadenopathy and hepatomegaly, typically seen with this disease. Monarticular and polyarticular involvement can occur. Cases of polyarthritis simulating RA in the setting of non-Hodgkin's lymphoma have been reported.[302] Although it is unusual to see direct involvement of the synovium, this has also been reported. Cases with radiographic evidence of bone destruction have been associated with non-Hodgkin's lymphomatous arthropathy.[303] Suspicion of lymphoma should be heightened in patients in whom severe constitutional symptoms seem out of proportion to the degree of arthritis, especially in patients who are negative for rheumatoid factor.

Angioimmunoblastic Lymphadenopathy

Angioimmunoblastic lymphadenopathy is a rare lymphoproliferative disorder marked by the clinical features of lymphadenopathy, hepatosplenomegaly, rash, and hypergammaglobulinemia. Patients can develop a nonerosive, symmetric, seronegative polyarthritis concurrent with other features, or as an initial complaint of the disease.[304-306] Similar features have been reported with intravascular lymphoma, with a report of a patient presenting with a symmetric polyarthritis accompanied by fever.[307] Table 122-6 lists musculoskeletal complaints reported with hematologic malignancy.

Graft-versus-Host Disease

Graft-versus-host disease is a complication of bone marrow transplantation and a major cause of morbidity and mortality in the transplant population. Numerous musculoskeletal complaints arise in the setting of acute graft-versus-host

Table 122-6 Musculoskeletal Manifestations of Hematologic Malignancy

Malignancy	Pathogenesis
Leukemia	Infiltration of synovium
Lymphoma	Metastases or invasion of bone, rarely joint
Angioblastic lymphadenopathy	Vasculitis, cryoglobulinemia
Multiple myeloma	Metastasis or invasion of bone, hyperuricemia

disease (lasting 0 to 3 months) and of chronic graft-versus-host disease (lasting >3 months after transplantation). The most frequent manifestation is involvement of the skin, which in many cases can progress to resemble the changes of systemic sclerosis. Skin changes consistent with eosinophilic fasciitis also have been reported.[290] Graft-versus-host disease can lead to symptoms of keratoconjunctivitis sicca and xerostomia resembling Sjögren's syndrome. Other features, including arthralgias, arthritis, myositis, Raynaud's phenomenon, and serositis, have also been reported.[290]

SUMMARY

A plethora of factors contribute to the development of musculoskeletal syndromes in the setting of autoimmune disease and malignancy. A great many autoimmune disorders are known, and for most, the underlying cause and pathogenesis have not been elucidated. This incredible diversity often makes understanding the relationships between associated symptoms difficult. To allow any generalizations regarding an association between an autoimmune disorder and the subsequent development of malignancy, large numbers of patients must be studied longitudinally for exceptionally long periods. Other confounders complicate the picture. Many of the agents used in the treatment of connective tissue and autoimmune disorders modulate the immune system. These agents may have direct carcinogenic potential, whereas others may affect the immune system in a way that may decrease tumor surveillance, subsequently leading to the development of a neoplasm. Intricately entwined are the unique differences among individual immune systems, not only in healthy individuals, but also in individuals whose immune systems are already altered because of an underlying autoimmune disorder. Although uncommon, it is plausible that virtually any of the autoimmune-based diseases and the agents used to treat them might be associated with malignancy in certain circumstances. Most important, when musculoskeletal symptoms arise, malignancy or paraneoplastic syndromes should be considered in the differential diagnosis, especially when patients present with atypical features of autoimmune disease or are refractory to conventional treatment. In addition, the potential for any agent to induce a neoplastic process must be weighed against its proposed benefits before it can be initiated as therapy.

Selected References

3. Zupanicic M, Annamalai A, Brenneman J, Ranatunga S: Migratory polyarthritis as a paraneoplastic syndrome, *J Gen Intern Med* 23:2136, 2008.

6. Gonzalez-Gay MA, Garcia-Porrua C, Salvarani C, et al: Cutaneous vasculitis and cancer: a clinical approach, *Clin Exp Rheumatol* 18:305, 2000.

7. Buggaini G, Krysenka A, Grazzini M, et al: Paraneoplastic vasculitis and paraneoplastic vascular syndromes, *Dermatol Ther* 23:597–605, 2010.

10. Bachmeyer C, Wetterwald E, Aractingi S: Cutaneous vasculitis in the course of hematologic malignancies, *Dermatology* 210:8, 2005.

11. Hamidou MA, Derenne S, Audrain MAP, et al: Prevalence of rheumatic manifestations and antineutrophil cytoplasmic antibodies in haematological malignancies: a prospective study, *Rheumatology (Oxford)* 39:417, 2000.

12. Hamidou MA, Boumalassa A, Larroche C, et al: Systemic medium-sized vessel vasculitis associated with chronic myelomonocytic leukemia, *Semin Arthritis Rheum* 31:119, 2001.

15. Knight AM, Ekbom A, Askling J: Cancer risk in a population based cohort of patients with Wegener's granulomatosis, *Arthritis Rheum* 44:S332, 2001 (abstract 1677).

17. Pankhurst T, Savage COS, Gordon C, et al: Malignancy is increased in ANCA-associated vasculitis, *Rheumatology (Oxford)* 43:1532, 2004.

19. Podjasek JO, Wetter DA, Pittelkow MR, Wada DA: Cutaneous small-vessel vasculitis associated with solid organ malignancies: the Mayo Clinic experience, 1996-2009, *J Am Acad Dermatol* 66:e55, 2012.

20. Dammacco F, Sansonno D, Piccoli C, et al: The cryoglobulins: an overview, *Eur J Clin Invest* 31:628, 2001.

21. Vallat L, Benhamou Y, Gutierrez M, et al: Clonal B cell populations in the blood and liver of patients with chronic hepatitis C virus infection, *Arthritis Rheum* 50:3668, 2004.

23. Ramos-Casals M, Garcia-Carrasco M, Trejo O, et al: Lymphoproliferative diseases in patients with cryoglobulinemia: clinical description of 27 cases, *Arthritis Rheum* 44:S58, 2001.

24. Monti G, Pioltelli P, Saccardo F, et al: Incidence and characteristics of non-Hodgkin lymphomas in a multicenter case file of patients with hepatitis C virus-related symptomatic mixed cryoglobulinemias, *Arch Intern Med* 165:101, 2005.

25. Bianco E, Marcucci F, Mele A, et al: Prevalence of hepatitis C virus infection in lymphoproliferative diseases other than B-cell non-Hodgkin's lymphoma, and in myeloproliferative diseases: an Italian multi-center case-control study, *Haematologica* 89:70, 2004.

29. Naschitz JE, Boss JH, Misselevich I, et al: The fasciitis-panniculitis syndromes: clinical and pathologic features, *Medicine (Baltimore)* 75:6, 1996.

32. Pfinsgraff J, Buckingham RB, Killian PJ, et al: Palmar fasciitis and arthritis with malignant neoplasms: a paraneoplastic syndrome, *Semin Arthritis Rheum* 16:118, 1986.

37. Mekhail N, Kapural L: Complex regional pain syndrome type I in cancer patients, *Curr Rev Pain* 4:227, 2000.

38. Michaels RM, Sorber JA: Reflex sympathetic dystrophy as a probable paraneoplastic syndrome: case report and literature review, *Arthritis Rheum* 27:1183, 1984.

42. Kalgaard OM, Seem E, Kvernebo K: Erythromelalgia: a clinical study of 87 cases, *J Intern Med* 242:191, 1997.

43. Kurzrock R, Cohen PR: Erythromelalgia and myeloproliferative disorders, *Arch Intern Med* 149:105, 1989.

48. Cohen JS: Erythromelalgia: new theories and new therapies, *J Am Acad Dermatol* 43(5 Pt 1):841, 2000.

49. Gonzalez-Gay MA, Garcia-Porrua C, Salvarani C, et al: Polymyalgia manifestations in different conditions mimicking polymyalgia rheumatica, *Clin Exp Rheumatol* 18:755, 2000.

53. Haugeberg G, Dovland H, Johnsen V: Increased frequency of malignancy found in patients presenting with new-onset polymyalgic symptoms suggested to have polymyalgia rheumatica, *Arthritis Rheum* 47:346, 2002.

54. Myklebust G, Wilsgaard T, Jacobsen BK, et al: No increased frequency of malignancy neoplasms in polymyalgia rheumatica and temporal arteritis: a prospective longitudinal study of 398 cases and matched population controls, *J Rheumatol* 29:2143, 2002.

58. Kermani TA, Schafer VS, Crowson CS, et al: Malignancy risk in patients with giant cell arteritis: a population-based cohort study, *Arthritis Care Res* 62:149, 2010.

59. DeCross AJ, Sahasrabudhe DM: Paraneoplastic Raynaud's phenomenon, *Am J Med* 92:571, 1992.

71. Olivieri I, Salvarani C, Cantini F: RS3PE syndrome: an overview, *Clin Exp Rheumatol* 18(4 Suppl 20):S53, 2000.

73. Russell EB: Remitting seronegative symmetrical synovitis with pitting edema syndrome: followup for neoplasia, *J Rheumatol* 32:1760, 2005.

75. Trotta F, Castellino G, Lo Monaco A: Multicentric reticulohistiocytosis, *Best Pract Res Clin Rheumatol* 18:759, 2004.

76. Snow JL, Muller SA: Malignancy-associated multicentric reticulohistiocytosis: a clinical, histological, and immunophenotypic study, *Br J Dermatol* 133:71, 1995.

82. Swissa M, Amital-Teplizki H, Haim N, et al: Autoantibodies in neoplasia: an unresolved enigma, *Cancer* 65:2554, 1990.

83. Armas JB, Dantas J, Mendonca D, et al: Anticardiolipin and antinuclear antibodies in cancer patients: a case control study, *Clin Exp Rheumatol* 18:227, 2000.

85. Solans-Laque R, Perez-Bocanegra C, Salud-Salvia A, et al: Clinical significance of antinuclear antibodies in malignant diseases: association with rheumatic and connective tissue paraneoplastic syndromes, *Lupus* 13:159, 2004.

86. Petri M: Epidemiology of the antiphospholipid antibody syndrome, *J Autoimmun* 15:145, 2000.

87. Asherson RA: Antiphospholipid antibodies, malignancy and paraproteinemias, *J Autoimmun* 15:117, 2000.

93. Bairey O, Blickstein D, Monselise Y, et al: Antiphospholipid antibodies may be a new prognostic parameter in aggressive non-Hodgkin's lymphoma, *Br J Haematol* 76:384, 2006.

95. Gomez-Puerta JA, Cervera R, Espinosa G, et al: Antiphospholipid antibodies associated with malignancies: clinical and pathological characteristics of 120 patients, *Semin Arthritis Rheum* 35:322, 2006.

98. Jan de Beur SM: Tumor-induced osteomalacia, *JAMA* 294:1260, 2005.

104. Bouros D, Hatzakis K, Labrakis H, et al: Association of malignancy with diseases causing interstitial pulmonary changes, *Chest* 121:1278, 2002.

106. Reich JM, Mullooly JP, Johnson RE: Linkage analysis of malignancy-associated sarcoidosis, *Chest* 107:605, 1995.

108. Ji J, Shu X, Li X, et al: Cancer risk in hospitalized sarcoidosis patients: a follow-up study in Sweden, *Ann Oncol* 20:1121, 2009.

110. Boffetta P, Rabkin CS, Gridley G: A cohort study of cancer among sarcoidosis patients, *Int J Cancer* 124:2697, 2009.

111. Katznenstein ALA, Doxtader E, Narendra S: Lymphomatoid granulomatosis: insights gained over 4 decades, *Am J Surg Pathol* 34:e35, 2010.

113. Jaffe ES, Wilson WH: Lymphomatoid granulomatosis: pathogenesis, pathology and clinical implications, *Cancer Surv* 30:233, 1997.

114. Katzenstein AA, Carrington CB, Liebow AA: Lymphomatoid granulomatosis: a clinicopathologic study of 152 cases, *Cancer* 43:360, 1979.

119. Madan V, Chinoy H, Griffiths CE, Cooper RG: Defining cancer risk in dermatomyositis. Part I, *Clin Exp Dermatol* 34:451, 2009.

120. Hill CL, Zhang Y, Sigurgeirsson B, et al: Frequency of specific cancer types in dermatomyositis and polymyositis: a population based study, *Lancet* 357:96, 2001.

121. Stockton D, Doherty VR, Brewster DH: Risk of cancer in patients with dermatomyositis or polymyositis, and follow-up implications: a Scottish population-based cohort study, *Br J Cancer* 85:41, 2001.

122. Buchbinder F, Forbes A, Hall S, et al: Incidence of malignant disease in biopsy-proven inflammatory myopathy, *Ann Intern Med* 134:1087, 2001.

123. Chen YJ, Wu CY, Shen JL: Predicting factors of malignancy in dermatomyositis and polymyositis: a case-control study, *Br J Dermatol* 144:825, 2001.

126. Boussen H, Megazaa A, Nasr C, et al: Dermatomyositis and nasopharyngeal carcinoma: report of 8 cases, *Arch Dermatol* 142:112, 2006.

127. Azuma K, Yamada H, Ohkubo M, et al: Incidence and predictive factors for malignancies in 136 Japanese patients with dermatomyositis, polymyositis, and clinically amyopathic dermatomyositis, *Mod Rheumatol* 21:178, 2011.

133. Sato S, Kuwana M: Clinically amyopathic dermatomyositis, *Curr Opin Rheumatol* 22:639, 2010.

138. Sparsa A, Liozon E, Herrmann F, et al: Routine versus extensive malignancy search for adult dermatomyositis and polymyositis: a study of 40 patients, *Arch Dermatol* 138:885, 2002.

140. Selva-O'Callaghan A, Grau JM, Gamez-Cenzano C, et al: Conventional cancer screening versus PET/CT in dermatomyositis/polymyositis, *Am J Med* 123:558, 2010.

141. Fardet L, Dupuy A, Gain M, et al: Factors associated with underlying malignancy in a retrospective cohort of 121 patients with dermatomyositis, *Medicine (Baltimore)* 88:91, 2009.

145. Hunger RE, Durr C, Brand CU: Cutaneous leukocytoclastic vasculitis in dermatomyositis suggests malignancy, *Dermatology* 202:123, 2001.

148. Talal N, Bunim J: The development of malignant lymphoma in the course of Sjögren's syndrome, *Am J Med* 36:529, 1964.

150. Sutcliffe N, Inanc M, Speight P, et al: Predictors of lymphoma development in primary Sjögren's syndrome, *Semin Arthritis Rheum* 28:80, 1998.

154. Ioannidis JPA, Vassiliou VA, Moutsopoulos HM: Long-term risk of mortality and lymphoproliferative disease and predictive classification of primary Sjögren's syndrome, *Arthritis Rheum* 46:741, 2002.

155. Baimpa E, Dahabreh IJ, Voulgarelis M, Moutsopoulos HM: Hematologic manifestations and predictors of lymphoma development in primary Sjögren syndrome, *Medicine (Baltimore)* 88:284, 2009.

156. Voulgarelis M, Moutsopoulos HM: Mucosa-associated lymphoid tissue lymphoma in Sjögren's syndrome: risks, management, and prognosis, *Rheum Dis Clin N Am* 34:921, 2008.

160. Smedby KE, Hjalgrim H, Askling J, et al: Autoimmune and chronic inflammatory disorders and risk of non-Hodgkin lymphoma by subtype, *J Natl Cancer Inst* 98:51, 2006.

161. Zintzaras E, Voulgarelis M, Moutsopoulos HM: The risk of lymphoma development in autoimmune diseases, *Arch Intern Med* 165:2337, 2005.

162. Engels EA, Cerhan JR, Linet MS, et al: Immune-related conditions and immune-modulating medications as risk factors for non-Hodgkin's lymphoma: a case-control study, *Am J Epidemiol* 162:1153, 2005.

163. Theander E, Henriksson G, Ljungbery O, et al: Lymphoma and other malignancies in primary Sjögren's syndrome, *Ann Rheum Dis* 65:796, 2006.

175. Isomaki HA, Hakulinen T, Joutsenlathi U: Excess risk of lymphomas, leukemia and myeloma in patients with rheumatoid arthritis, *J Chronic Dis* 31:691, 1978.

176. Mellemkjaer L, Linet MS, Gridley G, et al: Rheumatoid arthritis and cancer risk, *Eur J Cancer* 32:1753, 1996.

177. Gridley G, McLaughlin JK, Ekbom A, et al: Incidence of cancer among patients with rheumatoid arthritis, *J Natl Cancer Inst* 85:307, 1993.

178. Ekström K, Hjalgrim H, Brandt L, et al: Risk of malignant lymphomas in patients with rheumatoid arthritis and in their first-degree relatives, *Arthritis Rheum* 48:963, 2003.

179. Wolfe F, Michaud K: Lymphoma in rheumatoid arthritis: the effect of methotrexate and anti-tumor necrosis factor therapy in 18,572 patients, *Arthritis Rheum* 50:1740, 2004.

180. Setoguchi S, Solomon DH, Weinblatt ME, et al: Tumor necrosis factor α antagonist use and cancer in patients with rheumatoid arthritis, *Arthritis Rheum* 54:2757, 2006.

181. Franklin J, Lunt M, Bunn D, et al: Incidence of lymphoma in a large primary-care derived cohort of inflammatory polyarthritis, *Ann Rheum Dis* 65:617, 2006.

182. Thomas E, Brewster DH, Black RJ: Risk of malignancy among patients with rheumatic conditions, *Int J Cancer* 88:497, 2000.

183. Cibere J, Sibley J, Haga M: Rheumatoid arthritis and the risk of malignancy, *Arthritis Rheum* 40:1580, 1997.

188. Baecklund E, Backlin C, Iliadou A, et al: Characteristics of diffuse large B cell lymphomas in rheumatoid arthritis, *Arthritis Rheum* 54:3774, 2006.

189. Baecklund E, Ekbom A, Sparen P, et al: Disease activity and risk of lymphoma in patients with rheumatoid arthritis: nested case-control study, *BMJ* 317:180, 1998.

190. Baecklund E, Iliadou A, Askling J, et al: Association of chronic inflammation, not its treatment, with increased lymphoma risk in rheumatoid arthritis, *Arthritis Rheum* 54:692, 2006.

191. Hellgren K, Smedby KE, Feltelius N, et al: Do rheumatoid arthritis and lymphoma share risk factors? *Arthritis Rheum* 62:1252, 2010.

194. Tennis P, Andrews E, Bombardier C, et al: Record linkage to conduct an epidemiologic study on the association of rheumatoid arthritis and lymphoma in the province of Saskatchewan, Canada, *J Clin Epidemiol* 46:685, 1993.

196. Wolfe F, Michaud K: Biologic treatment of rheumatoid arthritis and the risk of malignancy, *Arthritis Rheum* 56:2886, 2007.

197. Smitten AL, Simon TA, Hochberg MC, Suissa S: A meta-analysis of the incidence of malignancy in adult patients with rheumatoid arthritis, *Arthritis Res Ther* 10:R45, 2008.

198. Askling J, Fored CM, Brandt L, et al: Risks of solid cancers in patients with rheumatoid arthritis and after treatment with tumour necrosis factor antagonists, *Ann Rheum Dis* 64:1421, 2005.

200. Khurana R, Wolf R, Berney S, et al: Risk of development of lung cancer is increased in patients with rheumatoid arthritis: a large case control study in US veterans, *J Rheumatol* 35:1704, 2008.

203. Buchbinder R, Barber M, Heuzenroeder L, et al: Incidence of melanoma and other malignancies among rheumatoid arthritis patients treated with methotrexate, *Arthritis Rheum* 59:794, 2008.

205. Pettersson T, Pukkala E, Teppo L, et al: Increased risk of cancer in patients with systemic lupus erythematosus, *Ann Rheum Dis* 51:437, 1992.

218. Sultan SM, Ioannou Y, Isenberg A: Is there an association of malignancy with systemic lupus erythematosus? An analysis of 276 patients under long-term review, *Rheumatology (Oxford)* 39:1147, 2000.

220. Bernatsky S, Clarke A, Ramsey-Goldman R: Malignancy and systemic lupus erythematosus, *Curr Rheum Rep* 4:351, 2002.

221. Bernatsky S, Boivin J, Clarke A, et al: Cancer risk in SLE: a meta-analysis, *Arthritis Rheum* 44:S244, 2001.

222. Bernatsky S, Boivin JF, Joseph L, et al: An international cohort study of cancer in systemic lupus erythematosus, *Arthritis Rheum* 52:1481, 2005.

226. Bernatsky S, Boivin JF, Joseph L, et al: Race/ethnicity and cancer occurrence in systemic lupus erythematosus, *Arthritis Rheum* 53:781, 2005.

232. Santana IU, Gomes AD, Lyrio LD, et al: Systemic lupus erythematosus, human papillomavirus infection, cervical pre-malignant and malignant disease: a systematic review, *Clin Rheumatol* 30:665, 2011.

233. Bernatsky S, Ramsey-Goldman R, Gordon C, et al: Factors associated with abnormal Pap results in systemic lupus erythematosus, *Rheumatology (Oxford)* 43:1386, 2004.

239. Bernatsky S, Joseph L, Boivin JF, et al: The relationship between cancer and medication exposures in systemic lupus erythaematosus: a case-cohort study, *Ann Rheum Dis* 67:74, 2008.

241. Wooten M: Systemic sclerosis and malignancy: a review of the literature, *South Med J* 101:59, 2008.

248. Hill CL, Nguyen AM, Roder D, et al: Risk of cancer in patients with scleroderma: a population based cohort study, *Ann Rheum Dis* 62:728, 2003.

249. Derk CT, Rasheed M, Artlett CM, et al: A cohort study of cancer incidence in systemic sclerosis, *J Rheumatol* 33:1123, 2006.

251. Pontifex EK, Hill CL, Roberts-Thompson P: Risk factors for lung cancer in patients with scleroderma: a nested case-control study, *Ann Rheum Dis* 66:551, 2007.

254. Chatterjee S, Dombi GW, Severson RK, et al: Risk of malignancy in scleroderma: a population-based cohort study, *Arthritis Rheum* 52:2415, 2005.

262. Arndt CA, Crist WM: Common musculoskeletal tumors of childhood and adolescence, *N Engl J Med* 341:342, 1999.

263. Hayden JB, Hoang BH: Osteosarcoma: basic science and clinical implications, *Orthop Clin North Am* 37:1, 2006.

265. Hadjipavlou A, Lander P, Srolovitz H, et al: Malignant transformation in Paget's disease of bone, *Cancer* 70:2802, 1992.

266. Mankin HJ, Hornicek FJ: Paget's sarcoma: a historical and outcome review, *Clin Orthop Relat Res* 438:97, 2005.

267. Terek RM: Recent advances in the basic science of chondrosarcoma, *Orthop Clin North Am* 37:9, 2006.

273. Stummvol GH, Aringer M, Machold KP, et al: Cancer polyarthritis resembling rheumatoid arthritis as a first sign of hidden neoplasms, *Scand J Rheumatol* 30:40, 2001.

278. Loprinzi CL, Duffy J, Ingle JN: Postchemotherapy rheumatism, *J Clin Oncol* 11:768, 1993.

279. Kim MJ, Ye YM, Park HS: Chemotherapy-related arthropathy, *J Rheumatol* 33:1364, 2006.

283. Sestak I, Cuzick J, Sapunar F, et al: Risk factors for joint symptoms in patients enrolled into the ATAC trial: a retrospective, exploratory analysis, *Lancet Oncol* 9:866, 2008.

284. Briot K, Tubiana-Hulin M, Bastit L, et al: Effect of a switch of aromatase inhibitors on musculoskeletal symptoms in postmenopausal

women with hormone receptor-positive breast cancer: the ATOLL (Articular Tolerance of Letrozole Study), *Breast Cancer Res Treat* 120:127, 2010.

286. Raanani P, Ben-Bassat I: Immune-mediated complications during interferon therapy in hematological patients, *Acta Haematol* 107:133, 2002.

291. Ehrenfeld M, Gur H, Shoenfeld Y: Rheumatologic features of hematologic disorders, *Curr Opin Rheumatol* 11:62, 1999.

294. Jones OY, Spencer CH, Bowyer SL: A multicenter case-control study on predictive factors distinguishing leukemia from juvenile rheumatoid arthritis, *Pediatrics* 117:840, 2006.

295. Gur H, Koren V, Ehrenfeld M, et al: Rheumatic manifestations preceding adult acute leukemia: characteristics and implication on course and prognosis, *Acta Haematol* 101:1, 1999.

296. Kai T, Ishii E, Matsuzaki A, et al: Clinical and prognostic implications of bone lesions in childhood leukemia at diagnosis, *Leuk Lymphoma* 23:119, 1996.

297. Lacy MZ, Gertz MA, Hanson CA, et al: Multiple myeloma associated with diffuse osteosclerotic bone lesions: a clinical entity distinct from osteosclerotic myeloma (POEMS syndrome), *Am J Hematol* 56:288, 1997.

306. Tsochatzis E, Vassilopoulos D, Deutsch M: Angioimmunoblastic T-cell lymphoma-associated arthritis: case report and literature review, *J Clin Rheumatol* 11:326, 2005.

Full references for this chapter can be found on www.expertconsult.com.

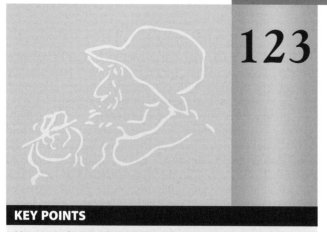

123 Tumors and Tumor-like Lesions of Joints and Related Structures

ANDREW E. ROSENBERG

KEY POINTS

Most mass lesions that involve joints and synovial-lined structures are benign; synovial cysts are the most common. They are not true cysts because they lack an epithelial lining. Synovial cysts may involve joints (Baker's cyst) or tendon sheaths (ganglion cysts). Treatment depends on the symptoms; observation is a reasonable course of action in many cases.

Synovial chondromatosis is an uncommon benign condition characterized by nodules of hyaline cartilage, often ossified, within the subsynovial connective tissue, most frequently involving the knee. Treatment is removal of the nodules.

Tenosynovial giant cell tumor of joints and tendon sheaths, previously known as giant cell tumor of tendon sheath and pigmented villonodular synovitis, affects both sexes equally, usually in the 3rd or 4th decade. Lesions are most often monoarticular, with the knee being involved in 80% of cases. The disease is due to a translocation that results in overexpression of colony-stimulating factor-1. Although they can be locally destructive, the tumors do not metastasize; treatment is removal.

The most common primary malignant tumor of joints is synovial sarcoma, which usually affects children and young adults. The disease has an aggressive course, with a long-term survival of around 50%.

Lymphoproliferative diseases, especially acute leukemia, may involve joints. Joint involvement is most common in children, for whom the reported incidence of joint involvement ranges from 12% to 65%. Arthritis can occur at any time in the course of the disease and can be the presenting complaint. It is due to leukemic infiltration into the synovium.

Joints and periarticular structures are often involved by non-neoplastic, mass-forming lesions, such as synovial cysts and loose bodies. These structures are affected infrequently, however, by benign or malignant neoplasms. Joint neoplasms can be divided into tumors that are primary or arise de novo within the joint and tumors that are secondary and access the joint by invading from neighboring bones and soft tissues, or by spreading from distant sites via the vascular system. Primary joint neoplasms are more common and tend to recapitulate the phenotype of tissues that normally construct the joint and synovial sheath—synovium, fat, blood vessels, fibrous tissue, and cartilage. Regardless of the histologic type, the benign variants greatly outnumber their malignant counterparts, and as a group these tumors tend to develop in the synovium, not in the other periarticular structures. These biologically and morphologically diverse lesions often pose significant challenges in diagnosis and treatment, and their clinicopathologic features are the focus of this chapter.

NON-NEOPLASTIC LESIONS

Synovial and Ganglion Cysts

Cysts are defined as closed compartments or sacs that are lined by epithelium and are frequently filled with fluid. Neither the synovial cyst nor the ganglion cyst is considered a true cyst because each lacks an epithelial lining.

Synovial cysts are common and are formed from the synovial lining of a joint, tendon, or bursa. They are non-neoplastic lesions and are caused by herniation of the synovium through the joint capsule or tendon sheath into neighboring tissues, or by expansion of a pre-existing bursa. In adults, synovial cysts frequently develop in association with a variety of joint disorders, including trauma, osteoarthritis, crystal arthropathies, infection, and rheumatoid arthritis or one of its variants. Most synovial cysts have an anatomic relationship to a joint, and most originate in the posterior aspect of the knee, where they are known as a popliteal or Baker's cyst, followed in frequency by the shoulder and hip. These lesions may also arise in the spine, where they develop from the facet joints, most commonly in the lower lumbar region. The posteromedial region of the knee may be prone to the development of synovial cysts because the synovium-lined joint capsule in this anatomic site may not provide adequate structural support.[1] Synovial cysts of the posterior knee joint are purported to affect 2.4% of children, who, in contrast to adults, are usually asymptomatic and have an otherwise normal knee joint.[2]

Synovial cysts can enlarge as they become increasingly distended with synovial fluid.[1-4] Consequently, they may manifest as a periarticular mass, produce progressive joint pain and swelling, limit joint mobility, and compress adjacent neurovascular structures. An example of the last-mentioned item occurs in the spine, where synovial cysts that arise from facet joints may impinge or extend into spinal nerves, causing radicular pain.[5-7] Other complications of synovial cysts, which sometimes can produce dramatic clinical findings, are acute rupture and secondary infection.

A variety of radiographic techniques have been used to image synovial cysts. Imaging modalities that provide the greatest quantity of diagnostic information include arthrography, ultrasonography, computed tomography (CT), and magnetic resonance imaging (MRI).[1-4] All of these modalities reveal synovial cysts to be simple or septated thin-walled structures associated with joints and periarticular

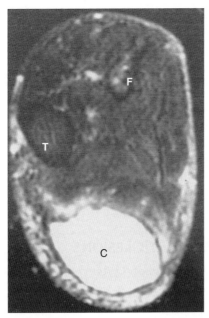

Figure 123-1 Magnetic resonance image shows a high T2 signal intensity, large, oval-shaped synovial cyst that extends from the knee joint into the posterior calf. C, synovial cyst; F, fibula; T, tibia.

structures and filled with fluid, whose density is similar to that of water (Figure 123-1).

Grossly, synovial cysts usually range in size from 1 to 10 cm. Their inner surface is smooth, glistening, and translucent; however, prior hemorrhage or secondary infection may distort this surface by virtue of attached blood clot and inflammatory debris or the generation of granulation tissue. The cyst wall comprises an inner surface lined by flattened or plump cuboidal synoviocytes arranged one or several cell layers thick, which are surrounded by an outer sheath of fibrous tissue (Figure 123-2). Sometimes the synovial lining cells may be hyperplastic and form papillary fronds, and occasionally scattered subsynovial collections of hemosiderin-laden macrophages are indicative of previous hemorrhage. Facet joint cysts often contain abundant amorphous debris surrounded by macrophages and are associated with severe changes of the ligamentum flavum.

Treatment of synovial cysts varies and depends on their location and associated symptoms. These cysts may be managed successfully with conservative therapy; however, in certain situations, surgical excision is required.[1-7]

Ganglion cysts have been recognized for centuries; Hippocrates described them as being composed of "mucoid flesh."[8] They are more common than synovial cysts and arise from tendon sheaths, ligaments, menisci, joint capsules, and bursae.[8] Occasionally, they develop de novo in the subchondral areas of bone, and rarely, they arise within nerve or skeletal muscle and lack communication with a joint. Intraneural ganglia have been shown to develop from dissection of joint fluid along an articular branch of a nerve.[9] Ganglion cysts are distinguished from synovial cysts by virtue of the fact that they lack a surface lining of synoviocytes. A variety of hypotheses have been proposed to explain their pathogenesis, but none have been proven.[8] The most accepted theory is that ganglia develop from mucoid cystic degeneration of periarticular structures. They are commonly associated with repetitive motion activities, inflammatory arthritides, and trauma.

Most ganglia arise along the dorsal and volar aspects of the wrists and fingers and the dorsum of the feet.[8,10] They usually are asymptomatic and typically manifest as a slowly growing, mobile, firm mass that moves with the structure from which it has arisen (Figure 123-3). Ganglia may be painful if traumatized and can compress adjacent neurovascular structures, producing a variety of symptoms. The radiographic characteristics of ganglia are similar to those of synovial cysts, and they appear on images as small, fluid-filled cystic structures.[1,10]

Macroscopically, most ganglia are round, but they may form elongate cylindrical structures if they track along a tendon sheath. Ganglia are uniloculated or multiloculated, have thin walls, and are filled with translucent mucoid fluid (Figure 123-4). The cyst lacks an inner cell lining, and the bulk of the wall consists of dense fibrous tissue, which is usually surrounded by areolar tissue (Figure 123-5). In many instances, the cyst wall is distorted by variable quantities of reactive myxoid tissue and muciphages, which result from small ruptures and extravasation of fluid.

When ganglion cysts form, they may remain stable for years or may spontaneously resolve, and ganglia that disappear may subsequently redevelop. Treatment is frequently conservative because of their innocuous nature. Ganglia

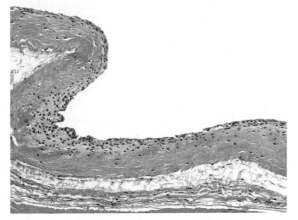

Figure 123-2 Wall of a synovial cyst, composed of an inner lining of synoviocytes overlaying a layer of dense, fibrous tissue.

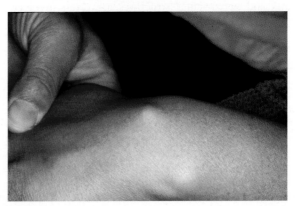

Figure 123-3 Round, firm ganglion cyst bulging from the dorsal aspect of the hand.

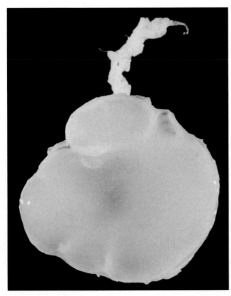

Figure 123-4 Intact ganglion cyst with thread-like pedicle that attaches to a periarticular structure.

Loose Bodies

Loose bodies and *joint mice* are generic terms for free-floating structures within a joint cavity. They are the most common tumor-like lesions of joints and may be exogenous, such as fragments of a bullet, or endogenous, such as pieces of articular cartilage, osteophytes, menisci, ligaments, or bone.[11-13] When not otherwise specified, the term *loose bodies* refers to detached pieces of articular cartilage or subchondral bone (osteoarticular loose bodies) or both that lie free within the joint, or that have become secondarily embedded in the synovium. Loose bodies can cause pain, crepitance, and locking, and they can limit joint range of motion.

Osteoarticular loose bodies are a secondary complication of a variety of conditions, including trauma, osteochondritis

occasionally require aspiration or surgical excision, however, especially if they are symptomatic.

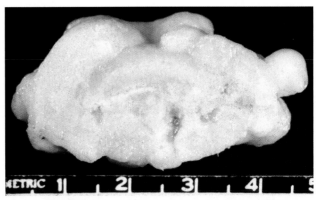

Figure 123-6 Large, nodular loose body formed from a semilunar-shaped piece of articular cartilage that is surrounded by newly formed cartilage.

dissecans, and arthritides of various causes. When dislodged, the sloughed articular cartilage remains viable because it receives its nourishment from the synovial fluid, but the bone dies because it derives its nutrition solely from blood vessels. Over time, as the loose body tumbles within the joint, its edges become rounded and smooth; however, it eventually becomes embedded within the synovium. When the synovium encompasses the loose body, it may digest and resorb it, or adjacent subsynovial connective tissue cells may undergo a proliferative and metaplastic response.

These cells produce layers of newly formed fibrocartilage and hyaline cartilage, which may undergo endochondral ossification and are deposited on the surface of the loose body (Figure 123-6). These layers of newly formed tissue surround the centrally located loose body, similar to the cambium layers of a tree, and provide a mechanism for the whole structure to increase gradually in size and become significantly larger than the initial osteochondral defect from which they originated (Figures 123-7 and 123-8). As the loose body enlarges, the innermost portion of original articular cartilage cannot be supported adequately by diffusion of synovial fluid, and it dies and calcifies. This combination of events causes the loose body to appear on x-rays as dense speckled and ring-like calcifications (Figure 123-9). Radiographically and histologically, the differential

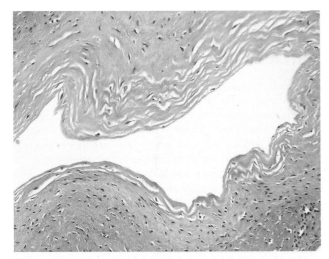

Figure 123-5 Ganglion cyst wall composed of scattered flattened fibroblasts on the luminal surface and a well-formed layer of fibrous tissue.

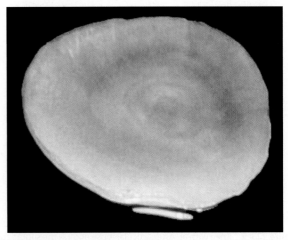

Figure 123-7 Loose body with visible layers of newly formed tissue.

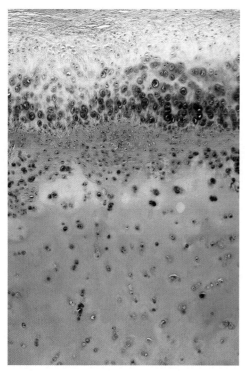

Figure 123-8 Loose body composed of sloughed articular hyaline cartilage *(bottom)* covered by consecutive layers of newly formed metaplastic hyaline cartilage and bone.

diagnosis includes synovial chondromatosis. Treatment is simple excision, which can be done arthroscopically.[12,13]

Intra-articular Ossicles

Small bony nodules normally occur in the knees of some rodents[14] and other mammals and may rarely occur in humans.[15-17] In rodents, they are constantly found in the

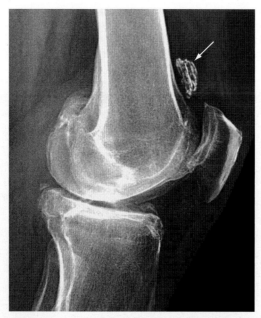

Figure 123-9 Knee with an osteoarticular loose body in the suprapatellar region *(arrow).*

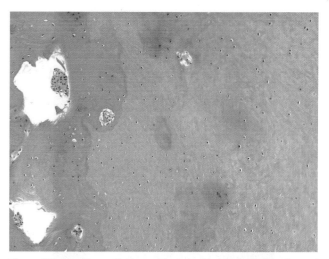

Figure 123-10 Intra-articular ossicle embedded in the fibrocartilage of the meniscus.

anterior portions of the joint and frequently in the posterior portions as well. In humans, nodules develop within the substance of the meniscus of the knee joint adjacent to its attachments to the tibia.

The exact origin of such structures is unknown, although they probably are true sesamoid bones, as seen in rodents, or they may represent ossification secondary to local injury. This latter possibility is supported by the fact that previous knee trauma has been noted in numerous reported cases. The main symptom of meniscal ossicles is pain after exertion, such as walking or prolonged standing, with relief when the knee is at rest. Radiographs may reveal an intra-articular calcification that can be confused with a loose body. MRI shows the ossicle to be a corticated marrow-containing structure that has increased signal intensity on T1-weighted images and decreased signal intensity on T2-weighted images.[15,17] The ossicle is located within the lateral or the medial meniscus and appears as a small ($\approx$1 cm in diameter), palpable bony nodule (Figure 123-10).[16] If the ossicle is symptomatic, it should be excised; however, if it is an incidental finding, it can be managed conservatively.[15,17]

NEOPLASMS

Fatty Lesions of the Synovium

Although the subsynovial connective tissue of diarthrodial joints is rich in fat, a true lipoma of the synovium is rare. When these rare tumors develop, they most frequently affect the knee joint and the synovial sheaths of tendons of the hands, ankles, and feet, where they are more common in the extensor than in the flexor synovial sheaths.[18,19] Synovial lipomas can be sessile or pedunculated, and when pedunculated, they may produce pain if they twist on their stalks and become secondarily ischemic. Synovial lipoma, similar to its subcutaneous counterpart, comprises lobules of mature white adipocytes that are delineated by a thin fibrous capsule.

A more common but still unusual fatty lesion of the joint is lipoma arborescens, also known as *villous lipomatous proliferation* and *lipomatosis of the synovium*.[20,21] This disorder is

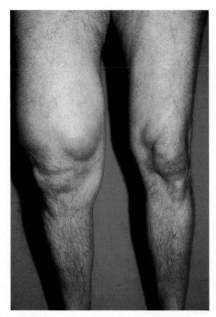

Figure 123-11 Lipoma arborescens manifesting as a suprapatellar mass.

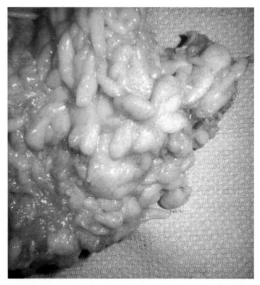

Figure 123-13 Lipoma arborescens composed of a villonodular mass of fatty tissue covered by glistening synovium.

characterized by a diffuse increase in the quantity of subsynovial fat, which bulges into the overlying synovial lining, producing a villous architecture. It is uncertain whether the proliferating fat is neoplastic (lipomatosis) or is a manifestation of a hyperplastic or reactive process. Affected patients are usually adults, but sometimes adolescents and rarely children develop the lesion.[22] Lipoma arborescens causes chronic effusions, pain, and swelling, and restricts joint motion.[21] The duration of symptoms is often long, and symptoms have been reported to be present for as long as 30 years; however, acute onset has been documented.

Lipoma arborescens most commonly arises in the knee (Figure 123-11), especially the suprapatellar portion, although it also has been observed in the hip, ankle, and wrist joints. It is typically localized to one joint, but several cases of bilateral knee involvement have been described.[21] Laboratory studies are unremarkable, and the joint fluid is clear and yellow.[21] Plain films show joint fullness, and findings of osteoarthritis are often present. Arthrography reveals multiple lobulated filling defects, which on CT represent a villonodular mass of low signal intensity that on MRI has the density of fat (Figure 123-12).[23] At surgery, the affected synovium has a prominent villous or villonodular architecture and is tan-yellow (Figure 123-13). Histologically, the lesion comprises sheets of mature adipocytes admixed with nutrient blood vessels, all of which are partially compartmentalized by fibrous septa, and is covered on its intra-articular surface by several layers of synovial cells (Figure 123-14). Synovectomy may relieve the symptoms and prevent effusions, but associated osteoarthritis may be progressive.[21]

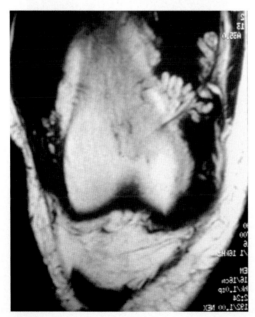

Figure 123-12 Magnetic resonance image of lipoma arborescens shows villonodular mass in the knee joint.

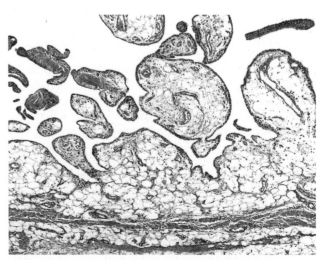

Figure 123-14 Lipoma arborescens with subsynovial compartment filled with mature adipocytes and covered by synoviocytes.

The clinicopathologic differential diagnosis includes diffuse tenosynovial giant cell tumor, synovial chondromatosis, and synovial hemangioma. These lesions can be distinguished easily from lipoma arborescens by their distinct histologic features. Another disorder that should be included in the differential diagnosis is Hoffa's disease—a condition of irritation, inflammation, and hyperplasia of the synovial lining in regions where fat is normally present, such as adjacent to the patella or patellar ligament.[24]

Vascular Lesions of the Synovium

Benign vascular tumors of the synovium are rare. Their growth pattern can be localized or diffuse. They tend to predominate in adolescence and young adulthood, but symptoms frequently can be traced back to childhood.[25] The joint most commonly involved is the knee, but hemangiomas also have been described in the elbow, the ankle, the tarsometatarsal and temporomandibular joints, and the tendon sheaths of the wrist and ankle.[26,27] Unusual complications of synovial hemangiomas include a secondary destructive arthritis and Kasabach-Merritt syndrome.

Synovial hemangiomas produce a variety of symptoms, including unilateral, intermittent joint pain and enlargement, which may result in limitation of motion, locking, buckling, and hemarthrosis, especially after minimal trauma.[26] Classically, the affected joint diminishes in size if sufficiently elevated to allow the blood to drain out of the lesion. On physical examination, the joint is swollen and doughy, and nearby cutaneous hemangiomas may be evident. Joint aspiration frequently yields bloody fluid. Preoperative diagnosis of localized hemangioma is difficult, and the differential diagnosis includes localized tenosynovial giant cell tumor, and in the knee includes discoid meniscus, meniscal tears, cysts, and ossicles.[21] The diffuse hemangioma is more easily identified, but it can mimic diffuse tenosynovial giant cell tumor and hemophilic arthropathy.

Radiographic evaluation may show nothing more than a vague soft tissue shadow indicative of a swollen synovium and a distended joint capsule or regional osteoporosis in patients who have had long-term symptoms and recurrent hemarthrosis. Rarely, calcified phleboliths are apparent; however, they are associated more often with a soft tissue arteriovenous malformation with secondary joint involvement than with an isolated intra-articular hemangioma (Figure 123-15). Arthrography may show an intra-articular filling defect, and arteriography may be negative in small localized capillary hemangiomas, but contrast material may collect in the more diffuse lesions that contain cavernous or large ectatic vascular spaces (Figure 123-16). CT reveals a lobulated soft tissue mass with mild enhancement after contrast injection.[21] MRI may show the tumor to have a low to isointense signal on T1-weighted images and high signal intensity on T2-weighted images.[28]

Macroscopically, the localized hemangioma tends to be small, but larger lesions (8 cm) have been documented.[28] It may be poorly defined, well circumscribed, sessile, or stalked, and ranges in color from red to dark blue-purple. Microscopically, the hemangioma is usually of the cavernous or venous type, with large dilated blood-filled vessels lined by cytologically benign endothelial cells. In arteriovenous

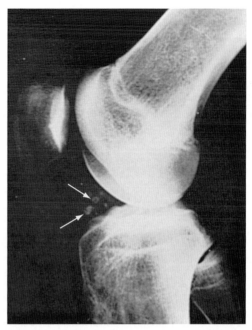

Figure 123-15 Localized synovial hemangioma with phleboliths prominently seen in the joint *(arrows)*. The patient is 16 years old with painful swelling for many years when standing and relief of this pain when the knee is flexed.

hemangioma, which grows in a diffuse fashion, the entire synovium may be edematous and beefy red or stained brown by hemosiderin, and consists of prominent tortuous, congested vessels that may penetrate the joint capsule and extend into neighboring soft tissues. Histologically, the vessels recapitulate architecturally abnormal arteries, veins,

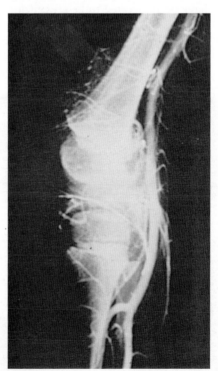

Figure 123-16 Arteriogram of an arteriovenous malformation in the soft tissues of the thigh and leg with involvement of the knee joint. The extensive vascular blush in the knee indicates aberrant synovial and capsular vasculature.

and capillaries; have abnormal interconnections; and are arranged in a disorganized tangle.

Therapy for a localized hemangioma is marginal surgical excision, which usually is curative. Diffuse lesions frequently are difficult to eradicate because of their extensive nature. Incomplete excision or debulking may be the only surgical option. Radiation therapy is not indicated.

Fibroma of Tendon Sheath

Fibroma of tendon sheath is an uncommon benign neoplasm that clinically mimics tenosynovial giant cell tumor but is morphologically distinct. Fibroma of tendon sheath first was identified as a clinicopathologic entity in 1936, and since that time, more than several hundred cases have been reported.[29,30] A translocation t(2;11) (q31-32;q12) that has been identified in this tumor is likely related to its molecular genesis.

Fibroma of tendon sheath usually arises from the tendons and sheaths of the flexor surfaces of the distal extremities; approximately 70% of cases involve the fingers or hand. Of the fingers, the thumb is affected most frequently, followed in descending order by the index and middle fingers.[29] Less commonly, large diarthrodial joints such as the knee and rarely the elbow and ankle are sites of origin.[29-31] Patients range in age from infants to the elderly, but the median age is the early 4th decade of life.[29,30] Most series report a male predominance, with the largest study of 138 cases having a male-to-female ratio of 3 : 1.[29] Patients present with a slow-growing, painless mass that usually has been noted for several months to a year.[30] In 6% to 10% of cases, a history of antecedent trauma is reported. Tumors developing in large joints can be painful, can restrict range of motion, and may be palpable.[32]

Plain x-rays show soft tissue fullness; rarely is evidence of bony erosion noted.[29] CT or MRI shows a solid, well-circumscribed mass of soft tissue density that usually has low signal intensity on T1-weighted and variable intensity on T2-weighted images. At surgery, the tumors are often attached directly to the tendon or tendon sheath. They are rubbery, oblong, well circumscribed, or encapsulated; average 1.5 to 1.8 cm in greatest dimension; and have a tan-white cut surface (Figure 123-17).[29,30]

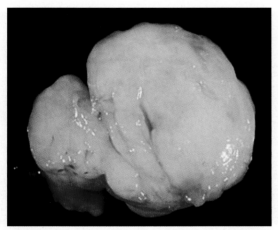

Figure 123-17 Fibroma of tendon sheath that formed a well-circumscribed, tan-white mass.

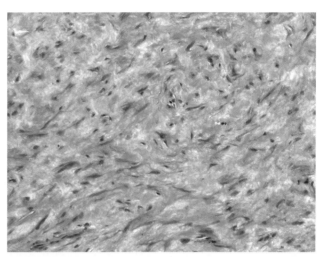

Figure 123-18 Fibroma of tendon sheath composed of a hypocellular collagenous mass.

Microscopically, fibroma of tendon sheath is multilobular, with clefts interposed between adjacent lobules. The lobules are composed of spindle and stellate fibroblasts enmeshed in a collagenous and sometimes myxoid stroma (Figure 123-18). Immunohistochemically, the tumor cells have the staining profile of myofibroblasts, and ultra-structurally, the cells have features of fibroblasts and myofibroblasts.[33]

The natural history of fibroma of tendon sheath consists of slow growth that eventually ceases. The treatment of choice is surgical excision, but a 24% recurrence rate has been reported.[29]

Synovial Chondromatosis

Synovial chondromatosis is an uncommon condition characterized by the formation of multiple nodules of hyaline cartilage within the subsynovial connective tissue. If the cartilage nodules undergo endochondral ossification, the term *synovial osteochondromatosis* is appropriate. It is unclear whether the proliferating cartilage is metaplastic or neoplastic; however, more recent cytogenetic abnormalities involving chromosome 6 found in the cartilage of these lesions support a neoplastic process.[34] Regardless, synovial chondromatosis is benign and does not metastasize.

Synovial chondromatosis most commonly affects middle-aged men, with an average age in the 5th decade of life.[35] Middle-aged women are more likely to develop the disease in the temporomandibular joint. The genders are equally affected with regard to hand and foot involvement, and patients with hand and foot involvement are usually in their 6th decade.

Patients commonly describe joint pain, swelling, stiffness, crepitance, and limitation of motion with a locking or grating sensation on movement.[35] Symptoms usually are long-standing, recurrent, and progressive.

Synovial chondromatosis typically arises in large diarthrodial joints. The knee is affected in more than 50% of cases, usually as a monoarticular condition.[35] Other common sites include the hip, elbow, shoulder, and ankle. Infrequently, synovial chondromatosis arises in the small joints of the hands and feet and in the temporomandibular joint.[36] When cartilage nodules develop in the synovial lining of bursae, tendons, and ligaments, this is known as *extra-articular synovial chondromatosis*.[32] The extra-articular variant most commonly affects the fingers, followed by the toes, hand, wrist, foot, and ankle, and more than one synovial sheath may be involved.[32]

Plain x-ray findings largely depend on whether the cartilage nodules are calcified or ossified, and whether they erode adjacent bony structures. Visible calcifications are absent in 5% to 33% of cases; however, most often, multiple oval intra-articular radiodensities range in size from a few millimeters to several centimeters (Figure 123-19).[37] The pattern of mineralization varies and may appear as irregular flecks that represent calcified cartilage or show a trabecular architecture, which is a manifestation of endochondral ossification. Lesions that are not mineralized can be seen on an arthrogram because they produce multiple filling defects. In approximately 11% of cases, nodules erode the neighboring skeleton, especially along the anterior aspect of the distal femur.

CT may show mass-like nodules in the synovium that have a density similar to skeletal muscle. CT also can detect small calcifications and erosions before they are apparent on plain films. MRI shows that the nodules of cartilage have low signal intensity on T1-weighted sequences and high intensity on T2-weighted sequences; this reflects the high water content of the hyaline cartilage.[37] Areas of calcification or mineralized bone have a low signal intensity on T1-weighted and T2-weighted sequences. CT and MRI scans are helpful in identifying the intra-articular source of the lesion and its anatomic extent. In long-standing disease, the bones adjacent to involved joints may be osteoporotic and may show changes of secondary osteoarthritis.

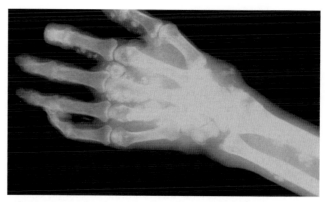

Figure 123-20 Synovial chondromatosis of the hand and forearm. Multiple calcified nodules of varying size are evident in the soft tissues of the fingers, wrist, and forearm.

The cartilage in extra-articular synovial chondromatosis has similar radiographic changes.[37] Nodules of cartilage are frequently mineralized and may appear as a linear arrangement of small calcific densities that are aligned along the sheath and that can span many joints (Figure 123-20).

The radiographic differential diagnosis of synovial chondromatosis includes osteochondritis dissecans, osteoarthritis with loose bodies, tuberculosis, hemopathic arthropathies, pseudogout with extensive synovial calcification, and synovial tumors. In many instances, the clinical presentation and the radiographic picture should lead to the correct diagnosis. However, in many cases, x-rays and the clinical picture are vague, so that only a biopsy specimen can remove all doubt about the diagnosis.

Characteristic of synovial chondromatosis is a thickened synovium containing numerous opalescent firm nodules of cartilage that bulge from the surface in a cobblestone pattern (Figure 123-21). These nodules usually measure less than 5 cm and may lose their attachment to the synovium and form loose bodies, sometimes hundreds of them. The calcified cartilage is white, and areas of ossification manifest as gritty tan trabeculae, which may house fatty marrow. The synovium adjacent to the cartilage may show reactive changes, such as edema, hyperemia, hyperplasia, and villous transformation.

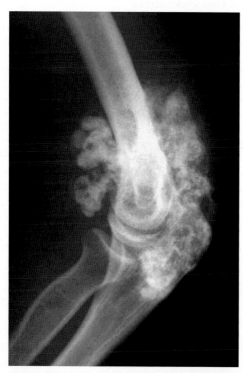

Figure 123-19 Synovial chondromatosis of the elbow. Multiple large calcified bodies fill the joint space and are adjacent to bone.

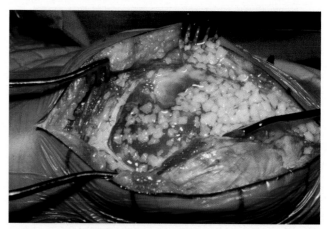

Figure 123-21 Intraoperative appearance of synovial chondromatosis. Innumerable nodules of cartilage fill the joint.

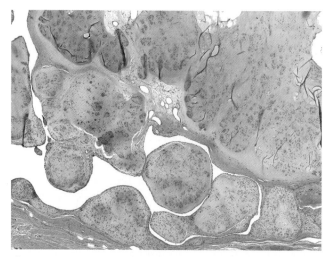

Figure 123-22 Synovial chondromatosis with nodules of hyaline cartilage in the synovium.

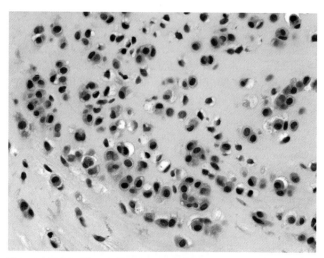

Figure 123-24 The cartilage in synovial chondromatosis can be cellular, and the chondrocytes may exhibit limited cytologic atypia.

Cartilage develops in the connective tissue of the subsynovial compartment (Figure 123-22). Neoplastic chondrocytes produce the hyaline matrix that eventually forms individual nodules, which peripherally abut surrounding tissues (Figure 123-23). Cartilage varies in its cellularity, and chondrocytes range from small to large; some may be binucleate and hyperchromatic, similar to the chondrocytes in intraosseous chondrosarcoma (Figure 123-24). Despite these histologic findings of concern, experience has shown that hypercellular variants with atypical chondrocytes usually behave in a benign fashion. Infrequently, the disease manifests as a single, solitary nodule of cartilage, which may be very large and may undergo partial endochondral ossification. Intra-articular osteochondroma can severely limit joint motion and may be confused clinically with other types of neoplasms.[38]

Over time, nodules of cartilage attached to the synovium are invaded by blood vessels. This invasion results in endochondral ossification, with woven and lamellar bone formation and the development of a medullary cavity with fatty marrow (Figure 123-25). If these nodules lose their synovial attachments and become free-floating, they may continue to increase in size, because the cartilage derives its nourishment from synovial fluid, although the osseous portion and the marrow die.

The treatment of choice for synovial chondromatosis consists of excision of the involved synovium and removal of all loose bodies. The prognosis is good, although recurrences may be noted if removal is incomplete. Most recurrences develop in the setting of diffuse involvement of the synovium.

Synovial chondromatosis rarely undergoes malignant transformation into chondrosarcoma, although in one series, this phenomenon occurred in 5% of cases. However, a significant percentage of the few reported cases of synovial chondrosarcomas have shown evidence of underlying synovial chondromatosis.[39-41] The chondrosarcomatous component exhibits dense hypercellularity, marked cytologic atypia, and mitotic activity; the stroma is often myxoid.

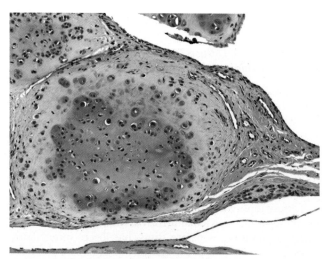

Figure 123-23 Nodules of hyaline cartilage merging with surrounding connective tissue in synovial chondromatosis.

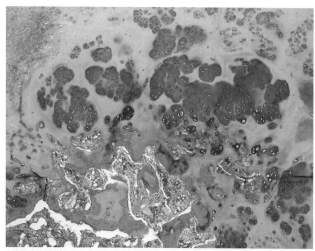

Figure 123-25 Nodules of cartilage in synovial chondromatosis undergoing endochondral ossification.

Chondroma of Tendon Sheath and Periarticular Structures

A solitary soft tissue chondroma is considered to be a benign neoplasm. It commonly arises in tendon sheaths and infrequently involves joint capsules or other periarticular structures.

Tendon sheath chondromas usually arise in the flexor tendon sheaths of the distal extremities and are about three times more common in the hands than in the feet.[42-44] They affect the sexes equally and are detected in early to mid-adulthood, presenting as a painless, slowly growing, firm mass. Radiographically, tendon sheath chondromas appear as an extraosseous, well-delineated soft tissue mass that contains calcifications, which are punctate or ring-like in 33% to 70% of cases.[45,46] Grossly, the tumors are ovoid, firm, blue-white, well-circumscribed masses of hyaline cartilage that are usually 1 to 2 cm in dimension and, in contrast to synovial chondromatosis, are solitary. Histologically, the hyaline cartilage is well formed with occasional small foci of myxoid change. The cartilage can be cellular, and chondrocytes may show limited cytologic atypia; this sometimes causes confusion with chondrosarcoma.[47] The treatment of choice is simple excision, which is infrequently associated with local recurrence.[43,44,47]

The intracapsular and periarticular regions are uncommon sites for soft tissue chondromas. When they occur, they usually originate in the anterior infrapatellar region of the knee (Figure 123-26).[48] In this location, chondromas can achieve a large size (8 cm) and may interfere with knee motion. Their morphology and biologic behavior are similar to those of soft tissue chondromas that arise elsewhere. Intracapsular chondromas have been reported in the knees of three members of a family with familial dysplasia epiphysealis hemimelica.[45] Two other cases have been described in which cartilaginous hamartomas of the volar plates of the proximal and distal interphalangeal joints of the hands and feet were associated with peculiar hypertrophic skin lesions of the hand and hemihypertrophy of the limb.

Tenosynovial Giant Cell Tumor

Tenosynovial giant cell tumor comprises a group of benign tumors that affect the synovial lining of joints, tendon sheaths, and bursae.[46] These lesions were previously known as *giant cell tumor of tendon sheath*, *localized nodular synovitis*, and *pigmented villonodular synovitis*. Tenosynovial giant cell tumor may be localized or diffuse and may be locally aggressive in that it may invade into bone, grow through joint capsules, extend along tendons, and infiltrate into adjacent soft tissues. Despite its destructive potential, this lesion does not have the capacity to metastasize.

The common histologic denominator of these lesions is the neoplastic proliferation of synovial-like cells that may form a localized mass or spread along the synovial surface and invade downward into subsynovial connective tissue. The growing cells expand the subsynovial compartment, producing finger-like extensions, villi, and redundant folds. These projections often fuse into nodules and form convoluted lobulated masses admixed with a tangle of hair-like villi. The process may be a local phenomenon involving only part of the synovial lining, or it may be extensive, with the whole synovial surface affected.

Until recently, the origin of tenosynovial giant cell tumor was unknown. Previously considered a reactive process, possibly in response to repeated hemorrhage, many tenosynovial giant cell tumors now have been shown to result from a translocation between chromosomes 1p13 and 2q35 in which the gene encoding colony-stimulating factor-1 is fused to the collagen VI alpha-3 (*COL6A3*) gene.[46,49,50] Consequently, overexpression of colony-stimulating factor-1 occurs in the neoplastic cells, which account for only 2% to 16% of cells in the mass.[49] The remaining cells largely represent non-neoplastic inflammatory cells that are recruited into the tumor because they contain the receptor for colony-stimulating factor.[49,51] This phenomenon has been termed a *landscape effect* and is also observed in certain types of lymphomas and sarcomas.

Tenosynovial Giant Cell Tumor of Joints and Tendon Sheaths: Diffuse Type (Synonym: Pigmented Villonodular Synovitis)

The diffuse type of tenosynovial giant cell tumor of the joint involves large areas of the synovial lining, although uninvolved areas are invariably present. Its incidence is approximately 1.8 per 1 million. Although it may occur in all age groups, spanning children to the elderly, most affect young adults are in the 3rd to 4th decade of life.[52] The sexes tend to be equally affected, although some series have reported a predominance of males or of females.[52-54]

Diffuse tenosynovial giant cell tumor of the joint usually manifests as monoarticular arthritis. Bilaterality or involvement of multiple separate sites has been infrequently reported. Some patients with polyarticular disease also have had significant congenital anomalies. Primary complaints include pain and mild intermittent or repeated bouts of

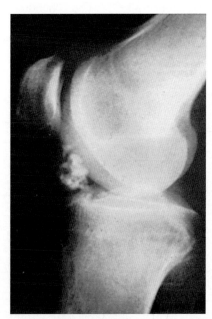

Figure 123-26 Intra-articular solitary chondroma of the knee in the infrapatellar region; it is a well-delineated mass with amorphous dense calcification, suggesting mineralized cartilage. *(Courtesy Dr. C. Campbell.)*

swelling. Symptoms develop insidiously and progress slowly over a long time, ranging from months to years.[52,54] The involved area may be stiff, swollen, and warm, and a palpable mass sometimes can be appreciated. Point tenderness can be detected in approximately 50% of patients. Anatomic instability of the involved joint is uncommon.

The knee joint is affected most commonly and is involved in about 80% of cases.[52,54] The next most frequent sites are the hip, ankle, calcaneocuboid joints, elbow, and tendon sheaths of fingers and sometimes toes. Occasionally, the palm, the sole of the foot, and unusual locations such as the temporomandibular joint and posterior elements of the spine are involved. Bursal involvement is rare, but if it happens, it usually occurs in the popliteal and iliopectineal bursae and the bursa anserina. Infrequently, the disease affects large tendon sheaths proximal to the ankle and wrist, and produces a periarticular soft tissue mass.[55,56] It is thought that some of these lesions dissect through a joint capsule or a tendon sheath and extend along fascial planes to produce a soft tissue mass.[55]

Invasion of bone on either side of a joint can be seen with intra-articular, bursal, or tendon sheath involvement. This most frequently occurs when the tumor involves "tight" joints, such as the hip, elbow, wrist, and feet, or when tendon sheaths are closely apposed to neighboring bones (Figure 123-27).[57,58] Rarely, only one bone may be invaded by an intra-articular lesion, and in this situation, it may be difficult to distinguish this type of lesion from a primary bone tumor (Figure 123-28).[59]

Joint aspiration frequently yields blood-tinged brown fluid that lacks diagnostic abnormalities.[60] Synovial fluid analysis may show a low glucose content, a minimally elevated protein level, and a fair mucin clot. The inflammatory cell count is usually low but may be elevated. Similar findings can be seen in trauma, Charcot's joint, bleeding disorders, sickle cell disease, and Ehlers-Danlos syndrome.

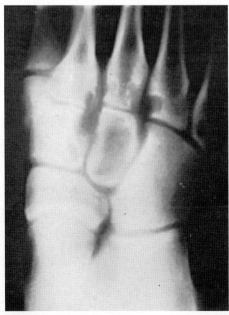

Figure 123-27 Pigmented villonodular synovitis involving the small joints of the foot with multiple bone erosions. No calcification is present in the lesion.

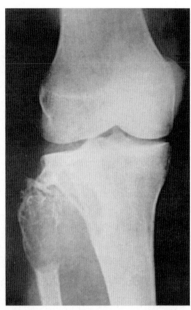

Figure 123-28 Pigmented villonodular synovitis involving the tibiofibular joint with an adjacent extensive soft tissue mass and eccentric erosion of both bones, simulating a primary bone tumor. The knee joint is normal.

In at least two-thirds of cases, a soft tissue density due to the tumor or effusion or both can be visualized on a plain film.[61-64] Joint narrowing or calcification is uncommon. Arthrography may show numerous nodular filling defects that extend into an expanded joint space. Arteriograms are unusually striking owing to the prominent vascularity of the tumor. There tends to be an inverse correlation between the degree of vascularity and the amount of fibrosis or scarring of the lesion.

CT and MRI are useful in delineating the extent of disease and can detect intralesional lipid and hemosiderin deposits, which are important diagnostic features.[61-63] The tumor has low signal intensity (equal to that of skeletal muscle) on T1-weighted images and is heterogeneous on T2-weighted images. Extension into the bone manifests radiographically as multiple, well-marginated, subchondral cyst–like lucencies or juxtacortical oval pressure erosions (see Figures 123-27 and 123-28).[58,59] In the knee, the femoral area adjacent to the intercondylar region is the site most frequently invaded as the tumor grows along the cruciate ligamentous insertions. Periarticular osteopenia, periosteal reactions, and joint destruction are unusual because the joint space is preserved until late in the course of the disease.[62,63] The radiographic differential diagnosis of a given case includes (1) tuberculosis, which generally involves more osteopenia and joint destruction; (2) hemophilia, which is also associated with more extensive joint destruction; (3) synovial chondromatosis, which frequently has calcified radiopaque bodies; and (4) rheumatoid arthritis, which shows more severe osteopenia and joint narrowing.

Grossly, the synovium in diffuse tenosynovial giant cell tumor is red-brown to mottled orange-yellow and looks like a plush Angora rug (Figure 123-29). Matted masses of villous projections and synovial folds are prominent and are admixed with sessile or pedunculated, rubbery-to-soft

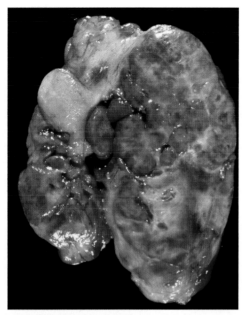

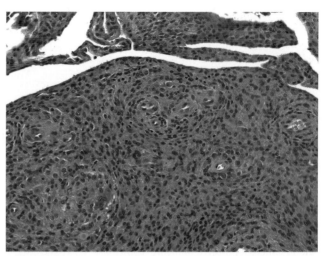

Figure 123-31 Synovial lining cells covering the mass of proliferating polyhedral cells admixed with multinucleated giant cells.

Figure 123-29 Diffuse type of tenosynovial giant cell tumor consisting of mottled brown-yellow-red villonodular mass.

nodules (0.5 to 2 cm in diameter). The synovial membrane is thick and succulent, and is often coated with a fibrinous exudate. Red-brown or golden brown tissue may extend deep into subsynovial structures or may invade the joint capsule. If a tendon sheath is involved, a sausage-shaped mass may be evident because the sheath is distended by the proliferating tumor. If the joint capsule is invaded, adjacent soft tissue structures, including nerves and vessels, may be covered by wispy, red-brown tissue. If soft tissue invasion is extensive, the lesion may appear as a soft-to-rubbery, red-brown mass with foci of hemorrhagic cysts. Similar tissue may be present near the chondro-osseous junction or may be wrapped around vascular and ligamentous attachments to bone surfaces, which represent entrance points into the interior of the bone. Although other conditions, such as hemochromatosis and hemosiderosis, also may discolor the

synovium brown, the nodular component is usually absent; in addition, microscopic features are definitive for separating these entities (see later).

Microscopic examination reveals marked synovial cell hyperplasia with surface proliferation and, more important, subsynovial invasion by masses of mitotically active polygonal or round cells with moderate amounts of eosinophilic cytoplasm and round nuclei (Figures 123-30 and 123-31). Included among the invading synovial cells are scattered lymphocytes, multinucleated giant cells (osteoclast, Touton, or foreign body type), hemosiderin-laden macrophages, and fibroblasts. Hemosiderin also can be seen between cells and in synovial lining cells and polygonal cells. Foci of hemorrhage are common and are surrounded peripherally by giant cells and macrophages (Figure 123-32). Scattered collections of foamy macrophages (xanthoma cells) filled with lipid also are a frequent finding. These different cell populations fill and distend the synovial villi, causing them to fuse with adjacent ones, forming nodules. In some nodules, abundant collagen deposition with hyalinization may cause confusion with neoplastic bone. Rarely, the tumor may contain focally calcified cartilaginous matrix.[65]

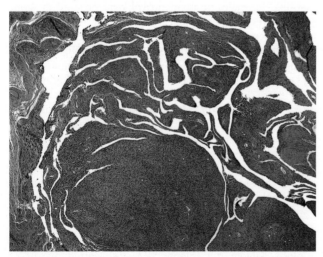

Figure 123-30 Diffuse type of tenosynovial giant cell tumor growing with a villonodular architecture. Invading cells produce the nodular configuration.

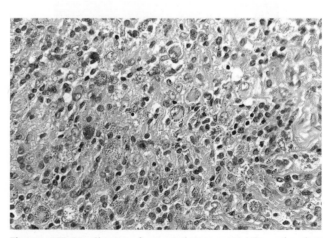

Figure 123-32 Sheets of macrophages containing abundant hemosiderin.

Immunohistochemical studies have been interpreted to support a synovial cell or fibrohistiocytic phenotype.[33,64] The tumor cells express clusterin, D2-40, and a minority of large cells stain with antibodies to desmin.[66] It is important to note that cells that harbor the translocation express colony-stimulating factor-1 (CSF1). Flow cytometric analyses have shown that some of these tumors, especially tumors that have large extra-articular soft tissue components, may be aneuploid and have high proliferative indices.[56] Although these flow cytometric findings may help predict which cases would be more locally aggressive, examples of diffuse tenosynovial cell tumors with these attributes have not metastasized.[56]

Treatment of diffuse tenosynovial giant cell tumor of the joint is not standardized and has included radiation therapy, total synovectomy, arthrodesis, bone grafting, and primary arthroplasty. Although no single therapy has been consistently successful, wide synovectomy is currently the recommended treatment.[52,54] It is difficult to perform an actual complete synovectomy, however; residual involved synovium frequently remains, causing a local recurrence rate of 16% to 48%.[67,68] Tumors arising in the knee have a higher rate of recurrence compared with tumors arising in other joints. Rarely, recurrent disease or tumors with large extra-articular components may require more radical surgery, such as ray resection or amputation.[56] Studies have shown that moderate doses of radiation may control and even cure patients with such extensive disease, possibly obviating the need for radical surgery or amputation. Finally, drugs targeting CSF1 are being tested to determine their efficacy in clinically challenging cases.[69]

Malignant Diffuse Tenosynovial Giant Cell Tumor

Malignant tenosynovial giant cell tumor is a rare lesion; only a handful of cases have been reported.[70-73] The knee is the joint that has been most commonly affected, and in many cases, coexisting benign-appearing, diffuse tenosynovial giant cell tumor is noted. In the malignant variant, the neoplastic cells may be spindle or polyhedral shaped and cytologically malignant. These tumors have the capacity to behave aggressively; almost 50% of patients die from metastatic disease.[70]

Localized Tenosynovial Giant Cell Tumor of the Joint (Synonyms: Benign Giant Cell Synovioma, Benign Synovioma, Localized Nodular Synovitis)

Localized tenosynovial giant cell tumor of the joint manifests as a solitary, well-circumscribed mass. It usually consists of a single sessile or pedunculated, sometimes lobulated, tumor that ranges from 1 to 8 cm in diameter (Figure 123-33). Most commonly, it is unilateral, arises in the knee, and is equally distributed between the sexes.[74]

Symptoms are similar to those of diffuse tenosynovial giant cell tumor, except that in the localized variant, a higher frequency of joint locking is reported because the mass interferes with motion.[74] A few patients may present with acute severe joint pain caused by torsion and infarction of the tumor. Effusions are common, but the synovial fluid tends to be less bloody than in the diffuse variant, and may be clear.

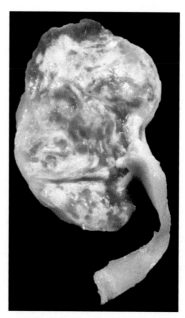

Figure 123-33 Localized tenosynovial giant cell tumor of the joint with attached pedicle. The mass is well circumscribed and brown-yellow.

Imaging studies show a heterogeneous nodular mass that contains lipid and hemosiderin deposits (Figure 123-34). In the knee joint, the tumor frequently arises in the suprapatellar notch, in the femoral notch, and between the meniscus and the joint capsule.[74] Usually, no bone invasion occurs. Marginal excision is usually curative. Small lesions can be extirpated arthroscopically.[74]

Histologically, localized tenosynovial giant cell tumor of the joint is identical to the nodules of the diffuse variant. The main difference is that the prominent synovial villi present in the diffuse variant are absent or sparse.

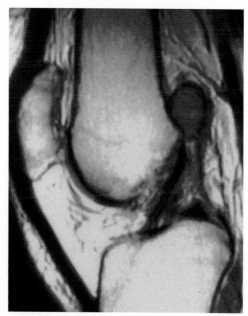

Figure 123-34 Magnetic resonance image shows well-delineated dark mass in posterior knee joint.

Localized Tenosynovial Giant Cell Tumor of the Tendon Sheath (Synonyms: Giant Cell Tumor of Tendon Sheath, Fibroxanthoma of Tendon Sheath)

Localized tenosynovial giant cell tumor of the tendon sheath usually involves the hand or wrist, and less frequently the foot or ankle.[53] It is the most common soft tissue tumor of the hand and usually arises from the flexor tendon sheaths of the finger; the index finger is affected most frequently, followed in descending order of frequency by the third, fourth, fifth, and first fingers.

Tumors of the digits predominate in females, with a male-to-female ratio of at least 2 : 1,[53,75] and tumors of the toes have an equal sex distribution.[53] On average, patients are in the 3rd to 5th decades of life and present with a painless, palpable, firm, mobile mass.

Clinically, the mass usually is solitary and is located on the flexor surface, but it may bulge into the extensor or lateral aspects of the digits (Figure 123-35). The tumors are slow growing, and the intervals between detection and surgical treatment have ranged from several weeks to longer than a decade, with an average interval of slightly longer than 2 years.[53,75]

Radiographically, the tumors appear as well-circumscribed soft tissue masses, and in about 25% of cases, adjacent extrinsic excavation of the cortical bone has a sclerotic margin (Figure 123-36).[53,75] MRI reveals the lesions to have a hypointense signal on T1-weighted images and either a hypointense or a hyperintense signal on T2-weighted images. These findings are helpful in distinguishing giant cell tumor of tendon sheath from other soft tissue tumors.[76]

The gross pathology is that of a well-circumscribed, multinodular, round, rubbery, variegated red-brown-tan-yellow mass, generally not larger than 5 cm in diameter, which is firmly attached but easily peeled off the involved tendon

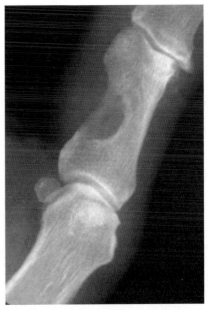

Figure 123-36 The cortex of the phalanx is eroded by the tenosynovial giant cell tumor.

(Figure 123-37). Sometimes at surgery, the lesion may "pop out" of the incision. The cut surface reveals a solid mass that ranges from hues of yellow to orange-red-brown, depending on the quantity of lipid and blood pigments present. Often bands or septa of white fibrous tissue subcompartmentalize the lesion. The morphology and immunophenotype of the cell types present are identical to those in the diffuse variant (Figure 123-38).[66,77] Ultrastructurally, proliferating cells have features similar to type A and type B synovial lining cells.[75-78] Flow cytometry has been performed on a few cases, and all have been diploid.[56] Cytogenetics shows that many of these tumors have a translocation between 1p13 and 2q35.[49,51,79]

These tumors are benign and do not metastasize. Rarely have malignant giant cell tumors of tendon sheath been reported.[70,80] The treatment of choice is conservative surgical excision, which is usually curative. Local recurrence may be noted if excision is incomplete.[53,75]

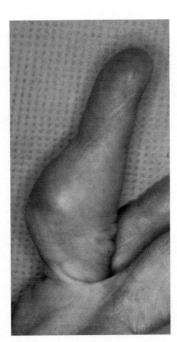

Figure 123-35 Tenosynovial giant cell tumor manifesting as a mobile, solid, firm mass.

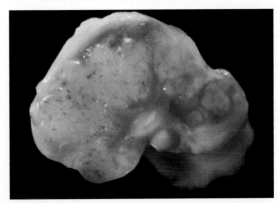

Figure 123-37 Well-delineated, white-yellow and focally brown tenosynovial giant cell tumor.

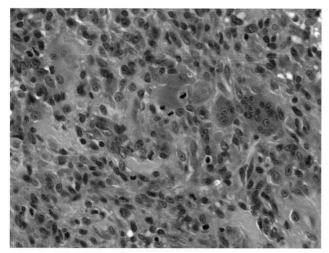

Figure 123-38 Mitotically active polyhedral cells and scattered osteoclast-type giant cells in tenosynovial giant cell tumor.

MALIGNANT TUMORS OF THE JOINT

Malignant tumors of joints are uncommon and are classified into primary and secondary types. Primary malignancies are virtually always sarcomas and usually arise within the synovium of large diarthrodial joints, especially the knee. Patients are adults, who present with chronic symptoms of pain, swelling, and effusion, and most tumors are chondrosarcomas or synovial sarcomas. Rarely, other sarcomas originate within a joint; our experience has included cases of intra-articular myxoinflammatory fibroblastic sarcoma, pleomorphic fibrosarcoma, extraskeletal myxoid chondrosarcoma, conventional chondrosarcoma, malignant tenosynovial giant cell tumor, and angiosarcoma (Figure 123-39). Secondary malignant tumors of joints, by definition, originate beyond the confines of the joint; most are sarcomas that extend from neighboring bone or surrounding soft

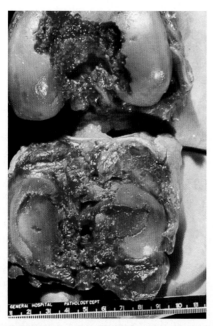

Figure 123-39 Angiosarcoma of synovium of the knee joint. The hemorrhagic tumor erodes into the distal femur and proximal tibia.

tissue. Although synovial tissue is highly vascular, metastases or involvement of the synovium by carcinoma, lymphoma, or leukemia is uncommon.

Primary Sarcomas of Joints

Conventional Chondrosarcoma

Conventional chondrosarcoma arising in the synovium is unusual; fewer than 50 cases have been reported in the English language.[39-41,71,81] In approximately 50% of cases, the chondrosarcoma arose in association with pre-existing synovial chondromatosis.[40-42,81,82] Patients are usually in the 5th to 7th decade of life and have an equal sex distribution.[81] Typically, patients present with a progressively enlarging mass in the joint that may cause mechanical dysfunction, pain, and stiffness. In patients who have pre-existing synovial chondromatosis, the duration of symptoms is usually long, and in some instances, symptoms may be present for 25 years.[81] Most chondrosarcomas arise in the knee joint, followed by the hip and elbow joints.

Radiographic studies usually show a periarticular soft tissue mass that may have dense irregular or ring-like calcifications. Occasionally, invasion into the medullary cavity of adjacent bone is evident. The radiographic differential diagnosis varies according to the presence of calcification and includes synovial chondromatosis, synovial sarcoma, diffuse tenosynovial giant cell tumor, and chronic synovitis.[81]

Grossly, the involved joint is filled with synovium massively thickened by innumerable nodules of opalescent blue-white cartilage. The nodules of cartilage vary in size and may be free-floating in the joint cavity. In several cases, the tumor has extended into adjacent soft tissue and bone.

Microscopically, the tumor is composed of malignant hyaline and myxoid cartilage. Rarely, the matrix is entirely myxoid and has features of extraskeletal myxoid chondrosarcoma.[82] The neoplastic cartilage is cellular and contains cytologically atypical chondrocytes. The periphery of the lobules of cartilage is typically the most cellular, and in this region, some of the tumor cells are spindled. Other findings include necrosis and permeation of invaded bone.[81] Coexisting synovial chondromatosis can be identified by its well-formed nodules of hyaline cartilage, which are less cellular, containing cytologically banal-appearing chondrocytes and a matrix that is frequently mineralized.

Treatment is usually surgical extirpation with consideration given for chemotherapy in high-grade lesions or lesions that have metastasized. Inadequate surgical removal virtually ensures local recurrence, which may necessitate subsequent radical excision. Metastases have occurred in approximately one-third of reported patients; the lung is the most common site for systemic spread.[81]

Synovial Sarcoma

Synovial sarcoma is a common sarcoma that accounts for approximately 6% to 10% of soft tissue sarcomas. It usually develops in the deep soft tissues and rarely arises in joints (Figure 123-40), but it may secondarily invade articular synovium from neighboring soft tissues. Earlier descriptions of this tumor attest to its wide spectrum of morphology

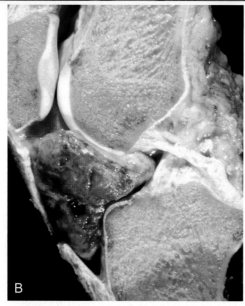

Figure 123-40 **A,** Magnetic resonance image of a rare example of intra-articular synovial sarcoma. The infrapatellar tumor is well circumscribed and has a focal inhomogeneous appearance. **B,** The gross specimen shows that the tan, hemorrhagic tumor bulges into the joint but is covered by synovium.

because such names as *adenosarcoma* and *synovial fibrosarcoma* were used until the term *synovial sarcoma*, first introduced in 1936, became commonplace. The morphology of synovial sarcoma mimics a joint in its early stage of development in that it contains cleft-like spaces and glands delineated by large polygonal (epithelioid) cells surrounded by fascicles of spindle cells. The clefts and glands simulate a microscopic "joint space" that is bounded by synovial lining cells and is supported by subsynovial mesenchymal cells. Because epithelial or spindle cells may predominate, synovial sarcoma has been subtyped into biphasic and monophasic spindle cell and epithelial types, although the latter type is very rare.

Synovial sarcoma commonly affects adolescents and young adults. In a series of 121 cases, the age range was 9 to 74 years, with a median age of 34 years; however, it occurs in children with significant frequency.[83,84]

The term *synovial sarcoma* implies that the tumor originates from the synovium; however, less than 10% of cases

are intra-articular or show continuity with a synovial lining.[85,86]

Approximately 60% to 70% of synovial sarcomas arise in the extremities, especially the lower limb, in the vicinity of large joints, particularly the popliteal areas of the knee and foot.[87,88] Regions of the thigh, hand, leg, and digits may be affected, and in the distal extremities, tumors are often adjacent to joint capsules or tendon sheaths or both. Tumors also have been reported in the neck, torso, craniofacial region, retroperitoneum, orbit, tongue, mediastinum, soft palate, heart, kidney, lung, pleura, and prostate.

No clinical features specific to synovial sarcoma distinguish it from other sarcomas. The most common complaint is the development of a slowly enlarging, deep-seated, palpable mass that is painful in about 50% of cases.[84,88] Symptoms may be present for an unusually long time, ranging from months to 25 years with an average of about 6 months to 2.5 years, before medical evaluation is sought.[84,88] Delay in diagnosis is more frequent with tumors that are located in the deep soft tissues than in tumors that are based in the more superficial and clinically noticeable regions. In some cases involving the knee region, vague mild pain over several months may occur before a mass is appreciated, and if the tumor reaches a large size, limitation of motion finally may be noted. Head and neck lesions produce symptoms related to their specific sites, such as hoarseness and breathing or swallowing difficulties. Rarely, a patient may present with a symptom secondary to pulmonary metastasis, such as hemoptysis.[88]

Classically, plain film findings of synovial sarcoma consist of a well-circumscribed, deep-seated soft tissue mass. Synovial sarcoma is one of the few primary soft tissue tumors that frequently calcify. Approximately 30% to 50% of cases reveal radiographically detectable calcifications that may have a fine, stippled, or dense appearance (Figure 123-41).[89] The calcification may be focal or may present throughout most of the tumor.[90] Periosteal reaction of adjacent bone is elicited in approximately 20% of cases, but bone is rarely invaded by the tumor.

CT is more sensitive than plain radiography in showing calcification or periosteal reaction. MRI is important in delineating the anatomic extent of the tumor and usually shows a large inhomogeneous mass with areas of hemorrhage. The radiographic differential diagnosis includes hemangioma, lipoma, synovial chondromatosis, soft tissue chondrosarcoma or osteosarcoma, myositis ossificans, aneurysm, and other sarcomas.

The gross pathology of synovial sarcoma reveals a well-demarcated, pink-tan, fleshy mass that easily detaches or "shells out" from its tumor bed (Figure 123-40B). The cut surface is usually uniform, gray-yellow, and rubbery. Calcified areas are gritty and hard. In larger tumors, areas of hemorrhage or necrosis or both with cystification and gelatinous breakdown of tissue may be seen. Synovial sarcoma sometimes grows between tendons, muscles, and fascial planes, or wraps around neurovascular bundles.

Synovial sarcoma is subtyped into three patterns on the basis of predominant microscopic findings: monophasic spindle cell, monophasic epithelial, and biphasic variants. Use of such a classification system requires some subjectivity because many of these tumors have a variable histologic picture. A useful differential observation is that marked

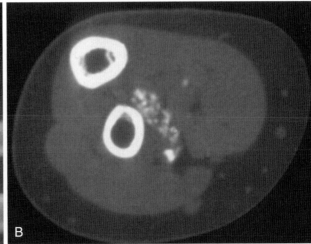

Figure 123-41 **A,** Focally mineralized synovial sarcoma in the deep soft tissues in the vicinity of the elbow joint. **B,** Axial computed tomography scan shows intratumoral calcification.

cellular pleomorphism and atypia usually are not present in synovial sarcoma and, when observed, tend to point to some other type of neoplasm, such as pleomorphic fibrosarcoma.

Microscopically, the hallmark of the more common biphasic synovial sarcoma is the two different populations of neoplastic cells consisting of epithelial and spindle cells (Figure 123-42). Epithelial cells may be cuboidal or columnar and, similar to true epithelium, may have well-defined cytoplasmic borders. These cells may form glandular spaces, line papillae or cleft-like spaces, or grow in cohesive groups (see Figure 123-42). Epithelial cells usually are surrounded by fascicles of uniform small and plump spindle cells. Spindle cell fascicles are densely cellular and frequently are arranged in a "herringbone" pattern. In most biphasic synovial sarcomas, the spindle cell component predominates, and calcification of hyalinized stroma most frequently occurs in spindle cell regions. Some tumors may show bone formation, which may be present in spindle or epithelial areas. In the monophasic variants, spindle or epithelial cells may predominate (Figure 123-43; see Figure 123-42).

Immunohistochemistry has shown that epithelial and the spindle cell components frequently stain with antibodies to keratin and epithelial membrane antigen, which usually are associated with epithelial neoplasms.[91-93] This pattern of reactivity has helped make it possible to separate synovial sarcoma from morphologically similar tumors, such as fibrosarcoma and malignant peripheral nerve sheath tumor.[93] It has also provided evidence that synovial sarcoma does not arise from or recapitulate the synovium, because normal synovial cells do not stain with these antibodies.[94]

Cytogenetic studies of synovial sarcomas have detected a consistent translocation t(X;18)(p11.2;q11.2) in almost all cases, regardless of whether the tumor is biphasic or monophasic.[87,95] This finding provides insight into the genesis of synovial sarcoma, which may be related to dysregulation of transcription and can be used as a diagnostic feature. No relationship between the location of the translocation breakpoint and the prognosis has been discerned.

The prognosis of synovial sarcoma is poor. In one study of 150 patients with nonmetastatic disease, 5-year, 10-year,

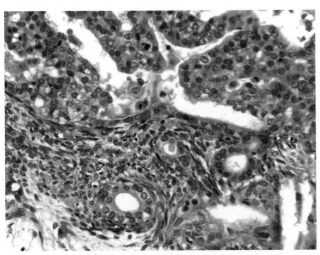

Figure 123-42 Biphasic synovial sarcoma with epithelial cells forming glands and papillary structures. The spindle cell component surrounds the glands.

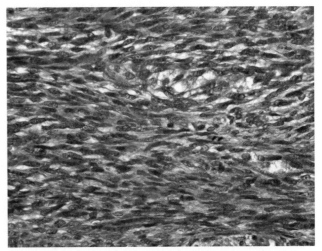

Figure 123-43 Monophasic spindle cell variant of synovial sarcoma with the fascicles of tumor cells forming a herringbone pattern.

and 15-year disease-free survival rates were 59%, 52%, and 52%.[90] Many factors influence prognosis; tumors that are small (<5 cm), that arise in patients younger than 25 years of age, and that lack poorly differentiated areas have a high rate of cure.[84] In contrast, large tumors (≥5 cm) that arise in patients 25 years old or older and that contain poorly differentiated areas have a dismal outcome.[84] The impact of histologic subtype has been controversial. Radiographically, the tumors appear as well-circumscribed soft tissue masses. However, in about 25% of cases they produce extrinsic erosion of the adjacent cortical bone, and when this occurs the margin of the excavation is sclerotic (see Figure 123-36).[53,75]

The natural history of synovial sarcoma consists of local recurrence, which may be repetitive. Most recurrences manifest within 2 years after initial treatment, but intervals longer than 10 years are not exceptional. Ultimately, metastases occur in many patients, and the most common site is the lungs; regional lymph node involvement has been reported in a few patients.[96] About 10% of patients die within 1 year after diagnosis with metastatic disease; 90% of these patients have massive pulmonary metastases.

Treatment must contend with issues involved with local and systemic therapy. Successful local control usually can be achieved by limb salvage surgery combined with radiation.[96,97] Because regional lymph nodes may be involved, their status should be evaluated carefully, and they should be treated if enlarged. Systemic treatment consists of various chemotherapy regimens, which have provided questionable benefit, although adjuvant chemotherapy usually is recommended for patients who are at high risk—patients with tumors larger than 5 cm.[98-101]

Secondary Malignant Tumors of the Joint

Sarcomas

Primary sarcomas of bone, such as osteosarcoma and chondrosarcoma, infrequently involve a joint because intact articular cartilage usually acts as a barrier to direct tumor extension. However, when it is observed, joint invasion usually occurs via a pathway created by a transarticular fracture, via growth along tendoligamentous structures, or through capsule insertion sites. This circumstance may make it difficult to distinguish on histologic grounds alone some forms of synovial chondromatosis from a low-grade intraosseous chondrosarcoma that has secondarily spread into the joint.

Similarly, primary soft tissue sarcomas gain access into the interior of a joint by growing through the joint capsule in conduits occupied by pre-existing vascular structures or along tendons and ligaments. This complication can make providing adequate therapy challenging because treatment may require en bloc resection of the joint.

Metastatic Carcinoma

The synovium, in contrast to other richly vascular tissues, is rarely the site of metastatic carcinoma; this may reflect the fact that only clinical cases in which joint symptoms prevail are reported because at autopsy, joints are not routinely examined. Most carcinomas that metastasize to the synovium originate in the lung, followed by the gastrointestinal tract and breast.[99-101] Affected patients are usually elderly, and the knee is the most frequently involved joint. In many reported cases, the underlying bone also contains metastatic deposits.

Malignant Lymphoproliferative Disease

The various types of malignant lymphoproliferative diseases, including leukemia, lymphoma, and myeloma, can involve the synovium and may produce osteoarticular symptoms.[102-104] This complication occurs most frequently in leukemia and is seen in both acute and chronic forms.[104] Joint symptoms have been observed in 12% to 65% of children and in 4% to 13% of adults with leukemia.[104] Arthritis can develop at any time during the disease course and can be the presenting complaint. Large joints are affected more commonly than small joints, and the arthritis is often pauciarticular, asymmetric, migratory, and severe. Symptoms may result from leukemic infiltration of the synovium or irritation of the neighboring periosteum. When arthritis is the major presenting symptom, it may cause confusion with septic arthritis, rheumatic fever, subacute bacterial endocarditis, or rheumatoid arthritis.

References

1. Fritschy D, Fasel J, Imbert JC, et al: The popliteal cyst, *Knee Surg Sports Traumatol Arthrosc* 14:623, 2006.
2. Seil R, Rupp S, Jochum P, et al: Prevalence of popliteal cysts in children: a sonographic study and review of the literature, *Arch Orthop Trauma Surg* 119:73, 1999.
3. Labropoulos N, Shifrin DA, Paxinos O: New insights into the development of popliteal cysts, *Br J Surg* 91:1313, 2004.
4. Beaman FD, Peterson JJ: MR imaging of cysts, ganglia, and bursae about the knee, *Magn Reson Imaging Clin N Am* 15:39, 2007.
5. Choudhri HF, Perling LH: Diagnosis and management of juxtafacet cysts, *Neurosurg Focus* 20:E1, 2006.
6. Boviatsis EJ, Staurinou LC, Kouyialis AT, et al: Spinal synovial cysts: pathogenesis, diagnosis and surgical treatment in a series of seven cases and literature review, *Eur Spine J* 17:831, 2008.
7. Spinner RJ, Hébert-Blouin MN, Maus TP, et al: Evidence that atypical juxtafacet cysts are joint derived, *J Neurosurg Spine* 12:96, 2010.
8. McEvedy BV: Simple ganglia, *Br J Surg* 49:40, 1962.
9. Spinner RJ, Scheithauer BW, Amrami KK: The unifying articular (synovial) origin of intraneural ganglia: evolution-revelation-revolution, *Neurosurgery* 65(4 Suppl):A115, 2009.
10. Nahra ME, Bucchieri JS: Ganglion cysts and other tumor related conditions of the hand and wrist, *Hand Clin* 20:249, 2004.
11. Milgram JW: The classification of loose bodies in human joints, *Clin Orthop Relat Res* 124:282, 1977.
12. Clarke HD, Scott WN: The role of debridement: through small portals, *J Arthroplasty* 18:10, 2003.
13. Adelani MA, Wupperman RM, Holt GE: Benign synovial disorders, *J Am Acad Orthop Surg* 16:268, 2008.
14. Cooper G, Schiller AL: *Anatomy of the guinea pig*, Cambridge, 1975, Harvard University Press.
15. Kato Y, Oshida M, Saito A, et al: Meniscal ossicles, *J Orthop Sci* 12:375, 2007.
16. Van Breuseghem I, Geusens E, Pans S, et al: The meniscal ossicle revisited, *JBR-BTR* 86:276, 2003.
17. Rohilla S, Yadav RK, Singh R, et al: Meniscal ossicle, *J Orthop Traumatol* 10:143, 2009.
18. Hirano K, Deguchi M, Kanamono T: Intra-articular synovial lipoma of the knee joint (located in the lateral recess): a case report and review of the literature, *Knee* 14:63, 2007.
19. Sonoda H, Takasita M, Taira H, et al: Carpal tunnel syndrome and trigger wrist caused by a lipoma arising from flexor tenosynovium: a case report, *J Hand Surg Am* 27:1056, 2002.

20. Allen PW: Lipoma arborescens. In *Tumors and proliferations of adipose tissue*, Chicago, 1981, Year Book Medical Publishers, p 129.

21. Kloen P, Keel SB, Chandler HP, et al: Lipoma arborescens of the knee, *J Bone Joint Surg Br* 80:298, 1998.

22. Bansal M, Changulani M, Shukla R, Sampath J: Synovial lipomatosis of the knee in an adolescent girl, *Orthopedics* 31:185, 2008.

23. Davies AP, Blewitt N: Lipoma arborescens of the knee, *Knee* 12:394, 2005.

24. Hoffa A: The influence of the adipose tissue with regard to the pathology of the knee joint, *JAMA* 43:795, 1904.

25. Devaney K, Vinh TN, Sweet DE: Synovial hemangioma: a report of 20 cases with differential diagnostic considerations, *Hum Pathol* 24:737, 1993.

26. Lichtenstein L: Tumors of synovial joints, bursae, and tendon sheaths, *Cancer* 8:816, 1955.

27. Greenspan A, Azouz EM, Matthews J 2nd, et al: Synovial hemangioma: imaging features in eight histologically proven cases, review of the literature, and differential diagnosis, *Skeletal Radiol* 24:583, 1995.

28. Sasho T, Nakagawa K, Matsuki K, et al: Two cases of synovial haemangioma of the knee joint: Gd-enhanced image features on MRI and arthroscopic excision, *Knee* 18:509, 2011.

29. Chung EB, Enzinger FM: Fibroma of tendon sheath, *Cancer* 44:1979, 1945.

30. Pulitzer DR, Martin PC, Reed RJ: Fibroma of tendon sheath: a clinicopathologic study of 32 cases, *Am J Surg Pathol* 13:472, 1989.

31. Moretti VM, de la Cruz M, Lackman RD, Fox EJ: Fibroma of tendon sheath in the knee: a report of three cases and literature review, *Knee* 17:306, 2010.

32. Sim FH, Dahlin DC, Ivins JC: Extra-articular synovial chondromatosis, *J Bone Joint Surg Am* 59:492, 1977.

33. Maluf HM, DeYoung BR, Swanson PE, et al: Fibroma and giant cell tumor of tendon sheath: a comparative histological and immunohistological study, *Mod Pathol* 8:155, 1995.

34. Buddingh EP, Naumann S, Nelson M, et al: Cytogenetic findings in benign cartilaginous neoplasms, *Cancer Genet Cytogenet* 141:164, 2003.

35. Davis RI, Hamilton A, Biggart JD: Primary synovial chondromatosis: a clinicopathologic review and assessment of malignant potential, *Hum Pathol* 29:683, 1998.

36. Guarda-Nardini L, Piccotti F, Ferronato G, Manfredini D: Synovial chondromatosis of the temporomandibular joint: a case description with systematic literature review, *Int J Oral Maxillofac Surg* 39:745, 2010.

37. Fetsch JF, Vinh TN, Remotti F, et al: Tenosynovial (extraarticular) chondromatosis: an analysis of 37 cases of an underrecognized clinicopathologic entity with a strong predilection for the hands and feet and a high local recurrence rate, *Am J Surg Pathol* 27:1260, 2003.

38. Veras E, Abadeer R, Khurana H, et al: Solitary synovial osteochondroma, *Ann Diagn Pathol* 14:94, 2010.

39. Sah AP, Geller DS, Mankin HJ, et al: Malignant transformation of synovial chondromatosis of the shoulder to chondrosarcoma: a case report, *J Bone Joint Surg Am* 89:1321, 2007.

40. Rybak LD, Khaldi L, Wittig J, Steiner GC: Primary synovial chondrosarcoma of the hip joint in a 45-year-old male: case report and literature review, *Skeletal Radiol* 40:1375, 2011.

41. Zamora EE, Mansor A, Vanel D, et al: Synovial chondrosarcoma: report of two cases and literature review, *Eur J Radiol* 72:38, 2009.

42. Dahlin DC, Salvador AH: Cartilaginous tumors of the soft tissues of the hands and feet, *Mayo Clin Proc* 49:721, 1974.

43. Chung EB, Enzinger FM: Chondroma of soft parts, *Cancer* 41:1414, 1978.

44. Lichtenstein L, Goldman RL: Cartilage tumors in soft tissues, particularly in the hand and foot, *Cancer* 17:1203, 1964.

45. Hensinger RN, Cowell HR, Ramsey PL, et al: Familial dysplasia epiphysealis hemimelica, associated with chondromas and osteochondromas: report of a kindred with variable presentations, *J Bone Joint Surg Am* 56:1513, 1974.

46. Rubin BP: Tenosynovial giant cell tumor and pigmented villonodular synovitis: a proposal for unification of these clinically distinct but histologically and genetically identical lesions, *Skeletal Radiol* 36:267, 2007.

47. Jones WA, Ghorbal MS: Benign tendon sheath chondroma, *J Hand Surg Br* 11:276, 1986.

48. Gonzalez-Lois C, Garcia-de-la-Torre P, SantosBriz-Terron A, et al: Intracapsular and para-articular chondroma adjacent to large joints: report of three cases and review of the literature, *Skeletal Radiol* 30:672, 2001.

49. West RB, Rubin BP, Miller MA, et al: A landscape effect in tenosynovial giant-cell tumor from activation of CSF1 expression by a translocation in a minority of tumor cells, *Proc Natl Acad Sci U S A* 103:690, 2006.

50. Möller E, Mandahl N, Mertens F, Panagopoulos I: Molecular identification of COL6A3-CSF1 fusion transcripts in tenosynovial giant cell tumors, *Genes Chromosomes Cancer* 47:21, 2008.

51. Möller E, Mandahl N, Mertens F, et al: Molecular identification of COL6A3-CSF1 fusion transcripts in tenosynovial giant cell tumors, *Genes Chromosomes Cancer* 47:21, 2008.

52. Tyler WK, Vidal AF, Williams RJ, et al: Pigmented villonodular synovitis, *J Am Acad Orthop Surg* 14:376, 2006.

53. Ravi V, Wang WL, Lewis VO: Treatment of tenosynovial giant cell tumor and pigmented villonodular synovitis, *Curr Opin Oncol* 23:361, 2011.

54. Mendenhall WM, Mendenhall CM, Reith JD, et al: Pigmented villonodular synovitis, *Am J Clin Oncol* 29:548, 2006.

55. Somerhausen NS, Fletcher CD: Diffuse-type giant cell tumor: clinicopathologic and immunohistochemical analysis of 50 cases with extraarticular disease, *Am J Surg Pathol* 24:479, 2000.

56. Abdul-Karim FW, el-Naggar AK, Joyce MJ, et al: Diffuse and localized tenosynovial giant cell tumor and pigmented villonodular synovitis: a clinicopathologic and flow cytometric DNA analysis, *Hum Pathol* 23:729, 1992.

57. Carpintero P, Gascon E, Mesa M, et al: Clinical and radiologic features of pigmented villonodular synovitis of the foot: report of eight cases, *J Am Podiatr Med Assoc* 97:415, 2007.

58. De Schepper AM, Hogendoorn PC, Bloem JL: Giant cell tumors of the tendon sheath may present radiologically as intrinsic osseous lesions, *Eur Radiol* 17:499, 2007.

59. Jergesen HE, Mankin HJ, Schiller AL: Diffuse pigmented villonodular synovitis of the knee mimicking primary bone neoplasms: a report of two cases, *J Bone Joint Surg Am* 60:825, 1978.

60. Myers BW, Masi AT: Pigmented villonodular synovitis and tenosynovitis: a clinical epidemiologic study of 166 cases and literature review, *Medicine (Baltimore)* 59:223, 1980.

61. Lin J, Jacobson JA, Jamadar DA, et al: Pigmented villonodular synovitis and related lesions: the spectrum of imaging findings, *AJR Am J Roentgenol* 172:191, 1999.

62. Murphey MD, Rhee JH, Lewis RB, et al: Pigmented villonodular synovitis: radiologic-pathologic correlation, *Radiographics* 28:1493, 2008.

63. Masih S, Antebi A: Imaging of pigmented villonodular synovitis, *Semin Musculoskel Radiol* 7:205, 2003.

64. O'Connell JX, Fanburg JC, Rosenberg AE: Giant cell tumor of tendon sheath and pigmented villonodular synovitis: immunophenotype suggests a synovial cell origin, *Hum Pathol* 26:771, 1995.

65. Hoch BL, Garcia RA, Smalberger GJ: Chondroid tenosynovial giant cell tumor: a clinicopathological and immunohistochemical analysis of 5 new cases, *Int J Surg Pathol* 19:180, 2011.

66. Boland JM, Folpe AL, Hornick JL, Grogg KL: Clusterin is expressed in normal synoviocytes and in tenosynovial giant cell tumors of localized and diffuse types: diagnostic and histogenetic implications, *Am J Surg Pathol* 33:1225, 2009.

67. Sharma H, Rana B, Mahendra A, et al: Outcome of 17 pigmented villonodular synovitis (PVNS) of the knee at 6 years mean follow-up, *Knee* 14:390, 2007.

68. Chiari C, Pirich C, Brannath W, et al: What affects the recurrence and clinical outcome of pigmented villonodular synovitis? *Clin Orthop Relat Res* 450:172, 2006.

69. Nielsen TO: Discovery research to clinical trial: a ten year journey, *Clin Invest Med* 33:E342, 2010.

70. Bertoni F, Unni KK, Beabout JW, et al: Malignant giant cell tumor of the tendon sheaths and joints (malignant pigmented villonodular synovitis), *Am J Surg Pathol* 21:153, 1997.

71. Bhadra AK, Pollock R, Tirabosco RP, et al: Primary tumours of the synovium: a report of four cases of malignant tumour, *J Bone Joint Surg Br* 89:1504, 2007.

72. Li CF, Wang JW, Huang WW, et al: Malignant diffuse-type tenosynovial giant cell tumors: a series of 7 cases comparing with 24 benign

lesions with review of the literature, *Am J Surg Pathol* 32:587, 2008.

73. Li CF, Wang JW, Huang WW, et al: Malignant diffuse-type tenosynovial giant cell tumors: a series of 7 cases comparing with 24 benign lesions with review of the literature, *Am J Surg Pathol* 32:587, 2008.

74. Dines JS, DeBerardino TM, Wells JL, et al: Long-term follow-up of surgically treated localized pigmented villonodular synovitis of the knee, *Arthroscopy* 23:930, 2007.

75. Ushijima M, Hashimoto H, Tsuneyoshi M, et al: Giant cell tumor of the tendon sheath (nodular tenosynovitis): a study of 207 cases to compare the large joint group with the common digit group, *Cancer* 57:875, 1986.

76. Kitagawa Y, Ito H, Amano Y, et al: MR imaging for preoperative diagnosis and assessment of local tumor extent on localized giant cell tumor of tendon sheath, *Skeletal Radiol* 32:633, 2003.

77. Monaghan H, Salter DM, Al-Nafussi A: Giant cell tumour of tendon sheath (localised nodular tenosynovitis): clinicopathological features of 71 cases, *J Clin Pathol* 54:404, 2001.

78. Alguacil-Garcia A, Unni KK, Goellner JR: Giant cell tumor of tendon sheath and pigmented villonodular synovitis: an ultrastructural study, *Am J Clin Pathol* 69:6, 1978.

79. Nilsson M, Hoglund M, Panagopoulos I, et al: Molecular cytogenetic mapping of recurrent chromosomal breakpoints in tenosynovial giant cell tumors, *Virchows Arch* 441:475, 2002.

80. Wu NL, Hsiao PF, Chen BF, et al: Malignant giant cell tumor of the tendon sheath, *Int J Dermatol* 4:543, 2004.

81. Bertoni F, Unni KK, Beabout JW, et al: Chondrosarcomas of the synovium, *Cancer* 67:155, 1991.

82. Gebhardt MC, Parekh SG, Rosenberg AE, et al: Extraskeletal myxoid chondrosarcoma of the knee, *Skeletal Radiol* 28:354, 1999.

83. Okcu MF, Munsell M, Treuner J, et al: Synovial sarcoma of childhood and adolescence: a multicenter, multivariate analysis of outcome, *J Clin Oncol* 21:1602, 2003.

84. Bergh P, Meis-Kindblom JM, Gherlinzoni F, et al: Synovial sarcoma: identification of low and high risk groups, *Cancer* 85:2596, 1999.

85. Dardick I, O'Brien PK, Jeans MT, et al: Synovial sarcoma arising in an anatomical bursa, *Virchows Arch A Pathol Anat Histol* 397:93, 1982.

86. McKinney CD, Mills SE, Fechner RE: Intraarticular synovial sarcoma, *Am J Surg Pathol* 16:1017, 1992.

87. Haldar M, Randall RL, Capecchi MR: Synovial sarcoma: from genetics to genetic-based animal modeling, *Clin Orthop Relat Res* 466:2156, 2008.

88. Cadman NL, Soule EH, Kelly PJ: Synovial sarcoma: an analysis of 134 tumors, *Cancer* 18:613, 1965.

89. Milchgrub S, Ghandur-Mnaymneh L, Dorfman HD, et al: Synovial sarcoma with extensive osteoid and bone formation, *Am J Surg Pathol* 17:357, 1993.

90. Varela-Duran J, Enzinger FM: Calcifying synovial sarcoma, *Cancer* 50:345, 1982.

91. Corson JM, Weiss LM, Banks-Schlegel SP, et al: Keratin proteins and carcinoembryonic antigen in synovial sarcomas: an immunohistochemical study of 24 cases, *Hum Pathol* 15:615, 1984.

92. Fisher C: Synovial sarcoma, *Diagn Pathol* 1:13, 1994.

93. Olsen SH, Thomas DG, Lucas DR: Cluster analysis of immunohistochemical profiles in synovial sarcoma, malignant peripheral nerve sheath tumor, and Ewing sarcoma, *Mod Pathol* 19:659, 2006.

94. Miettinen M, Virtanen I: Synovial sarcoma—a misnomer, *Am J Pathol* 117:18, 1984.

95. Amary MF, Berisha F, Bernardi F, et al: Detection of SS18-SSX fusion transcripts in formalin-fixed paraffin-embedded neoplasms: analysis of conventional RT-PCR, qRT-PCR and dual color FISH as diagnostic tools for synovial sarcoma, *Mod Pathol* 20:482, 2007.

96. Guadagnolo BA, Zagars GK, Ballo MT, et al: Long-term outcomes for synovial sarcoma treated with conservation surgery and radiotherapy, *Int J Radiat Oncol Biol Phys* 69:1173, 2007.

97. Brecht IB, Ferrari A, Int-Veen C, et al: Grossly-resected synovial sarcoma treated by the German and Italian Pediatric Soft Tissue Sarcoma Cooperative Groups: discussion on the role of adjuvant therapies, *Pediatr Blood Cancer* 46:11, 2006.

98. Al-Hussaini H, Hogg D, Blackstein ME, et al: Clinical features, treatment, and outcome in 102 adult and pediatric patients with localized high-grade synovial sarcoma, *Sarcoma* 2011:231789, 2011.

99. Younes M, Hayem G, Brissaud P, et al: Monoarthritis secondary to joint metastasis: two case reports and literature review, *Joint Bone Spine* 69:495, 2002.

100. Capovilla M, Durlach A, Fourati E, et al: Chronic monoarthritis and previous history of cancer: think about synovial metastasis, *Clin Rheumatol* 26:60, 2007.

101. Vandecandelaere P, Sciot R, Westhovens R, et al: Malignant involvement of the knee synovium in a patient with metastatic oesophageal adenocarcinoma, *Acta Clin Belg* 65:48, 2010.

102. Ehrenfeld M, Gur H, Shoenfeld Y: Rheumatologic features of hematologic disorders, *Curr Opin Rheumatol* 11:62, 1999.

103. Acree SC, Pullarkat ST, Quismorio FP Jr, et al: Adult leukemic synovitis is associated with leukemia of monocytic differentiation, *J Clin Rheumatol* 17:130, 2011.

104. Evans TI, Nercessian BM, Sanders KM: Leukemic arthritis, *Semin Arthritis Rheum* 24:48, 1994.

The references for this chapter can also be found on www.expertconsult.com.

Page numbers followed by f indicate figures;
t, tables; b, boxes.

Antibodies *(Continued)*
 molecule, schematic, 192f
 monomer, chain molecules, 192f
 profiles, morbidity/mortality patterns
  (association), 1437-1438
 response, 1435
  non-self-protein, impact, 1435
 5D4, 482
Antibody-dependent cell-mediated
 cytotoxicity (ADCC), 124
Anti-CAM targeting, 363
Anticardiolipin ELISA, sensitivity, 1335
Anti-CCP autoantibodies, RA development
 predictor, 807
Anti-CCP+ RA, immune complexes, 813
Anti-CD20 antibody rituximab treatment,
 variable tissue response, 484f
Anti-CD20 therapy, peripheral blood B cell
 depletion, 983-984
Anti-CD40L treatment, 1313-1314
Anticentromere antibody, 797
 patients, characteristics, 1371-1372
Antichemokines, studies, 364
Anticipatory property, 255
Anticitrullinated protein antibody (ACPA),
 129-130, 240, 505, 804, 807-808,
 1059-1060, 1068-1069, 1110
 discovery, timeline, 805f
 disease prediction, 1069
 genetic associations, 811
 local targets, 808
 pathogenic potential, 1069
 presence, 1069
Anticonvulsants, 1025-1028
 action, mechanism, 1026-1027
  list, 1027t
 suicidal ideation, risk, 1028
Anticyclic citrullinated protein (anti-CCP)
 antibody, 1110
 appearance, kinetics, 807
 clinical relevance, 807-808
 detection, 1182
 genetic associations, 811
 specificity, 807
Anticytokine therapy, usage, 365, 1314
Anti-deoxyribonucleic acid (anti-DNA)
 antibodies, 796
Antidepressants, 1023-1025
 analgesic efficacy, 1023t
 chemical structures, 1024f
 tricyclic antidepressants (TCAs), 1023-1024
Antidiuretic hormone (ADH), synthesis,
 1020-1022
Anti-DNA antibody tests, usage, 793-794
Anti-DNA autoantibodies, elution, 1269-1271
Anti-double-stranded DNA (anti-dsDNA)
 antibodies, 1274
 cause, 1280
Antiendothelial antibody (AECA), AECA-
 mediated vascular injury/regeneration,
 358
Antiendothelial cell antibodies, levels
 (elevation), 1443
Antifungal chemotherapy, improvement,
 1846
Anti-GBM disease (Goodpasture's disease),
 1455
Antigen-activated B cells
 clonal expansion, 202
 markers, 204t
Antigen-independent activation, 205-206
Antigen-induced arthritis, 407
Antigen-presenting cells (APCs), 117
 adaptive immune system, 1745
 co-stimulatory molecules, 179

Antigen-presenting cells (APCs) *(Continued)*
 germline-encoded receptors, 140
 implication, 134
 interactions, 989f
 membrane receptors, involvement, 149
 MHC molecules, expression, 1045
 uptake, 1433-1434
Antigen-processing pathways, 146f
Antigens (Ags)
 acquisition, 121-124
 binding, 191-192
 capture, 422
 definition, 269t
 endocytosis, 124f
 immune exclusion, secretory antibodies
  function (provision), 1256f
 presence, 1072
 presentation, 124-126, 294
  enhancement, CLRs (usage), 122-123
 processing, 145-146
 recognition, 102-103, 121-124
 retrieval methods, availability, 759
 T cells, cross-presentation, 107-108
 transport, catecholamines (role), 422
Antigen-specific interactions (maintenance),
 immunologic synapses (usage), 270-271
Antigen-specific T cells
 DC contact, 272
 recognition, 299
Anti-G6PI antibodies, presence, 811
Anti-hen egg lysozyme (HEL) antibody, 207
Antihistone (nucleosome), 796
Anti-HMGCR antibodies, presence,
 1406-1407
Anti-IFN-α monoclonal antibody (MEDI-
 545), usage, 1292
Anti-IgE therapy, 172
Anti-IL-5 antibodies (mepolizumab), usage,
 172
Anti-IL-6 therapy, 1314
Anti-IL-10 murine monoclonal antibody
 (BN10), 1314
Anti-IL-10 therapy, 1314
Anti-inflammatory analgesic therapy, 889-890
 selection, complexity, 889-890
Anti-inflammatory arachidonic acid
 metabolites, 1084
Anti-inflammatory cells, mast cell role,
 238-239
Anti-inflammatory drugs, usage, 396
Anti-inflammatory lipids, biosynthesis, 874f
Anti-inflammatory lipoxins, generation, 161f
Anti-inflammatory prophylaxis, ULT
 administration (usage), 1003
Anti-Jo-1 antibody levels, disease activity
 (correlation), 798
Antikeratin antibodies (AKAs), presence, 805
Antikinetochore (centromere), presence, 797
Anti-La/SSB antibodies, pathogenic role
 (absence), 1177
Antimalarials, 932-935
 absorption, 934
 action mechanism, 925t
 anti-inflammatory properties, 933
 benefits, 933-934
 bioavailability, 934
 chemical structures, 933
  illustration, 933f
 distribution, 934
 elimination, 934
 half-life, 934
 hydroxychloroquine, actions, 933-934
 indications, 934
 inhibitory effects, 933
 pharmacology, 934

Antimetabolites, usage, 521
Antimicrobial peptides, 263
 production, 263
 release, 130
Antineuronal antibody-mediated CNS
 pathology, type II process, 293
Antineutrophil cytoplasmic antibody
 (ANCA)
 ANCA-associated crescentic
  glomerulonephritis, 1487f
 ANCA-associated disease, spectrum, 1483
 ANCA-associated vasculitis, nonmelanoma
  (association), 520
 ANCA-positive pauci-immune focal
  necrotizing glomerulonephritis, 292
 immune mechanisms, involvement
  (schematic representation), 1486f
 immunofluorescence, 1482f
 levels (decrease), rituximab treatment
  (usage), 1492
Antineutrophil cytoplasmic antibody-
 associated vasculitides (AAVs), 164, 1481
 adjuvant therapy, 1493
 adverse events, 1494
 agents, alternatives, 1493
 cardiovascular disease, 1494-1495
 clinical features, 1485-1490
 CYCAZAREM trial, 1492
 diagnosis, 1490-1491
 diagnostic tests, 1490-1491
 differential diagnostic features, 1490t
 end-stage kidney disease (ESKD), presence,
  1494
 environmental factors, 1484
 epidemiology, 1482-1484
 genetics, 1484-1485
 immunosuppressants, usage, 1492
 IMPROVE study, 1492
 incidence, determination, 1482-1483
 induction therapy, cyclophosphamide
  (usage), 1491
 intravenous immunoglobulin (IVIG), usage,
  1493
 laboratory results, 1490
 management, EULAR recommendations,
  1493t
 MEPEX study, 1493
 methotrexate, usage, 1492
 natural history, 1491
 NORAM trial, 1492
 outcome, 1494-1495
 prevalence, 1482-1483
 prognosis, 1494-1495
 remission
  induction, 1491-1492
  maintenance, 1492-1493
 small case series, 1492
 treatment, 1491-1494
  algorithm, 1491f
Antineutrophil cytoplasmic antibody
 (ANCA) vasculitis, 1789-1791
 classification, 1790
 clinical presentation, 1790
 definition, 1790
 diagnosis, 1790
 diagnostic tests, 1790
 epidemiology, 1790
 outcome, 1791
 treatment, 1790-1791
Antinuclear antibodies (ANAs)
 ANA-related phenomenon, description,
  789-790
 anti-DNA antibody tests, 793-794
 assays, 794
 chromatin-associated antigens, 796